Apley's
System of Orthopaedics and Fractures

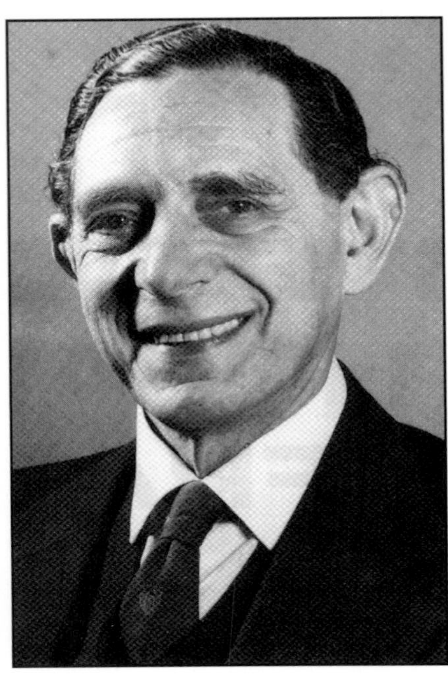

Alan Graham Apley 1914–1996
Inspired teacher, wise mentor and joyful friend

Louis Solomon MD FRCS
Emeritus Professor of Orthopaedics
University of Bristol
Bristol
UK

David Warwick MD FRCS FRCSOrth Eur Dip Hand Surg
Consultant Hand Surgeon
Reader in Orthopaedic Surgery
University of Southampton
Southampton
UK

Selvadurai Nayagam BSc MChOrth
FRCSOrth
Consultant Orthopaedic Surgeon
Royal Liverpool Children's Hospital
and
The Royal Liverpool University
Hospital
Liverpool
UK

Apley's System of Orthopaedics and Fractures

Ninth Edition

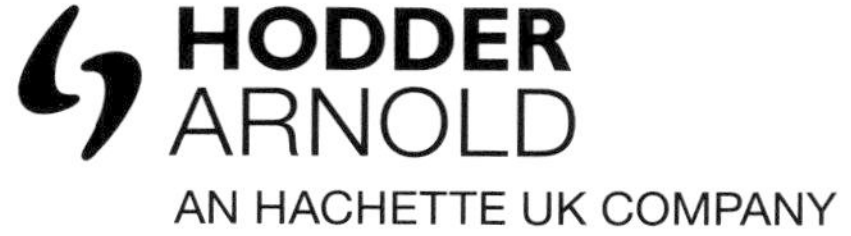

First published in Great Britain in 1959 by Butterworths Medical Publications
Second edition 1963
Third edition 1968
Fourth edition 1973
Fifth edition 1977
Sixth edition 1982
Seventh edition published in 1993 by Butterworth Heineman.
Eight edition published in 2001 by Arnold.
This ninth edition published in 2010 by
Hodder Arnold, an imprint of Hodder Education, an Hachette UK Company,
338 Euston Road, London NW1 3BH

http://www.hodderarnold.com

British Library Cataloguing in Publication Data
A catalogue record for this book is available from the British Library

Library of Congress Cataloging-in-Publication Data
A catalog record for this book is available from the Library of Congress

ISBN-13 978 0 340 942 055
ISBN-13 [ISE] 978 0 340 942 086 (International Students' Edition, restricted territorial availability)

1 2 3 4 5 6 7 8 9 10

Commissioning Editor: Gavin Jamieson
Project Editor: Francesca Naish
Production Controller: Joanna Walker
Cover Designer: Helen Townson
Indexer: Laurence Errington
Additional editorial services provided by
Naughton Project Management.

Cover image © Linda Bucklin/stockphoto.com

Typeset in 10 on 12pt Galliard by Phoenix Photosetting, Chatham, Kent
Printed and bound in India by Replika Press

Dedication

To our students, trainees and patients, all of whom have helped to make our lives interesting, stimulating and worthwhile; and also to our wives and children (and grand-children) who have tolerated our absences – both material and spiritual – while preparing this new edition.

Contents

Contributors

Principal Authors

Louis Solomon MD FRCS Eng FRCS Ed
Emeritus Professor of Orthopaedic Surgery
University of Bristol
Honorary Consultant Orthopaedic Surgeon
Bristol Royal Infirmary, Bristol, UK

Selvadurai Nayagam BSc, MChOrth FRCSOrth
Consultant Orthopaedic Surgeon
Royal Liverpool Children's Hospital and
The Royal Liverpool University Hospital
Liverpool, UK

David Warwick MD BM FRCS FRCS (Orth) Eur Dip Hand Surg
Consultant Hand Surgeon
Reader in Orthopaedic Surgery
University of Southampton, Southampton, UK

Contributing Authors

Will Aston BSc, MBBS, FRCS Ed(TR&Orth)
Consultant Orthopaedic Surgeon
Royal National Orthopaedic Hospital
Stanmore, UK
Tumours

Gavin William Bowyer MA MChir FRCS(Orth)
Consultant Trauma and Orthopaedic Surgeon
and Honorary Senior Lecturer
Southampton University Hospitals
Southampton, UK
The Ankle and Foot
Injuries of the ankle and foot

Felicity Briggs MA(Oxon) UK
Research Assistant and Graduate Medical Student
Epilogue: Global Orthopaedics

Timothy William Roy Briggs MD(Res) MCh(Orth) FRCS FRCS Ed
Professor and Consultant Orthopaedic Surgeon
Joint Medical Director
Joint Training Programme Director
Royal National Orthopaedic Hospital
Stanmore, UK
Tumours

Andrew Spencer Cole BSc MBBS FRCS(TR&Orth)
Consultant Orthopaedic Surgeon
Southampton University Hospitals
Southampton, UK
The Shoulder and Pectoral Girdle
Injuries of the Shoulder and Upper Arm and elbow

Roderick Dunn MBBS DMCC FRCS(Plast)
Consultant Plastic, Reconstructive and Hand
Surgeon, Odstock Centre for Burns, Plastic and
Maxillofacial Surgery, Salisbury District Hospital
Salisbury, UK
The Wrist and The Hand: Congenital Variations

Deborah Eastwood FRCS
Consultant Orthopaedic Surgeon and
Hon Senior Lecturer
University College London;
Great Ormond Street Hospital for Children
London, UK
Genetic Disorders, Dysplasias and Malformations
Neuromuscular Disorders

Christopher J Edwards BSc MBBS FRCP MD
Consultant Rheumatologist & Honorary Senior
Lecturer
Associate Director
Wellcome Trust Clinical Research Facility
Southampton University Hospitals NHS Trust
Southampton General Hospital, UK
Inflammatory Rheumatic Disorders

Stephen Eisenstein PhD FRCS(Ed)
Hon Professor, Keele University; Emeritus Director Centre for Spinal Studies;
The Robert Jones and Agnes Hunt Orthopaedic Hospital, Shropshire, UK
The Neck
The Back
Injuries of the Spine

Reinhold Ganz MD
Professor and Chairman Emeritus
Orthopaedic Department Inselspital
University of Bern, Switzerland
The Hip: Femoro-acetabular Impingement

Shunmugam Govender MBBS MD FRCS FC(Orth) (SA)
Professor and Head of Department of Orthopaedics;
Director of Spinal Services King George V Hospital;
Nelson R Mandela School of Medicine
Durban, South Africa
Infection
The Back: Infections of the Spine

Max Jonas MBBS FRCA
Consultant and Senior Lecturer in Critical Care
Southampton University Hospitals NHS Trust
Southampton, UK
The Management of Major Injuries

Theo Karachalios MD DSc
Associate Professor in Orthopaedics,
School of Health Sciences, University of Thessalia
University General Hospital of Larissa
Hellenic Republic
The Knee

Christopher Lavy OBE MD MCh FRCS
Hon Professor and Consultant,
Nuffield Department of Orthopaedic Surgery,
University of Oxford, UK
Epilogue: Global Orthopaedics

Ian Douglas Learmonth MB ChB FRCS Ed FRCS FCS(SA)Orth
Emeritus Professor, University of Bristol;
Honorary Consultant, University Hospitals, Bristol;
Honorary Consultant, North Bristol Trust, UK
Total Hip Replacement

Michael Leunig MD
Head of Orthopaedics, Lower Extremities
Schulthess Klinik, Zurich, Switzerland
The Hip: Femoro-Acetabular Impingement

Wagih S El Masry FRCS FRCP
Consultant Surgeon in Spinal Injuries;
Director, Midlands Centre for Spinal Injuries
President International Spinal Cord Society (ISCOS)
RJ & AH Orthopaedic Hospital, Oswestry, UK
Injuries of the Spine

Fergal P Monsell MSc FRCS FRCS(Orth)
Consultant Paediatric Orthopaedic Surgeon
Bristol Royal Hospital for Children
Bristol, UK
The Hip: Disorders in Children

Paul Pavlou BSc (Hons) MB BS MRCS
Orthopaedic Registrar, Wessex training scheme
The Shoulder and Pectoral Girdle
Injuries of the Shoulder

H. Srinivasan MB BS FRCS FRCS Ed DSc (Hon)
Formerly Senior Orthopaedic Surgeon
Central Leprosy Teaching & Research Institute
Chengalpattu (Tamil Nadu), India;
Director Central JALMA Institute for Leprosy (ICMR), Agra (UP), India; and Editor Indian Journal of Leprosy
Infection and Peripheral Nerve Disorders: Leprosy

Thomas G Staunton MB FRCP(C) FRCP
Consultant Neurologist
Norfolk and Norwich University Hospital;
Consultant Clinical Neurophysiologist
Robert Jones and Agnes Hunt Orthopaedic Hospital, Shropshire, UK
Neuromuscular Disorders: Neurophysiological Studies

David Sutton BM DA FRCA
Department of Anaesthetics
Southampton General Hospital
Southampton, UK
Management of Major Injuries

Surendar Mohan Tuli MBBS MS PhD
Senior Consultant in Spinal Diseases and Orthopaedics, Vimhans Hospital, New Delhi, India
Infection: Tuberculosis of Bones and Joints
The Back

Charles J Wakeley BSc MBBS FRCS FRCS Ed FRCR
Consultant Radiologist, Department of Radiology
University Hospital Bristol NHS Foundation Trust
Bristol, UK
Diagnosis in Orthopaedics: Imaging

Preface

When Alan Apley produced the first edition of his System of Orthopaedics and Fractures 50 years ago he saw it as an aid to accompany the courses that he conducted for aspiring surgeons who were preparing for the FRCS exams. With characteristic humour, he called the book 'a prophylactic against writer's cramp'. Pictures were unnecessary: if you had any sense (and were quick enough to get on the heavily oversubscribed Apley Course) you would be treated to an unforgettable display of clinical signs by one of the most gifted of teachers.

You also learnt how to elicit those signs by using a methodical clinical approach – the Apley System. The Fellowship exam was heavily weighted towards clinical skills. Miss an important sign or stumble over how to examine a knee or a finger and you could fail outright. What Apley taught you was how to order the steps in physical examination in a way that could be applied to every part of the musculoskeletal system. *'Look, Feel, Move'* was the mantra. He liked to say that he had a preference for four-letter words. And always in that order! Deviate from the System by grasping a patient's leg before you look at it minutely, or by testing the movements in a joint before you feel its contours and establish the exact site of tenderness and you risked becoming an unwilling participant in a theatrical comedy.

Much has changed since then. With each new edition the System has been expanded to accommodate new tests and physical manoeuvres developed in the tide of super-specialisation. Laboratory investigations have become more important and imaging techniques have advanced out of all recognition. Clinical classifications have sprung up and attempts are now made to find a numerical slot for every imaginable fracture. No medical textbook is complete without its 'basic science' component, and advances are so rapid that changes become necessary within the period of writing a single edition. The present volume is no exception: new bits were still being added right up to the time of proof-reading.

For all that, we have retained the familiar structure of the Apley System. As in earlier editions, the book is divided into three sections: General Orthopaedics, covering the main types of musculoskeletal disorder; Regional Orthopaedics, where we engage with these disorders in specific parts of the body; and thirdly Fractures and Joint Injuries. In a major departure from previous editions, we have enlisted the help of colleagues who have particular experience of conditions with which we as principal authors are less familiar. Their contributions are gratefully acknowledged. Even here, though, we have sought their permission to 'edit' their material into the Apley mould so that the book still has the sound and 'feel' of a single authorial voice.

For the second edition of the book, in 1963, Apley added a new chapter: 'The Management of Major Accidents'. Typically frank, he described the current arrangements for dealing with serious accidents as "woefully inadequate" and offered suggestions based on the government's Interim Report on Accident Services in Great Britain and Ireland (1961). There has been a vast improvement since then and the number of road accident deaths today is half of what it was in the 1960's (Department of Transport statistics). So important is this subject that the relevant section has now been re-written by two highly experienced Emergency and Intensive Care Physicians and is by far the longest chapter in the present edition.

Elsewhere the text has been brought completely up to date and new pictures have been added. In most cases the illustrations appear as composites – a series of images that tell a story rather than a single 'typical' picture at one moment in the development of some disorder. At the beginning of each Regional chapter, in a run of pictures we show the method of examining that region: where to stand, how to confront the patient and where to place our hands. For the experienced reader this may seem like old hat; but then we have designed this book for orthopaedic surgeons of all ages and all levels of experience. We all have something to learn from each other.

As before, operations are described only in outline, emphasising the principles that govern the choice of treatment, the indications for surgery, the design of the operation, its known complications and the likely outcome. Technical procedures are learnt in simulation courses and, ultimately, in the operating theatre. Written instructions can only ever be a guide. Drawings are usually too idealised and 'in theatre' photographs are usually intelligible only to someone who has already performed that operation. Textbooks that grapple with these impediments tend to run to several volumes.

The emphasis throughout is on *clinical* orthopaedics. We acknowledge the value of a more academic approach that starts with embryology, anatomy, biomechanics, molecular biology, physiology and pathology before introducing any patient to the reader. Instead we have chosen to present these 'basic' subjects in small portions where they are relevant to the clinical disorder under discussion: bone growth and metabolism in the chapter on metabolic bone disease, genetics in the chapter on osteodystrophies, and so forth.

In the preface to the last edition we admitted our doubts about the value of exhaustive lists of references at the end of each chapter. We are even more divided about this now, what with the plethora of 'search engines' that have come to dominate the internet. We can merely bow our heads and say we still have those doubts and have given references only where it seems appropriate to acknowledge where an old idea started or where something new is being said that might at first sight be questioned.

More than ever we are aware that there is a dwindling number of orthopaedic surgeons who grew up in the Apley era, even fewer who experienced his thrilling teaching displays, and fewer still who worked with him. Wherever they are, we trust that they will recognise the Apley flavour in this new edition. Our chief concern, however, is for the new readers who – we hope – will glean something that helps them become the next generation of teachers and mentors.

LS
SN
DJW

Acknowledgements

Fifty years ago Apleys' System of Orthopaedics and Fractures was written by one person – the eponymous Apley. As the years passed and new editions became ever larger, a second author appeared and then a third. Throughout those years we have always been able to get help (and sometimes useful criticism) from willing colleagues who have filled the gaps in our knowledge. Their words and hints are scattered among the pages of this book and we are forever grateful to them.

For the present edition we have gone a step further and enlisted a number of those colleagues as nominated Contributing Authors. In some cases they have brought up to date existing chapters; in others they have added entirely new sections to a book that has now grown beyond the scope of two or three specialists. Their names are appropriately listed elsewhere but here we wish to thank them again for joining us. They have allowed us to mould their words into the style of the Apley System so that the text continues to carry the flavour of a unified authorial voice.

We are also grateful to those colleagues who have supplied new pictures where our own collections have fallen short. In particular we want to thank Dr Santosh Rath and Dr G.N. Malaviya for pictures of peripheral deformities in leprosy, Mr Evert Smith for pictures (and helpful descriptions) of modern implants in hip replacement operations, Dr Peter Bullough who allowed us to reprint two of the excellent illustrations in his book on Orthopaedic Pathology, and Dr Asif Saifuddin for permission to use some images from his book on Musculoskeletal MRI. Others who gave us generous assistance with pictures are Fiona Daglish, Colin Duncan, Neeraj Garg, Nikolaos Giotakis, Jagdeep Nanchahal and Badri Narayan.

We have been fortunate in having friends and family around us who have given us helpful criticism on the presentation of this work. Caryn Solomon, a tireless internet traveller, found the picture for the cover and Joan Solomon gave expert advice on layout and design. James Crabtree stepped in as a model for some 'clinical' pictures. We are grateful to all of them.

Throughout the long march to completion of this work we have enjoyed the constant help and collaboration of Francesca Naish, Gavin Jamieson, Joanna Walker and Helen Townson (our Editorial Manager, Commissioning Editor, Production Manager and Design Manager respectively) at Hodder Arnold. No problem was too complex and no obstacle too great to withstand their tireless efforts in driving this work forward.

Nora Naughton and Aileen Castell (Naughton Project Management) were in the background setting up the page copies, patiently enduring the many amendments that came in over the internet. Their attention to detail has been outstanding.

Finally, we want to express our deepest thanks to those nearest to us who added not a word to the text but through their support and patience made it possible for us to take so much time beyond the everyday occupations of family life to produce a single book.

L. S.
D.W.
S. N.

List of abbreviations used

ACA angulation correction axis
ACE angiotensin-converting enzyme
ACL anterior cruciate ligament
ACTH adrenocorticotropic hormone
AFP alpha-fetoprotein
AIDP acute inflammatory demyelinating polyneuropathy
AIDS acquired immune deficiency syndrome
AL anterolateral
ALI acute lung injury
AM anteromedial
AMC arthrogryposis multiplex congenita
ANA antinuclear antibodies
anti-CCP anti-cyclic citrullinated peptide antibodies
AP anteroposterior
APC antigen-presenting cell
APC anteroposterior compression (injuries)
ARCO Association Research Circulation Osseous
ARDS adult respiratory distress syndrome
ARDS acute respiratory distress syndrome
ARM awareness, recognition, management
AS ankylosing spondylitis
ATLS advanced trauma life support
AVN avascular necrosis
BASICS British Association for Immediate Care
BCP basic calcium phosphate
BMD bone mineral density
BMP bone morphogenetic protein
BSA body surface area
BVM bag-valve-mask
CDH congenital dislocation of the hip
CFD congenital femoral deficiency
CMAP compound muscle action potential
CMC carpo-metacarpal
CMI cell-mediated immunity
CNS central nervous system
COMP cartilage oligometric matrix protein
CORA centre of rotation of angulation
CPM continuous passive motion
CPPD calcium pyrophosphate dihydrate
CRP C-reactive protein
CRPS complex regional pain syndrome
CSF cerebrospinal fluid
CT computed tomography
CVP central venous pressure
DDH developmental dysplasia of the hip
dGEMRIC delayed gadolinium-enhanced MRI of cartilage
DIC disseminated intravascular coagulation
DIP distal interphalangeal (joint)
DISH diffuse idiopathic skeletal hyperostosis
DISI dorsal intercalated segment instability
DMARDs disease-modifying antirheumatic drugs
DRUJ distal radio-ulnar joint
DTH delayed type hypersensitivity
DVT deep vein thrombosis
DXA dual-energy x-ray absorptiometry
ECRB extensor carpi radialis brevis
ECRL extensor carpi radialis longus
EDF elongation-derotation-flexion
EDG extensor diversion graft
EEG electroencephalography
EMG electromyography
EMS emergency medical service
ENL erythema nodosum leprosum
ESR erythrocyte sedimentation rate
ETA estimated time of arrival
FAI femoro-acetabular impingement
FAST focussed assessment sonography in trauma
FDP flexor digitorum profundus
FDS flexor digitorum superficialis
FFOs functional foot orthoses
FPB flexor pollicis brevis
FPE fatal pulmonary embolism
FPL flexor pollicis longus
GABA gamma-aminobutryic acid
GAGs glycosaminoglycans
GCS Glasgow Coma Scale
GMFCS gross motor function classification system
GPI general paralysis of the insane
HA hydroxyapatite

HEMS	helicopter emergency medical service
HGPRT	hypoxanthine-guanine phosphoribosyltransferase
HHR	humeral head replacement
HIV	human immunodeficiency virus
HLA	human leucocyte antigen
HMSN	hereditary motor and sensory neuropathy
HRT	hormone replacement therapy
ICP	intracerebral pressure
ICU	intensive care unit
IL	interleukin
INR	international normalized ratio
IP	interphalangeal
IRMER	Ionising Radiation Medical Exposure Regulations
ITAP	intra-osseous transcutaneous amputation prosthesis
IVF	in vitro fertilization
JIA	juvenile idiopathic arthritis
LCL	lateral collateral ligament
LMA	laryngeal mask airway
LMN	lower motor neuron
LMWH	low molecular weight heparin
MCL	medial collateral ligament
MCP	metacarpo-phalangeal (joint)
M-CSF	macrophage colony-stimulating factor
MED	multiple epiphyseal dysplasia
MHC	major histocompatibility complex
MIC	minimal inhibitory concentration
MIPO	minimally invasive percutaneous osteosynthesis
MIS	minimally invasive surgery
MODS	multiple organ failure or dysfunction syndrome
MPM	mortality prediction model
MPS	mucopolysaccharidoses
MRI	magnetic resonance imaging
MRSA	methicillin-resistant *Staphylococcus aureus*
MTP	metatarsophalangeal (joint)
NCV	nerve conduction velocity
NP	nasopharyngeal
NSAIDs	non-steroidal anti-inflammatory drugs
OA	osteoarthritis
OI	osteogenesis imperfecta
OP	oropharyngeal
OPG	osteoprotegerin
OPLL	ossification of the posterior longitudinal ligament
PA	posteroanterior
PACS	Picture Archiving and Communication System
PAFC	pulmonary artery flotation catherization
PAOP	pulmonary artery occlusion pressure
PCL	posterior cruciate ligament
PCR	polymerase chain reaction
PD	proton density
PE	pulmonary embolism
PEA	pulseless electrical activity
PEEP	positive end-expiratory pressure
PET	positron emission tomography
PFFD	proximal focal femoral deficiency
PIP	proximal interphalangeal (joint)
PL	posterolateral
PM	posteromedial
PMMA	polymethylmethacrylate
PNS	peripheral nervous system
PPE	personal protective equipment
PPS	post-polio syndrome
PTH	parathyroid hormone
PTS	post-thrombotic syndrome
PVNS	pigmented villonodular synovitis
QCT	quantitative computed tomography
QUS	quantitative ultrasonometry
RA	radiographic absorptiometry *and* rheumatoid arthritis
RANKL	receptor activator of nuclear factor-ligand
RF	rheumatoid factor
RR	reversal reaction
RSD	reflex sympathetic dystrophy
RSI	rapid sequence induction
SACE	serum angiotensin converting enzyme
SAMU	Services de l'Aide Medical Urgente
SAPHO	for synovitis, acne, pustulosis, hyperostosis and osteitis
SCFE	slipped capital femoral epiphysis
SCIWORA	spinal cord injury without obvious radiographic abnormality
SDD	digestive tract
SE	spin echo
SED	spondyloepiphyseal dysplasia
SEMLS	single event multi-level surgery
SIRS	systemic inflammatory response
SLAP	superior labrum, anterior and posterior (tear)
SLE	systemic lupus erythematosus
SMR	standardized mortality ratio
SMUR	Services Mobile d'Urgence et de Reamination
SNAP	sensory nerve action potential
SNPs	single nucleotide polymorphisms
SONK	'spontaneous' osteonecrosis of the knee
SOPs	standard operating procedure
SPECT	single photon emission computed tomography
SSEP	somatosensory evoked responses
STIR	short-tau inversion recovery
STT	scaphoid-trapezium-trapezoid arthritis
SCIWORA	spinal cord injury without radiographic abnormality

TAR	prompts one to remember *t*hrombocytopaenia with *a*bsent *r*adius syndrome
TB	tuberculosis
^{99m}Tc-MDP	^{99m}Tc-methyl diphosphonate
TE	time to echo
TFCC	triangular fibrocartilage complex
TIP	terminal interphalangeal (joint)
TNF	tumour necrosis factor
TR	repetition time
TSR	total shoulder replacement
UHMWPE	ultra-high molecular weight polyethylene
UMN	upper motor neuron
US	ultrasound
VACTERLS	refers to the systems involved and the defects identified: *v*ertebral, *a*nal, *c*ardiac, *t*racheal, *e*sophageal, *r*enal, *l*imb and *s*ingle umbilical artery.
VCT	voluntary counselling and testing
VISI	volar intercalated segment instability
VP	ventriculo-peritoneal
VS	vertical shear
VTE	venous thromboembolism
VQC	ventilation-perfusion
WBC	white blood cell
XLPE	highly cross-linked polyethylene

Section 1

General Orthopaedics

Orthopaedic diagnosis

1

Louis Solomon, Charles Wakeley

Orthopaedics is concerned with bones, joints, muscles, tendons and nerves – the skeletal system and all that makes it move. Conditions that affect these structures fall into seven easily remembered pairs:

1. Congenital and developmental abnormalities.
2. Infection and inflammation.
3. Arthritis and rheumatic disorders.
4. Metabolic and endocrine disorders.
5. Tumours and lesions that mimic them.
6. Neurological disorders and muscle weakness.
7. Injury and mechanical derangement.

Diagnosis in orthopaedics, as in all of medicine, is the identification of disease. It begins from the very first encounter with the patient and is gradually modified and fine-tuned until we have a picture, not only of a pathological process but also of the functional loss and the disability that goes with it. Understanding evolves from the systematic gathering of information from the history, the physical examination, tissue and organ imaging and special investigations. Systematic, but never mechanical; behind the enquiring mind there should also be what D. H. Lawrence has called 'the intelligent heart'. It must never be forgotten that the patient has a unique personality, a job and hobbies, a family and a home; all have a bearing upon, and are in turn affected by, the disorder and its treatment.

HISTORY

'Taking a history' is a misnomer. The patient tells a story; it is we the listeners who construct a history. The story may be maddeningly disorganized; the history has to be systematic. Carefully and patiently compiled, it can be every bit as informative as examination or laboratory tests.

As we record it, certain key words and phrases will inevitably stand out: injury, pain, stiffness, swelling, deformity, instability, weakness, altered sensibility and loss of function or inability to do certain things that were easily accomplished before.

Each symptom is pursued for more detail: we need to know when it began, whether suddenly or gradually, spontaneously or after some specific event; how it has changed or progressed; what makes it worse; what makes it better.

While listening, we consider whether the story fits some pattern that we recognize, for we are already thinking of a diagnosis. Every piece of information should be thought of as part of a larger picture which gradually unfolds in our understanding. The surgeon-philosopher Wilfred Trotter (1870–1939) put it well: 'Disease reveals itself in casual parentheses'.

SYMPTOMS

Pain

Pain is the most common symptom in orthopaedics. It is usually described in metaphors that range from inexpressively bland to unbelievably bizarre – descriptions that tell us more about the patient's state of mind than about the physical disorder. Yet there are clearly differences between the throbbing pain of an abscess and the aching pain of chronic arthritis, between the 'burning pain' of neuralgia and the 'stabbing pain' of a ruptured tendon.

Severity is even more subjective. High and low pain thresholds undoubtedly exist, but to the patient pain is as bad as it feels, and any system of 'pain grading' must take this into account. The main value of estimating severity is in assessing the progress of the disorder or the response to treatment. The commonest method is to invite the patient to mark the severity on an analogue scale of 1–10, with 1 being mild and easily ignored and 10 being totally unbearable. The problem about this type of grading is that patients who have never experienced very severe pain simply do not know what 8 or 9 or 10 would feel like. The following is suggested as a simpler system:

- Grade I (mild) Pain that can easily be ignored.
- Grade II (moderate) Pain that cannot be ignored, interferes with function and needs attention or treatment from time to time.

- Grade III (severe) Pain that is present most of the time, demanding constant attention or treatment.
- Grade IV (excruciating) Totally incapacitating pain.

Identifying the site of pain may be equally vague. Yet its precise location is important, and in orthopaedics it is useful to ask the patient to point to – rather than to say – where it hurts. Even then, do not assume that the site of pain is necessarily the site of pathology; 'referred' pain and 'autonomic' pain can be very deceptive.

Referred pain Pain arising in or near the skin is usually localized accurately. Pain arising in deep structures is more diffuse and is sometimes of unexpected distribution; thus, hip disease may manifest with pain in the knee (so might an obturator hernia). This is not because sensory nerves connect the two sites; it is due to inability of the cerebral cortex to differentiate clearly between sensory messages from separate but embryologically related sites. A common example is 'sciatica' – pain at various points in the buttock, thigh and leg, supposedly following the course of the sciatic nerve. Such pain is not necessarily due to pressure on the sciatic nerve or the lumbar nerve roots; it may be 'referred' from any one of a number of structures in the lumbar spine, the pelvis and the posterior capsule of the hip joint.

Autonomic pain We are so accustomed to matching pain with some discrete anatomical structure and its known sensory nerve supply that we are apt to dismiss any pain that does not fit the usual pattern as 'atypical' or 'inappropriate' (i.e. psychologically determined). But pain can also affect the autonomic nerves that accompany the peripheral blood vessels and this is much more vague, more widespread and often associated with vasomotor and trophic changes. It is poorly understood, often doubted, but nonetheless real.

Stiffness

Stiffness may be generalized (typically in systemic disorders such as rheumatoid arthritis and ankylosing spondylitis) or localized to a particular joint. Patients often have difficulty in distinguishing localized stiffness from painful movement; limitation of movement should never be assumed until verified by examination.

Ask when it occurs: regular early morning stiffness of many joints is one of the cardinal symptoms of rheumatoid arthritis, whereas transient stiffness of one or two joints after periods of inactivity is typical of osteoarthritis.

Locking 'Locking' is the term applied to the sudden inability to complete a particular movement. It suggests a mechanical block – for example, due to a loose

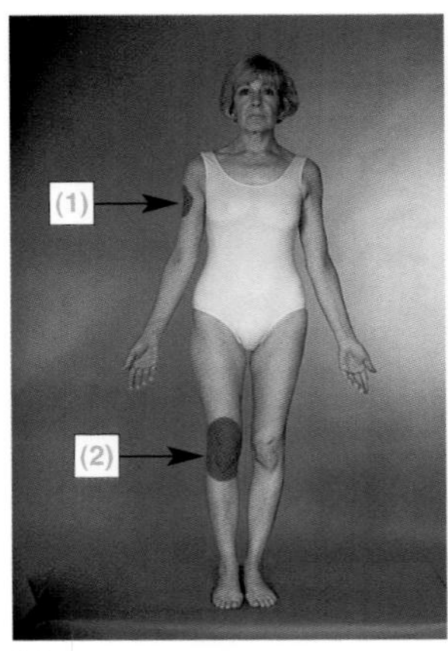

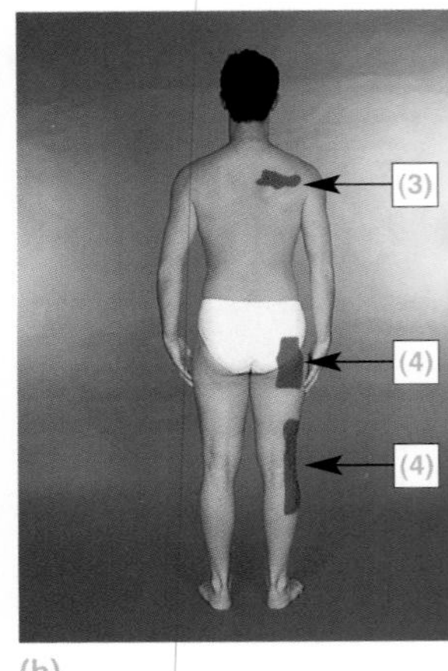

(a) (b)

1.1 Referred pain Common sites of referred pain: (1) from the shoulder; (2) from the hip; (3) from the neck; (4) from the lumbar spine.

body or a torn meniscus becoming trapped between the articular surfaces of the knee. Unfortunately, patients tend to use the term for any painful limitation of movement; much more reliable is a history of 'unlocking', when the offending body slips out of the way.

Swelling

Swelling may be in the soft tissues, the joint or the bone; to the patient they are all the same. It is important to establish whether it followed an injury, whether it appeared rapidly (think of a haematoma or a haemarthrosis) or slowly (due to inflammation, a joint effusion, infection or a tumour), whether it is painful (suggestive of acute inflammation, infection or a tumour), whether it is constant or comes and goes, and whether it is increasing in size.

Deformity

The common deformities are described by patients in terms such as round shoulders, spinal curvature, knock knees, bow legs, pigeon toes and flat feet. Deformity of a single bone or joint is less easily described and the patient may simply declare that the limb is 'crooked'.

Some 'deformities' are merely variations of the normal (e.g. short stature or wide hips); others disappear spontaneously with growth (e.g. flat feet or bandy legs in an infant). However, if the deformity is progressive, or if it affects only one side of the body while the opposite joint or limb is normal, it may be serious.

Weakness

Generalized weakness is a feature of all chronic illness, and any prolonged joint dysfunction will inevitably

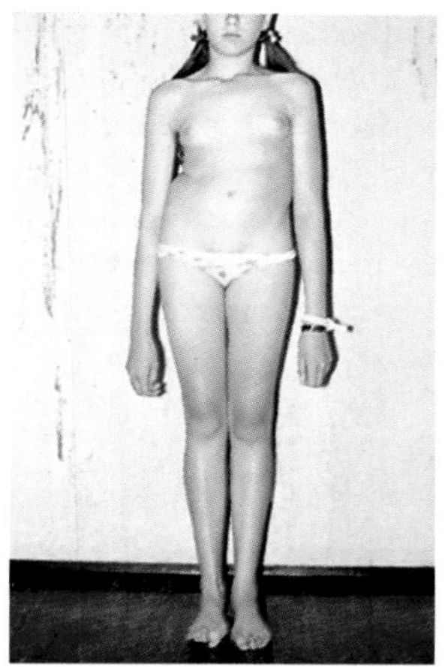
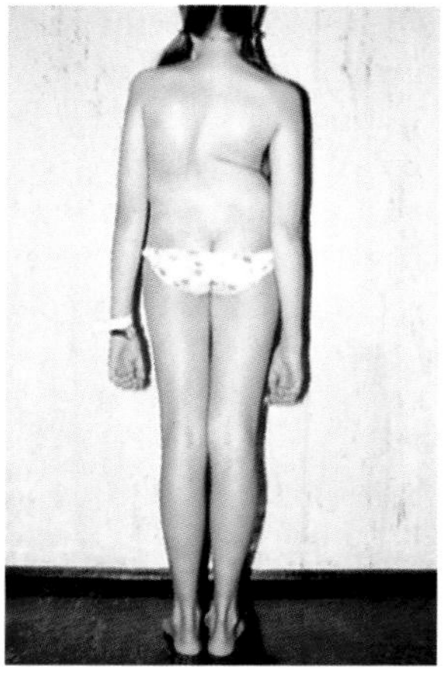

1.2 Deformity This young girl complained of a prominent right hip; the real deformity was scoliosis.

lead to weakness of the associated muscles. However, pure muscular weakness – especially if it is confined to one limb or to a single muscle group – is more specific and suggests some neurological or muscle disorder. Patients sometimes say that the limb is 'dead' when it is actually weak, and this can be a source of confusion. Questions should be framed to discover precisely which movements are affected, for this may give important clues, if not to the exact diagnosis at least to the site of the lesion.

Instability

The patient may complain that the joint 'gives way' or 'jumps out of place'. If this happens repeatedly, it suggests abnormal joint laxity, capsular or ligamentous deficiency, or some type of internal derangement such as a torn meniscus or a loose body in the joint. If there is a history of injury, its precise nature is important.

Change in sensibility

Tingling or numbness signifies interference with nerve function – pressure from a neighbouring structure (e.g. a prolapsed intervertebral disc), local ischaemia (e.g. nerve entrapment in a fibro-osseous tunnel) or a peripheral neuropathy. It is important to establish its exact distribution; from this we can tell whether the fault lies in a peripheral nerve or in a nerve root. We should also ask what makes it worse or better; a change in posture might be the trigger, thus focussing attention on a particular site.

Loss of function

Functional disability is more than the sum of individual symptoms and its expression depends upon the needs of that particular patient. The patient may say 'I can't stand for long' rather than 'I have backache'; or 'I can't put my socks on' rather than 'My hip is stiff'. Moreover, what to one patient is merely inconvenient may, to another, be incapacitating. Thus a lawyer or a teacher may readily tolerate a stiff knee provided it is painless, but to a plumber or a parson the same disorder might spell economic or spiritual disaster. One question should elicit the important information: 'What can't you do now that you used to be able to do?'

Past history

Patients often forget to mention previous illnesses or accidents, or they may simply not appreciate their relevance to the present complaint. They should be asked specifically about childhood disorders, periods of incapacity and old injuries. A 'twisted ankle' many years ago may be the clue to the onset of osteoarthritis in what is otherwise an unusual site for this condition. Gastrointestinal disease, which in the patient's mind has nothing to do with bones, may be important in the later development of ankylosing spondylitis or osteoporosis. Similarly, certain rheumatic disorders may be suggested by a history of conjunctivitis, iritis, psoriasis or urogenital disease. Metastatic bone disease may erupt many years after a mastectomy for breast cancer. Patients should also be asked about previous medication: many drugs, and especially corticosteroids, have long-term effects on bone. Alcohol and drug abuse are important, and we must not be afraid to ask about them.

Family history

Patients often wonder (and worry) about inheriting a disease or passing it on to their children. To the doctor, information about musculoskeletal disorders in the patient's family may help with both diagnosis and counselling.

When dealing with a suspected case of bone or joint infection, ask about communicable diseases, such as tuberculosis or sexually transmitted disease, in other members of the family.

Social background

No history is complete without enquiry about the patient's background. There are the obvious things such as the level of care and nutrition in children; dietary constraints which may cause specific deficiencies; and, in certain cases, questions about smoking habits, alcohol consumption and drug abuse, all of which call for a special degree of tact and non-judgemental enquiry.

Find out details about the patient's work practices, travel and recreation: could the disorder be due to a particular repetitive activity in the home, at work or on the sportsfield? Is the patient subject to any unusual occupational strain? Has he or she travelled to another country where tuberculosis is common?

Finally, it is important to assess the patient's home circumstances and the level of support by family and friends. This will help to answer the question: 'What has the patient lost and what is he or she hoping to regain?'

EXAMINATION

In *A Case of Identity* Sherlock Holmes has the following conversation with Dr Watson.

> Watson: *You appeared to read a good deal upon [your client] which was quite invisible to me.*
>
> Holmes: *Not invisible but unnoticed, Watson.*

Some disorders can be diagnosed at a glance: who would mistake the facial appearance of acromegaly or the hand deformities of rheumatoid arthritis for anything else? Nevertheless, even in these cases systematic examination is rewarding: it provides information about the patient's particular disability, as distinct from the clinicopathological diagnosis; it keeps reinforcing good habits; and, never to be forgotten, it lets the patient know that he or she has been thoroughly attended to.

The examination actually begins from the moment we set eyes on the patient. We observe his or her general appearance, posture and gait. Can you spot any distinctive feature: Knock-knees? Spinal curvature? A short limb? A paralysed arm? Does he or she appear to be in pain? Do their movements look natural? Do they walk with a limp, or use a stick? A tell-tale gait may suggest a painful hip, an unstable knee or a foot-drop. The clues are endless and the game is played by everyone (qualified or lay) at each new encounter throughout life. In the clinical setting the assessment needs to be more focussed.

When we proceed to the structured examination, the patient must be suitably undressed; no mere rolling up of a trouser leg is sufficient. If one limb is affected, both must be exposed so that they can be compared.

We examine the good limb (for comparison), then the bad. There is a great temptation to rush in with both hands – a temptation that must be resisted. Only by proceeding in a purposeful, orderly way can we avoid missing important signs.

Alan Apley, who developed and taught the system used here, shied away from using long words where short ones would do as well. (He also used to say 'I'm neither an inspector nor a manipulator, and I am definitely not a palpator'.) Thus the traditional clinical routine, inspection, palpation, manipulation, was replaced by *look, feel, move*. With time his teaching has been extended and we now add *test*, to include the special manoeuvres we employ in assessing neurological integrity and complex functional attributes.

Look

Abnormalities are not always obvious at first sight. A systematic, step by step process helps to avoid mistakes.

Shape and posture The first things to catch one's attention are the shape and posture of the limb or the body or the entire person who is being examined. Is the patient unusually thin or obese? Does the overall posture look normal? Is the spine straight or unusually curved? Are the shoulders level? Are the limbs normally positioned? It is important to look for deformity in three planes, and always compare the affected part with the normal side. In many joint disorders and in most nerve lesions the limb assumes a characteristic posture. In spinal disorders the entire torso may be deformed. Now look more closely for swelling or wasting – one often enhances the appearance of the other! Or is there a definite lump?

Skin Careful attention is paid to the colour, quality and markings of the skin. Look for bruising, wounds and ulceration. Scars are an informative record of the past – surgical archaeology, so to speak. Colour reflects vascular status or pigmentation – for example the pallor of ischaemia, the blueness of cyanosis, the redness of inflammation, or the dusky purple of an old bruise. Abnormal creases, unless due to fibrosis, suggest underlying deformity which is not always obvious; tight, shiny skin with no creases is typical of oedema or trophic change.

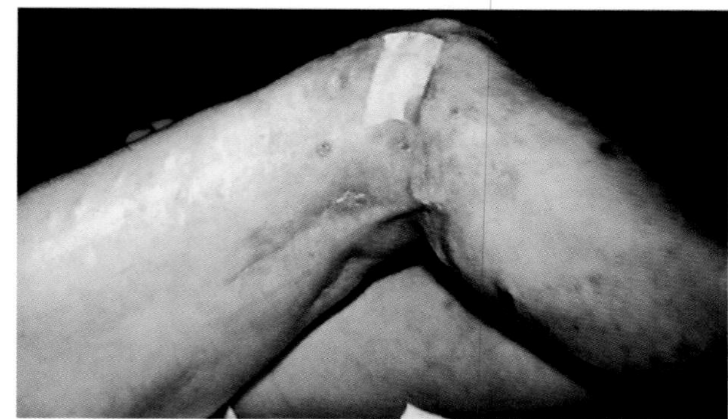

1.3 Look Scars often give clues to the previous history. The faded scar on this patient's thigh is an old operation wound – internal fixation of a femoral fracture. The other scars are due to postoperative infection; one of the sinuses is still draining.

General survey Attention is initially focussed on the symptomatic or most obviously abnormal area, but we must also look further afield. The patient complains of the joint that is hurting now, but we may see at a glance that several other joints are affected as well.

Feel

Feeling is exploring, not groping aimlessly. Know your anatomy and you will know where to feel for the landmarks; find the landmarks and you can construct a virtual anatomical picture in your mind's eye.

The skin Is it warm or cold; moist or dry; and is sensation normal?

The soft tissues Can you feel a lump; if so, what are its characteristics? Are the pulses normal?

The bones and joints Are the outlines normal? Is the synovium thickened? Is there excessive joint fluid?

Tenderness Once you have a clear idea of the structural features in the affected area, feel gently for tenderness. Keep your eyes on the patient's face; a grimace will tell you as much as a grunt. Try to localize any tenderness to a particular structure; if you know precisely *where* the trouble is, you are halfway to knowing *what* it is.

Move

'Movement' covers several different activities: active movement, passive mobility, abnormal or unstable movement, and provocative movement.

Active movement Ask the patient to move without your assistance. This will give you an idea of the degree of mobility and whether it is painful or not. Active movement is also used to assess muscle power.

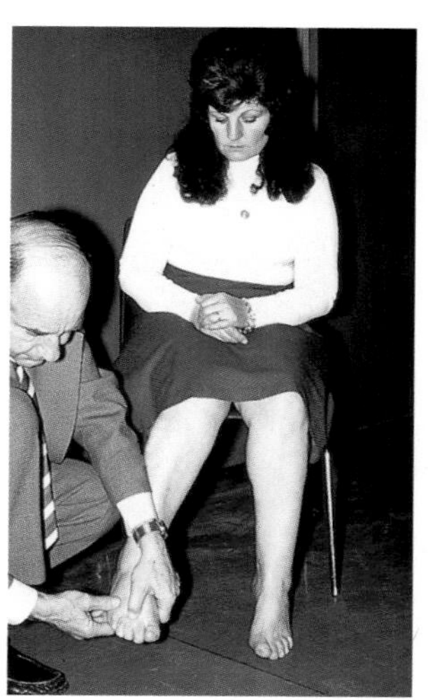

(a)

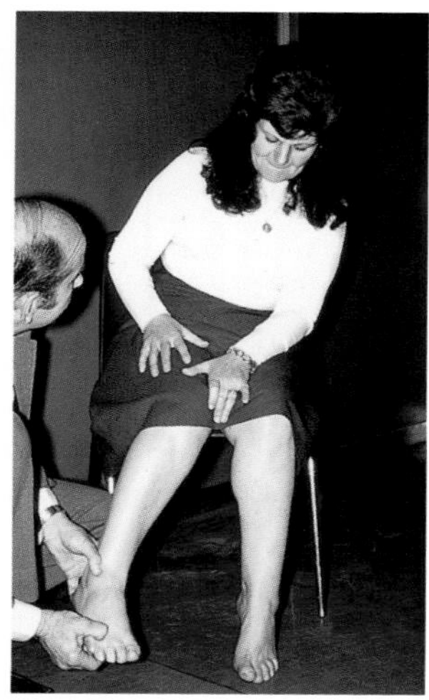

(b)

1.4 Feeling for tenderness (a) The wrong way – there is no need to look at your fingers, you should know where they are. (b) It is much more informative to look at the patient's face!

Passive movement Here it is the examiner who moves the joint in each anatomical plane. Note whether there is any difference between the range of active and passive movement.

Range of movement is recorded in degrees, starting from zero which, by convention, is the neutral or anatomical position of the joint and finishing where movement stops, due either to pain or anatomical limitation. Describing the range of movement is often made to seem difficult. Words such as 'full', 'good', 'limited' and 'poor' are misleading. Always cite the range or span, from start to finish, in degrees. For example, 'knee flexion 0–140°' means that the range of flexion is from zero (the knee absolutely straight) through an arc of 140 degrees (the leg making an acute angle with the thigh). Similarly, 'knee flexion 20–90°' means that flexion begins at 20 degrees (i.e. the joint cannot extend fully) and continues only to 90 degrees.

For accuracy you can measure the range of movement with a goniometer, but with practice you will learn to estimate the angles by eye. Normal ranges of movement are shown in chapters dealing with individual joints. What is important is always to compare the symptomatic with the asymptomatic or normal side.

While testing movement, feel for crepitus. Joint crepitus is usually coarse and fairly diffuse; tenosynovial crepitus is fine and precisely localized to the affected tendon sheath.

Unstable movement This is movement which is inherently unphysiological. You may be able to shift or angulate a joint out of its normal plane of movement, thus demonstrating that the joint is unstable. Such abnormal movement may be obvious (e.g. a wobbly knee); often, though, you have to use special manoeuvres to pick up minor degrees of instability.

Provocative movement One of the most telling clues to diagnosis is reproducing the patient's symptoms by applying a specific, provocative movement. Shoulder pain due to impingement of the subacromial structures may be 'provoked' by moving the joint in a way that is calculated to produce such impingement; the patient recognizes the similarity between this pain and his or her daily symptoms. Likewise, a patient who has had a previous dislocation or subluxation can be vividly reminded of that event by stressing the joint in such a way that it again threatens to dislocate; indeed, merely starting the movement may be so distressing that the patient goes rigid with anxiety at the anticipated result – this is aptly called the *apprehension test.*

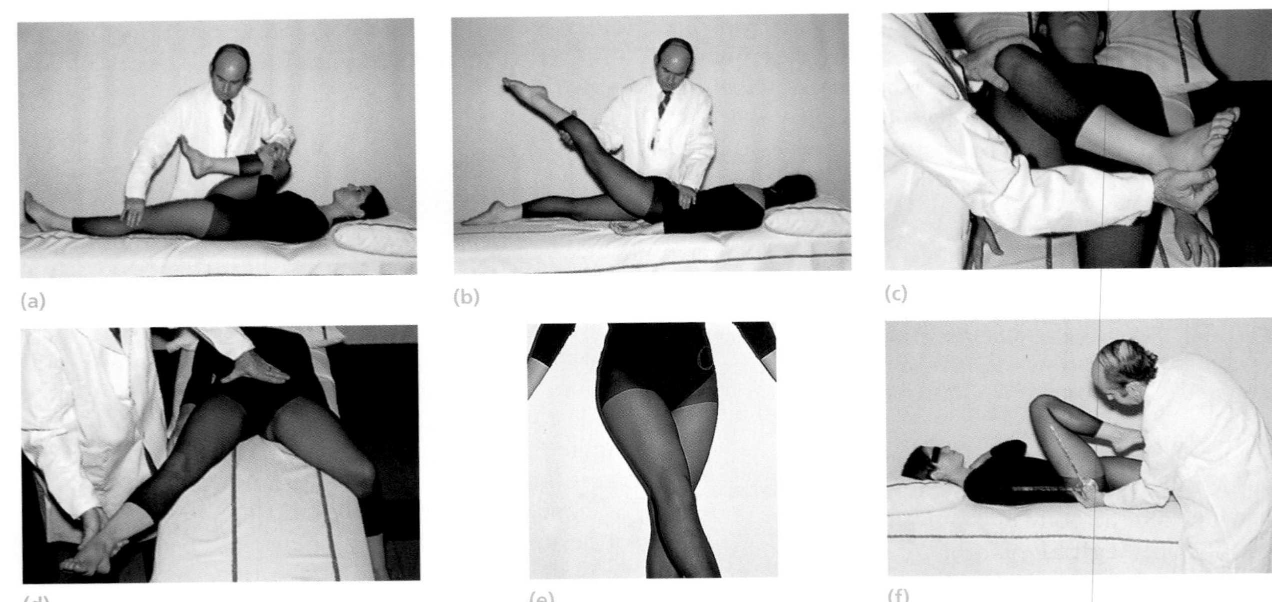

1.5 Testing for movement (a) Flexion, (b) extension, (c) rotation, (d) abduction, (e) adduction. The range of movement can be estimated by eye or measured accurately using a goniometer (f).

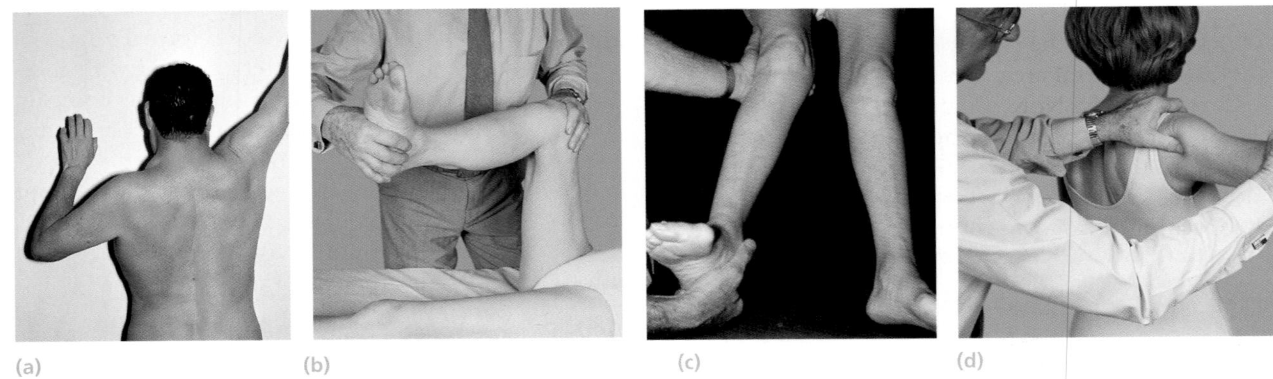

1.6 Move (a) Active movement – the patient moves the joint. The right shoulder is normal; the left has restricted active movement. (b) Passive movement – the examiner moves the joint. (c) Unstable movement – the joint can be moved across the normal planes of action, in this case demonstrating valgus instability of the right knee. (d) Provocative movement – the examiner moves (or manipulates) the joint so as to provoke the symptoms of impending pain or dislocation. Here he is reproducing the position in which an unstable shoulder is likely to dislocate.

Test

The apprehension test referred to in the previous paragraph is one of several clinical tests that are used to elicit suspected abnormalities: some examples are *Thomas' test* for flexion deformity of the hip, *Trendelenburg's test* for instability of the hip, *McMurray's test* for a torn meniscus of the knee, *Lachman's test* for cruciate ligament instability and various tests for intra-articular fluid. These and others are described in the relevant chapters in Section 2.

Tests for muscle tone, motor power, reflexes and various modes of sensibility are part and parcel of neurological examination, which is dealt with on page 10.

Caveat

We recognize that the sequence set out here may sometimes have to be modified. We may need to 'move' before we 'look': an early scoliotic deformity of the spine often becomes apparent only when the patient bends forwards. The sequence may also have to be altered because a patient is in severe pain or disabled: you would not try to move a limb at all in someone with a suspected fracture when an x-ray can provide the answer. When examining a child you may have to take your chances with look or feel or move whenever you can!

Terminology

Colloquial terms such as front, back, upper, lower, inner aspect, outer aspect, bow legs, knock knees have the advantage of familiarity but are not applicable to every situation. Universally acceptable anatomical definitions are therefore necessary in describing physical attributes.

Bodily surfaces, planes and positions are always described in relation to the **anatomical position** – as if the person were standing erect, facing the viewer, legs together with the knees pointing directly forwards, and arms held by the sides with the palms facing forwards.

The principal planes of the body are named **sagittal, coronal and transverse**; they define the direction across which the body (or body part) is viewed in any description. **Sagittal planes**, parallel to each other, pass vertically through the body from front to back; the **midsagittal** or **median plane** divides the body into right and left halves. **Coronal planes** are also orientated vertically, corresponding to a frontal view, at right angles to the saggital planes; **transverse planes** pass horizontally across the body.

Anterior signifies the frontal aspect and **posterior** the rear aspect of the body or a body part. The terms **ventral** and **dorsal** are also used for the front and the back respectively. Note, though, that the use of these terms is somewhat confusing when it comes to the foot: here the upper surface is called the **dorsum** and the sole is called the **plantar surface**.

Medial means facing towards the median plane or midline of the body, and **lateral** away from the median plane. These terms are usually applied to a limb, the clavicle or one half of the pelvis. Thus the inner aspect of the thigh lies on the medial side of the limb and the outer part of the thigh lies on the lateral side. We could also say that the little finger lies on the medial or **ulnar side** of the hand and the thumb on the lateral or **radial side** of the hand.

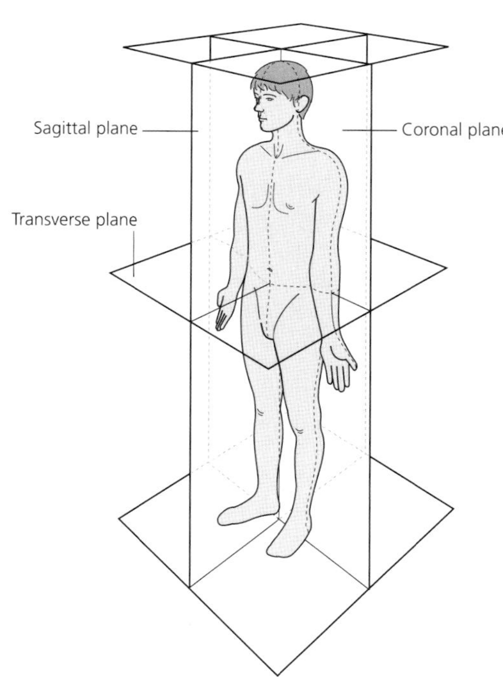

1.7 The principal planes of the body, as viewed in the anatomical position: sagittal, coronal and transverse.

Proximal and **distal** are used mainly for parts of the limbs, meaning respectively the upper end and the lower end as they appear in the anatomical position. Thus the knee joint is formed by the distal end of the femur and the proximal end of the tibia.

Axial alignment describes the longitudinal arrangement of adjacent limb segments or parts of a single bone. The knees and elbows, for example, are normally angulated slightly outwards (**valgus)** while the opposite – 'bow legs' – is more correctly described as **varus** (see on page 13, under Deformity). Angulation in the middle of a long bone would always be regarded as abnormal.

Rotational alignment refers to the tortile arrangement of segments of a long bone (or an entire limb) around a single longitudinal axis. For example, in the anatomical position the patellae face forwards while the feet are turned slightly outwards; a marked difference in rotational alignment of the two legs is abnormal.

Flexion and extension are joint movements in the sagittal plane, most easily imagined in hinge joints like the knee, elbow and the joints of the fingers and toes. In elbows, knees, wrists and fingers flexion means bending the joint and extension means straightening it. In shoulders and hips flexion is movement in an anterior direction and extension is movement posteriorwards. In the ankle flexion is also called **plantarflexion** (pointing the foot downwards) and extension is called **dorsiflexion** (drawing the foot upwards). Thumb movements are the most complicated and are described in Chapter 16.

Abduction and adduction are movements in the coronal plane, away from or towards the median plane. Not quite for the fingers and toes, though: here abduction and adduction mean away from and towards the longitudinal midline of the hand or foot!

Lateral rotation and medial rotation are twisting movements, outwards and inwards, around a longitudinal axis.

Pronation and supination are also rotatory movements, but the terms are applied only to movements of the forearm and the foot.

Circumduction is a composite movement made up of a rhythmic sequence of all the other movements. It is possible only for ball-and-socket joints such as the hip and shoulder.

Specialized movements such as opposition of the thumb, lateral flexion and rotation of the spine, and inversion or eversion of the foot, will be described in the relevant chapters.

NEUROLOGICAL EXAMINATION

If the symptoms include weakness or incoordination or a change in sensibility, or if they point to any disorder of the neck or back, a complete neurological examination of the related part is mandatory.

Once again we follow a systematic routine, first looking at the general appearance, then assessing motor function (muscle tone, power and reflexes) and finally testing for sensory function (both skin sensibility and deep sensibility).

Appearance

Some neurological disorders result in postures that are so characteristic as to be diagnostic at a glance: the claw hand of an ulnar nerve lesion; drop wrist following radial nerve palsy; or the 'waiter's tip' deformity of the arm in brachial plexus injury. Usually, however, it is when the patient moves that we can best appreciate the type and extent of motor disorder: the dangling arm following a brachial plexus injury; the flail lower limb of poliomyelitis; the symmetrical paralysis of spinal cord lesions; the characteristic drop-foot gait following sciatic or peroneal nerve damage; and the jerky, 'spastic' movements of cerebral palsy.

Concentrating on the affected part, we look for trophic changes that signify loss of sensibility: the smooth, hairless skin that seems to be stretched too tight; atrophy of the fingertips and the nails; scars that tell of accidental burns; and ulcers that refuse to heal. Muscle wasting is important; if localized and asymmetrical, it may suggest dysfunction of a specific motor nerve.

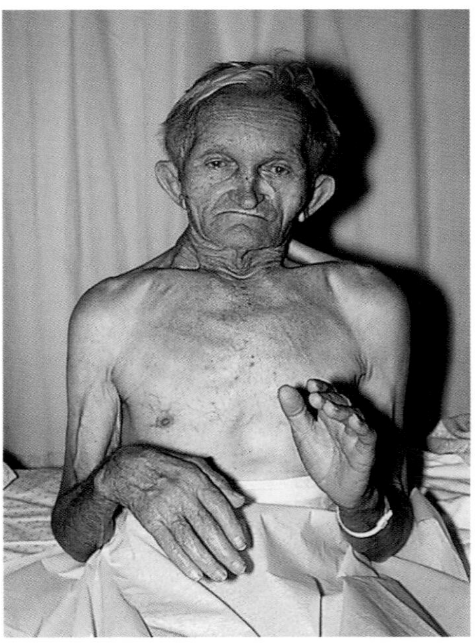

1.8 Posture Posture is often diagnostic. This patient's 'drop wrist' – typical of a radial nerve palsy – is due to carcinomatous infiltration of the supraclavicular lymph nodes on the right.

Muscle tone

Tone in individual muscle groups is tested by moving the nearby joint to stretch the muscle. Increased tone (spasticity) is characteristic of upper motor neuron disorders such as cerebral palsy and stroke. It must not be confused with rigidity (the 'lead-pipe' or 'cogwheel' effect) which is seen in Parkinson's disease. Decreased tone (flaccidity) is found in lower motor neuron lesions; for example, poliomyelitis. Muscle power is diminished in all three states; it is important to recognize that a 'spastic' muscle may still be weak.

Power

Motor function is tested by having the patient perform movements that are normally activated by specific nerves. We may learn even more about composite movements by asking the patient to perform specific tasks, such as holding a pen, gripping a rod, doing up a button or picking up a pin.

Testing for power is not as easy as it sounds; the difficulty is making ourselves understood. The simplest way is to place the limb in the 'test' position, then ask the patient to hold it there as firmly as possible and resist any attempt to change that position. The normal limb is examined first, then the affected limb, and the two are compared. Finer muscle actions, such as those of the thumb and fingers, may be reproduced by first demonstrating the movement yourself, then testing it in the unaffected limb, and then in the affected one.

Muscle power is usually graded on the Medical Research Council scale:

Grade 0 No movement.
Grade 1 Only a flicker of movement.
Grade 2 Movement with gravity eliminated.
Grade 3 Movement against gravity.
Grade 4 Movement against resistance.
Grade 5 Normal power.

It is important to recognize that muscle weakness may be due to muscle disease rather than nerve disease. In muscle disorders the weakness is usually more widespread and symmetrical, and sensation is normal.

Tendon reflexes

A deep tendon reflex is elicited by rapidly stretching the tendon near its insertion. A sharp tap with the tendon hammer does this well; but all too often this is performed with a flourish and with such force that the finer gradations of response are missed. It is better to employ a series of taps, starting with the most forceful and reducing the force with each successive tap until there is no response. Comparing the two sides in this way, we can pick up fine differences showing that a reflex is 'diminished' rather than 'absent'. In the upper limb we test biceps, triceps and brachioradialis; and in the lower limb the patellar and Achilles tendons.

The tendon reflexes are monosynaptic segmental reflexes; that is, the reflex pathway takes a 'short cut' through the spinal cord at the segmental level. Depression or absence of the reflex signifies interruption of the pathway at the posterior nerve root, the anterior horn cell, the motor nerve root or the peripheral nerve. It is a reliable pointer to the segmental level of dysfunction: thus, a depressed biceps jerk suggests pressure on the fifth or sixth cervical (C5 or 6) nerve roots while a depressed ankle jerk signifies a similar abnormality at the first sacral level (S1). An unusually brisk reflex, on the other hand, is characteristic of an upper motor neuron disorder (e.g. cerebral palsy, a stroke or injury to the spinal cord); the lower motor neuron is released

Table 1.1 Nerve root supply and actions of main muscle groups

Sternomastoids	Spinal accessory C2, 3, 4
Trapezius	Spinal accessory C3, 4
Diaphragm	C3, 4, 5
Deltoid	C5, 6
Supra- and infraspinatus	C5, 6
Serratus anterior	C5, 6, 7
Pectoralis major	C5, 6, 7, 8
Elbow flexion	C5, 6
extension	C7
Supination	C5, 6
Pronation	C6
Wrist extension	C6, (7)
flexion	C7, (8)
Finger extension	C7
flexion	C7, 8, T1
ab- and adduction	C8, T1
Hip flexion	L1, 2, 3
extension	L5, S1
adduction	L2, 3, 4
abduction	L4, 5, S1
Knee extension	L(2), 3, 4
flexion	L5, S1
Ankle dorsiflexion	L4, 5
plantarflexion	S1, 2
inversion	L4, 5
eversion	L5, S1
Toe extension	L5
flexion	S1
abduction	S1, 2

from the normal central inhibition and there is an exaggerated response to tendon stimulation. This may manifest as ankle clonus: a sharp upward jerk on the foot (dorsiflexion) causes a repetitive, 'clonic' movement of the foot; similarly, a sharp downward push on the patella may elicit patellar clonus.

Superficial reflexes

The superficial reflexes are elicited by stroking the skin at various sites to produce a specific muscle contraction; the best known are the abdominal (T7–T12), cremasteric (L1, 2) and anal (S4, 5) reflexes. These are corticospinal (upper motor neuron) reflexes. Absence of the reflex indicates an upper motor neuron lesion (usually in the spinal cord) above that level.

The plantar reflex

Forceful stroking of the sole normally produces flexion of the toes (or no response at all). An extensor response (the big toe extends while the others remain in flexion) is characteristic of upper motor neuron disorders. This is the *Babinski sign* – a type of withdrawal reflex which is present in young infants and normally disappears after the age of 18 months.

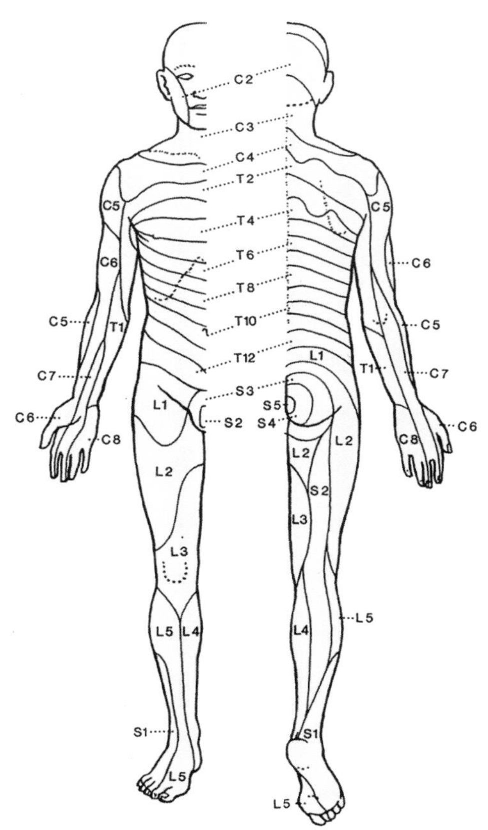

1.9 Examination Dermatomes supplied by the spinal nerve roots.

Sensibility

Sensibility to touch and to pinprick may be increased (hyperaesthesia) or unpleasant (dysaesthesia) in certain irritative nerve lesions. More often, though, it is diminished (hypoaesthesia) or absent (anaesthesia), signifying pressure on or interruption of a peripheral nerve, a nerve root or the sensory pathways in the spinal cord. The area of sensory change can be mapped out on the skin and compared with the known segmental or dermatomal pattern of innervation. If the abnormality is well defined it is an easy matter to establish the level of the lesion, even if the precise cause remains unknown.

Brisk percussion along the course of an injured nerve may elicit a tingling sensation in the distal distribution of the nerve (*Tinel's sign*). The point of hypersensitivity marks the site of abnormal nerve sprouting: if it progresses distally at successive visits this signifies regeneration; if it remains unchanged this suggests a local neuroma.

Tests for temperature recognition and two-point discrimination (the ability to recognize two touch-points a few millimetres apart) are also used in the assessment of peripheral nerve injuries.

Deep sensibility can be examined in several ways. In the vibration test a sounded tuning fork is placed over a peripheral bony point (e.g. the medial malleolus or the head of the ulna); the patient is asked if he or she can feel the vibrations and to say when they disappear. By comparing the two sides, differences can be noted. Position sense is tested by asking the patient to find certain points on the body with the eyes closed – for example, touching the tip of the nose with the forefinger. The sense of joint posture is tested by grasping the big toe and placing it in different positions of flexion and extension. The patient (whose eyes are closed) is asked to say whether it is 'up' or 'down'. Stereognosis, the ability to recognize shape and texture by feel alone, is tested by giving the patient (again with eyes closed) a variety of familiar objects to hold and asking him or her to name each object.

The pathways for deep sensibility run in the posterior columns of the spinal cord. Disturbances are, therefore, found in peripheral neuropathies and in spinal cord lesions such as posterior column injuries or tabes dorsalis. The sense of balance is also carried in the posterior columns. This can be tested by asking the patient to stand upright with his or her eyes closed; excessive body sway is abnormal (*Romberg's sign*).

Cortical and cerebellar function

A staggering gait may imply an unstable knee – or a disorder of the spinal cord or cerebellum. If there is no musculoskeletal abnormality to account for the sign, a full examination of the central nervous system will be necessary.

EXAMINING INFANTS AND CHILDREN

Paediatric practice requires special skills. You may have no first-hand account of the symptoms; a baby screaming with pain will tell you very little, and over-anxious parents will probably tell you too much. When examining the child, be flexible. If he or she is moving a particular joint, take your opportunity to examine movement then and there. You will learn much more by adopting methods of play than by applying a rigid system of examination. And leave any test for tenderness until last!

INFANTS AND SMALL CHILDREN

The baby should be undressed, in a warm room, and placed on the examining couch. Look carefully for birthmarks, deformities and abnormal movements – or absence of movement. If there is no urgency or distress, take time to examine the head and neck, including facial features which may be characteristic of specific dysplastic syndromes. The back and limbs are then examined for abnormalities of position or shape. Examining for joint movement can be difficult. Active movements can often be stimulated by gently stroking the limb. When testing for passive mobility, be careful to avoid frightening or hurting the child.

In the neonate, and throughout the first two years of life, examination of the hips is mandatory, even if the child appears to be normal. This is to avoid missing the subtle signs of developmental dysplasia of the hips (DDH) at the early stage when treatment is most effective.

It is also important to assess the child's general development by testing for the normal milestones which are expected to appear during the first two years of life.

NORMAL DEVELOPMENTAL MILESTONES	
Newborn	Grasp reflex present Morrow reflex present
3–6 months	Holds head up unsupported
6–9 months	Able to sit up
9–12 months	Crawling and standing up
9–18 months	Walking
18–24 months	Running

OLDER CHILDREN

Most children can be examined in the same way as adults, though with different emphasis on particular physical features. Posture and gait are very important; subtle deviations from the norm may herald the appearance of serious abnormalities such as scoliosis or neuromuscular disorders, while more obvious 'deformities' such as knock knees and bow legs may be no more than transient stages in normal development; similarly with mild degrees of 'flat feet' and 'pigeon toes'. More complex variations in posture and gait patterns, when the child sits and walks with the knees turned inwards (medially rotated) or outwards (laterally rotated) are usually due to anteversion or retroversion of the femoral necks, sometimes associated with compensatory rotational 'deformities' of the femora and tibiae. Seldom need anything be done about this; the condition usually improves as the child approaches puberty and only if the gait is very awkward would one consider performing corrective osteotomies of the femora.

PHYSICAL VARIATIONS AND DEFORMITIES

JOINT LAXITY

Children's joints are much more mobile than those of most adults, allowing them to adopt postures that would be impossible for their parents. An unusual degree of joint mobility can also be attained by adults willing to submit to rigorous exercise and practice, as witness the performances of professional dancers and athletes, but in most cases, when the exercises stop, mobility gradually reverts to the normal range.

Persistent generalized joint hypermobility occurs in about 5% of the population and is inherited as a simple mendelian dominant. Those affected describe themselves as being 'double-jointed': they can hyperextend their metacarpophalangeal joints beyond a right angle, hyperextend their elbows and knees and bend over with knees straight to place their hands flat on the ground; some can even 'do the splits' or place their feet behind their neck!

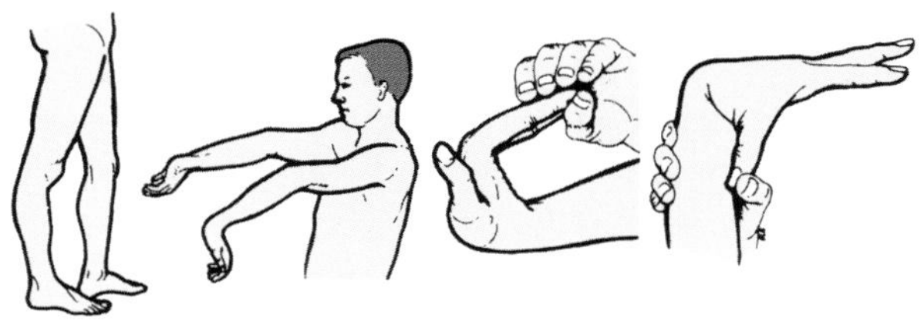

1.10 Tests for joint hypermobility Hyperextension of knees and elbows; metacarpophalangeal joints extending to 90 degrees; thumb able to touch forearm.

It is doubtful whether these individuals should be considered 'abnormal'. However, epidemiological studies have shown that they do have a greater than usual tendency to recurrent dislocation (e.g. of the shoulder or patella). Some experience recurrent episodes of aching around the larger joints; however, there is no convincing evidence that hypermobility by itself predisposes to osteoarthritis.

Generalized hypermobility is not usually associated with any obvious disease, but severe laxity is a feature of certain rare connective tissue disorders such as Marfan's syndrome, Ehlers–Danlos syndrome, Larsen's disease and osteogenesis imperfecta.

Deformity

The boundary between variations of the normal and physical deformity is blurred. Indeed, in the development of species, what at one point of time might have been seen as a deformity could over the ages have turned out to be so advantageous as to become essential for survival.

So too in humans. The word 'deformity' is derived from the Latin for 'misshapen', but the range of 'normal shape' is so wide that variations should not automatically be designated as deformities, and some undoubted 'deformities' are not necessarily pathological; for example, the generally accepted cut-off points for 'abnormal' shortness or tallness are arbitrary and people who in one population might be considered abnormally short or abnormally tall could, in other populations, be seen as quite ordinary. However, if one leg is short and the other long, no-one would quibble with the use of the word 'deformity'!

Specific terms are used to describe the 'position' and 'shape' of the bones and joints. Whether, in any particular case, these amount to 'deformity' will be determined by additional factors such as the extent to which they deviate from the norm, symptoms to which they give rise, the presence or absence of instability and the degree to which they interfere with function.

Varus and valgus It seems pedantic to replace 'bow legs' and 'knock knees' with 'genu varum' and 'genu valgum', but comparable colloquialisms are not available for deformities of the elbow, hip or big toe; and, besides, the formality is justified by the need for clarity and consistency. Varus means that the part distal to the joint in question is displaced towards the median plane, valgus away from it.

Kyphosis and lordosis Seen from the side, the normal spine has a series of curves: convex posteriorly in the thoracic region (kyphosis), and convex anteriorly in the cervical and lumbar regions (lordosis). Excessive curvature constitutes kyphotic or lordotic deformity (also sometimes referred to as hyperkyphosis and

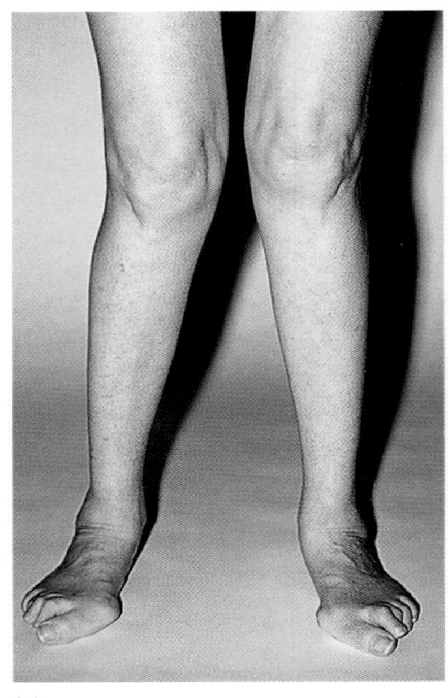

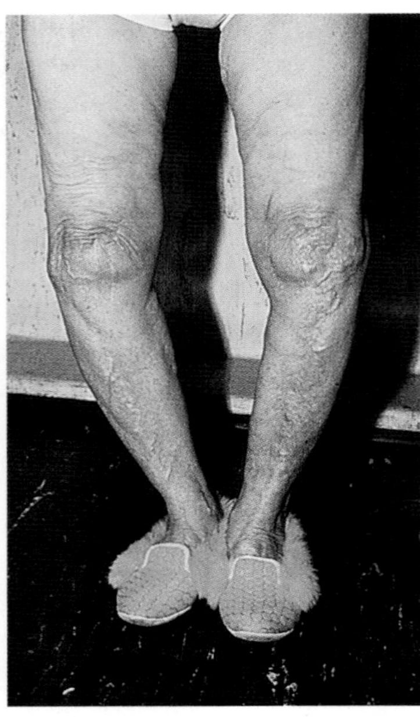

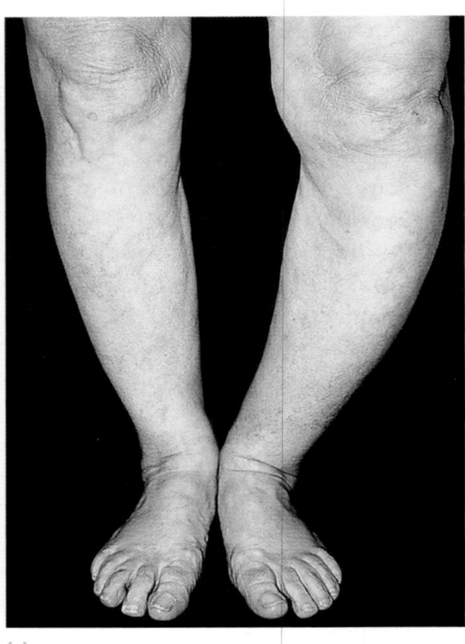

(a) (b) (c)

1.11 Varus and valgus (a) Valgus knees in a patient with rheumatoid arthritis. The toe joints are also valgus. (b) Varus knees due to osteoarthritis. (c) Another varus knee? No – the deformity here is in the left tibia due to Paget's disease.

hyperlordosis). Colloquially speaking, excessive thoracic kyphosis is referred to as 'round-shouldered'.

Scoliosis Seen from behind, the spine is straight. Any curvature in the coronal plane is called scoliosis. The position and direction of the curve are specified by terms such as thoracic scoliosis, lumbar scoliosis, convex to the right, concave to the left, etc.

Postural deformity A postural deformity is one which the patient can, if properly instructed, correct voluntarily: e.g. thoracic 'kyphosis' due to slumped shoulders. Postural deformity may also be caused by temporary muscle spasm.

Structural deformity A deformity which results from a permanent change in anatomical structure cannot be voluntarily corrected. It is important to distinguish postural scoliosis from structural (fixed) scoliosis. The former is non-progressive and benign; the latter is usually progressive and may require treatment.

'Fixed deformity' This term is ambiguous. It seems to mean that a joint is deformed and unable to move. Not so – it means that one particular movement cannot be completed. Thus the knee may be able to flex fully but not extend fully – at the limit of its extension it is still 'fixed' in a certain amount of flexion. This would be called a 'fixed flexion deformity'.

CAUSES OF JOINT DEFORMITY

There are six basic causes of joint deformity:

1. ***Contracture of the overlying skin*** This is seen typically when there is severe scarring across the flexor aspect of a joint, e.g. due to a burn or following surgery.
2. ***Contracture of the subcutaneous fascia*** The classical example is Dupuytren's contracture in the palm of the hand.
3. ***Muscle contracture*** Fibrosis and contracture of muscles that cross a joint will cause a fixed deformity of the joint. This may be due to deep infection or fibrosis following ischaemic necrosis (Volkmann's ischaemic contracture).
4. ***Muscle imbalance*** Unbalanced muscle weakness or spasticity will result in joint deformity which, if not corrected, will eventually become fixed. This is seen most typically in poliomyelitis and cerebral palsy. Tendon rupture, likewise, may cause deformity.
5. ***Joint instability*** Any unstable joint will assume a 'deformed' position when subjected to force.
6. ***Joint destruction*** Trauma, infection or arthritis may destroy the joint and lead to severe deformity.

CAUSES OF BONE DEFORMITY

Bone deformities in small children are usually due to genetic or developmental disorders of cartilage and bone growth; some can be diagnosed in utero by special imaging techniques (e.g. achondroplasia); some become apparent when the child starts to walk, or later still during one of the growth spurts (e.g. hereditary multiple exostosis); and some only in early adulthood (e.g. multiple epiphyseal dysplasia). There are a myriad genetic disorders affecting the skeleton, yet any one of these conditions is rare. The least unusual of them are described in Chapter 8.

Acquired deformities in children may be due to fractures involving the physis (growth plate); ask about previous injuries. Other causes include rickets, endocrine disorders, malunited diaphyseal fractures and tumours.

Acquired deformities of bone in adults are usually the result of previous malunited fractures. However, causes such as osteomalacia, bone tumours and Paget's disease should always be considered.

Bony lumps

A bony lump may be due to faulty development, injury, inflammation or a tumour. Although x-ray examination is essential, the clinical features can be highly informative.

Size A large lump attached to bone, or a lump that is getting bigger, is nearly always a tumour.

Site A lump near a joint is most likely to be a tumour (benign or malignant); a lump in the shaft may be fracture callus, inflammatory new bone or a tumour.

Margin A benign tumour has a well-defined margin; malignant tumours, inflammatory lumps and callus have a vague edge.

Consistency A benign tumour feels bony hard; malignant tumours often give the impression that they can be indented.

Tenderness Lumps due to active inflammation, recent callus or a rapidly growing sarcoma are tender.

Multiplicity Multiple bony lumps are uncommon: they occur in hereditary multiple exostosis and in Ollier's disease.

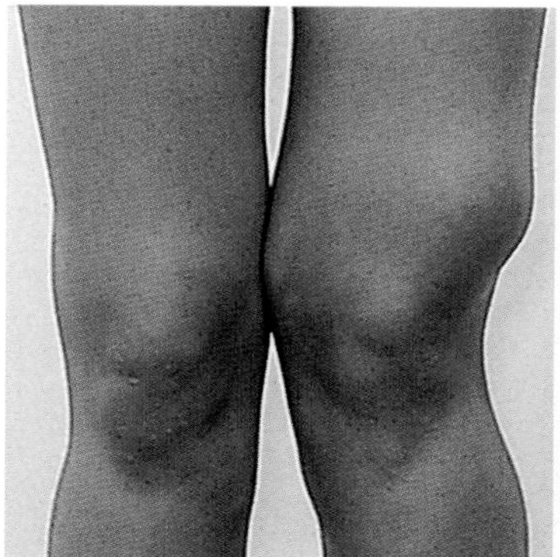
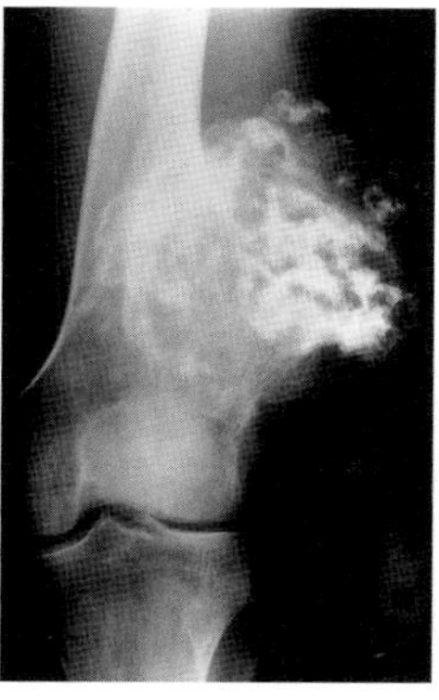

1.12 Bony lumps The lump above the left knee is hard, well-defined and not increasing in size. The clinical diagnosis of cartilage-capped exostosis (osteochondroma) is confirmed by the x-rays.

Joint stiffness

The term 'stiffness' covers a variety of limitations. We consider three types of stiffness in particular: (1) all movements absent; (2) all movements limited; (3) one or two movements limited.

All movements absent Surprisingly, although movement is completely blocked, the patient may retain such good function that the restriction goes unnoticed until the joint is examined. Surgical fusion is called 'arthrodesis'; pathological fusion is called 'ankylosis'. Acute suppurative arthritis typically ends in bony ankylosis; tuberculous arthritis heals by fibrosis and causes fibrous ankylosis – not strictly a 'fusion' because there may still be a small jog of movement.

All movements limited After severe injury, movement may be limited as a result of oedema and bruising. Later, adhesions and loss of muscle extensibility may perpetuate the stiffness.

With active inflammation all movements are restricted and painful and the joint is said to be 'irritable'. In acute arthritis spasm may prevent all but a few degrees of movement.

In osteoarthritis the capsule fibroses and movements become increasingly restricted, but pain occurs only at the extremes of motion.

Some movements limited When one particular movement suddenly becomes blocked, the cause is usually mechanical. Thus a torn and displaced meniscus may prevent extension of the knee but not flexion.

Bone deformity may alter the arc of movement, such that it is limited in one direction (loss of abduction in coxa vara is an example) but movement in the opposite direction is full or even increased.

These are all examples of 'fixed deformity'.

DIAGNOSTIC IMAGING

The map is not the territory

Alfred Korzybski

Plain film radiography

Plain film x-ray examination is over 100 years old. Notwithstanding the extraordinary technical advances of the last few decades, it remains the most useful method of diagnostic imaging. Whereas other methods may define an inaccessible anatomical structure more accurately, or may reveal some localized tissue change, the plain film provides information simultaneously on the size, shape, tissue 'density' and bone architecture – characteristics which, taken together, will usually suggest a diagnosis, or at least a range of possible diagnoses.

The radiographic image

X-rays are produced by firing electrons at high speed onto a rotating anode. The resulting beam of x-rays is attenuated by the patient's soft tissues and bones, casting what are effectively 'shadows' which are displayed as images on an appropriately sensitized plate or stored as digital information which is then available to be transferred throughout the local information technology (IT) network.

The more dense and impenetrable the tissue, the greater the x-ray attenuation and therefore the more blank, or white, the image that is captured. Thus, a metal implant appears intensely white, bone less so and soft tissues in varying shades of grey depending on their 'density'. Cartilage, which causes little attenuation, appears as a dark area between adjacent bone ends; this 'gap' is usually called the joint space, though of course it is not a space at all, merely a radiolucent zone filled with cartilage. Other 'radiolucent' areas are produced by fluid-filled cysts in bone.

One bone overlying another (e.g. the femoral head inside the acetabular socket) produces superimposed images; any abnormality seen in the resulting combined image could be in either bone, so it is important to obtain several images from different projections in order to separate the anatomical outlines. Similarly, the bright image of a metallic foreign body superimposed upon that of, say, the femoral condyles could mean that the foreign body is in front of, inside or behind the bone. A second projection, at right angles to the first, will give the answer.

Picture Archiving and Communication System (PACS) This is the system whereby all digitally coded images are filed, stored and retrieved to enable the images to be sent to work stations throughout the hospital, to other hospitals or to the Consultant's personal computer.

Radiographic interpretation

Although *radiograph* is the correct word for the plain image which we address, in the present book we have chosen to retain the old-fashioned term '*x-ray*', which has become entrenched by long usage.

The process of interpreting this image should be as methodical as clinical examination. It is seductively easy to be led astray by some flagrant anomaly; systematic study is the only safeguard. A convenient sequence for examination is: *the patient – the soft tissues – the bone – the joints.*

THE PATIENT

Make sure that the name on the film is that of your patient; mistaken identity is a potent source of error. The clinical details are important; it is surprising how much more you can see on the x-ray when you know the background. Similarly, when requesting an x-ray examination, give the radiologist enough information from the patient's history and the clinical findings to help in guiding his or her thoughts towards the diagnostic possibilities and options. For example, when considering a malignant bone lesion, simply knowing the patient's age may provide an important clue: under the age of 10 it is most likely to be a Ewing's sarcoma; between 10 and 20 years it is more likely to be an osteosarcoma; and over the age of 50 years it is likely to be a metastatic deposit.

THE SOFT TISSUES

Generalized change Muscle planes are often visible and may reveal wasting or swelling. Bulging outlines around a hip, for example, may suggest a joint effusion; and soft-tissue swelling around interphalangeal joints may be the first radiographic sign of rheumatoid arthritis. Tumours tend to displace fascial planes, whereas infection tends to obliterate them.

Localized change Is there a mass, soft tissue calcification, ossification, gas (from penetrating wound or gas-forming organism) or the presence of a radio-opaque foreign body?

THE BONES

Shape The bones are well enough defined to allow one to check their general anatomy and individual shape. For example, for the spine, look at the overall

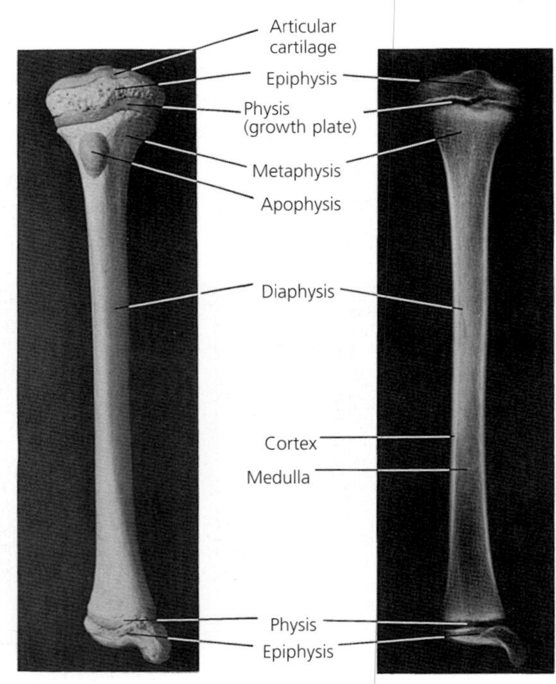

1.13 The radiographic image X-ray of an anatomical specimen to show the appearance of various parts of the bone in the x-ray image.

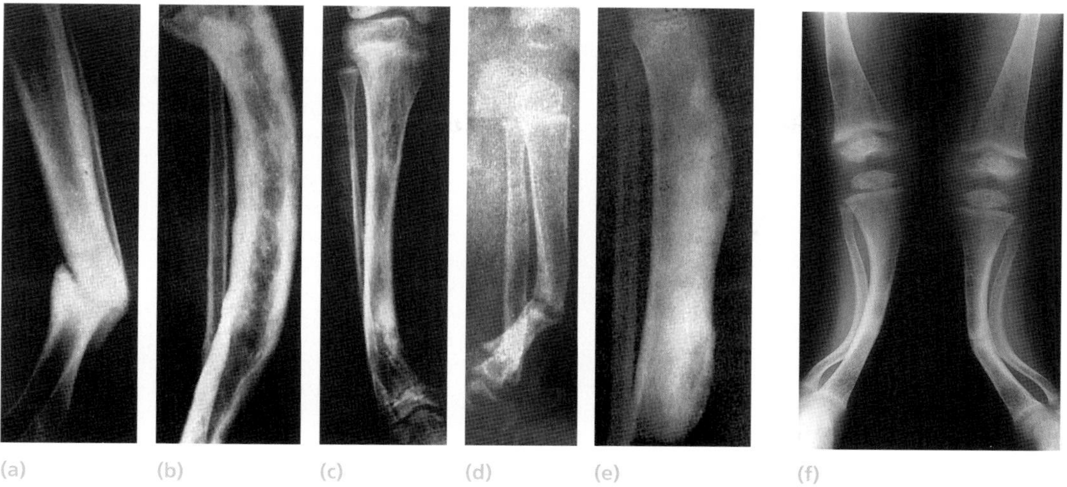

1.14 X-rays – bent bones (a) Mal-united fracture. (b) Paget's disease. (c) Dyschondroplasia. (d) Congenital pseudarthrosis. (e) Syphilitic sabre tibia. (f) Osteogenesis imperfecta.

vertebral alignment, then at the disc spaces, and then at each vertebra separately, moving from the body to the pedicles, the facet joints and finally the spinous appendages. For the pelvis, see if the shape is symmetrical with the bones in their normal positions, then look at the sacrum, the two innominate bones, the pubic rami and the ischial tuberosities, then the femoral heads and the upper ends of the femora, always comparing the two sides.

Generalized change Take note of changes in bone 'density' (osteopaenia or osteosclerosis). Is there abnormal trabeculation, as in Paget's disease? Are there features suggestive of diffuse metastatic infiltration, either sclerotic or lytic? Other polyostotic lesions include fibrous dysplasia, histiocyotis, multiple exostosis and Paget's disease. With aggressive looking polyostotic lesions think of metastases (including myeloma and lymphoma) and also multifocal infection. By contrast, most primary tumours are monostotic.

Localized change Focal abnormalities should be approached in the same way as one would conduct a clinical analysis of a soft tissue abnormality. Start describing the abnormality from the centre and move outwards. Determine the lesion's size, site, shape, density and margins, as well as adjacent periosteal changes and any surrounding soft tissue changes. Remember that benign lesions are usually well defined with sclerotic margins (Fig. 1.15b) and a smooth periosteal reaction. Ill-defined areas with permeative bone destruction (Fig. 1.15c) and irregular or spiculated periosteal reactions (Fig. 1.15d) suggest an aggressive lesion such as infection or a malignant tumour.

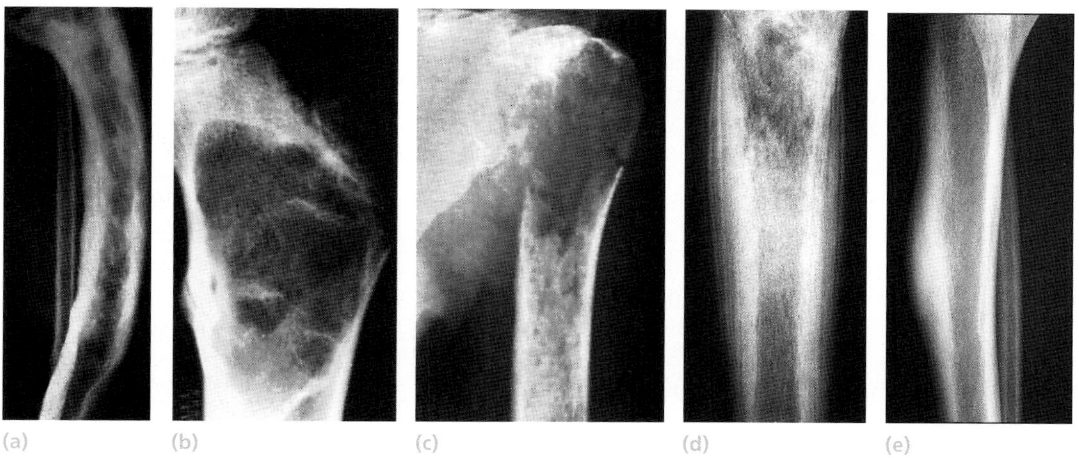

1.15 X-rays – important features to look for (a) *General shape and appearance*, in this case the cortices are thickened and the bone is bent (Paget's disease). (b,c) *Interior density*, a vacant area may represent a true cyst (b), or radiolucent material infiltrating the bone, like the metastatic tumour in (c). (d) *Periosteal reaction*, typically seen in healing fractures, bone infection and malignant bone tumours – as in this example of Ewing's sarcoma. Compare this with the smooth periosteal new bone formation shown in (e).

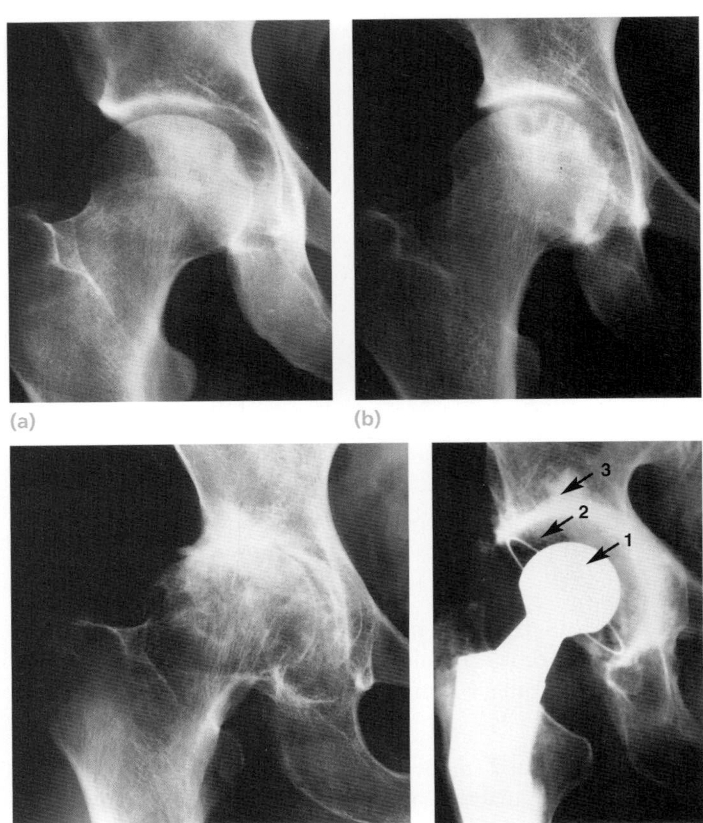

1.16 Plain x-rays of the hip Stages in the development of osteoarthritis (OA). (a) Normal hip: anatomical shape and position, with joint 'space' (articular cartilage) fully preserved. (b) Early OA, showing joint space slightly decreased and a subarticular cyst in the femoral head. (c) Advanced OA: joint space markedly decreased; osteophytes at the joint margin. (d) Hip replacement: the cup is radiolucent but its position is shown by a circumferential wire marker. Note the differing image 'densities': (1) the metal femoral implant; (2) the polyethylene cup (radiolucent); (3) acrylic cement impacted into the adjacent bone.

THE JOINTS

The radiographic 'joint' consists of the articulating bones and the 'space' between them.

The 'joint space' The joint space is, of course, illusory; it is occupied by a film of synovial fluid plus radiolucent articular cartilage which varies in thickness from 1 mm or less (the carpal joints) to 6 mm (the knee). It looks much wider in children than in adults because much of the epiphysis is still cartilaginous and therefore radiolucent. Lines of increased density within the radiographic articular 'space' may be due to calcification of the cartilage or menisci (chondrocalcinosis). Loose bodies, if they are radio-opaque, appear as rounded patches overlying the normal structures.

Shape Note the general orientation of the joint and the congruity of the bone ends (actually the subarticular bone plates), if necessary comparing the abnormal with the normal opposite side. Then look for narrowing or asymmetry of the joint 'space': narrowing signifies loss of hyaline cartilage and is typical of infection, inflammatory arthropathies and osteoarthritis. Further stages of joint destruction are revealed by irregularity of the radiographically visible bone ends and radiolucent cysts in the subchondral bone. Bony excrescences at the joint margins (osteophytes) are typical of osteoarthritis.

Erosions Look for associated bone erosions. The position of erosions and symmetry help to define various types of arthropathy. In rheumatoid arthritis and psoriasis the erosions are peri-articular (at the bare area where the hyaline cartilage covering the joint has ended and the intracapsular bone is exposed to joint fluid). In gout the erosions are further away from the articular surfaces and are described as juxta-articular. Rheumatoid arthritis is classically symmetrical and predominantly involves the metacarpophalangeal and proximal interphalangeal joints in both hands. The erosions in psoriasis are usually more feathery with ill-defined new bone at their margins. Ill-defined erosions suggest active synovitis whereas corticated erosions indicate healing and chronicity.

Diagnostic associations

However carefully the individual x-ray features are observed, the diagnosis will not leap ready-made off the x-ray plate. Even a fracture is not always obvious. It is the pattern of abnormalities that counts: if you see one feature that is suggestive, look for others that are commonly associated.

- Narrowing of the joint space + subchondral sclerosis and cysts + osteophytes = osteoarthritis.
- Narrowing of the joint space + osteoporosis + periarticular erosions = inflammatory arthritis. Add to this the typical distribution, more or less symmetrically in the proximal joints of both hands, and you must think of rheumatoid arthritis.

- Bone destruction + periosteal new bone formation = infection or malignancy until proven otherwise.
- Remember: the next best investigation is either the previous radiograph or the subsequent follow-up radiograph. Sequential films demonstrate either progression of changes in active pathology or status quo in longstanding conditions.

Limitations of conventional radiography

Conventional radiography involves exposure of the patient to ionizing radiation, which under certain circumstances can lead to radiation-induced cancer. The Ionising Radiation Medical Exposure Regulations (IRMER) 2000 are embedded in European Law, requiring all clinicians to justify any exposure of the patient to ionizing radiation. It is a criminal offence to breach these regulations. Ionizing radiation can also damage a developing foetus, especially in the first trimester.

As a diagnostic tool, conventional radiography provides poor soft-tissue contrast: for example, it cannot distinguish between muscles, tendons, ligaments and hyaline cartilage. Ultrasound (US), computed tomography (CT) and magnetic resonance imaging (MRI) are now employed to complement plain x-ray examination. However, in parts of the world where these techniques are not available, some modifications of plain radiography still have a useful role.

X-RAYS USING CONTRAST MEDIA

Substances that alter x-ray attenuation characteristics can be used to produce images which contrast with those of the normal tissues. The contrast media used in orthopaedics are mostly iodine-based liquids which can be injected into sinuses, joint cavities or the spinal theca. Air or gas also can be injected into joints to produce a 'negative image' outlining the joint cavity.

Oily iodides are not absorbed and maintain maximum concentration after injection. However, because they are non-miscible, they do not penetrate well into all the nooks and crannies. They are also tissue irritants, especially if used intrathecally. Ionic, water-soluble iodides permit much more detailed imaging and, although also somewhat irritant and neurotoxic, are rapidly absorbed and excreted.

Sinography

Sinography is the simplest form of contrast radiography. The medium (usually one of the ionic water-soluble compounds) is injected into an open sinus; the film shows the track and whether or not it leads to the underlying bone or joint.

Arthrography

Arthrography is a particularly useful form of contrast radiography. Intra-articular loose bodies will produce filling defects in the opaque contrast medium. In the knee, torn menisci, ligament tears and capsular ruptures can be shown. In children's hips, arthrography is a useful method of outlining the cartilaginous (and therefore radiolucent) femoral head. In adults with avascular necrosis of the femoral head, arthrography may show up torn flaps of cartilage. After hip replacement, loosening of a prosthesis may be revealed by seepage of the contrast medium into the cement/bone interface. In the hip, ankle, wrist and

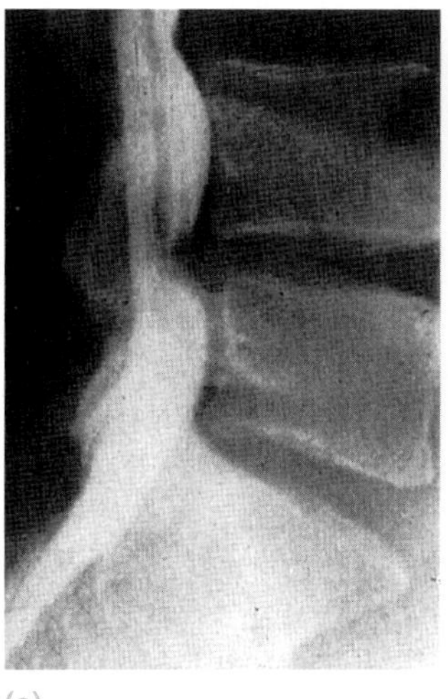
(a)

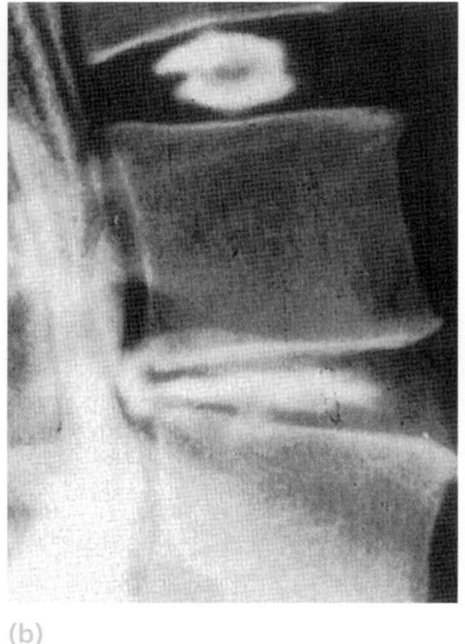
(b)

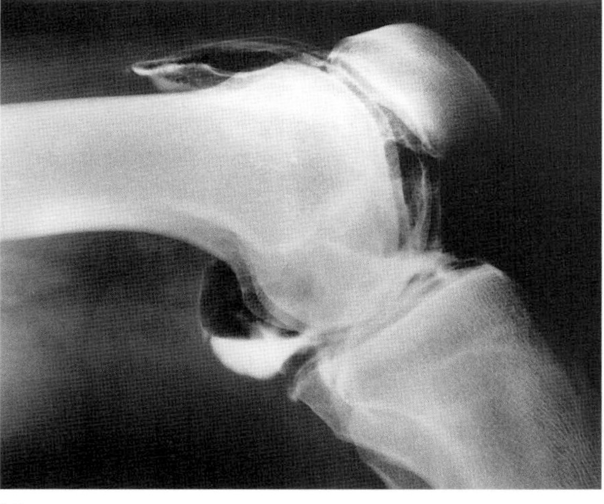
(c)

1.17 Contrast radiography (a) Myelography shows the outline of the spinal theca. Where facilities are available, myelography has been largely replaced by CT and MRI. (b) Discography is sometimes useful: note the difference between a normal intervertebral disc (upper level) and a degenerate disc (lower level). (c) Contrast arthrography of the knee shows a small popliteal herniation.

shoulder, the injected contrast medium may disclose labral tears or defects in the capsular structures. In the spine, contrast radiography can be used to diagnose disc degeneration (discography) and abnormalities of the small facet joints (facetography).

Myelography

Myelography was used extensively in the past for the diagnosis of disc prolapse and other spinal canal lesions. It has been largely replaced by non-invasive methods such as CT and MRI. However, it still has a place in the investigation of nerve root lesions and as an adjunct to other methods in patients with back pain.

The oily media are no longer used, and even with the ionic water-soluble iodides there is a considerable incidence of complications, such as low-pressure headache (due to the lumbar puncture), muscular spasms or convulsions (due to neurotoxicity, especially if the chemical is allowed to flow above the mid-dorsal region) and arachnoiditis (which is attributed to the hyperosmolality of these compounds in relation to cerebrospinal fluid). Precautions, such as keeping the patient sitting upright after myelography, must be strictly observed.

Metrizamide has low neurotoxicity and at working concentrations it is more or less isotonic with cerebrospinal fluid. It can therefore be used throughout the length of the spinal canal; the nerve roots are also well delineated (radiculography). A bulging disc, an intrathecal tumour or narrowing of the bony canal will produce characteristic distortions of the opaque column in the myelogram.

Plain tomography

Tomography provides an image 'focused' on a selected plane. By moving the tube and the x-ray film in opposite directions around the patient during the exposure, images on either side of the pivotal plane are deliberately blurred out. When several 'cuts' are studied, lesions obscured in conventional x-rays may be revealed. The method is useful for diagnosing segmental bone necrosis and depressed fractures in cancellous bone (e.g. of the vertebral body or the tibial plateau); these defects are often obscured in the plain x-ray by the surrounding intact mass of bone. Small radiolucent lesions, such as osteoid osteomas and bone abscesses, can also be revealed.

A useful procedure in former years, conventional tomography has been largely supplanted by CT and MRI.

Computed tomography (CT)

Like plain tomography, CT produces sectional images through selected tissue planes – but with much greater resolution. A further advance over conventional tomography is that the images are trans-axial (like transverse anatomical sections), thus exposing anatomical planes that are never viewed in plain film x-rays. A general (or 'localization') view is obtained, the region of interest is selected and a series of cross-sectional images is produced and digitally recorded. 'Slices' through the larger joints or tissue masses may be 5–10 mm apart; those through the small joints or intervertebral discs have to be much thinner.

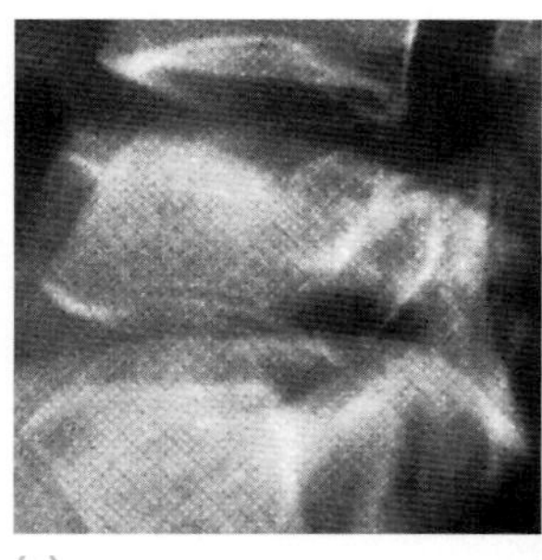

(a)

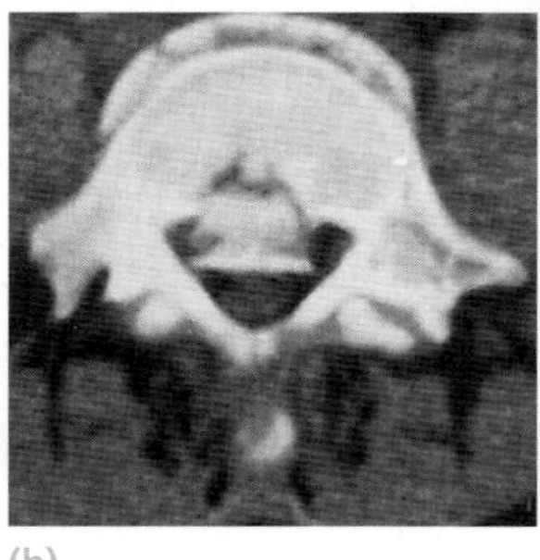

(b)

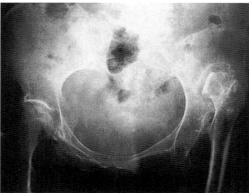

(c)

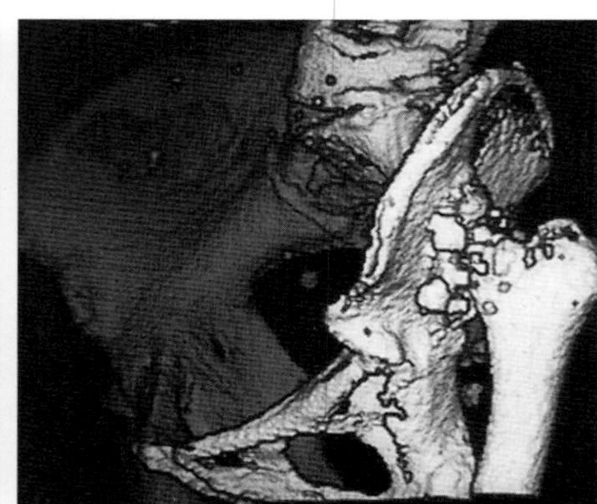

(d)

1.18 Computed tomography (CT) The plain x-ray (a) shows a fracture of the vertebral body but one cannot tell precisely how the bone fragments are displaced. The CT (b) shows clearly that they are dangerously close to the cauda equina. (c) Congenital hip dislocation, defined more clearly by (d) three-dimensional CT reconstruction.

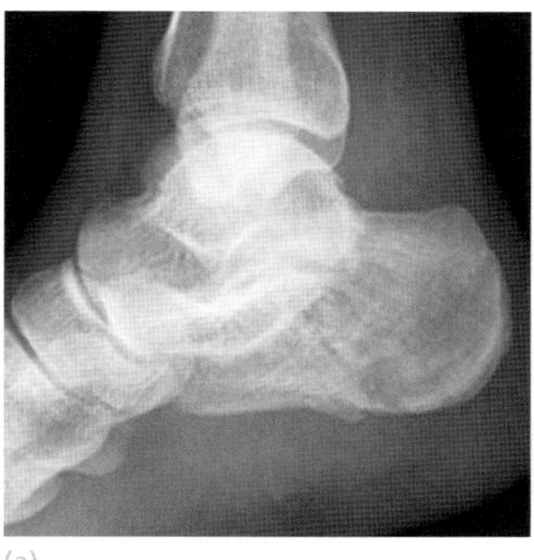
(a)

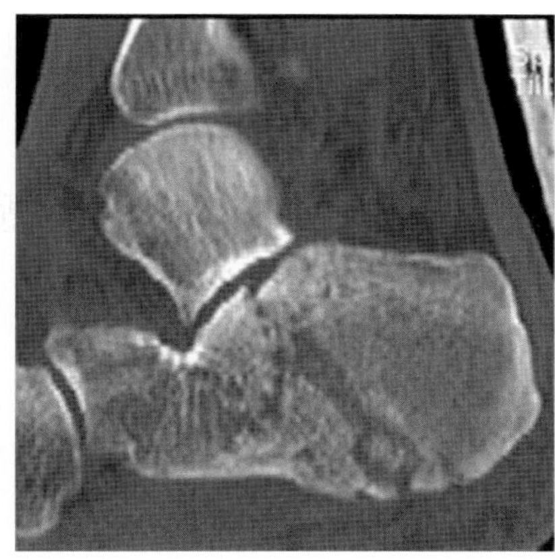
(b)

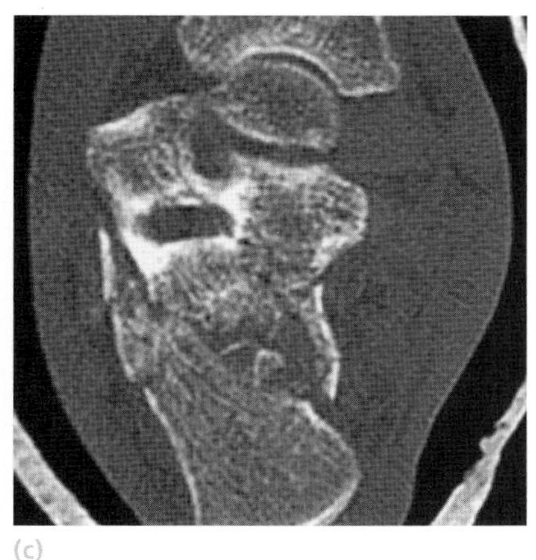
(c)

1.19 CT for complex fractures (a) A plain x-ray shows a fracture of the calcaneum but the details are obscure. CT sagittal and axial views (b,c) give a much clearer idea of the seriousness of this fracture.

New multi-slice CT scanners provide images of high quality from which multi-planar reconstructions in all three orthogonal planes can be produced. Three-dimensional surface rendered reconstructions and volume rendered reconstructions may help in demonstrating anatomical contours, but fine detail is lost in this process.

Clinical applications

Because CT achieves excellent contrast resolution and spatial localization, it is able to display the size, shape and position of bone and soft-tissue masses in transverse planes. Image acquisition is extremely fast. The technique is therefore ideal for evaluating acute trauma to the head, spine, chest, abdomen and pelvis. It is better than MRI for demonstrating fine bone detail and soft-tissue calcification or ossification.

Computed tomography is also an invaluable tool for assisting with pre-operative planning in secondary fracture management. It is routinely used for assessing injuries of the vertebrae, acetabulum, proximal tibial plateau, ankle and foot – indeed complex fractures and fracture-dislocations at any site.

It is also useful in the assessment of bone tumour size and spread, even if it is unable to characterize the tumour type. It can be employed for guiding soft-tissue and bone biopsies.

Limitations

An important limitation of CT is that it provides relatively poor soft-tissue contrast when compared with MRI.

A major disadvantage of this technique is the relatively high radiation exposure to which the patient is subjected. It should, therefore, be used with discretion.

Magnetic resonance imaging (MRI)

Magnetic resonance imaging produces cross-sectional images of any body part in any plane. It yields superb soft-tissue contrast, allowing different soft tissues to be clearly distinguished, e.g. ligaments, tendons, muscle and hyaline cartilage. Another big advantage of MRI is that it does not use ionizing radiation. It is, however, contra-indicated in patients with pacemakers and possible metallic foreign bodies in the eye or brain, as these could potentially move when the patient is introduced into the scanner's strong magnetic field. Approximately 5% of patients cannot tolerate the scan due to claustrophobia, but newer scanners are being developed to be more 'open'.

MRI physics

The patient's body is placed in a strong magnetic field (between 5 and 30 000 times the strength of the earth's magnetic field). The body's protons have a positive charge and align themselves along this strong external magnetic field. The protons are spinning and can be further excited by radiofrequency pulses, rather like whipping a spinning top. These spinning positive charges will not only induce a small magnetic field of their own, but will produce a signal as they relax (slow down) at different rates.

A proton density map is recorded from these signals and plotted in x, y and z coordinates. Different speeds of tissue excitation with radiofrequency pulses (repetition times, or TR) and different intervals between recording these signals (time to echo, or TE) will yield anatomical pictures with varying 'weighting' and characteristics. T_1 weighted (T_1W) images have a high spatial resolution and provide good anatomical-looking pictures. T_2 weighted (T_2W) images give more information about the physiological characteristics of the tissue. Proton density (PD) images are also described as

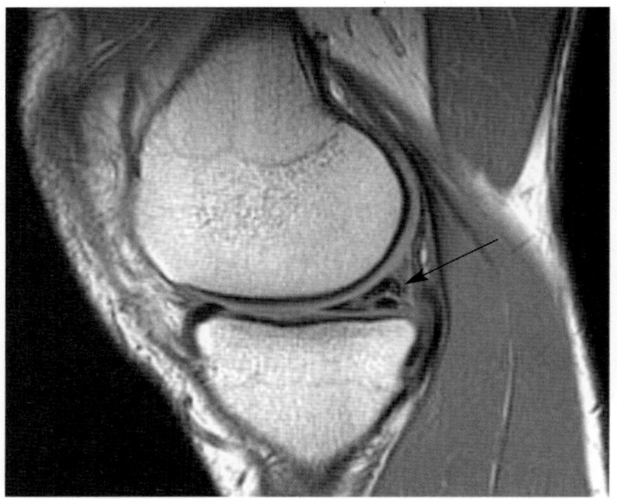

1.20 Magnetic resonance imaging MRI is ideal for displaying soft-tissue injuries, particularly tears of the menisci of the knee; this common injury is clearly shown in the picture.

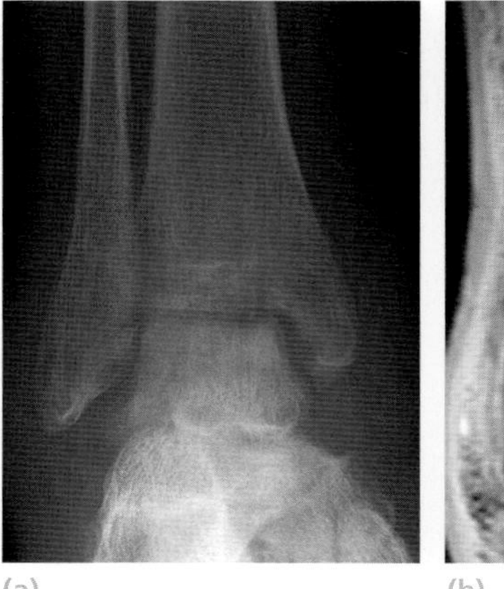

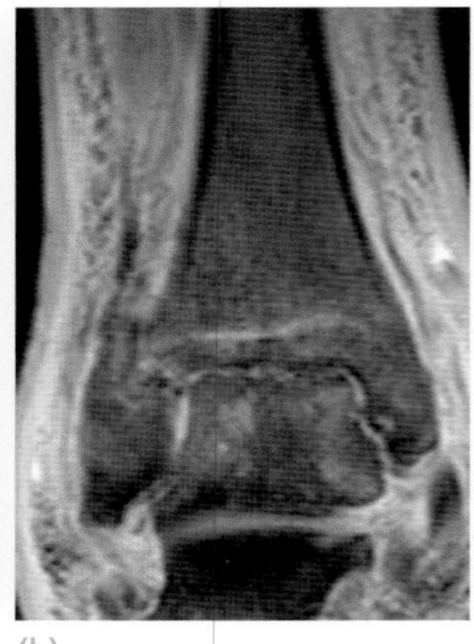

(a) (b)

1.21 MRI A case of septic arthritis of the ankle, suspected from the plain x-ray (a) and confirmed by MRI (b).

'balanced' or 'intermediate' as they are essentially a combination of T_1 and T_2 weighting and yield excellent anatomical detail for orthopaedic imaging. Fat suppression sequences allow highlighting of abnormal water, which is particularly useful in orthopaedics when assessing both soft tissue and bone marrow oedema.

Intravenous contrast

Just as in CT, enhancement by intravenous contrast relies on an active blood supply and leaky cell membranes. Areas of inflammation and active tumour tissue will be highlighted. Gadolinium compounds are employed as they have seven unpaired electrons and work by creating local magnetic field disturbances at their sites of accumulation.

Indirect arthrography

Gadolinium compounds administered intravenously will be secreted through joint synovium into joint effusions resulting in indirect arthrography. However, there is no additional distension of the joint, which limits its effect.

Direct arthrography

Direct puncture of joints under image guidance with a solution containing dilute gadolinium (1:200 concentration) is routinely performed. This provides a positive contrast within the joint and distension of the joint capsule, thereby separating many of the closely applied soft-tissue structures that can be demonstrated on the subsequent MRI scan.

Clinical applications

Magnetic resonance imaging is becoming cheaper and more widely available. Its excellent anatomical detail, soft-tissue contrast and multi-planar capability make it ideal for non-invasive imaging of the musculoskeletal system. The multi-planar capability provides accurate cross-sectional information and the axial images in particular will reveal detailed limb compartmental anatomy. The excellent soft-tissue contrast allows identification of similar density soft tissues, for example in distinguishing between tendons, cartilage and ligaments. By using combinations of T_1W, T_2W and fat suppressed sequences, specific abnormalities can be further characterized with tissue specificity, so further extending the diagnostic possibilities.

In orthopaedic surgery, MRI of the hip, knee, ankle, shoulder and wrist is now fairly commonplace. It can detect the early changes of bone marrow oedema and osteonecrosis before any other imaging modality. In the knee, MRI is as accurate as arthroscopy in diagnosing meniscal tears and cruciate ligament injuries. Bone and soft-tissue tumours should be routinely examined by MRI as the intraosseous and extra-osseous extent and spread of disease, as well as the compartmental anatomy, can be accurately assessed. Additional use of fat suppression sequences determines the extent of peri-lesional oedema and intravenous contrast will demonstrate the active part of the tumour.

Intravenous contrast is used to distinguish vascularized from avascular tissue, e.g. following a scaphoid fracture, or in defining active necrotic areas of tumour, or in demonstrating areas of active inflammation.

Direct MRI arthrography is used to distend the joint capsule and outline labral tears in the shoulder and the hip. In the ankle, it provides the way to demonstrate anterolateral impingement and assess the integrity of the capsular ligaments.

Limitations

Despite its undoubted value, MRI (like all singular methods of investigation) has its limitations and it must be seen as one of a group of imaging techniques, none of which by itself is appropriate in every situation. Conventional radiographs and CT are more sensitive to soft-tissue calcification and ossification, changes which can easily be easily overlooked on MRI. Conventional radiographs should, therefore, be used in combination with MRI to prevent such errors.

Diagnostic ultrasound

High-frequency sound waves, generated by a transducer, can penetrate several centimetres into the soft tissues; as they pass through the tissue interfaces some of these waves are reflected back (like echoes) to the transducer, where they are registered as electrical signals and displayed as images on a screen. Unlike x-rays, the image does not depend on tissue density but rather on reflective surfaces and soft-tissue interfaces. This is the same principle as applies in sonar detection for ships or submarines.

Depending on their structure, different tissues are referred to as highly echogenic, mildly echogenic or echo-free. Fluid-filled cysts are echo-free; fat is highly echogenic; and semi-solid organs manifest varying degrees of 'echogenicity', which makes it possible to differentiate between them.

Real-time display on a monitor gives a dynamic image, which is more useful than the usual static images. A big advantage of this technique is that the equipment is simple and portable and can be used almost anywhere; another is that it is entirely harmless.

Clinical applications

Because of the marked echogenic contrast between cystic and solid masses, ultrasonography is particularly useful for identifying hidden 'cystic' lesions such as haematomas, abscesses, popliteal cysts and arterial aneurysms. It is also capable of detecting intra-articular fluid and may be used to diagnose a synovial effusion or to monitor the progress of an 'irritable hip'.

Ultrasound is commonly used for assessing tendons and diagnosing conditions such as tendinitis and partial or complete tears. The rotator cuff, patellar ligament, quadriceps tendon, Achilles tendon, flexor tendons and peroneal tendons are typical examples.

The same technique is used extensively for guiding needle placement in diagnostic and therapeutic joint and soft-tissue injections.

Another important application is in the screening of newborn babies for congenital dislocation (or dysplasia) of the hip; the cartilaginous femoral head and acetabulum (which are, of course, 'invisible' on x-ray) can be clearly identified, and their relationship to each other shows whether the hip is normal or abnormal.

Ultrasound imaging is quick, cheap, simple and readily available. However, the information obtained is highly operator dependent, relying on the experience and interpretation of the technician.

Doppler ultrasound

Blood flow can be detected by using the principle of a change in frequency of sound when material is moving towards or away from the ultrasound transducer. This is the same principle as the change in frequency of the noise from a passing fire engine when travelling towards and then away from an observer. Abnormal increased blood flow can be observed in areas of inflammation or in aggressive tumours. Different flow rates can be shown by different colour representations ('colour Doppler').

Radionuclide imaging

Photon emission by radionuclides taken up in specific tissues can be recorded by a gamma camera to produce an image which reflects physiological activity in that tissue or organ. The radiopharmaceutical used for radionuclide imaging has two components: a chemical compound that is chosen for its metabolic uptake in the target tissue or organ, and a radioisotope tracer that will emit photons for detection.

Isotope bone scans

For bone imaging the ideal isotope is technetium-99m (^{99m}Tc): it has the appropriate energy characteristics for gamma camera imaging, it has a relatively short half-life (6 hours) and it is rapidly excreted in the urine. A bone-seeking phosphate compound is used as the substrate as it is selectively taken up and concentrated in bone. The low background radioactivity means that any site of increased uptake is readily visible.

Technetium-labelled hydroxymethylene diphosphonate (^{99m}Tc-HDP) is injected intravenously and its activity is recorded at two stages: (1) the early perfusion phase, shortly after injection, while the isotope is still in the blood stream or the perivascular space thus reflecting local blood flow difference; and (2) the delayed bone phase, 3 hours later, when the isotope has been taken up in bone tissue. Normally, in the early perfusion phase the vascular soft tissues around the joints produce the sharpest (most active) image; 3 hours later this activity has faded and the bone outlines are shown more clearly, the greatest activity appearing in the cancellous tissue at the ends of the long bones.

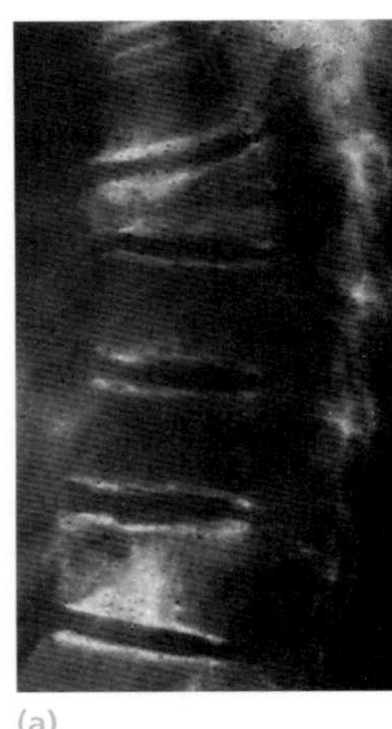

(a)

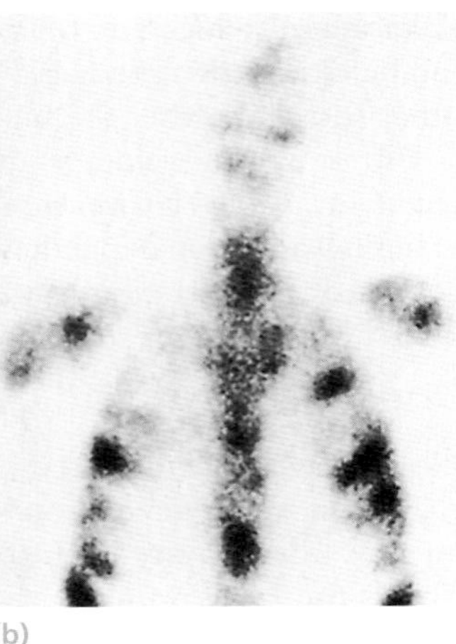

(b)

1.22 Radionuclide scanning (a) The plain x-ray showed a pathological fracture, probably through a metastatic tumour. (b) The bone scan revealed generalized secondaries, here involving the spine and ribs.

Changes in radioactivity are most significant when they are localized or asymmetrical. Four types of abnormality are seen:

Increased activity in the perfusion phase This is due to increased soft-tissue blood flow, suggesting inflammation (e.g. acute or chronic synovitis), a fracture, a highly vascular tumour or regional sympathetic dystrophy.

Decreased activity in the perfusion phase This is much less common and signifies local vascular insufficiency.

Increased activity in the delayed bone phase This could be due either to excessive isotope uptake in the osseous extracellular fluid or to more avid incorporation into newly forming bone tissue; either would be likely in a fracture, implant loosening, infection, a local tumour or healing after necrosis, and nothing in the bone scan itself distinguishes between these conditions.

Diminished activity in the bone phase This is due to an absent blood supply (e.g. in the femoral head after a fracture of the femoral neck) or to replacement of bone by pathological tissue.

CLINICAL APPLICATIONS

Radionuclide imaging is useful in many situations: (1) the diagnosis of stress fractures or other undisplaced fractures that are not detectable on the plain x-ray; (2) the detection of a small bone abscess, or an osteoid osteoma; (3) the investigation of loosening or infection around prostheses; (4) the diagnosis of femoral head ischaemia in Perthes' disease or avascular necrosis in adults; (5) the early detection of bone metastases. The scintigraphic appearances in these conditions are described in the relevant chapters. In most cases the isotope scan serves chiefly to pinpoint the site of abnormality and it should always be viewed in conjunction with other modes of imaging.

Bone scintigraphy is relatively sensitive but non-specific. One advantage is that the whole body can be imaged to look for multiple sites of pathology (occult metastases, multi-focal infection and multiple occult fractures). It is also one of the only techniques to give information about physiological activity in the tissues being examined (essentially osteoblastic activity). However, the technique carries a significant radiation burden (equivalent to approximately 200 chest x-rays) and the images yielded make anatomical localization difficult (poor spatial resolution). For localized problems MRI has superseded bone scintigraphy as it yields much greater specificity due to its superior anatomical depiction and tissue specificity.

Other radionuclide compounds

Gallium-67 (^{67}Ga) Gallium-67 concentrates in inflammatory cells and has been used to identify sites of hidden infection: for example, in the investigation of prosthetic loosening after joint replacement. However, it is arguable whether it gives any more reliable information than the ^{99m}Tc bone scan.

Indium-111-labelled leucocytes (^{111}I) The patient's own white blood cells are removed and labelled with indium-111 before being re-injected into the patient's blood stream. Preferential uptake in areas of infection is expected, thereby hoping to distinguish sites of active infection from chronic inflammation. For example, white cell uptake is more likely to be seen with an infected total hip replacement as opposed to mechanical loosening. However, as this technique is expensive and still not completely specific, it is seldom performed.

SINGLE PHOTON EMISSION COMPUTED TOMOGRAPHY

Single photon emission computed tomography (SPECT) is essentially a bone scan in which images are recorded and displayed in all three orthogonal planes. Coronal, sagittal and axial images at multiple levels make spatial localization of pathology possible: for example, activity in one side of a lumbar vertebra on the planar images can be further localized to the body, pedicle or lamina of the vertebra on the SPECT images.

POSITRON EMISSION TOMOGRAPHY

Positron emission tomography (PET) is an advanced nuclear medicine technique that allows functional imaging of disease processes. Positron-emitting isotopes with short half-lives are produced on site at specialist centres using a cyclotron. Various radiopharmaceuticals can be employed, but currently the most commonly used is 18-fluoro-2-deoxy-D-glucose (^{18}FDG). The ^{18}FDG is accumulated in different parts of the body where it can effectively measure the rate of consumption of glucose. Malignant tumours metabolize glucose at a faster rate than benign tumours and PET scanners are extremely useful in looking for occult sites of disease around the body on this basis.

PET/CT is a hybrid examination performing both PET and CT on the patient in order to superimpose the two images produced. The combination of these two techniques uses the sensitivity of PET for functional tissue changes and the cross-sectional anatomy detail of CT to localize the position of this activity.

PET is useful in oncology to identify occult malignant tumours and metastases and more accurately 'stage' the disease. Furthermore, activity levels at known sites of disease can be used to assess treatment and distinguish 'active' residual tumour or tumour recurrence from 'inactive' post-surgical scarring and necrotic tumour.

BONE MINERAL DENSITOMETRY

Bone mineral density (BMD) measurement is now widely used in identifying patients with osteoporosis and an increased risk of osteoporotic fractures.

Various techniques have been developed, including radiographic absorptiometry (RA), quantitative computed tomography (QCT) and quantitative ultrasonometry (QUS). However, the most widely used technique is dual energy x-ray absorptiometry (DXA).

RA uses conventional radiographic equipment and measures bone density in the phalanges. QCT measures trabecular bone density in vertebral bodies, but is not widely available and involves a higher dose of ionizing radiation than DXA. QUS assesses bone mineral density in the peripheral skeleton (e.g. the wrist and calcaneus) by measuring both the attenuation of ultrasound and the variation of speed of sound through the bone.

DXA employs columnated low-dose x-ray beams of two different energy levels in order to distinguish the density of bone from that of soft tissue. Although this involves the use of ionizing radiation, it is an extremely low dose. A further advantage of DXA is the development of a huge international database that allows expression of bone mineral density values in comparison to both an age and sex matched population (Z score) and also to the peak adult bone mass (T score). The T score in particular allows calculation of relative fracture risk. Individual values for both the lumbar spine and hips are obtained as there is often a discrepancy between these two sites and the fracture risk is more directly related to the value at the target area. By World Health Organization (WHO) criteria, T scores of <–1.0 indicate 'osteopenia' and T scores of <–2.5 indicate 'osteoporosis'.

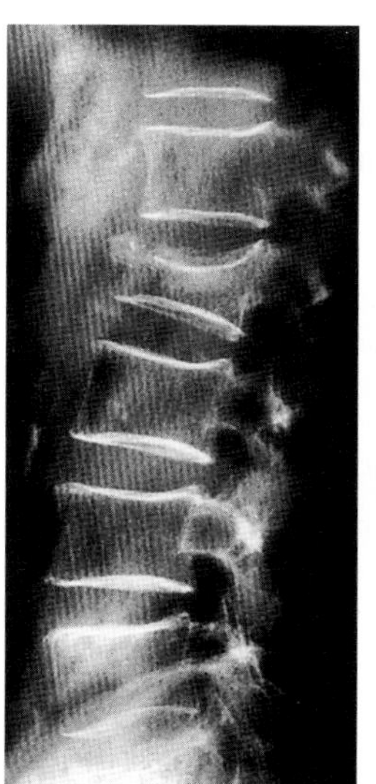

(a)

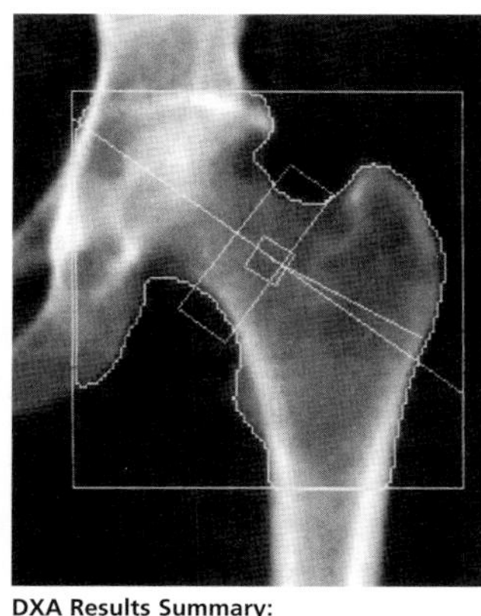

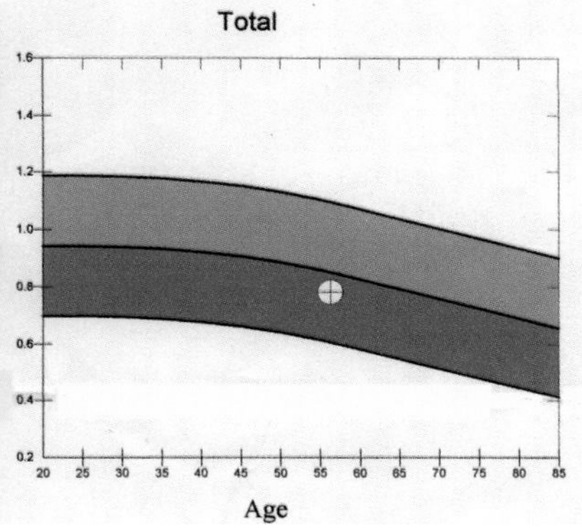

DXA Results Summary:

Region	Area (cm²)	BMC (g)	BMD (g/cm²)	T - score	PR(%)	Z - score	AM(%)
Neck	5.37	3.62	0.675	–1.6	79	–0.5	93
Troch	12.48	7.10	0.569	–1.3	81	–0.6	90
Inter	20.07	18.92	0.943	–1.0	86	–0.5	92
Total	**37.92**	**29.64**	**0.782**	**–1.3**	**83**	**–0.6**	**92**
Ward's	1.03	0.54	0.527	–1.8	72	0.0	100

Total BMD CV 1.)%
WHO Classification: Osteopenia
Fracture Risk: Increased

(b)

1.23 Measurement of bone mass (a) X-ray of the lumbar spine shows a compression fracture of L2. The general loss of bone density accentuates the cortical outlines of the vertebral body end-plates. These features are characteristic of diminished bone mass, which can be measured accurately by dual energy x-ray absorptiometry. (b) DXA scan from another woman who attended for monitoring at the onset of the menopause.

BLOOD TESTS

Non-specific blood tests

Non-specific blood abnormalities are common in bone and joint disorders; their interpretation hinges on the clinical and x-ray findings.

Hypochromic anaemia is usual in rheumatoid arthritis, but it may also be a consequence of gastrointestinal bleeding due to the anti-inflammatory drugs.

Leucocytosis is generally associated with infection, but a mild leucocytosis is not uncommon in rheumatoid arthritis and during an attack of gout.

The erythrocyte sedimentation rate (ESR) is usually increased in acute and chronic inflammatory disorders and after tissue injury. However, patients with low-grade infection may have a normal ESR and this should not be taken as a reassuring sign. The ESR is strongly affected by the presence of monoclonal immunoglobulins; a high ESR is almost mandatory in the diagnosis of myelomatosis.

C-reactive protein (and other acute phase proteins) may be abnormally increased in chronic inflammatory arthritis and (temporarily) after injury or operation. The test is often used to monitor the progress and activity of rheumatoid arthritis and chronic infection.

Plasma gamma-globulins can be measured by protein electrophoresis. Their precise characterization is helpful in the assessment of certain rheumatic disorders, and more particularly in the diagnosis of myelomatosis.

Rheumatoid factor tests

Rheumatoid factor, an IgM autoantibody, is present in about 75% of adults with rheumatoid arthritis. However, it is not pathognomonic: some patients with undoubted rheumatoid arthritis remain 'seronegative', while rheumatoid factor is found in some patients with other disorders such as systemic lupus erythematosus and scleroderma.

Ankylosing spondylitis, Reiter's disease and psoriatic arthritis characteristically test negative for rheumatoid factor; they have been grouped together as the 'seronegative spondarthritides'.

Tissue typing

Human leucocyte antigens (HLA) can be detected in white blood cells and they are used to characterize individual tissue types. The seronegative spondarthritides are closely associated with the presence of HLA-B27 on chromosome 6; this is frequently used as a confirmatory test in patients suspected of having ankylosing spondylitis or Reiter's disease, but it should not be regarded as a specific test because it is positive in about 8% of normal western Europeans.

Biochemistry

Biochemical tests are essential in monitoring patients after any serious injury. They are also used routinely in the investigation of rheumatic disorders and abnormalities of bone metabolism. Their significance is discussed under the relevant conditions.

SYNOVIAL FLUID ANALYSIS

Arthrocentesis and synovial fluid analysis is a much-neglected diagnostic procedure; given the correct indications it can yield valuable information. It should be considered in the following conditions.

Acute joint swelling after injury The distinction between synovitis and bleeding may not be obvious; aspiration will settle the question immediately.

Acute atraumatic synovitis in adults Synovial fluid analysis may be the only way to distinguish between infection, gout and pseudogout. Characteristic crystals can be identified on polarized light microscopy.

Suspected infection Careful examination and laboratory investigations may provide the answer, but they take time. Joint aspiration is essential for early diagnosis.

Chronic synovitis Here joint aspiration is less urgent, and is only one of many diagnostic procedures in the investigation of suspected tuberculosis or atypical rheumatic disorders.

Technique

Joint aspiration should always be performed under strict aseptic conditions. After infiltrating the skin with a local anaesthetic, a 20-gauge needle is introduced and a sample of joint fluid is aspirated; even a small quantity of fluid (less than 0.5 mL) is enough for diagnostic analysis.

The volume of fluid and its appearance are immediately noted. Normal synovial fluid is clear and slightly yellow. A cloudy or turbid fluid is due to the presence of cells, usually a sign of inflammation. Blood-stained fluid may be found after injury, but is also seen in acute inflammatory disorders and in pigmented villonodular synovitis.

A single drop of fresh synovial fluid is placed on a glass slide and examined through the microscope. Blood cells are easily identified; abundant leucocytes may suggest infection. Crystals may be seen, though this usually requires a careful search; they are better characterized by polarized light microscopy (see Chapter 4).

Dry smears are prepared with heparinized fluid; more concentrated specimens can be obtained if the

Table 1.2 Examination of synovial fluid

Suspected condition	Appearance	Viscosity	White cells	Crystals	Biochemistry	Bacteriology
Normal	Clear yellow	High	Few	–	As for plasma	–
Septic arthritis	Purulent	Low	+	–	Glucose low	+
Tuberculous arthritis	Turbid	Low	+	–	Glucose low	+
Rheumatoid arthritis	Cloudy	Low	++	–	–	–
Gout	Cloudy	Normal	++	Urate	–	–
Pseudogout	Cloudy	Normal	+	Pyrophosphate	–	–
Osteoarthritis	Clear yellow	High	Few	Often+	–	–

fluid is centrifuged. After suitable staining (Wright's and Gram's), the smear is examined for pus cells and organisms. Remember, though, that negative findings do not exclude infection.

Laboratory tests

If enough fluid is available, it is sent for full laboratory investigation (cells, biochemistry and bacteriological culture). A simultaneous blood specimen allows comparison of synovial and blood glucose concentration; a marked reduction of synovial glucose suggests infection.

A high white cell count (more than 10 000/mm^3) is usually indicative of infection, but a moderate leucocytosis is also seen in gout and other types of inflammatory arthritis.

Bacteriological culture and tests for antibiotic sensitivity are essential in any case of suspected infection.

BONE BIOPSY

Bone biopsy is often the crucial means of making a diagnosis or distinguishing between local conditions that closely resemble one another. Confusion is most likely to occur when the x-ray or MRI discloses an area of bone destruction that could be due to a compression fracture, a bone tumour or infection (e.g. a collapsed vertebral body). In other cases it is obvious that the lesion is a tumour – but what type of tumour? Benign or malignant? Primary or metastatic? Radical surgery should never be undertaken for a suspected neoplasm without first confirming the diagnosis histologically, no matter how 'typical' or 'obvious' the x-ray appearances may be.

In bone infection, the biopsy permits not only histological proof of acute inflammation but also bacteriological typing of the organism and tests for antibiotic sensitivity.

The investigation of metabolic bone disease sometimes calls for a tetracycline-labelled bone biopsy to show: (a) the type of abnormality (osteoporosis, osteomalacia, hyperparathyroidism), and (b) the severity of the disorder.

Open or closed?

Open biopsy, with exposure of the lesion and excision of a sizeable portion of the bone, seems preferable, but it has several drawbacks. (1) It requires an operation, with the attendant risks of anaesthesia and infection. (2) New tissue planes are opened up, predisposing to spread of infection or tumour. (3) The biopsy incision may jeopardize subsequent wide excision of the lesion. (4) The more inaccessible lesions (e.g. a tumour of the acetabular floor) can be reached only by dissecting widely through healthy tissue.

A carefully performed 'closed' biopsy, using a needle or trephine of appropriate size to ensure the removal of an adequate sample of tissue, is the procedure of choice except when the lesion cannot be accurately localized or when the tissue consistency is such that a sufficient sample cannot be obtained. Solid or semi-solid tissue is removed intact by the cutting needle or trephine; fluid material can be aspirated through the biopsy needle.

Precautions

- The biopsy site and approach should be carefully planned with the aid of x-rays or other imaging techniques.
- If there is any possibility of the lesion being malignant, the approach should be sited so that the wound and biopsy track can be excised if later radical surgery proves to be necessary.
- The procedure should be carried out in an operating theatre, under anaesthesia (local or general) and with full aseptic technique.
- For deep-seated lesions, fluoroscopic control of the needle insertion is essential.
- The appropriate size of biopsy needle or cutting trephine should be selected.

- A knowledge of the local anatomy and of the likely consistency of the lesion is important. Large blood vessels and nerves must be avoided; potentially vascular tumours may bleed profusely and the means to control haemorrhage should be readily to hand. More than one surgeon has set out to aspirate an 'abscess' only to plunge a wide-bore needle into an aneurysm!
- Clear instructions should be given to ensure that the tissue obtained at the biopsy is suitably processed. If infection is suspected, the material should go into a culture tube and be sent to the laboratory as soon as possible. A smear may also be useful. Whole tissue is transferred to a jar containing formalin, without damaging the specimen or losing any material. Aspirated blood should be allowed to clot and can then be preserved in formalin for later paraffin embedding and sectioning. Tissue thought to contain crystals should not be placed in formalin as this may destroy the crystals; it should either be kept unaltered for immediate examination or stored in saline.
- No matter how careful the biopsy, there is always the risk that the tissue will be too scanty or too unrepresentative for accurate diagnosis. Close consultation with the radiologist and pathologist beforehand will minimize this possibility. In the best hands, needle biopsy has an accuracy rate of over 95%.

DIAGNOSTIC ARTHROSCOPY

Arthroscopy is performed for both diagnostic and therapeutic reasons. Almost any joint can be reached but the procedure is most usefully employed in the knee, shoulder, wrist, ankle and hip. If the suspect lesion is amenable to surgery, it can often be dealt with at the same sitting without the need for an open operation. However, arthroscopy is an invasive procedure and its mastery requires skill and practice; it should not be used simply as an alternative to clinical examination and imaging.

Technique

The instrument is basically a rigid telescope fitted with fibreoptic illumination. Tube diameter ranges from about 2 mm (for small joints) to 4–5 mm (for the knee). It carries a lens system that gives a magnified image. The eyepiece allows direct viewing by the arthroscopist, but it is far more convenient to fit a small, sterilizable solid-state television camera which produces a picture of the joint interior on a television monitor.

The procedure is best carried out under general anaesthesia; this gives good muscle relaxation and permits manipulation and opening of the joint compartments. The joint is distended with fluid and the arthroscope is introduced percutaneously. Various instruments (probes, curettes and forceps) can be inserted through other skin portals; they are used to help expose the less accessible parts of the joint, or to obtain biopsies for further examination. Guided by the image on the monitor, the arthroscopist explores the joint in a systematic fashion, manipulating the arthroscope with one hand and the probe or forceps with the other. At the end of the procedure the joint is washed out and the small skin wounds are sutured. The patient is usually able to return home later the same day.

Diagnosis

The knee is the most accessible joint. The appearance of the synovium and the articular surfaces usually allows differentiation between inflammatory and non-inflammatory, destructive and non-destructive lesions. Meniscal tears can be diagnosed and treated immediately by repair or removal of partially detached segments. Cruciate ligament deficiency, osteocartilaginous fractures, cartilaginous loose bodies and synovial 'tumours' are also readily visualized.

Arthroscopy of the shoulder is more difficult, but the articular surfaces and glenoid labrum can be adequately explored. Rotator cuff lesions can often be diagnosed and treated at the same time.

Arthroscopy of the wrist is useful for diagnosing torn triangular fibrocartilage and interosseous ligament ruptures.

Arthroscopy of the hip is less widely used, but it is proving to be useful in the diagnosis of unexplained hip pain. Labral tears, synovial lesions, loose bodies and articular cartilage damage (all of which are difficult to detect by conventional imaging techniques) have been diagnosed with a reported accuracy rate of over 50%.

Complications

Diagnostic arthroscopy is safe but not entirely free of complications, the commonest of which are haemarthosis, thrombophlebitis, infection and joint stiffness. There is also a significant incidence of algodystrophy following arthroscopy.

REFERENCES AND FURTHER READING

Apley AG, Solomon L. Physical Examination in Orthopaedics. Oxford, Butterworth Heinemann, 1997.

Resnick D. Diagnosis of Bone and Joint Disorders, Edn 4. Philadelphia, WB Saunders, 2002.

Infection 2

Louis Solomon, H. Srinivasan, Surendar Tuli, Shunmugam Govender

Micro-organisms may reach the musculoskeletal tissues by (a) *direct introduction* through the skin (a pinprick, an injection, a stab wound, a laceration, an open fracture or an operation), (b) *direct spread from a contiguous focus* of infection, or (c) *indirect spread via the blood stream* from a distant site such as the nose or mouth, the respiratory tract, the bowel or the genitourinary tract.

Depending on the type of invader, the site of infection and the host response, the result may be a pyogenic osteomyelitis, a septic arthritis, a chronic granulomatous reaction (classically seen in tuberculosis of either bone or joint), or an indolent response to an unusual organism (e.g. a fungal infection). Soft-tissue infections range from superficial wound sepsis to widespread cellulitis and life-threatening necrotizing cellulitis. Parasitic lesions such as hydatid disease also are considered in this chapter, although these are infestations rather than infections.

GENERAL ASPECTS OF INFECTION

Infection – as distinct from mere residence of micro-organisms – is a condition in which pathogenic organisms multiply and spread within the body tissues. This usually gives rise to an acute or chronic *inflammatory reaction*, which is the body's way of combating the invaders and destroying them, or at least immobilizing them and confining them to a single area. The signs of inflammation are recounted in the classical mantra: *redness, swelling, heat, pain* and *loss of function*. In one important respect, bone infection differs from soft-tissue infection: since bone consists of a collection of rigid compartments, it is more susceptible than soft tissues to vascular damage and cell death from the build-up of pressure in acute inflammation. Unless it is rapidly suppressed, bone infection will inevitably lead to necrosis.

Host susceptibility to infection is increased by (a) *local factors* such as trauma, scar tissue, poor circulation, diminished sensibility, chronic bone or joint disease and the presence of foreign bodies, as well as (b) *systemic factors* such as malnutrition, general illness, debility, diabetes, rheumatoid disease, corticosteroid administration and all forms of immunosuppression, either acquired or induced. Resistance is also diminished in the very young and the very old.

Bacterial colonization and resistance to antibiotics is enhanced by the ability of certain microbes (including *Staphylococcus*) to adhere to avascular bone surfaces and foreign implants, protected from both host defences and antibiotics by a protein-polysaccharide slime (*glycocalyx*).

Acute pyogenic bone infections are characterized by the formation of pus – a concentrate of defunct leucocytes, dead and dying bacteria and tissue debris – which is often localized in an abscess. Pressure builds up within the abscess and infection may then extend into a contiguous joint or through the cortex and along adjacent tissue planes. It may also spread further afield via lymphatics (causing lymphangitis and lymphadenopathy) or via the blood stream (bacteraemia and septicaemia). An accompanying systemic reaction varies from a vague feeling of lassitude with mild pyrexia to severe illness, fever, toxaemia and shock. The generalized effects are due to the release of bacterial enzymes and endotoxins as well as cellular breakdown products from the host tissues.

Chronic pyogenic infection may follow on unresolved acute infection and is characterized by persistence of the infecting organism in pockets of necrotic tissue. Purulent material accumulates and may be discharged through sinuses at the skin or a poorly healed wound. Factors which favour this outcome are the presence of damaged muscle, dead bone or a foreign implant, diminished local blood supply and a weak host response. Resistance is likely to be depressed in the very young and the very old, in states of malnutrition or immunosuppression, and in certain diseases such as diabetes and leukaemia.

Table 2.1 Factors predisposing to bone infection

Malnutrition and general debility
Diabetes mellitus
Corticosteroid administration
Immune deficiency
Immunosuppressive drugs
Venous stasis in the limb
Peripheral vascular disease
Loss of sensibility
Iatrogenic invasive measures
Trauma

Chronic non-pyogenic infection may result from invasion by organisms that produce a cellular reaction leading to the formation of granulomas consisting largely of lymphocytes, modified macrophages and multinucleated giant cells; this type of granulomatous infection is seen most typically in tuberculosis. Systemic effects are less acute but may ultimately be very debilitating, with lymphadenopathy, splenomegaly and tissue wasting.

The principles of treatment are: (1) to provide analgesia and general supportive measures; (2) to rest the affected part; (3) to identify the infecting organism and administer effective antibiotic treatment or chemotherapy; (4) to release pus as soon as it is detected; (5) to stabilize the bone if it has fractured; (6) to eradicate avascular and necrotic tissue; (7) to restore continuity if there is a gap in the bone; and (8) to maintain soft-tissue and skin cover. Acute infections, if treated early with effective antibiotics, can usually be cured. Once there is pus and bone necrosis, operative drainage will be needed.

ACUTE HAEMATOGENOUS OSTEOMYELITIS

Aetiology and pathogenesis

Acute haematogenous osteomyelitis is mainly a disease of children. When adults are affected it is usually because their resistance is lowered. Trauma may determine the site of infection, possibly by causing a small haematoma or fluid collection in a bone, in patients with concurrent bacteraemia.

The incidence of acute haematogenous osteomyelitis in western European children is thought to have declined in recent years, probably a reflection of improving social conditions. A study from Glasgow, Scotland, covering the period 1990–99, suggests that it is less than 3 cases per 100 000 per year (Blyth et al., 2001). However, it is almost certainly much higher among less affluent populations.

The causal organism in both adults and children is usually *Staphylococcus aureus* (found in over 70% of cases), and less often one of the other Gram-positive cocci, such as the Group A beta-haemolytic streptococci (*Streptococcus pyogenes*) which is found in chronic skin infections, as well as Group B streptococcus (especially in new-born babies) or the alpha-haemolytic diplococcus S. *pneumoniae*.

In children between 1 and 4 years of age the Gram-negative *Haemophilus influenzae* used to be a fairly common pathogen for osteomyelitis and septic arthritis, but the introduction of *H. influenzae* type B vaccination about 20 years ago has been followed by a much reduced incidence of this infection in many countries. In recent years its place has been taken by

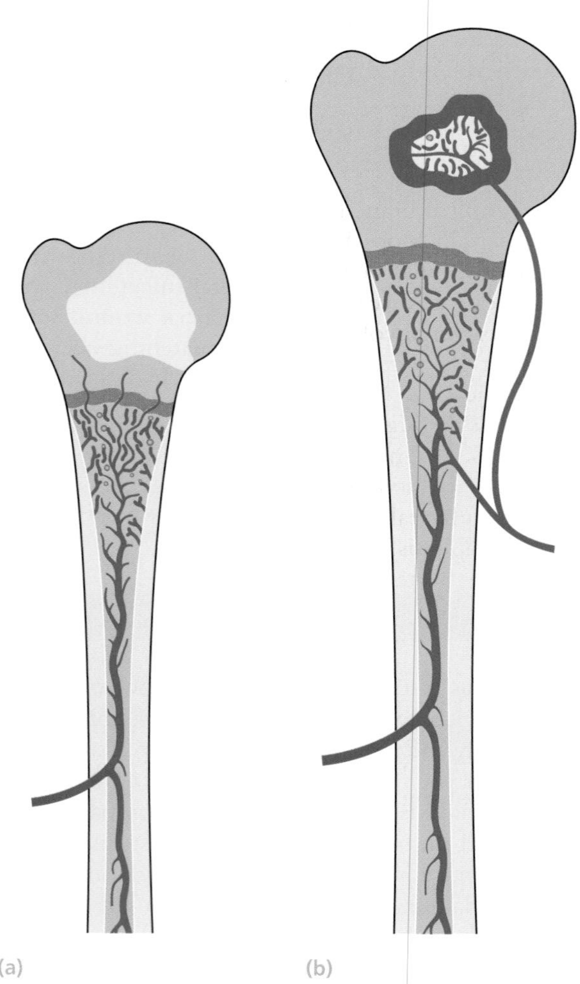

2.1 Epiphyseal and metaphyseal blood supply **(a)** In new-born infants some metaphyseal arterioles from the nutrient artery penetrate the physis and may carry infection directly from the metaphysis to the epiphysis. **(b)** In older children the physis acts as a barrier and the developing epiphysis receives a separate blood supply from the epiphyseal and peri-articular blood vessels.

Kingella kingae, mainly following upper respiratory infection in young children. Other Gram-negative organisms (e.g. *Escherichia coli, Pseudomonas aeruginosa, Proteus mirabilis* and the anaerobic *Bacteroides fragilis*) occasionally cause acute bone infection. Curiously, patients with sickle-cell disease are prone to infection by *Salmonella typhi.*

Anaerobic organisms (particularly *Peptococcus magnus*) have been found in patients with osteomyelitis, usually as part of a mixed infection. Unusual organisms are more likely to be found in heroin addicts and as opportunistic pathogens in patients with compromised immune defence mechanisms.

The blood stream is invaded, perhaps from a minor skin abrasion, treading on a sharp object, an injection point, a boil, a septic tooth or – in the newborn – from an infected umbilical cord. In adults the source of infection may be a urethral catheter, an indwelling arterial line or a dirty needle and syringe.

In children the infection usually starts in the vascular metaphysis of a long bone, most often in the proximal tibia or in the distal or proximal ends of the femur. Predilection for this site has traditionally been attributed to the peculiar arrangement of the blood vessels in that area (Trueta, 1959): the non-anastomosing terminal branches of the nutrient artery twist back in hairpin loops before entering the large network of sinusoidal veins; the relative vascular stasis and consequent lowered oxygen tension are believed to favour bacterial colonization. It has also been suggested that the structure of the fine vessels in the hypertrophic zone of the physis allows bacteria more easily to pass through and adhere to type 1 collagen in that area (Song and Sloboda, 2001). In infants, in whom there are still anastomoses between metaphyseal and epiphyseal blood vessels, infection can also reach the epiphysis.

In adults, haematogenous infection accounts for only about 20% of cases of osteomyelitis, mostly affecting the vertebrae. *Staphylococcus aureus* is the commonest organism but *Pseudomonas aeruginosa* often appears in patients using intravenous drugs. Adults with diabetes, who are prone to soft-tissue infections of the foot, may develop contiguous bone infection involving a variety of organisms.

Pathology

Acute haematogenous osteomyelitis shows a characteristic progression marked by *inflammation, suppuration, bone necrosis, reactive new bone formation* and, ultimately, *resolution and healing* or else *intractable chronicity.* However, the pathological picture varies considerably, depending on the patient's age, the site of infection, the virulence of the organism and the host response.

Acute osteomyelitis in children The 'classical' picture is seen in children between 2 and 6 years. The earliest change in the metaphysis is an acute inflammatory reaction with vascular congestion, exudation of fluid and infiltration by polymorphonuclear leucocytes. The intraosseous pressure rises rapidly, causing intense pain, obstruction to blood flow and intravascular thrombosis. Even at an early stage the bone tissue is threatened by impending ischaemia and resorption due to a combination of phagocytic activity and the local accumulation of cytokines, growth factors, prostaglandin and bacterial enzymes. By the second or third day, pus forms within the bone and forces its way along the Volkmann canals to the surface where it produces a subperiosteal abscess. This is much more evident in children, because of the relatively loose attachment of the periosteum, than in adults. From the subperiosteal abscess pus can spread along the shaft, to re-enter the bone at another level or burst into the surrounding soft tissues. The developing physis acts as a barrier to direct spread towards the epiphysis, but where the metaphysis is partly intracapsular (e.g. at the hip, shoulder or elbow) pus may discharge through the periosteum into the joint.

The rising intraosseous pressure, vascular stasis, small-vessel thrombosis and periosteal stripping

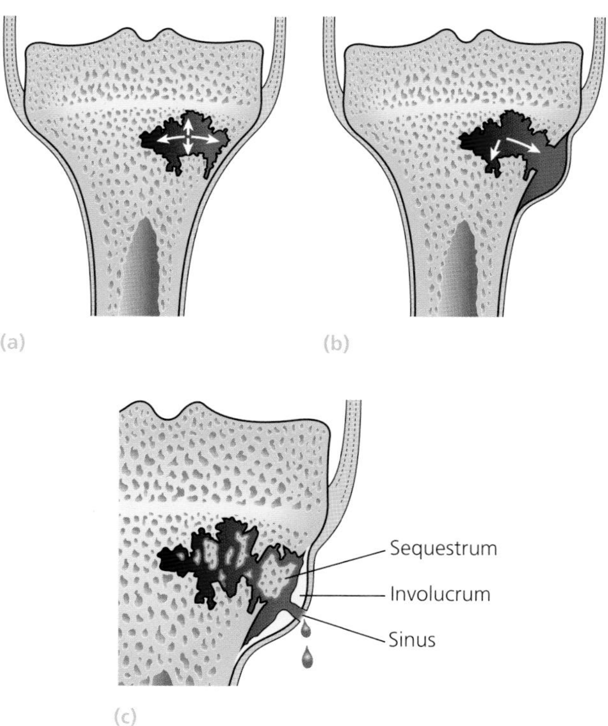

2.2 Acute osteomyelitis (a) Infection in the metaphysis may spread towards the surface, to form a subperiosteal abscess (b). Some of the bone may die, and is encased in periosteal new bone as a sequestrum (c). The encasing involucrum is sometimes perforated by sinuses.

increasingly compromise the blood supply; by the end of a week there is usually microscopic evidence of bone death. Bacterial toxins and leucocytic enzymes also may play their part in the advancing tissue destruction. With the gradual ingrowth of granulation tissue the boundary between living and devitalized bone becomes defined. Pieces of dead bone may separate as *sequestra* varying in size from mere spicules to large necrotic segments of the cortex in neglected cases.

Macrophages and lymphocytes arrive in increasing numbers and the debris is slowly removed by a combination of phagocytosis and osteoclastic resorption. A small focus in cancellous bone may be completely resorbed, leaving a tiny cavity, but a large cortical or cortico-cancellous sequestrum will remain entombed, inaccessible to either final destruction or repair.

Another feature of advancing acute osteomyelitis is new bone formation. Initially the area around the infected zone is porotic (probably due to hyperaemia and osteoclastic activity) but if the pus is not released, either spontaneously or by surgical decompression, new bone starts forming on viable surfaces in the bone and from the deep layers of the stripped periosteum. This is typical of pyogenic infection and fine streaks of subperiosteal new bone usually become apparent on x-ray by the end of the second week. With time this new bone thickens to form a casement, or *involucrum*, enclosing the sequestrum and infected tissue. If the infection persists, pus and tiny sequestrated spicules of bone may discharge through perforations (*cloacae*) in the involucrum and track by sinuses to the skin surface.

If the infection is controlled and intraosseous pressure released at an early stage, this dire progress can be halted. The bone around the zone of infection becomes increasingly dense; this, together with the periosteal reaction, results in thickening of the bone. In some cases the normal anatomy may eventually be reconstituted; in others, though healing is sound, the bone is left permanently deformed.

If healing does not occur, a nidus of infection may remain locked inside the bone, causing pus and sometimes bone debris to be discharged intermittently through a persistent sinus (or several sinuses). The infection has now lapsed into *chronic osteomyelitis*, which may last for many years.

Acute osteomyelitis in infants The early features of acute osteomyelitis in infants are much the same as those in older children. However, a significant difference, during the first year of life, is the frequency with which the metaphyseal infection spreads to the epiphysis and from there into the adjacent joint. In the process, the physeal anlage may be irreparably damaged, further growth at that site is severely retarded and the joint will be permanently deformed. How this comes about is still argued over. Following Trueta (1957) it has long been held that, during the first 6–9 months of life, small metaphyseal vessels penetrate the physeal cartilage and this permits the infection to spread into the cartilaginous epiphysis. Others have disagreed with this hypothesis (Chung, 1976), but what is indisputable is that during infancy osteomyelitis and septic arthritis often go together. Another feature in infants is an unusually exuberant periosteal reaction resulting in sometimes bizarre new bone formation along the diaphysis; fortunately, with longitudinal growth and remodelling the diaphyseal anatomy is gradually restored.

Acute osteomyelitis in adults Bone infection in the adult usually follows an open injury, an operation or spread from a contiguous focus of infection (e.g. a neuropathic ulcer or an infected diabetic foot). True haematogenous osteomyelitis is uncommon and when it does occur it usually affects one of the vertebrae (e.g. following a pelvic infection) or a small cuboidal bone. A vertebral infection may spread through the end-plate and the intervertebral disc into an adjacent vertebral body.

If a long bone is infected, the abscess is likely to spread within the medullary cavity, eroding the cortex and extending into the surrounding soft tissues. Periosteal new bone formation is less obvious than in childhood and the weakened cortex may fracture. If the bone end becomes involved there is a risk of the infection spreading into an adjacent joint. The outcome is often a gradual slide towards subacute and chronic osteomyelitis.

Clinical features

Clinical features differ in the three groups described above.

Children The patient, usually a child over 4 years, presents with severe pain, malaise and a fever; in neglected cases, toxaemia may be marked. The parents will have noticed that he or she refuses to use one limb or to allow it to be handled or even touched. There may be a recent history of infection: a septic toe, a boil, a sore throat or a discharge from the ear.

Typically the child looks ill and feverish; the pulse rate is likely to be over 100 and the temperature is raised. The limb is held still and there is acute tenderness near one of the larger joints (e.g. above or below the knee, in the popliteal fossa or in the groin). Even the gentlest manipulation is painful and joint movement is restricted ('pseudoparalysis'). Local redness, swelling, warmth and oedema are later signs and signify that pus has escaped from the interior of the bone. Lymphadenopathy is common but non-specific. *It is important to remember that all these features may be attenuated if antibiotics have been administered.*

Infants In children under a year old, and especially in the newborn, the constitutional disturbance can be misleadingly mild; the baby simply fails to thrive and is drowsy but irritable. Suspicion should be aroused by a history of birth difficulties, umbilical artery catheterization or a site of infection (however mild) such as an inflamed intravenous infusion point or even a heel puncture. Metaphyseal tenderness and resistance to joint movement can signify either osteomyelitis or septic arthritis; indeed, both may be present, so the distinction hardly matters. Look for other sites – multiple infection is not uncommon, especially in babies who acquire the infection in hospital. Radionuclide bone scans may help to discover additional sites.

Adults The commonest site for haematogenous infection is the thoracolumbar spine. There may be a history of some urological procedure followed by a mild fever and backache. Local tenderness is not very marked and it may take weeks before x-ray signs appear; when they do appear the diagnosis may still need to be confirmed by fine-needle aspiration and bacteriological culture. Other bones are occasionally involved, especially if there is a background of diabetes, malnutrition, drug addiction, leukaemia, immunosuppressive therapy or debility.

In the very elderly, and *in those with immune deficiency*, systemic features are mild and the diagnosis is easily missed.

Diagnostic imaging

PLAIN X-RAY

During the first week after the onset of symptoms the plain x-ray shows no abnormality of the bone. Displacement of the fat planes signifies soft-tissue swelling, but this could as well be due to a haematoma or soft-tissue infection. By the second week there may be a faint extra-cortical outline due to periosteal new bone formation; this is the classic x-ray sign of early pyogenic osteomyelitis, but treatment should not be delayed while waiting for it to appear. Later the periosteal thickening becomes more obvious and there is patchy rarefaction of the metaphysis; later still the ragged features of bone destruction appear.

An important late sign is the combination of regional osteoporosis with a localized segment of apparently increased density. Osteoporosis is a feature of metabolically active, and thus living, bone; the segment that fails to become osteoporotic is metabolically inactive and possibly dead.

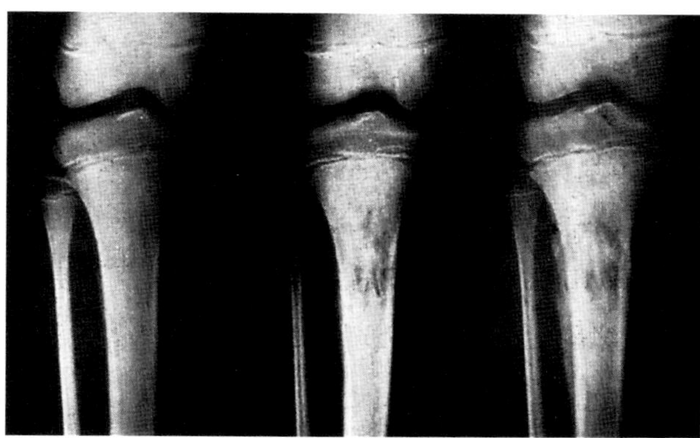

2.3 Acute osteomyelitis The first x-ray, 2 days after symptoms began, is normal – it always is; metaphyseal mottling and periosteal changes were not obvious until the second film, taken 14 days later; eventually much of the shaft was involved.

ULTRASONOGRAPHY

Ultrasonography may detect a subperiosteal collection of fluid in the early stages of osteomyelitis, but it cannot distinguish between a haematoma and pus.

RADIONUCLIDE SCANNING

Radioscintigraphy with ^{99m}Tc-HDP reveals increased activity in both the perfusion phase and the bone phase. This is a highly sensitive investigation, even in the very early stages, but it has relatively low specificity and other inflammatory lesions can show similar changes. In doubtful cases, scanning with ^{67}Ga-citrate or ^{111}In-labelled leucocytes may be more revealing.

MAGNETIC RESONANCE IMAGING

Magnetic resonance imaging can be helpful in cases of doubtful diagnosis, and particularly in suspected infection of the axial skeleton. It is also the best method of demonstrating bone marrow inflammation. It is extremely sensitive, even in the early phase of bone infection, and can therefore assist in differentiating between soft-tissue infection and osteomyelitis. However, specificity is too low to exclude other local inflammatory lesions.

Laboratory investigations

The most certain way to confirm the clinical diagnosis is to aspirate pus or fluid from the metaphyseal subperiosteal abscess, the extraosseous soft tissues or an adjacent joint. This is done using a 16- or 18-gauge trocar needle. Even if no pus is found, a smear of the aspirate is examined immediately for cells and organisms; a simple Gram stain may help to identify the type of infection and assist with the initial choice of antibiotic. A sample is also sent for detailed microbiological examination and tests for sensitivity to antibiotics. *Tissue aspiration* will give a positive result in over 60% of cases; *blood cultures* are positive in less than half the cases of proven infection.

The *C-reactive protein (CRP) values* are usually elevated within 12–24 hours and the *erythrocyte sedimentation rate (ESR)* within 24–48 hours after the onset

CARDINAL FEATURES OF ACUTE OSTEOMYELITIS IN CHILDREN
Pain
Fever
Refusal to bear weight
Elevated white cell count
Elevated ESR
Elevated CRP

of symptoms. The *white blood cell (WBC) count* rises and the haemoglobin concentration may be diminished. *In the very young and the very old these tests are less reliable and may show values within the range of normal.*

Antistaphylococcal antibody titres may be raised. This test is useful in atypical cases where the diagnosis is in doubt.

Osteomyelitis in an unusual site or with an unusual organism should alert one to the possibility of heroin addiction, sickle-cell disease (*Salmonella* may be cultured from the faeces) or deficient host defence mechanisms including HIV infection.

Differential diagnosis

Cellulitis This is often mistaken for osteomyelitis. There is widespread superficial redness and lymphangitis. The source of skin infection may not be obvious and should be searched for (e.g. on the sole or between the toes). If doubt remains about the diagnosis, MRI will help to distinguish between bone infection and soft-tissue infection. The organism is usually staphylococcus or streptococcus. Mild cases will respond to high dosage oral antibiotics; severe cases need intravenous antibiotic treatment.

Acute suppurative arthritis Tenderness is diffuse, and movement at the joint is completely abolished by muscle spasm. In infants the distinction between metaphyseal osteomyelitis and septic arthritis of the adjacent joint is somewhat theoretical, as both often coexist. A progressive rise in C-reactive protein values over 24–48 hours is said to be suggestive of concurrent septic arthritis (Unkila-Kallis et al., 1994).

Streptococcal necrotizing myositis Group A beta-haemolytic streptococci (the same organisms which are responsible for the common 'sore throat') occasionally invade muscles and cause an acute myositis which, in its early stages, may be mistaken for cellulitis or osteomyelitis. Although the condition is rare, it should be kept well to the foreground in the differential diagnosis because it may rapidly spiral out of control towards muscle necrosis, septicaemia and death. Intense pain and board-like swelling of the limb in a patient with fever and a general feeling of illness are warning signs of a medical emergency. MRI will reveal muscle swelling and possibly signs of tissue breakdown. Immediate treatment with intravenous antibiotics is essential. Surgical debridement of necrotic tissue – and sometimes even amputation – may be needed to save a life.

Acute rheumatism The pain is less severe and it tends to flit from one joint to another. There may also be signs of carditis, rheumatic nodules or erythema marginatum.

Sickle-cell crisis The patient may present with features indistinguishable from those of acute osteomyelitis. In areas where *Salmonella* is endemic it would be wise to treat such patients with suitable antibiotics until infection is definitely excluded.

Gaucher's disease 'Pseudo-osteitis' may occur with features closely resembling those of osteomyelitis. The diagnosis is made by finding other stigmata of the disease, especially enlargement of the spleen and liver.

Treatment

If osteomyelitis is suspected on clinical grounds, blood and fluid samples should be taken for laboratory investigation and then treatment started immediately without waiting for final confirmation of the diagnosis. There are four important aspects to the management of the patient:

- Supportive treatment for pain and dehydration.
- Splintage of the affected part.
- Appropriate antimicrobial therapy.
- Surgical drainage.

GENERAL SUPPORTIVE TREATMENT

The distressed child needs to be comforted and treated for pain. Analgesics should be given at repeated intervals without waiting for the patient to ask for them. Septicaemia and fever can cause severe dehydration and it may be necessary to give fluid intravenously.

SPLINTAGE

Some type of splintage is desirable, partly for comfort but also to prevent joint contractures. Simple skin traction may suffice and, if the hip is involved, this also helps to prevent dislocation. At other sites a plaster slab or half-cylinder may be used but it should not obscure the affected area.

ANTIBIOTICS

Blood and aspiration material are sent immediately for examination and culture, but the prompt intravenous administration of antibiotics is so vital that treatment should not await the result.

Initially the choice of antibiotics is based on the findings from direct examination of the pus smear and the clinician's experience of local conditions – in other words, a 'best guess' at the most likely pathogen. *Staphylococcus aureus* is the most common at all ages, but treatment should provide cover also for other bacteria that are likely to be encountered in each age group; a more appropriate drug which is also capable of good bone penetration can be substituted, if necessary, once the infecting organism is identified and its antibiotic sensitivity is known. Factors such as the patient's age, general state of resistance, renal function, degree of toxaemia and previous history of allergy must be taken into account. The following recommendations are offered as a guide.

- *Neonates and infants up to 6 months of age* Initial antibiotic treatment should be effective against penicillin-resistant *Staphylococcus aureus*, Group B streptococcus and Gram-negative organisms. Drugs of choice are flucloxacillin plus a third-generation cephalosporin like cefotaxime. Alternatively, effective empirical treatment can be provided by a combination of flucloxacillin (for penicillin-resistant staphylococci), benzylpenicillin (for Group B streptococci) and gentamicin (for Gram-negative organisms).
- *Children 6 months to 6 years of age* Empirical treatment in this age group should include cover against *Haemophilus influenzae,* unless it is known for certain that the child has had an anti-haemophilus vaccination. This is best provided by a combination of intravenous flucloxacillin and cefotaxime or cefuroxime.
- *Older children and previously fit adults* The vast majority in this group will have a staphylococcal infection and can be started on intravenous flucloxacillin and fusidic acid. Fusidic acid is preferred to benzylpenicillin partly because of the high prevalence of penicillin-resistant staphylococci and because it is particularly well concentrated in bone. However, for a known streptococcal infection benzylpenicillin is better. Patients who are allergic to penicillin should be treated with a second- or third-generation cephalosporin.
- *Elderly and previously unfit patients* In this group there is a greater than usual risk of Gram-negative infections, due to respiratory, gastro-intestinal, or urinary disorders and the likelihood of the patient needing invasive procedures. The antibiotic of choice would be a combination of flucloxacillin and a second- or third-generation cephalosporin.
- *Patients with sickle-cell disease* These patients are prone to osteomyelitis, which may be caused by a staphylococcal infection but in many cases is due to salmonella and/or other Gram-negative organisms. Chloramphenicol, which is effective against Gram-positive, Gram-negative and anaerobic organisms, used to be the preferred antibiotic, though there were always worries about the rare complication of aplastic anaemia. Nowadays the antibiotic of choice is a third-generation cephalosporin or a fluoroquinolone like ciprofloxacin.
- *Heroin addicts and immunocompromised patients* Unusual infections (e.g. with *Pseudomonas aeruginosa*, *Proteus mirabilis* or anaerobic *Bacteroides* species) are likely in these patients. Infants with human immunodeficiency virus (HIV) infection may also have picked up other sexually transmitted organisms during birth. All patients with this type of background are therefore best treated empirically with a broad-spectrum antibiotic such as one of the third-generation cephalosporins or a fluoroquinolone preparation, depending on the results of sensitivity tests.
- *Patients considered to be at risk of meticillin-resistant Staphylococcus aureus (MRSA) infection* Patients admitted with acute haematogenous osteomyelitis and who have a previous history of MRSA infection, or any patient with a bone infection admitted to a hospital or a ward where MRSA is endemic, should be treated with intravenous vancomycin (or similar antibiotic) together with a third-generation cephalosporin.

The usual programme is to administer the drugs intravenously (if necessary adjusting the choice of antibiotic once the results of antimicrobial sensitivity become available) until the patient's condition begins to improve and the CRP values return to normal levels – which usually takes 2–4 weeks depending on the virulence of the infection and the patient's general degree of fitness. By that time the most appropriate antibiotic would have been prescribed, on the basis of sensitivity tests; this can then be administered orally for another 3–6 weeks, though if bone destruction is marked the period of treatment may have to be longer. While patients are on oral antibiotics it is important to track the serum antibiotic levels in order to ensure that the minimal inhibitory concentration (MIC) is maintained or exceeded. CRP, ESR and WBC values are also checked at regular intervals and treatment can be discontinued when these are seen to remain normal.

DRAINAGE

If antibiotics are given early (within the first 48 hours after the onset of symptoms) drainage is often unnecessary. However, if the clinical features do not improve within 36 hours of starting treatment, or even earlier if there are signs of deep pus (swelling, oedema, fluctuation), and most certainly if pus is

When treating patients with bone or joint infection it is wise to maintain continuous collaboration with a specialist in microbiology

aspirated, the abscess should be drained by open operation under general anaesthesia. If pus is found – and released – there is little to be gained by drilling into the medullary cavity. If there is no obvious abscess, it is reasonable to drill a few holes into the bone in various directions. There is no evidence that widespread drilling has any advantage and it may do more harm than good; if there is an extensive intramedullary abscess, drainage can be better achieved by cutting a small window in the cortex. The wound is closed without a drain and the splint (or traction) is reapplied. Once the signs of infection subside, movements are encouraged and the child is allowed to walk with the aid of crutches. Full weightbearing is usually possible after 3–4 weeks.

At present about one-third of patients with confirmed osteomyelitis are likely to need an operation; adults with vertebral infection seldom do.

Complications

A lethal outcome from septicaemia is nowadays extremely rare; with antibiotics the child nearly always recovers and the bone may return to normal. But morbidity is common, especially if treatment is delayed or the organism is insensitive to the chosen antibiotic.

Epiphyseal damage and altered bone growth In neonates and infants whose epiphyses are still entirely cartilaginous, metaphyseal vessels penetrate the physis and may carry the infection into the epiphysis. If this happens, the physeal growth plate can be irrevocably damaged and the cartilaginous epiphysis may be destroyed, leading to arrest of growth and shortening of the bone. At the hip joint, the proximal end of the femur may be so badly damaged as to result in a pseudarthrosis.

Suppurative arthritis This may occur: (1) in very young infants, in whom the growth disc is not an impenetrable barrier; (2) where the metaphysis is intracapsular, as in the upper femur; or (3) from metastatic infection. In infants it is so common as almost to be taken for granted, especially with osteomyelitis of the femoral neck. Ultrasound will help to demonstrate an effusion, but the definitive diagnosis is given by joint aspiration.

Metastatic infection This is sometimes seen – generally in infants – and may involve other bones, joints, serous cavities, the brain or lung. In some cases the infection may be multifocal from the outset. It is easy to miss secondary sites of infection when attention is focussed on one particular area; it is important to be alert to this complication and to examine the child all over and repeatedly.

Pathological fracture Fracture is uncommon, but it may occur if treatment is delayed and the bone is weakened either by erosion at the site of infection or by overzealous debridement.

Chronic osteomyelitis Despite improved methods of diagnosis and treatment, acute osteomyelitis sometimes fails to resolve. Weeks or months after the onset of acute infection a sequestrum appears in the follow-up x-ray and the patient is left with a chronic infection and a draining sinus. This may be due to late or inadequate treatment but is also seen in debilitated patients and in those with compromised defence mechanisms.

SUBACUTE HAEMATOGENOUS OSTEOMYELITIS

This condition is no longer rare, and in some countries the incidence is equal to that of acute osteomyelitis. Its relative mildness is presumably due to the organism being less virulent or the patient more resistant (or both). It is more variable in skeletal distribution than acute osteomyelitis, but the distal femur and the proximal and distal tibia are the favourite sites. The anatomical classification suggested by Roberts et al. (1982) is useful in comparing features in various reported series of cases.

Pathology

Typically there is a well-defined cavity in cancellous bone – usually in the tibial metaphysis – containing glairy seropurulent fluid (rarely pus). The cavity is lined by granulation tissue containing a mixture of acute and chronic inflammatory cells. The surrounding bone trabeculae are often thickened. The lesion sometimes encroaches on and erodes the bony cortex. Occasionally it appears in the epiphysis and, in adults, in one of the vertebral bodies.

Clinical features

The patient is usually a child or adolescent who has had pain near one of the larger joints for several weeks or even months. He or she may have a limp and often there is slight swelling, muscle wasting and local tenderness. The temperature is usually normal and there is little to suggest an infection.

The WBC count and blood cultures usually show no abnormality but the ESR is sometimes elevated.

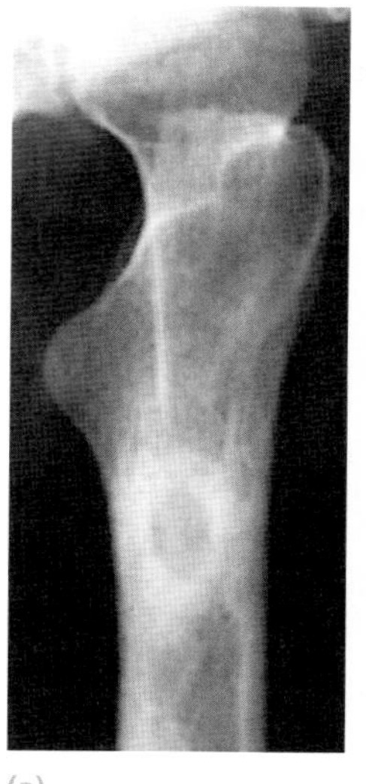
(a)

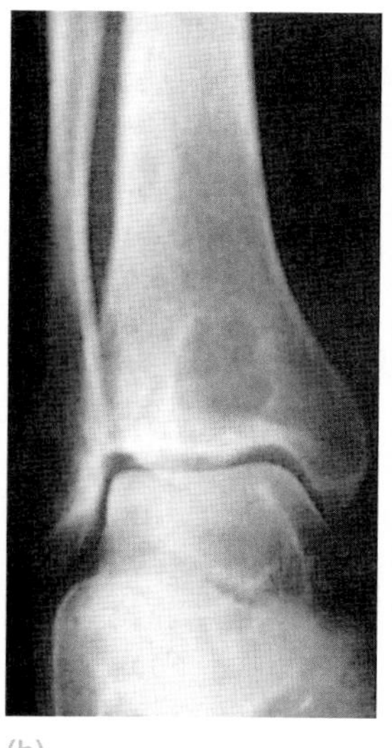
(b)

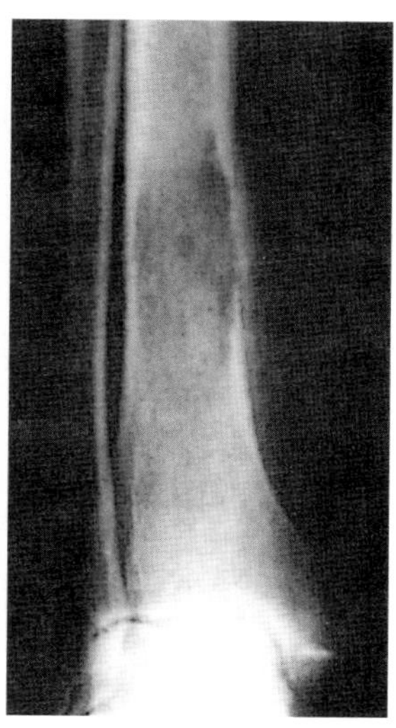
(c)

2.4 Subacute osteomyelitis (a,b) The classic Brodie's abscess looks like a small walled-off cavity in the bone with little or no periosteal reaction; (c) sometimes rarefaction is more diffuse and there may be cortical erosion and periosteal reaction.

Imaging

The typical radiographic lesion is a circumscribed, round or oval radiolucent 'cavity' 1–2 cm in diameter. Most often it is seen in the tibial or femoral metaphysis, but it may occur in the epiphysis or in one of the cuboidal bones (e.g. the calcaneum). Sometimes the 'cavity' is surrounded by a halo of sclerosis (the classic *Brodie's abscess*); occasionally it is less well defined, extending into the diaphysis.

Metaphyseal lesions cause little or no periosteal reaction; diaphyseal lesions may be associated with periosteal new bone formation and marked cortical thickening. If the cortex is eroded the lesion may be mistaken for a malignant tumour.

The radioisotope scan shows markedly increased activity.

Diagnosis

The clinical and x-ray appearances may resemble those of cystic tuberculosis, eosinophilic granuloma or osteoid osteoma; occasionally they mimic a malignant bone tumour like Ewing's sarcoma. Epiphyseal lesions are easily mistaken for chondroblastoma. The diagnosis often remains in doubt until a biopsy is performed.

If fluid is encountered, it should be sent for bacteriological culture; this is positive in about half the cases and the organism is almost always *Staphylococcus aureus.*

Treatment

Treatment may be conservative if the diagnosis is not in doubt. Immobilization and antibiotics (flucloxacillin and fusidic acid) intravenously for 4 or 5 days and then orally for another 6 weeks usually result in healing, though this may take up to 12 months. If the diagnosis is in doubt, an open biopsy is needed and the lesion may be curetted at the same time. Curettage is also indicated if the x-ray shows that there is no healing after conservative treatment; this is always followed by a further course of antibiotics.

POST-TRAUMATIC OSTEOMYELITIS

Open fractures are always contaminated and are therefore prone to infection. The combination of tissue injury, vascular damage, oedema, haematoma, dead bone fragments and an open pathway to the atmosphere must invite bacterial invasion even if the wound is not contaminated with particulate dirt. *This is the most common cause of osteomyelitis in adults.*

Staphylococcus aureus is the usual pathogen, but other organisms such as *E. coli, Proteus mirabilis* and *Pseudomonas aeruginosa* are sometimes involved. Occasionally, anaerobic organisms (clostridia, anaerobic streptococci or *Bacteroides*) appear in contaminated wounds.

Clinical features

The patient becomes feverish and develops pain and swelling over the fracture site; the wound is inflamed and there may be a seropurulent discharge. Blood tests reveal increased CRP levels, leucocytosis and an elevated ESR; it should be remembered, though, that these inflammatory markers are non-specific and may be affected by tissue trauma.

X-ray appearances may be more difficult than usual to interpret because of bone fragmentation. *MRI* can be helpful in differentiating between bone and soft-tissue infection, but is less reliable in distinguishing between longstanding infection and bone destruction due to trauma.

Microbiological investigation

A wound swab should be examined and cultured for organisms which can be tested for antibiotic sensitivity. Unfortunately, though, standard laboratory methods still yield negative results in about 20 per cent of cases of overt infection.

Treatment

The essence of treatment is prophylaxis: thorough cleansing and debridement of open fractures, the provision of drainage by leaving the wound open, immobilization of the fracture and antibiotics. In most cases a combination of flucloxacillin and benzylpenicillin (or sodium fusidate), given 6-hourly for 48 hours, will suffice. If the wound is clearly contaminated, it is wise also to give metronidazole for 4 or 5 days to control both aerobic and anaerobic organisms.

Pyogenic wound infection, once it has taken root, is difficult to eradicate. The presence of necrotic soft tissue and dead bone, together with a mixed bacterial flora, conspire against effective antibiotic control. Treatment calls for regular wound dressing and repeated excision of all dead and infected tissue.

Traditionally it was recommended that stable implants (fixation plates and medullary nails) should be left in place until the fracture had united, and this advice is still respected in recognition of the adage that even worse than an infected fracture is an *infected unstable* fracture. However, advances in external fixation techniques have meant that almost all fractures can, if necessary, be securely fixed by that method, with the added advantage that the wound remains accessible for dressings and superficial debridement.

If these measures fail, the management is essentially that of chronic osteomyelitis.

POSTOPERATIVE OSTEOMYELITIS

This subject is dealt with in Chapter 12.

CHRONIC OSTEOMYELITIS

This used to be the dreaded sequel to acute haematogenous osteomyelitis; nowadays it more frequently follows an open fracture or operation.

The usual organisms (and with time there is always a mixed infection) are *Staphylococcus aureus, Escherichia coli, Streptococcus pyogenes, Proteus mirabilis* and *Pseudomonas aeruginosa*; in the presence of foreign implants *Staphylococcus epidermidis*, which is normally non-pathogenic, is the commonest of all.

Predisposing factors

Acute haematogenous osteomyelitis, if left untreated – and provided the patient does not succumb to septicaemia – will subside into a chronic bone infection which lingers indefinitely, perhaps with alternating 'flare-ups' and spells of apparent quiescence. The host defences are inevitably compromised by the presence of scar formation, dead and dying bone around the focus of infection, poor penetration of new blood vessels and non-collapsing cavities in which microbes can thrive. Bacteria covered in a protein–polysaccharide slime (*glycocalyx*) that protects them from both the host defences and antibiotics have the ability to adhere to inert surfaces such as bone sequestra and metal implants, where they multiply and colonize the area. There is also evidence that bacteria can survive inside osteoblasts and osteocytes and be released when the cells die (Ellington et al., 2003).

These processes are evident in patients who have been inadequately treated (perhaps 'too little too late'), but in any event certain patients are at greater risk than others: those who are very old or debilitated, those suffering from substance abuse and those with diabetes, peripheral vascular disease, skin infections, malnutrition, lupus erythematosus or any type of immune deficiency. The commonest of all predisposing factors is local trauma, such as an open fracture or a prolonged bone operation, especially if this involves the use of a foreign implant.

Pathology

Bone is destroyed or devitalized, either in a discrete area around the focus of infection or more diffusely along the surface of a foreign implant. Cavities containing pus and pieces of dead bone (sequestra) are surrounded by vascular tissue, and beyond that by areas of sclerosis – the result of chronic reactive new bone formation – which may take the form of a distinct bony sheath (involucrum). In the worst cases a sizeable length of the diaphysis may be devitalized and encased in a thick involucrum.

Sequestra act as substrates for bacterial adhesion in much the same way as foreign implants, ensuring the persistence of infection until they are removed or discharged through perforations in the involucrum and sinuses that drain to the skin. A sinus may seal off for weeks or even months, giving the appearance of

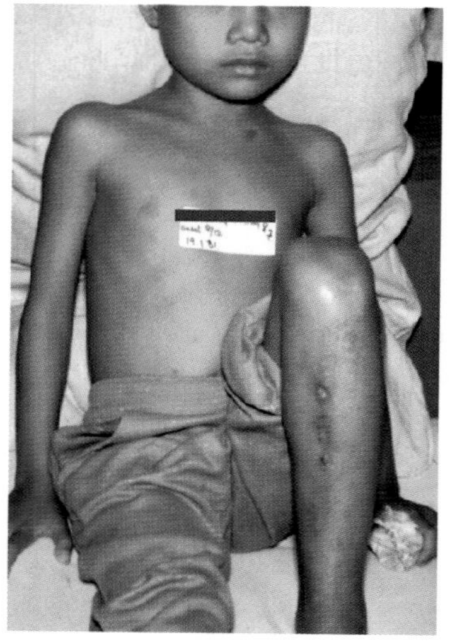
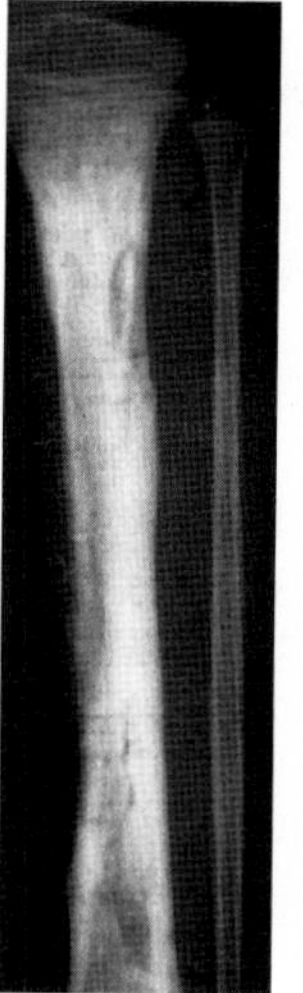
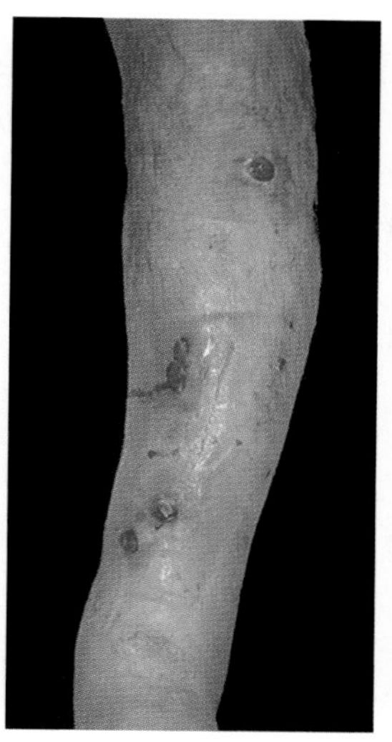
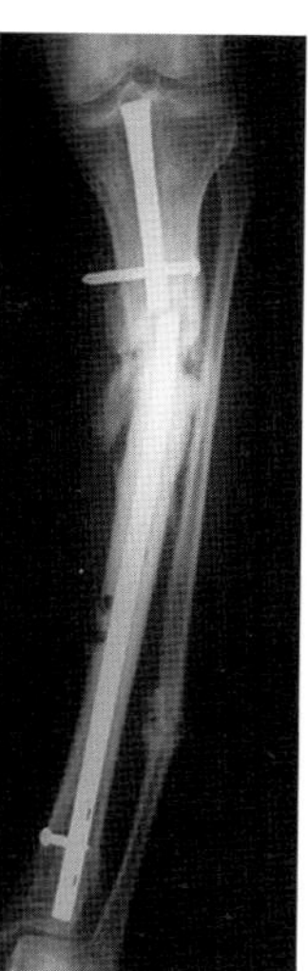

(a) (b)

2.5 Chronic osteomyelitis Chronic osteomyelitis may follow acute. The young boy (a) presented with draining sinuses at the site of a previous acute infection. The x-ray shows densely sclerotic bone. (b) In adults, chronic osteomyelitis is usually a sequel to open trauma or operation.

healing, only to reopen (or appear somewhere else) when the tissue tension rises. Bone destruction, and the increasingly brittle sclerosis, sometimes results in a pathological fracture.

The histological picture is one of chronic inflammatory cell infiltration around areas of acellular bone or microscopic sequestra.

Clinical features

The patient presents because pain, pyrexia, redness and tenderness have recurred (a 'flare'), or with a discharging sinus. In longstanding cases the tissues are thickened and often puckered or folded inwards where a scar or sinus adheres to the underlying bone. There may be a seropurulent discharge and excoriation of the surrounding skin. In post-traumatic osteomyelitis the bone may be deformed or ununited.

Imaging

X-ray examination will usually show bone resorption – either as a patchy loss of density or as frank excavation around an implant – with thickening and sclerosis of the surrounding bone. However, there are marked variations: there may be no more than localized loss of trabeculation, or an area of osteoporosis, or periosteal thickening; sequestra show up as unnaturally dense fragments, in contrast to the surrounding osteopaenic bone; sometimes the bone is crudely thickened and misshapen, resembling a tumour. A *sinogram* may help to localize the site of infection.

Radioisotope scintigraphy is sensitive but not specific. ^{99m}Tc-HDP scans show increased activity in both the perfusion phase and the bone phase. Scanning with ^{67}Ga-citrate or ^{111}In-labelled leucocytes is said to be more specific for osteomyelitis; such scans are useful for showing up hidden foci of infection.

CT and *MRI* are invaluable in planning operative treatment: together they will show the extent of bone destruction and reactive oedema, hidden abscesses and sequestra.

Investigations

During acute flares the CSR, ESR and WBC levels may be increased; these non-specific signs are helpful in assessing the progress of bone infection but they are not diagnostic.

Organisms cultured from discharging sinuses should be tested repeatedly for antibiotic sensitivity; with time, they often change their characteristics and become resistant to treatment. Note, however, that a superficial swab sample may not reflect the really persistent infection in the deeper tissues; sampling from deeper tissues is important.

The most effective antibiotic treatment can be applied only if the pathogenic organism is identified and tested for sensitivity. Unfortunately standard bacterial cultures still give negative results in about 20% of cases of overt infection. In recent years more sophisticated molecular techniques have been developed, based on the amplification of bacterial DNA or RNA fragments (the polymerase chain reaction or PCR) and their subsequent identification by gel electrophoresis. However, although this has been shown to reveal unusual and otherwise undetected organisms in a significant percentage of cases, the technique is not widely available for routine testing.

A range of other investigations may also be needed to confirm or exclude suspected systemic disorders (such as diabetes) that could influence the outcome.

Staging of chronic osteomyelitis in long bones

'Staging' the condition helps in risk–benefit assessment and has some predictive value concerning the outcome of treatment. The system popularized by Cierny et al. (2003) is based on both the local pathological anatomy and the host background (Table 2.2). The least serious, and most likely to benefit, are patients classified as Stage 1 or 2, Type A, i.e. those with localized infection and free of compromising disorders. Type B patients are somewhat compromised by a few local or systemic factors, but if the infection is localized and the bone still in continuity and stable (Stage 1–3) they have a reasonable chance of recovery. Type C patients are so severely compromised that the prognosis is considered to be poor. If the lesion is also classified as Stage 4 (e.g. intractable diffuse infection in an ununited fracture), operative treatment may be contraindicated and the best option may be long-term palliative treatment. Occasionally one may have to advise amputation.

Table 2.2 Staging for adult chronic osteomyelitis

LESION	TYPE
Stage 1	Medullary
Stage 2	Superficial
Stage 3	Localized
Stage 4	Diffuse
HOST CATEGORY	
Type A	Normal
Type B	Compromised by local or systemic conditions
Type C	Severely compromised by local and systemic conditions

Treatment

ANTIBIOTICS

Chronic infection is seldom eradicated by antibiotics alone. Yet bactericidal drugs are important (a) to suppress the infection and prevent its spread to healthy bone and (b) to control acute flares. The choice of antibiotic depends on microbiological studies, but the drug must be capable of penetrating sclerotic bone and should be non-toxic with long-term use. Fusidic acid, clindamycin and the cephalosporins are good examples. Vancomycin and teicoplanin are effective in most cases of meticillin-resistant *Staphylococcus aureus* infection (MRSA).

Antibiotics are administered for 4–6 weeks (starting from the beginning of treatment or the last debridement) before considering operative treatment. During this time serum antibiotic concentrations should be measured at regular intervals to ensure that they are kept at several times the minimal bactericidal concentration. *Continuous collaboration with a specialist in microbiology is important.* If surgical clearance fails, antibiotics should be continued for another 4 weeks before considering another attempt at full debridement.

LOCAL TREATMENT

A sinus may be painless and need dressing simply to protect the clothing. Colostomy paste can be used to stop excoriation of the skin. An acute abscess may need urgent incision and drainage, but this is only a temporary measure.

OPERATION

A waiting policy, punctuated by spells of bed rest and antibiotics to control flares, may have to be patiently endured until there is a clear indication for radical surgery: for *chronic haematogenous infections* this means intrusive symptoms, failure of adequate antibiotic treatment, and/or clear evidence of a sequestrum or dead bone; for *post-traumatic infections*, an intractable wound and/or an infected ununited fracture; for *postoperative infection*, similar criteria and evidence of bone erosion.

The presence of a *foreign implant* is a further incentive to operate. Traditionally it was felt that internal fixation devices (plates, screws and intramedullary nails) should be retained, even though infected, in order to maintain stability. Nowadays, however, a range of ingenious external fixation systems are available and it is possible to immobilize almost any fracture by this method, thus bypassing the fracture and allowing earlier removal of infected material at that site.

When undertaking operative treatment, collaboration with a plastic surgeon is strongly recommended.

Debridement At operation all infected soft tissue and dead or devitalized bone, as well as any infected implant, must be excised. After three or four days the wound is inspected and if there are renewed signs of tissue death the debridement may have to be repeated – several times if necessary. Antibiotic cover is continued for at least 4 weeks after the last debridement.

Dealing with the 'dead space' There are several ways of dealing with the resulting 'dead space'. *Porous antibiotic-impregnated beads* can be laid in the cavity and left for 2 or 3 weeks and then replaced with *cancellous bone grafts*. Bone grafts have also been used on their own; in the *Papineau technique* the entire cavity is packed with small cancellous chips (preferably autogenous) mixed with an antibiotic and a fibrin sealant. Where possible, the area is covered by adjacent muscle and the skin wound is sutured without tension. An alternative approach is to employ a *muscle flap transfer*: in suitable sites a large wad of muscle, with its blood supply intact, can be mobilized and laid into the cavity; the surface is later covered with a split-skin graft. In areas with too little adjacent muscle (e.g. the distal part of the leg), the same objective can be achieved by transferring a myocutaneous island flap on a long vascular pedicle. A free vascularized bone graft is considered to be a better option, provided the site is suitable and the appropriate facilities for microvascular surgery are available.

A different approach is the one developed and refined by Lautenbach in South Africa. This involves radical excision of all avascular and infected tissue followed by closed irrigation and suction drainage of the bed using double-lumen tubes and an appropriate antibiotic solution in high concentration (based on microbiological tests for bacterial sensitivity). The 'dead space' is gradually filled by vascular granulation tissue. The tubes are removed when cultures remain negative in three consecutive fluid samples and the cavity is obliterated. The technique, which has been used with considerable success, is described in detail by Hashmi et al. (2004).

In refractory cases it may be possible to excise the infected and/or devitalized segment of bone completely and then close the gap by the *Ilizarov method* of 'transporting' a viable segment from the remaining diaphysis. This is especially useful if infection is associated with an ununited fracture (see Chapter 12).

Soft-tissue cover Last but not least, the bone must be adequately covered with skin. For small defects split-thickness skin grafts may suffice; for larger wounds local musculocutaneous flaps, or free vascularized flaps, are needed.

Aftercare Success is difficult to measure; a minute focus of infection might escape the therapeutic onslaught, only to flare into full-blown osteomyelitis many years later. Prognosis should always be guarded; local trauma must be avoided and any recurrence of symptoms, however slight, should be taken seriously and investigated. The watchword is 'cautious optimism' – a 'probable cure' is better than no cure at all.

GARRÉ'S SCLEROSING OSTEOMYELITIS

Garré, in 1893, described a rare form of non-suppurative osteomyelitis which is characterized by marked sclerosis and cortical thickening. There is no abscess, only a diffuse enlargement of the bone at the affected site – usually the diaphysis of one of the tubular bones or the mandible. The patient is typically an adolescent or young adult with a long history of aching and slight swelling over the bone. Occasionally there are recurrent attacks of more acute pain accompanied by malaise and slight fever.

X-rays show increased bone density and cortical thickening; in some cases the marrow cavity is completely obliterated. There is no abscess cavity.

Diagnosis can be difficult. If a small segment of bone is involved, it may be mistaken for an osteoid osteoma. If there is marked periosteal layering of new bone, the lesion resembles a Ewing's sarcoma. The biopsy will disclose a low-grade inflammatory lesion with reactive bone formation. Micro-organisms are seldom cultured but the condition is usually ascribed to a staphylococcal infection.

Treatment is by operation: the abnormal area is excised and the exposed surface thoroughly curetted. Bone grafts, bone transport or free bone transfer may be needed.

MULTIFOCAL NON-SUPPURATIVE OSTEOMYELITIS

This obscure disorder – it is not even certain that it is an infection – was first described in isolated cases in the 1960s and 70s, and later in a more comprehensive report on 20 patients of mixed age and sex (Björkstén and Boquist, 1980). It is now recognized that: (1) it is not as rare as initially suggested; (2) it comprises several different syndromes which have certain features in common; and (3) there is an association with chronic skin infection, especially pustular lesions of the palms and soles (palmo-plantar pustulosis) and pustular psoriasis.

In children the condition usually takes the form of multifocal (often symmetrical), recurrent lesions in the long-bone metaphyses, clavicles and anterior rib-cage; in adults the changes appear predominantly in the sterno-costo-clavicular complex and the vertebrae. In recent years the various syndromes have been drawn together under the convenient acronym SAPHO – standing for synovitis, acne, pustulosis, hyperostosis and osteitis (Boutin and Resnick, 1998).

Early osteolytic lesions show histological features suggesting a subacute inflammatory condition; in longstanding cases there may be bone thickening and round cell infiltration. The aetiology is unknown. Despite the local and systemic signs of inflammation, there is no purulent discharge and micro-organisms have seldom been isolated.

The two most characteristic clinical syndromes will be described.

SUBACUTE RECURRENT MULTIFOCAL OSTEOMYELITIS

This appears as an inflammatory bone disorder affecting mainly children and adolescents. Patients develop recurrent attacks of pain, swelling and tenderness around one or other of the long-bone metaphyses (usually the distal femur or the proximal or distal tibia), the medial ends of the clavicles or a vertebral segment. Over the course of several years multiple sites are affected, sometimes symmetrically and sometimes simultaneously; with each exacerbation the child is slightly feverish and may have a raised ESR.

X-ray changes are characteristic. There are small lytic lesions in the metaphysis, usually closely adjacent to the physis. Some of these 'cavities' are surrounded by sclerosis; others show varying stages of healing. The clavicle may become markedly thickened. If the spine is affected, it may lead to collapse of a vertebral body. *Radioscintigraphy* shows increased activity around the lesions.

Biopsy of the lytic focus is likely to show the typical histological features of acute or subacute inflammation. In longstanding lesions there is a chronic inflammatory reaction with lymphocyte infiltration. Bacteriological cultures are almost invariably negative.

Treatment is entirely palliative; antibiotics have no effect on the disease. Although the condition may run a protracted course, the prognosis is good and the lesions eventually heal without complications.

STERNO-COSTO-CLAVICULAR HYPEROSTOSIS

Patients are usually in their forties or fifties, and men are affected more often than women. Clinical and radiological changes are usually confined to the sternum and adjacent bones and the vertebral column. As with recurrent multifocal osteomyelitis, there is a curious association with cutaneous pustulosis. The usual complaint is of pain, swelling and tenderness around the sternoclavicular joints; sometimes there is also a slight fever and the ESR may be elevated. Patients with vertebral column involvement may develop back pain and stiffness.

X-rays show hyperostosis of the medial ends of the clavicles, the adjacent sternum and the anterior ends of the upper ribs, as well as ossification of the sternoclavicular and costoclavicular ligaments. Vertebral changes include sclerosis of individual vertebral bodies, ossification of the anterior longitudinal ligament, anterior intervertebral bridging, end-plate erosions, disc space narrowing and vertebral collapse. *Radioscintigraphy* shows increased activity around the sternoclavicular joints and affected vertebrae.

The condition usually runs a protracted course with recurrent 'flares'. There is no effective treatment but in the long term symptoms tend to diminish or disappear; however, the patient may be left with ankylosis of the affected joints.

INFANTILE CORTICAL HYPEROSTOSIS (CAFFEY'S DISEASE)

Infantile cortical hyperostosis is a rare disease of infants and young children. It usually starts during the first few months of life with painful swelling over the tubular bones and/or the mandible. The child may be feverish and irritable, refusing to move the affected limb. Infection may be suspected but, apart from the swelling, there are no local signs of inflammation. The ESR, though, is usually elevated.

X-rays characteristically show periosteal new-bone formation resulting in thickening of the affected bone.

After a few months the local features may resolve spontaneously, only to reappear somewhere else. Flat bones, such as the scapula and cranial vault, may also be affected.

Other causes of hyperostosis (osteomyelitis, scurvy) must be excluded. The cause of Caffey's disease is

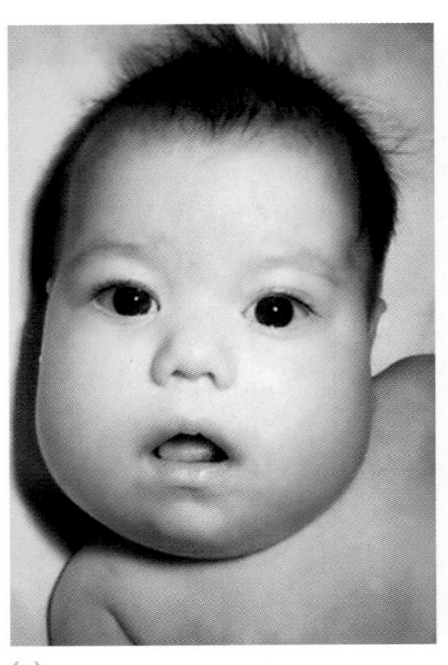
(a)

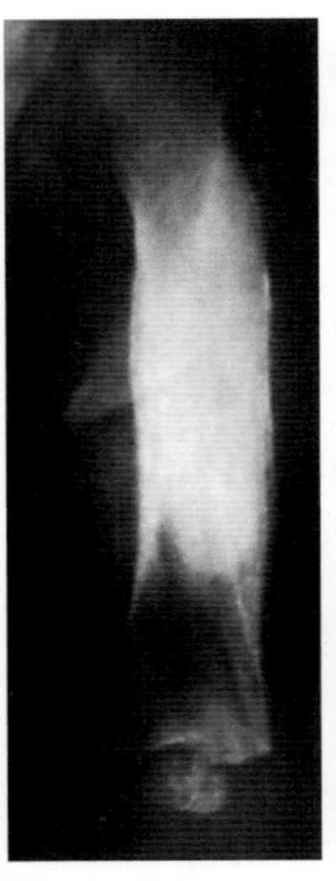
(b)

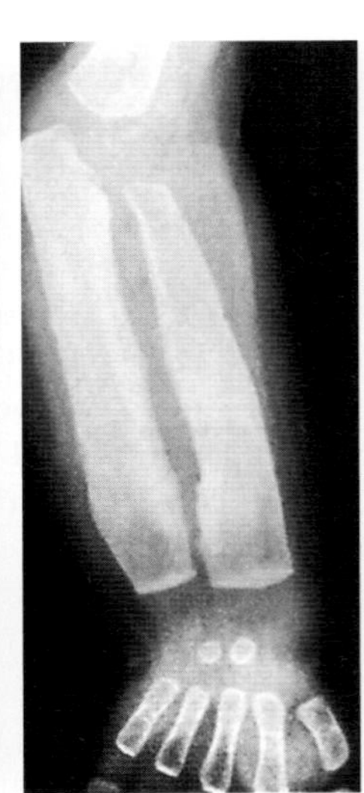
(c)

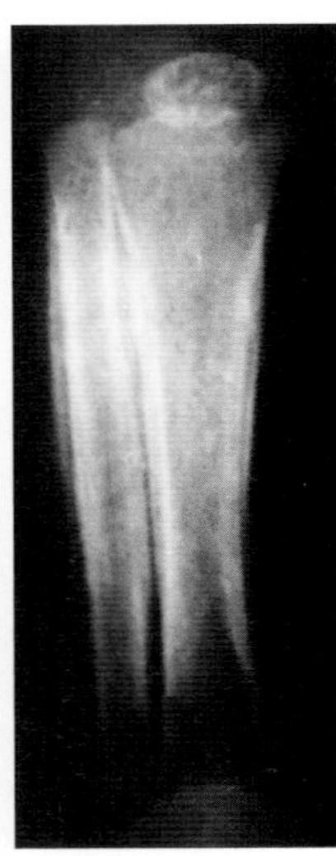
(d)

2.6 Caffey's disease This infant with Caffey's disease developed marked thickening of the mandible and long bones. The lesions gradually cleared up, leaving little or no trace of their former ominous appearance.

unknown but a virus infection has been suggested. Antibiotics are sometimes employed; it is doubtful whether they have any effect.

ACUTE SUPPURATIVE ARTHRITIS

A joint can become infected by: (1) direct invasion through a penetrating wound, intra-articular injection or arthroscopy; (2) direct spread from an adjacent bone abscess; or (3) blood spread from a distant site. In infants it is often difficult to tell whether the infection started in the metaphyseal bone and spread to the joint or vice versa. In practice it hardly matters and in advanced cases it should be assumed that the entire joint and the adjacent bone ends are involved.

The causal organism is usually *Staphylococcus aureus*; however, in children between 1 and 4 years old, *Haemophilus influenzae* is an important pathogen unless they have been vaccinated against this organism. Occasionally other microbes, such as *Streptococcus, Escherichia coli* and *Proteus*, are encountered.

Predisposing conditions are rheumatoid arthritis, chronic debilitating disorders, intravenous drug abuse, immunosuppressive drug therapy and acquired immune deficiency syndrome (AIDS).

Pathology

The usual trigger is a haematogenous infection which settles in the synovial membrane; there is an acute inflammatory reaction with a serous or seropurulent exudate and an increase in synovial fluid. As pus appears in the joint, articular cartilage is eroded and destroyed, partly by bacterial enzymes and partly by proteolytic enzymes released from synovial cells, inflammatory cells and pus. In infants the entire epiphysis, which is still largely cartilaginous, may be severely damaged; in older children, vascular occlusion may lead to necrosis of the epiphyseal bone. In adults the effects are usually confined to the articular cartilage, but in late cases there may be extensive erosion due to synovial proliferation and ingrowth.

If the infection goes untreated, it will spread to the underlying bone or burst out of the joint to form abscesses and sinuses.

With healing there may be: (1) complete resolution and a return to normal; (2) partial loss of articular cartilage and fibrosis of the joint; (3) loss of articular cartilage and bony ankylosis; or (4) bone destruction and permanent deformity of the joint.

Clinical features

The clinical features differ somewhat according to the age of the patient.

In new-born infants the emphasis is on septicaemia rather than joint pain. The baby is irritable and refuses to feed; there is a rapid pulse and sometimes a fever. Infection is often suspected, but it could be anywhere! The joints should be carefully felt and moved to elicit the local signs of warmth, tenderness and resistance to movement. The umbilical cord should be examined for a source of infection. An inflamed intravenous infusion site should always excite suspicion. The baby's chest, spine and abdomen should be carefully examined to exclude other sites of infection.

Special care should be taken not to miss a concomitant osteomyelitis in an adjacent bone end.

In children the usual features are acute pain in a single large joint (commonly the hip or the knee) and reluctance to move the limb ('pseudoparesis'). The child is ill, with a rapid pulse and a swinging fever. The overlying skin looks red and in a superficial joint swelling may be obvious. There is local warmth and marked tenderness. All movements are restricted, and

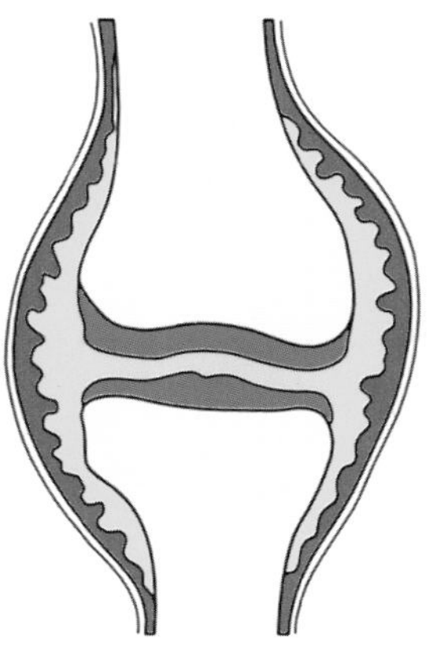
(a)

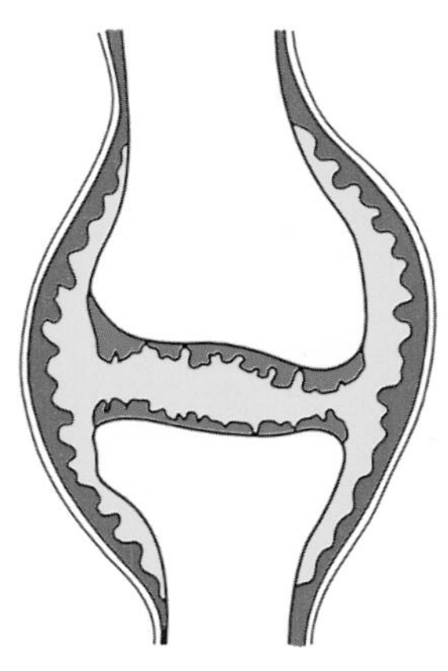
(b)

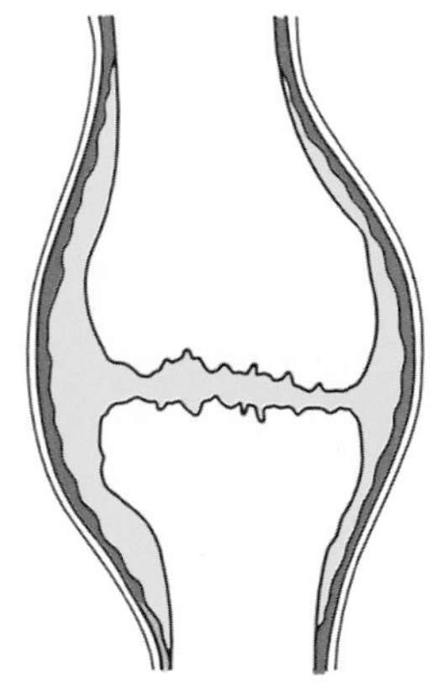
(c)

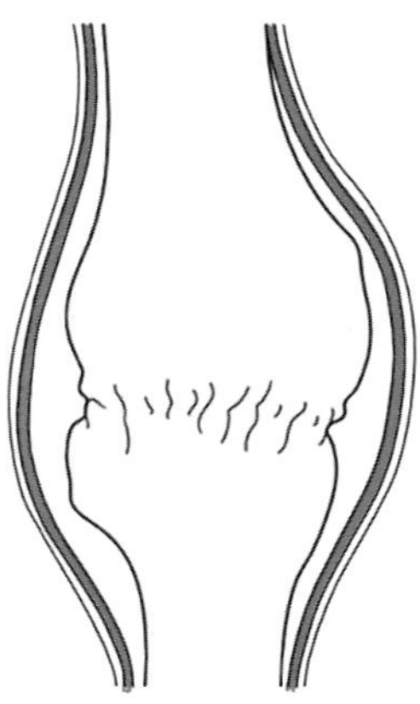
(d)

2.7 Acute suppurative arthritis – pathology In the early stage (a), there is an acute synovitis with a purulent joint effusion. (b) Soon the articular cartilage is attacked by bacterial and cellular enzymes. If the infection is not arrested, the cartilage may be completely destroyed (c). Healing then leads to bony ankylosis (d).

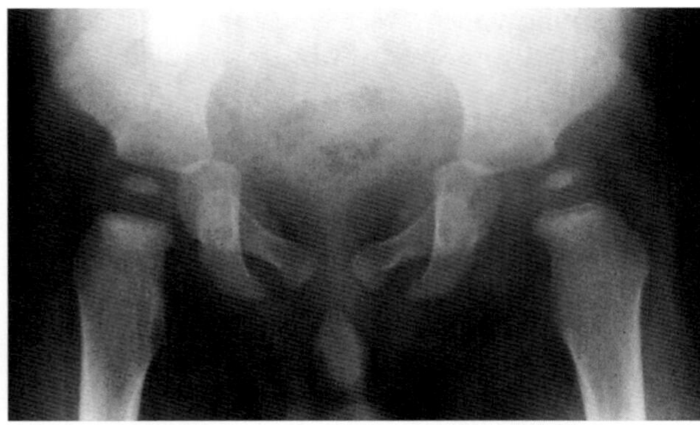

(a)

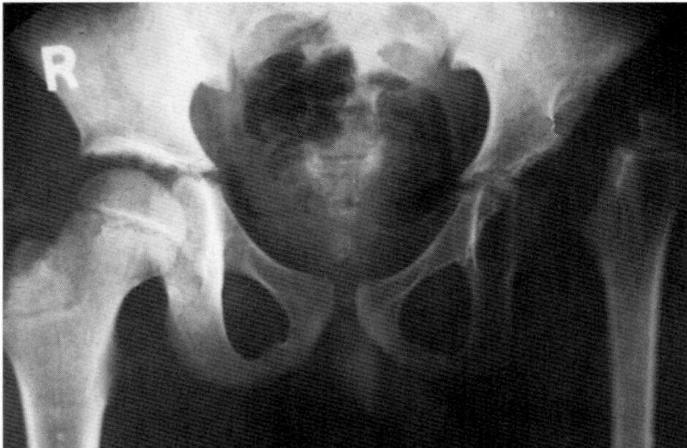

(b)

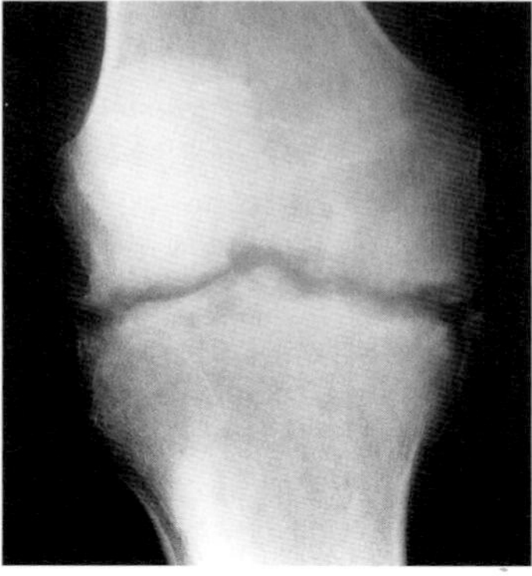

(c)

2.8 Suppurative arthritis – x-ray (a) In this child the left hip is subluxated and the soft tissues are swollen. (b) If the infection persists untreated, the cartilaginous epiphysis may be entirely destroyed, leaving a permanent pseudarthrosis. (c) Septic arthritis in an adult knee joint.

often completely abolished, by pain and spasm. It is essential to look for a source of infection – a septic toe, a boil or a discharge from the ear.

In adults it is often a superficial joint (knee, wrist, a finger, ankle or toe) that is painful, swollen and inflamed. There is warmth and marked local tenderness, and movements are restricted. The patient should be questioned and examined for evidence of gonococcal infection or drug abuse. Patients with rheumatoid arthritis, and especially those on corticosteroid treatment, may develop a 'silent' joint infection. Suspicion may be aroused by an unexplained deterioration in the patient's general condition; every joint should be carefully examined.

Imaging

Ultrasonography is the most reliable method for revealing a joint effusion in early cases. Both hips should be examined for comparison. Widening of the space between capsule and bone of more than 2 mm is indicative of an effusion, which may be echo-free (perhaps a transient synovitis) or positively echogenic (more likely septic arthritis).

X-ray examination is usually normal early on but signs to be watched for are soft-tissue swelling, loss of tissue planes, widening of the radiographic 'joint space' and slight subluxation (because of fluid in the joint). With *E. coli* infections there is sometimes gas in the joint. Narrowing and irregularity of the joint space are late features.

MRI and *radionuclide imaging* are helpful in diagnosing arthritis in obscure sites such as the sacroiliac and sternoclavicular joints.

Investigations

The white cell count and ESR are raised and blood culture may be positive. However, special investigations take time and it is much quicker (and usually more reliable) to aspirate the joint and examine the fluid. It may be frankly purulent but beware! – in early cases the fluid may look clear. A white cell count and Gram stain should be carried out immediately: the normal synovial fluid leucocyte count is under 300 per mL; it may be over 10 000 per mL in non-infective inflammatory disorders, but counts of over 50 000 per mL are highly suggestive of sepsis. Gram-positive cocci are probably *S. aureus*; Gram-negative cocci are either *H. influenzae* or *Kingella kingae* (in children) or *Gonococcus* (in adults). Samples of fluid are also sent for full microbiological examination and tests for antibiotic sensitivity.

Differential diagnosis

Acute osteomyelitis In young children, osteomyelitis may be indistinguishable from septic arthritis; often one must assume that both are present.

Other types of infection *Psoas abscess* and local *infection of the pelvis* must be kept in mind. Systemic features will obviously be the same as those of septic arthritis.

Trauma Traumatic synovitis or haemarthrosis may be associated with acute pain and swelling. A history of injury does not exclude infection. Diagnosis may remain in doubt until the joint is aspirated.

Irritable joint At the onset the joint is painful and lacks some movement, but the child is not really ill and there are no signs of infection. Ultrasonography may help to distinguish septic arthritis from transient synovitis.

Haemophilic bleed An acute haemarthrosis closely resembles septic arthritis. The history is usually conclusive, but aspiration will resolve any doubt.

Rheumatic fever Typically the pain flits from joint to joint, but at the onset one joint may be misleadingly inflamed. However, there are no signs of septicaemia.

Juvenile rheumatoid arthritis This may start with pain and swelling of a single joint, but the onset is usually more gradual and systemic symptoms less severe than in septic arthritis.

Sickle-cell disease The clinical picture may closely resemble that of septic arthritis – and indeed the bone nearby may actually be infected! – so this condition should always be excluded in communities where the disease is common.

Gaucher's disease In this rare condition acute joint pain and fever can occur without any organism being found ('pseudo-osteitis'). Because of the predisposition to true infection, antibiotics should be given.

Gout and pseudogout *In adults*, acute crystal-induced synovitis may closely resemble infection. On aspiration the joint fluid is often turbid, with a high white cell count; however, microscopic examination by polarized light will show the characteristic crystals.

Treatment

The first priority is to aspirate the joint and examine the fluid. Treatment is then started without further delay and follows the same lines as for acute osteomyelitis. Once the blood and tissue samples have been obtained, there is no need to wait for detailed results before giving antibiotics. If the aspirate looks purulent, the joint should be drained without waiting for laboratory results (see below).

GENERAL SUPPORTIVE CARE

Analgesics are given for pain and intravenous fluids for dehydration.

SPLINTAGE

The joint should be rested, and for neonates and infants this may mean light splintage; with hip infection, the joint should be held abducted and 30 degrees flexed, on traction to prevent dislocation.

ANTIBIOTICS

Antibiotic treatment follows the same guidelines as presented for acute haematogenous osteomyelitis (see page 35). The initial choice of antibiotics is based on judgement of the most likely pathogens.

Neonates and infants up to the age of 6 months should be protected against staphylococcus and Gram-negative streptococci with one of the penicillinase-resistant penicillins (e.g. flucloxacillin) plus a third-generation cephalosporin.

Children from 6 months to puberty can be treated similarly. Unless they had been immunized there is a risk of *Haemophilus* infection.

Older teenagers and adults can be started on flucloxacillin and fusidic acid. If the initial examination shows Gram-negative organisms a third-generation cephalosporin is added. More appropriate drugs can be substituted after full microbiological investigation.

Antibiotics should be given intravenously for 4–7 days and then orally for another 3 weeks.

DRAINAGE

Under anaesthesia the joint is opened through a small incision, drained and washed out with physiological saline. A small catheter is left in place and the wound is closed; suction–irrigation is continued for another 2 or 3 days. This is the safest policy and is certainly advisable (1) in very young infants, (2) when the hip is involved and (3) if the aspirated pus is very thick. For the knee, arthroscopic debridement and copious irrigation may be equally effective. Older children with early septic arthritis (symptoms for less than 3 days) involving any joint except the hip can often be treated successfully by repeated closed aspiration of the joint; however, if there is no improvement within 48 hours, open drainage will be necessary.

AFTERCARE

Once the patient's general condition is satisfactory and the joint is no longer painful or warm, further damage is unlikely. If articular cartilage has been preserved, gentle and gradually increasing active movements are encouraged. If articular cartilage has been destroyed the aim is to keep the joint immobile while ankylosis is awaited. Splintage in the optimum position is therefore continuously maintained, usually by plaster, until ankylosis is sound.

Complications

Infants under 6 months of age have the highest incidence of complications, most of which affect the hip. The most obvious risk factors are a delay in diagnosis and treatment (more than 4 days) and concomitant osteomyelitis of the proximal femur.

Subluxation and dislocation of the hip, or instability of the knee should be prevented by appropriate posturing or splintage.

Damage to the cartilaginous physis or the epiphysis in the growing child is the most serious complication. Sequelae include *retarded growth, partial* or *complete destruction of the epiphysis, deformity of the joint, epiphyseal osteonecrosis, acetabular dysplasia* and *pseudarthrosis of the hip.*

Articular cartilage erosion (chondrolysis) is seen in

older patients and this may result in restricted movement or complete *ankylosis of the joint*.

GONOCOCCAL ARTHRITIS

Neisseria gonorrhoeae is the commonest cause of septic arthritis in sexually active adults, especially among poorer populations. Even in affluent communities the incidence of sexually transmitted diseases has increased (probably related to the increased use of non-barrier contraception) and with it the risk of gonococcal and syphilitic bone and joint diseases and their sequelae. The infection is acquired only by direct mucosal contact with an infected person – carrying a risk of greater than 50% after a single contact!

Clinical features

Two types of clinical disorder are recognized: (a) *disseminated gonococcal infection* – a triad of polyarthritis, tenosynovitis and dermatitis – and (b) *septic arthritis of a single joint* (usually the knee, ankle, shoulder, wrist or hand). Both syndromes may occur in the same patient. There may be a slight pyrexia and the ESR and WBC count will be raised. If the condition is suspected, the patient should be questioned about possible contacts during the previous days or weeks and they should be examined for other signs of genitourinary infection (e.g. a urethral discharge or cervicitis).

Joint aspiration may reveal a high white cell count and typical Gram-negative organisms, but bacteriological investigations are often disappointing. Samples should also be taken from the various mucosal surfaces and tests should be performed for other sexually transmitted infections.

Treatment

Treatment is similar to that of other types of pyogenic arthritis. Patients will usually respond fairly quickly to a third-generation cephalosporin given intravenously or intramuscularly. However, bear in mind that many patients with gonococcal infection also have chlamydial infection, which is resistant to cephalosporins; both are sensitive to quinolone antibiotics such as ciprofloxacin and ofloxacin. If the organism is found to be sensitive to penicillin (and the patient is not allergic), treatment with ampicillin or amoxicillin and clavulanic acid is also effective.

SEPTIC ARTHRITIS AND HIV-1 INFECTION

Septic arthritis has been encountered quite frequently in HIV-positive intravenous drug users, HIV-positive haemophiliacs and other patients with AIDS. The usual organisms are *Staphylococcus aureus* and *Streptococcus*; however, opportunistic infection by unusual organisms is not uncommon.

The patient may present with an acutely painful, inflamed joint and marked systemic features of bacteraemia or septicaemia. In some cases the infection is confined to a single, unusual site such as the sacroiliac joint; in others several joints may be affected simultaneously. Opportunistic infection by unusual organisms may produce a more indolent clinical picture.

Treatment follows the general principles outlined before. Patients with staphylococcal and streptococcal infections usually respond well to antibiotic treatment and joint drainage; opportunistic infections may be more difficult to control.

SPIROCHAETAL INFECTION

Two conditions which are likely to be encountered by the orthopaedic surgeon are dealt with here: *syphilis* and *yaws*. *Lyme disease*, which also originates with a spirochaetal infection, is better regarded as due to a systemic autoimmune response and is dealt with in Chapter 3.

SYPHILIS

Syphilis is caused by the spirochaete *Treponema pallidum*, generally acquired during sexual activity by direct contact with infectious lesions of the skin or mucous membranes. The infection spreads to the regional lymph nodes and thence to the blood stream. The organism can also cross the placental barrier and enter the foetal blood stream directly during the latter half of pregnancy, giving rise to congenital syphilis.

In acquired syphilis a *primary* ulcerous lesion, or *chancre*, appears at the site of inoculation about a month after initial infection. This usually heals without treatment but, a month or more after that, the disease enters a *secondary phase* characterized by the appearance of a maculopapular rash and bone and joint changes due to periostitis, osteitis and osteochondritis. After a variable length of time, this phase is followed by a *latent period* which may continue for many years. The term is somewhat deceptive because in about half the cases pathological lesions continue to appear in various organs and 10–30 years later the patient may present again with *tertiary syphilis*, which takes various forms including the appearance of large granulomatous gummata in bones and joints and neuropathic disorders in which the loss of sensibility gives rise to joint breakdown (*Charcot joints*).

In congenital syphilis the primary infection may be

so severe that the foetus is either still-born or the infant dies shortly after birth. The ones who survive manifest pathological changes similar to those described above, though with modified clinical appearances and a contracted timescale.

Clinical features of acquired syphilis

Early features The patient usually presents with pain, swelling and tenderness of the bones, especially those with little soft-tissue covering, such as the frontal bones of the skull, the anterior surface of the tibia, the sternum and the ribs. *X-rays* may show typical features of *periostitis* and *thickening of the cortex* in these bones, as well as others that are not necessarily symptomatic. *Osteitis* and *septic arthritis* are less common. Occasionally these patients develop polyarthralgia or polyarthritis. Enquiry may reveal a history of sexually transmitted disease.

Late features The typical late feature, which may appear only after many years, is the syphilitic *gumma*, a dense granulomatous lesion associated with local bone resorption and adjacent areas of sclerosis. Sometimes this results in a pathological fracture. *X-rays* may show thick periosteal new bone formation at other sites, especially the tibia.

The other well-recognized feature of tertiary syphilis is a neuropathic arthropathy due to loss of sensibility in the joint – most characteristically the knee (see page 98).

Other neurological disorders, the early signs of which may only be discovered on careful examination, are tabes dorsalis and 'general paralysis of the insane' (GPI). With modern treatment these late sequelae have become rare.

Clinical features of congenital syphilis

Early congenital syphilis Although the infection is present at birth, bone changes do not usually appear until several weeks afterwards (Rasool and Govender, 1989). The baby is sick and irritable and examination may show skin lesions, hepatosplenomegaly and anaemia. Serological tests are usually positive in both mother and child.

The first signs of skeletal involvement may be joint swelling and 'pseudoparalysis' – the child refuses to move a painful limb. Several sites may be involved, often symmetrically, with slight swelling and tenderness at the ends or along the shafts of the tubular bones. The characteristic *X-ray changes* are of two kinds: *osteochondritis ('metaphysitis')* – trabecular erosion in the juxta-epiphyseal regions of tubular bones showing first as a lucent band near the physis and later as frank bone destruction which may result in epiphyseal separation; and, less frequently, *periostitis* – diffuse periosteal new bone formation along the diaphysis, usually of mild degree but sometimes producing an 'onion-peel' effect. The condition must be distinguished from scurvy (rare in the first 6 months of life), multifocal osteomyelitis, the battered baby syndrome and Caffey's disease (see page 42).

Late congenital syphilis Bone lesions in older children and adolescents resemble those of acquired syphilis and some features occurring 10 or 15 years after birth may be manifestations of tertiary disease, the result of gumma formation and endarteritis. Gummata appear

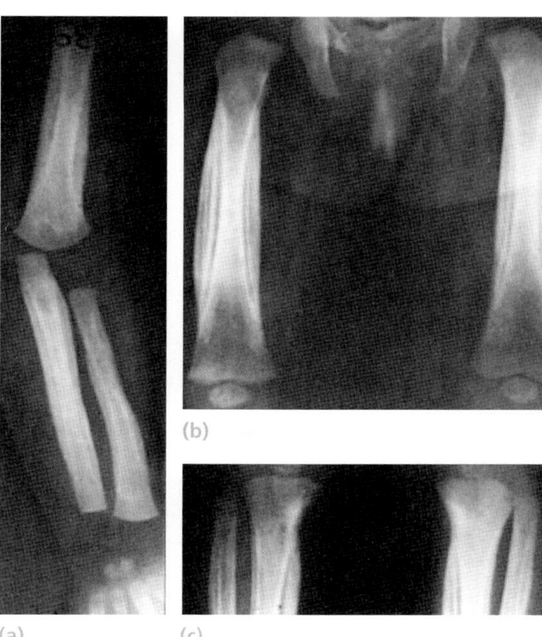

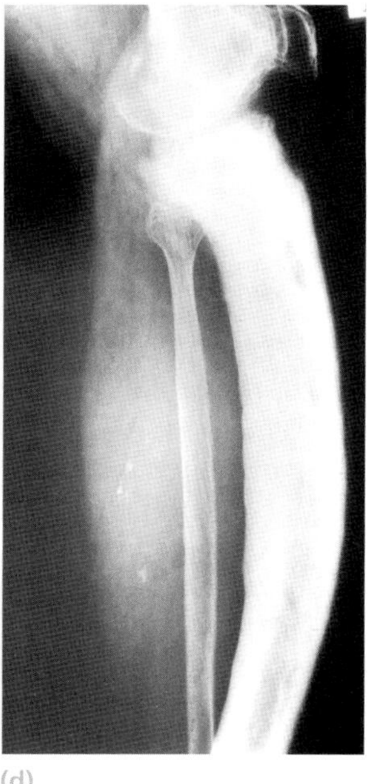

(a) (b) (c) (d)

2.9 Syphilis (a–c) Congenital syphilis, with diffuse periostitis of many bones. (d) Acquired syphilitic periostitis of the tibia.

either as discrete, punched-out radiolucent areas in the medulla or as more extensive destructive lesions in the cortex. The surrounding bone is thick and sclerotic. Sometimes the predominant feature is dense endosteal and periosteal new bone formation affecting almost the entire bone (the classic *'sabre tibia'*).

Other abnormalities which have come to be regarded as 'classic' features in older children are dental malformations ('Hutchinson's teeth'), erosion of the nasal bones, thickening and expansion of the finger phalanges (dactylitis) and painless effusions in the knees or elbows ('Clutton's joints').

Treatment

Early lesions will usually respond to intramuscular injections of benzylpenicillin given weekly for 3 or 4 doses. Late lesions will require high-dosage intravenous penicillin for a week or 10 days, but some forms of tertiary syphilis will not respond at all. An alternative would be treatment with one of the third-generation cephalosporins.

Yaws

Yaws is a non-venereal spirochaetal infection caused by *Treponema pertenue*. It is seen mainly in the poorer tropical parts of Africa, Asia and South America. Though considered – at least in Europe – to be a 'rare' disease, several thousand cases a year are reported in Indonesia.

The infection is contracted by skin-to-skin contact. A knobbly ulcer covered by a scab (the *primary* or *'mother' yaw*), usually develops on the face, hands or feet. Secondary skin lesions appear 1–4 months later and successive lesions may go on to pustular ulceration; as each one heals it leaves a pale tell-tale scar. This *secondary stage* is followed by a long *latent period*, merging into a *tertiary stage* during which skeletal changes similar to those of syphilis develop – periosteal new bone formation, cortical destruction and osteochondritis.

Clinical features

Children under 10 years old are the usual victims. In areas where the disease is endemic the typical skin lesions and an associated lymphadenopathy are quickly recognized. Elsewhere further investigations may be called for – serological tests and dark-field examination of scrapings from one of the skin lesions.

At a later stage deformities and bone tenderness may become apparent. *X-rays* show features such as cortical erosion, joint destruction and periosteal new bone formation; occasionally thickening of a long bone may be so marked as to resemble the 'sabre tibia' of late congenital syphilis.

Treatment

Treatment with benzylpenicillin, preferably given by intramuscular injection, is effective. For those who are hypersensitive to penicillin, erythromycin is a satisfactory alternative.

TROPICAL ULCER

Tropical ulcer, though the name sounds vague and non-specific, is a distinct entity that is seen frequently in tropical and subtropical regions, particularly in parts of Africa, where people walk bare-legged through rough terrain or long grass. It almost always occurs on the leg and men make up the majority of patients (probably because they are out and about more often than women). The initial lesion is a small split in the skin (a cut, thorn-scratch, insect bite or other minor abrasion), which is then contaminated with all kinds of dirt or stagnant water. The most likely infecting organisms are *Fusiformis fusiformis* and *Borrelia vincentii* (both common in faeces). This results in an indolent ulcer which defies most forms of topical treatment (and certainly traditional remedies native to those parts of the world). The ulcer may eventually bore its way into the soft tissues and the underlying bone; occa-

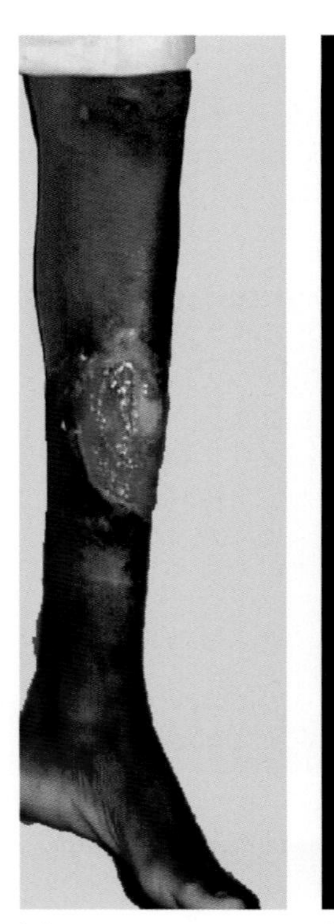

(a)

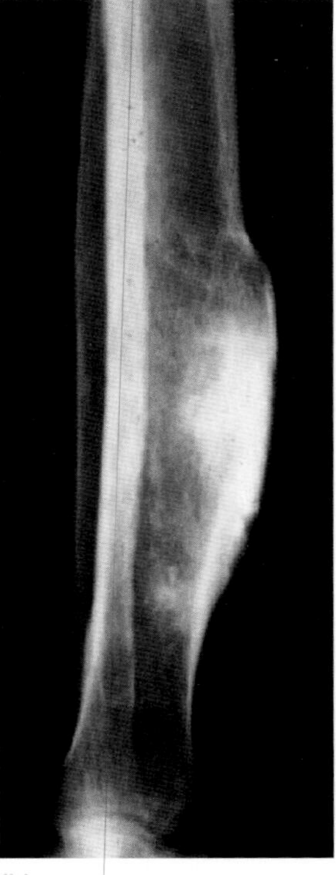

(b)

2.10 Tropical ulcer What started as a small ulcer has turned into a large spreading lesion. The x-ray shows the typical marked periosteal reaction in the underlying bone.

sionally, after many years, it gives rise to a locally invasive squamous-cell carcinoma.

Clinical features

What starts as a small inflamed scratch or cut develops over a few days into a large pustule. By the time the patient attends for medical treatment the pustule has usually ruptured, leaving a foul-smelling, discharging ulcer with hard rolled edges on the leg, the ankle or foot. In some cases the ulcer has already started to spread and after 4–6 weeks it may be several centimetres in diameter! Two or three adjacent ulcers may join up to form a large sloughing mass that erodes tendons, ligaments and the underlying bone. Even if the bone is not directly involved, x-ray examination may show a marked periosteal reaction to the overlying infection. With time that segment of the bone may become thickened and sclerotic, or there may be erosion of the cortex. With healing, soft-tissue scarring sometimes causes joint contractures at the knee, the ankle or the foot.

Occasionally an invasive squamous cell carcinoma develops in a chronic ulcer.

Treatment

'*Prevention* is better than cure.' For people living or working in the tropics, the chance of infection can be reduced by wearing shoes and any type of covering for the legs. Scratches and abrasions should be cleaned and kept clean until they heal.

Early cases of tropical ulcer may respond to benzylpenicillin or erythromycin given daily for a week. If this is not effective, a broad-spectrum antibiotic will be needed (e.g. a third-generation cephalosporin). Ulcers should be cleansed every day and kept covered with moist or non-adherent dressings. Topical treatment with metronidazole gel is advisable.

Late cases of ulceration will require painstaking cleansing and de-sloughing together with broad-spectrum antibiotics effective against the causative anaerobic Gram-negative organisms as well as secondary infecting microbes cultured from swab samples. Soft-tissue and bone destruction may be severe enough to require extensive debridement and skin-grafting. Occasionally amputation is the best option.

TUBERCULOSIS

Once common throughout the world, tuberculosis showed a steady decline in its prevalence in developed countries during the latter half of the twentieth century, due mainly to the effectiveness of public health programmes, a general improvement in nutritional status and advances in chemotherapy. In the last two decades, however, the annual incidence (particularly of extrapulmonary tuberculosis) has risen again, a phenomenon which has been attributed variously to a general increase in the proportion of elderly people, changes in population movements, the spread of intravenous drug abuse and the emergence of AIDS.

The skeletal manifestations of the disease are seen chiefly in the spine and the large joints, but the infection may appear in any bone or any synovial or bursal sheath. Predisposing conditions include chronic debilitating disorders, diabetes, drug abuse, prolonged corticosteroid medication, AIDS and other disorders resulting in reduced defence mechanisms.

Pathology

Mycobacterium tuberculosis (usually human, sometimes bovine) enters the body via the lung (droplet infection) or the gut (swallowing infected milk products) or, rarely, through the skin. In contrast to

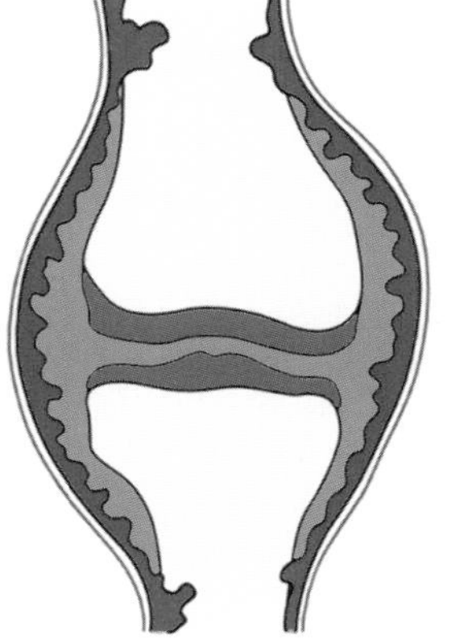
(a)

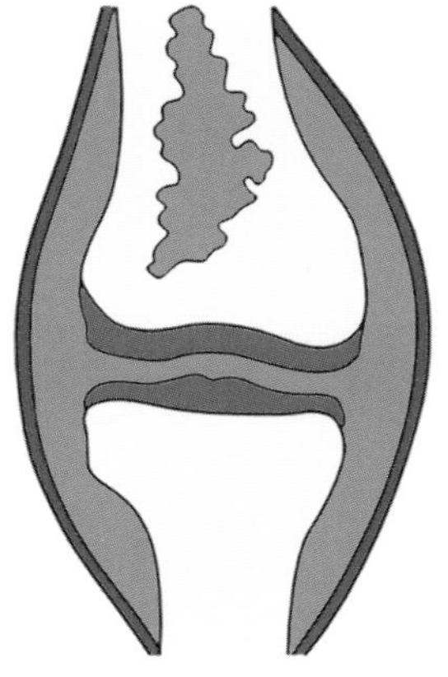
(b)

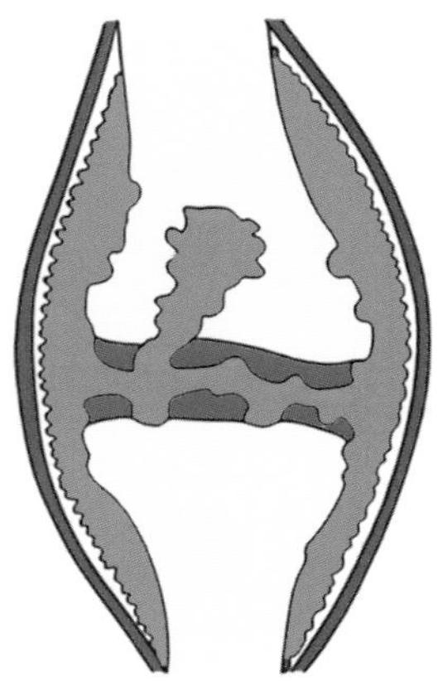
(c)

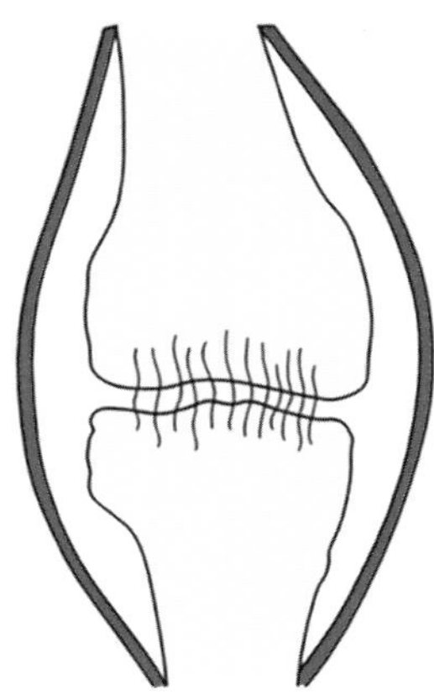
(d)

2.11 Tuberculous arthritis – pathology The disease may begin as synovitis (a) or osteomyelitis (b). From either, it can extend to become a true arthritis (c); not all the cartilage is destroyed, and healing is usually by fibrous ankylosis (d).

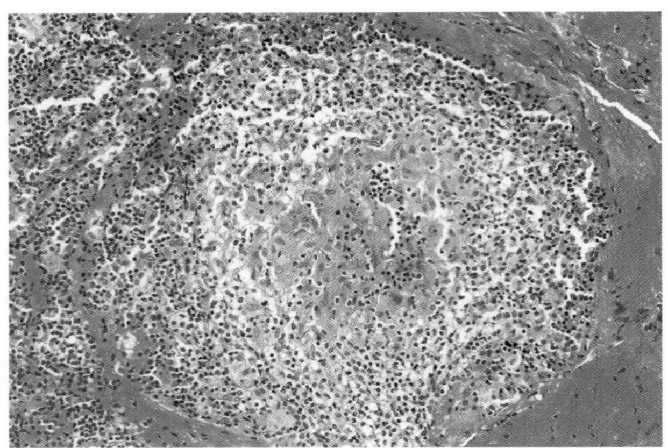

2.12 Tuberculosis – histology A typical tuberculous granuloma, with central necrosis and scattered giant cells surrounded by lymphocytes and histiocytes.

pyogenic infection, it causes a granulomatous reaction which is associated with tissue necrosis and caseation.

Primary complex The initial lesion in lung, pharynx or gut is a small one with lymphatic spread to regional lymph nodes; this combination is the primary complex. Usually the bacilli are fixed in the nodes and no clinical illness results, but occasionally the response is excessive, with enlargement of glands in the neck or abdomen.

Even though there is often no clinical illness, the initial infection has two important sequels: (1) within nodes which are apparently healed or even calcified, bacilli may survive for many years, so that a reservoir exists; (2) the body has been sensitized to the toxin (a positive Heaf test being an index of sensitization) and, should reinfection occur, the response is quite different, the lesion being a destructive one which spreads by contiguity.

Secondary spread If resistance to the original infection is low, widespread dissemination via the blood stream may occur, giving rise to miliary tuberculosis, meningitis or multiple tuberculous lesions. More often, blood spread occurs months or years later, perhaps during a period of lowered immunity, and bacilli are deposited in extrapulmonary tissues. Some of these foci develop into destructive lesions to which the term 'tertiary' may be applied.

Tertiary lesion Bones or joints are affected in about 5 per cent of patients with tuberculosis. There is a predilection for the vertebral bodies and the large synovial joints. Multiple lesions occur in about one-third of patients. In established cases it is difficult to tell whether the infection started in the joint and then spread to the adjacent bone or vice versa; synovial membrane and subchondral bone have a common blood supply and they may, of course, be infected simultaneously.

Once the bacilli have gained a foothold, they elicit a chronic inflammatory reaction. The characteristic microscopic lesion is the tuberculous granuloma (or 'tubercle') – a collection of epithelioid and multinucleated giant cells surrounding an area of necrosis, with round cells (mainly lymphocytes) around the periphery.

Within the affected area, small patches of caseous necrosis appear. These may coalesce into a larger yellowish mass, or the centre may break down to form an abscess containing pus and fragments of necrotic bone.

Bone lesions tend to spread quite rapidly. Epiphyseal cartilage is no barrier to invasion and soon the infection reaches the joint. Only in the vertebral bodies, and more rarely in the greater trochanter of the femur or the metatarsals and metacarpals, does the infection persist as a pure chronic osteomyelitis.

If the synovium is involved, it becomes thick and oedematous, giving rise to a marked effusion. A pannus of granulation tissue may extend from the synovial reflections across the joint; articular cartilage is

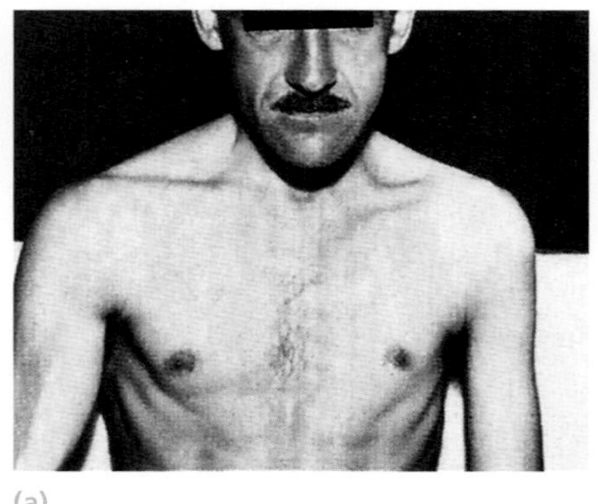

(a)

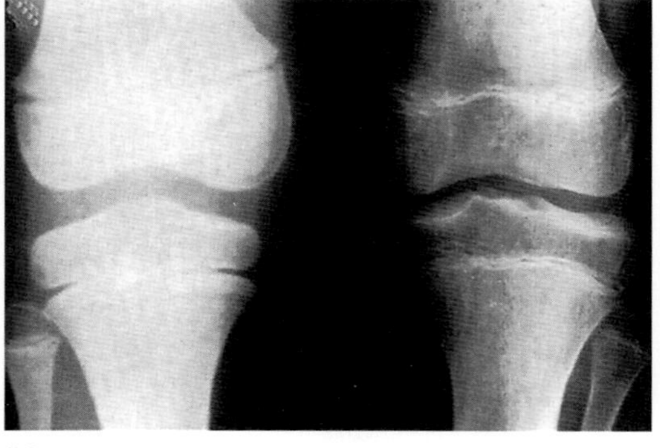

(b)

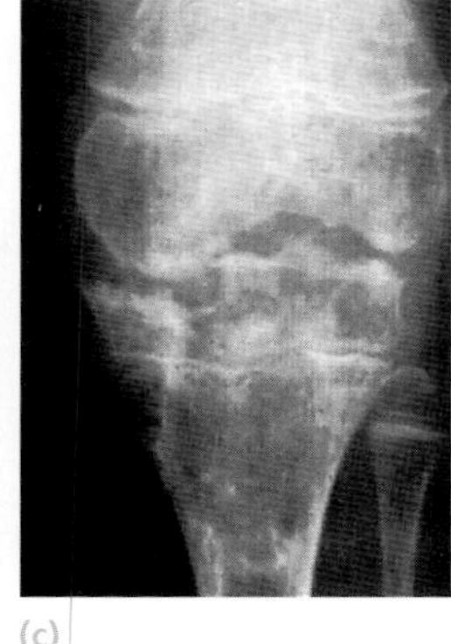

(c)

2.13 Tuberculosis – clinical and x-ray features (a) Generalized wasting used to be a common feature of all forms of tuberculosis. Nowadays, skeletal tuberculosis occurs in deceptively healthy-looking individuals. An early feature is peri-articular osteoporosis due to synovitis – the left knee in (b). This often resolves with treatment, but if cartilage and bone are destroyed (c), healing occurs by fibrosis and the joint retains a 'jog' of painful movement.

slowly destroyed, though the rapid and complete destruction elicited by pyogenic organisms does not occur in the absence of secondary infection. At the edges of the joint, along the synovial reflections, there may be active bone erosion. In addition, the increased vascularity causes local osteoporosis.

If unchecked, caseation and infection extend into the surrounding soft tissues to produce a 'cold' abscess ('cold' only in comparison to a pyogenic abscess). This may burst through the skin, forming a sinus or tuberculous ulcer, or it may track along the tissue planes to point at some distant site. Secondary infection by pyogenic organisms is common. If the disease is arrested at an early stage, healing may be by resolution to apparent normality. If articular cartilage has been severely damaged, healing is by fibrosis and incomplete ankylosis, with progressive joint deformity. Within the fibrocaseous mass, mycobacteria may remain imprisoned, retaining the potential to flare up into active disease many years later.

Clinical features

There may be a history of previous infection or recent contact with tuberculosis. The patient, usually a child or young adult, complains of pain and (in a superficial joint) swelling. In advanced cases there may be attacks of fever, night sweats, lassitude and loss of weight. Relatives tell of 'night cries': the joint, splinted by muscle spasm during the waking hours, relaxes with sleep and the inflamed or damaged tissues are stretched or compressed, causing sudden episodes of intense pain. Muscle wasting is characteristic and synovial thickening is often striking. Regional lymph nodes may be enlarged and tender. Movements are limited in all directions. As articular erosion progresses the joint becomes stiff and deformed.

In tuberculosis of the spine, pain may be deceptively slight – often no more than an ache when the spine is jarred. Consequently the patient may not present until there is a visible abscess (usually in the groin or the lumbar region to one side of the midline) or until collapse causes a localized kyphosis. Occasionally the presenting feature is weakness or instability in the lower limbs.

Multiple foci of infection are sometimes found, with bone and joint lesions at different stages of development. This is more likely in people with lowered resistance.

X-ray

Soft-tissue swelling and peri-articular osteoporosis are characteristic. The bone ends take on a 'washed-out' appearance and the articular space is narrowed. In children the epiphyses may be enlarged, probably the result of long-continued hyperaemia. Later on there is erosion of the subarticular bone; characteristically this is seen *on both sides of the joint*, indicating an inflammatory process starting in the synovium. Cystic lesions may appear in the adjacent bone ends but there is little or no periosteal reaction. In the spine the characteristic appearance is one of bone erosion and collapse around a diminished intervertebral disc space; the soft-tissue shadows may define a paravertebral abscess.

Investigations

The ESR is usually increased and there may be a relative lymphocytosis. The Mantoux or Heaf test will be positive: these are sensitive but not specific tests; i.e. a negative Mantoux virtually excludes the diagnosis, but a positive test merely indicates tuberculous infection, now or at some time in the past.

If synovial fluid is aspirated, it may be cloudy, the protein concentration is increased and the white cell count is elevated.

Acid-fast bacilli are identified in synovial fluid in 10–20 per cent of cases, and cultures are positive in over half. A synovial biopsy is more reliable: sections will show the characteristic histological features and acid-fast bacilli may be identified; cultures are positive in about 80 per cent of patients who have not received antimicrobial treatment.

Diagnosis

Except in areas where tuberculosis is common, diagnosis is often delayed simply because the disease is not suspected. Features that should trigger more active investigation are:

- a long history of pain or swelling
- involvement of only one joint
- marked synovial thickening
- severe muscle wasting
- enlarged and matted regional lymph nodes
- periarticular osteoporosis on x-ray
- a positive Mantoux test.

Synovial biopsy for histological examination and culture is often necessary. Joint tuberculosis must be differentiated from the following.

Transient synovitis This is fairly common in children. At first it seems no different from any other low-grade inflammatory arthritis; however, it always settles down after a few weeks' rest in bed. If the synovitis recurs, further investigation (even a biopsy) may be necessary.

Monarticular rheumatoid arthritis Occasionally rheumatoid arthritis starts in a single large joint. This is clinically indistinguishable from tuberculosis and the diagnosis may have to await the results of synovial biopsy.

Subacute arthritis Diseases such as amoebic dysentery or brucellosis are sometimes complicated by arthritis. The history, clinical features and pathological investigations usually enable a diagnosis to be made.

Haemorrhagic arthritis The physical signs of blood in a joint may resemble those of tuberculous arthritis. If the bleeding has followed a single recent injury, the history and absence of marked wasting are diagnostic. Following repeated bleeding, as in haemophilia, the clinical resemblance to tuberculosis is closer, but there is also a history of bleeding elsewhere.

Pyogenic arthritis In longstanding cases it may be difficult to exclude an old septic arthritis.

Treatment

REST

Hugh Owen Thomas long ago urged that tuberculosis should be treated by rest – which had to be 'prolonged, uninterrupted, rigid and enforced'. This often involved splintage of the joint and traction to overcome muscle spasm and prevent collapse of the articular surfaces. With modern chemotherapy this is no longer mandatory; rest and splintage are varied according to the needs of the individual patient. Those who are diagnosed and treated early are kept in bed only until pain and systemic symptoms subside, and thereafter are allowed restricted activity until the joint changes resolve (usually 6 months to a year). Those with progressive joint destruction may need a longer period of rest and splintage to prevent ankylosis in a bad position; however, as soon as symptoms permit, movements are again encouraged.

CHEMOTHERAPY

The most effective treatment is a combination of antituberculous drugs, which should always include rifampicin and isoniazid. During the last decade the incidence of drug resistance has increased and this has led to the addition of various 'potentiating' drugs to the list. The following is one of several recommended regimens.

Initial, *'intensive phase treatment'*, consists of isoniazid 300–400 mg, rifampicin 450–600 mg and fluoroquinolones 400–600 mg daily for 5 or 6 months. All replicating sensitive bacteria are likely to be killed by this bactericidal attack. This is followed by a *'continuation phase treatment'* lasting 9 months, the purpose of which is to eliminate the 'persisters', slow-growing, intermittently-growing, dormant or intracellular mycobacteria. This involves the use of isoniazid and pyrazinamide 1500 mg per day for 4½ months and isoniazid and rifampicin for another 4½ months. Then a *'prophylactic phase'*, consisting of isoniazid and ethambutol 1200 mg per day for a further 3 or 4 months.

During the entire treatment period drugs and dosage may have to be adjusted and modified, depending on the individual patient's age, size, general health and drug reactions.

OPERATION

Operative drainage or clearance of a tuberculous focus is seldom necessary nowadays. However, a cold abscess may need immediate aspiration or draining.

Once the condition is controlled and arthritis has completely subsided, normal activity can be resumed, though the patient must report any renewed symptoms. If, however, the joint is painful and the articular surface is destroyed, arthrodesis or replacement arthroplasty may be considered. The longer the period of quiescence, the less the risk of reactivation of the disease; there is always some risk and it is essential to give chemotherapy for 3 months before and after the operation.

BRUCELLOSIS

Brucellosis is an unusual but nonetheless important cause of subacute or chronic granulomatous infection in bones and joints. Three species of organism are seen in humans: *Brucella melitensis, B. abortus* (from cattle) and *B. suis* (from pigs). Infection usually occurs from drinking unpasteurized milk or from coming into contact with infected meat (e.g. among farmers and meat packers). In the past it has been more common in countries around the Mediterranean and in certain parts of Africa and India. About 50 per cent of patients with chronic brucellosis develop arthritis.

Pathology

The organism enters the body with infected milk products or, occasionally, directly through the skin or mucosal surfaces. It is taken up by the lymphatics and then carried by the blood stream to distant sites. Foci of infection may occur in bones (usually the vertebral bodies) or in the synovium of the larger joints. The characteristic lesion is a chronic inflammatory granuloma with round-cell infiltration and giant cells. There may be central necrosis and caseation leading to abscess formation and invasion of the surrounding tissues.

Clinical features

The patient usually presents with fever, headache and generalized weakness, followed by joint pains and backache. The initial illness may be acute and alarming; more often it begins insidiously and progresses until the symptoms localize in a single large joint (usually the hip or knee) or in the spine. The joint becomes painful, swollen and tender; movements are restricted in all directions. If the spine is affected, there is usually local tenderness and back movements are restricted.

The systemic illness follows a fluctuating course, with alternating periods of fever and apparent improvement (hence the older term 'undulant fever'). Diagnosis is often long delayed and may not be resolved until destructive changes are advanced.

X-rays

The picture is that of a subacute arthritis, with loss of articular space, slowly progressive bone erosion and peri-articular osteoporosis. In the spine there may be destruction and collapse of adjacent vertebral bodies with obliteration of the disc.

Investigations

A positive agglutination test (titre above 1/80) is diagnostic. Joint aspiration or biopsy may allow the organism to be cultured and identified.

Diagnosis

Diagnosis is usually delayed while other types of subacute arthritis are excluded.

Tuberculosis and brucellosis have similar clinical and radiological features. The distinction is often difficult and may have to await the results of agglutination tests, synovial biopsy and bacteriological investigation.

Reiter's disease and other forms of reactive arthritis often follow an initial systemic illness. However, fever is not so marked and joint erosion is usually late and mild.

Treatment

Antibiotics The infection usually responds to a combined onslaught with tetracycline and streptomycin for 3–4 weeks. Alternative drugs, which are equally effective and which may be used as 'combination therapy', are rifampicin and the newer cephalosporins.

Operation An abscess will need drainage, and necrotic bone and cartilage should be meticulously excised. If the joint is destroyed, arthrodesis or arthroplasty may be necessary once the infection is completely controlled.

LEPROSY

Leprosy is a mildly infectious chronic inflammatory disease caused by acid-fast *Mycobacterium leprae*. It is characterized by granulomatous lesions in the peripheral nerves, the skin and the mucosa of the upper respiratory tract.

Leprosy was once common throughout the world. Today it is rarely seen outside parts of South Asia, Africa, Latin America and some of the Pacific Islands. While the disease is easily cured with drugs, its crippling effects persist in a cumulative number of people.

The infection is acquired mainly by respiratory transmission; unbroken skin to skin contact is thought not to be dangerous. Several years may elapse before clinical features appear.

Pathology

Most people infected with *M. leprae* develop protective immunity and get rid of the infection. Some develop a few skin lesions, appearing as vague hypopigmented macules (*indeterminate leprosy*), that recover spontaneously. If the condition progresses, it takes one of several forms, depending on the host's immune response.

Tuberculoid leprosy occurs where there is delayed type hypersensitivity (DTH) to *M. leprae* antigens, combined with some decrease in cell-mediated immunity (CMI). The granuloma in tuberculoid leprosy is focal and circumscribed and is made up of epithelioid cells, with a few scattered giant cells and a cuff of lymphocytes, very similar to tuberculosis.

Lepromatous leprosy is seen in patients who are unable to mount effective CMI against *M. leprae*. Here the granuloma is diffuse and extensive and it consists of macrophages, many loaded with acid-fast bacilli. There may be a sprinkling of round cells in the lepromatous granuloma. The entire body skin may thus be affected.

Borderline types are intermediate forms that show some features of both of the above conditions. Without treatment, they tend to progress increasingly towards the lepromatous form.

Peripheral nerves are always affected in leprosy. Dermal nerve twigs, cutaneous nerves as well as major nerve trunks may thus be involved. The affected nerves become thickened. Besides the granuloma there is hypertrophy of the epineurium and perineurium, demyelination, axonal degeneration and endoneurial fibrosis. A thickened nerve trunk may be strangulated by its own sheath or by the rigid walls of a fibro-osseous tunnel through which it passes (e.g. the ulnar nerve at the elbow). Sometimes, a tuberculoid granuloma in a nerve undergoes caseation. An important factor contributing to nerve damage is that medication is less likely to reach the segment of the nerve thus rendered ischaemic.

The chronic course of leprosy is often punctuated by acute inflammatory episodes – so-called *'reactions'* – which are due to the deposition of immune complexes (erythema nodosum leprosum or ENL or Type

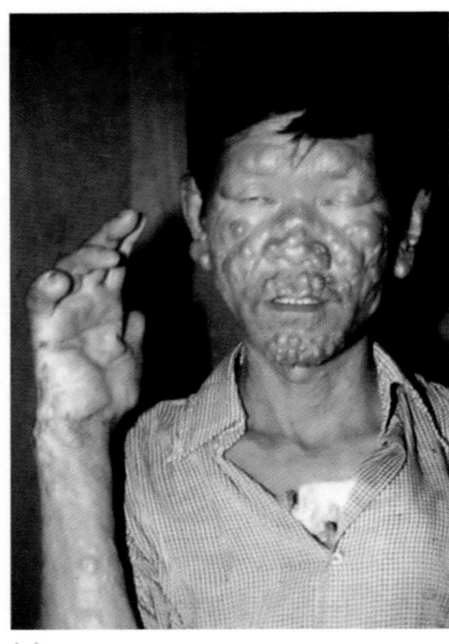

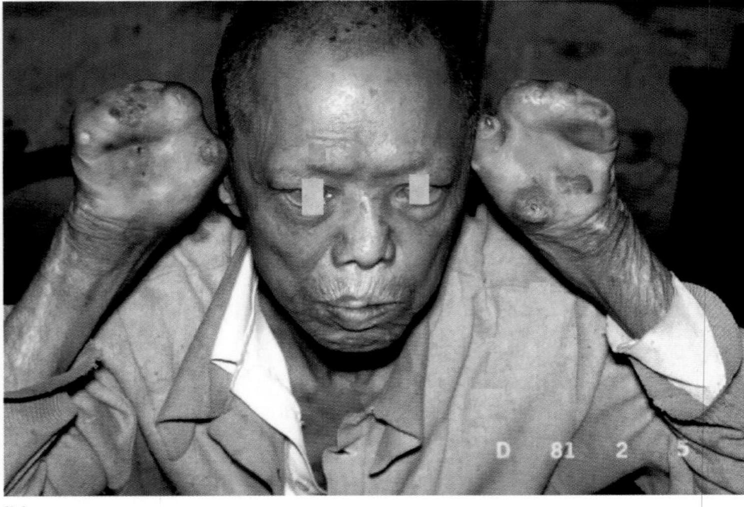

(a) (b)

2.14 Leprosy – late features (a) Patient showing typical ulnar claw-hand deformity. (b) This patient was even worse off, having lost all the fingers of both hands.

II reaction) or due to an increase in CMI and DTH levels (reversal reaction or RR or Type I reaction). Reactions occurring in the nerves (acute neuritis) greatly increase the risk of nerve damage.

Clinical features

Hypopigmented skin patches with impaired sensibility develop in all types of leprosy. Thickened cutaneous nerves may be seen and thickened nerve trunks may be felt where they are superficial, especially where they cross a bone (typically behind the medial condyle of the humerus at the elbow). Irrecoverable nerve damage with characteristic patterns of muscle weakness and deformities of the hands and feet may also be seen. Trophic ulcers, causing progressive destruction of the affected part, appear in the hands and feet.

Skin lesions in *tuberculoid leprosy* are sparse, well-demarcated, hypopigmented and anaesthetic. In contrast, in *lepromatous leprosy*, the skin is affected diffusely and extensively and the lesions present as multiple, symmetrically distributed macular patches with some sensory impairment. Plaques and nodules develop in advanced stages. Coarsening of the facial skin and loss of eyebrows may produce typical leonine features. Lepromatous ulceration of the nasal mucosa leads to destruction of the nasal septum and nasal deformity.

Peripheral nerves are affected extensively in *lepromatous leprosy* whereas in *tuberculoid leprosy* the neural lesions are few and focal in distribution. Cutaneous nerves as well as major nerve trunks of the upper and lower limbs are usually involved. Except for the Vth and VIIth nerves, the cranial nerves are not affected. Clinical defects in nerve function appear early in *tuberculoid leprosy* but much later in *lepromatous leprosy*.

Nerve lesions in tuberculoid leprosy may undergo caseation and liquefaction resulting in an intraneural 'cold abscess' mimicking an intraneural tumour, or the pus may break through the epineurium to present as a chronic collar-stud abscess.

Diagnosis

In countries where the disease is common the clinical diagnosis is seldom in doubt. Suggestive signs are the appearance of skin lesions with loss of sensibility, palpably or even visibly thickened nerves which may also be tender, areas of anaesthesia, chronic ulcers of the feet and typical deformities of hands and feet due to muscle weakness and imbalance. In countries where the disease is not endemic, diagnosis may have to await the results of skin smear examination, serological tests and skin or nerve biopsy.

Patterns of nerve involvement

Nerve trunks of the upper limbs are involved more often than those of the lower limbs. There is a pattern in the selection, site of involvement, risk of damage and chances of recovery (see Table 2.3). In the upper limb ulnar nerve paralysis is the most common and combined ulnar and median nerve paralysis is seen less frequently. Occasionally, triple nerve paralysis (paralysis of ulnar, median and radial nerves) may occur. Any other pattern is extremely rare.

Treatment

For purposes of treatment, patients are categorized as having *paucibacillary* (cases of indeterminate and

Table 2.3 Features of nerve trunk involvement in leprosy

Nerve affected	Preferred site	Involvement[a]	Motor paralysis	Recovery
Ulnar[c]	Above elbow/wrist	++++	++++	+
Median	Above wrist	++	++	++
Common peroneal	Back of knee	+++	+	++
Tibial	Behind ankle	+++	+++	b
Radial	Cutaneous division	+++	NA	NA
	Radial groove	++	(forearm muscles only)	+++

[a] Thickening; [b] tenderness/pain; [c] most commonly involved nerve trunk; + uncommon; ++ common; +++ quite common; ++++ very common; NA, not applicable.

tuberculoid leprosy) or *multibacillary* (cases of lepromatous and borderline leprosy) leprosy.

MULTIDRUG THERAPY

Combined chemotherapy with rifampicin as one of the drugs is the mainstay of treatment; however, the choice of drugs and duration of treatment depend on the type of disease. Following the recommendations of the World Health Organization, patients with *paucibacillary disease* are treated with rifampicin 600 mg once monthly and dapsone 100 mg once daily, for 6 months; and patients with *multibacillary disease* are given rifampicin 600 mg and clofazimine 300 mg once monthly and dapsone 100 mg and clofazimine 50 mg once daily, for 12 months. Reactions, especially acute neuritis, are treated with anti-inflammatory medication, of which prednisolone is the most important, and other supportive therapy.

NERVE DECOMPRESSION

Surgical decompression of a nerve trunk is sometimes required in order to improve perfusion of the nerve and allow the anti-leprosy and anti-inflammatory drugs to reach the affected segment and thus prevent or abort nerve damage. Surgical decompression is indicated: (a) in acute neuritis when, even while under treatment with corticosteroids, there is increasing neurological deficit; and (b) in cases of severe, unresponsive nerve pain, for relief of pain. Decompression involves tunnel release (often with excision of the medial epicondyle for the ulnar nerve) combined with incision of the epineurium over the entire sclerosed segment of the nerve. *Stripping the epineurium should not be done.*

TREATMENT OF NERVE ABSCESS

Cold abscesses associated with deteriorating neurological function and those that are likely to burst through the skin need to be excised or surgically evacuated. If there is no associated neural deficit it is not necessary to intervene immediately, provided the patient can be reviewed periodically.

MANAGEMENT OF RESIDUAL PARALYSIS AND TROPHIC LESIONS

The long-term neuropathic complications of leprosy are dealt with in Chapter 11. The notorious deformities and disablement result from: (a) *local leprous granulomas* (as in the face); (b) *damage to nerves* of the hands and feet and consequent muscle paralysis; and (c) so-called '*trophic lesions*' (ulcers, shortening of digits and mutilations) arising from injuries to insensitive hands and feet. These conditions are prevented by early treatment of the disease, adequate treatment of neuritis and protection of anaesthetic hands and feet.

Paresis and established deformities can usually be corrected or at least improved by surgery (see Chapter 11). Although this is done mainly to improve function, restoration of normal appearance is also important for leprosy patients. Deformities such as claw-fingers and drop-foot stigmatize affected individuals as 'leprosy patients', with dire social consequences.

Those requiring surgery should have had anti-leprosy treatment and should not have had acute neuritis of any nerve trunk for at least 6 months prior to surgery. They must be well motivated and there should be proper pre-operative preparation with appropriate physiotherapy. Absence of facilities for pre- and post-operative therapy is an absolute contraindication for corrective surgery.

MYCOTIC INFECTIONS

Mycotic or fungal infection causes an indolent granulomatous reaction, often leading to abscess formation, tissue destruction and ulceration. When the musculoskeletal system is involved, it is usually by direct spread from the adjacent soft tissues. Occasionally, however, a bone or joint may be infected by haematogenous spread from a distant site.

These disorders are conveniently divided into 'superficial' and 'deep' infections.

Superficial mycoses These are primarily infections of the skin or mucous surfaces which spread into the adjacent soft tissues and bone. The more common examples are the *maduromycoses* (a group consisting of several species), *Sporothrix* and various species of *Candida*.

The *actinomycoses* are usually included with the superficial fungal infections. The causal organisms, of which *Actinomyces israelii* is the commonest in humans, are not really fungi but anaerobic bacilli with fungus-like appearance and behaviour.

Deep mycoses This group comprises infections by *Blastomyces, Histoplasma, Coccidioides, Cryptococcus, Aspergillus* and other rare fungi. The organisms, which occur in rotting vegetation and bird droppings, gain entry through the lungs and, in humans, may cause an influenza-like illness. Bone or joint infection is uncommon except in patients with compromised host defences.

Maduromycosis

This chronic fungal infection is seen mainly in northern Africa and the Indian subcontinent. The organisms usually enter through a cut in the foot; from there they spread through the subcutaneous tissues and along the tendon sheaths. The bones and joints are infected by direct invasion; local abscesses form and break through the skin as multiple sinuses. The patient may present at an early stage with a tender subcutaneous nodule (when the diagnosis is seldom entertained); more often he or she is seen when the foot is swollen and indurated, with discharging sinuses and ulcers. X-rays may show multiple bone cavities or progressive bone destruction. The organism can be identified in the sinus discharge or in tissue biopsies.

Treatment is unsatisfactory as there is no really effective chemotherapy. Intravenous amphotericin B is advocated, but it is fairly toxic and causes side effects such as headaches, vomiting and fever. Necrotic tissue should be widely excised. Even then it is sometimes difficult to stop further invasion, and amputation is sometimes necessary.

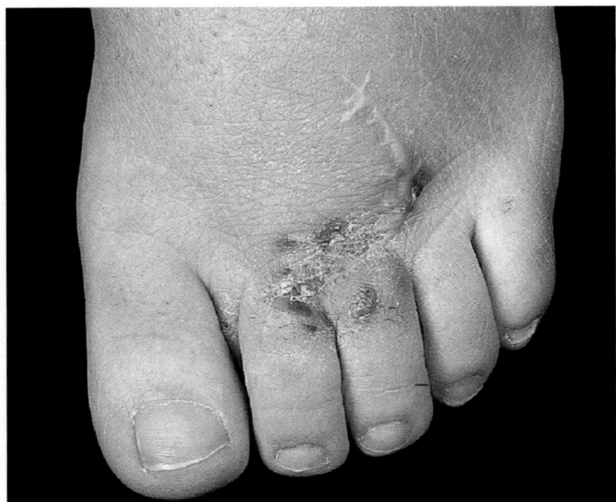

2.15 Maduromycosis This Mediterranean market-worker was perpetually troubled by tiny abscesses and weeping sinuses in her foot. X-rays showed that bone destruction had already spread to the tarsal bones, and after 2 years of futile treatment the foot had to be amputated.

Candidiasis

Candida albicans is a normal commensal in humans and it often causes superficial infection of the skin or mucous membranes. Deep and systemic infections are rare except under conditions of immunosuppression.

Candida osteomyelitis and arthritis may follow direct contamination during surgery or other invasive procedures such as joint aspiration or arthroscopy. The diagnosis is usually made only after tissue sampling and culture.

Treatment consists of thorough joint irrigation and curettage of discrete bone lesions, together with intravenous amphotericin B.

Actinomycosis

Infection is usually by *Actinomyces israelii*, an anaerobic Gram-positive bacillus. Although rare, it is important that it should be diagnosed because the organism is sensitive to antibiotics.

The most common site of infection is the mandible (from the mouth and pharynx), but bone lesions are also seen in the vertebrae (spreading from the lung or gut) and the pelvis (spreading from the caecum or colon). Peripheral lesions may occur by direct infection of the soft tissues and later extension to the bones. There may be a firm, tender swelling in the soft tissues, going on to form an abscess and one or more chronic discharging sinuses. X-rays may show cyst-like areas of bone destruction. The organism can be readily identified in the sinus discharge, but only on anaerobic culture.

Treatment, by large doses of benzylpenicillin G, tetracycline or erythromycin, has to be continued for several months.

The deep mycoses

Histoplasmosis, blastomycosis and coccidioidomycosis are rare causes of bone and joint infection, but they should always be considered in patients on immunosuppressive therapy who develop arthritis of one of the large joints or osteomyelitis in an unusual site. Diagnosis is usually delayed and often involves specialized microbiological investigations to identify the organism.

Treatment with intravenous amphotericin B is moderately effective. Operation may be necessary to drain an abscess or to remove necrotic tissue.

HYDATID DISEASE

Hydatid disease is caused by the tapeworm *Echinococcus*. Parasitic infestation is common among sheep farmers, but bone lesions are rare.

The organism, a cestode worm, has a complicated life-cycle. The definitive host is the dog or some other carnivore that carries the tapeworm in its bowel. Segments of worm and ova pass out in the faeces and are later ingested by one of the intermediate hosts – usually sheep or cattle or man. Here the larvae are carried via the portal circulation to the liver, and occasionally beyond to other organs, where they produce cysts containing numerous scolices. Infested meat is then eaten by dogs (or humans), giving rise to a new generation of tapeworm.

Scolices carried in the blood stream occasionally settle in bone and produce hydatid cysts that slowly enlarge with little respect for cortical or epiphyseal boundaries. The bones most commonly affected are the vertebrae, pelvis, femur, scapula and ribs.

Clinical features

The patient may complain of pain and swelling, or may present for the first time with a pathological fracture or compression of the spinal cord. Infestation sometimes starts in childhood but the cysts take so long to enlarge that clinical symptoms and signs may not become apparent for many years. The diagnosis is more likely if the patient comes from a sheep-farming district.

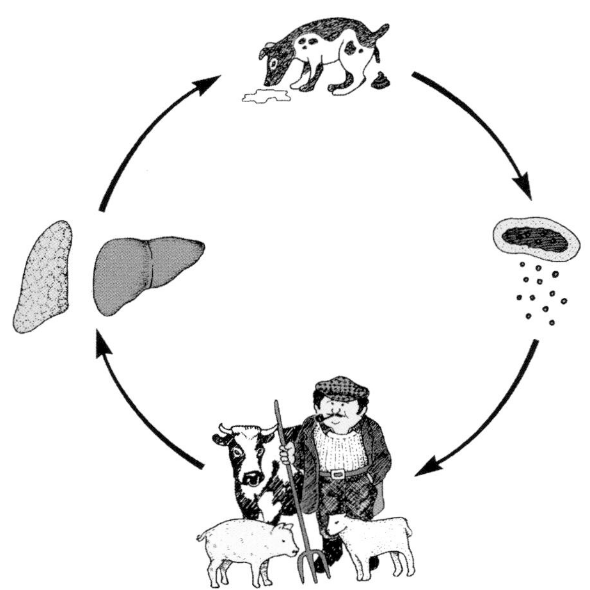

2.16 Hydatid disease The life-cycle of the tapeworm which causes hydatid disease.

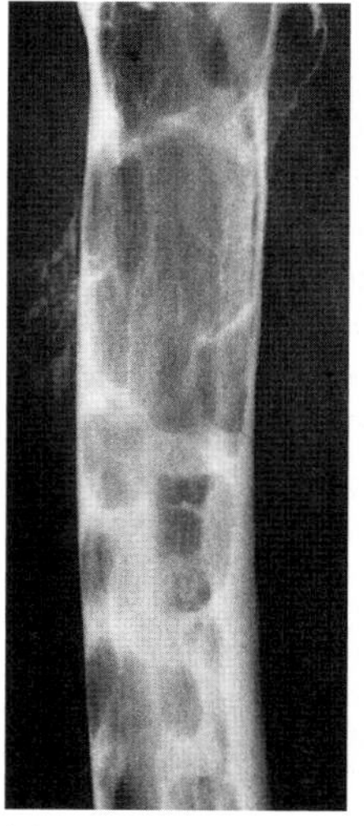

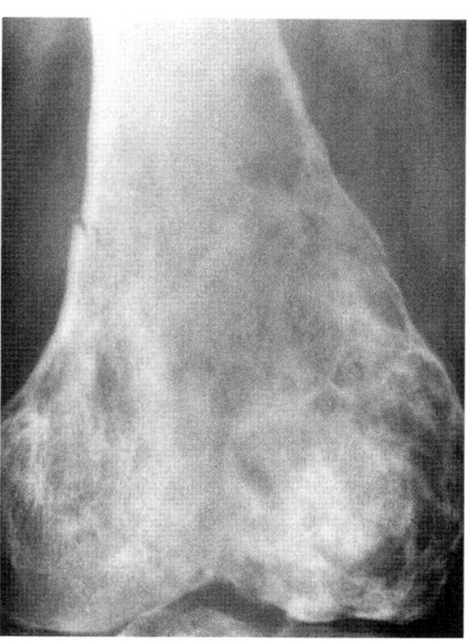

(a) (b)

2.17 Hydatid disease of bone Two examples of hydatid involvement of bone: there is no expansion of the cortex in (a) and very little in (b).

Imaging

X-rays show solitary or multiloculated bone cysts, but only moderate expansion of the cortices. However, cortical thinning may lead to a pathological fracture. In the spine, hydatid disease may involve adjacent vertebrae, with large cysts extending into the paravertebral soft tissues. These features are best seen on *CT* and *MRI*, which should always be performed if operative excision of the lesion is contemplated.

Investigations

Casoni's (complement fixation) test may be positive, especially in longstanding cases.

Diagnosis

Hydatid disease must be included in the differential diagnosis of benign and malignant bone cysts and cyst-like tumours. If the clinical and radiological features are not conclusive, needle biopsy should be considered, though there is a risk of spreading the disease.

Treatment

The anthelminthic drug albendazole is moderately effective in destroying the parasite. It has to be given in repeated courses: a recommended programme is oral administration of 10 mg per kg per day for 3 weeks, repeated at least 4 times with a one-week 'rest' between courses. Liver, renal and bone marrow function should be monitored during treatment.

However, the bone cysts do not heal and recurrence is common. The indications for surgery are continuing enlargement or spread of the lesion, a risk of fracture, invasion of soft tissues and pressure on important structures. Curettage and bone grafting will lessen the risk of pathological fracture; at operation the cavity can be 'sterilized' with copious amounts of hypertonic saline, alcohol or formalin to lessen the risk of recurrence.

Radical resection, with the margin at least 2 cm beyond the cyst, is more certain, but also much more challenging. In a long bone the space can sometimes be filled with a tumour-prosthesis, to include an arthroplasty if necessary. Large cysts of the vertebral column, or the pelvis and hip joint, are particularly difficult to manage in this way and in some cases surgical excision is simply impractical or impossible.

REFERENCES AND FURTHER READING

Blyth MJG, Kinkaid R, Craigen MAC, Bennet GC. The changing epidemiology of acute and subacute haematogenous osteomyelitis in children. *J Bone Joint Surg* 2001; **83B:** 99–102.

Björkstén B & Boquist L. Histopathological aspects of chronic recurrent multifocal osteomyelitis. *J Bone Joint Surg* 1980; **62B:** 276–380.

Boutin RD & Resnick D. The SAPHO syndrome: an evolving concept for unifying several idiopathic disorders of bone and skin. *Am J Roentgenol* 1998; **170:** 585–91.

Carr AJ, Cole WG, Robertson DM, Chow CW. Chronic multifocal osteomyelitis. *J Bone Joint Surg* 1993; **75B:** 582–91.

Chung SMK. The articular supply of the developing proximal end of the human femur. *J Bone Joint Surg* 1976; **58A:** 961–70,

Cierny G 3rd, Mader JT, Penninck JJ. A clinical staging system for adult osteomyelitis. *Clin Orthop Relat Res* 2003; **414:** 7–24.

Ebong WW. Acute osteomyelitis in Nigerians with sickle-cell disease. *Ann Rheum Dis* 1986; **45:** 911–5.

Ellington JK, Harris M, Webb L, *et al.* Intracellular Staphylococcus aureus. A mechanism for the indolence of osteomyelitis. *J Bone Joint Surg* 2003; **85B:** 918–21.

Gristina AG. Biomaterial-centred infection: microbial adhesion versus tissue integration. *Science* 1988; **237:** 437–51

Hashmi MA, Norman P, Saleh M. The management of chronic osteomyelitis using the Lautenbach method. *J Bone Joint Surg* 2004; **86B:** 269–75.

Lidwell OM. Clean air at operation and subsequent sepsis in the joint. *Clin Orthop Relat Res* 1986; **211:** 91–102.

Perez-Stable EJ & Hopewell PC. Current tuberculosis treatment regimens: choosing the right one for your patient. *Clin Chest Med*, 1989; **10:** 323–39.

Rasool MN & Govender S. The skeletal manifestations of congenital syphilis. *J Bone Joint Surg* 1989; **71B:** 752–5.

Roberts JM, Drummond DS, Breed AL, *et al.* Subacute haematogenous osteomyelitis in children: a retrospective study. *J Paediatr Orthop* 1982; **2:** 249–54.

Song Kit M, Sloboda John F. Acute hematogenous osteomyelitis in children. *J Am Acad Orthop Surg* 2001; **9:** 166–75.

Trueta J. The normal vascular anatomy of the human femoral head during growth. *J Bone Joint Surg* 1957; **39B:** 358–94.

Trueta J. Three types of acute haematogenous osteomyelitis. *J Bone Joint Surg* 1959; **41B:** 671–80.

Unkila-Kallis L, Kallis MJT, Peltola H. The usefulness of C-reactive protein levels in the identification of concurrent septic arthritis in children who have acute haematogenous osteomyelitis. *J Bone Joint Surg*, 1994; **76A:** 848–53.

Whalen JL, Fitzgeral RH Jr, Morrissy RT. A histological study of acute haematogenous osteomyelitis following physeal injuries in rabbits. *J Bone Joint Surg* 1988; **70A:** 1383–92.

Inflammatory rheumatic disorders

3

Christopher Edwards, Louis Solomon

The term 'inflammatory rheumatic disorders' covers a number of diseases that cause chronic pain, stiffness and swelling around joints and tendons. In addition, they are commonly associated with extra-articular features including skin rashes and inflammatory eye disease. Individuals with these diseases tend to die younger than their peers as a result of the effects of chronic inflammation. Many – perhaps all – are due to a faulty immune reaction resulting from a combination of environmental exposures against a background of genetic predisposition.

RHEUMATOID ARTHRITIS

Rheumatoid arthritis (RA) is the most common cause of chronic inflammatory joint disease. The most typical features are a symmetrical polyarthritis and tenosynovitis, morning stiffness, elevation of the erythrocyte sedimentation rate (ESR) and the appearance of autoantibodies that target immunoglobulins (*rheumatoid factors*) in the serum. Rheumatoid arthritis is a systemic disease and changes can be widespread in a number of tissues of the body. Individuals with RA tend to die younger than their peers as a result of the effects of chronic inflammation on a number of organ systems. Chief among these is early ischaemic heart disease secondary to the effects of inflammation on the cardiovascular system.

The reported prevalence of RA in most populations is 1–3 per cent, with a peak incidence in the fourth or fifth decades. Women are affected 3 or 4 times more commonly than men. Both the prevalence and the clinical expression vary between populations; the disease is more common (and generally more severe) in Caucasians living in the urban communities of Europe and North America than in the rural populations of Africa.

Cause

The cause of RA is still incompletely worked out. However, a great deal is now known about the circumstances in which RA develops, and hypotheses about its aetiology and pathogenesis have been suggested. Important factors in the evolution of RA are: (1) genetic susceptibility; (2) an immunological reaction, possibly involving a foreign antigen, preferentially focussed on synovial tissue; (3) an inflammatory reaction in joints and tendon sheaths; (4) the appearance of rheumatoid factors (RF) in the blood and synovium; (5) perpetuation of the inflammatory process; and (6) articular cartilage destruction.

Genetic susceptibility A genetic association is suggested by the fact that RA is more common in first-degree relatives of patients than in the population at large; furthermore twin studies have revealed a concordance rate of around 30 per cent if one of the pair is affected. The human leucocyte antigen (HLA) DR4 occurs in about 70 per cent of people with RA, compared to a frequency of less than 30 per cent in normal controls. HLA-DR4 is encoded in the major histocompatibility complex (MHC) region on chromosome 6. There are strong associations between HLA-DR4 and RA. In particular a key structural conformation within the HLA-DR4 binding groove called the 'shared epitope' seems important. This may suggest that a particular antigen that fits into this may be playing a part.

HLA Class II molecules appear as surface antigens on cells of the immune system (B lymphocytes, macrophages, dendritic cells), which can act as antigen-presenting cells (APCs). In some T-cell immune reactions, the process is initiated only when the antigenic peptide is presented in association with a specific HLA allele. It has been suggested that this is the case in people who develop RA; the idea is even more attractive if one proposes that the putative antigen has a special affinity for synovial tissue. So far no such antigen has been discovered.

The inflammatory reaction Once the APC/T-cell interaction is initiated, various local factors come into play and lead to a progressive enhancement of the immune response. There is a marked proliferation of cells in the synovium, with the appearance of new blood vessel formation. Immune cells coordinate their action by the use of 'short-range hormones' (cytokines), which can activate inflammatory cells such as macrophages and B cells. Some cytokines called chemokines attract other inflammatory cells to the area.

Over recent years it has become clear that certain cytokines are important in RA. These include tumour necrosis factor (TNF), interleukin-1 (IL-1) and interleukin-6 (IL-6). The resulting synovitis, both in joints and in tendon sheath linings, is the hallmark of early RA.

Rheumatoid factor B-cell activation in RA leads to the production of anti-IgG autoantibodies, which are detected in the blood as 'rheumatoid factor' (RF). Low levels of RF can be found in many 'normal' individuals but when the levels are high an inflammatory disease is likely. Other autoimmune conditions such as systemic lupus erythematosus (SLE) and Sjögren's syndrome are also associated with the presence of RF.

In recent years other autoantibodies associated with RA have been identified. The most important are anti-cyclic citrullinated peptide antibodies (anti-CCP). The presence of anti-CCP is very specific for RA. Patients with a positive RF test tend to be more severely affected than those with a negative test.

Chronic synovitis and joint destruction Chronic rheumatoid synovitis is associated with the production of proteolytic enzymes, prostaglandins and the cytokines TNF and IL-1. Immune complexes are deposited in the synovium and on the articular cartilage, where they appear to augment the inflammatory process. This combination of factors leads to depletion of the cartilage matrix and, eventually, damage to cartilage and underlying bone. Vascular proliferation and osteoclastic activity, most marked at the edges of the articular surface, may contribute further to cartilage destruction and peri-articular bone erosion.

Pathology

Rheumatoid arthritis is a systemic disease but the most characteristic lesions are seen in the synovium or within rheumatoid nodules. The synovium is engorged with new blood vessels and packed full of inflammatory cells.

JOINTS AND TENDONS

The pathological changes, if unchecked, proceed in four stages. Previously it was felt that having gone through these stages the disease activity could be 'burnt out'. This does not appear to be the case. In any one joint features of different stages can be occurring simultaneously and even when joints are very badly destroyed the ongoing inflammation can continue to seriously damage systemic health by accelerating other disease processes such as ischaemic heart disease.

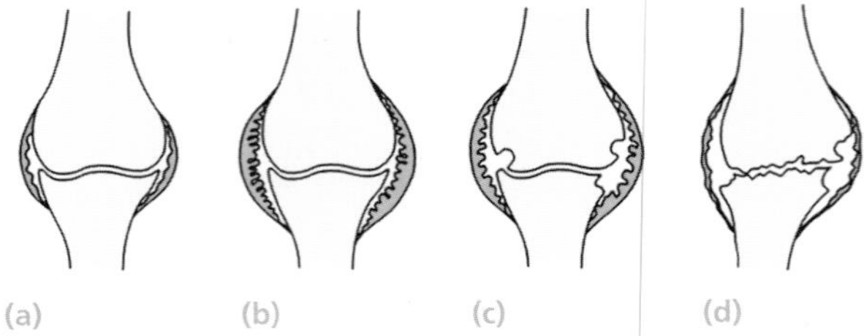

3.1 Rheumatoid arthritis – pathology (a) Stage 1 – pre-clinical. (b) Stage 2 – synovitis and joint swelling. (c) Stage 3 – early joint destruction with peri-articular erosions. (d) Stage 4 – advanced joint destruction and deformity.

Stage 1 – pre-clinical Well before RA becomes clinically apparent the immune pathology is already beginning. Raised ESR, C-reactive protein (CRP) and RF may be detectable years before the first diagnosis.

Stage 2 – synovitis Early changes are vascular congestion with new blood vessel formation, proliferation of synoviocytes and infiltration of the subsynovial layers by polymorphs, lymphocytes and plasma cells. There is thickening of the capsular structures, villous formation of the synovium and a cell-rich effusion into the joints and tendon sheaths. Although painful, swollen and tender, these structures are still intact and mobile, and the disorder is potentially reversible.

Stage 3 – destruction Persistent inflammation causes joint and tendon destruction. Articular cartilage is eroded, partly by proteolytic enzymes, partly by vascular tissue in the folds of the synovial reflections, and partly due to direct invasion of the cartilage by a pannus of granulation tissue creeping over the articular surface. At the margins of the joint, bone is eroded by granulation tissue invasion and osteoclastic resorption.

Similar changes occur in tendon sheaths, causing tenosynovitis, invasion of the collagen bundles and, eventually, partial or complete rupture of tendons.

A synovial effusion, often containing copious amounts of fibrinoid material, produces swelling of the joints, tendons and bursae.

Stage 4 – deformity The combination of articular destruction, capsular stretching and tendon rupture leads to progressive instability and deformity of the joints. The inflammatory process usually continues but the mechanical and functional effects of joint and tendon disruption now become vital.

EXTRA-ARTICULAR TISSUES

Rheumatoid nodules The rheumatoid nodule is a small granulomatous lesion consisting of a central necrotic zone surrounded by a radially disposed palisade of local histiocytes, and beyond that by inflammatory

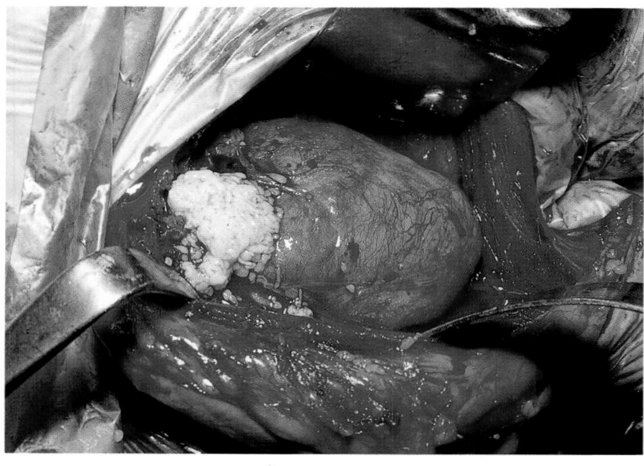

(a)

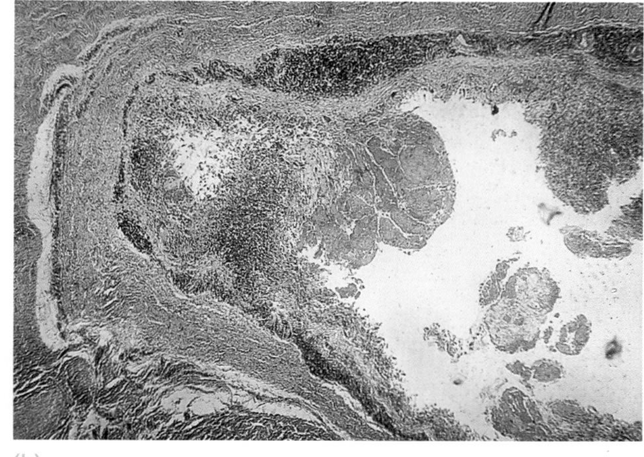

(b)

3.2 Rheumatoid synovitis (a) The macroscopic appearance of rheumatoid synovitis with fibrinoid material oozing through a rent in the capsule. (b) Histology shows proliferating synovium with round-cell infiltration and fibrinoid particles in the joint cavity (x120).

granulation tissue. Nodules occur under the skin (especially over bony prominences), in the synovium, on tendons, in the sclera and in many of the viscera.

Lymphadenopathy Not only the nodes draining inflamed joints, but also those at a distance such as the mediastinal nodes, can be affected. This, as well as a mild *splenomegaly*, is due to hyperactivity of the reticuloendothelial system. More severe splenomegaly can also be associated with neutropaenia as part of *Felty's syndrome*.

Vasculitis This can be a serious and life-threatening complication of RA. Involvement of the skin, including nailfold infarcts, is common but organ infarction can occur.

Muscle weakness Muscle weakness is common. It may be due to a generalized *myopathy* or *neuropathy*, but it is important to exclude spinal cord disease or cord compression due to vertebral displacement (atlanto-axial subluxation). Sensory changes may be part of a neuropathy, but localized sensory and motor symptoms can also result from *nerve compression* by thickened synovium (e.g. carpal tunnel syndrome).

Visceral disease The lungs, heart, kidneys, gastrointestinal tract and brain are sometimes affected. *Ischaemic heart disease* and *osteoporosis* are common complications.

Clinical features

The onset of RA is usually insidious, with symptoms emerging over a period of months. Occasionally the disease starts quite suddenly.

In the early stages the picture is mainly that of a polysynovitis, with soft-tissue swelling and stiffness. Typically, a woman of 30–40 years complains of pain, swelling and loss of mobility in the proximal joints of the fingers. There may be a previous history of 'muscle pain', tiredness, loss of weight and a general lack of well-being. As time passes, the symptoms 'spread' to other joints – the wrists, feet, knees and shoulders in order of frequency. Another classic feature is generalized stiffness after periods of inactivity, and especially after rising from bed in the early morning. This early morning stiffness typically lasts longer than 30 minutes.

Physical signs may be minimal, but usually there is symmetrically distributed swelling and tenderness of the metacarpophalangeal joints, the proximal interphalangeal joints and the wrists. Tenosynovitis is common in the extensor compartments of the wrist and the flexor sheaths of the fingers; it is diagnosed by feeling thickening, tenderness and crepitation over the back of the wrist or the palm while passively moving the fingers. If the larger joints are involved, local warmth, synovial hypertrophy and intra-articular effusion may be more obvious. Movements are often limited but the joints are still stable and deformity is unusual.

In the later stages joint deformity becomes increasingly apparent and the acute pain of synovitis is replaced by the more constant ache of progressive joint destruction. The combination of joint instability and tendon rupture produces the typical 'rheumatoid' deformities: ulnar deviation of the fingers, radial and volar displacement of the wrists, valgus knees, valgus feet and clawed toes. Joint movements are restricted and often very painful. About a third of all patients develop pain and stiffness in the cervical spine. Function is increasingly disturbed and patients may need help with grooming, dressing and eating.

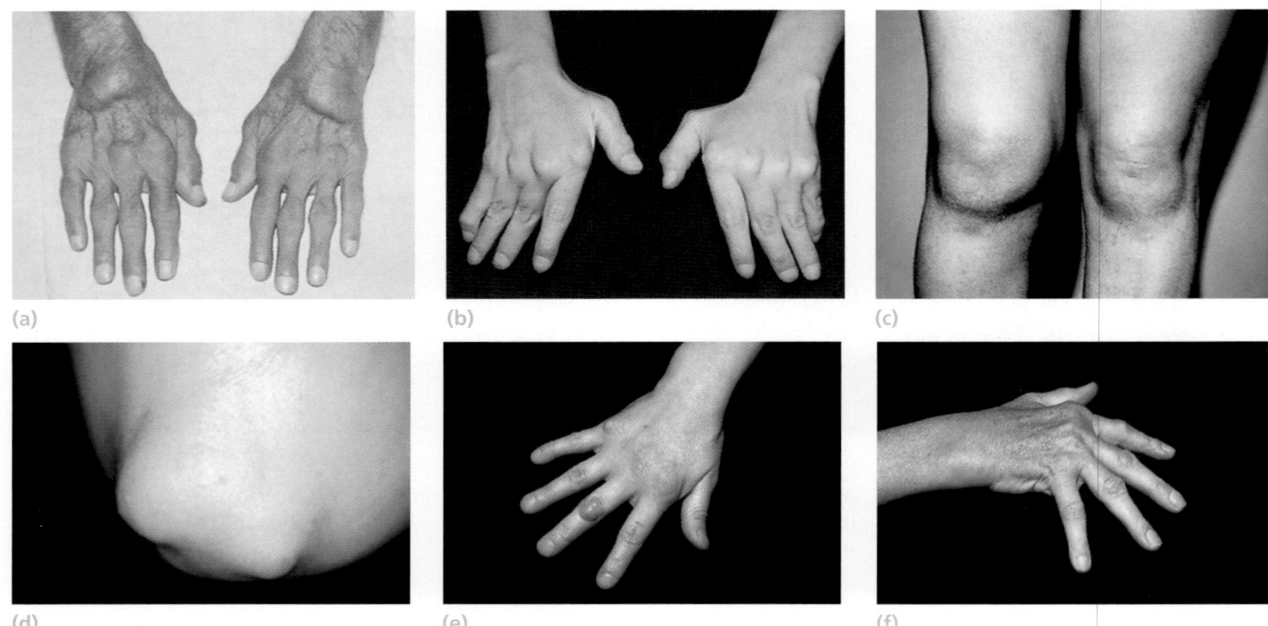

(a) (b) (c) (d) (e) (f)

3.3 Rheumatoid arthritis – clinical features (a) Early features of swelling and stiffness of the proximal finger joints and the wrists. (b) The late hand deformities are so characteristic as to be almost pathognomonic. (c) Occasionally rheumatoid disease starts with synovitis of a single large joint (in this case the right knee). Extra-articular features include subcutaneous nodules (d,e) and tendon ruptures (f).

Extra-articular features These often appear in patients with severe disease. The most characteristic is the appearance of *nodules*. They are usually found as small subcutaneous lumps, rubbery in consistency, at the back of the elbows, but they also develop in tendons (where they may cause 'triggering' or rupture), in the viscera and the eye. They are pathognomonic of RA, but occur in only 25% of patients.

Less specific features include *muscle wasting, lymphadenopathy, scleritis, nerve entrapment syndromes, skin atrophy* or *ulceration, vasculitis* and *peripheral sensory neuropathy*. Marked visceral disease, such as *pulmonary fibrosis*, is rare.

Imaging

X-rays Early on, x-rays show only the features of synovitis: soft-tissue swelling and peri-articular osteoporosis. The later stages are marked by the appearance of marginal bony erosions and narrowing of the articular space, especially in the proximal joints of the hands and feet. However, most individuals have evidence of erosions within 2 years. In advanced disease, articular destruction and joint deformity are obvious. Flexion and extension views of the cervical spine often show subluxation at the atlanto-axial or mid-cervical levels; surprisingly, this causes few symptoms in the majority of cases.

Ultrasound scanning and MRI The use of other imaging techniques to look at soft-tissue changes and early erosions within joints has become more common. Ultrasound can be particularly useful in defining the presence of synovitis and early erosions. Additional information on vascularity can be obtained if Doppler techniques are used.

Blood investigations

Normocytic, hypochromic anaemia is common and is a reflection of abnormal erythropoiesis due to disease activity. It may be aggravated by chronic gastrointestinal blood loss caused by non-steroidal anti-inflammatory drugs. In active phases the ESR and CRP concentration are usually raised.

Serological tests for rheumatoid factor are positive in about 80 per cent of patients and antinuclear factors are present in 30 per cent. Neither of these tests is specific and neither is required for a diagnosis of rheumatoid arthritis. Newer tests such as those for anti-CCP antibodies have added much greater specificity but at the expense of sensitivity.

Synovial biopsy

Synovial tissue may be obtained by needle biopsy, via the arthroscope, or by open operation. Unfortunately, most of the histological features of rheumatoid arthritis are non-specific.

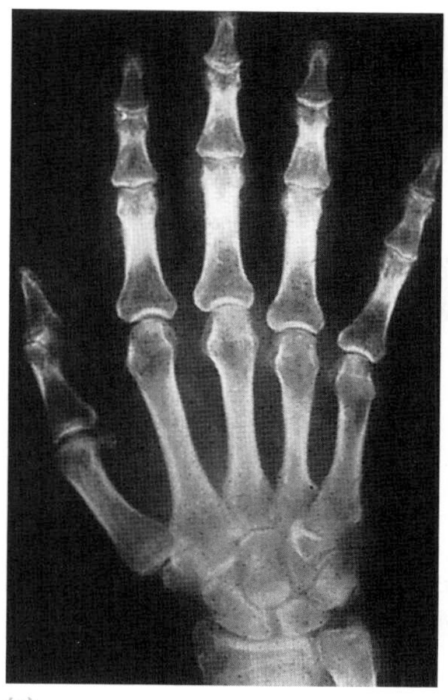

(a)

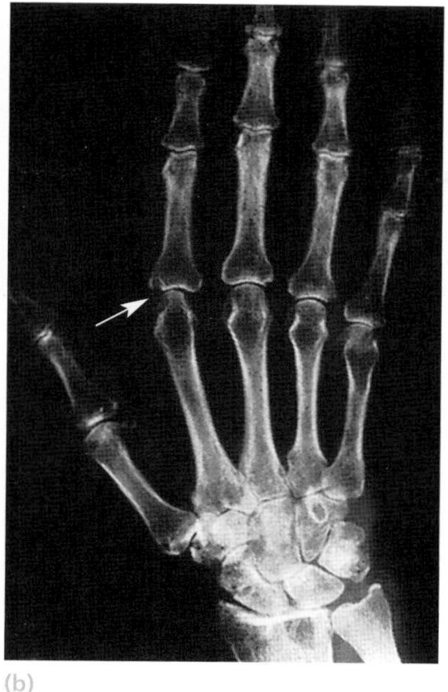

(b)

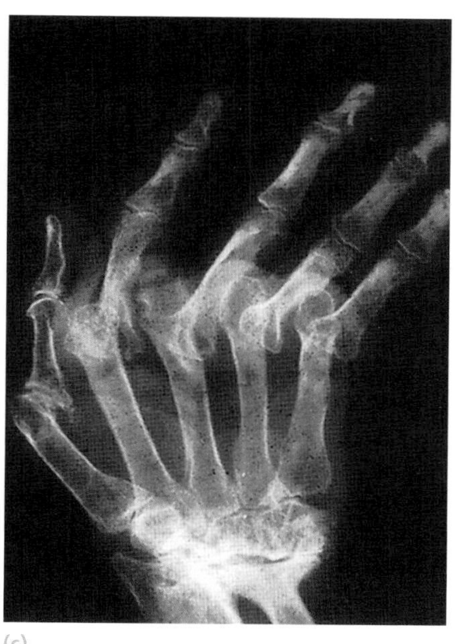

(c)

3.4 Rheumatoid arthritis – x-ray changes The progress of disease is well shown in this patient's x-rays. First, there was only soft-tissue swelling and peri-articular osteoporosis; later juxta-articular erosions appeared (arrow); ultimately, the joints became unstable and deformed.

Diagnosis

The usual criteria for diagnosing rheumatoid arthritis are the presence of a bilateral, symmetrical polyarthritis involving the proximal joints of the hands or feet, and persisting for at least 6 weeks. If there are subcutaneous nodules or x-ray signs of peri-articular erosions, the diagnosis is certain. *A positive test for rheumatoid factor in the absence of the above features is not sufficient evidence of rheumatoid arthritis, nor does a negative test exclude the diagnosis if the other features are all present.* The chief value of the rheumatoid factor tests is in the assessment of prognosis: persistently high titres herald more serious disease including extra-articular features.

Atypical forms of presentation are not uncommon. The early stages may be punctuated by spells of quiescence, during which the diagnosis is doubted, but sooner or later the more characteristic features appear. Occasionally, in older people, the onset is explosive, with the rapid appearance of severe joint pain and stiffness; paradoxically these patients have a relatively good prognosis. Now and then (more so in young women) the disease starts with chronic pain and swelling of a single large joint and it may take months or years before other joints are involved.

The presence of tenderness on squeezing across all metacarpophalangeal or metatarsophalangeal joints, early morning stiffness of at least 30 minutes and a raised ESR are highly suggestive of a diagnosis of rheumatoid arthritis. A rapid diagnosis is vital so that early treatment can be started with disease-modifying antirheumatic drugs.

In the differential diagnosis of polyarthritis several disorders must be considered.

Seronegative inflammatory polyarthritis Polyarthritis is a feature of a number of conditions including psoriatic arthritis, adult Still's disease, systemic lupus erythematosus and other connective-tissue diseases. These are considered in later sections.

Ankylosing spondylitis This is primarily an inflammatory disease of the sacroiliac and intervertebral joints, causing back pain and progressive stiffness; however, it may also involve the peripheral joints.

Reiter's disease The larger joints and the lumbosacral spine are the main targets. There is usually a history of urethritis or colitis and often also conjunctivitis.

Polyarticular gout Tophaceous gout affecting multiple joints can, at first sight, be mistaken for rheumatoid arthritis. On x-ray the erosions are quite different from those of rheumatoid arthritis; the diagnosis is clinched by identifying typical birefringent urate crystals in the joint fluid or a nodular tophus.

It is a curious fact that, although both gout and RA are fairly common, the two conditions are rarely seen in the same patient. The reason for this is unknown.

Calcium pyrophosphate deposition disease This condition is usually seen in older people. Typically it affects large joints, but it may occur in the wrist and metacarpophalangeal joints as well. X-ray signs are fairly characteristic and crystals may be identified in synovial fluid or synovium.

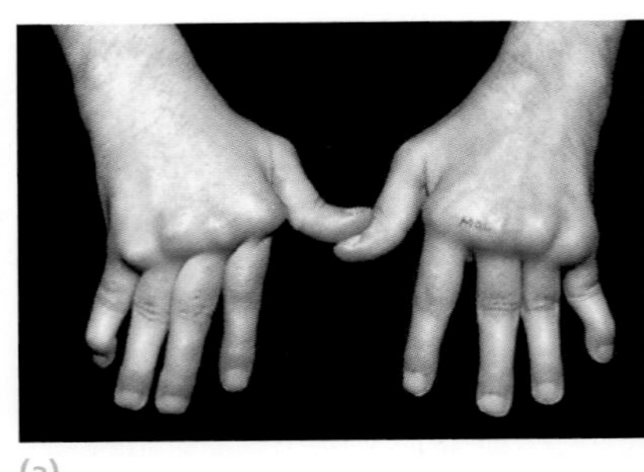
(a)

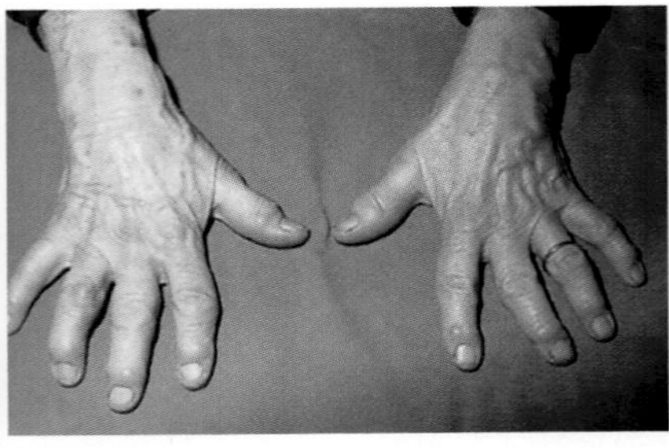
(b)

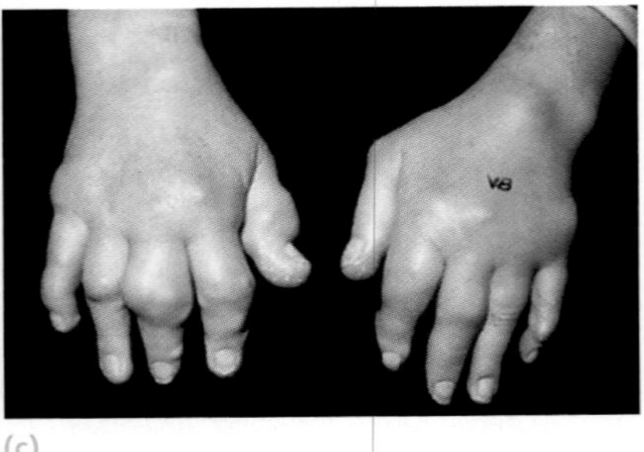
(c)

3.5 Rheumatoid arthritis – differential diagnosis All three patients presented with painful swollen fingers. In (a) mainly the proximal joints were affected (rheumatoid arthritis); in (b) the distal joints were the worst (Heberden's osteoarthritis); in (c) there were asymmetrical nodular swellings around the joints (gouty tophi).

Sarcoidosis Sarcoid disease sometimes presents with a symmetrical small-joint polyarthritis and no bone involvement; in other cases a large joint such as the knee or ankle may be involved. Erythema nodosum and hilar lymphadenopathy on chest x-ray are clues to the diagnosis.

Acute sarcoidosis usually subsides spontaneously within 6 months. *Chronic sarcoidosis* produces granulomatous infiltration of lungs, bone, synovium and other organs and is more common in Afro-Caribbean than Caucasian peoples. In addition to polyarthritis and tenosynovitis, there are usually x-ray features of punched-out 'cysts' and cortical erosions in the bones of the hands and feet. The ESR and serum angiotensin converting enzyme (SACE) may be raised. Biopsy of affected tissue shows typical non-caseating granulomas. Treatment with non-steroidal anti-inflammatory drugs (NSAIDs) may be adequate but in more intractable cases corticosteroids or other immunosuppressive preparations are necessary.

Lyme disease This tick-borne spirochaetal infection usually starts with a skin lesion and flu-like symptoms and then spreads to multiple organs. If the initial lesions are missed or left untreated, patients may present with an asymmetrical inflammatory polyarthritis affecting mainly the larger joints. It is most likely to be encountered in known endemic areas in North America, Europe and Asia. In late cases serological tests may be positive. Treatment with doxycycline or one of the newer cephalosporins is usually effective for the arthritic features.

Viral arthritis Viral infections are often associated with a transient polyarthralgia; flu-like illness and a rash will suggest the diagnosis. However, some infections – most typically parvovirus B19 – occasionally cause a symmetrical polysynovitis (including the finger joints) and early morning stiffness, symptoms which may last for several months or may recur over a few years. The absence of 'rheumatoid' x-ray features and subcutaneous nodules will raise suspicions about the diagnosis.

Polymyalgia rheumatica This condition, which is seen mainly in the middle-aged or elderly, is characterized by aching discomfort around the pectoral and pelvic girdles, post-inactivity stiffness and muscular weakness. The joints are not tender but the muscles may be. The ESR and CRP are almost always elevated. Corticosteroids (as little as 10 mg a day) provide rapid and dramatic relief of all symptoms, and this response is often used as a diagnostic test. The condition may be associated with, and certainly carries the risk of, temporal arteritis resulting in blindness.

Osteoarthritis Polyarticular osteoarthritis (OA), which typically involves the finger joints, is often mistaken for RA. A moment's reflection will usually dispel any doubt: OA always involves the *distal* interphalangeal joints and causes a nodular arthritis with radiologically obvious osteophytes, whereas RA affects the *proximal* joints of the hand and causes predominantly erosive features.

Some confusion may arise from the fact that RA, in its later stages, is associated with loss of articular cartilage and *secondary OA*. Enquiry into the early history will usually untangle the diagnosis. Sometimes, however, RA atypically affects only a few of the larger joints and it is then very difficult to distinguish from OA; x-ray features such as loss of articular cartilage throughout the entire joint and lack of hypertrophic bone changes (sclerosis and osteophytes) should suggest an inflammatory arthritis.

Treatment

There is no cure for rheumatoid arthritis. However, advances in therapy have revolutionized the treatment approach with associated major improvements in outcome (Kennedy et al., 2005). Medical treatment is guided by the principle that inflammation should be reduced rapidly and aggressively. A multidisciplinary approach is needed from the beginning: ideally the therapeutic team should include a rheumatologist, orthopaedic surgeon, physiotherapist, occupational therapist, orthotist and social worker. Their deploy-

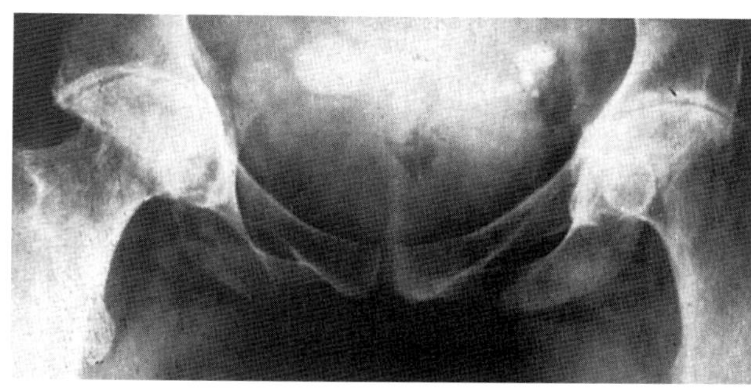

(a)

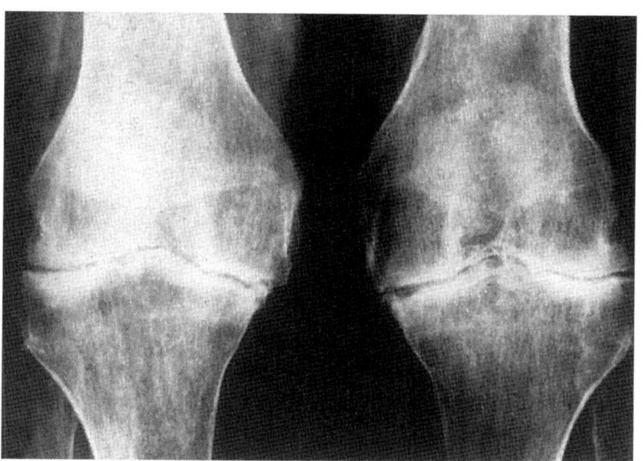

(b)

3.6 Rheumatoid arthritis – aftermath After the acute inflammatory phase has passed, the patient may be left with features of secondary osteoarthritis, especially in the hips (a) and the knees (b).

ment and priorities will vary according to the individual and stage of the disease.

At the onset of the disease both the patient and the doctor will be uncertain about the likely rate of progress. An attempt should be made to determine the likely prognosis. Poor prognosis is associated with female sex, multiple joint involvement, high ESR and CRP, positive RF and anti-CCP, younger age and the presence of erosions at diagnosis.

PRINCIPLES OF MEDICAL MANAGEMENT

Treatment should be aimed at controlling inflammation as rapidly as possible. This is likely to require the use of corticosteroids for their rapid onset (initially oral doses of 30 mg of prednisolone or 120 mg i.m. methylprednisolone may be used). Steroids should be rapidly tapered to prevent significant side effects.

In addition, disease-modifying antirheumatic drugs (DMARDs) should be started at this time. The first choice is now methotrexate at doses of 10–25 mg/week. This may be used initially alone or in combination with sulfasalazine and hydroxychloroquine. Leflunomide can also be considered if methotrexate is not tolerated. Gold and penicillamine are now used rarely.

Control of pain and stiffness with non-steroidal anti-inflammatory drugs (NSAIDs) may be needed, maintaining muscle tone and joint mobility by a balanced programme of exercise, and general advice on coping with the activities of daily living.

If there is no satisfactory response to DMARDs, it is wise to progress rapidly to biological therapies such as the TNF inhibitors infliximab, etanercept and adalimumab (Scott & Kingsley, 2006; Deighton et al., 2006).

Additional measures include the injection of long-acting corticosteroid preparations into inflamed joints and tendon sheaths. It is sometimes feared that such injections may themselves cause damage to articular cartilage or tendons. However, there is little evidence that they are harmful, provided they are used sparingly and with full precautions against infection.

Prolonged rest and immobility is likely to weaken muscles and lead to a worse prognosis. However, some splinting can be helpful at any stage of the disease.

KEY ELEMENTS IN MEDICAL TREATMENT

- Identify patients with RA as early as possible
- Start disease-modifying antirheumatic drugs (DMARDs) immediately
- Consider combination therapy with multiple DMARDs
- If DMARDs fail, progress rapidly to biological therapies such as the TNF inhibitors infliximab, etanercept and adalimumab

PHYSIOTHERAPY AND OCCUPATIONAL THERAPY

Preventative splinting and orthotic devices may delay the march of events; however, it is important to encourage activity. If these fail to restore and maintain function, operative treatment is indicated.

SURGICAL MANAGEMENT

At first this consists mainly of soft-tissue procedures (synovectomy, tendon repair or replacement and joint stabilization); in some cases osteotomy may be more appropriate.

In late rheumatoid disease, severe joint destruction, fixed deformity and loss of function are clear indications for reconstructive surgery. Arthrodesis, osteotomy and arthroplasty all have their place and are considered in the appropriate chapters. However, it should be recognized that patients who are no longer suffering the pain of active synovitis and who are contented with a limited pattern of life may not want or need heroic surgery merely to improve their anatomy. Careful assessment for occupational therapy, the provision of mechanical aids and adjustments to their home environment may be much more useful. It appears safe to continue methotrexate during elective orthopaedic surgery. However, doses of corticosteroids should be as low as possible and biological therapies such as the TNF inhibitors should be stopped prior to surgery where possible.

Complications

Fixed deformities The perils of rheumatoid arthritis are often the commonplace ones resulting from ignorance and neglect. Early assessment and planning should prevent postural deformities, which will result in joint contractures.

Muscle weakness Even mild degrees of myopathy or neuropathy, when combined with prolonged inactivity, may lead to profound muscle wasting and weakness. This should be prevented by control of inflammation, physiotherapy and pain control, if possible; if not, the surgeon must be forewarned of the difficulty of postoperative rehabilitation.

Joint rupture Occasionally the joint lining ruptures and synovial contents spill into the soft tissues. Treatment is directed at the underlying synovitis, i.e. splintage and injection of the joint, with synovectomy as a second resort.

Infection Patients with rheumatoid arthritis – and even more so those on corticosteroid therapy – are susceptible to infection. Sudden clinical deterioration, or increased pain in a single joint, should alert one to the possibility of septic arthritis and the need for joint aspiration.

Spinal cord compression This is a rare complication of cervical spine (atlanto-axial) instability. The onset of weakness and upper motor neuron signs in the lower limbs is suspicious. If they occur, immobilization of the neck is essential and spinal fusion should be carried out as soon as possible.

Systemic vasculitis Vasculitis is a rare but potentially serious complication. Corticosteroids and immunosuppressives such as intravenous cyclophosphamide may be required.

Amyloidosis This is another rare but potentially lethal complication of longstanding rheumatoid arthritis. The patient presents with proteinuria and progressive renal failure. Finding amyloid in a rectal or renal biopsy makes the diagnosis. Aggressive control of inflammation has reduced this complication significantly.

Prognosis

Rheumatoid arthritis runs a variable course. When the patient is first seen it is difficult to predict the outcome, but high titres of rheumatoid factor, peri-articular erosions, rheumatoid nodules, severe muscle wasting, joint contractures and evidence of vasculitis are bad prognostic signs. Women, on the whole, fare somewhat worse than men. Without effective treatment about 10 per cent of patients improve steadily after the first attack of active synovitis; 60 per cent have intermittent phases of disease activity and remission, but with a slow downhill course over many years; 20 per cent have severe joint erosion, which is usually evident within the first 5 years; and 10 per cent end up completely disabled. In addition, a reduction in life expectancy by 5–10 years is common and is often due to premature ischaemic heart disease. However, early aggressive medical treatment appears to reduce the morbidity and mortality.

SERONEGATIVE SPONDYLOARTHROPATHIES

ANKYLOSING SPONDYLITIS

Like rheumatoid arthritis, this is a generalized chronic inflammatory disease, but its effects are seen mainly in the spine and sacroiliac joints. It is characterized by pain and stiffness of the back, with variable involvement of the hips and shoulders and (more rarely) the peripheral joints. Its reported prevalence is 0.1 to 0.2 per cent in western Europe and North America, but is much lower in Japanese and African peoples. Males are affected more frequently than females (estimates vary from 2:1 to 10:1) and the usual age at onset is between 15 and 25 years. There is a strong tendency to familial aggregation and association with the genetic marker HLA-B27.

Cause

There is considerable evidence for regarding ankylosing spondylitis (AS) as a genetically determined immunopathological disorder. The disease is much more common in family members of patients than in the general population – HLA-B27 is present in over 95 per cent of Caucasian patients and in half of their first-degree relatives (as compared with 8 per cent of the general population); and racial groups with an unusually low prevalence of AS also show a very low prevalence of HLA-B27 (e.g. less than 1 per cent in Japanese people).

There are various theories about the 'triggering factor' that initiates the abnormal immune response. It may be a bacterial antigen, which closely resembles HLA-B27 that induces an antibody response, which also targets the HLA-B27 positive cells; or, as in the case of RA, the HLA-B27 molecule may be involved in the presentation of a specific antigen to the T cells, which then react with the antigen-presenting cells. Since classic ankylosing spondylitis is sometimes associated with genitourinary or bowel infection, and disorders such as Reiter's disease and ulcerative colitis cause vertebral and sacroiliac changes indistinguishable from those of ankylosing spondylitis, it has been suggested that the putative organism may be carried to the spine by local lymphatic drainage.

Pathology

There are two basic lesions: synovitis of diarthrodial joints and inflammation at the fibro-osseous junctions of syndesmotic joints and tendons. The preferential involvement of the insertion of tendons and ligaments (the entheses) has resulted in the unwieldy term *enthesopathy*.

Synovitis of the sacroiliac and vertebral facet joints causes destruction of articular cartilage and peri-articular bone. The costovertebral joints also are frequently involved, leading to diminished respiratory excursion. When peripheral joints are affected the same changes occur.

Inflammation of the fibro-osseous junctions affects the intervertebral discs, sacroiliac ligaments, symphysis pubis, manubrium sterni and the bony insertions of large tendons. Pathological changes proceed in three stages: (1) an inflammatory reaction with cell infiltration, granulation tissue formation and erosion of adjacent bone; (2) replacement of the granulation tissue by fibrous tissue; and (3) ossification of the fibrous tissue, leading to ankylosis of the joint.

Ossification across the surface of the disc gives rise to small bony bridges or syndesmophytes linking adjacent vertebral bodies. If many vertebrae are involved the spine may become absolutely rigid.

Clinical features

The disease starts insidiously: a teenager or young adult complains of backache and stiffness recurring at intervals over a number of years. This is often diagnosed as 'simple mechanical back pain', but the symptoms are worse in the early morning and after inactivity. Referred pain in the buttocks and thighs may appear as 'sciatica' and some patients are mistakenly treated for intervertebral disc prolapse. Gradually pain and stiffness become continuous and other symptoms begin to appear: general fatigue, pain and swelling of joints, tenderness at the insertion of the Achilles tendon, 'foot strain', or intercostal pain and tenderness.

Occasionally the disease starts with pain and slight swelling in a peripheral joint such as the ankle, or pain and stiffness of the hip. Sooner or later, though, backache will come to the fore. In women the axial skeletal disease may remain restricted to the sacroiliac joints making diagnosis challenging.

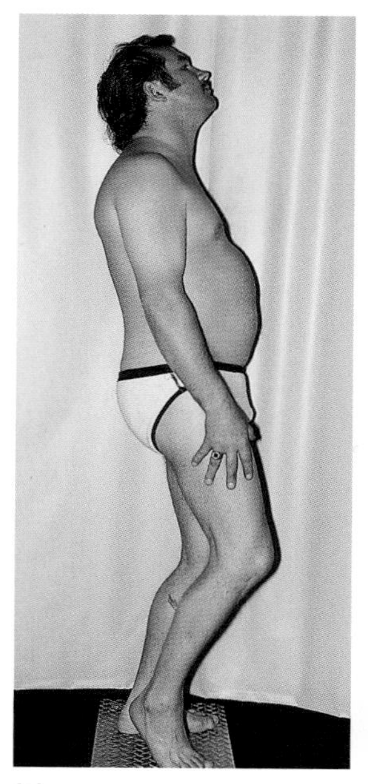

(a)

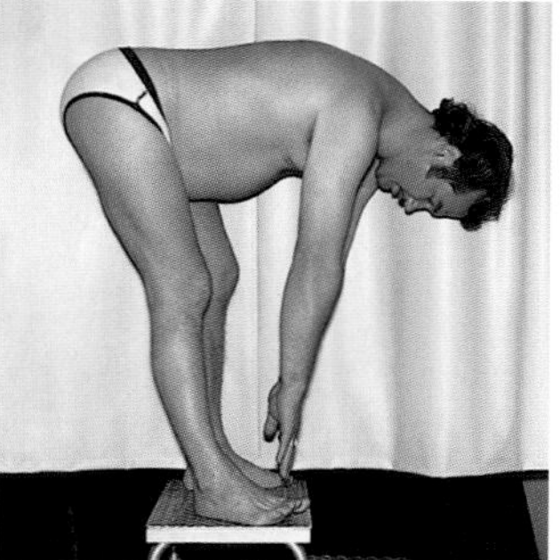

(b)

3.7 Ankylosing spondylitis – early The cardinal clinical feature is marked stiffness of the spine. (a) This patient manages to stand upright by keeping his knees slightly flexed. (b) It looks as if he can bend down to touch his toes, but his back is rigid and all the movement takes place at his hips.

Early on there is little to see apart from slight flattening of the lower back and limitation of extension in the lumbar spine. There may be diffuse tenderness over the spine and sacroiliac joints, or (occasionally) swelling and tenderness of a single large joint.

In established cases the posture is typical: loss of the normal lumbar lordosis, increased thoracic kyphosis and a forward thrust of the neck; upright posture and balance are maintained by standing with the hips and knees slightly flexed, and in late cases these may become fixed deformities. Spinal movements are diminished in all directions, but loss of extension is always the earliest and the most severe disability. It is revealed dramatically by the 'wall test': the patient is asked to stand with his back to the wall; heels, buttocks, scapulae and occiput should all be able to touch the wall simultaneously. If extension is seriously diminished the patient will find this impossible. In the most advanced stage the spine may be completely ankylosed from occiput to sacrum – sometimes in positions of grotesque deformity. Marked loss of cervical extension may restrict the line of vision to a few paces.

Chest expansion, which should be at least 7 cm in young men, is often markedly decreased. In old people, who may have pulmonary disease, this test is unreliable.

Peripheral joints (usually shoulders, hips and knees) are involved in over a third of the patients; they show the features of inflammatory arthritis – swelling, tenderness, effusion and loss of mobility. There may also be tenderness of the ligament and tendon insertions close to a large joint or under the heel.

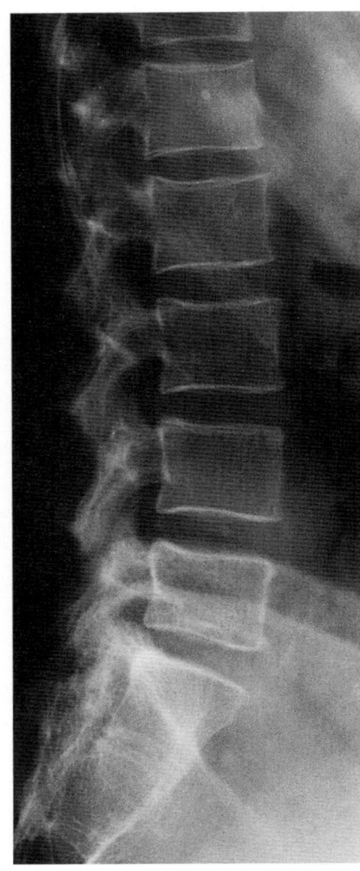

(a)

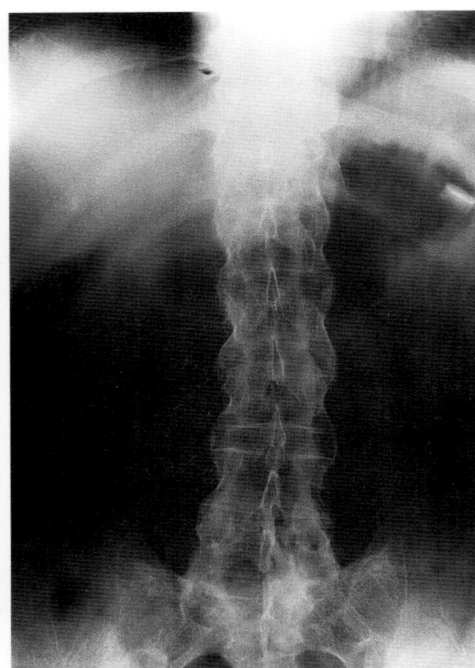

(b)

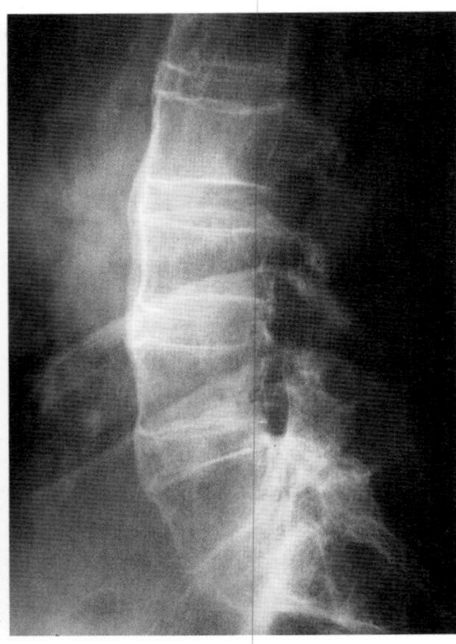

(c)

3.8 Ankylosing spondylitis – x-rays (a) An early sign is 'squaring' of the lumbar vertebrae. (b,c) Bony bridges (syndesmophytes) between the vertebral bodies convert the spine into a rigid column.

Extraskeletal manifestations General fatigue and loss of weight are common. Acute anterior uveitis occurs in about 25 per cent of patients; it usually responds well to treatment but, if neglected, may lead to permanent damage including glaucoma. Other extraskeletal disorders, such as aortic valve disease, carditis and pulmonary fibrosis (apical), are rare and occur very late in the disease.

Imaging

X-rays The cardinal sign – and often the earliest – is erosion and fuzziness of the sacroiliac joints. Later there may be peri-articular sclerosis, especially on the iliac side of the joint and finally bony ankylosis.

The earliest vertebral change is flattening of the normal anterior concavity of the vertebral body ('squaring'). Later, ossification of the ligaments around the intervertebral discs produces delicate bridges (syndesmophytes) between adjacent vertebrae. Bridging at several levels gives the appearance of a 'bamboo spine'.

Osteoporosis is common in longstanding cases and there may be hyperkyphosis of the thoracic spine due to wedging of the vertebral bodies.

Peripheral joints may show erosive arthritis or progressive bony ankylosis.

MRI MRI allows detailed investigation of sacroiliac joints and may show typical erosions and features of inflammation such as bone oedema. Various techniques including gadolinium contrast can be used to demonstrate inflammatory lesions in other areas of the spine.

Special investigations

The ESR and CRP are usually elevated during active phases of the disease. HLA-B27 is present in 95 per cent of cases. Serological tests for rheumatoid factor are usually negative.

Diagnosis

Diagnosis is easy in patients with spinal rigidity and typical deformities, but it is often missed in those with early disease or unusual forms of presentation. In over 10 per cent of cases the disease starts with an asymmetrical inflammatory arthritis – usually of the hip, knee or ankle – and it may be several years before back pain appears. Atypical onset is more common in women, who may show less obvious changes in the sacroiliac joints. A history of AS in a close relative is strongly suggestive.

Mechanical disorders Low back pain in young adults is usually attributed to one of the more common disorders such as muscular strain, facet joint dysfunction or spondylolisthesis. These conditions differ from AS in several ways: the onset of pain is related to specific physical activities, stiffness is less pronounced and symptoms are eased rather than aggravated by inactivity. Tenderness is also more localized and the peripheral joints are normal.

Diffuse idiopathic hyperostosis (Forestier's disease) This is a fairly common disorder, predominantly of older men, characterized by widespread ossification of ligaments and tendon insertions. X-rays show pronounced but asymmetrical intervertebral spur formation and bridging throughout the dorsolumbar spine (see Fig. 5.13b). Although it bears a superficial resemblance to AS, it is not an inflammatory disease, spinal pain and stiffness are seldom severe, the sacroiliac joints are not eroded and the ESR is normal.

Other seronegative spondyloarthropathies A number of disorders are associated with vertebral and sacroiliac lesions indistinguishable from those of ankylosing spondylitis. They are *Reiter's disease, psoriatic arthritis, ulcerative colitis, Crohn's disease, Whipple's disease* and *Behçet's syndrome*. In each there are certain characteristic features: the rash or nail changes of psoriasis, intestinal ulceration in inflammatory bowel disease, genitourinary and ocular inflammation in Reiter's disease, buccal and genital ulceration in Behçet's syndrome. Yet there is considerable overlap between them; all show some familial aggregation and all are associated with the histocompatibility antigen, HLA-B27. Patients with one of these disorders (including AS) often have close relatives with another, or with a positive HLA-B27.

Treatment

The disease is not usually as damaging as rheumatoid arthritis and many patients continue to lead an active life. Treatment consists of: (1) general measures to maintain satisfactory posture and preserve movement; (2) anti-inflammatory drugs to counteract pain and stiffness; (3) the use of TNF inhibitors for severe disease; and (4) operations to correct deformity or restore mobility (Manadan et al., 2007; Siridopoulos et al., 2008).

General measures Patients are encouraged to remain active and follow their normal pursuits as far as possible. They should be taught how to maintain satisfactory posture and urged to perform spinal extension exercises every day. Swimming, dancing and gymnastics are ideal forms of recreation. Rest and immobilization are contraindicated because they tend to increase the general feeling of stiffness.

Non-steroidal anti-inflammatory drugs It is doubtful whether these drugs prevent or retard the progress to ankylosis, but they do control pain and counteract soft-tissue stiffness, thus making it possible to benefit from exercise and activity. They may have to be continued for many years.

TNF inhibitors With the introduction of the TNF inhibitors it has become possible to treat the underlying inflammatory processes active in AS. This can result in significant improvement in disease activity including remission. These therapies are generally reserved for individuals who have failed to be controlled with non-steroidal anti-inflammatory drugs.

Operation Significantly damaged hips can be treated by joint replacement, though this seldom provides more than moderate mobility. Moreover, the incidence of infection is higher than usual and patients may need prolonged rehabilitation.

Deformity of the spine may be severe enough to warrant lumbar or cervical osteotomy. These are difficult and potentially hazardous procedures; fortunately, with improved activity and exercise programmes, they are seldom needed. If spinal deformity is combined with hip stiffness, hip replacements (permitting full extension) often suffice.

Complications

Spinal fractures The spine is often both rigid and osteoporotic; fractures may be caused by comparatively mild injuries. The commonest site is C5–7, but it is prudent to x-ray the entire spine in accident

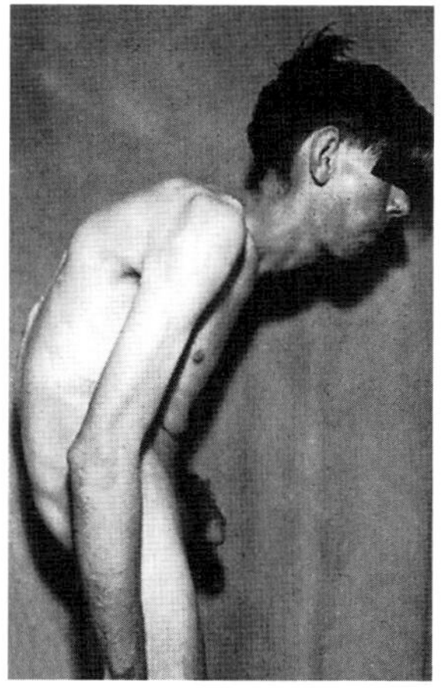
(a)

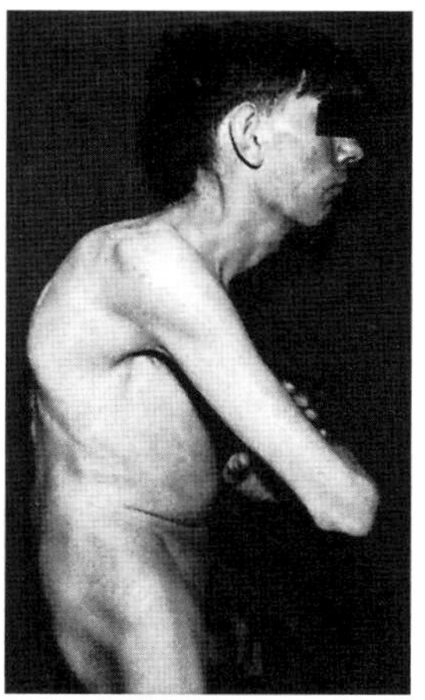
(b)

3.9 Ankylosing spondylitis – operative treatment Spinal osteotomy is occasionally performed to correct a severe, rigid deformity. (a) Before operation this man could see only a few paces ahead; (b) after osteotomy his back is still rigid but his posture, function and outlook are improved.

victims who have AS. Treatment in these cases is directed at preventing further deformity.

Hyperkyphosis In longstanding cases the spine may become severely kyphotic, so much so that the patient has difficulty lifting his head to see in front of his feet.

Spinal cord compression This is uncommon, but it should be thought of in patients who develop long-tract symptoms and signs. It may be caused by atlanto-axial subluxation or by ossification of the posterior longitudinal ligament.

Lumbosacral nerve root compression Patients may occasionally develop root symptoms, including lower limb weakness and paraesthesia, in addition to their 'usual' pelvic girdle symptoms.

Reiter's syndrome and reactive arthritis

The syndrome described by Hans Reiter in 1916 (and 100 years before that by Benjamin Brodie) is a clinical triad of *urethritis, arthritis* and *conjunctivitis* occurring some weeks after either *dysentery* or *genitourinary infection*. It is now recognized that this is one of the classic forms of reactive arthritis, i.e. an aseptic inflammatory arthritis associated with non-specific infection (often urogenital or bowel).

Its prevalence is difficult to assess, but it is probably the commonest type of large-joint polyarthritis in young men. It is thought to occur in 1–3 per cent of all people who develop either non-specific urogenital infection or *Shigella* dysentery, but its incidence may be as high as 25 per cent in those who are HLA-B27 positive. Men are affected more often than women (the ratio is about 10:1), but this may simply reflect the difficulty of diagnosing the genitourinary infection in women. The usual age at onset is between 20 and 40 years, but children are affected too – perhaps after an episode of diarrhoea.

Cause

Familial aggregation, overlap with other forms of seronegative spondyloarthropathy in first-degree relatives and a close association with HLA-B27 point to a genetic predisposition, the bowel or genitourinary infection acting as a trigger. Gut pathogens include *Shigella flexneri*, *Salmonella, Campylobacter* species and *Yersinia enterocolitica*. *Lymphogranuloma venereum* and *Chlamydia trachomatis* have been implicated as sexually transmitted infections. All these bacteria can survive in human cells; assuming that either the bacterium or a peptide bacterial fragment acts as the antigen, the pathogenesis could be the same as that suggested for ankylosing spondylitis.

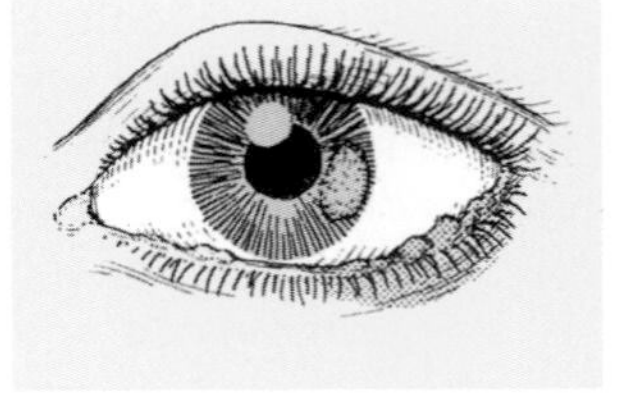

(a)

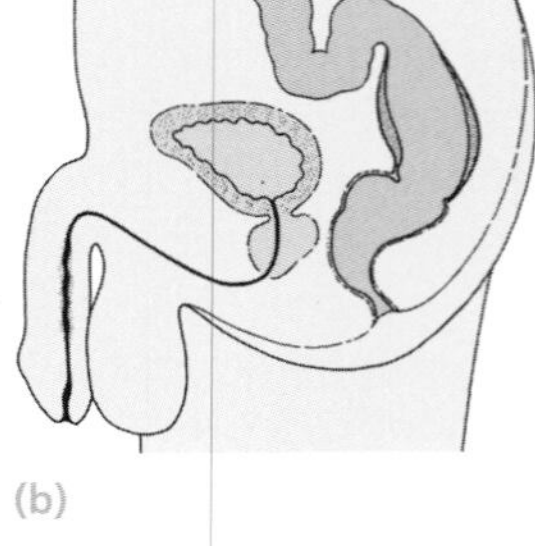

(b)

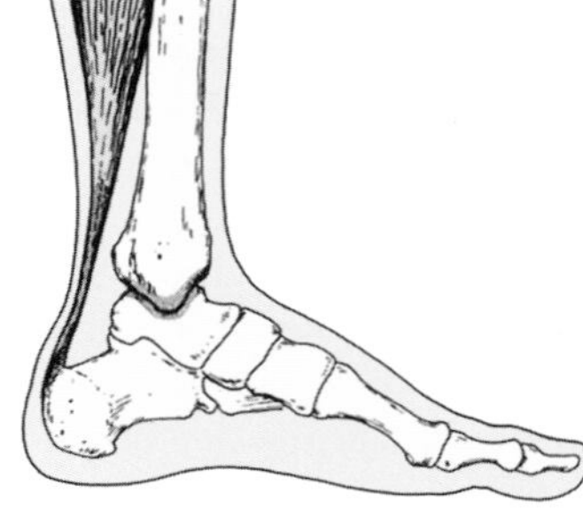

(c)

3.10 Reiter's syndrome – the classic 'Reiter's triad' consists of conjunctivitis (a), urethritis (b) (sometimes colitis) and arthritis (c). Tenderness of the tendo Achilles and the plantar fascia is also common.

Pathology

The pathological changes are essentially the same as those in ankylosing spondylitis, with the emphasis first on subacute large-joint synovitis and in some individuals with a chronic disease course tending towards sacroiliitis and spondylitis.

Clinical features

The acute phase of the disease is marked by an asymmetrical inflammatory arthritis of the lower limb joints – usually the knee and ankle but often the tarsal and toe joints as well. The joint may be acutely painful, hot and swollen with a tense effusion, suggesting gout or infection. Tendo Achilles tenderness and plantar fasciitis (evidence of enthesopathy) are common, and the patient may complain of backache even in the early stage. Conjunctivitis, urethritis and bowel infections are often mild and easily missed; the patient should be carefully questioned about symptoms during the previous few weeks. Cystitis and cervicitis may occur in women.

Less frequent, but equally characteristic, features are a vesicular or pustular dermatitis of the feet (keratoderma blennorrhagica), balanitis and mild buccal ulceration.

The acute disorder usually lasts for a few weeks or months and then subsides, but most patients have either recurrent attacks of arthritis or other features of chronic disease.

The chronic phase is more characteristic of a spondyloarthropathy. Over half of the patients with Reiter's disease complain of mild, recurrent episodes of polyarthritis (including upper limb joints). About half of those again develop sacroiliitis and spondylitis with

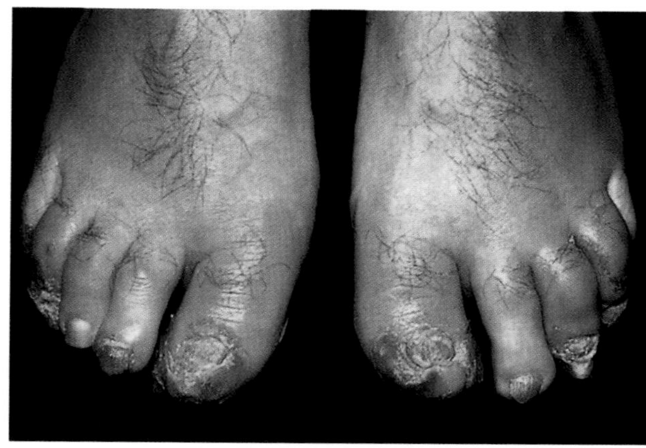

3.11 Reiter's disease – other features The characteristic pustular dermatitis of the feet – keratoderma blennorrhagicum.

features resembling those of ankylosing spondylitis. Uveitis is also fairly common and may give rise to posterior synechiae and glaucoma.

X-rays

Sacroiliac and vertebral changes are similar to those of ankylosing spondylitis. If peripheral joints are involved, they may show features of erosive arthritis.

Special investigations

Tests for HLA-B27 are positive in 75 per cent of patients with sacroiliitis. The ESR may be high in the active phase of the disease. The causative organism can sometimes be isolated from urethral fluids or faeces, and tests for antibodies may be positive.

Diagnosis

The diagnosis should be considered in any young adult who presents with an acute or subacute arthritis in the lower limbs. It is more likely to be missed in women, in children and in those with very mild (and often forgotten) episodes of genitourinary or bowel infection. Some patients never develop the full syndrome and one should be alert to the *formes fruste* with large-joint arthritis alone.

Gout and infective arthritis Reiter's disease, gout and infection should all be considered in the differential diagnosis of inflammation in a large peripheral joint. Examination of synovial fluid for organisms and crystals may provide important clues.

Gonococcal arthritis Gonococcal arthritis takes two forms: (1) bacterial infection of the joint; and (2) a reactive arthritis with sterile joint fluid. A history of genitourinary infection further complicates the distinction from Reiter's disease, and diagnosis may depend on identifying the organism or gonococcal antibodies.

Enteropathic arthritis Ulcerative colitis and Crohn's disease may be associated with subacute synovitis, causing pain and swelling of one or more of the peripheral joints. These subside when the intestinal disease is controlled.

Treatment

Initial treatment for Reiter's disease should be aimed at ensuring the infectious organism responsible has been cleared. This is particularly important for sexually transmitted infections such as *Chlamydia trachomatis.*

Even if the triggering infection is identified, treating it will have no effect on the reactive arthritis. However, there is some evidence that treatment of *Chlamydia* infection with tetracycline for periods of up to 3 months can reduce the risk of recurrent joint disease.

Symptomatic treatment could include the use of analgesia and non-steroidal anti-inflammatory drugs. If the inflammatory response is aggressive then local injection of corticosteroids or even intramuscular methylprednisolone may be useful. If symptoms and signs do not resolve then DMARDs used in the treatment of RA may be needed. Topical steroids may be used for uveitis.

PSORIATIC ARTHRITIS

Polyarthritis and psoriasis are often seen together. Usually this is simply a chance concurrence of two fairly common disorders. In some cases, however, the patient has a true psoriatic arthritis – a distinct entity characterized by seronegative polysynovitis, erosive (sometimes very destructive) arthritis, and a significant incidence of sacroiliitis and spondylitis.

The prevalence of psoriasis is 1–2 per cent, but only about 5 per cent of those affected will develop psoriatic arthritis. The usual age at onset is 30–50 years (often later than the skin lesions).

Cause

As with the other seronegative spondyloarthropathies, there is a strong genetic component: patients often give a family history of psoriasis; there is a significantly increased incidence of other spondyloarthropathies in close relatives; and 60 per cent of those with psoriatic spondylitis or sacroiliitis have HLA-B27.

Psoriatic skin lesions may well be a reactive phenomenon, and the joint lesions a form of 'reactive arthritis'. However, no specific trigger agent has thus far been identified.

Pathology

The joint changes are similar to those in rheumatoid arthritis – chronic synovitis with cell infiltration and exudate, going on to fibrosis. Cartilage and bone destruction may be unusually severe ('arthritis mutilans'). However, rheumatoid nodules are not seen.

Sacroiliac and spine changes, which occur in about 30 per cent of patients, are similar to those in ankylosing spondylitis.

Clinical features

The patient may present with one of several patterns of joint involvement. These include: arthritis of distal interphalangeal joints, 'arthritis mutilans', asymmetrical large joint oligoarthritis and patterns mimicking rheumatoid arthritis or ankylosing spondylitis. Psoriasis of the skin or nails usually precedes the arthritis, but hidden lesions (in the natal cleft or umbilicus) are easily overlooked.

The condition can progress slowly or very rapidly and may become quiescent. Sometimes (particularly in women) joint involvement is more symmetrical, and in these cases the condition may be indistinguishable from seronegative rheumatoid arthritis. Asymmetrical swelling of two or three fingers may be due to a combination of interphalangeal arthritis and tenosynovitis.

Sacroiliitis and spondylitis are seen in about one-third of patients, and occasionally this is the predominant change with a clinical picture resembling ankylosing spondylitis. As in the other spondyloarthropathies, heel pain (*enthesitis*) is not uncommon.

In the worst cases both the spine and the peripheral joints may be involved. Fingers and toes are severely deformed due to erosion and instability of the interphalangeal joints (*arthritis mutilans*).

Ocular inflammation occurs in about 30 per cent of patients.

Imaging

X-ray examination may show severe destruction of the interphalangeal joints of the hands and feet; changes in the large joints are similar to those of rheumatoid disease. Sacroiliac erosion is fairly common; if the spine is involved the appearances are identical to those of ankylosing spondylitis.

Ultrasound scanning and *MRI* may show greater definition of the extent and activity of synovitis.

Special investigations

Tests for rheumatoid factor are almost always negative. HLA-B27 occurs in 50–60 per cent, especially in those with overt sacroiliitis.

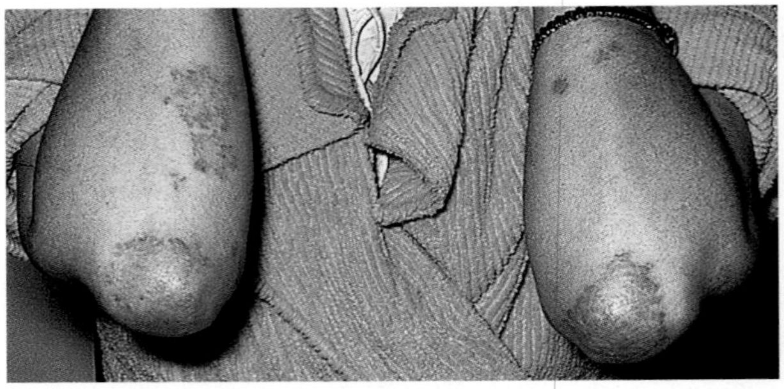

(a)

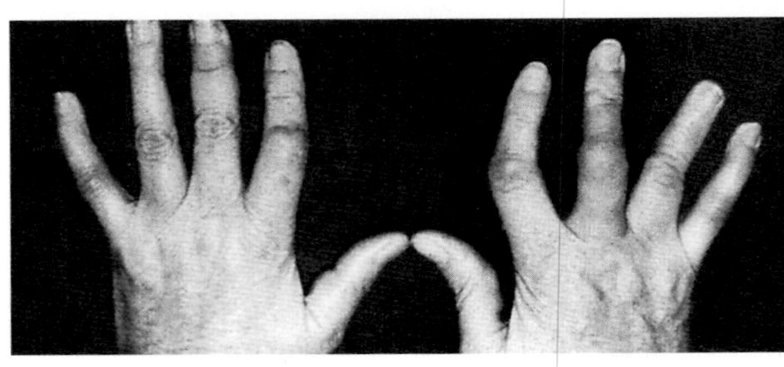

(b)

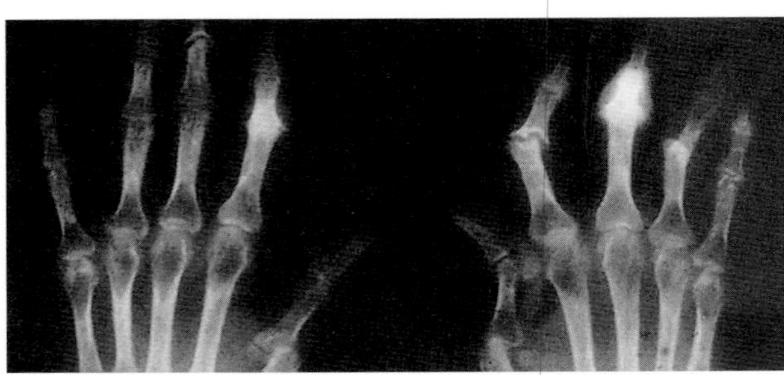

(c)

3.12 Psoriatic arthritis (1) (a) Psoriasis of the elbows and forearms; (b) typical finger deformities, and (c) x-rays show distal joint involvement – clearly the disease is not simply rheumatoid arthritis in a patient with psoriasis.

Diagnosis

The main difficulty is to distinguish 'psoriatic arthritis' from 'psoriasis with seronegative RA'. The important distinguishing features of psoriatic arthritis are: (1) asymmetrical joint distribution; (2) involvement of distal finger joints; (3) the presence of sacroiliitis or spondylitis; and (4) the absence of rheumatoid nodules.

Treatment

In mild disease no more than topical preparations to control the skin disease and NSAIDs for the arthritis are needed. In resistant forms of arthritis, immunosuppressive agents (methotrexate) and TNF inhibitors (infliximab, etanercept and adalimumab) have proved effective.

Surgery may be needed for unstable joints. Arthrodesis of the distal interphalangeal joints may greatly improve function.

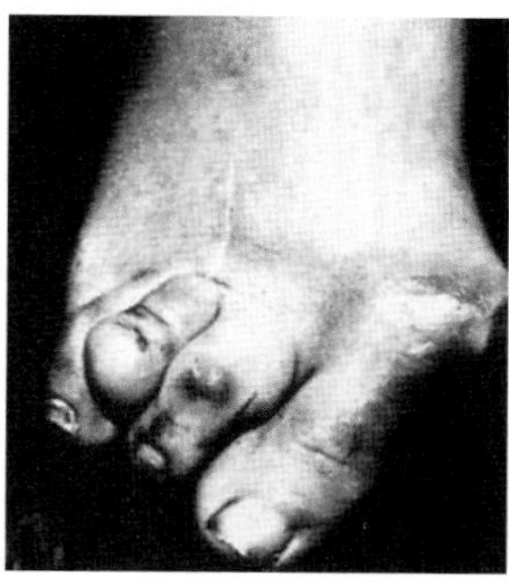

(a)

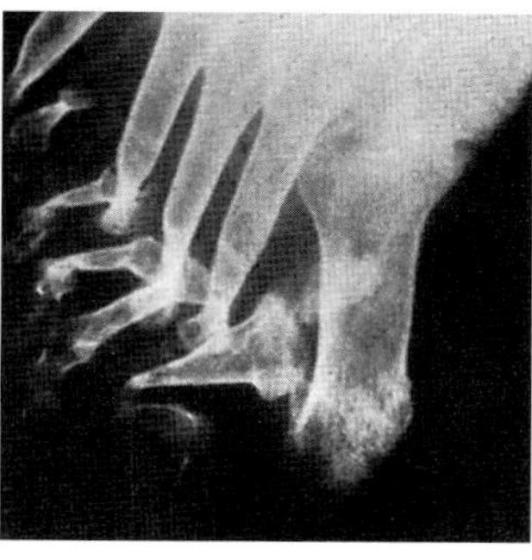

(b)

3.13 Psoriatic arthritis (2) The feet and toes are often involved. In this case the patient developed a severely destructive form of the disease (arthritis mutilans).

ENTEROPATHIC ARTHRITIS

Both Crohn's disease and ulcerative colitis may be associated with either peripheral arthritis or sacroiliitis and spondylitis.

Peripheral arthritis

Peripheral arthritis is fairly common, occurring in about 15 per cent of patients with inflammatory bowel disease. Typically one or perhaps a few of the larger joints are involved. Pain and swelling may appear quite suddenly and last for 2–3 months before subsiding. Synovitis is usually the only feature but joint erosion can occur. Men and women are affected with equal frequency and there is no particular association with HLA-B27.

Treatment is directed at the underlying disorder: attacks of arthritis are often triggered by a flare-up of bowel disease and when the latter is brought under control the arthritis can disappear. Anti-inflammatory drugs should not generally be used as they may have a deleterious effect on the bowel disease. Other treatment options are local corticosteroid injection and disease-modifying treatments such as methotrexate. This may also improve the bowel disease. In severe cases TNF inhibitors may be needed.

Sacroiliitis and spondylitis

This pattern is seen in about 10 per cent of patients with inflammatory bowel disease, and in half of these patients the clinical picture closely resembles that of ankylosing spondylitis. HLA-B27 is positive in 60 per cent and there is an increased incidence of ankylosing spondylitis in close relatives. Unlike the peripheral arthritis, sacroiliitis shows no temporal relationship to gastrointestinal inflammation and its course is unaffected by treatment of the bowel disease. Management is the same as that of ankylosing spondylitis.

Complications

In addition to spondyloarthritis, there are several unusual but important complications of inflammatory bowel disease that may confuse the clinical picture.

Septic arthritis of the hip Infection may spread directly from the bowel. The patient presents with a fever and pain in the groin. Hip movements are limited and there may be swelling due to an abscess. Treatment is by antibiotics and operative drainage.

Psoas abscess In Crohn's disease a posterior fistula may track into the psoas sheath. The patient complains of back pain and may develop a typical psoas abscess with pain in the hip, limitation of movement and a tender mass in the groin. Treatment is by operative drainage of the abscess.

Osteopaenia Patients with chronic bowel disease often develop osteoporosis and osteomalacia – partly due to malabsorption and partly as a consequence of treatment with corticosteroids. Compression fractures of the spine may cause severe back pain.

JUVENILE IDIOPATHIC ARTHRITIS

Juvenile idiopathic arthritis (JIA) is the preferred term for non-infective inflammatory joint disease of more than 3 months' duration in children under 16 years of age. It embraces a group of disorders in all of which pain, swelling and stiffness of the joints are common features. The prevalence is about 1 per 1000 children, and boys and girls are affected with equal frequency.

The cause is similar to that of rheumatoid arthritis: an abnormal immune response to some antigen in children with a particular genetic predisposition. However, rheumatoid factor is usually absent.

The pathology, too, may be like that of rheumatoid arthritis: primarily a synovial inflammation leading to fibrosis and ankylosis. Stiffening tends to occur in whatever position the joint is allowed to assume; thus flexion deformities are a common and characteristic feature. Chronic inflammation and alterations in the local blood supply may affect the epiphyseal growth plates, leading to both local bone deformities and an overall retardation of growth. However, cartilage erosion is less marked than in rheumatoid arthritis and severe joint instability is uncommon.

Clinical features

Children with JIA present in several characteristic ways. About 15 per cent have a *systemic illness*, and arthritis only develops somewhat later; the majority (60–70 per cent) have a *pauciarticular arthritis*

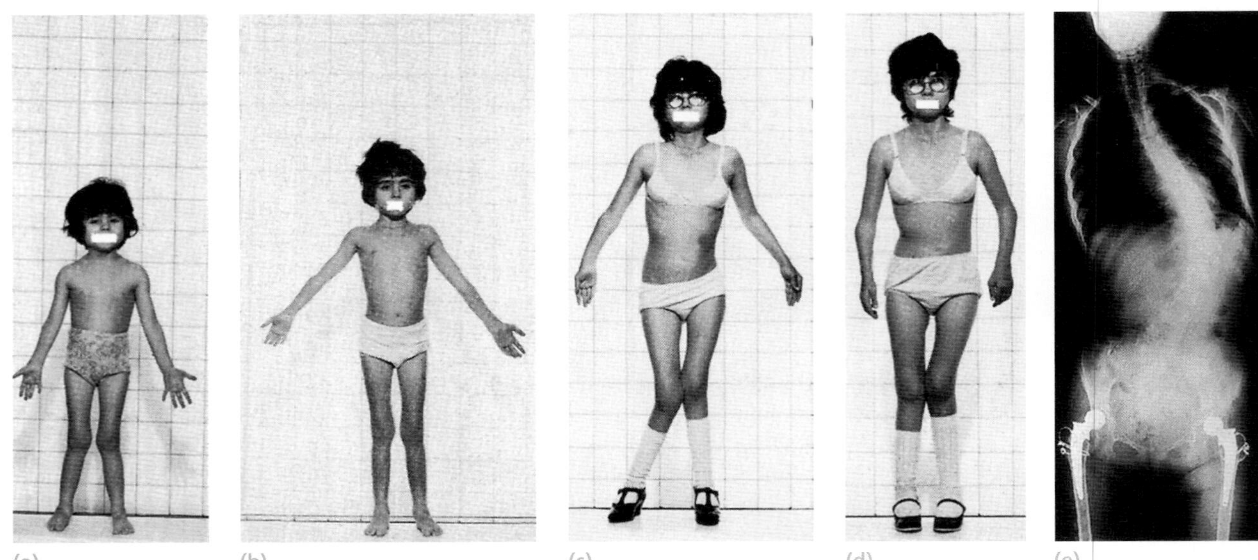

(a) (b) (c) (d) (e)

3.14 Juvenile idiopathic arthritis (a–d) This young girl developed JIA when she was 5 years old. Here we see her at 6, 9 and 14 years of age. The arthritis has become inactive, leaving her with a knee deformity which was treated by osteotomy. Her eyes, too, were affected by iridocyclitis. (Courtesy of Mr Malcolm Swann and Dr Barbara Ansell). (e) X-ray of another young girl who required hip replacements at the age of 14 years and, later, surgical correction of her scoliosis.

affecting a few of the larger joints; about 10 per cent present with *polyarticular arthritis*, sometimes closely resembling RA; the remaining 5–10 per cent develop a *seronegative spondyloarthritis*.

SYSTEMIC JIA

This, the classic *Still's disease*, is usually seen below the age of 3 years and affects boys and girls equally. It starts with intermittent fever, rashes and malaise; during these episodes, which occur almost daily, the child appears to be quite ill but after a few hours the clinical condition improves again. Less constant features are lymphadenopathy, splenomegaly and hepatomegaly. Joint swelling occurs some weeks or months after the onset; fortunately, it usually resolves when the systemic illness subsides but it may go on to progressive seronegative polyarthritis, leading to permanent deformity of the larger joints and fusion of the cervical apophyseal joints. By puberty there may be stunting of growth, often abetted by the earlier use of corticosteroids.

PAUCIARTICULAR JIA

This is by far the commonest form of JIA. It usually occurs below the age of 6 years and is much more common in girls; occasionally older children are affected. Only a few joints are involved and there is no systemic illness. The child presents with pain and swelling of medium-sized joints (knees, ankles, elbows and wrists); sometimes only one joint is affected. Rheumatoid factor tests are negative but antinuclear antibodies (ANA) may be positive. A serious complication is chronic iridocyclitis, which occurs in about 50 per cent of patients. The arthritis often goes into remission after a few years but by then the child is left with asymmetrical deformities and growth defects that may be permanent.

POLYARTICULAR JIA

Polyarticular arthritis, typically with involvement of the temporomandibular joints and the cervical spine, is usually seen in older children, mainly girls. The hands and wrists are often affected, but the classic deformities of rheumatoid arthritis are uncommon and rheumatoid factor is usually absent. In some cases, however, the condition is indistinguishable from adult rheumatoid arthritis, with a positive rheumatoid factor test; these probably warrant the designation 'juvenile rheumatoid arthritis'.

SERONEGATIVE SPONDYLOARTHROPATHY

In older children – usually boys – the condition may take the form of sacroiliitis and spondylitis; hips and knees are sometimes involved as well. Tests for HLA-B27 are often positive and this should probably be regarded as 'juvenile ankylosing spondylitis'.

X-rays

In early disease non-specific changes such as soft-tissue swelling may be seen, but x-ray is mainly useful to exclude other painful disorders. Later there may be signs of progressive joint erosion and deformity.

Investigations

The white cell count and ESR are markedly raised in systemic JIA, less so in the other forms. Rheumatoid factor tests are positive only in juvenile RA. Joint aspiration and synovial fluid examination may be essential to exclude infection or haemarthrosis.

Diagnosis

In the early stages, before chronic arthritis is fully established, diagnosis may be difficult. Systemic JIA may start with an illness resembling a viral infection. Pauciarticular JIA, especially if only one joint is involved, is indistinguishable from *Reiter's disease* or *septic arthritis* (if the signs are acute) or *tuberculous synovitis* (if they are more subdued).

Other conditions that need to be excluded are *rheumatic fever*, one of the *bleeding disorders* and *leukaemia*.

In most cases the problem is resolved once the full pattern of joint involvement is established, but blood investigations, joint aspiration and synovial biopsy may be required to clinch the diagnosis.

Treatment

General treatment Systemic treatment is similar to that of rheumatoid arthritis, including the use of second-line drugs such as hydroxychloroquine, sulfasalazine or low-dose methotrexate for those with seropositive juvenile RA. Corticosteroids should be used only for severe systemic disease and for chronic iridocyclitis unresponsive to topical therapy. Severe inflammatory disease may need to be treated with cytokine inhibitors such as anti-TNF therapies.

Children and parents alike need sympathetic counselling to help them cope with the difficulties of social adjustments, education and training.

Local treatment The priorities are to prevent stiffness and deformity. Night splints may be useful for the wrists, hands, knees and ankles; prone lying for some period of each day may prevent flexion contracture of the hips. Between periods of splinting, active exercises are encouraged; these are started by the physiotherapist but the parents must be taught how to continue the programme.

Fixed deformities may need correction by serial plasters or by a spell in hospital on a continuous passive motion (CPM) machine; when progress is no longer being made, joint capsulotomy may help. For painful eroded joints, useful procedures include custom-designed arthroplasties of the hip and knee (even in children), and arthrodesis of the wrist or ankle.

Complications

Ankylosis While most patients recover good function, some loss of movement is common. Hips, knees and elbows may be unable to extend fully, and in the spondylitic form of JIA the spine, hips and knees may be almost rigid. Temporomandibular ankylosis and stiffness of the cervical spine can make general anaesthesia difficult and dangerous.

Growth defects There is a general retardation of growth, aggravated by prolonged corticosteroid therapy. In addition, epiphyseal disturbances lead to characteristic deformities: external torsion of the tibia, dysplasia of the distal ulna, underdevelopment of the mandible, shortness of the neck and scoliosis.

Fractures Children with chronic joint disease may suffer osteoporosis and they are prone to fractures.

Iridocyclitis This is most common in ANA-positive pauciarticular disease; untreated it may lead to blindness.

Amyloidosis In children with longstanding active disease there is a serious risk of amyloidosis, which may be fatal.

Prognosis

Fortunately, most children with JIA recover from the arthritis and are left with only moderate deformity and limitation of function. However, 5–10 per cent (and especially those with juvenile rheumatoid arthritis) are severely crippled and require treatment throughout life.

A significant number of children with JIA (about 3 per cent) still die – usually as a result of renal failure due to amyloidosis, or following overwhelming infection.

CONNECTIVE TISSUE DISEASES

This term is applied to a group of closely related conditions that have features which overlap with those of rheumatoid arthritis. Like RA, these are 'autoimmune disorders', probably triggered by environmental exposures, such as viral infections, in genetically predisposed individuals. They include systemic lupus erythematosus, scleroderma, Sjögren's syndrome, polymyositis, dermatomyositis and a number of overlap syndromes with features of more than one disease.

SYSTEMIC LUPUS ERYTHEMATOSUS (SLE)

Systemic lupus occurs mainly in young females and may be difficult to differentiate from RA. Although joint pain is usual, it is often overshadowed by systemic symptoms such as malaise, anorexia, weight loss and fever. Characteristic clinical features are skin rashes (especially the 'butterfly rash' of the face), Raynaud's phenomenon, peripheral vasculitis, splenomegaly, and disorders of the kidney, heart, lung, eye and central nervous system. Anaemia, leucopaenia and elevation of the ESR are common. Tests for ANA are usually positive.

Treatment Corticosteroids are indicated for severe systemic disease and may have to be continued for life. Progressive joint deformity is unusual and the arthritis can almost always be controlled.

Complications A curious complication of SLE is avascular necrosis (usually of the femoral head). This may be due in part to the corticosteroid treatment, but the disease itself seems to predispose to bone ischaemia, possibly as a manifestation of the antiphospholipid (Hughes) syndrome which sometimes accompanies SLE.

REFERENCES AND FURTHER READING

Deighton CM, George E, Kiely PDW, Ledingham, J *et al.* Updating the British Society for Rheumatology guidelines for anti-tumour necrosis factor therapy in adult rheumatoid arthritis (again). *Rheumatology* 2006; **45:** 649–52.

Kennedy T, McCabe C, Struthers G, *et al.* BSR guidelines on standards of care for persons with rheumatoid arthritis. *Rheumatology* 2005; **44:** 553–6

Manadan AM, James N, Block JA. New therapeutic approaches for spondyloarthritis. *Curr Opin Rheumatol* 2007; **19:** 259–64.

Scott DL, Kingsley GH. Tumor necrosis factor inhibitors for rheumatoid arthritis. *N Engl J Med* 2006; **355:** 704–12.

Sidiropoulos PI, Hatemi G, Song M, *et al.* Evidence-based recommendations for the management of ankylosing spondylitis: systematic literature search of the 3E Initiative in Rheumatology involving a broad panel of experts and practising rheumatologists. *Rheumatology* 2008; **47:** 355–61.

Crystal deposition disorders

4

Louis Solomon

The crystal deposition disorders are a group of conditions characterized by the presence of crystals in and around joints, bursae and tendons. Although many different crystals are found, three clinical conditions in particular are associated with this phenomenon:

- gout
- calcium pyrophosphate dihydrate (CPPD) deposition disease
- calcium hydroxyapatite (HA) deposition disorders.

Characteristically, in each of the three conditions, crystal deposition has three distinct consequences: (1) it may be totally *inert and asymptomatic*; (2) it may induce an *acute inflammatory reaction*; or (3) it may result in *slow destruction* of the affected tissues.

GOUT

Gout is a disorder of purine metabolism characterized by hyperuricaemia, deposition of monosodium urate monohydrate crystals in joints and peri-articular tissues and recurrent attacks of acute synovitis. Late changes include cartilage degeneration, renal dysfunction and uric acid urolithiasis.

The clinical disorder was known to Hippocrates and its association with hyperuricaemia was recognized well over 100 years ago. The prevalence of symptomatic gout varies from 1 to over 10 per 1000, depending on the race, sex and age of the population studied: it is much commoner in Caucasian than in Negroid peoples; it is more widespread in men than in women (the ratio may be as high as 20:1); and it is rarely seen before the menopause in females.

Although the risk of developing clinical features of gout increases with increasing levels of serum uric acid, only a fraction of those with hyperuricaemia develop symptoms. However, 'hyperuricaemia' and 'gout' are generally regarded as part and parcel of the same disorder.

Pathology

Hyperuricaemia Nucleic acid and purine metabolism normally proceeds, through complex pathways, to the production of hypoxanthine and xanthine; the final breakdown to uric acid is catalysed by the enzyme xanthine oxidase. Monosodium urate appears in ionic form in all the body fluids; about 70 per cent is derived from endogenous purine metabolism and 30 per cent from purine-rich foods in the diet. It is excreted (as uric acid) mainly by the kidneys and partly in the gut.

Urate is poorly soluble, with a plasma saturation value of only 7 mg/dL (0.42 mmol/L). This concentration is commonly exceeded in normal individuals and epidemiological studies have identified entire populations (for example the Maoris of New Zealand) who have unusually high levels of serum uric acid. The term 'hyperuricaemia' is therefore generally reserved for individuals with a serum urate concentration which is significantly higher than that of the population to which they belong (more than two standard deviations above the mean); this is about 0.42 mmol/L for men and 0.35 mmol/L for women in western Caucasian peoples. By this definition, about 5 per cent of men and less than 1 per cent of women have hyperuricaemia; the majority suffer no pathological consequences and they remain asymptomatic throughout life.

Gout Urate crystals are deposited in minute clumps in connective tissue, including articular cartilage; the commonest sites are the small joints of the hands and feet. For months, perhaps years, they remain inert. Then, possibly as a result of local trauma, the needle-like crystals are dispersed into the joint and the surrounding tissues where they excite an acute inflammatory reaction. Individual crystals may be phagocytosed by synovial cells and polymorphs or may float free in the synovial fluid.

With the passage of time, urate deposits may build up in joints, peri-articular tissues, tendons and bursae;

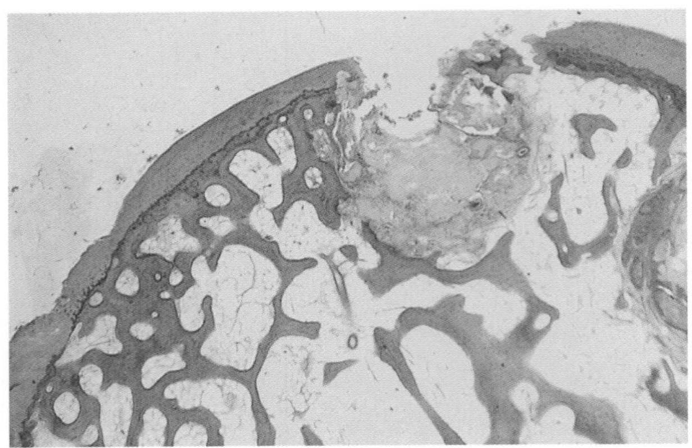

4.1 Gout - pathology Histological section through a gouty MTP joint, showing the urate tophus occupying a cavity in the articular surface.

Table 4.1 Some factors predisposing to hyperuricaemia

Older age, male gender
Genetic enzyme defects, hyperparathyroidism
Haemolytic disorders, myeloproliferative disorders
Obesity, diabetes, hypertension
High consumption of red meat, hyperlipidaemia
Chronic inflammatory diseases
Long-term use of aspirin or diuretics
Alcohol abuse

common sites are around the metatarsophalangeal joints of the big toes, the Achilles tendons, the olecranon bursae and the pinnae of the ears. These clumps of chalky material, or tophi (L. *tophus* = porous stone), vary in size from less than 1 mm to several centimetres in diameter. They may ulcerate through the skin or destroy cartilage and peri-articular bone.

Classification

Gout is often classified into 'primary' and 'secondary' forms. *Primary gout* (95 per cent) occurs in the absence of any obvious cause and may be due to constitutional under-excretion (the vast majority) or overproduction of urate. *Secondary gout* (5 per cent) results from prolonged hyperuricaemia due to acquired disorders such as myeloproliferative diseases, administration of diuretics or renal failure.

This division is somewhat artificial; people with an initial tendency to 'primary' hyperuricaemia may develop gout only when secondary factors are introduced – for example obesity, alcohol abuse, or treatment with diuretics or salicylates which increase tubular reabsorption of uric acid.

Clinical features

Patients are usually men over the age of 30 years; women are seldom affected until after the menopause. Often there is a family history of gout.

The gouty stereotype is obese, rubicund, hypertensive and fond of alcohol. However, many patients have none of these attributes and some are nudged into an attack by the uncontrolled administration of diuretics or aspirin.

THE ACUTE ATTACK

The sudden onset of severe joint pain which lasts for a week or two before resolving completely is typical of acute gout. The attack usually comes out of the blue but may be precipitated by minor local trauma, operation, intercurrent illness, unaccustomed exercise or alcohol consumption. The commonest sites are the metatarsophalangeal joint of the big toe, the ankle and finger joints, and the olecranon bursa. Occasionally, more than one site is involved. The skin looks red and shiny and there is considerable swelling. The joint feels hot and extremely tender, suggesting a cellulitis or septic arthritis. Sometimes the only feature is acute pain and tenderness in the heel or the sole. Hyperuricaemia is present at some stage, though not necessarily during an acute attack. However, while a low serum uric acid makes gout unlikely, hyperuricaemia is not 'diagnostic' and is often seen in normal middle-aged men.

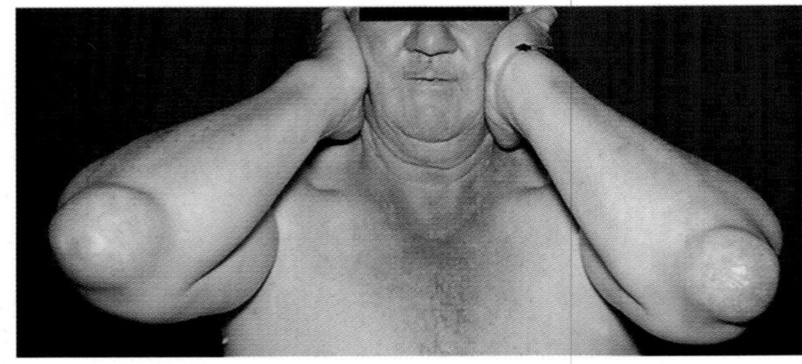

(a)

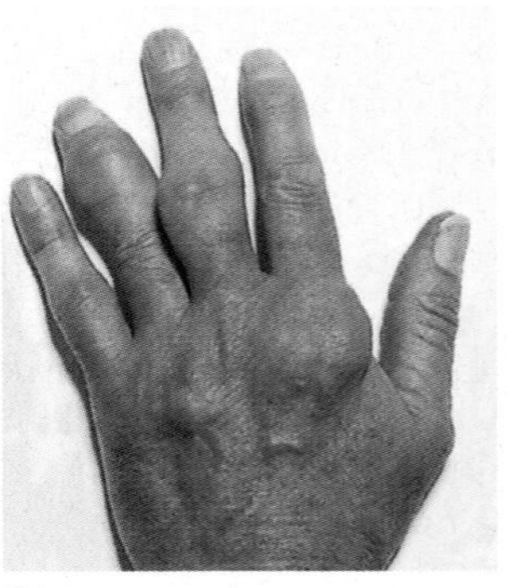

(b)

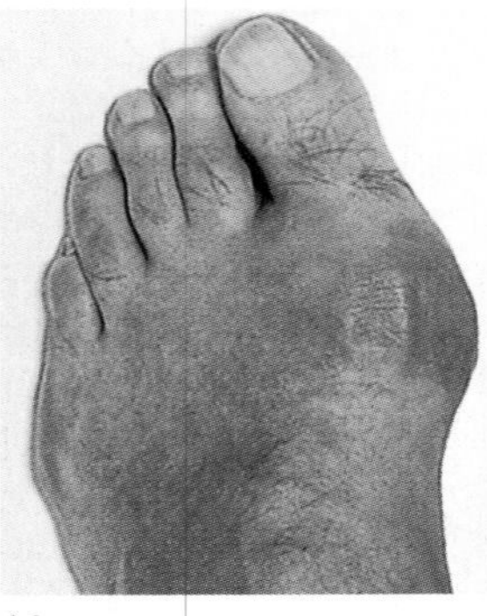

(c)

4.2 Gout (a) This is the typical 'gouty type', with his rubicund face, large olecranon bursae and small subcutaneous tophi over the elbows. (b,c) Tophaceous gout affecting the hands and feet; the swollen big toe joint is particularly characteristic.

The true diagnosis can be established beyond doubt by finding the characteristic negatively birefringent urate crystals in the synovial fluid. A drop of fluid on a glass slide is examined by polarizing microscopy. Crystals may be sparse but if the fluid specimen is centrifuged a concentrated pellet may be obtained for examination.

CHRONIC GOUT

Recurrent acute attacks may eventually merge into polyarticular gout. Joint erosion causes chronic pain, stiffness and deformity; if the finger joints are affected, this may be mistaken for rheumatoid arthritis. Tophi may appear around joints over the olecranon, in the pinna of the ear and – less frequently – in almost any other tissue. A large tophus can ulcerate through the skin and discharge its chalky material. Renal lesions include calculi, due to uric acid precipitation in the urine, and parenchymal disease due to deposition of monosodium urate from the blood.

X-rays

During the acute attack x-rays show only soft-tissue swelling. Chronic gout may result in joint space narrowing and secondary osteoarthritis. Tophi appear as characteristic punched-out 'cysts' or deep erosions in the para-articular bone ends; these excavations are larger and slightly further from the joint margin than the typical rheumatoid erosions. Occasionally, bone destruction is more marked and may resemble neoplastic disease (see Fig. 9.1).

Differential diagnosis

Infection Cellulitis, septic bursitis, an infected bunion or septic arthritis must all be excluded, if necessary by immediate joint aspiration. Remember that crystals and sepsis may coexist, so always send fluid for both culture and crystal analysis.

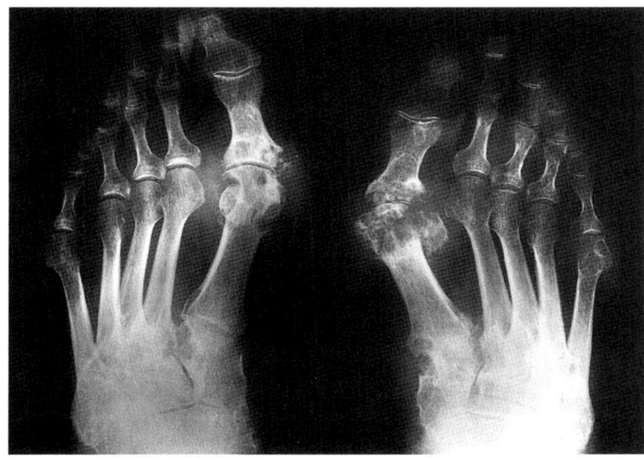

4.3 Gout – x-rays The typical picture is of large periarticular excavations – tophi consisting of uric acid deposits.

Reiter's disease This may present with acute pain and swelling of a knee or ankle, but the history is more protracted and the response to anti-inflammatory drugs less dramatic.

Pseudogout Pyrophosphate crystal deposition may cause an acute arthritis indistinguishable from gout – except that it tends to affect large rather than small joints and is somewhat more common in women than in men. Articular calcification may show on x-ray. Demonstrating the crystals in synovial fluid establishes the diagnosis.

Rheumatoid arthritis (RA) Polyarticular gout affecting the fingers may be mistaken for rheumatoid arthritis, and elbow tophi for rheumatoid nodules. In difficult cases biopsy will establish the diagnosis. RA and gout seldom occur together.

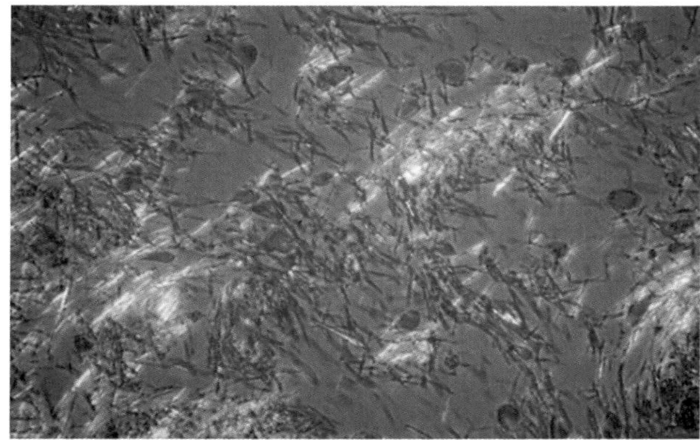

(a)

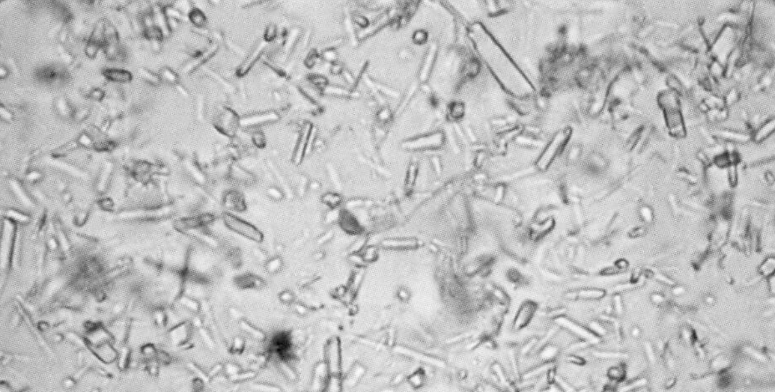

(b)

4.4 Crystals In polarized light, crystals appear bright on a dark background. If a compensator is added to the optical system, the background appears in shades of mauve and birefringent crystals as yellow or blue, depending on their spatial orientation. In these two specimens (obtained from crystal deposits in cartilage) there are differences in shape, size and type of birefringence of the crystals. (a) Urate crystals are needle-like, 5–20 μm long and exhibit strong negative birefringence. (b) Pyrophosphate crystals are rhomboid-shaped, slightly smaller than urate crystals and show weak positive birefringence. (Courtesy of Professor P. A. Dieppe).

Treatment

The acute attack The acute attack should be treated by resting the joint, applying ice packs if pain is severe, and giving full doses of a non-steroidal anti-inflammatory drug (NSAID). Colchicine, one of the oldest of medications, is less effective and may cause diarrhoea, nausea and vomiting. A tense joint effusion may require aspiration and intra-articular injection of corticosteroids. Oral corticosteroids are sometimes used for patients who cannot tolerate NSAIDs or in whom NSAIDs are contraindicated. *The sooner treatment is started the sooner is the attack likely to end.*

Interval therapy Between attacks, attention should be given to simple measures such as losing weight, cutting out alcohol and eliminating diuretics. Urate-lowering drug therapy is indicated if acute attacks recur at frequent intervals, if there are tophi or if renal function is impaired. It should also be considered for asymptomatic hyperuricaemia if the plasma urate concentration is persistently above 6 mg/dL (0.36 mmol/L). However, one must remember that this starts a life-long commitment and many clinicians feel that people who have never had an attack of gout and are free of tophi or urinary calculi do not need treatment.

Uricosuric drugs (probenecid or sulfinpyrazone) can be used if renal function is normal. However, allopurinol, *a xanthine oxidase inhibitor*, is usually preferred, and for patients with renal complications or chronic tophaceous gout allopurinol is definitely the drug of choice.

Urate-lowering drugs should never be started before the acute attack has completely subsided, and they should always be covered by an anti-inflammatory preparation or colchicine, otherwise they may actually prolong or precipitate an acute attack. Patients who suffer an acute attack of gout while already on a constant dose of urate-lowering treatment should be advised to continue taking the drug at the usual dosage while the acute episode is being treated.

Surgery With prolonged urate-lowering therapy, adjusted to maintain a normal serum uric acid level (less than 0.36 mmol/L), tophi may gradually dissolve. However, ulcerating tophi that fail to heal with conservative treatment can be evacuated by curettage; the wound is left open and dressings are applied until it heals.

CALCIUM PYROPHOSPHATE DIHYDRATE ARTHROPATHY (PSEUDOGOUT)

'CPPD deposition' encompasses three overlapping conditions: (1) *chondrocalcinosis* – the appearance of calcific material in articular cartilage and menisci; (2) *pseudogout* – a crystal-induced synovitis; and (3) *chronic pyrophosphate arthropathy* – a type of degenerative joint disease. Any one of these conditions may occur on its own or in any combination with the others (Dieppe et al., 1982). In contrast to classic gout, serum biochemistry shows no consistent abnormality.

CPPD crystal deposition is known to occur in certain metabolic disorders (e.g. hyperparathyroidism and haemochromatosis) that cause a critical change in ionic calcium and pyrophosphate equilibrium in cartilage. The rare familial forms of chondrocalcinosis are probably due to a similar biochemical defect. However, in the vast majority of cases chondrocalcinosis follows some local change in the cartilage due to ageing, degeneration, enzymatic degradation or trauma.

Pathology

The incidence of CPPD arthropathy rises with increasing age; men and women are equally affected and in some cases the disease runs in families

Pyrophosphate is probably generated in abnormal cartilage by enzyme activity at chondrocyte surfaces; it combines with calcium ions in the matrix where crystal nucleation occurs on collagen fibres. The crystals grow into microscopic 'tophi', which appear as nests of amorphous material in the cartilage matrix.

Chondrocalcinosis is most pronounced in fibrocartilaginous structures (e.g. the menisci of the knee, triangular ligament of the wrist, pubic symphysis and intervertebral discs) but may also occur in hyaline articular cartilage, tendons and peri-articular soft tissues. From time to time CPPD crystals are extruded into the joint where they excite *an inflammatory reaction* similar to gout. The longstanding presence of CPPD crystals also appears to influence the development of *osteoarthritis* in joints not usually prone to this condition (e.g. shoulders, elbows and ankles). Characteristically, there is a hypertrophic reaction with marked osteophyte formation. Synovitis is more obvious than in 'ordinary' osteoarthritis.

Clinical features

The clinical disorder takes several forms, all of them appearing with increasing frequency in relation to age.

Asymptomatic chondrocalcinosis Calcification of the menisci is common in elderly people and is usually asymptomatic. When it is seen in association with osteoarthritis, this does not necessarily imply cause and effect. Both are common in elderly people and they are bound to be seen together in some patients; x-rays may reveal chondrocalcinosis in other, asymptomatic, joints. Chondrocalcinosis in patients under

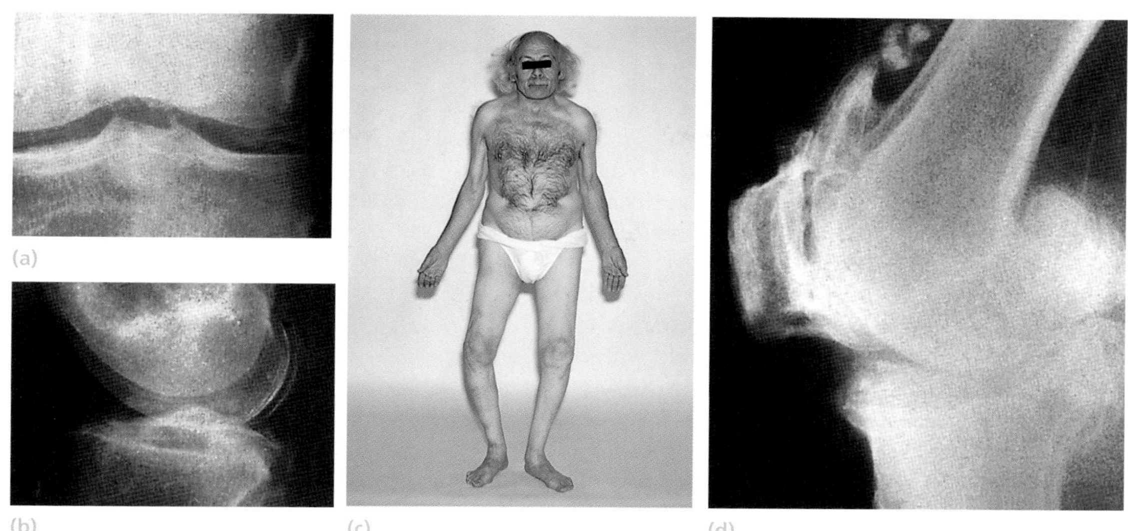

(a) (b) (c) (d)

4.5 Chondrocalcinosis and pyrophosphate arthropathy Calcium pyrophosphate crystals may be deposited in cartilage, causing (a) calcification of menisci and (b) a thin, dense line within the articular cartilage. (c,d) Chronic calcium pyrophosphate arthropathy, on the other hand, is much more serious, as seen in this man who presented with osteoarthritis in several of the larger joints, including unusual sites such as the elbow and ankle. X-ray of the right knee showed the characteristic features of articular calcification, loose bodies in the joint and large trailing osteophytes around the patellofemoral joint.

50 years of age should suggest the possibility of an underlying metabolic disease or a familial disorder.

Acute synovitis (pseudogout) The patient, typically a middle-aged woman, complains of acute pain and swelling in one of the larger joints – usually the knee. Sometimes the attack is precipitated by a minor illness or operation. The joint is tense and inflamed, though usually not as acutely as in gout. Untreated the condition lasts for a few weeks and then subsides spontaneously. *X-rays* may show signs of chondrocalcinosis, and the diagnosis can be confirmed by finding *positively birefringent crystals* in the synovial fluid.

Chronic pyrophosphate arthropathy The patient, usually an elderly woman, presents with polyarticular 'osteoarthritis' affecting the larger joints (hips, knees) and – more helpfully – unusual joints, such as the ankles, shoulders, elbows and wrists where osteoarthritis is seldom seen. There are the usual features of pain, stiffness, swelling, joint crepitus and loss of movement. It is often diagnosed, simply, as 'generalized osteoarthritis', but the x-ray features are distinctive. Sometimes alternating bouts of acute synovitis and chronic arthritis may mimic rheumatoid disease.

X-rays

The characteristic x-ray features arise from a combination of (1) intra-articular and peri-articular calcification, and (2) degenerative arthritis in distinctive sites (Resnick and Resnick, 1983).

GOUT AND PSEUDOGOUT

GOUT	PSEUDOGOUT
Smaller joints	Large joints
Pain intense	Pain moderate
Joint inflamed	Joint swollen
Hyperuricaemia	Chondrocalcinosis
Uric acid crystals	Ca pyrophosphate crystals

Calcification is usually seen in and around the knees, wrists, shoulders, hips, pubic symphysis and intervertebral discs; it is often bilateral and symmetrical. In articular cartilage it appears as a thin line parallel to the joint. In the fibrocartilaginous menisci and discs it produces cloudy, irregular opacities. Less common sites are the joint synovium, capsule, ligaments, tendons and bursae.

Degenerative changes are similar to those of straightforward osteoarthritis but notably involving unusual sites such as the non-weightbearing joints, the isolated patellofemoral compartment in the knee and the talonavicular joint in the foot. In advanced cases joint destruction may be marked, with the formation of loose bodies.

Diagnosis

THE ACUTE ATTACK

'Pseudogout' must be distinguished from other acute inflammatory disorders.

Acute gout usually occurs in men, and typically in smaller joints or in the olecranon bursa. The final word often lies with joint aspiration and identification of the characteristic crystals.

Post-traumatic haemarthrosis can be misleading; pseudogout is often precipitated by trauma. A clear history and aspiration of blood-stained fluid will solve the problem.

Septic arthritis must not be missed; a delay of 24 hours can mean the difference between successful and unsuccessful treatment. Systemic features are more evident, but blood tests and joint aspiration are essential to clinch the diagnosis; joint fluid should be submitted with a request for both crystal analysis and bacteriological culture.

Reiter's disease can start in a single large joint; always enquire about (and look for) signs of conjunctivitis, urethritis and colitis.

CHRONIC CPPD ARTHROPATHY

Chronic pyrophosphate arthropathy usually affects multiple joints and it has to be distinguished from other types of polyarticular arthritis.

Osteoarthritis and joint calcification are both common in older people; the two together do not necessarily make it a CPPD arthropathy. The distinctive x-ray features, and especially the involvement of unusual joints (the elbow, wrist and ankle), point to a CPPD disorder rather than a simple concurrence of two common conditions.

Inflammatory polyarthritis usually involves the smaller joints as well, and systemic features of inflammation are more marked.

Metabolic disorders such as *hyperparathyroidism, haemochromatosis* and *alkaptonuria* may be associated with calcification of articular cartilage and fibrocartilage as well as joint symptoms. It is important to exclude such generalized disorders before labelling a patient as 'just another case of chondrocalcinosis'.

Haemochromatosis is an uncommon disorder of middle-aged people (usually men), resulting from chronic iron overload. The clinical features are those of cirrhosis and diabetes, with a typical bronze pigmentation of the skin. About half of the patients develop joint symptoms (particularly in the hands and fingers); some also have chronic backache. X-rays reveal chondrocalcinosis and a destructive arthropathy, typically in the metacarpophalangeal joints. The plasma iron and iron-binding capacity are raised.

Alkaptonuria is a rare, heritable disorder characterized by the appearance of homogentisic acid in the urine, dark pigmentation of the connective tissues (*ochronosis*) and calcification of hyaline and fibrocartilage. The inborn error is an absence of homogentisic acid oxidase in the liver and kidney. Those affected usually remain asymptomatic until the third or fourth decade when they present with pain and stiffness of the spine and (later) larger joints. There may also be dark pigmentation of the ear cartilage and the sclerae, and clothes may become stained by homogentisic acid in the sweat. X-rays reveal narrowing and calcification of the intervertebral discs at multiple levels, and spinal osteoporosis. At a later stage the large peripheral joints may show chondrocalcinosis and severe osteoarthritis. The feature which gives the condition its name is that the urine turns dark brown when it is alkalinized or if it is left to stand for some hours.

Hyperparathyroidism is described on page 140.

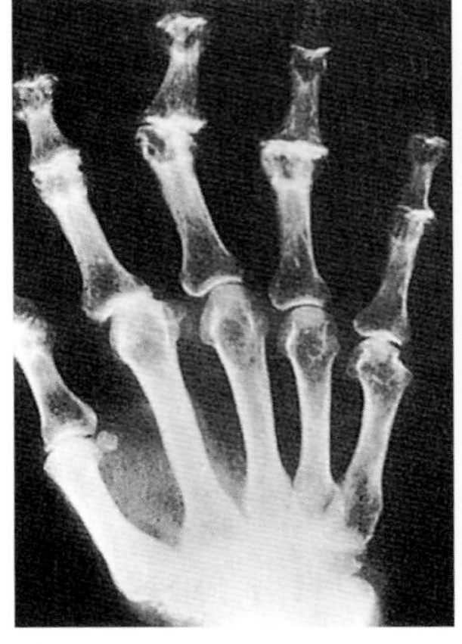

(a)

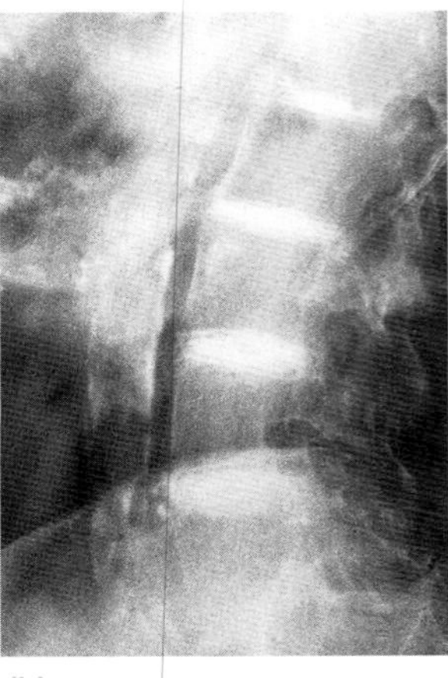

(b)

4.6 Haemochromatosis and alkaptonuria
(a) Haemochromatosis: the degenerative arthritis of the proximal finger joints is typical. (b) Alkaptonuria: the intervertebral discs are calcified – this man has backache.

Treatment

The treatment of *pseudogout* is the same as that of acute gout: rest and high-dosage anti-inflammatory therapy. In elderly patients, joint aspiration and intra-articular corticosteroid injection is the treatment of choice as these patients are more vulnerable to the side effects of non-steroidal anti-inflammatory drugs.

Chronic chondrocalcinosis appears to be irreversible. Fortunately it usually causes few symptoms and little disability. When it is associated with *progressive joint degeneration* the treatment is essentially that of advanced osteoarthritis.

BASIC CALCIUM PHOSPHATE CRYSTAL DEPOSITION DISEASE

Basic calcium phosphate (BCP) is a normal component of bone mineral, in the form of calcium hydroxyapatite crystals. It also occurs abnormally in dead or damaged tissue. Minute deposits in joints and peri-articular tissues can give rise to either an acute reaction (synovitis or tendinitis) or a chronic, destructive arthropathy.

Prolonged hypercalcaemia or hyperphosphataemia, of whatever cause, may result in widespread metastatic calcification. However, by far the most common cause of BCP crystal deposition in and around joints is local tissue damage – strained or torn ligaments, tendon attrition and cartilage damage or degeneration.

Pathology

The minute (less than 1 mm) BCP crystals are deposited around chondrocytes in articular cartilage and in relatively avascular or damaged parts of tendons and ligaments – most notably around the shoulder and knee. The deposits grow by crystal accretion and eventually may be detectable by x-ray in the peri-articular tendons or ligaments. Calcification of the posterior longitudinal ligament of the cervical spine may also be associated with BCP crystal deposition.

Sometimes the calcific deposit has a creamy consistency but in longstanding cases it is more like chalk. The mini-tophus may be completely inert, but in symptomatic cases it is surrounded by an acute vascular reaction and inflammation. Crystal shedding into joints may give rise to synovitis. More rarely this is complicated by the development of a rapidly destructive, erosive arthritis. Bits of articular cartilage and bone or fragments of a meniscus may be found in the synovial cavity.

Clinical features

Two clinical syndromes are associated with BCP crystal deposition: (1) an acute or subacute peri-arthritis; and (2) a chronic rapidly destructive arthritis.

ACUTE OR SUBACUTE PERI-ARTHRITIS

This is by far the commonest form of BCP crystal deposition disorder affecting joints. The patient, usually an adult between 30 and 50 years, complains of pain close to one of the larger joints – most commonly the shoulder or the knee. Symptoms may start suddenly, perhaps after minor trauma, and rise to a crescendo during which the tissues around the joint are swollen, warm and exquisitely tender – but tender near the joint in relation to a tendon or ligament, rather than in the joint.

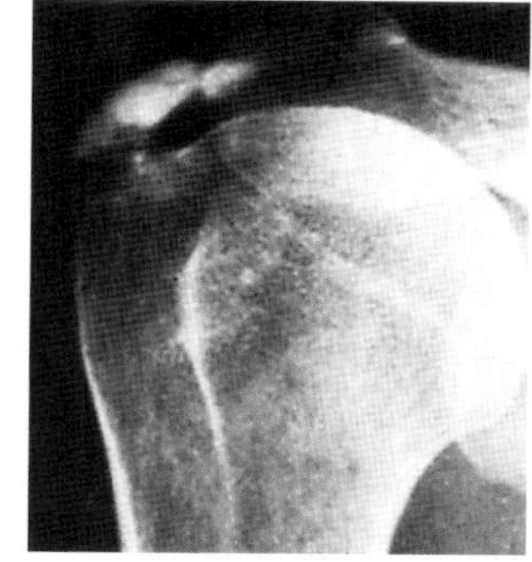

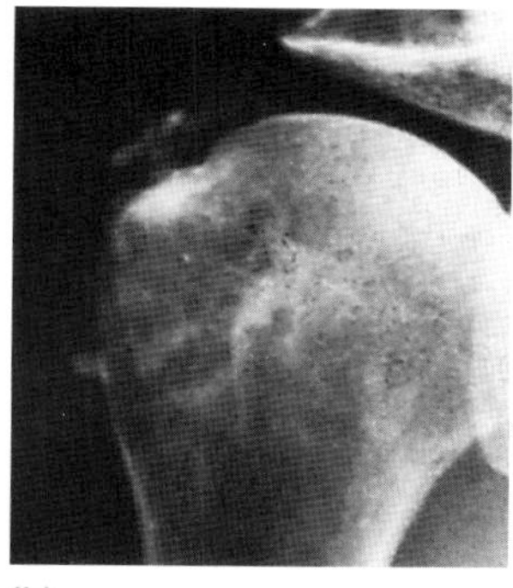

(a) (b)

4.7 Acute calcification of supraspinatus (a) Dense mass in the tendon. (b) Following the 'reaction' some calcium has escaped into the subdeltoid bursa.

At other times the onset is more gradual and it is easier to localize the area of tenderness to one of the peri-articular structures. Both forms of the condition are seen most commonly in rotator cuff lesions of the shoulder. Symptoms usually subside after a few weeks or months; sometimes they are aborted only when the calcific deposit is removed or the surrounding tissues are decompressed. In acute cases, operation may

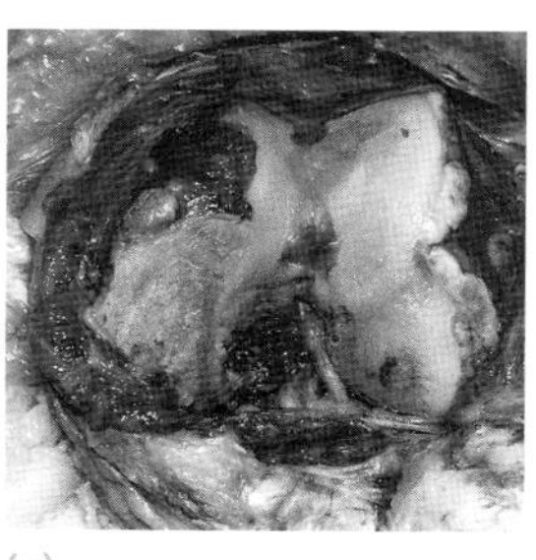

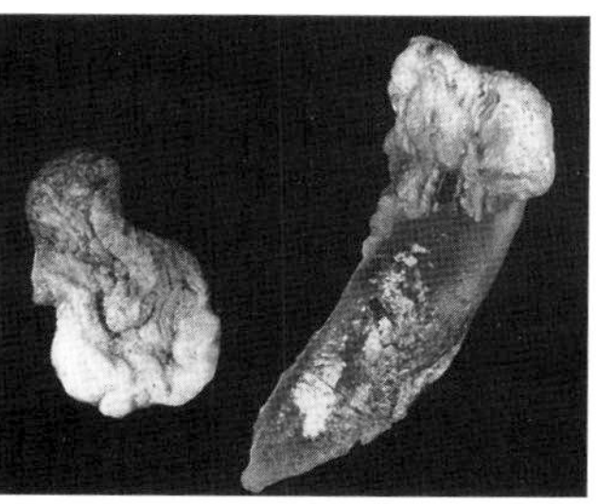

(a) (b)

4.8 BCP destructive arthropathy (a) Knee joint exposed at operation. The articular surface is severely eroded. (b) Fragments of meniscus. Note the white crystalline material on the large meniscal fragment.

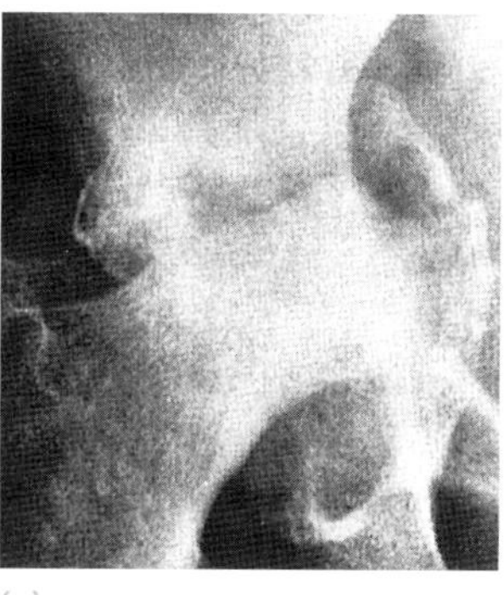

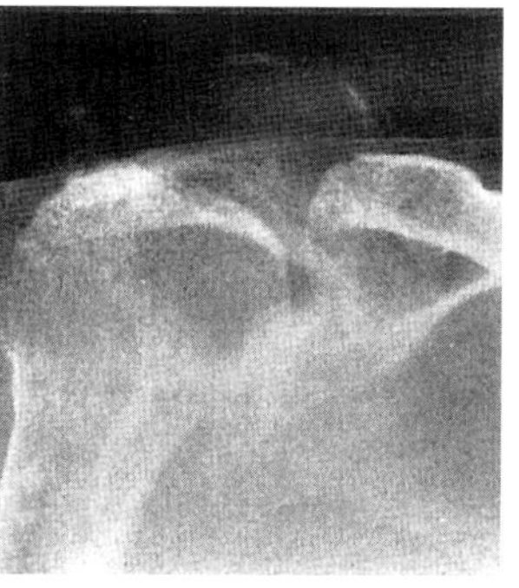

(a) (b)

4.9 Rapidly destructive OA X-rays of two patients with rapidly destructive OA of a large joint, (a) the hip in one and (b) the shoulder in the other. Common features are rapid progression to joint disruption, crumbling of the sub-articular bone and peri-articular ossification.

disclose a tense globule of creamy material oozing from between the frayed fibres of tendon or ligament.

CHRONIC DESTRUCTIVE ARTHRITIS

BCP crystals are sometimes found in association with a chronic erosive arthritis; whether they cause the arthritis or modify a pre-existing disorder remains uncertain.

A more dramatic type of rapidly destructive arthritis of the shoulder is occasionally seen in elderly patients with rotator cuff lesions. This was described in 1981 by McCarty and his colleagues from Milwaukee and acquired the sobriquet 'Milwaukee shoulder'. Similar conditions affect the hip and knee. They have been attributed to BCP crystal (or mixed BCP and CPPD crystal) shedding into the joint.

X-rays

With peri-arthritis, calcification may be seen in tendons or ligaments close to the joint, most commonly in the rotator cuff around the shoulder.

Articular cartilage and fibrocartilaginous menisci and discs never show the type of calcification seen in CPPD deposition disease, but 'loose bodies' may be seen in synovial joints. Erosive arthritis causes loss of the articular space, with little or no sclerosis or osteophyte formation. The typical picture of rapidly destructive arthritis is one of severe erosion and destruction of subchondral bone. In advanced cases the joint may become unstable and, eventually, dislocated.

Investigations

There is little help from special investigations. Serum biochemistry is usually normal, except in those patients with hypercalcaemia or hyperphosphataemia. Synovial fluid examination may reveal high counts of polymorphonuclear leucocytes, but this hardly serves to distinguish the condition from other types of subacute synovitis. BCP crystals are too small to be seen by light microscopy but can be identified by electron probe or transmission electron microscopy.

Treatment

Acute peri-arthritis should be treated by rest and non-steroidal anti-inflammatory drugs. Resistant cases may respond to local injection of corticosteroids; this treatment should be used only to weather the acute storm – repeated injections for lesser pain may dampen the repair process in damaged tendons or ligaments and thus predispose to recurrent attacks. Persistent pain and tenderness may call for operative removal of the calcific deposit or 'decompression' of the affected tendon or ligament.

Erosive arthritis is treated like osteoarthritis. However, rapidly progressive bone destruction calls for early operation: in the case of the shoulder, synovectomy and soft-tissue repair; for the hip, usually total joint replacement.

REFERENCES AND FURTHER READING

Dieppe PA, Alexander GJM., Jones HE, *et al.* Pyrophosphate arthropathy: a clinical and radiological study of 105 cases. *Ann Rheum Dis* 1982; **41:** 371–6.

McCarty DJ, Halverson PB, Carrera GF, *et al.* 'Milwaukee shoulder' – association of microspheroids containing hydroxyapatite crystals, active collagenase and neutral protease with rotator cuff defects. *Arth Rheum* 1981; **24:** 464–73.

Resnick CS, Resnick D. Crystal deposition disease. *Semin Arthritis Rheum* 1983; **12:** 390–403.

Osteoarthritis

5

Louis Solomon

THE PHYSIOLOGY OF SYNOVIAL JOINTS

ARTICULAR CARTILAGE

Hyaline cartilage, the pearly gristle which covers the bone ends in every diarthrodeal joint, is supremely adapted to transmit load and movement from one skeletal segment to another. It increases the area of the articular surfaces and helps to improve their adaptability and stability; it changes its shape under load and distributes compressive forces widely to the subarticular bone; and, covered by a film of synovial fluid, it is more slippery than any man-made material, offering very little frictional resistance to movement and surface gliding.

This specialized connective tissue has a gel-like matrix consisting of a proteoglycan ground substance in which are embedded an architecturally structured collagen network and a relatively sparse scattering of specialized cells, the chondrocytes, which are responsible for producing all the structural components of the tissue. It has a high water content (60–80 per cent), most of which is exchangeable with the synovial fluid.

Chondrocytes of adult hyaline cartilage have little capacity for cell division in vivo and direct damage to the articular surface is poorly repaired, or repaired only with fibrocartilage. The fact that the normal wear of daily joint activity does not result in degradation of the articular surface is due to the highly effective lubricating mechanisms bestowed by synovial fluid. In another sense, though, chondrocytes do undertake repair: in the early stages of cartilage degradation, matrix molecular constituents will be replenished by increased chondrocyte activity.

The proteoglycans exist mainly in the form of aggrecan, a large aggregating molecule with a protein core along which are arranged up to 100 chondroitin sulphate and keratan sulphate glycosaminoglycans (GAGs), rather like the bristles on a bottlebrush.

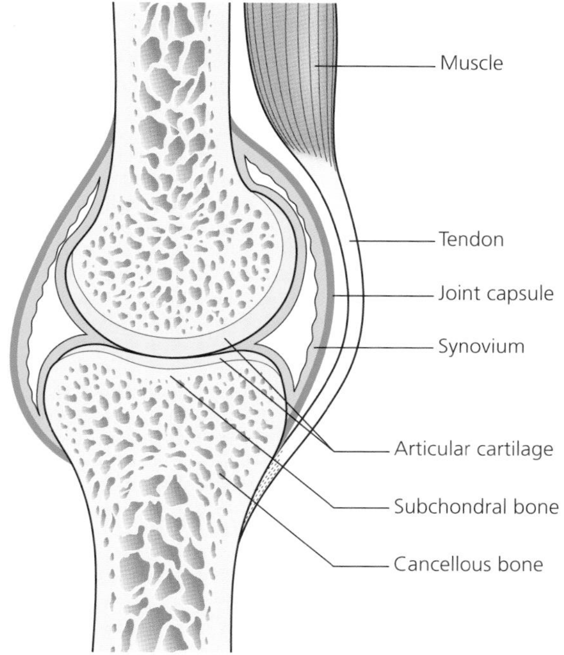

5.1 Diagram showing the components of a synovial joint

Hundreds of aggrecan molecules are linked, in turn, to a long unbranched hyalurinate chain (hyaluronan), to form an even larger molecule with a molecular weight of over 100 million daltons. These negatively charged macromolecules are responsible for the stiffness and springiness of articular cartilage.

The fibrillar component of articular cartilage is mainly type II collagen. The collagen bundles are arranged in structured patterns, parallel to the articular surface in the superficial zones and perpendicular to the surface in the deeper layers where they anchor the articular cartilage to the subchondral bone.

The main functions of aggrecan are to absorb changes in load and mitigate deformation, while the collagen network copes with tensile forces. There is considerable interaction between the molecules of each component and between the molecules of the different components of cartilage: if these links are degraded or broken, the cartilage will tend to unravel. This happens to some degree with ageing, but much more so in pathological states leading to osteoarthritis.

Proteoglycan has a strong affinity for water, resulting in the collagen network being subjected to considerable tensile stresses. With loading, the cartilage deforms and water is slowly squeezed onto the surface where it helps to form a lubricating film. When loading ceases, the surface fluid seeps back into the cartilage up to the point where the swelling pressure in the cartilage is balanced by the tensile force of the collagen network. As long as the network holds and the proteoglycans remain intact, cartilage retains its compressibility and elasticity. If the collagen network is degraded or disrupted, the matrix becomes waterlogged and soft; this, in turn, is followed by loss of proteoglycans, cellular damage and splitting ('fibrillation') of the articular cartilage. Trouble mounts up further as the damaged chondrocytes begin to release matrix-degrading enzymes.

THREATS TO CARTILAGE INTEGRITY
Loss of joint stability
Localized increase in loading stress
Increased stiffness of the cartilage
Inflammatory (enzymatic) degradation
Restriction of free joint movement
Sclerosis in the subchondral bone

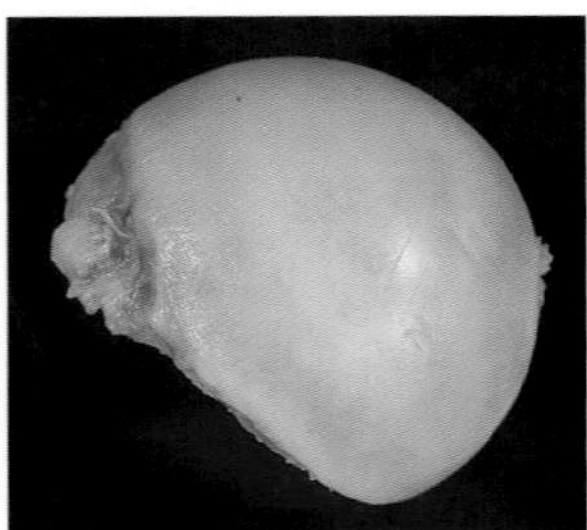

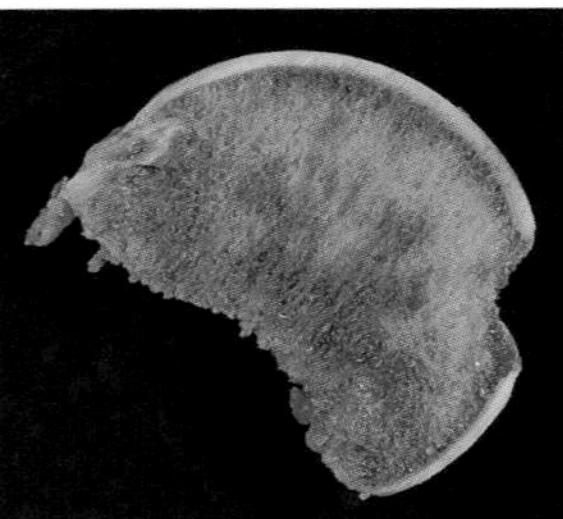

5.2 Normal articular cartilage Normal articular cartilage, smooth and glistening, is well preserved into old age. These specimens were taken from elderly patients with fractures of the femoral neck.

Capsule and ligaments

The soft tissues enclosing the joint consist of a fibrous *capsule* with tough condensations on its surface – the *ligaments* – which, together with the overlying muscles, help to provide stability. The ligaments running from one bone to another are inelastic and have a fixed length. Not surprisingly, therefore, they are under different degrees of tension in different positions of the joint. When the joint assumes a position where the ligaments are fully taut, they provide maximum stability and may keep the joint 'locked' even without the assistance of muscles; when less taut they permit a certain degree of laxity in the joint; and when they are overstretched or torn the joint becomes unstable.

Non-pathological ligamentous laxity is a fairly common heritable trait which is employed to astonishing (and sometimes bizarre) effect by acrobatic performers; stability is maintained by highly developed muscle power and the articular cartilage is not necessarily damaged.

Inflamed or injured joints that need splinting should always be held in the position where the ligaments are fully taut; if the ligaments are allowed to fibrose and shorten in the 'relaxed' position it may take months (or be impossible) to regain full passive movement afterwards.

Synovium and synovial fluid

The interior surface of the capsule is lined by a thin membrane, the synovium, which is richly supplied with blood vessels, lymphatics and nerves. It provides a non-adherent covering for the articular surfaces and it produces synovial fluid, a viscous plasma dialysate laced with hyaluronan. This fluid nourishes the avascular articular cartilage, plays an important part in reducing friction during movement and has slight adhesive properties which assist in maintaining joint stability.

In normal life the volume of synovial fluid in any particular joint remains fairly constant, regardless of movement. When a joint is injured fluid increases (as in any bruised or oedematous connective tissue) and this appears as a joint effusion. Synovium is also the target tissue in joint infections and autoimmune disorders such as rheumatoid arthritis.

MECHANISMS FOR MAINTAINING JOINT STABILITY
Alignment of joint components
Shape and fit of articular surfaces
Adhesive property of synovial fluid
Integrity of capsule and ligaments
Muscle tone and power
Neurological control of balance

Joint lubrication

The coefficient of friction in the normal joint is extremely low – one reason why, barring trauma or disease, there is little difference in the amount of wear on articular surfaces between young adults and old people. This extraordinary slipperiness of cartilage surfaces is produced by a highly efficient combination of lubricating systems.

Boundary layer lubrication at the bearing surfaces is mediated by a large, water soluble glycoprotein fraction, *lubricin*, in the viscous synovial fluid. A single layer of molecules attaches to each articular surface and these glide upon each other in a manner that has been likened to surfaces rolling on miniscule ball-bearings. This is most effective at points of direct contact.

Fluid film lubrication is provided by the hydrodynamic mechanism described earlier (see under Articular cartilage). During movement and loading fluid is squeezed out of the proteoglycan-rich cartilage and forms a thin 'cushion' where contact is uneven, then seeps back into the cartilage when loading ceases.

Lubrication between synovial folds is provided by *hyalurinate* molecules in the synovial fluid.

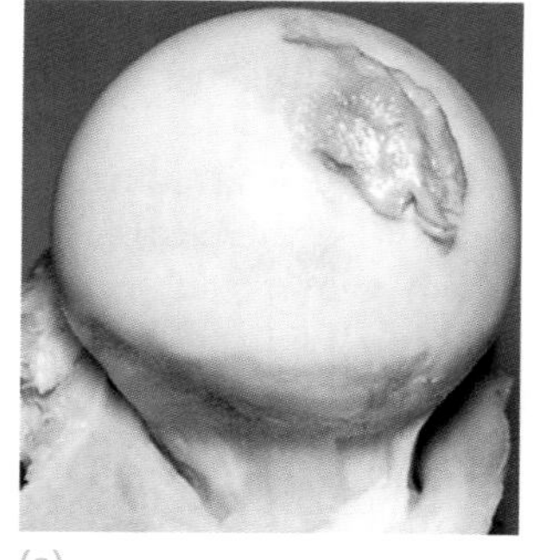

(a)

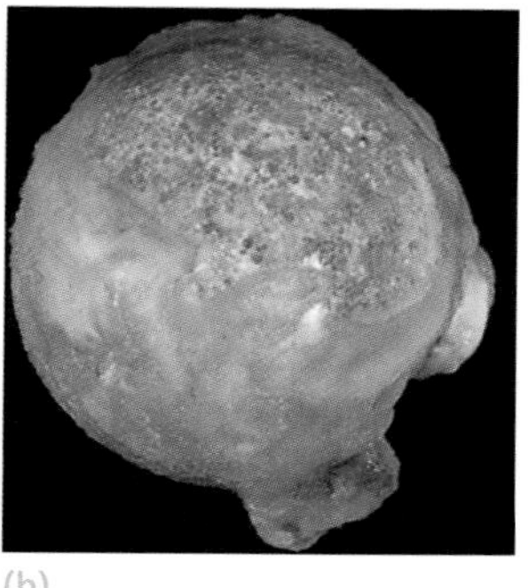

(b)

5.3 Osteoarthritis: non-progressive and progressive (a) Non-progressive OA changes are common in older people; here we see them along the inferomedial edge of the femoral head, while the articular cartilage over the rest of the head looks perfect. (b) Progressive OA changes are seen characteristically in the maximal load-bearing area; in the hip this is the superior part of the joint. Articular cartilage has been destroyed, leaving a bald patch on the dome of the femoral head.

OSTEOARTHRITIS

Osteoarthritis (OA) is a chronic disorder of synovial joints in which there is progressive softening and disintegration of articular cartilage accompanied by new growth of cartilage and bone at the joint margins (osteophytes), cyst formation and sclerosis in the subchondral bone, mild synovitis and capsular fibrosis. It differs from simple wear and tear in that it is asymmetrically distributed, often localized to only one part of a joint and often associated with abnormal loading rather than frictional wear.

In its most common form, it is unaccompanied by any systemic illness and, although there are sometimes local signs of inflammation, it is not primarily an inflammatory disorder.

It is also not a purely degenerative disorder, and the term 'degenerative arthritis' – which is often used as a synonym for OA – is a misnomer. Osteoarthritis is a dynamic phenomenon; it shows features of both destruction and repair. Cartilage softening and disintegration are accompanied from the very outset by hyperactive new bone formation, osteophytosis and remodelling. The final picture is determined by the relative vigour of these opposing processes. In addition, there are various secondary factors which influence the progress of the disorder: the appearance of calcium-containing crystals in the joint; ischaemic changes (especially in elderly people) which result in areas of osteonecrosis in the subchondral bone; the appearance of joint instability; and the effects of prolonged anti-inflammatory medication.

Aetiology

The most obvious thing about OA is that it increases in frequency with age. This does not mean that OA is simply an expression of senescence. Cartilage does 'age', showing diminished cellularity, reduced proteoglycan concentration, loss of elasticity and a decrease in breaking strength with advancing years. These factors may well predispose to OA, but it is significant that the progressive changes which are associated with clinical and radiological deterioration are restricted to certain joints, and to specific areas of those joints, while other areas show little or no progression with age (Byers et al., 1970).

Primary changes in cartilage matrix might (theoretically) weaken its structure and thus predispose to cartilage breakdown; crystal deposition disease and ochronosis are well-known examples.

'Inheritance' has for many years been thought to play a role in the development of OA. A number of studies have demonstrated a significant increase in the prevalence of generalized OA in first-degree relatives of patients with OA as compared with controls (Kellgren, 1963) and others have published similar observations for OA of the hip (Lanyon et al., 2000). However, one should bear in mind that OA of large joints is often attributable to anatomical variations, e.g. acetabular dysplasia and other forms of epiphyseal dysplasia, and it is these that are inherited rather than any tendency to develop OA as a primary abnormality. At the molecular level, genetic defects in type II collagen have been demonstrated in some cases

(Palotie et al., 1989; Knowlton et al., 1990), but it is unlikely that this is a major aetiological factor in the majority of cases.

Articular cartilage may be damaged by trauma or previous inflammatory disorders. Enzymes released by synovial cells and leucocytes can cause leaching of proteoglycans from the matrix, and synovial-derived interleukin-1 (IL-1) may suppress proteoglycan synthesis. This could explain the appearance of 'secondary' OA in patients with rheumatoid diseases; whether similar processes operate in 'primary' ('idiopathic') OA is unknown.

In most cases the precipitating cause of OA is increased mechanical stress in some part of the articular surface. This may be due to increased load (e.g. in deformities that affect the lever system around a joint) or to a reduction of the articular contact area (e.g. with joint incongruity or instability). Both factors operate in varus deformity of the knee and in acetabular dysplasia – common precursors of OA. Changes in the subchondral bone may also increase stress concentration in the overlying cartilage, either by altering the shape of the articular surface or by an increase in bone density (e.g. following fracture healing) which reduces the shock-absorbing effect of the supporting cancellous bone.

From the foregoing outline it should be apparent that the division of osteoarthritis into *'primary'* (when there is no obvious antecedent factor) and *'secondary'* (when it follows a demonstrable abnormality) is somewhat artificial. This is borne out in clinical practice: patients with 'secondary' OA of the knee following meniscectomy have been found also to have a higher than usual incidence of 'primary' OA in other joints (Doherty et al., 1983). Perhaps primary, generalized factors (genetic, metabolic or endocrine) alter the physical properties of cartilage and thereby determine who is likely to develop OA, while secondary factors such as anatomical defects or trauma specify when and where it will occur. OA is, ultimately, more process than disease, occurring in any condition which causes a disparity between the mechanical stress to which articular cartilage is exposed and the ability of the cartilage to withstand that stress.

Pathogenesis

The initial stages of OA have been studied in animal models with induced joint instability and may not be representative of all types of OA.

The earliest changes, while the cartilage is still morphologically intact, are an increase in water content of the cartilage and easier extractability of the matrix proteoglycans; similar findings in human cartilage have been ascribed to failure of the internal collagen network that normally restrains the matrix gel. At a slightly later stage there is loss of proteoglycans and

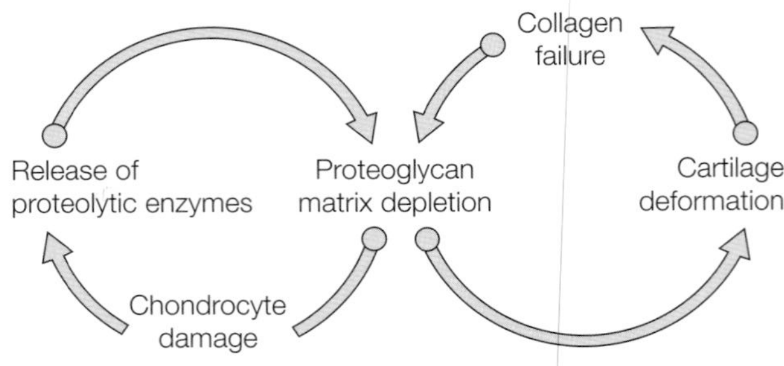

5.4 The cycle of articular cartilage deformation and collagen failure

defects appear in the cartilage. As the cartilage becomes less stiff, secondary damage to chondrocytes may cause release of cell enzymes and further matrix breakdown. Cartilage deformation may also add to the stress on the collagen network, thus amplifying the changes in a cycle that leads to tissue breakdown.

Articular cartilage has an important role in distributing and dissipating the forces associated with joint loading. When it loses its integrity these forces are increasingly concentrated in the subchondral bone. The result: focal trabecular degeneration and cyst formation, as well as increased vascularity and reactive sclerosis in the zone of maximal loading.

What cartilage remains is still capable of regeneration, repair and remodelling. As the articular surfaces become increasingly malapposed and the joint unstable, cartilage at the edges of the joint reverts to the more youthful activities of growth and endochondral ossification, giving rise to the bony excrescences, or osteophytes, that so clearly distinguish osteoarthritis (once called 'hypertrophic arthritis') from 'atrophic' disorders such as rheumatoid disease.

Pathology

The cardinal features are: (1) progressive cartilage destruction; (2) subarticular cyst formation, with (3) sclerosis of the surrounding bone; (4) osteophyte formation; and (5) capsular fibrosis.

Initially the cartilaginous and bony changes are confined to one part of the joint – the most heavily loaded part. There is softening and fraying, or fibrillation, of the normally smooth and glistening cartilage. The term *chondromalacia* (Gr = cartilage softening) seems apt for this stage of the disease, but it is used only of the patellar articular surfaces where it features as one of the causes of anterior knee pain in young people.

With progressive disintegration of cartilage, the underlying bone becomes exposed and some areas may be polished, or burnished, to ivory-like smoothness (eburnation). Sometimes small tufts of fibrocartilage may be seen growing out of the bony surface. At

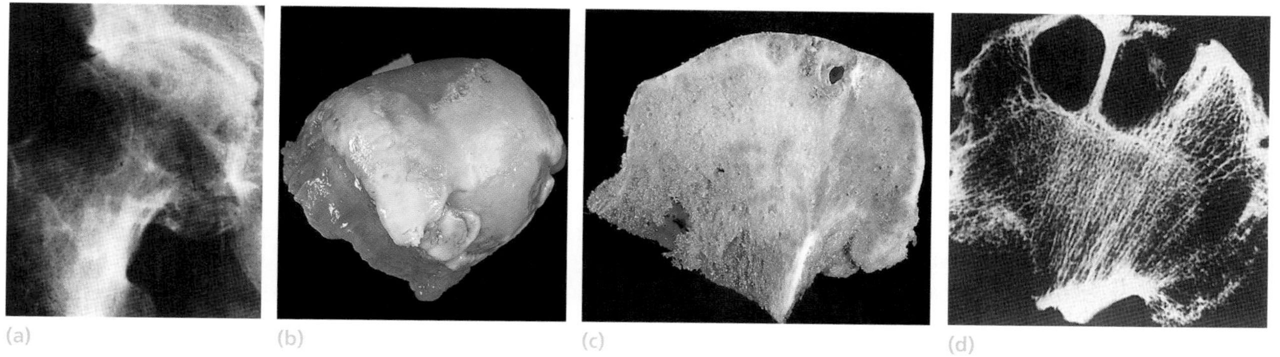

5.5 Osteoarthritis – pathology (a) The x-ray shows loss of articular cartilage at the superior pole and cysts in the underlying bone; the specimen (b) shows that the top of the femoral head was completely denuded of cartilage and there are large osteophytes around the periphery. In the coronal section (c) the subarticular cysts are clearly revealed. (d) A fine-detail x-ray shows the extent of the subarticular bone destruction.

a distance from the damaged area the articular cartilage looks relatively normal, but at the edges of the joint there is remodelling and growth of osteophytes covered by thin, bluish cartilage.

Beneath the damaged cartilage the bone is dense and sclerotic. Often within this area of subchondral sclerosis, and immediately subjacent to the surface, are one or more cysts containing thick, gelatinous material.

The joint capsule usually shows thickening and fibrosis, sometimes of extraordinary degree. The synovial lining, as a rule, looks only mildly inflamed; sometimes, however, it is thick and red and covered by villi.

The *histological appearances* vary considerably, according to the degree of destruction. Early on, the cartilage shows small irregularities or splits in the surface, while in the deeper layers there is patchy loss of metachromasia (obviously corresponding to the depletion of matrix proteoglycans). Most striking, however, is the increased cellularity, and the appearance of clusters, or clones, of chondrocytes – 20 or more to a batch. In later stages, the clefts become more extensive and in some areas cartilage is lost to the point where the underlying bone is completely denuded. The biochemical abnormalities corresponding to these changes were described by Mankin et al. (1971).

The subchondral bone shows marked osteoblastic activity, especially on the deep aspect of any cyst. The cyst itself contains amorphous material; its origin is mysterious – it could arise from stress disintegration of small trabeculae, from local areas of osteonecrosis or from the forceful pumping of synovial fluid through cracks in the subchondral bone plate. As in all types of arthritis, small areas of osteonecrosis are quite common. The osteophytes appear to arise from cartilage hyperplasia and ossification at the edge of the articular surface.

The capsule and synovium are often thickened but cellular activity is slight; however, sometimes there is marked inflammation or fibrosis of the capsular tissues.

A feature of OA that is difficult to appreciate from the morbid anatomy is the marked vascularity and

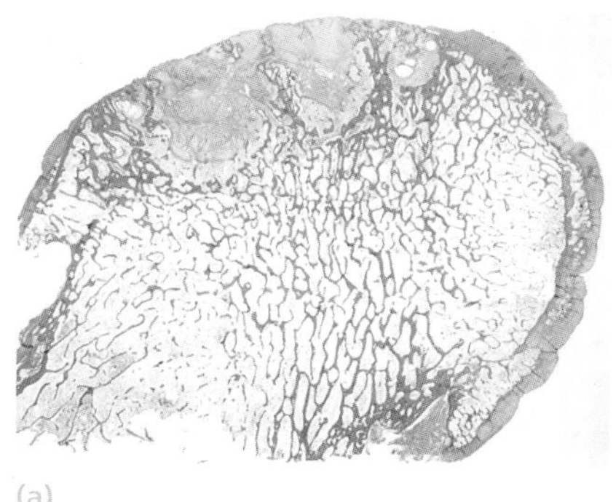

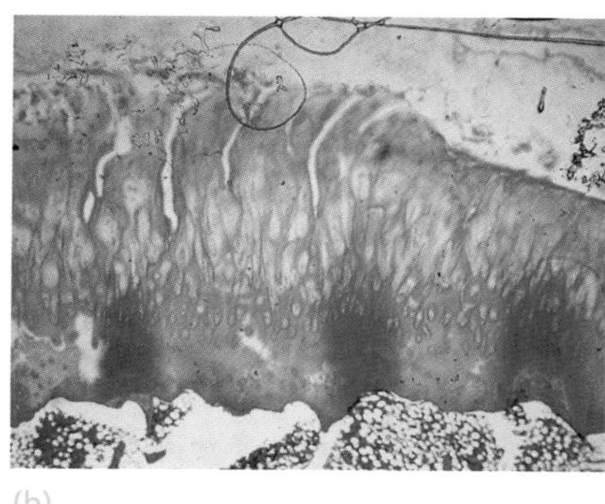

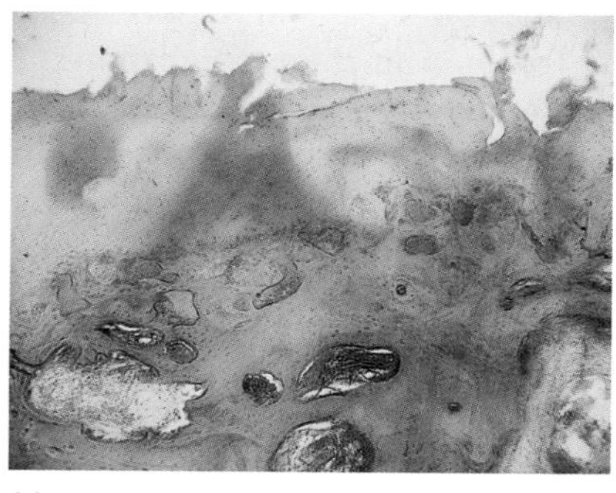

5.6 Osteoarthritis – histology (a) Destructive changes (loss of articular cartilage and cyst formation) are most marked where stress is greatest; reparative changes are represented by sclerosis around the cysts and new bone formation (osteophytes) in less stressed areas. (b) In this high-power view, the articular cartilage shows loss of metachromasia and deep clefts in the surface (fibrillation). Attempts at repair result in (c) subarticular sclerosis and buds of fibrocartilage mushrooming where the articular surface is destroyed.

venous congestion of the subchondral bone. This can be shown by angiographic studies and the demonstration of increased intraosseous pressure. It is also apparent from the intense activity around osteoarthritic joints on radionuclide scanning.

Prevalence

Osteoarthritis is the commonest of all joint diseases. It is a truly universal disorder, affecting both sexes and all races; everyone who lives long enough will have it somewhere, in some degree. However, there are significant differences in its rate of occurrence in different ethnic groups, in the different sexes within any group, and in the different joints.

Reports of prevalence rates vary, depending on the method of evaluation. Autopsy studies show OA changes in everyone over the age of 65 years. Radiographic surveys suggest that the prevalence rises from 1 per cent below the age of 30 years to over 50 per cent in people above the age of 60. Osteoarthritis of the finger joints is particularly common in elderly women, affecting more than 70 per cent of those over 70 years.

Men and women are equally likely to develop OA, but more joints are affected in women than in men.

Osteoarthritis is much more common in some joints (the fingers, hip, knee and spine) than in others (the elbow, wrist and ankle). This may simply reflect the fact that some joints are more prone to predisposing abnormalities than others.

A similar explanation may account for certain geographical and ethnic differences in prevalence. For example, the female-to-male ratio for OA of the hip is about 1:1 in northern Europe but is nearer 2:1 in southern Europe where there is a high incidence of acetabular dysplasia in girls. Even more striking is the virtual absence of hip OA in southern Chinese and African blacks (Hoagland et al., 1973; Solomon, 1976); this may simply be because predisposing disorders such as developmental displacement of the hip, Perthes' disease and slipped femoral epiphysis are uncommon in these populations. That they have no inherent resistance to OA is shown by the fact that they often develop the condition in other joints, for example the knee.

Risk factors

Joint dysplasia Disorders such as congenital acetabular dysplasia and Perthes' disease presage a greater than normal risk of OA in later life. It is not always easy to spot minor degrees of dysplasia and careful studies may have to be undertaken if these are not to be missed.

Trauma Fractures involving the articular surface are obvious precursors of secondary OA, so too lesser injuries which result in joint instability. What is less certain is whether malunion of a long-bone fracture predisposes to OA by causing segmental overload in a joint above or below the healed fracture (for example, in the knee or ankle after a tibial fracture). Contrary to popular belief, research has shown that moderate angular deformities of the tibia (up to 15 degrees) are not associated with an increased risk of OA (Merchant and Dietz, 1989). This applies to mid-shaft fractures; malunion close to a joint may well predispose to secondary OA.

Occupation There is good evidence of an association between OA and certain occupations which cause repetitive stress, for example OA of the knees in workers engaged in knee-bending activities (Felson, 1991), OA in the upper limbs in people working with heavy vibrating tools (Schumacher et al., 1972) and OA of the hands in cotton mill workers (Lawrence, 1961). More controversial is the relationship of OA to sporting activity. Boxers are certainly prone to developing OA of the hands but this may be due to trauma. The same applies to footballers with OA of the knees and baseball pitchers with OA of the shoulder. More convincing evidence of a causative relationship comes from recent studies which have shown a significant increase in the risk of hip and knee OA in athletes (Harris et al., 1994; Kulkala et al., 1994).

Bone density It has long been known that women with femoral neck fractures seldom have OA of the hip. This negative association between OA and osteoporosis is reflected in more recent studies which have demonstrated a significant increase in bone mineral density in people with OA compared to those without (Hannan et al., 1992; Hart et al., 1994). However, this may not be simple cause and effect: bone density is determined by a variety of genetic, hormonal and metabolic factors which may also influence cartilage metabolism independently of any effect due to bone density.

Obesity The simple idea that obesity causes increased joint loading and therefore predisposes to OA may be correct – at least in part. The association is closer in women than in men and therefore (as with bone density) it may reflect other endocrine or metabolic factors in the pathogenesis of OA.

Family history Women whose mothers had generalized OA are more likely to develop the same condition. The particular trait responsible for this is not known (see above under Aetiology).

Symptoms

Patients usually present after middle age. Joint involvement follows several different patterns: symptoms centre either on one or two of the weightbearing joints (hip or knee), on the interphalangeal joints (especially in women) or on any joint that has suffered a previous affliction (e.g. congenital dysplasia, osteonecrosis or intra-articular fracture). A family history is common in patients with polyarticular OA.

Pain is the usual presenting symptom. It is often quite widespread, or it may be referred to a distant site – for example, pain in the knee from OA of the hip. It starts insidiously and increases slowly over months or years. It is aggravated by exertion and relieved by rest, although with time relief is less and less complete. In the late stage the patient may have pain in bed at night. There are several possible causes of pain: mild synovial inflammation, capsular fibrosis with pain on stretching the shrunken tissue; muscular fatigue; and, perhaps most important of all, bone pressure due to vascular congestion and intraosseous hypertension.

Stiffness is common; characteristically it occurs after periods of inactivity, but with time it becomes constant and progressive.

Swelling may be intermittent (suggesting an effusion) or continuous (with capsular thickening or large osteophytes).

Deformity may result from capsular contracture or joint instability, but be aware that the deformity may actually have preceded and contributed to the onset of OA.

Loss of function, though not the most dramatic, is often the most distressing symptom. A limp, difficulty in climbing stairs, restriction of walking distance, or progressive inability to perform everyday tasks or enjoy recreation may eventually drive the patient to seek help.

Typically, the symptoms of OA follow an intermittent course, with periods of remission sometimes lasting for months.

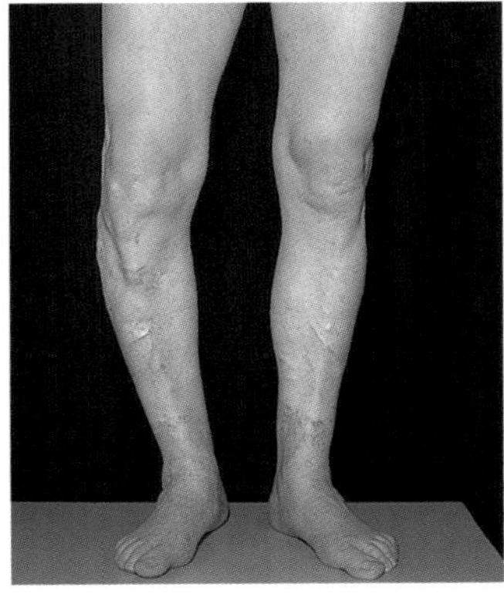

(a)

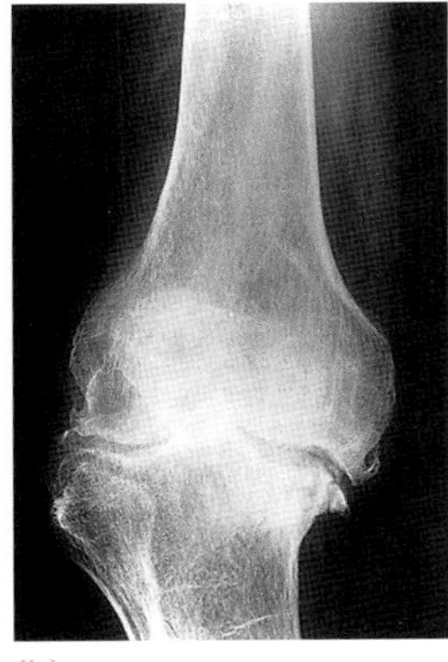

(b)

5.7 Osteoarthritis – clinical and x-ray (a) Varus deformity of the right knee due to osteoarthritis. (b) The x-ray shows the classic features: disappearance of the joint 'space', subarticular sclerosis and osteophyte formation at the margins of the joint.

Signs

Joint swelling may be the first thing one notices in peripheral joints (especially the fingers, wrists, knees and toes). This may be due to an *effusion*, but hard ('knobbly') ridges around the margins of the distal interphalangeal, the first metatarsophalangeal or knee joints can be just as obvious.

Tell-tale scars denote previous abnormalities, and *muscle wasting* suggests longstanding dysfunction.

Deformity is easily spotted in exposed joints (the knee or the large-toe metatarsophalangeal joint), but deformity of the hip can be masked by postural adjustments of the pelvis and spine.

Local tenderness is common, and in superficial joints fluid, synovial thickening or osteophytes may be felt.

Limited movement in some directions but not others is usually a feature, and is sometimes associated with pain at the extremes of motion.

Crepitus may be felt over the joint (most obvious in the knee) during passive movements.

Instability is common in the late stages of articular destruction, but it may be detected much earlier by special testing. Instability can be due to loss of cartilage and bone, asymmetrical capsular contracture and/or muscle weakness.

Other joints should always be examined; they may show signs of a more generalized disorder. It is also helpful to know whether problems in other joints add to the difficulties in the one complained of (e.g. a stiff lumbar spine or an unstable knee making it more difficult to cope with restricted movement in an osteoarthritic hip).

Function in everyday activities must be assessed. X-ray appearances do not always correlate with either the degree of pain or the patient's actual functional capacity. Can the patient with an arthritic knee walk up and down stairs, or rise easily from a chair? Does he or she limp? Or use a walking stick?

Detailed examination of specific joints is dealt with in Section 2 of the book.

Imaging

X-rays X-ray appearances are so characteristic that other forms of imaging are seldom necessary for ordinary clinical assessment. The cardinal signs are asymmetrical loss of cartilage (narrowing of the 'joint space'), sclerosis of the subchondral bone under the area of cartilage loss, cysts close to the articular surface, osteophytes at the margins of the joint and remodelling of the bone ends on either side of the joint. Late features may include joint displacement and bone destruction.

Look carefully for signs of previous disorders (e.g. congenital defects, old fractures, Perthes' disease or rheumatoid arthritis). Such cases are usually designated

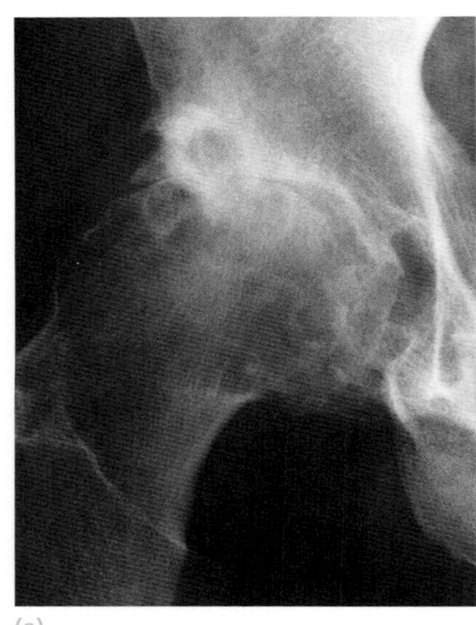
(a)

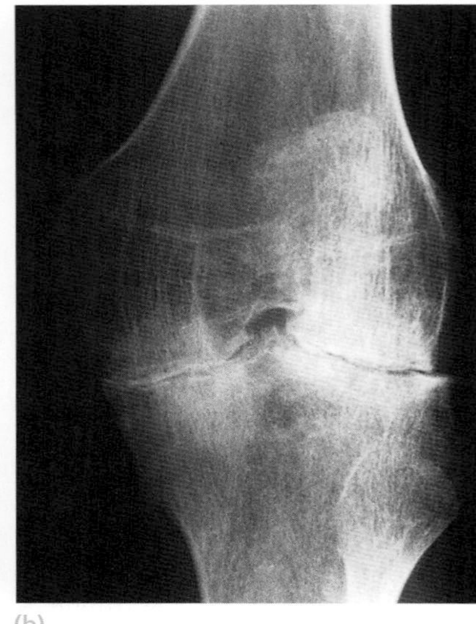
(b)

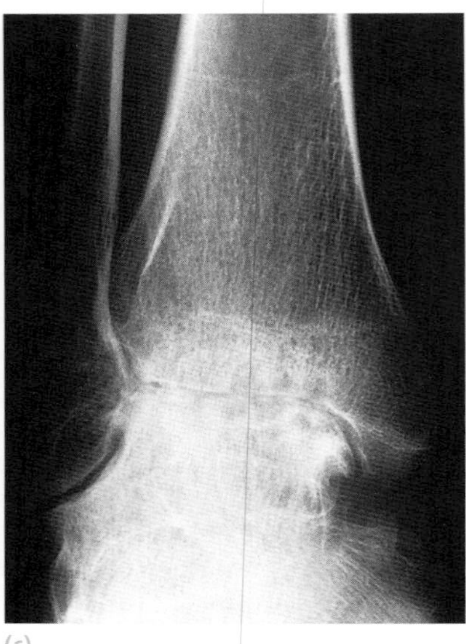
(c)

5.8 Osteoarthritis – x-rays The cardinal features of osteoarthritis are remarkably constant whether in (a) the hip, (b) the knee or (c) the ankle: loss of articular cartilage seen as narrowing of the 'joint space', subarticular cyst formation and sclerosis, osteophyte formation and bone remodelling.

THE CARDINAL SIGNS OF OSTEOARTHRITIS

Narrowing of the 'joint space'

Subchondral sclerosis

Marginal osteophytes

Subchondral cysts

Bone remodelling

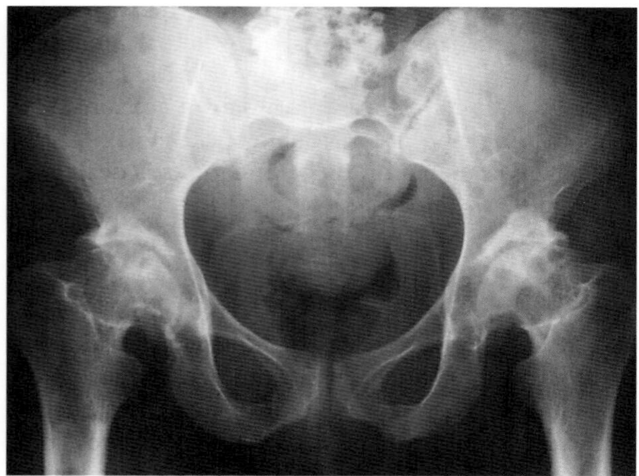

5.9 Secondary osteoarthritis The flattened femoral heads and shortened femoral necks are tell-tale signs of multiple epiphyseal dysplasia in this patient with secondary OA. Her mother had an almost identical x-ray picture.

as *'secondary osteoarthritis'*, though in a certain sense OA is always secondary to some previous abnormality if only we could discover what it was!

Radionuclide scanning Scanning with ^{99m}Tc-HDP shows increased activity during the bone phase in the subchondral regions of affected joints. This is due to increased vascularity and new bone formation.

CT and MRI Advanced imaging is sometimes needed to elucidate a specific problem, e.g. early detection of an osteocartilaginous fracture, bone oedema or avascular necrosis. These methods are also used for severity grading in clinical trials.

Arthroscopy

Arthroscopy may show cartilage damage before x-ray changes appear. The problem is that it reveals too much, and the patient's symptoms may be ascribed to chondromalacia or OA when they are, in fact, due to some other disorder.

Natural history

Osteoarthritis usually evolves as a slowly progressive disorder. However, symptoms characteristically wax and wane in intensity, sometimes disappearing for several months.

The x-rays show no such fluctuation. However, there is considerable variation between patients in the degrees of destruction and repair. Most of the men and half of the women have a *hypertrophic* reaction, with marked sclerosis and large osteophytes. In about 20 per cent of cases – most of them women – reactive changes are more subdued, inviting descriptions such as *atrophic* or *osteopaenic* OA. Occasionally OA takes the form of a *rapidly progressive* disorder (Solomon, 1976; Solomon, 1984).

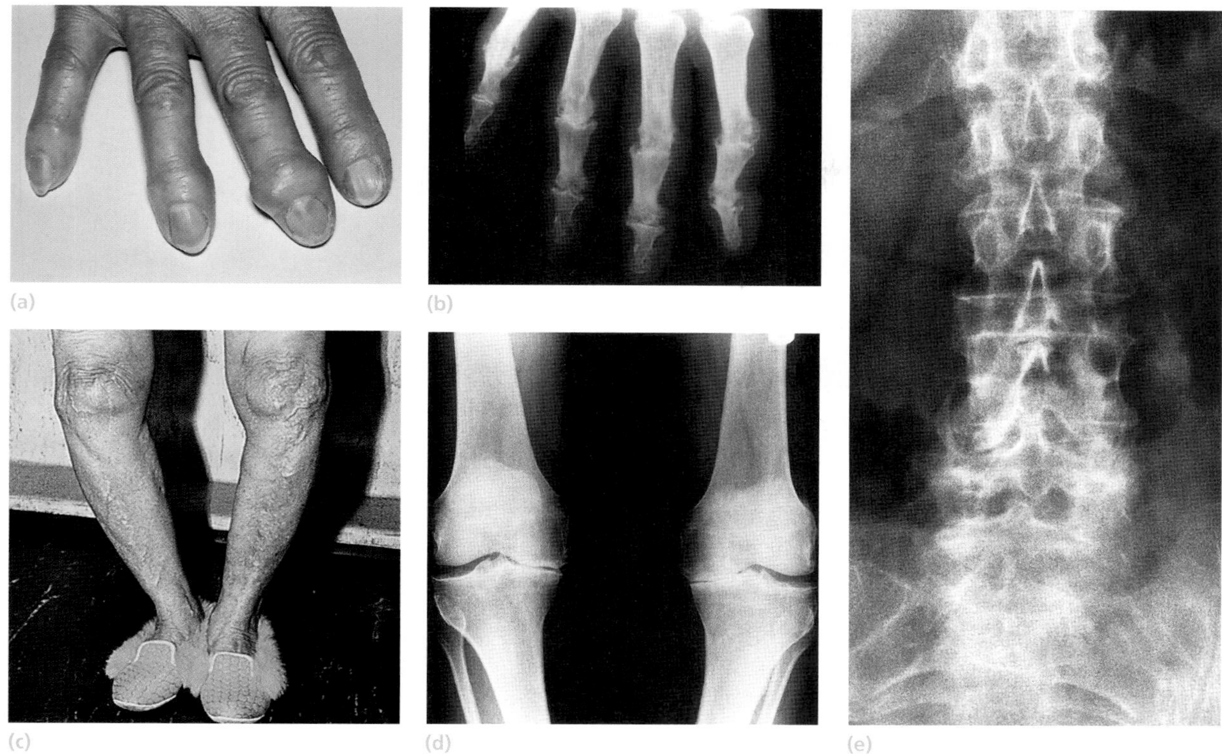

5.10 Polyarticular (generalized) osteoarthritis (a,b) An almost invariable feature of polyarticular OA is involvement of the terminal finger joints – Heberden's nodes. There is a strong association with OA of the knees (c,d) and the lumbar facet joints (e).

Complications

Capsular herniation Osteoarthritis of the knee is sometimes associated with a marked effusion and herniation of the posterior capsule (Baker's cyst).

Loose bodies Cartilage and bone fragments may give rise to loose bodies, resulting in episodes of locking.

Rotator cuff dysfunction Osteoarthritis of the acromioclavicular joint may cause rotator cuff impingement, tendinitis or cuff tears.

Spinal stenosis Longstanding hypertrophic OA of the lumbar apophyseal joints may give rise to acquired spinal stenosis. The abnormality is best demonstrated by CT and MRI.

Spondylolisthesis In patients over 60 years of age, destructive OA of the apophyseal joints may result in severe segmental instability and spondylolisthesis (so-called 'degenerative' spondylolisthesis, which almost always occurs at L4/5).

Clinical variants of osteoarthritis

Although the features of OA in any particular joint are fairly consistent, the overall clinical picture shows variations which define a number of subgroups.

MONARTICULAR AND PAUCIARTICULAR OSTEOARTHRITIS

In its 'classic' form, OA presents with pain and dysfunction in one or two of the large weightbearing joints. There may be an obvious underlying abnormality: multiple epiphyseal dysplasia, localized acetabular dysplasia, old Perthes' disease, previous slipped epiphysis, inflammatory joint disease, avascular necrosis, a previous fracture or damage to ligaments or menisci. In the majority, however, the abnormality is more subtle and may come to light only with special imaging techniques.

POLYARTICULAR (GENERALIZED) OSTEOARTHRITIS

This is by far the most common form of OA, though most of the patients never consult an orthopaedic surgeon. The patient is usually a middle-aged woman who presents with pain, swelling and stiffness of the finger joints. The first carpometacarpal and the big toe metatarsophalangeal joints, the knees and the lumbar facet joints may be affected at more or less the same time.

The changes are most obvious in the hands. The interphalangeal joints become swollen and tender, and in the early stages they often appear to be inflamed. Over a period of years osteophytes and soft-tissue swelling produce a characteristic knobbly

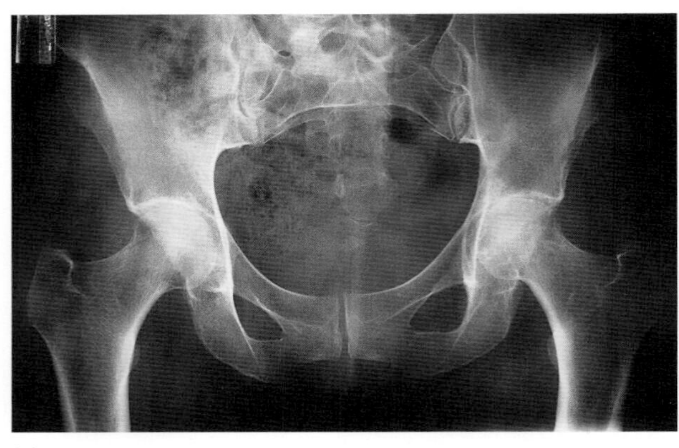

(a)

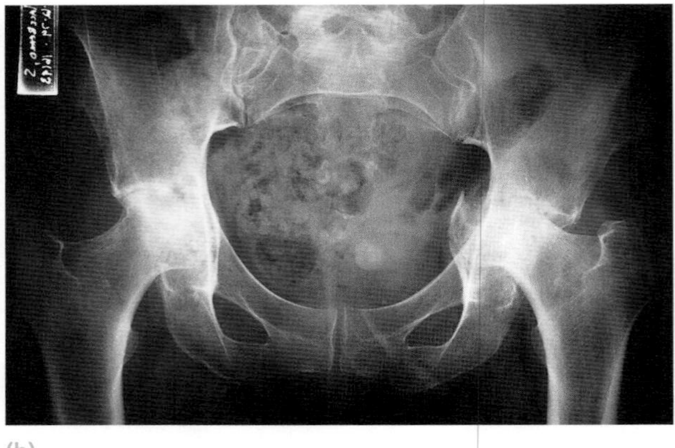

(b)

5.11 Rapidly destructive osteoarthritis (a) X-ray obtained when the patient was first seen, complaining of pain in the left hip. This shows the typical features of an atrophic form of osteoarthritis on the painful side. (b) Eleven months later there is marked destruction of the left hip, with crumbling of both the femoral head and the acetabular floor, and similar features are beginning to appear on the right side.

appearance of the distal interphalangeal joints (Herberden's nodes) and, less often, the proximal interphalangeal joints (Bouchard's nodes); pain may later disappear but stiffness and deformity persist. Some patients present with painful knees or backache and the knobbly fingers are noticed only in passing. There is a strong association with carpal tunnel syndrome and isolated tenovaginitis.

X-rays show the characteristic features of OA, usually maximal in the distal interphalangeal joints of the fingers.

OSTEOARTHRITIS IN UNUSUAL SITES

Osteoarthritis is uncommon in the shoulder, elbow, wrist and ankle. If any of these joints is affected one should suspect a previous abnormality – congenital or traumatic – or an associated generalized disease such as a crystal arthropathy.

RAPIDLY DESTRUCTIVE OSTEOARTHRITIS (see also page 84)

Every so often a patient with apparently straightforward OA shows rapid and startling progression of bone destruction. The condition was at one time thought to be due to the dampening of pain impulses by powerful anti-inflammatory drugs – a notional type of 'analgesic arthropathy'. It is now recognized that it occurs mainly in elderly women and that it is associated with the deposition of calcium pyrophosphate dihydrate crystals, though whether this is the cause of the condition or a consequence thereof is still undecided.

Differential diagnosis of osteoarthritis

A number of conditions may mimic OA, some presenting as a monarthritis and some as a polyarthritis affecting the finger joint.

Avascular necrosis 'Idiopathic' osteonecrosis causes joint pain and local effusion. Early on the diagnosis is made by MRI. Later x-ray appearances are usually pathognomonic; however, once bone destruction occurs the x-ray changes can be mistaken for those of OA. The cardinal distinguishing feature is that in osteonecrosis the 'joint space' (articular cartilage) is preserved in the face of progressive bone collapse and deformity, whereas in OA articular cartilage loss precedes bone destruction.

Inflammatory arthropathies Rheumatoid arthritis, ankylosing spondylitis and Reiter's disease may start in one or two large joints. The history is short and there are local signs of inflammation. X-rays show a predominantly atrophic or erosive arthritis. Sooner or later other joints are affected and systemic features appear.

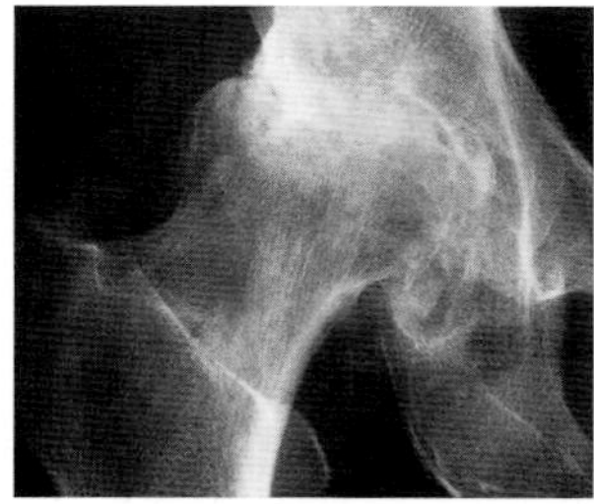

(a)

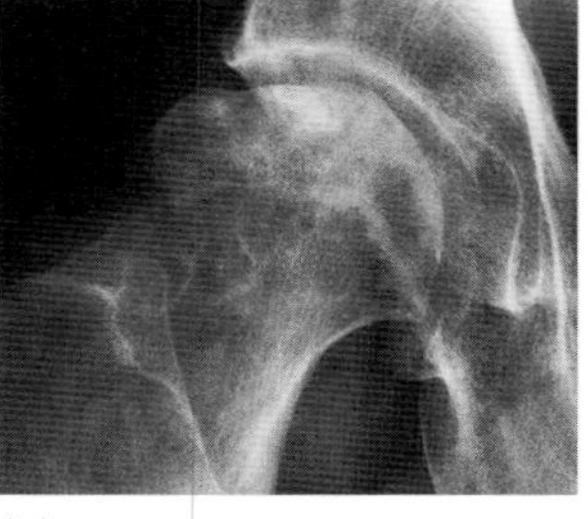

(b)

5.12 Differential diagnosis – osteoarthritis and osteonecrosis (a) Osteoarthritis with marked subarticular bone collapse is sometimes mistaken for osteonecrosis. The clue to the diagnosis is that in OA the articular 'space' (cartilage) is progressively reduced before bone collapse occurs, whereas in primary osteonecrosis (b) articular cartilage is preserved even while the underlying bone crumbles.

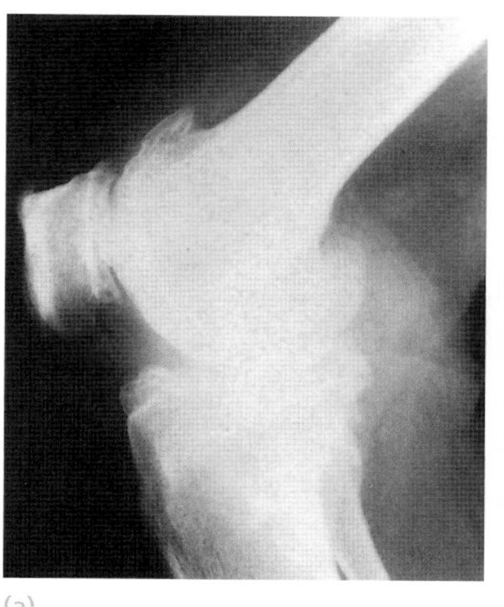
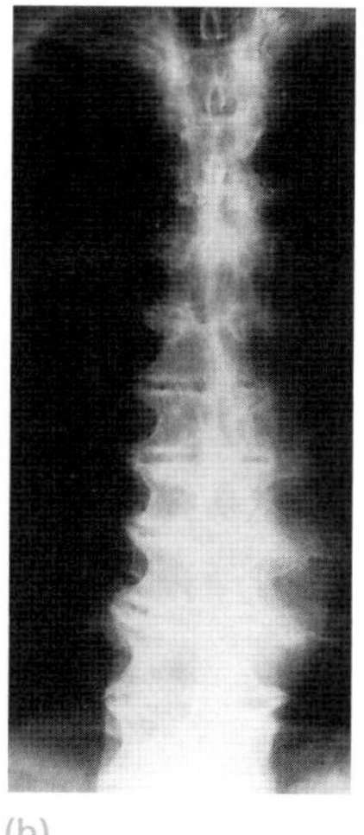

(a) (b)

5.13 Diffuse idiopathic skeletal hyperostosis – DISH (a) The large bony outgrowths around the knee suggest something more than the usual OA. X-rays of the spine (b) show the typical features of DISH. The spinal condition is also known as Forestier's disease.

Polyarthritis of the fingers Polyarticular OA may be confused with other disorders which affect the finger joints (see Fig. 5.10). Close observation shows several distinguishing features. *Nodal OA* affects predominantly the distal joints, *rheumatoid arthritis* the proximal joints. *Psoriatic arthritis* is a purely destructive arthropathy and there are no interphalangeal 'nodes'. *Tophaceous gout* may cause knobbly fingers, but the knobs are tophi, not osteophytes. X-rays will show the difference.

Diffuse idiopathic skeletal hyperostosis (DISH) This is a fairly common disorder of middle-aged people, characterized by bone proliferation at the ligament and tendon insertions around peripheral joints and the intervertebral discs (Resnick et al., 1975). On x-ray examination the large bony spurs are easily mistaken for osteophytes. DISH and OA often appear together, but DISH is not OA: the bone spurs are symmetrically distributed, especially along the pelvic apophyses and throughout the vertebral column. When DISH occurs by itself it is usually asymptomatic.

Multiple diagnosis Osteoarthritis is so common after middle age that it is often found in patients with other conditions that cause pain in or around a joint. Before jumping to the conclusion that the symptoms are due to the OA features seen on x-ray, be sure to exclude peri-articular disorders as well as more distant abnormalities giving rise to referred pain.

Management

The management of OA depends on the joint (or joints) involved, the stage of the disorder, the severity of the symptoms, the age of the patient and his or her functional needs. Three observations should be borne in mind: (1) symptoms characteristically wax and wane, and pain may subside spontaneously for long periods; (2) some forms of OA actually become less painful with the passage of time and the patient may need no more than reassurance and a prescription for pain killers; (3) at the other extreme, the recognition (from serial x-rays) that the patient has a rapidly progressive type of OA may warrant an early move to reconstructive surgery before bone loss compromises the outcome of any operation.

EARLY TREATMENT

There is, as yet, no drug that can modify the effects of OA. Treatment is, therefore, symptomatic. The principles are: (1) maintain movement and muscle strength; (2) protect the joint from 'overload'; (3) relieve pain; and (4) modify daily activities.

Physical therapy The mainstay of treatment in the early case is physical therapy, which should be directed at maintaining joint mobility and improving muscle strength. The programme can include aerobic exercise, but care should be taken to avoid activities which increase impact loading. Other measures, such as massage and the application of warmth, may reduce pain but improvement is short-lived and the treatment has to be repeated.

Load reduction Protecting the joint from excessive load may slow down the rate of cartilage loss. It is also effective in relieving pain. Common sense measures such as weight reduction for obese patients, wearing shock-absorbing shoes, avoiding activities like climbing stairs and using a walking stick are worthwhile.

Analgesic medication Pain relief is important, but not all patients require drug therapy and those who do may not need it all the time. If other measures do not provide symptomatic improvement, patients may respond to a simple analgesic such as paracetamol. If this fails to control pain, a non-steroidal anti-inflammatory preparation may be better.

INTERMEDIATE TREATMENT

Joint debridement (removal of loose bodies, cartilage tags, interfering osteophytes or a torn or impinging acetabular or glenoid labrum) may give some improvement. This may be done either by arthroscopy or by open operation.

If appropriate radiographic images suggest that symptoms are due to localized articular overload arising from joint malalignment (e.g. varus deformity of the knee) or incongruity (e.g. acetabular and femoral head dysplasia), a corrective osteotomy may prevent or delay progression of the cartilage damage. These techniques are discussed in the relevant chapters in Section 2.

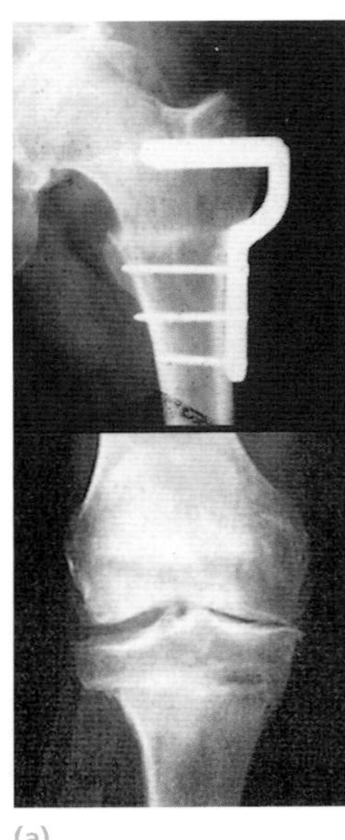
(a)

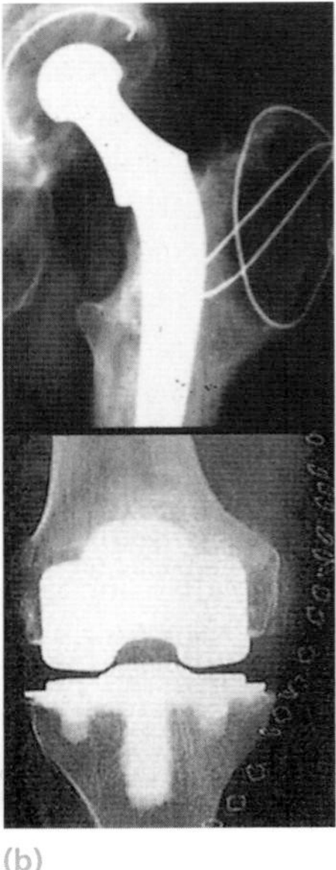
(b)

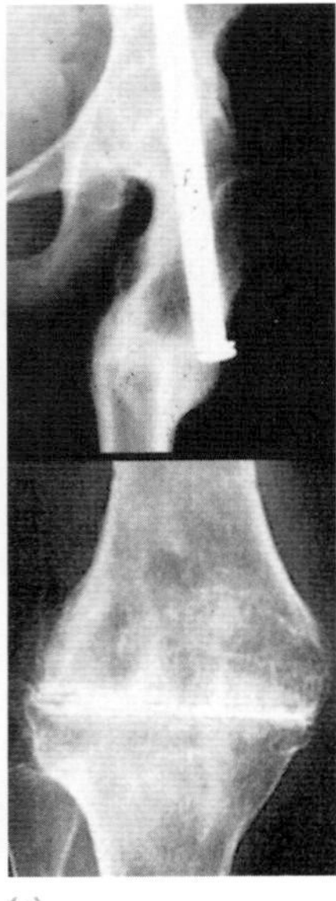
(c)

5.14 Operative treatment The three basic operations: (a) osteotomy, (b) arthroplasty, (c) athrodesis – at the hip.

LATE TREATMENT

Progressive joint destruction, with increasing pain, instability and deformity (particularly of one of the weightbearing joints), usually requires reconstructive surgery. Three types of operation have, at different times, held the field: realignment osteotomy, arthroplasty and arthrodesis.

Realignment osteotomy Until the development of joint replacement surgery in the 1970s, realignment osteotomy was widely employed. Refinements in techniques, fixation devices and instrumentation led to acceptable results from operations on the hip and knee, ensuring that this approach has not been completely abandoned. High tibial osteotomy is still considered to be a viable alternative to partial joint replacement for unicompartmental OA of the knee, and intertrochanteric femoral osteotomy is sometimes preferred for young patients with localized destructive OA of the hip. These operations should be done while the joint is still stable and mobile and x-rays show that a major part of the articular surface (the radiographic 'joint space') is preserved. Pain relief is often dramatic and is ascribed to (1) vascular decompression of the subchondral bone, and (2) redistribution of loading forces towards less damaged parts of the joint. After load redistribution, fibrocartilage may grow to cover exposed bone.

Joint replacement Joint replacement, in one form or another, is nowadays the procedure of choice for OA in patients with intolerable symptoms, marked loss of function and severe restriction of daily activities. For OA of the hip and knee in middle-aged and older patients, total joint replacement by modern techniques promises improvement lasting for 15 years or longer. Similar operations for the shoulder, elbow and ankle are less successful but techniques are improving year by year. However, joint replacement operations are highly dependent on technical skills, implant design, appropriate instrumentation and postoperative care – requirements that cannot always be met, or may not be cost-effective, in all parts of the world.

Arthrodesis Arthrodesis is still a reasonable choice if the stiffness is acceptable and neighbouring joints are not likely to be prejudiced. This is most likely to apply to small joints that are prone to OA, e.g. the carpal and tarsal joints and the large toe metatarsophalangeal joint.

ENDEMIC OSTEOARTHRITIS

Osteoarthritis occasionally occurs as an endemic disorder affecting entire communities. This phenomenon may be due either to an underlying generalized dysplasia in a genetically isolated community or some environmental factor peculiar to that region.

Kashin–Beck disease

In 1859 Kashin, a Russian physician, reported the occurrence of an unusual form of polyarticular osteoarthritis associated with stunted growth in a Siberian population. It is now known that the condition affects large numbers of children and adults (estimates vary from 1 to 6 million!) in the area stretching from Northern China across Eastern Siberia to North Korea (Allander, 1994).

Clinical features

The condition starts in childhood with joint pain and progressive signs of polyarticular swelling, deformity and shortness of stature. Adults with this condition may be severely crippled.

X-rays show distortion of the epiphyses in tubular bones during growth, and increasing signs of osteoarthritis in affected joints during adult life.

Pathogenesis

There is, as yet, no agreement about the aetiology and pathogenesis of this condition. Hypothetical causes that have received the most attention are (a) deficiency of trace elements such as selenium and iodine in the soil and (b) contamination of the staple grain product by mycotoxins during storage. This combination could lead to an accumulation of free radicals and subsequent damage to growing chondrocytes in the exposed community. There are, however, some arguments against a purely environmental causation: first, there is no consistent correlation between local selenium and iodine levels and the prevalence of Kashin–Beck disease; second, the condition may be common in one village and completely absent in another only 30–50 miles away (Allender, 1994). The early radiographic changes appear only in the epiphyses and the adjacent growth plates and not in other parts of the tubular bones which must, at an earlier stage, have consisted largely of cartilage. This, as well as the clinical appearances and the tendency for the condition to appear in familial clusters, are reminiscent of a genetic disorder such as spondylo-epiphyseal dysplasia, a recognized cause of stunted growth, bone deformities and 'secondary' polyarticular OA. The most likely explanation for this endemic disorder is that it is either an expression of a straightforward genetic defect causing a type of chondrodysplasia or that the genetic defect causes an increased susceptibility to the toxic effects of certain trace element deficiencies.

Treatment

There is no specific treatment for this condition. Preventive measures consist mainly of selenium supplementation in children's diet or added to agricultural fertilizer. In iodine-deficient areas, iodine is given as well. Dosage should be monitored since selenium excess can cause unpleasant side effects and, in some cases, severe illness.

Patients with established arthritis will need treatment as for other forms of OA.

Mseleni joint disease

For many years visitors travelling along the eastern seaboard of South Africa have known about a crippling type of polyarticular OA that was common among the Tsonga people living around the Mseleni Mission Station in Northern Zululand (now Kwazulu). The first report in the medical literature appeared in 1970 (Wittman and Fellingham, 1970). Further studies suggested an overall prevalence rate of at least 5 per cent, with women affected more often than men and relatives of affected individuals much more commonly than relatives of unaffected people (Fellingham et al., 1973; Yach and Botha, 1985). A later radiographic survey showed that the polyarthropathy actually comprises two distinct disorders: one with features of multiple epiphyseal dysplasia affecting males and females in equal proportions and another with typical features of protrusio acetabuli occurring almost exclusively in females (Solomon et al., 1986).

Clinical features

In the first group, symptoms such as joint discomfort, slight deformity and stunting of growth start to appear in both boys and girls during childhood. When x-ray changes appear they are those of symmetrically

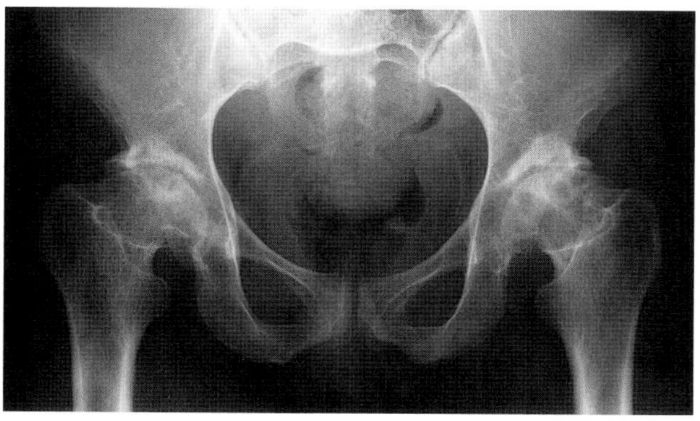

(a)

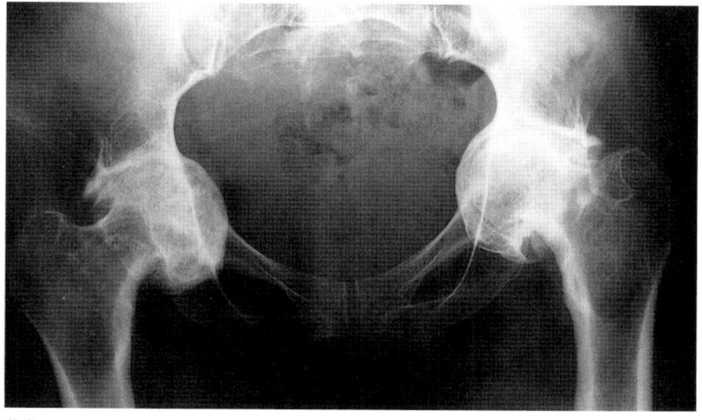

(b)

5.15 Endemic osteoarthritis – Mseleni disease X-rays showing the two forms of osteoarthritis endemic in the African population of eastern Kwazulu: (a) generalized epiphyseal dysplasia and (b) bilateral protrusio acetabuli.

distributed epiphyseal dysplasia affecting particularly the hips, knees and ankles; sometimes the vertebral bodies also develop abnormally. During adulthood the affected joints develop secondary OA: they become painful and swollen, unstable and increasingly deformed.

The second group consists mainly of girls at puberty or a year or two later. Their main complaint is of pain in the hip joints and even at that age x-ray features of early protrusio acetabuli can be discerned. During adulthood those with the most marked changes develop typical features of secondary OA.

Causation

Various studies on the aetiology of Mseleni joint disease have failed to identify a convincing nutritional or other environmental cause for this condition. There seems little doubt that the group with typical features of epiphyseal changes represent a heritable form of multiple epiphyseal dysplasia or spondylo-epiphyseal dysplasia.

It is uncertain whether those with protrusio acetabuli have been fully investigated as a separate entity. However, what is well recognized is that features of calcium deficiency rickets are found in African children from this area (Pettifor, 2008) and that (at least in the past) young girls in Kwazulu were the ones who traditionally were given the work of carrying the loads of water and other foodstuffs needed by their families – often over long distances. Young boys were not expected to do this work. Could this combination of factors affecting girls have caused some distortion of the acetabular socket before closure of the triradiate cartilage? Whether a changing cultural milieu will improve the situation remains to be seen.

Treatment

In the past the people of Mseleni lived as a fairly isolated group without intermarrying among neighbouring peoples and thereby changing the gene pool. As with other endemic disorders, Mseleni disease is in part a social problem and one can expect its prevalence to fall with increasing social mobility and improved living conditions. Meanwhile, patients are treated as are those with other types of OA, i.e. by employing a mixture of analgesic medication, physical therapy and reconstructive surgery where necessary and feasible.

Handigodu joint disease

This is yet another endemic polyosteoarthopathy, similar to that of Mseleni joint disease, which was encountered some 30 years ago in a Dalit community in Handigodu, South-Western India. It evidently starts in childhood and by early adulthood patients appear with painful, swollen joints (mainly the hips and knees), deformities and stunting of growth. In the most severe cases they have great difficulty walking and are reduced to crawling. As with Mseleni joint disease in the past, this community is isolated from the general population and patients appear in family clusters. It is, in all probability, a heritable form of multiple epiphyseal dysplasia.

NEUROPATHIC JOINT DISEASE

Charcot, in 1868, described a type of destructive arthropathy associated with disease of the central nervous system. Almost all his patients had tabes dorsalis, but the name *'Charcot's joint disease'* came to be applied to any destructive arthropathy arising from loss of pain sensibility and position sense.

Nowadays the most common cause is diabetic neuropathy, which occurs in 0.2–0.5 per cent of patients with diabetes mellitus; other causes are tabes dorsalis, leprosy (affecting mainly the lower limb joints), syringomyelia (upper and lower limbs), multiple sclerosis, myelomeningocele, spinal cord compression and congenital indifference to pain. The term is also applied (less accurately) to rapidly destructive forms of osteoarthritis where there is no neurological lesion.

Pathogenesis and pathology

Neuropathic joints lack the normal reflex safeguards against abnormal stress or injury and the subchondral bone disintegrates with alarming speed. Unlike the usual forms of osteoarthritis, this is a mainly destructive condition and there are few signs of repair. Some cases show increased vascularity and osteoclastic activity in the subchondral bone; in others, capsular and ligamentous laxity and joint instability go hand in hand with articular disintegration.

The early changes are similar to those of osteoarthritis. However, it soon becomes apparent that this is a rapidly destructive process; the articular surface breaks up, fragments of bone and cartilage appear in the joint or embedded in the synovium, and there is thickening of the synovial membrane and marked joint effusion. In the late stages, there is complete loss of articular cartilage, fragmentation of the subchondral bone and joint subluxation.

Clinical features

The patient complains of weakness, instability, swelling, laxity and progressive deformity of the joint: usually the tarsal or ankle joints in diabetics, the large

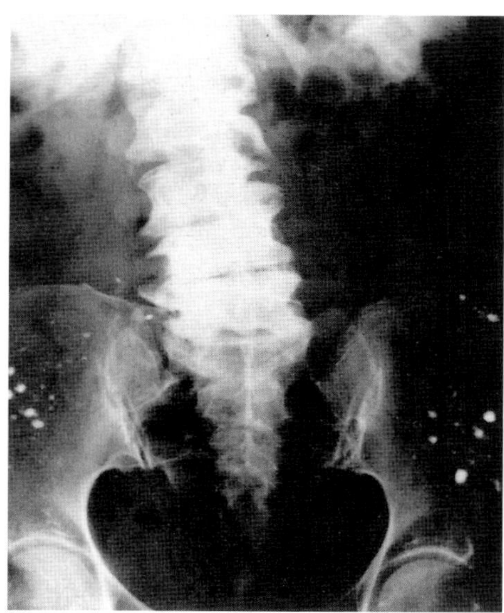
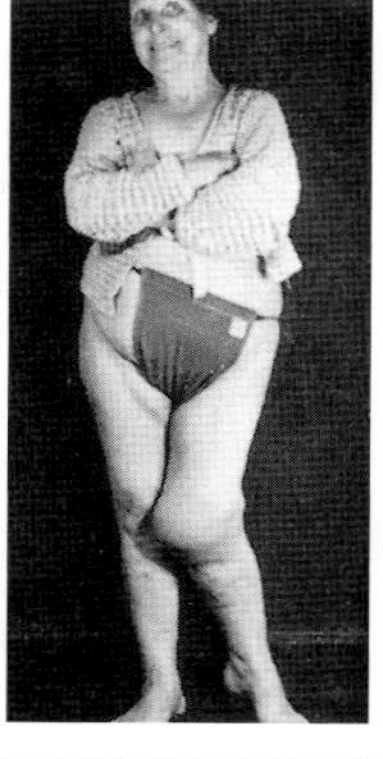
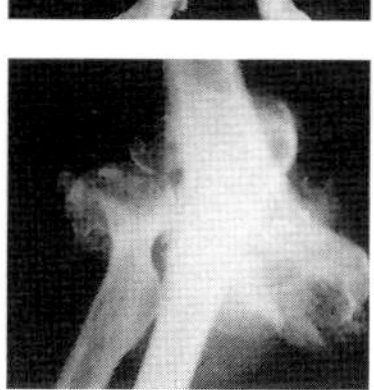
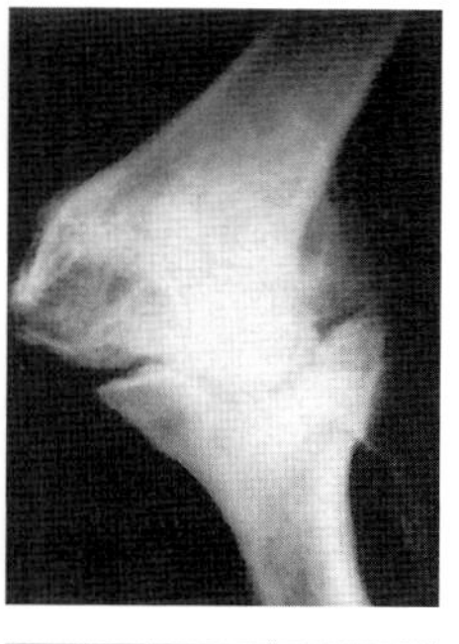
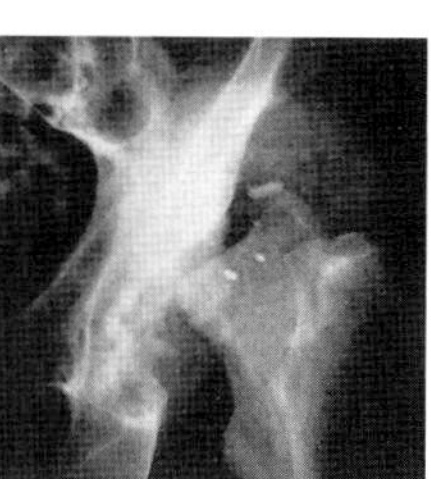

5.16 Charcot's disease The vertebrae are distorted and dense, the buttocks show the radio-opaque remains of former injections; the knee, elbow and hip joints look grotesque. Moral: 'If it's bizarre, do a "WR"'. Note also the happy smile (though not all Charcot joints are tabetic nor are they always painless).

lower limb joints in leprosy and tabes dorsalis and the upper limb joints (especially the shoulder) in syringomyelia. The joint is neither warm nor particularly tender, but swelling is marked, fluid is greatly increased and in the late stages bits of bone may be felt everywhere. There is always some instability and in the worst cases the joint is flail. The appearances suggest that movement would be agonizing and yet it is often painless. The paradox is diagnostic. General examination may reveal features of the underlying neurological disorder.

A fracture or dislocation may initiate the destructive process and in those cases clinical deterioration is more rapid and more painful than usual.

X-rays

The radiogaphic changes may at first be mistaken for those of osteoarthritis. However, thinning of the articular space is unusually rapid and there is little in the way of osteophyte formation. Joint swelling and the appearance of intra-articular 'calcification' are further clues. Ultimately there is gross erosion of the articular surfaces and displacement of the joint.

Treatment

There is no way of halting or slowing the destructive process. Treatment is usually conservative and consists of splintage of the unstable joint. Despite the bizarre appearances, patients often seem to manage well. Some patients complain of pain and may need analgesic medication.

Weightbearing joints are sometimes so unstable that splintage is useless. Arthrodesis may be attempted, but the patient should be warned that there is only a small chance of success.

HAEMOPHILIC ARTHROPATHY

Recurrent intra-articular bleeding may lead to chronic synovitis and progressive articular destruction. Clinically this is seen only in classic haemophilia, in which there is a deficiency of clotting factor VIII, and Christmas disease, due to deficiency of factor IX. Both are X-linked recessive disorders manifesting in males but carried by females. Their incidence is about 1 per 10 000 male births. Plasma clotting factor levels above 40 per cent of the normal are compatible with normal control of haemorrhage. Patients with clotting factor levels above 5 per cent ('mild haemophilia') may have prolonged bleeding after injury or operation; those with levels below 1 per cent ('severe haemophilia') have frequent spontaneous joint and muscle haemorrhages.

Pathology

Haemorrhage into the joint causes synovial irritation, inflammation and subsynovial fibrosis. Haemosiderin appears in the synovial cells and macrophages and after repeated bleeds the synovium becomes thick and heavily pigmented. A vascular pannus creeps over the articular surface and the cartilage is gradually eroded. The subchondral bone may be exposed and penetrated, and occasionally large cysts develop at the bone ends. These changes are attributed to cartilage-degrading enzymes released by the proliferative synovitis and by cells that have accumulated iron, but an additional factor may be the interference with normal cartilage nutrition due to prolonged or repeated joint immobilization.

Bleeding into muscles is less common but equally harmful. Increased tension may lead to muscle necro-

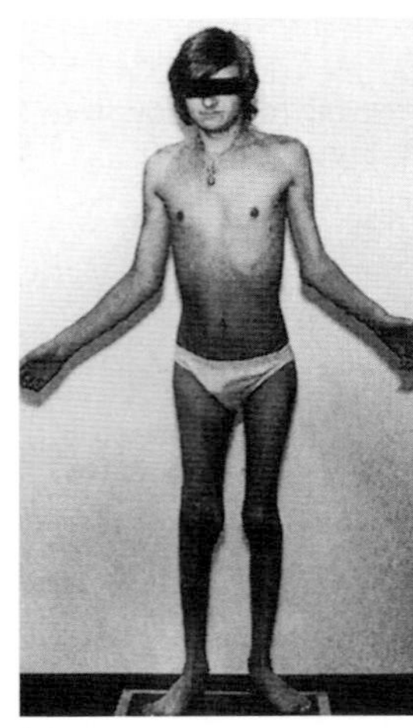

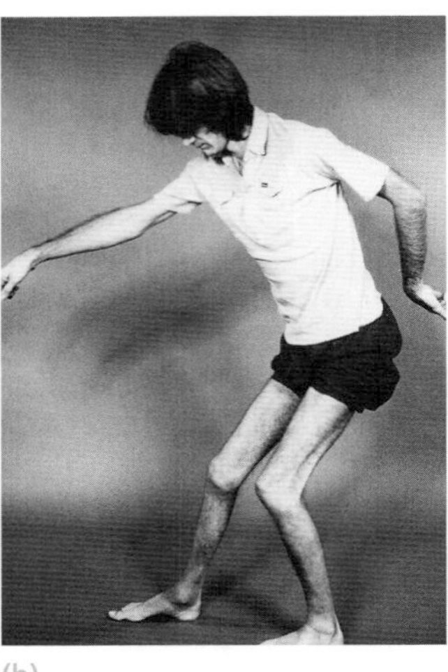

(a) (b)

5.17 Haemophilic arthropathy – clinical features (a) Recurrent haemarthrosis and chronic synovitis led to contractures of the elbow joints and deformities of the knees and ankles. (b) This man had difficulty staying upright, let alone walking, without support.

sis, reactive fibrosis and joint contractures. Sometimes nerves are compressed, causing a neurapraxia; temporary weakness may contribute further to the development of joint deformity.

Cysts and pseudotumours are rare phenomena. A large soft-tissue haematoma may become encapsulated before it is absorbed, and may then draw in more fluid by osmosis to produce a slowly expanding 'cyst'. A subperiosteal haematoma occasionally stimulates cystic resorption of bone resembling a tumour.

Clinical features

Only males are affected and in severe haemophilia joint bleeds usually begin when the child starts to walk. The clinical picture depends on the severity of the disorder, the site of bleeding and the efficacy of long-term treatment. The commonest features are acute bleeding into joints or muscles, chronic arthritis and joint contractures. The sites most frequently involved are the knees, ankles, elbow, shoulders and hips.

ACUTE BLEEDING INTO A JOINT, MUSCLE OR NERVE

With trivial injury a joint (usually the knee, elbow or ankle) may rapidly fill with blood. Pain, warmth, boggy swelling, tenderness and limited movement are the outstanding features. The resemblance to a low-grade inflammatory joint is striking, but the history is diagnostic.

Acute bleeding into muscles (especially the forearm, calf or thigh) is less common. A painful swelling appears and movement of the related joint is resisted. The distinction from a haemarthosis may be difficult (e.g. with groin pain due to iliopsoas haemorrhage); usually only those movements that stretch the affected muscles are painful, whereas in haemarthrosis all movements are painful.

Bleeding into a peripheral nerve causes intense pain followed by a variable degree of sensory change and muscle weakness. Nerve function usually recovers after several months.

Neurological symptoms and signs may also be caused by a large soft-tissue haematoma. Following effective treatment, the haematoma is usually resorbed within 10–14 days but full movement may take longer to return.

Bleeding into the forearm or leg may give rise to a classical compartment syndrome. The tell-tale signs of acute pain and tissue tension should be heeded before sensory and motor impairment are obvious.

JOINT DEGENERATION

This, the sequel to repeated bleeding, usually begins before the age of 15 years. Chronic synovitis is followed by cartilage degeneration. An affected joint shows wasting, limitation of movement and fixed deformity not unlike a tuberculous or rheumatoid joint. In longstanding cases, articular destruction may lead to instability.

X-ray changes vary according to the stage of the disorder. A useful classification is that of Arnold and Hilgartner (1977): *Stage I* – soft-tissue swelling; *Stage II* – osteoporosis and epiphyseal overgrowth; *Stage III* – slight narrowing of the articular space and squaring of the bone ends; *Stage IV* – marked narrowing of the articular space; and *Stage V* – joint disintegration.

Cysts and pseudotumours are rare complications.

Treatment

The most important aspect of treatment is to counteract bleeding as soon as it occurs, or better still to prevent recurrent bleeds. Patients are taught to recognize the early symptoms of bleeding and to administer the appropriate clotting factor concentrate themselves. In some centres factor concentrate is administered prophylactically two or three times a week; this is given intravenously, if necessary by indwelling catheter. It is essential to establish the precise diagnosis: factor VIII or IX is effective only for the specific disorder.

In former years (and probably still in some parts of the world) fresh-frozen plasma or concentrates that had not undergone viral inactivation were used for factor replacement, but this carried the risk of HIV contamination. These products are no longer recommended and have been replaced by virally inactivated factor concentrates.

The acute bleed Bleeding into the tissues is treated by

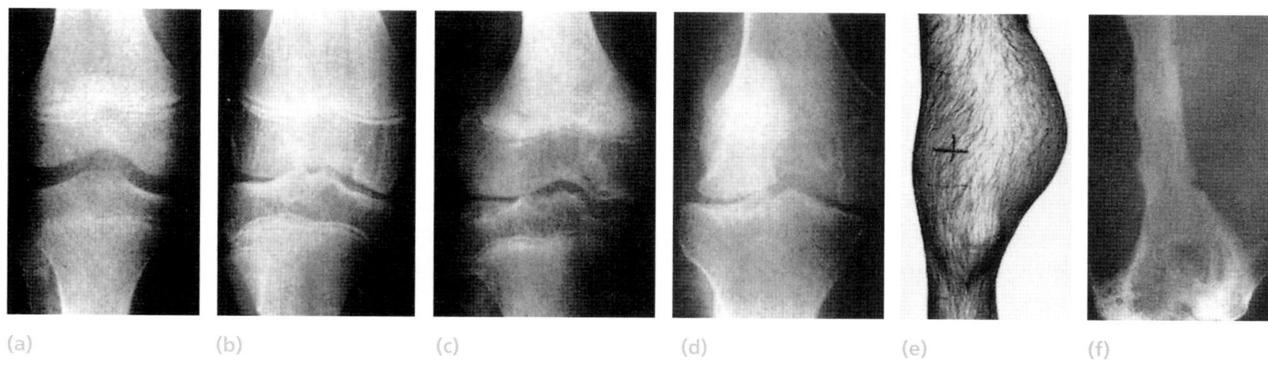

(a) (b) (c) (d) (e) (f)

5.18 Haemophilic arthritis (a) At first, there is blood in the joint but the surfaces are intact; (b) later the cartilage is attacked and the joint 'space' narrows; (c) bony erosions appear and eventually the joint becomes deformed and unstable; in (d) early subluxation is obvious. (e,f) This large pseudotumour was extirpated and, at the same time, massive bone grafts were inserted – no light undertaking in a haemophilic.

immediate factor replacement. Analgesics are given for pain and the limb is immobilized in a splint – but not for more than a day or two. Once the acute episode has passed, movement is encouraged, under continuing cover with factor concentrate. Aspiration is avoided unless distension is severe or there is a strong suspicion of infection. Nerve palsy may require intermittent splintage and physiotherapy until the neurapraxia recovers, and during this time the skin must be protected from injury.

Chronic arthropathy The aim is to prevent the development of joint contractures, stiffness and progressive muscle weakness. Under cover of factor infusions the patient is given physiotherapy, and impending contractures are managed by intermittent splintage and, if necessary, traction or passive correction by an inflatable splint.

Operative treatment has become safer since the introduction of clotting factor concentrates. However, patients who develop anti-factor antibodies are unsuitable for any form of surgery. It is also important to screen patients for hepatitis B virus and HIV antibodies, as their presence demands special precautions during the operation.

The clotting factor concentration should be raised to above 25 per cent for factor VIII and above 15 per cent for factor IX, and it should be kept at those levels throughout the postoperative period. It goes without saying that operative treatment should be carried out in a hospital with the appropriate multidisciplinary expertise on site.

Useful procedures are tendon lengthening (to correct contractures), osteotomy (for established deformity) and arthrodesis of the knee or ankle (for painful joint destruction). Synovectomy is sometimes performed but the benefits are dubious. Total hip replacement is technically feasible, but tissue dissection should be kept to a minimum and meticulous haemostasis is needed. Not surprisingly, the complication rate is higher than for hip replacement in non-bleeders (Nelson et al., 1992).

REFERENCES AND FURTHER READING

Allander E. Kashin–Beck disease. An analysis of research and public health activities based on a bibliography 1849–1992. *Scand J Rheumat* 1994; **23**(suppl 99): 1–36.

Arnold WD, Hilgartner MW. Hemophilic arthropathy. *J Bone Joint Surg*, 1977; **59A:** 287–305.

Byers PD, Contepomi CA, Farkas TA. A post mortem study of the hip joint including the prevalence of features on the right side. *Ann Rheum Dis* 1970; **29:** 15–31.

Doherty M, Holt M, MacMillan P *et al.* A reappraisal of 'analgesic hip'. *Ann Rheum Dis* 1986; **45:** 272–6.

Doherty M, Watt I, Dieppe P. Influence of primary generalised osteoarthritis on development of secondary osteoarthritis. *Lancet* 1983; **2:** 8–11.

Fellingham SA, Elphinstone RD, Wittman W. Mseleni joint disease: background and prevalence. *S Afr Med J* 1973; **47:** 2173–80.

Felson DT, Anderson JJ, Namack A *et al.* Obesity and symptomatic knee osteoarthritis. *Arthr Rheum* 1987; **30:** S130.

Felson DT, Hannan MT, Naimark A, *et al.* Occupational physical demands, knee bending, and knee osteoarthritis: results from the Framingham Study. *J Rheumatol*, 1991; **18:** 1587–92.

Hannan MT, Zhang Y, Anderson JJ, *et al.* Bone mineral density and knee osteoarthritis in elderly men and women: The Framingham Study. *Arthr Rheum* 1992; **35:** S1 (S40).

Harris PA, Hart DJ, Jawad S *et al.* Risk of osteoarthritis (OA) associated with running: A radiological survey. *Arthr Rheum* 1994; **37:** S369.

Hart DJ, Mootoosamy I, Doyle DV, *et al.* The relationship between osteoarthritis and osteoporosis in the general population: The Chingford Study. *Ann Rheum Dis* 1994; **53:** 158–62.

Hoaglund FT, Yau ACMC, Wong WL. Osteoarthritis of the hip and other joints in Southern Chinese in Hong Kong. *J Bone Joint Surg* 1973; **55A:** 545–7.

Kellgren JH. Genetic factors in generalized osteoarthrosis. *Ann Rheum Dis* 1963; **22:** 237–55.

Knowlton RG, Katzenstein PL, Moskowitz RW *et al.* Genetic linkage of a polymorphism in the type II procollagen gene (COL2A1) to primary osteoarthritis associated with mild chondrodysplasia. *N Eng J Med* 1990; **322:** 526.

Kulkala UM, Kaprio J, Sarno S. Osteoarthritis of weight bearing joints of lower limbs in former elite male athletes. *BMJ* 1994; **308:** 231.

Lanyon P, Doherty S, Doherty M. Assessment of a genetic contribution to osteoarthritis of the hip: sibling study. *BMJ* 2000; **321(7270):** 1179–83.

Lawrence, JS. Rheumatism in cotton operatives. *Br J of Ind Med* 1961; **18:** 270–6.

Mankin HJ, Dorfman DD, Lippiello L, Zarins A. Biochemical and metabolic abnormalities in articular cartilage from osteoarthritic human hips. II. Correlation of morphology with metabolic data. *J Bone Joint Surg* 1971; **53A:** 523–37.

Merchant TC, Dietz FR. Long-term follow-up after fractures of the tibial and fibular shafts. *J Bone Joint Surg* 1989; **71A:** 599.

Nelson IW, Sivamerugan S, Latham PD *et al.* Total hip arthroplasties for haemophilic arthropathies. *Clin Orthop Relat Res* 1992; **276:** 210–13.

Palotie A, Vaisanen P, Ott J *et al.* Predisposition to familial osteoarthrosis linked to type II collagen gene. *Lancet* 1989; **2:** 924.

Pettifor JM. Vitamin D and/or calcium deficiency rickets in infants and children: a global perspective. *Indian J Med Res* 2008; **127:** 245–9.

Resnick D, Shaul SR, Robins JM. Diffuse idiopathic skeletal hyperostosis (DISH): Forestier's disease with extraspinal manifestations. *Radiology* 1975; **115:** 513–24.

Schumacher HR, Agudelo C, Labowitz R. Jackhammer arthropathy. *J Occup Med* 1972; **14:** 563.

Sokoloff, L. Endemic forms of osteoarthritis. *Clin Rheum Dis* 1985; **11:** 187–202.

Solomon L. Patterns of osteoarthritis of the hip. *J Bone Joint Surg* 1976; **58B:** 176–83.

Solomon L. Geographical and anatomical patterns of osteoarthritis. *Br J Rheumatol* 1984; **23:** 177–180.

Solomon L, McLaren P, Irwig L *et al.* Distinct types of hip disorder in Mselini joint disease. *S Afr Med J* 1986; **69:** 15–17.

Wittman W, Fellingham S. Unusual hip disease in remote part of Zululand. *Lancet* 1970; **1:** 842–3.

Yach D, Botha JL. Mseleni joint disease in 1981: decreased prevalence rates, wider geographical location than before, and socioeconomic impact of an endemic osteoarthrosis in an underdeveloped community in South Africa. *Int J Epidemiol* 1985; **14:** 276–84.

Osteonecrosis and related disorders

6

Louis Solomon

Avascular necrosis has long been recognized as a complication of femoral head fractures, the usual explanation being traumatic severance of the blood supply to the femoral head. Segmental osteonecrosis also appears as a distinctive feature in a number of non-traumatic disorders: joint infection, Perthes' disease, caisson disease, Gaucher's disease, systemic lupus erythematosus (SLE), high-dosage corticosteroid administration and alcohol abuse, to mention only the more common ones. Whatever the cause, the condition, once established, may come to dominate the clinical picture, demanding attention in its own right.

MAIN CONDITIONS ASSOCIATED WITH NON-TRAUMATIC OSTEONECROSIS

Infections
- Osteomyelitis
- Septic arthritis

Haemoglobinopathy
- Sickle cell disease

Storage disorders
- Gaucher's disease

Caisson disease
- Dysbaric osteonecrosis

Coagulation disorders
- Familial thrombophilia
- Hypofibrinolysis
- Hypolipoproteinaemia
- Thrombocytopenic purpura

Other
- Perthes' disease
- Cortisone administration
- Alcohol abuse
- SLE (? increase in antiphospholipid antibodies)
- Pregnancy (? decreased fibrinolysis; ? fatty liver)
- Anaphylactic shock
- Ionizing radiation

SLE, systemic lupus erythematosus.

Aetiology and pathogenesis

Sites which are peculiarly vulnerable to ischaemic necrosis are the femoral head, the femoral condyles, the head of the humerus, the capitulum and the proximal parts of the scaphoid and talus. These subarticular regions lie at the most distant parts of the bone's vascular territory, and they are largely enclosed by cartilage, giving restricted access to local blood vessels. The subchondral trabeculae are further compromised in that they are sustained largely by a system of endarterioles with limited collateral connections.

Another factor which needs to be taken into account is that the vascular sinusoids which nourish the marrow and bone cells, unlike arterial capillaries, have no adventitial layer and their patency is determined by the volume and pressure of the surrounding marrow tissue, which itself is encased in unyielding bone. The system functions essentially as a closed compartment within which one element can expand

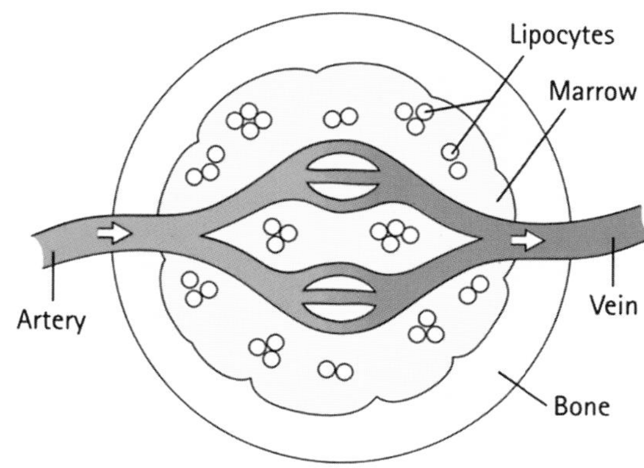

6.1 Avascular necrosis – pathogenesis The medullary cavity of bone is virtually a closed compartment containing myeloid tissue, marrow fat and capillary blood vessels. Any increase in fat cell volume will reduce capillary circulation and may result in bone ischaemia.

only at the expense of the others. Local changes such as decreased blood flow, haemorrhage or marrow swelling can, therefore, rapidly spiral to a vicious cycle of ischaemia, reactive oedema or inflammation, marrow swelling, increased intraosseous pressure and further ischaemia.

The process described above can be initiated in at least four different ways: (1) severance of the local blood supply; (2) venous stasis and retrograde arteriolar stoppage; (3) intravascular thrombosis; and (4) compression of capillaries and sinusoids by marrow swelling. *Ischaemia, in the majority of cases, is due to a combination of several of these factors.*

TRAUMATIC OSTEONECROSIS

In traumatic osteonecrosis the vascular anatomy is particularly important. In fractures and dislocations of the hip the retinacular vessels supplying the femoral head are easily torn. If, in addition, there is damage to or thrombosis of the ligamentum teres, osteonecrosis is inevitable. Little wonder that displaced fractures of the femoral neck are complicated by osteonecrosis in over 20 per cent of cases. Undisplaced fractures, or lesser injuries, also sometimes result in subchondral necrosis; this may be due to thrombosis of intraosseous capillaries or sinusoidal occlusion due to marrow oedema.

Other injuries which are prone to osteonecrosis are fractures of the scaphoid and talus. Significantly, in these cases it is always the proximal fragment which suffers. This is because the principal vessels enter the bones near their distal ends and take an intraosseous course from distal to proximal.

Impact injuries and osteoarticular fractures at any of the convex articular surfaces behave in the same way and often develop localized ischaemic changes. These small lesions are usually referred to as 'osteochondroses' and many of them have acquired eponyms which are firmly embedded in orthopaedic history.

NON-TRAUMATIC OSTEONECROSIS

The mechanisms here are more complex and may involve several pathways to intravascular stasis or thrombosis, as well as extravascular swelling and capillary compression.

Intravascular thrombosis Various mechanisms leading to capillary thrombosis have been demonstrated in patients with non-traumatic osteonecrosis. Over 80 per cent of cases are associated with high-dosage corticosteroid medication or alcohol abuse (or both, acting cumulatively). These conditions give rise to hyperlipidaemia and fatty degeneration of the liver. Jones (1994) has favoured the idea that fat embolism plays a part, giving rise to capillary endothelial damage, platelet aggregation and thrombosis. Glueck et al. (1996, 1997a) have suggested that thrombophilia and hypofibrinolysis are important aetiological factors in both adult osteonecrosis and Perthes' disease. Other coagulopathies have been implicated, e.g. antiphospholipid deficiency in SLE (Asherson et al., 1993) and enhanced coagulability in sickle-cell disease (Francis, 1991), and it now seems likely that coagulation abnormalities of one sort or another play at least a contributory role in some of the disorders associated with non-traumatic osteonecrosis.

Extravascular marrow swelling High-dosage corticosteroid administration and alcohol overuse cause fat cell swelling in the marrow, a feature which is very obvious in bone specimens obtained during joint replacement. There is a demonstrable rise in intraosseous pressure and contrast venography shows slowing of venous blood flow from the bone. Ficat and Arlet (1980) posited that the increase in marrow fat volume in the femoral head caused sinusoidal compression, venous stasis and retrograde ischaemia leading to trabecular bone death; in other words, the establishment of a compartment syndrome.

Whichever of these mechanisms offers the primary pathway to non-traumatic bone ischaemia, it is almost certain that both intravascular and extravascular factors come into play at a fairly early stage and each enhances the effect of the other.

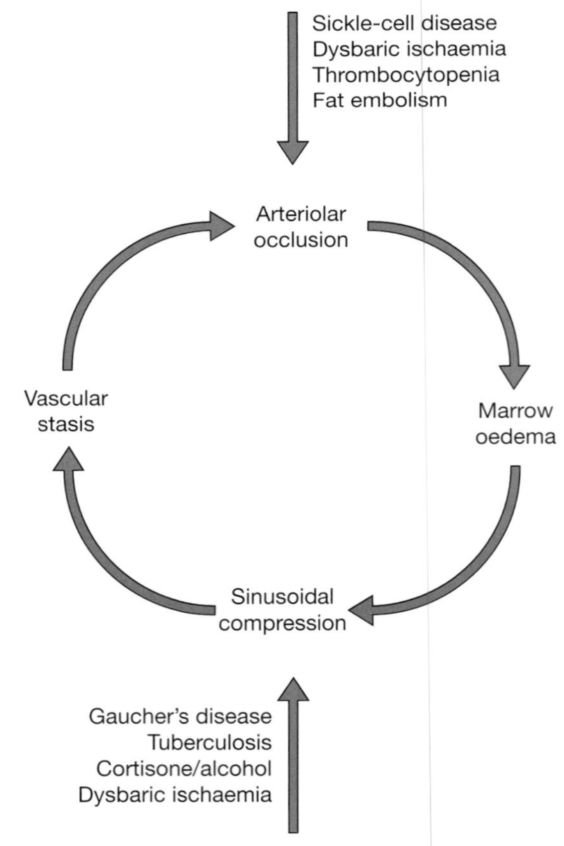

6.2 Avascular necrosis Algorithm showing how various disorders may enter the vicious cycle of capillary stasis and marrow engorgement.

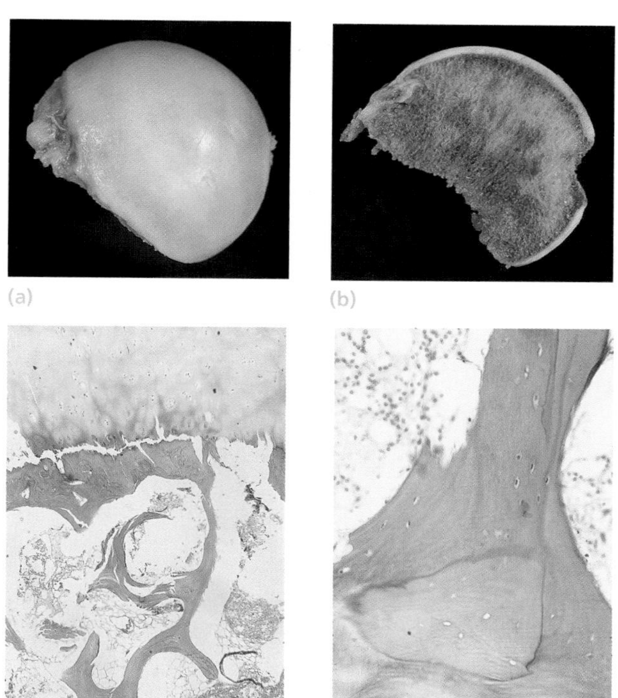

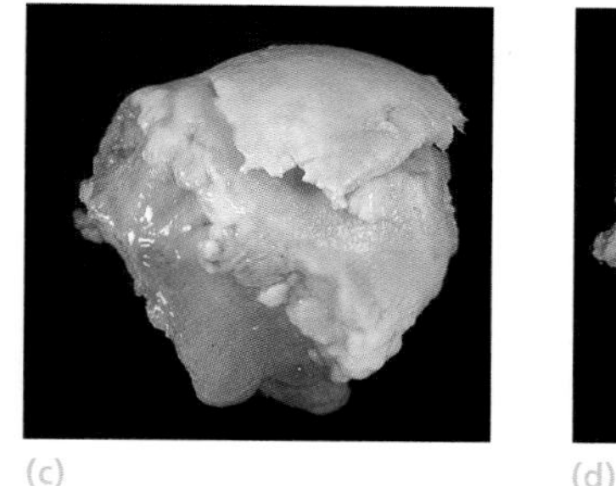

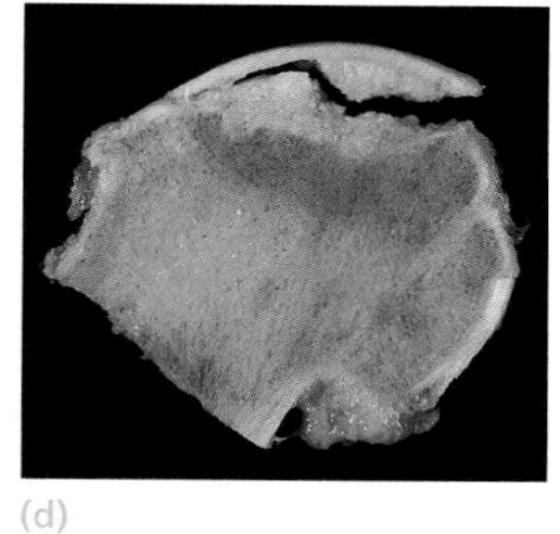

(a) (b) (c) (d) (e) (f)

6.3 Osteonecrosis – pathology (a,b) Normal femoral head and cut section. The articular cartilage is obviously intact and the subchondral bone is well vascularized. (c,d) In this femoral head with osteonecrosis the articular cartilage is lifted off the bone; the coronal section in (d) shows that this is due to a subarticular fracture through the necrotic segment in the dome of the femoral head. (e) Histological section across the junction between articular cartilage and bone showing living cartilage cells but necrotic subchondral marrow and bone. (f) High power view showing islands of dead bone with empty osteocytic lacunae enfolded by new, living bone.

Pathology and natural history

Bone cells die after 12–48 hours of anoxia, yet for days or even weeks the gross appearance of the affected segment remains unaltered. During this time the most striking histological changes are seen in the marrow: loss of fat cell outlines, inflammatory cell infiltration, marrow oedema, the appearance of tissue histiocytes, and eventual replacement of necrotic marrow by undifferentiated mesenchymal tissue.

A characteristic feature of ischaemic segmental necrosis is the tendency to bone repair, and within a few weeks one may see new blood vessels and osteoblastic proliferation at the interface between ischaemic and live bone. As the necrotic sector becomes demarcated, vascular granulation tissue advances from the surviving trabeculae and new bone is laid down upon the dead; it is this increase in mineral mass that later produces the radiographic appearance of increased density or 'sclerosis'.

Reparative new bone formation proceeds slowly and probably does not advance for more than 8–10 mm into the necrotic zone. With time, structural failure begins to occur in the most heavily stressed part of the necrotic segment. Usually this takes the form of a linear tangential fracture close to the articular surface, possibly due to shearing stress. The crack may break through the articular cartilage and at operation it may be possible to lift the 'lid' off the necrotic segment like the cracked shell of a hard-boiled egg. However, until very late the articular cartilage retains its thickness and viability. In the final stages, fragmentation of the necrotic bone leads to progressive deformity and destruction of the joint surface.

In the past, when diagnosis was based entirely on x-ray changes, it was thought that osteonecrosis always progressed to bone collapse. Now that it is possible to detect the earliest signs by MRI, it has become apparent that this is not the case.

The size of the necrotic segment, as defined by the hypo-intense band in the T_1 weighted MRI, is usually established at the time of the initiating ischaemic event, and from then on it rarely increases; indeed, there is evidence that non-traumatic lesions sometimes diminish in size and occasionally even disappear (Sakamoto et al., 1997). In persistent lesions, the rate of bone collapse depends largely on the site and extent of the necrotic segment: lesions which lie outside the normal stress trajectories may remain structurally intact while those that involve large segments of the load-bearing surface usually collapse within 3 years (see under Staging).

Clinical features

The earliest stage of bone death is asymptomatic; by the time the patient presents, the lesion is usually well advanced. Pain is a common complaint. It is felt in or near a joint, and perhaps only with certain movements. Some patients complain of a 'click' in the joint, probably due to snapping or catching of a loose articular fragment. In the later stages the joint becomes

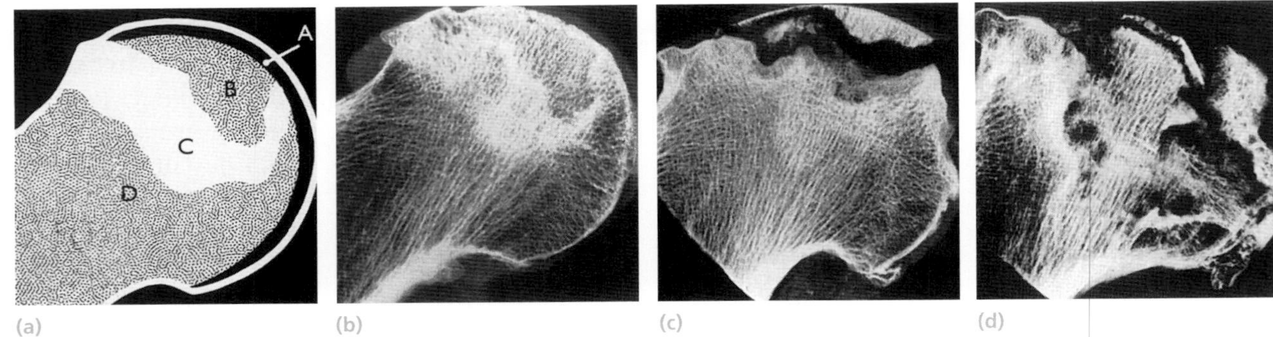

(a) (b) (c) (d)

6.4 Avascular necrosis of bone – pathology (a) This is a diagramatic guide to the fine-detail x-rays of necrotic femoral heads (b–d) which show the progress of osteonecrosis. The articular cartilage (A) remains intact for a long time. The necrotic segment (B) has a texture similar to that of normal bone, but it may develop fine cracks. New bone surrounds the dead trabeculae and causes marked sclerosis (C). Beyond this the bone remains unchanged (D). In the later stages the necrotic bone breaks up and finally the joint surface is destroyed.

stiff and deformed. Local tenderness may be present and, if a superficial bone is affected, there may be some swelling. Movements – or perhaps one particular movement – may be restricted; in advanced cases there may be fixed deformities.

Imaging

X-ray The early signs of ischaemia are confined to the bone marrow and cannot be detected by plain x-ray examination. X-ray changes, when they appear (seldom before 3 months after the onset of ischaemia), are due to (a) reactive new bone formation at the boundary of the ischaemic area and (b) trabecular failure in the necrotic segment. An area of increased radiographic density appears in the subchondral bone; soon afterwards, suitable views may show a thin tangential fracture line just below the articular surface – the *'crescent sign'*. In the late stages there is distortion of the articular surface and more intense 'sclerosis', now partly due to bone compression in a collapsed segment.

Occasionally the necrotic portion separates from the parent bone as a discrete fragment. However, it is now recognized that in the case of the femoral head and the medial femoral condyle such necrotic fragments may have resulted from small osteo-articular fractures which only later failed to unite and lost their blood supply.

With all the changes described here (and this is the cardinal feature distinguishing primary avascular necrosis from the sclerotic and destructive forms of osteoarthritis) the 'joint space' retains its normal width because the articular cartilage is not destroyed until very late.

Radioscintigraphy Radionuclide scanning with ^{99m}Tc-sulphur colloid, which is taken up in myeloid tissue,

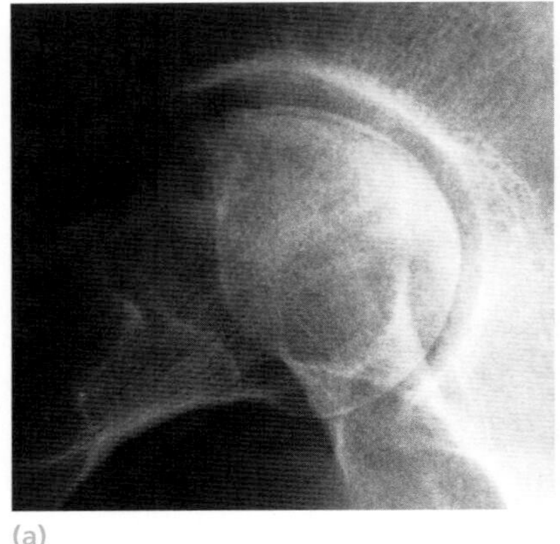

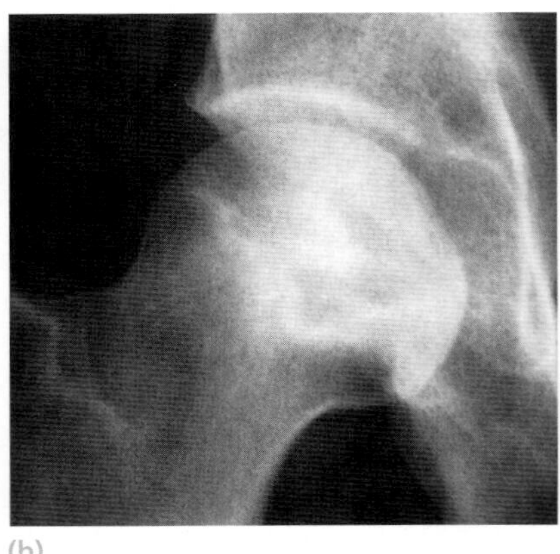

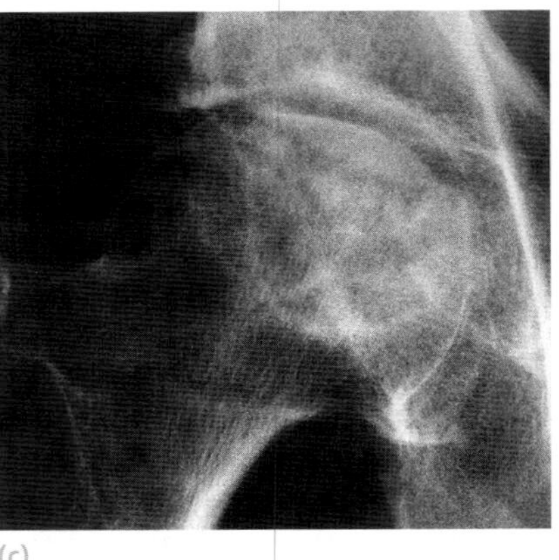

(a) (b) (c)

6.5 Avascular necrosis – x-ray (a) The earliest x-ray sign is a thin radiolucent crescent just below the convex articular surface where load bearing is at its greatest. This represents an undisplaced subarticular fracture in the early necrotic segment. (b) At a later stage the avascular segment is defined by a band of increased density due to vital new bone formation. At this stage the femoral head may still be spherical and (unlike osteoarthritis) the articular space is still well-defined. (c) In late cases there is obvious collapse and distortion of the articular surface.

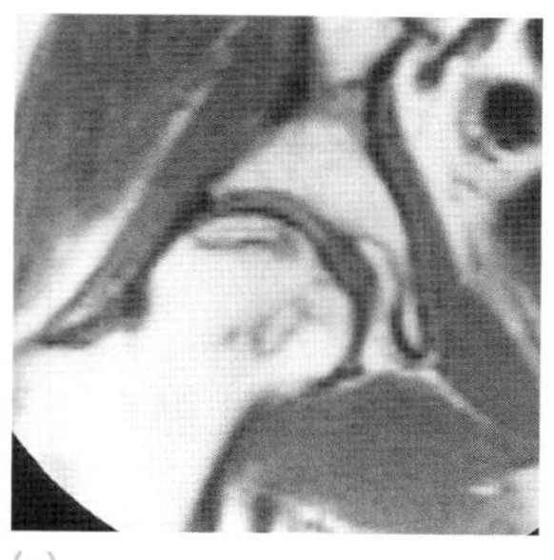
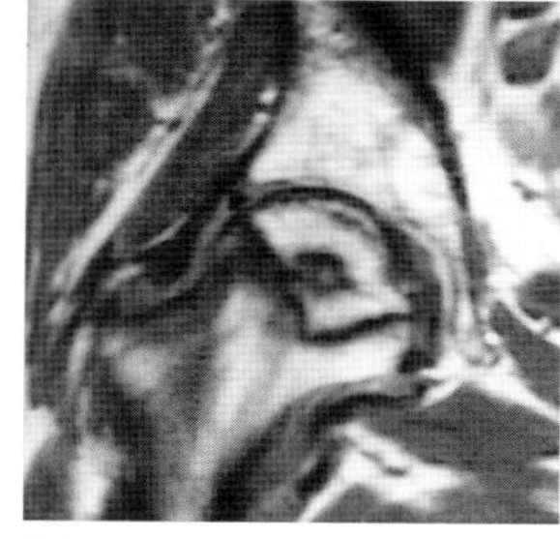

(a) (b)

6.6 Osteonecrosis – MRI (a) Before any change is discernible on the plain x-ray, MRI will show a typical hypo-intense band in the T_1 weighted image, outlining the ischaemic segment beneath the articular surface. (b) In this case the size of the ischaemic segment is much larger – and the likelihood of bone crumbling much greater.

may reveal an avascular segment. This is most likely in traumatic avascular necrosis, where a large segment of bone is involved, or in sickle-cell disease where a 'cold' area contrasts significantly with the generally high nuclide uptake due to increased erythroblastic activity. ^{99m}Tc-HDP scans (in the bone phase) may also show a 'cold' area, particularly if a large segment of bone is avascular (e.g. after fracture of the femoral neck). More often, however, the picture is dominated by *increased* activity, reflecting hyperaemia and new bone formation in the area around the infarct.

Magnetic resonance imaging MRI is the most reliable way of diagnosing marrow changes and bone ischaemia at a comparatively early stage. The first sign is a band-like low-intensity signal on the T_1 weighted spin echo (SE) image (and a similar but high-intensity signal on the short-tau inversion recovery (STIR) image), corresponding to the interface between ischaemic and normal bone. The site and size of the demarcated necrotic zone have been used to predict the progress of the lesions (see Chapter 19).

Computed tomography CT involves considerable radiation exposure and it is not very useful for diagnosing osteonecrosis. However, it does show the area of bone destruction very clearly and it may be useful in planning surgery.

Tests for haemodynamic function

During the early stage of ischaemic necrosis the intramedullary pressure is often markedly raised. This phenomenon is most easily demonstrated in the femoral head. A cannula introduced into the metaphysis enables measurements to be taken (1) at rest and (2) after rapid injection of saline. The normal resting pressure is 10–20 mmHg, rising by about 15 mm after saline injection; in early osteonecrosis both the intramedullary pressure and the response to saline injection may be increased three- or four-fold. Venous stasis can also be demonstrated by venography after injection of radio-opaque medium into the bone.

Similar findings have been recorded in osteoarthritis, but the change is not nearly as marked as in osteonecrosis.

Staging the lesion

Ficat and Arlet (1980) introduced the concept of *radiographic staging* for osteonecrosis of the hip to distinguish between early (pre-symptomatic) signs and later features of progressive demarcation and collapse of the necrotic segment in the femoral head. *Stage 1* showed no

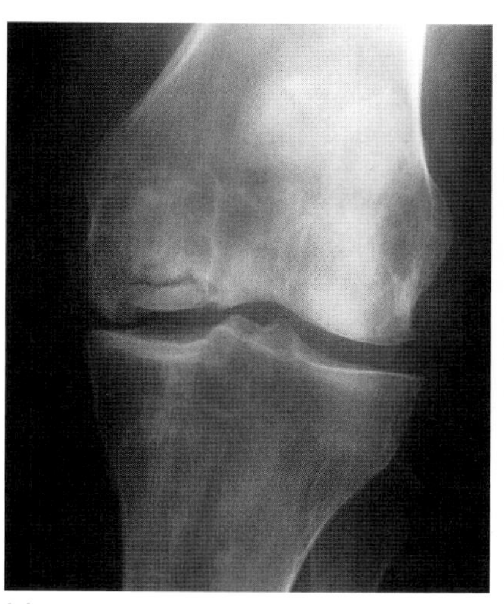
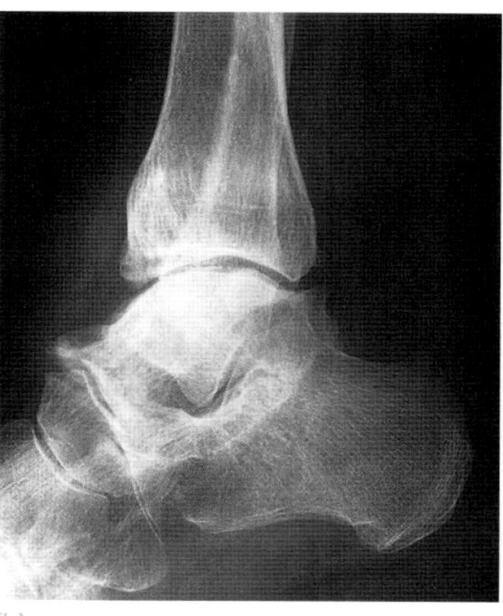
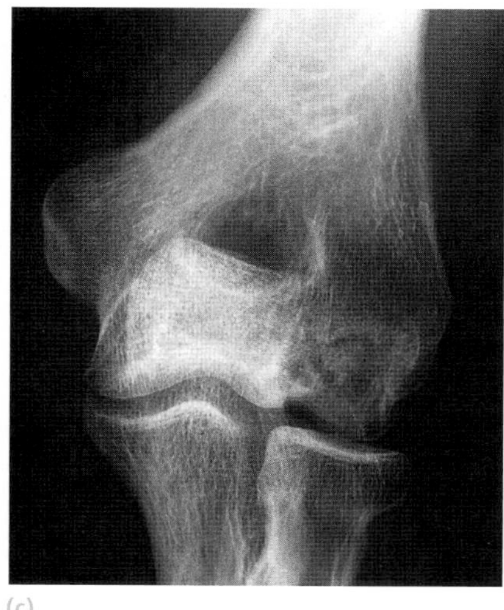

(a) (b) (c)

6.7 Osteonecrosis – distribution The most common sites for osteonecrosis are the head of the femur, the head of the humerus and, as shown here, the medial condyle of the femur, the talus and the capitulum. All these areas are located beneath convex articular surfaces; osteonecrosis is seldom seen beneath a concave articular surface.

x-ray change and the diagnosis was based on measurement of intraosseous pressure and histological features of bone biopsy (or nowadays on MRI). In *Stage 2* the femoral head contour was still normal but there were early signs of reactive change in the subchondral area. *Stage 3* was defined by clearcut x-ray signs of osteonecrosis with evidence of structural damage and distortion of the bone outline. In *Stage 4* there were collapse of the articular surface and signs of secondary OA.

Later modifications involving assessment of both *the extent* and *the location* of the early changes on plain x-ray and MRI have proved to be more reliable as predictors of outcome, at least in relation to femoral head necrosis (Shimizu et al., 1994; Steinberg et al., 1995).

The location and size of the necrotic segment in Ficat stages 1–3 are defined by the hypo-intense band on the T_1 weighted MRI. Two general observations can be made: (1) the size of the ischaemic segment is determined at a very early stage and it rarely increases after that; (2) small lesions which do not involve the maximally loaded zone of the articular surface tend not to collapse, whereas large lesions extending under the maximally loaded articular surface break down in over 60 per cent of cases. Shimizu's classification is particularly useful in planning treatment; this is discussed in Chapter 19.

Table 6.1 ARCO staging of osteonecrosis

Stage 0	Patient asymptomatic and all clinical investigations 'normal' Biopsy shows osteonecrosis
Stage 1	X-rays normal. MRI or radionuclide scan shows osteonecrosis
Stage 2	X-rays and/or MRI show early signs of osteonecrosis but no distortion of bone shape or subchondral 'crescent sign' Subclassification by area of articular surface involved: A = less than 15 per cent B = 15–30 per cent C = more than 30 per cent
Stage 3	X-ray shows 'crescent sign' but femoral head still spherical Subclassification by length of 'crescent'/articular surface: A = less than 15 per cent B = 15–30 per cent C = more than 30 per cent
Stage 4	Signs of flattening or collapse of femoral head A = less than 15 per cent of articular surface B = 15–30 per cent of articular surface C = more than 30 per cent of articular surface
Stage 5	Changes as above plus loss of 'joint space' (secondary OA)
Stage 6	Changes as above plus marked destruction of articular surfaces

The most widely used system, which permits comparison between series from different participating centres, is the one promoted by the International Association of Bone Circulation and Bone Necrosis (*Association Research Circulation Osseous – ARCO*) which applies mainly to femoral head necrosis (Table 6.1).

Diagnosis of the underlying disorder

In many cases of osteonecrosis an underlying disorder will be obvious from the history: a known episode of trauma, an occupation such as deep-sea diving or working under compressed air, a family background of Gaucher's disease or sickle-cell disease. There may be a record of high-dosage corticosteroid administration; for example, after renal transplantation where the drug is used for immunosuppression. However, smaller doses (e.g. as short-term treatment for asthma or as an adjunct in neurosurgical emergencies) and even topical steroid preparations can also be dangerous in patients with other risk factors (Solomon and Pearse, 1994). Combinations of drugs (e.g. corticosteroids and azathioprine, or corticosteroids after a period of alcohol abuse) also can be potent causes of osteonecrosis; occasionally corticosteroids have been given without the patient's knowledge.

Alcohol abuse is often difficult to determine because patients tend to hide the information. There is no biochemical marker that is specific for high alcohol intake but elevation of three or four of the following is suggestive: aspartate transaminase, γ-glutamyl transpeptidase, serum urate, serum triglyceride and mean red cell volume (Whitehead et al., 1978).

Ideally patients with very early non-traumatic osteonecrosis, and children with early Perthes' disease, should undergo laboratory tests for coagulopathies; this is justified by reports of cases in which the condition has been halted or reversed by treatment with antithrombotic preparations such as warfarin and stanozolol (Glueck et al., 1997b). Unfortunately the tests are very expensive and there is understandable resistance to adopting this approach in routine management.

In cases of suspected SLE, antiphospholipid antibodies may be measured.

Prevention

Where risk factors for osteonecrosis are recognized, preventive steps can be taken especially in the management of corticosteroid medication and alcohol abuse. Corticosteroids should be used only when essential and in minimal effective dosage. *It is important also to be aware of the cumulative effect of even moderate doses of corticosteroids in patients with a history of alcohol abuse.* Anoxia must be prevented in

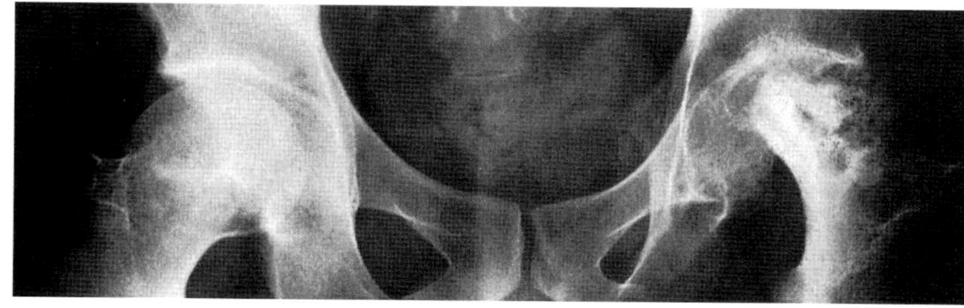

(a)

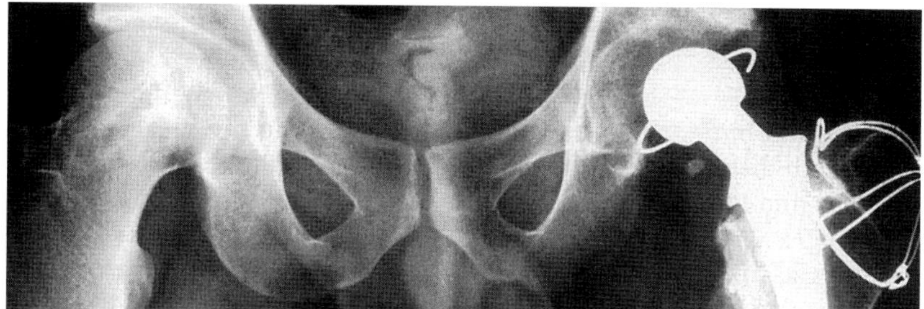

(b)

6.8 Osteonecrosis – treatment
(a) Alcohol abuse has led to bilateral femoral head necrosis, advanced on the left but detectable only by MRI on the right. (b) The left hip had to be replaced; at the same time the right side was treated by drilling of the femoral neck (medullary decompression). This x-ray was taken 8 years later.

patients with haemoglobinopathies. Decompression procedures for divers and compressed-air workers should be rigorously applied.

Treatment

In planning treatment, all the factors that influence the natural course of the condition must be taken into account: the general medical background, the type of ischaemic necrosis, the site and extent of the necrotic segment, its stage of development, the patient's age and capacity for bone repair, the persistence or otherwise of the aetiological agent and its effect on bone turnover.

Only general principles will be discussed here; the treatment of osteonecrosis in specific sites is dealt with in the appropriate chapters on regional orthopaedics.

EARLY OSTEONECROSIS

While the bone contour is intact there is always the hope that structural failure can be prevented. Some lesions heal spontaneously and with minimal deformity; this is seen especially in areas which are not severely stressed: the non-weightbearing joints, the superomedial part of the femoral head and the non-weightbearing surfaces of the femoral condyles and talus. Here one can afford to pursue a waiting policy.

In the past, various types of medication failed to show convincing evidence of preventing collapse of the subchondral bone in cases of early osteonecrosis. Recently, however, there have been promising reports of the effect of bisphosphonates in these cases. In a controlled study of the patients (54 femoral heads) with ARCO stage 2 or 3 osteonecrosis, those treated with oral alendronate for 25 weeks were found after 2 years to show a significantly lower rate of femoral head collapse than untreated controls (Lai et al., 2005). Other studies have shown similar results (Nishii et al., 2006). However, it is still too early to comment on the long-term success of this treatment.

Lesions in heavily loaded joints have a poor prognosis and will probably end in structural failure if left untreated. Simple measures to reduce loading of weight-bearing joints may help, though their value has not been proven. If the bone contour is still intact, an 'unloading' osteotomy will help to preserve the anatomy while remodelling proceeds. This approach is applicable especially to the hip and knee.

Medullary decompression and bone grafting may have a place in ARCO stage 1 and 2 osteonecrosis of the femoral head (Chapter 19).

INTERMEDIATE STAGE OSTEONECROSIS

Once there is structural damage and distortion of the articular surface, conservative operations are inappropriate. However, the joint may still be salvageable and in this situation realignment osteotomy – either alone or combined with curettage and bone grafting of the necrotic segment – has a useful role.

If mobility can be sacrificed without severe loss of function (e.g. in the ankle or wrist), arthrodesis will relieve pain and restore stability.

LATE STAGE OSTEONECROSIS

Destruction of the articular surface may be give rise to pain and severe loss of function. Three options are available: (1) non-operative management, concentrating on pain control, modification of daily activities and, where appropriate, splintage of the joint; (2) arthrodesis of the joint, e.g. the ankle or wrist; or (3) partial or total joint replacement, the preferred option for the shoulder, hip and knee.

SYSTEMIC DISORDERS ASSOCIATED WITH OSTEONECROSIS

Drug-induced necrosis

Alcohol, corticosteroids, immunosuppressives and cytotoxic drugs, either singly or in combination, are the commonest causes of non-traumatic osteonecrosis. 'At risk' doses for these drugs have not been established; the threshold depends not only on the total intake but also on the time over which the intake is spread and the presence or absence of associated disorders which themselves may predispose to osteonecrosis. A cumulative dose of 2000 mg of prednisone equivalent administered over several years (for example in the treatment of rheumatoid arthritis) is less likely to cause osteonecrosis than the same dose given over a period of a few months (e.g. after organ transplantation). It is important to bear in mind that multiple causative agents have an additive effect; thus, osteonecrosis has been encountered after comparatively short courses and low doses of corticosteroids (totals of 800 mg or less), but in these cases an additive factor can almost always be identified (Solomon and Pearse, 1994).

The threshold dose for alcohol is equally vague. However, based on the known dose relationship of alcohol-induced fatty degeneration of the liver, we would set it at around 150 mg of ethanol per day (for men) – the equivalent of 300 mL of spirits, 1.2 litres of table wine or 3 litres of beer – continuing for over 2 years. The dose for women is considerably less. Asking patients 'How much do you drink?' is unlikely to elicit an accurate response. However, the presence of raised serum triglyceride and γ-GT levels, together with an increased mean corpuscular volume (MCV), is suggestive of excessive alcohol intake.

Sickle-cell disease

Sickle-cell disease is a genetic disorder in which the red cells contain abnormal haemoglobin (HbS). In deoxygenated blood there is increased aggregation of the haemoglobin molecules and distortion of the red cells, which become somewhat sickle-shaped. At first this is reversible and the cells reacquire their normal shape when the blood is oxygenated. Eventually, however, the red cell membrane becomes damaged and the cells are permanently deformed.

The sickle-cell trait, which originated in West and Central Africa centuries ago, is an example of natural selection for survival in areas where malaria was endemic. From there the gene was carried to countries along the Mediterranean, the Persian Gulf, parts of India and across the Atlantic where it appears in people of Afro-American descent. In recent years it has spread more widely in Europe but it is rarely encountered south of the equator.

Sickle-cell disease is most likely in homozygous offspring (those with HbS genes from both mother and father), but it may also occur in heterozygous children with HbS/C haemoglobinopathy and HbS/thalassaemia. Inheritance of one HbS gene and one normal β-globin gene confers the (heterozygous) *sickle-cell trait*; HbS concentration is low and sickling occurs only under conditions of hypoxia (e.g. under inefficient anaesthesia, in extreme cold, at very high altitudes and when flying in unpressurized aircraft).

In the established disorder, the main clinical features are due to a combination of chronic haemolytic anaemia and a tendency to clumping of the sickle-shaped cells which results in diminished capillary flow and recurrent episodes of intracapillary thrombosis. Secondary changes such as trabecular coarsening, infarctions of the marrow, periostitis and osteonecrosis are common. Complications include hyperuricaemia (due to increased red cell turnover) and an increased susceptibility to bacterial infection.

Clinical features

Children during the first two years of life may present with swelling of the hands and feet. X-rays at first seem normal, but later there may be suggestive features such as marrow densities and periosteal new bone formation ('dactylitis'). These changes are usually transient, but treatment is required for pain.

In older children a typical feature is recurrent episodes of severe pain, sometimes associated with fever. These 'crises', which may affect almost any part of the body, are thought to be due to infarcts.

Osteonecrosis of the femoral head is common, both in children (when it is sometimes mistaken for Perthes' disease) and in young adults, in whom other causes of non-traumatic osteonecrosis have to be excluded (Iwegbu and Fleming, 1985). Males and females are affected with almost equal frequency. The child develops a painful limp and movements are restricted.

X-rays may show no more than a diffuse increase in density of the epiphysis; however, in most cases the changes are very similar to those of Perthes' disease, usually going on to flattening of the epiphysis. In young adults there are both destructive lesions and diffuse sclerosis of the femoral head. The head of the humerus and the femoral condyles may be similarly affected.

Other bone changes are due to a combination of marrow hyperplasia and medullary infarctions. Trabecular coarsening and thickening of the cortices may be mistaken for signs of infection.

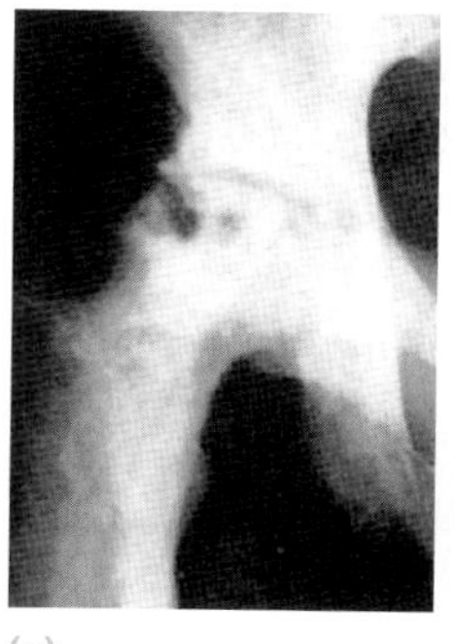

(a)

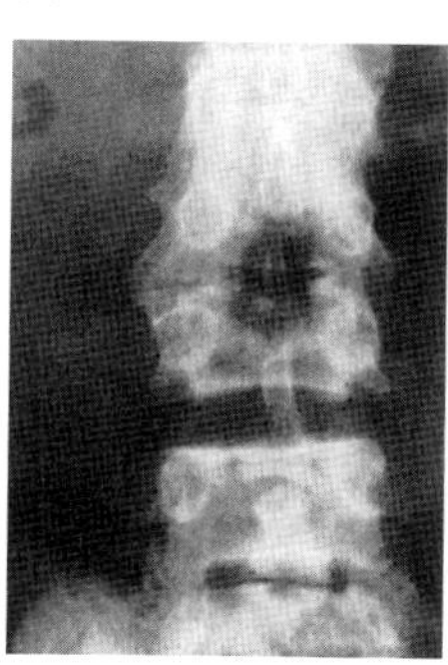

(b)

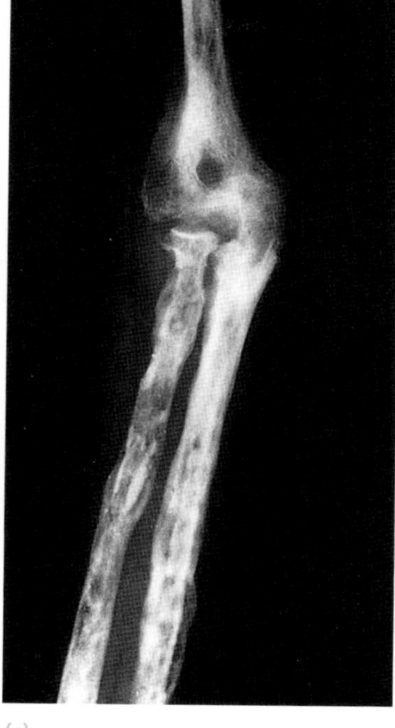

(c)

6.9 Sickle-cell disease (a) Typical features of osteonecrosis are seen in the femoral head, often accompanied by patchy areas of bone destruction and endosteal sclerosis in the femoral shaft. (b) The spine also may be involved, producing appearances similar to those of bone infection. (c) In severe cases infarctions of tubular bones may resemble osteomyelitis, with sequestra and a marked periosteal reaction.

Bacterial osteomyelitis and septic arthritis, sometimes involving multiple sites, are serious complications, particularly in children. In over 50 per cent of cases the organism is *Salmonella*.

Treatment

A follow-up study of untreated children with femoral head necrosis due to sickle-cell disease showed that 80 per cent of them had permanently damaged hips with severe loss of function (Hernigou et al., 1991). This may be due to recurrent infarction and inflammatory changes in the joint.

Hypoxic conditions favouring the occurrence of crises should be avoided. If episodes of bone pain are frequent, transfusions may be necessary to reduce the concentration of HbS. During a crisis the patient should be given adequate analgesia and should be kept fully oxygenated. Infections should be guarded against, or treated promptly with the appropriate antibiotics.

Femoral head necrosis in children should be treated in the same way as Perthes' disease (see page 511). Adults are treated along the lines described on page 531. The emphasis in all cases should be on conservatism. Anaesthesia carries definite risks; failure to maintain adequate oxygenation may precipitate vascular occlusion in the central nervous system, lungs or kidneys. Prophylactic antibiotics are advisable as the risk of postoperative infection is high.

Caisson disease and dysbaric osteonecrosis

Decompression sickness (caisson disease) and osteonecrosis are important causes of disability in deep-sea divers and compressed-air workers building tunnels or underwater structures. Under increased air pressure the blood and other tissues (especially fat) become supersaturated with nitrogen; if decompression is too rapid the gas is released as bubbles, which cause local tissue damage, generalized embolic phenomena and intracapillary coagulation. Prolonged compression may also cause swelling of marrow fat cells and decreased intramedullary blood flow, possibly due to oxygen toxicity (Pooley and Walder, 1984).

The symptoms of decompression sickness, which may develop within minutes, are pain near the joints ('the bends'), breathing difficulty and vertigo ('the staggers'). In the most acute cases there can be circulatory and respiratory collapse, severe neurological changes, coma and death. Only 10 per cent of patients with bone necrosis give a history of decompression sickness.

Radiological bone lesions have been found in 17 per cent of compressed-air workers in the UK; almost half the lesions are juxta-articular – mainly in the humeral head and femoral head – but microscopic bone death is much more widespread than x-rays suggest.

Clinical and x-ray features The necrosis may cause pain and loss of joint movement, but many lesions remain 'silent' and are found only on routine x-ray examination. Medullary infarcts cause mottled calcification or areas of dense sclerosis. Juxta-articular changes are similar to those in other forms of osteonecrosis.

Management The aim is prevention; the incidence of osteonecrosis is proportional to the working pressure, the length of exposure, the rate of decompression and the number of exposures. Strict enforcement of suitable working schedules has reduced the risks considerably. The treatment of established lesions follows the principles already outlined.

Gaucher's disease (see also page 177)

In this familial disorder lack of a specific enzyme results in the abnormal storage of glucocerebroside in the macrophages of the reticuloendothelial system.

The effects are seen chiefly in the liver, spleen and bone marrow, where the large polyhedral 'Gaucher cells' accumulate. Bone complications are common and osteonecrosis is among the worst of them. The hip is most frequently affected, but lesions also appear in the distal femur, the talus and the head of the humerus. Bone ischaemia is usually attributed to the increase in medullary cell volume and sinusoidal compression, but it is likely that other effects (abnormal cell emboli and increased blood viscosity) are equally important.

Clinical features

Bone necrosis may occur at any age and causes pain around one of the larger joints (usually the hip). In longstanding cases movements are restricted. There is a tendency for the Gaucher deposits to become infected and the patient may present with septicaemia. Blood tests reveal anaemia, leucopenia and thrombocytopaenia. A diagnostic, though inconstant, finding is a raised serum acid phosphatase level.

X-ray

The appearances resemble those in other types of osteonecrosis, and 'silent' lesions may be found in a number of bones. A special feature (due to replacement of myeloid tissue by Gaucher cells) is expansion of the tubular bones, especially the distal femur, producing the Erlenmeyer flask appearance. Cortical thinning and osteoporosis may lead to pathological fracture.

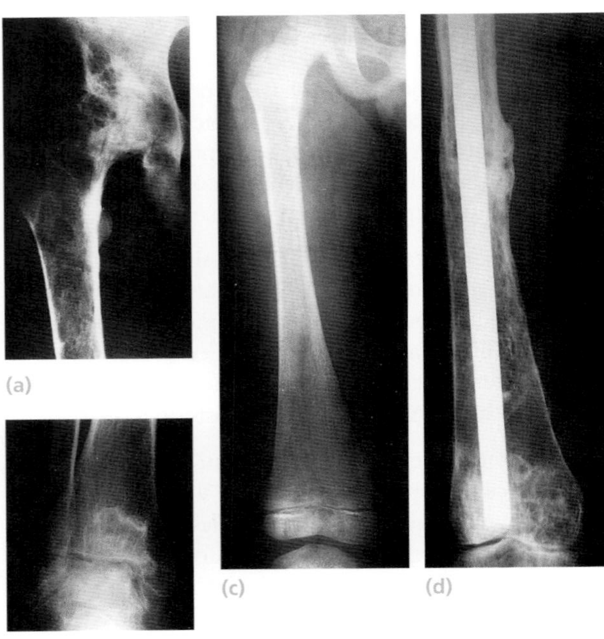

(a) (b) (c) (d)

6.10 Gaucher's disease (a) Gaucher deposits are seen throughout the femur. The cortices are thin and there is osteonecrosis of the femoral head. (b) Bone infarction is seen in the distal end of the tibia and the talus. (c) The typical Erlenmeyer flask appearance is seen in the x-ray of this teenager. (d) Ten years later the bone changes are much more marked, the cortices are extremely thin and the patient has obviously suffered a pathological fracture.

Treatment

The condition can now be treated by replacement of the missing enzyme and there is evidence that this will reduce the incidence of bone complications.

The management of established osteonecrosis follows the principles outlined earlier. However, there is a greater risk of infection following operation and suitable precautions should be taken. For adults, total joint replacement is probably preferable to other procedures.

Radiation necrosis

Ionizing radiation, if sufficiently intense or prolonged, may cause bone death. This is due to the combined effects of damage to small blood vessels, marrow cells and bone cells. Such changes, which are dose-related, often occurred in the past when low-energy radiation was in use. Nowadays, with megavoltage apparatus and more sophisticated planning techniques, long-term bone damage is much less likely; patients who present with osteonecrosis are usually those who were treated some years ago. Areas affected are mainly the shoulder and ribs (after external irradiation for breast cancer), the sacrum, pelvis and hip (after irradiation of pelvic lesions) and the jaws (after treatment of tumours around the head and neck).

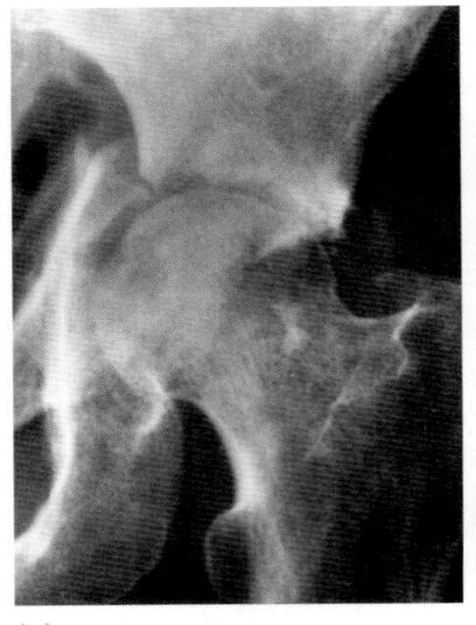

(a)

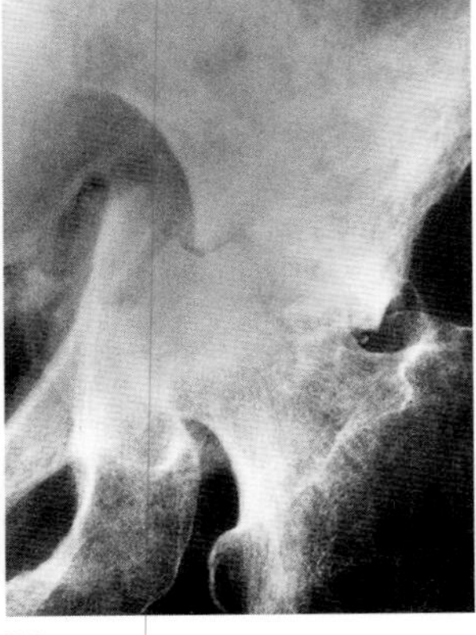

(b)

6.11 Radiation necrosis – x-rays This patient received radiation therapy for carcinoma of the bladder. One year later he developed pain in the left hip and x-ray showed (a) a fracture of the acetabulum. Diagnosis of radiation necrosis was confirmed when (b) the fracture failed to heal and the joint crumbled.

Pathology

Unlike the common forms of ischaemic necrosis, which always involve subchondral bone, radiation necrosis is more diffuse and the effects more variable. Marrow and bone cells die, but for months or even years there may be no structural change in the bone. Gradually, however, stress fractures appear and may result in widespread bone destruction. A striking feature is the absence of repair and remodelling. The surrounding bone is usually osteoporotic; in the jaw, infection may follow tooth extraction.

Clinical features

The patient usually presents with pain around the shoulder, the hip, the sacrum or the pubic symphysis. There will always be a history of previous treatment by ionizing radiation, though this may not come to light unless appropriate questions are asked.

There may be local signs of irradiation, such as skin pigmentation, and the area is usually tender. Movements in the nearby joint are restricted. General examination may reveal scars or other evidence of the original lesion.

X-rays show areas of bone destruction and patchy sclerosis; in the hip there may be an unsuspected fracture of the acetabulum or femoral neck, or collapse of the femoral head.

Treatment

Treatment depends on the site of osteonecrosis, the quality of the surrounding bone and the life expectancy of the patient. If a large joint is involved (e.g. the hip), replacement arthroplasty may be considered; however, bone quality is often poor and there is a high risk of early implant loosening. Nevertheless, if pain cannot be adequately controlled, and if the patient has a reasonable life expectancy, joint replacement is justified.

Osteochondrosis (osteochondritis)

The terms 'osteochondrosis' or 'osteochondritis' have for many years been applied to a group of conditions in which there is demarcation, and sometimes separation and necrosis, of a small segment of articular cartilage and bone. The affected area shows many of the features of ischaemic necrosis, including death of bone cells in the osteoarticular fragment and reactive vascularity and osteogenesis in the surrounding bone. The disorder occurs mainly in adolescents and young adults, often during phases of increased physical activity, and may be initiated by trauma or repetitive stress.

The pathogenesis of these lesions is still not completely understood. Impact injuries can cause oedema or bleeding in the subarticular bone, resulting in capillary compression or thrombosis and localized ischaemia. The critical event may well be a small osteochondral fracture, too faint to show up on plain x-ray examination but often visible on MRI. If the crack fails to unite, the isolated fragment may lose its blood supply and become necrotic. Traction injuries may similarly damage the blood supply to an apophysis. However, it is thought that there must be other predisposing factors, for the condition is sometimes multifocal and sometimes runs in families.

Clinical presentation

The classic example of this disorder is the condition known as *osteochondritis dissecans*. This occurs typically in young adults, usually men, and affects particular sites: the inner (medial) surface of the medial femoral condyle in the knee, the anteromedial corner of the talus in the ankle, the superomedial part of the femoral head, the humeral capitulum and the head of the second metatarsal bone. (Note that these are all slightly bulbous areas with convex articular surfaces). The patient usually complains of intermittent pain; sometimes there is swelling and a small effusion in the joint. If the necrotic fragment becomes completely

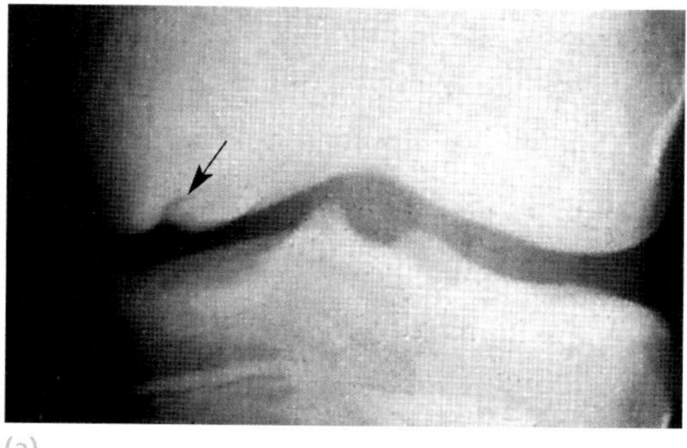
(a)

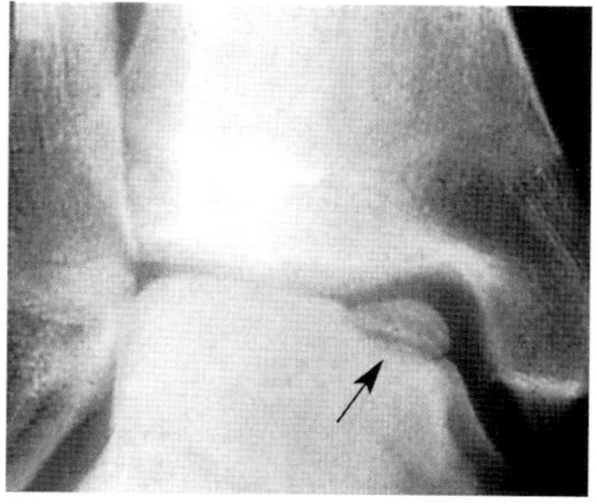
(b)

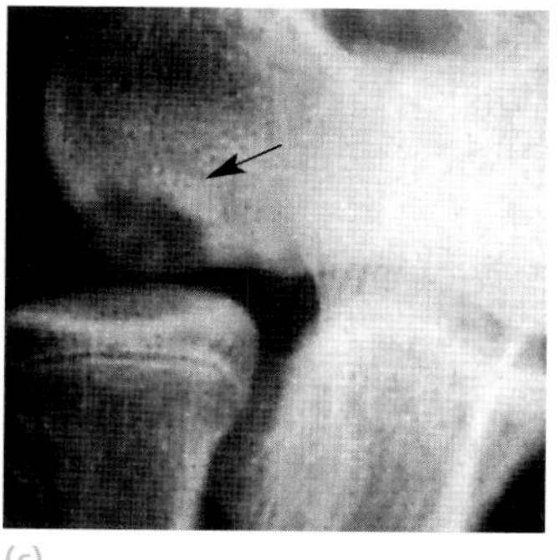
(c)

6.12 Osteochondritis dissecans The osteochondral fragment usually remains in place at the articular surface. The most common sites are (a) the medial femoral condyle, (b) the talus and (c) the capitulum.

detached it may cause locking of the joint, or unexpected episodes of 'giving way' in the knee or ankle.

Imaging

X-rays must be taken with the joint in the appropriate position to show the affected part of the articular surface in tangential projection. The dissecting fragment is defined by a radiolucent line of demarcation. When it separates, the resulting 'crater' may be obvious.

The early changes (i.e. before demarcation of the dissecting fragment) are better shown by MRI: there is decreased signal intensity in the area around the affected osteochondral segment.

Radionuclide scanning with ^{99m}Tc-HDP shows markedly increased activity in the same area.

Treatment

Treatment in the early stage consists of load reduction and restriction of activity. In young people complete healing may occur, though it can take up to two years. For a large joint like the knee, it is generally recommended that partially detached fragments be pinned back in position after roughening of the base, while completely detached fragments should be pinned back only if they are fairly large and completely preserved. These procedures may be carried out by arthroscopy. If the fragment becomes detached and causes symptoms, it should be fixed back in position or else completely removed.

Treatment of osteochondrosis at the elbow, wrist and metatarsal head is discussed in the relevant chapters.

'Spontaneous' osteonecrosis of the knee ('SONK')

This condition is similar to osteochondritis dissecans of the medial femoral condyle, but is distinguished by three important features: it appears in *elderly people* (usually women) who are *osteoporotic* and the lesion invariably appears on the *highest part* of the medial femoral condyle. A detailed description appears in Chapter 20.

BONE MARROW OEDEMA SYNDROME

In 1959 Curtiss and Kincaid described an uncommon clinical syndrome characterized by pain and *transient osteoporosis* of one or both hips affecting women in the last trimester of pregnancy. It is now recognized that the condition can occur in patients of either sex and at all ages from late adolescence onwards. Although quite distressing at its onset, the condition typically lasts for only 6–12 months, after which the symptoms subside and radiographic bone density is restored. Sometimes successive joints are affected ('regional migratory osteoporosis'), with similar symptoms occurring at each site.

The aetiology of this condition is obscure. The intense activity shown on radionuclide scanning suggests a neurovascular abnormality akin to that of reflex sympathetic dystrophy (RSD). However, there are no trophic changes in the soft tissues and no long-term effects, such as one sees in RSD. The demonstration of diffuse changes on MRI – low signal intensity on T_1 weighted images and matching high signal intensity on T_2 weighted images – corresponding to the areas of increased scintigraphic activity are characteristic of *bone marrow oedema* (Wilson et al., 1988), and this is now thought to be an important aspect of transient osteoporosis. What causes it is still unknown.

Similar 'marrow oedema changes' are sometimes seen in areas around typical lesions of osteonecrosis and it has been suggested that transient osteoporosis is due to a sub-lethal, reversible episode of ischaemia associated with reactive hyperaemia in the surrounding bone (Hofmann et al., 1993). Many would disagree with this hypothesis; the most significant differences between the two conditions are listed in Table 6.2. The issue is important because transient osteoporosis has until now been regarded as a reversible disorder which requires only symptomatic treatment while osteonecrosis often calls for operative intervention.

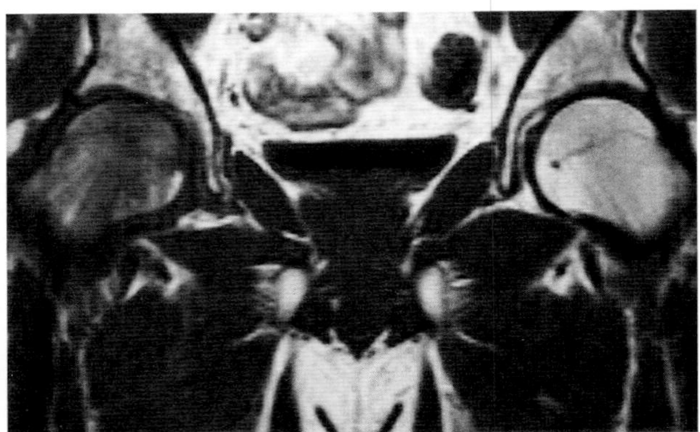

6.13 Bone marrow oedema MRI showing the typical diffuse area of low signal intensity in the right femoral head in the T_1 weighted image.

Table 6.2 Differences between transient bone marrow oedema and osteonecrosis

	Bone marrow oedema	Osteonecrosis
Sex distribution (M:F)	1:3	1:1
Predisposing factors	Pregnancy	Systemic disorders
		Corticosteroids
Onset	Acute	Gradual
Clinical progress	Self-limiting	Progressive
X-ray	Osteopaenia	Sclerosis
Scintigraphy	Increased activity	Reduced activity
MRI	Diffuse changes	Focal changes
Histology	Marrow oedema	Marrow necrosis
	Minimal bone death	Bone necrosis

REFERENCES AND FURTHER READING

Asherson RA, Lioté F, Page B *et al.* Avascular necrosis of bone and antiphospholipid antibodies in systemic lupus erythematosus. *J Rheum* 1993; **20:** 284–8.

Curtiss PH, Kincaid WE. Transitory demineralization of the hip in pregnancy: A report of three cases. *J Bone Joint Surg* 1959; **41A:** 1327–33.

Ficat RP. Idiopathic bone necrosis of the femoral head: Early diagnosis and treatment. *J Bone Joint Surg* 1985; **67B:** 3–9.

Ficat RP, Arlet J. *Ischemia and Necroses of Bone* (edited and adapted by DS Hungerford), Williams & Wilkins, Baltimore, 1980.

Francis RB Jr. Platelets, coagulation and fibrinolysis in sickle-cell disease: Their possible role in vascular occlusion. *Blood Coagul Fibrinolysis* 1991; **2:** 341–53.

Glueck CJ, Crawford A, Roy D *et al.* Association of antithrombotic factor deficiencies and hypofibrinolysis with Legg-Perthes' disease. *J Bone Joint Surg* 1996; **78A:** 3–13.

Glueck CJ, Freiberg R, Tracy T et al. Thrombophilia and hypofibrinolysis. Pathophysiologies of osteonecrosis. *Clin Orthop* 1997a; **334:** 43–56.

Glueck CJ, Crawford A, Roy D *et al.* Correspondence. *J Bone Joint Surg* 1997b; **79A:** 1114–15.

Guerra JJ, Steinberg ME. Distinguishing transient osteoporosis from avascular necrosis of the hip. *J Bone Joint Surg* 1995; **77A:** 616–24.

Hernigou P, Galacteros F, Bachir D, *et al.* Deformities of the hip in adults who have sickle-cell disease and had avascular necrosis in childhood. *J Bone Joint Surg* 1991; **73A:** 81–92.

Hofmann S, Engel A, Neuhold A, *et al.* Bone-marrow oedema syndrome and transient osteoporosis of the hip. *J Bone Joint Surg* 1993; **75B:** 210–16.

Iwegbu CF, Fleming AF. Avascular necrosis of the femoral head in sickle-cell disease. *J Bone Joint Surg* 1985; **67B:** 29–32.

Jones JP Jr. Concepts of etiology and early pathogenesis of osteonecrosis. In Schafer IM (ed.). *Instructional Course Lectures, Am Acad Orthop Surg* 1994; **43:** 499–512.

Lai KA, Shen WJ, Yang CY *et al.* The use of alendronate to prevent early collapse of the femoral head in patients with nontraumatic osteonecrosis. *J Bone Joint Surg* 2005; **87A:** 2155–59.

Nishii T, Sugano N, Miki H *et al.* Does alendronate prevent collapse in osteonecrosis of the femoral head? *Clin Orthop Relat Res* 2006; **443:** 273–9.

Pooley J, Walder DN. The effect of compressed air on bone marrow blood flow and its relationship to caisson disease of bone. In *Bone Circulation* eds Arlet J, Ficat RP, Hungerford DS. Baltimore, Williams & Wilkins, pp 63–67, 1984.

Sakamoto M, Shimizu K, Iida S, *et al.* Osteonecrosis of the femoral head. A prospective study with MRI. *J Bone Joint Surg* 1997; **79B:** 213–19.

Shimizu K, Moriya H, Akita T. Prediction of collapse with magnetic resonance imaging of avascular necrosis of the femoral head. *J Bone Joint Surg* 1994; **76A:** 215–23.

Solomon L, Pearse MF. Osteonecrosis following low-dose short-course corticosteroids. *J Orthop Rheumatol* 1994; **7:** 203–5.

Steinberg ME, Hayken GD, Steinberg DR. A quantitative system for staging avascular necrosis. *J Bone Joint Surg* 1995; **77B:** 34–41.

Whitehead TP, Clarke CA, Whitfield AGW. Biochemical and haematological markers of alcohol intake. *Lancet* 1978; **1:** 978–81.

Wilson AJ, Murphy WA, Hardy DC, *et al.* Transient osteoporosis: transient bone marrow oedema? *Radiology* 1988; **167:** 757–60.

Yamamoto T, Bullough PG. Spontaneous osteonecrosis of the knee: the result of spontaneous insufficiency fracture. *J Bone Joint Surg* 2000; **82A:** 858–66.

Yamamoto T, Kubo T, Hirasawa Y, *et al.* A clinicopathologic study of transient osteoporosis of the hip. *Skeletal Radiol* 1999; **28:** 621–7.

Metabolic and endocrine disorders

7

Louis Solomon

Metabolic bone disorders are associated with critical alterations in the regulation of bone formation, bone resorption and distribution of minerals in bone. Clinical features arise from both systemic responses to changes in mineral exchange and local effects of abnormal bone structure and composition. Orthopaedic surgeons deal mainly with the bone abnormalities (e.g. rickety deformities in growing bones or insufficiency fractures in the elderly) but it is important also to be aware of the systemic disorders that may lie behind apparently straightforward 'orthopaedic' defects and to understand the unseen metabolic changes that influence the outcome of many of our surgical interventions.

BONE AND BONES

Understanding of disorders of the musculoskeletal system begins with a basic knowledge of the anatomical structure and physiology of the bones and joints – the framework that supports the body, protects the soft tissues, transmits load and power from one part of the body to another and mediates movement and locomotion.

Embryonic development of the limbs begins with the appearance of the arm buds at about 4 weeks from ovulation and the leg buds shortly afterwards. These at first have the appearance of miniature paddles but by around 5 weeks the finger and toe rays become differentiated. By then primitive skeletal elements and pre-muscle masses have begun to differentiate in the limbs. From about 6 weeks after ovulation the primitive cartilaginous bone-models start to become vascularized and primary ossification centres appear in the chondroid anlage. By now spinal nerves would be growing into the limbs. At 7 or 8 weeks cavitation occurs where the joints will appear and during the next few weeks the cartilaginous epiphyseal precursors become vascularized. Between 8 and 12 weeks the primitive joints and synovium become defined.

From then onwards further development goes hand in hand with growth. Bone formation in the cartilaginous model progresses along the diaphysis but the epiphyseal ends remain unossified until after birth. The entire sequence has been aptly summarized as *condensation → chondrification → ossification.*

Soon after birth secondary ossification centres begin to appear in the still cartilaginous ends of the tubular bones, a process that will occur during childhood in all the *endochondrial bones* (bones formed in cartilage). By then each bone end is defined as an *epiphysis*, the still-growing cartilage beyond that as the *physis* and the shaft as the *diaphysis.*

Longitudinal growth continues through adolescence until the epiphysis is fully ossified and fused to the diaphysis. At the same time an increase in bone girth occurs by a different process – *appositional bone formation* by generative cells in the deepest layer of the periosteum. The small cuboidal bones also grow by interstitial cartilage proliferation and appositional (periosteal) bone formation.

After the end of bone growth (which varies for different bones) no further increase in size occurs, but bone and joint remodelling continues throughout life.

Where bones connect with each other, i.e. at the joints, the contact surfaces remain cartilaginous. In *diarthrodial joints* (freely movable, synovial joints) this is *hyaline cartilage*, which is ideally suited to permit low-friction movement and to accommodate both compressive and tensile forces. In *synarthroses*, where greater resistance to shearing forces is needed, the interface usually consists of tough *fibrocartilage* (e.g. the pubic symphysis).

BONE STRUCTURE AND PHYSIOLOGY

Bones as structural organs have three main functions: *support, protection* and *leverage*. They support every part of the body in a wide variety of positions and

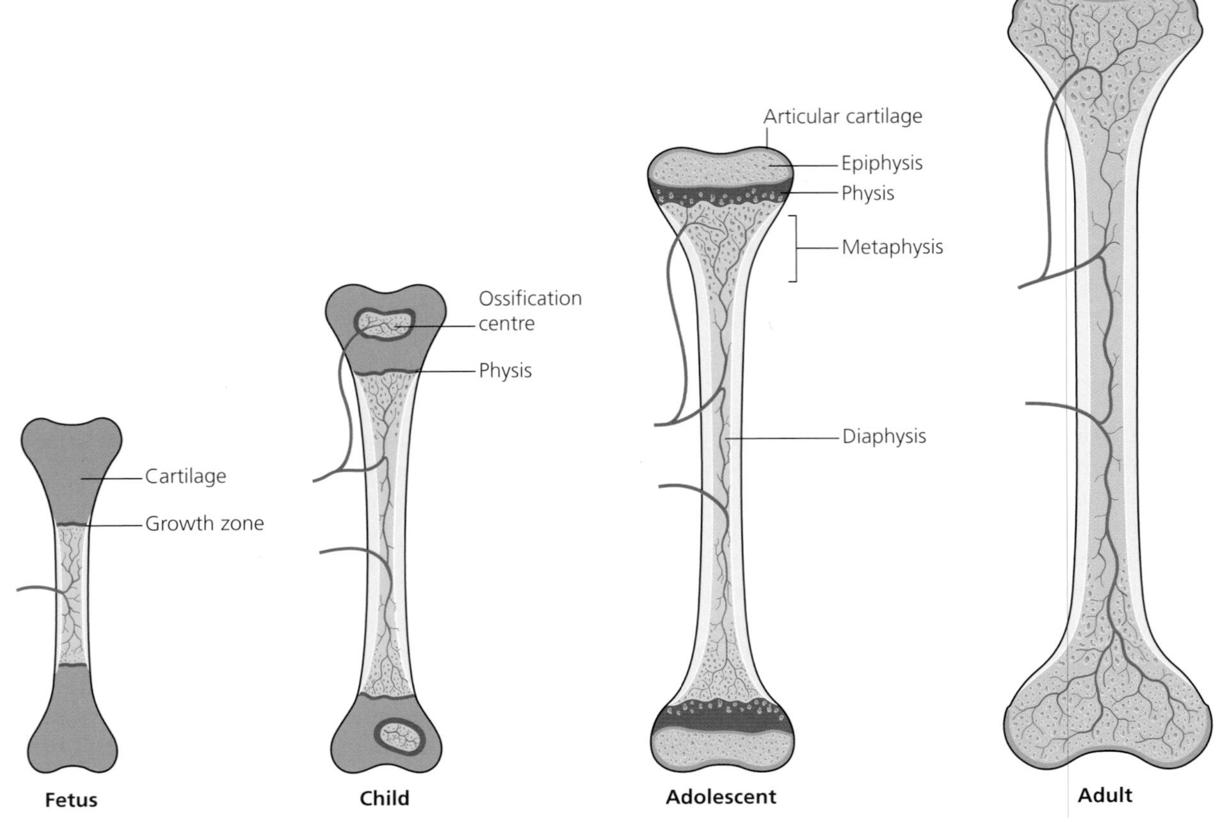

7.1 Stages in bone development Schematic representation of the stages in the development of a tubular bone showing the progress from diaphyseal ossification, through endochondral growth at the physis and increase in width of the diaphysis by sub-periosteal appositional bone formation.

load-bearing; they protect important soft tissues such as the brain, the spinal cord, the heart and the lungs; and they act as jointed levers that facilitate a range of movements from straightforward locomotion to the breathtaking feats of musical virtuosos, ballet dancers and Olympic athletes.

Bone as tissue has an equally important role: it is a mineral reservoir which helps to regulate the composition – and in particular the calcium ion concentration – of the extracellular fluid. For all its solidity, it is in a continuous state of flux, its internal shape and structure changing from moment to moment in concert with the normal variations in mechanical function and mineral exchange.

All modulations in bone structure and composition are brought about by cellular activity, which is regulated by hormones and local factors; these agents, in turn, are controlled by alterations in mineral ion concentrations. Disruption of this complex interactive system results in systemic changes in mineral metabolism and generalized skeletal abnormalities.

BONE COMPOSITION

Bone consists of a largely collagenous matrix which is impregnated with mineral salts and populated by cells (osteoblasts and osteoclasts).

The matrix

Type I collagen fibres, derived from tropocollagen molecules produced by osteoblasts, make up over 80 per cent of the unmineralized matrix. They form a network which embodies a *mucopolysaccharide* (*proteoglycans*) ground substance and also acts as a scaffold on which the mineral component – crystalline hydroxyapatite – is deposited.

Other non-collagenous proteins exist in small amounts in the mineralized matrix – mainly *sialoproteins (osteopontin), osteonectin, osteocalcin (bone Gla protein)* and *alkaline phosphatases.* Their functions have not been fully elucidated but they appear to be involved in the regulation of bone cells and matrix mineralization. Osteocalcin is produced only by osteoblasts and its concentration in the blood is, to some extent, a measure of osteoblastic activity.

A number of *growth factors* have now been identified; they are produced by the osteoblasts and some of them, acting in combination, have a regulatory effect on bone cell development, differentiation and metabolism.

Bone morphogenetic protein (BMP) – a collection of growth factor proteins – has attracted a great deal of attention. It was originally found by Marshall Urist in 1964 (Urist, 1965) and is now produced in purified form from bone matrix. It has been shown to have the important property of inducing the differentiation of progenitor cells into cartilage and thereafter into bone. It is now produced commercially and is being used to enhance osteogenesis in bone fusion operations (Rihn et al., 2008).

Bone mineral

Almost half the bone volume is mineral matter – mainly *calcium* and *phosphate* in the form of *crystalline hydroxyapatite* which is laid down in osteoid at the calcification front. The interface between bone and osteoid can be labelled by administering tetracycline, which is taken up avidly in newly mineralized bone and shows as a fluorescent band on ultraviolet light microscopy. In mature bone the proportions of calcium and phosphate are constant and the molecule is firmly bound to collagen. It is important to appreciate that in life *'demineralization' of bone occurs only by resorption of the entire matrix.*

While the collagenous component lends tensile strength to bone, the crystalline mineral enhances its ability to resist compression.

Unmineralized matrix is known as *osteoid*; in normal life it is seen only as a thin layer on surfaces where active new bone formation is taking place, but the proportion of osteoid to mineralized bone increases significantly in rickets and osteomalacia.

Bone cells

There are three types of bone cell: osteoblasts, osteocytes and osteoclasts.

Osteoblasts Osteoblasts are concerned with bone formation and osteoclast activation. They are derived from mesenchymal precursors in the bone marrow and the deep layer of the periosteum. Differentiation is controlled by a number of interacting growth factors, including bone morphogenetic proteins.

Mature osteoblasts form rows of small (20 μm) mononuclear cells along the free surfaces of trabeculae and haversian systems where *osteoid* is laid down prior to calcification. They are rich in alkaline phosphatase and are responsible for the production of type I collagen as well as the non-collagenous bone proteins and for the mineralization of bone matrix (Peck and Woods, 1988). Stimulated by parathyroid hormone (PTH), they play a critical role in the initiation and control of osteoclastic activity (page 122).

At the end of each bone remodelling cycle the osteoblasts either remain on the newly formed bone surface as quiescent lining cells or they become embedded in the matrix as 'resting' osteocytes. During advanced ageing their numbers decrease.

Osteocytes These cells can be regarded as spent osteoblasts; however, they are by no means inactive. Lying in their bony lacunae, they communicate with each other and with the surface lining cells by slender cytoplasmic processes. Their function is obscure: they may, under the influence of PTH, participate in bone resorption ('osteocytic osteolysis') and calcium ion transport (Peck and Woods, 1988). It has also been suggested that they are sensitive to mechanical stimuli and communicate information and changes in stress and strain to the active osteoblasts (Skerry et al., 1989) which can then modify their osteogenic activity accordingly. Ultimately the ageing osteocytes are phagocytosed during osteoclastic bone resorption and remodelling.

Osteoclasts These large multinucleated cells are the principal mediators of bone resorption. They develop from mononuclear precursors in the haemopoietic marrow (the same lineage as macrophages) under the influence of local osteoblastic stromal cells that generate an essential osteoclast differentiating factor –

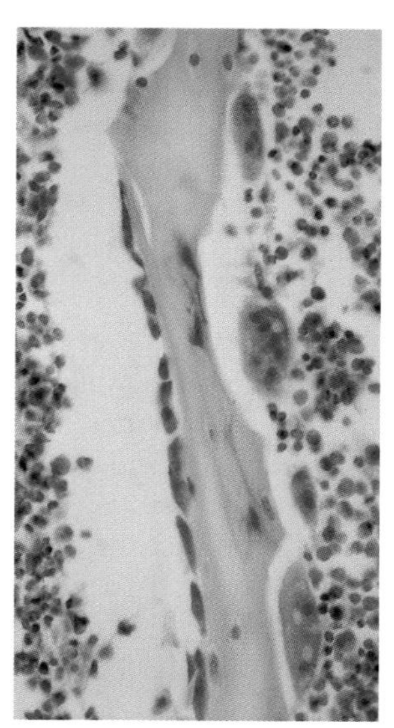

(a)

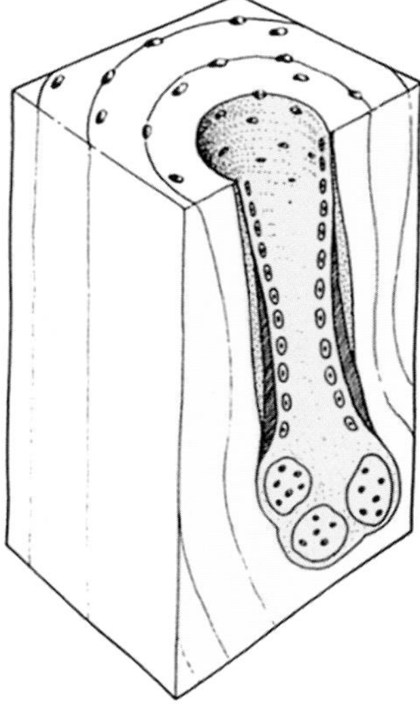

(b)

7.2 Bone cells (a) Histological section showing a trabecula lined on one surface by excavating osteoclasts and on the other surface by a string of much smaller osteoblasts. These two types of cell, working in concert, continuously remodel the internal bone structure. (b) In compact bone the osteoclasts burrow deeply into the existing bone, with the osteoblasts following close behind to re-line the cavity with new bone.

receptor activator of nuclear factor-κβ ligand (RANKL) – which binds with a specific receptor site *(RANK)* on the osteoclast precursors.

Mature osteoclasts have a foamy appearance, due to the presence of numerous vesicles in the cytoplasm. In response to appropriate stimuli the osteoclast forms a sealed attachment to a bone surface, where the cell membrane develops a ruffled border within which bone resorption takes place. This process, and the important interactions between RANKL and RANK, are discussed further on page 122.

Following resorption of the bone matrix, the osteoclasts are left in shallow excavations – Howship's lacunae – along free bone surfaces. By identifying these excavations one can distinguish 'resorption surfaces' from the smooth 'formation surfaces' or 'resting surfaces' in histological sections.

Bone structure

Bone in its immature state is called *woven bone*; the collagen fibres are arranged haphazardly and the cells have no specific orientation. Typically it is found in the early stages of fracture healing, where it acts as a temporary weld before being replaced by mature bone.

The mature tissue is *lamellar bone*, in which the collagen fibres are arranged parallel to each other to form multiple layers (or laminae) with the osteocytes lying between the lamellae. Unlike woven bone, which is laid down in fibrous tissue, lamellar bone forms only on existing bone surfaces.

Lamellar bone exists in two structurally different forms, c*ompact (cortical) bone* and *cancellous (trabecular) bone.*

Compact bone

Compact (cortical) bone is dense to the naked eye. It is found where support matters most: the outer walls of all bones but especially the shafts of tubular bones, and the subchondral plates supporting articular cartilage. It is made up of compact units – haversian systems or osteons – each of which consists of a central canal (the haversian canal) containing blood vessels, lymphatics and nerves and enclosed by closely packed, more or less concentric lamellae of bone. Between the lamellae lie osteocytes, bedded in lacunae which appear to be discrete but which are in fact connected by a network of fine canaliculi. The haversian canal offers a free surface lined by bone cells; its size varies, depending on whether the osteon is in a phase of resorption or formation. During resorption osteoclasts eat into the surrounding lamellae and the canal widens out; during formation osteoblasts lay down new lamellae on the inner surface and the canal closes down again.

Cancellous bone

Cancellous (trabecular) bone has a honeycomb appearance; it makes up the interior meshwork of all bones and is particularly well developed in the ends of the tubular bones and the vertebral bodies. The structural units of trabecular bone are flattened sheets or spars that can be thought of as unfolded osteons. Three-dimensionally the trabecular sheets are interconnected (like a honeycomb) and arranged according to the mechanical needs of the structure, the thickest and strongest along trajectories of compressive stress and the thinnest in the planes of tensile stress. The interconnectedness of this meshwork lends added strength to cancellous bone beyond the simple effect of tissue mass. The spaces between trabeculae – the 'opened out' vascular spaces – contain the marrow and fine sinusoidal vessels that course through the tissue, nourishing both marrow and bone.

Trabecular bone is obviously more porous than cortical bone. Although it makes up only one-quarter of the total skeletal mass, it provides two-thirds of the total bone surface. Add to this the fact that it is covered with marrow and it is easy to understand why the effects of metabolic disorders are usually seen first in trabecular bone.

Haversian system

Bones vary greatly in size and shape. At the most basic level, however, they are similar: compact on the outside and spongy on the inside. Their outer surfaces (except at the articular ends) are covered by a tough *periosteal membrane*, the deepest layer of which consists of potentially bone-forming cells. The inner, endosteal, surfaces are irregular and lined by a fine *endosteal membrane* in close contact with the marrow spaces.

The osteonal pattern in the cortex is usually depicted from two-dimensional histological sections. A three-dimensional reconstruction would show that the *haversian canals* are long branching channels running in the longitudinal axis of the bone and connecting extensively with each other and with the endosteal and periosteal surfaces by smaller channels (*Volkmann canals*). In this way the vessels in the haversian canals form a rich anastomotic network between the medullary and periosteal blood supply. Blood flow in this capillary network is normally centrifugal – from the medullary cavity outwards – and it has long been held that the cortex is supplied entirely from this source. However, it seems likely that at least the outermost layers of the cortex are normally also supplied by periosteal vessels, and if the medullary vessels are blocked or destroyed the periosteal circulation can take over entirely and the direction of blood flow is reversed.

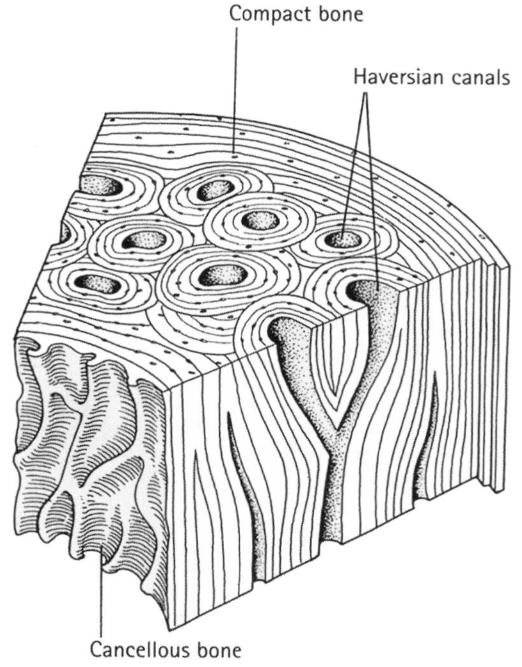

(a)

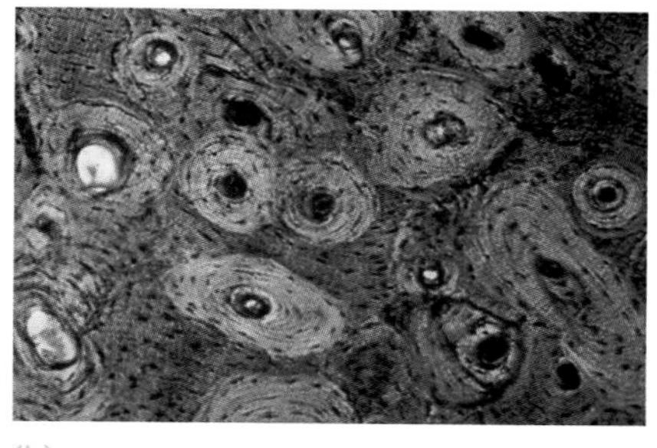

(b)

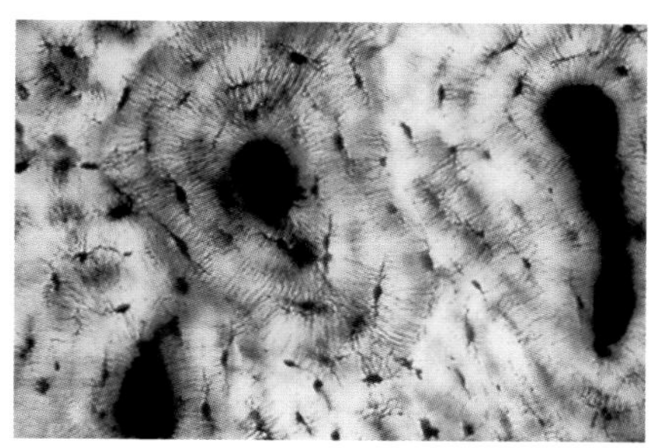

(c)

7.3 The haversian systems (a) A schematic diagram representing a wedge taken from the cortex of a long bone. It shows the basic elements of compact bone: densely packed osteons, each made up of concentric layers of bone and osteocytes around a central haversian canal which contains the blood vessels; outer laminae of sub-periosteal bone; and similar laminae on the interior surface (endosteum) merging into a lattice of cancellous bone. (b,c) Low- and high-power views showing the osteons in various stages of formation and resorption.

BONE DEVELOPMENT AND GROWTH

Bones develop in two different ways: by ossification of a prior cartilage model or framework (*endochondral ossification)* and by direct *intramembranous ossification.*

ENDOCHONDRAL OSSIFICATION

This is the usual manner in which tubular bones develop. At birth the cartilage model is complete and ossification has already begun at the centre of the diaphysis. After secondary ossification of the epiphyseal ends has begun, further growth in length takes place in the still cartilaginous zone between the extending area of diaphyseal bone and the epiphysis. In this way the still-cartilaginous zone between the ossifying diaphysis and the epiphysis gradually narrows down but does not disappear until late adolescence. This actively growing cartilage disc is called the *physis,* seated as it is between the epiphysis and the diaphysis.

The physis (or what used to be known as the 'growth plate') consists of four distinct zones. Coextensive with the epiphysis is a *zone of resting chondrocytes* in haphazard array. This merges into a *proliferative zone* in which the chondrocytes are lined up longitudinally; being capable of interstitial growth, they add progressively to the overall length of the bone. The older cells in this zone (those 'left behind' nearest the advancing new bone of the diaphysis) gradually enlarge and constitute a *hypertrophic zone.* Close to the interface between cartilage and bone the cartilage becomes calcified (probably with the involvement of alkaline phosphatase produced by the hypertrophic cells); this *zone of calcified cartilage* finally undergoes osteoclastic resorption and, with the ingrowth of new blood vessels from the metaphysis, ossification. Woven bone is laid down on the calcified scaffolding and this in turn is replaced by lamellar bone which forms the newest part of the bone shaft, now called the *metaphysis.*

It should be noted that a similar process takes place in the late stage of fracture repair.

INTRAMEMBRANOUS OSSIFICATION

With the growth in length, the bone also has to increase in girth and, since a tubular bone is an open cylinder, this inevitably demands that the medullary cavity increase in size proportionately. New bone is added to the outside by direct ossification at the deepest layer of the

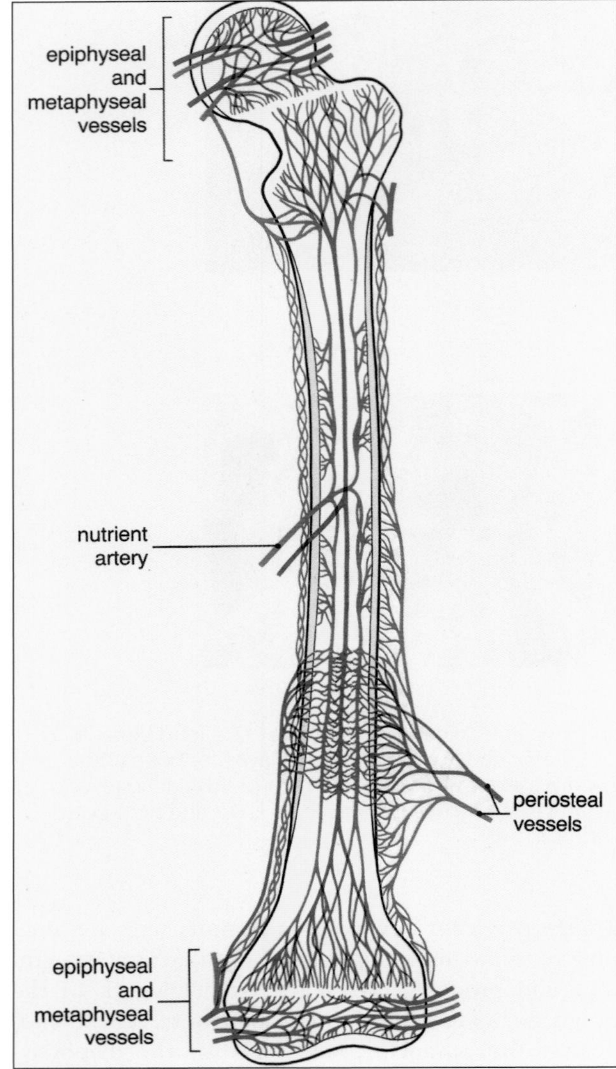

7.4 Blood supply to bone Schematic presentation of blood supply in tubular bones. (Reproduced from Bullough PG. Atlas of Orthopaedic Pathology: With Clinical and Radiological Correlations (2nd edition). Baltimore: University Park Press, 1985. By kind permission of Dr Peter G Bullough and Elsevier.)

periosteum where mesenchymal cells differentiate into osteoblasts (*intramembranous, or 'appositional', bone formation*) and old bone is removed from the inside of the cylinder by osteoclastic *endosteal resorption*.

Intramembranous periosteal new bone formation also occurs as a response to periosteal stripping due to trauma, infection or tumour growth, and its appearance is a useful radiographic pointer.

Bone resorption

Bone resorption is carried out by the *osteoclasts* under the influence of stromal cells (including *osteoblasts*) and both local and systemic activators. Although it has long been known that PTH promotes bone resorption, osteoclasts have no receptor for PTH but the hormone acts indirectly through its effect on the vitamin D metabolite 1,25-dihydroxycholecalciferol [$1,25(OH)_2D_3$] and osteoblasts.

Proliferation of osteoclastic progenitor cells requires the presence of an osteoclast differentiating factor produced by the stromal osteoblasts after stimulation by (for example) PTH, glucocorticoids or pro-inflammatory cytokines. It is now known that this 'osteoclast differentiating factor' is the receptor activator of nuclear factor-κβ ligand (RANKL for short), and that it has to bind with a RANK receptor on the osteoclast precursor in the presence of a macrophage colony-stimulating factor (M-CSF) before full maturation and osteoclastic resorption can begin.

It is thought that osteoblasts first 'prepare' the resorption site by removing osteoid from the bone surface while other matrix constituents act as osteoclast attractors. During resorption each osteoclast forms a sealed attachment to the bone surface where the cell membrane folds into a characteristic ruffled border within which hydrochloric acid and proteolytic enzymes are secreted. At this low pH minerals in the matrix are dissolved and the organic components are destroyed by lysosomal enzymes. Calcium and phosphate ions are absorbed into the osteoclast vesicles from where they pass into the extracellular fluid and, ultimately, the blood stream.

In cancellous bone this process results in thinning (and sometimes actual perforation) of existing trabeculae. In cortical bone the cells either enlarge an existing haversian canal or else burrow into the compact bone to create a *cutting cone* – like miners sinking a new shaft in the ground. During hyperactive bone resorption these processes are reflected in the appearance of hydroxyproline in the urine and a rise in serum calcium and phosphate levels.

Bone modelling and remodelling

The sequential process of bone resorption and formation has been likened to sculpting and is, in fact, known as bone modelling and remodelling. During growth each bone has continuously to be 'sculpted' into the normal shape of that particular part of the skeleton. How else can a long bone retain its basic shape as the flared ends are constantly re-formed further and further from the midshaft during growth?

The internal architecture of the bone is also subject to remodelling, not only during growth but throughout life. This serves several crucial purposes: 'old bone' is continually replaced by 'new bone' and in this way the skeleton is protected from exposure to cumulative loading frequencies and the risk of stress failure; bone turnover is sensitive to the demands of function

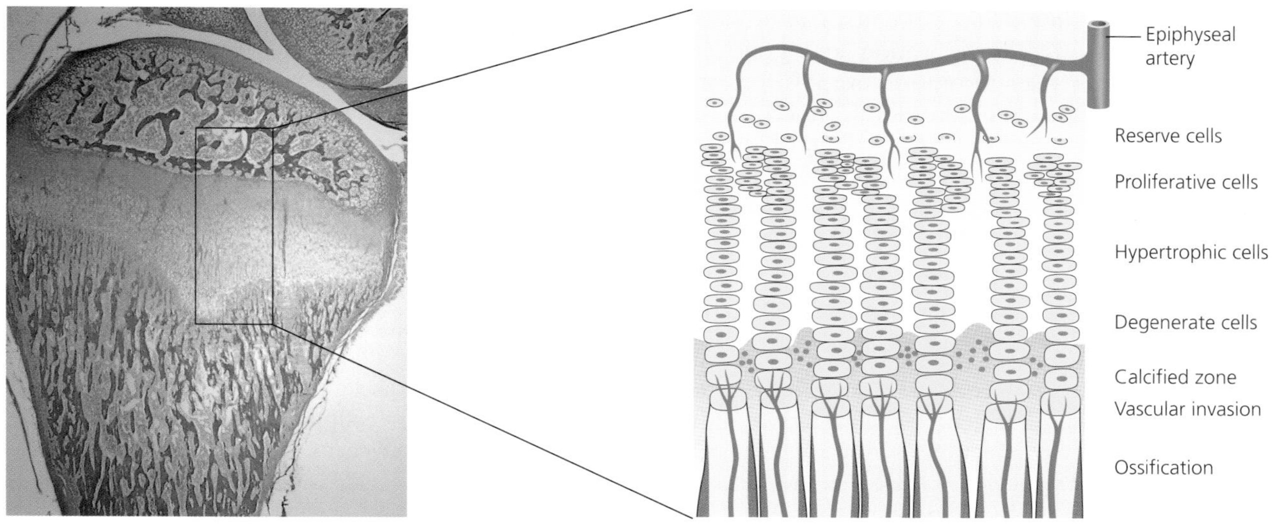

7.5 Endochondral ossification Histological section of a growing endochondral bone with a schematic figure showing the layers of the growth disc (physis). (Reproduced from Bullough PG. Atlas of Orthopaedic Pathology: With Clinical and Radiological Correlations (2nd edition). Baltimore: University Park Press, 1985. Second figure by kind permission of Dr Peter G Bullough and Elsevier.)

and trabeculae are fashioned (or refashioned) in accordance with the stresses imposed upon the bone, the thicker and stronger trabeculae following the trajectories of compressive stress and the finer trabeculae lying in the planes of tensile stress; besides, the maintenance of calcium homeostasis requires a constant turnover of the mineral deposits which would otherwise stay locked in bone.

7.6 Wolff's Law Wolff's Law is beautifully demonstrated in the trabecular pattern at the upper end of the femur. The thickest trabeculae are arranged along the trajectories of greatest stress.

At each *remodelling site* work proceeds in an orderly sequence. Prompted by the osteoblasts, osteoclasts gather on a free bone surface and proceed to excavate a cavity. After 2–4 weeks resorption ceases; the osteoclasts undergo apoptosis and are phagocytosed. There is a short quiescent period, then the excavated surface is covered with osteoblasts and for the next 3 months osteoid is laid down and mineralized to leave a new 'packet' of bone (or *osteon*). The entire *remodelling cycle* takes from 4 to 6 months and at the end the boundary between 'old' and 'new' bone is marked by a histologically identifiable 'cement line'.

The osteoblasts and osteoclasts participating in each cycle of bone turnover work in concert, together acting as a *bone remodelling unit* (of which there are more than a million at work in the adult skeleton at any time). Resorption and formation are *coupled*, the one ineluctably following the other. Systemic hormones and local growth factors are involved in coordinating this process; indeed it is likely that PTH and 1,25-$(OH)_2D$ are involved in initiating both formation and resorption. This ensures that (at least over the short term) a balance is maintained though at any moment and at any particular site one or other phase may predominate.

In the long term, change does occur. The annual rate of bone turnover in healthy adults has been estimated as 4 per cent for cortical bone and 25 per cent for trabecular bone (Parfitt, 1988). The rate may be increased or decreased either by alterations in the number of remodelling units at work or by changes in the remodelling time. During the first half of life formation slightly exceeds resorption and bone mass increases; in later years resorption exceeds formation and bone mass steadily diminishes. Connecting spars may be perforated or lost, further diminishing bone strength and increasing the likelihood of fragility fractures. Rapid bone loss is usually due to excessive resorption rather than diminished formation.

Local regulation of bone remodelling

The coordinated interaction between osteoblastic bone formation and osteoclastic resorption has been explained to a large extent by elucidation of the RANKL/RANK connection. However, another cytokine – osteoprotegerin (OPG) – comes into play in the regulatory mechanism of this system. OPG, which is also expressed by osteoblasts, is able to inhibit the differentiation of osteoclast precursors by preferentially binding with RANKL (acting as a 'decoy' receptor) and so reducing bone resorption by preventing RANKL from binding with its receptor on the osteoclast precursor.

Bone remodelling is, therefore, influenced continuously by an array of hormones, cytokine systems, dietary elements, medication and signals from mechanical stresses that impinge on any part of the RANKL/RANK/OPG triad. Already explanations involving this system have been advanced for the occurrence of osteoporosis in metastatic bone disease, myelomatosis, rheumatoid arthritis and other inflammatory conditions. There is promise also that down-regulation of osteoclastogenesis may offer an effective treatment for age-related osteoporosis.

It has been said, with good reason, that the RANKL/RANK/OPG signalling system is '...one of the most important discoveries in bone biology in the past decade' (Boyce and Xing, 2007).

MINERAL EXCHANGE AND BONE TURNOVER

Calcium and phosphorus have an essential role in a wide range of physiological processes. Over 98 per cent of the body's calcium and 85 per cent of its phosphorus are tightly packed as hydroxyapatite crystals in bone and capable of only very slow exchange. A small amount exists in a rapidly exchangeable form, either in partially formed crystals or in the extracellular fluid and blood where their concentration is maintained within very narrow limits by an efficient homeostatic mechanism involving intestinal absorption, renal excretion and mineral exchange in bone.

The control of calcium is more critical than that of phosphate. Transient alterations in blood levels are rapidly compensated for by changes in renal tubular absorption. A more persistent fall in extracellular calcium concentration can be accommodated by increasing bone resorption.

All these adjustments are regulated by PTH, 1,25-$(OH)_2$ D and an array of systemic and local growth factors.

Calcium

Calcium is essential for normal cell function and physiological processes such as blood coagulation, nerve conduction and muscle contraction. An uncompensated fall in extracellular calcium concentration (hypocalcaemia) may cause tetany; an excessive rise (hypercalcaemia) can lead to depressed neuromuscular transmission.

The main sources of calcium are dairy products, green vegetables and soya (or fortified foods). The recommended daily intake for adults is 800–1000 mg (20–25 mmol), and ideally this should be increased to 1200 mg during pregnancy and lactation. Children need less, about 200–400 mg per day.

About 50 per cent of the dietary calcium is absorbed (mainly in the upper gut) but much of that is secreted back into the bowel and only about 200 mg (5 mmol) enters the circulation. The normal concentration in plasma and extracellular fluid is 2.2–2.6 mmol/l (8.8–10.4 mg/dL). Much of this is bound to protein; about half (1.1 mmol) is ionized and effective in cell metabolism and the regulation of calcium homoeostasis.

Calcium absorption in the intestine is promoted by vitamin D metabolites, particularly 1,25-$(OH)_2$ vitamin D, and requires a suitable calcium/phosphate ratio. Absorption is inhibited by excessive intake of phosphates (common in soft drinks), oxalates (found in tea and coffee), phytates (chapatti flour) and fats, by the administration of certain drugs (including corticosteroids) and in malabsorption disorders of the bowel.

Urinary excretion varies between 2.5 and 5 mmol (100–200 mg) per 24 hours. If the plasma ionized calcium concentration falls, PTH is released and causes (a) increased renal tubular reabsorption of calcium and (b) a switch to increased 1,25-$(OH)_2$ vitamin D production and enhanced intestinal calcium absorption. If the calcium concentration remains low, calcium is drawn from the skeleton by increased bone resorption, which again is under the indirect influence of PTH.

Hypocalcaemia The classic feature of hypocalcaemia is the development of tetany. Patients may complain of loss of sensation, paraesthesiae and muscle spasms. More severe signs are convulsions and laryngeal spasm.

Hypercalcaemia Clinical features vary with the degree of hypercalcaemia: a mild elevation of serum calcium concentration may cause no more than general lassitude, polyuria and polydipsia. With plasma levels between 3 and 3.5 mmol/L, patients may complain of anorexia, nausea, muscle weakness and fatigue. Those with severe hypercalcaemia (more than 3.5 mmol/L) have a plethora of symptoms including abdominal pain, nausea, vomiting, severe fatigue and depression. In longstanding cases patients may develop kidney stones or nephrocalcinosis due to chronic hypercalciuria; some complain of joint symptoms, due to chondrocalcinosis. The clinical picture is aptly (though unkindly) summarized in the old adage 'moans, groans, bones and stones'.

There may also be symptoms and signs of the underlying cause, which should always be sought (in the vast majority this will be hyperparathyroidism, metastatic bone disease, myelomatosis, Paget's disease or renal failure).

Phosphorus

Apart from its role (with calcium) in the composition of hydroxyapatite crystals in bone, phosphorus is needed for many important metabolic processes, including energy transport and intracellular cell signalling. It is abundantly available in the diet and is absorbed in the small intestine, more or less in proportion to the amount ingested; however, absorption is reduced in the presence of antacids such as aluminium hydroxide, which binds phosphorus in the gut. Phosphate excretion is extremely efficient, but 90 per cent is reabsorbed in the proximal tubules. Plasma concentration – almost entirely in the form of ionized inorganic phosphate (Pi) – is normally maintained at 0.9–1.3 mmol/L (2.8–4.0 mg/dL).

The solubility product of calcium and phosphate is held at a fairly constant level; any increase in the one will cause the other to fall. The main regulators of plasma phosphate concentration are PTH and 1,25-$(OH)_2D$. If the Pi rises abnormally, a reciprocal fall in calcium concentration will stimulate PTH secretion which in turn will suppress urinary tubular reabsorption of Pi, resulting in increased Pi excretion and a fall in plasma Pi. High Pi levels also result in diminished 1,25-$(OH)_2D$ production, causing reduced intestinal absorption of phosphorus.

In recent years interest has centred on another group of hormones or growth factors which also have the effect of suppressing tubular reabsorption of phosphate independently of PTH. These so-called 'phosphotonins' are associated with rare phosphate-losing disorders and tumour-induced osteomalacia. Their exact role in normal physiology is still under investigation.

Magnesium

Magnesium plays a small but important part in mineral homeostasis. The cations are distributed in the cellular and extracellular compartments of the body and appear in high concentration in bone. Magnesium is necessary for the efficient secretion and peripheral action of parathyroid hormone. Thus, if hypocalcaemia is accompanied by hypomagnesaemia it cannot be fully corrected until normal magnesium concentration is restored.

Vitamin D

Vitamin D, through its active metabolites, is principally concerned with calcium absorption and transport and (acting together with PTH) bone remodelling. Target organs are the small intestine and bone.

Naturally occurring vitamin D (cholecalciferol) is derived from two sources: directly from the diet and indirectly by the action of ultraviolet light on the precursor 7-dehydrocholesterol in the skin. For people who do not receive adequate exposure to bright sunlight, the recommended daily requirement for adults is 400–800 IU (10–20 μg) per day – the higher dose for people over 70 years of age. In most countries this is obtained mainly from exposure to sunlight; those who lack such exposure are likely to suffer from vitamin D deficiency unless they take dietary supplements.

Vitamin D itself is inactive. Conversion to active metabolites (which function as hormones) takes place first in the liver by 25-hydroxylation to form 25-hydroxycholecalciferol [25-OHD], and then in the kidneys by further hydroxylation to 1,25-dihydroxycholecalciferol [1,25-$(OH)_2D$]. The enzyme responsible for this conversion is activated mainly by PTH, but also by other hormones (including oestrogen and prolactin) or by an abnormally low concentration of phosphate. If the PTH concentration falls and phosphate remains high, 25-OHD is converted alternatively to 24,25-$(OH)_2D$ which is inactive. On the other hand, during negative calcium balance production switches to 1,25-$(OH)_2D$ in response to PTH secretion (see below); the increased 1,25-$(OH)_2D$ then helps to restore the serum calcium concentration.

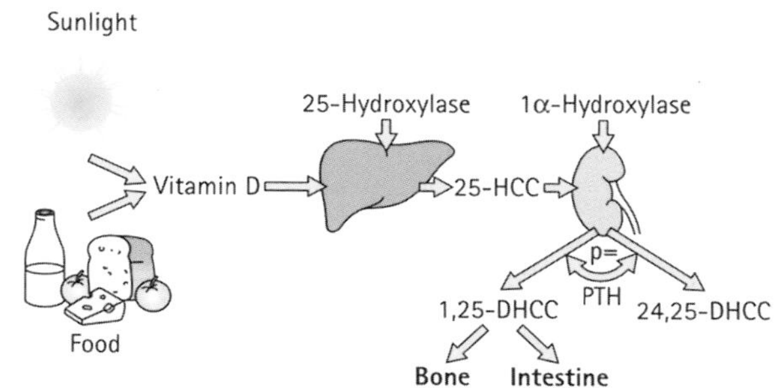

7.7 Vitamin D metabolism The active vitamin D metabolites are derived either from the diet or by conversion of precursors when the skin is exposed to sunlight. The inactive 'vitamin' is hydroxylated, first in the liver and then in the kidney, to form the active metabolites 25-HCC and 1,25-DHCC.

The terminal metabolite, 1,25-$(OH)_2D$ (*calcitriol*) acts on the *lining cells of the small intestine* to increase the absorption of calcium and phosphate. *In bone* it promotes osteoclastic resorption; it also enhances calcium transport across the cell membrane and indirectly assists with osteoid mineralization.

Some antiepileptic drugs interfere with the vitamin D metabolic pathway and may cause vitamin D deficiency.

The concentration of all the active metabolites can be measured in serum samples, the best indicator of vitamin D status being 25-OHD concentration (serum 1,25-$(OH)_2D$ has a half-life of only 15 hours and is therefore not as good an indicator). The recommended serum concentration is 25–30 ng/L, a level which is often not achieved in elderly people, especially in northern climes.

Parathyroid hormone

Parathyroid hormone (PTH) is the fine regulator of calcium exchange, controlling the concentration of extracellular calcium between critical limits by either direct or indirect action on the renal tubules, the renal parenchyma, the intestine and bone.

Production and release are stimulated by a fall and suppressed (up to a point) by a rise in plasma ionized calcium. The active terminal fragment of the PTH molecule can be readily estimated in blood samples.

Acting on the *renal tubules*, PTH increases phosphate excretion by restricting its reabsorption, and conserves calcium by increasing its reabsorption. These responses rapidly compensate for any change in plasma ionized calcium.

Acting on the *kidney parenchyma*, PTH controls hydroxylation of the vitamin D metabolite 25-OHD; a rise in PTH concentration stimulates conversion to the active metabolite 1,25-$(OH)_2D$ and a fall in PTH causes a switch towards the inactive metabolite 24,25-$(OH)_2D$.

In the *intestine* PTH has the indirect effect of stimulating calcium absorption by promoting the conversion of 25-OHD to 1,25-$(OH)_2D$ in the kidney.

In *bone* PTH acts to promote osteoclastic resorption and the release of calcium and phosphate into the blood. This it does not by direct action on osteoclasts but by stimulating osteoblastic activity, increased expression of RANKL and diminished production of OPG, thus leading to enhanced osteoclast differentiation and maturation (see page 124). Furthermore, the PTH-induced rise in 1,25$(OH)_2D$ also has the effect of stimulating osteoclastogenesis. The net effect of these complex interactions is a prolonged rise in plasma calcium.

Calcitonin

Calcitonin, which is secreted by the C cells of the thyroid, does more or less the opposite of PTH: it binds to receptors on the osteoclasts, suppresses osteoclastic bone resorption and increases renal calcium excretion. This occurs especially when bone turnover is high, as in Paget's disease. Its secretion is stimulated by a rise in serum calcium concentration above 2.25 mmol/L (9 mg/dL).

Gonadal hormones

In addition to their effects on bone growth, gonadal hormones have an important role in maintaining bone mass and trabecular integrity. *Oestrogen* appears to act on both osteoblasts and osteoclasts and is now believed to work via the RANKL/RANK/OPG system. It increases the production and activity of OPG, thereby interfering with osteoclast differentiation and bone resorption. Oestrogen is also thought to enhance calcium absorption by the intestine. It is well known that bone loss accelerates after the menopause and a similar effect is seen in amenorrhoeic young women

Table 7.1 Regulation of mineral metabolism by PTH and 1,25-$(OH)_2$ vitamin D

	Source	Secretion increased by	Secretion decreased by	Effects on intestine	Effects on kidney	Effects on bone	Effect on serum Ca and Pi
PTH	Parathyroid gland	Fall in serum Ca	Rise in serum Ca Increase in 1,25-$(OH)_2D$	No direct effect but Ca absorption increased through 1,25-$(OH)_2D$	Increase in 1,25-$(OH)_2D$ Increased reabsorption of Ca Increased excretion of phosphate	No direct effect but resorption increased via action on 1,25-$(OH)_2D$	Rise in serum Ca Fall in serum Pi
1,25$(OH)_2$ vitamin D	Kidney tubule	Fall in serum Ca Fall in serum Pi Rise in serum PTH	Rise in serum Ca Rise in serum Pi Fall in PTH	Increased absorption of Ca Increased absorption of phosphate		Osteoclastogenesis and increased bone resorption	Rise in serum Ca+Pi

who may actually lose bone at a time when their peers are building up to peak bone mass.

Androgens also retard bone resorption, though the signalling pathway is somewhat uncertain. Bone loss increases after the male climacteric, which occurs 15–20 years later than the female menopause.

Glucocorticoids

Corticosteroids in excess cause a pernicious type of osteoporosis due to a combination of factors: diminished osteoblastic bone formation (the most important effect), an adverse effect on collagen, decreased intestinal calcium absorption and increased calcium excretion. RANKL expression by osteoblasts is enhanced and OPG expression is opposed, leading to increased osteoclastogenesis and bone resorption.

Thyroxine

Thyroxine increases both formation and resorption, but more so the latter; hyperthyroidism is associated with high bone turnover and osteoporosis.

Local factors

The intimate processes of signalling between osteoblasts and osteoclasts, cell recruitment and activation, spatial organization and mineral transport are mediated by local factors derived from bone cells, matrix components and cells of the immune system. Some serve as messengers between systemic and local agents, or between the various cells that are responsible for bone remodelling; others are important in promoting bone resorption in inflammatory disorders and fractures and may also account for the bone destruction and hypercalcaemia in metastatic bone disease and myelomatosis.

Mechanical stress

It is well known that the direction and thickness of trabeculae in cancellous bone are related to regional stress trajectories. This is recognized in Wolff's Law (1896), which says that the architecture and mass of the skeleton are adjusted to withstand the prevailing forces imposed by functional need or deformity. Physiological stress is supplied by gravity, load-bearing, muscle action and vascular pulsation. If a continuous bending force is applied, more bone will form on the concave surfaces (where there is compression) and bone will thin down on the convex surfaces (which are under tension). Weightlessness, prolonged bed rest, lack of exercise, muscular weakness and limb immobilization are all associated with osteoporosis. How physical signals are transmitted to bone cells is not known, but they almost certainly operate through local growth factors.

Electrical stimulation

When bone is loaded or deformed, small electrical potentials are generated – negative on compressed surfaces and positive on surfaces under tension (Brighton and McCluskey, 1986). This observation led to the idea that stress-generated changes in bone mass may be mediated by electrical signals; from this it was a logical step to suggest that induced electrical potentials can affect bone formation and resorption. How, precisely, this is mediated remains unknown. Electromagnetic field potentials have been used for the treatment of delayed fracture union and regional osteoporosis, so far with inconclusive results.

Other environmental factors

Moderate rises in temperature or oxygen tension have been shown experimentally to increase bone formation. *Acid–base balance* affects bone resorption, which is increased in chronic acidosis and decreased in alkalosis.

Increased dietary phosphates or pyrophosphates tend to inhibit bone resorption. Pyrophosphate analogues (*bisphosphonates*) are used in the treatment of osteoporosis, where they appear to inhibit both resorption and formation.

Fluoride has complex effects on bone, the most important being direct stimulation of osteoblastic activity, the formation of fluorapatite crystals (which are resistant to osteoclastic resorption) and an apparent increase in mineral density without a concomitant gain in strength; there is also evidence of calcium retention and secondary hyperparathyroidism. *Fluorosis* occurs as an endemic disorder in India and some other parts of the world due to an excess of fluoride in the drinking water.

AGE-RELATED CHANGES IN BONE

During childhood each bone increases in size and changes somewhat in shape. At the epiphyseal growth plate (physis), new bone is added by endochondral ossification; on the surface, bone is formed directly by sub-periosteal appositional ossification; the medullary cavity is expanded by endosteal bone resorption; bulbous bone ends are re-formed and sculpted continuously by coordinated formation and resorption. Although during childhood each bone gets longer and wider, the bone tissue of which it is made remains quite porous.

Between puberty and 30 years of age the haversian canals and intertrabecular spaces are to some extent filled in and the cortices increase in overall thickness; i.e. the bones become heavier and stronger. Bone mass increases at the rate of about 3 per cent per year and dur-

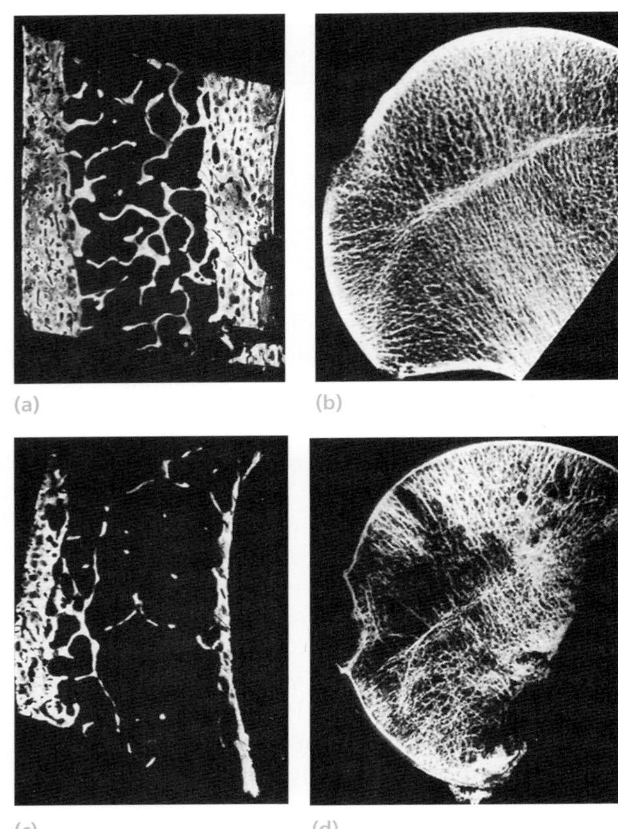

(a) (b) (c) (d)

7.8 Age-related changes in bone These fine-detail x-rays of iliac crest biopsies and femoral head slices show the marked contrast between trabecular density in a healthy 40-year-old woman (a,b) and one of 75 years (c,d).

ing the third decade each individual attains a state of *peak bone mass*, the level of which is determined by genetic, hormonal, nutritional and environmental factors. By the end of bone growth, mean bone mass is about 5–10 per cent greater in young men than in young women, due mainly to increased appositional bone formation when androgen levels rise after puberty (Seeman, 2003). At the other end of the scale, young women with amenorrhoea due to prolonged and intensive exercise or anorexia nervosa tend to have lower than normal bone mass. The greater the peak bone mass, the less marked will be the effects of the inevitable depletion which occurs in later life.

From 30 years onwards there is a slow but inexorable loss of bone; haversian spaces enlarge, trabeculae become thinner, the endosteal surface is resorbed and the medullary space expands, i.e. year by year the bones become slightly more porous. The diminution in bone mass proceeds at a rate of about 0.3 per cent per year in men and 0.5 per cent per year in women up to the menopause.

From the onset of the menopause and for the next 10 years the rate of bone loss in women accelerates to about 3 per cent per year, occurring predominantly in trabecular bone. This steady depletion is due mainly to excessive resorption – osteoclastic activity seeming to be released from the restraining influence of gonadal hormone. (Similar changes are seen in younger women about 5 years after oophorectomy). About 30 per cent of white women will lose bone to the extent of developing postmenopausal osteoporosis. For reasons that are not yet fully understood, the degree of bone depletion is less marked in blacks than in whites (Solomon 1968).

From the age of 65 or 70 years the rate of bone loss in women gradually tails off and by the age of 75 years it is about 0.5 per cent per year. This later phase of depletion is due mainly to diminishing osteoblastic activity (Parfitt, 1988).

Men are affected in a similar manner, but the phase of rapid bone loss occurs 15 or 20 years later than in women, at the climacteric.

Bone mass and bone strength

It is important to recognize that throughout life, and regardless of whether *bone mass* increases or decreases, the degree of *mineralization* in normal people varies very little from age to age or from one person to another.

With advancing years the loss of bone mass is accompanied by a *disproportionate loss of bone strength*, which is explained in a number of ways. (1) The absolute diminution in bone mass is the most important, but not the only, factor. (2) With increased postmenopausal bone resorption, perforations and gaps appear in the plates and cross-spars of trabecular bone; not all these defects are repaired and the loss of structural connectivity further reduces the overall strength of the bone. (3) In old age the decrease in bone cell activity makes for a slower remodelling rate; old bone takes longer to be replaced and microtrauma to be repaired, thus increasing the likelihood of stress failure.

This tendency to increased bone fragility with age is counteracted to some extent, in tubular bones, by the fact that as their cortices become thinner they actually increase in diameter; i.e. during each remodelling cycle resorption exceeds formation on the endosteal surface while formation slightly exceeds resorption on the periosteal surface. Simple mechanics can show that, of two cylinders with equal mass, the one with a greater diameter and thin walls is stronger than one with thicker walls but lesser diameter.

The boundary between 'normal' age-related bone loss and a clinical disorder (*osteoporosis*) is poorly defined. Factors that have an adverse influence on bone mass are shown in Table 7.2. Ageing individuals also often have some degree of *osteomalacia* due to lack of dietary vitamin D and poor exposure to sunlight, and this added to the normal age-related bone depletion

Table 7.2 Factors adversely affecting bone mass

Early onset of menopause
General nutritional deficiency and ill health
Lack of vitamin D, calcium and phosphate
Chronic illness
High consumption of alcohol
Smoking
Inactivity
Long-term medication (anti-inflammatory drugs, diuretics, glucocorticoids, antiepileptic drugs, thyroid hormone)

makes them more vulnerable than usual to insufficiency fractures (Schnitzler and Solomon, 1983).

METABOLIC BONE DISORDERS

Patients with metabolic bone disorders usually appear to the orthopaedic surgeon in one of the following guises: a child with bone deformities (*rickets*); an elderly person with a fracture of the femoral neck or a vertebral body following comparatively minor trauma (*postmenopausal or post-climacteric osteoporosis*); an elderly patient with bone pain and multiple compression fractures of the spine (*osteomalacia*); a middle-aged person with hypercalcaemia and pseudogout (*hyperparathyroidism*); or someone with multiple fractures and a history of prolonged *corticosteroid treatment*.

X-rays may show *stress fractures, vertebral compression, cortical thinning, loss of trabecular structure* or merely an ill-defined loss of radiographic density – *osteopaenia* – which can signify either osteomalacia or osteoporosis.

These appearances are so common in old people that they seldom generate a call for detailed investigation. However, in patients under the age of 50, those with repeated fractures or bone deformities and those with associated systemic features, a full clinical, radiological and biochemical evaluation is essential.

History

Children are likely to be brought for examination because of failure to thrive, below-normal growth or deformity of the lower limbs. Adults may complain of back pain, the sudden onset of bone pain near one of the large joints or symptoms suggesting a full-blown fracture following some comparatively modest injury. Generalized muscle weakness is common in osteomalacia.

Details such as the patient's sex, age, race, onset of menopause, nutritional background, level of physical activity, previous illnesses, medication and operations are important. The onset and duration of symptoms and their relationship to previous disease or trauma should be carefully considered, especially in older people who may have suffered insufficiency fractures. Other causal associations are retarded growth, malnutrition, dietary fads, intestinal malabsorption, alcohol abuse and cigarette smoking.

A careful family history may yield clues to heritable disorders associated with osteoporosis and vulnerability to fracture.

Examination

The patient's appearance may be suggestive of an endocrine or metabolic disorder: the moon face and cushingoid build of hypercortisonism; the smooth, hairless skin of testicular atrophy; physical underdevelopment and bone deformities in rickets. Thoracic kyphosis is a non-specific feature of vertebral osteoporosis.

X-rays

Decreased skeletal radiodensity is a late and unreliable sign of bone loss; it becomes apparent only after a 30 per cent reduction in mineral or skeletal mass, and even then one cannot tell whether this is due to *osteoporosis* (a decrease in bone mass) or *osteomalacia* (insufficient mineralization of bone) or a combination of both. Sometimes the term *osteopaenia* is used to describe a mild or moderate loss of radiodensity in bone x-rays without implying whether this is pathological or not.

A more reliable sign of osteoporosis is a loss of the horizontal trabeculae in vertebral bodies; the remaining vertical trabeculae seem, by contrast, to be more conspicuous and the vertebral cortices are sharply etched around the faded interiors. The presence of obvious fractures – new and old – especially in the spine, ribs, pubic rami or corticocancellous junctions of the long bones, is suggestive of severe osteoporosis. Small stress fractures are more difficult to detect: they may be found in the femoral neck, the proximal part of the femur or the upper end of the tibia.

In addition to these general signs of reduced bone mass or defective mineralization, there may be specific features of bone disorders such as rickets, hyperparathyroidism, metastatic bone disease or myelomatosis.

Measurement of bone mass

The investigation of bone-losing disorders has been greatly advanced by the development of methods for measuring bone mineral density and bone mass. Measurement is based on the principle that a beam of energy is attenuated as it passes through bone, and the degree of attenuation is related to the mass and mineral content of the bone. Bone mineral density (BMD) is ex-

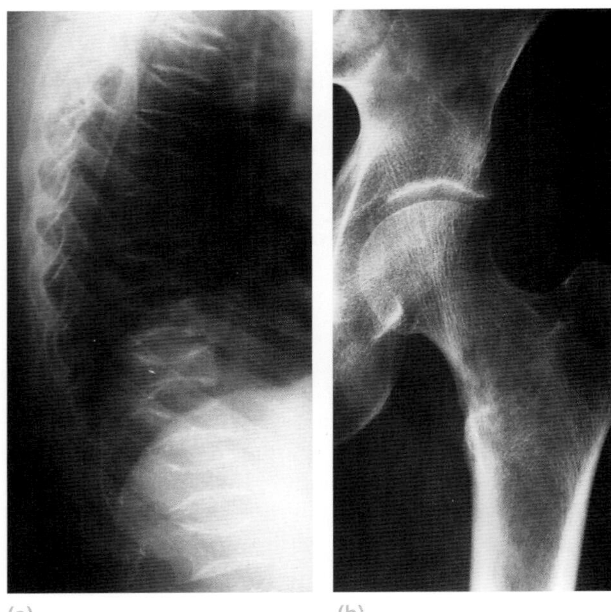

(a) (b)

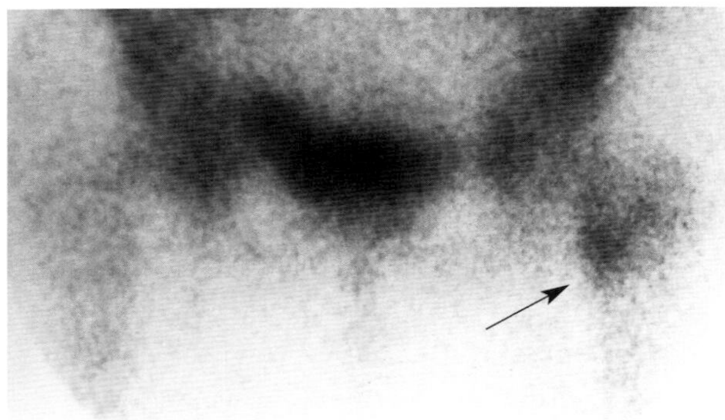

(c)

7.9 Clinical and x-ray features An elderly patient known to have spinal osteoporosis (a) presents with sudden onset of pain in the left groin. The plain x-ray (b) shows a suspicious feature at the base of the femoral neck. This is enough to call for a bone scan (c) which reveals increased activity at the suspicious site, confirming the diagnosis of a spontaneous stress fracture.

pressed in grams per unit area (or unit volume in the case of quantitative computed tomography) and is recorded in comparison to the sex and age specific distribution of these values in the general population. The measurements are specific for each location (lumbar spine, femoral neck, distal radius, etc).

Radiographic absorptiometry Density is measured using standard radiographs and comparing the values against those of an aluminium reference wedge. The method is applicable only to appendicular sites such as the hand or calcaneum and values do not necessarily correlate to findings in the femoral neck or vertebrae.

Single-energy x-ray absorptiometry This measures the attenuation of a collimated photon beam as it passes through bone. The method is simple and not very expensive. However, it is applicable only to the appendicular skeleton, and measuring the BMD at the wrist (for example) does not accurately reflect bone density in the spine or femoral neck.

Dual-energy x-ray absorptiometry (DXA) This is now the method of choice (see Fig. 1.23). Precision and accuracy are excellent, x-ray exposure is not excessive and measurements can be obtained anywhere in the skeleton (Mirsky and Einhorn, 1998). Normative graphs and tables are provided to show where the obtained measurement falls in relation to age and gender matched controls; a value of 2.5 standard deviations or more below the norm is usually taken as indicative of abnormal loss of bone mass.

Some investigators have reported good correlation between measurements in the appendicular and axial skeleton. However, the risk of fracture at any particular site is best gauged by measuring bone density at the target site, though it should be noted that the presence of vertebral spurs or osteophytes and intervertebral bone bridges can make density measurements less reliable for that region. DXA can also provide a lateral view of the entire spine in one image; while lacking the higher definition of conventional x-rays, this is a helpful screening method for identifying vertebral compression fractures.

Quantitative computed tomography (QCT) Quantitative CT permits measurement of mineral content per unit volume of bone, which is a three-dimensional expression of bone density. It also provides separate values for cortical and cancellous bone. Its main drawback is the high radiation exposure (compared to DXA), and there is as yet no evidence that it is more accurately predictive of fracture than DXA.

Indications for bone densitometry

The main indications for using bone densitometry are: (a) to assess the degree and progress of bone loss in patients with clinically diagnosed metabolic bone disease or conditions such as hyperparathyroidism, corticosteroid-induced osteoporosis, gonadal deficiency or other endocrine disorders; (b) as a screening procedure for perimenopausal women with multiple risk factors for osteoporotic fractures; and (c) to monitor the effect of treatment for osteoporosis. Other indications are mentioned in Table 7.3.

Biochemical tests

Serum calcium and phosphate concentrations should be measured in the fasting state, and it is the ionized calcium fraction that is important.

Serum bone alkaline phosphatase concentration is an index of osteoblastic activity; it is raised in osteomala-

Table 7.3 Indications for BMD measurement

All postmenopausal women under the age of 65
Young women following oophorectomy
Men with testosterone deficiency
Perimenopausal women with fractures of wrist, ribs, vertebral bodies or hip
Women or men with x-ray features of osteopaenia
Patients with hyperparathyroidism, hyperthyroidism, renal insufficiency or rheumatoid arthritis
Patients on long-term glucocorticoids, thyroid hormone, thiazide diuretics
Patients with dietary deficiencies
Some experts would add all women over the age of 65 regardless of risk factors

cia and in disorders associated with high bone turnover (hyperparathyroidism, Paget's disease, bone metastases).

Osteocalcin (Gla protein) is a more specific marker of bone formation; elevated serum levels suggest increased bone turnover.

Parathyroid hormone activity can be estimated from serum assays of the COOH terminal fragment. However, in renal failure the test is unreliable because there is reduced clearance of the COOH fragment.

Vitamin D activity is assessed by measuring the serum 25-OHD concentration. Serum 1,25-$(OH)_2D$ levels do not necessarily reflect vitamin uptake but are reduced in advanced renal disease.

Urinary calcium and phosphate excretion can be measured. Significant alterations are found in malabsorption disorders, hyperparathyroidism and other conditions associated with hypercalcaemia.

Urinary hydroxyproline excretion is a measure of bone resorption. It may be increased in high-turnover conditions such as Paget's disease but it is not sensitive enough to reflect lesser increases in bone resorption.

Excretion of pyridinium compounds and telopeptides derived from bone collagen cross-links is a much more sensitive index of bone resorption (Rosen et al., 1994). This may be useful in monitoring the progress of hyperparathyroidism and other types of osteoporosis. However, excretion is also increased in chronic arthritis associated with bone destruction.

NB: Laboratory reports should always state the normal range for each test, which may be different for infants, children and adults.

Bone biopsy

Standardized bone samples are easily obtained from the iliac crest and can be examined (without prior

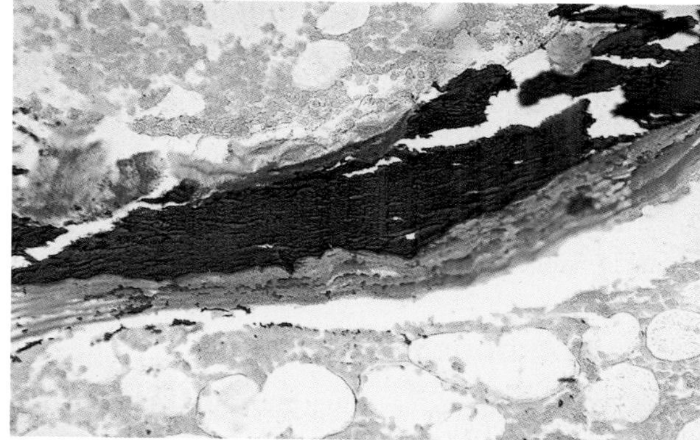

7.10 Bone biopsy von Kossa stain showing the unusually wide osteoid layer (in red) in a patient with osteomalacia.

decalcification) for histological bone volume, osteoid formation and the relative distribution of formation and resorption surfaces. The rate of bone remodelling can also be gauged by labelling the bone with tetracycline on two occasions (2 weeks apart) before obtaining the biopsy. Tetracycline is taken up in new bone and produces a fluorescent strip on ultraviolet light microscopy. By measuring the distance between the two labels, the rate of new bone formation can be calculated. Characteristically in osteomalacia there is a decrease in the rate of bone turnover and an increase in the amount of uncalcified osteoid.

OSTEOPOROSIS

Osteoporosis as a clinical disorder is characterized by an abnormally low bone mass and defects in bone structure, a combination which renders the bone unusually fragile and at greater than normal risk of fracture in a person of that age, sex and race. Although the cancellous regions are more porous and the cortices thinner than normal, the existing bone is fully mineralized.

Bone depletion may be brought about by predominant bone resorption, decreased bone formation or a combination of the two. It seems self-evident that the main reason for the loss of bone strength is the reduction in bone mass; however, in the remaining trabecular bone there may also be a loss of structural connectivity between bone plates, and this so alters the mechanical properties that the loss of strength is out of proportion to the diminution in bone mass. As a consequence, the bone – particularly around the diaphyseo-metaphyseal junctions in tubular bones and in the mainly cancellous vertebral bodies – eventually reaches a state in which a comparatively modest stress or strain causes a fracture. For reasons that are not fully understood, black African peoples are considerably less prone to these effects and have a low incidence of 'osteoprotic fractures' (Solomon, 1968).

This section deals with *generalized osteoporosis*, but it should not be forgotten that osteoporosis is sometimes confined to a particular bone or group of bones – *regional osteoporosis* (for example due to disuse, immobilization or inflammation) – which is usually reversible once the local cause is addressed.

X-rays and bone densitometry

The term *osteopaenia* is sometimes used to describe bone which appears to be less 'dense' than normal on x-ray, without defining whether the loss of density is due to *osteoporosis* or *osteomalacia*, or indeed whether it is sufficiently marked to be regarded as at all pathological. More characteristic signs of osteoporosis are loss of trabecular definition, thinning of the cortices and insufficiency fractures. Compression fractures of the vertebral bodies, wedging at multiple levels or biconcave distortion of the vertebral end-plates due to bulging of intact intervertebral discs are typical of severe postmenopausal osteoporosis.

The clinical and radiographic diagnosis should be backed up by assessment of BMD as measured by DXA of the spine and hips, using the lower value of the two. In otherwise 'normal' women over the age of 50 years, anything more than 2 standard deviations below the average for the relevant population group may be taken as indicative of osteoporosis.

POSTMENOPAUSAL OSTEOPOROSIS

Symptomatic postmenopausal osteoporosis is an exaggerated form of the physiological bone depletion that normally accompanies ageing and loss of gonadal activity. Two overlapping phases are recognized: an

RISK FACTORS FOR POSTMENOPAUSAL OSTEOPOROSIS

Caucasoid (white) or Asiatic ethnicity

Family history of osteoporosis

History of anorexia nervosa and/or amenorrhoea

Low peak bone mass in the third decade

Early onset of menopause

Unusually slim or emaciated build

Oophorectomy

Early hysterectomy

Nutritional insufficiency

Chronic lack of exercise

Cigarette smoking

Alcohol abuse

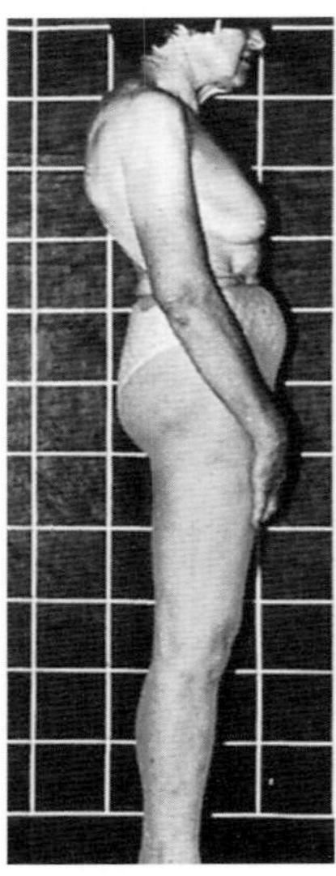
(a)

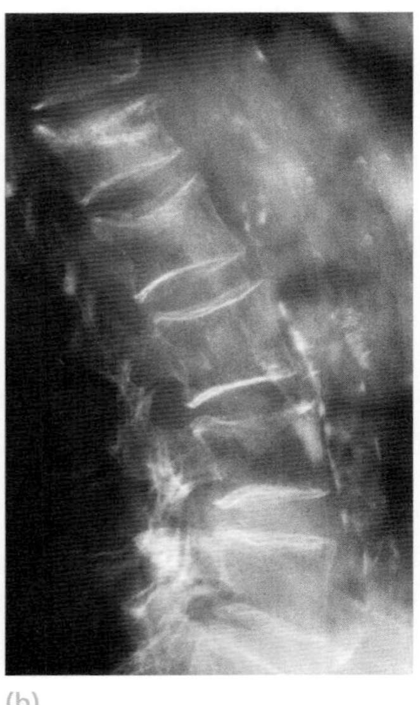
(b)

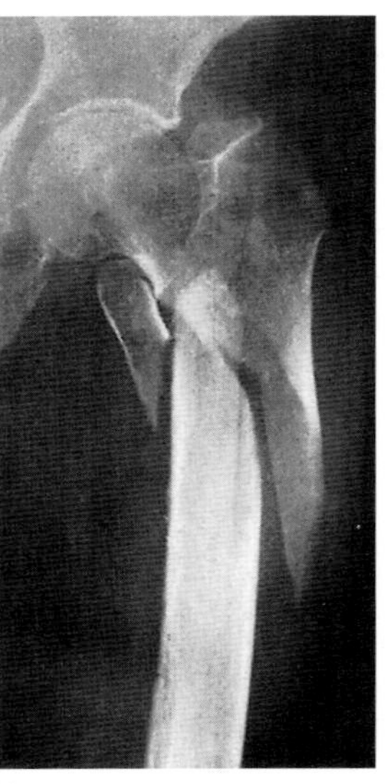
(c)

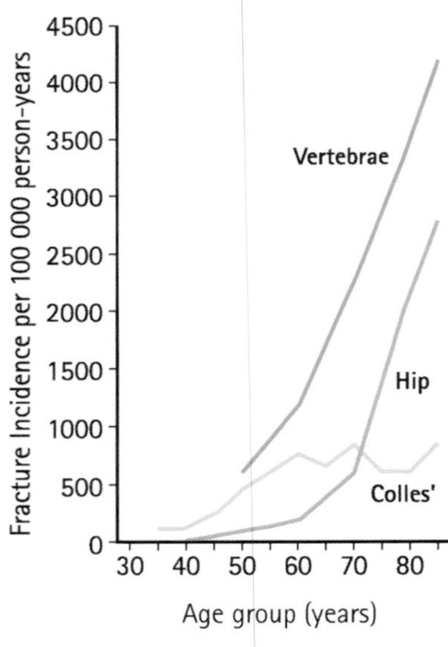

(d)

7.11 Osteoporosis – clinical features (a) This woman noticed that she was becoming increasingly round-shouldered; she also had chronic backache and her x-rays (b) show typical features of postmenopausal osteoporosis: loss of bone density in the vertebral bodies giving relative prominence to the vertebral end-plates, ballooning of the disc spaces associated with marked compression of several vertebral bodies and obvious compression fractures of T12 and L1. An additional feature commonly seen in osteoporotic patients is calcification of the aorta. (c) The next most common feature in these patients is a fracture of the proximal end of the femur. (d) The incidence of fractures of the vertebrae, hip and wrist rises progressively after the menopause.

early postmenopausal syndrome characterized by rapid bone loss due predominantly to increased osteoclastic resorption (high-turnover osteoporosis) and a less well-defined syndrome which emerges in elderly people and is due to a gradual slow-down in osteoblastic activity and the increasing effects of dietary insufficiencies, chronic ill health and reduced mobility (low-turnover osteoporosis).

Around the menopause, and for the next 10 years, bone loss normally accelerates to about 3 per cent per year compared with 0.3 per cent during the preceding two decades. This is due mainly to increased bone resorption, the withdrawal of oestrogen having removed one of the normal restraints on osteoclastic activity. Genetic influences play an important part in determining when and how this process becomes exaggerated, but a number of other risk factors have been identified (see Box on page 132).

Clinical features and diagnosis

A woman at or near the menopause develops back pain and increased thoracic kyphosis; she, or someone in the family, may have noticed that her height has diminished. *X-rays* of the spine may show wedging or compression of one or more vertebral bodies and often the lateral view also shows calcification of the aorta.

This is the typical picture, but sometimes the first clinical event is a low-energy fracture of the distal radius (Colles' fracture), the hip or the ankle. Women who have had one low-energy fracture have twice the normal risk of developing another.

DXA may show significantly reduced bone density in the vertebral bodies or femoral neck.

The rate of bone turnover is either normal or slightly increased; measurement of excreted collagen cross-link products and telopeptides may suggest a high-turnover type of bone loss.

Once the clinical diagnosis has been established, screening tests should be performed to rule out other causes of osteoporosis (e.g. hyperparathyroidism, malignant disease or hypercortisonism).

Prevention and treatment

Bone densitometry can be used to identify women who are at more than usual risk of suffering a fracture at the menopause, and prophylactic treatment of this group is sensible. However, routine DXA screening (even in countries where it is available) is still not universally employed; for practical purposes, it is usually reserved for women with multiple risk factors and particularly those with suspected oestrogen deficiency (premature or surgically induced menopause) or some other bone-losing disorder, and those who have already suffered previous low-energy fractures at the menopause.

Women approaching the menopause should be advised to maintain adequate levels of dietary calcium and vitamin D, to keep up a high level of physical activity and to avoid smoking and excessive consumption of alcohol. If necessary, the recommended daily requirements should be met by taking calcium and vitamin D supplements; these measures have been shown to reduce the risk of low-energy fractures in elderly women (Chapuy et al., 1994).

Hormone replacement therapy (HRT) Until the beginning of the twenty-first century HRT was the most widely used medication for postmenopausal osteoporosis. Taking oestrogen (or a combination of oestrogen and progesterone) for 5–10 years was shown convincingly to reduce the risk of osteoporotic fractures, though after stopping the medication the BMD gradually falls to the usual low level. Moreover there was growing concern about the apparent increased risks of thromboembolism, stroke, breast cancer and uterine cancer. As more experience has been gained with other antiresorptive drugs, the preference for HRT has waned.

Bisphosphonates Bisphosphonates are now regarded as the preferred medication for postmenopausal osteoporosis. They act by reducing osteoclastic bone resorption and the general rate of bone turnover. The newer preparations have been shown to prevent bone loss and to reduce the risk of vertebral and hip fractures. Alendronate can be administered by mouth in once-weekly doses for both prevention and treatment of osteoporosis. Gastrointestinal side effects are a bother and suitable precautions should be taken; for patients who cannot tolerate the drug, pamidronate has been given intravenously at 3-monthly intervals.

Parathyroid hormone Trials of *parathyroid hormone*, either by itself or in combination with alendronate, have shown good results in obtaining a rise in BMD in patients with postmenopausal osteoporosis (Black et al., 2005). This could be a way of managing patients with severe osteoporosis who do not respond to bisphosphonates alone.

Recent advances in drug treatment A novel way of reducing osteoclastic activity and bone resorption is to interrupt the RANKL–RANK interaction which is essential for prompting osteoclastogenesis (see page 122). Phase 3 trials are now being conducted using *denosumab*, an antibody to RANKL, which holds out the promise of an effective new line of treatment for postmenopausal osteoporosis (McClung et al., 2006).

Management of fractures Femoral neck and other long-bone fractures may need operative treatment. Methods are described in the relevant chapters in Section 3.

Vertebral fractures are painful and patients will need

analgesic treatment, partial rest and assistance with personal care for about 6 weeks. Physiotherapy should initially be aimed at maintaining muscle tone and movement in all unaffected areas; if pain is adequately controlled, patients should be encouraged to walk and when symptoms allow they can be introduced to postural training. Spinal orthoses may be needed for support and pain relief, but they cannot be expected to correct any structural deformity. Operative measures are occasionally called for to treat severe compression fractures.

INVOLUTIONAL OSTEOPOROSIS

In advanced age the rate of bone loss slowly decreases but the incidence of femoral neck and vertebral fractures rises steadily; by around 75 years of age almost a third of white women will have at least one vertebral fracture. For reasons that are not completely known, age-related fractures are much less common in black people.

BMD measurements in this age group show that there is considerable overlap between those who suffer fractures and those who do not; the assumption is that qualitative changes contribute increasingly to bone fragility in old age. Causes include a rising incidence of chronic illness, mild urinary insufficiency, dietary deficiency, lack of exposure to sunlight, muscular atrophy, loss of balance and an increased tendency to fall. Many old people suffer from vitamin D deficiency and develop some degree of osteomalacia on top of the postmenopausal osteoporosis (Solomon, 1973).

Treatment Initially, treatment is directed at management of the fracture. This will often require internal fixation; the sooner these patients are mobilized and rehabilitated the better. Patients with muscle weakness and/or poor balance may benefit from gait training and, if necessary, the use of walking aids and rail fittings in the home.

Thereafter the question of general treatment must be considered. Obvious factors such as concurrent illness, dietary deficiencies, lack of exposure to sunlight and lack of exercise will need attention. If the patient is not already on vitamin D and calcium as well as antiresorptive medication, this should be prescribed; although bone mass will not be restored, at least further loss may be slowed.

POST-CLIMACTERIC OSTEOPOROSIS IN MEN

With the gradual depletion in androgenic hormones, men eventually suffer the same bone changes as postmenopausal women, only this occurs about 15 years later unless there is some specific cause for testicular failure. *Osteoporotic fractures in men under 60 years of age should arouse the suspicion of some underlying disorder – notably hypogonadism, metastatic bone disease, multiple myeloma, liver disease, renal hypercalciuria, alcohol abuse, malabsorption disorder, malnutrition, glucocorticoid medication or anti-gonadal hormone treatment for prostate cancer.* Other causes of secondary osteoporosis are shown in Table 7.4.

Treatment is much the same as for postmenopausal osteoporosis. Vitamin D and calcium supplementation is important; alendronate is the antiresorptive drug of choice. If testosterone levels are unusually low, hormone treatment should be considered.

SECONDARY OSTEOPOROSIS

Among the numerous causes of secondary osteoporosis, hypercortisonism, gonadal hormone deficiency, hyperthyroidism, multiple myeloma, chronic alcoholism and immobilization will be considered further.

Hypercortisonism

Glucocorticoid overload occurs in endogenous Cushing's disease or after prolonged treatment with corticosteroids. This often results in severe osteoporosis, especially if the condition for which the drug is administered is itself associated with bone loss – for example, rheumatoid arthritis.

Glucocorticoids have a complex mode of action. The deleterious effect on bone is mainly by suppression of osteoblast function, but it also causes reduced calcium absorption, increased calcium excretion and stimulation of PTH secretion (Hahn, 1980). There is now evidence that it also depresses OPG expression and this would have an enhancing effect on osteoclastogenesis and bone resorption.

Treatment presents a problem, because the drug may be essential for the control of some generalized disease. However, forewarned is forearmed: corticosteroid dosage should be kept to a minimum, and it should not be forgotten that intra-articular preparations and cortisone ointments are absorbed and may have systemic effects if given in high dosage or for prolonged periods. Patients on long-term glucocorticoid treatment should, ideally, be monitored for bone density.

Preventive measures include the use of calcium supplements (at least 1500 mg per day) and vitamin D metabolites. In postmenopausal women and elderly men bisphosphonates may be effective in reducing bone resorption.

In late cases general measures to control bone pain may be required. Fractures are treated as and when they occur.

Gonadal hormone insufficiency

Oestrogen lack is an important factor in postmenopausal osteoporosis. It also accounts for osteoporosis in younger women who have undergone oophorectomy, and in pubertal girls with ovarian agenesis and primary amenorrhoea (Turner's syndrome). Treatment is the same as for postmenopausal osteoporosis.

Amenorrhoeic female athletes, and adolescents with anorexia nervosa, may become osteoporotic; fortunately these conditions are usually self-limiting.

A decline in testicular function probably contributes to the continuing bone loss and rising fracture rate in men over 70 years of age. A more obvious relationship is found in young men with overt hypogonadism; this may require long-term treatment with testosterone.

Hyperthyroidism

Thyroxine speeds up the rate of bone turnover, but resorption exceeds formation. Osteoporosis is quite common in hyperthyroidism, but fractures usually occur only in older people who suffer the cumulative effects of the menopause and thyroid overload. In the worst cases osteoporosis may be severe with spontaneous fractures, a marked rise in serum alkaline phosphatase, hypercalcaemia and hypercalciuria. Treatment is needed for both the osteoporosis and the thyrotoxicosis.

Multiple myeloma and carcinomatosis

Generalized osteoporosis, anaemia and a high ESR are characteristic features of myelomatosis and metastatic bone disease. Bone loss is due to overproduction of local osteoclast-activating factors. Treatment with bisphosphonates may reduce the risk of fracture.

Alcohol abuse

This is a common (and often neglected) cause of osteoporosis at all ages, with the added factor of an increased tendency to falls and other injuries. Bone changes are due to a combination of decreased calcium absorption, liver failure and a toxic effect on osteoblast function. Alcohol also has a mild glucocorticoid effect.

Immobilization

The worst effects of stress reduction are seen in states of weightlessness; bone resorption, unbalanced by formation, leads to hypercalcaemia, hypercalciuria and severe osteoporosis. Lesser degrees of osteoporosis are seen in bedridden patients, and regional osteoporosis is common after immobilization of a limb. The effects can be mitigated by encouraging mobility, exercise and weightbearing.

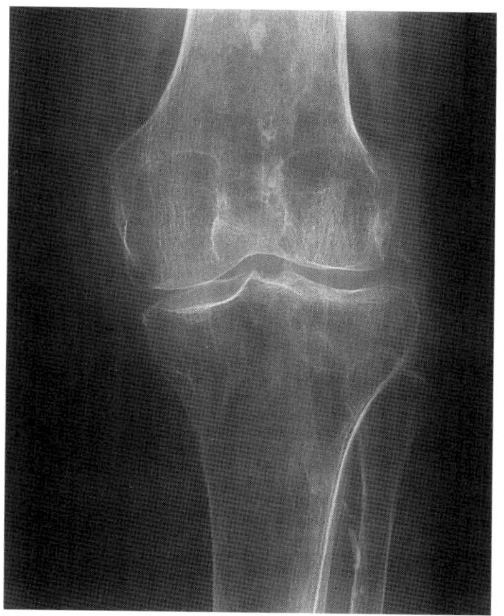

7.12 Disuse osteoporosis X-ray of the knee after prolonged immobilization. Note the extremely thin cortices and the loss of trabecular pattern in the metaphyses.

Table 7.4 Causes of secondary osteoporosis

Nutritional	**Endocrine disorders**
Malabsorption	Gonadal insufficiency
Malnutrition	Hyperparathyroidism
Scurvy	Thyrotoxicosis
	Cushing's disease
Inflammatory disorders	**Malignant disease**
Rheumatoid disease	Carcinomatosis
Ankylosing spondylitis	Multiple myeloma
Tuberculosis	Leukaemia
Drug induced	**Other**
Corticosteroids	Smoking
Excessive alcohol consumption	Chronic obstructive pulmonary disease
Anticonvulsants	Osteogenesis imperfecta
Heparin	Chronic renal disease
Immunosuppressives	

Other conditions

There are many other causes of secondary osteoporosis, including hyperparathyroidism (which is considered below), rheumatoid arthritis, ankylosing spondylitis and subclinical forms of osteogenesis imperfecta. The associated clinical features usually point to the diagnosis.

RICKETS AND OSTEOMALACIA

Rickets and osteomalacia are different expressions of the same disease: inadequate mineralization of bone. Osteoid throughout the skeleton is incompletely calcified, and the bone is therefore 'softened' (*osteomalacia*). In children there are additional effects on physeal growth and ossification, resulting in deformities of the endochondral skeleton (*rickets*).

The inadequacy may be due to defects anywhere along the metabolic pathway for vitamin D: nutritional lack, underexposure to sunlight, intestinal malabsorption, decreased 25-hydroxylation (liver disease, anticonvulsants) and reduced 1α-hydroxylation (renal disease, nephrectomy, 1α-hydroxylase deficiency). The pathological changes may also be caused by calcium deficiency or hypophosphataemia.

Pathology

The characteristic pathological changes in *rickets* arise from the inability to calcify the intercellular matrix in the deeper layers of the physis. The proliferative zone is as active as ever, but the cells, instead of arranging themselves in orderly columns, pile up irregularly; the entire physeal plate increases in thickness, the zone of calcification is poorly mineralized and bone formation is sparse in the zone of ossification. The new trabeculae are thin and weak, and with joint loading the juxta-epiphyseal metaphysis becomes broad and cup-shaped.

Away from the physis the changes are essentially those of *osteomalacia*. Sparse islands of bone are lined by wide osteoid seams, producing unmineralized ghost trabeculae that are not very strong. The cortices also are thinner than normal and may show signs of new or older stress fractures. If the condition has been present for a long time there may be stress deformities of the bones: indentation of the pelvis, bending of the femoral neck (coxa vara) and bowing of the femora and tibiae.

Remember that even mild osteomalacia can increase the risk of fracture if it is superimposed on post-menopausal or senile osteoporosis.

Clinical features of rickets and osteomalacia

In the past the vast majority of cases of rickets and osteomalacia were due to dietary vitamin D deficiency and/or insufficient exposure to sunlight. These patients still embody the classical picture of the disorder.

Children The infant with *rickets* may present with tetany or convulsions. Later the parents may notice that there is a failure to thrive, listlessness and muscular flaccidity. Early bone changes are deformity of the skull (craniotabes) and thickening of the knees, ankles and wrists from physeal overgrowth. Enlargement of the costochondral junctions ('rickety rosary') and lateral indentation of the chest (Harrison's sulcus) may also appear. Distal tibial bowing has been attributed to sitting or lying cross-legged. Once the child stands, lower limb de-

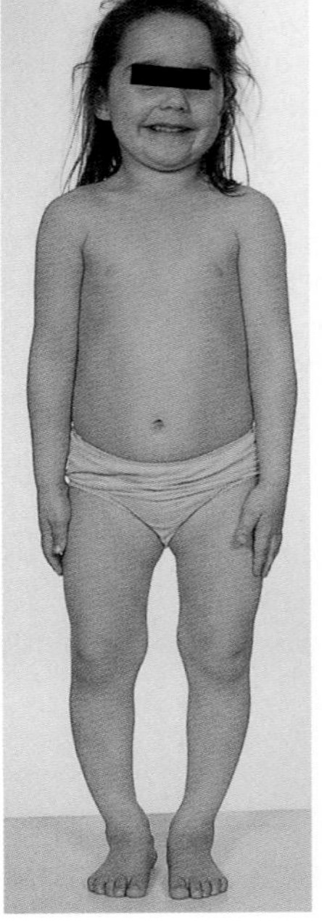

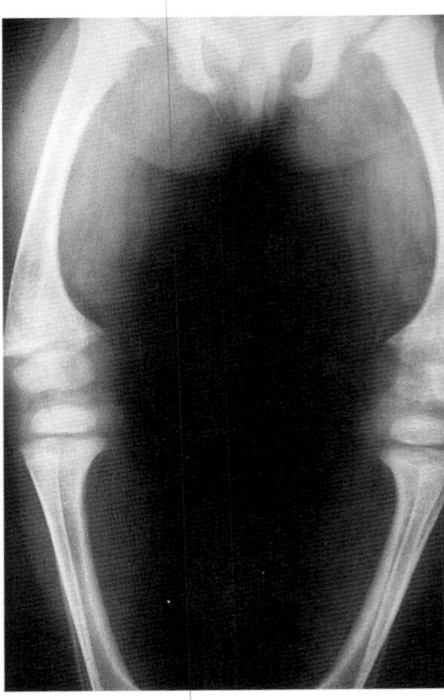

(a) (b)

7.13 Rickets In countries with advanced health systems nutritional rickets is nowadays uncommon. This 5-year-old girl, after investigation, was found to have familial hypophosphataemic rickets. In addition to the obvious varus deformities on her legs, (a) her lower limbs are disproportionately short compared to her upper body. (b) X-ray of another child with classical nutritional rickets, showing the well-marked physes, the flared metaphyses and the bowing deformities of the lower limb bones.

formities increase, and stunting of growth may be obvious. In severe rickets there may be spinal curvature, coxa vara and bending or fractures of the long bones.

Adults *Osteomalacia* has a much more insidious course and patients may complain of bone pain, backache and muscle weakness for many years before the diagnosis is made. Vertebral collapse causes loss of height, and existing deformities such as mild kyphosis or knock knees – themselves perhaps due to childhood rickets – may increase in later life. Unexplained pain in the hip or one of the long bones may presage a stress fracture.

X-rays

Children In active *rickets* there is thickening and widening of the growth plate, cupping of the metaphysis and, sometimes, bowing of the diaphysis. The metaphysis may remain abnormally wide even after healing has occurred. If the serum calcium remains persistently low there may be signs of *secondary hyperparathyroidism*: sub-periosteal erosions are at the sites of maximal remodelling (medial borders of the proximal humerus, femoral neck, distal femur and proximal tibia, lateral borders of the distal radius and ulna).

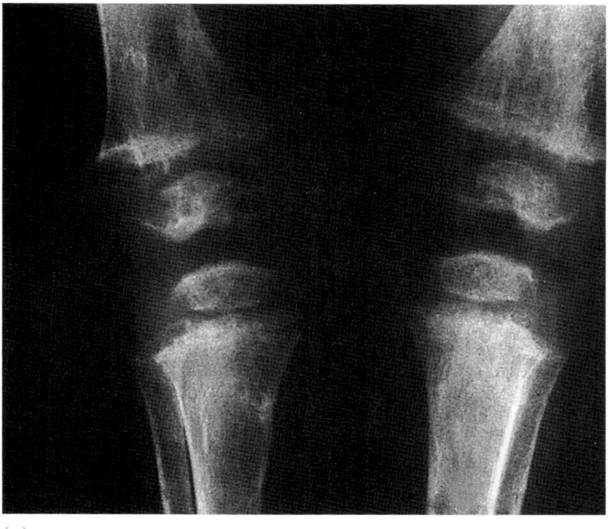

(a)

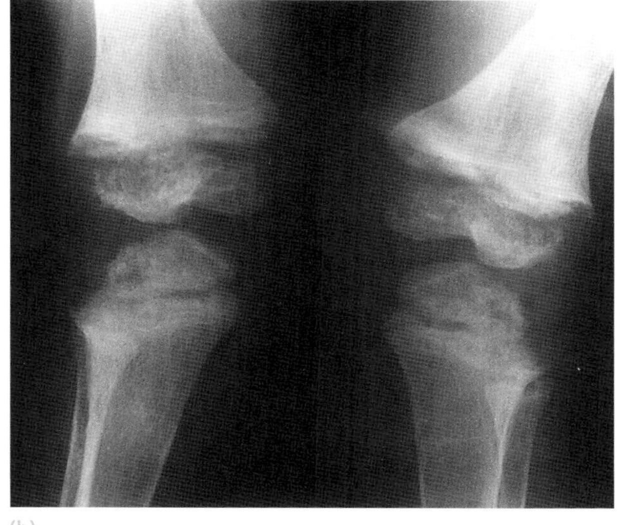

(b)

7.14 Rickets – x-rays X-rays obtained at two points during growth in a child with nutritional rickets. The typical features such as widening of the physis and flaring of the metaphysis are well marked (a). After treatment the bones have begun to heal but the bone deformities are still noticeable (b).

Adults The classical lesion of *osteomalacia* is the Looser zone, a thin transverse band of rarefaction in an otherwise normal-looking bone. These zones, seen especially in the shafts of long bones and the axillary edge of the scapula, are due to incomplete stress fractures which heal with callus lacking in calcium. More often, however, there is simply a slow fading of skeletal structure, resulting in biconcave vertebrae (from disc pressure), lateral indentation of the acetabula ('trefoil' pelvis) and spontaneous fractures of the ribs, pubic rami, femoral neck or the metaphyses above and below the knee. Features of *secondary hyperparathyroidism* characteristically appear in the middle phalanges of the fingers, and in severe cases so-called *'brown tumours'* are seen in the long bones.

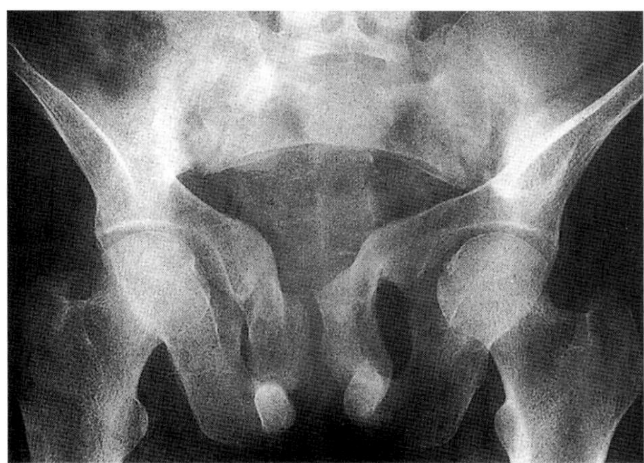

(a)

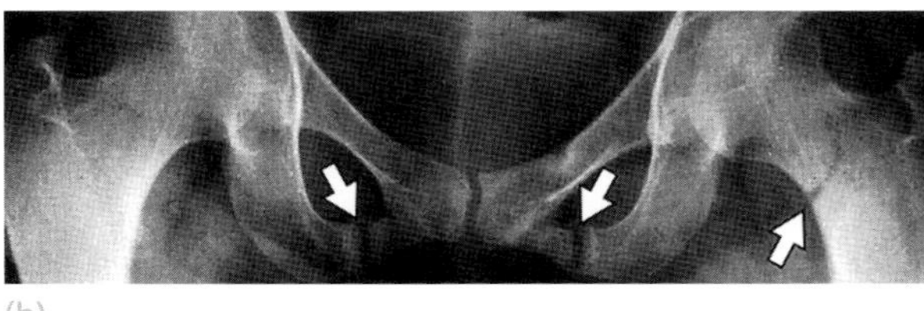

(b)

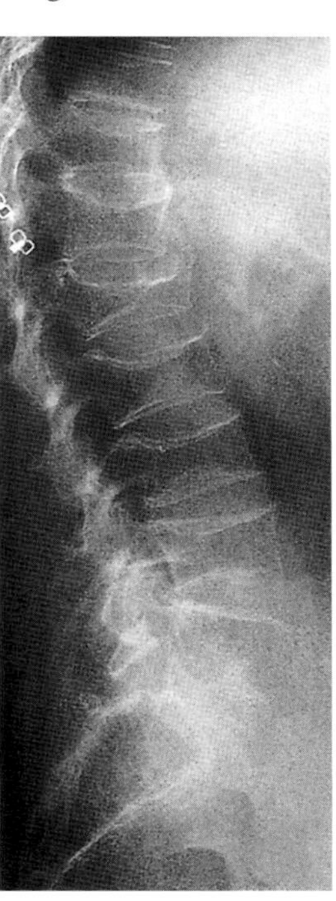

(c)

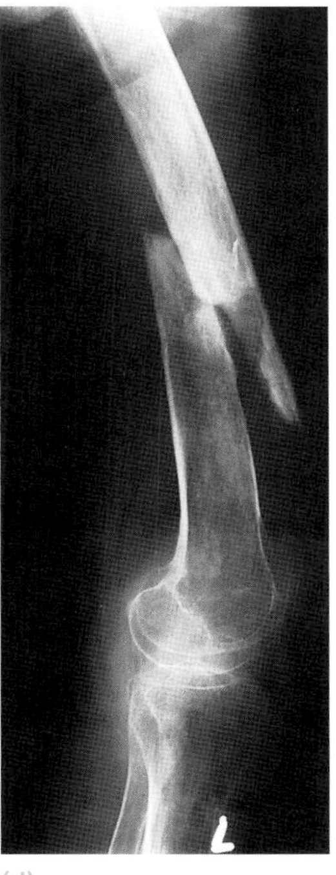

(d)

7.15 Osteomalacia Four characteristic features of osteomalacia: (a) indentation of the acetabula producing the trefoil or champagne glass pelvis; (b) Looser's zones in the pubic rami and left femoral neck; (c) biconcave vertebrae; and (d) fracture in the mid-diaphysis of a long bone following low-energy trauma (the femoral cortices in this case are egg-shell thin).

Biochemistry

Changes common to almost all types of vitamin D related rickets and osteomalacia are diminished levels of serum calcium and phosphate, increased alkaline phosphatase and diminished urinary excretion of calcium. In vitamin D deficiency 25-OH D levels also are low. The 'calcium phosphate product' (derived by multiplying calcium and phosphorus levels expressed in mmol/L), normally about 3, is diminished in rickets and osteomalacia, and values of less than 2.4 are diagnostic.

Bone biopsy

With clearcut clinical and x-ray features the diagnosis is obvious. In less typical cases a bone biopsy will provide the answer. Osteoid seams are both wider and more extensive, and tetracycline labelling shows that mineralization is defective.

Treatment

Dietary lack of vitamin D (less than 100 IU per day) is common in strict vegetarians, in old people who often eat very little and even in entire populations whose traditional foods contain very little vitamin D. If there is also reduced exposure to sunlight, rickets or osteomalacia may result. The use of sun-blocking lotions, or overall cover by clothing, may seriously reduce exposure to ultraviolet light. Some of these problems can be corrected by simple social adjustments.

Treatment with vitamin D (400–1000 IU per day) and calcium supplements is usually effective; however, elderly people often require larger doses of vitamin D (up to 2000 IU per day).

Intestinal malabsorption – especially fat malabsorption – can cause vitamin D deficiency (fat and vitamin D absorption go hand in hand). If vitamin D supplements are administered they have to be given in large doses (50 000 IU per day).

Surgery Established long-bone deformities may need bracing or operative correction once the metabolic disorder has been treated.

OSTEOMALACIA AND OSTEOPOROSIS	
Common in ageing women Prone to pathological fracture Decreased bone density	
Osteomalacia	**Osteoporosis**
Unwell	Well
Generalized chronic ache	Pain only after fracture
Muscles weak	Muscles normal
Looser's zones	No Looser's zones
Alkaline phosphatase increased	Normal
Serum phosphorus decreased	Normal
Ca × P <2.4 mmol/L	Ca × P >2.4 mmol/L

VITAMIN D RESISTANT RICKETS AND OSTEOMALACIA

There are several types of rickets and osteomalacia that do not respond to physiological doses of vitamin D. Although some are uncommon, they should be borne in mind in dealing with resistant cases.

Inadequacy of hepatic 25-OHD

Defective conversion to (or too-rapid breakdown of) 25-OHD in the liver may result from long-term administration of anticonvulsants or rifampicin, and if these drugs are prescribed it is wise to give adequate amounts of vitamin D at the same time. Occasionally the condition is also seen in severe liver failure. Treatment in these cases requires vitamin D in very large doses.

Abnormalities of 1,25-$(OH)_2$D metabolism

Renal failure Patients with early renal failure sometimes develop osteomalacia; this is thought to be due to reduced 1α-hydroxylase activity resulting in deficiency of 1,25-$(OH)_2$D. The condition can be treated with 1,25-$(OH)_2$D (or else with very large doses of vitamin D).

Patients with advanced renal disease treated by haemodialysis develop a more complex syndrome – renal osteodystrophy. This is considered on page 141.

Vitamin D dependent rickets and osteomalacia Rare causes of 1,25-$(OH)_2$D failure are two heritable (autosomal recessive) disorders.

Type I (pseudo vitamin D deficient rickets) is due to deficiency of 1α-hydroxylase; children develop very severe rickets and secondary hyperparathyroidism causing multiple fractures and generalized myopathy, as well as dental enamel hypoplasia. They need lifelong treatment with 1-(OH) D.

Type II vitamin D dependent rickets and osteomalacia is resistant to treatment with both vitamin D and calcitriol (1,25-$(OH)_2$D). Plasma 1,25-$(OH)_2$D levels are elevated but vitamin D receptors at the target organs (intestine and bone) are defective. Bone changes usually appear during childhood but adults also are affected. There is hypocalcaemia and secondary hyperparathyroidism. Neither vitamin D nor any of its metabolites is curative and patients may need long-term parenteral calcium.

NB: Patients treated with supra-physiological doses of calcitriol run the risk of developing hypercalcaemia, hypercalciuria and nephrocalcinosis; plasma calcium concentration should be measured regularly and ideally treatment should be conducted under the supervision of a specialist in this field.

Hypophosphataemic rickets and osteomalacia

Chronic hypophosphataemia occurs in a number of disorders in which there is impaired renal tubular reabsorption of phosphate. Calcium levels are normal and there are no signs of hyperparathyroidism, but bone mineralization is defective.

Familial hypophosphataemic rickets In many countries this is the commonest form of rickets seen today. It is an X-linked genetic disorder with dominant inheritance, starting in infancy or soon after and causing bony deformity of the lower limbs if it is not recognized and treated.

During infancy the children look normal but deformities of the lower limbs (genu valgum or genu varum) develop when they begin to walk, and growth is below normal. There is no myopathy. X-rays may show marked epiphyseal changes but, because the serum calcium is normal, there are no signs of secondary hyperparathyroidism.

During adulthood there is a tendency to develop heterotopic bone formation around some of the larger joints and in the longitudinal ligaments of the spinal canal (which may give rise to neurological symptoms).

Table 7.5 Characteristics of different types of rickets

	Vitamin D deficiency	Renal tubular	Renal glomerular
Family history	–	+	–
Myopathy	+	–	+
Growth defect	±	++	++
Serum:			
Ca	↓	N	↓
P	↓	↓	↑
Alk. phos.	↑	↑	↑
Urine:			
Ca	↓	↓	↓
P	↓	↑	↓
Osteitis fibrosa	±	+	++
Other	Dietary deficiency or malabsorption	Amino-aciduria	Renal failure Anaemia

N = normal; Ca = calcium; P = phosphorus; Alk. Phos. = alkaline phosphatase.

Treatment requires the use of phosphate (up to 3 g per day, to replace that which is lost in the urine) and large doses of vitamin D (to prevent secondary hyperparathyroidism due to phosphate administration). *If calcitriol is given instead, plasma calcium concentration should be monitored in order to forestall the development of hypercalciuria and nephrocalcinosis.* Treatment is continued until growth ceases.

Bony deformities may require bracing or osteotomy. If the child needs to be immobilized, vitamin D must be stopped temporarily to prevent hypercal-

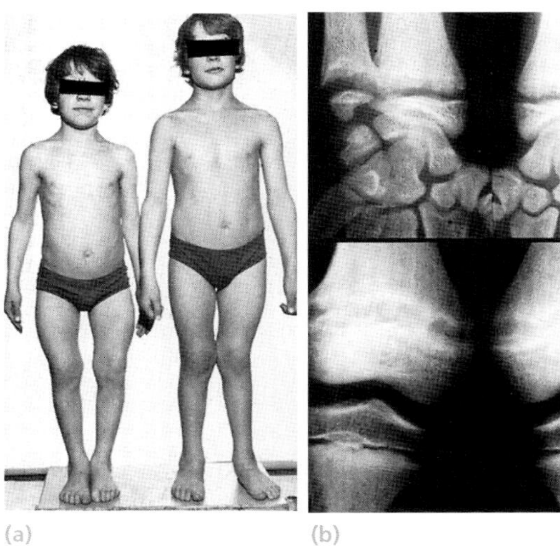

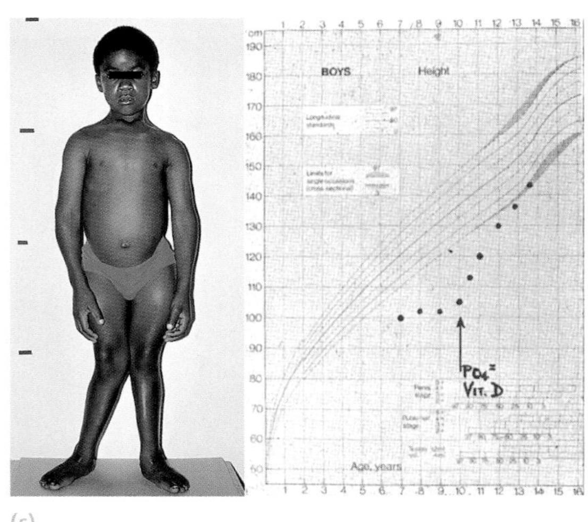

(a) (b) (c)

7.16 Renal tubular rickets – familial hypophosphataemia (a) These brothers presented with knee deformities; their x-rays (b) show defective juxta-epiphyseal calcification. (c) Another example of hypophosphataemic rickets; his growth chart shows that he was well below the normal range in height, but improved dramatically on treatment with vitamin D and inorganic phosphate.

caemia from the combined effects of treatment and disuse bone resorption.

Adult-onset hypophosphataemia Although rare, this must be remembered as a cause of unexplained bone loss and joint pains in adults. The condition responds dramatically to treatment with phosphate, vitamin D and calcium.

More severe *renal tubular defects* can produce a variety of biochemical abnormalities, including chronic phosphate depletion and osteomalacia. If there is acidosis, this must be corrected; in addition, patients may need phosphate replacement, together with calcium and vitamin D.

Oncogenic osteomalacia Hypophosphataemic vitamin D resistant rickets or osteomalacia may be induced by certain tumours, particularly vascular tumours like haemangiopericytomas, and also fibrohistiocytic lesions such as giant cell tumours and pigmented villonodular synovitis. The patient is usually an adult and osteomalacia may appear before the tumour is discovered. Clinical and biochemical features are similar to those of other types of hypophosphataemic disorder and (as in the latter) the condition is believed to be mediated by phosphatonin (Sundaram and McCarthy, 2000). Removal of the tumour will reverse the bone changes; if this cannot be done, treatment is the same as outlined above.

HYPERPARATHYROIDISM

Excessive secretion of PTH may be *primary* (usually due to an adenoma or hyperplasia), *secondary* (due to persistent hypocalcaemia) or *tertiary* (when secondary hyperplasia leads to autonomous overactivity).

Pathology

Overproduction of PTH enhances calcium conservation by stimulating tubular absorption, intestinal absorption and bone resorption. The resulting hypercalcaemia so increases glomerular filtration of calcium that there is hypercalciuria despite the augmented tubular reabsorption. Urinary phosphate also is increased, due to suppressed tubular reabsorption. The main effects of these changes are seen in the kidney: calcinosis, stone formation, recurrent infection and impaired function. There may also be calcification of soft tissues.

There is a general loss of bone substance. In severe cases, osteoclastic hyperactivity produces subperiosteal erosions, endosteal cavitation and replacement of the marrow spaces by vascular granulations and fibrous tissue (osteitis fibrosa cystica). Haemorrhage and giant-cell reaction within the fibrous stroma may give rise to brownish, tumour-like masses, whose liquefaction leads to fluid-filled cysts.

PRIMARY HYPERPARATHYROIDISM

Primary hyperparathyroidism is usually caused by a solitary adenoma in one of the small glands. Patients are middle-aged (40–65 years) and women are affected twice as often as men. Many remain asymptomatic and are diagnosed only because routine biochemistry tests unexpectedly reveal a raised serum calcium level.

Clinical features

Symptoms and signs are mainly due to *hypercalcaemia*: anorexia, nausea, abdominal pain, depression,

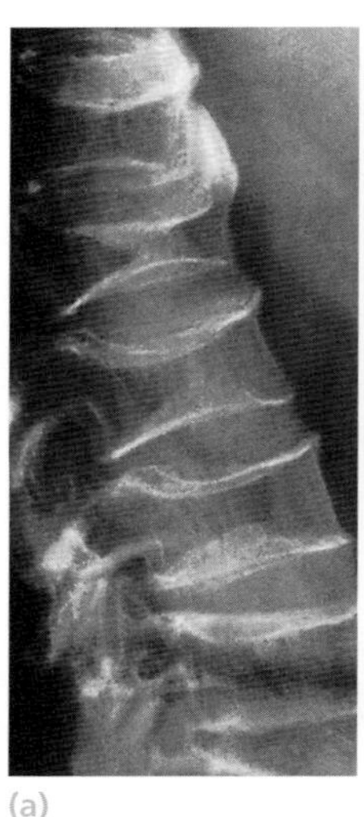
(a)

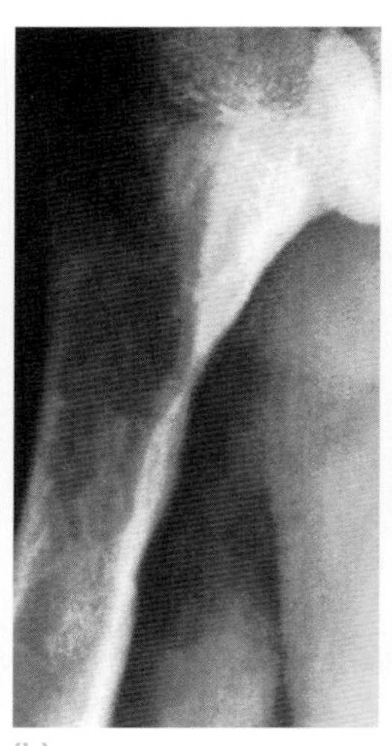
(b)

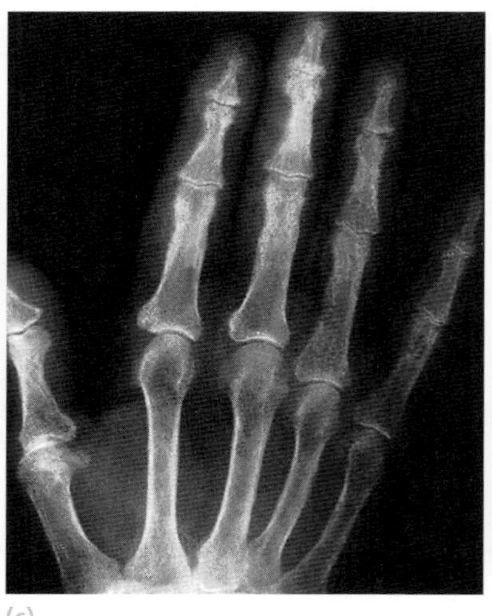
(c)

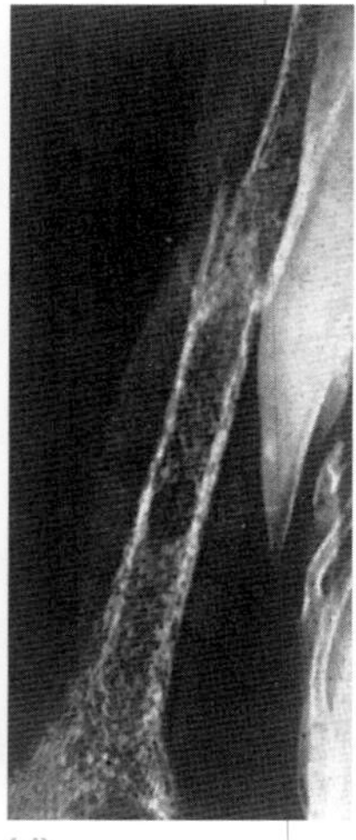
(d)

7.17 Hyperparathyroidism (a) This hyperparathyroid patient with spinal osteoporosis later developed pain in the right arm; an x-ray (b) showed cortical erosion of the humerus; he also showed (c) typical erosions of the phalanges. (d) Another case, showing 'brown tumours' of the humerus and a pathological fracture.

fatigue and muscle weakness. Patients may develop polyuria, kidney stones or nephrocalcinosis due to chronic hypercalciuria. Some complain of joint symptoms, due to chondrocalcinosis. Only a minority (probably less than 10 per cent) present with bone disease; this is usually generalized osteoporosis rather than the classic features of osteitis fibrosa, bone cysts and pathological fractures.

X-rays

Typical x-ray features are osteoporosis (sometimes including vertebral collapse) and areas of cortical erosion. Hyperparathyroid 'brown tumours' should be considered in the differential diagnosis of atypical cyst-like lesions of long bones. The classical – and almost pathognomonic – feature, which should always be sought, is sub-periosteal cortical resorption of the middle phalanges. Non-specific features of hypercalcaemia are renal calculi, nephrocalcinosis and chondrocalcinosis.

Biochemical tests

There may be hypercalcaemia, hypophosphataemia and a raised serum PTH concentration. Serum alkaline phosphatase is raised with osteitis fibrosa.

Diagnosis

It is necessary to exclude other causes of hypercalcaemia (multiple myeloma, metastatic disease, sarcoidosis) in which PTH levels are usually depressed. Hyperparathyroidism also comes into the differential diagnosis of all types of osteoporosis and osteomalacia.

Treatment

Treatment is usually conservative and includes adequate hydration and decreased calcium intake. The indications for parathyroidectomy are marked and unremitting hypercalcaemia, recurrent renal calculi, progressive nephrocalcinosis and severe osteoporosis.

Postoperatively there is a danger of severe hypocalcaemia due to brisk formation of new bone (the 'hungry bone syndrome'). This must be treated promptly, with one of the fast-acting vitamin D metabolites.

SECONDARY HYPERPARATHYROIDISM

Parathyroid oversecretion is a predictable response to chronic hypocalcaemia. Secondary hyperparathyroidism is seen, therefore, in various types of rickets and osteomalacia, and accounts for some of the radiological features in these disorders. Treatment is directed at the primary condition.

RENAL OSTEODYSTROPHY

Patients with chronic renal failure and lowered glomerular filtration rate are liable to develop diffuse bone changes which resemble those of other conditions that affect bone formation and mineralization. Thus the dominant picture may be that of secondary hyperparathyroidism [due to phosphate retention, hypocalcaemia and diminished production of 1,25-$(OH)_2D$], osteoporosis, osteomalacia or – in advanced cases – a combination of these. In older

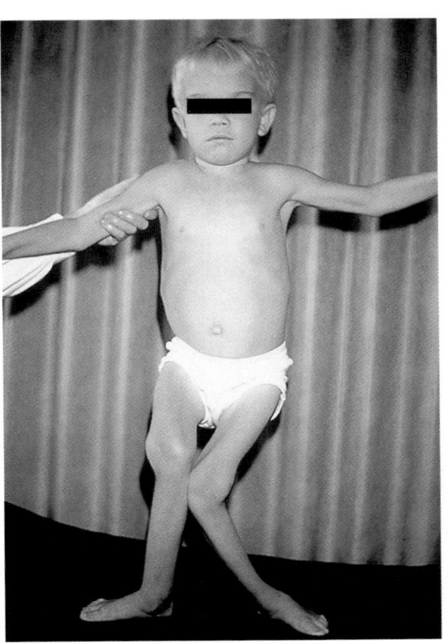

(a)

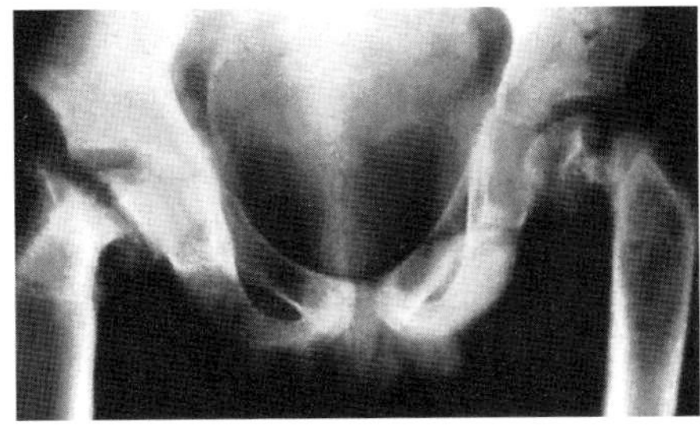

(b)

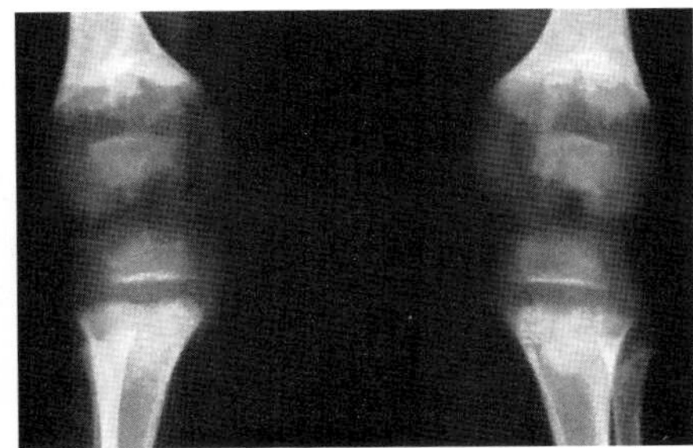

(c)

7.18 Renal glomerular osteodystrophy (a) This young boy with chronic renal failure developed severe deformities of (b) the hips and (c) the knees. Note the displacement of the upper femoral epiphyses.

patients the effects of postmenopausal osteoporosis may be superimposed; in some there are concomitant changes due to glucocorticoid medication; and in patients with end-stage renal failure bone changes can be aggravated by aluminium retention or contamination of dialysing fluids.

Clinical features

Renal abnormalities usually precede the bone changes by several years. Children are more severely affected than adults: they are usually stunted, pasty-faced and have marked rachitic deformities associated with myopathy. *X-rays* show widened and irregular epiphyseal plates.

In older children with longstanding disease there may be displacement of the epiphyses (epiphyseolysis). Osteosclerosis is seen mainly in the axial skeleton and is more common in young patients: it may produce a 'rugger jersey' appearance in lateral x-rays of the spine, due to alternating bands of increased and decreased bone density.

In all patients signs of secondary hyperparathyroidism may be widespread and severe. *Biochemical features* are low serum calcium, high serum phosphate and elevated alkaline phosphatase levels. Urinary excretion of calcium and phosphate is diminished. Plasma PTH levels may be raised.

Diagnosis

Precise diagnosis, differentiation from other metabolic bone disorders and attribution to a specific category of change requires painstaking biochemical investigation and bone biopsy for quantitative tetracycline histomorphometry. It is important that the underlying metabolic changes be established as this will determine the choice of treatment.

Treatment

Hyperphosphataemia and secondary hyperparathyroidism can be treated by restricting the intake of phosphorus (e.g. by taking phosphate binders) and administering vitamin D or one of its analogues. More recently a calcimimetic drug, cinacalcet, has been introduced; this acts directly on the parathyroid glands increasing the sensitivity of calcium receptors and inducing a reduction in serum PTH levels. However, the biochemical changes are usually more complex and treatment should always be managed by a specialist in this field.

Renal failure, if irreversible, may require haemodialysis or renal transplantation.

Epiphyseolysis may need internal fixation and residual deformities can be corrected once the disease is under control.

SCURVY

Vitamin C (ascorbic acid) deficiency causes failure of collagen synthesis and osteoid formation. The result is osteoporosis, which in infants is most marked in the juxta-epiphyseal bone. Spontaneous bleeding is common.

The infant is irritable and anaemic. The gums may be spongy and bleeding. Sub-periosteal haemorrhage

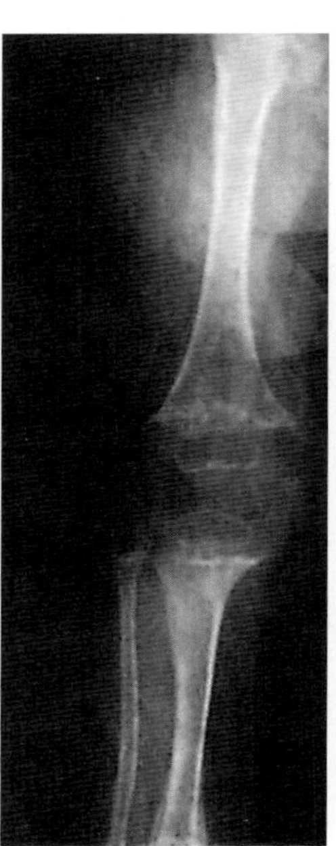
(a)

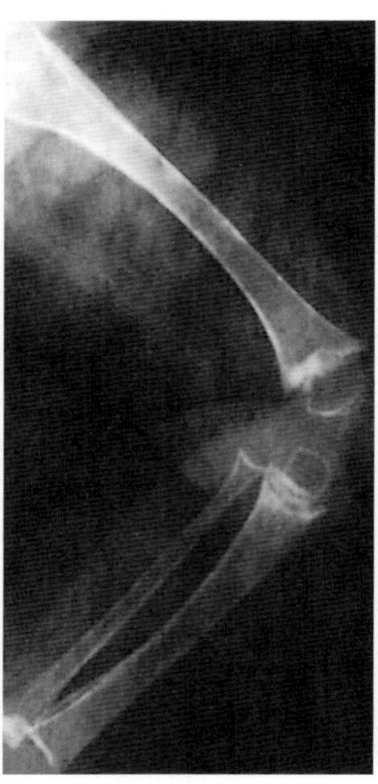
(b)

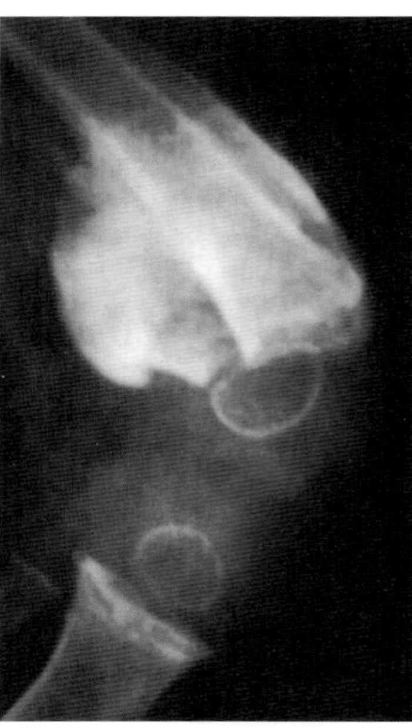
(c)

7.19 Scurvy (a,b) The epiphyseal ring sign and small sub-periosteal haemorrhages; (c) the femoral epiphysis has displaced and the sub-periosteal haemorrhage has calcified.

causes excruciating pain and tenderness near the large joints. Fractures or epiphyseal separations may occur.

X-rays show generalized bone rarefaction, most marked in the long-bone metaphyses. The normal calcification in growing cartilage produces dense transverse bands at the juxta-epiphyseal zones and around the ossific centres of the epiphyses (the 'ring sign'). The metaphyses may be deformed or fractured. Sub-periosteal haematomas show as soft-tissue swellings or peri-osseous calcification.

Treatment is with large doses of vitamin C.

HYPERVITAMINOSIS

Hypervitaminosis A occurs in children following excessive dosage; in adults it seldom occurs except in explorers who eat polar bear livers. There may be bone pain, and headache and vomiting due to raised intracranial pressure. X-ray shows increased density in the metaphyseal region and sub-periosteal calcification.

Hypervitaminosis D occurs if too much vitamin D is given. It exerts a PTH-like effect and so, as in the underlying rickets, calcium is withdrawn from bones; but metastatic calcification occurs. In treatment the dose of vitamin D must be properly regulated and the infant given a low-calcium diet but plentiful fluids.

FLUOROSIS

Fluorine in very low concentration – 1 part per million (ppm) or less – has been used to reduce the incidence of dental caries. At slightly higher levels (2–4 ppm) it may produce mottling of the teeth, a condition which is fairly common in those parts of the world where fluorine appears in the soil and drinking water. In some areas – notably parts of India and Africa where fluorine concentrations in the drinking water may be above 10 ppm – chronic fluorine intoxication (fluorosis) is endemic and widespread skeletal abnormalities are occasionally encountered in the affected population. Mild bone changes are also sometimes seen in patients treated with sodium fluoride for osteoporosis.

Fluorine directly stimulates osteoblastic activity; fluoroapatite crystals are laid down in bone and these are unusually resistant to osteoclastic resorption. Other effects are thought to be due to calcium retention, impaired mineralization and secondary hyperparathyroidism. The characteristic pathological features in severe cases are sub-periosteal new-bone accretion and osteosclerosis, most marked in the vertebrae, ribs, pelvis and the forearm and leg bones, together with hyperostosis at the bony attachments of ligaments, tendons and fascia in these areas. Despite the apparent thickening and 'density' of the skeleton, tensile strength is reduced and the bones fracture more easily under bending and twisting loads.

Patients complain of backache, bone pain and joint stiffness. Examination may show thickening of the tubular bones. Sometimes the first clinical manifestation is a stress fracture. In the worst cases there may be deformities of the spine and lower limbs; hyperostosis can lead to vertebral canal encroachment and resultant neurological defects.

The typical x-ray features are osteosclerosis, osteophytosis and heterotopic ossification of ligamentous and fascial attachments. Changes are most marked in the spine and pelvis, where the bones become densely opaque.

In a full-blown case the diagnosis should be obvious, but the rarity of the condition leads to it being overlooked. X-ray features at individual sites can be mistaken for those of Paget's disease, idiopathic skeletal hyperostosis, renal osteodystrophy or osteopetrosis.

There is no specific treatment for this condition. After exposure ceases it still takes years for bone fluoride to be excreted. If there is evidence of osteomalacia and secondary hyperparathyroidism, this can be treated with calcium and vitamin D.

PAGET'S DISEASE (OSTEITIS DEFORMANS)

Paget's disease is characterized by increased bone turnover and enlargement and thickening of the bone, but the internal architecture is abnormal and the bone is unusually brittle. The condition has a curious ethnic and geographical distribution, being relatively common (a prevalence of more than 3 per cent in people aged over 40) in North America, Britain, western Europe and Australia but rare in Asia, Africa and the Middle East. There is a tendency to familial aggregation. The cause is unknown, although the discovery of inclusion bodies in the osteoclasts has suggested a viral infection (Rebel et al., 1980).

Pathology

The disease may appear in one or several sites; in the tubular bones it starts at one end and progresses slowly towards the diaphysis, leaving a trail of altered architecture behind. The characteristic cellular change is a marked increase in osteoclastic and osteoblastic activity. Bone turnover is accelerated, plasma alkaline phosphatase is raised (a sign of osteoblastic activity) and there is increased excretion of hydroxyproline in

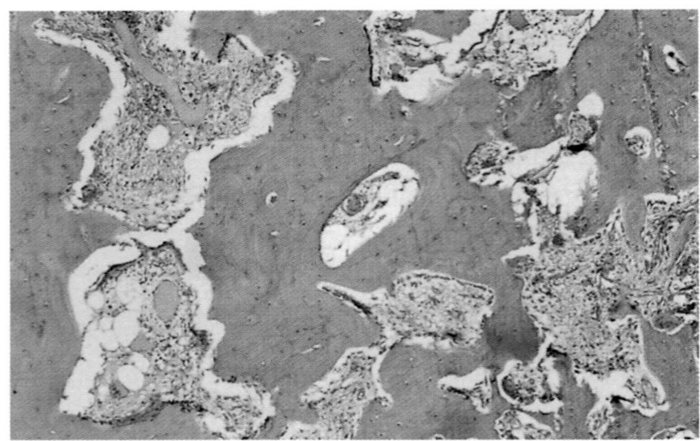

7.20 Paget's disease – histology Section from pagetic bone, showing the mosaic pattern due to overactive bone resorption and bone formation. The trabeculae are thick and patterned by cement lines. Some surfaces are excavated by osteoclastic activity whilst others are lined by rows of osteoblasts. The marrow spaces contain fibrovascular tissue.

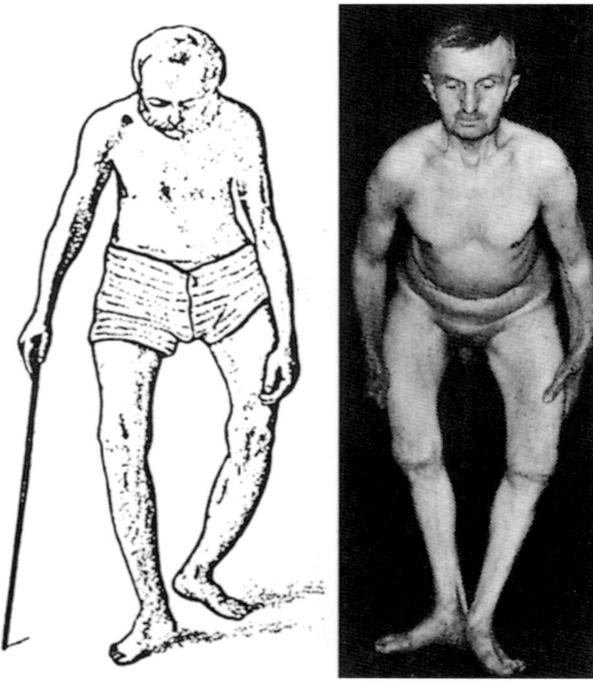

7.21 Paget's disease Paget's original case compared with a modern photograph.

the urine (due to osteoclastic activity).

In the osteolytic (or 'vascular') stage there is avid resorption of existing bone by large osteoclasts, the excavations being filled with vascular fibrous tissue. In adjacent areas osteoblastic activity produces new woven and lamellar bone, which in turn is attacked by osteoclasts. This alternating activity extends on both endosteal and periosteal surfaces, so the bone increases in thickness but is structurally weak and easily deformed. Gradually, osteoclastic activity abates and the eroded areas fill with new lamellar bone, leaving an irregular pattern of cement lines that mark the limits of the old resorption cavities; these 'tidemarks' produce a marbled or mosaic appearance on microscopy. In the late, osteoblastic, stage the thickened bone becomes increasingly sclerotic and brittle.

Clinical features

Paget's disease affects men and women equally. Only occasionally does it present in patients under 50, but from that age onwards it becomes increasingly common. The disease may for many years remain localized to part or the whole of one bone – the pelvis and tibia being the commonest sites, and the femur, skull, spine and clavicle the next commonest.

Most people with Paget's disease are asymptomatic, the disorder being diagnosed when an x-ray is taken for some unrelated condition or after the incidental discovery of a raised serum alkaline phosphatase level. When patients do present, it is usually because of pain or deformity, or some complication of the disease.

The pain is a dull constant ache, worse in bed when the patient warms up, but rarely severe unless a fracture occurs or sarcoma supervenes.

Deformities are seen mainly in the lower limbs. Long bones bend across the trajectories of mechanical stress; thus the tibia bows anteriorly and the femur anterolaterally. The limb looks bent and feels thick, and the skin is unduly warm – hence the term 'osteitis deformans'. If the skull is affected, it enlarges; the patient may complain that old hats no longer fit. The skull base may become flattened (platybasia), giving the appearance of a short neck. In generalized Paget's disease there may also be considerable kyphosis, so the patient becomes shorter and ape-like, with bent legs and arms hanging in front of him.

Cranial nerve compression may lead to impaired vision, facial palsy, trigeminal neuralgia or deafness. Another cause of deafness is otosclerosis. Vertebral thickening may cause spinal cord or nerve root compression.

Steal syndromes, in which blood is diverted from internal organs to the surrounding skeletal circulation, may cause cerebral impairment and spinal cord ischaemia. If there is also spinal stenosis the patient develops typical symptoms of 'spinal claudication' and lower limb weakness.

X-rays

The appearances are so characteristic that the diagnosis is seldom in doubt. During the resorptive phase there may be localized areas of osteolysis; most typical is the flame-shaped lesion extending along the shaft of

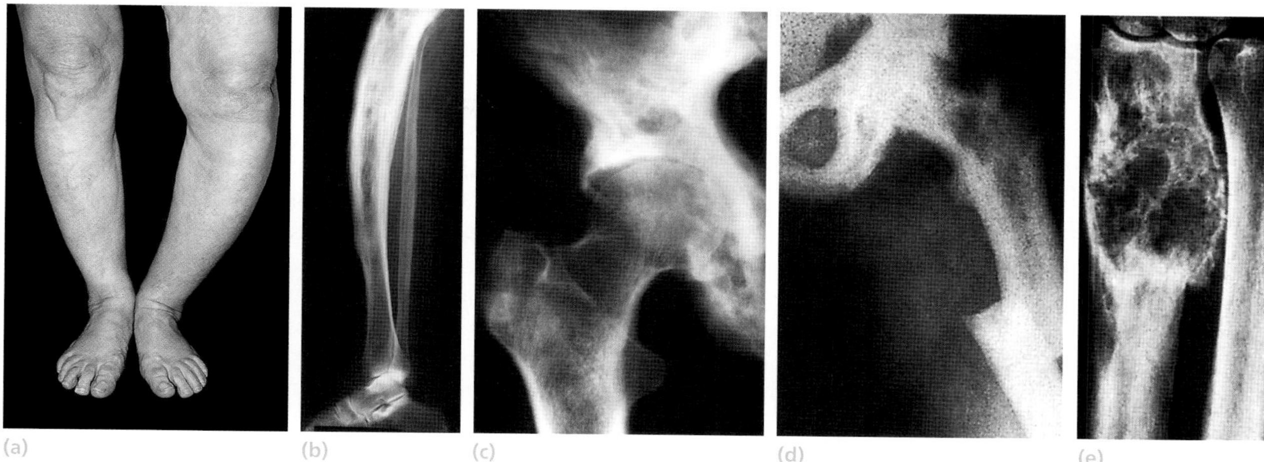

7.22 Paget's disease (a) Deformity of the tibia due to Paget's disease. (b) X-ray shows that the bone is thickened, coarsened and bent. Complications include (c) erosive arthritis in a nearby joint; (d) fracture; and (e) osteosarcoma of the affected bone.

the bone, or a circumscribed patch of osteoporosis in the skull (osteoporosis circumscripta). Later the bone becomes thick and sclerotic, with coarse trabeculation. The femur or tibia sometimes develops fine cracks on the convex surface – stress fractures that heal with increasing deformity of the bone. Occasionally the diagnosis is made only when the patient presents with a pathological fracture. Silent lesions are revealed by increased activity in the radionuclide scan.

Biochemical investigations

Serum calcium and phosphate levels are usually normal, though patients who are immobilized may develop hypercalcaemia. The most useful routine tests are measurement of the serum alkaline phosphatase concentration (which reflects osteoblastic activity and extent of the disease) and 24-hour urinary hydroxyproline (which correlates with bone resorption). Urinary N-telopeptide is a sensitive marker of bone resorption and is helpful in gauging the response to treatment.

Complications

Fractures Fractures are common, especially in the weightbearing long bones. In the femoral neck they are often vertical; elsewhere the fracture line is usually partly transverse and partly oblique, like the line of section of a felled tree. In the femur there is a high rate of non-union; for femoral neck fractures prosthetic replacement and for shaft fractures early internal fixation are recommended. Small stress fractures may be very painful; they resemble Looser's zones on x-ray, except that they occur on convex surfaces.

Osteoarthritis Osteoarthritis of the hip or knee is not merely a consequence of abnormal loading due to bone deformity; in the hip it seldom occurs unless the

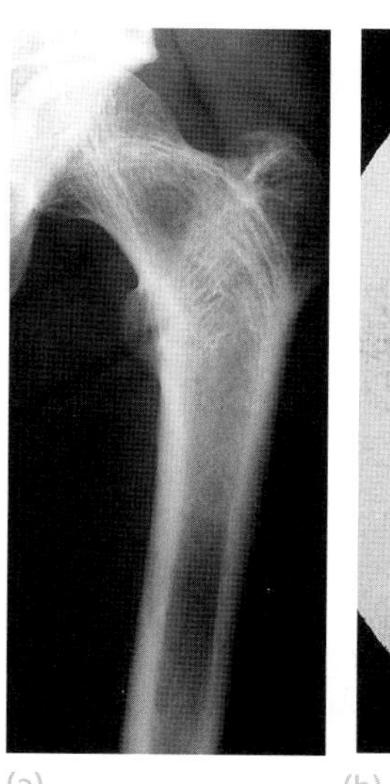

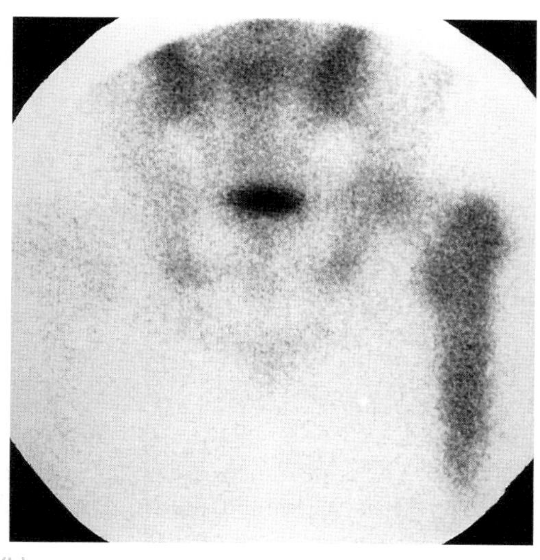

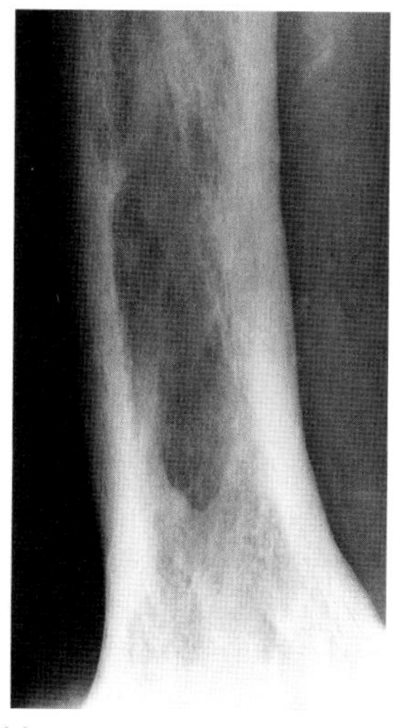

7.23 Paget's disease (a,b) In this early case the x-ray is almost normal, but the radionuclide scan of the same femur shows increased activity. (c) Flame-shaped area of osteopaenia.

innominate bone is involved. The x-ray appearances suggest an atrophic arthritis with sparse remodelling, and at operation joint vascularity is increased.

Nerve compression and spinal stenosis Occasionally this is the first abnormality to be detected, and may call for definitive surgical treatment. Local bone hypertrophy may cause hearing loss.

Bone sarcoma Osteosarcoma arising in an elderly patient is almost always due to malignant transformation in Paget's disease. The frequency of malignant change is probably around 1 per cent. It should always be suspected if a previously diseased bone becomes more painful, swollen and tender. Occasionally it presents as the first evidence of Paget's disease. The prognosis is extremely grave.

High-output cardiac failure Though rare, this is an important general complication. It is due to prolonged, increased bone blood flow.

Hypercalcaemia Hypercalcaemia may occur if the patient is immobilized for long.

In spite of all these complications, patients with Paget's disease usually come to terms with the condition and live to a ripe old age.

Treatment

Most patients with Paget's disease never have any symptoms and require no treatment. Sometimes pain is due to an associated arthritis rather than bone disease, and this may respond to non-steroidal anti-inflammatory therapy.

The indications for specific treatment are: (1) persistent bone pain; (2) repeated fractures; (3) neurological complications; (4) high-output cardiac failure; (5) hypercalcaemia due to immobilization; and (6) for some months before and after major bone surgery where there is a risk of excessive haemorrhage.

Drugs that suppress bone turnover, notably calcitonin and bisphosphonates, are most effective when the disease is active and bone turnover is high.

Calcitonin is the most widely used. It reduces bone resorption by decreasing both the activity and the number of osteoclasts; serum alkaline phosphatase and urinary hydroxyproline levels are lowered. Salmon calcitonin is more effective than the porcine variety; subcutaneous injections of 50–100 MRC units are given daily until pain is relieved and the alkaline phosphatase levels are reduced and stabilized. Maintenance injections once or twice weekly may have to be continued indefinitely, but some authorities advocate stopping the drug and resuming treatment if symptoms recur. Calcitonin can also be administered in a nasal spray.

Bisphosphonates bind to hydroxyapatite crystals, inhibiting their rate of growth and dissolution. It is claimed that the reduction in bone turnover following their use is associated with the formation of lamellar rather than woven bone and that, even after treatment is stopped, there may be prolonged remission of disease (Bickerstaff et al., 1990). Etidronate can be given orally (always on an empty stomach) but dosage should be kept low (e.g. 5 mg/kg per day for up to 6 months) and vitamin D and calcium should also be given lest impaired bone mineralization results in osteomalacia. The newer bisphosphonates (e.g. alendronate or pamidronate) do not have this disadvantage, so they should be used as the treatment of choice; they produce remissions even with short courses of 1 or 2 weeks.

Surgery The main indication for operation is a pathological fracture, which (in a long bone) usually requires internal fixation. When the fracture is treated the opportunity should be taken to straighten the bone. Other indications for surgery are painful osteoarthritis (total joint replacement), nerve entrapment (decompression) and severe spinal stenosis (decompression). *Beware – blood loss is likely to be excessive in these cases.*

An osteosarcoma, if detected early, may be resectable, but generally the prognosis is grave.

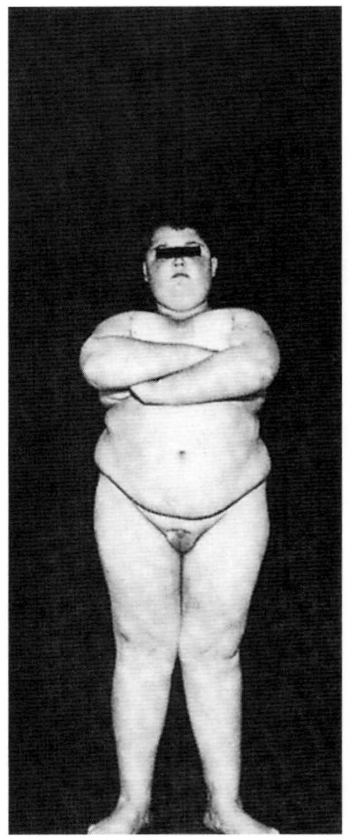

(a)

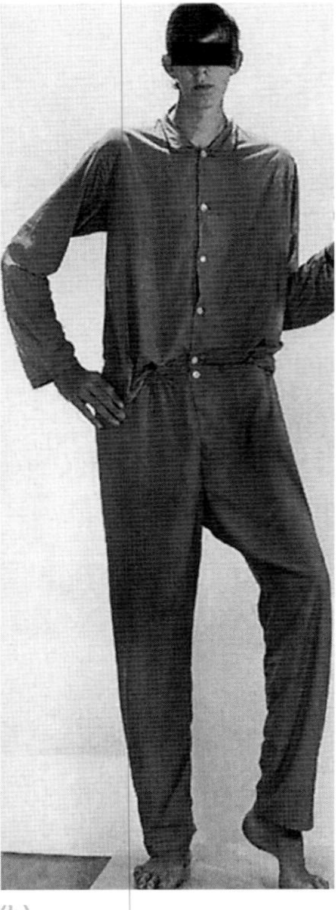

(b)

7.24 Endocrine disorders (a) *Hypopituitarism:* a boy of 12 with the unmistakable build of Frölich's syndrome. (b) *Hyperpituitarism:* this 16-year-old giant suffered from a pituitary adenoma.

ENDOCRINE DISORDERS

The endocrine system plays an important part in skeletal growth and maturation, as well as the maintenance of bone turnover. The anterior lobe of the pituitary gland directly affects growth; it also controls the activities of the thyroid, the gonads and the adrenal cortex, each of which has its own influence on bone; and the pituitary itself is subject to feedback stimuli from the other glands. The various mechanisms are, in fact, part of an interactive system in which balance is more important than individual activity. For example: pituitary growth hormone stimulates cell proliferation and growth at the physes. Gonadal hormone promotes growth plate maturation and fusion. While pituitary activity is in the ascendant, the bones elongate; after sexual maturation, the rise in gonadal hormone activity simultaneously 'feeds back' on the pituitary and also directly closes down further physeal growth.

When the system goes out of balance abnormalities occur. They are often complex, with several levels of dysfunction, due to (a) the local effects of the lesion which upsets the endocrine gland (e.g. pressure on cranial nerves from a pituitary adenoma); (b) oversecretion or undersecretion by the gland affected; and (c) over- or under-activity of other glands that are dependent on the primary dysfunctional gland.

The descriptions which follow have been somewhat simplified.

PITUITARY DYSFUNCTION

The *posterior lobe* of the pituitary gland has no influence on the musculoskeletal system.

The *anterior lobe* is responsible for the secretion of pituitary growth hormone, as well as the thyrotropic, gonadotropic and adrenocorticotropic hormones. Abnormalities may affect the production of some of these hormones and not others; thus there is no single picture of 'pituitary deficiency' or 'pituitary excess'. Moreover, the clinical effects are determined in part by the stage in skeletal maturation at which the abnormality occurs.

Hypopituitarism

Anterior pituitary hyposecretion may be caused by *intrinsic disorders* such as infarction or haemorrhage in the pituitary, infection and intrapituitary tumours, or by *extrinsic lesions* (such as a craniopharyngioma) which press on the anterior lobe of the pituitary. In some cases there may also be features due to posterior lobe dysfunction (e.g. diabetes insipidus); and space-occupying lesions are likely to have other intracranial pressure effects, such as headache or visual field defects.

CLINICAL FEATURES

Children In childhood and adolescence two distinct clinical disorders are encountered. In the *Lorain syndrome* the predominant effect is on growth. The body proportions are normal but the child fails to grow (proportionate dwarfism). Sexual development may be unaffected. The condition must be distinguished from other causes of short stature: hereditary or constitutional shortness, which is not as marked; childhood illness or malnutrition; rickets; and the various bone dysplasias, which generally result in disproportionate dwarfism.

In *Fröhlich's adiposogenital syndrome* the effects include those of gonadal hormone deficiency. There is delayed skeletal maturation associated with adiposity and immaturity of the secondary sexual characteristics. Weakness of the physes combined with disproportionate adiposity may result in epiphyseal displacement (epiphysiolysis or 'slipped epiphysis') at the hip or knee.

Adults Panhypopituitarism causes a variety of symptoms and signs, including those of cortisol and sex hormone deficiency. The only important skeletal effect is premature osteoporosis.

INVESTIGATIONS

Laboratory investigations should include direct assays and tests for hormone function.

X-rays of the skull may show expansion of the pituitary fossa and erosion of the adjacent bone.

CT and MRI may reveal the tumour.

TREATMENT

Treatment will depend on the cause and the degree of dwarfism. If a tumour is identified, it can be removed or ablated. A word of warning: the sudden reactivation of pituitary function after removal of a tumour may result in slipping of the proximal femoral epiphysis. Awareness of this risk will make for early diagnosis and, if necessary, surgical treatment of the epiphysiolysis.

Growth hormone deficiency has been successfully treated by the administration of biosynthetic growth hormone (somatotropin). The response should be checked by serial plots on the growth chart.

Hyperpituitarism

Oversecretion of pituitary growth hormone is usually due to an acidophil adenoma. However, there are rare cases of growth hormone secretion by pancreatic (and other) tumours. The effects vary according to the age of onset.

Gigantism Growth hormone oversecretion in childhood and adolescence causes excessive growth of the entire skeleton. The condition may be suspected quite early, and it is important to track the child's development by regular clinical and x-ray examination. In addition to being excessively tall, patients may develop deformity of the hip due to epiphyseal displacement (epiphysiolysis). There may be mental retardation and sexual immaturity.

Treatment is directed at early removal of the pituitary tumour.

Acromegaly Oversecretion of pituitary growth hormone in adulthood causes enlargement of the bones and soft tissues, but without the very marked elongation which is seen in gigantism. The bones are thickened, rather than lengthened, due to appositional growth; there is also hypertrophy of articular cartilage, which leads to enlargement of the joints. Bones such as the mandible, the clavicles, ribs, sternum and scapulae, which develop secondary growth centres in late adolescence or early adulthood, may go on growing longer than usual. Thickening of the skull, prominence of the orbital margins, overgrowth of the jaw and enlargement of the nose, lips and tongue produce the characteristic facies of acromegaly. The chest is broad and barrel-shaped and the hands and feet are large. Thickening of the bone ends may cause secondary osteoarthritis. About 10 per cent of acromegalics develop diabetes and cardiovascular disease is more common than usual.

Treatment is sometimes possible; the indications for operation are the presence of a tumour in childhood and cranial nerve pressure symptoms at any age. Trans-sphenoidal surgery has a high rate of success, provided the diagnosis is made reasonably early and the tumour is not too large. Mild cases of acromegaly can be treated by administering growth hormone suppressants (a somatostatin analogue or bromocriptine, a dopamine agonist).

Adrenocortical dysfunction

The adrenal cortex secretes both mineralocorticoids (aldosterone) and glucocorticoids (cortisol). The latter has profound effects on bone and mineral metabolism, causing suppression of osteoblast activity, reduced calcium absorption, increased calcium excretion and enhanced PTH activity. Bone resorption is increased and formation is suppressed.

Hypercortisonism (Cushing's syndrome)

Glucocorticoid excess may be caused by increased pituitary secretion of adrenocorticotropic hormone (ACTH) (the original Cushing's disease), by independent oversecretion by the adrenal cortex (usually due to a steroid-secreting tumour) or by excessive

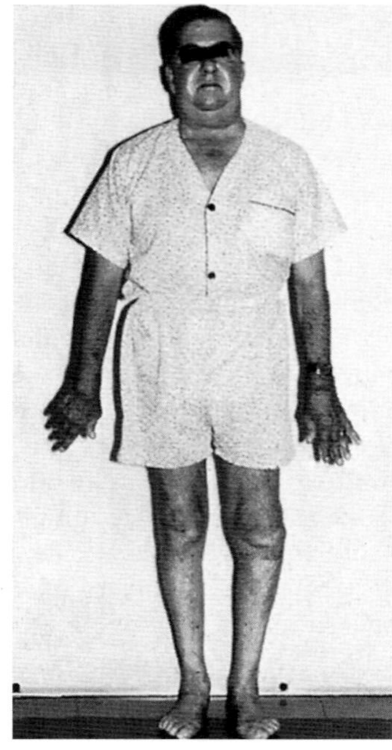

(a)

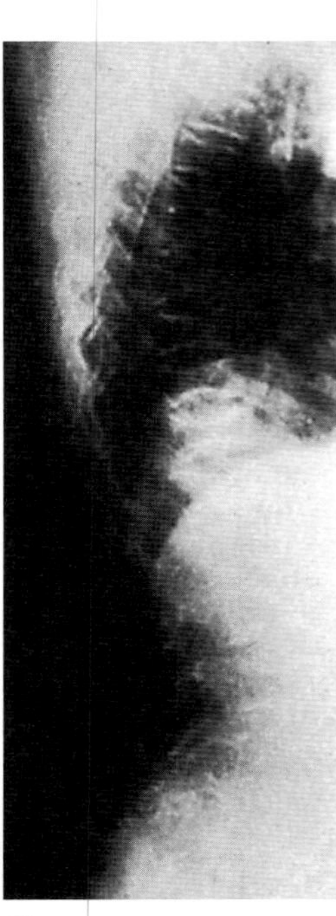

(b)

7.25 Cushing's syndrome (a) A patient with rheumatoid arthritis on long-term corticosteroid treatment. (b) On x-ray, the bones look washed-out and there are compression fractures at multiple levels.

treatment with glucocorticoids (probably the commonest cause). Whatever the cause, the clinical picture is much the same and is generally referred to as Cushing's syndrome.

Patients have a characteristic appearance: the face is rounded and looks somewhat puffy ('moon face') and the trunk is distinctly obese, often with abdominal striae. However, the legs are quite thin and there may be proximal wasting and weakness.

X-rays show generalized osteoporosis; fractures of the vertebrae and femoral neck are common. A CT scan may show an adrenal tumour.

Biochemical tests are usually normal, but there may be a slight increase in urinary calcium.

Problems for the orthopaedic surgeon are manifold: fractures and wounds heal slowly, bones provide little purchase for internal fixation, wound breakdown and infection are more common than usual, and the patients are generally less fit.

Prevention means using systemic corticosteroids only when essential and in low dosage. If treatment is prolonged, calcium supplements (at least 1500 mg per day) and vitamin D should be given. In postmenopausal women and elderly men, hormone replacement therapy is important. Bisphosphonates may also be effective in slowing the rate of bone loss and preventing further fractures.

Treatment includes the management of fractures and general measures to control bone pain. If a tumour is found, this will need surgical removal.

THYROID DYSFUNCTION

Hypothyroidism

Hypothyroidism takes various forms, depending on the age of onset.

Congenital hypothyroidism (cretinism) may be caused by developmental abnormalities of the thyroid, but it also occurs in endemic form in areas of iodine deficiency. Unless the condition is treated immediately (and diagnosis at birth is not easy!) the child becomes severely dwarfed and may have learning disabilities. X-rays may show irregular epiphyseal ossification. Treatment with thyroid hormone is essential.

Juvenile hypothyroidism is usually less severe than the congenital type. Growth and sexual development are retarded and the child may be mentally subnormal. X-rays show the typical epiphyseal 'fragmentation' appearance. Treatment with thyroid hormone may reverse these changes.

Adult hypothyroidism (myxoedema) may result from some primary disorder of thyroid function (including Hashimoto's disease) or from iatrogenic suppression following treatment for hyperthyroidism. The onset is slow and there may be a long period of non-specific symptoms such as weight increase, a general lack of energy and depression. Later complications include deafness, thinning of the hair, muscle weakness, nerve entrapment syndromes and joint pain, sometimes associated with CPPD crystal deposition.

Treatment with thyroxine is effective and will have to be continued for life.

Hyperthyroidism

Hyperthyroidism is an important cause of osteoporosis. This is dealt with on page 135.

PREGNANCY

Pregnancy can hardly be described as an endocrine disorder. However, pregnant women often develop musculoskeletal symptoms, some of which have been ascribed to hormonal changes; others are due to the increased weight and unusual posture.

Backache is common during the later months. The lordotic posture may be to blame and postural exercises are a help. But there is also increased laxity of the pelvic joints due to secretion of relaxin, and this may play a part. Back pain may persist after childbirth and x-rays sometimes show increased sclerosis near the sacroiliac joint – *osteitis condensans ilii*. This is, in all probability, due to increased stress or minor trauma to the bone associated with sacroiliac laxity.

Carpal tunnel syndrome is common; it is probably due to fluid retention and soft-tissue swelling. Operation should be avoided; symptoms can be controlled with a wrist splint and the condition does not recur after the end of pregnancy.

Rheumatic disorders respond in unusual ways. Patients with rheumatoid arthritis often improve dramatically, while those with systemic lupus erythematosus sometimes develop a severe exacerbation of the disease.

REFERENCES AND FURTHER READING

Bickerstaff DR, Douglas DL, Burke PH *et al.* Improvement in the deformity of the face in Paget's disease treated with diphosphonates. *J Bone Joint Surg* 1990; **72B:** 132–6.

Black DM, Cummings SR, Karpf DB *et al.* Randomised trial of effect of alendronate on risk of fracture in women with existing vertebral fractures. *Lancet* 1996; **348:** 1535–41.

Black DM, Bilezikian JP, Ensrud KE *et al.* One year of alendronate after one year of parathyroid hormone. *N Engl J Med* 2005; **353:** 555–65.

Boyce BF, Xing L. Biology of RANK, RANKL and osteoprotegerin. *Arthritis Res Ther* 2007; **9(Suppl 1):S1**.

Brighton CT, McCluskey WP. Cellular response and mechanisms of action of electrically induced osteogenisis. In *Bone and Mineral Research* 4th ed Peck WA. Elsevier, Amsterdam 1986.

Chapuy MC, Arlot ME, Delmas PD *et al.* Effect of calcium and cholecalciferol treatment for three years on hip fractures in elderly women. *BMJ* 1994; **308:** 1081–2.

Cummings SR, Black DM, Nevitt MC *et al.* Bone density at various sites for prediction of hip fractures. *Lancet* 1993; **341:** 72–5.

El Hajj Fuleihan G, Testa MA, Angell JE *et al.* Reproducibility of DXA absorptiometry: a model for bone loss estimates. *J Bone Miner Res* 1995; **10:** 1004–14.

Geneant HK, Engelke K, Fuerst T *et al.* Noninvasive assessment of bone mineral and structure: State of the art. *J Bone Miner Res* 1996; **11:** 707–30.

Hahn TJ. Drug-induced disorders of vitamin D and mineral metabolism. *Clin Endocrinol Metab* 1980; **9:** 107–29.

Horowitz MC. Cytokines and estrogen in bone: anti-osteoporotic effects. *Science* 1993; **260:** 626–27.

HYP Consortium. A gene (PEX) with homologies to endopeptidases is mutated in patients with X-linked hypophosphatemic rickets. *Nat Genet* 1995; **11:** 130–6.

Liberman UA, Downs RW Jr, Dequeker J *et al.* Effect of oral alendronate on bone mineral density and the incidence of fractures in postmenopausal osteoporosis. *N Engl J Med* 1995; **333:** 1437–43.

Lindsay R, Hart DM, Clark DM. The minimum effective dose of estrogen for prevention of postmenopausal bone loss. *Obstet Gynecol* 1984; **63:** 759–63.

Masud T, Mootoosamy I, McCloskey EV *et al.* Assessment of osteopenia from spinal radiographs using two different methods: the Chingford study. *Br J Radiol* 1996; **69:** 451–6.

McClung MR, Lewiecki ME, Cohen S *et al.* Denosumab in postmenopausal women with low bone mineral density. *N Engl J Med* 2006; **354:** 821–31.

Mirsky EC, Einhorn TA. Bone densitometry in orthopaedic practice. *J Bone Joint Surg* 1998; **80A:** 1687–98.

Nesbitt T, Drezner MK. Hepatocyte production of phosphatonin in HYP mice. *J Bone Miner Res* 1996; **(Supplement 1)**:S136.

Pak CYC, Sakhall K, Adams-Huet B. Treatment of postmenopausal osteoporosis with slow-release sodium fluoride. *Ann Intern Med* 1995; **123:** 401–8.

Parfitt AM. Bone remodelling: relationship to the amount and structure of bone, and the pathogenesis and prevention of fractures. In Osteoporosis eds Riggs BL, Nelton LJ III, Raven Press, New York, pp. 45–93 1988.

Peck WA, Woods WL. The cells of bone. In *Osteoporosis* eds Riggs BL, Melton LJ III, Raven Press, New York, pp. 1–44 1988.

Rebel A, Basle M, Poulard A *et al.* Towards a viral aetiology for Paget's disease of bone. *Metab Bone Dis Relat Res* 1980; **3:** 235–8.

Rihn JA, Gates C, Glassman SD *et al.* The use of bone morphogenetic protein in lumbar spine surgery. *J Bone Joint Surg* 2008; **90A:** 2014–25.

Rosen HN, Dresner-Pollak R, Moses AC *et al.* Specificity of urinary excretion of cross-linked N-telopeptides of type I collagen as a marker of bone turnover. *Calcif Tiss Int* 1994; **54:** 26–9.

Schnitzler CM, Solomon L. Osteomalacia in elderly white South African women. *S Afr Med J* 1983; **64:** 527–30.

Seeman E. Periosteal bone formation – a neglected determinant of bone strength. *N Engl J Med* 2003; **349:** 320–23.

Skerry TM, Bitensky L, Chayen J, Lanyon LE. Early strain-related changes in enzyme activity in osteocytes following bone loading in vivo. *J Bone Miner Res* 1989; **4:** 783–788.

Solomon L. Fracture of the femoral neck in the elderly. Bone ageing or disease? *S Afr J Surg* 1973; **11:** 269–79.

Solomon L. Osteoporosis and fracture of the femoral neck in the South African Bantu. *J Bone Joint Surg* 1968; **50B:** 2–13.

Sundaram M, McCarthy M. Oncogeneic osteomalacia. *Skeletal Radiol,* 2000; **29:** 117–124.

Urist MR. Bone: formation by induction. *Science* 1965; **150:** 893–9.

Genetic disorders, skeletal dysplasias and malformations

8

Deborah Eastwood, Louis Solomon

There can be few diseases in which genetic factors do not play a role – if only in creating a background favourable to the operation of some more proximate pathogen. Sometimes, however, a genetic defect is the major – or the only – determinant of an abnormality that is either present at birth (e.g. achondroplasia) or evolves over time (e.g. Huntington's chorea). Such conditions can be broadly divided into three categories: *chromosome disorders*, *single gene disorders* and *polygenic* or *multifactorial disorders*. Various anomalies may also result from *injury to the formed embryo*. Many of these conditions affect the musculoskeletal system, producing cartilage and bone dysplasia (abnormal bone growth and/or modelling), *malformations* (e.g. absence or duplication of certain parts) or *structural defects of connective tissue*. In some a specific *metabolic abnormality* has been identified.

Genetic influences also contribute to the development of many *acquired disorders*. Osteoporosis, for example, is the result of a multiplicity of endocrine, dietary and environmental factors, yet twin studies have shown a significantly closer concordance in bone mass between identical twins than between non-identical twins.

Before considering the vast range of developmental disorders, it may be helpful to review certain general aspects of genetic abnormalities.

THE HUMAN GENOME

Each cell (apart from germ cells) in the human body contains within its nucleus 46 *chromosomes*, each of which consists of a single molecule of *deoxyribonucleic acid (DNA)*; unravelled, this life-imparting molecule would be several centimetres long, a double-stranded chain along which thousands of segments are defined and demarcated as *genes*. A small amount of DNA is also found within the mitochondria of the cell and this is termed the mitochondrial DNA.

Each gene consists of a group of nucleotides and every nucleotide contains a deoxyribose sugar, a phosphate molecule and either a purine base (adenine or guanine) or a pyrimidine (thymine or cytosine) base. Some genes are comparatively large and some much smaller. They are the basic units of inherited biological information, each one coding for the synthesis of a specific protein. Working as a set (*or genome*) they 'tell' the cells how to develop, differentiate and function in specialized ways.

Chromosomes can be identified and numbered by microscopic examination of suitably prepared blood cells or tissue samples; the *cell karyotype* defines its chromosomal complement. *Somatic (diploid) cells* should have 46 chromosomes: 44 (numbers 1–22), called *autosomes*, are disposed in 22 homologous pairs – one of each pair being derived from the mother and one from the father, both carrying the same type of genetic information; the remaining 2 chromosomes are the *sex chromosomes*, females having two X chromosomes (one from each parent) and males having one X chromosome from the mother and one Y chromosome from the father. *Germ line cells* (eggs and sperm) have a *haploid* number of chromosomes (22 plus either an X or a Y). This is the *euploidic* situation; abnormalities of chromosome number would lead to an *aneuploidic* state.

Gene studies are complicated and involve the mapping of molecular sequences by specialized techniques after fragmenting the chains of DNA by means of restriction enzymes. Each gene occurs at a specific point, or *locus*, on a specific chromosome. The chromosomes being paired, there will be two forms, or *alleles*, of each gene (one maternal, one paternal) at each locus; if the two alleles coding for a particular trait are identical, the person is said to be *homozygous* for that trait; if they are not identical, the individual is *heterozygous*. Some chromosomes contain only a few genes (e.g. chromosomes 13, 18 and 21) whereas others contain many more (e.g. 17, 19 and 22).

The full genetic make-up of an individual is called the *genotype*. The finished person – a product of inherited traits and environmental influences – is the *phenotype*.

An important part of the unique human genotype is the *major histocompatibility complex (MHC)*, also known as the *HLA system* (after human leucocyte antigen). This is a cluster of genes on chromosome 6 that is responsible for immunological specificity. The proteins for which they code are attached to cell surfaces and act as 'chaperones' for foreign antigens which have to be accompanied by HLA before they are recognized and engaged by the body's T-cells. HLA proteins can be identified by serological tests and are registered according to their corresponding genetic loci on the short arm of chromosome 6. HLA typing is particularly important in tissue transplantation: acceptance or rejection of the transplant hinges on the degree of matching between the HLA genes of donor and recipient.

Genetic mutation

A mutation is any permanent change in DNA sequencing or structure. Such changes in a somatic cell are characteristic of malignancy. In a germ-line cell, mutations contribute to generational diversity. Some genes have many forms (or mutations) and the Human Genome Project has identified thousands of single nucleotide polymorphisms (SNPs).

Point mutations The substitution of one nucleotide for another is the most common type of mutation. The effect varies from production of a more useful protein to a new but functionless protein, or an inability to form any protein at all; the result may be compatible with an essentially normal life or it may be lethal.

Deletions/Insertions Deletion or insertion of a segment in the gene chain can result in an unusual protein being synthesized, perhaps a more advantageous one but maybe one that is non-functional or one that has a dire effect on tissue structure and function (e.g. production of a shortened dystrophin protein in the Becker variant of muscular dystrophy).

GENETIC DISORDER

Any serious disturbance of either the quantity or the arrangement of genetic material may result in disease. Three broad categories of abnormality are recognized: chromosome disorders, single gene disorders and polygenic or multifactorial disorders.

Chromosome disorders Additions, deletions and changes in chromosomal structure usually have serious effects; affected fetuses are either still-born or become infants with severe physical and mental abnormalities. In live-born children there are a few chromosome disorders with significant orthopaedic abnormalities: *Down's syndrome*, in which there is one extra chromosome 21 (trisomy 21), *Turner's syndrome*, in which one of the X chromosomes is lacking (monosomy X), and *Klinefelter's syndrome*, in which there is one Y but several X chromosomes.

Single gene disorders Gene mutation may occur by insertion, deletion, substitution or fusion of amino-acids or nucleotides in the DNA chain. This can have profound consequences for cartilage growth, collagen structure, matrix patterning and marrow cell metabolism. The abnormality is then passed on to future generations according to simple mendelian rules (see below). There are literally thousands of single gene disorders, accounting for over 5 per cent of child deaths, yet it is rare to see any one of them in a lifetime of orthopaedic practice.

Polygenic and multifactorial disorders Many normal traits (body build, for example) derive from the interaction of multiple genetic and environmental influences. Likewise, certain diseases have a polygenic background, and some occur only when a genetic predisposition combines with an appropriate environmental 'trigger'. *Gout*, for example, is more common than usual in families with hyperuricaemia: the uric acid level is a polygenic trait, reflecting the interplay of multiple genes; it is also influenced by diet and may be more than usually elevated after a period of overindulgence; finally, a slight bump on the toe acts as the proximate trigger for an acute attack of gout.

NON-GENETIC DEVELOPMENTAL DISORDERS

Many developmental abnormalities occur sporadically and have no genetic background. Most of these are of unknown aetiology, but some have been linked to specific teratogenic agents which damage the embryo or the placenta during the first few months of gestation. Suspected or known teratogens include viral infections (e.g. rubella), certain drugs (e.g. thalidomide) and ionizing radiation. The clinical features are usually asymmetrical and localized, ranging from mild morphological defects to severe malformations such as spina bifida or phocomelia ('congenital amputations').

PATTERNS OF INHERITANCE

The single gene disorders have characteristic patterns of inheritance, which may be *autosomal* or *X-linked*, and *dominant* or *recessive*.

Autosomal dominant disorders Autosomal dominant disorders are inherited even if only one of a pair of alleles on a non-sex chromosome is abnormal; the condition is said to be *heterozygous*. A typical example is hereditary multiple exostoses. Either parent may be

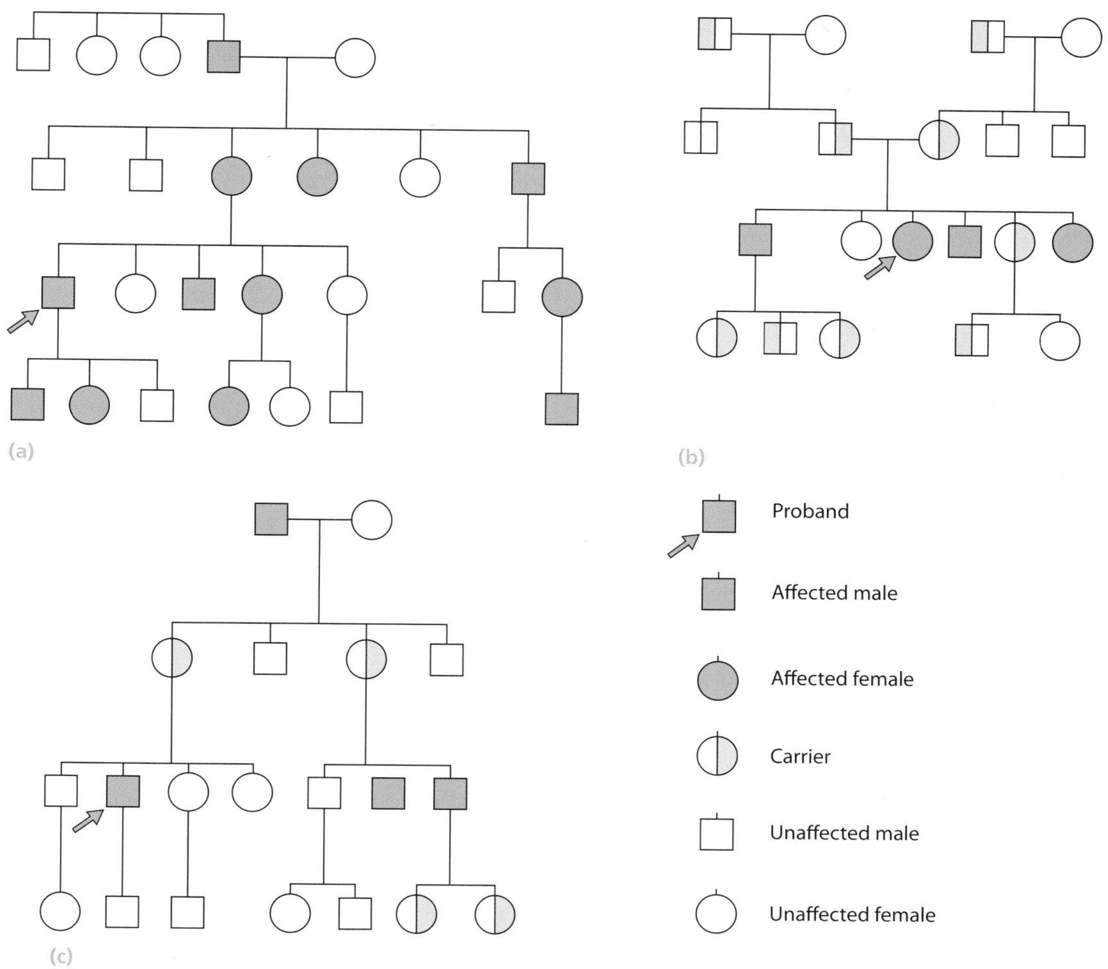

8.1 Patterns of inheritance (a) Autosomal dominant. (b) Autosomal recessive. (c) X-linked recessive.

affected and half the children of both sexes develop exostoses. The pedigree shows a 'vertical' pattern of inheritance, with several affected siblings in successive generations (Fig. 8.1a)

Sometimes both parents appear to be normal: the patient may be the first member of the family to suffer the effects of a mutant gene; or (as often happens) the disease shows variable expressivity, some members of the family (in the above example) developing many large exostoses and severe bone deformities, while others have only a few small and well-disguised nodules.

Autosomal recessive disorders These disorders appear only when both alleles of a pair are abnormal – i.e. the condition is always *homozygous*. Each parent contributes a faulty gene, though if both are heterozygous they themselves will be clinically normal. Theoretically 1 in 4 of the children will be homozygous and will therefore develop the disease; 2 out of 4 will be *heterozygous carriers* of the faulty gene. The typical pedigree shows a 'horizontal' pattern of inheritance: several siblings in one generation are affected but neither their parents nor their children have the disease (Fig. 8.1b).

X-linked disorders These conditions are caused by a faulty gene in the X chromosome. Characteristically, therefore, they never pass directly from father to son because the father's X chromosome inevitably goes to the daughter and the Y chromosome to the son. *X-linked dominant disorders* (e.g. hypophosphataemic rickets) pass from an affected mother to half of her daughters and half of her sons, or from an affected father to all of his daughters but none of his sons. Not surprisingly, they are twice as common in girls as in boys. *X-linked recessive disorders* – of which the most notorious is haemophilia – have a highly distinctive pattern of inheritance (Fig. 8.1c): an affected male will pass the gene only to his daughters, who will become unaffected heterozygous carriers; they, in turn, will transmit it to half of their daughters (who will likewise be carriers) and half of their sons (who will be bleeders).

In-breeding

All types of genetic disease are more likely to occur in the children of consanguineous marriages or in closed communities where many people are related to each other. The rare recessive disorders, in particular, are seen in these circumstances, where there is an increased risk of a homozygous pairing between two mutant genes.

Genetic heterogenicity

The same phenotype (i.e. a patient with a characteristic set of clinical features) can result from widely different gene mutations. For example, there are four different types of osteogenesis imperfecta (brittle bone disease), some showing autosomal dominant and some autosomal recessive inheritance. Where this occurs, the recessive form is usually the more severe. Subtleties of this kind must be borne in mind when counselling parents.

Genetic markers

Many common disorders show an unusually close association with certain blood groups, tissue types or other serum proteins that occur with higher than expected frequency in the patients and their relatives. These are referred to as genetic markers; they arise from gene sequences that do not cause the disease but are either 'linked' to other (abnormal) loci or else express some factor that predisposes the individual to a harmful environmental agent. A good example is ankylosing spondylitis: over 90 per cent of patients, and 60 per cent of their first-degree relatives, are positive for HLA-B27. In this case (as in other autoimmune diseases) the HLA marker gene may provide the necessary conditions for invasion by a foreign viral fragment.

Gene mapping

With advancing recombinant DNA technology, the genetic disorders are gradually being mapped to specific loci. In some cases (e.g. Duchenne muscular dystrophy) the mutant gene itself has been cloned, holding out the possibility of effective treatment in the future.

PRE-NATAL DIAGNOSIS

Many genetic disorders can be diagnosed before birth, thus improving the chances of treatment or, at worst, giving the parents the choice of selective abortion. Ultrasound imaging is harmless and is now done almost routinely. On the other hand, tests that involve amniocentesis or chorionic villus sampling carry a risk of injury to the fetus and are therefore used only when there is reason to suspect some abnormality. Indications are: (1) maternal age over 35 years (increased risk of Down's syndrome) or an unduly high paternal age (increased risk of achondroplasia); (2) a previous history of chromosomal abnormalities (e.g. Down's syndrome) or genetic abnormalities amenable to biochemical diagnosis (neural tube defects, or inborn errors of metabolism) which will benefit from prompt neonatal treatment; or (3) to confirm non-invasive tests suggesting an abnormality.

Maternal screening

Fetal neural tube defects are associated with increased levels of alpha-fetoprotein (AFP) in the amniotic fluid and, to a lesser extent, the maternal blood. Women with positive blood tests may be given the option of further investigation by amniocentesis. It has also been noted that abnormally low levels of AFP are associated with Down's syndrome.

Fetal cells may be present in maternal plasma and in the near future it is possible that genetic testing of these cells will be possible.

Amniocentesis

Under local anaesthesia, a small amount (about 20 ml) of fluid is withdrawn from the amniotic sac with a needle and syringe. (It is best to determine the position of the fetus beforehand by ultrasonography.) The procedure is usually carried out between the 12th and 15th weeks of pregnancy. The fluid can be examined directly for AFP and desquamated fetal cells can be collected and cultured for chromosomal studies and biochemical tests for enzyme disorders. It is well to remember that this procedure carries a small risk (0.5–0.75 per cent of cases) of losing the fetus.

Chorionic villus sampling

Under ultrasound screening, a fine catheter is passed through the cervix and a small sample of chorion is sucked out. This is usually done between the 10th and 12th weeks of pregnancy. Mesenchymal fibroblasts can be cultured and used for *chromosomal studies, biochemical tests* and DNA *analysis.* Rapid advances in DNA technology have made it possible to diagnose sickle-cell anaemia and haemophilia (among other disorders) during early pregnancy, but spina bifida cannot be tested for. The procedure-related fetal loss rate is about 1 per cent.

Pre-implantation genetic diagnosis

With assisted reproductive technologies such as *in vitro* fertilization (IVF), genetic abnormalities in the embryos can be detected prior to implantation, thus allowing only 'healthy' embryos (as far as technology can tell) to be implanted into the mother.

Fetal imaging

High resolution ultrasonography should provide images of all the long bones and joint movements by 11 weeks of gestation. Bone lengths increase linearly with time and by 18–23 weeks all three segments of each limb are clearly visible; a single measurement of one bone can be used to estimate growth. A femoral length that is normal for the fetal age is very significant in excluding many of the skeletal dysplasias or malformations; even with mesomelic abnormalities where the lower leg is most affected, the femur is likely to be short. By the 18th week of pregnancy anatomical abnormalities such as open neural tube defects and short limbs should be visible.

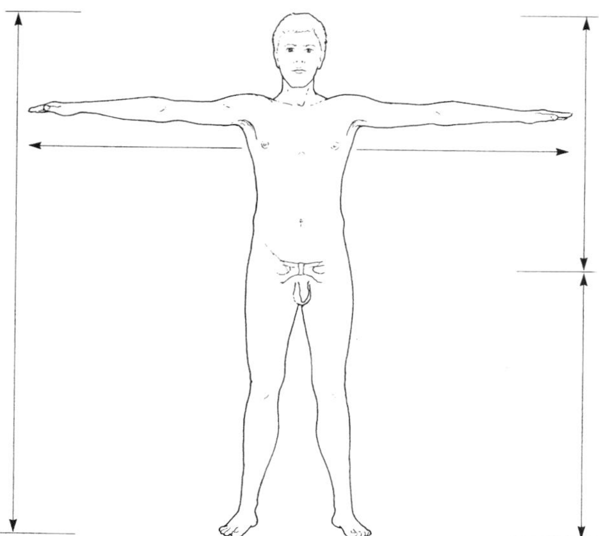

8.2 Normal proportions Upper segment = lower segment. Total height = span.

DIAGNOSIS IN CHILDHOOD

Clinical features

Tell-tale features suggesting skeletal dysplasia are:

- retarded growth and shortness of stature
- disproportionate length of trunk and limbs
- localized malformations (dysmorphism)
- soft-tissue contractures
- childhood deformity.

All the skeletal dysplasias affect growth, although this may not be obvious at birth. Children should be measured at regular intervals and a record kept of height, length of lower segment (top of pubic symphysis to heel), upper segment (pubis to cranium), span, head circumference and chest circumference. Failure to reach the expected height for the local population group should be noted, and marked shortness of stature is highly suspicious.

Bodily proportion is as important as overall height. The normal upper segment:lower segment ratio changes gradually from about 1.5:1 at the end of the first year to about 1:1 at puberty. *Shortness of stature with normal proportions* is not necessarily abnormal, but it is also seen in endocrine disorders which affect the different parts of the skeleton more or less equally (e.g. hypopituitarism). By contrast, *small stature with disproportionate shortness of the limbs* is characteristic of skeletal dysplasia, the long bones being more markedly affected than the axial skeleton.

The different segments of the limbs also may be disproportionately affected. The subtleties of dysplastic growth are reflected in terms such as *rhizomelia* – unusually short proximal segments (humeri and femora), *mesomelia* – short middle segments (forearms and legs) and *acromelia* – stubby hands and feet.

Dysmorphism (a misshapen part of the body) is most obvious in the face and hands. There is a remarkable consistency about these changes, which makes for a disturbing similarity of appearance in members of a particular group.

Local deformities – such as kyphosis, valgus or varus knees, bowed forearms and ulnar deviated wrists – result from disturbed bone growth.

X-rays

The presence of any of the above features calls for a limited radiographic survey: a posteroanterior view of the chest, anteroposterior views of the pelvis, knees and hands, additional views of one arm and one leg, a lateral view of the thoracolumbar spine and standard views of the skull. Fractures, bent bones, exostoses, epiphyseal dysplasia and spinal deformities may be obvious, especially in the older child. Sometimes a complete survey is needed and it is important to note which portion of the long bones (epiphysis, metaphysis or diaphysis) is affected. With severe and varied changes in the metaphyses, periosteal new bone formation or epiphyseal separation, always consider the possibility of non-accidental injuries – the 'battered baby' syndrome.

Special investigations

In many cases the diagnosis can be made without laboratory tests; however, *routine blood* and *urine analysis* may be helpful in excluding metabolic and endocrine disorders such as rickets and pituitary or thyroid dysfunction. Special tests are also available to identify specific excretory metabolites in the storage disorders, and specific enzyme activity can be measured in serum, blood cells or cultured fibroblasts.

Bone biopsy is occasionally helpful in disorders of bone density.

Direct testing for gene mutations is already available for a number of conditions and is rapidly being extended to others. It is a useful adjunct to clinical diagnosis. Still somewhat controversial is its application to pre-clinical diagnosis of late-onset disorders and neonatal screening for potentially dangerous conditions such as sickle-cell disease.

Previous medical history

Always ask whether the mother was exposed to teratogenic agents (x-rays, cytotoxic drugs or virus infections) during the early months of pregnancy.

The family history

A careful family history should always be obtained. This should include information about similar disorders in parents and close relatives, previous deaths in the family (and the cause of death), abortions and consanguineous marriages. However, the fact that parents or relatives are said to be 'normal' does not exclude the possibility that they are either very mildly affected or have a biochemical defect without any physical abnormality. Many developmental disorders have characteristic patterns of inheritance which may be helpful in diagnosis.

Racial background is sometimes important: some diseases are particularly common in certain communities, for example, sickle-cell disease in Negroid peoples and Gaucher's disease in Ashkenazi Jews.

DIAGNOSIS IN ADULTHOOD

It is unusual for a patient to present in adulthood with a condition that has been present since birth but in milder cases the abnormality may not have been recognized, particularly when several members of the family are similarly affected.

In the worst of the genetic disorders the fetus is still-born or survives for only a short time. Individuals who reach adulthood, though recognizably abnormal, may lead active lives, marry and have children of their own. Nevertheless, they often seek medical advice for several reasons:

- short stature – especially disproportionate shortness of the lower limbs
- local bone deformities or exostoses
- spinal stenosis
- repeated fractures
- secondary osteoarthritis (e.g. due to epiphyseal dysplasia)
- joint laxity or instability.

The clinical approach is similar to that employed with children.

PRINCIPLES OF MANAGEMENT

Management of the individual patient depends on the diagnosis, the pattern of inheritance, the type and severity of deformity or disability, mental capacity and social aspirations. However, it is worth noting some general principles.

Communication

Once the diagnosis has been made, the next step is to explain as much as possible about the disorder to the patient (if old enough) and the parents without causing unnecessary distress. This is a skill that the orthopaedic surgeon must develop. Nowadays, with quick and easy access to the internet, it is relatively easy to obtain useful information about almost any condition, which the clinician can pass on in simple language.

Rare developmental disorders are best treated in a centre that offers a 'special interest' team consisting of a paediatrician, medical geneticist, orthopaedic surgeon, psychologist, social worker, occupational therapist, orthotist and prosthetist.

Counselling

Patients and families may need expert counselling about (1) the likely outcome of the disorders; (2) what will be required of the family; and (3) the risk of siblings or children being affected. Where there are severe deformities or mental disability, the entire family may need counselling.

Maintaining an independent lifestyle

Parents are often anxious about having their child grow up as 'normal' as possible, yet 'normality' may mean something different for the child. For example, it is expected that children will become independently mobile only by learning to walk in a safe and effective manner, but some children with genetic disorders may be equally independently mobile with the use of a wheelchair. Management must be influenced by goals for adult life and not just the short-term goals of childhood.

Intrauterine surgery

The concept of operating on the unborn fetus is already a reality and is likely to be extended in the future. At present, however, it is still too early to say whether the advantages (e.g. prenatal skin closure for dysraphism) will outweigh the risks.

Prevention and correction of deformities

Realignment of the limb, correction of ligamentous laxity and/or joint reconstruction can improve the stability and efficiency of gait and reduce the risk of secondary joint degenerative change.

Anomalies such as coxa vara, genu valgum, club foot, radial club hand or scoliosis (and many others outside the field of orthopaedics) are amenable to corrective surgery. In recent years, with advances in methods of limb lengthening, many short-limbed patients have benefited from this operation; however, the risks should be carefully explained and the expected benefits should not be exaggerated.

Several developmental disorders are associated with potentially dangerous spinal anomalies: for example, spinal stenosis and cord compression in achondroplasia; atlantoaxial instability, due to odontoid aplasia, in any disorder causing vertebral dysplasia; or severe kyphoscoliosis, which occurs in a number of conditions. Cord decompression or occipitocervical fusion are perfectly feasible, but surgical correction of congenital kyphoscoliosis carries considerable risks and should be undertaken only in specialized units.

When considering the need for surgery, it must be remembered that some of these patients have a significantly reduced walking tolerance and hence improvements in limb alignment or length, for example, may not bring about any significant functional change. Conservative measures such as physiotherapy and splinting still have an important role to play.

Gene therapy

Gene therapy is still at the experimental stage. A carrier molecule or vector (often a virus that has been genetically modified to carry some normal human genetic material) is used to deliver the therapeutic (i.e. normal) material into the abnormal target cells where the DNA is 'uploaded' allowing, for example, functional protein production to be resumed. There have been considerable concerns that the viral 'infection' may trigger an immune reaction and this is one of several factors affecting the development of this line of therapy in the human 'model'.

CLASSIFICATION OF DEVELOPMENTAL DISORDERS

There is no completely satisfactory classification of developmental disorders. The same genetic abnormality may be expressed in different ways, while a variety of gene defects may cause almost identical clinical syndromes. The grouping used in Table 8.1 lists only the least rare of the developmental disorders that come within the sphere of orthopaedic surgery and offers no more than a convenient way of remembering and dividing the various clinical syndromes.

THE CHONDRO-OSTEODYSTROPHIES

The chondro-osteodystrophies, or skeletal dysplasias, are a large group of disorders characterized by abnormal cartilage and bone growth. Since the various conditions are caused by different gene defects, it would be scientifically correct to classify them according to their basic molecular pathology. However, the orthopaedic surgeon faced with a patient will seek first to categorize the disorder according to recognizable clinical and x-ray appearances; it is with this in mind that the conditions are presented here in clinical rather than etiological groups, as follows:

- those with predominantly epiphyseal changes
- those with predominantly physeal and metaphyseal changes
- those with mainly diaphyseal changes; and
- those with a mixture of abnormalities.

DYSPLASIAS WITH PREDOMINANTLY EPIPHYSEAL CHANGES

This group of disorders is characterized by abnormal development and ossification of the epiphyses. Limb length may be reduced, though not as severely as in conditions where the physis is affected.

MULTIPLE EPIPHYSEAL DYSPLASIA

Multiple epiphyseal dysplasia (MED) varies in severity from a trouble-free disorder with mild anatomical abnormalities to a severe crippling condition. There is widespread involvement of the epiphyses but the vertebrae are not at all, or only mildly, affected.

Table 8.1 A practical grouping of generalized developmental disorders

1 Disorders of cartilage and bone growth	2 Connective tissue disorders
1.1 Dysplasias with predominantly physeal and metaphyseal changes	2.1 Generalized joint laxity
1.1.1 Hereditary multiple exostosis	2.2 Ehlers–Danlos syndrome
1.1.2 Achondroplasia	2.3 Larsen's syndrome
1.1.3 Hypochondroplasia	2.4 Osteogenesis imperfecta (brittle bones)
1.1.4 Metaphyseal chondrodysplasia	2.4.1 Mild
1.1.5 Dyschondroplasia (enchodromatosis, Ollier's disease)	2.4.2 Lethal
1.2 Dysplasias with predominantly epiphyseal changes	2.4.3 Severe
1.2.1 Multiple epiphyseal dysplasia	2.4.4 Moderate
1.2.2 Spondyloepiphyseal dysplasia	2.5 Fibrodysplasia ossificans progressive
1.2.3 Dysplasia epiphysealis hemimlica (Trevor's disease)	**3 Storage disorders and other metabolic defects**
1.2.4 Chondrodysplasia punctata (stippled epiphysis)	3.1 Mucopolysaccharidoses
1.3 Dysplasias with predominantly metaphyseal and diaphyseal changes	3.1.1 Hurler's syndrome (MPS I)
1.3.1 Metaphyseal dysplasia (Pyle's disease)	3.1.2 Hunter's syndrome (MPS II)
1.3.2 Craniometaphyseal dysplasia	3.1.3 Morquio–Brailsford syndrome (MPS IV)
1.3.3 Diaphyseal dysplasia (Engelmann's disease, Cumurati's disease)	3.2 Gaucher's disease
1.3.4 Craniodiaphyseal dysplasia	3.3 Homocystinuria
1.3.5 Osteopetrosis (marble bones, Albers–Shönbert disease)	3.4 Alkaptonuria
1.3.6 Pyknodysostosis	3.5 Congenital hyperuricaemia
1.3.7 Candle bones, spotted bones and striped bones	**4 Chromosome disorders**
1.4 Combined and mixed dysplasias	4.1 Down's syndrome
1.4.1 Spondylometaphyseal	4.2 Thoracospinal anomalies
1.4.2 Pseudoachondroplasia	4.3 Elevation of the scapula (Sprengel's deformity)
1.4.3 Diastrophic dysplasia	4.4 Limb anomalies
1.4.4 Cleidocranial dysplasia	
1.4.5 Nail–patella syndrome	
1.4.6 Craniofacial dysplasia	

Clinical features

Children are below average height and the parents may have noticed that the lower limbs are disproportionately short compared to the trunk. They sometimes walk with a waddling gait and they may complain of hip or knee pain. Some develop progressive deformities of the knees and/or ankles. The hands and feet may be short and broad. The face, skull and spine are normal.

In some cases only one or two pairs of joints are involved, while in others the condition is widespread; these are probably expressions of several different disorders.

In adult life, residual epiphyseal defects may lead to joint incongruity and secondary osteoarthritis. If the anatomical changes are mild, the underlying abnormality may be missed and the patient is regarded as 'just another case of OA' (see Fig. 5.9 page 92).

X-ray

Changes are apparent from early childhood. Epiphyseal ossification is delayed, and when it appears it is irregular or abnormal in outline. In the growing child the epiphyses are misshapen; in the hips this may be mistaken for bilateral Perthes' disease, but the symmetrical nature

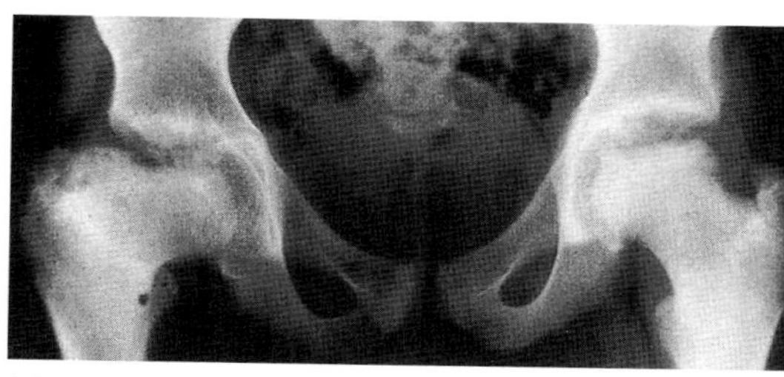

(a)

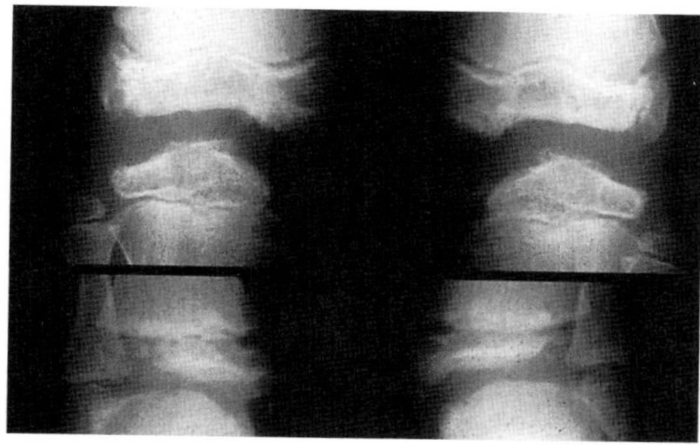

(b)

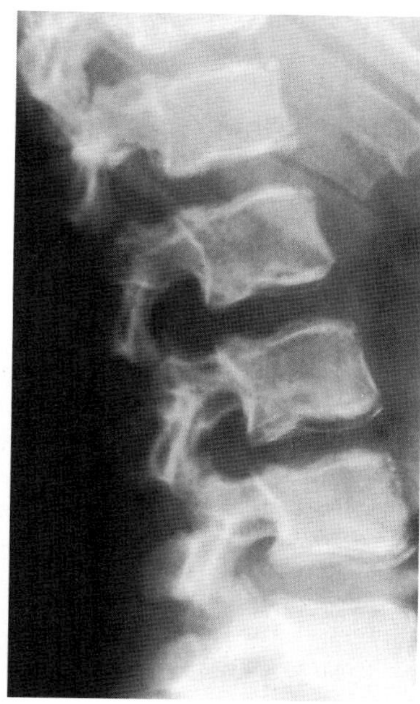

(c)

8.3 Multiple epiphyseal dysplasia (a,b) X-rays show epiphyseal distortion and flattening at multiple sites, in this case the hips, knees and ankles. (c) The ring epiphyses of the vertebral bodies also may be affected; in spondyloepiphyseal dysplasia this is the dominant feature.

of the changes and the presence of changes in other epiphyses usually define the condition as MED. The vertebral ring epiphyses may be affected, but only mildly. At maturity the femoral heads, femoral condyles and humeral heads are flattened; secondary osteoarthritis may ensue and, if many joints are involved, the patient can be severely crippled.

Genetics

This appears to be a heterogeneous disorder but most cases have an autosomal dominant pattern of inheritance.

The abnormality identified in some cases is in the gene which codes for cartilage oligometric matrix protein (COMP). In ways which are not fully understood, this results in defective chondrocyte function.

Diagnosis

MED is often confused with other childhood disorders which are associated with either lower-limb shortness or Perthes-like changes in the epiphyses.

Achondroplasia and hypochondroplasia should not be difficult to exclude. The former is marked by a more severe shortening in height and characteristic facial changes; the latter by the absence of epiphyseal changes. *Dyschondrosteosis*, likewise, is associated with normal epiphyses.

Pseudoachondroplasia shows widespread epiphyseal abnormalities. However, the skeletal deformities are more severe than those of MED and they also involve the spine.

Perthes' disease is confined to the hips and shows a typical cycle of changes from epiphyseal irregularity to fragmentation, flattening and healing.

Hypothyroidism, if untreated, causes progressive and widespread epiphyseal dysplasia. However, these children have other clinical and biochemical abnormalities and have learning difficulties.

Management

Children may complain of slight pain and limp, but little can (or need) be done about this. At maturity, deformities around the hips, knees or ankles sometimes require corrective osteotomy.

In later life, secondary osteoarthritis may call for reconstructive surgery.

Spondyloepiphyseal dysplasia

The term 'spondyloepiphyseal dysplasia' (SED) encompasses a heterogeneous group of disorders in which multiple epiphyseal dysplasia is associated with well-marked vertebral changes – delayed ossification, flattening of the vertebral bodies (platyspondyly), irregular ossification of the ring epiphyses and indentations of the end-plates (Schmorl's nodes). The mildest of these disorders is indistinguishable from MED; the more severe forms have characteristic appearances.

Clinical features

SED congenita

This autosomal dominant disorder can be diagnosed in infancy: the limbs are short, but the trunk is even

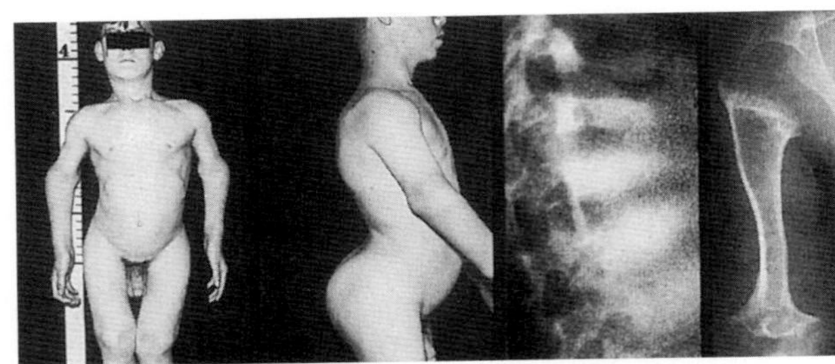

(a)

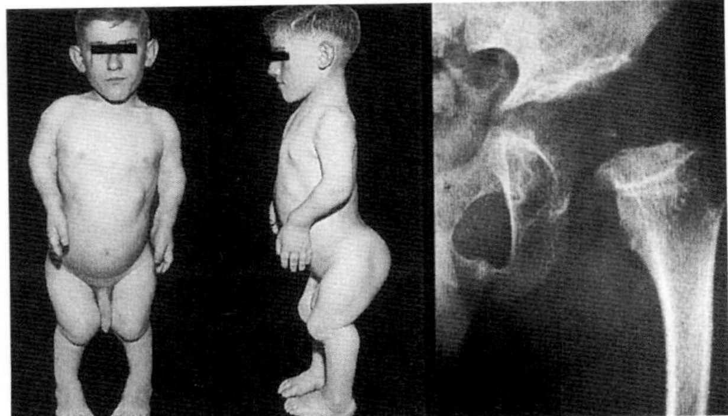

(b)

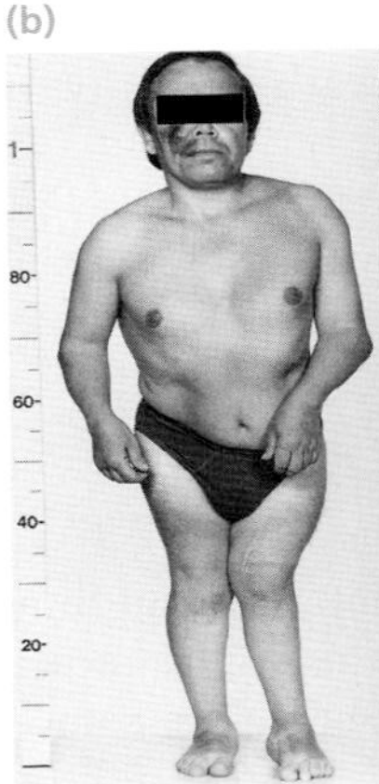

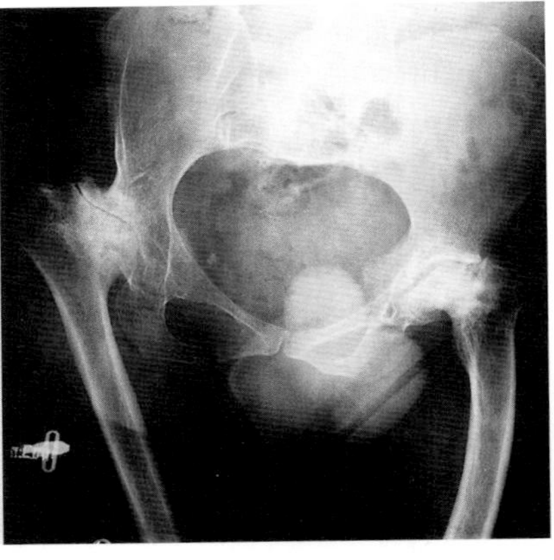

(c)

8.4 Spondyloepiphyseal dysplasia (a,b) Adolescent boys with marked lumbar lordosis, vertebral deformities, flexed hips and epiphyseal dysplasia affecting all the limbs. (c) Widespread deformities and barrel chest in adulthood. X-rays show severe secondary osteoarthritis of the hips.

shorter and the neck hardly there. Older children develop a dorsal kyphosis and a typical barrel-shaped chest; they stand with the hips flexed and the lumbar spine in marked lordosis. By adolescence they often have scoliosis.

X-rays show widespread epiphyseal dysplasia and the characteristic vertebral changes. Odontoid hypoplasia is common and may lead to atlantoaxial subluxation and cord compression.

Diagnosis is not always easy; there are obvious similarities to Morquio's disease but, in the latter, shortening is in the distal limb segments and urinalysis shows increased excretion of keratan sulphate.

Management may involve corrective osteotomies for severe coxa vara or knee deformities. Odontoid hypoplasia increases the risks of anaesthesia; if there is evidence of subluxation, atlantoaxial fusion may be advisable.

SED TARDA

An X-linked recessive disorder, SED tarda is much less severe and may become apparent only after the age of 5 years when the child fails to grow normally and develops a kyphoscoliosis. Adult men tend to be more severely affected than women, showing a disproportionate shortening of the trunk and a tendency to barrel chest. They may develop backache or secondary osteoarthritis of the hips.

X-rays show the characteristic platyspondyly and abnormal ossification of the ring epiphyses, together with more widespread dysplasia.

Treatment may be needed for backache or (in older adults) for secondary osteoarthritis of the hips.

DYSPLASIA EPIPHYSEALIS HEMIMELICA (TREVOR'S DISEASE)

This is a curious 'hemidysplasia' affecting just one half (medial or lateral) of one or more epiphyses on one

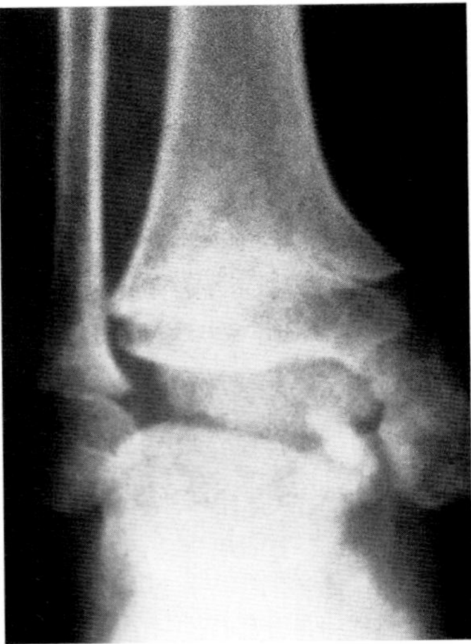

(a)

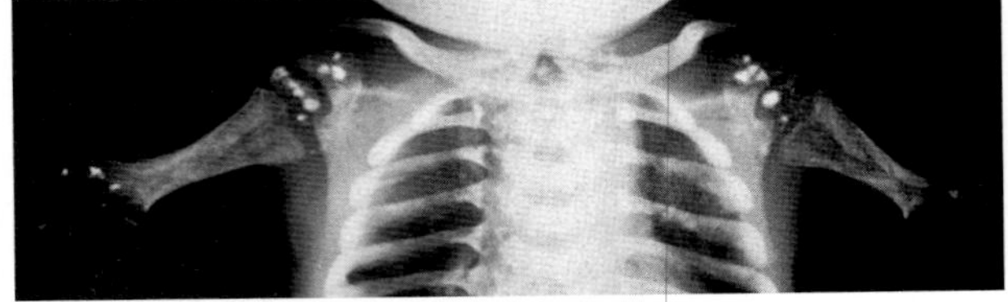

(b)

8.5 Epiphyseal dysplasia (a) Trevor's disease. (b) Conradi's disease – the 'spots' disappeared later.

side of the body. It is a sporadic disorder which usually appears at the ankle or knee. The child (most often a boy) presents with a bony swelling on one side of the joint; several sites may be affected – all on the same side in the same limb, but rarely in the upper limb.

X-rays show an asymmetrical enlargement of the bony epiphysis and distortion of the adjacent joint. At the ankle, this may give the appearance of an abnormally large medial malleolus.

Treatment is called for if the deformity interferes with joint function. The excess bone is removed, taking care not to damage the articular cartilage or ligaments.

CHONDRODYPLASIA PUNCTATA (STIPPLED EPIPHYSES)

Chondrodysplasia punctata (or Conradi's disease) is a generalized, multisystem disorder producing facial abnormalities, vertebral anomalies, asymmetrical epiphyseal changes and bone shortening. In severe cases there may also be cardiac anomalies, congenital cataracts and learning difficulties; some of these children die during infancy.

The characteristic *x-ray* feature is a punctate stippling of the cartilaginous epiphyses and apophyses. This disappears by the age of 4 years but is often followed by epiphyseal irregularities and dysplasia. It is unlikely that these changes will be confused with those of MED, Down's syndrome or hypothyroidism.

Orthopaedic management is directed at the deformities that develop in older children: joint contractures, limb length inequality or scoliosis.

DYSPLASIAS WITH PREDOMINANTLY PHYSEAL AND METAPHYSEAL CHANGES

In these disorders there is abnormal physeal growth, defective metaphyseal modelling and shortness of the tubular bones. The axial skeleton is affected too, but the limbs are disproportionately short compared to the spine.

HEREDITARY MULTIPLE EXOSTOSIS (DIAPHYSEAL ACLASIS)

Multiple exostosis is the most common, and least disfiguring, of the skeletal dysplasias.

Clinical Features

The condition is usually discovered in childhood; hard lumps appear at the ends of the long bones and along the apophyseal borders of the scapula and pelvis. As the child grows, these lumps enlarge and some may become hugely visible, especially around the knee. The more severely affected bones are abnormally short; this is seldom very marked but on measurement the lower body segment is shorter than the upper and span is less than height (Solomon, 1963). In the forearm and leg, the thinner of the two bones (the ulna or fibula) is usually the more defective, resulting in typical deformities: ulnar deviation of the wrist, bowing of the radius, subluxation of the radial head, valgus knees and valgus ankles. Bony lumps may cause pressure on nerves or vessels. Occasionally one of the cartilage-capped exostoses goes on growing into adult life and transforms to a chondrosarcoma; this is said to occur in 1–2 per cent of patients.

X-RAY

Typically the long-bone metaphyses are broad and poorly modelled, with sessile or pedunculated exostoses arising from the cortices – almost as if longitudinal growth has been squandered in profligate lateral expansion. A mottled appearance around a bony excrescence indicates calcification in the cartilage cap. The distal end of the ulna is sometimes tapered or carrot-shaped and the bone may be markedly reduced in length; in these cases the radius is usually bowed, or the discrepancy in length may lead to subluxation of the radiohumeral joint.

The cuboidal carpal and tarsal bones show little or no change on x-ray. This is simply because the ossified parts of these bones (which is all that is visible on x-ray) are completely surrounded by cartilage during early development, and any cartilage irregularities are subsumed in the overall expansion of the bone.

Pathology

The underlying fault in multiple exostosis is unrestrained transverse growth of the cartilaginous physis (growth plate). The condition affects only the endochondral bones. Cartilaginous excrescences appear at the periphery of the physes and proceed, in the usual way, to endochondral ossification. If the abnormal physeal proliferation ceases at that point, but the bone continues to grow in length, the exostosis is left behind where it arose (now part of the metaphysis) but its cartilage cap is still capable of autonomous growth. If the physeal abnormality persists, further growth proceeds in the new abnormal mould, without remodelling of the broadened and misshapen metaphysis. The process finally comes to a stop when endochondral proliferation

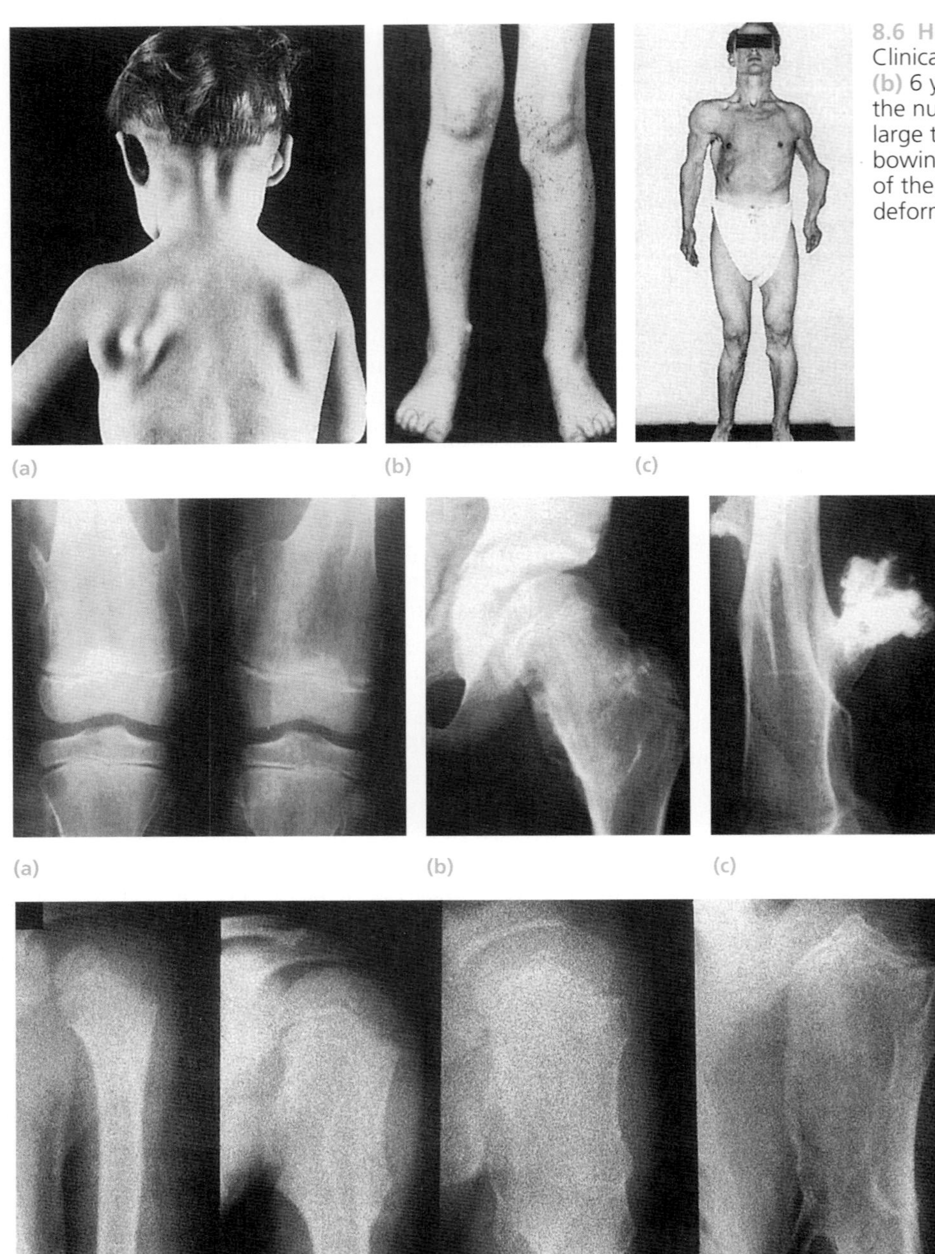

8.6 Hereditary multiple exostoses Clinical presentation at (a) 3 years (b) 6 years and (c) 28 years. In (c) note the numerous small 'bumps', the one large tumour near the right shoulder, bowing of the left radius, shortening of the left forearm and valgus deformity of the right knee.

8.7 Hereditary multiple exostoses – x-rays (a) Typical x-ray appearances of the knees. (b) Sessile exostoses of the femoral neck. (c) A large pedunculated exostosis of the distal femur. (d) Evolution of the wide metaphysis during growth.

ceases at the end of the normal period of growth for that bone; any further growth of the exostotic cartilage cap after that suggests neoplastic change.

Genetics

The condition is acquired by autosomal dominant transmission; half the children are affected, boys and girls equally. However, expression is variable and some people are so mildly affected as to be unaware of the disorder. In some cases the condition appears to be due to a spontaneous mutation but this may be because the parent is so mildly affected as to seem normal.

Abnormalities have been identified on chromosomes 8, 11 and 19, referred to as EXT 1, 2 and 3, the differing sites being responsible for different phenotypes. The molecular basis of this condition is not yet understood.

Management

Exostoses may need removal because of pressure on a nerve or vessel, because of their unsightly appearance, or because they tend to get bumped during everyday activities. Care must be taken not to damage the physes. Deformities of the legs or forearms may be severe enough to warrant treatment by corrective osteotomy or concomitant correction and lengthening by the Ilizarov technique (see Chapter 12). Physeal stapling or plating may be used to direct longitudinal growth.

Exostoses should stop growing when the parent bone does; any subsequent enlargement suggests malignant change and calls for advanced imaging and wide local resection.

ACHONDROPLASIA

This is the commonest form of abnormally short stature; adult height is usually around 122 cm (48 inches). Disproportionate shortening of the limb bones is detectable *in utero* by ultrasound scan.

Clinical Features

The abnormality is obvious in childhood: growth is severely stunted; the limbs – particularly the proximal segments – are disproportionately short (rhizomelic shortening) and the skull is quite large with prominent forehead and saddle-shaped nose. Frontal bossing and mid-face hypoplasia contribute to the characteristic appearance of people with achondroplasia. The fingers appear stubby and somewhat splayed (trident hands). A thoracolumbar kyphos is often present in infancy but this almost always disappears in a year or two. Mental development is normal.

By early childhood the trunk is obviously disproportionately long in comparison with the limbs. Joint laxity is common and contributes to the characteristic standing posture: flat feet, bowed legs, flexed hips, prominent buttocks, lordotic spine and elbows slightly flexed.

Relative stenosis of the foramen magnum can be a problem in infancy. During adulthood, shortening of the vertebral pedicles may lead to lumbar spinal stenosis and disc prolapse (which is quite common) has exceptionally severe neurological effects. Cervical spine stenosis may cause typical features of cord compression.

X-Rays

All bones that are formed by endochondral ossification are affected, so the facial bones and skull base are abnormal but the cranial vault is not. The foramen magnum is smaller than usual. The tubular bones are short but thick, the metaphyses flared and the physeal lines somewhat irregular; sites of muscle attachment, such as the tibial tubercle and the greater trochanter of the femur, are prominent. Although the proximal limb bones are disproportionately affected (rhizomelia), changes are also seen in the wrists and hands, where the metaphyses are broad and cup-shaped. The epiphyses are surprisingly normal and hence joint degeneration is uncommon.

The pelvic cavity is small (too small for normal delivery) and the iliac wings are flared, producing an almost horizontal acetabular roof. The vertebral interpedicular distance often diminishes from L1 to L5 and the spinal canal is reduced in size. These features are best defined on CT or MRI.

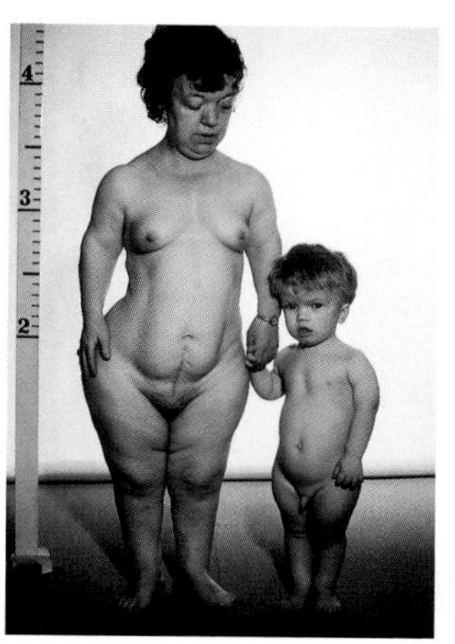
(a)

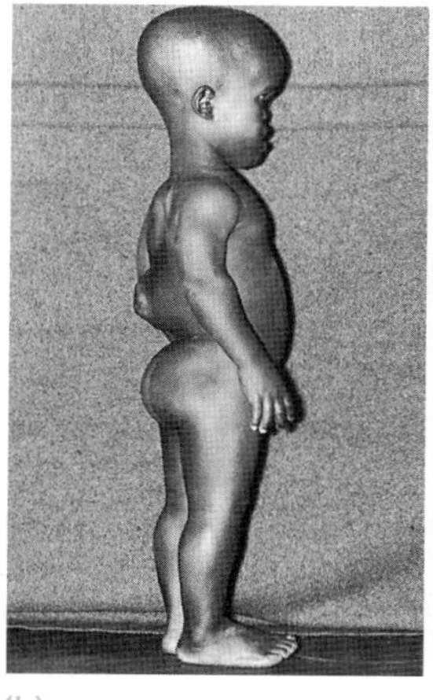
(b)

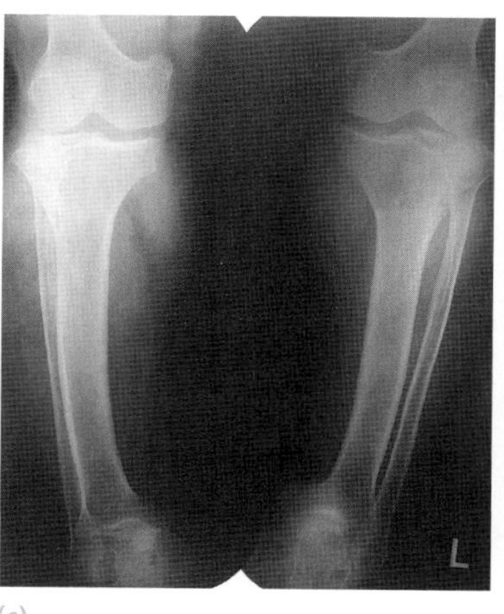

(c)

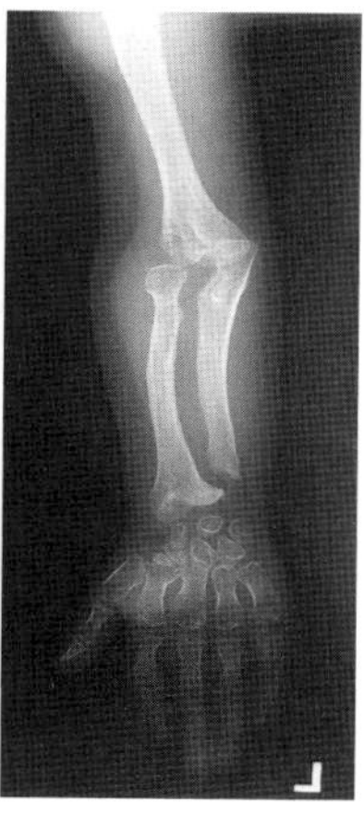
(d)

8.8 Achondroplasia (a) Mother and child with achondroplasia, showing the typical disproportionate shortening of the tubular bones, particularly the proximal segments of the upper and lower limbs. (b) Other features are seen in this child: lumbar lordosis, a prominent thoracolumbar gibbus and bossing of the forehead. (c,d) X-rays show the short, thick bones (including the metacarpals).

Diagnosis

Achondroplasia should not be confused with other types of short-limbed 'dwarfism'. In some (e.g. Morquio's disease) the shortening affects distal segments more than proximal and there may be widespread associated abnormalities. Others (e.g. pseudoachondroplasia and the epiphyseal dysplasias) are distinguished by the fact that the head and face are quite normal whereas the epiphyses show characteristic changes on x-ray examination.

Pathology

This is essentially an abnormality of endochondral longitudinal growth resulting in diminished length of the tubular bones. Membrane bone formation is unaffected, hence the normal growth of the skull vault and the periosteal contribution to bone width.

Genetics

Achondroplasia occurs in about 1 in 30,000 births. Inheritance is by autosomal dominant transmission; however, because few achondroplastic people have children, over 80 per cent of cases are sporadic.

The fault has been shown to be a gain-in-function mutation in the gene encoding for the growth-suppressing fibroblast growth factor receptor 3 (FGFR-3) on chromosome 4. The effect on the proliferative zone of the physis is increased inhibition of growth, and the thickness of the hypertrophic cell zone is reduced; this accounts for the diminution in endochondral bone growth.

Management

During childhood, operative treatment may be needed for lower limb deformities (usually genu varum). Occasionally the thoracolumbar kyphosis fails to correct itself; if there is significant deformity (angulation of more than 40°) by the age of 5 years, there is a risk of cord compression and operative correction may be needed.

During adulthood, spinal stenosis may call for decompression. Intervertebral disc prolapse superimposed on a narrow spinal canal should be treated as an emergency.

Advances in methods of external fixation have made leg lengthening a feasible option. This is achieved by distraction osteogenesis (see Chapter 12). However, there are drawbacks: complications, including non-union, infection and nerve palsy, may be disastrous; and the cosmetic effect of long legs and short arms may be less pleasing than anticipated. It is essential that the details of the operation, its aims and limitations and the potential complications be fully discussed with the patient (and, where appropriate, with the parents).

Anaesthesia carries a greater than usual risk and requires expert supervision.

HYPOCHONDROPLASIA

This has been described as a very mild form of achondroplasia. However, apart from shortness of stature (with the emphasis on proximal limb segments) and noticeable lumbar lordosis, there is little to suggest any abnormality; the head and face are not affected and many of those with hypochondroplasia pass for normal stocky individuals. X-rays may show slight pelvic flattening and thickening of the long bones. The condition is transmitted as autosomal dominant, hence several members of the same family may be affected.

Those affected sometimes ask for limb lengthening; after careful discussion, this may be done with a considerable chance of success.

DYSCHONDROSTEOSIS (LEHRI–WEILL SYNDROME)

In this disorder there is also disproportionate shortening of the limbs, but it is mainly the middle segments (forearms and legs) which are affected. It is the commonest of the mesomelic dysplasias and is transmitted as an autosomal dominant defect. Stature is reduced but not as markedly as in achondroplasia. The most characteristic x-ray changes are shortening of the forearms and leg bones, bowing of the radius and Madelung's deformity of the wrist, which may require operative treatment (see page 390).

METAPHYSEAL CHONDRODYSPLASIA (DYSOSTOSIS)

This term describes a type of short-limbed dwarfism in which the bony abnormality is virtually confined to the metaphyses. The epiphyses are unaffected but the metaphyseal segments adjacent to the growth plates are broadened and mildly scalloped, somewhat resembling rickets. There may be bilateral coxa vara and bowed legs; patients tend to walk with a waddling gait. Apart from a lordotic posture, the spine is normal. The main deformities are around the hips and knees.

There are several forms of metaphyseal chondrodysplasia. The best known (Schmid type) has the classic features described above, with autosomal dominant inheritance. Another group (McKusick type) is associated with sparse hair growth and is sometimes complicated by Hirschsprung's disease; inheritance shows an autosomal recessive pattern. It is thought that these cases may represent an entirely distinct entity. The

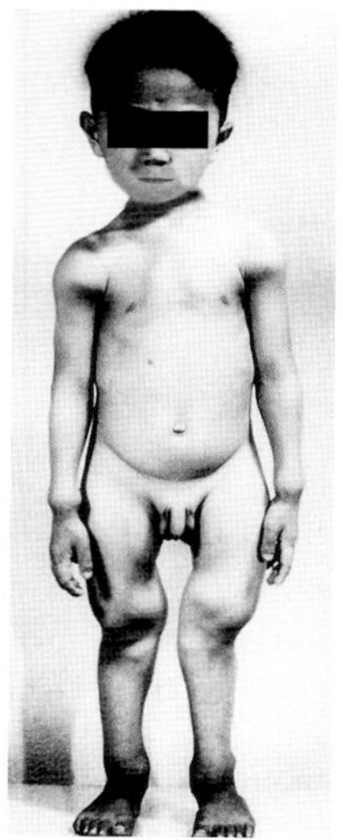
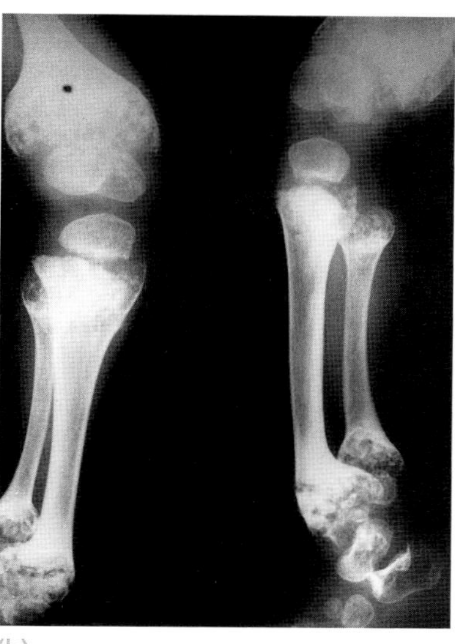

(a) (b)

8.9 Metaphyseal chondrodysplasia This boy with the rare Jansen type shows the typical shortening of the lower limbs and metaphyseal enlargement of the long bones. The x-rays show that the changes are confined to the metaphyses.

rarest (and most severe) of all (Jansen type) is usually sporadic and may be associated with deafness.

Operative correction (osteotomy) may be needed for coxa vara or tibia vara.

DYSCHONDROPLASIA (ENCHONDROMATOSIS; OLLIER'S DISEASE)

This is a rare, but easily recognized, disorder in which there is defective transformation of physeal cartilage columns into bone. No consistent inheritance pattern has been identified.

Clinical Features

Typically the disorder is unilateral; indeed only one limb or even one bone may be involved. An affected limb is short, and if the growth plate is asymmetrically involved the bone grows bent; bowing of the distal end of the femur or tibia is not uncommon and the patient may present with valgus or varus deformity at the knee and ankle. Shortening of the ulna may lead to bowing of the radius and, sometimes, dislocation of the radial head. The fingers or toes frequently contain *multiple enchondromata*, which are characteristic of the disease and may be so numerous that the hand is crippled. A rare variety of dyschondroplasia is associated with *multiple haemangiomata (Maffucci's disease)*; this is described below.

The condition is not inherited; indeed, it is probably an embryonal rather than a genetic disorder.

X-Rays

The characteristic change in the long bones is radiolucent streaking extending from the physis into the metaphysis – the appearance of persistent, incompletely ossified cartilage columns trapped in bone. If only half the physis is affected, growth is asymmetrically retarded and the bone becomes curved. With maturation the radiolucent columns eventually ossify but the deformities remain. In the hands and feet the cartilage islands characteristically produce *multiple enchondromata*. Beware of any change in the appearance of the lesions after the end of normal growth; this may be a sign of *malignant change*, which occurs in 5–10 per cent of cases.

Treatment

Bone deformity may need correction, but this should be deferred until growth is complete; otherwise it is likely to recur.

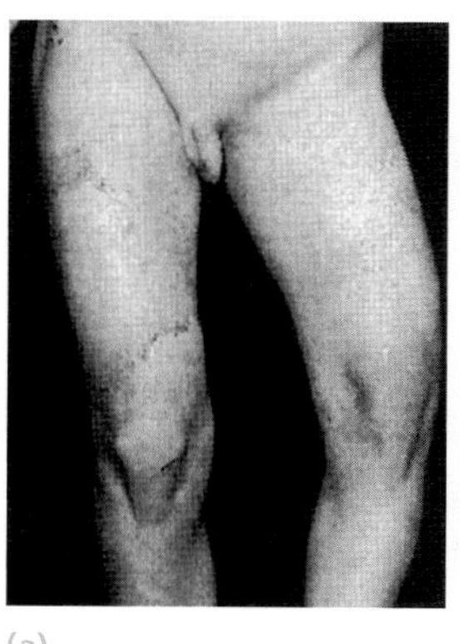
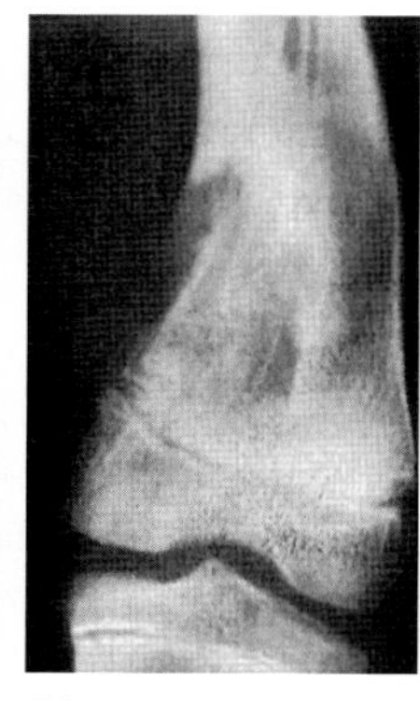
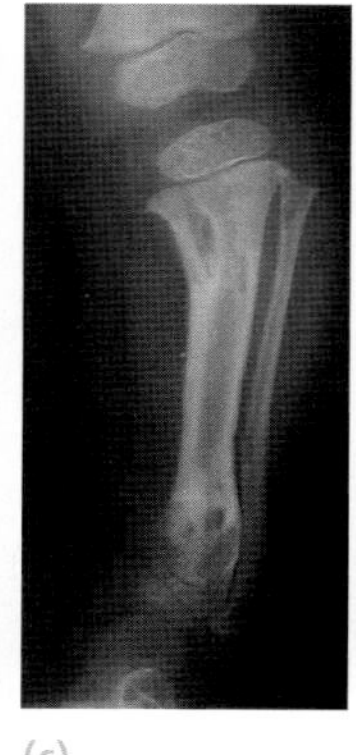
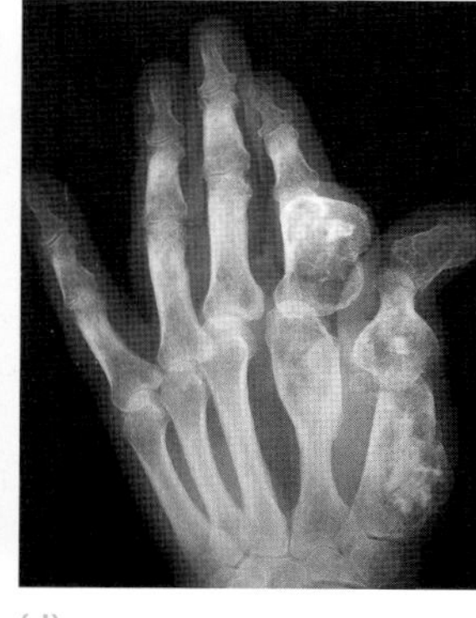
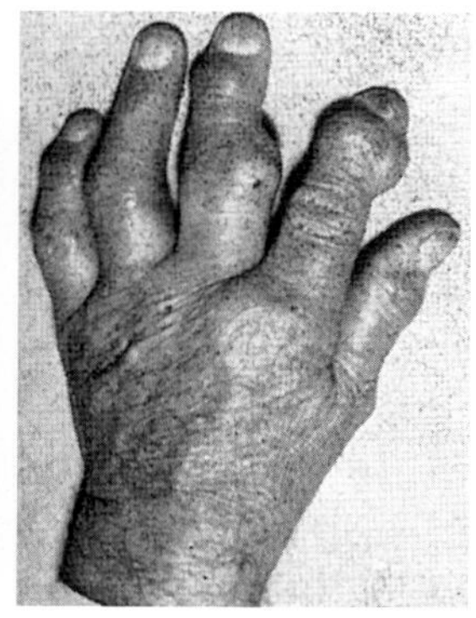

(a) (b) (c) (d) (e)

8.10 Dyschondroplasia (a,b) The bent femur in this boy is due to slow growth of half the lower femoral physis. (c) Incomplete ossification of the cartilage columns accounts for the curious metaphyseal appearance. (d,e) Two patients with multiple chondromas.

Maffucci's disease

This rare disorder is characterized by the development of multiple enchondromas and soft-tissue haemangiomas of the skin and viscera. Lesions appear during childhood; boys and girls are affected with equal frequency.

There is a strong tendency for malignant change to occur in both soft-tissue and bone lesions; the incidence of sarcomatous transformation in one of the enchondromas is probably greater than 50 per cent, but fortunately these tumours are not highly malignant.

Patients with Mafucci's disease should be monitored regularly throughout life for any change in either the bone or visceral lesions.

Metaphyseal dysplasia (Pyle's disease)

The only significant clinical feature in this disorder is genu valgum – or rather valgus angulation of the bones on either side of the knee. X-rays show a typical 'bottle shape' of the distal femur or proximal tibia – the so-called Erlenmeyer flask deformity – suggesting a failure of bone modelling. Inheritance pattern is autosomal recessive. Treatment is seldom needed.

Other conditions – notably Gaucher's disease and thalassaemia – are also associated with Ehlenmeyer flask deformities of the femur.

Craniometaphyseal dysplasia

This condition, of autosomal dominant inheritance, is similar to Pyle's disease, but here the tubular defect is associated with progressive thickening of the skull and mandible resulting in a curiously prominent forehead, a large jaw and a squashed-looking nose. Foraminal occlusion may cause cranial nerve compression – sometimes severe enough to require operative treatment.

Dysplasias with predominantly diaphyseal changes

Most of the 'metaphyseal' and 'diaphyseal dysplasias' appear to be the result of defective bone modelling. Unlike the physeal and epiphyseal disorders, dwarfing is not a feature. There may be associated thickening of the skull bones, with the risk of foraminal occlusion and cranial nerve entrapment.

Fibrous dysplasia is dealt with in Chapter 9.

Osteopetrosis (marble bones, Albers–Schönberg disease)

Osteopetrosis is one of several conditions which are characterized by sclerosis and thickening of the bones which appear with increased radiographic density. This is the result of an imbalance between bone formation and bone resorption; in the most common form, osteopetrosis, there is failed bone resorption due to a defect in osteoclast production and/or function.

Osteopetrosis tarda

The common form of osteopetrosis is a fairly benign, autosomal dominant disorder that seldom causes symptoms and may only be discovered in adolescence or adulthood after a pathological fracture or when an x-ray is taken for other reasons – hence the designation *tarda*. Appearance and function are unimpaired, unless there are complications: pathological fracture

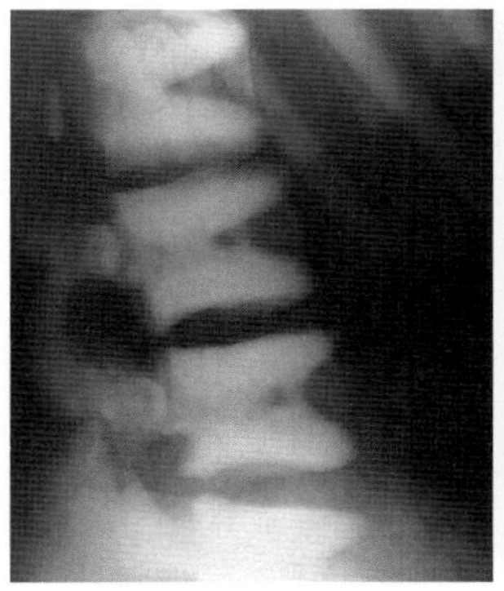
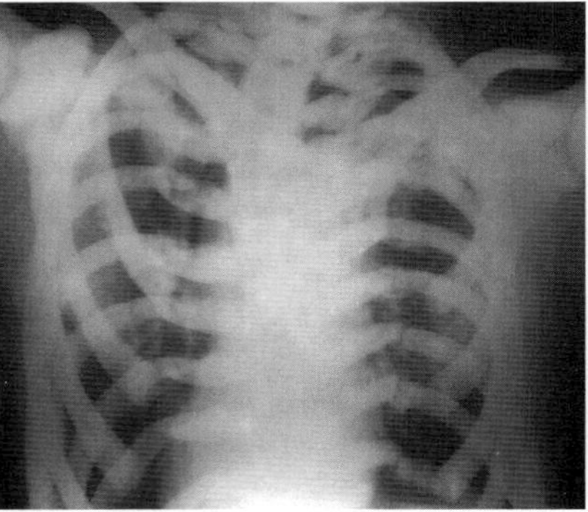
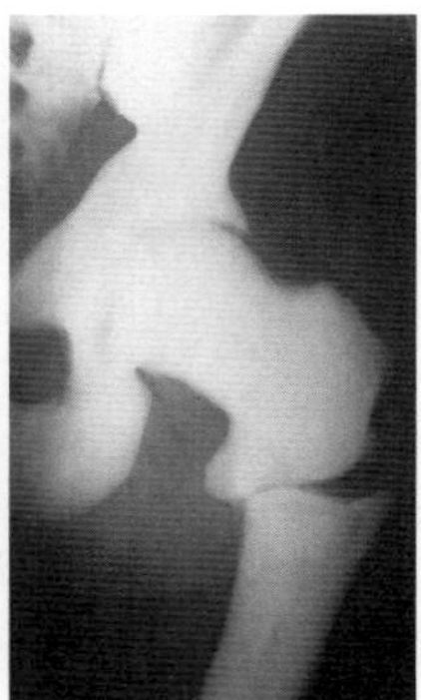
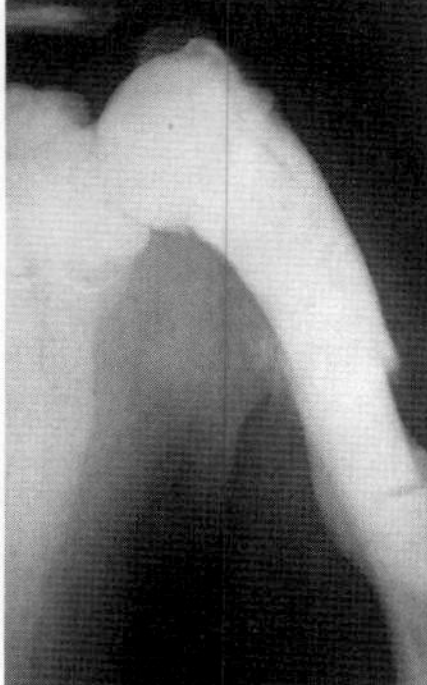

8.11 Marble bones Despite the remarkable density, the bones break easily; but, as in this humerus, union occurs, although rather slowly.

or cranial nerve compression due to bone encroachment on foramina. Sufferers are also prone to bone infection, particularly of the mandible after tooth extraction.

X-rays show increased density of all the bones: cortices are widened, leaving narrow medullary canals; sclerotic vertebral end-plates produce a striped appearance ('football-jersey spine'); the skull is thickened and the base densely sclerotic.

Treatment is required only if complications occur.

Osteopetrosis congenita

This rare, autosomal recessive form of osteopetrosis is present at birth and causes severe disability. Bone encroachment on marrow results in pancytopenia, haemolysis, anaemia and hepatosplenomegaly. Foraminal occlusion may cause optic or facial nerve palsy. Osteomyelitis following, for example, tooth extraction or internal fixation of a fracture is quite common. Repeated haemorrhage or infection usually leads to death in early childhood.

Treatment, in recent years, has focused on methods of enhancing bone resorption and haematopoeisis, e.g. by transplanting marrow from normal donors and by long-term treatment with gamma-interferon.

DIAPHYSEAL DYSPLASIA (ENGELMANN'S OR CAMURATI'S DISEASE)

This is another rare childhood disorder in which x-rays show fusiform widening and sclerosis of the shafts of the long bones, and sometimes thickening of the skull. The condition is notable because of its association with muscle pain and weakness. Children complain of 'tired legs' and have a typical wide-based or waddling gait. There may be muscle wasting and failure to thrive.

Muscle pain may need symptomatic treatment. Milder cases usually clear up spontaneously by the age of 25 years.

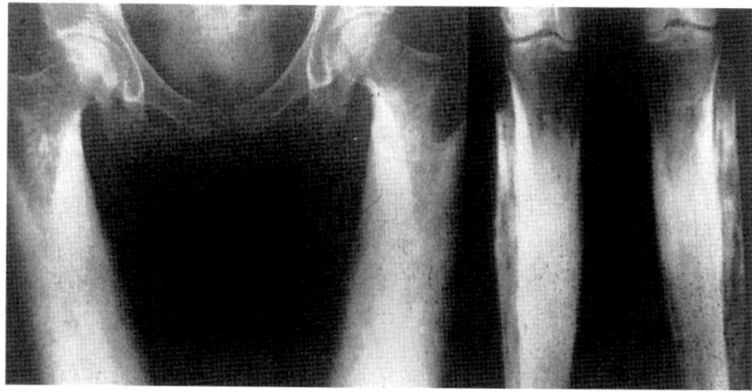

8.12 Engelmann's disease This patient had considerable discomfort from her long bones – all of which were wide and looked dense on x-ray.

CRANIODIAPHYSEAL DYSPLASIA

This rare autosomal recessive disorder is characterized by cylindrical expansion of the long bones and gross thickening of the skull and facial bones. Prominent facial contours may appear in early childhood and are the most striking feature of the condition – giving rise to the name *'leontiasis'*. Foraminal occlusion may cause deafness or visual impairment.

PYKNODYSOSTOSIS

Interest in this rare disorder owes something to the suggestion that the French impressionist, Toulouse-Lautrec, was a victim. Clinical features are shortness of stature, frontal bossing, underdevelopment of the mandible and abnormal dentition. The presence of blue sclerae and propensity to fracture may cause confusion with osteogenesis imperfecta. The condition is inherited as an autosomal recessive trait.

On *x-ray* the bones are dense; the skull is enlarged, with wide suture lines and open fontanelles, but the facial bones and mandible are hypoplastic, thus accounting for the typical 'triangular' facies.

Despite appearances, it causes little trouble (apart from the odd pathological fracture) and needs no treatment.

CANDLE, SPOTTED AND STRIPED BONES

Candle bones (melorheostosis, Leri's disease) This rare, non-familial, condition is sometimes discovered (almost accidentally) in patients who complain of pain and stiffness in one limb. *X-rays* show irregular patches of sclerosis, usually distributed in a linear fashion through the limb; the appearance is reminiscent of wax that congeals on the side of a burning candle. Some patients also develop scleroderma and joint contractures.

Spotted bones (osteopoikilosis) Routine x-rays sometimes show (quite incidentally) numerous white spots distributed throughout the skeleton. Closer examination occasionally reveals whitish spots in the skin (disseminated lenticular dermatofibrosis). The condition is inherited as an autosomal dominant trait.

Striped bones (osteopathia striata) X-rays show lines of increased density parallel to the shafts of long bones, but radiating like a fan in the pelvis. The condition is symptomless. Some cases show autosomal dominant inheritance.

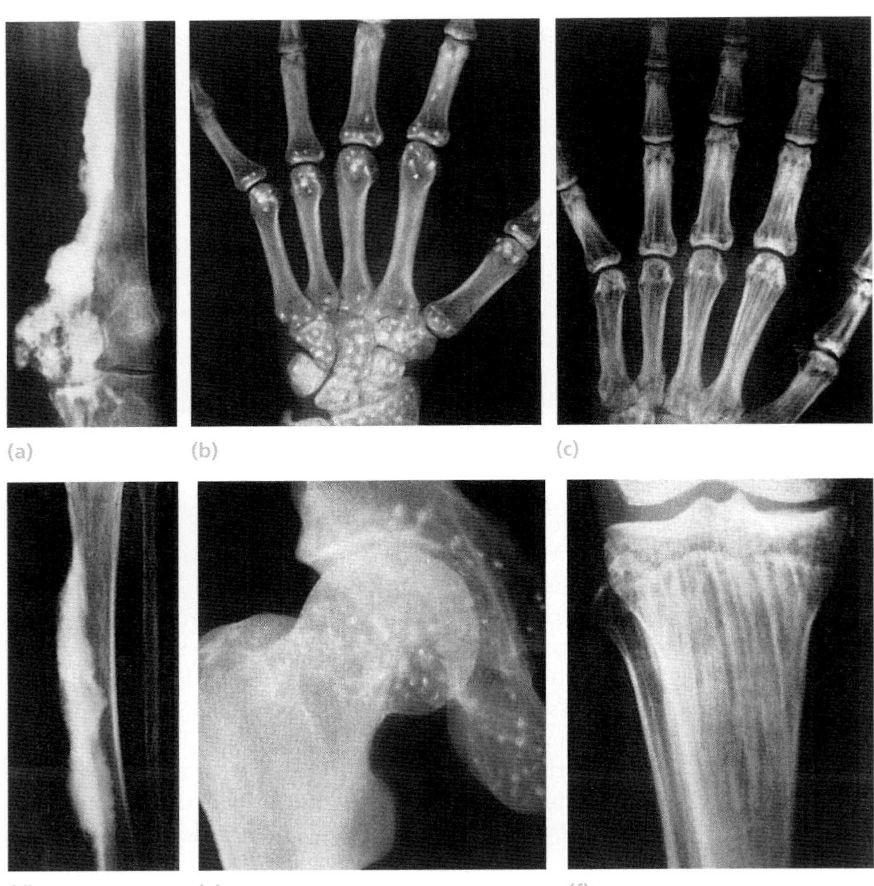

(a) (b) (c) (d) (e) (f)

8.13 Candle bones, spotted bones and striped bones (a,b) Melorheostosis (c,d) Osteopoikilosis (e,f) Osteopathia striatia.

COMBINED AND MIXED DYSPLASIAS

A number of disorders show a mixture of epiphyseal, physeal, metaphyseal and vertebral defects – i.e. dwarfism combined with epiphyseal maldevelopment, abnormal modelling of the metaphyses and platyspondyly.

SPONDYLOMETAPHYSEAL DYSPLASIA

This is the commonest of the 'mixed' dysplasias. There may be severe vertebral flattening and kyphoscoliosis. Epiphyseal changes are usually mild but the metaphyses are broad and ill-formed. Patients may need treatment for spinal deformity or malalignment of the hip or knee.

PSEUDOACHONDROPLASIA

This rare autosomal dominant disorder resembles achondroplasia in that it is characterized by short-limbed dwarfism associated with ligamentous laxity, exaggerated lumbar lordosis and bow-leg deformities. *In contrast to achondroplasia, clinical features are not evident at birth but become apparent only a year or two later; the head and face look normal and spinal stenosis is not a feature.*

Ligamentous laxity (particularly noticeable in the wrists) as much as anything has a significant effect on restricting function and also walking tolerance.

The characteristic x-ray features are underdevelopment and flattening of the epiphyses, widening of the metaphyses, shortening of the tubular bones and oval-shaped vertebral bodies. By the end of growth, the hips may be dysplastic and the vertebral bodies often show defects of the bony end-plates. Spinal stenosis is not a feature.

Deformities sometimes require surgical correction. In adults, secondary osteoarthritis may call for reconstructive surgery.

DIASTROPHIC DYSPLASIA

This autosomal recessive disorder affects all types of cartilage. Infants are severely dwarfed and distorted, with deformities of the hands ('hitch-hiker's thumb'), club feet, joint contractures, dislocations, 'cauliflower' ears and cleft palate. Softening of the laryngeal cartilage may produce respiratory distress. In older children the main problems are scoliosis and joint contractures.

X-rays show epiphyseal hypoplasia and maldevelopment, metaphyseal thickening, flattening of the pelvis and kyphoscoliosis. Odontoid hypoplasia is usual.

Management involves early correction of joint contractures and treatment of club foot and hand deformities. Scoliosis may require correction and spinal fusion.

CLEIDOCRANIAL DYSPLASIA

This disorder, of autosomal dominant inheritance, is characterized by hypoplasia of the clavicles and flat bones. In a typical case the patient is somewhat short, with a large head, frontal prominence, a flat-looking face and drooping shoulders. The teeth appear late and develop poorly. Because the clavicles are hypoplastic or absent, the chest seems narrow and the patient can bring his shoulders together anteriorly. The pelvis is narrow but the symphysis pubis may be unduly wide and there may be some disproportion of the forearm or finger bones.

X-rays show a brachycephalic skull and persistence of wormian bones. Characteristically there is underdevelopment of the clavicles, scapulae and pelvis. Much of the clavicle may be missing, leaving a nubbin of bone at the medial or lateral end. Scoliosis and coxa vara are common.

Treatment is unnecessary unless the patient develops severe coxa vara or scoliosis; dental anomalies may need attention.

NAIL–PATELLA SYNDROME

This curious condition is relatively common and is inherited as an autosomal dominant trait. The nails are hypoplastic and the patellae unusually small or absent. The radial head is subluxed laterally and the elbows may lack full extension. Congenital nephropathy may be associated. The characteristic *x-ray* features are hypoplastic or absent patellae and the presence of bony protuberances ('horns') on the lateral aspect of the iliac blades.

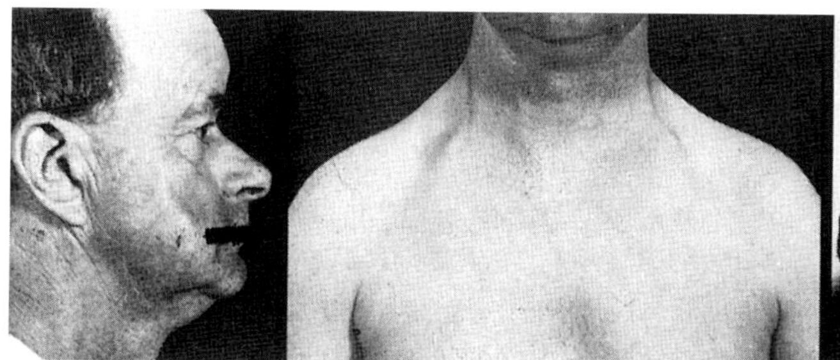
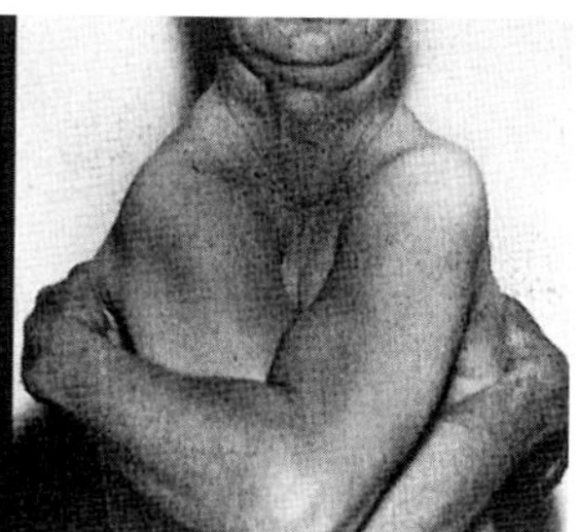

8.14 Cleidocranial dysplasia The 'squashed face' and sloping shoulders which can be brought together anteriorly are pathognomonic.

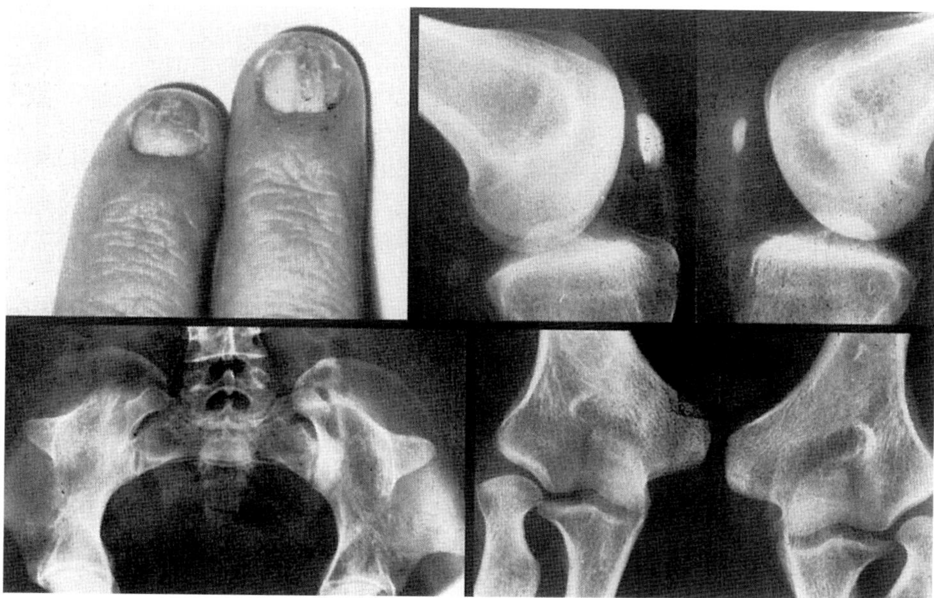

8.15 The nail–patella syndrome The dystrophic nails, minute patellae, pelvic 'horns' and subluxed radii combine to give an unmistakable picture.

Craniofacial dysplasia

Many disorders – some inherited, some not – are distinguished primarily by the abnormal appearance of the face and skull. Other bones may be affected as well, but it is the odd facial appearance that is most striking. Premature fusion of the cranial sutures may lead to exophthalmos and learning difficulties. Orthopaedic problems arise from the associated anomalies of the hands and feet.

The best-known of these conditions is *Apert's syndrome* (acrocephalosyndactyly). The head is somewhat egg-shaped: flat at the back, narrow anteroposteriorly, with a broad, towering forehead, depressed face, bulging eyes and prominent jaw. The hands and feet are misshapen, with syndactyly or synostosis of the medial rays. The condition sometimes shows autosomal dominant inheritance, but most cases are sporadic.

Cerebral compression can be prevented by early craniotomy and the facial appearance may be improved by maxillofacial reconstruction. Syndactyly usually needs operative treatment.

CONNECTIVE TISSUE DISORDERS

Collagen is the commonest form of body protein, making up 90 per cent of the non-mineral bony matrix and 70 per cent of the structural tissue in ligaments and tendons. Some 20 types of collagen, produced by 30 or more genes, have been identified; those distributed most abundantly in the musculoskeletal system are *type I* (in bone, ligament, tendon and skin), *type II* (in cartilage) and *type III* (in blood vessels, muscle and skin).

Heritable defects of collagen synthesis give rise to a number of disorders involving either the soft connective tissues or bone, or both. In many cases the specific collagen defect can now be identified.

Benign joint hypermobility (Generalized familial joint laxity)

About 5 per cent of normal people have joint hypermobility, as defined by a positive score of more than 5 (the Beighton score) in the following tests:

1. Passive hyperextension of the metacarpophalangeal joint of the fifth finger to beyond 90° (score 2);
2. Passive stretching of the thumb to touch the radial border of the forearm (score 2);
3. Hyperextension of the elbows (score 2);
4. Hyperextension of the knees (score 2);
5. Ability to bend forward and place the hands flat on the floor with the knees held perfectly straight (score 1).

The trait runs in families and is inherited as a mendelian dominant. The condition is not in itself disabling but it may predispose to congenital dislocation of the hip in the newborn or recurrent dislocation of the patella or shoulder in later life. Transient joint pains are common and there is an increased risk of ankle sprains.

A more florid hypermobility syndrome characterized by lax connective tissues and joint subluxations may be associated with other conditions such as gastro-oesophageal reflux, irritable bowel syndrome and bowel or uterine prolapse, sometimes merging with variants of Ehlers–Danlos syndome (see below).

Marfan's syndrome

This is a generalized disorder affecting the skeleton, joint ligaments, eyes and cardiovascular structures. It is thought to be due to a cross-linkage defect in collagen and elastin. The genetic abnormality has been mapped to the fibrillin gene on chromosome 15. It is transmitted as autosomal dominant but sporadic cases also occur. Males and females are affected equally.

Clinical Features

Patients tend to be tall, with disproportionately long legs and arms, and often with flattening or hollowing of the chest (pectus excavatum). Typically, the upper body segment is shorter than the lower (a ratio of less than 0.8 is suggestive) and arm span exceeds height by 5 cm or more. The digits are unusually long, giving rise to the term 'arachnodactyly' (spider fingers). Spinal abnormalities include spondylolisthesis and scoliosis. There is an increased incidence of slipped upper femoral epiphysis. Generalized joint laxity is

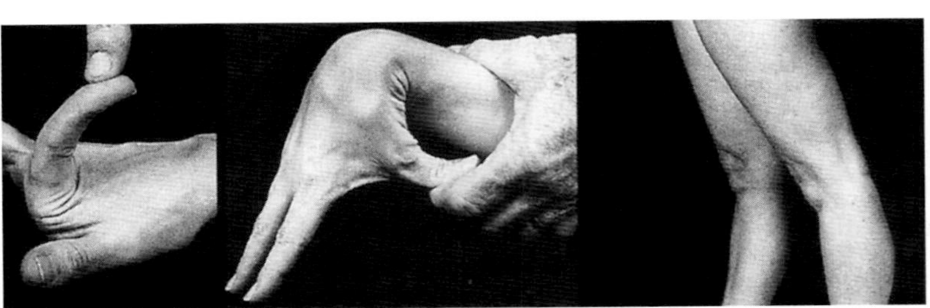

8.16 Generalized joint laxity Simple tests for joint hypermobility.

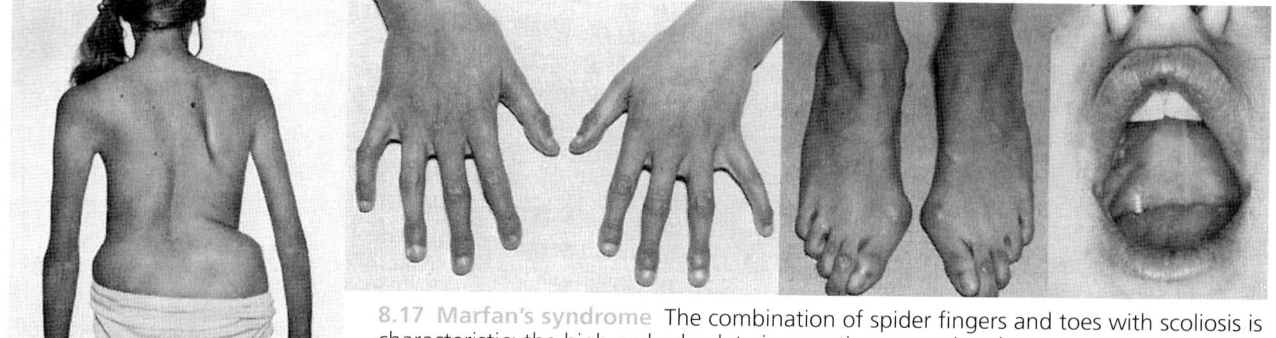

8.17 Marfan's syndrome The combination of spider fingers and toes with scoliosis is characteristic; the high-arched palate is sometimes associated.

usual and patients may develop flat feet or dislocation of the patella or shoulder.

Associated abnormalities include a high arched palate, hernias, lens dislocation, retinal detachment, aortic aneurysm and mitral or aortic incompetence. Cardiovascular complications are particularly serious and account for most of the deaths in severe cases.

X-rays

Bone structure appears normal (apart from excessive length), but x-rays may reveal complications such as scoliosis, spondylolisthesis or slipped epiphysis.

Diagnosis

'Marfanoid' features are quite common and it is now thought that there are several variants of the underlying condition. Mild cases are easily missed or mistaken for uncomplicated joint laxity; it is important to look for ophthalmic and cardiovascular defects.

Homocystinuria, an inborn error of methionine metabolism; has in the past been confused with Marfan's syndrome.

Management

Patients occasionally need treatment for progressive scoliosis or flat feet. The heart should be carefully checked before operation.

Ehlers–Danlos syndrome

This syndrome comprises a collection of 6 major but heterogenous subtypes with a common phenotype of unusual skin elasticity, joint hypermobility and vascular fragility, expressions of underlying abnormalities of elastin and collagen formation. Sub-grouping is based on clinical findings, genetic cause and inheritance pattern. Of the many types of EDS so far described over 90 per cent show autosomal dominant inheritance.

Clinical Features

Babies may show marked hypotonia and joint laxity. Hypermobility persists and older patients are often capable of bizarre feats of contortion. The skin is soft and hyperextensible; it is easily damaged and vascular fragility may give rise to 'spontaneous' bruising. Joint laxity, recurrent dislocations and scoliosis are common.

Management

Complications (e.g. recurrent dislocation or scoliosis) may need treatment. However, if joint laxity is marked, soft-tissue reconstruction usually fails to cure the tendency to dislocation. Beware! Blood vessel fragility may cause severe bleeding at operation or afterwards. Wound healing is often poor, leaving 'cigarette paper' scars.

Joint instability may lead to osteoarthritis in later life.

Larsen's syndrome

This is a heterogeneous condition, the more severe (recessive) forms presenting in infancy with marked joint laxity and dislocation of the hips, instability of the knees, subluxation of the radial head, equinovarus deformities of the feet and 'dish-face' appearance. Spinal deformities are common in older children. Mild forms of the same condition show autosomal dominant inheritance.

Operative treatment may be needed for joint instability and dislocation.

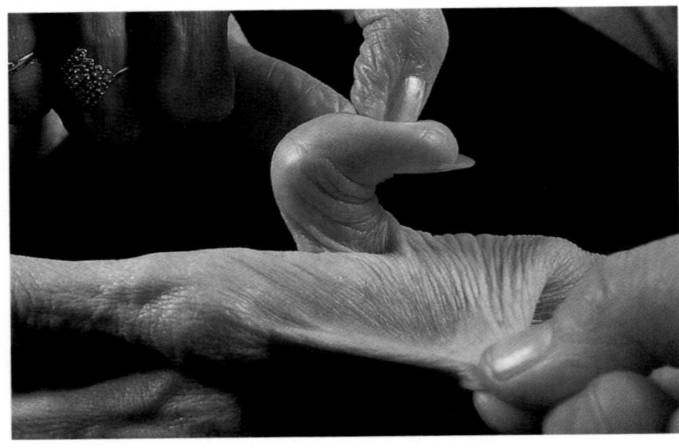

(a)

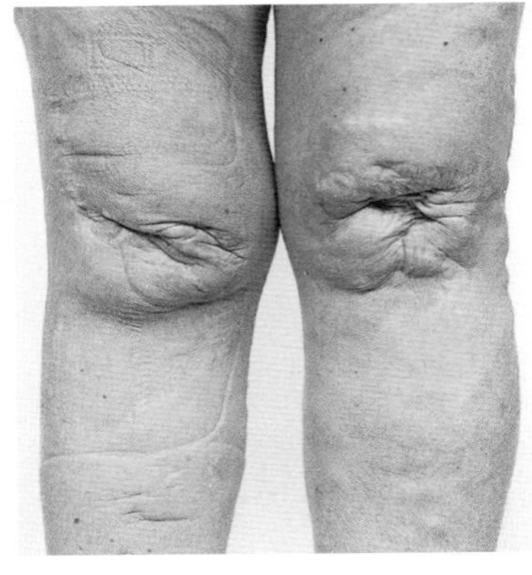

(b)

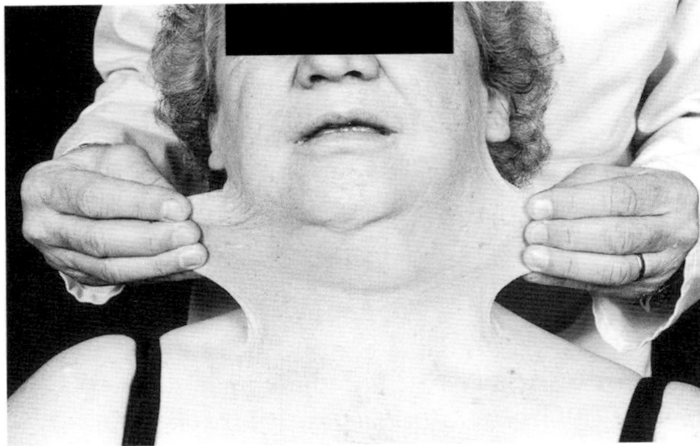

(c)

8.18 Ehlers–Danlos syndrome (a) Typical features of Ehlers–Danlos syndrome: marked joint hypermobility and skin laxity. (b) Characteristic tissue-paper scarring of the knees and (c) the usual remarkable skin hyperextensibility.

Osteogenesis imperfecta (brittle bones)

Osteogenesis imperfecta (OI) is one of the commonest of the genetic disorders of bone, with an estimated incidence of 1 in 20 000. Abnormal synthesis and structural defects of type I collagen result in abnormalities of the bones, teeth, ligaments, sclerae and skin. The defining clinical features are (1) osteopenia, (2) liability to fracture, (3) laxity of ligaments, (4) blue coloration of the sclerae and (5) dentinogenesis imperfecta ('crumbling teeth'). However, there are considerable variations in the severity of expression of these features and in the pattern of inheritance and it is now recognized that the condition embraces a heterogeneous group of collagen abnormalities resulting from many different genetic mutational defects (Kocher and Shapiro, 1998).

Pathology

The genetic abnormality in OI expresses itself as an alteration in the structural integrity, or a reduction in the total amount of type I collagen, one of the major components of fibrillar connective tissue in skin, ligaments and bone. Even small alterations in the composition of type I collagen can lead to weakening of these tissues and imperfect ossification in all types of bone. Bone formation is initiated in the normal way but it progresses abnormally, the fully formed tissue consisting of a mixture of woven and lamellar bone, and in the worst cases almost entirely of immature woven bone. There is thinning of the dermis, laxity of ligaments, increased corneal translucency and (in some cases) loss of dentin leading to tooth decay.

Clinical features

The clinical features vary considerably, according to the severity of the condition. The most striking abnormality is the propensity to fracture, generally after minor trauma and often without much pain or swelling. In the classic case fractures are discovered during infancy and they recur frequently throughout childhood. Callus formation is florid, so much so that the lump has occasionally been mistaken for an osteosarcoma; however, the new bone is also abnormal and it remains 'pliable' for a long time, thus predisposing to malunion and an increased risk of further fracture. By the age of 6 years there may be severe deformities of the long bones, and vertebral compression fractures often lead to kyphoscoliosis. After puberty fractures occur less frequently.

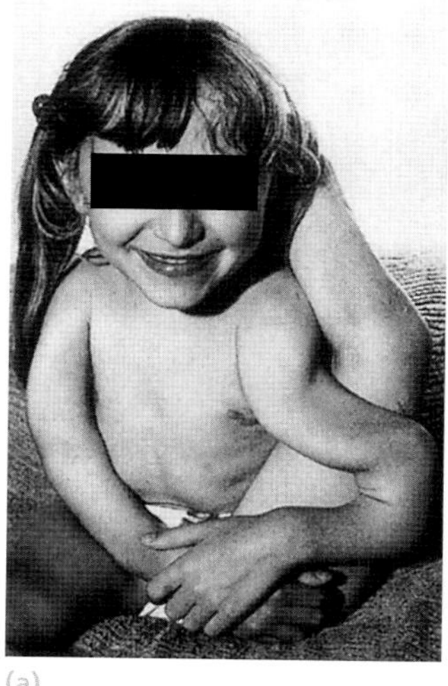
(a)

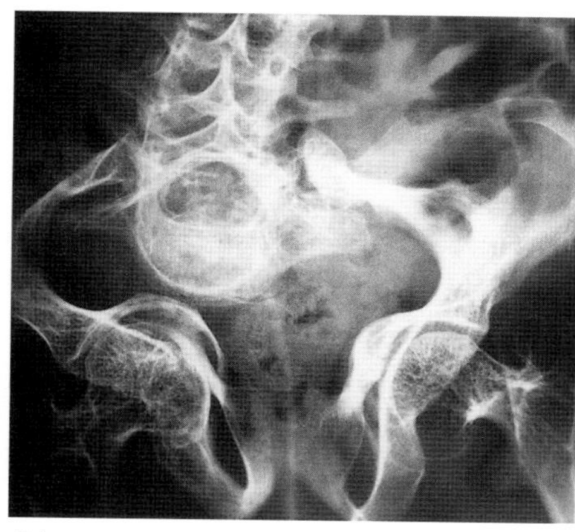
(b)

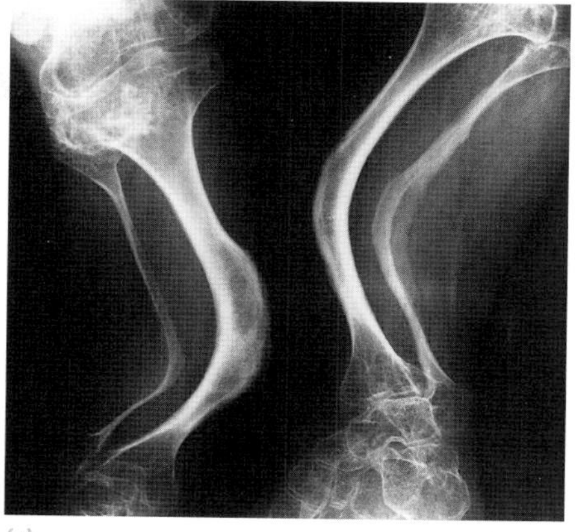
(c)

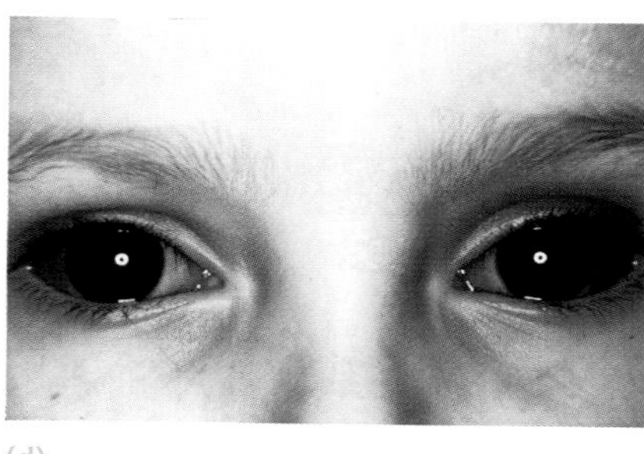
(d)

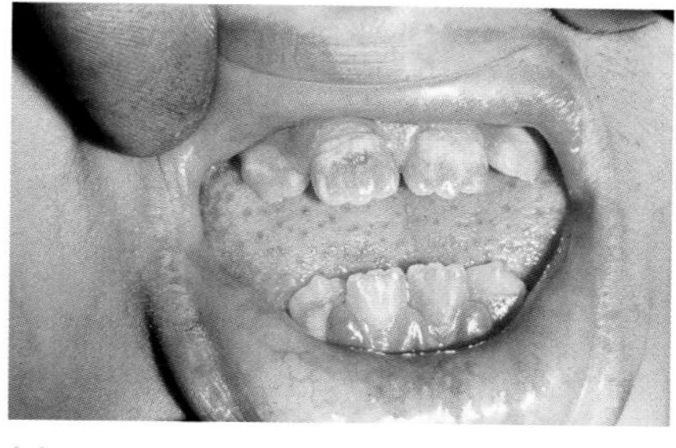
(e)

8.19 Osteogenesis imperfecta (a) This young girl had severe deformities of all her limbs, the result of multiple mini-fractures of the long bones over time. This is the classic (type III) form of OI. (b,c) X-ray features in a slightly older patient with the same condition. (d) The typical deep blue sclerae in type I disease. (e) Faulty dentine in a patient with type IV disease.

The skin is thin and somewhat loose and the joints are hypermobile. Blue or grey sclerae, when they occur, are due to uveal pigment showing through the hypertranslucent cornea. The teeth may be discoloured and carious.

In milder cases fractures develop a year or two after birth – perhaps when the child starts to walk; they are also less frequent and deformity is not a marked feature.

In the most severe types of OI, fractures are present before birth and the infant is either stillborn or lives only for a few weeks, death being due to respiratory failure, basilar indentation or intracranial haemorrhage following injury.

X-rays

There is generalized osteopenia, thinning of the long bones, fractures in various stages of healing, vertebral compression and spinal deformity. The type of abnormality varies with the severity of the disease. The skull may be enlarged and shows the presence of wormian bones – areas of vicarious ossification in the calvarium. After puberty, fractures occur less frequently, but in those who survive the incidence rises again after the climacteric. It is thought that very mild ('subclinical') forms of OI may account for some cases of recurrent fractures in adults.

Diagnosis

In most cases the clinical and radiological features are so distinctive that the diagnosis is not in doubt. However, mistakes have been made and rare disorders causing multiple fractures may have to be excluded by laboratory tests. In hypophosphatasia, for example, the serum alkaline phosphatase level is very low. In older children with atypical features it is essential to look for evidence of physical abuse.

Classification

The clinical variants of OI can be divided into subgroups showing well-defined differences in the pattern of inheritance, age of presentation and severity of changes in the bones and extra-skeletal tissues. This is helpful in assessing the prognosis and planning treatment for any particular patient.

The most widely used classification is that of Sillence (1981), which defines four clinical types of OI. The principal features can be summarized as follows:

OI TYPE I (MILD)

- The commonest variety; over 50 per cent of all cases.
- Fractures usually appear at 1–2 years of age.
- Healing is reasonably good and deformities are not marked.

- Sclerae deep blue
- Teeth usually normal but some have dentinogenesis imperfecta.
- Impaired hearing in adults.
- Quality of life good; normal life expectancy.
- Autosomal dominant inheritance.

OI TYPE II (LETHAL)

- 5–10 per cent of cases.
- Intra-uterine and neonatal fractures.
- Large skull and wormian bones.
- Sclerae grey.
- Rib fractures and respiratory difficulty.
- Stillborn or survive for only a few weeks.
- Most due to new dominant mutations; some autosomal recessive.

OI TYPE III (SEVERE DEFORMING)

- The 'classic', but not the most common, form of OI.
- Fractures often present at birth.
- Large skull and wormian bones; pinched-looking face.
- Marked deformities and kyphoscoliosis by 6 years.
- Sclerae grey, becoming white.
- Dentinogenesis imperfecta.
- Marked joint laxity.
- Respiratory problems.
- Poor quality of life; few survive to adulthood.
- Sporadic, or autosomal recessive inheritance.

OI TYPE IV (MODERATELY SEVERE).

- Uncommon; less than 5 per cent of cases.
- Frequent fractures during early childhood.
- Deformities common.
- Sclerae pale blue or normal.
- Dentinogenesis imperfecta.
- Survive to adulthood with fairly good function.
- Autosomal dominant inheritance.

Management

There is no medical treatment which will counteract the effects of this abnormality, and genetic manipulation is no more than a promise for the future.

Conservative treatment is directed at preventing fractures – if necessary by using lightweight orthoses during physical activity – and treating fractures when they occur. However, splintage should not be overdone as this may contribute further to the prevailing osteopenia. General measures to prevent recurrent trauma, maintain movement and encourage social adaptation are very important. Children with severe OI may be treated medically with cyclical bisphosphonates to increase bone mineral density and reduce the tendency to fracture.

Most of the long-term orthopaedic problems are encountered in types III and IV. Fractures are treated conservatively, but immobilization must be kept to a minimum. Long-bone deformities are common, due either to malunion of complete fractures or breaking of recurrent incomplete fractures; these may require operative correction, usually by 4 or 5 years of age. Multiple osteotomies are performed and the bone fragments are then realigned on a straight intramedullary rod; the same effect can be achieved by closed osteoclasis. The problem of the bone outgrowing the rod has been addressed by using telescoping nails; however, these carry a fairly high complication rate.

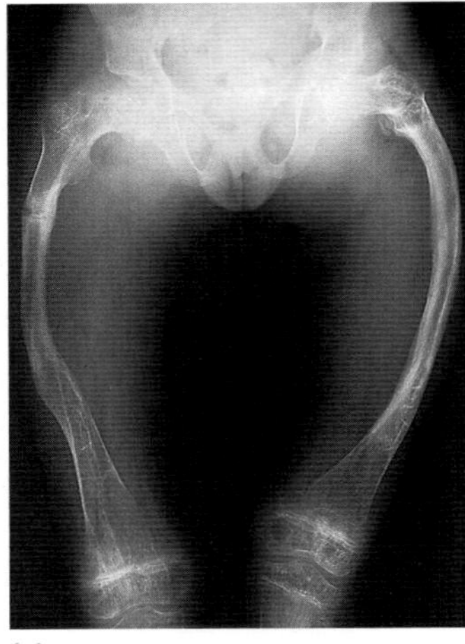

(a)

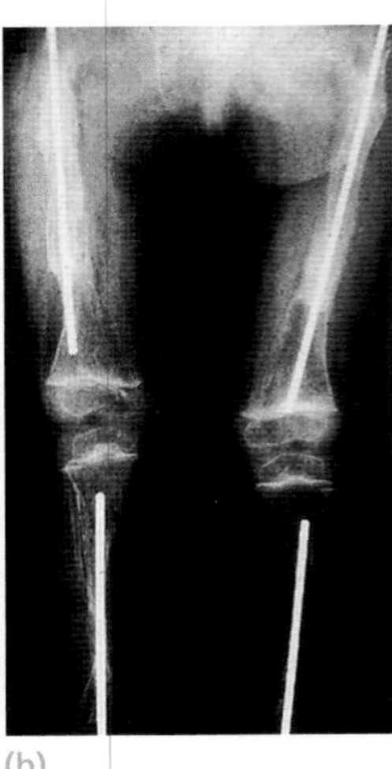

(b)

8.20 Osteogenesis imperfecta (a) Moderately severe (type IV) disease. These deformities can be corrected by multiple osteotomies and 'rodding' (b).

Spinal deformity is also common and is particularly difficult to treat. Bracing is ineffectual and progressive curves require operative instrumentation and spinal fusion.

After adolescence, fractures are much less common and patients may pursue a reasonably comfortable and useful life.

FIBRODYSPLASIA OSSIFICANS PROGRESSIVA

This rare condition, formerly known as myositis ossificans progressiva, is characterized by widespread ossification of the connective tissue of muscle, mainly in the trunk. It starts in early childhood with episodes of fever and soft-tissue inflammation around the shoulders and trunk. As this subsides the tissues harden and plaques of ossification extend throughout the affected areas. In the worst cases movements are restricted and the patient is severely disabled. Associated anomalies are shortening of the big toe and thumb. The condition is probably transmitted as an autosomal dominant but, since affected individuals seldom have children, most

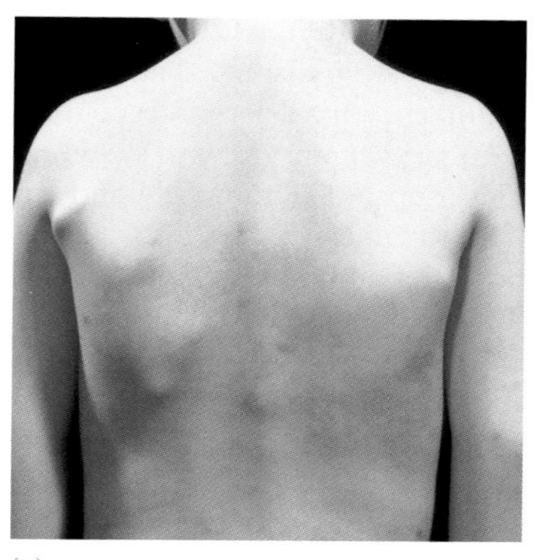
(a)

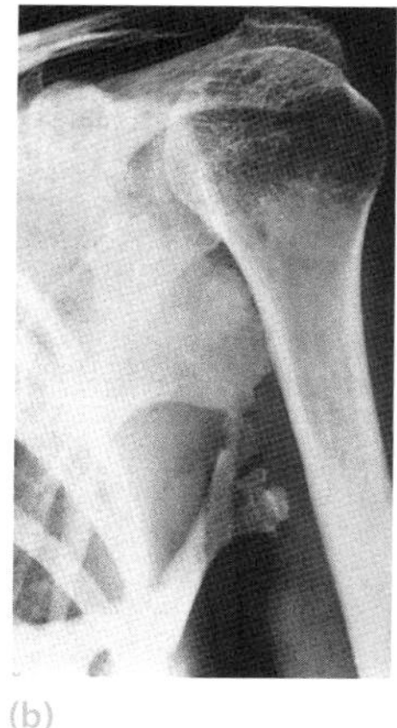
(b)

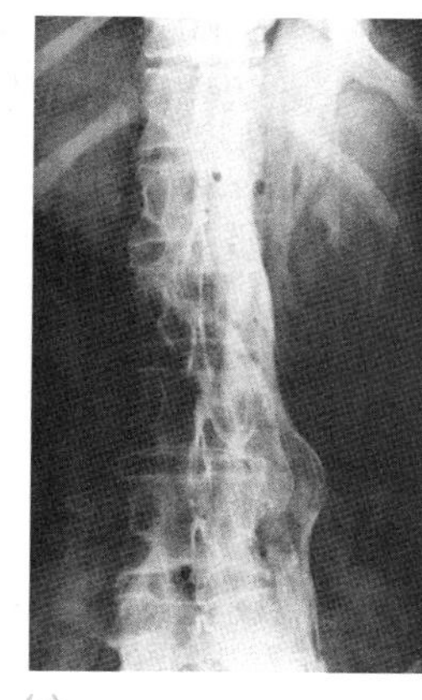
(c)

8.21 Fibrodysplasia ossificans progressive (a) The lumps in this boy's back were hard and his back movements were limited. (b,c) This adult shows the extensive soft-tissue ossification.

cases result from new mutations. Treatment with bisphosphonates may prevent progression.

Neurofibromatosis

Neurofibromatosis is one of the commonest single gene disorders affecting the skeleton. Two types are recognized:

Type 1 (NF-1) – also known as von Recklinghausen's disease – has an incidence of about 1 in 3500 live births. The abnormality is located in the gene which codes for neurofibromin, on chromososme 17. It is transmitted as autosomal dominant, with almost 100 per cent penetrance, but more than 50 per cent of cases are due to new mutation. The most characteristic lesions are neurofibromata (Schwann cell tumours) and patches of skin pigmentation (*café au lait* spots), but other features are remarkably protean and musculoskeletal abnormalities are seen in almost half of those affected.

Type 2 (NF-2) is much less common, with an incidence of 1 in 50 000 births. It is associated with the gene which codes for schwannomin, located on chromosome 22. Like NF-1, it is transmitted as autosomal dominant. Unlike NF-1, intracranial lesions (e.g. acoustic neuromas and meningiomas) are usual while musculoskeletal manifestations are rare.

Clinical features of NF-1

Almost all patients have the typical widespread patches of skin pigmentation and multiple cutaneous neurofibromata which usually appear before puberty. Less common is a single large plexiform neurofibroma, or an area of soft-tissue overgrowth in one of the limbs.

The orthopaedic surgeon is most likely to encounter the condition in a child or adolescent who presents with *scoliosis* (the most suggestive deformity is a very short, sharp curve) or with *localized vertebral abnormalities* such as scalloping of the posterior aspects of the verte-

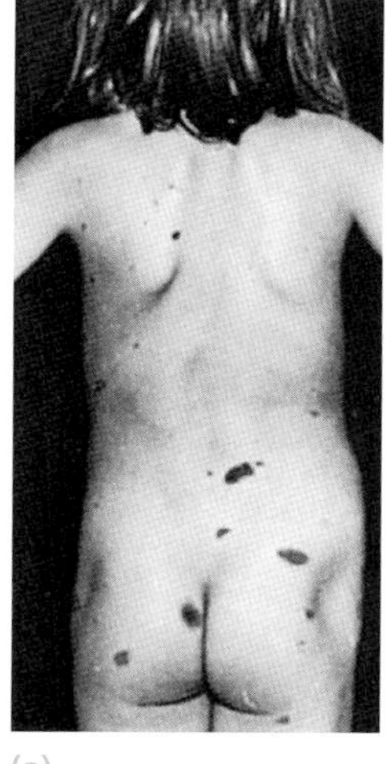
(a)

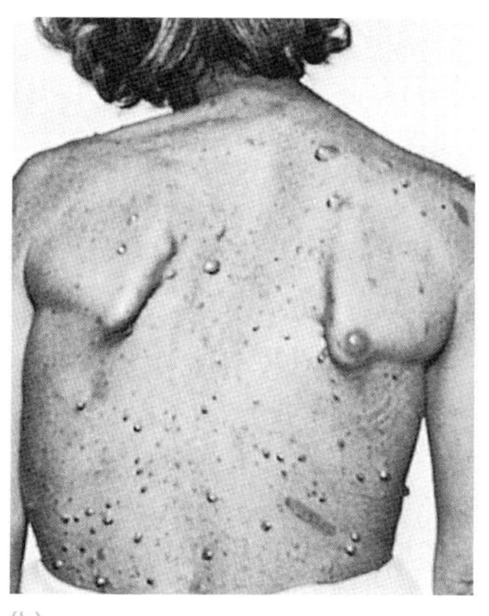
(b)

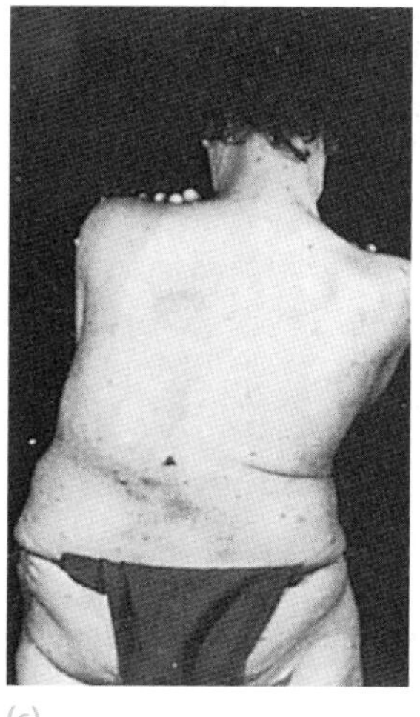
(c)

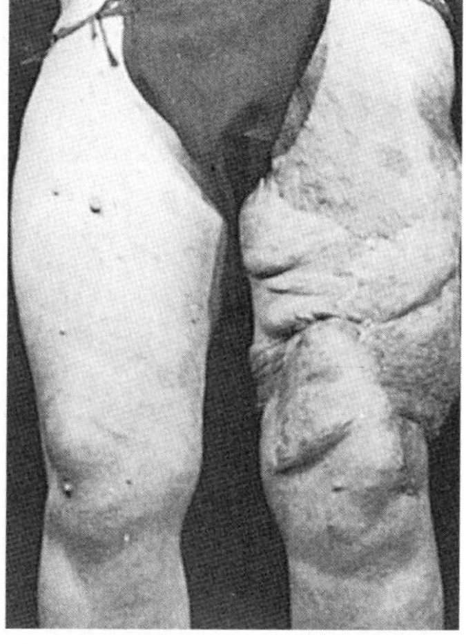
(d)

8.22 Neurofirbromatosis (a) Café-au-lait spots; (b) multiple neurofibromata and slight scoliosis; (c,d) a patient with scoliosis and soft-tissue overgrowth ('elephantiasis').

bral bodies, erosion of the pedicles, intervertebral foraminal enlargement and pencilling of the ribs at affected levels. *Dystrophic spinal deformities*, including deformities of the cervical spine, are also seen.

Congenital tibial dysplasia and pseudarthrosis are rare conditions, but almost 50 per cent of patients with these lesions have some evidence of neurofibromatosis (see page 185).

Malignant change occurs in 2–5 per cent of affected individuals and is the most common complication in older patients.

Treatment

The orthopaedic conditions associated with neurofibromatosis are dealt with on page 184 of this chapter and in the section on scoliosis in Chapter 18.

STORAGE DISORDERS AND METABOLIC DEFECTS

Many single gene disorders are expressed as undersecretion of an enzyme that controls a specific stage in the metabolic chain; the undegraded substrate accumulates and may be stored, with harmful effects, in various tissues or be excreted in the urine. Conditions involving the musculoskeletal system are the mucopolysaccharidoses (MPS), Gaucher's disease, homocystinuria, alkaptonuria and congenital hyperuricaemia. All these inborn errors of metabolism are inherited as recessive traits.

MUCOPOLYSACCHARIDOSES

The polysaccharide glycosaminoglycans (GAGs) form the side-chains of macromolecular proteoglycans, a major component of the matrix in bone, cartilage, intervertebral discs, synovium and other connective tissues. Defunct proteoglycans are degraded by lysosomal enzymes. Deficiency of any of these enzymes causes a hold-up on the degradative pathway. Partially degraded GAGs accumulate in the lysosomes in the liver, spleen, bones and other tissues, and spill over in the blood and urine where they can be detected by suitable biochemical tests. Confirmation of the enzyme lack can be obtained by tests on cultured fibroblasts or leucocytes.

Clinical Features

Depending on the specific enzyme deficiency and the type of GAG storage, at least six clinical syndromes have been defined. All except Hunter's syndrome (an X-linked recessive disorder) are transmitted as autosomal recessive. As a group they have certain recognizable features: significantly short stature with vertebral deformity, coarse facies, hepatosplenomegaly and (in some cases) learning difficulties. X-rays show bone dysplasia affecting the vertebral bodies, epiphyses and metaphyses; typically the bones have a spatulate appearance.

There is a superficial similarity to spondyloepiphyseal and spondylometaphyseal dysplasia. However, careful observation reveals several points of difference, and the diagnosis can be confirmed by testing for abnormal GAG excretion or demonstrating the enzyme deficiency in blood cells or cultured fibroblasts.

At least 10 different disorders are recognized; here only the three most common conditions will be described.

HURLER'S SYNDROME (MPS I)

Infants look normal at birth but over the next 2–3 years they gradually develop a typical appearance: they are undersized, with increasing kyphosis, hepatosplenomegaly, coarse facies, protruding tongue, defective hearing and learning difficulty. Speech is very poor. Joints are stiff and walking is delayed. There may be corneal opacities, respiratory difficulty and cardiac anomalies.

X-rays usually show unmistakable features such as hypoplastic epiphyses and vertebral bodies, poorly modelled metaphyses, short but wide metacarpals, underdeveloped mandible, spatulate ribs and clavicles, flared iliac blades, shallow acetabuli and coxa valga.

Cardiac or respiratory complications usually cause death in later childhood.

HUNTER'S SYNDROME (MPS II)

This is also a recessive disorder, but X-linked – so all patients are male. Clinical features are similar to those of Hurler's syndrome, but less severe. Suspicious features usually appear at about 3 years, cardiorespiratory complications gradually become more severe and death usually occurs in the middle or late teens.

MORQUIO–BRAILSFORD SYNDROME (MPS IV)

Development seems normal for the first year or two, although walking may be delayed. Thereafter the child beings to look dwarfed, with a moderate kyphosis,

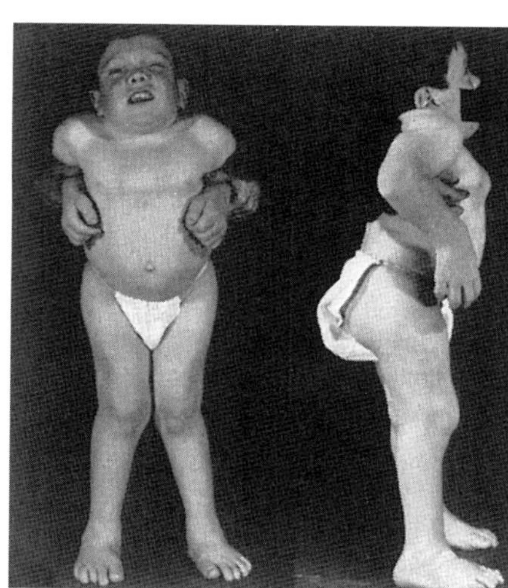

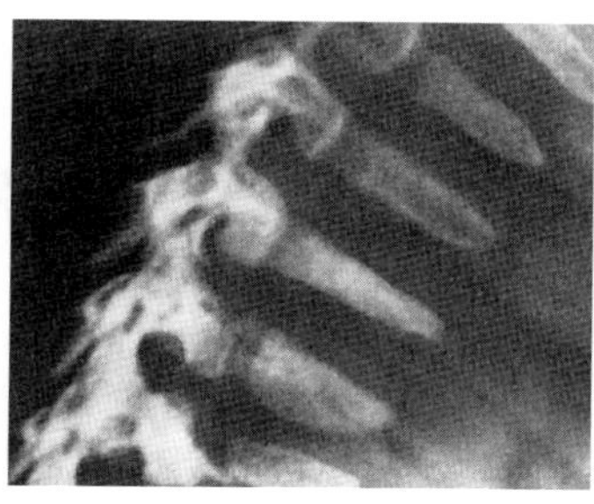

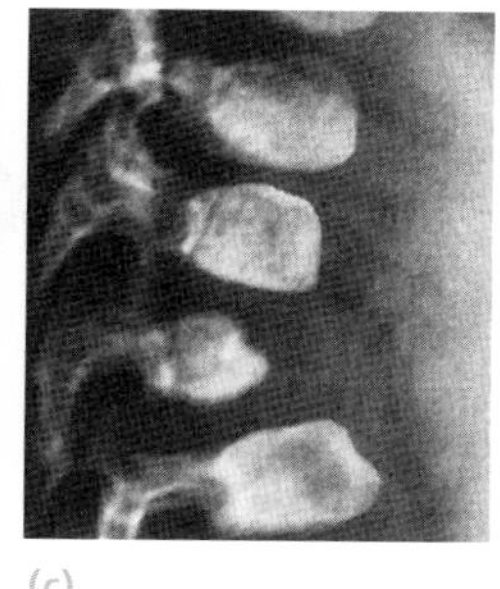

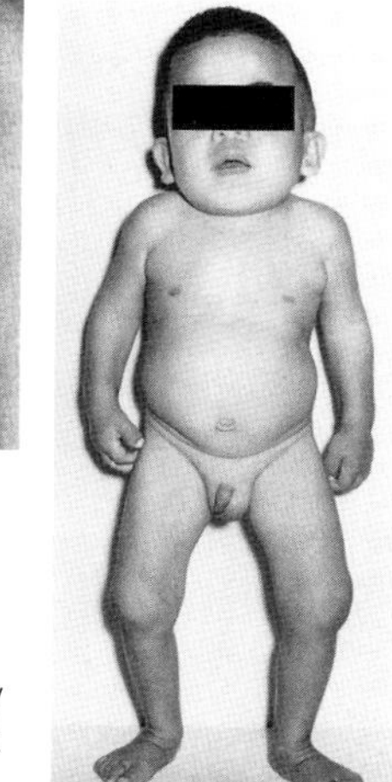

(a) (b) (c) (d)

8.23 Mucopolysaccharidoses (a) Morquio-Brailsford syndrome – note the manubriosternal angle. (b) Platyspondyly in a similar patient, contrasted with (c) the sabot appearance in Hurler's syndrome. (d) A boy with Hunter's syndrome; his appearance is similar to that in Hurler's syndrome.

short neck and protuberant sternum. There is marked joint laxity and progressive genu valgum. Suitable tests will reveal a conductive hearing loss. However, the face is unaffected and intelligence is normal.

X-rays of the spine show the typical ovoid, hypoplastic vertebral bodies, which end up abnormally flat (platyspondyly) and peculiarly pointed anteriorly. Odontoid hypoplasia is usual. A marked manubriosternal angle (almost 90°) is pathognomonic. By the age of 5 years the femoral head epiphyses are underdeveloped and flat, and the acetabula abnormally shallow. The long bones are of normal width but the metacarpals may be short and broad, and pointed at their proximal ends.

Management

There is, as yet, no specific treatment for the mucopolysaccharide disorder. However, enzyme replacement and gene manipulation are possible in the future.

Bone marrow transplantation has been used for the last 20–30 years; when successful it halts progression of CNS disease and some of the clinical features of the condition but it cannot reverse neurological damage that has already developed and it does not prevent progression of bone and joint disease. Enzyme replacement therapy is successful in mild cases of MPS I but it does not cross the blood-brain barrier.

Hurler's syndrome has a very poor prognosis but the complications (e.g. respiratory infection) may need treatment.

Morquio's syndrome presents several orthopaedic problems. Genu valgum may need correction by femoral osteotomy, though this should be delayed till growth has ceased. Coxa valga and subluxation of the hips, if symmetrical, may cause little disability; unilateral subluxation may need femoral or acetabular osteotomy. Atlantoaxial instability may threaten the cord and require occipitocervical fusion. All the 'spondylodysplasias' carry a risk of atlantoaxial subluxation during anaesthesia and intubation, and special precautions are needed during operation.

GAUCHER'S DISEASE

The genetic disorder first described by Gaucher over 100 years ago is now known to be caused by lack of a specific enzyme which is responsible for the breakdown of and excretion of cell membrane products from defunct cells. This is a classic example of a lipid storage disease for which the pathogenesis has been painstakingly worked out, leading to the development of effective treatment.

Each time one of the cells in the body dies, a glucocerebroside is released from the cell membrane; before it can be excreted, the glycoside bond holding the glucose molecule has to be split by a specific enzyme – glucosylceramide β-glucosidase. If this enzyme is lacking, the glucocerebroside cannot be excreted and instead is stored in the lysosomal bodies of macrophages of the reticuloendothelial system, notably in the marrow, spleen and liver. Accumulation of these abnormal macrophages leads to enlargement of the spleen and liver, and secondary changes in the marrow and bone.

Most patients suffer from a chronic form of the disorder, with changes predominantly in the marrow, bone and spleen, and varying degrees of pancytopenia (Type I). A rare form of the disease affecting the central nervous system (Type II) appears in infancy and usually causes death within a

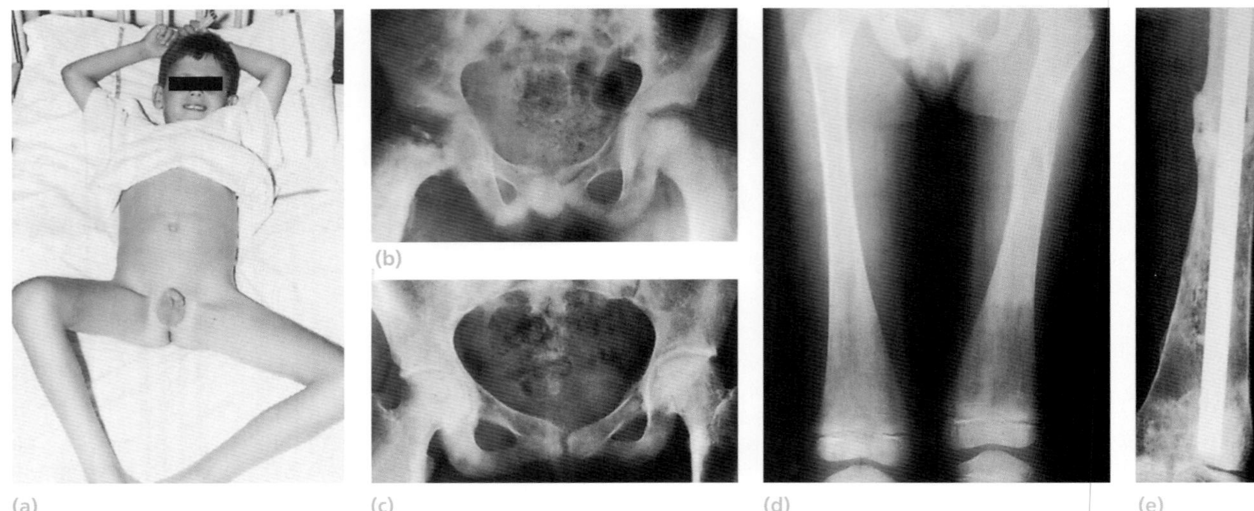

8.24 Gaucher's disease (a) A distressed young boy during an acute Gaucher crisis. The right hip is intensely painful and abduction is restricted. The x-ray (b) shows avascular necrosis of the right femoral head. (c) X-ray of an older patient with a sclerotic left femoral head, the result of previous ischaemic necrosis. (d) Bilateral failure of femoral tubularization (the Erlenmeyer flask appearance). (e) Pathological fractures sometimes occur and can be treated by internal fixation. The sclerotic patches in the interior part of the bone are typical of old medullary infarcts.

year. Type III is a subacute disorder characterized by the appearance of hepatosplenomegaly in childhood and skeletal and neurological abnormalities during adolescence.

Like other storage disorders, Gaucher's disease is acquired by autosomal recessive transmission. The genetic abnormality accountable for the lack of the specific enzyme glucosylceramide β-glucosidase is located on the long arm of chromosome 1 (1q21) where around 80 mutations of 3 basic types have been identified.

Clinical Features

In the commonest form of the disease (Type I), patients present in childhood or adult life with bone pain and, sometimes, loss of movement in one of the larger joints. The spleen may be enlarged, or it may already have been removed. Older patients may develop back pain, due to vertebral osteopenia and compression fractures. Femoral neck fractures also are not uncommon; however, diaphyseal fractures are rare. The haematocrit and platelet count are usually diminished. A suggestive finding (when positive) is elevation of the serum acid phosphatase level.

A common complication is osteonecrosis, usually of the femoral head but sometimes in the femoral condyles, the proximal end of the humerus or the bones around the ankle. The patient (usually a child or adolescent) may present with an acute 'bone crisis': unrelenting pain, local tenderness and restriction of movement accompanied by pyrexia, leucocytosis and an elevated ESR. The clinical features resemble those of osteomyelitis or septic arthritis; indeed, Gaucher's disease predisposes to bone infection and this may be a source of confusion.

Imaging

X-rays show a variable pattern of radiolucency or patchy density, more marked in cancellous bone. The distal end of the femur may be expanded, producing the Erlenmeyer flask appearance. A skeletal survey may reveal osteonecrosis of the femoral head, femoral condyles, talus or humeral head.

A radioisotope bone scan may help to distinguish a crisis episode from infection: the former is usually 'cold', the latter 'hot'.

MRI is the most reliable way of defining marrow involvement.

Treatment

Bone pain may need symptomatic treatment and bisphosphonates have been used for osteoporosis. For the acute crisis, analgesic medication and bed rest followed by non-weightbearing walking with crutches is recommended.

Specific therapy is available (albeit costly) in the form of the replacement enzyme, alglucerase. This has been shown to reverse the blood changes and reduce the size of the liver and spleen. The bone complications also are diminished.

Osteonecrosis of the femoral head usually results in progressive deformity of the hip. However most patients manage quite well with symptomatic treatment and surgery should be deferred for as long as possible (Katz *et al*, 1996).

HOMOCYSTINURIA

This rare disorder is due to deficiency of the enzyme cystathionine β-synthetase and accumulation of homocysteine and methionine. Patients are tall and thin and may develop features reminiscent of Marfan's disease (page 170). However, unlike Marfan's disease, homocystinuria is of autosomal recessive inheritance and is associated with marked osteoporosis and learning difficulty. Joint laxity is unusual but there may be muscle weakness. Thromboembolic disease is common and may be fatal. Homocysteine levels are raised in the blood and urine. The enzyme deficiency may be detected in fibroblast cultures. Though rare, the condition should be diagnosed because it can be treated: about half the patients are 'cured' by pyridoxine (vitamin B6) administered from early childhood. Others may be helped by a low methionine, cysteine-supplemented diet.

ALKAPTONURIA

Deficiency of the enzyme homogentisic acid oxidase leads to accumulation of homogentisic acid, which is deposited in connective tissue and excreted in the urine. On standing the urine turns dark (hence the name, alkaptonuria); cartilage and other connective tissues are stained grey – a condition referred to as ochronosis. Clinical problems arise from degenerative changes in articular cartilage with the development of osteoarthritis, and from calcification of the intervertebral discs.

CONGENITAL HYPERURICAEMIA

The Lesch–Nyhan syndrome is a rare, X-linked recessive disorder causing absence of the enzyme hypoxanthine-guanine phosphoribosyltransferase (HGPRT). This enzyme controls a 'salvage pathway' in the complex purine metabolic chain; absence of HGPRT results in excessive uric acid formation and gout. The young boys have learning difficulties and are prone to self-mutilation (gnawing the ends of their fingers). Milder cases present simply as early-onset severe gout. Diagnosis can be confirmed by measuring HGPRT in red cell preparations.

CHROMOSOME DISORDERS

Chromosome disorders are common but usually result in fetal abortion. Of the non-lethal conditions, several produce bone or joint abnormalities.

DOWN'S SYNDROME (TRISOMY 21)

This condition results, in 95 per cent of cases, from having an extra copy of chromosome 21. It is much more common than any of the skeletal dysplasias, with an overall incidence of 1 per 800 live births – and 1 in 250 if the mother is over 37 years of age.

Clinical features

Affected infants can be recognized at birth: the head is foreshortened and the eyes slant upwards, with prominent epicanthic folds; the nose is flattened, the lips are parted and the tongue protrudes. There may be abnormal palmar creases, clinodactyly and spreading of the first and second toes. The babies are unusually floppy (hypotonic) and skeletal development is delayed. Children are short and, because of their characteristic facial appearance, they tend to resemble each other. They show varying degrees of learning difficulty. Joint laxity may lead to sprains or subluxation (e.g. of the patella). Plano-valgus feet are common and some children develop developmental dysplasia of the hip. Up to 50 per cent of these children – and particularly those more severely affected – will develop idiopathic scoliosis. Despite these physical drawbacks, functional performance is surprisingly good and overtreatment must be resisted.

Adults have a significant incidence of atlantoaxial instability, though fortunately this seldom causes neurological complications. Associated anomalies, particularly cardiac defects, are common, and there is diminished resistance to infection. Life expectancy is about 35 years.

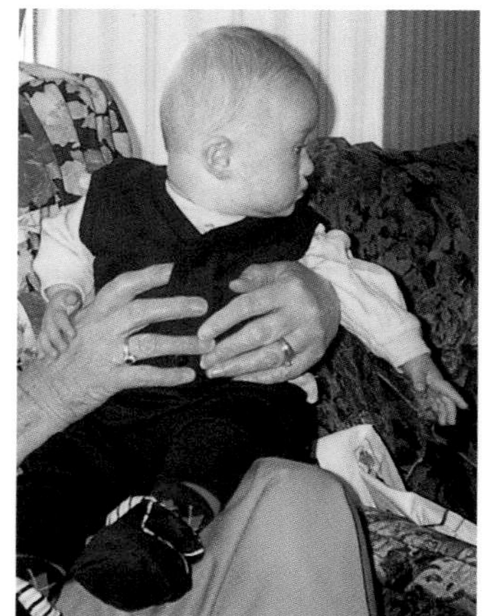

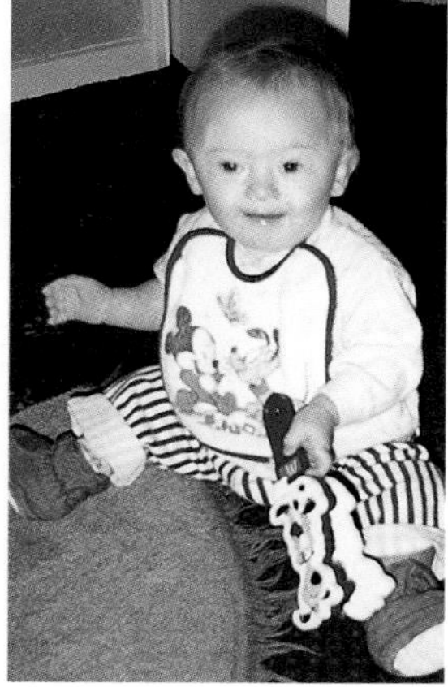

8.25 Down's syndrome Head shape and facial features in an eleven-month old child with Down's syndrome.

Treatment

There is no specific treatment but surgery can offer considerable cosmetic improvement; there is now an increasing trend towards offering these children maxillo-facial surgery to alter their characteristic facial appearance. Atlantoaxial fusion is occasionally needed for patients with neurological symptoms.

Attentive care will allow many of these people to pursue a pleasant and productive life.

TURNER'S SYNDROME

Congenital female hypogonadism is a rare abnormality caused by a defective or non-functioning X chromosome. Those affected are phenotypically female, with a normal vagina and uterus, but the ovaries are markedly hypoplastic or absent. Patients are short, with webbing of the neck, barrel chest and increased carrying angle of the elbows. Cardiovascular and renal abnormalities are common. They have primary amenorrhoea, and hypogonadism leads to early-onset osteoporosis. Treatment consists of oestrogen replacement from puberty onwards.

KLINEFELTER'S SYNDROME

Klinefelter's syndrome, a form of male hypogonadism, occurs in about 1 per 1000 males. Those affected have more than one X chromosome (as well as the usual Y chromosome). They are recognizably male, but they have eunuchoid proportions, with gynaecomastia and underdeveloped testicles. The condition should be borne in mind as a cause of osteoporosis in men. Treatment with androgens may improve bone mass.

LOCALIZED MALFORMATIONS

Localized congenital malformations of the vertebrae or limbs are common. The majority cause no disability and may be discovered incidentally during investigation of some other disorder. Some have a genetic background and similar malformations are seen in association with generalized skeletal dysplasia. Most are sporadic and probably non-genetic – i.e. caused by injury to the developing embryo, especially during the first 3 months of pregnancy. In some cases there is a known teratogenic agent; for example, maternal infection or drug administration. Usually, however, the exact cause is unknown.

VERTEBRAL ANOMALIES

These are of three main kinds of vertebral anomaly:

1. *Agenesis* – complete absence of one or more vertebrae;
2. *Dysgenesis* – hemivertebrae or with vertebrae fused together (sometimes called errors of segmentation);
3. *Dysraphism* – deficiencies of the neural arch. These are considered in the sections on spinal deformity and spina bifida.

Corresponding sacral anomalies are also encountered and associated visceral anomalies (lower intestinal and urogenital defects) are common in sacral dysgenesis and dysraphism.

Congenital short neck (Klippel–Feil syndrome)

In this condition there is a failure of vertebral segmentation. The patient has an unusually short neck,

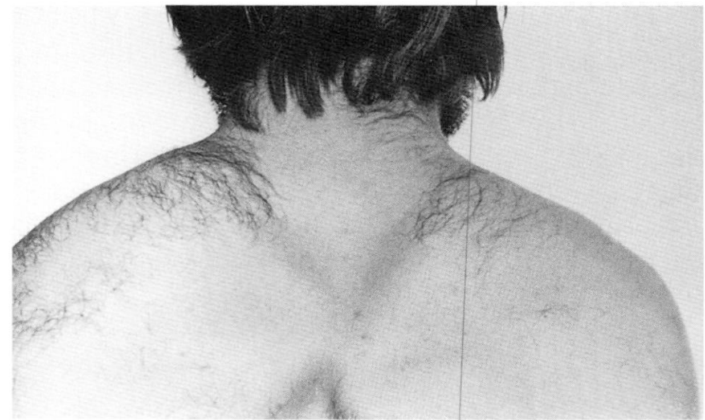

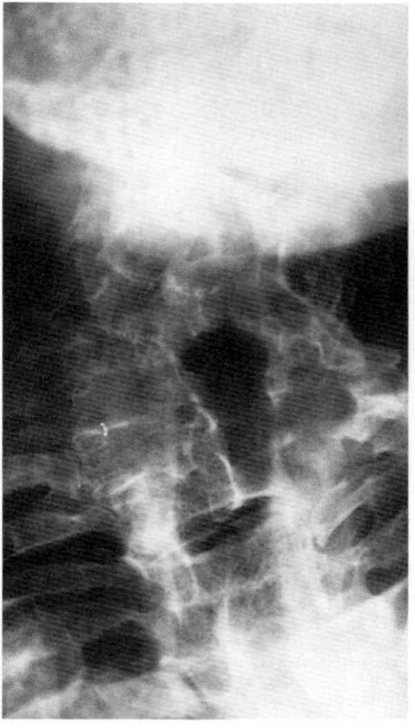

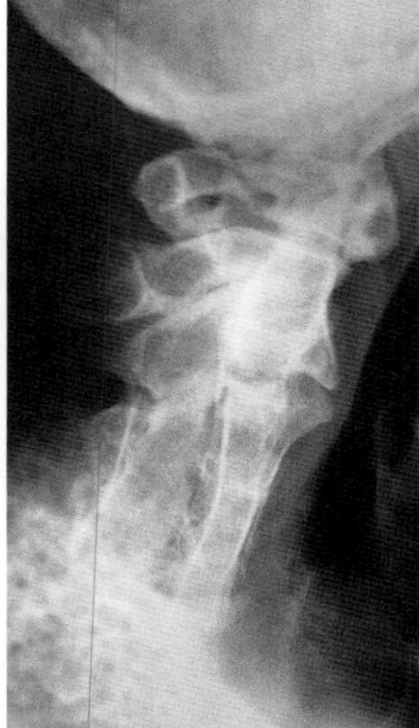

8.26 Klippel–Feil syndrome The short neck and vertebral anomalies in a typical patient.

and neck movements are restricted or absent. Prominence of the trapezius muscles gives the appearance of webbing at the base of the neck. The posterior hairline is much lower than normal. Associated anomalies are common and include hemivertebra, posterior arch defects, cervical meningomyelocele, thoracic defects, scapular elevation and visceral abnormalities involving the renal and cardio-respiratory systems. Occasionally, a familial pattern of inheritance is noted suggesting a genetic aetiology.

X-rays may show fusion of the lower cervical vertebrae and various combinations of the associated disorders, together with scoliosis or kyphosis.

The natural history of the condition often depends on the severity of the visceral anomalies.

Orthopaedic treatment is usually unnecessary. However cervical instability, with the risk of neurological injury, may develop in the relatively hypermobile segment adjacent to the fusion mass and surgical fusion with or without cord decompression may be warranted. Contact sports should be avoided.

Elevation of the scapula (Sprengel's deformity)

Mild degrees of congenital elevation of the scapula are common. In the full-blown Sprengel deformity the child has obvious asymmetry of the shoulders, with elevation and underdevelopment of the affected side. The scapula is abnormally small and too high. Sometimes the clavicle is affected as well. Shoulder movements may be restricted and on abduction or elevation the scapula moves very little or not at all. Occasionally both sides are involved.

Sprengel's deformity may be associated with other defects of the cervical spine (e.g. Klippel–Feil syndrome), and high thoracic kyphosis or scoliosis is quite common.

This condition, which usually occurs sporadically, represents a failure of scapular descent from the cervical spine. The high scapula may still be attached to the spine by a tough fibrous band or a cartilaginous bar (the omovertebral bar). Associated vertebral or rib anomalies are quite common.

Treatment is required only if shoulder movements are severely limited or if the deformity is particularly unsightly. Operation is best performed before the age of 6 years. The vertebroscapular muscles are released from the spine, the supraspinous part of the scapula is excised together with the omovertebral bar and the scapula is repositioned by tightening the lower muscles. Great care is needed as there is a risk of injury to the accessory nerve or the brachial plexus.

Thoracospinal anomalies

Segmentation defects in the thoracic region usually involve the ribs as well; for example, hemivertebrae may be associated with fusion of adjacent ribs or other types of dysplasia. Some of these disorders are of autosomal dominant inheritance.

Clinically, patients present in childhood with scoliosis or kyphoscoliosis, sometimes leading to paraplegia. *X-rays* may show various combinations of thoracic vertebral fusion or dysgenesis and rib anomalies, together with scoliosis and marked distortion of the thorax.

Operative treatment may be needed for threatened cord compression.

Sacral Agenesis

This term describes a group of conditions in which part or all of the distal spine is missing. Variable motor deficiencies are noted below the lowest level of normal spine but sensation is often preserved more distally. Other deformities of the lower limb may be

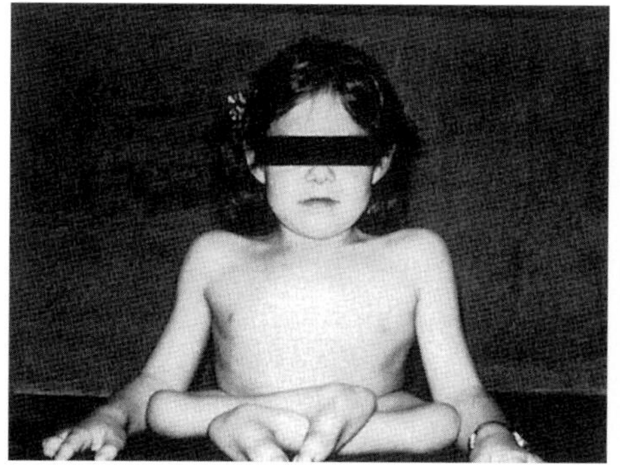

(a)

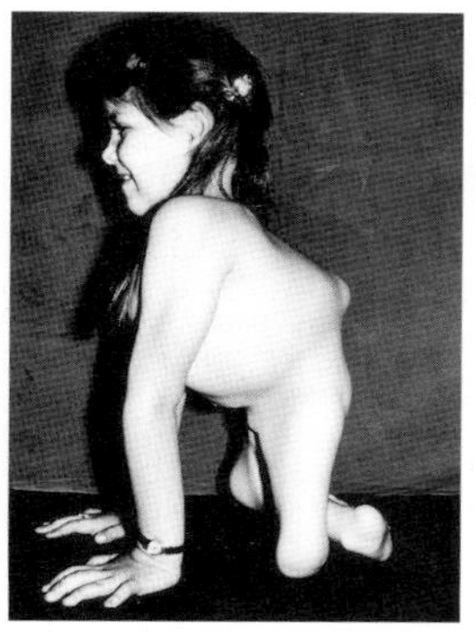

(b)

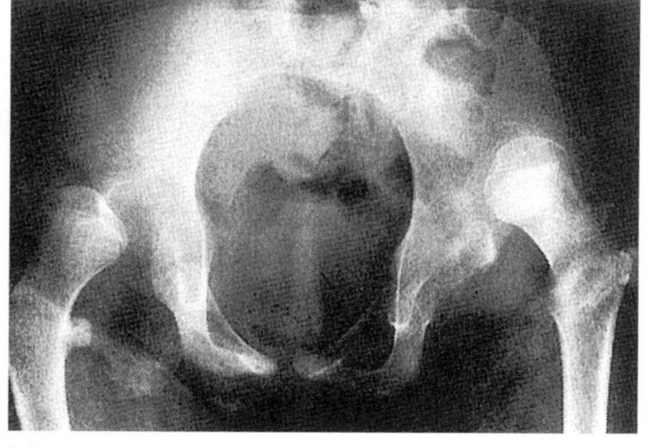

(c)

8.27 Sacral agenesis This girl shows (a) the characteristic sitting posture and (b) the spinal hump. (c) The sacrum is absent and the hips are dislocated.

present and, as with congenital scoliosis, there may be associated cardiac, visceral and renal abnormalities. Some cases of sacral agenesis appear to be inherited in either an autosomal or sex-linked dominant fashion.

LIMB ANOMALIES

Localized malformations of the limbs include extra bones, absent bones, hypoplastic bones and fusions. Complete absence of a limb is called *amelia*, almost complete absence (a mere stub remaining) *phocomelia* and partial absence *ectromelia*; defects may be transverse or axial. In the hands and feet *brachydactyly*, *syndactyly*, *polydactyly* and *symphalangism* are among the many possibilities.

The embryonal limb buds appear at about the 26th day of gestation; by the 30th day the upper limb has started differentiating into its three segments (upper arm, forearm and hand) and in the lower limb the same process occurs shortly afterwards. By the end of the 6th week the embryo has acquired a recognizable human form. The upper limb is fully formed by 12 weeks and the lower limb by 14 weeks. During this period the muscles and nerves also develop and by the 20th week joint movement is possible.

Most of the malformations involving limb reductions are due to embryonal insults between the 4th and 6th weeks of gestation. Some are genetically determined and these usually have an autosomal dominant pattern of inheritance.

Classification

Various classifications of limb deficiencies have been proposed; none is completely satisfactory. Some veer towards the purely descriptive; others go into almost obsessive detail based on topographical and morphological features. Their usefulness lies in the elaboration of an agreed terminology which will aid communication and permit sensible auditing of the results of various forms of treatment.

Some of the important and less rare disorders are described below and further details appear in the section on Regional Orthopaedics.

UPPER LIMB

When dealing with upper limb deficiencies it is important to remember that hand function may be very satisfactory (albeit not ideal) even if the appearance is not. Before any surgical treatment is considered, it is important to decide what the aims of treatment are, what side effects there might be and how to achieve the most acceptable balance between *function*, *appearance* and *pain*. A hand that functions better but hurts more may not be more useful to a particular patient. Hand dominance and whether or not the abnormality is bilateral are also important factors to note when planning treatment.

Radial deficiency

Absence or hypoplasia of the radius may occur alone or in association with visceral anomalies or (more rarely) certain blood dyscrasias. Two acronyms may help to keep this in mind. 'VACTERLS' refers to the systems involved and the defects identified: vertebral, anal, cardiac, tracheal, esophageal, renal, limb and single umbilical artery. 'TAR' prompts one to remember thrombocytopaenia with absent radius syndrome. Fanconi's anaemia and the Holt–Oram syndrome are also sometimes associated with radial deficiency.

The forearm is short and bowed; the hand is underdeveloped and markedly deviated towards the radial side (*radial club hand*) and the thumb may be missing. The elbow too is often abnormal. In about half the cases the condition is bilateral.

The clinical deformity may look bizarre but children often acquire excellent function. If this seems unlikely, operative reconstruction may be advisable. This could involve pollicisation of a digit and other complex reconstructive procedures. In the young child simple stretching and splinting may help to

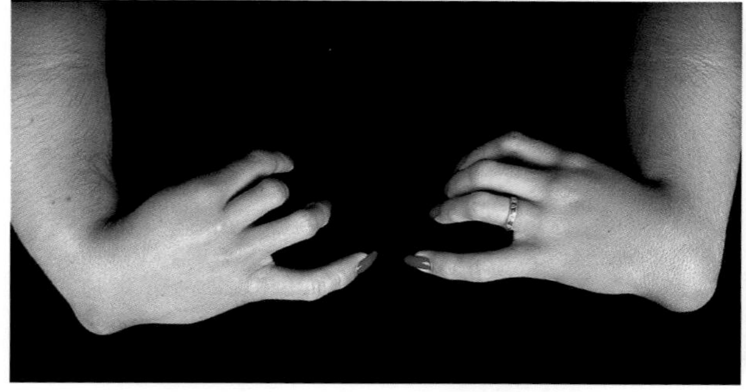

(a)

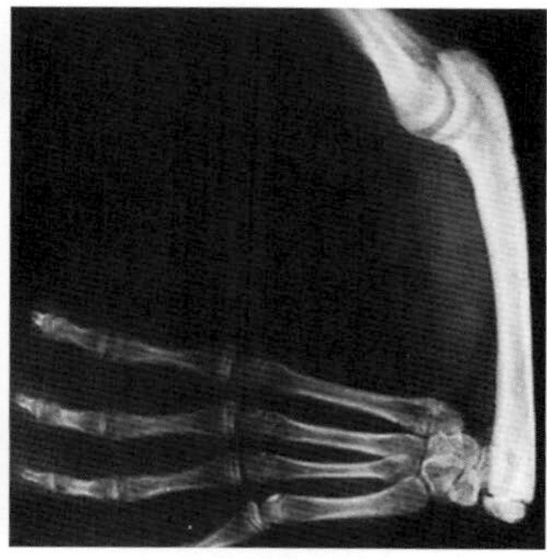

(b)

8.28 Radial dysplasia (a) Bilateral. (b) X-ray showing that the entire radius is absent.

Tumours

9

Will Aston, Timothy Briggs, Louis Solomon

Tumours, tumour-like lesions and cysts are considered together, partly because their clinical presentation and management are similar and partly because the definitive classification of bone tumours is still evolving and some disorders may yet move from one category to another. Benign lesions are quite common, primary malignant ones rare; yet so often do they mimic each other, and so critical are the decisions on treatment, that a working knowledge of all the important conditions is necessary.

CLASSIFICATION

Most classifications of bone tumours are based on the recognition of the dominant tissue in the various lesions (Table 9.1). Knowing the cell line from which the tumour has sprung may help with both diagnosis and planning of treatment. There are, however, pitfalls in this approach:

Table 9.1 A classification of bone tumours. Modified after Revised WHO Classification – Schajowicz (1994)

Predominant tissue	Benign	Malignant
Bone forming	Osteoma Osteoid osteoma Osteoblastoma	Osteosarcoma: central peripheral parosteal
Cartilage forming	Chondroma Osteochondroma Chondroblastoma ?Chondromyxoid fibroma	Chondrosarcoma: central peripheral juxtacortical clear-cell mesenchymal
Fibrous tissue	Fibroma Fibromatosis	Fibrosarcoma
Mixed	?Chondromyxoid fibroma	
Giant-cell tumours	Benign osteoclastoma	Malignant osteoclastoma
Marrow tumours		Ewing's tumour Myeloma
Vascular tissue	Haemangioma Haemangiopericytoma Haemangioendothelioma	Angiosarcoma Malignant haemangiopericytoma
Other connective tissue	Fibroma Fibrous histiocytoma Lipoma	Fibrosarcoma Malignant fibrous histiocytoma Liposarcoma
Other tumours	Neurofibroma Neurilemmoma	Adamantinoma Chordoma

- the most pervasive tissue is not necessarily the tissue of origin
- there is not necessarily any connection between conditions in one category
- there is often no relationship between benign and malignant lesions with similar tissue elements (e.g. osteoma and osteosarcoma)
- the commonest malignant lesions in bone – metastatic tumours – are not, strictly speaking, 'bone' tumours, i.e. not of mesenchymal origin.

CLINICAL PRESENTATION

HISTORY

The history is often prolonged, and this unfortunately results in a delay in obtaining treatment. Patients may be completely *asymptomatic* until the abnormality is discovered on x-ray. This is more likely with benign lesions; and, since some of these (e.g. non-ossifying fibroma) are common in children but rare after the age of 30, they must be capable of spontaneous resolution. Malignant tumours, too, may remain silent if they are slow-growing and situated where there is room for inconspicuous expansion (e.g. the cavity of the pelvis).

Age may be a useful clue. Many benign lesions present during childhood and adolescence – but so do some primary malignant tumours, notably Ewing's tumour and osteosarcoma. Chondrosarcoma and fibrosarcoma typically occur in older people (fourth or sixth decades); and myeloma, the commonest of all primary malignant bone tumours, is seldom seen before the sixth decade. *In patients over 70 years of age, metastatic bone lesions are more common than all primary tumours together.*

Pain is a common complaint and gives little indication of the nature of the lesion; however, progressive and unremitting pain is a sinister symptom. It may be caused by rapid expansion with stretching of surrounding tissues, central haemorrhage or degeneration in the tumour, or an incipient pathological fracture. However, even a tiny lesion may be very painful if it is encapsulated in dense bone (e.g. an osteoid osteoma).

Swelling, or the appearance of a *lump*, may be alarming. Often, though, patients seek advice only when a mass becomes painful or continues to grow.

A *history of trauma* is offered so frequently that it cannot be dismissed as having no significance. Yet, whether the injury initiates a pathological change or merely draws attention to what is already there remains unanswered.

Neurological symptoms (paraesthesiae or numbness) may be caused by pressure upon or stretching of a peripheral nerve. Progressive dysfunction is more ominous and suggests invasion by an aggressive tumour.

Pathological fracture may be the first (and only) clinical signal. Suspicion is aroused if the injury was slight; in elderly people, whose bones usually fracture at the cortico-cancellous junctions, any break in the mid-shaft should be regarded as pathological until proved otherwise.

EXAMINATION

If there is a *lump*, where does it arise? Is it discrete or ill-defined? Is it soft or hard, or pulsatile? And is it tender? *Swelling* is sometimes diffuse, and the overlying skin warm and inflamed; it can be difficult to distinguish a tumour from infection or a haematoma.

If the tumour is near a joint there may be an *effusion* and/or *limitation of movement*. Spinal lesions, whether benign or malignant, often cause *muscle spasm* and *back stiffness*, or a *painful scoliosis*.

The examination will focus on the symptomatic part, but it should include the area of lymphatic drainage and, often, the pelvis, abdomen, chest and spine.

IMAGING

X-RAYS

Plain x-rays are still the most useful of all imaging techniques. There may be an obvious abnormality in the bone – cortical thickening, a discrete lump, a 'cyst' or ill-defined destruction. Where is the lesion: in the metaphysis or the diaphysis? Is it solitary or are there multiple lesions? Are the margins well-defined or ill-defined?

Remember that 'cystic' lesions are not necessarily hollow cavities: any radiolucent material (e.g. a fibroma or a chondroma) may look like a cyst. If the boundary of the 'cyst' is sharply defined it is probably

QUESTIONS TO ASK WHEN STUDYING AN X-RAY

Is the lesion solitary or are there multiple lesions?

What type of bone is involved?

Where is the lesion in the bone?

Are the margins of the lesion well- or ill-defined?

Are there flecks of calcification in the lesion?

Is the cortex eroded or destroyed?

Is there any periosteal new-bone formation?

Does the tumour extend into the soft tissues?

benign; if it is hazy and diffuse it suggests an invasive tumour. Stippled calcification inside a cystic area is characteristic of cartilage tumours.

Look carefully at the bone surfaces: periosteal new-bone formation and extension of the tumour into the soft tissues are suggestive of malignant change.

Look also at the soft tissues: Are the muscle planes distorted by swelling? Is there calcification?

For all its informative detail, the x-ray alone can seldom be relied on for a definitive diagnosis. With some notable exceptions, in which the appearances are pathognomonic (osteochondroma, non-ossifying fibroma, osteoid osteoma), further investigations will be needed. *If other forms of imaging are planned (bone scans, CT or MRI), they should be done before undertaking a biopsy, which itself may distort the appearances.*

RADIONUCLIDE SCANNING

Scanning with ^{99m}Tc-methyl diphosphonate (^{99m}Tc-MDP) shows non-specific reactive changes in bone; this can be helpful in revealing the site of a small tumour (e.g. an osteoid osteoma) that does not show up clearly on x-ray. Skeletal scintigraphy is also useful for detecting skip lesions or 'silent' secondary deposits.

COMPUTED TOMOGRAPHY

CT extends the range of x-ray diagnosis; it shows more accurately both intraosseous and extraosseous extension of the tumour and the relationship to surrounding structures. It may also reveal suspected lesions in inaccessible sites, like the spine or pelvis; and it is a reliable method of detecting pulmonary metastases.

MAGNETIC RESONANCE IMAGING

MRI provides further information. Its greatest value is in the assessment of tumour spread: (a) within the bone, (b) into a nearby joint and (c) into the soft tissues. Blood vessels and the relationship of the tumour to the perivascular space are well defined. MRI is also useful in assessing soft-tissue tumours and cartilaginous lesions.

LABORATORY INVESTIGATIONS

Blood tests are often necessary to exclude other conditions, e.g. infection or metabolic bone disorders, or a 'brown tumour' in hyperparathyroidism. *Anaemia*, increased *ESR* and elevated *serum alkaline phosphatase* levels are non-specific findings, but if other causes are excluded they may help in differentiating between benign and malignant bone lesions. *Serum protein electrophoresis* may reveal an abnormal globulin fraction and the urine may contain *Bence Jones protein* in patients with myeloma. A raised *serum acid phosphatase* suggests prostatic carcinoma.

BIOPSY

Needle biopsy Needle biopsy should be performed either by the surgeon planning definitive treatment or by an experienced radiologist. Often it is carried out with the help of ultrasound or CT guidance (Stoker et al., 1991; Saifuddin et al., 2000). A large bore biopsy needle, such as a Jamshidi or a Trucut needle, is used. It is important to ensure that a representative sample of the tumour is taken and that it is adequate to make a histological diagnosis; a frozen section can be used in order to confirm this. If infection is suspected then a sample should be sent for microbiology. It is also essential that the biopsy is carried out in the line of any further surgical incision so that the tract can be excised at the time of definitive surgery.

Open biopsy This is a more reliable way of obtaining a representative sample, however it is associated with significant morbidity (Mankin et al., 1982). It is often performed if a needle biopsy would place the neurovascular structures at risk or if a diagnosis has not been made after needle biopsy. The site is selected so that it can be included in any subsequent operation. As little as possible of the tumour is exposed and a block of tissue is removed – ideally in the boundary zone, so as to include normal tissue, pseudocapsule and abnormal tissue. If bone is removed the raw area is covered with bone wax or methylmethacrylate cement. If a tourniquet is used, it should be released and *full haemostasis* achieved before closing the wound. Drains should be avoided, so as to minimize the risk of tumour contamination.

An experienced histopathologist should be on hand and the specimens should be delivered fresh, unfixed and uncrushed.

For tumours that are almost certainly benign, an *excisional biopsy* is permissible (the entire lesion is removed); with cysts that need operations, representative tissue can be obtained by careful curettage. In either case, histological confirmation of the diagnosis is essential.

Biopsy should never be regarded as a 'minor' procedure. Complications include haemorrhage, wound breakdown, infection and pathological fracture (Mankin at al., 1982, 1996; Springfield and Rosenberg, 1996). The person doing the biopsy should have a clear idea of what may be done next and where operative incisions or skin flaps will be placed. Errors and complications are far less likely if the procedure is performed in a specializing centre.

A last word of warning: When dealing with tumours that could be malignant, there is a strong temptation to perform the biopsy as soon as possible; as this may alter the CT and MRI appearances, it is important to delay the procedure until all the imaging studies have been completed.

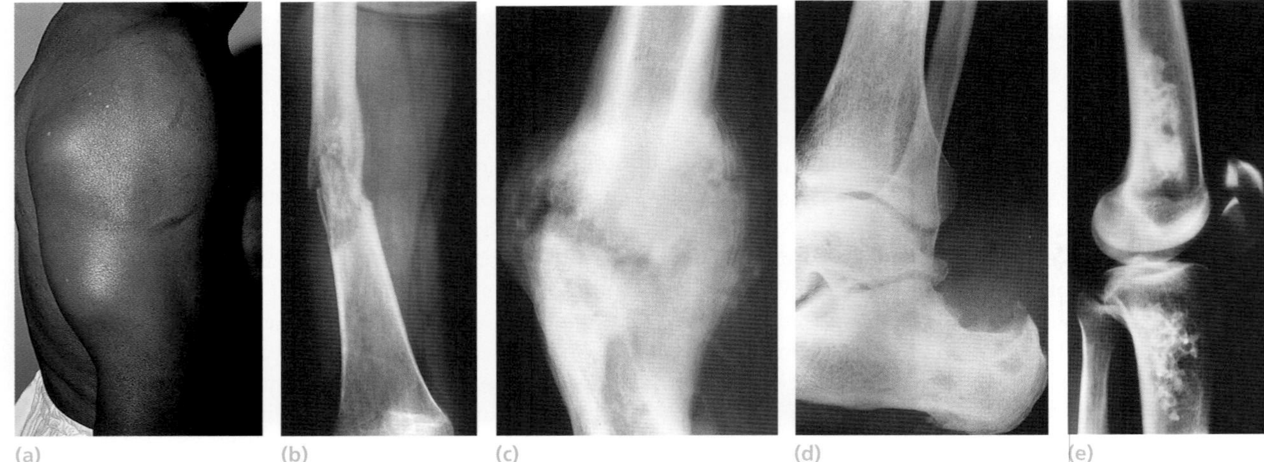

9.1 Tumours – differential diagnosis (a) This huge swelling was simply a clotted haematoma. (b) Bone infection with pathological fracture. (c) Florid callus in an un-united fracture. (d) Large erosion in the calcaneum by a gouty tophus. (e) Bone infarcts.

Differential diagnosis

A number of conditions may mimic a tumour, either clinically or radiologically, and the histopathology may be difficult to interpret. It is important not to be misled by the common dissemblers.

Soft-tissue haematoma A large, clotted sub-periosteal or soft-tissue haematoma may present as a painful lump in the arm or lower limb. Sometimes the x-ray shows an irregular surface on the underlying bone. Important clues are the history and the rapid onset of symptoms.

Myositis ossificans Although rare, this may be a source of confusion. Following an injury the patient develops a tender swelling in the vicinity of a joint; the x-ray shows fluffy density in the soft tissue adjacent to bone. Unlike a malignant tumour, however, the condition soon becomes less painful and the new bone better defined and well demarcated.

Stress fracture Some of the worst mistakes have been made in misdiagnosing a stress fracture. The patient is often a young adult with localized pain near a large joint; x-rays show a dubious area of cortical 'destruction' and overlying periosteal new bone; if a biopsy is performed the healing callus may show histological features resembling those of osteosarcoma. If the pitfall is recognized, and there is adequate consultation between surgeon, radiologist and pathologist, a serious error can be prevented.

Tendon avulsion injuries Children and adolescents – especially those engaged in vigorous sports – are prone to avulsion injuries at sites of tendon insertion, particularly around the hip and knee (Donnelly et al., 1999). The best known example is the tibial apophyseal stress lesion of Osgood–Schlatter's disease (see page 565), but lesions at less familiar sites (the iliac crest, the ischial tuberosity, the lesser trochanter of the femur, the hamstring insertions, the attachments of adductor magnus and longus and the distal humeral apophyses) may escape immediate recognition.

Bone infection Osteomyelitis typically causes pain and swelling near one of the larger joints; as with primary bone tumours, the patients are usually children or young adults. X-rays may show an area of destruction in the metaphysis, with periosteal new bone. Systemic features, especially if the patient has been treated with antibiotics, may be mild. If the area is explored, tissue should be submitted for both bacteriological and histological examination.

Gout Occasionally a large gouty tophus causes a painful swelling at one of the bone ends, and x-ray shows a large, poorly defined excavation. If it is kept in mind the diagnosis will be easily confirmed – if necessary by obtaining a biopsy from the lump.

Other bone lesions Non-neoplastic bone lesions such as fibrous cortical defects, medullary infarcts and 'bone islands' are occasionally mistaken for tumours.

STAGING OF BONE TUMOURS

In treating tumours we strive to reconcile two conflicting principles: the lesion must be removed widely enough to ensure that it does not recur, but damage must be kept to a minimum. The balance between

Table 9.2 Staging of benign bone tumours as described by Enneking

Latent	Well-defined margin. Grows slowly and then stops Remains static/heals spontaneously E.g. Osteoid osteoma
Active	Progressive growth limited by natural barriers Not self-limiting. Tendency to recur E.g. Aneurysmal bone cyst
Aggressive	Growth not limited by natural barriers (e.g. giant cell tumour)

these objectives depends on knowing (a) how the tumour usually behaves (i.e. how aggressive it is), and (b) how far it has spread. The answers to these two questions are embodied in the staging system developed by Enneking (1986).

AGGRESSIVENESS

Tumours are graded not only on their cytological characteristics but also on their clinical behaviour, i.e. the likelihood of recurrence and spread after surgical removal.

Benign lesions, by definition, occupy the lowest grade, though even in this group there are important differences in behaviour calling for further subdivision into *latent*, *active* and *aggressive* lesions (Table 9.2). The least aggressive tumours may disappear spontaneously (e.g. non-osteogenic fibroma); the most aggressive are difficult to distinguish from a low-grade sarcoma and sometimes undergo malignant change (e.g. aggressive osteoblastoma). Most are amenable to local (marginal) excision with little risk of recurrence.

Malignant tumours are divided into 'low-grade' and 'high-grade': the former are only moderately aggressive and take a long time to metastasize (e.g. secondary chondrosarcoma or parosteal osteosarcoma), while the latter are usually very aggressive and metastasize early (e.g. osteosarcoma or fibrosarcoma).

SPREAD

Assuming that there are no metastases, the local extent of the tumour is the most important factor in deciding how much tissue has to be removed. Lesions that are confined to an enclosed tissue space (e.g. a bone, a joint cavity or a muscle group within its fascial envelope) are called '*intracompartmental*'. Those that extend into interfascial or extrafascial planes with no natural barrier to proximal or distal spread (e.g. perivascular sheaths, pelvis, axilla) are designated '*extracompartmental*'. The extent of the tumour and adjacent 'contaminated' tissue are best shown by CT and MRI; skip lesions can be detected by scintigraphy.

SURGICAL STAGE

'Staging' the tumour is an important step towards selecting the operation best suited to that particular patient, and carrying a low risk of recurrence. Locally recurrent sarcomas tend to be more aggressive, more often extracompartmental and more likely to metastasize than the original tumour.

Bone sarcomas are broadly divided as follows:

- *Stage I* All low-grade sarcomas.
- *Stage II* Histologically high-grade lesions.
- *Stage III* Sarcomas which have metastasized.

Table 9.3 Surgical stages as described by Enneking

Stage	Grade	Site	Metastases
IA	Low	Intracompartmental	No
IB	Low	Extracompartmental	No
IIA	High	Intracompartmental	No
IIB	High	Extracompartmental	No
IIIA	Low	Intra- or extracompartmental	Yes
IIIA	High	Intra- or extracompartmental	Yes

Following Enneking's original classification, each category is further subdivided into *Type A* (intracompartmental) and *Type B* (extracompartmental) (Fig. 9.3). Thus, a localized chondrosarcoma arising in a cartilage-capped exostosis would be designated IA, suitable for wide excision without exposing the tumour. An osteosarcoma confined to bone would be IIA – operable by wide excision or amputation with a low risk of local recurrence; if it has spread into the soft tissues it would be IIB – less suitable for wide excision and preferably treated by radical resection or disarticulation through the proximal joint. If there are pulmonary metastases it would be classified as stage III.

STAGING OF SOFT-TISSUE TUMOURS

Soft-tissue tumours are staged using the American Joint Committee for Cancer Staging System, according to their histological grade (G), size (T), lymph node involvement (N) and whether they have metastasized (M) (Russell et al., 1977). The main differences between this and the Enneking system are the increased number of histological grades (from low and high to 1, 2 and 3) and use of the size of the tumour (less than or greater than 5 cm), rather than whether it is intra- or extracompartmental.

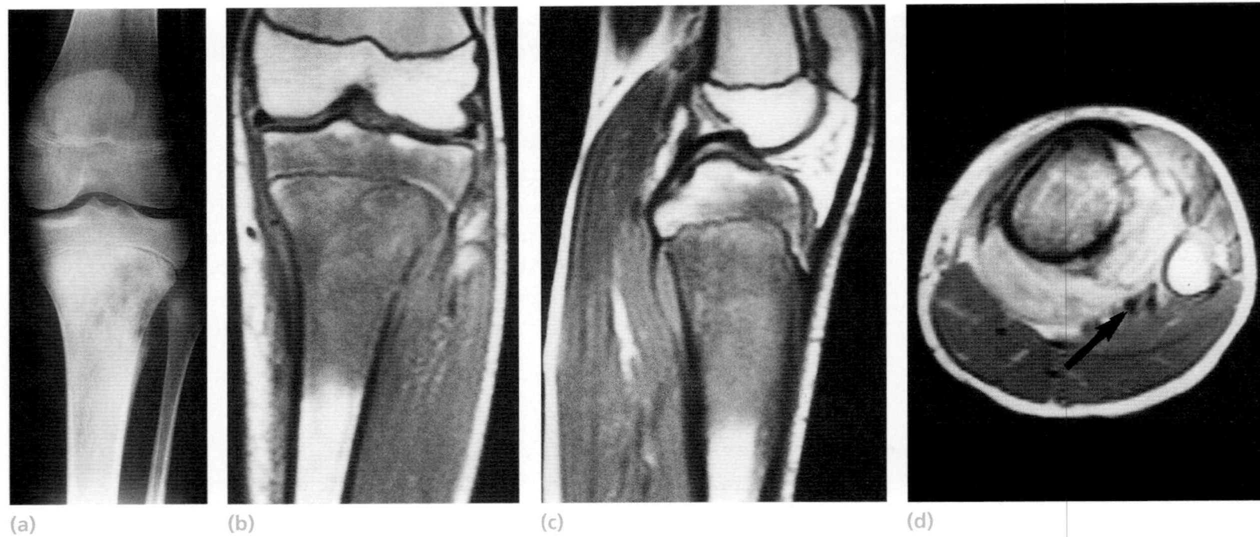

(a) (b) (c) (d)

9.2 Staging (a) Plain x-ray shows a destructive lesion of the proximal tibia, almost certainly an osteosarcoma; but is it locally resectable? (b,c) Coronal and sagittal MR images show the tumour extending medially, laterally and posteriorly into the soft tissue. (d) Transectional MRI shows that the abnormal tissue extends posteriorly right up to the vascular compartment (arrow). This tumour would be assessed as Stage IIB.

PRINCIPLES OF MANAGEMENT

For all but the simplest and most obvious of benign tumours, management calls for a multidisciplinary team approach and is best conducted in a tertiary centre specializing in the treatment of bone and soft-tissue tumours. Consultation and cooperation between the orthopaedic surgeon, radiologist, pathologist and (certainly in the case of malignant tumours) the oncologist is essential in the initial management. In many cases physiotherapists, occupational therapists and prosthetists will also be involved.

Once clinical and radiological examination have suggested the most likely diagnosis, further management proceeds as follows.

Benign, asymptomatic lesions If the diagnosis is beyond doubt (e.g. a non-ossifying fibroma or a small osteochondroma) one can afford to temporize; treatment may never be needed. However, if the appearances are not pathognomonic, a biopsy is advisable and this may take the form of excision or curettage of the lesion.

Benign, symptomatic or enlarging tumours Painful lesions, or tumours that continue to enlarge after the end of normal bone growth, require biopsy and confirmation of the diagnosis. Unless they are unusually aggressive, they can generally be removed by local (marginal) excision or (in the case of benign cysts) by curettage.

Suspected malignant tumours If the lesion is thought to be a primary malignant tumour, the patient is admitted for more detailed examination, blood tests, chest x-ray, further imaging (including pulmonary CT) and biopsy. This should allow a firm diagnosis and staging to be established. The various treatment options can then be discussed with the patient (or the parents, in the case of a young child). A choice needs to be made between amputation, limb-sparing operations and different types of adjuvant therapy, and the patient must be fully informed about the pros and cons of each.

METHODS OF TREATMENT

TUMOUR EXCISION

The more aggressive the lesion the more widely does it need to be excised, in order to ensure that the tumour as well as any dubious marginal tissue is completely removed.

Intracapsular (intralesional) excision and *curettage* are incomplete forms of tumour ablation and therefore applicable only to benign lesions with a very low risk of recurrence, or to incurable tumours which need debulking to relieve local symptoms. Adjunctive treatment such as the use of acrylic cement after curettage decreases the risk of local recurrence.

Marginal excision goes beyond the tumour, but only just. If the dissection of a malignant lesion is carried through the reactive zone, there is a significant risk of recurrence (up to 50 per cent). For benign lesions, however, this is a suitable method; the resulting cavity can be filled with graft bone.

Wide excision implies that the dissection is carried out well clear of the tumour, through normal tissue. This is appropriate for low-grade intracompartmental lesions (grade IA), providing a risk of local recurrence

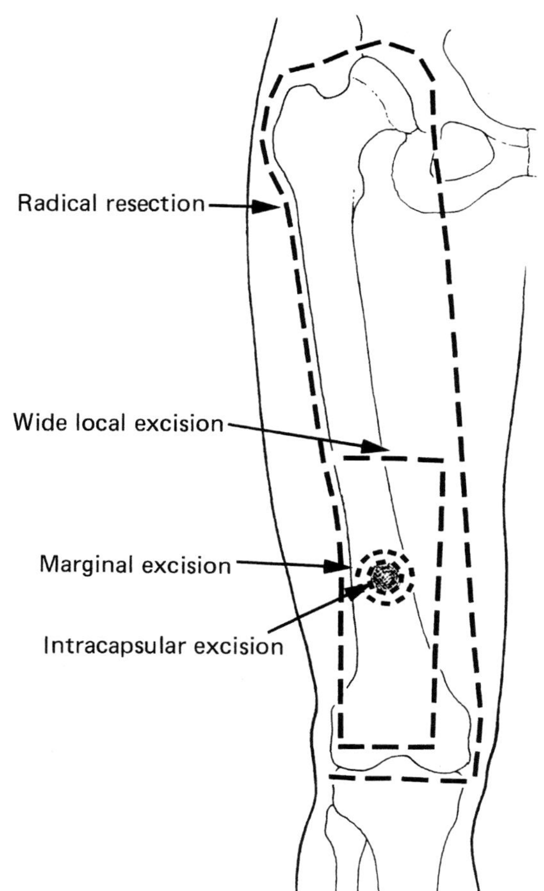

9.3 Tumour excision The more aggressive a tumour is, and the wider it has spread, the more widely it needs to be excised. Local excision is suitable only for low-grade tumours that are confined to a single compartment. Radical resection may be needed for high-grade tumours and this often means amputation at a level above the compartment involved.

below 10 per cent. However, wide excision is also used *in conjunction with chemotherapy* for grade IIA lesions.

Radical resection means that the entire compartment in which the tumour lies is removed *en bloc* without exposing the lesion. It may be possible to do this while still sparing the limb, but the surrounding muscles, ligaments and connective tissues will have to be sacrificed; in some cases a true radical resection can be achieved only by amputating at a level above the compartment involved. This method is required for high-grade tumours (IIA or IIB).

LIMB SALVAGE

Amputation is no longer the automatic choice for grade II sarcomas. Improved methods of imaging and advances in chemotherapy have made limb salvage the treatment of choice for many patients. However, this option should be considered only if the local control of the tumour is likely to be as good as that obtained by amputation, if it is certain that there are no skip lesions and if a functional limb can be preserved. The ongoing debate around limb sparing versus amputation is addressed in an excellent paper by DiCaprio and Friedlaender (2003).

Advanced surgical facilities for bone grafting and endoprosthetic replacement at various sites must be available. The first step consists of wide excision of the tumour with preservation of the neurovascular structures. The resulting defect is then dealt with in one of several ways. Short diaphyseal segments can be replaced by *vascularized or non-vascularized bone grafts*. Longer gaps may require *custom-made implants*. Osteo-articular segments can be replaced by *large allografts*, *endoprostheses* or *allograft–prosthetic composites*. It is recognized, however, that the use of large allografts carries a high risk of infection and fracture; this has led to them not being used as widely as in the past. Endoprostheses used to be custom-made but nowadays modular systems for tumour reconstruction are available.

In growing children, *extendible implants* have been used in order to avoid the need for repeated operations; however, they may need to be replaced at the end of growth. Other procedures, such as *grafting and arthrodesis* or *distraction osteosynthesis*, are suitable for some situations.

Sarcomas around the hip and shoulder present special problems. Complete excision is difficult and reconstruction involves complex grafting and replacement procedures (O'Connor et al., 1996).

Outcome Tumour replacement by massive endoprosthesis carries a high risk of complications such as wound breakdown and infection; the 10-year survival rate of these prostheses with mechanical failure as the end point is 75 per cent and for failure due to any cause is 58 per cent. The limb salvage rate at 20 years is 84 per cent (Jeys et al., 2008).

AMPUTATION

Considering the difficulties of limb-sparing surgery – particularly for high-grade tumours or if there is doubt about whether the lesion is intracompartmental – amputation and early rehabilitation may be the wisest option. Preoperative planning and the definitive operation are best carried out in a specialized unit, so as to minimize the risk of complications and permit early rehabilitation.

Amputation may be curative but it is sometimes performed essentially to achieve local control of a tumour which is resistant to chemotherapy and radiation therapy.

MULTI-AGENT CHEMOTHERAPY

Multi-agent chemotherapy is now the preferred neoadjuvant and adjuvant treatment for malignant bone and soft-tissue tumours. There is good evidence to show that, for sensitive tumours, modern chemotherapy regimens effectively reduce the size of the primary lesion, prevent metastatic seeding and improve the chances of survival. When combined with surgery for osteosarcoma and Ewing's tumours, the long-term disease-free survival rate in the best series is now about 60 per cent.

Drugs currently in use are methotrexate, doxorubicin (Adriamycin), cyclophosphamide, vincristine and *cis*-platinum. Treatment is started 8–12 weeks preoperatively and the effect is assessed by examining the resected tissue for tumour necrosis; greater than 90 per cent necrosis is taken as a good response. If there is little or no necrosis, a different drug may be selected for postoperative treatment. Maintenance chemotherapy is continued for another 6–12 months.

RADIOTHERAPY

High-energy irradiation has long been used to destroy radiosensitive tumours or as adjuvant therapy before operation. Nowadays the indications are more restricted. For highly sensitive tumours (such as Ewing's sarcoma) it offers an alternative to amputation; it is then combined with adjuvant chemotherapy. The same combination can be used as adjunctive treatment for high-grade tumours, for tumours in inaccessible sites, lesions that are inoperable because of their size, proximity to major blood vessels or advanced local spread, for marrow-cell tumours such as myeloma and malignant lymphoma, for metastatic deposits and for palliative local tumour control where no surgery is planned. Radiotherapy may also be employed postoperatively when a marginal or intralesional excision has occurred, so as to 'sterilize' the tumour bed.

The main *complications* of this treatment are the occurrence of post-irradiation spindle-cell sarcoma and pathological fracture in weightbearing bones, particularly in the proximal half of the femur.

BENIGN BONE LESIONS

NON-OSSIFYING FIBROMA (FIBROUS CORTICAL DEFECT)

This, the commonest benign lesion of bone, is a developmental defect in which a nest of fibrous tissue appears within the bone and persists for some years before ossifying. It is asymptomatic and is almost always encountered in children as an incidental finding on x-ray. The commonest sites are the metaphyses of long bones; occasionally there are multiple lesions.

The *x-ray* appearance is unmistakable. There is a more or less oval radiolucent area surrounded by a thin margin of dense bone; views in different planes may show that a lesion that appears to be 'central' is actually adjacent to or within the cortex, hence the alternative name 'fibrous cortical defect'.

Pathology Although it looks cystic on x-ray, it is a solid lesion consisting of unremarkable fibrous tissue with a few scattered giant cells.

As the bone grows the defect becomes less obvious and it eventually heals spontaneously. However, it sometimes enlarges to several centimetres in diameter and there may be a pathological fracture. There is no risk of malignant change.

Treatment Treatment is usually unnecessary. If the defect is very large or has led to repeated fractures, it can be treated by curettage and bone grafting. Recurrence is rare.

FIBROUS DYSPLASIA

Fibrous dysplasia is a developmental disorder in which areas of trabecular bone are replaced by cellular fibrous tissue containing flecks of osteoid and woven bone. It may affect one bone (monostotic), one limb

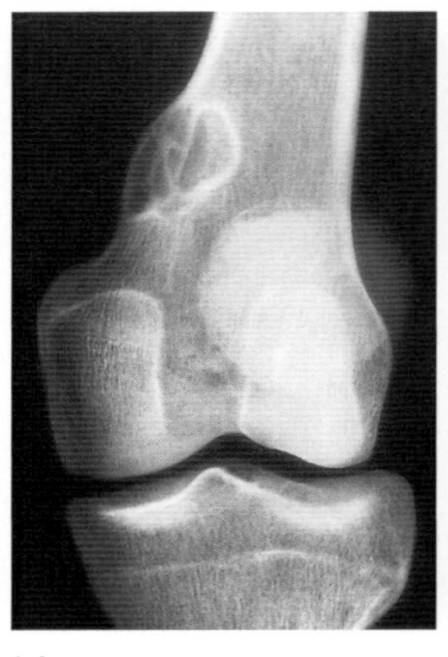

(a)

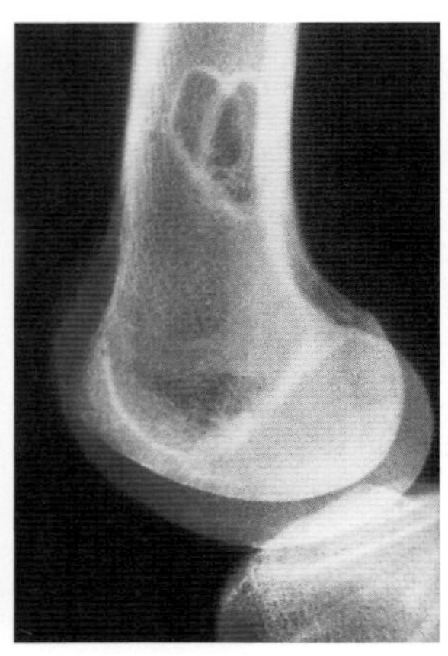

(b)

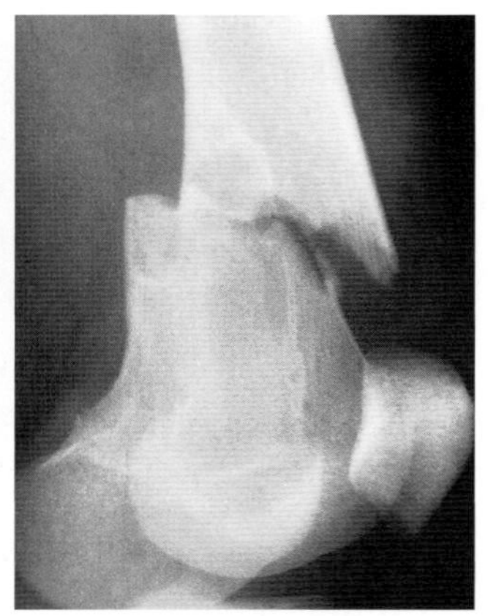

(c)

9.4 Non-ossifying fibroma (a) The x-ray shows a cortical defect, although in some projection planes this looks deceptively like a medullary lesion (b). The bone may fracture through the weakened area (c).

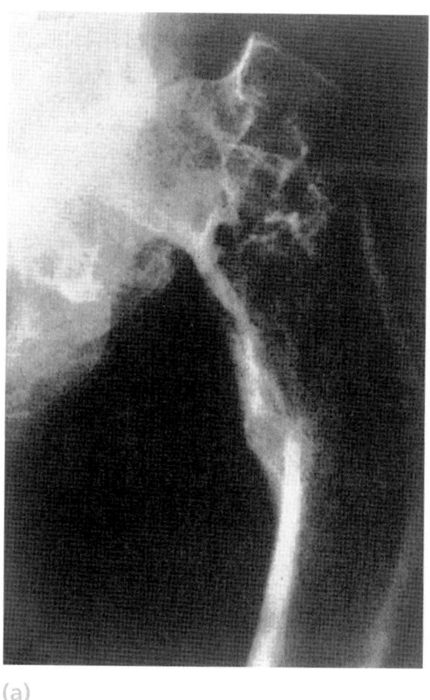
(a)

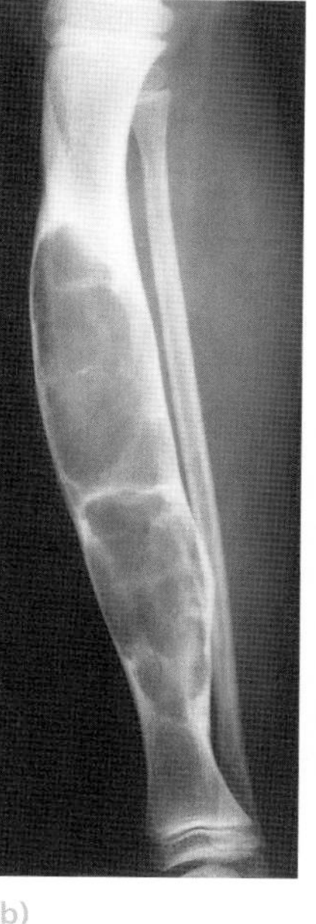
(b)

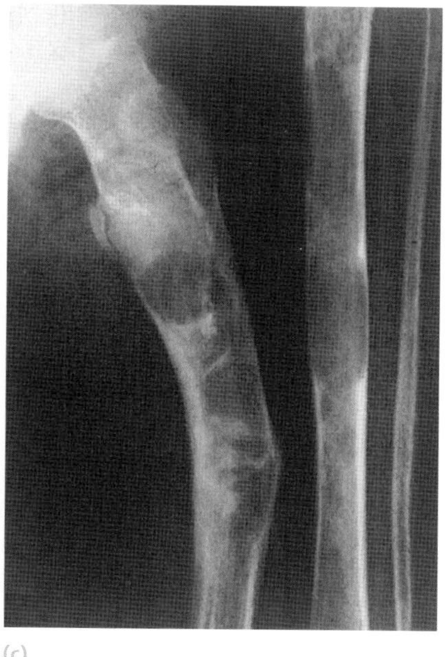
(c)

9.5 Fibrous dysplasia Monostotic fibrous dysplasia of (a) the upper femur (with the so-called 'shepherd's crook' appearance) and (b) of the tibia. (c) Polyostotic fibrous dysplasia.

(monomelic) or many bones (polyostotic). If the lesions are large, the bone is considerably weakened and pathological fractures or progressive deformity may occur.

The most common sites of occurrence are the proximal femur, tibia, humerus, ribs and cranio-facial bones. Small, single lesions are asymptomatic. Large, monostotic lesions may cause pain or may be discovered only when the patient develops a pathological fracture. Patients with polyostotic disease present in childhood or adolescence with pain, limp, bony enlargement, deformity or pathological fracture. Untreated, the characteristic deformities persist through adult life.

Occasionally the bone disorder is associated with *café-au-lait* patches on the skin and (in girls) precocious sexual development (*Albright's syndrome*).

X-rays show radiolucent 'cystic' areas in the metaphysis or shaft; because they contain fibrous tissue with diffuse spots of immature bone, the lucent patches typically have a slightly hazy or 'ground-glass' appearance. The weightbearing bones may be bent, and one of the classic features is the 'shepherd's crook' deformity of the proximal femur. *Radioscintigraphy* shows marked activity in the lesion.

Pathology At operation the lesional tissue has a coarse, gritty feel (due to the specks of immature bone). The histological picture is of loose, cellular fibrous tissue with widespread patches of woven bone and scattered giant cells.

Both clinically and histologically the monostotic condition may resemble either a bone-forming tumour or hyperparathyroidism. However, detailed x-ray and laboratory studies will exclude these disorders.

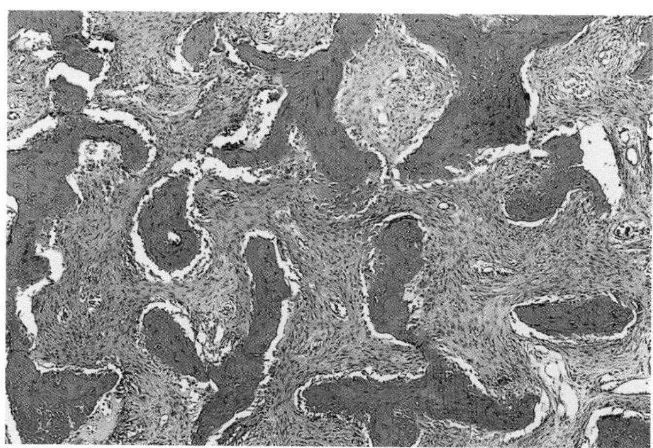

9.6 Fibrous dysplasia – histology Microscopic islands of metaplastic bone lie scattered in a bed of cellular fibrous tissue. Occasional giant cells are seen. (x120)

Malignant transformation to fibrosarcoma occurs in 0.5 per cent of patients with monostotic lesions and up to 5 per cent of patients with Albright's syndrome.

Treatment Treatment depends on the extent of the defect and the presence or absence of deformities. Small lesions need no treatment. Those that are large and painful or threatening to fracture (or have fractured) can be curetted and grafted, but there is a strong tendency for the abnormality to recur. A mixture of cortical and cancellous bone grafts may provide added strength even if the lesion is not eradicated. For very large lesions, the grafts can be supplemented by methylmethacrylate cement. Deformities may need correction by suitably designed osteotomies.

With large cysts, the bone often bleeds profusely at operation: forewarned is forearmed.

Osteoid osteoma

This tiny bone tumour (less than 1 cm in diameter) causes symptoms out of all proportion to its size. Patients are usually under 30 years of age and males predominate. Any bone except the skull may be affected, but over half the cases occur in the femur or tibia. The patient complains of persistent pain, sometimes well localized but sometimes referred over a wide area. Typically the pain is relieved by salicylates. If the diagnosis is delayed, other features appear: a limp or muscle wasting and weakness; spinal lesions may cause intense pain, muscle spasm and scoliosis.

The important *x-ray* feature is a small radiolucent area, the so-called 'nidus'. Lesions in the diaphysis are surrounded by dense sclerosis and cortical thickening; this may be so marked that the nidus can be seen only in fine cut CT scans. Lesions in the metaphysis show less cortical thickening. Further away the bone may be osteoporotic. ^{99m}Tc-MDP scintigraphy reveals intense, localized activity.

It is sometimes difficult to distinguish an osteoid osteoma from a small Brodie's abscess without biopsy. Ewing's sarcoma and chronic periostitis must also be excluded.

Pathology The excised lesion appears as a dark-brown or reddish 'nucleus' surrounded by dense bone; the central area consists of unorganized sheets of osteoid and bone cells.

There is no risk of malignant transformation.

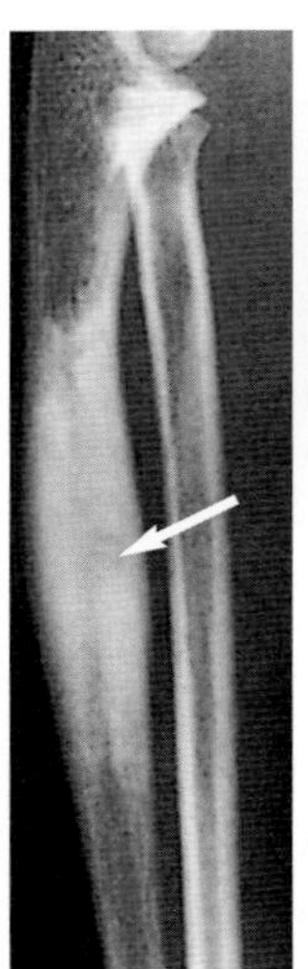

(a)

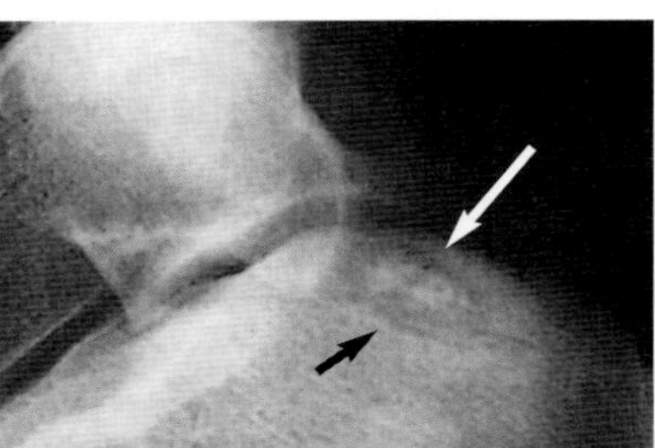

(b)

9.7 Osteoid osteoma The x-ray appearance depends on the site of the lesion. (a) With cortical tumours there is marked reactive bone thickening leaving a small lucent nidus, which may itself have a central speck of ossification. (b) Lesions in cancellous bone produce far less periosteal reaction and are easily mistaken for a Brodie's abscess.

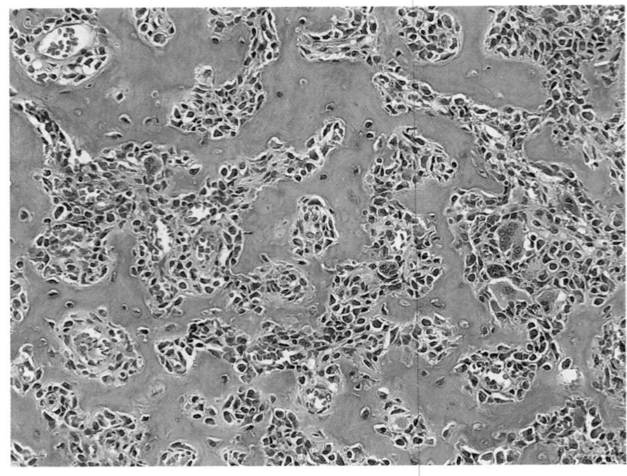

9.8 Osteoid osteoma – histology The histological features are characteristic: the nidus consists of sheets of pink-staining osteoid in a fibrovascular stroma. Giant cells and osteoblasts are prominent. (×300)

Treatment The only effective treatment is complete removal or destruction of the nidus. The lesion is carefully localized by x-ray and/or CT and then excised in a small block of bone or destroyed by CT-localized radio-ablation. The specimen should be x-rayed immediately to confirm that it does contain the little tumour. If the excision is likely to weaken the host bone (especially in the vulnerable medial cortex of the femoral neck), prophylactic internal fixation may be needed.

Osteoblastoma (giant osteoid osteoma)

This tumour is similar to an osteoid osteoma but it is larger (more than 1 cm in diameter), more cellular and sometimes more ominous in appearance. It is usually seen in young adults, more often in men than in women. It tends to occur in the spine and the flat bones; patients present with pain and local muscle spasm.

X-ray shows a well-demarcated osteolytic lesion which may contain small flecks of ossification. There is surrounding sclerosis but this is not always easy to see, especially with lesions in the flat bones or the vertebral pedicle. A *radioisotope scan* will reveal the 'hot' area. Larger lesions may appear cystic, and sometimes a typical aneurysmal bone cyst appears to have arisen in an osteoblastoma.

Pathology When the tumour is exposed it has a somewhat fleshy appearance. Histologically it resembles an osteoid osteoma, but the cellularity is more striking. Occasionally the picture may suggest a low-grade osteosarcoma.

Treatment Treatment consists of excision and bone grafting. With lesions in the vertebral pedicle or the floor of the acetabulum, this is not always easy and removal may be incomplete; local recurrence is common and malignant transformation has been reported (McLeod et al., 1976).

Compact osteoma (ivory exostosis)

This rare benign 'tumour' appears as a localized thickening on the outer or inner surface of compact bone. An adolescent or young adult presents with a painless, ivory-hard lump, usually on the outer surface of the skull, occasionally on the subcutaneous surface of the tibia. If it occurs on the inner table of the skull it may cause focal epilepsy; sometimes it protrudes into the paranasal sinuses. On x-ray a sessile plaque of exceedingly dense bone with a well-circumscribed edge is seen. This might suggest a parosteal osteosarcoma, but the long history, the absence of pain and the smooth outline will dispel this suspicion.

Treatment Unless the tumour impinges on important structures, it need not be removed. However, the patient may want to be rid of it; excision is easier if a margin of normal bone is taken with it.

Chondroma (enchondroma)

Islands of cartilage may persist in the metaphyses of bones formed by endochondral ossification; sometimes they grow and take on the characteristics of a benign tumour. Chondromas are usually asymptomatic and are discovered incidentally on x-ray or after a pathological fracture. They are seen at any age (but mostly in young people) and in any bone preformed in cartilage (most commonly the tubular bones of the hands and feet). Lesions may be solitary or multiple and part of a generalized dysplasia.

X-ray shows a well-defined, centrally placed radiolucent area at the junction of metaphysis and diaphysis; sometimes the bone is slightly expanded. In mature lesions there are flecks or wisps of calcification within the lucent area; when present, this is a pathognomonic feature.

Pathology When it is exposed the lesion is seen to consist of pearly-white cartilaginous tissue, often with a central area of degeneration and calcification. Histologically the appearances are those of simple hyaline cartilage.

Complications There is a small but significant risk of *malignant change* – probably less than 2 per cent (and hardly ever in a child) for patients with solitary lesions but as high as 30 per cent in those with multiple lesions (Ollier's disease) and up to 100 per cent in patients with associated haemangiomas (Maffucci's syndrome).

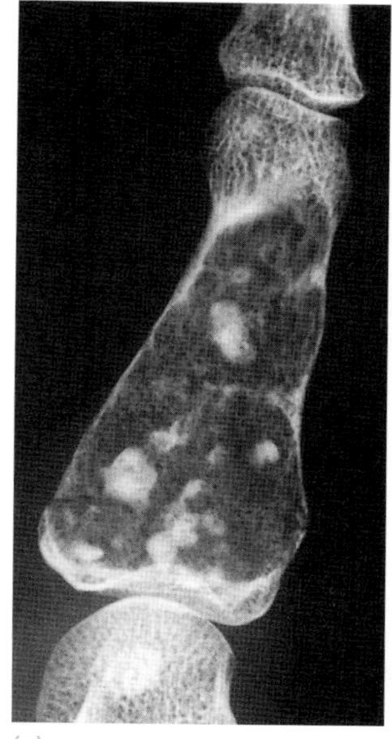

(a)

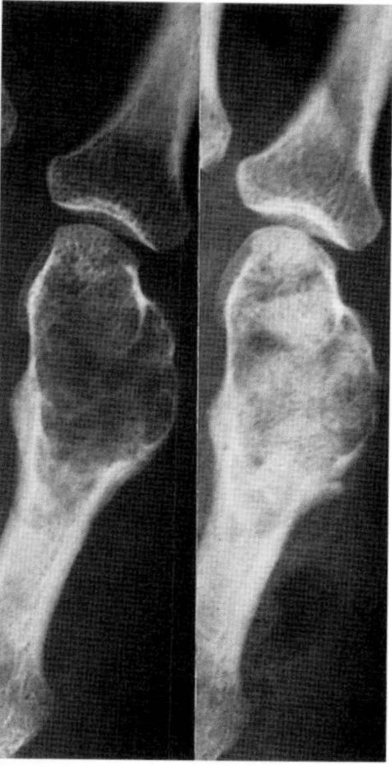

(b)

9.9 Chondroma (a) The hand is a common site. (b) Another chondroma before and after curettage and bone grafting.

Signs of malignant transformation in patients over 30 years are: (1) the onset of pain; (2) enlargement of the lesion; and (3) cortical erosion. Unfortunately, biopsy is of little help in this regard as the cartilage usually looks benign during the early stages of malignant transformation. If the other features are present, and especially in older patients, the lesion should be treated as a stage IA malignancy; the biopsy then serves chiefly to confirm the fact that it is a cartilage tumour.

Treatment Treatment is not always necessary, but if the tumour appears to be enlarging, or if it presents as a pathological fracture, it should be removed as thoroughly as possible by curettage; the defect is filled with bone graft or bone cement. There is a fairly high recurrence rate and the tissue may be seeded in adjacent bone or soft tissues. Chondromas in expendable sites are better removed *en bloc*.

Periosteal chondroma

These are rare developmental lesions arising in the deep layer of the periosteum, usually around the proximal humerus, femur or phalanges. A cartilaginous lump bulges from the bone into the soft tissues and causes some alarm when it is discovered by the patient.

Because the cartilage remains uncalcified, the lesion itself does not show on x-ray, but the surface of the bone may be irregular or scalloped. MRI may reveal the full extent of the tumour. Histologically the lesion is composed of highly cellular cartilage.

Treatment Because of its propensity to recur, it is best removed by marginal excision (taking a rim of normal bone). Recurrent lesions may look more aggressive but the lesion probably does not undergo malignant change.

CHONDROBLASTOMA

This benign tumour of immature cartilage cells is one of the few lesions to appear primarily in the epiphysis, usually of the proximal humerus, femur or tibia. Patients are affected around the end of the growth period or in early adult life; there is a predilection for males. The presenting symptom is a constant ache in the joint; the tender spot is actually in the adjacent bone.

X-ray shows a rounded, well-demarcated radiolucent area in the epiphysis with no hint of central calcification; this site is so unusual that the diagnosis springs readily to mind. However, sometimes the lesion extends across the physeal line. Occasionally the articular surface is breached. Like osteoblastoma, the lesion sometimes expands and acquires the features of an aneurysmal bone cyst.

Pathology The histological appearances are fairly typical – there are large collections of chondroblasts set off by the surrounding matrix of immature fibrous tissue. Within the stroma are scattered giant cells. In expansile lesions, the edge may resemble that of an aneurysmal bone cyst. These tumours do not undergo malignant change but they may be locally aggressive and extend into the joint.

Treatment In children the risk of damage to the physis makes one hesitate to remove the lesion. After the end of the growth period the lesion can be removed – by marginal excision wherever possible or (less satisfactorily) by curettage and alcohol or phenol cauterization – and replaced with autogenous bone grafts. There is a high risk of recurrence after incomplete removal, and if this happens repeatedly there may be serious damage to the nearby joint. Occasionally one is forced to excise the recurrent lesion with an adequate margin of bone and accept the inevitable need for joint reconstruction.

CHONDROMYXOID FIBROMA

Like other benign cartilaginous lesions, this is seen mainly in adolescents and young adults. It may occur in any bone but is more common in those of the lower limb.

Patients seldom complain and the lesion is usually discovered by accident or after a pathological fracture.

X-rays are very characteristic: there is a rounded or ovoid radiolucent area placed eccentrically in the metaphysis; in children it may extend up to or even slightly across the physis. The endosteal margin may be scalloped, but is almost always bounded by a dense zone of reactive bone extending tongue-like towards the diaphysis. The cortex may be asymmetrically expanded. Sometimes there is calcification in the 'vacant' area.

Pathology Although the lesion looks 'cystic' on x-ray, it contains mucinous material and bits of cartilage. Histologically three types of tissue can usually be identified: patches of myxomatous tissue with delicate, stellate cells; islands of hyaline cartilage; and

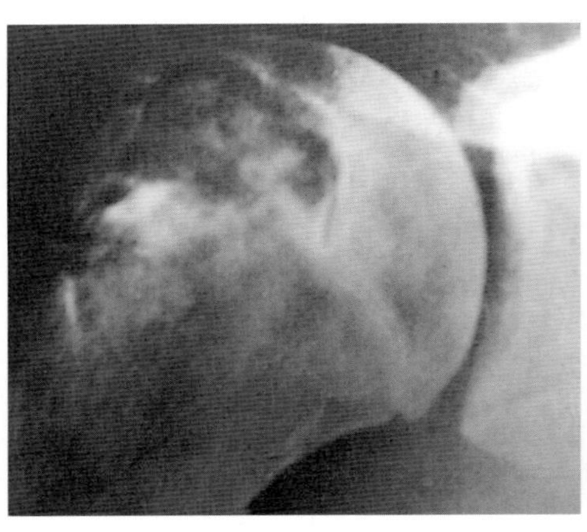

(a)

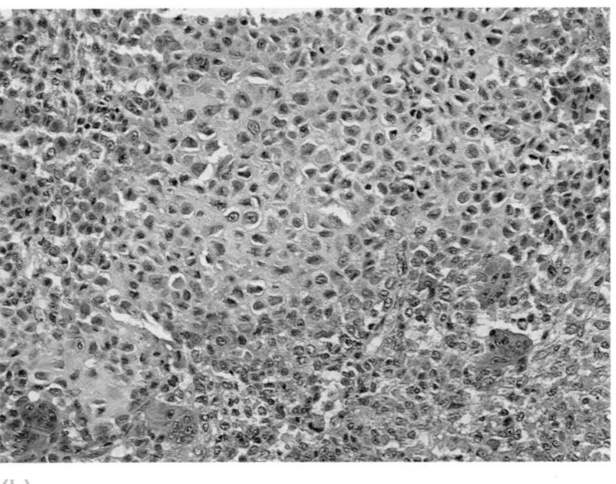

(b)

9.10 Chondroblastoma (a) X-ray shows a cyst-like lesion occupying the epiphysis, and sometimes extending across the physis into the adjacent bone. (b) The characteristic features in this photomicrograph are the more faintly staining islands of chondroid tissue composed of round cells ('chondroblasts') and scattered multinucleated giant cells. (×300)

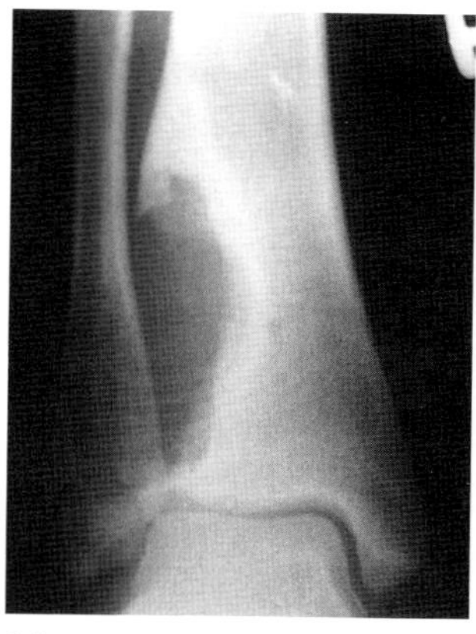

(a)

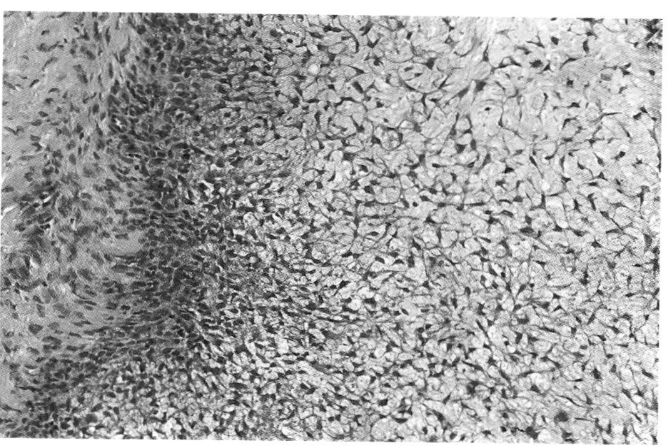

(b)

9.11 Chrondromyxoid fibroma (a) The x-ray is quite typical: there is an eccentric cyst-like lesion with a densely sclerotic endosteal margin often extending like a tongue towards the diaphysis. (b) The section shows predominantly myxomatous cells and fibrous tissue; elsewhere chondroid tissue and giant cells are more obvious. (×300)

areas of fibrous tissue with cells of varying degrees of maturity.

Malignant change has been recorded but this is extremely rare.

Treatment Where feasible, the lesion should be excised but often one can do no more than a thorough curettage followed by autogenous bone grafting. There is a considerable risk of recurrence; if repeated operations are needed, care should be taken to prevent damage to the physis (in children) or the nearby joint surface.

Osteochondroma (cartilage-capped exostosis)

This, one of the commonest 'tumours' of bone, is a developmental lesion which starts as a small overgrowth of cartilage at the edge of the physeal plate and develops by endochondral ossification into a bony protuberance still covered by the cap of cartilage. Any bone that develops in cartilage may be involved; the commonest sites are the fast-growing ends of long bones and the crest of the ilium. In long bones, growth leaves the bump stranded further down the metaphysis. Here it may go on growing but at the end of the normal growth period for that bone it stops enlarging. *Any further enlargement after the end of the growth period is suggestive of malignant transformation.*

The patient is usually a teenager or young adult when the lump is first discovered. Occasionally there is pain due to an overlying bursa or impingement on soft tissues, or, rarely, paraesthesia due to stretching of an adjacent nerve.

The *x-ray* appearance is pathognomonic. There is a well-defined exostosis emerging from the metaphysis, its base co-extensive with the parent bone. It looks smaller than it feels because the cartilage cap is usually invisible on x-ray; however, large lesions undergo cartilage degeneration and calcification and then the x-ray shows the bony exostosis surrounded by clouds of calcified material.

Multiple lesions may develop as part of a heritable disorder – *hereditary multiple exostosis* – in which there are also features of abnormal bone growth resulting in characteristic deformities (see Chapter 8).

Pathology At operation the cartilage cap is seen surmounting a narrow base or pedicle of bone. The cap consists of simple hyaline cartilage; in a growing exostosis the deeper cartilage cells are arranged in columns, giving rise to the formation of endochondral new bone. Large lesions may have a 'cauliflower' appearance, with degeneration and calcification in the centre of the cartilage cap.

Complications The incidence of *malignant transformation* is difficult to assess because troublesome lesions are so often removed before they show histological features of malignancy. Figures usually quoted are 1 per cent for solitary lesions and 6 per cent for multiple.

Features suggestive of malignant change are: (1) enlargement of the cartilage cap in successive examinations; (2) a bulky cartilage cap (more than 1 cm in thickness); (3) irregularly scattered flecks of calcification within the cartilage cap; and (4) spread into the surrounding soft tissues. MRI may be needed to reveal these changes.

Treatment If the tumour causes symptoms it should be excised; if, in an adult, it has recently become bigger or painful then operation is urgent, for these features suggest malignancy. This is seen most often with pelvic exostoses – not because they are inherently different but because considerable enlargement may, for long periods, pass unnoticed. If there are suspicious features, further imaging and staging should be carried out before doing a biopsy. If the histology is that of 'benign' cartilage but the tumour is known for

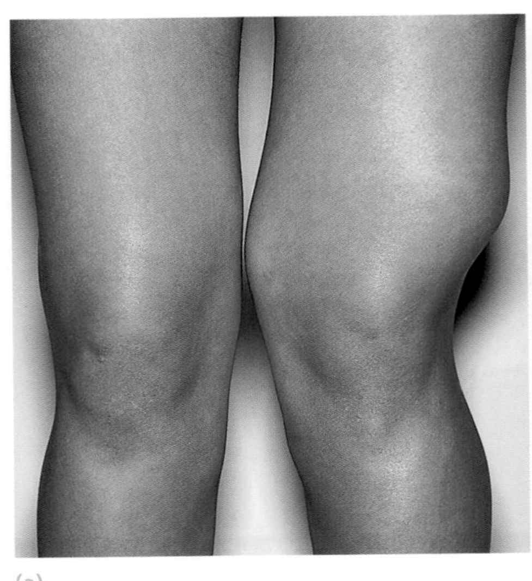

(a)

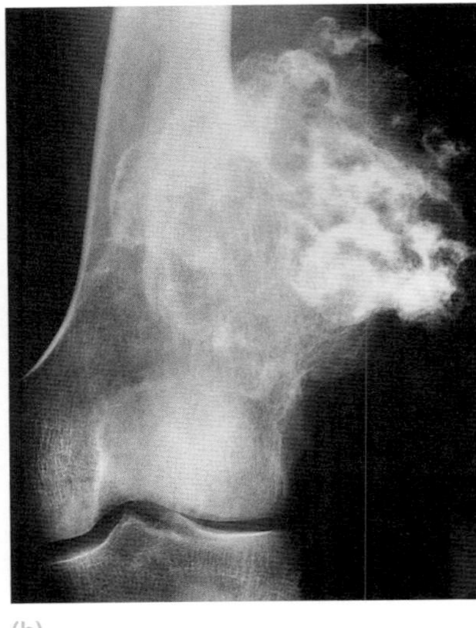

(b)

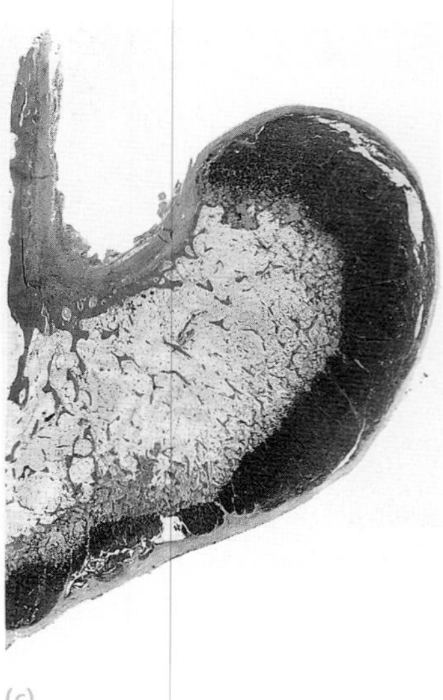

(c)

9.12 Osteochondroma (a) A young girl presented with this lump on her leg. It felt bony hard. (b) X-ray examination showed the typical features of a large cartilage-capped exostosis; of course the cartilage cap does not show on x-ray unless it is calcified. The bony part may be sessile, pedunculated or cauliflower-like. (c) Histological sections show that the exostosis is always covered by a hyaline cartilage cap from which the bony excrescence grows.

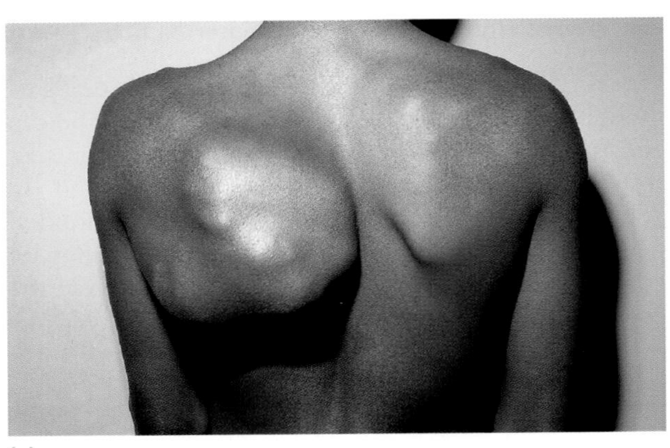

(a)

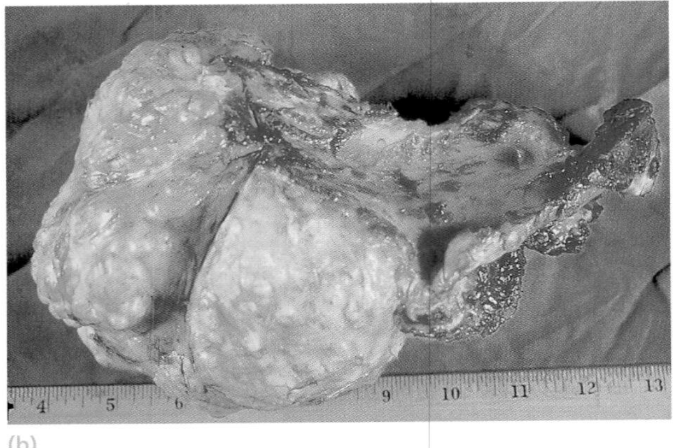

(b)

9.13 Osteochondroma – treatment (a) This 20-year-old man had known about the lump on his left scapula for many years. He stopped growing at the age of 18 but the tumour continued to enlarge. (b) Despite the benign histology in the biopsy, the tumour together with most of the scapula was removed; sections taken from the depths of the lesion showed atypical cells suggestive of malignant change.

certain to be enlarging after the end of the growth period, it should be treated as a chondrosarcoma.

SIMPLE BONE CYST

This lesion (also known as a *solitary cyst* or *unicameral bone cyst*) appears during childhood, typically in the metaphysis of one of the long bones and most commonly in the proximal humerus or femur. It is not a tumour, it tends to heal spontaneously and it is seldom seen in adults. The condition is usually discovered after a pathological fracture or as an incidental finding on x-ray.

X-rays show a well-demarcated radiolucent area in the metaphysis, often extending up to the physeal plate; the cortex may be thinned and the bone expanded.

Diagnosis is usually not difficult but other cyst-like lesions may need to be excluded. Non-osteogenic fibroma, fibrous dysplasia and the benign cartilage tumours are solid and merely look cystic on x-ray. In doubtful cases a needle can be inserted into the lesion under x-ray control: with a simple cyst, straw-coloured fluid will be withdrawn. Very seldom will there be any need for biopsy. However, if curettage is thought to be necessary, material from the cyst should be submitted for examination.

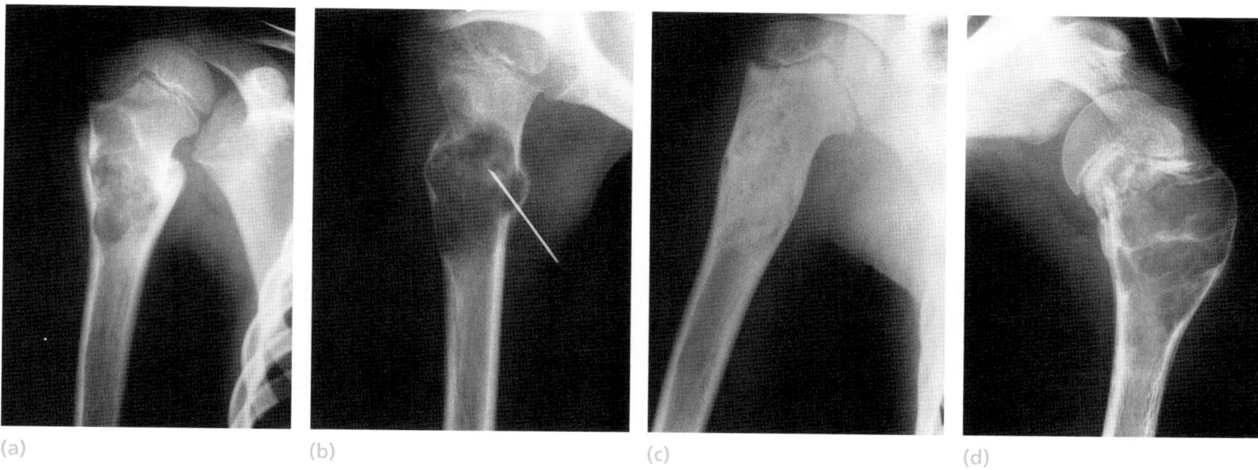

(a) (b) (c) (d)

9.14 Simple bone cysts (a) A typical solitary (or unicameral) cyst – on the shaft side of the physis and expanding the cortex. (b) Injection with methylprednisolone, and (c) healing. (d) Fracture through a cyst.

Pathology The lining membrane consists of flimsy fibrous tissue, often containing giant cells. In an actively growing cyst, there is osteoclastic resorption of the adjacent bone.

Treatment Treatment depends on whether the cyst is symptomatic, actively growing or involved in a fracture. *Asymptomatic lesions* in older children can be left alone but the patient should be cautioned to avoid injury which might cause a fracture. *'Active' cysts* (those in young children, usually abutting against the physeal plate and obviously enlarging in sequential x-rays) should be treated, in the first instance, by aspiration of fluid and injection of 80–160 mg of methylprednisolone or autogenous bone marrow. This often stops further enlargement and leads to healing of the cyst.

If the cyst goes on enlarging, or if there is a *pathological fracture*, the cavity should be thoroughly cleaned by curettage and then packed with bone chips, but great care should be taken not to damage the nearby physeal plate. If the risk of fracture is thought to be high, prophylactic internal fixation should be applied.

There is always the risk that the cyst will recur and more than one operation may be needed.

Aneurysmal bone cyst

Aneurysmal bone cyst may be encountered at any age and in almost any bone, though more often in young adults and in the long-bone metaphyses. Usually it arises spontaneously but it may appear after degeneration or haemorrhage in some other lesion.

With expanding lesions, patients may complain of pain. Occasionally, a large cyst may cause a visible or palpable swelling of the bone.

X-rays show a well-defined radiolucent cyst, often trabeculated and eccentrically placed. In a growing tubular bone it is always situated in the metaphysis and therefore may resemble a simple cyst or one of the other cyst-like lesions. Occasional sites include vertebrae and the flat bones. In an adult an aneurysmal bone cyst may be mistaken for a giant-cell tumour

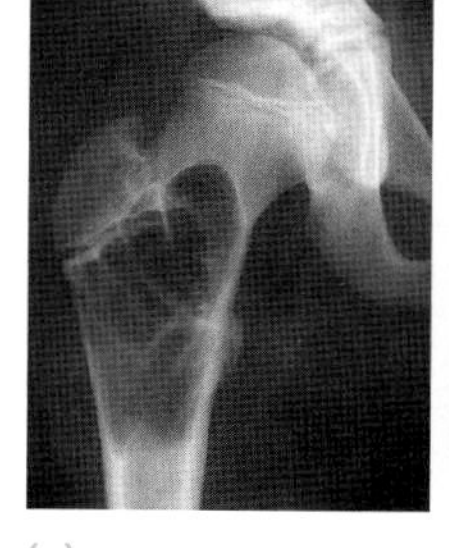

(a)

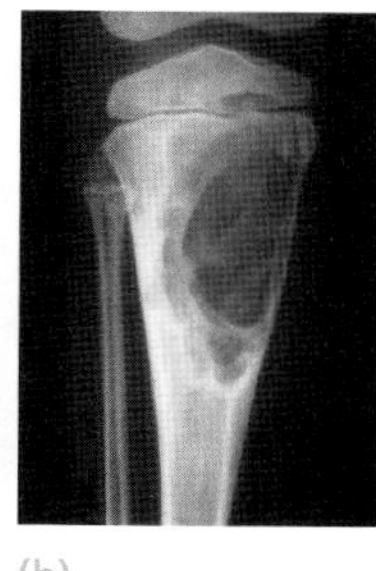

(b)

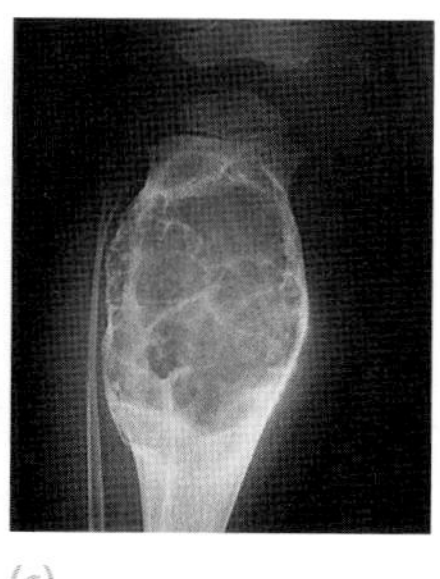

(c)

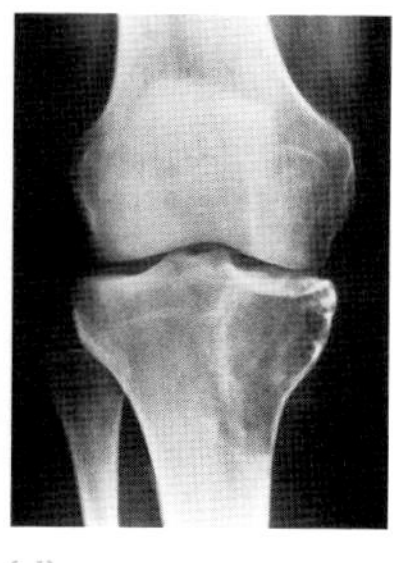

(d)

9.15 Cyst-like lesions (a) *Simple bone cyst*. Fills the medullary cavity but does not expand the bone. (b) *Chondromyxoid fibroma*. Looks cystic but it is actually a radiolucent benign tumour; always in the metaphysis; hard boundary tailing off towards the diaphysis. (c) *Aneurysmal bone cyst*. Expansile cystic tumour, always on the metaphyseal side of the physis. (d) *Giant-cell tumour*. Hardly ever appears before epiphysis has fused, the pathognomonic feature is that it extends right up to the subarticular bone plate; sometimes malignant.

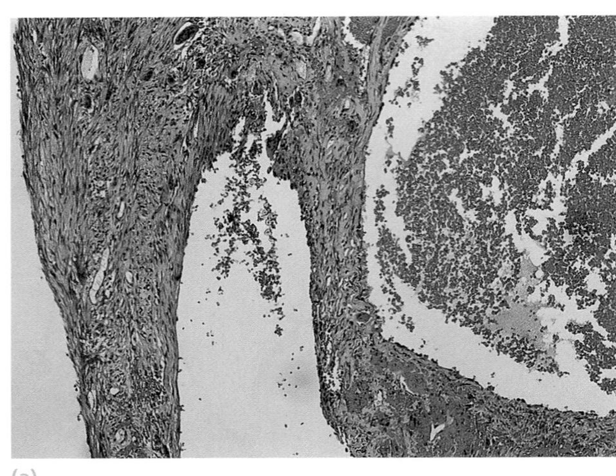

(a)

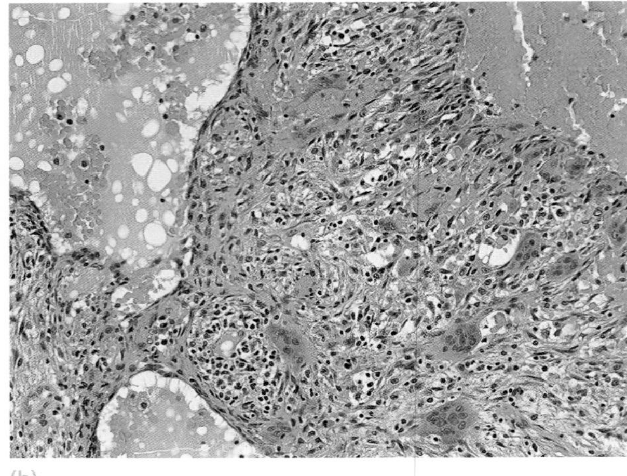

(b)

9.16 Aneurysmal bone cyst – histology (a) The cyst contained blood and was lined by loose fibrous tissue containing numerous giant cells. (×120) (b) A high-power view of the same. (×300)

but, unlike the latter, it usually does not extend right up to the articular margin. Occasionally it causes marked ballooning of the bone end.

Pathology When the cyst is opened it is found to contain clotted blood, and during curettage there may be considerable bleeding from the fleshy lining membrane. Histologically the lining consists of fibrous tissue with vascular spaces, deposits of haemosiderin and multinucleated giant cells. Occasionally the appearances so closely resemble those of giant-cell tumour that only the most experienced pathologists can confidently make the diagnosis. Malignant transformation does not occur.

Treatment The cyst should be carefully opened, thoroughly curetted and then packed with bone grafts. Sometimes the graft is resorbed and the cyst recurs, necessitating a second or third operation. In these cases, packing with methylmethacrylate cement may be more effective. However, if the cyst is in a 'safe' area (i.e. where there is no risk of fracture) there is no hurry to re-operate; the lesion occasionally heals spontaneously (Malghem et al., 1989).

9.17 Giant-cell tumours The tumour always abuts against the joint margin.

GIANT-CELL TUMOUR

Giant-cell tumour, which represents 5 per cent of all primary bone tumours, is a lesion of uncertain origin that appears in mature bone, most commonly in the distal femur, proximal tibia, proximal humerus and distal radius, though other bones also may be affected. It is hardly ever seen before closure of the nearby physis and characteristically it extends right up to the subarticular bone plate. Rarely, there are multiple lesions.

The patient is usually a young adult who complains of pain at the end of a long bone; sometimes there is slight swelling. A history of trauma is not uncommon

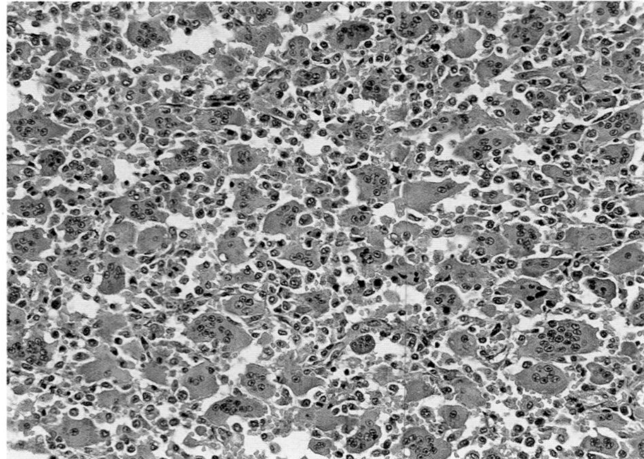

9.18 Giant-cell tumour – histology A low-power view of the biopsy shows the abundant multinucleated giant cells lying in a stroma composed of round and polyhedral tumour cells. There are numerous mitotic figures.

and pathological fracture occurs in 10–15 per cent of cases. On examination there may be a palpable mass with warmth of the overlying tissues.

X-rays show a radiolucent area situated eccentrically at the end of a long bone and bounded by the subchondral bone plate. The endosteal margin may be quite obvious, but in aggressive lesions it is ill-defined. The centre sometimes has a soap-bubble appearance due to ridging of the surrounding bone. The cortex is thin and sometimes ballooned; aggressive lesions extend into the soft tissue. The appearance of a 'cystic' lesion in mature bone, extending right up to the subchondral plate, is so characteristic that the diagnosis is seldom in doubt. However, it is prudent to obtain estimations of blood calcium, phosphate and alkaline phosphatise concentrations so as exclude an unusual 'brown tumour' associated with hyperparathyroidism.

Because of the tumour's potential for aggressive behaviour, *detailed staging procedures* are essential. CT scans and MRI will reveal the extent of the tumour, both within the bone and beyond. It is important to establish whether the articular surface has been breached.

Biopsy is essential. This can be done either as a frozen section before proceeding with operative treatment or (especially if a more extensive operation is contemplated) as a separate procedure.

Pathology The tumour has a reddish, fleshy appearance; it comes away in pieces quite easily when curetted but is difficult to remove completely from the surrounding bone. Aggressive lesions have a poorly defined edge and extend well into the surrounding bone. Histologically the striking feature is an abundance of multinucleated giant cells scattered on a background of stromal cells with little or no visible intercellular tissue. Aggressive lesions tend to show more cellular atypia and mitotic figures, but histological grading is unreliable as a predictor of tumour behaviour.

Rarely metastases are discovered in the lungs. The tumour has the potential to transform into an osteosarcoma.

Treatment Well-confined, slow-growing lesions with benign histology can safely be treated by thorough curettage and 'stripping' of the cavity with burrs and gouges, followed by swabbing with hydrogen peroxide or by the application of liquid nitrogen; the cavity is then packed with bone chips. More aggressive tumours, and recurrent lesions, should be treated by excision followed, if necessary, by bone grafting or prosthetic replacement. Tumours in awkward sites (e.g. the spine) may be difficult to eradicate; supplementary radiotherapy is sometimes recommended, but it carries a significant risk of causing malignant transformation.

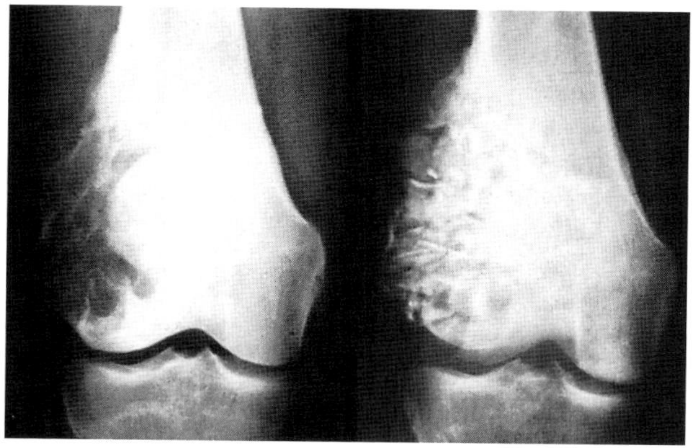

(a)

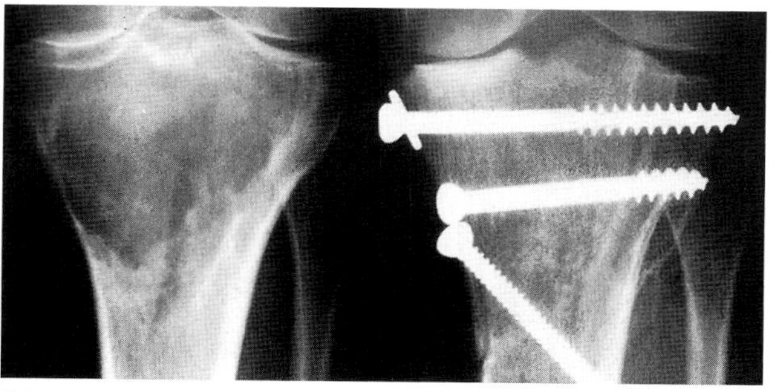

(b)

9.19 Giant-cell tumour – treatment (a) Excision and bone grafts. (b) Block resection and replacement with a large allograft.

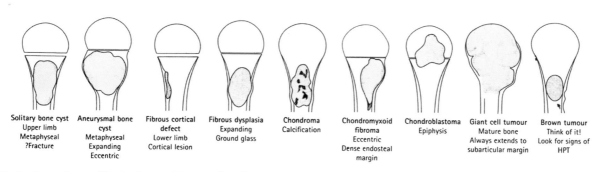

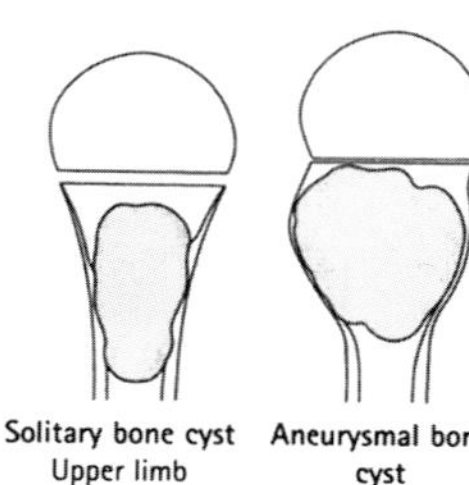
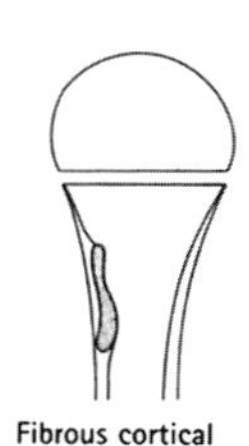
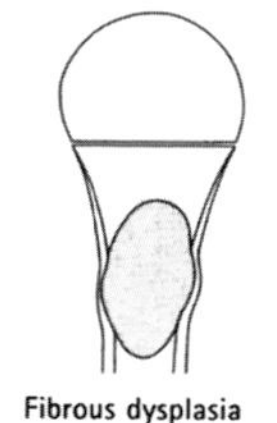
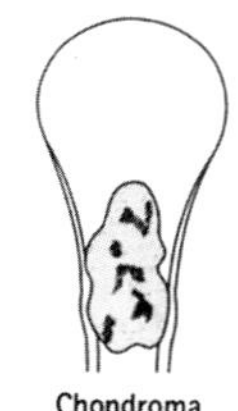
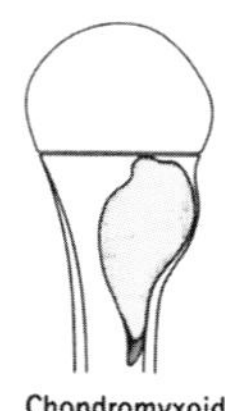
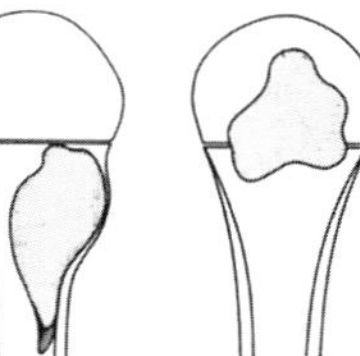
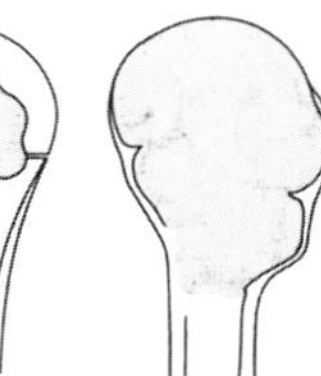
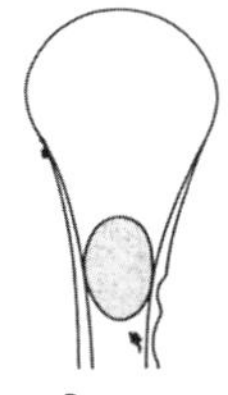

9.20 Cysts and cyst-like lesions of bone Thumb-nail sketches of lesions which appear as 'cysts' on x-ray examination.

GIANT-CELL SARCOMA

Giant-cell sarcoma is an unequivocally malignant lesion with x-ray features like those of a highly aggressive benign giant-cell tumour. There is a high risk of metastasis and treatment requires wide, or even radical, resection.

Eosinophilic granuloma and histiocytosis

Histiocytosis-X defines an unusual group of disorders in which cells of the reticuloendothelial system (histiocytes and eosinophils) form granulomatous collections which may cause osteolytic lesions resembling bone tumours.

Eosinophilic granuloma is the commonest of these conditions, and the only one presenting as a pure bone lesion. Marrow-containing bone is resorbed and one or more lytic lesions may appear in the flat bones or the metaphyses of long bones. The patient is usually a child; there is seldom any complaint of pain and the condition is discovered incidentally or after a pathological fracture.

X-ray shows a well-demarcated oval area of radiolucency within the bone; sometimes this is associated with marked reactive sclerosis. There may be multiple lesions and in the skull they have a characteristic punched-out appearance. Vertebral collapse may result in a flat wedge (*vertebra plana*) which is pathognomonic.

The condition usually heals spontaneously and is therefore rarely seen in adults. Occasionally, however, a solitary lesion may herald the onset of one of the generalized disorders (see below). Operation is usually done to obtain a biopsy; if the lesion is easily accessible it may be completely excised or curetted; if not, radiotherapy is effective.

Hand–Schüller–Christian disease is a disseminated form of the same condition. The patient is a child, usually with widespread lesions involving the skull, vertebral bodies, liver and spleen. There may be anaemia and a tendency to recurrent infection.

Individual lesions can be treated by curettage or radiotherapy; however, complete remission is very unlikely.

Letterer–Siwe disease is an extremely rare (and severe) form of histiocytosis. It is seen in infants and usually progresses rapidly to a fatal outcome.

Haemangioma

Osseous haemangiomas consist of vascular channels (capillary, venous or cavernous) and are usually seen in middle-aged patients, the spine being the commonest site. They are usually symptomless and discovered accidentally when the back is x-rayed for some other reason. However, if the patient does have backache, the haemangioma is likely to be blamed.

The *x-ray* shows coarse vertical trabeculation (the so-called 'corduroy appearance') in the vertebral body. Other sites include the skull and pelvis where the appearance occasionally suggests malignancy, but there is no associated cortical or medullary destruction. Rarely the presenting feature may be a pathological fracture.

If operation is needed there is a risk of profuse bleeding, and embolization may be a useful preliminary.

Osteolysis ('disappearing bones')

In massive osteolysis (Gorham's disease) there is progressive disappearance of bone, associated with hae-

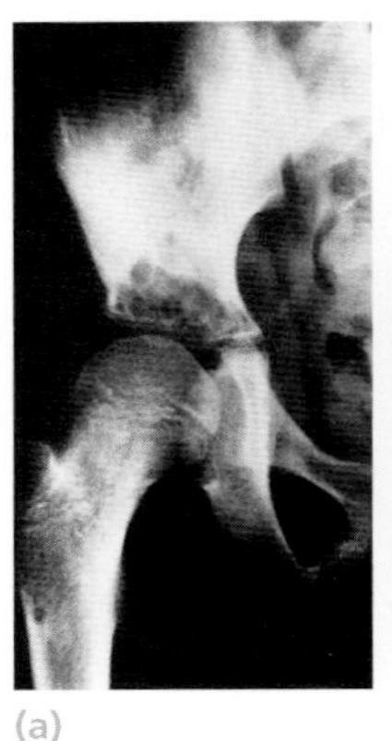
(a)

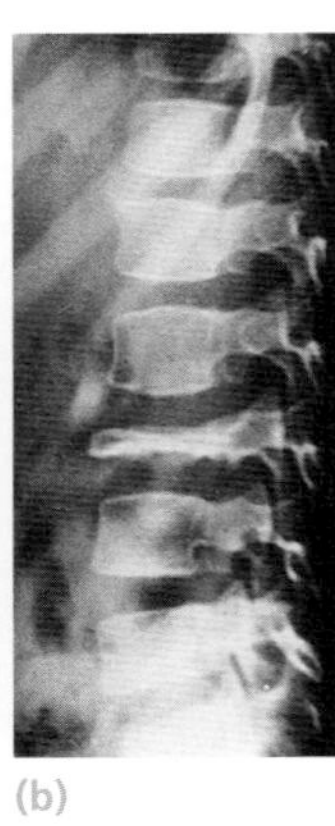
(b)

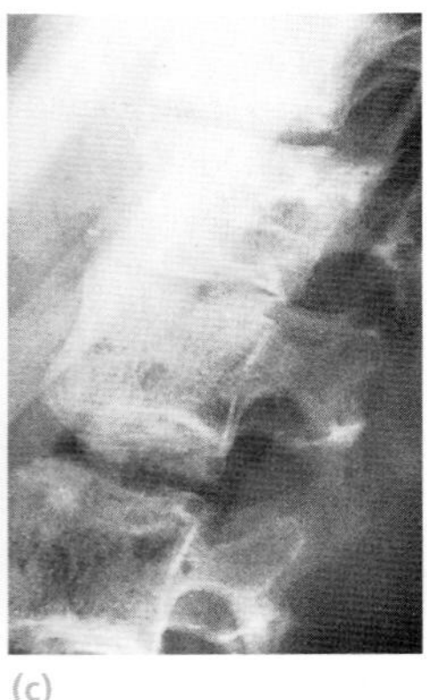
(c)

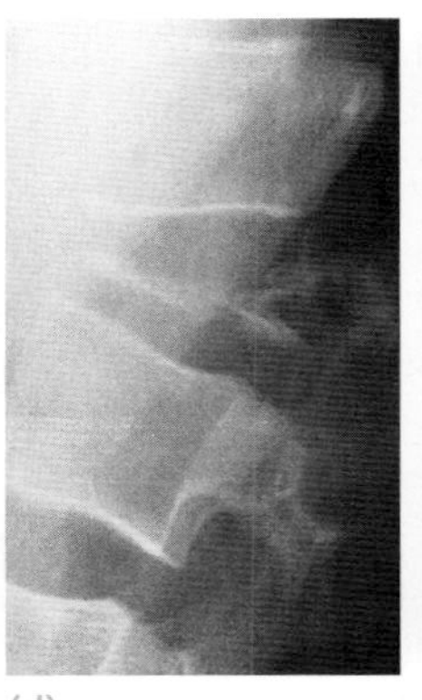
(d)

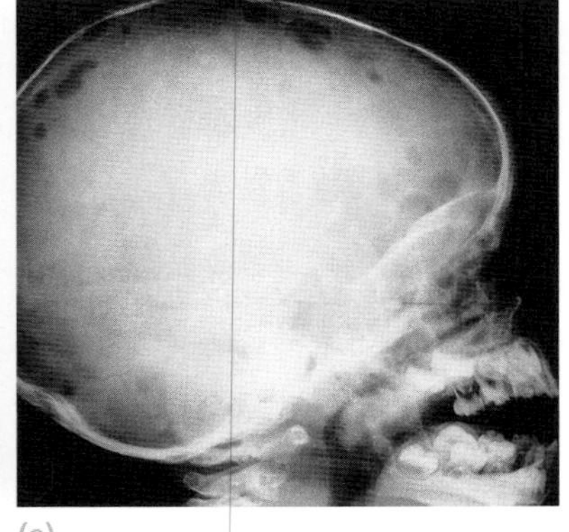
(e)

9.21 Histiocytosis-X (a) An eosinophilic granuloma of the ischium which went on to spontaneous healing. (b) Completely flattened vertebral body with discs of normal height, probably due to eosinophilic granuloma. (c,d) Two stages in the development of vertebral flattening from an eosinophilic granuloma. (e) Hand–Schüller–Christian disease, which typically affects the skull.

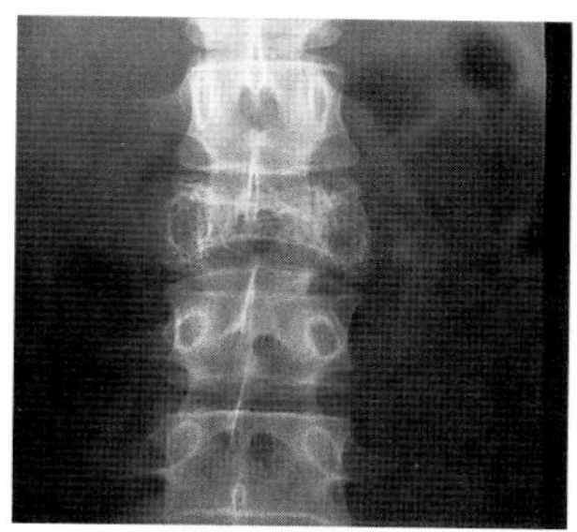
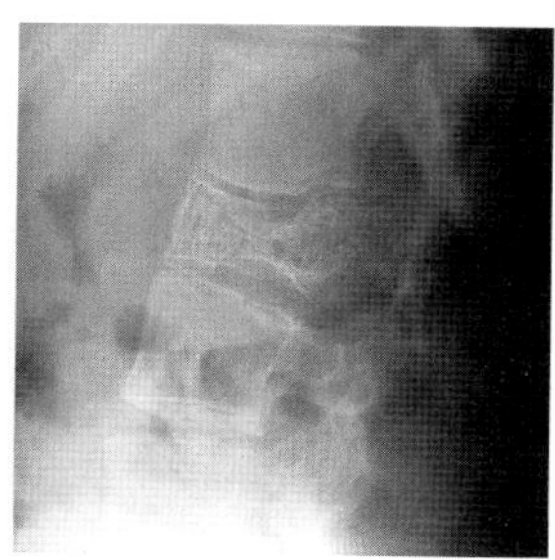

9.22 Haemangioma Most of these tumours are symptomless and discovered accidentally during x-ray examination for another reason, but in this case the vertebra collapsed and the patient presented with back pain.

mangiomatosis or multiple lymphangiectases. Usually the progression involves contiguous bones, but occasionally multiple sites are affected. Patients may present with mild pain or with a pathological fracture. No effective treatment is known, but spontaneous arrest has been described. Occasionally, however, the process spreads to vital structures and the outcome is fatal.

PRIMARY MALIGNANT BONE TUMOURS

CHONDROSARCOMA

Chondrosarcoma is one of the commonest malignant tumours originating in bone. The highest incidence is in the fourth and fifth decades and men are affected more often than women.

These tumours are slow-growing and are usually present for many months before being discovered. Patients may complain of a dull ache or a gradually enlarging lump. Medullary lesions may present as a pathological fracture.

Although chondrosarcoma may develop in any of the bones that normally develop in cartilage, almost 50 per cent appear in the metaphysis of one of the long tubular bones, mostly in the lower limbs. The next most common sites are the pelvis and the ribs. Despite the relatively frequent occurrence of benign cartilage tumours in the small bones of the hands and feet, malignant lesions are rare at these sites.

Chondrosarcomas take various forms, usually designated according to: (a) their location in the bone (*central* or *peripheral*); (b) whether they develop without precedent (*primary chondrosarcoma*) or by malignant change in a pre-existing benign lesion (*secondary chondrosarcoma*); and (c) the predominant *cell type* in the tumour.

By far the majority of chondrosarcomas fall into two well-defined categories: *central tumours* occupying the medullary cavity of the bone, and so-called *'peripheral tumours'* growing out from the cortex. Less common varieties are *juxtacortical chondrosarcoma*, *clear-cell chondrosarcoma* and *mesenchymal chondrosarcoma*.

Central chondrosarcoma The tumour develops in the medullary cavity of either tubular or flat bones, most commonly at the proximal end of the femur or in the innominate bone of the pelvis. *X-rays* show an expanded, somewhat radiolucent area in the bone, with flecks of increased density due to calcification within the tumour. Aggressive lesions may take on a globular appearance with scalloping or destruction of the cortex.

When a benign medullary chondroma (enchondroma) undergoes malignant transformation, it is difficult to be sure that the lesion was not a slowly evolving sarcoma from the outset.

Peripheral chondrosarcoma This tumour usually arises in the cartilage cap of an exostosis (osteochondroma) that has been present since childhood. Exostoses of the pelvis and scapula seem to be more susceptible than others to malignant change, but perhaps this is simply because the site allows a tumour to grow without being detected and removed at an early stage. *X-rays* show the bony exostosis, often surmounted by clouds of patchy calcification in the otherwise unseen lobulated cartilage cap. A tumour that is very large and calcification that is very fluffy and poorly outlined are suspicious features, but the clearest sign of malignant change is a demonstrable progressive enlargement of an osteochondroma after the end of normal bone growth. MRI is the best means of showing the size and internal features of the cartilage cap.

Juxtacortical (periosteal) chondrosarcoma Here the lesion appears as an excrescence on the surface of one of the tubular bones – usually the femur. It arises from the outermost layers of the cortex, deep to the periosteum. *X-ray changes* comprise features of both a chondrosarcoma and a periosteal osteosarcoma: an outgrowth from the bone surface, often containing flecks of calcification, as well as 'sunray' streaks and new-bone formation at the margins of the stripped periosteum. The dominant cell type is chondroblastic but there may also be sparse osteoid formation, leading one to doubt whether this is a cartilage tumour or a non-aggressive osteosarcoma.

Clear-cell chondrosarcoma There is some doubt as to whether this rare tumour is really a chondrosarcoma. In some respects the tumour resembles an aggressive chondroblastoma (e.g. its typical location in the head of the femur rather than the metaphysis). However, despite the fact that it is very slow-growing, it does eventually metastasize.

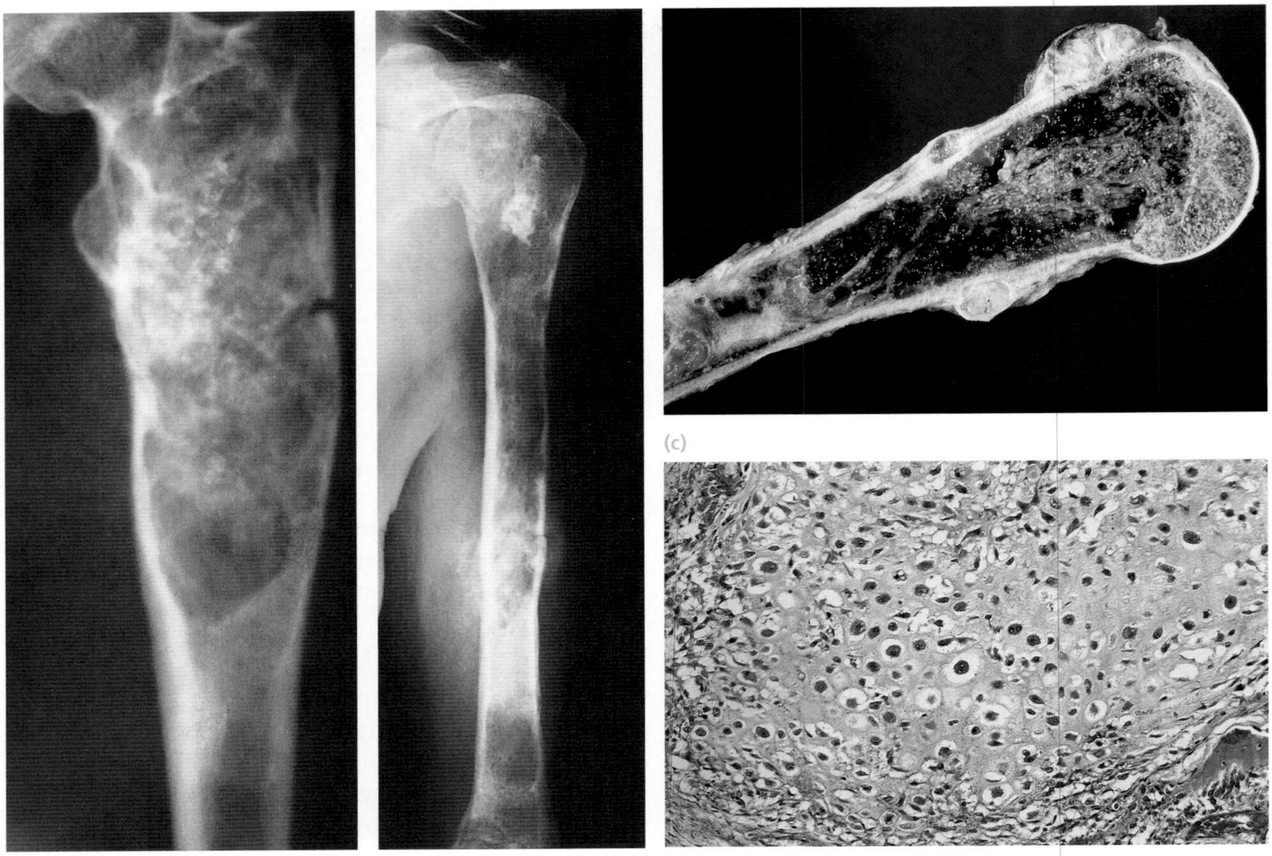

(a) (b) (c) (d)

9.23 Central chondrosaroma (a) Typical x-ray of a central chondrosarcoma of the femur. (b) In this case the patient presented with a pathological fracture of the humerus. X-rays showed rarefaction of the bone with central flecks of calcification. At the fracture site the lesion extends into the soft tissues. (c) Radical resection was carried out. Pale glistening cartilage tissue was found in the medullary cavity and, in several places, spreading beyond the cortex. Much of the bone is occupied by haemorrhagic tissue. (d) The histological sections show lobules of highly atypical cartilage cells, including binucleate cells.

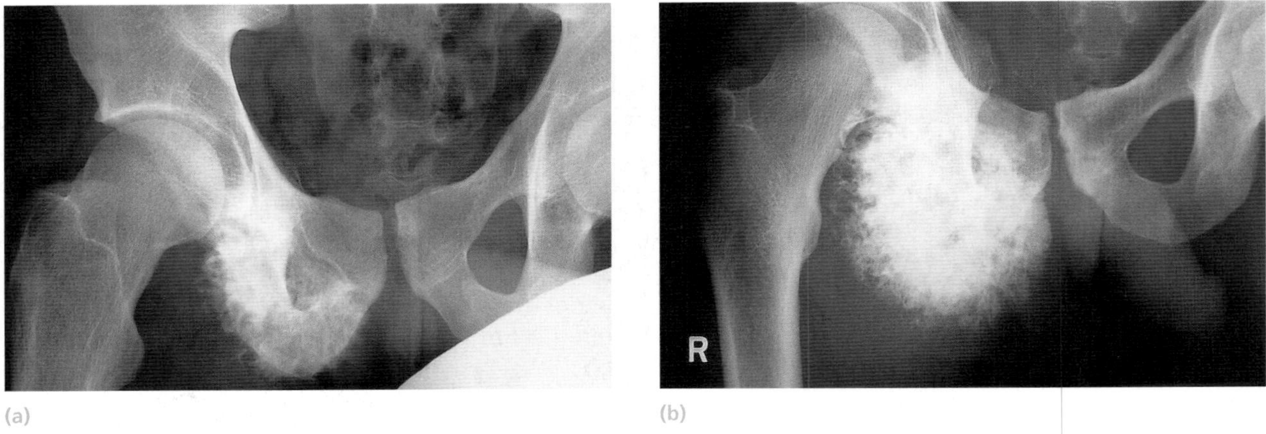

(a) (b)

9.24 Chondrosarcoma At the age of 20 years, this young man complained of pain in the right groin; x-ray showed an osteochondroma of the right inferior pubic ramus. (a) A biopsy showed 'benign' cartilage but a year later the tumour had doubled its size (b), a clear sign that it was malignant.

Mesenchymal chondrosarcoma This is an equally controversial entity. It tends to occur in younger individuals and in about 50 per cent of cases the tumour lies in the soft tissues outside an adjacent bone. The x-ray appearances are similar to those of the common types of chondrosarcoma but the clinical behaviour of the tumour is usually more aggressive. Histology shows a mixture of mesenchymal cells and chondroid tissue.

Staging

If a chondrosarcoma is suspected, full staging procedures should be employed. CT scans and MRI must be carried out before performing a biopsy.

Pathology

A biopsy is essential to confirm the diagnosis. However, low-grade chondrosarcoma may show histological features no different from those of an aggressive benign cartilaginous lesion. High-grade tumours are more cellular, and there may be obvious abnormal features of the cells, such as plumpness, hyperchromasia and mitoses.

Treatment

Since most chondrosarcomas are slow-growing and metastasize late, they present the ideal case for wide excision and prosthetic replacement, provided it is certain that the lesion can be completely removed without exposing the tumour and without causing an unacceptable loss of function; in that case amputation may be preferable. In some cases isolated pulmonary metastases can be resected. The tumour does not respond to either radiotherapy or chemotherapy.

Prognosis is determined largely by the cellular grade and the resection margin. There is a tendency for these tumours to recur late and the patient should therefore be followed up for 10 years or longer.

OSTEOSARCOMA

In its classic (intramedullary) form, osteosarcoma is a highly malignant tumour arising within the bone and spreading rapidly outwards to the periosteum and surrounding soft tissues. It is said to occur predominantly in children and adolescents, but epidemiological studies suggest that between 1972 and 1981 the age of presentation rose significantly (Stark et al., 1990). It may affect any bone but most commonly involves the long-bone metaphyses, especially around the knee and at the proximal end of the humerus.

Pain is usually the first symptom; it is constant, worse at night and gradually increases in severity. Sometimes the patient presents with a lump. Pathological fracture is rare. On examination there may be little to find except local tenderness. In later cases there is a palpable mass and the overlying tissues may appear swollen and inflamed. The ESR is usually raised and there may be an increase in serum alkaline phosphatase.

X-rays

The x-ray appearances are variable: hazy osteolytic areas may alternate with unusually dense osteoblastic areas. The endosteal margin is poorly defined. Often the cortex is breached and the tumour extends into

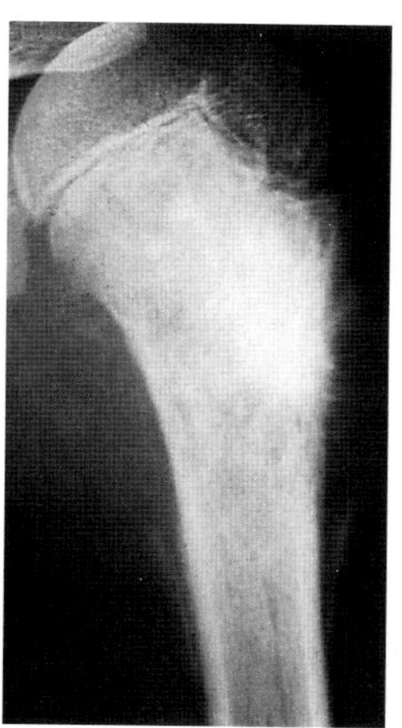
(a)

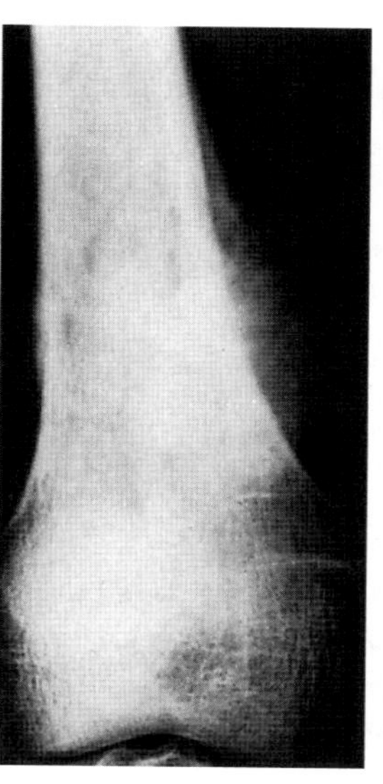
(b)

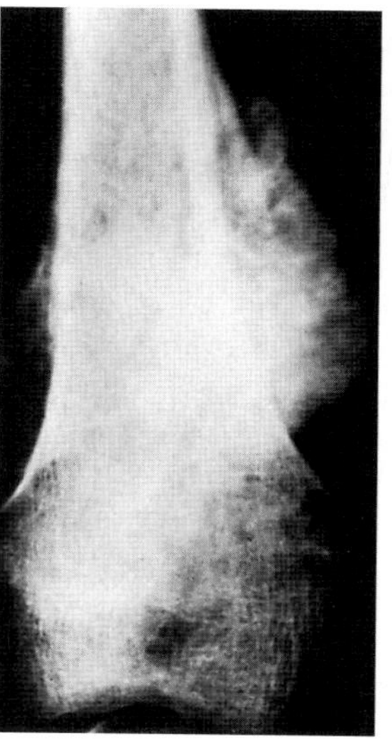
(c)

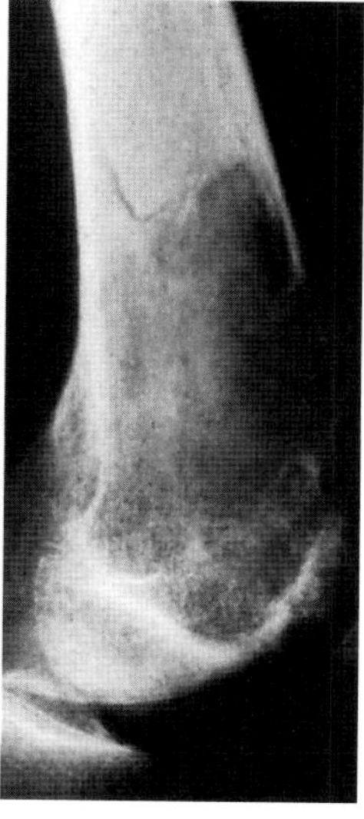
(d)

9.25 Osteosarcoma (a) The metaphyseal site; increased density, cortical erosion and periosteal reaction are characteristic. (b) Sunray spicules and Codman's triangle; (c) the same patient after radiotherapy. (d) A predominantly osteolytic tumour.

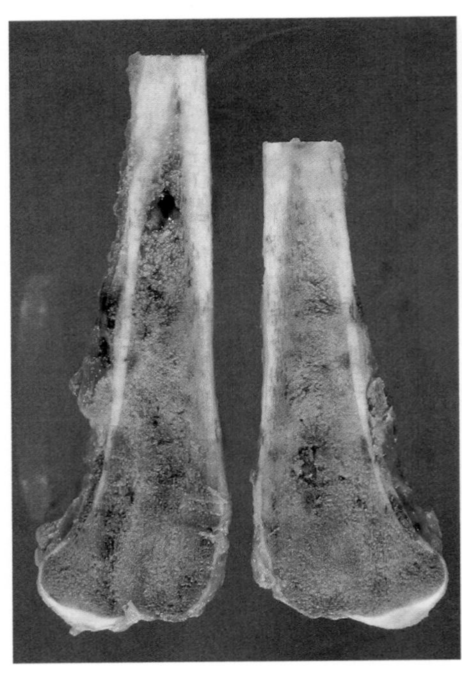

(a)

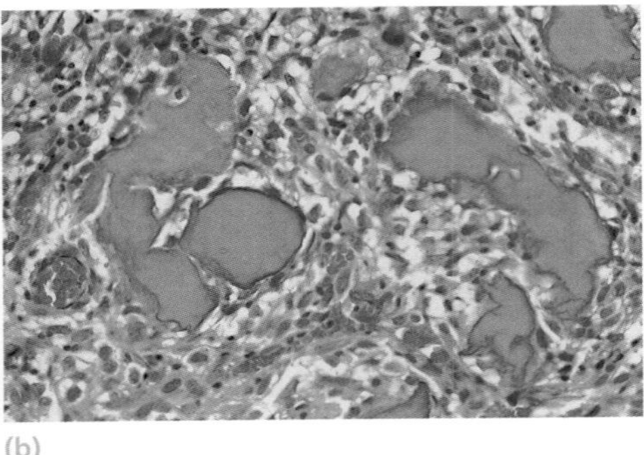

(b)

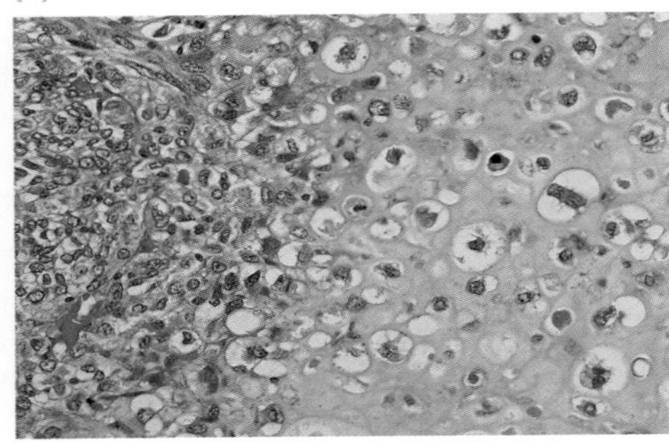

(c)

9.26 Osteosarcoma – pathology (a) After resection this lesion was cut in half; pale tumour tissue is seen occupying the distal third of the femur and extending through the cortex. **(b)** The dominant features in the histological sections were malignant stromal tissue showing osteoid formation (pink masses). (×480) **(c)** The same tumour showed areas of chondroblastic differentiation. (×480)

the adjacent tissues; when this happens, streaks of new bone appear, radiating outwards from the cortex – the so-called 'sunburst' effect. Where the tumour emerges from the cortex, reactive new bone forms at the angles of periosteal elevation (Codman's triangle). While both the sunburst appearance and Codman's triangle are typical of osteosarcoma, they may occasionally be seen in other rapidly growing tumours.

Diagnosis and staging

In most cases the diagnosis can be made with confidence on the x-ray appearances. However, atypical lesions can cause confusion. Conditions to be excluded are post-traumatic swellings, infection, stress fracture and the more aggressive 'cystic' lesions.

Other imaging studies are essential for staging purposes. Radioisotope scans may show up skip lesions, but a negative scan does not exclude them. CT and MRI reliably show the extent of the tumour. Chest x-rays are done routinely, but pulmonary CT is a much more sensitive detector of lung metastases. About 10 per cent of patients have pulmonary metastases by the time they are first seen.

A biopsy should always be carried out before commencing treatment; it must be carefully planned to allow for complete removal of the tract when the tumour is excised.

Pathology

The tumour is usually situated in the metaphysis of a long bone, where it destroys and replaces normal bone. Areas of bone loss and cavitation alternate with dense patches of abnormal new bone. The tumour extends within the medulla and across the physeal plate. There may be obvious spread into the soft tissues with ossification at the periosteal margins and streaks of new bone extending into the extraosseous mass.

The histological appearances show considerable variation: some areas may have the characteristic spindle cells with a pink-staining osteoid matrix; others may contain cartilage cells or fibroblastic tissue with little or no osteoid. Several samples may have to be examined; pathologists are reluctant to commit themselves to the diagnosis unless they see evidence of osteoid formation.

Treatment

The appalling prognosis that formerly attended this tumour has markedly improved, partly as a result of better diagnostic and staging procedures, and possibly because the average age of the patients has increased, but mainly because of advances in chemotherapy to control metastatic spread. However, it is still important to eradicate the primary lesion completely; the mortality rate after local recurrence is far worse than following effective ablation at the first encounter.

The principles of treatment are outlined on page 192. After clinical assessment and advanced imaging, the patient is admitted to a special centre for biopsy. The lesion will probably be graded IIA or IIB. Multi-agent neoadjuvant chemotherapy is given for 8–12 weeks and then, provided the tumour is resectable and there are no skip lesions, a wide resection is car-

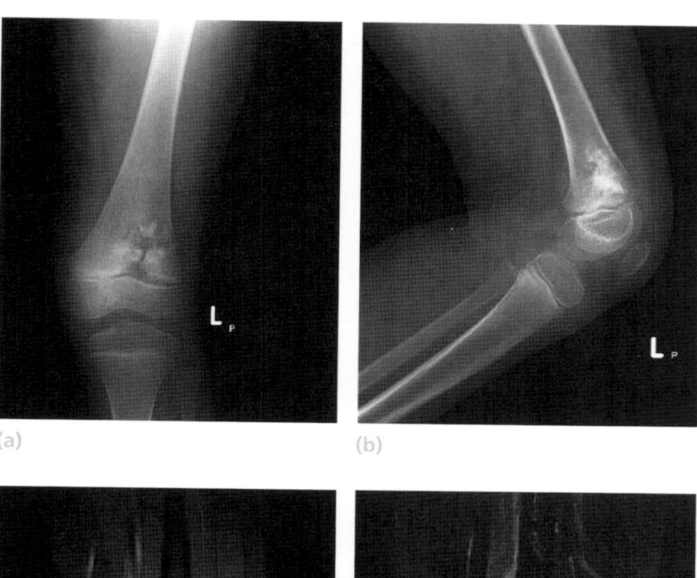

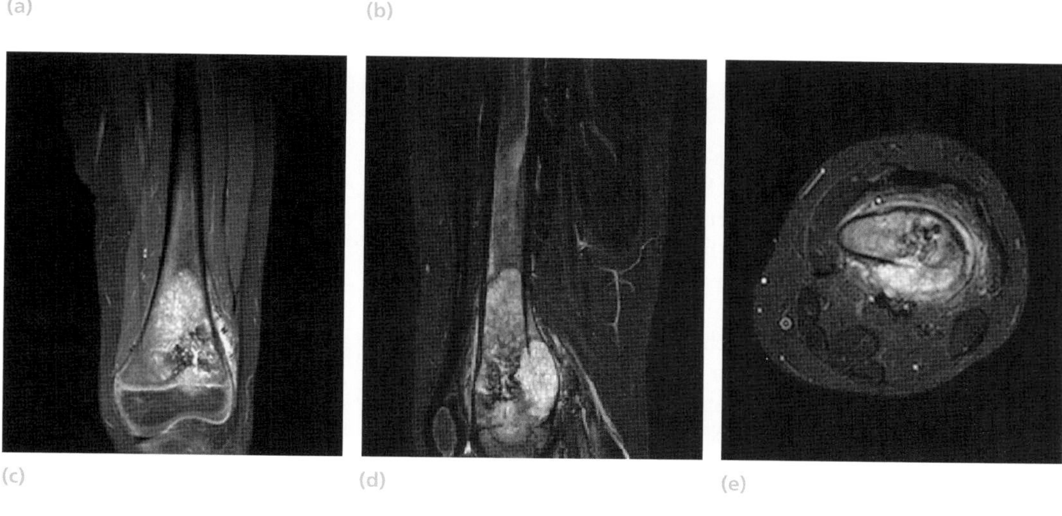

9.27 Osteosarcoma – imaging (a,b) X-rays of a distal femoral osteosarcoma in a child. (c,d,e) MRI examination: coronal, sagittal and axial scans showing the intra-and extra-osseous extensions of the tumour and its proximity to the neurovascular bundle.

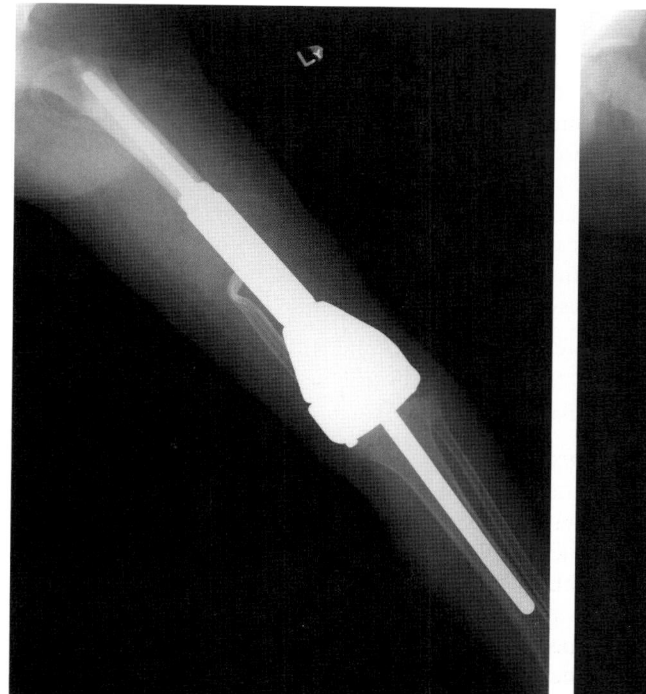

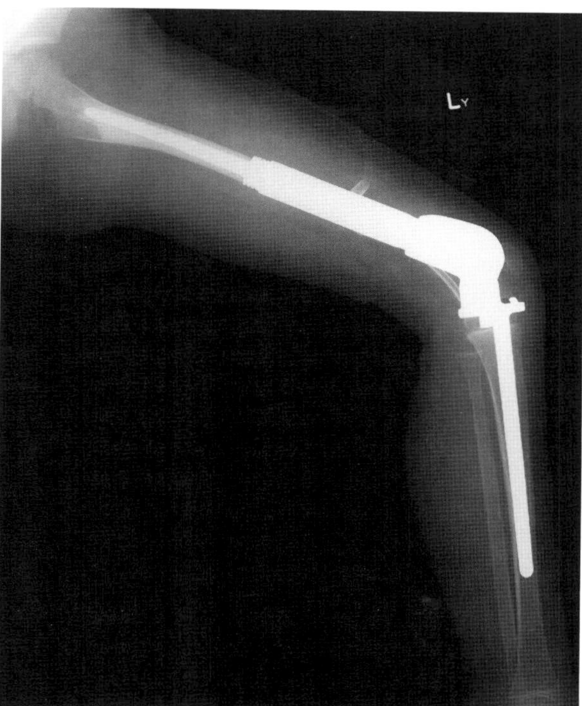

9.28 Osteosarcoma – operative treatment Postoperative x-rays showing an endoprosthetic replacement following wide resection of the lesion (Stanmore Implants Worldwide).

ried out. Depending on the site of the tumour, preparations would have been made to replace that segment of bone with either a large bone graft or a custom-made implant; in some cases an amputation may be more appropriate.

The pathological specimen is examined to assess the response to preoperative chemotherapy. If tumour necrosis is marked (more than 90 per cent), chemotherapy is continued for another 6–12 months; if the response is poor, a different chemotherapeutic regime is substituted.

Pulmonary metastases, especially if they are small and peripherally situated, may be completely resected with a wedge of lung tissue.

Outcome

Long-term survival after wide resection and chemotherapy has improved from around 50 per cent in 1980 (Rosen et al., 1982; Carter et al., 1991) to over 60 per cent in recent years (Smeland et al., 2004). Tumour-replacement implants usually function well. There is a fairly high complication rate (mainly wound breakdown and infection) but, in patients who survive, 10-year survival with mechanical failure as the end point is 75 per cent and for failure for any cause is 58 per cent. The limb salvage rate at 20 years is 84 per cent (Jeys et al., 2008) Aseptic loosening is more prevalent in younger patients.

Variants of osteosarcoma

PAROSTEAL OSTEOSARCOMA

This is a low-grade sarcoma situated on the surface of one of the tubular bones, usually at the distal femoral or proximal tibial metaphysis. The patient is a young adult who presents with a slowly enlarging mass near the bone end.

X-ray shows a dense bony mass on the surface of the bone or encircling it; the cortex is not eroded and usually a thin gap remains between cortex and tumour. The picture is easily mistaken for that of a benign bone lesion and the diagnosis is often missed until the tumour recurs after local excision. *CT* and *MRI* will show the boundary between tumour and surrounding soft tissues. Although the lesion is outside the bone, it does not spread into the adjacent muscle compartment until fairly late. Staging, therefore, often defines it as a low-grade intracompartmental tumour (stage IA).

Pathology At biopsy the tumour appears as a hard mass. On microscopic examination the lesion consists of well-formed bone but without any regular trabecular arrangement. The spaces between trabeculae are filled with cellular fibroblastic tissue; a few atypical cells and mitotic figures can usually be found. Occasionally the tumour has a much more aggressive appearance (***dedifferentiated parosteal osteosarcoma***).

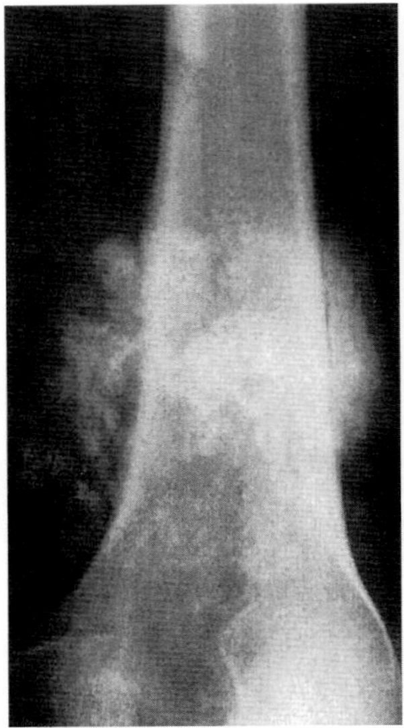
(a)

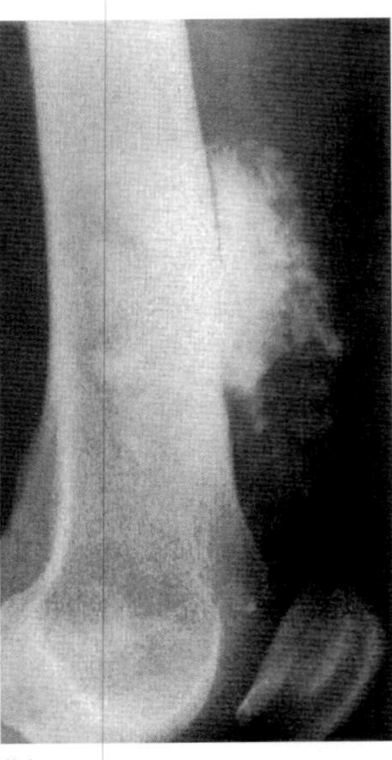
(b)

9.29 Parosteal osteosarcoma (a,b) X-rays show an ill-defined extraosseous tumour – note the linear gap between cortex and tumour.

Treatment For a low-grade parosteal osteosarcoma, wide excision without adjuvant therapy is sufficient to ensure a recurrence rate below 10 per cent. Dedifferentiated parosteal osteosarcoma should be treated in the same way as intramedullary sarcoma.

PERIOSTEAL OSTEOSARCOMA

This rare tumour is quite distinct from parosteal osteosarcoma. It is more like an intramedullary osteosarcoma, but situated on the surface of the bone. It occurs in young adults and causes local pain and swelling.

X-ray shows a superficial defect of the cortex, but *CT* and *MRI* may reveal a larger soft-tissue mass. The appearances sometimes suggest a periosteal chondroma and the diagnosis may not be certain until a biopsy is performed.

Pathology Histologically this is a true osteosarcoma, but characteristically the sections show a prominent cartilaginous element.

Treatment Treatment is the same as that of classic osteosarcoma.

PAGET'S SARCOMA

Paget's disease affects about 2 per cent of western Europeans. Although malignant transformation is a rare complication of this disease, most osteosarcomas appearing after the age of 50 years fall into this category. Warning signs are the appearance of pain or swelling in a patient with longstanding Paget's disease. In late cases, pathological fracture may occur.

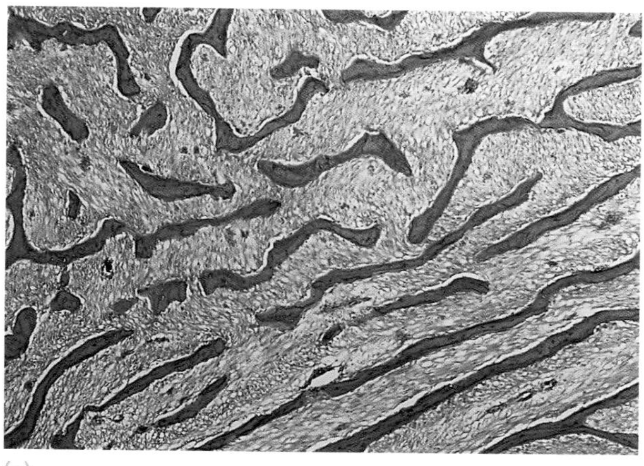

(a)

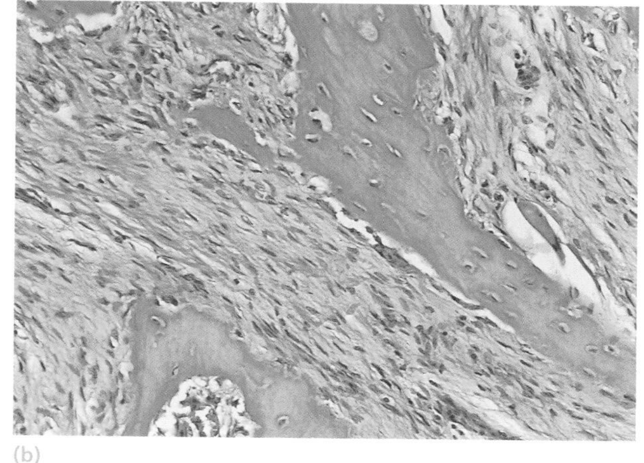

(b)

9.30 Parosteal osteosarcoma – histology (a) Histologically there are bony trabeculae and spindle-shaped, well-differentiated fibrous tissue cells with occasional mitotic figures. (×120) (b) High-power view of the same. (×300)

X-ray shows the usual features of Paget's disease, but with areas of bone destruction and soft-tissue invasion.

This is a high-grade tumour – if anything even more malignant than classic osteosarcoma. Staging usually shows that extracompartmental spread has occurred; most patients have pulmonary metastases by the time the tumour is diagnosed.

Treatment Even with radical resection or amputation and chemotherapy the 5-year survival rate is low. If the lesion is definitely extracompartmental, palliative treatment by radiotherapy may be preferable; chemotherapy is usually difficult because of the patient's age and uncertainty about renal and cardiac function.

Fibrosarcoma of bone

Fibrosarcoma is rare in bone; it is more likely to arise in previously abnormal tissue (a bone infarct, fibrous dysplasia or after irradiation). The patient – usually an adult – complains of pain or swelling; there may be a pathological fracture.

X-ray shows an undistinctive area of bone destruction. *CT* or *MRI* will reveal the soft-tissue extension.

Pathology Histologically the lesion consists of masses of fibroblastic tissue with scattered atypical and mitotic cells. Appearances vary from well-differentiated to highly undifferentiated, and the tumours are sometimes graded accordingly.

Treatment Low-grade, well-confined tumours (stage IA) can be treated by wide excision with prosthetic replacement. High-grade lesions (IIA or IIB) require radical resection or amputation; if this cannot be achieved, local excision must be combined with radiation therapy. The value of adjuvant chemotherapy is still uncertain.

Malignant fibrous histiocytoma

Like fibrosarcoma, this tumour tends to occur in previously abnormal bone (old infarcts or Paget's disease). Patients are usually middle-aged adults and x-rays may reveal a destructive lesion adjacent to an

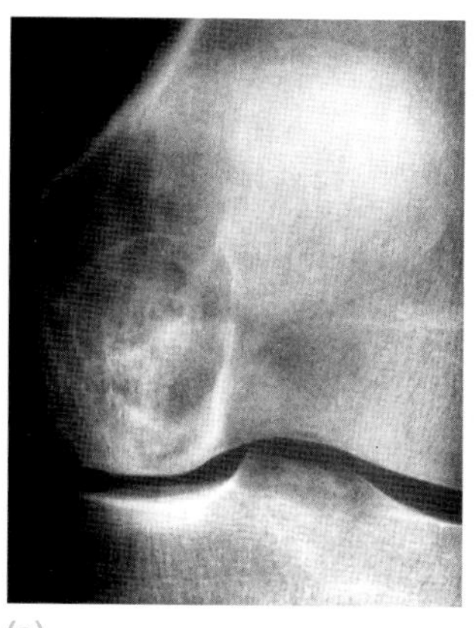

(a)

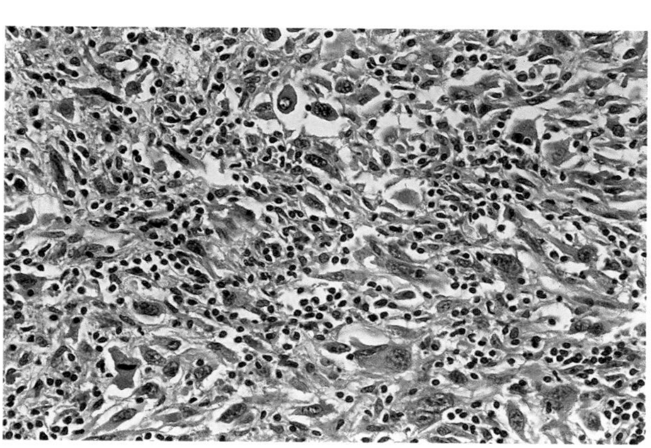

(b)

9.31 Fibrosarcoma (a) The area of bone destruction in the femoral condyle has no special distinguishing features. (b) The biopsy showed highly atypical fibroblastic tissue.

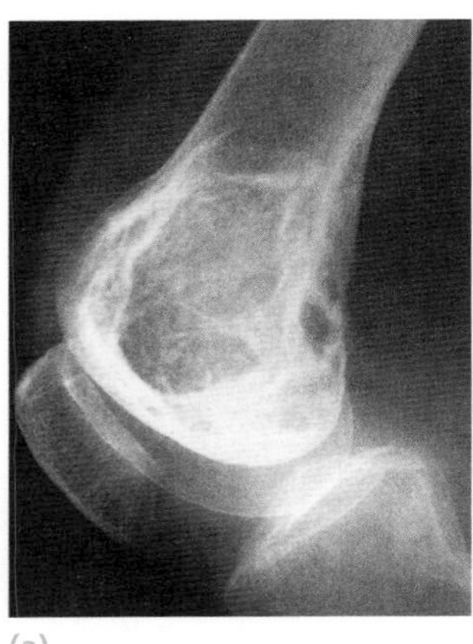
(a)

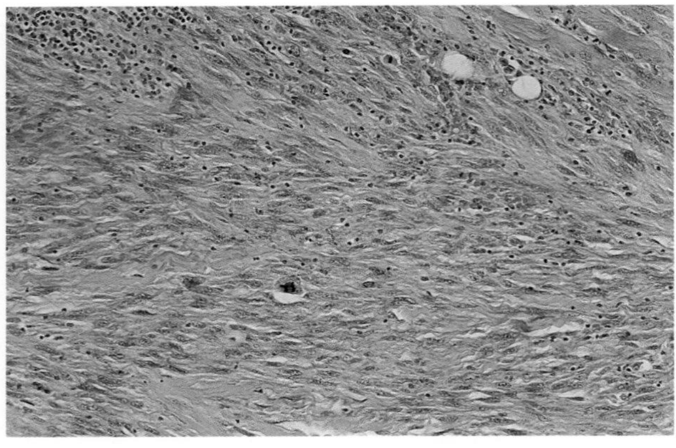
(b)

9.32 Malignant fibrous histiocytoma (a) X-ray showing a large 'cystic' lesion in the distal femur. The lesion may occur in an area of old bone 'infarct', which may account for the flecks of increased density in this x-ray. (b) Histology shows abnormal fibrohistiocytic cells, many of which are unusually large and some of which are binucleate or multinucleate. (×480)

old area of medullary infarction. Staging studies almost invariably show that the tumour has spread beyond the bone.

Histologically it is a fibrous tumour, but the arrangement of the tissue is in interweaving bundles, and the presence of histiocytes and of giant cells distinguishes it from the more uniform fibrosarcoma.

Treatment Treatment consists of wide or radical resection and adjuvant chemotherapy. For inaccessible lesions, local radiotherapy may be needed.

Ewing's sarcoma

Ewing's sarcoma is believed to arise from endothelial cells in the bone marrow. It occurs most commonly between the ages of 10 and 20 years, usually in a tubular bone and especially in the tibia, fibula or clavicle.

The patient presents with pain – often throbbing in character – and swelling. Generalized illness and pyrexia, together with a warm, tender swelling and a raised ESR, may suggest a diagnosis of osteomyelitis.

Imaging

X-rays usually show an area of bone destruction which, unlike that in osteosarcoma, is predominantly in the mid-diaphysis. New bone formation may extend along the shaft and sometimes it appears as fusiform layers of bone around the lesion – the so-called 'onion-peel' effect. Often the tumour extends into the surrounding soft tissues, with radiating streaks of ossification and reactive periosteal bone at the proximal and distal margins. These features (the 'sunray' appearance and Codman's triangles) are usually associated with osteosarcoma, but they are just as common in Ewing's sarcoma.

CT and *MRI* reveal the large extraosseous component. *Radioisotope scans* may show multiple areas of activity in the skeleton.

Pathology

Macroscopically the tumour is lobulated and often fairly large. It may look grey (like brain) or red (like redcurrant jelly) if haemorrhage has occurred into it. Microscopically, sheets of small dark polyhedral cells with no regular arrangement and no ground substance are seen.

Diagnosis

The condition which should be excluded as rapidly as possible is bone infection. On biopsy the essential step is to recognize this as a malignant round-cell tumour, distinct from osteosarcoma. Other round-cell tumours that may resemble Ewing's are reticulum-cell sarcoma (see below) and metastatic neuroblastoma.

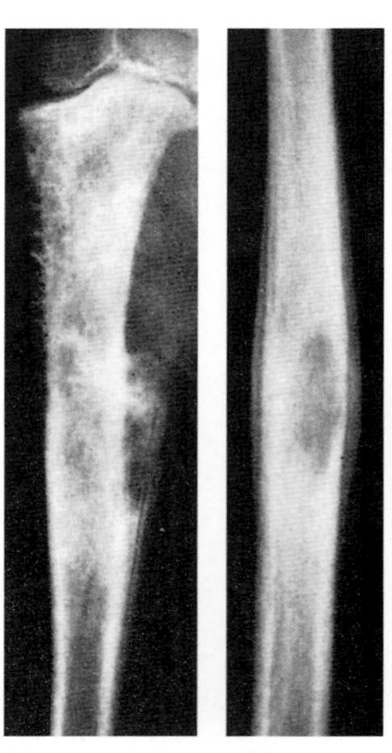
(a)

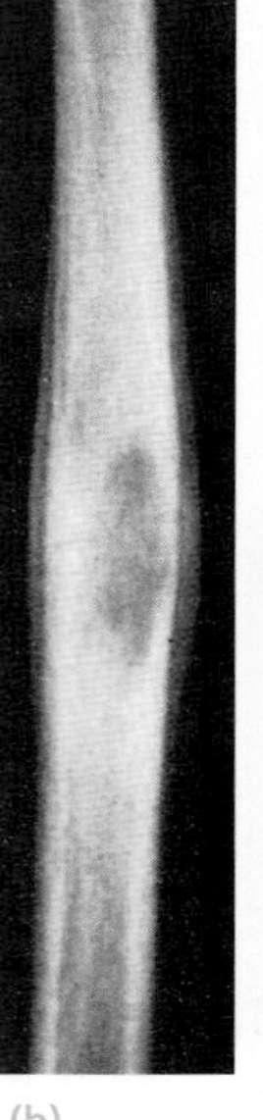
(b)

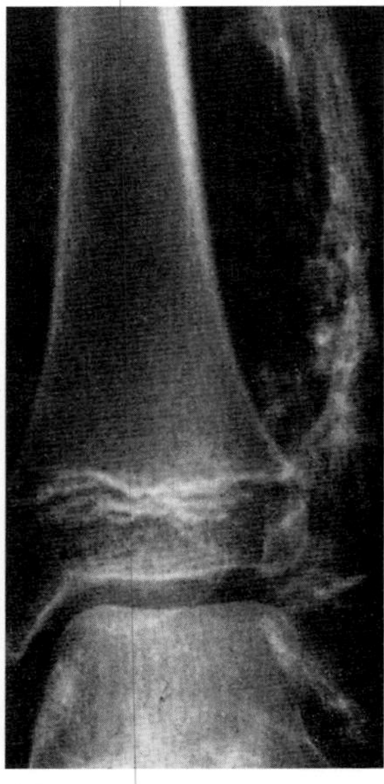
(c)

9.33 Ewing's tumour Examples of Ewing's tumour in (a) the humerus, (b) the mid-shaft of the fibula and (c) the lower end of the fibula.

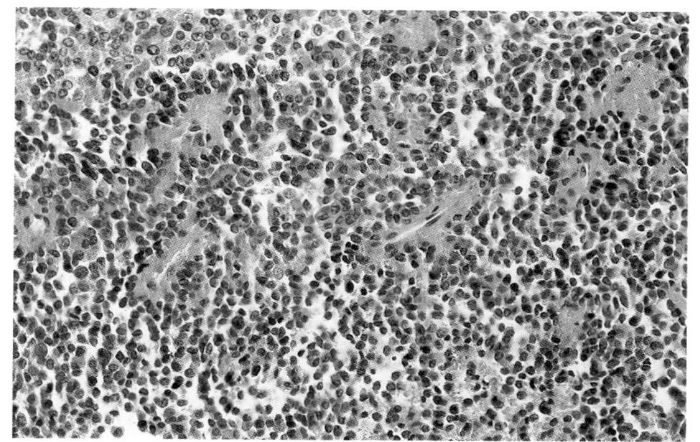

9.34 Ewing's tumour – histology There is a monotonous pattern of small round cells clustered around blood vessels. (×480)

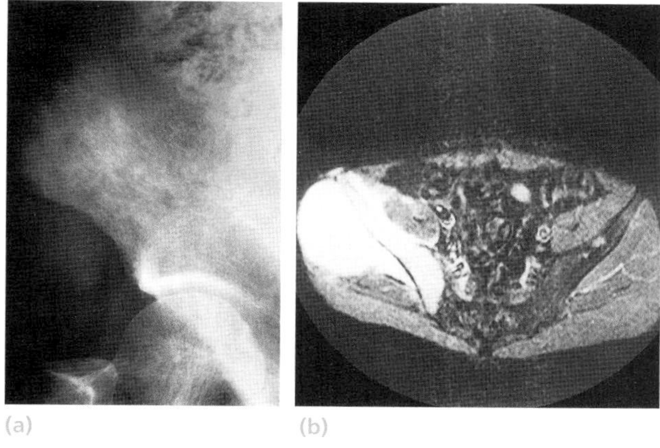

(a) (b)

9.35 Non-Hodgkin's lymphoma (a) X-ray showing a rather nondescript moth-eaten appearance of the ilium. (b) MRI reveals the extent of the soft-tissue lesion.

Treatment

The prognosis is always poor and surgery alone does little to improve it. Radiotherapy has a dramatic effect on the tumour but overall survival is not much enhanced. Chemotherapy is much more effective, offering a 5-year survival rate of about 50 per cent (Souhami and Craft, 1988; Damron et al., 2007).

The best results are achieved by a combination of all three methods: a course of preoperative neoadjuvant chemotherapy; then wide excision if the tumour is in a favourable site, or radiotherapy followed by local excision if it is less accessible; and then a further course of chemotherapy for 1 year. Postoperative radiotherapy may be added if the resected specimen is found not to have a sufficiently wide margin of normal tissue.

The prognosis for these tumours has improved dramatically since the introduction of multi-agent chemotherapy – from an erstwhile 10 per cent survival rate to the current 70 per cent for patients with non-metastatic Ewing's sarcoma.

NON-HODGKIN'S LYMPHOMA (RETICULUM-CELL SARCOMA)

Like Ewing's sarcoma, this is a round-cell tumour of the reticuloendothelial system. It is usually seen in sites with abundant red marrow: the flat bones, the spine and the long-bone metaphyses. The patient, usually an adult of 30–40 years, presents with pain or a pathological fracture.

X-ray shows a mottled area of bone destruction in areas that normally contain red marrow; the *radioisotope scan* may reveal multiple lesions.

Pathology Histologically this is a marrow-cell tumour with collections of abnormal lymphocytes. Special reticulin stains are needed to show the fine fibrillar network that helps to distinguish the picture from that of Ewing's sarcoma.

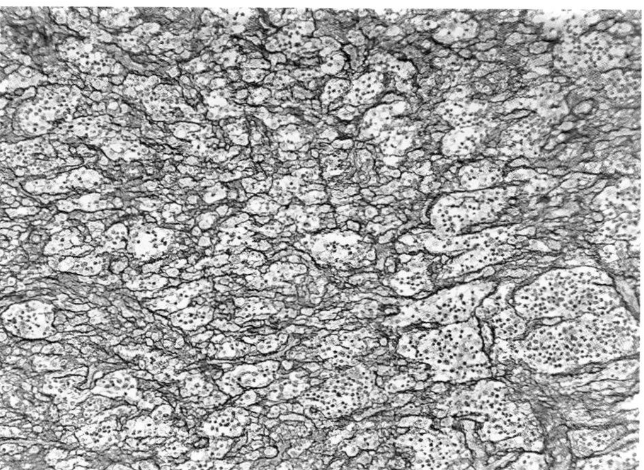

9.36 Non-Hodgkin's lymphoma – histology There is dense infiltration of abnormal lymphoid cells (a typical 'round-cell tumour'), which is distinguished from Ewing's by the characteristic distribution of reticulin around collections of cells and between individual cells. (×200; special reticulin stain)

Treatment The preferred treatment is by chemotherapy and radical resection; radiotherapy is reserved for less accessible lesions.

MULTIPLE MYELOMA

Multiple myeloma is a malignant B-cell lymphoproliferative disorder of the marrow, with plasma cells predominating. The effects on bone are due to marrow cell proliferation and increased osteoclastic activity, resulting in *osteoporosis* and the appearance of discrete *lytic lesions* throughout the skeleton. A particularly large colony of plasma cells may form what appears to be a solitary tumour *(plasmacytoma)* in one of the bones, but sooner or later most of these cases turn out to be unusual examples of the same widespread disease.

Associated features of the marrow-cell disorder are plasma protein abnormalities, increased blood viscosity and anaemia. Bone resorption leads to hypercalcaemia in about one-third of cases. Late secondary features are due to renal dysfunction and spinal cord or root compression caused by vertebral collapse.

The patient, typically aged 45–65, presents with weakness, backache, bone pain or a pathological fracture. Hypercalcaemia may cause symptoms such as thirst, polyuria and abdominal pain. Clinical signs (apart from a pathological fracture) are often unremarkable. Localized tenderness and restricted hip movements could be due to a plasmacytoma in the proximal femur. In late cases there may be signs of cord or nerve root compression, chronic nephritis and recurrent infection.

X-rays

X-rays often show nothing more than generalized osteoporosis; but remember that *myeloma is one of the commonest causes of osteoporosis and vertebral compression fracture in men over the age of 45 years.* The 'classical' lesions are multiple punched-out defects with 'soft' margins (lack of new bone) in the skull, pelvis and proximal femur, a crushed vertebra, or a solitary lytic tumour in a large-bone metaphysis.

Investigations

Mild anaemia is common, and an almost constant feature is a high ESR. Blood chemistry may show a raised creatinine level and hypercalcaemia. Over half the patients have Bence Jones protein in their urine, and serum protein electrophoresis shows a characteristic abnormal band. A sternal marrow puncture may show plasmacytosis, with typical 'myeloma' cells.

Diagnosis

If the only x-ray change is osteoporosis, the differential diagnosis must include all the *other causes of bone loss.* If there are lytic lesions, the features can be similar to those of *metastatic bone disease.*

Paraproteinaemia is a feature of other (benign) *gammopathies*; it is wise to seek the help of a haematologist before reaching a clinical diagnosis.

Pathology

At operation the affected bone is soft and crumbly. The typical microscopic picture is of sheets of plasma-

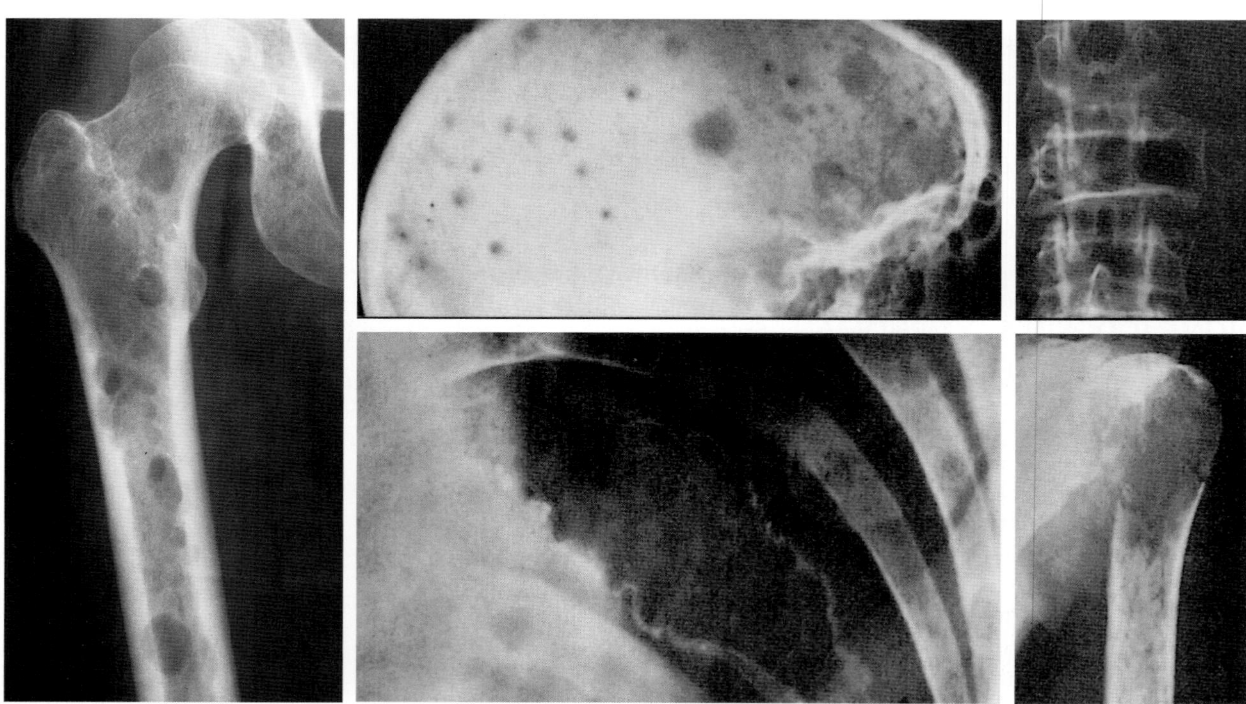

9.37 Myeloma The characteristic x-ray features are bone rarefaction, vertebral compression fractures, expanding lesions (typically in the ribs and pelvis) and punched-out areas in the skull and the long bones.

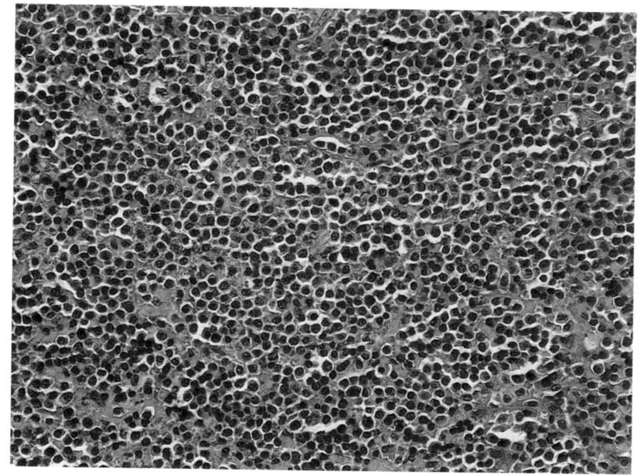

9.38 Myeloma – histology There are dense sheets of plasma cells with eccentric nuclei. (×480)

cytes with a large eccentric nucleus containing a spoke-like arrangement of chromatin.

Treatment

The immediate need is for pain control and, if necessary, treatment of pathological fractures. General supportive measures include correction of fluid balance and (in some cases) hypercalcaemia.

Limb fractures are best managed by internal fixation and packing of cavities with methylmethacrylate cement (which also helps to staunch the profuse bleeding that sometimes occurs). Perioperative antibiotic prophylaxis is important as there is a higher than usual risk of infection and wound breakdown.

Spinal fractures carry the risk of cord compression and need immediate stabilization – either by effective bracing or by internal fixation. Unrelieved cord pressure may need decompression.

Solitary plasmacytomas can be treated by radiotherapy.

Specific therapy is with alkylating cytotoxic agents (e.g. melphalan). Corticosteroids are also used – especially if bone pain is marked – but this probably does not alter the course of the disease. Treatment should be carried out in a specialized unit where dosages and response parameters can be properly monitored.

The *prognosis* in established cases is poor, with a median survival of between 2 and 5 years.

Chordoma

This rare malignant tumour arises from primitive notochordal remnants. It affects young adults and usually presents as a slow-growing mass in the sacrum; however, it may occur elsewhere along the spine.

The patient complains of longstanding backache. The tumour expands anteriorly and, if it involves the sacrum, may eventually (after months or even years) cause rectal or urethral obstruction; rectal examination may disclose the presacral mass. In late cases there may also be neurological signs.

X-ray shows a radiolucent lesion in the sacrum. *CT* and *MRI* reveal the extent of intrapelvic enlargement.

Treatment This is a low-grade tumour, though often with extracompartmental spread. After wide excision there is little risk of recurrence. However, attempts to prevent damage to the pelvic viscera usually result in inadequate surgery (intralesional or close marginal excision) and consequently a greater risk of recurrence. If there are doubts in this regard, operation should be combined with local radiotherapy.

Adamantinoma

This rare tumour has a predilection for the anterior cortex of the tibia but is occasionally found in other long bones. The patient is usually a young adult who complains of aching and mild swelling in the front of the leg. On examination there is thickening and tenderness along the subcutaneous border of the tibia.

X-ray shows a typical bubble-like defect in the anterior tibial cortex; sometimes there is thickening of the surrounding bone.

Adamantinoma is a low-grade tumour which metastasizes late – and usually only after repeated and inadequate attempts at removal. Early on it is confined to bone; later, *CT* may show that the tumour has extended inwards to the medullary canal or outwards beyond the periosteum.

Pathology The histological picture varies considerably but the most typical features are islands of epithelial-like cells in a densely-populated stroma of spindle cells; the 'epithelial' nests may have an acinar arrangement.

Treatment If the diagnosis is made reasonably early, wide local excision with a substantial margin of normal bone is adequate. Preoperative CT and MRI are essential to determine how deep the tumour penetrates; if it is confined to the anterior cortex, the posterior cortex can be preserved and this makes reconstruction much easier. If the lesion extends to the endosteal surface, a full segment of bone must be excised; the gap is filled with a vascularized graft or a suitable endoprosthesis, or managed by distraction osteogenesis (see Chapter 12).

If there has been more than one recurrence, or if the tumour extends into the surrounding soft tissues, radical resection or amputation is advisable.

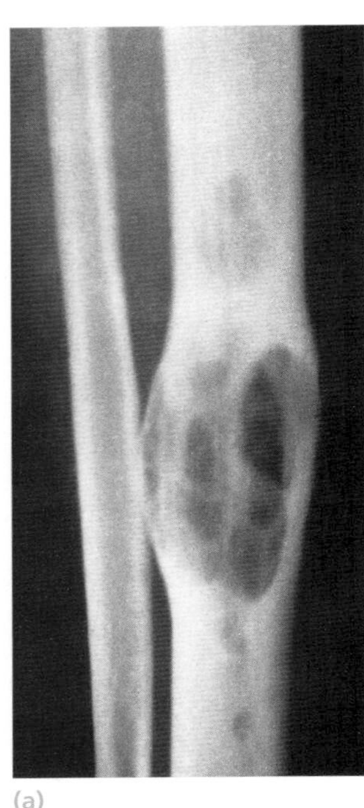

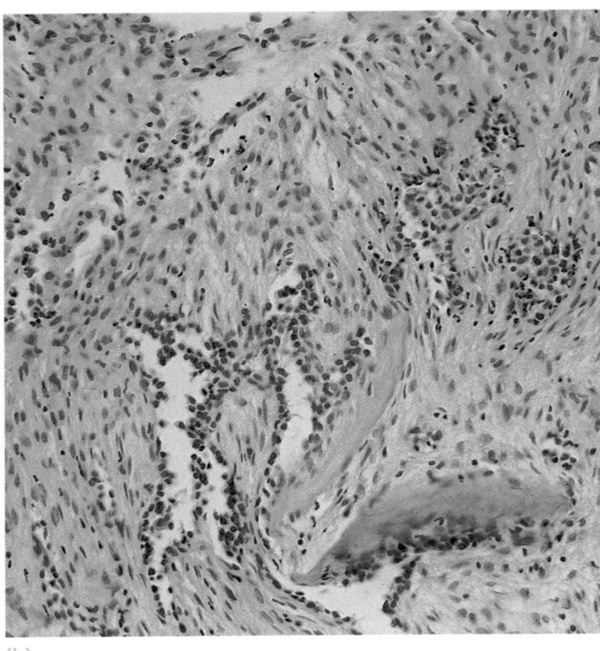

(a) (b)

9.39 Adamantinoma (a) The bubble-like appearance in the mid-shaft of the tibia is typical. (b) Histology shows clusters of epithelial-like cells, sometimes with an acinar arrangement in a moderately cellular fibrous stroma. (×300)

METASTATIC BONE DISEASE

The skeleton is one of the commonest sites of secondary cancer; *in patients over 50 years bone metastases are seen more frequently than all primary malignant bone tumours together*. The commonest source is carcinoma of the breast; next in frequency are carcinomas of the prostate, kidney, lung, thyroid, bladder and gastrointestinal tract. In about 10 per cent of cases no primary tumour is found.

The commonest sites for bone metastases are the vertebrae, pelvis, the proximal half of the femur and the humerus. Spread is usually via the blood stream; occasionally, visceral tumours spread directly to adjacent bones (e.g. the pelvis or ribs).

Metastases are usually osteolytic, and pathological fractures are common. Bone resorption is due either to the direct action of tumour cells or to tumour-derived factors that stimulate osteoclastic activity. Osteoblastic lesions are uncommon; they usually occur in prostatic carcinoma.

Clinical features

The patient is usually aged 50–70 years; with any destructive bone lesion in this age group, the differential diagnosis must include metastasis.

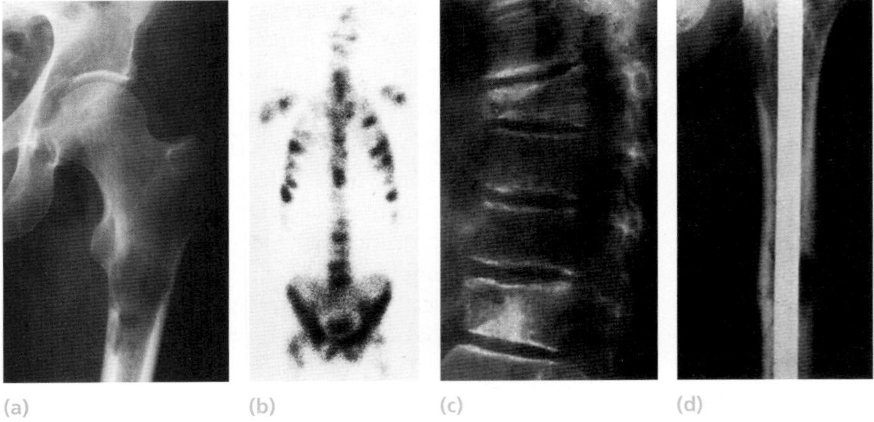

(a) (b) (c) (d)

9.40 Metastatic tumours (a,b) This patient presented with pain in the right upper thigh. X-ray showed what appeared to be a single metastasis in the upper third of the femur. However, the radioisotope scan revealed many deposits in other parts of the skeleton. (c) Patients over 60 with vertebral compression fractures may simply be very osteoporotic, but they should always be investigated for metastatic bone disease and myelomatosis. (d) Prophylactic nailing for a femoral metastasis which might otherwise have resulted in a pathological fracture.

Pain is the commonest – and often the only – clinical feature. The sudden appearance of backache or thigh pain in an elderly person (especially someone known to have been treated for carcinoma in the past) is always suspicious. If x-rays do not show anything, a radionuclide scan might.

Some deposits remain clinically silent and are discovered incidentally on x-ray examination or bone scanning, or after a pathological fracture. Sudden collapse of a vertebral body or a fracture of the mid-shaft of a long bone in an elderly person are ominous signs; if there is no history and no clinical clue pointing to a primary carcinoma, a biopsy of the fracture area is essential.

Symptoms of hypercalcaemia may occur (and are often missed) in patients with skeletal metastases. These include anorexia, nausea, thirst, polyuria, abdominal pain, general weakness and depression.

In children under 6 years of age, metastatic lesions are most commonly from adrenal neuroblastoma. The child presents with bone pain and fever; examination reveals the abdominal mass.

Imaging

X-rays Most skeletal deposits are osteolytic and appear as rarified areas in the medulla or produce a moth-eaten appearance in the cortex; sometimes there is marked bone destruction, with or without a pathological fracture. Osteoblastic deposits suggest a prostatic carcinoma; the pelvis may show a mottled increase in density which has to be distinguished from Paget's disease or lymphoma.

Radioscintigraphy Bone scans with ^{99m}Tc-MDP are the most sensitive method of detecting 'silent' metastatic deposits in bone; areas of increased activity are selected for x-ray examination.

Special investigations

The ESR may be increased and the haemoglobin concentration is usually low. The serum alkaline phosphatase concentration is often increased, and in prostatic carcinoma the acid phosphatase also is elevated.

Patients with breast cancer can be screened by measuring blood levels of tumour-associated antigen markers.

Treatment

By the time a patient has developed secondary deposits the prognosis for survival is poor. Occasionally, radical treatment (combined chemotherapy, radiotherapy and surgery) targeted at a solitary secondary deposit and the parent primary lesion may be rewarding and even apparently curative. This applies particularly to solitary renal cell, breast and thyroid tumour metastases; but in the great majority of cases, and certainly in those with multiple secondaries, treatment is entirely symptomatic. For that reason, elaborate witch-hunts to discover the source of an occult primary tumour are avoided, though it may be worthwhile investigating for tumours that are amenable to hormonal manipulation.

Prognosis

Bauer (1995) has suggested useful criteria for assessing prognosis (see Box). In his series of patients, survivorship at 1 year was as follows:

- of patients with 4 or 5 of Bauer's criteria 50 per cent were alive
- of patients with 2 or 3 criteria 25 per cent were alive
- of patients with only 1 or none of the criteria, the majority survived for less than 6 months and none were alive at 1 year.

Palliative care

Despite a poor prognosis, patients deserve to be made comfortable, to enjoy (as far as possible) their remaining months or years, and to die in a peaceful and dignified way. The active treatment of skeletal metastases contributes to this in no small measure. In addition, patients need sympathetic counselling and practical assistance with their material affairs.

Control of pain and metastatic activity Most patients require *analgesics*, but the more powerful narcotics should be reserved for the terminally ill.

Unless specifically contraindicated, *radiotherapy* is used both to control pain and to reduce metastatic growth. This is often combined with other forms of treatment (e.g. internal fixation).

Secondary deposits from breast or prostate can often be controlled by *hormone therapy:* stilboestrol for prostatic secondaries and androgenic drugs or oestrogens for breast carcinoma. Disseminated secondaries from breast carcinoma are sometimes treated by oophorectomy combined with adrenalectomy or by hypophyseal ablation.

BAUER'S POSITIVE CRITERIA FOR SURVIVAL
A solitary metastasis
No pathological fracture
No visceral metastases
Renal or breast primary
No lung cancer

Hypercalcaemia may have serious consequences, including renal acidosis, nephrocalcinosis, unconsciousness and coma. It should be treated by ensuring adequate hydration, reducing the calcium intake and, if necessary, administering bisphosphonates.

Treatment of limb fractures Surgical timidity may condemn the patient to a painful lingering death, so shaft fractures should almost always be treated by internal fixation and (if necessary) packing with methylmethacrylate cement. If there are multiple fractures, more than one bone may be fixed at the same sitting, though one must bear in mind that the risk of fat embolism increases with multiple intramedullary nailing. Pain is immediately relieved, nursing is made easier and the patient can get up and about or attend for other types of treatment without unnecessary discomfort. Shaft fractures usually unite satisfactorily.

In most cases intramedullary nailing is the most effective method; fractures near joints (e.g. the distal femur or proximal tibia) may need fixation with plates or blade-plates, and sometimes replacement by an endoprosthesis.

Fractures of the femoral neck rarely, if ever, unite. They are best treated by prosthetic replacement: a hemiarthroplasty if the pelvis is intact, or total joint replacement if the acetabulum is involved. If the pelvic wall is destroyed, it can be reconstructed by large bone grafts, a reconstruction cage or a custom-made prosthesis; however, if such extensive surgery is contraindicated, one may have to settle for a simple excisional arthroplasty.

Postoperative irradiation is essential to prevent further extension of the metastatic lesion.

Prophylactic fixation Large deposits that threaten to result in fracture should be treated by internal fixation while the bone is still intact. As a rule of thumb, where 50 per cent of a single cortex of a long bone (in any radiological view) has been destroyed, pathological fracture should be regarded as inevitable. In addition, avulsion of the lesser trochanter is an indication of imminent hip fracture.

Mirels devised a scoring system (Table 9.4) to evaluate fracture risk and therefore act as a guide as to whether (and when) a fracture should be fixed or not. A score of 8 or more indicates a high risk and a need for internal fixation to be carried out prior to radiotherapy (Mirels, 1989).

The principles of fixation are the same as for the management of fractures in general. A preoperative radionuclide scan will show whether other lesions are present in that bone, thus calling for more extensive fixation and postoperative radiotherapy.

Treatment of metastatic spinal disease Metastatic spinal disease is 40 times more common than all primary tumours of the spine together (Galasko et al., 2000).

Table 9.4 Mirel's scoring system for metastatic bone disease

Score	1	2	3
Site	Upper limb	Lower limb	Peritrochanteric
Pain	Mild	Moderate	Functional
Lesion	Blastic	Mixed	Lytic
Size*	<1/3	1/3–2/3	>2/3

*As seen on plain x-ray, maximum destruction of cortex in any view. Maximum possible score is 12. If the lesion scores 8 or above, then prophylactic fixation is recommended prior to radiotherapy.

Between 41 and 70 per cent of all malignant tumours have a spinal metastasis, mostly in the thoracic spine and mainly in the vertebral body. The aims of intervention are to decrease pain, preserve the ability to walk, maintain urinary and faecal continence and prolong survival.

Pathological fractures usually require some form of support. If the spine is still completely stable, a well-fitting brace may be sufficient. However, spinal instability may cause severe pain, making it almost impossible for the patient to sit or stand – with or without a brace. For these patients, operative stabilization is indicated – either posterior or anterior spinal fusion, depending on the individual need. Preoperative assessment should include CT or MRI to establish whether the cord is threatened; if it is, spinal decompression should be carried out at the same time. *If there are overt symptoms and signs of cord compression, treatment is urgent.*

Other forms of surgery sometimes called for are debulking of the tumour or removal of a solitary metastasis by vertebrectomy and reconstruction.

Operative intervention appears to provide a better functional outcome than radiotherapy. Patients remain ambulatory and continent for longer and the 5-year survival rate is around 18 per cent. In general, radiotherapy alone is reserved for patients with soft-tissue compression and as palliation for inoperable cases.

It is well to remember that radiotherapy used as a preoperative adjunct has been shown to increase the postoperative infection rate (Jeys et al., 2005).

SOFT-TISSUE TUMOURS

Benign soft-tissue tumours are common, malignant ones rare. The distinction between these two groups is not always easy, and some lesions, treated confidently as 'benign', recur in more aggressive form after inadequate removal. Features suggestive of malignancy are: pain in a previously painless lump; a rapid increase in size; a lump deep to the fascia; size greater than 5 cm; poor demarcation; and attachment to the surrounding structures.

As with bone tumours, special imaging and staging should be carried out before the field is disturbed by operation. Chest x-rays and blood investigations may also be necessary. If the imaging is conclusive then the lesion can be removed with either a marginal or wide excision biopsy, dependent on the diagnosis. Alternatively, a biopsy to confirm the diagnosis should be undertaken prior to excision.

The role of chemotherapy for soft-tissue sarcomas is uncertain, except in the treatment of rhabdomyosarcoma and synovial sarcoma.

Radiotherapy is indicated for all high-grade lesions and for tumours that are removed with poor margins or by intralesional excision. If margins are contaminated then re-operation with wide resection of that margin must be performed.

The account that follows is intended as a summary of those soft-tissue tumours likely to be encountered in orthopaedics.

Fatty tumours

LIPOMA

A lipoma, one of the commonest of all tumours, may occur almost anywhere; sometimes there are multiple lesions. The tumour usually arises in the subcutaneous layer. It consists of lobules of fat with a surrounding capsule which may become tethered to neighbouring structures. The patient, usually aged over 50, complains of a painless swelling. The lump is soft and almost fluctuant; the well-defined edge and lobulated surface distinguish it from a chronic abscess. Fat is notably radiotranslucent, a feature that betrays the occasional sub-periosteal lipoma.

If the lump is troublesome it may be removed by marginal excision. Prior biopsy is usually unnecessary; however, one should never be complacent about a 'lipoma' and if there are any atypical features, preoperative staging and biopsy are essential in order to avoid the risk of performing a marginal excision and then discovering that the lesion was malignant.

LIPOSARCOMA

Liposarcoma is rare but should be suspected if a fatty tumour (especially in the buttock, the thigh or the popliteal fossa) goes on growing and becomes painful. The lump may feel quite firm and is usually not translucent. CT or MRI is essential to determine the extent of the tumour.

Treatment depends on the degree of malignancy. Low-grade lesions can be removed by wide excision; high-grade tumours need radical resection. For liposarcomas in inaccessible sites, radiation therapy is often effective.

Fibrous tumours

FIBROMA

The common fibroma is a solitary, benign tumour of fibrous tissue. It is usually discovered as a small asymptomatic nodule or lump. Treatment is not essential; if it is removed, a marginal excision is adequate.

FIBROMATOSIS

This term encompasses a group of well-differentiated fibrous lesions that typically infiltrate the tissues, sometimes in an aggressive manner. They have a strong tendency to recur after local excision but they do not metastasize.

The lesions appear in various forms, divided broadly into *superficial fibromatoses* (comprising clinical

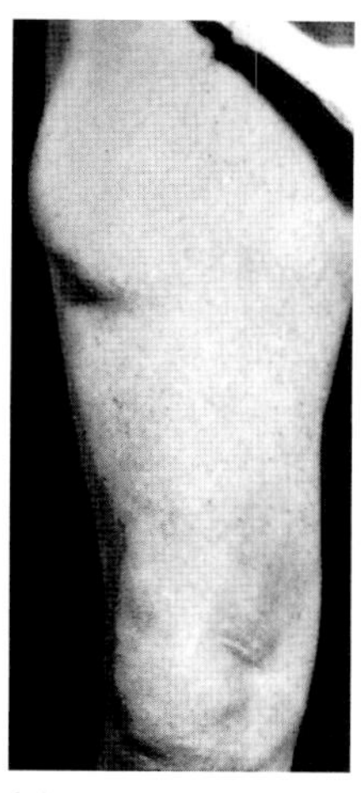
(a)

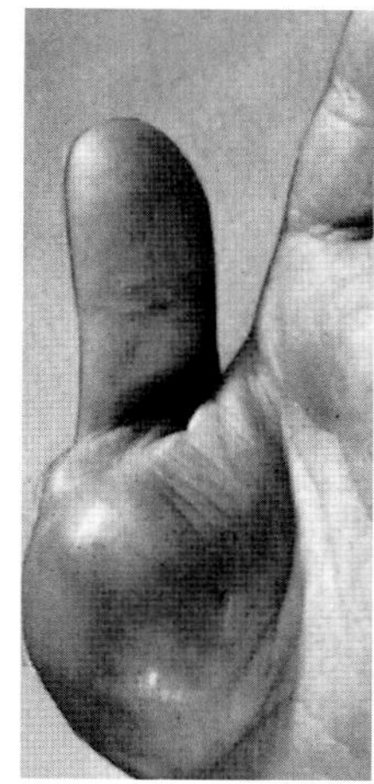
(b)

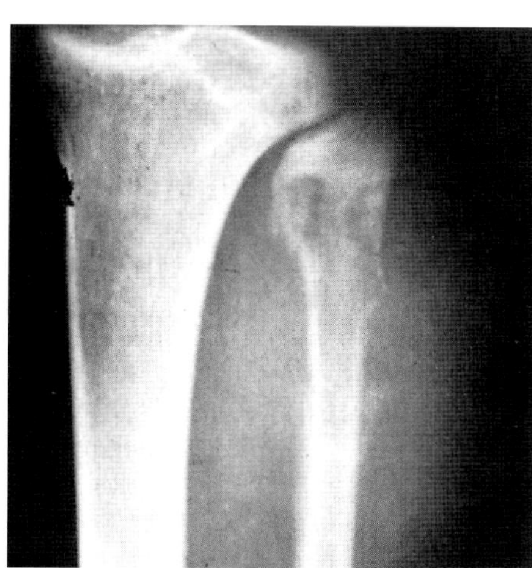
(c)

9.41 Fatty tumours (a) Subcutaneous lipoma in the thigh. Like so many lipomas, this one felt almost fluctuant; (b) intramuscular lipoma; (c) liposarcoma – the cortex of the fibula has been eroded.

entities as diverse as Dupuytren's contracture, Peyronie's disease and thickened fibrous plaques elsewhere in superficial mesenchymal tissues), and more aggressive but comparatively rare *deep fibromatoses*, or *desmoid tumours*, which usually appear in young adults as thick cords or plaques in the subcutaneous tissues of the limbs or trunk where they grow into featureless masses with ill-defined margins. CT and MRI are useful to show the extent of this invasive tumour.

After local excision, desmoid tumours often recur in increasingly invasive form, threatening nearby neurovascular structures. Pressure on nerves may cause paraesthesiae. A particularly hazardous situation arises when the tumour, after several attempts at eradication, infiltrates into the axilla or pelvis; once this occurs, complete removal may be impossible.

Pathology Microscopically these lesions vary from those with clearly benign cells to some whose appearance suggests malignancy (multinucleated cells with many mitoses). Differentiation from fibrosarcoma may be difficult and demands considerable histological expertise, but it is important because fibromatosis does not metastasize and can be eradicated if surgery is sufficiently thorough.

Treatment Although the tumour sometimes regresses spontaneously, the most predictable results are achieved by a combination of wide excision and radiation therapy (Pritchard et al., 1996). The risk of local recurrence is strongly related to the adequacy of the margin of resection. Intralesional and marginal resections result in more than twice the recurrence rate following resection well beyond the tumour margins.

Non-operative treatment has been tried for lesions that are inaccessible or where several attempts at surgical removal have failed. The most promising results thus far reported have been achieved by the use of hormonal agents (e.g. tamoxifen, an anti-oestrogen preparation) and cytotoxic chemotherapy (Janinis et al., 2003).

FIBROSARCOMA

Fibrosarcoma may occur in any area of connective tissue but is more common in the extremities. It presents as an ill-defined, painless mass and may grow to a considerable size. The diagnosis is usually made only after biopsy and histological examination. Local extension can be shown on MRI. There may be metastases in the lungs.

High-grade lesions showing atypical spindle cells are usually easy to diagnose. Low-grade lesions may be difficult to distinguish from fibromatosis.

For *low-grade lesions*, wide excision is usually sufficient. For *high-grade lesions*, wide excision should be supplemented by preoperative and postoperative radiation therapy.

SYNOVIAL TUMOURS

PIGMENTED VILLONODULAR SYNOVITIS AND GIANT-CELL TUMOUR OF TENDON SHEATH

These are two forms of the same condition – a benign disorder that occurs wherever synovial membrane is found: in joints, tendon sheaths or bursae.

Pigmented villonodular synovitis (PVNS) presents as a longstanding boggy swelling of the joint – usually the hip, knee or ankle – in an adolescent or young adult. X-ray may show excavations in the juxta-articular bone on either side of the joint. When the joint is opened, the synovium is swollen and hyperplastic, often covered with villi and golden-brown in colour – the effect of haemosiderin deposition. The juxta-articular excavations contain clumps of friable synovial material.

Tendon sheath lesions are seen mainly in the hands and feet, where they cause nodular thickening of the affected sheath. X-ray may show pressure erosion of an adjacent bone surface – for example, on one of the phalanges. At operation the boggy synovial tissue is often yellow; this type of lesion is sometimes called *xanthoma of tendon sheath*.

Pathology Histologically, joint and tendon sheath lesions are identical. There is proliferation and hypertrophy of the synovium, which contains fibroblastic tissue with foamy histiocytes and multinucleated giant cells. These features have engendered yet another name for the same condition: *giant-cell tumour of tendon sheath*.

Treatment The only effective treatment is synovectomy. Although the tumour does not undergo malignant change, the recurrence rate is high unless excision is complete. This may be unattainable and subtotal synovectomy is then sometimes combined with local radiotherapy. If, despite such aggressive treatment, there are repeated recurrences, it may be necessary to sacrifice the joint and carry out arthroplasty or arthrodesis.

SYNOVIAL SARCOMA

This malignant tumour usually develops near synovial joints in adolescents and young adults. However, only about 20 per cent involve the joint itself and the term 'synovioma' is a misnomer because this is not a tumour of synovium, though the histological appearance may resemble that of synovium.

The patient usually complains of rapid enlargement of a lump around one of the larger joints – the hip, the knee or the shoulder. Occasionally the tumour presents as a small swelling in the hand or foot and the histological diagnosis comes as a complete surprise. Pain is a common feature and many lesions are present for years before they are diagnosed. *X-rays* show a soft-tissue mass, sometimes with extensive calcification. *MRI* will help to outline the tumour.

Biopsy reveals a fleshy lesion composed of prolifera-

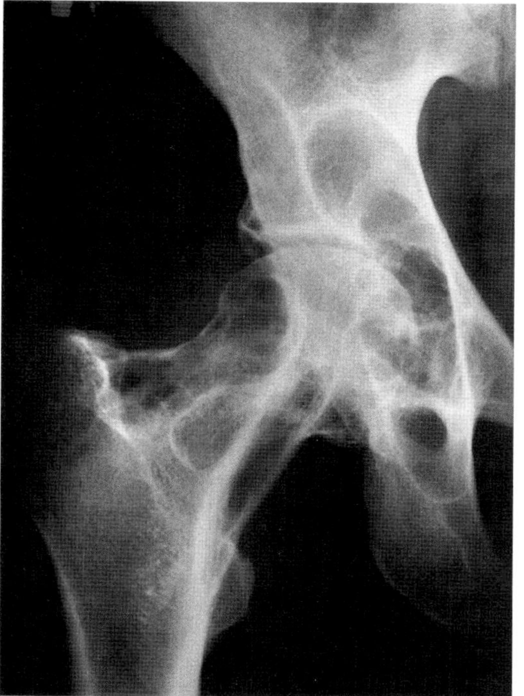
(a)

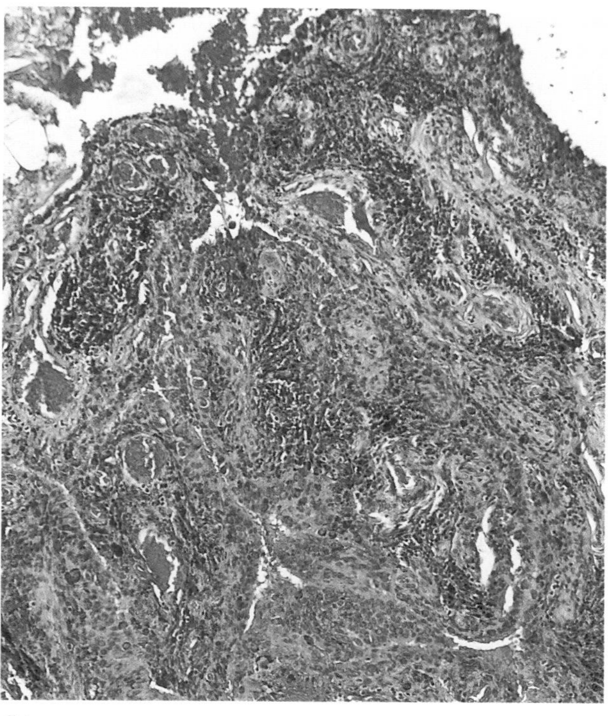
(b)

9.42 Pigmented villonodular synovitis (a) A farmer presented with pain in the hip. The x-rays showed cystic excavations on both sides of the joint and at first suggested tuberculosis. However, there were no signs of infection. At operation the synovium was thick and golden in colour. (b) The biopsy showed dense proliferation of the synovium with scattered multinucleated giant cells and haemosiderin. (×120)

tive 'synovial' cells and fibroblastic tissue; characteristically the cellular areas are punctured by vacant slits that give the tissue an acinar appearance. Cellular abnormality and mitoses reflect the degree of malignancy.

Small, well-defined lesions can be treated by wide excision. High-grade lesions, which usually have ill-defined margins, require radical resection – and this may mean radical amputation. Resection may be combined with radiotherapy and occasionally chemotherapy.

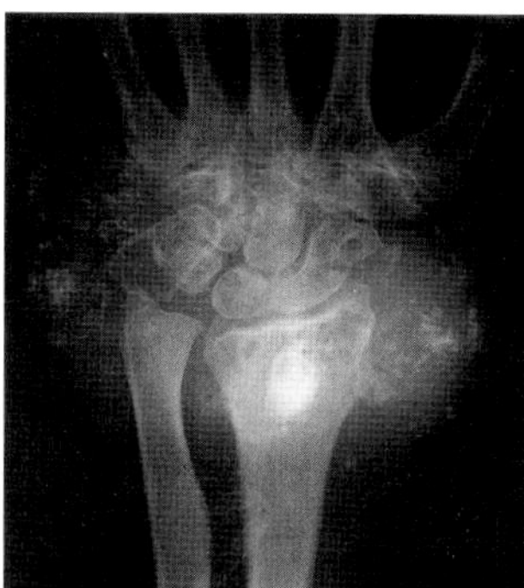
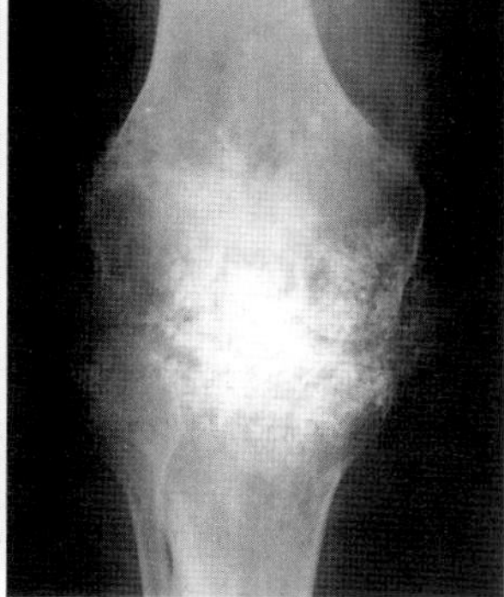

9.43 Malignant synoviomas X-rays showing the so-called 'snowstorm' appearance.

Blood vessel tumours

HAEMANGIOMA

This benign lesion, probably a hamartoma, is usually seen during childhood but may be present at birth. It occurs in two forms. The *capillary haemangioma* is more common; it usually appears as a reddish patch on the skin, and the congenital naevus or 'birthmark' is a familiar example. A *cavernous haemangioma* consists of a sponge-like collection of blood spaces; superficial lesions appear as blue or purple skin patches, sometimes overlying a soft subcutaneous mass; deep lesions may extend into the fascia or muscles, and occasionally an entire limb is involved. X-rays may show calcified phleboliths in the cavernous lesions.

There is no risk of malignant change and treatment is needed only if there is significant discomfort or disability. Local excision carries a high risk of recurrence, but more radical procedures seem unnecessarily destructive. Preoperative embolization of feeding vessels may reduce intra-operative bleeding.

GLOMUS TUMOUR

This rare tumour usually occurs around fine peripheral neurovascular structures, and especially in the nail beds of fingers or toes. A young adult presents with recurrent episodes of intense pain in the fingertip. A small bluish nodule may be seen under the nail; the area is sensitive to cold and exquisitely tender. X-rays sometimes show erosion of the underlying phalanx. Treatment is excision; the tumour, never larger than a pea, is easily shelled out of its fibrous capsule.

NERVE TUMOURS

NEUROMA

A neuroma is not a tumour but an overgrowth of fibrous tissue and randomly sprouting nerve fibrils following injury to a nerve. It is often tender and local percussion may induce distal paraesthesiae, thus indicating the level of the lesion (Tinel's sign).

Treatment can be frustrating. If the neuroma is excised (or as a prophylactic measure during amputation) the epineural sleeve can be freed from the nerve fascicles and sealed with a synthetic tissue adhesive.

NEURILEMMOMA

Neurilemmoma is a benign tumour of the nerve sheath. It is seen in the peripheral nerves and in the spinal nerve roots. The patient complains of pain or paraesthesiae; sometimes there is a small palpable swelling along the course of the nerve.

Growth on a spinal nerve root is a rare cause of 'sciatica', and x-rays of the spine may show erosion of the intervertebral foramen at that level. MRI will demonstrate the eccentric swelling on a peripheral nerve.

With careful dissection the tumour can be removed from its capsule without damage to the nerve.

NEUROFIBROMA

This is a benign tumour of fibrous and neural elements; its origin in a peripheral nerve may be obvious, but it is also seen as a nodule in the skin or subcutaneous tissues where it presumably originates in fine nerve fibrils. Occasionally it arises directly in bone; more often it causes pressure erosion of an adjacent surface.

Lesions may be solitary or multiple. Curiously, they are sometimes associated with skeletal abnormalities (scoliosis, pseudarthrosis of the tibia) or overgrowth of a digit or an entire limb, in which there is no obvious neural pathology.

The patient may present with a lump overlying one of the peripheral nerves, or with neurological symptoms such as paraesthesiae or muscle weakness. If a nerve root is involved, symptoms can mimic those of a disc prolapse; x-rays may show erosion of a vertebral pedicle or enlargement of the intervertebral foramen.

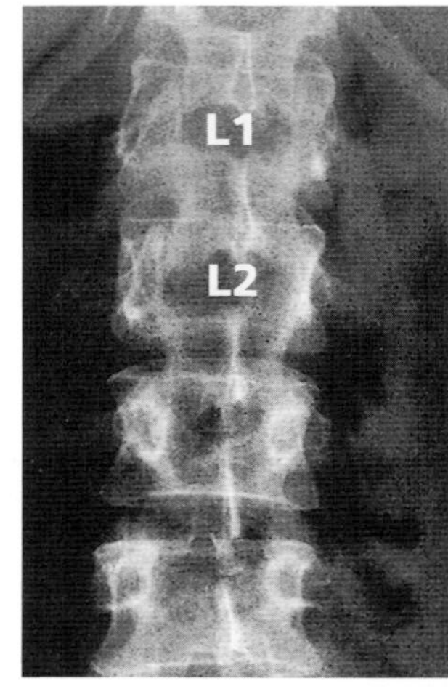

(a)

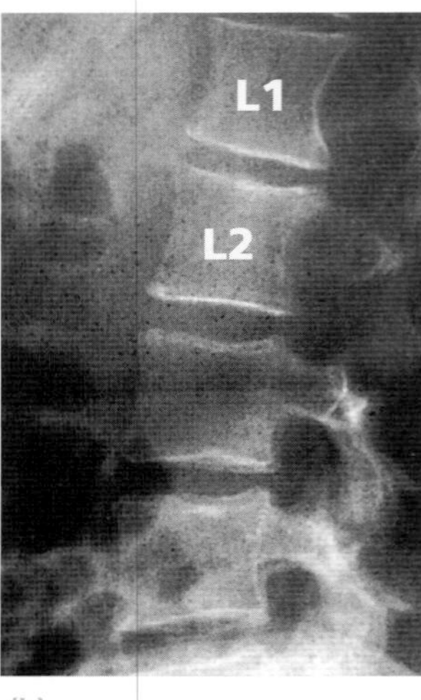

(b)

9.44 Neurofibromatosis (a) The anteroposterior x-ray shows erosion of the pedicles of L1 and L2. Compare the appearance with the well-marked pedicles (like staring eyes) at L3 and L4. (b) The lateral view shows scalloping of the backs of L1 and L2.

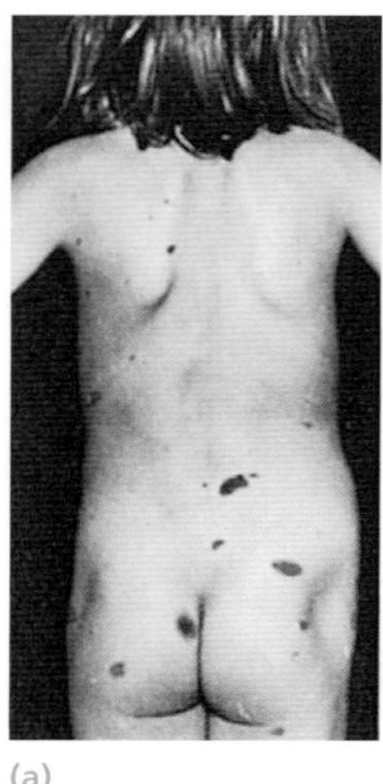

(a)

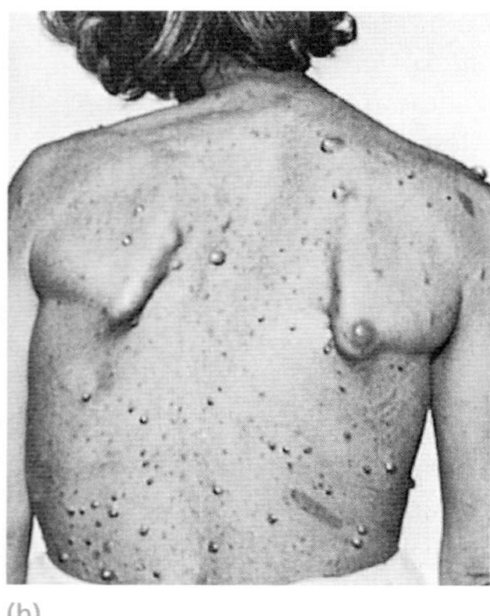

(b)

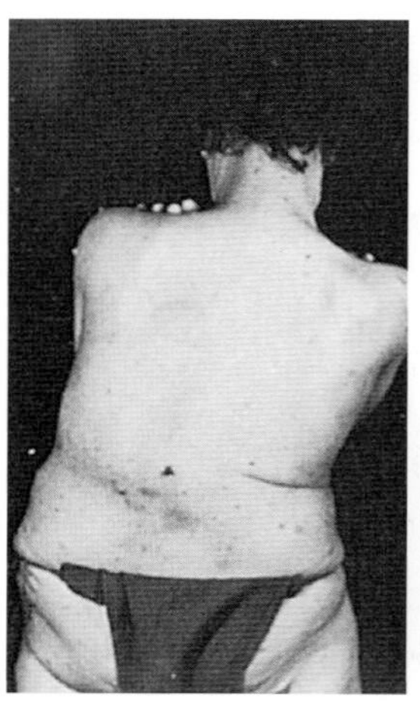

(c)

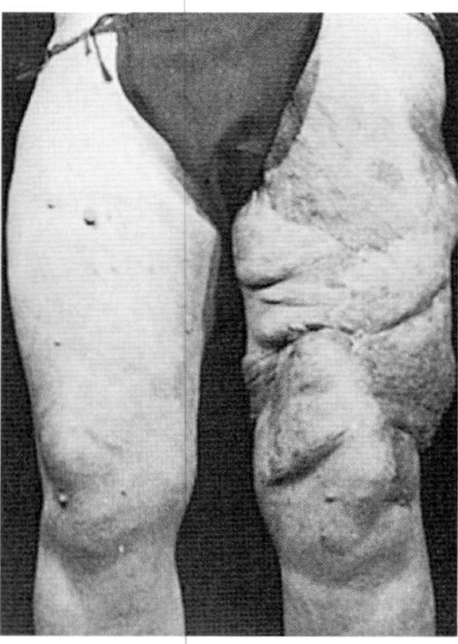

(d)

9.45 Neurofibromatosis (a) Café-au-lait spots, (b) multiple fibromata and slight scoliosis; (c,d) a patient with scoliosis and elephantiasis.

Multiple neurofibromatosis (von Recklinghausen's disease) is transmitted by autosomal dominant inheritance (see page 175). Patients (usually children) develop numerous skin nodules and *café-au-lait* patches; there may be associated skeletal abnormalities. Malignant transformation is said to occur in 5–10 per cent of cases.

Pathology The pathological appearance of the individual tumour is characteristic: on cross-section the lesion consists of pale fibrous tissue with nerve elements running into and through the substance of the tumour. Microscopically, the fibrillar and cellular elements are arranged in a wavy pattern.

Treatment Treatment is needed only if pain or paraesthesiae become troublesome, or if a tumour becomes very large. However, the tumour cannot be completely separated from intact nerve fibres; if it involves an unimportant nerve, it can be excised *en bloc*; if nerve damage is not acceptable, intracapsular shelling out is preferable, notwithstanding the risk of recurrence.

NEUROSARCOMA (MALIGNANT SCHWANNOMA)

Malignant tumours may arise from the cells of the nerve sheath or from a pre-existing neurofibroma. Symptoms are due to local pressure. There may be a visible or palpable swelling and percussion causes distal paraesthesiae.

Histologically this is a cellular fibrous lesion.

If the tumour arises in the neurovascular bundle, spread is inevitable and local excision is not feasible without severe damage to important structures. For this reason, treatment usually involves amputation.

MUSCLE TUMOURS

Tumours of muscle are rare; only those that occur in the striped muscle of the extremities are considered here.

RHABDOMYOMA

Rhabdomyoma is a rare cause of a lump in the muscle. It is occasionally confused with the 'lump' that appears after muscle rupture: both are in the line of a muscle, can be moved across but not along it, and harden with muscle contraction. However, with muscle rupture symptoms appear quite suddenly, there is a depression proximal or distal to the lump and the swelling does not grow any bigger. If a tumour is suspected, early exploration and biopsy are advisable because malignant change may occur. If the diagnosis is confirmed, the tumour should be excised.

RHABDOMYOSARCOMA

Malignant tumours are occasionally seen in the muscles around the shoulder or hip. The patient – usually a young adult – presents with ache and an enlarging, ill-defined lump that moves with the affected muscle. CT and MRI show that the mass is in the muscle, but the edge may be poorly demarcated because the tumour tends to spread along the fascial planes. At biopsy the tissue looks and feels different from normal muscle and microscopic examination shows clusters of highly abnormal muscle cells.

This is a high-grade lesion which requires radical resection of the affected muscle, i.e. from its origin to its insertion. If this cannot be assured or if the tumour has spread beyond the fascial sheath, amputation is advisable. Recurrent lesions are also treated by amputation. If complete removal is impossible, adjunctive radiotherapy may lessen the risk of recurrence.

REFERENCES AND FURTHER READING

American Joint Committee on Cancer. Bone: In *AJCC Cancer Staging Manual*, 5th Edn, eds Fleming ID *et al.* Lippincott-Raven, Philadelphia 1997.

Bauer HCF. Posterior decompression and stabilization for spinal metastases. Analysis of sixty-seven consecutive patients. *J Bone Joint Surg* 1997; **79A:** 514–22.

Bauer HCF, Wedin R. Survival after surgery for spinal and extremity metastases. Prognostication in 241 patients. *Acta Orthop Scand* 1995; **66:** 143–6.

Damron TA, Ward WG, Stewart A. Osteosarcoma, chondrosarcoma, and Ewing's sarcoma: National Cancer Data Base Report. *Clin Orthop Relat Res* 2007; **459:** 40–7.

Carter SR, Grimer RJ, Sneath RS. A review of 13 years experience of osteosarcoma. *Clin Orthop Relat Res* 1991; **270:** 45–51.

DiCaprio MR, Friedlaender GE. Malignant bone tumours: Limb sparing versus amputation. *J Amer Med Assoc* 2003; **11:** 25–37.

Donnelly LF, Bisset GF, Helms CA *et al.* Chronic avulsive injuries of childhood. *Skeletal Radiol* 1999; **28:** 138–44.

Enneking WF. A system of staging musculoskeletal neoplasms. *Clin Orthop Relat Res* 1986; **204:** 9–24.

Galasko CS, Norris HE, Crank S. Spinal instability secondary to metastatic cancer. *J Bone Joint Surg* 2000; **82A:** 570–94.

Horowitz SM, Glasser DB, Lane JM, Healy JH Prosthetic and extremity survivorship after limb salvage for sarcoma. *Clin Orthop* 1993; **295:** 280–6.

Janinis J, Patriki M, Vini L *et al.* The pharmacological treatment of aggressive fibromatosis: a systematic review. *Ann Oncol* 2003; **14:** 181–90.

Jeys LM, Grimer RJ, Carter SR, Tillman RM. Periprosthetic infection in patients treated for an orthopaedic oncological condition. *J Bone Joint Surg* 2005; **87A:** 842–9.

Jeys LM, Kulkarni A, Grimer RJ, Carter SR, *et al.* Endoprosthetic reconstruction for the treatment of musculoskeletal tumors of the appendicular skeleton and pelvis. *J Bone Joint Surg* 2008; **90A:** 1265–71.

Lange TA, Austin CW, Siebert JJ *et al.* Ultrasound imaging as a screening study for malignant soft tissue tumors. *J Bone Joint Surg* 1987; **69A:** 100–105.

Malghem J, Maldague B, Esselinckx W *et al.* Spontaneous healing of aneurysmal bone cysts. *J Bone Joint Surg* 1989; **71B:** 645–50.

Mankin HJ, Gebhardt MC. Advances in the management of bone tumours. *Clin Orthop Relat Res* 1985; **200:** 73–84.

Mankin HJ, Lange TA, Spanier SS. The hazards of biopsy in patients with malignant primary bone and soft-tissue tumors. *J Bone Joint Surg* 1982; **64A:** 1121–7.

Mankin HJ, Mankin CJ, Simon MA. The hazards of biopsy, revisited. *J Bone Joint Surg* 1996; **78A:** 656–63

McLeod RA, Dahlin DC, Beabout JW. The spectrum of osteoblastoma. *Am J Roentgenol* 1976; **126:** 321–35.

Mirels H. Metastatic disease in long bones: A proposed scoring system for diagnosing impending pathological fractures. *Clin Orthop Relat Res* 1989; **249:** 256–64.

O'Connor MI, Sim FH, Chao EYS. Limb salvage for neoplasms around the shoulder girdle. *J Bone Joint Surg* 1996; **78A:** 1872–88.

Peabody TD, Gibbs CP, Simon MA. Evaluation and staging of musculoskeletal neoplasms. *J Bone Joint Surg* 1998; **80A:** 1204–18.

Pettersson H, Gillespy T, Hamlin DJ *et al.* Primary musculoskeletal tumors: examination with MR imaging compared with conventional modalities. *Radiology* 1987; **164:** 237–41.

Pritchard DJ, Nascimento AG, Petersen IA. Local control of extra-abdominal desmoid tumors. *J Bone Joint Surg* 1996; **78A:** 848–54.

Roberts P, Chan D, Grimer RJ *et al.* Prosthetic replacement of the distal femur for primary bone tumours. *J Bone Joint Surg* 1991; **73B:** 762–9.

Rosen G. Neoadjuvant chemotherapy for osteogenic sarcoma. In *Limb Salvage in Musculoskeletal Oncology* ed. Enneking WF, Churchill Livingstone, New York, p. 260, 1987.

Rosen G, Caparrow B, Huvos AG *et al.* Pre-operative chemotherapy for osteogenic sarcoma: selection of post-operative chemotherapy based on the response of the primary tumor to pre-operative chemotherapy. *Cancer* 1982; **49:** 1221–30.

Saifuddin A, Mitchell R, Burnett S. *et al.* Ultrasound guided needle biopsy of primary bone tumours. *J Bone Joint Surg* 2000; **82B:** 505–4.

Russell WO, Cohen J, Enzinger F, *et al.* A clinical and pathological staging system for soft tissue sarcoma. *Cancer* 1977; **40:** 1562–70.

Schajowicz F. Tumors and tumorlike lesions of bone, 2nd ed., Berlin: Springer–Verlag; 1994.

Sim FH, Frassica FJ, Frassica DA. Soft-tissue tumours: Diagnosis, evaluation, and management. *J Am Acad Orthop Surg* 1994; **2:** 202–11.

Smeland S, WiebeT, Böhling T, *et al.* Chemotherapy in osteosarcoma. The Scandinavian Sarcoma Group experience. *Acta Orthop Scand* 2004; **(Suppl 311):** 75

Souhami RL, Craft AW. Annotation. Progress in management of malignant bone tumours. *J Bone Joint Surg* 1988; **70B:** 345–7.

Springfield DS, Rosenberg A. Biopsy: complicated and risky. *J Bone Joint Surg* 1996; **78A:** 639–43.

Stark A, Kreicbergs A, Nilsonne U, Sillvensward L. The age of osteosarcoma patients is increasing. *J Bone Joint Surg* 1990; **72:** 89–93.

Stoker DJ, Cobb JP, Pringle JAS. Needle biopsy of musculoskeletal lesions. A review of 208 procedures. *J Bone Joint Surg* 1991; **37B:** 498–500.

Watt, I. Radiology in the diagnosis and management of bone tumours. *J Bone Joint Surg* 1985; **67B:** 520–9.

Neuromuscular disorders

10

Deborah Eastwood, Thomas Staunton, Louis Solomon

NERVES AND MUSCLES

NEURONS

The neuron is the defining unit of the nervous system. It is a specialized cell, capable of electrical excitation and conduction of electrochemical impulses (*action potentials*) along its thread-like extensions. Its basic structure consists of a cell body, 5–25 μm in diameter, with branching processes – *dendrites* – that are capable of receiving signals from other neuronal terminals. A finer, longer branch – the *axon* – carries the action potentials along its length to or from excitable target organs. Further signal transmission to the dendrites of another neuron, or neuro-excitable tissue like muscle, occurs at a *synapse* where the axon terminal releases a chemical neurotransmitter – typically acetylcholine.

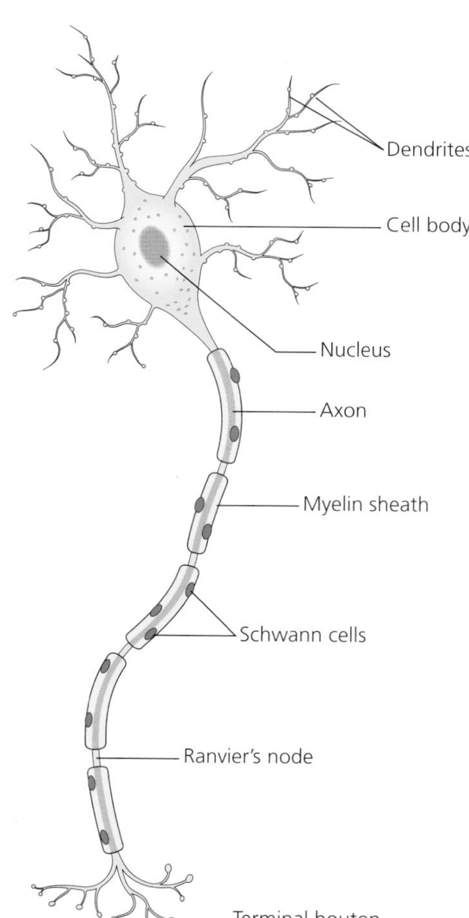

10.1 Diagram of a typical neuron

All motor axons and the larger sensory axons serving touch, pain and proprioception are covered by a sheath – *the neurilemma* – and coated with *myelin*, a multilayered lipoprotein substance derived from the accompanying Schwann cells (or oligodendrocytes in the central nervous system). Every few millimetres the myelin sheath is interrupted, leaving short segments of bare axon called the *nodes of Ranvier*. In these nerves the myelin coating serves as an insulator, which allows the impulse to be propagated by electromagnetic conduction from node to node, much faster than is the case in unmyelinated nerves. Consequently, depletion of the myelin sheath causes slowing – and eventually complete blocking – of axonal conduction.

Most axons, in particular the small-diameter fibres carrying crude sensation and efferent sympathetic fibres, are not myelinated but wrapped in Schwann cell cytoplasm. Damage to these axons causes unpleasant or bizarre sensations and abnormal sudomotor and vasomotor effects.

NERVOUS PATHWAYS

Anatomically, neurological structures can be divided into the *central nervous system* (the CNS, comprising the brain and tracts of the spinal cord) and the *peripheral nervous system* (PNS) which includes the cranial and spinal nerves. In terms of physiological function, both the CNS and the PNS have a somatic component and an autonomic component.

The *somatic nervous system* provides efferent motor and afferent sensory pathways to and from peripheral parts of the body serving, respectively, voluntary muscle contraction and sensibility.

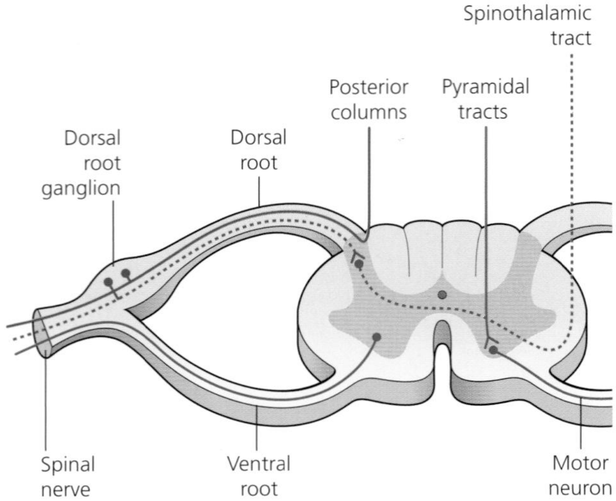

10.2 Main nerve pathways Simplified diagram showing the main neurological pathways to and from a typical thoracic spinal cord segment. Fibres carrying touch, sharp pain and temperature impulses (-------) decussate, in some cases over several spinal segments, and ascend in the contralateral spinothalamic tracts; those carrying vibration and proprioceptive impulses (——) enter the ipsilateral posterior columns. Motor neurons (——) arise in the anterior horn of the grey matter and innervate ipsilateral muscles.

The *autonomic system* controls involuntary reflex and homeostatic activities of the cardiovascular system, visceral organs and glands. Its two components, sympathetic and parasympathetic divisions, serve more or less opposing functions.

SOMATIC MOTOR SYSTEM

Efferent impulses are conducted along axons in the corticospinal or pyramidal tracts (upper motor neurons – UMN) and along peripheral nerves from cell bodies in the anterior horn of the spinal cord to striated muscle fibres (lower motor neurons – LMN). The terminal synapses are situated at the neuromuscular junctions. Each large α-motor neuron innervates from a few to several hundred muscle fibres (together forming a *motor unit*) and stimulates muscle fibre contraction. In large muscles of the lower limb, power is adjusted by recruiting more or fewer motor units. Smaller γ-motor neurons connect to sensors (muscle spindles) that control proprioceptive feedback from muscle fibres.

SOMATIC SENSORY SYSTEM

Axons conveying afferent impulses from receptors in the skin and other peripheral structures enter the dorsal nerve roots, with their cell bodies in the dorsal root (or cranial nerve) ganglia, and end in synapses within the central nervous system. Myelinated fibres carrying sensory stimuli from touch, pressure, pain and temperature (*exteroceptive sensation*) decussate and enter the contralateral spinothalamic tracts running up the spinal cord to the brain. Fibres from sensors in the joints, ligaments, tendons and muscle carrying the sense of movement and bodily position in space (*proprioceptive sensation*) join the ipsilateral posterior columns in the spinal cord.

Sensory areas (dermatomes) corresponding to the spinal nerve roots are shown in Figure 10.5. However, it should be remembered that there is considerable overlap of the boundaries shown in these body maps; furthermore, some parts, such as the hands and lips, are more sensitive and discriminatory than others.

REFLEX ACTIVITY AND TONE

Sudden stretching of a muscle (e.g. by tapping sharply over the tendon) induces an involuntary muscle contraction – *the stretch reflex*. The sharp change in muscle fibre length is detected by the muscle spindle; the impulse is transmitted rapidly along myelinated afferent (sensory) neurons which synapse directly with the corresponding segmental α-motor neurons in the spinal cord, triggering efferent signals which stimulate the muscle to contract. This is the basis of the familiar clinical tests for tendon reflexes, and is also the mechanism for maintaining normal *muscle tone*.

Segmental reflex activity is normally regulated by motor impulses passing from the brain down the spinal cord. Interruption of the UMN pathways results in undamped reflex muscle contraction (clinically hyperactive tendon reflexes) and spastic paralysis. Damage to either afferent or efferent neurons in the reflex arc causes hypotonia; interruption of the LMN pathway results in flaccid LMN paralysis.

AUTONOMIC SYSTEM

The autonomic system is involved with the regulation of involuntary activities of cardiac muscle and smooth (unstriated) muscle of the lungs, gastrointestinal tract, kidneys, bladder, genital organs, sweat glands and small blood vessels, with afferent (sensory) and efferent (motor) pathways constituting a continuously active reflex arc (though there is also some input from higher centres). In addition afferent fibres also convey visceral pain sensation.

The system is divided into *sympathetic* and *parasympathetic* pathways, both of which comprise efferent and afferent neurons.

Preganglionic *sympathetic neurons* leave the spinal cord with the ventral nerve roots at all levels from T1 to L1, enter the paravertebral sympathetic chain of ganglia and synapse with postganglionic neurons that spread out to all parts of the body; they may also run up or down the sympathetic chain to synapse in other ganglia or pass on to become splanchnic nerves. Important functions are the reflex control of heart rate, blood flow and sweating, as well as other responses associated with conditions of 'fight and flight'.

Parasympathetic neurons leave the CNS (from the brain-stem) with cranial nerves III, VII, IX, X and with the nerve roots of S2, 3 and 4 to reach ganglia where they synapse with postganglionic neurons close to their target organs.

Peripheral nerves

Peripheral nerves are bundles of axons conducting efferent (motor) impulses from cells in the anterior horn of the spinal cord to the muscles, and afferent (sensory) impulses from peripheral receptors via cells in the posterior root ganglia to the cord. They also convey sudomotor and vasomotor fibres from ganglion cells in the sympathetic chain. Some nerves are predominantly motor, some predominantly sensory; the larger trunks are mixed, with motor and sensory axons running in separate bundles. Detailed peripheral nerve structure is described in Chapter 11.

Skeletal muscle

Each skeletal muscle belly, held within a connective tissue *epimysium*, consists of thousands of muscle fibres, separated into bundles (or *fascicles*). Each fascicle is surrounded by a flimsy *perimysium* which envelops anything up to about 100 muscle fibres; large muscles concerned with mass movement, like the glutei or quadriceps, have a large number of fibres in each fascicle, while muscles used for precision movements (like those of the hand) have a much smaller number in each bundle.

The muscle fibre is the important unit of all striated muscle. Lying in a barely discernable connective tissue cover, or *endomysium*, it is in actuality a single cell with a cell membrane (the *sarcolemma*), a type of cytoplasm (or sarcoplasm), mitochondria and many thousands of nuclei; its diameter is about 10 μm at birth and 60–80 μm in mature adults.

The fibre itself consists of many tiny (1 μm diameter) *myofibrils*, each of which is striated: dark bands consisting of thick myosin filaments alternate with light bands of thin actin filaments (A and I bands respectively). In the middle of each A band is a lighter H zone and in the middle of the I band there is a dark thin Z line. The portion of the myofibril between two Z lines is the sarcomere, representing a single contractile unit.

The α-motor neuron and the group of muscle fibres it supplies constitute a single motor unit; the number of muscle fibres in the unit may be less than five in muscles concerned with fine manipulatory movements or more than 100 in those employed in gross power movements.

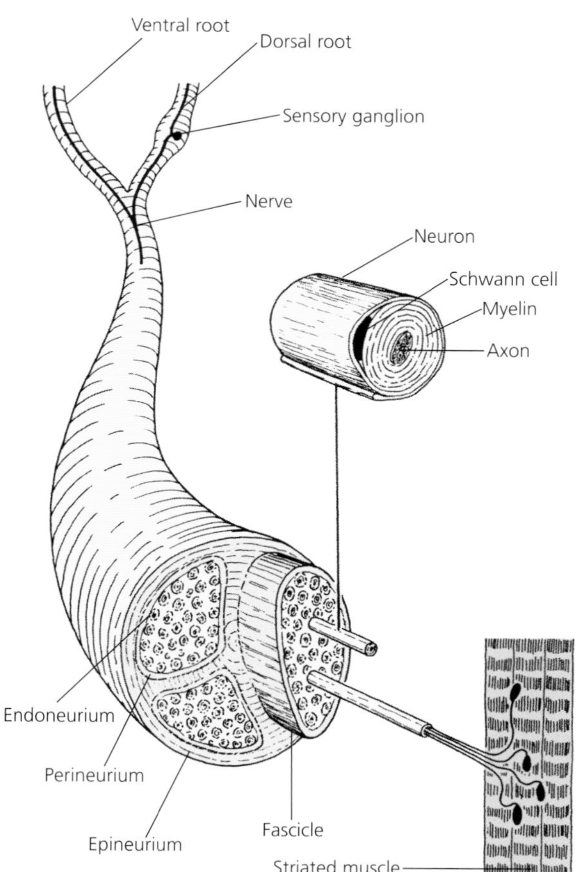

10.3 Nerve structure Diagram of the structural elements of a peripheral nerve.

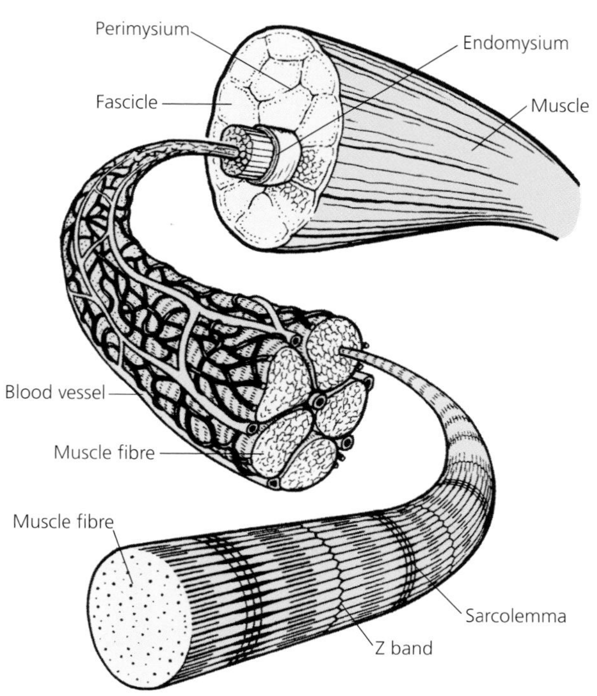

10.4 Muscle structure Diagram showing the structural elements of striated muscle.

Muscle fibres are also of different types, which can be distinguished by histochemical staining. *Type I fibres* contract slowly and are not easily fatigued; their prime function is postural control. *Type II fibres* are fast contracting but they fatigue rapidly; hence they are ideally suited to intense activities of short duration. All muscles consist of a mixture of fibre types, the balance depending on anatomical site, basic muscle function, degree of training, genetic disposition and response to previous injury or illness. Long-distance runners have a greater proportion of type I fibres than the average in age- and sex-matched individuals.

Muscle contraction is a complex activity. Individual myofibrils respond to electrical stimuli in much the same way as do motor neurons. However, muscle fibres, and the muscle as a whole, are activated by overlap and summation of contractile responses. When the fibres contract, internal tension in the muscle increases. In *isometric contraction* there is increased tension without actual shortening of the muscle or movement of the joint controlled by that muscle. In *isotonic contraction* the muscle shortens and moves the joint, but tension within the muscle fibres remains constant.

Muscle tone is the state of tension in a resting muscle when it is passively stretched; characteristically tone is increased in upper motor neuron (UMN) lesions (spastic paralysis) and decreased in lower motor neuron (LMN) lesions (flaccid paralysis).

Muscle contracture (as distinct from contraction) is the adaptive change which occurs when a normally innervated muscle is held immobile in a shortened position for some length of time. If a joint is allowed to be held flexed for a long time, it may be impossible to straighten it passively without injuring the muscle. Active exercise will eventually overcome the muscle contracture, unless the muscle has been permanently damaged.

Muscle wasting follows either disuse or denervation; in the former, the fibres are intact but thinner; in the latter, they degenerate and are replaced by fibrous tissue or fat.

Muscle fasciculation – or muscle twitch – is a local involuntary muscle contraction of a small bundle of muscle fibres. It is usually benign but can be due to motor neuron disease or dysfunction.

CLINICAL ASSESSMENT

History

Age at presentation is important. Certain congenital or syndromic neuromuscular disorders are obvious at birth (e.g. spina bifida and arthrogryposis). Others, while undoubtedly caused by perinatal problems, may not actually manifest themselves until later in childhood; cerebral palsy is the prime example. Conditions such as poliomyelitis may affect anyone although children are most commonly afflicted. In contrast, spinal cord lesions and peripheral neuropathies are more common in adults. The orthopaedic surgeon must be ready to diagnose and treat neuromuscular disease throughout life.

Past medical history may be relevant in terms of previous trauma (accidental or surgical), previous illnesses and their treatment (chemotherapy).

Muscle weakness may be due to upper or lower motor neuron lesions (spastic versus flaccid paralysis) but it may also be due to a primary muscle problem. The type and degree of weakness, the rate of onset, whether it affects part of a limb, a whole limb, upper or lower limb, one side of the body or both sides – all these details should be enquired into and help to give an insight into the aetiology.

Numbness and *paraesthesiae* may be the main complaints. It is important to establish their exact distribution to help localize the anatomical nature and level of the lesion accurately. The rate of onset and the relationship to posture may, similarly, suggest the cause. A history of trauma, including recent surgical procedures, or the use of a tourniquet must be noted.

Deformity is a common complaint in longstanding disorders. It arises as a result of muscle imbalances that may be very subtle and the deformity (such as 'claw toes') may not be recognized until it is pointed out to the patient.

Non-orthopaedic problems should also be discussed. It can be particularly important to note 'throw-away' comments regarding problems such as headaches, dizziness, falls, feeding problems, hearing difficulties or visual disturbances in addition to the more obvious complaints of cognitive impairment, speech disorders or incontinence. Some symptoms will only be disclosed on direct questioning as the patient may not consider them relevant; other symptoms, such as incontinence or impotence, may be too embarrassing to mention. Symptoms may also have been present for so long that they are considered to be 'normal'.

Family history may reveal clues to the underlying aetiology of the patient's symptoms.

Examination

Neurological examination is described in Chapter 1. Particular attention should be paid to the patient's mental state, natural posture, gait, sense of balance, involuntary movements, muscle wasting, muscle tone and power, reflexes, skin changes, the various modes of sensibility and autonomic functions such as sphincter control, peripheral blood flow and sweating. *The back* should always be carefully examined as it holds the key to many causes of neurological disorder.

Table 10.1 Nerve root supply and actions of main muscle groups

Sternomastoids	Spinal accessory C2, 3, 4
Trapezius	Spinal accessory C3, 4
Diaphragm	C3, 4, 5
Deltoid	C5, 6
Supra- and infraspinatus	C5, 6
Serratus anterior	C5, 6, 7
Pectoralis major	C5, 6, 7, 8
Elbow flexion	C5, 6
extension	C7
Supination	C5, 6
Pronation	C6
Wrist flexion	C6, (7)
extension	C6, 7, (8)
Finger flexion	C7, 8, T1
extension	C7, 8, T1
ab- and adduction	C8, T1
Hip flexion	L1, 2, 3
extension	L5,S1
adduction	L2, 3, 4
abduction	L4, 5, S1
Knee extension	L(2), 3, 4
flexion	L5, S1
Ankle dorsiflexion	L4, 5
plantarflexion	S1, 2
inversion	L4, 5
eversion	L5, S1
Toe extension	L5
flexion	S1
abduction	S1, 2

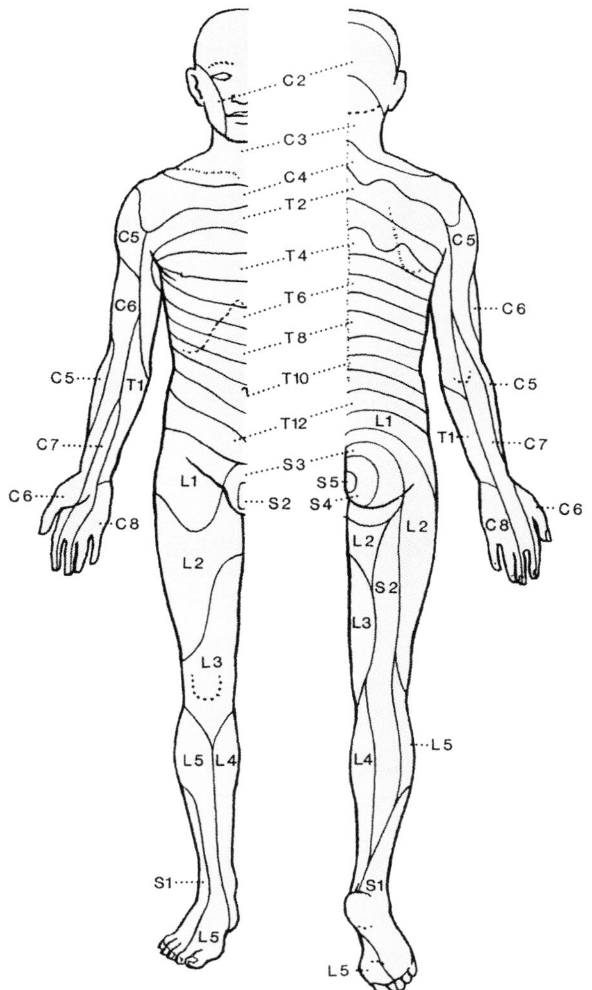

10.5 Examination Dermatomes supplied by the spinal nerve roots.

GAIT AND POSTURE

A single gait cycle consists of a stance phase (60 per cent) and a swing phase (40 per cent) and each full cycle represents the stride length. Many parameters of each phase at each joint and in all three planes (coronal, sagittal and transverse) can be analysed, often using a *computerized gait analysis* facility. However, much can be learnt by carefully studying the way the patient walks and moves; clinical gait analysis improves with experience and allows distinctive movement patterns to be recognized:

- *Dystonia* – This term refers to abnormal posturing (focal or generalized) that may affect any part of the body and is often aggravated when the patient is concentrating on a particular motor task such as walking.
- *Antalgic gait* – A markedly shortened stance phase on one side. Pain makes the patient move off the affected limb as quickly as possible.
- *Spastic gait* – A stiff-legged gait, often with a crouching posture (flexed hips and knees and feet in equinus) and 'scissoring' (legs crossing each other), due to muscle imbalance.
- *Drop-foot gait* – During swing, the foot 'drops' into equinus; if the foot was not lifted higher than usual the toes would drag along the floor. This is caused by disorder or damage to the peripheral nerves supplying the foot dorsiflexors.
- *High-stepping gait* – This could be due to a bilateral foot drop or it may signify problems with balance or proprioception.
- *Waddling (Trendelenburg) gait* – The trunk is thrown from side to side with each step. The

MRC GRADING OF MUSCLE POWER

Grade	Description
0	No muscle action – total paralysis
1	Minimal muscle contraction
2	Power insufficient to overcome gravity
3	Anti-gravity muscle power
4	Less than full power
5	Full power

mechanics are similar to those that produce a positive Trendelenburg test (see page 493), as seen in patients with functionally weak abductor muscles (or dislocation) of the hip.

- *Ataxic gait* – Ataxia produces a more obvious and irregular loss of balance, which is compensated for by a broad-based gait, or sometimes uncontrollable staggering.

MOTOR POWER AND TONE

It is important to examine not only individual muscles but also functional groups. In flaccid paralysis, grading muscle power is important; in spastic paralysis, the spasticity often obscures the inherent weakness and testing specific muscles can be difficult due to the patient's inability to isolate individual movements. Muscle power is usually graded as shown in the accompanying Box. Repeated muscle charting allows an objective measure of progressive disease or recovery to be documented.

WEAKNESS

When patients complain of 'weakness' they often fail to distinguish between true loss of muscle power and difficulties due to pain or instability. When testing for muscle power it is essential to address individual muscles and muscle groups as well as mass movements.

Different patterns of weakness will be encountered. Weakness may be partial (*paresis*) or complete (*paralysis*).

- *Monoplegia* (weakness of one limb) is usually indicative of a lower motor neuron defect, most commonly a peripheral nerve or nerve root; the movements affected on clinical testing will suggest the likely anatomical location. However, if only the lower limb is affected the lesion could be in the distal part of the spinal cord.
- *Hemiparesis* (weakness of either the right or the left side of the body) usually denotes pathology somewhere between the cerebral cortex and the cervical segment of the spinal cord; this will be an upper motor neuron (spastic) type of weakness. Complete loss of power is called *hemiplegia*.
- *Diplegia* (weakness in both upper or both lower limbs) can be due to either UMN or LMN disorder. In some cases the apparently unaffected limbs may show minimal degrees of weakness which could easily be missed.
- *Quadriplegia* (all four limbs affected) could be due to either UMN or LMN pathology, e.g. cerebral palsy, high cord damage or anterior horn cell pathology like poliomyelitis.

DEFORMITY

In *unbalanced paralysis*, one group of muscles is too weak to balance the pull of the antagonists. At first this produces a deformity that can be corrected passively (*dynamic deformity*); over time the active muscles and the soft tissues of the joints contract and the deformity becomes *fixed* or *structural*.

In *balanced paralysis*, the joint assumes the position imposed on it by gravity and it may feel floppy or flail.

In a dynamic deformity, rebalancing of the muscle forces may be possible with a tendon transfer. If the deformity is fixed, soft-tissue releases, and possibly osteotomies, may be needed to correct the deformity before rebalancing can be considered.

Paralysis occurring in childhood seriously affects growth. Bones are thinner and shorter than usual and in the absence of normal mechanical stresses (imposed by normal muscle pull) bone modelling can be defective (e.g. a valgus femoral neck–shaft angle, which is often seen in neuromuscular disorders).

SENSATION

All sensory modalities must be tested over all dermatomes. Any sensory disturbance must be mapped to see if it fits a particular distribution pattern: dermatomal, glove and stocking or peripheral nerve distribution.

AUTONOMIC SYSTEM

A basic assessment of autonomic nervous system function is useful: colour, warmth and sudomotor function can be assessed quickly and easily.

Imaging

Plain x-rays of the skull and/or spine are routine for all disorders of the central nervous system. If the diagnosis is not obvious, further studies by CT or MRI may be necessary.

Spinal imaging is usually directed at identifying compression of the cord or the nerve roots, the level of compression and its cause. *Fractures and dislocations* usually show on the plain x-rays but a CT scan will reveal the exact relationship of bone fragments to nerve structures. *Prolapsed intervertebral disc* is usually diagnosed on clinical examination, but myelography, CT and MRI will help to establish the extent of the lesion and its exact site. *Narrowing of the spinal canal* is best demonstrated by CT; the commonest cause is osteophytic overgrowth following disc degeneration and osteoarthritis of the facet joints. This is even worse when the spinal canal is congenitally narrow or trefoil-shaped (spinal stenosis).

Destructive lesions of the bones may be due to infection or tumour (usually metastatic lesions). These may show on plain x-rays but CT, MRI and myelography are helpful.

Imaging of the brain is usually by MRI. Functional scans such as positron emission tomography (PET scan) that can isolate specific areas of brain activity are also gaining in popularity and are used in conjunction with MRI and CT.

Other investigations

Blood and *cerebrospinal fluid* investigations may be necessary, depending on the working diagnosis.

Muscle biopsy, to be reliable, calls for great care: the biopsy must be taken from a muscle that is affected but still functioning; local anaesthetic infiltration must be avoided; the specimen must be handled gently; and, depending on the tests required, it must be kept at its resting fibre length. Biopsies must be placed in special transport medium or frozen immediately.

Audiological and *ophthalmic testing* and *assessment of mental capacity* are also helpful in certain cases.

NEUROPHYSIOLOGICAL STUDIES

Neurodiagnostic techniques comprising *nerve conduction studies* and needle *electromyography* have an important role in the investigation of peripheral nerve and muscle disorders. Theoretically, any motor or sensory nerve can be studied, but in everyday clinical practice most of these investigations are involved in studying the median, ulnar and radial motor and sensory responses in the upper limb, and the sciatic nerve as well as the posterior tibial and peroneal divisions, motor and sensory, in the lower limbs.

Needle electromyography (EMG) of individual muscles is used as a complementary technique, which gives information about the nature and number of the activated or denervated motor units from the specific nerve root that innervates the muscle being tested. This can be used for anatomical clarification and separation of radiculopathy from peripheral neuropathy and myopathy.

Nerve conduction studies

Motor nerve conduction

The nerve under study (usually a mixed motor and sensory nerve) is stimulated electrically at an easily accessible subcutaneous site (e.g. the forearm or wrist for the median nerve or behind the medial malleolus for the posterior tibial nerve), until it propagates an action potential which travels to the innervated muscle where a surface electrode records the response. Measurements are displayed on an oscilloscope screen, the most informative being the time it takes in milliseconds (ms) for the impulse to reach the muscle, called the *latency*, and the magnitude of the response in millivolts (mV), called the *amplitude* of the evoked compound muscle action potential (CMAP). By measuring the distance from the stimulating electrode to the recording electrode, and setting this against the latency, one can deduce the *nerve conduction velocity* (NCV) in metres per second between those two points.

In practice it is more useful (and more accurate) to stimulate the nerve at two points, first at a distal site and then at a proximal site, and subtract the distal latency from the proximal latency to obtain a truer measurement for the intervening segment of the nerve. Thus, to measure the NCV of the median nerve in the carpal tunnel, one would take readings with the stimulating electrode first distal to the carpal tunnel and then in the upper forearm; this would allow one to deduce the NCV in the particular segment of the nerve at the carpal tunnel.

Similarly with measurement of amplitude, which is proportional to the number of motor units stimulated: if a patient has lost one-half of the nerve fibres in a peripheral nerve (e.g. due to compression, trauma

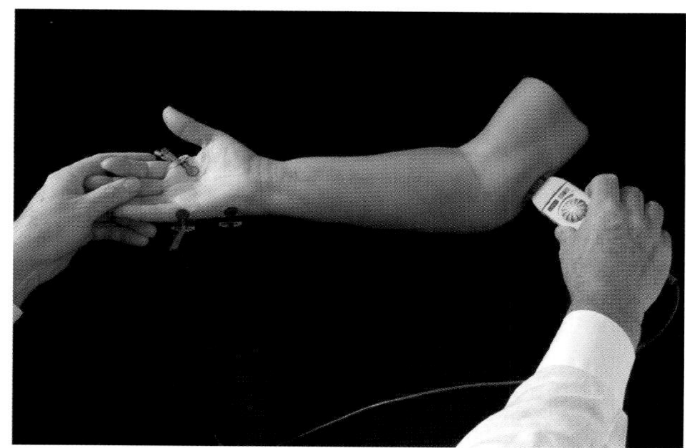

10.6 Ulnar motor nerve conduction The ulnar nerve is stimulated above the elbow, posterior to the medial epicondyle, and the CMAP is recorded from the abductor digiti minimi.

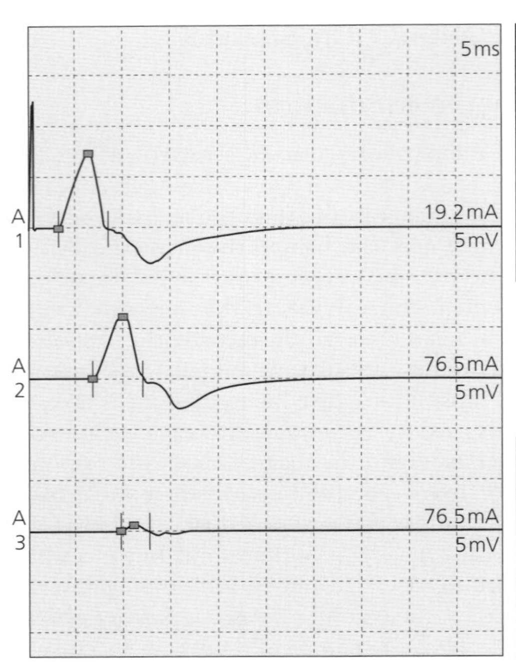

Stimulus site	Lat1 ms	Dur ms	Amp mV	Area mVms
A1: Wrist	2.9	5.2	7.7	21.1
A2: Below elbow	6.5	5.3	6.3	17.5
A3: Above elbow	9.5	3.0	0.6	1.1
A4: Axilla				
A5: Erb's point				

Segment	Dist mm	Diff ms	CV m/s
Wrist-Below elbow	220	3.6	61
Below elbow-Above elbow	80	3.0	27
Above elbow-axilla			
AxillaErb's point-			

10.7 Nerve conduction velocity Oscillographic recordings of nerve conduction studies in a case of acute ulnar nerve palsy due to compression of the patient's arm while undergoing surgery under general anaesthesia. These tracings show an acute motor nerve conduction block at the elbow, with normal distal CMAPs when stimulating below the elbow (tracings A1 and A2) and a reduced amplitude CMAP when stimulating above the elbow (A3). There is severe focal conduction slowing across the elbow at 27 m/s, compared to 61 m/s in the segment below the elbow.

or vascular insufficiency) the size of the elicited CMAP will be reduced by approximately 50 per cent compared to the contralateral normal limb. When a nerve is stimulated at two sites, distally and then proximally, the evoked CMAPs should be of similar amplitudes. However, if the CMAP on proximal stimulation is observed to be smaller than the CMAP on distal stimulation, one assumes that a reduced number of motor units have conducted the action potential over the intervening segment of the nerve: this is referred to as *conduction block* and is a feature of a potentially recoverable neuropraxic lesion.

Common investigations are measurement of the NCV for the median nerve at the wrist or the ulnar nerve at the elbow in suspected cases of carpal tunnel syndrome or cubital tunnel syndrome respectively. In a focal entrapment neuropathy one will find focal slowing with normal velocities on either side of the lesion.

Conduction slowing of uniform degree along the whole length of the nerve suggests a demyelinating neuropathy, e.g. Charcot–Marie–Tooth syndrome.

Sensory nerve conduction

In a similar manner, a sensory nerve action potential (SNAP) may be recorded by stimulating a suitable subcutaneous sensory nerve and recording with surface electrodes on the skin over a measured distance along the same sensory nerve, e.g. from the index and middle fingers of the *median* nerve. SNAP is much smaller in amplitude than CMAP and is measured in microvolts.

NOTE: Clinical nerve conduction studies estimate the population of large myelinated sensory or motor nerves. Type C fibres (small myelinated fibres serving pain and temperature appreciation) have an amplitude below the sensitivity of recording techniques, as well as slowed velocity (5–10 metres/second) and cannot be tested with standard clinical techniques.

Electromyography (EMG)

To record the electrical discharge of motor units in a muscle, a concentric needle electrode, the shape of a small hypodermic needle, is inserted into the muscle and connected to an oscilloscopic screen and a loudspeaker. This will provide both a visual pattern on the

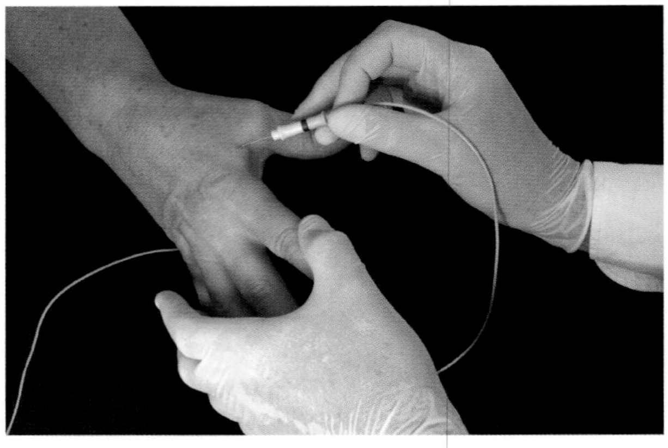

10.8 Needle electromyography (EMG) The first dorsal interosseus muscle (C8–T1 ulnar nerve) is being sampled during voluntary contraction against resistance.

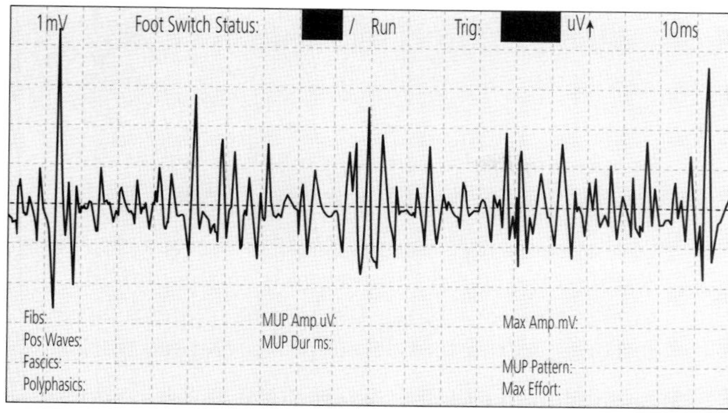

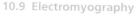

10.9 Electromyography
Normal recruitment of motor units on needle EMG of the biceps muscle, to full interference/recruitment pattern. (Amplitude 1 mV/division)

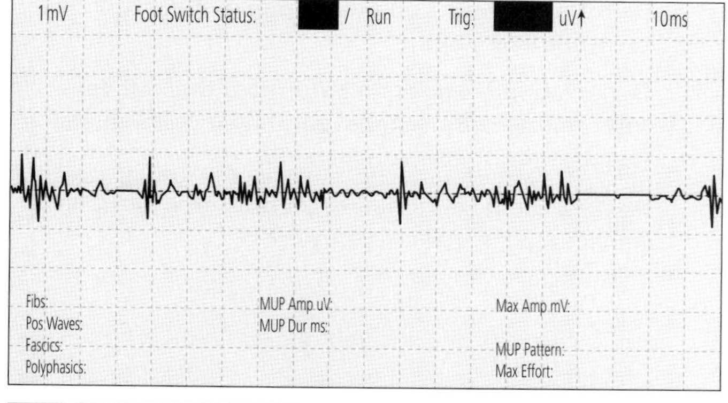

Myopathic recruitment pattern in a patient with polymyositis. There are multiple small amplitude motor units. (Amplitude 1 mV/division)

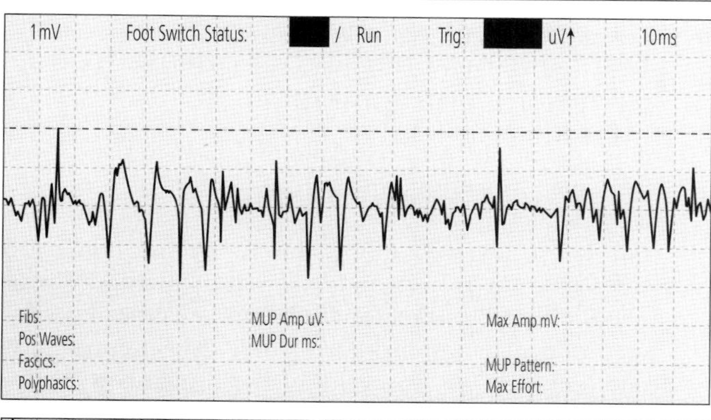

Acute denervation pattern, characterized by florid low amplitude fibrillation potentials recorded from tibialis anterior (resting state).

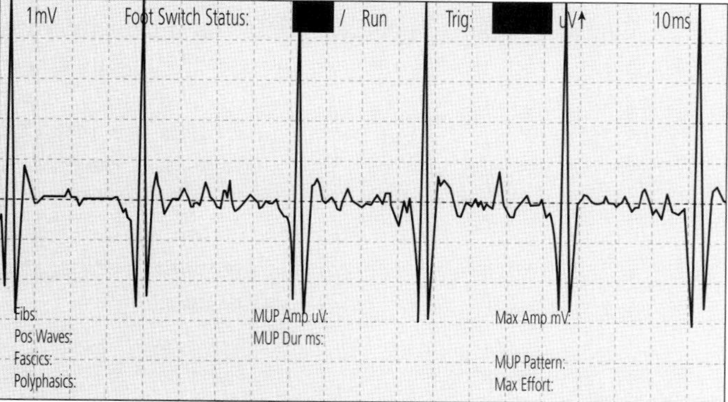

Severe neurogenic abnormality. Single rapidly firing giant motor potential, typical of severe motor unit loss in a patient with old poliomyelitis. A similar pattern is seen in motor neuron disease. (Amplitude 1 mV/division)

screen and, simultaneously, crackling sounds from the loudspeaker.

At rest, a normal muscle is silent. As the patient slowly contracts the muscle there is recruitment of one, then more and then multiple motor units (a motor unit being defined as the anterior horn cell in the spinal cord, with its motor axon and the variable number of muscle fibres it innervates in the muscle). This is reflected first as a progressive increase in the number and then also as increased amplitude of motor unit action potentials, with recognizable patterns. A full *recruitment pattern* usually looks and sounds like 'white noise', with so many motor units firing that both the spikes on the screen and the crackles from the speakers overlap each other – a so-called *'interference pattern'*.

In nerve disorders the muscle may not be silent at rest and may manifest increased insertional activity (activity during insertion of the needle electrode). There are changes of active denervation, referred to as *fibrillation potentials* and *positive sharp waves*, produced by denervated muscle fibres firing spontaneously. This signifies motor nerve fibre loss or disruption. It takes 7–12 days for the changes of active denervation to develop after axonal disruption.

In a denervated muscle (e.g. the result of spinal root entrapment) the number of motor units recruited will be reduced proportional to disrupted axons. Instead of the white noise of full recruitment one sees a reduced pattern of muscle potentials.

In muscle disease similar changes to the above may be seen, but the pattern of action potentials differs and the full interference pattern appears at lower levels of active contraction.

A chronic neuropathy, with re-sprouting of remaining viable nerve fibres, results in longer re-innervated motor units with a polyphasic or higher amplitude profile.

Diagnostic evaluation of the patient

Which nerves are studied in any patient, and the interpretation of the electrophysiological findings, will depend upon the clinical presentation and the provisional diagnosis. Appropriate nerve conduction studies and EMG can confirm or refute the clinical diagnosis. *Comprehensive study of all nerves without a diagnostic plan is usually unhelpful.*

When investigating a specific nerve root syndrome, nerve conduction and EMG studies are concentrated in the appropriate anatomical territory and the findings are compared to those in other nerve root territories in the same as well as the contralateral (usually asymptomatic) limb. For example, in a patient with a weak arm and radial distribution paraesthesiae due to a C5/6 disc prolapse, one would study the median nerve motor and sensory potentials at the carpal tunnel, the radial sensory potentials at the wrist and EMG of C6 innervated muscles (e.g. biceps and brachioradialis). The findings are then compared to those in the C7 muscles such as extensor digitorum communis and triceps.

In a *mononeuropathy* or *plexopathy* one needs to compare conduction values (amplitude and velocity) in one limb to those in the other.

In a disorder such as a *focal entrapment* one may demonstrate a reduced amplitude on proximal stimulation compared to distal stimulation, representing conduction block, or significant focal conduction slowing.

NEUROPHYSIOLOGICAL SIGNS OF NEUROPATHIC DISORDER

Reduced motor or sensory potentials reflect non-functioning (perhaps transected) nerves

Loss of sensory responses (SNAP) reflects a disorder *distal* to the spinal foramen (e.g. in the plexus); intact SNAP in a hypaesthetic limb suggests disease *proximal* to the foramen (e.g. a prolapsed disc)

Conduction block (i.e. intact distal motor response with focal conduction block) implies a neuropraxic recoverable injury

Denervation changes on EMG more than 10 days after injury confirm significant nerve damage and loss of motor nerve function

Any recruited volitional motor units in a weak limb implies a potential for recovery

Distinguishing nerve root disease from peripheral entrapment

The major anatomical defining characteristic of a proximal root entrapment (e.g. due to a prolapsed disc) is the preservation of the sensory action potential in the involved limb. This is because the lesion interrupts the nerve root proximal to the dorsal root ganglion which is anatomically (and electrically) situated outside the spinal cord where it is in continuity, and maintains the integrity of the distal axon; hence the SNAP remains normal.

The CMAP may be reduced as the motor nerve is separated from the anterior horn cell in the spinal cord. For example, in a wrist drop from a C7 root entrapment, the radial motor potentials are reduced or even absent, there is gross denervation on EMG, but the radial sensory potentials are preserved and entirely normal! *The presence of an intact sensory potential is what distinguishes root and proximal disease from peripheral entrapment and plexus disease.*

Intraoperative neurophysiological techniques

Spinal monitoring: somatosensory evoked responses (SSEP)

Neurophysiological tests are sometimes necessary during corrective spinal operations to obviate injury to the cord. These techniques use the basic principles defined above, often combining them with techniques employed in electroencephalography (EEG), such as *averaging*. A peripheral nerve in the upper or the lower limb (usually the median or posterior tibial) is stimulated but, instead of recording from the nerve or the muscle twitch, one records from the scalp overlying the patient's sensory parietal cortex.

The evoked responses from the recorded cortex are miniscule and one must therefore *average* the obtained responses from at least 100–200 stimuli in order to differentiate the time-linked evoked response from the background brain EEG activity. Averaging 200 or more responses at a stimulus rate of 3 per second to demonstrate a reproducible response may take 2 minutes or longer, assuming all other factors are even and perfect. The surgeon should be aware of this drawback. One can also measure potentials developed in the cervical spinal cord at C7 level and the L1 level as well as distally in the brachial plexus at Erb's point, resulting from peripheral nerve stimulation.

The important measured parameter is usually the *latency* of the response, e.g. the N20 response from median nerve stimulation (a brain response occurring at approximately 20 milliseconds after stimulating the median nerve at the wrist). Accidental nerve injury during surgery around the spinal cord will produce a delay in the latency or a sudden loss of the evoked response.

Other intraoperative techniques

Various techniques are used, tailor-made according to the procedure involved. These may include *nerve or nerve root stimulation* at various sites and measurement of either the distal nerve or muscle impulse. This can demonstrate conduction block or slowing or normal continuity of the nerve.

Intraoperative EMG is performed with the needle in situ in the appropriate muscle (e.g. the quadriceps for L4 root procedures, abductor hallucis for the S1 root) to assess the muscle contraction when the nerve is stimulated, either intentionally or otherwise.

Cord-to-cord stimulation and *cord-to-cortical potential measurement* are usually resolved as averaged recordings to reveal intraoperative evidence of spinal pathway disruption.

CEREBRAL PALSY

The term 'cerebral palsy' includes a group of disorders that result from non-progressive brain damage during early development and are characterized by abnormalities of movement and posture. The incidence is about 2 per 1000 live births, with the highest rates in premature babies and those of multiple births. Known causal factors are maternal toxaemia, prematurity, perinatal anoxia, kernicterus and postnatal brain infections or injury; birth injury, though often blamed, is a distinctly unusual cause. These factors may also cause damage to other areas of the developing brain and thus many children with cerebral palsy have associated problems such as epilepsy, perceptual problems, behavioural problems and learning difficulties.

The main consequence is the development of neuromuscular incoordination, dystonia, weakness and spasticity. Oro-facial motor incoordination may make speech and swallowing difficult and drooling is a frequent problem; none of these defects, however, implies a poor intellect although, even these days, far too frequently the wrong conclusions are drawn.

Classification

Cerebral palsy is usually classified according to the type of motor disorder, with subdivisions referring to the topographical distribution of the clinical signs.

TYPE OF MOTOR DISORDER

- *Spasticity* is the commonest muscle movement disorder and is associated with damage to the pyramidal system in the CNS. It is characterized by increased muscle tone and hyper-reflexia. The resistance to passive movement may obscure a basic weakness of the affected muscles.
- *Hypotonia* is usually a phase, lasting several years during early childhood before the features of spasticity become obvious.
- *Athetosis* manifests as continuous, involuntary, writhing movements which may be exacerbated when the child is frightened. It is caused by damage to the extrapyramidal systems of the CNS. In pure athetoid cerebral palsy, joint contractures are unusual and muscle tone is not increased.
- *Dystonia* may occur with athetosis. There is a more generalized increase in muscle tone and abnormal positions induced by activity.
- *Ataxia* appears in the form of muscular incoordination during voluntary movements. It is usually due to cerebellar damage. Balance is poor and the patient walks with a characteristic wide-based gait.
- *Mixed palsy* appears as a combination of spasticity and athetosis. The presence of both types of motor disorder can make the results of surgical intervention unpredictable.

NOTE: In some types of cerebral palsy there is considerable variability in the 'tone' and 'posture' from day to day or situation to situation. If surgical treatment is being considered, it should never be based on a single assessment when, due to stress, the child appears to have abnormally high tone and muscle contractures.

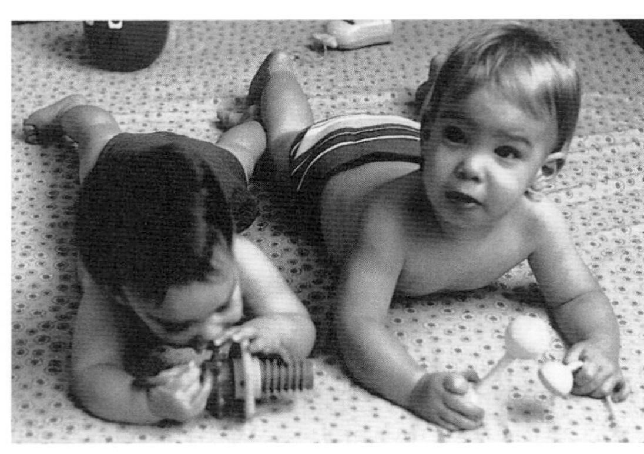
(a)

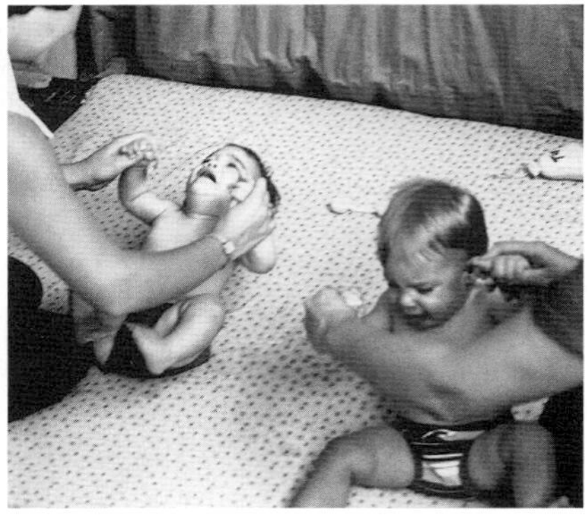
(b)

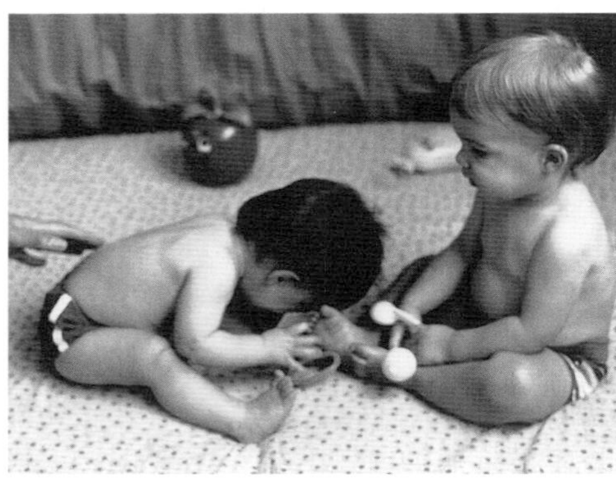
(c)

10.10 Cerebral palsy – early diagnosis By 6 months these twin brothers had developed quite differently, the one being smaller and showing (a) lack of head and arm control, (b) lack of body control when helped to the sitting position and (c) inability to sit unaided.

TOPOGRAPHIC DISTRIBUTION (see Fig. 10.12)

- *Hemiplegia* is the commonest. This usually appears as a spastic palsy on one side of the body with the upper limb more severely affected than the lower. Most of these children can walk and they respond reasonably well to treatment.
- *Diplegia* involves both sides of the body, with the lower limbs always most severely affected. Some disorder of upper limb function is invariably present but signs may be subtle. Side to side involvement may be asymmetrical and the terms *asymmetric diplegia* and occasionally *bilateral hemiplegia* are used. Many cases are secondary to prematurity and periventricular leucomalacia is seen on brain MRI. Intelligence is often normal. The less severely affected children can have reasonable mobility but the non-walking diplegic patient may be similar to the total body involvement group discussed below.
- *Total body involvement* describes a general and often more severe disorder affecting all four limbs, the trunk, neck and face with varying degrees of severity. Patients usually have a low IQ, they may have epilepsy, they are often unable to walk and the response to treatment is poor.
- *Monoplegia* occasionally appears in an upper limb; careful examination will often show that other areas are involved as well. True monoplegia is so unusual that other diagnoses should be considered, e.g. a neonatal brachial plexopathy.

Diagnosis in infancy

The full-blown clinical picture may take months or even years to develop. A history of prenatal toxaemia, haemorrhage, premature birth, difficult labour, foetal distress or kernicterus should arouse suspicion. A neonatal ultrasound scan of the head may identify intracerebral bleeding that would increase the likelihood of later problems.

Early symptoms include difficulty in sucking and swallowing, with dribbling at the mouth. The mother may notice that the baby feels stiff or wriggles awkwardly. Gradually it becomes apparent that the motor milestones are delayed. The normal child holds up its head at 3 months, sits up at 6 months and begins walking at about 1 year.

Diagnosis in later childhood

Most children presenting to the orthopaedic surgeon have already had the diagnosis made. Occasionally, for example with a mild hemiplegia or a symmetrical mild diplegia, the diagnosis has not been made and the child is simply referred for advice about their gait or their tendency to trip and fall. A familiarity and knowledge of the normal developmental milestones and gait patterns helps the clinician identify the child who is outside the normal range.

Bleck (1987) has described seven tests for children

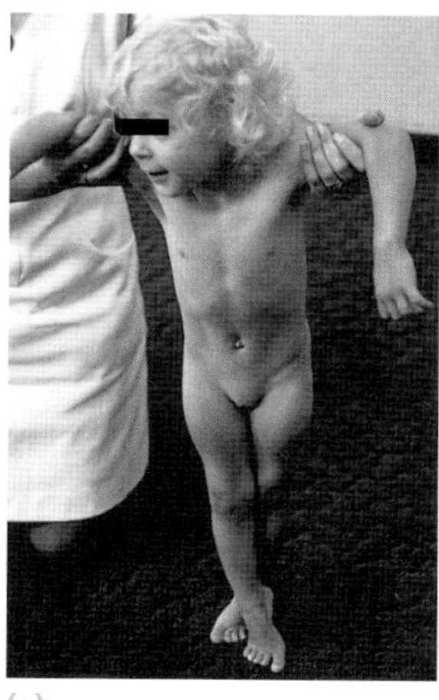
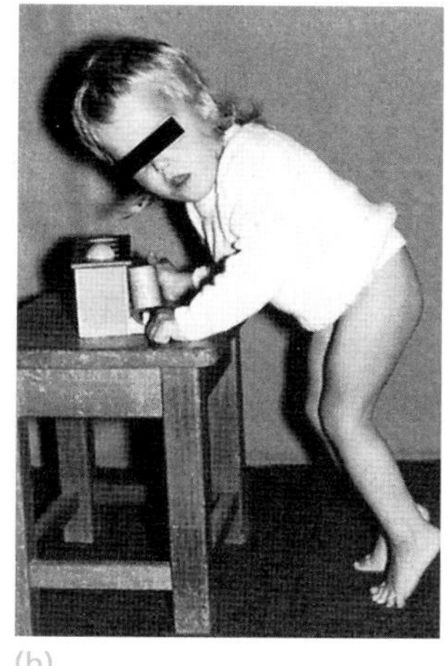
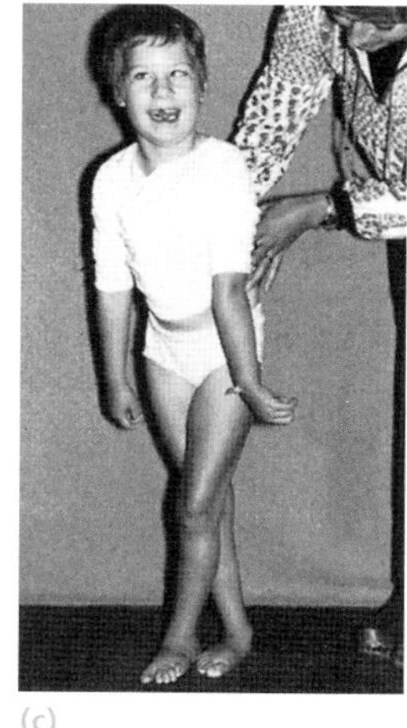
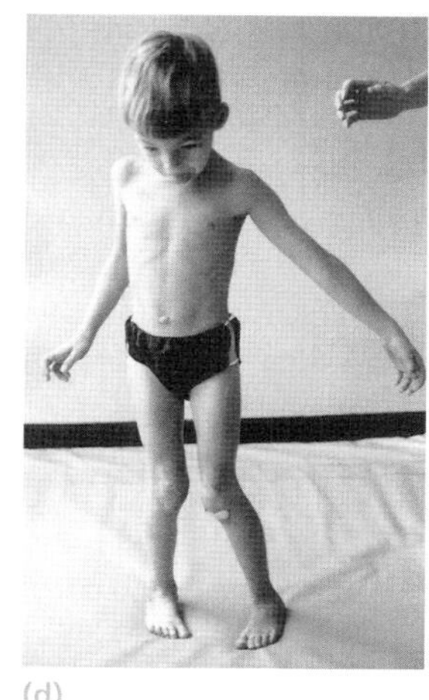

(a) (b) (c) (d)

10.11 Cerebral palsy (a) Adductor spasm (scissor stance); (b) flexion deformity of hips and knees with equinus of the feet; (c) general posture and characteristic facial expression; (d) ataxic type of palsy.

over 1 year; these give an idea of severity and of the prognosis for walking. The primitive neck-righting reflex, asymmetrical and symmetrical tonic neck reflexes, the Moro reflex and the extensor thrust response should all have disappeared at 1 year of age. Children who retain more than two primitive reflexes after that age, cannot sit unsupported by 4 years and cannot walk unaided by 8 years are unlikely ever to walk independently.

Ideally the child should be reviewed by a multidisciplinary team so that speech, hearing, visual acuity, intelligence and motivation can also be assessed.

Since cerebral palsy is essentially a disorder of posture and movement, the child should be carefully observed sitting, standing, walking and lying. His or her condition should then be evaluated according to the gross motor function classification system (GMFCS) which categorizes the child, relative to their age, in terms of mobility and bases this on their average function, not the best that they can achieve on a given occasion (Palisano et al., 2008). The system is reliable and valid; it aids in communication between members of the multidisciplinary team and is a useful guide to management.

SITTING POSTURE

The child may find it difficult or impossible to sit unsupported: children with a hypotonic trunk may slump into a kyphotic posture and others may always 'fall' to one side. In attempting to sit, the lower limbs may be thrust into extension. There may be an obvious scoliosis or pelvic obliquity.

STANDING POSTURE

In the typical case of a spastic diplegia, the child stands with hips flexed, adducted and internally rotated, the knees are also flexed and the feet are in equinus. With tight hamstrings, the normal lumbar lordosis may be obliterated and the child may have difficulty standing unsupported. Often attempts to correct one deformity may aggravate another and it is important to establish which deformity is the primary one and which are compensatory. Many patients show pelvic obliquity and a scoliosis. Asking the child to 'stand tall' and watching their response often gives some insight into the dynamic nature of the posture and muscle strength and, of course, intellectual ability.

Balance reactions are often poor and a gentle push that would force a normal child to take a step in the appropriate direction to maintain his or her balance may simply knock over a child with cerebral palsy.

GAIT

If a child can walk, the elements of gait are analysed taking note of the use of walking aids and orthotic devices. Gait should be observed with and without

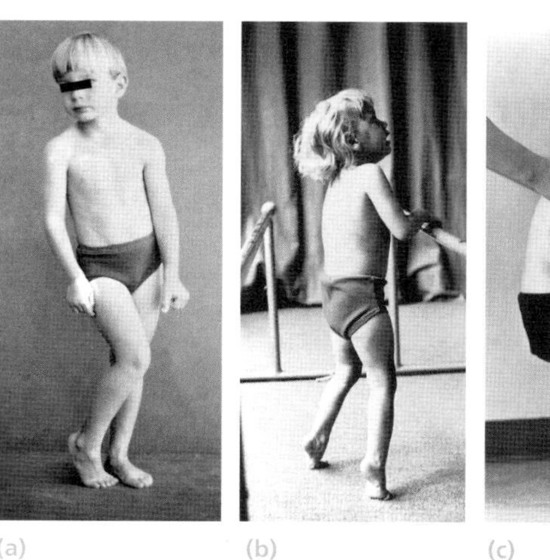
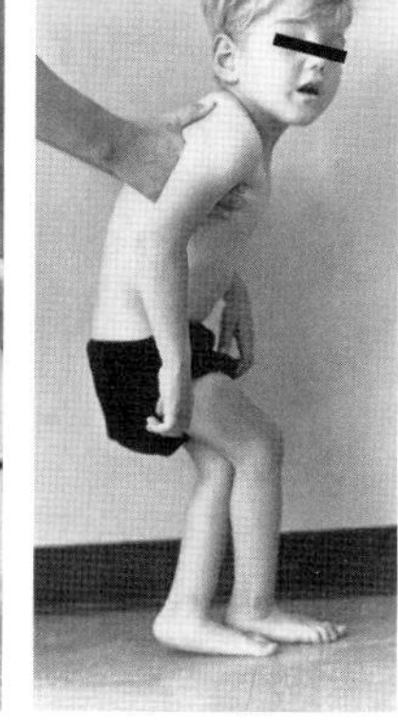

(a) (b) (c)

10.12 Spastic palsy Common types of spastic palsy: (a) hemiplegic, (b) diplegic, (c) whole body.

shoes or orthotic supports and the differences (if any) noted. Dystonic, athetoid and ataxic movements may become more noticeable during walking. Every opportunity must be taken to observe gait so that differences between 'normal' and 'best behaviour' walking can be identified. In hemiplegics, best behaviour walking may demonstrate a flat foot pattern with the heel coming down most of the time while the more normal or representative pattern will highlight the asymmetric flexed knee and toe-walking pattern.

Clinical gait analysis is difficult but improves with practice. Each limb must be observed in both the stance and swing phases of gait and in the coronal, sagittal and transverse planes. In the spastic diplegic patient, the standing posture mentioned above is influential in defining their walking pattern too. The lack of free rotation at the hip means that the trunk has to move from side to side as each leg swings through and with the adduction it leads to a 'scissoring' action (one leg crossing in front of the other). This results in a narrow walking base and, when combined with the hip and knee flexion and foot equinus, there is a strong tendency to fall; this can be helped by the use of walking aids such as crutches.

Computerized gait analysis ideally supplements observational gait analysis. Kinematics (joint and limb segment movement), kinetics (joint moments and powers), EMG (identification of the phases in which muscles are firing), pedobarography (foot pressures) and metabolic energy analysis (assessment of the 'cost' of walking) are all part of the analysis, as is a video recording which can be viewed from any direction and at any speed. Interpretation of all this data requires skill and experience and the application of the information to an individual child also requires a degree of common sense. Pattern recognition is important (in both forms of gait analysis). Perhaps its main role is to help the clinician distinguish between dynamic and fixed tightness and in the identification of dyskinesia.

A good account of gait patterns in cerebral palsy is given by Sutherland and Davids (1993).

NEUROMUSCULAR EXAMINATION

Examination of the limbs shows the typical features of upper motor neuron or spastic paresis. Passive movements are resisted, the reflexes are exaggerated and there is a positive Babinski response. However, spasticity may obscure the fact that muscle power is actually weak. By the end of the examination the clinician should have a clear idea of the *muscle tone*, *muscle power* and *range of movement* at each joint.

In children with cerebral palsy the physical signs often vary from day to day or even minute to minute depending on factors such as the emotional state of the patient and the temperature of the room. It takes time to examine a child and get a representative 'feel' for the tone, the muscle strength and the degree of deformity present. The physiotherapist has often seen the child more often and in more relaxed circumstances than is the case in the orthopaedic clinic and can therefore identify whether today's examination is truly representative.

DEFORMITY ASSESSMENT

It is important to assess the degree of deformity present at each joint and relate it to muscle-tendon length. Deformity at one level may be markedly affected by the position of the joints above and below. For example, ankle equinus with the knee extended often disappears when the knee is flexed; thus one can differentiate between tightness in the soleus and tightness in the gastrocnemius muscle. In the *Silfverskiöld* test, with the child lying supine on the examination couch, the knee is flexed to a right angle and the ankle is dorsiflexed; this tests soleus tightness. The knee is then fully extended on the couch and ankle dorsiflexion is repeated; now it is mainly gastrocnemius tightness that is being tested. Similarly, tight hamstrings may limit knee extension more with the hips flexed than when the hips are extended and hip adduction may be easier in flexion than in extension due to a tight gracilis. If hip abduction is restricted, order an x-ray to look for subluxation of the joint.

In the upper limb, finger flexors may be tight with the wrist extended but if the wrist is allowed to flex the fingers can extend. Children can use these fixed-length reactions to manipulate their hand and finger function using 'trick' movements.

In the patient with total body involvement, spinal deformity is common; usually this is a scoliosis, often associated with pelvic obliquity. Kyphosis and lordosis also occur.

SENSATION

Sensation is often not entirely normal and problems with stereognosis (as well as with perception) may be important factors contributing to upper limb disability.

MUSCLE CONTRACTURE

A degree of muscle contracture is almost inevitable with all forms of cerebral palsy where longstanding spasticity leads to relative shortening of the muscles and hence fixed contractures and changes in joint congruity. There is still some debate as to whether the changes are due to a true shortening of the muscle or a failure to grow along with skeletal growth. Certainly most of the effects are seen during the period of growth; after skeletal maturity the changes in muscle-tendon length and joint contracture are much less progressive.

BONY DEFORMITY

Normal bone growth is influenced by muscle pull. Hence in children with persistent abnormal muscle pull there may be a failure of normal modelling and new deformities can develop. The normal degree of femoral neck anteversion persists and sometimes even increases with growth rather than improving – and significant external tibial torsion may also be present.

Bony deformities may, in turn, engender new problems. Persistent adduction of the hip leads to valgus of the femoral neck, acetabular dysplasia and subluxation of the joint. Flexion deformity of the knee is associated with upward displacement of the patella and patello-femoral pain. External tibial torsion may give rise to planovalgus deformity of the foot.

STRUCTURAL SCOLIOSIS

Flexible curves are common, but unfortunately many become structural; this is especially likely in patients with total body involvement.

Management

There is no single 'blueprint' for the management of all patients with cerebral palsy; each patient and his or her family provides a different challenge. This section will aim to discuss first some basic principles that are applicable to all children and then some more specific principles that relate to various types of cerebral palsy.

GOAL SETTING

It is human nature for a parent to want and indeed expect the best for their child and it is the role of the healthcare professionals to support them in their wishes. However, it is also important for the professionals to ensure that the difference between hopeful optimism and pragmatic realism is understood by all involved in the child's care. Few patients with total body involvement will ever walk. The prognosis for walking in the patient with spastic diplegia may be assessed by looking at Bleck's (1975) criteria and those of Beals (1966). The definition of walking must also be conveyed to the parents along with an explanation that many children with cerebral palsy reach their peak of physical function in late childhood and with the increase in size and weight that comes with puberty weak muscles may no longer be able to maintain walking ability.

For all patients with cerebral palsy the priorities are: (1) an ability to communicate with others; (2) an ability to cope with the activities of daily living (including personal hygiene); and (3) independent mobility – which may mean a motorized wheelchair rather than walking.

For the child who from an early age is recognized to be 'non-walking' realistic goals should be: (1) a straight spine with a level pelvis; (2) located, mobile and painless hips that flex to 90 degrees (for comfortable sitting) and extend sufficiently to allow comfortable sleeping and participation in standing/swivel transfers; (3) knees that are mobile enough for sitting, sleeping and transferring; and (4) plantigrade feet that fit into shoes and rest on the footplates of the wheelchair comfortably.

For all children good medical care is also essential as is access to good quality orthotic supports, walking aids and/or wheelchairs as appropriate. Unfortunately these basic needs are still not met for children in many disadvantaged communities.

TONE MANAGEMENT

Tone management is one of the most important aspects of patient care and it underpins all other forms of treatment.

Medical treatment The most generally effective medications are ***anticonvulsants*** for seizures, ***short-term benzodiazepine*** use for postoperative pain and ***trihexyphenadryl*** for dystonia.

Baclofen, an agonist of gamma-aminobutryic acid (GABA), acts by inhibiting reflex activity. In oral form it does not cross the blood–brain barrier well. When effective, it reduces muscle tone/spasticity generally. This may have a negative effect on head and trunk control and combined with the side effects of drowsiness means that its use may be limited. Intrathecal baclofen is administered via a refillable, subcutaneous implanted pump and the dose administered can be titrated according to the child's response. Long-term studies of its use are not yet available but it appears that it may be most effective in those with severe spasticity or dystonia. It is not effective in all patients and test doses and assessment of its benefits are required in all prospective patients.

Dantrolene produces weakness without much reduction in spasticity and hence it is rarely used in cerebral palsy.

Analgesic medication is needed for the reduction of pain associated with musculoskeletal problems, constipation and gastro-oesophageal reflux.

Botulinum toxin This potent neurotoxin is produced by *Clostridium botulinum*; it acts by blocking acetyl choline release at the neuromuscular junction. The preparation is injected into the 'spastic' muscle at (or as near as possible to) the motor end point. The usual targets are the hip adductors, hamstrings, gastrocnemius and tibialis posterior. The weakness/paralysis that it causes takes a few days to become obvious; the effect is temporary and as new nerve terminals form there is a return of muscle tone at around 10–12 weeks.

Botulinum toxin must not be used on its own but rather as part of a package of care in the overall tone management programme. Thus injections are followed by increased physiotherapy input and often an alteration in orthotic/splinting regimens. This means that the overall benefits attributed to the injections may last considerably longer than the 10–12 weeks of true neuromuscular blockade.

It is precisely because the toxin is never used on its own that it has been difficult to prove what the true benefits of this form of treatment are but it is considered useful as a focal treatment for a dynamic muscle imbalance that is interfering with function, producing deformity or causing pain. It is perhaps more effective in younger children who are less likely to have fixed deformity. Multilevel injections may be required but the overall dose per child must be kept within safe limits.

There is also a role for botulinum toxin in the management of postoperative pain and spasm although for optimal effect the injections need to be given some days prior to surgery.

Selective dorsal rhizotomy Division of selected dorsal nerve roots from L1 to S2 has only recently gained wide acceptance, perhaps as the indications for its use have been refined and the techniques for performing the procedure have improved. In cerebral palsy, the normal inhibitory influences on muscle tone from the higher centres are deficient. This technique aims to reduce spasticity and rebalance muscle tone by selectively reducing the input from the muscle spindles, thus leading to less excitation of the anterior horn cells. Long-term studies are not yet available but good results have been obtained in children aged 3–8 years who meet the following criteria: they are walking but have significant spasticity; they were born prematurely; they have good intellectual function and good voluntary control. The presence of fixed contractures is a relative contraindication and may need surgical correction.

Physical therapy Cerebral palsy affects motor function in several ways. There is a dependence on immature or primitive reflexes and a loss of selective muscle control. Physiotherapy attempts to reduce or prevent the problems arising from abnormal muscle tone, imbalance between opposing muscle groups and abnormal body balance mechanisms. To this end various structured approaches or 'schools' have been popularized. No single method has been shown to be significantly better than another but all have good points and all can work well in individual cases. In addition to these programmed approaches, there is a philosophy that a range of regular movement exercises will prevent or (perhaps more realistically) reduce the degree of muscle/joint contracture.

Physiotherapy is considered to be most helpful in early childhood up to the age of 7 or 8 years but there is surprisingly little evidence to guide us in knowing what type of physiotherapy to prescribe and how often to do so in any particular case. However, postoperative physiotherapy is essential in order to maximize the effects of surgery and overcome the immediate pain, stiffness and weakness that follow surgery.

Positioning and splinting Care must be taken at all times to ensure that the child both sits and sleeps, works and eats in a good position and with good posture. Adjustments may need to be made to chairs, wheelchair and the child's sleep system so as to limit disadvantageous positions such as hip adduction.

Splints are used to prevent muscle contracture, maintain joint position and improve movement and hence function. They also have an important role in maintaining position following surgery. Splints may be corrective – in that they aim to hold a passively correctable deformity – or 'adoptive', e.g. when the splint adopts the shape of the foot and simply aims to prevent further loss of position. A badly fitting splint at best does nothing and at worst provokes pain and spasm and increasing deformity.

Manipulation and serial casting These methods may have a limited role in improving muscle/joint contractures, but relapse is frequent.

Operative treatment

The indications for surgery are: (1) a spastic deformity which cannot be controlled by conservative measures; (2) fixed deformity that interferes with function; and (3) secondary complications such as bony deformities, dislocation of the hip and joint instability.

It is important to remember that in cerebral palsy all muscles are weak: thus, muscle-lengthening surgery is also muscle-weakening surgery unless by improving the mechanical alignment of the limb, and hence the muscle, you allow it to work more efficiently. Correction of bony deformity may be important in this respect and although the surgery may be more 'aggressive' it may actually be more appropriate.

Weak muscles can be augmented by tendon transfers but the muscle being transferred is weak already and may have a limited ability to function in its new role; on the other hand it may produce an unwanted overcorrection because of its increased tone. The role of gravity plays an important part in guiding the choice of tendon transfers.

The timing of surgical intervention is often crucial. Development of the CNS and the gait pattern matures around the age of 7–8 years and thus many orthopaedic surgeons advocate delaying surgery until this age and then doing all the necessary operations at one or two sittings. Our preferred approach is to avoid *'little and often'* surgery in favour of the *'all or none'* philosophy, but as always some patients require the former and some the latter. Earlier operation may be called for if the hip threatens to dislocate.

REGIONAL SURVEY

Upper limb

Upper limb deformities are seen most typically in the child with spastic hemiplegia or total body involvement and consist of flexion of the elbow, pronation of the forearm, flexion of the wrist, clenched fingers and adduction of the thumb. In the mildest cases, spastic postures emerge only during exacting activities. Proprioception is often disturbed and this may preclude any marked improvement of function, whatever the kind of treatment. Operative treatment is usually delayed until after the age of 8 years and is aimed at improving the resting position of the limb and restoring grasp.

Elbow flexion deformity Provided the elbow can extend to a right angle, no treatment is needed. Occasionally it may be necessary to treat a more marked flexion contracture by fractional lengthening of the biceps and brachialis tendons with release of the brachialis origin.

Forearm pronation deformity This is fairly common and may give rise to subluxation or dislocation of the radial head. Simple release of pronator teres may improve the position, or the tendon can be rerouted round the back of the forearm in the hope that it may act as a supinator.

Wrist flexion deformity Wrist flexion is usually in an ulnar direction; it can be improved by lengthening or releasing flexor carpi ulnaris. If extension is weak, the released flexor tendon is transferred into one of the wrist extensors. In severe cases wrist arthrodesis with excision of the proximal carpal row may be of cosmetic rather than functional benefit. *N.B. Before operating on the wrist it is essential to consider what effect this will have on finger movements.*

Flexion deformity of the fingers Spasticity of the long flexor muscles may give rise to clawing. The flexor tendons can be lengthened individually, but if the deformity is severe a forearm muscle slide may be more appropriate. Ideally these operations should be undertaken by a specialist in hand surgery. *If the fingers can be unclenched only by simultaneously flexing the wrist, it is obviously important not to extend the wrist by tendon transfer or fusion.*

Thumb-in-palm deformity This is due to spasticity of the thumb adductors or flexors (or both), but later there is also contracture of flexor pollicis longus. In mild cases, function can be improved by splinting the thumb away from the palm, or by operative release of the adductor pollicis and first dorsal interosseus muscles. Resistant deformity may need combined lengthening of flexor pollicis longus and release of the thenar muscles, followed by tendon transfers to reinforce abduction and extension. Here again the operations should be performed by a specialist in this field.

Lower limb

The functional effects of lower limb spasticity differ considerably, depending on whether the patient has hemiplegia, diplegia or whole-body involvement; this will obviously influence the lines of surgical treatment.

SPASTIC HEMIPLEGIA

Four subtypes of hemiplegia have been identified and the most common lower limb problem is with foot deformity.

Foot/ankle Tibialis anterior is invariably weak and the patient develops an *equinovarus foot deformity.* Active plantar flexion is required to assist knee extension during the stance phase of gait so care must be taken when considering a lengthening of the gastrocnemius/soleus complex. The trend is to perform a muscle recession rather than a tendon lengthening procedure.

A *dynamic varus deformity* can be treated by a split tibialis anterior tendon transfer to the outer side of the foot (only half the tendon is transferred so as to avoid the risk of overcorrection into valgus). In older children with fixed deformity, formal muscle lengthening with or without a calcaneal osteotomy may be required.

Pes valgus (pronated foot deformity) may require subtalar arthrodesis.

Hip/knee Surgery is not usually required but if it is it follows the principles outlined below for the walking diplegic patient.

Leg length discrepancy Due to discrepancies in growth, the hemiplegic limb is often short irrespective of any joint contractures. An epiphyseodesis of the contralateral distal femoral and/or proximal tibial physes may be considered. This can improve some aspects of the gait pattern.

SPASTIC DIPLEGIA

Most patients with cerebral palsy have a spastic diplegia and treatment is concentrated on the lower limbs. In the very young child, this consists of physiotherapy and splintage to prevent fixed contractures. Surgery is indicated either to correct structural defects (e.g. a fixed contracture or hip subluxation) or to improve gait. By 3–4 years of age the sitting and walking patterns can be observed, and particular attention should be paid to the interrelationship between the various postural defects, especially lumbar lordosis/hip flexion and knee flexion/ankle equinus.

Most children will walk but they are delayed in learning to master this – a child who is not walking by the age of 6 or 7 is unlikely to do so. Non-ambulant children often have orthopaedic problems similar to those with total body involvement (see below).

In walking diplegics, observational gait analysis is important and computerized gait analysis may have a role in guiding treatment. Affected children are often relatively symmetrical in their gait pattern but in some asymmetry is very marked with one limb maintaining a hemiplegic posture and one more consistent with a diplegic gait. Each limb must be assessed independently.

Hip adduction deformity The child walks with the thighs together and sometimes even with the knees crossing ('scissors gait'). This may be combined with spastic internal rotation. Adductor release is indicated if passive abduction is less than 20 degrees on each side. If medial hamstring lengthening is planned (see below) it should be done first because this alone may restore some hip abduction.

For most patients open tenotomy of adductor longus and division of gracilis will suffice. Only if this fails to restore passive abduction (a rare occurrence) should the other adductors be released. Anterior branch obturator neurectomy should not be performed.

Hip flexion deformity This is often associated with fixed knee flexion (the child walks with a 'sitting' posture) or else hyperextension of the lumbar spine. Operative correction is indicated if the hip deformity is more than 30 degrees. In the walking child, it is important not to weaken hip flexion too much and thus intramuscular lengthening of the psoas tendon at the pelvic brim is advocated. (In the non-walking child, psoas release at the level of the lesser trochanter is allowed). An associated fixed flexion deformity of the knee may require medial hamstring lengthening as well.

Hip internal rotation deformity Internal rotation is usually associated with flexion and adduction. If so, adductor release and psoas lengthening will be helpful. If, after a few years, rotation is still excessive, a derotation osteotomy of the femur (subtrochanteric or supracondylar) may be considered; however, be warned that this may have to be followed by compensatory rotation osteotomy of the tibia.

Hip subluxation Subluxation of the hip occurs in about 30 per cent of children with cerebral palsy. A persistent flexion-adduction deformity leads to femoral neck anteversion. If the abductors are weak and the child is not fully weightbearing, there is a risk of acetabular dysplasia and subluxation of the joint; in non-walkers there may be complete dislocation. *Correction of flexion and adduction deformities (see above) before the age of 6 years* may have a role in *preventing subluxation*. Older children may need varus-derotation osteotomy of the femur, perhaps combined with acetabular reconstruction. Longstanding dislocation in a non-walker may be impossible to reconstruct; if discomfort makes operation imperative, the proximal end of the femur can be excised. In the adult walking diplegic patient, total hip replacement can be considered in selected cases where painful degenerative change is affecting function.

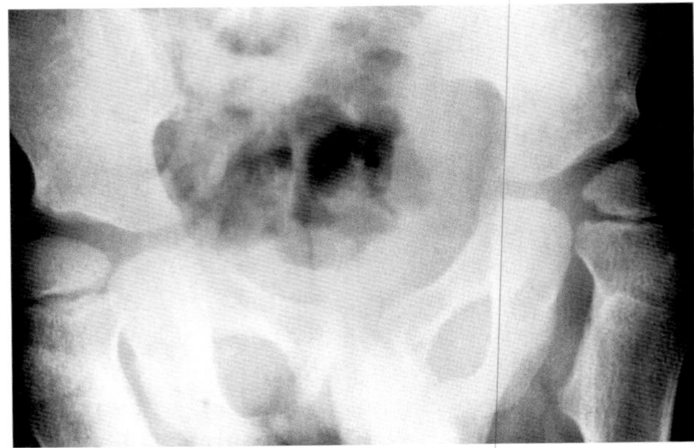

10.13 Spastic hips X-ray of a boy with spastic adducted hips showing acetabular dysplasia and coxa valga, worse on the left side.

Knee flexion deformity This is one of the commonest deformities; it is usually due to functional hamstring tightness but is often aggravated by hip flexion or weakness of ankle plantar flexion. Spastic flexion deformity may be revealed only when the hip is flexed to 90 degrees so that the hamstrings are tightened.

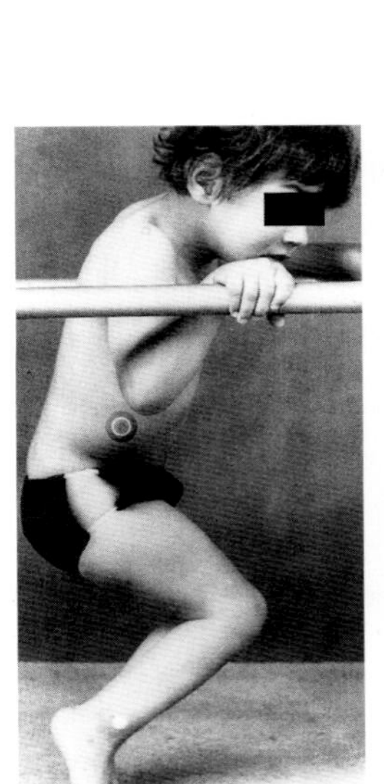

(a)

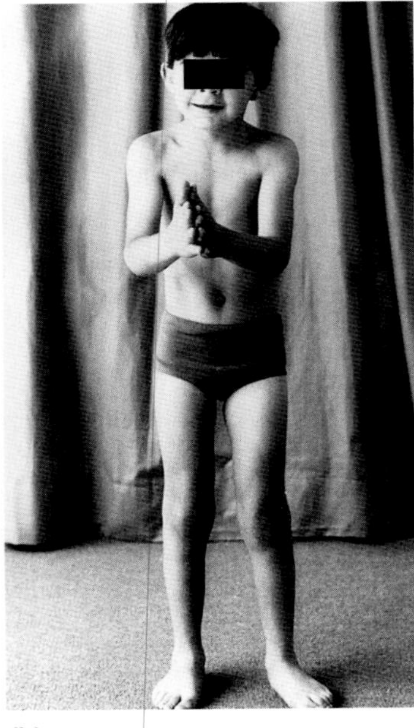

(b)

10.14 Spastic knee flexion deformity (a) This boy has spastic flexion of the knees due to tight hamstrings. (b) Here he is after hamstring release.

Capsular contracture of the knee joint is uncommon. Gait analysis can be helpful in deciding whether the hamstrings are truly short or only functionally short.

Fractional lengthening of the hamstrings (medial more often than medial and lateral combined) reliably improves gait mechanics but risks weakening hip extension and exacerbating hip flexion/lumbar lordosis; this is because the hamstrings normally assist with hip extension. Fractional lengthening of semimembranosus can be combined with detachment and transfer of semitendinosus to the adductor tubercle at the distal end of the femur. Good results have been reported by Ma et al. (2006) in children with bilateral spastic flexion deformities of more than 15 degrees combined with a flexed-knee posture when standing or walking and ability to stand and walk only with support.

Severe flexion deformities (more than 25 or 30 degrees) have also been treated by extension osteotomy of the distal femur or by physeal plating anteriorly.

Remember that knee extension is aided by plantarflexion of the foot in walking, so it is important not to weaken the triceps surae by overzealous lengthening of the Achilles tendon (see below).

Spastic knee extension This can usually be corrected by simple tenotomy of the proximal end of rectus femoris.

External tibial torsion This is easily corrected by supramalleolar osteotomy, but before doing this first ensure that the deformity is not actually advantageous in compensating for an ankle/hindfoot deformity (see below).

Equinus of the foot The child with spastic diplegia usually toe-walks. This triggers an excessive plantarflexion–knee extension couple that may be manifested as knee hyperextension. In children with limited dorsiflexion, the gastrocnemius is often more affected than the soleus. Selective fractional lengthening of the fascia/muscle is gaining favour but judicious percutaneous lengthening of the Achilles tendon is still popular. Relative overlengthening is a problem, particularly when associated knee flexion contractures exist.

If a *varus deformity* is present, treatment is as for the hemiplegic patient described above. The more common deformity is, however, one of *equinovalgus and a 'rocker-bottom' foot*. It makes the use of splints difficult and disrupts the plantarflexion–knee extension couple, exacerbating a knee flexion posture. It is important to note whether the hindfoot deformity is reducible or not. Correction can be achieved by either a calcaneal lengthening or displacement osteotomy but often a subtalar fusion is required. Such surgery must be combined with a release of tight structures (such as the Achilles tendon) and possibly peroneal lengthening and plication of the medial structures when appropriate.

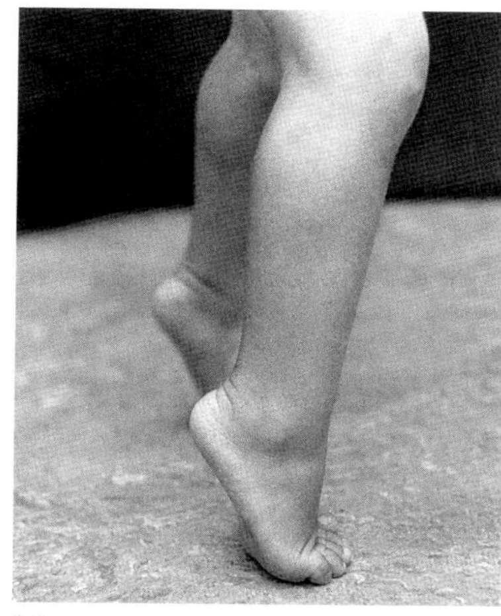

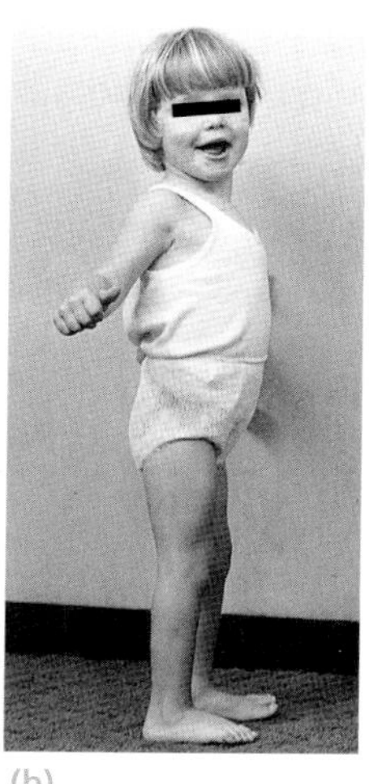

(a) (b)

10.15 Spastic equinus (a) Standing posture of a young girl with bilateral spastic equinus deformities. (b) Tendo Achillis lengthening resulted in complete correction and a balanced posture.

External tibial torsion may be corrected by a supramalleolar osteotomy but remember that an externally rotated gait pattern may be compensating for an inability of the foot to clear the ground when walking because of weak muscles/stiff joints.

Single event multi-level surgery (SEMLS) The diplegic patient usually has problems at all levels and often the most appropriate way to improve gait and overall function is to enhance the mechanical efficiency of gait by combining changes at hip, knee and ankle. Soft-tissue and bony surgery to both limbs can be performed at one sitting or staged over a few weeks. Postoperative rehabilitation is complex and time-consuming but the results can be very rewarding.

A good review of management of lower limb deformities in children with cerebral palsy is presented by Karol (2004).

Total body involvement

All parts of the body are affected; function is generally poor and the aims of surgical intervention differ significantly from those for the hemiplegic or walking diplegic patient.

HIP

Hip subluxation progressing to dislocation is common. The adduction and flexion contractures outlined above are more frequent and more severe in this group of patients, leaving the hip at risk of developing subluxation with acetabular dysplasia. Hips are often 'windswept' (one hip lying adducted, flexed and internally rotated while the other lies in abduction and external rotation and often more extended).

The hip at risk of subluxation must be watched closely and, if necessary, treated by adductor and psoas releases as outlined above (a psoas tenotomy at the lesser trochanter is appropriate). Hip subluxation, defined as more than 30 per cent uncovering of the femoral head, may require a femoral varus derotation (and shortening) osteotomy as well as an acetabular procedure for correction in addition to the soft-tissue releases. If the hip has dislocated, open reduction, release of soft tissues and bony realignment will be necessary. The alternative is to consider a proximal femoral resection.

The opposite hip may require similar surgery, or in the case of a windswept deformity, it may benefit from a release of the hip abductors and extensors, mainly the gluteus maximus and the iliotibial band.

This is complex surgery and the complication rates are high. Some families, and indeed some surgeons, opt for no active treatment of the subluxed or dislocated hip particularly if it is relatively pain-free and care of the child is not compromised significantly. Others feel that hip subluxation/dislocation should be prevented at all costs and although recent reports from Scandinavia suggest that hip dislocation is 'preventable' this is only true with an aggressive regimen of tone management and surgery which many people feel causes unnecessary suffering to the child concerned. Obviously, the management of such cases brings up moral dilemmas which are best dealt with by maintaining good communication with the families and therapists at all stages and being clear about the aims of any intervention.

SPINE/PELVIS

Scoliosis is very common (probably appearing in more than 50 per cent) in this group of patients. The deformity is often a long C-shaped thoracolumbar curve and it frequently incorporates the pelvis which is tilted obliquely so that one hip is abducted and the other adducted and threatening to dislocate. Of course the adducted hip may be the primary problem with pelvic obliquity and scoliosis following; in essence, trunk muscle involvement due to the cerebral palsy must be a major determinant of developing deformity.

Various forms of non-operative treatment (as described on page 239) have been used, and in some cases patients opt for long-term use of an adapted wheelchair.

Where facilities and surgical expertise are available, operative correction and spinal stabilization are often advocated. Indications are a progressive curve of more than 40 degrees in a child over 10 years, inability to sit without support, and a range of hip movement that will allow the child to sit after spinal stabilization. Fixation is achieved with pedicle screws and rods extending from the thoracic spine to the pelvis; there is an attempt to recreate a lumbar lordosis but in so doing it may, at least temporarily, exacerbate hamstring tightness making sitting more difficult.

Careful preoperative evaluation is essential to ensure that the child is fit for a long and difficult operation that is known to carry a high complication rate, including neurological defects, problems with wound healing and implant failure. This type of spinal surgery has been shown to increase life expectancy, but demonstrating a concurrent improvement in quality of life has been more difficult to prove.

A good review of this subject is presented by McCarthy et al., 2006.

OTHER JOINTS

Surgery to other joints may be required and follows the principles outlined above for the hemiplegic and diplegic patient.

ADULT ACQUIRED SPASTIC PARESIS

Cerebral damage following a *stroke* or *head injury* may cause persistent spastic paresis in the adult; this can be accompanied by disturbance of proprioception and stereognosis.

In the early recuperative stage, physiotherapy and splintage are used to prevent fixed deformities; all affected joints should be put through a full range of movement every day. The use of botulinum toxin (as for children with cerebral palsy) may be beneficial in resistant cases (see page 239).

Deformities that are passively correctible should be splinted in the neutral position until controlled muscle power returns; proprioception and coordination can be improved by occupational therapy. Yet even with the best attention, these measures may fail to prevent the development of fixed deformities. Once maximal motor recovery has been achieved – usually by 9 months after a stroke but more than a year after a brain injury – residual deformities or joint instability should be considered for operative treatment. The patient should have sufficient cognitive ability, awareness of body position in space and good psychological impetus if a lasting result is to be expected.

In the lower limbs the principal deformities requiring correction are equinus or equinovarus of the foot, flexion of the knee and adduction of the hip. In the upper limb (where the chances of regaining controlled movement are less) the common residual deformities are adduction and internal rotation of the shoulder (often accompanied by shoulder pain), and flexion of the elbow, wrist and metacarpo-phalangeal joints. Treatment is similar to that of spastic deformity in the child, and is summarized in Table 10.2.

Table 10.2 Treatment of the principal deformities of the limbs

	Deformity	Splintage	Surgery
Foot	Equinus Equinovarus	Spring-loaded dorsiflexion Bracing in eversion and dorsiflexion	Lengthen tendo Achillis Lengthen tendo Achillis and transfer lateral half of tibialis anterior to cuboid
Knee	Flexion	Long caliper	Hamstring release
Hip	Adduction	–	Obturator neurectomy Adductor muscle release
Shoulder	Adduction	–	Subscapularis release
Elbow	Flexion	–	Release elbow flexors
Wrist	Flexion	Wrist splint	Lengthen or release wrist flexors; may need fusion or carpectomy
Fingers	Flexion	–	Lengthen or release flexors

FRIEDREICH'S ATAXIA

Friedreich's ataxia, though rare itself (1–2/50 000 in the UK) is the most common of the hereditary ataxias. It is an autosomal recessive condition which can be detected on genetic testing, the defect being a triplet expansion localized to chromosome 9. In the USA, about 1 in 90 adults is a carrier for this condition.

The condition presents in childhood (rarely adulthood) and all patients develop progressive ataxia of the limbs and of their gait with associated extensor plantar responses but absent knee and ankle reflexes and sensory disturbances such as loss of vibration sense and two-point discrimination. Dysarthria appears within 5 years of disease onset.

The neurological degeneration is seen in the spinocerebellar tracts, the corticospinal tracts, the posterior columns of the spinal cord and parts of the cerebellum itself. Nerve conduction studies demonstrate slowed motor velocities in both median and tibial nerves with absent sensory action potentials in the sural and digital nerves.

Painful muscle spasms occur in some patients and if so they tend to worsen with time. The more common orthopaedic complaints are a progressive cavo-varus foot deformity that is usually rigid, the development of clawed toes and a scoliosis. In general, the earlier the onset of the disease the greater is the risk of significant curve progression. In the more severe cases, functional and neurological deterioration may be rapid with the development of a cardiomyopathy and death in early to mid adulthood. In other more mild cases, surgical correction of foot and spine deformities may be worthwhile.

LESIONS OF THE SPINAL CORD

The three major pathways in the spinal cord are the corticospinal tracts (in the anterior columns) carrying motor neurons, the spinothalamic tracts carrying sensory neurons for pain, touch and temperature, and the posterior column tracts serving deep sensibility (joint position and vibration) (see Fig. 10.2).

Clinical features

True lesions of the spinal cord present with a UMN spastic paresis and often a fairly precise sensory level that suggests the level of cord involvement. However, extradural compressive lesions will often involve the nerve roots as well resulting in a combination of UMN and LMN signs.

Patients often complain of weakness and numbness with loss of balance and possibly alteration in bowel or bladder control and, in men, impotence. The symptoms may be of variable severity and the speed of onset is similarly variable depending mainly on the aetiological factor.

Several 'classical' patterns are recognized.

Cervical cord compression The patient typically presents with UMN symptoms in the lower limbs (stiffness and a change in gait pattern) and LMN signs in the upper limbs (complaints of numbness and clumsiness). Pain is a variable feature. Bladder symptoms are of frequency and incontinence more commonly than retention.

A central cord syndrome may be caused by a hyperextension injury in a middle-aged patient with longstanding cervical spondylosis, or may develop in syringomyelia. In these cases there is disproportionately more UMN weakness in the upper limbs compared to the lower limbs with bladder dysfunction and a variable sensory loss below the lesion.

Thoracic cord compression This typically presents as a UMN paralysis affecting the lower limbs, together with variable sensory loss depending on the degree of involvement of the dorsal columns or the spinothalamic tracts.

Lumbar cord compression The spinal cord terminates around the level of L1 so compression here may involve the conus medullaris or the cauda equina or both, giving a mixture of UMN and LMN signs. The typical *cauda equina syndrome* consists of lower limb weakness, absent reflexes, impaired sensation and urinary retention (with overflow perhaps mimicking incontinence).

Brown-Séquard lesion The pure form of this syndrome is very unusual but less pure forms are common and serve as a reminder that careful assessment of the neurological symptoms and signs is important in helping the clinician to localize the pathology and understand its aetiology. The pure lesion is defined as an incomplete hemispherical cord lesion: below the lesion there is ipsilateral UMN weakness and posterior column dysfunction, with contralateral loss of skin sensibility; at the level of the lesion there is ipsilateral loss of sensibility.

Spinal shock Acute cord lesions at any level may present with a flaccid paralysis which resolves over time, usually to reveal the more typical UMN signs associated with cord injury.

Diagnosis and management

The more common causes of spinal cord dysfunction are listed in Table 10.3. Traumatic and compressive lesions are the ones most likely to be seen by orthopaedic surgeons. Plain x-rays will show structural abnormalities of the spine; cord compression can be visualized by myelography, alone or combined with CT. Intrinsic lesions of the cord require further investigation by blood tests, CSF examination and MRI.

Table 10.3 Causes of spinal cord dysfunction

Acute injury
Vertebral fractures
Fracture-dislocation
Infection
Epidural abscess
Poliomyelitis
Intervertebral disc prolapsed
Sequestrated disc
Disc prolapse in spinal stenosis
Vertebral canal stenosis
Congenital stenosis
Acquired stenosis
Spinal cord tumours
Neurofibroma
Meningioma
Intrinsic cord lesions
Tabes dorsalis
Syringomyelia
Other degenerative disorders
Miscellaneous
Spina bifida
Vascular lesions
Multiple lesions
Multiple sclerosis
Haemorrhagic disorders

Acute compressive lesions require urgent diagnosis and treatment if permanent damage is to be prevented. Bladder dysfunction is ominous: whereas motor and sensory signs may improve after decompression, loss of bladder control, if present for more than 24 hours, is usually irreversible.

Spinal injury is dealt with in Chapter 25 but a few important points deserve mention here.

- Any spinal injury may be associated with cord damage, and great care is needed in transporting and examining the patient.
- In the early period of 'spinal shock' the usual picture is one of flaccid paralysis, with or without priapism.
- Plain x-rays seldom show the full extent of bone displacement, which is much better displayed by CT or MRI.
- Unstable injuries usually need operative decompression and/or stabilization; stable injuries can be treated conservatively.

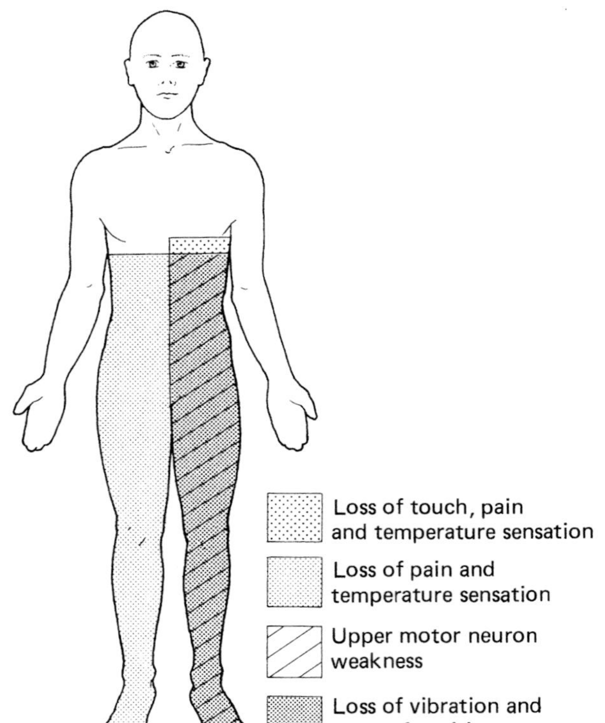

10.16 The Brown-Séquard syndrome

- Many centres consider the use of corticosteroids beneficial in terms of reducing the degree of permanent neurological damage but the side effects of gastrointestinal haemorrhage and avascular necrosis are potentially serious.

Epidural abscess is a surgical emergency. The patient rapidly develops acute pain and muscle spasm, with fever, leucocytosis and elevation of the ESR. X-rays may show disc space narrowing and bone erosion. Treatment is by immediate decompression and antibiotics.

Acute disc prolapse usually causes unilateral symptoms and signs. However, complete lumbar disc prolapse may present as a cauda equina syndrome with urinary retention and overflow; spinal canal obstruction is demonstrated by MRI.

Operative discectomy is urgent.

Chronic discogenic disease is often associated with narrowing of the intervertebral foramina and compression of nerve roots (radiculopathy), and occasionally with bony hypertrophy and pressure on the spinal cord (myelopathy). Diagnosis is usually obvious on x-ray and MRI.

Operative decompression may be needed.

Spinal stenosis produces a typical clinical syndrome, due partly to direct pressure on the cord or nerve roots and partly to vascular obstruction and ischaemic neuropathy during hyperextension of the lumbar spine. The patient complains of 'tiredness', weakness and sometimes aching or paraesthesia in the lower limbs after standing or walking for a few minutes, symptoms that are relieved by bending forward, sitting or crouching so as to flex the lumbar spine.

Congenital narrowing of the spinal canal is rare, except in developmental disorders such as achondroplasia, but even a moderately reduced canal may be further narrowed by osteophytes, thus compromising the cord and nerve roots.

Treatment calls for bony decompression of the nerve structures.

Vertebral disease, such as tuberculosis or metastatic disease, may cause cord compression and paraparesis. The diagnosis is usually obvious on x-ray, but a needle biopsy may be necessary for confirmation.

Management is usually by anterior decompression and, if necessary, internal stabilization. However, in metastatic disease, if the prognosis is poor it may be wise also to use radiotherapy and corticosteroids, plus narcotics for pain.

Spinal cord tumours are a comparatively rare cause of progressive paraparesis. X-rays may show bony erosion, widening of the spinal canal or flattening of the vertebral pedicles. Widening of the intervertebral foramina is typical of neurofibromatosis. Treatment usually involves operative removal of the tumour.

Intrinsic lesions of the cord produce slowly progressive neurological signs. Two conditions in particular – tabes dorsalis and syringomyelia – may present with orthopaedic problems because of neuropathic joint destruction.

Tabes dorsalis is a late manifestation of syphilis causing degeneration ('tabes' means wasting) of the posterior columns of the spinal cord. A pathognomonic feature is 'lightning pains' in the lower limbs. Much later other neurological features appear: sensory ataxia, which causes a stamping gait; loss of position sense and sometimes of pain sensibility; trophic lesions in the lower limbs; progressive joint instability; and almost painless destruction of joints (Charcot joints). There is no treatment for the cord disorder.

Syringomyelia In syringomyelia a long cavity (the syrinx) filled with CSF develops within the spinal cord, most commonly in the cervical region. Usually the cause is unknown but the condition is sometimes associated with tumours, or spinal cord injury in adults and congenital anomalies with hydrocephalus and herniation of the cerebellar tonsils in children.

Symptoms and signs are most noticeable in the upper limbs. The expanding cyst presses on the anterior horn cells, producing weakness and wasting of the hand muscles. Also, destruction of the decussating spinothalamic fibres in the centre of the cord produces a characteristic dissociated sensory loss in the upper limbs: impaired response to pain and temperature but preservation of touch. There may be trophic lesions in the fingers and neuropathic arthropathy ('Charcot joints') in the upper limbs. CT may reveal an expanded cord and the syrinx can be defined on MRI.

Deterioration may be slowed down by decompression of the foramen magnum.

SPINA BIFIDA

Spina bifida is a congenital disorder in which the two halves of the posterior vertebral arch fail to fuse at one or more levels. This neural tube defect, or spinal dysraphism, which occurs within the first month of foetal life, usually affects the lumbar or lumbosacral segments of the spine. In its most severe form, the condition is associated with major neurological problems in the lower limbs together with incontinence.

Pathology

Spina bifida occulta In the mildest forms of dysraphism there is a midline defect between the laminae and nothing more; hence the term 'occulta'. Most cases are discovered incidentally on spine x-rays (usually affecting L5). However, in some cases – and especially if several vertebrae are affected – there are telltale defects in the overlying skin, for example, a dimple, a pit or a tuft of hair. Occasionally there are associated intraspinal anomalies, such as tethering of the conus medullaris below L1, splitting of the spinal cord (diastematomyelia) and cysts or lipomas of the cauda equina.

Spina bifida cystica In the more overt forms of dysraphism the vertebral laminae are missing and the contents of the vertebral canal prolapse through the defect. The abnormality takes one of several forms.

The least disabling is a *meningocele*, which accounts for about 5 per cent of cases of spina bifida cystica. The dura mater is open posteriorly but the meninges are intact and a CSF-filled meningeal sac protrudes under the skin. The spinal cord and nerve roots remain inside the vertebral canal and there is usually no neurological abnormality.

The most common and most serious abnormality is a *myelomeningocele*, which usually occurs in the lower thoracic spine or the lumbosacral region. Part of the spinal cord and nerve roots prolapse into the meningeal sac. In some cases the neural tube is fully formed and the sac is covered by a membrane and/or skin – a *'closed' myelomeningocele*. In others the cord is in a more primitive state, the unfolded neural plate forming the roof of the sac – an *'open' myelomeningocele* which is always associated with a neurological deficit distal to the level of the lesion. If neural tissue is exposed to the air, it may become infected, leading to more severe abnormality and even death.

Hydrocephalus Distal tethering of the cord may cause herniation of the cerebellum and brain-stem through the foramen magnum, resulting in obstruction to CSF circulation and hydrocephalus. The ventricles dilate and the skull enlarges by separation of the cranial sutures. Persistently raised intracranial pressure may cause cerebral atrophy and learning difficulties.

Incidence and screening

Isolated laminar defects are seen in over 5 per cent of lumbar spine x-rays but cystic spina bifida is rare at 2–3 per 1000 live births. However, if one child is affected the risk for future siblings is significantly higher.

Neural tube defects are associated with high levels of alpha-fetoprotein (AFP) in the amniotic fluid and serum. This offers an effective method of antenatal screening during the 15th to 18th week of pregnancy.

Maternal blood testing is performed routinely at 15–18 weeks and followed by an amniocentesis if necessary. A mid-term high resolution ultrasound scan will detect 95 per cent of cases of spina bifida and, in many countries, counselling regarding a termination is offered. If the pregnancy is continued, arrangements should be made to ensure that appropriate services are available at birth and in the neonatal period to minimize the risk of further neurological damage.

Folic acid, 400 micrograms daily taken before conception and continuing through the first 12 weeks of pregnancy, has been shown to reduce the risk of neural tube defects in the fetus.

Clinical features

EARLY DIAGNOSIS

The major neural tube defects can easily be detected on antenatal scans or identified immediately at birth.

Spina bifida occulta is often encountered in normal people, and can usually be ignored. However, a posterior midline dimple, a tuft of hair or a pigmented naevus signifies the potential for something more serious. Children may present with mild neurological symptoms: enuresis, urinary frequency or intermittent incontinence; neurological examination may reveal weakness and some loss of sensibility in the lower limbs. Plain x-rays may show the laminar defect and any associated vertebral anomalies; a midline ridge of bone suggests bifurcation of the cord (diastematomyelia). Intraspinal anomalies are best shown by MRI.

Spina bifida cystica is usually obvious at birth in the shape of a saccular lesion overlying the lumbar spine. It may be covered only with membrane, or with membrane and skin. In open myelomeningoceles the

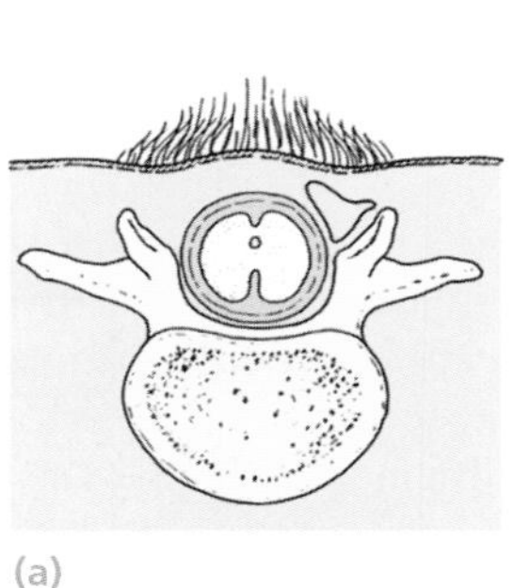
(a)

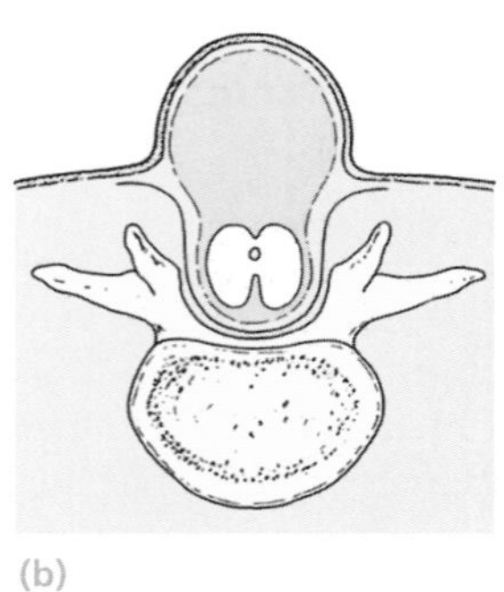
(b)

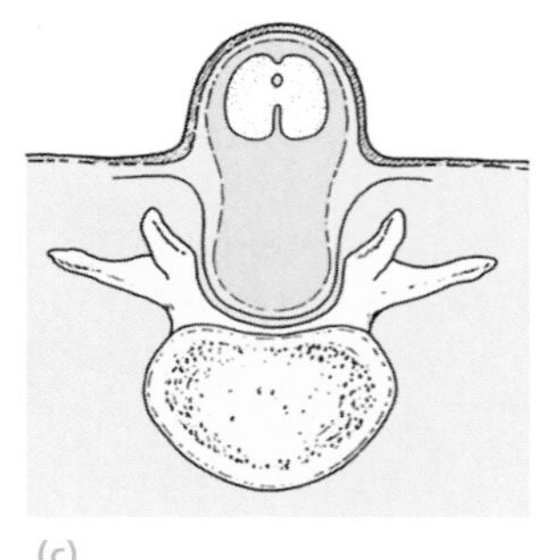
(c)

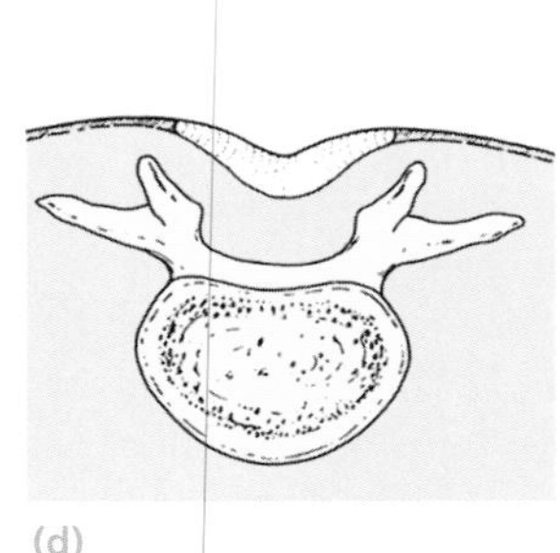
(d)

10.17 Dysraphism (a) Spina bifida occulta. (b) Meningocele. (c) Myelomeningocele. (d) Open myelomeningocele.

neural elements form the roof of the cyst, which merges into plum-coloured skin at its base. Meningoceles are covered by normal looking skin.

Hydrocephalus may be present at birth; with a communicating hydrocephalus the intracranial pressure may not be elevated until leakage from the spinal lesion is arrested by surgical closure of the lesion.

The baby's posture may suggest some type of paralysis, or even the neurological level of the lesion. Deformities of the lower limbs such as equinovarus or calcaneovalgus of the feet, recurvatum of the knee and hip dislocation are common and probably due to a combination of factors such as muscle imbalance, lack of movement and abnormal limb position in utero, or to associated anomalies that are independent of the paralysis.

Muscle charting, although difficult, is possible in the neonate and should be performed so that neurological deterioration can be identified promptly. In about one-third of infants with myelomeningocele there is complete LMN paralysis and loss of sensation and sphincter control below the affected level; in one-third there is a complete lesion at some level but a distal segment of cord is preserved, giving a mixed neurological picture with intact segmental reflexes and spastic muscle groups; in the remaining third the cord lesion is incomplete and some movement and sensation are preserved.

X-rays and CT will show the extent of the bony lesion as well as other vertebral anomalies. MRI may be helpful to define the neurological defects.

CLINICAL FEATURES IN OLDER CHILDREN

The minor forms of spina bifida may present clinically at any age. The physical signs mentioned above may have been noted previously and the child (or teenager) now presents with clawing of the toes, a change in gait pattern, incontinence or abnormal sensation. This delayed presentation is often attributed to the *tethered cord syndrome*. Tethering may be secondary to the early surgical reconstruction of the major defect or to conditions such as a diastematomyelia, and with growth there is progressive damage to the cord and/or nerve roots. MRI with gadolinium enhancement is the investigation of choice and neurosurgical release the treatment of choice before any further neurological damage occurs.

Older children with neurological lesions are liable to suffer fractures after minor injuries. These may not always be obvious but suspicion should be raised by the appearance of swelling, warmth and redness in the limb.

Treatment

In recent years intrauterine surgery has been attempted: closure of the defect is possible but a reduction in neurological disability has not yet been identified.

After birth, care must be taken to dress the 'wound' and prevent infection of these vulnerable tissues. Formal neurosurgical closure of the defect should take place within 48 hours of birth in order to prevent drying and ulceration, or infection of the lesion. All neural tissue should be carefully preserved and covered with dura; the skin is then widely undercut to facilitate complete closure. However some centres avoid urgent operation if the neurological level is high (above L1), if spinal deformities are very severe or if there is marked hydrocephalus.

A few weeks later, when the back has healed, the degree of *hydrocephalus* is assessed. Almost all children also have the *Arnold–Chiari* malformation with displacement of the posterior fossa structures through the foramen magnum. Thus, around 90 per cent of children will require active management of their real or potential hydrocephalus in the form of a ventriculo-peritoneal shunt (VP shunt) to reduce the risk of further damage to their CNS. A chronically raised intracranial pressure may be associated with learning difficulties and other problems. Similarly, if a child's neurological status changes unexpectedly, shunt

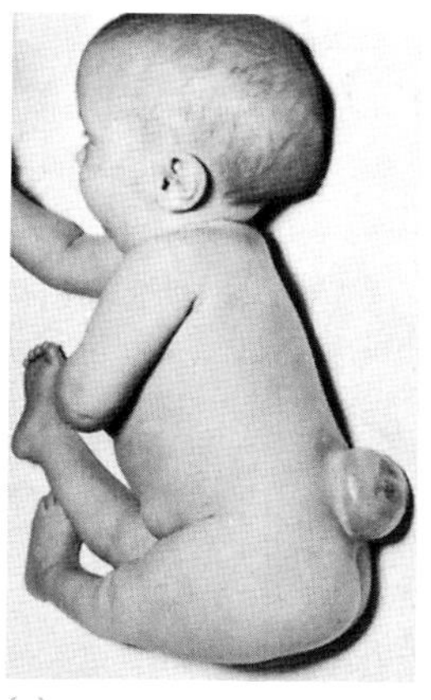
(a)

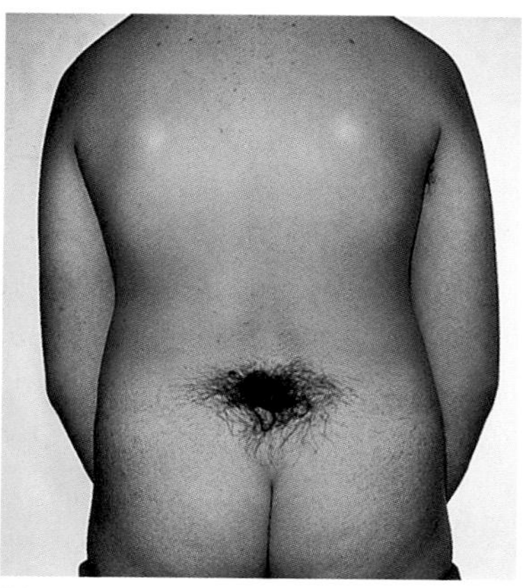
(b)

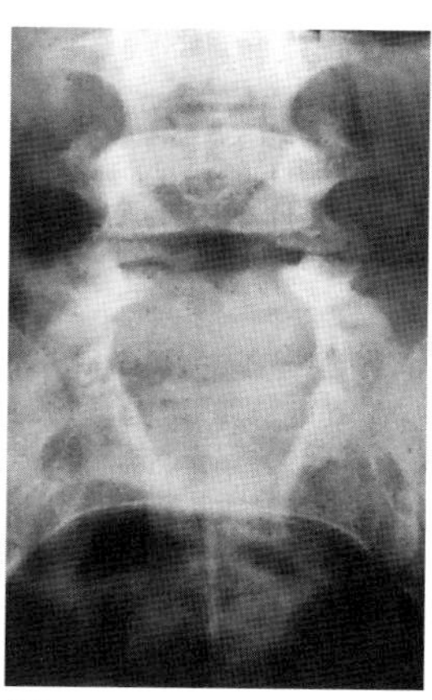
(c)

10.18 Spina bifida (a) Baby with spina bifida cystica (myelomeningocele). (b) Tuft of hair over the lumbosacral junction. X-ray in this case showed a sacral defect (c).

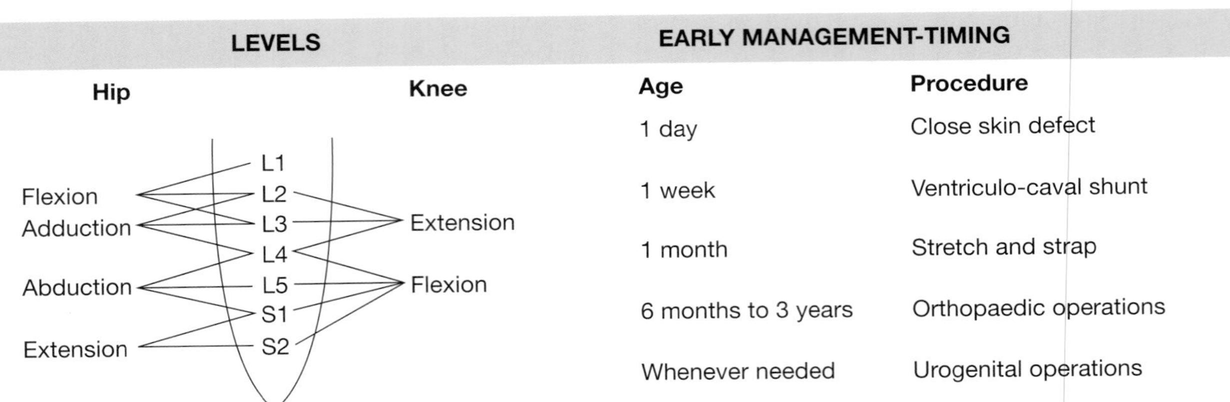

LEVELS
EARLY MANAGEMENT-TIMING
Hip
Knee
L1
L2
L3
L4
L5
S1
S2
Flexion
Adduction
Abduction
Extension
Extension
Flexion
Age
Procedure
1 day
Close skin defect
1 week
Ventriculo-caval shunt
1 month
Stretch and strap
6 months to 3 years
Orthopaedic operations
Whenever needed
Urogenital operations

10.19 Spina bifida The diagram shows the root levels concerned with hip and knee movements. The table is a simple guide to the timing of operations.

problems such as infection/blockage should be considered.

Ventriculo-peritoneal drainage can be maintained (if necessary, by changing the valve as the baby grows) for 5 or 6 years, by which time the tendency to hydrocephalus usually ceases.

Management of neonatal deformities will vary depending on the overall clinical picture, but physiotherapy and/or splinting will be the mainstays of early treatment. It must be remembered that the skin is likely to be insensate and pressure area care is essential.

In the more severe forms of spina bifida, there must be a multidisciplinary approach to treatment from early infancy through to adulthood. Orthopaedic management is important but so is the management of the neurological lesion in terms of urological function and bladder/bowel control. The vast majority of patients have urological problems necessitating the use of catheters or urinary diversion. Botulinum toxin injections may increase capacity and improve continence.

The psychosocial aspects of the condition must also be borne in mind; they can be overwhelming to the child and his or her family and require patient attention.

ORTHOPAEDIC MANAGEMENT

The orthopaedic surgeon, working as part of a team, must identify the important treatment goals while bearing in mind some basic observations:

- Except in the mildest cases, the late functional outcome cannot be predicted until the child is assessed both intellectually and in terms of neuromuscular function around the age of 3–4 years.
- Most patients with myelomeningocele will never be functionally independent.
- The maintenance and development of intellectual skills and upper limb function are often more important for independence in the activities of daily living than walking and, for many patients, the ability to sit comfortably is more important than the ability to stand awkwardly.
- The best predictor of walking ability and function is the motor level of the paralysis. Children with lesions below L4 will have quadriceps control and active knee extension and should be encouraged to walk. Children with higher lesions may start off walking with the aid of orthotic devices but they are likely to opt for a wheelchair with time.
- Immobilization and muscle imbalance both lead to joint deformity and the risk of pathological fracture. Physiotherapists working to correct, or indeed prevent, joint deformity must understand the risk of fracture, and orthotists must take into consideration the need for lightweight appliances and beware the risk of pressure sores when using splints.
- *Latex allergy* is present in some children with spina bifida and a history of allergic reactions should be noted. All treatment, including surgery, must be conducted in a latex-free environment. If a positive history is identified, antihistamines and/or corticosteroids should be given.

REGIONAL SURVEY

Spine

Spinal deformity (scoliosis and/or kyphosis) is common in children with myelomeningocele, due to a combination of muscle weakness and imbalance, associated congenital vertebral anomalies (in about 20 per cent of cases) and the tethered cord syndrome.

Distal tethering of the cord or other neural elements is almost inevitable after repair of a myelomeningocele; this may be harmless, but it can cause pain and progression of neurological dysfunction during phases of rapid growth, and in some cases it gives rise to scoliosis. Diagnosis may be aided by CT and MRI. Indications for operative release of the tethered cord are increasing pain and neurological dysfunction or progressive spinal deformity.

Kyphosis may result in stretching and breakdown, or chronic ulceration, of the overlying skin posteriorly and compression of the abdominal and thoracic viscera anteriorly. Treatment is difficult and may require localized vertebral resection and arthrodesis. However, the cord at the affected level is often non-functioning and therefore the risks of further neurological insult influencing the outcome are small.

Paralytic scoliosis appears as a long C-shaped curve which is usually progressive and makes sitting particularly difficult. It is unlikely to respond to a brace. Molded seat inserts for the wheelchair are essential to aid sitting balance and independence and may help reduce the rate of curve deterioration. Surgery via an anterior, a posterior or a combined approach is often necessary and fusion to the pelvis may be required, although this tends to reduce walking ability in ambulant patients – at least temporarily. The operation is always difficult and carries a high risk of complications, particularly postoperative infection and implant failure.

Hip

Patients with spina bifida present a wide spectrum of hip problems, the management of which is still being debated. In our approach the general aim is to secure hips that have enough movement to enable the child both to stand up in calipers and to sit comfortably.

If the neurological level of the lesion is above L1, all muscle groups are flaccid and splintage is the only option; in the long term, the child will probably use a wheelchair. With lesions below S1 a hip flexion contracture is the most likely problem and this can be corrected by elongation of the psoas tendon combined with detachment of the flexors from the ilium (the Soutter operation).

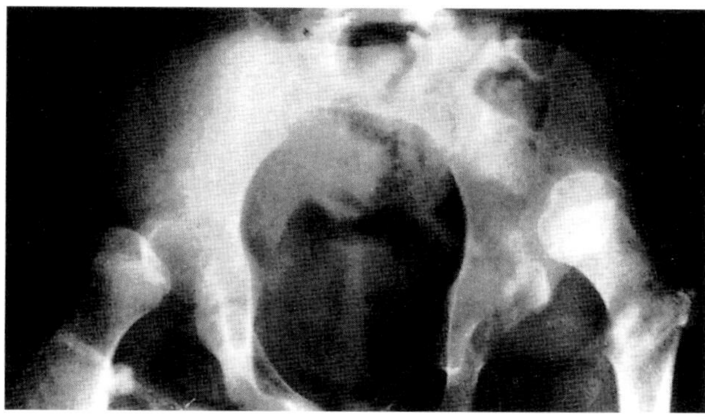

10.20 Spina bifida Muscle imbalance may lead to bilateral hip dislocation.

For children with 'in between' lesions, muscle imbalance is the main problem and many hips (up to 50 per cent) will sublux or dislocate by early childhood. The effect of hip joint subluxation or dislocation (and its associated pelvic obliquity) on spinal development is unclear, but the natural history of hip joint function in these children can be surprisingly good. This has led to the recognition that retaining hip movement may be more useful than striving for hip reduction by multiple operations, with their attendant complications and uncertain prognosis. There is, as yet, a lack of convincing evidence to suggest that function is improved significantly by operative hip relocation.

Knee

Unlike the hip, the knee usually presents no problem, because the aim is simple – a straight knee suitable for wearing callipers and using gait-training devices. In older children fixed flexion may follow prolonged sitting. If stretching (by distraction) fails to correct this deformity, one or more of the hamstrings may be lengthened, divided or reinserted into the femur or patella; this may have to be combined with a posterior capsular release. However, if the likely prognosis is that the patient will be wheelchair dependent, flexion contractures are, of course, less of a problem.

Some children are born with a hyperextension contracture and on occasion the hamstring tendons are subluxed anteriorly. Physiotherapy and sometimes serial casting are the treatments of choice initially but a V–Y quadricepsplasty and hamstring lengthening may be required in order to achieve enough knee flexion to facilitate standing.

Walking patients often develop a valgus knee, in some cases with torsional abnormalities in the lower limb. Secondary joint instability can further exacerbate the problems of walking, with patients relying more and more on the use of forearm crutches and a swing-through gait.

Foot

Foot deformities are among the most common problems in children with spina bifida. The aim of treatment is a mobile foot, with healthy skin and soft tissues that will not break down easily, that can be held or braced in a plantigrade position.

A flail foot or one that has a balanced paralysis or weakness is relatively easy to treat and only requires the use of accurately made orthoses (e.g. an ankle–foot orthosis) or occasionally simply well-fitting ankle boots.

Equinovarus deformity is likely to be more severe (and more resistant to treatment) than the 'ordinary' clubfoot. The standard treatment has been an aggressive soft-tissue release, but increasingly there have been reports of success with the Ponseti technique of gentle manipulation towards progressive correction, holding the feet in well-moulded plaster casts which are changed every week for about 8–10 weeks; in some cases a subcutaneous tendo achillis tenotomy is needed to fully correct the equinus (Ponseti and Smoley, 1963). This primary treatment may have to be followed later by further release of tight tendons and/or a tendon transfer. Bony procedures are reserved for residual or recurrent deformity in the older child.

A vertical talus deformity can be treated in a similar way by a 'reverse Ponseti' regimen and transfer of the tibialis anterior tendon to the neck of the talus, but surgical correction of this deformity is often required.

Toe deformities sometimes cause concern because of pressure points and difficulty fitting shoes. 'Orthopaedic shoes' with a high toe box may be needed and could be more appropriate than surgical intervention.

Poliomyelitis

Poliomyelitis is an acute infectious viral disease, spread by the oropharyngeal route, that passes through several distinct phases. Only around 10 per cent of patients exhibit any symptoms at all and involvement of the CNS occurs in less than 1 per cent of cases with effects on the anterior horn cells of the spinal cord and brain-stem, leading to LMN (flaccid) paralysis of the affected muscle groups. The poliomyelitis viruses have varying virulence and in countries where vaccination is encouraged it has become a rare disease; however, the effects of previous infection are still with us today.

Clinical features

Poliomyelitis typically passes through several clinical phases, from an acute illness resembling meningitis to paralysis, then slow recovery or convalescence and finally the long period of residual paralysis. The disease strikes at any age but most commonly in children.

The acute illness Early symptoms are fever and headache; in about one-third of cases the patient gives a history of a minor illness with sore throat, mild headache and slight pyrexia 5–7 days before. As the symptoms increase in severity, neck stiffness appears and meningitis may be suspected. The patient lies curled up with the joints flexed; the muscles are painful and tender and passive stretching provokes painful spasms.

Paralysis Soon muscle weakness appears; it reaches a peak in the course of 2–3 days and may give rise to difficulty with breathing and swallowing. If the patient does not succumb from respiratory paralysis, pain and pyrexia subside after 7–10 days and the patient enters the convalescent stage. However, he or she should be considered to be infective for at least 4 weeks from the onset of illness.

Recovery and convalescence A return of muscle power is most noticeable within the first 6 months, but there may be continuing improvement for up to 2 years.

Residual paralysis In some patients the illness does not progress beyond the early stage of meningeal irritation; some, again, who develop muscle weakness recover completely; in others recovery is incomplete and they are left with some degree of asymmetric flaccid (LMN) paralysis or unbalanced muscle weakness that in time leads to joint deformities and growth defects. Although sensation is intact, the limb often appears cold and blue.

Post-polio syndrome Although it was generally held that the pattern of muscle weakness became firmly established by 2 years, it is now recognized that in up to 50 per cent of cases reactivation of the virus results in progressive muscle weakness in both old and new muscle groups, giving rise to unaccustomed fatigue. If this occurs in patients with a confirmed history of poliomyelitis and a period of neurological stability of at least 15 years then the diagnosis of post-polio syndrome (PPS) must be considered. PPS is, however, a diagnosis of exclusion and care must be taken to investigate for other medical diagnoses that might explain the new symptoms. The older the child was at the onset of disease, the more severe the disease was

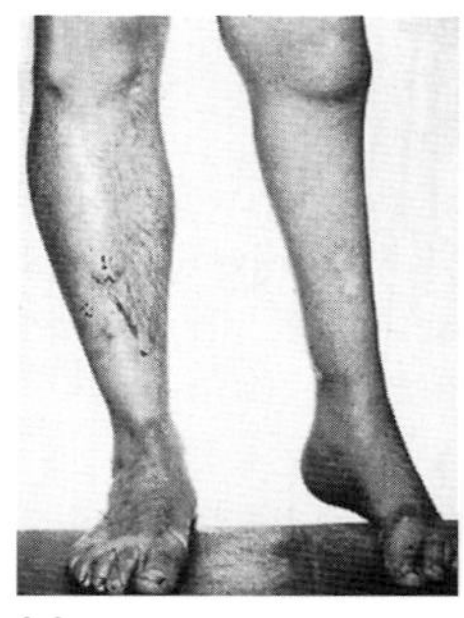
(a)

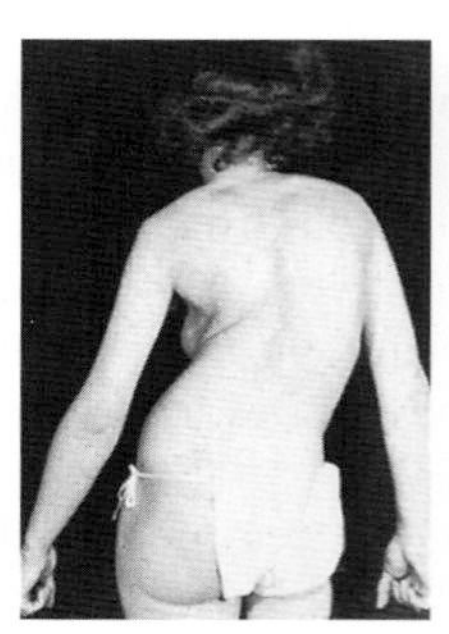
(b)

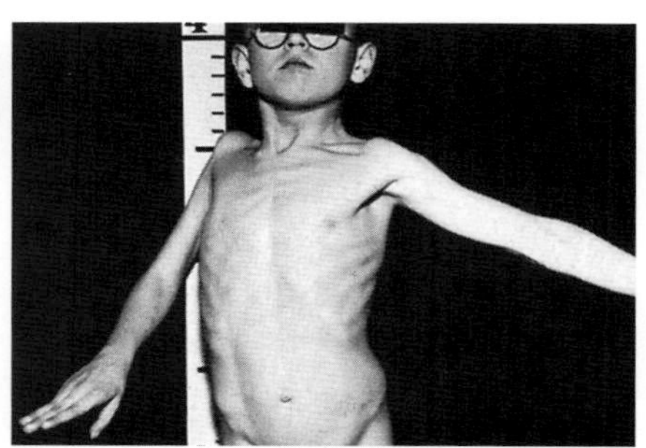
(c)

10.21 Poliomyelitis (a) Shortening and wasting of the left leg, with equinus of the ankle. (b) This long curve is typical of a paralytic scoliosis. (c) Paralysis of the right deltoid and supraspinatus makes it impossible for this boy to abduct his right arm.

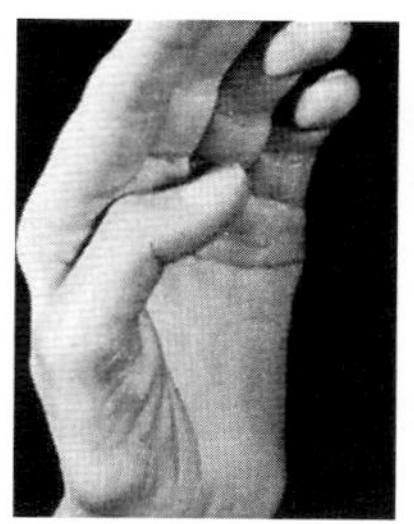
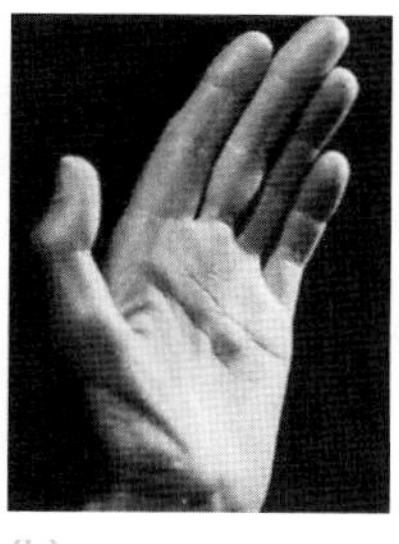
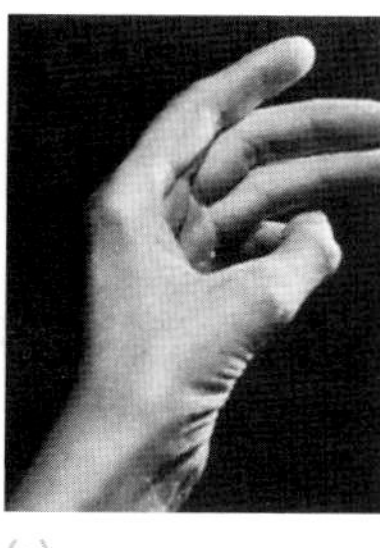

(a) (b) (c)

10.22 Poliomyelitis – treatment Opponens paralysis has been treated by superficialis tendon transfer. In (b) the tendon can be seen in action at the start of thumb opposition. (c) Full opposition achieved.

likely to have been and the more likely is it that the adult would develop PPS.

Early treatment

During the acute phase the patient is isolated and kept at complete rest, with symptomatic treatment for pain and muscle spasm. Active movement is avoided but gentle passive stretching helps to prevent contractures. Respiratory paralysis calls for artificial respiration.

Once the acute illness settles, physiotherapy is stepped up, active movements are encouraged and every effort is made to regain maximum power. Between exercise periods, splintage may be necessary to maintain joint and limb alignment and prevent fixed deformities.

Muscle charting (see page 230) is carried out at regular intervals until no further recovery is detected.

Late treatment

Once the severity of residual paralysis has been established, there are a number of basic problems that need to be addressed.

Isolated muscle weakness without deformity Isolated muscle weakness, even in the absence of joint deformity, may cause instability (e.g. quadriceps paralysis which makes weightbearing and walking impossible without some type of brace) or loss of complex function (e.g. thumb opposition, which can be treated by tendon transfer).

Passively correctible deformity Any unbalanced paralysis (i.e. muscle weakness on one aspect of a joint and greater power in the antagonists) can lead to deformity. At first this is passively correctable and can be counteracted by a splint (a calliper or lightweight brace). However, an appropriate tendon transfer may solve the problem permanently. It is here that muscle charting is particularly important. A muscle usually loses one grade of power when it is transferred; therefore, to be really useful, it should have grade 4 or 5 power, although a grade 3 muscle may act as a sort of tenodesis and reduce the deformity caused by gravity.

Fixed deformity Fixed deformities cannot be corrected by either splintage or tendon transfer alone; it is important also to restore alignment operatively and to stabilize the joint, if necessary, by arthrodesis. This is especially applicable to fixed deformities of the ankle and foot, but the same principle applies in treating paralytic scoliosis.

Occasionally a fixed deformity is beneficial. Thus, an equinus foot may help to compensate mechanically for quadriceps weakness; if so, it should not be corrected.

Flail joint Balanced paralysis, because it causes no deformity, may need no treatment. However, if the joint is unstable or flail it must be stabilized, either by permanent splintage or by arthrodesis.

Shortening Normal bone growth depends on normal muscle activity; thus many children who have been affected with poliomyelitis in their early years can be expected to develop a difference in leg length. Discrepancies of up to 3–5 cm can, in theory, be compensated for with a shoe raise although this tends to make the shorter (and weaker) leg clumsier. While leg lengthening is always an option, the fact that the increase in length discrepancy with growth can be calculated fairly accurately from growth tables means it

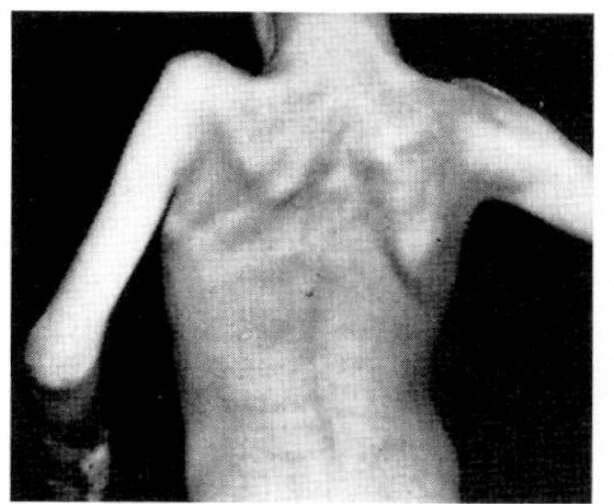
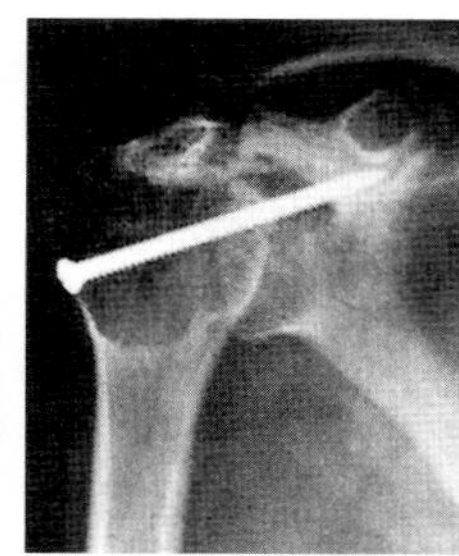
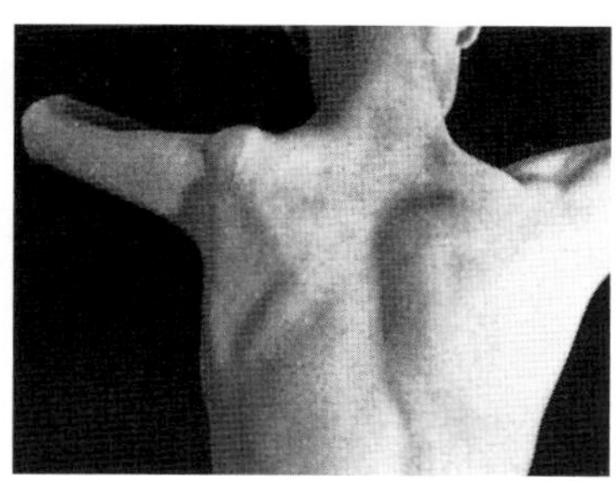

(a) (b) (c)

10.23 Poliomyelitis – arthrodesis (a) This patient had paralysis of the left deltoid: after arthrodesis (b) he could lift his arm (c) by using his scapular muscles.

can also be mitigated by a well-timed epiphyseodesis in the normal limb.

Disturbance of skeletal modelling As with all childhood paralytic disorders, the effects of muscle imbalance on the growing skeleton must be anticipated. Changes may become obvious with growth, appearing as torsional deformities or angular deformities in either the sagittal or the coronal plane. Moreover, muscle and joint contractures may aggravate the effects of any bone distortion. Any changes that interfere with function should be prevented or treated as soon as possible.

Vascular dysfunction Sensation is intact but the paralysed limb is often cold and blue. Large chilblains sometimes develop and sympathectomy may be needed.

Regional survey

Treatment is often concentrated on the lower limbs but this should not be at the expense of upper limb function. For children who are dependent on walking aids and/or wheelchairs, obtaining and maintaining bimanual function can be very important.

Shoulder

Provided the scapular muscles are strong, abduction at the shoulder can be restored by arthrodesing the gleno-humeral joint (50 degrees abducted and 25 degrees flexed). Contracted adductors may need division.

Elbow and forearm

At the elbow, *flexion* can be restored in one of two ways. If there is normal power in the anterior forearm muscles (wrist and finger flexors) the common flexor origin can be moved more proximally on the distal humerus to provide better leverage across the elbow. Alternatively, if the pectoralis major is strong, the lower half of the muscle can be detached at its origin on the rib-cage, swung down and joined to the biceps tendon.

Pronation of the forearm can be strengthened by transposing an active flexor carpi ulnaris tendon across the front of the forearm to the radial border. Loss of *supination* may be countered by transposing flexor carpi ulnaris across the back of the forearm to the distal radius.

Wrist and hand

Wrist deformity or instability can be markedly improved by arthrodesis. Any active muscles can then be used to restore finger movement.

In the thumb, weakness of opposition can be overcome by a flexor superficialis transfer. The tendon (usually of the ring finger) is wound round that of flexor carpi ulnaris (which acts as a pulley), threaded across the palm and fixed to the distal end of the first metacarpal.

Trunk

Unbalanced paralysis causes scoliosis, frequently a long thoracolumbar curve which may involve the lumbosacral junction, causing pelvic obliquity. Operative treatment is often needed, the most effective being a combination of anterior and posterior instrumentation and fusion (see page 463).

Hip

Hip deformities are usually complex and difficult to manage; the problem is often aggravated by the gradual development of subluxation or dislocation due either to muscle imbalance (abductors weaker than adductors) or pelvic obliquity associated with scoliosis. Furthermore, since paralysis usually occurs before the age of 5 years, growth of the proximal femur is abnormal and this may result in secondary deformities such as persistent anteversion of the femoral neck, coxa valga and underdevelopment of the acetabular socket – all of which will increase the tendency to instability and dislocation.

The keys to successful treatment are: (1) to reduce any scoliotic pelvic obliquity by correcting or improving the scoliosis; (2) to overcome or improve the muscle imbalance by suitable tendon transfer; (3) to correct the proximal femoral deformities by intertrochanteric or subtrochanteric osteotomy; and (4) to deepen the acetabular socket, if necessary, by an acetabuloplasty which will prevent posterior displacement of the femoral head.

Fixed flexion can be treated by Soutter's muscle slide operation or by transferring psoas to the greater trochanter. For fixed abduction with pelvic obliquity the fascia lata and iliotibial band may need division; occasionally, for severe deformity, proximal femoral osteotomy may be required as well. With this type of obliquity the 'higher' hip tends to be unstable and the 'lower' hip to have fixed abduction; if the abducted hip is corrected first the pelvis may level and the other hip become normal.

Knee

Instability due to relative weakness of the knee extensors is a major problem. Unaided walking may still be possible provided the hip has good extensor power and the foot good plantarflexion power (or fixed equinus); with this combination the knee is stabilized by being thrust into hyperextension as body weight comes onto the leg. The patient has often learnt to help this manoeuvre by placing a hand on the front of the thigh and pushing the thigh backwards with every stance phase of gait. If the hip or ankle joints are also weak, a full-length calliper will be required, or a supracondylar extension osteotomy of the femur must be considered.

Fixed flexion with flexors stronger than extensors is more common and must be corrected. Flexor-to-extensor transfer (e.g. hamstring muscles to the patella or the quadriceps tendon) is feasible if the flexor muscles are normal; however, quadriceps power is unlikely to be improved by more than one grade. If the flexors are not strong enough, the deformity can be corrected by supracondylar extension osteotomy.

Marked hyperextension (genu recurvatum) sometimes occurs, either as a primary deformity or secondary to fixed equinus. It can be improved by supracondylar flexion osteotomy; an alternative is to excise the patella and slot it into the upper tibia where it acts as a bone block (Hong-Xue Men et al., 1991).

Foot

Instability and *foot-drop* can be controlled by an ankle–foot orthosis or a below-knee calliper. Often there is imbalance causing varus, valgus or calcaneocavus *deformity*; fusion in the corrected position should be combined with tendon re-routing to restore balance, otherwise there is risk of the deformity recurring.

For varus or valgus the simplest procedure is to slot bone grafts into vertical grooves on each side of the sinus tarsi (Grice); alternatively, a triple arthrodesis (Dunn) of subtalar and mid-tarsal joints is performed, relying on bone carpentry to correct deformity. With associated foot-drop, Lambrinudi's modification is valuable; triple arthrodesis is performed but the fully plantarflexed talus is slotted into the navicular with the forefoot in only slight equinus: foot-drop is corrected because the talus cannot plantarflex further, and slight equinus helps to stabilize the knee. With calcaneocavus deformity, Elmslie's operation is useful: triple arthrodesis is performed in the calcaneus position, but corrected at a second stage by posterior wedge excision combined with tenodesis using half of the tendo achillis.

There is a low incidence of secondary osteoarthritis in the joints adjacent to the arthrodesed joint because of the relatively low demands placed on the paralytic limb.

Claw toes, if the deformity is mobile, are corrected by transferring the toe flexors to the extensors; if the deformity is fixed, the interphalangeal joints should be arthrodesed in the straight position and the long extensor tendons reinserted into the metatarsal necks.

MOTOR NEURON DISORDERS

Rare degenerative disorders of the large motor neurons may cause progressive and sometimes fatal paralysis.

Motor neuron disease (amyotrophic lateral sclerosis)

This is a degenerative disease of unknown aetiology. It affects both cortical (upper) motor neurons and the anterior horn cells of the cord, causing widespread UMN and LMN symptoms and signs. Patients usually present in middle age with dysarthria and difficulty in swallowing or, if the limbs are affected, with muscle weakness (e.g. clumsy hands or unexplained foot-drop) and wasting in the presence of exaggerated reflexes. Muscle cramps are troublesome; muscle atrophy and fasciculations may be obvious. Sensation and bladder control are normal. Some of these features are also seen in spinal cord compression, which can be excluded by MRI.

The disease is progressive and incurable. Patients usually end up in a wheelchair and have increasing difficulty with speech and eating. Cognitive function is usually spared although some patients have associated frontotemporal dementia or a pseudobulbar effect causing emotional lability. Most of them die within 5 years from a combination of respiratory weakness and aspiration pneumonia.

Spinal muscular atrophy

In this rare group of heritable disorders (a defect on the long arm of chromosome 5 has been identified) there is widespread degeneration of the anterior horn cells in the cord, leading to progressive LMN weakness. The commonest form (*Werdnig–Hoffman disease*) is inherited as an autosomal recessive and is diagnosed at birth or soon afterwards. The baby is floppy and weak, feeding is difficult and breathing is shallow. Death occurs, usually within a year.

A less severe form (*Kugelberg–Welander disease*), of either dominant or recessive inheritance, is usually seen in adolescents or young adults who present with limb weakness, proximal muscle wasting and 'paralytic' scoliosis. However, it sometimes appears in early childhood as a cause of delayed walking. Patients may live to 30–40 years of age but are usually confined to a wheelchair. Spinal braces are used to improve sitting ability; if this cannot prevent the spine from collapsing, operative instrumentation and fusion is advisable.

PERIPHERAL NEUROPATHIES

Disorders of the peripheral nerves may affect motor, sensory or autonomic functions, may be localized to a short segment or may involve the full length of the nerve fibres including their cell bodies in the anterior horn (motor neurons), posterior root ganglia (sensory neurons) and autonomic ganglia. In some cases spinal cord tracts are involved as well. There are over 100 types of neuropathy; in this section we consider those conditions that are most likely to come within the ambit of the orthopaedic surgeon.

Classification

Classification by anatomical level and distribution is probably the simplest. Although it does not fully cover pathological causation, it does relate to clinical presentation and provides a framework for further investigations. It is well to remember that in over 40 per cent of cases no specific cause is found!

1. *Radiculopathy* – involvement of nerve roots, most commonly by vertebral trauma, intervertebral disc herniation or bony spurs, space-occupying lesions of the spinal canal and root infections like herpes zoster.
2. *Plexopathy* – direct trauma (e.g. brachial plexus traction injuries), compression by local tumours (Pancoast's tumour), entrapment in thoracic outlet syndrome, and viral infection such as neuralgic amyotrophy.
3. *Distal neuronopathy* – involvement of neurons in distinct peripheral nerves, which is usually subdivided into:
    a. *Mononeuropathy* – involvement of a single nerve, usually mixed sensorimotor (e.g. nerve injury, nerve compression, entrapment syndromes and nerve tumours).
    b. *Multiple mononeuropathy* – involvement of several isolated nerves (e.g. leprosy and some cases of diabetes or vasculitis).
    c. *Polyneuropathy* – widespread symmetrical dysfunction (e.g. diabetic neuropathy, alcoholic neuropathy, vitamin deficiency, Guillain–Barré syndrome and a host of less common disorders (see Table 10.4).

Abnormalities may be predominantly sensory (e.g. diabetic polyneuropathy), predominantly motor (e.g. peroneal muscular atrophy) or mixed. Chronic motor loss with no sensory component is usually due to anterior horn cell disease rather than more esoteric pathology like lead poisoning.

Pathology

In general terms, large nerve fibres (those over 4 μm in diameter, which includes α-motor neurons, γ-motor neurons to the muscle spindles and sensory neurons serving touch and pressure) are myelinated whereas small fibres (less than 4 μm in diameter, mainly sensory neurons serving pain sensibility and autonomic neurons effecting vasomotor control, piloerection and neuroendocrine functions) are unmyelinated.

There are three basic types of peripheral neuronal pathology: (1) acute interruption of axonal continuity; (2) axonal degeneration; and (3) demyelination. In all three, conduction is disturbed or completely blocked, with consequent loss of motor and/or sensory and/or autonomic functions.

Table 10.4 Causes of polyneuropathy

Hereditary
Hereditary motor and sensory neuropathy
Friedreich's ataxia
Hereditary sensory neuropathy
Infections
Viral infections
Herpes zoster
Neuralgic amyotrophy
Leprosy
Inflammatory
Acute inflammatory polyneuropathy
Guillain–Barré syndrome
Systemic lupus erythematosus
Nutritional and metabolic
Vitamin deficiencies
Diabetes
Myxoedema
Amyloidosis
Neoplastic
Primary carcinoma
Myeloma
Toxic
Alcohol
Lead
Drugs
Various

ACUTE AXONAL INTERRUPTION

This occurs most typically after nerve division and is described in Chapter 11. Loss of motor and sensory functions is immediate and complete. The distal segments of axons that are crushed or severed will degenerate – as will the muscle fibres which are supplied by motor neurons if nerve conduction is not restored within two years. These changes are detectable at an early stage by nerve conduction studies and EMG. Axonal regeneration, when it occurs, is slow – the new axon grows by about 1 mm per day – and is often incomplete.

CHRONIC AXONAL DEGENERATION

In non-traumatic neuronal neuropathies the changes are slower and progressive. Most *large-fibre disorders* affect both sensory and motor neurons causing 'stocking' and 'glove' numbness, altered postural reflexes and ataxia as well as muscle weakness and wasting, beginning distally and progressing proximally. Symptoms tend to appear in the feet and legs before the hands and arms. Some disorders are predominantly either motor or sensory. Nerve conduction studies show a reduction in the size of CMAP and SNAP responses proportionate to the loss of peripheral nerve fibres, but relatively little conduction slowing (in contrast to the demyelinating neuropathies). EMG may demonstrate denervation changes in distal muscles and confirm the extent and severity of nerve loss.

Small-fibre neuropathies may cause orthostatic hypotension, cardiac arrhythmias, reduced peripheral limb perfusion, ischaemia and a predisposition to limb infection. Small nerve fibres also convey pain, heat and cold sensibility and when disturbed give rise to burning dysaesthesias. Neurophysiological tests are not sensitive enough to distinguish small-fibre disturbances.

DEMYELINATING NEUROPATHIES

Focal demyelination occurs most commonly in nerve entrapment syndromes and blunt soft-tissue trauma. The main effects are slowing of conduction and sometimes complete nerve block, causing sensory and/or motor dysfunction distal to the lesion. These changes are potentially reversible; recovery usually takes less than 6 weeks, and in some cases only a few days.

Demyelinating polyneuropathies are rare, with the exception of Guillain–Barré syndrome. Other conditions are the heritable motor and sensory neuropathies and some inherited metabolic disorders, but most of these show a mixture of axonal degeneration and demyelination.

Clinical features

Patients usually complain of sensory symptoms: 'pins and needles', numbness, a limb 'going to sleep', 'burning', shooting pains or restless legs. They may also notice weakness or clumsiness, or loss of balance in walking. Occasionally (in the predominantly motor neuropathies) the main complaint is of progressive deformity, for example, claw hand or cavus foot. The onset may be rapid (over a few days) or very gradual (over weeks or months). Sometimes there is a history of injury, a recent infective illness, a known disease such as diabetes or malignancy, alcohol abuse or nutritional deficiency.

Examination may reveal motor weakness in a particular muscle group. In the polyneuropathies the limbs are involved symmetrically, usually legs before arms and distal before proximal parts. Reflexes are usually depressed, though in small-fibre neuropathies (e.g. diabetes) this occurs very late. In mononeuropathy, sensory loss follows the 'map' of the affected nerve. In polyneuropathy, there is a symmetrical 'glove' or 'stocking' distribution. Trophic skin changes may be present. Deep sensation is also affected and some patients develop ataxia. If pain sensibility and proprioception are depressed there may be joint instability or breakdown of the articular surfaces ('Charcot' joints).

Clinical examination alone may establish the diagnosis. Further help is provided by electromyography (which may suggest the type of abnormality) and nerve conduction studies (which may show exactly where the lesion is).

The *mononeuropathies* – mainly nerve injuries and entrapment syndromes – are dealt with in Chapter 11. The more common polyneuropathies are listed in Table 10.4 and some are described below. In over 40 per cent of cases no specific cause is found.

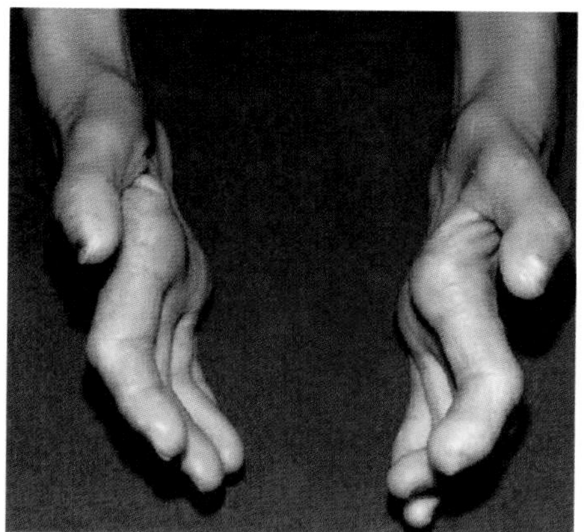
(a)

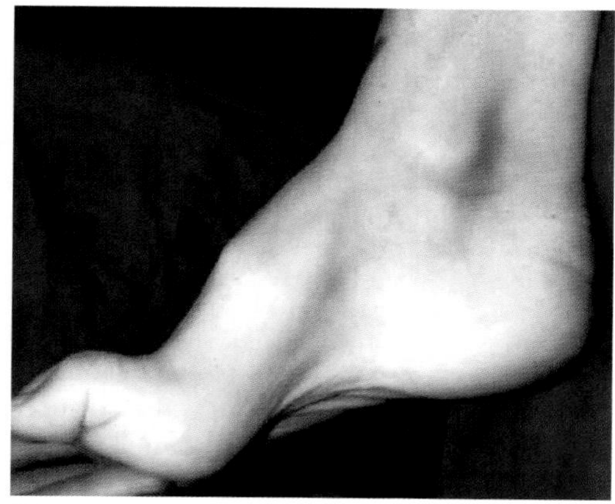
(b)

10.24 Peripheral neuropathy Two typical deformities in patients with peripheral neuritis: (a) ulnar claw hands and (b) pes cavus and claw toes.

Hereditary neuropathies

These rare disorders present in childhood and adolescence, usually with muscle weakness and deformity.

Hereditary sensory neuropathy

Congenital insensitivity to pain and temperature is inherited as either a dominant or a recessive trait. Patients develop neuropathic joint disease and ulceration of the feet. The cycle of painless injury and progressive deformity can lead to severe disability.

Hereditary motor and sensory neuropathy (HMSN)

This is the preferred name for a group of conditions which includes *peroneal muscular atrophy, Charcot–Marie–Tooth disease* and some *benign forms of spinal muscular atrophy.* They are the commonest of the inherited neuropathies, which are usually passed on as autosomal dominant disorders.

HMSN type I is seen in children who have difficulty walking and develop claw toes and pes cavus or cavovarus. There may be severe wasting of the legs and (later) the upper limbs, but often the signs are quite subtle. Spinal deformity may occur in severe cases. This is a demyelinating disorder and nerve conduction velocity is markedly slowed. The diagnosis can be confirmed by finding demyelination on sural nerve biopsy or (if the facilities are available) by genetic testing of blood samples.

HMSN type II occurs in adolescents and young adults and is much less disabling than type I; it affects only the lower limbs, causing mild pes cavus and wasting of the peronei. Nerve conduction velocity is only slightly reduced, indicating primary axonal degeneration.

Treatment In the early stages foot and ankle orthoses are helpful. If the deformities are progressive or disabling, operative correction may be indicated (see Chapter 21). Claw toes (due to intrinsic muscle weakness) can be corrected by transferring the toe flexors to the extensors, with or without fusion of the interphalangeal joints. Clawing of the big toe is best corrected by the Robert Jones procedure – transfer of the extensor hallucis longus to the metatarsal neck and fusion of the interphalangeal joint. The cavus deformity often needs no treatment, but if it causes pain it can be improved by calcaneal or dorsal mid-tarsal osteotomy or (in severe cases) triple arthrodesis.

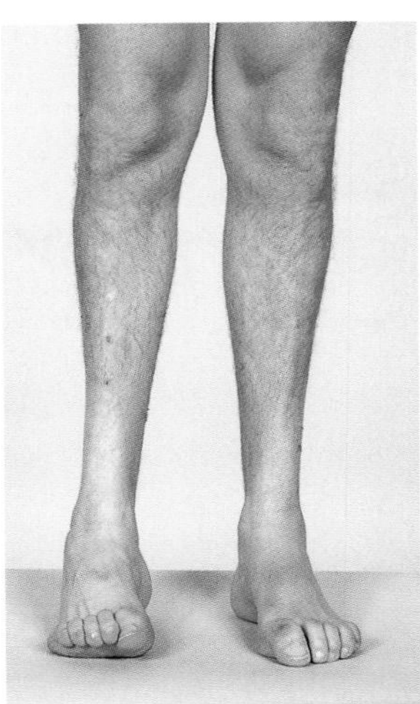

10.25 Hereditary neuropathies – peroneal muscular atrophy This patient has the typical wasting of the legs, cavus feet and claw toes associated with peroneal muscular atrophy.

Familial liability to pressure palsy (HNPP)

This is a relatively common, dominant disorder which often presents as multiple mixed entrapment mononeuropathies (e.g. carpal tunnel syndrome and ulnar nerve palsy), even in young patients.

Friedreich's ataxia

This autosomal recessive condition is the classic archetype of a large group of genetic disorders – the *spinocerebellar ataxias* – characterized by spinocerebellar dysfunction, but there may also be degeneration of the posterior root ganglia and peripheral nerves. Many of these disorders have now been genotypically defined. Patients generally present at around the age of 6 years with gait ataxia, lower limb weakness and deformities similar to those of severe Charcot–Marie–Tooth disease. The muscle weakness, which may also involve the upper limbs and the trunk, is progressive; by the age of 20 years the patient has usually taken to a wheelchair and is likely to die of cardiomyopathy before the age of 45. Despite the potentially poor prognosis, surgical correction of deformities is worthwhile.

Metabolic neuropathies

Diabetic neuropathy

Diabetes is one of the commonest causes of peripheral neuropathy. The metabolic disturbance associated with hyperglycaemia interferes with axonal and Schwann cell function, leading to mixed patterns of demyelination and axonal degeneration. Autonomic dysfunction and vascular disturbance also play a part.

The onset is insidious and the condition often goes undiagnosed until patients start complaining of numbness and paraesthesiae in the feet and lower legs. Even at that early stage there may be areflexia and diminished vibration sense. Another suspicious pattern is an increased susceptibility to nerve entrapment syndromes. Later, muscle weakness becomes more noticeable in proximal parts of the limbs. In advanced cases trophic complications can arise: neuropathic ulcers of the feet, regional osteoporosis, insufficiency fractures of the foot bones, or Charcot joints in the ankles and feet. Another late feature is loss of balance. Autonomic dysfunction may produce postural hypotension and abnormal sphincter control, and may also account for an increased susceptibility to infection.

Treatment It is vital to ensure that the underlying disorder is properly controlled. Local treatment consists of skin care, management of fractures and splintage or arthrodesis of grossly unstable or deformed joints. Management of the diabetic foot is discussed in Chapter 21.

Alcoholic neuropathy

Axonal degeneration may be due to some toxic effect of the alcohol, but the main cause is the accompanying nutritional deficiency, especially thiamine deficiency.

Presenting symptoms are, typically, 'burning' paraesthesiae, numbness and muscle weakness in the feet and legs. The calf muscles are tender to pressure and reflexes are depressed or absent. Men are likely to complain of urinary difficulty and impotence.

Treatment Early cases may respond to nutritional supplementation and administration of thiamine. Patients should be protected from trauma. Of course, steps should also be taken to deal with the alcohol abuse.

INFECTIVE NEUROPATHY

Herpes zoster (shingles)

This common disorder is caused by the varicella (chickenpox) virus. The virus, having lain dormant for many years in the dorsal root ganglia, is then reactivated and migrates down the nerve. The exact cause of the reactivation is unknown but immunocompromise, age and stress are contributory factors; thus elderly or immunosuppressed patients are particularly susceptible.

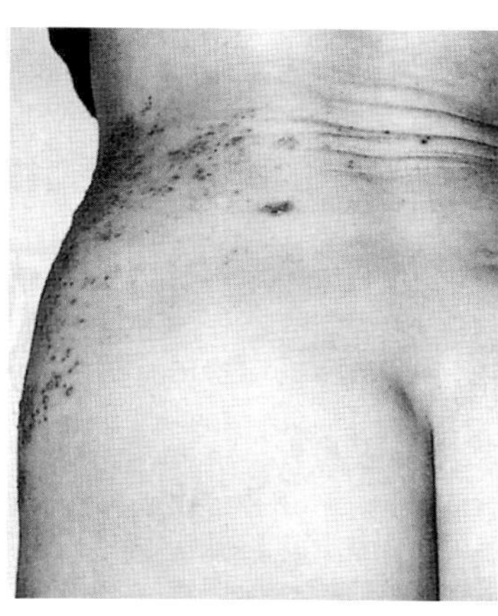

10.26 Herpes zoster This patient was treated for several weeks for 'sciatica' – then the typical rash of shingles appeared.

Following an injury or intercurrent illness, the patient develops severe unilateral pain in the distribution of several adjacent nerve roots. Motor roots and even the spinal cord may (rarely) be affected and involvement of the lumbar roots can closely mimic sciatica. Days or weeks later an irritating vesicular rash appears; characteristically it trails out along the dermatomes corresponding to affected nerves. The condition usually subsides spontaneously but post-herpetic neuralgia may persist for months or years.

Treatment is symptomatic, though in severe cases systemic antiviral therapy may be justified.

Neuralgic amyotrophy (acute brachial neuritis)

This unusual cause of severe shoulder girdle pain and weakness is believed to be due to a para-infectious disorder of one or more of the cervical nerve roots and the brachial plexus, sometimes producing a pseudo-mononeuropathic pattern (e.g. scapular winging or wrist-drop). There is often a history of an antecedent viral infection or antiviral inoculation; sometimes a small epidemic occurs among several inmates of an institution.

The history alone often suggests the diagnosis. Pain in the shoulder and arm is typically sudden in onset, intense and unabating; the patient can often recall the exact hour when symptoms began. Pain may extend into the neck and down as far as the hand; usually it lasts for two or three weeks. Other symptoms are paraesthesiae in the arm or hand and weakness of the muscles of the shoulder, forearm and hand.

Winging of the scapula (due to serratus anterior weakness), wasting of the shoulder girdle muscles,

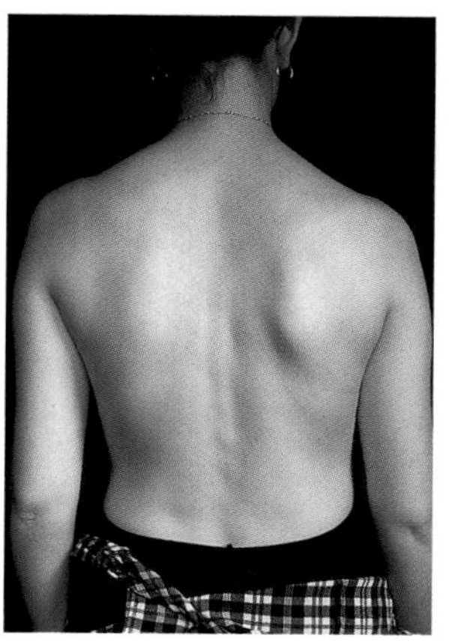

(a)

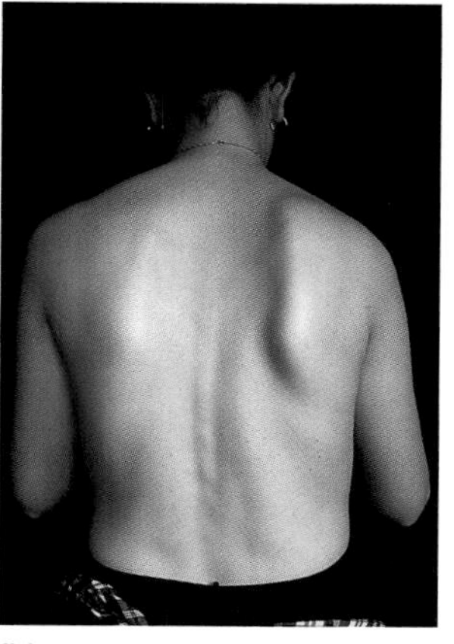

(b)

10.27 Neuralgic amyotrophy A common feature of neuralgic amyotrophy is winging of the scapula due to serratus anterior weakness. Even at rest (a) the right scapula is prominent in this young woman. When she thrusts her arms forwards against the wall (b) the abnormality is more pronounced.

and occasionally involvement of more distal arm muscles may be profound, becoming evident as the pain improves. Shoulder movement is initially limited by pain but this is superseded by weakness due to muscle atrophy. Sensory loss and paraesthesiae in one or more of the cervical dermatomes is not uncommon. Involvement of overlapping root territories of the brachial plexus is a feature that helps to distinguish neuralgic amyotrophy from an acute cervical disc herniation which is monoradicular.

There is no specific treatment; pain is controlled with analgesics. The prognosis is usually good but full neurological recovery may take months or years.

Guillain–Barré syndrome (acute inflammatory demyelinating polyneuropathy – AIDP)

Guillain–Barré syndrome describes an acute demyelinating motor and sensory (though mainly motor) polyneuropathy. It can occur at any age and usually appears two or three weeks after an upper respiratory or gastrointestinal infection – probably as an autoimmune reaction.

The typical history is of aching and weakness in the legs, often accompanied by numbness and paraesthesiae, which steadily progresses upwards over a period of hours, a few days or a few weeks. Symptoms may stop when the thigh and pelvic muscles are reached, and then gradually retreat, or may go on ascending to involve the upper limbs, facial muscles and diaphragm, resulting in quadriplegia and respiratory failure. In the established case there will be areflexia and loss of position sense. In severe cases patients may develop features of autonomic dysfunction. Unsurprisingly, the condition is also known as 'ascending paralysis'.

Cerebrospinal fluid analysis may show a characteristic pattern: elevated protein concentration in the presence of a normal cell count (unlike an infection, in which the cell count would also be elevated).

Nerve conduction studies may show conduction slowing or block; in severe cases there may be EMG signs of axonal damage.

Treatment Treatment consists essentially of bed rest, pain-relieving medication and supportive management to monitor, prevent and deal with complications such as respiratory failure and difficulty with swallowing. In severe cases specific treatment with intravenous immunoglobulins or plasmapheresis should be started as soon as possible. Once the acute disorder is under control, physiotherapy and splintage will help to prevent deformities and improve muscle power.

Most patients recover completely, though this may take 6 months or longer; about 10 per cent are left with long-term disability and about 3 per cent are likely to die.

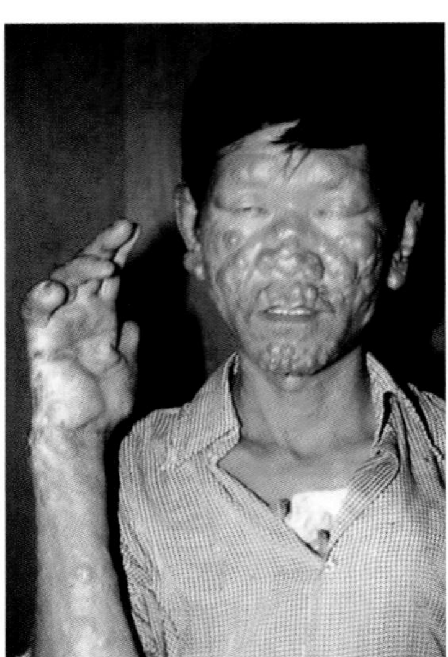

10.28 Leprosy – ulnar nerve paralysis Ulnar nerve paralysis is relatively common in longstanding leprosy. This patient has the typical ulnar claw-hand deformity.

Leprosy

Although uncommon in Europe and North America, this is still a frequent cause of peripheral neuropathy in Africa and Asia.

Mycobacterium leprae, an acid-fast organism, causes a diffuse inflammatory disorder of the skin, mucous membranes and peripheral nerves. Depending on the host response, several forms of disease may evolve.

The most severe neurological lesions are seen in *tuberculoid leprosy*. Anaesthetic skin patches develop over the extensor surfaces of the limbs; loss of motor function leads to weakness and deformities of the hands and feet. Thickened nerves may be felt as cords under the skin or where they cross the bones (e.g. the ulnar nerve behind the medial epicondyle of the elbow). Trophic ulcers are common and may predispose to osteomyelitis.

Lepromatous leprosy is associated with a symmetrical polyneuropathy, which occurs late in the disease.

Treatment by combined chemotherapy (mainly rifampicin and dapsone) is continued for 6 months to 2 years, depending on the response. Muscle weakness, particularly intrinsic muscle paralysis due to ulnar nerve involvement, may require multiple tendon transfers.

The condition is discussed in greater detail in Chapter 2 and the peripheral nerve complications are dealt with in Chapter 11.

PAIN

Many – perhaps most – musculoskeletal disorders are accompanied by pain. Whatever the nature of the underlying condition, pain usually requires treatment in its own right; sometimes it becomes the main focus of attention even after the initiating factors have disappeared or subsided.

Pain perception

Pain is confounding. The same receptors that appreciate discomfort also respond to tickling with feelings of pleasure. The electrical discharge in 'mild' pain is no different from that in 'severe' pain. That the degree of discomfort is related to the magnitude of the physical stimulus cannot be doubted, but ultimately both the severity of the pain and its character are experienced subjectively and cannot be measured.

Pain receptors Nociceptors in the form of free nerve endings are found in almost all tissues. They are stimulated by mechanical distortion, by chemical, thermal or electrical irritation, or by ischaemia. Musculoskeletal pain associated with trauma or inflammation is due to both tissue distortion and chemical irritation (local release of kinins, prostaglandins and serotonin). Visceral nociceptors respond to stretching and anoxia. In nerve injuries the regenerating axons may be hypersensitive to all stimuli.

Pain transmission Pain sensation is transmitted via both myelinated axons (large-diameter fibres), which carry well-defined and well-localized sensation, and the far more numerous unmyelinated fibres which are responsible for crude, poorly defined pain. From the dorsal horn synapses in the cord, some fibres participate in ipsilateral reflex motor and autonomic activities while others connect with axons in the contralateral spinothalamic tracts that run to the thalamus and cortex (where pain is appreciated and localized) as well as the reticular system, which may be responsible for reflex autonomic and motor responses to pain.

Pain modulation Pain impulses may be suppressed or inhibited by (1) simultaneous sensory impulses travelling via adjacent axons or (2) impulses descending from the brain. Thus, it is posited that pain impulses are 'sorted out' – some of them blocked, some allowed through – in the dorsal horn of the cord (the 'gate-control' theory of Melzak and Wall, 1965). This could explain why counter-stimulation sometimes reduces pain perception. In addition, certain morphine-like compounds (endorphins and enkephalins), normally elaborated in the brain and spinal cord, can inhibit pain sensibility. These neurotransmitters are activated by a variety of agents, including severe pain itself, other neurological stimuli, psychological messages and placebos.

Pain threshold The so-called 'pain threshold' is the level of stimulus needed to induce pain. There is no fixed threshold for any individual; pain perception is the result of all the factors mentioned above, operating against a complex and changing psychological background. The threshold is lowered by fear, anxiety, depression, lack of self-esteem and mental or physical fatigue; and it is elevated by relaxation, diversion, reduction of anxiety and general psychological support. The management of pain involves not only the elimination of noxious stimuli, or the administration of painkillers, but also the care of the whole person.

Acute pain

Severe acute pain, as seen typically after injury, is accompanied by an autonomic 'fight or flight' reaction: increased pulse rate, peripheral vasoconstriction, sweating, rapid breathing, muscle tension and anxiety. Similar features are seen in pain associated with acute neurological syndromes or in malignant disease. Lesser degrees of pain may have negligible side effects.

Treatment is directed at: (1) removing or counteracting the painful disorder; (2) splinting the painful area; (3) making the patient feel comfortable and secure; (4) administering analgesics, anti-inflammatory drugs or – if necessary – narcotic preparations; and (5) alleviating anxiety.

Chronic pain

Chronic pain usually occurs in degenerative and arthritic disorders or in malignant disease and is accompanied by vegetative features such as fatigue and depression. Treatment again involves alleviation of the underlying disorder if possible and general analgesic therapy, but there is an increased need for rehabilitative and psychologically supportive measures.

Complex regional pain syndrome (CRPS)

A number of clinical syndromes appear under this heading, including *Sudeck's atrophy, reflex sympathetic dystrophy, algodystrophy, shoulder–hand syndrome* and – particularly after a nerve injury – *causalgia*. What they have in common is pain out of proportion (in both intensity and duration) to the precipitating cause, vasomotor instability, trophic skin changes, regional osteoporosis and functional impairment.

Precipitating causes are trauma (often trivial), operation or arthroscopy, a peripheral nerve lesion, myocardial infarction, stroke and hemiplegia. The incidence of post-traumatic CRPS is unknown, largely because there are no agreed criteria for diagnosing mild cases. However, the condition is more common than is generally recognized and it has been suggested that as many as 30 per cent of patients with fractures of the extremities develop features of this condition – fortunately short-lived in the majority of cases. Adults are the usual sufferers but the condition occasionally occurs in children.

PATHOGENESIS

The pathophysiology of this condition has been argued over since it was first described a hundred years ago. Since many of the features involve autonomic pathways it was usually regarded as a type of sympathetic 'overactivity' – hence the earlier name 'reflex sympathetic dystrophy' – though this never explained why the abnormal activity was maintained for so long (sometimes indefinitely). It is now recognized that multiple mechanisms are involved: abnormal cytokine release, neurogenic inflammation, sympathetic-mediated enhancement of pain responses and as yet poorly understood cortical reactions to noxious stimuli (Gibbs et al., 2000; Birklein, 2005). For the time being, the purely descriptive term 'complex regional pain syndrome' will have to suffice.

CLINICAL FEATURES

Following some precipitating event, the patient complains of burning pain, and sometimes cold intolerance, in the affected area – usually the hand or foot, sometimes the knee or hip, and sometimes the shoulder in hemiplegia. In the mild or early case there may be no more than slight swelling, with tenderness and stiffness of the nearby joints. More suspicious are local redness and warmth, sometimes changing to cyanosis with a blotchy, cold and sweaty skin. X-rays are at first usually normal but triple-phase radionuclide scanning at this stage shows increased activity.

Later, or in more severe cases, trophic changes become apparent: a smooth shiny skin with scanty hair and atrophic, brittle nails. Swelling and tenderness persist and there may be marked loss of movement. X-rays now show patchy osteoporosis, which may be quite diffuse (Fig. 10.29).

In the most advanced stage, there can be severe joint stiffness and fixed deformities. The acute symptoms may subside after a year or 18 months, but some degree of pain often persists indefinitely.

Causalgia is a severe form of regional pain, usually seen after a nerve injury. Pain is intense, often 'burning' or 'penetrating' and exacerbated by touching, jarring or sometimes even by a loud noise. Symptoms may start distally and progress steadily up the limb to involve an entire quadrant of the body.

TREATMENT

Treatment should be started as early as possible; if the condition is allowed to persist for more than a few weeks it may become irreversible.

Mild cases often respond to a simple regimen of reassurance, anti-inflammatory drugs and physiotherapy. Other conservative measures include the administration of corticosteroids, calcium channel blockers and tricyclic antidepressants.

If there is no improvement after a few weeks, and as a first measure in severe cases, sympathetic blockade often helps. This can be done by one or more local anaesthetic injections to the stellate or the appropriate lumbar sympathetic ganglia, or by regional block with guanethidine given intravenously to the affected limb. However, the effectiveness of these measures is unpredictable and somewhat doubtful.

A small percentage of patients go on complaining of pain and impaired function almost indefinitely. Psychological treatment may help them to deal with the emotional distress and anxiety and to develop better coping strategies.

'Chronic pain syndrome'

In a minority of patients with chronic pain there is an apparent mismatch between the bitterness of complaint and the degree of physical abnormality. The most common example is the patient with discogenic disease and prolonged, unresponsive, disabling low back pain. Labels such as 'functional overlay', 'compensitis', 'supratentorial reaction' and 'illness behaviour' are introduced and both patient and doctor are overtaken by a sense of hopelessness. Sometimes there are well-marked features of depression, or complaints of widespread somatic illness (pain in various parts of the body, muscular weakness, paraesthesiae, palpitations and impotence).

Treatment is always difficult and should, ideally, be managed by a team that includes a specialist in pain control, a psychotherapist, a rehabilitation specialist and a social worker. Pain may be alleviated by a variety of measures: (1) analgesics and anti-inflammatory drugs; (2) local injections to painful areas; (3) local counter-irritants; (4) acupuncture; (5) transcutaneous nerve stimulation; (6) sympathetic block; and, occasionally, (7) surgical interruption of pain pathways. These methods, as well as psychosocial assessment and therapy, are best applied in a dedicated pain clinic.

FIBROMYALGIA

Fibromyalgia is not so much a diagnosis as a descriptive term for a condition in which patients complain of pain and tenderness in the muscles and other soft tissues around the back of the neck and shoulders and across the lower part of the back and the upper parts of the buttocks. What sets the condition apart from other 'rheumatic' diseases is the complete absence of demonstrable pathological changes in the affected tissues. Indeed, it is often difficult to give credence to the patient's complaints, an attitude which is encouraged by the fact that similar symptoms are encountered in some patients who have suffered trivial injuries in a variety of accidents; a significant number also develop psychological depression and anxiety.

The criteria for making the diagnosis were put forward by the American College of Rheumatology in

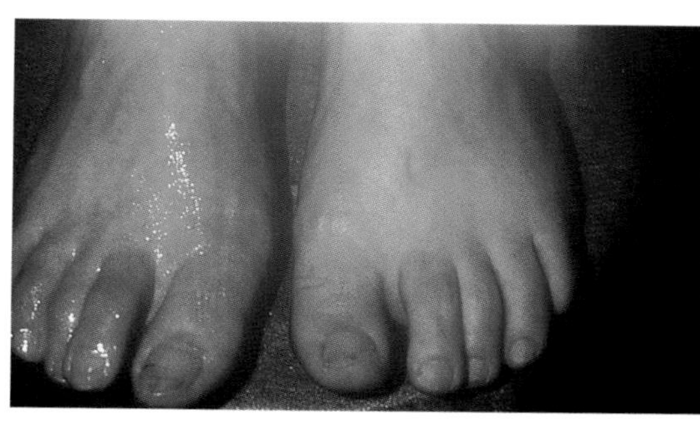

(a)

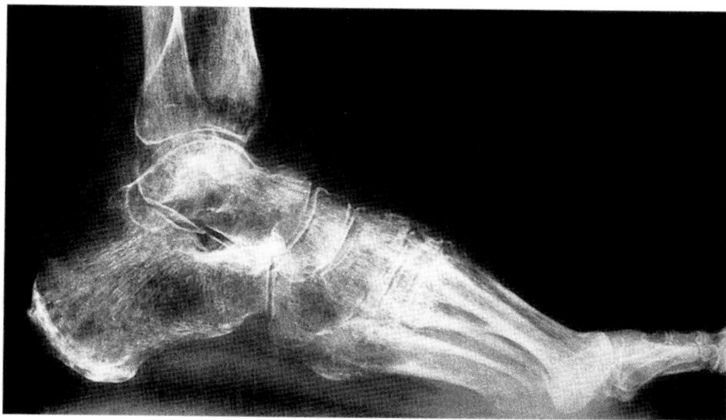

(b)

10.29 Complex regional pain syndrome (a) A 53-year old woman suffered an undisplaced fracture of her right tibia. The fracture healed but her foot became swollen, warm to the touch and tender, the skin reddish-purple and sweaty. (b) X-rays showed an unusual degree of osteoporosis.

1990. These included symptoms of widespread pain in all four quadrants of the body, together with at least 9 pairs of designated 'tender points' on physical examination. In practice, however, the diagnosis is often made in patients with much more localized symptoms and signs, and it is now quite common to attach this label to almost any condition associated with myofascial pain where no specific underlying disorder can be identified.

The cause of fibromyalgia remains unknown; no pathology has been found in the 'tender spots'. It has been suggested that this is an abnormality of 'sensory processing', which is perhaps another way of saying that the sufferers have a 'low pain threshold'; in fact they often do display increased sensitivity to pain in other parts of the body. There are also suggestions that the condition is related to stress responses which can be activated by sudden accidents or traumatic life events. This does not mean that such patients will necessarily show other features of psychological dysfunction and the condition cannot be excluded merely by psychological testing.

In mild cases, treatment can be limited to keeping up muscle tone and general fitness (hence the advice to have physiotherapy and then continue with daily exercises on their own), perhaps together with injections into the painful areas simply to reduce the level of discomfort. Patients with more persistent and more disturbing symptoms may benefit from various types of psychotherapy.

ARTHROGRYPOSIS

'Arthrogryposis' is a broad term used to describe a large group of congenital disorders – all of them rare – in which children are born with multiple non-progressive soft-tissue contractures and restriction of joint movement. In other respects these conditions differ widely in terms of pathological change and clinical appearance. In the most common form – *arthrogryposis multiplex congenita* (nowadays known as *amyoplasia*) – all joints of the upper and lower limbs are involved; at the extremes of the range there are some patients in whom only a few joints are affected (and not very severely at that) and others in whom all joints are severely affected. In the very rare myopathic form of the disease, children may develop spinal deformities.

The incidence is said to be about 1 in 3000 live births; in some cases a genetic linkage has been demonstrated. A more proximate cause may be an intrauterine lack of sufficient room for movement (for whatever reason) during foetal development. Joint capsules are often fibrotic.

The deformities are associated with unbalanced muscle weakness which follows a neurosegmental distribution, and necropsy specimens show sparseness of anterior horn cells in the cervical and lumbar cord. Deformities and contractures develop in utero and remain largely unchanged throughout life. Myopathic and neuropathic features may coexist in the same muscle.

Classification

Considering arthrogryposis as a whole, the conditions can be placed in three major categories:

1. *Those with total body involvement*: typified by the condition formerly known as *arthrogryposis multiplex congenita* and now termed *amyoplasia*, but also including other congenital disorders showing widespread joint contractures. In the rarer myopathic form of the disease, children may develop spinal deformities.
2. *Those with predominantly hand or foot involvement*: conditions with joint features similar to those of amyoplasia but usually limited to distal joints (wrists, hands, feet) and therefore termed *distal arthrogryposis*; included also are more severe types of distal myopathy such as the Freeman–Sheldon syndrome in which there are, in addition, abnormal facial features (the 'whistling face syndrome').

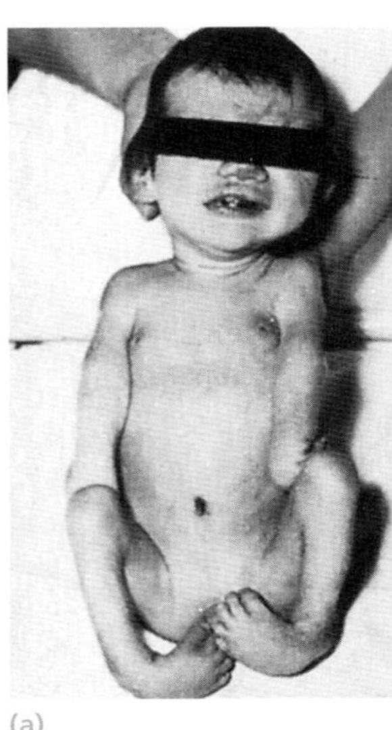

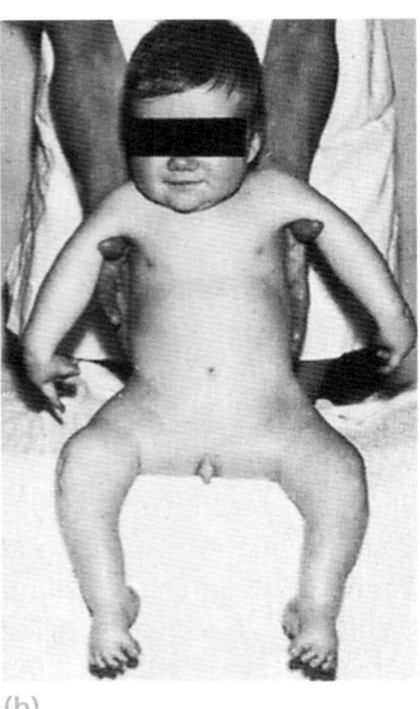

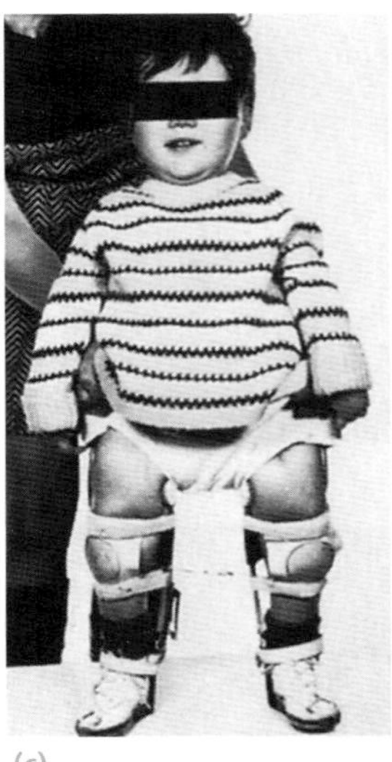

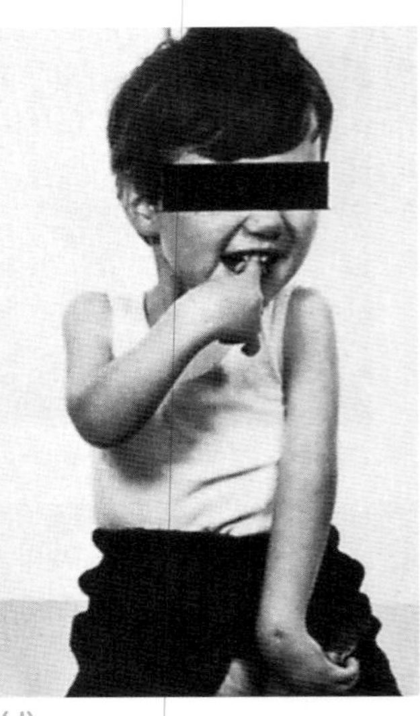

(a) (b) (c) (d)

10.30 Arthrogryposis multiplex congenita (a,b) Severe deformities are present at birth. In this case all four limbs are affected. (c,d) Operative treatment is often worthwhile. In this young boy the lower limbs were tackled first and the feet and knees are held in splints. In the upper limbs, the minimum aim is to enable a hand to reach the mouth.

3. *Pterygia syndromes*: conditions characterized by arthrogrypotic joint contractures with identifiable soft-tissue webs, usually across the flexor aspects of the knees and ankles.

Clinical features

Clinical examination is still the best way of making the diagnosis: involved joints are tubular and featureless and although the normal skin creases are missing there are often deep dimples over the joints. Muscle mass is markedly reduced. In some cases there is true muscle weakness.

In the *classic form of amyoplasia* the shoulders are adducted and internally rotated, the elbows usually extended and the wrists/hands flexed and deviated ulnarwards. In the lower limbs, the hips are flexed and abducted, the limbs externally rotated, the knees usually extended and the feet showing equinovarus or vertical talus deformities. Secondary problems include feeding difficulties due to the stiff jaw and immobile tongue.

Distal arthrogryposis often manifests an autosomal dominant pattern of inheritance. Common hand deformities are ulnar deviation of the metacarpo-phalangeal joints, fixed flexion of the PIP joints and tightly adducted thumbs. Foot deformities are likely to be resistant forms of equinovarus or vertical talus.

Treatment

The condition is unlikely to improve spontaneously and it is essentially incurable. Treatment of the individual joint begins shortly after birth and may follow basic principles with manipulation, stretching and splinting forming the mainstays of initial management. A few cautionary words: check for neonatal fractures before starting treatment, and avoid forceful manoeuvres.

In the pterygia syndromes, physiotherapy can be tried but early release of the popliteal contractures should be considered. Great care is needed to avoid injury to tight neurovascular structures.

In general, if progress is slow, tendon releases, tendon transfers and osteotomies may become necessary. Rigid equinovarus is particularly difficult to treat and operative correction is often necessary. Displacement or dislocation of the hip, likewise, often defies conservative treatment and open reduction is then needed. Unfortunately, recurrences of deformity are common.

Before surgical intervention is considered, it should be noted that children often cope surprisingly well with their deformities and a holistic approach to the child is essential in order to ensure that the interaction of all the involved joints is understood; changing the position of one joint can have a significant adverse effect on overall function. If both elbows are rigidly extended, function may be improved by leaving one elbow in extension and the other in partial flexion.

MUSCULAR DYSTROPHIES

The muscular dystrophies are a group of about 30 rare inherited disorders characterized by progressive muscle weakness and wasting. Pathological changes include malformation of muscle fibres, death of muscle cells and replacement of muscle by fibrous tissue and fat. They have been grouped according to their various inheritance patterns, age of onset, distribution of affected musculature and severity of the muscle weakness. Those most likely to be encountered in orthopaedic practice are:

- *Duchenne's muscular dystrophy* – a severe, generalized sex-linked disorder affecting only boys in early childhood. Becker's muscular dystrophy is similar but less severe, starts somewhat later and progresses more slowly.
- *Limb girdle dystrophies* – a mixed group, usually of autosomal recessive inheritance, with more localized changes, affecting boys and girls in later childhood.
- *Facioscapulohumeral dystrophy* – an autosomal dominant condition of variable severity, usually appearing in early adulthood.

Duchenne muscular dystrophy

This is a progressive disease of sex-linked inheritance with recessive transmission. It is therefore seen only in boys (or in girls with sex chromosome disorders), affecting 1 in 3500 male births. Some women are 'manifesting carriers' who have slight muscle weakness and cramps.

A defect at locus p21 on the X chromosome results in failure to code for the dystrophin gene, which is essential for maintaining the integrity of cardiac and skeletal muscle cells. Absence of functional dystrophin leads to cell membrane leakage, muscle fibre damage and replacement by fat and fibrous tissue.

Clinical features

The condition is usually unsuspected until the child starts to walk. He has difficulty standing and climbing stairs, he cannot run properly and he falls frequently. Weakness begins in the proximal muscles of the lower limbs and progresses distally, affecting particularly the glutei, the quadriceps and the tibialis anterior, giving rise to a wide-based stance and gait with the feet in equinus, the pelvis tilted forwards, the back arched in lordosis and the neck extended. The calf muscles look bulky, but much of this is due to fat and the pseudohypertrophy belies the obvious weakness. A characteristic feature is the child's method of rising from the floor by climbing up his own legs (Gowers' sign); this is due to weakness of the gluteus maximus and thigh muscles.

Shoulder girdle weakness follows around 5 years after the clinical onset of the disease, making it difficult for the patient to use crutches. Facial muscle involvement follows later. By the age of 10 years the child has usually lost the ability to walk and becomes dependent on a wheelchair; from then on there is rapid deterioration in spinal posture with the development of scoliosis and, subsequently, further deterioration in lung function. Cardiopulmonary failure is the usual cause of death, generally before the age of 30 years.

Investigations

The diagnosis is usually based on the clinical features and family history and by testing for serum creatinine phosphokinase levels which are 200–300 times the normal in the early stages of the disease (and also elevated, but less so, in female carriers). Confirmation is achieved by muscle biopsy and genetic testing with a DNA polymerase chain reaction.

Treatment

While the child can still walk, physiotherapy and splintage or tendon operations may help to prevent or correct joint deformities and so prolong the period of mobility.

Corticosteroids are useful in preserving muscle strength but there are significant side effects such as osteoporosis, increased risk of fractures and cataract formation.

Research studies in which dystrophin in the form of myoblasts is introduced into diseased muscle have been successful in animal models but not so far in humans. Gene therapy has also been tried but there have been difficulties with the viral vectors and associated immunological responses.

If scoliosis is marked (more than 30 degrees), instrumentation and spinal fusion helps to maintain pulmonary function and improves quality of life although not necessarily lifespan. Preoperative cardiac and pulmonary function evaluation should be performed.

Family counselling is important. Up to 20 per cent of families already have a younger affected sibling by the time the proband is diagnosed.

Becker muscular dystrophy

This condition, also an X-linked recessive disease, is similar to but milder than Duchenne's dystrophy. Dystrophin is decreased and/or abnormal in character. Affected boys retain the ability to walk into their teens and patients may survive until middle age. The muscles of facial expression are not affected and neither are the muscles controlling bowel or bladder function or swallowing.

Limb girdle dystrophy

This form of muscular dystrophy, characterized by weakness of the pelvic and shoulder girdle muscles, represents a heterogeneous group of conditions, most of which show an autosomal recessive inheritance pattern affecting both sexes.

Symptoms usually start in late adolescence. Pelvic girdle weakness causes a waddling gait and difficulty in rising from a low chair; pectoral girdle weakness makes it difficult to raise the arms above the head. However, the muscles of facial expression are spared. Disease progression is usually slow. (NB: These features can be mistaken for those of a mild form of spinal muscular atrophy.)

Treatment consists of physiotherapy and splintage to prevent contractures, and operative correction when necessary. Because the deltoid muscles are spared, shoulder movements can sometimes be improved by fixing the scapula to the ribs posteriorly, so improving deltoid leverage.

Facioscapulohumeral dystrophy

This is an autosomal dominant condition with very variable expression. In general, males are more severely affected than females and from a younger age. Characteristically, muscle weakness is first seen in the face (inability to purse the lips or close the eyes tightly). This is followed by weakness of scapular muscles causing winging of the scapula and difficulty with shoulder abduction. There may also be weakness of the anterior tibial muscles.

The condition is due to gene deletion on the long arm of chromosome 4; genetic testing to confirm the diagnosis is highly sensitive and specific.

MYOTONIA

Myotonia – persistent muscle contraction after cessation of voluntary effort – is a prominent feature in certain genetic disorders. The two least rare of these conditions are considered here: *dystrophia myotonica*, in which myotonia is part of a more widespread systemic disorder, and *myotonia congenita*, in which myotonia is usually the only abnormal clinical feature.

Dystrophia myotonica

Myotonic dystrophy is an autosomal dominant disorder with an incidence of about 1 in 7000. Patients usually present in adult life with distal muscle weakness and wasting. The defining feature, what the patient perceives as 'muscle stiffness', may have been present for some years; myotonia is most easily demonstrated by asking the patient to flex and extend the fingers rapidly. Some patients are only mildly affected while others develop more widespread muscle weakness; the face and tongue may be involved, causing ptosis and difficulty with chewing. EMG changes may be diagnostic. Enquiry will almost always reveal that a relative has been affected as well.

With time, systemic features appear – diabetes, cataracts and cardiorespiratory problems – and by middle age patients are often severely disabled.

Treatment is essentially palliative but foot deformities may need manipulation and splintage. Affected women who are planning to become pregnant should be warned that there is a risk of them giving birth to a floppy baby with feeding difficulties.

Myotonia congenita

The usual form of congenital myotonia is inherited by autosomal recessive transmission. Symptoms due to 'muscle stiffness' appear in childhood and usually progress slowly. Common complaints are that walking and climbing stairs are difficult; typically this is worse after periods of inactivity and is relieved by exercise. Symptoms tend also to be triggered by exposure to cold and can cause pain ('muscle cramps'). By adulthood there may be muscle weakness, though the forearms and calves are unusually bulky. There is no specific treatment for this condition. Patients are advised about avoiding aggravating activities.

In a more rare subgroup, showing autosomal dominant inheritance, symptoms appear in infancy or early childhood but do not progress and are usually mild enough not to need treatment. Other very rare subgroups have also been identified and their diagnosis can be difficult. The best advice is that children with 'atypical' features of congenital myotonia should be referred to a centre specializing in muscle disorders.

REFERENCES AND FURTHER READING

Banta JV, Lubicky JP. Orthopaedic aspects of myelomeningocele: spinal deformities. *J Bone Joint Surg* 1990; **72A:** 628–9.

Beals RK. Spastic paraplegia and diplegia: an evaluation of non-surgical and surgical factors influencing the prognosis for ambulation. *J Bone Joint Surg* 1966; **48A:** 827–46.

Beaty, JH, Canale JT. Orthopaedic aspects of myelomeningocele. Current concepts review. *J Bone Joint Surg* 1990; **72A:** 626–30.

Birklein F. Complex regional pain syndrome. *Neurology* 2005; **252:** 131–8.

Bleck EE. Locomotor prognosis in cerebral palsy. *Dev Med Child Neurol*, 1975; **17:** 18–25.

Bleck EE. *Orthopaedic Management in Cerebral Palsy.* Blackwell Scientific, Oxford; Lippincott, Philadelphia, 1987.

Gibbs GF, Drummond PD, Finch PM *et al.* Unravelling the pathophysiology of complex regional pain syndrome: focus on sympathetically maintained pain. *Clin Exp Pharmacol Physiol* 2000; **35:** 717–24.

Hoffer MM. Management of the hip in cerebral palsy. *J Bone Joint Surg* 1986; **68A:** 629–31.

Hong-Xue Men, Chan-Hua Bian, Chan-Dou Yang, *et al.* Surgical treatment of the flail knee after poliomyelitis. *J Bone Joint Surg* 1991; **73B:** 195–9.

Karol LA. Surgical management of the lower extremity in ambulatory children with CP. *J Am Acad Orthop Surg* 2004; **12:** 196–203.

Lau JHK, Parker JC, Hsu LCS, *et al.* Paralytic hip instability in poliomyelitis. *J Bone Joint Surg* 1986; **68B:** 528–33.

Louis DS, Hensinger RM, Fraser BA, *et al.* Surgical management of the severely multiply handicapped individual. *J Pediatr Orthop* 1989; **9:** 15–18.

Ma FY, Selber P, Nattrass GR, *et al.* Lengthening and transfer of the hamstrings for flexion a deformity of the knee in children with bilateral cerebral palsy: Technique and preliminary results. *J Bone Joint Surg* 2006; **88B:** 248–54.

Melzack R, Wall PD. Pain mechanisms: a new theory. *Science* 1965; **150:** 971–9

Mazur JM, Shurtleff D, Merelaus M, *et al.* Orthopaedic management of high level spina bifida. *J Bone Joint Surg* 1989; **71A:** 56–61.

McCarthy JJ, D'Andrea LP, Betz RR, Clements DH. Scoliosis in the child with cerebral palsy. *J Am Acad Orthop Surg* 2006; **14:** 367–75.

Palisano RJ, Rosenbaum P, Bartlett D, Livingston MH. Gross Motor Function Classification System. *Dev Med Child Neurol* 2008; **50(10):** 744 –50.

Ponseti IV, Smoley EN. Congenital club foot: The results of treatment. *J Bone Joint Surg* 1963; **45A:** 261–75.

Rang M, Wright J. What have 30 years of medical progress done for cerebral palsy? *Clin Orthop Relat Res* 1989; **247:** 55–60.

Roper BA, Tibrewal SB. Soft tissue surgery in Charcot-Marie-Tooth disease. *J Bone Joint Surg* 1989; **71B:** 17–20.

Scrutton D. The early management of hips in cerebral palsy. *Dev Med Child Neurol* 1989; **31:** 108–16.

Sutherland DH, Davids JR. Common gait abnormalities of the knee in cerebral palsy. *Clin Orthop Rel Res* 1993; **288:** 139–47.

Sutherland DH, Ohlson R, Cooper L, Woo SK. The development of mature gait. *J Bone Joint Surg* 1980; **62A:** 336–53.

Trail IA, Galasko CSB. The matrix seating system. *J Bone Joint Surg* 1990; **73B:** 666–9.

Peripheral nerve disorders

11

David Warwick, H. Srinivasan, Louis Solomon

NERVE STRUCTURE AND FUNCTION

Peripheral nerves are bundles of *axons* conducting efferent (motor) impulses from cells in the anterior horn of the spinal cord to the muscles, and afferent (sensory) impulses from peripheral receptors via cells in the posterior root ganglia to the cord. They also convey sudomotor and vasomotor fibres from ganglion cells in the sympathetic chain. Some nerves are predominantly motor, some predominantly sensory; the larger trunks are mixed, with motor and sensory axons running in separate bundles.

Each axon is, in reality, an extension or elongated process of a nerve cell, or *neuron* (see Chapter 10). The cell bodies of the motor neurons supplying the peripheral muscles are clustered in the anterior horn of the spinal cord; a single motor neuron with its axon may, therefore, be more than a metre long. The cell bodies of the sensory neurons serving the trunk and

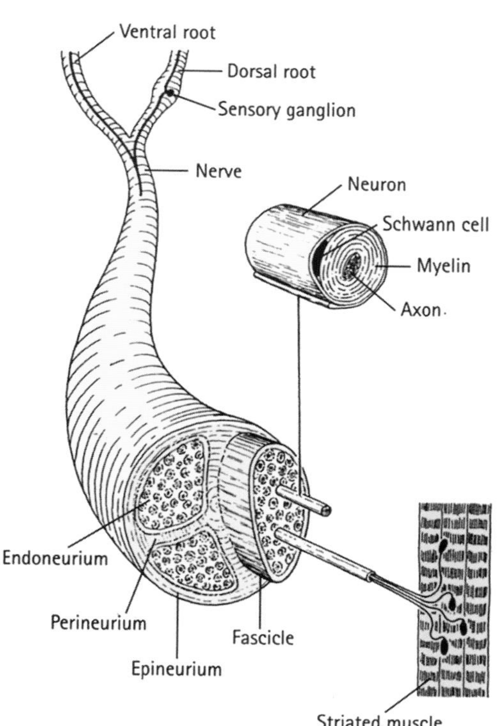

(a)

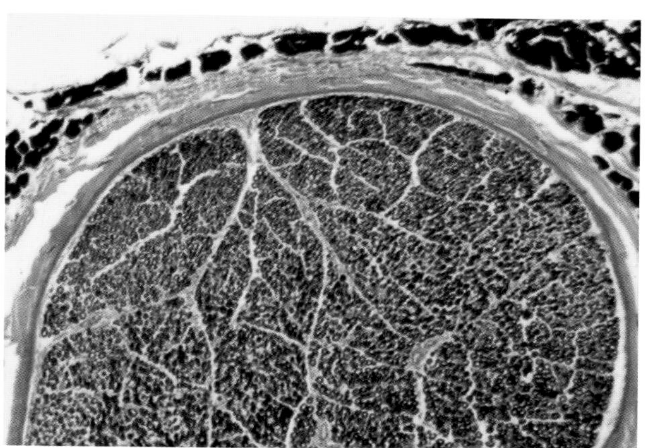

(b)

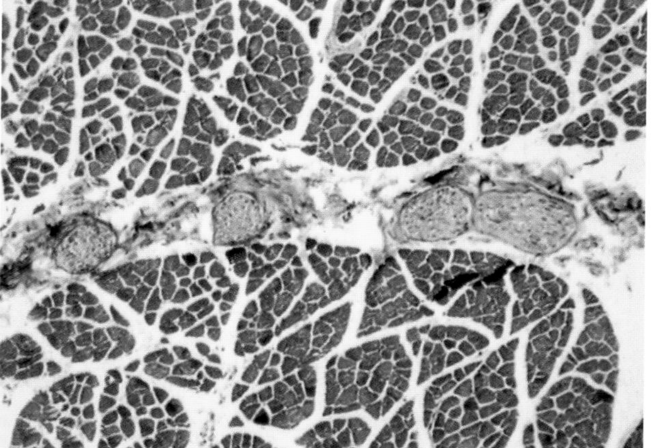

(c)

11.1 Nerve structure (a) Diagram of the structural elements of a peripheral nerve. (b) Histological section through a large nerve. (c) High-power view of the same, showing blood vessels in the perineurium.

limbs are situated in the dorsal root ganglia and each neuron has one process (axon) extending from the periphery to the cell body and another from the cell body up the spinal cord.

The peripheral ends of all the neurons are branched. A single motor neuron may supply anything from 10 to several thousand muscle fibres, the ratio depending on the degree of dexterity demanded of the particular muscle (the smaller the ratio, the finer the movement). Similarly, the peripheral branches of each sensory neuron may serve anything from a single muscle spindle to a comparatively large patch of skin; here again, the fewer the end receptors served the greater the degree of discrimination.

The signal, or action potential, carried by motor neurons is transmitted to the muscle fibres by the release of a chemical transmitter, acetylcholine, at the terminal bouton of the nerve. Sensory signals are similarly conveyed to the dorsal root ganglia and from there up the ipsilateral column of the spinal cord, through the brain-stem and thalamus, to the opposite (sensory) cortex. Proprioceptive impulses from the muscle spindles and joints bypass this route and are carried to the anterior horn cells as part of a local reflex arc. The economy of this system ensures that 'survival' mechanisms like balance and sense of position in space are activated with great speed.

In the peripheral nerves, all motor axons and the large sensory axons serving touch, pain and proprioception are coated with *myelin*, a multilayered lipoprotein membrane derived from the accompanying *Schwann cells*. Every few millimetres the myelin sheath is interrupted, leaving short segments of bare axon called the *nodes of Ranvier*. Nerve impulses leap from node to node at the speed of electricity, much faster than would be the case if these axons were not insulated by the myelin sheaths. Consequently, depletion of the myelin sheath causes slowing – and eventually complete blocking – of axonal conduction.

Most axons – in particular the small-diameter fibres carrying crude sensation and the efferent sympathetic fibres – are unmyelinated but wrapped in Schwann cell cytoplasm. Damage to these axons causes unpleasant or bizarre sensations and various sudomotor and vasomotor effects.

Outside the Schwann cell membrane the axon is covered by a connective tissue stocking, the *endoneurium*. The axons that make up a nerve are separated into bundles (fascicles) by fairly dense membranous tissue, the *perineurium*. In a transected nerve, these fascicles are seen pouting from the cut surface, their perineurial sheaths well defined and strong enough to be grasped by fine instruments during operations for nerve repair. The groups of fascicles that make up a nerve trunk are enclosed in an even thicker connective tissue coat, the *epineurium*. The epineurium varies in thickness and is particularly strong where the nerve is subjected to movement and traction, for example near a joint.

The nerve is richly supplied by *blood vessels* that run longitudinally in the epineurium before penetrating the various layers to become the *endoneurial capillaries*. These fine vessels may be damaged by stretching or rough handling of the nerve; however, they can withstand extensive mobilization of the nerve, making it feasible to repair or replace damaged segments by operative transposition or neurotization. The tiny blood vessels have their own *sympathetic nerve supply* coming from the parent nerve, and stimulation of these fibres (causing intraneural vasoconstriction) may be important in conditions such as reflex sympathetic dystrophy and other unusual pain syndromes.

PATHOLOGY

Nerves can be injured by ischaemia, compression, traction, laceration or burning. Damage varies in severity from transient and quickly recoverable loss of function to complete interruption and degeneration. There may be a mixture of types of damage in the various fascicles of a single nerve trunk.

Transient ischaemia

Acute nerve compression causes numbness and tingling within 15 minutes, loss of pain sensibility after 30 minutes and muscle weakness after 45 minutes. Relief of compression is followed by intense paraesthesiae lasting up to 5 minutes (the familiar 'pins and needles' after a limb 'goes to sleep'); feeling is restored within 30 seconds and full muscle power after about 10 minutes. These changes are due to transient endoneurial anoxia and they leave no trace of nerve damage.

Neurapraxia

Seddon (1942) coined the term 'neurapraxia' to describe a reversible physiological nerve conduction block in which there is loss of some types of sensation and muscle power followed by spontaneous recovery after a few days or weeks. It is due to mechanical pressure causing segmental demyelination and is seen typically in 'crutch palsy', pressure paralysis in states of drunkenness (*'Saturday night palsy'*) and the milder types of tourniquet palsy.

Axonotmesis

This is a more severe form of nerve injury, seen typically after closed fractures and dislocations. The term means, literally, axonal interruption. There is loss of conduction but the nerve is in continuity and the neural tubes are intact. Distal to the lesion, and for a few millimetres

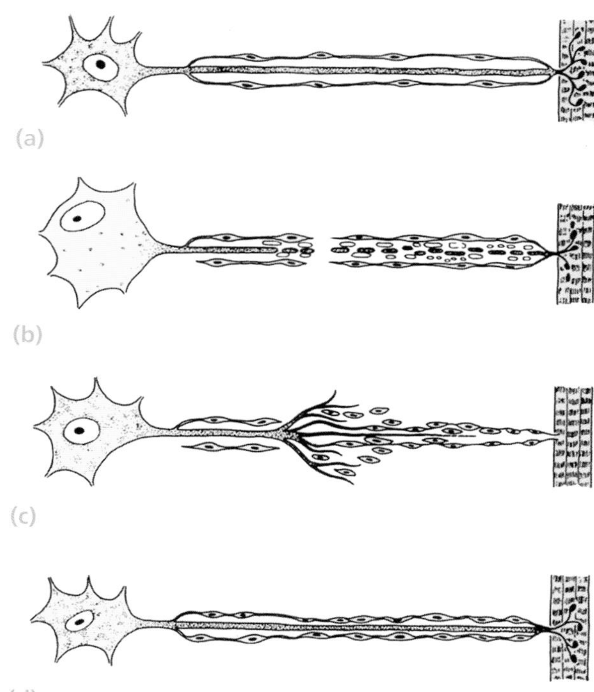

11.2 Nerve injury and repair (a) Normal axon and target organ (striated muscle). (b) Following nerve injury the distal part of the axon disintegrates and the myelin sheath breaks up. The nerve cell nucleus becomes eccentric and Nissl bodies are sparse. (c) New axonal tendrils grow into the mass of proliferating Schwann cells. One of the tendrils will find its way into the old endoneurial tube and (d) the axon will slowly regenerate.

retrograde, axons disintegrate and are resorbed by phagocytes. This *wallerian degeneration* (named after the physiologist, Augustus Waller, who described the process in 1851) takes only a few days and is accompanied by marked proliferation of Schwann cells and fibroblasts lining the endoneurial tubes. The denervated target organs (motor end-plates and sensory receptors) gradually atrophy, and if they are not re-innervated within 2 years they will never recover.

Axonal *regeneration* starts within hours of nerve damage, probably encouraged by neurotropic factors produced by Schwann cells distal to the injury. From the proximal stumps grow numerous fine unmyelinated tendrils, many of which find their way into the cell-clogged endoneurial tubes. These axonal processes grow at a speed of 1–2 mm per day, the larger fibres slowly acquiring a new myelin coat. Eventually they join to end-organs, which enlarge and start functioning again.

Neurotmesis

In Seddon's original classification, neurotmesis meant division of the nerve trunk, such as may occur in an open wound. It is now recognized that severe degrees of damage may be inflicted without actually dividing the nerve. If the injury is more severe, whether the nerve is in continuity or not, recovery will not occur. As in axonotmesis, there is rapid wallerian degeneration, but here the endoneurial tubes are destroyed over a variable segment and scarring thwarts any hope of regenerating axons entering the distal segment and regaining their target organs. Instead, regenerating fibres mingle with proliferating Schwann cells and fibroblasts in a jumbled knot, or 'neuroma', at the site of injury. Even after surgical repair, many new axons fail to reach the distal segment, and those that do may not find suitable Schwann tubes, or may not reach the correct end-organs in time, or may remain incompletely myelinated. Function may be adequate but is never normal.

The 'double crush' phenomenon

There is convincing evidence that proximal compression of a peripheral nerve renders it more susceptible to the effects of a second, more peripheral injury. This may explain why peripheral entrapment syndromes are often associated with cervical or lumbar spondylosis. A similar type of 'sensitization' is seen in patients with peripheral neuropathy due to diabetes or alcoholism.

CLASSIFICATION OF NERVE INJURIES

Seddon's description of the three different types of nerve injury (neurapraxia, axonotmesis and neurotmesis) served as a useful classification for many years. Increasingly, however, it has been recognized that many cases fall into an area somewhere between axonotmesis and neurotmesis. Therefore, following Sunderland (1978), a more practical classification is offered here.

First degree injury This embraces transient ischaemia and neurapraxia, the effects of which are reversible.

Second degree injury This corresponds to Seddon's axonotmesis. Axonal degeneration takes place but, because the endoneurium is preserved, regeneration can lead to complete, or near complete, recovery without the need for intervention.

Third degree injury This is worse than axonotmesis. The endoneurium is disrupted but the perineurial sheaths are intact and internal damage is limited. The chances of the axons reaching their targets are good, but fibrosis and crossed connections will limit recovery.

Fourth degree injury Only the epineurium is intact. The nerve trunk is still in continuity but internal damage is

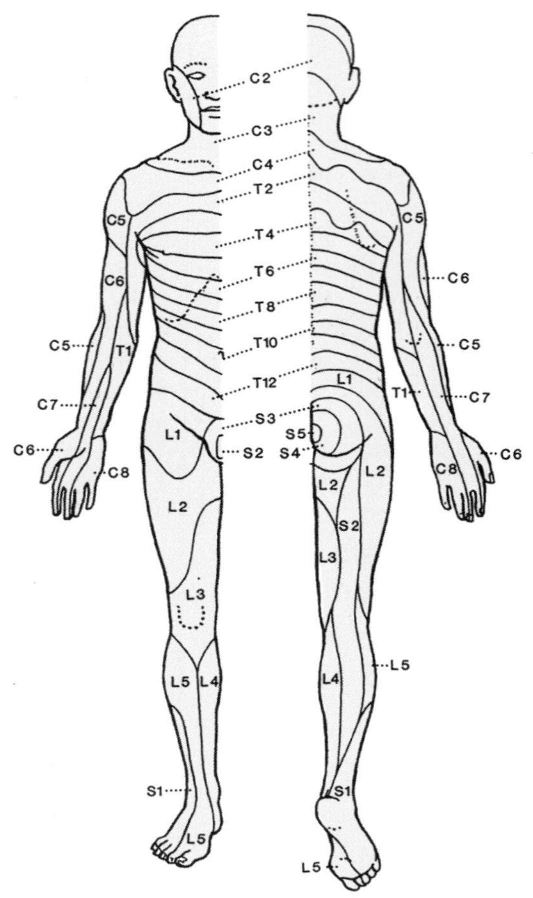

11.3 Examination Dermatomes supplied by spinal nerve roots. The sensory distribution of peripheral nerves is illustrated in the relevant sections.

severe. Recovery is unlikely; the injured segment should be excised and the nerve repaired or grafted.

Fifth degree injury The nerve is divided and will have to be repaired.

CLINICAL FEATURES

Acute nerve injuries are easily missed, especially if associated with fractures or dislocations, the symptoms of which may overshadow those of the nerve lesion. *Always test for nerve injuries following any significant trauma.* If a nerve injury is present, it is crucial also to look for an accompanying vascular injury.

Ask the patient if there is numbness, paraesthesia or muscle weakness in the related area. Then examine the injured limb systematically for signs of abnormal posture (e.g. a wrist drop in radial nerve palsy), weakness in specific muscle groups and changes in sensibility.

Areas of altered sensation should be accurately mapped. Each spinal nerve root serves a specific dermatome (see Fig. 11.3) and peripheral nerves have more or less discrete sensory territories which are illustrated in the relevant sections of this chapter. Despite the fact that there is considerable overlap in sensory boundaries, the area of altered sensibility is usually sufficiently characteristic to provide an anatomical diagnosis. Sudomotor changes may be found in the same topographic areas; the skin feels dry due to lack of sweating. If this is not obvious, the

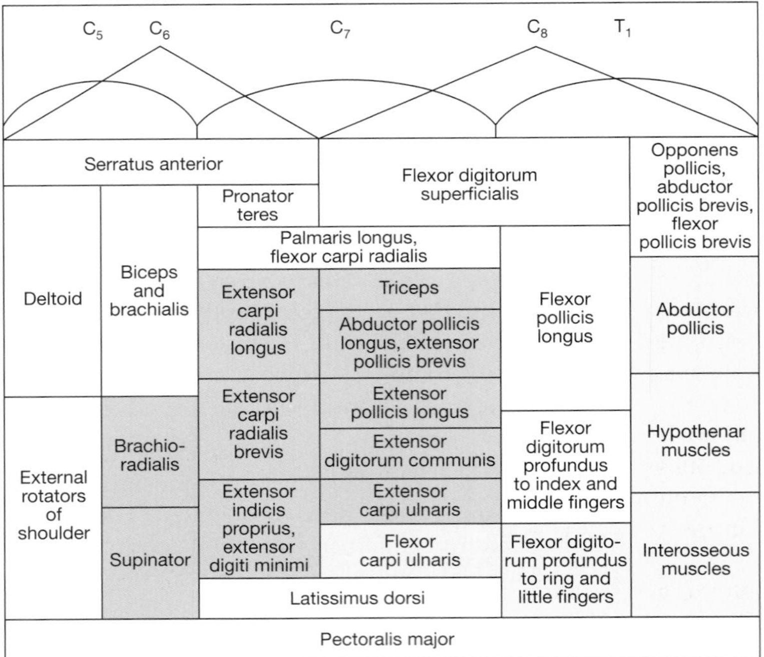

11.4 Examination Type of form used for recording muscle power in new and recovering nerve lesions (after Merle d'Aubigné). Power is recorded in individual blocks on the MRC Scale 1–5.

'plastic pen test' may help. The smooth barrel of the pen is brushed across the palmar skin: normally there is a sense of slight stickiness, due to the thin layer of surface sweat, but in denervated skin the pen slips along smoothly with no sense of stickiness in the affected area.

The neurological examination must be repeated at intervals so as not to miss signs which appear hours after the original injury, or following manipulation or operation.

In chronic nerve injuries there are other characteristic signs. The anaesthetic skin may be smooth and shiny, with evidence of diminished sensibility such as cigarette burns of the thumb in median nerve palsy or foot ulcers with sciatic nerve palsy. Muscle groups will be wasted and postural deformities may become fixed. Beware of trick movements which give the appearance of motor activity where none exists.

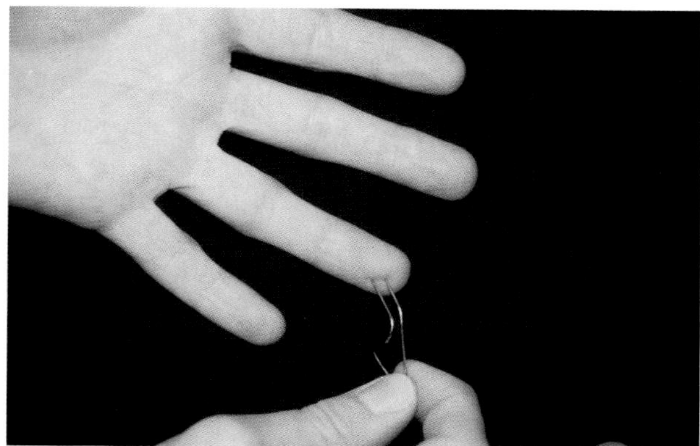

11.5 Two-point discrimination

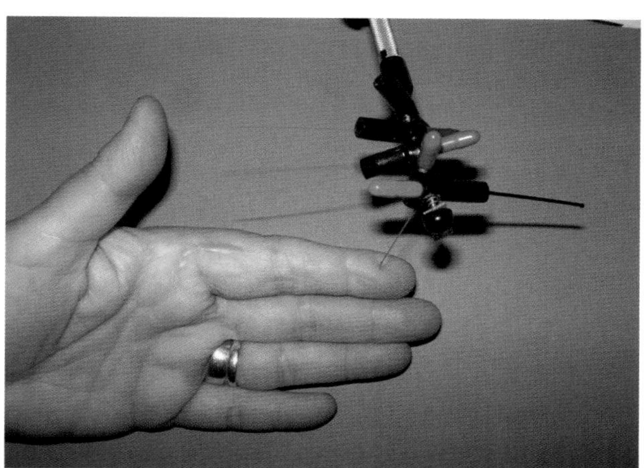

11.6 Monofilament assessment

Assessment of nerve recovery

The presence or absence of distal nerve function can be revealed by simple clinical tests of muscle power and sensitivity to light touch and pin-prick. Remember that after nerve injury motor recovery is slower than sensory recovery. More specific assessment is required to answer two questions: How severe was the lesion? How well is the nerve functioning now?

THE DEGREE OF INJURY

The history is most helpful. A low energy injury is likely to have caused a neurapraxia; the patient should be observed and recovery anticipated. A high energy injury is more likely to have caused axonal and endoneurial disruption (Sunderland third and fourth degree) and so recovery is less predictable. An open injury, or a very high energy closed injury, will probably have divided the nerve and early exploration is called for.

Tinel's sign – peripheral tingling or dysaesthesia provoked by percussing the nerve – is important. In a neurapraxia, Tinel's sign is negative. In axonotmesis, it is positive at the site of injury because of sensitivity of the regenerating axon sprouts. After a delay of a few days or weeks, the Tinel sign will then advance at a rate of about 1 mm each day as the regenerating axons progress along the Schwann-cell tube. *Motor activity* also should progress down the limb. Failure of Tinel's sign to advance suggests a fourth or fifth degree injury and the need for early exploration. If the Tinel sign proceeds very slowly, or if muscle groups do not sequentially recover as expected, then a good recovery is unlikely and here again exploration must be considered.

Electromyography (EMG) studies can be helpful. If a muscle loses its nerve supply, the EMG will show denervation potentials by the third week. This excludes neurapraxia but of course it does not distinguish between axonotmesis and neurotmesis; this remains a clinical distinction, but if one waits too long to decide then the target muscle may have failed irrecoverably and the answer hardly matters.

ASSESSMENT OF NERVE FUNCTION

Two-point discrimination is a measure of innervation density. After nerve regeneration or repair, a proportion of proximal sensory axons will fail to reach their appropriate sensory end-organ; they will either have regenerated down the wrong Schwann-cell tube or will be entangled in a neuroma at the site of injury.

Therefore, two-point discrimination (measured with a bent paper clip and compared with the opposite normal side) gives an indication of how completely the nerve has recovered. Static two-point discrimination measures slowly adapting sensors (Merkel cells) and moving two-point discrimination measures rapidly adapting sensors (Meissner corpuscles and pacinian corpuscles). Moving two-point discrimination is more sensitive and returns earlier. Normal static two-point discrimination is about 6 mm and moving is about 3 mm.

Threshold tests measure the threshold at which a sensory receptor is activated. They are more useful in nerve-compression syndromes, where individual receptors fail to send impulses centrally; two-point discrimination is preserved because the innervation density is not affected. Fine nylon monofilaments of varying widths are placed perpendicularly on the skin and the size of the lightest perceptible filament is recorded.

Locognosia is the ability to localize touch and can be tested with a standardized hand map.

The Moberg pick-up test measures tactile gnosis. The patient is blindfolded and instructed to pick up and identify nine objects as rapidly as possible.

Motor power is graded on the Medical Research Council scale as:

0 No contraction.
1 A flicker of activity.
2 Muscle contraction but unable to overcome gravity.
3 Contraction able to overcome gravity.
4 Contraction against resistance.
5 Normal power.

Principles of treatment

Nerve exploration

Closed low energy injuries usually recover spontaneously and it is worth waiting until the most proximally supplied muscle should have regained function. Exploration is indicated: (1) if the nerve was seen to be divided and needs to be repaired; (2) if the type of injury (e.g. a knife wound or a high energy injury) suggests that the nerve has been divided or severely damaged; (3) if recovery is inappropriately delayed and the diagnosis is in doubt.

Vascular injuries, unstable fractures, contaminated soft tissues and tendon divisions should be dealt with before the nerve lesion. The incision will be long, as the nerve must be widely exposed above and below the lesion before the lesion itself is repaired. The nerve must be handled gently with suitable instruments. Bipolar diathermy and magnification are essential. An operating microscope is ideal but magnifying loupes are better than nothing. A nerve stimulator is essential if scarring makes recognition uncertain. If microsurgical equipment and expertise are not available, then the nerve lesion should be identified and the wound closed pending transferral to an appropriate facility.

Primary repair

A divided nerve is best repaired as soon as this can be done safely. Primary suture at the time of wound toilet has considerable advantages: the nerve ends have not retracted much; their relative rotation is usually undisturbed; and there is no fibrosis.

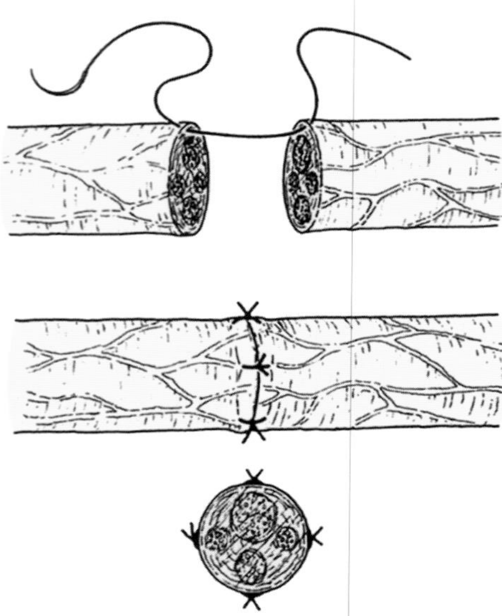

11.7 Nerve repair The stumps are correctly orientated and attached by fine sutures through the epineurium.

A clean cut nerve is sutured without further preparation; a ragged cut may need paring of the stumps with a sharp blade, but this must be kept to a minimum. The stumps are anatomically orientated and fine (10/0) sutures are inserted in the epineurium. There should be no tension on the suture line. Opinions are divided on the value of fascicular repair with perineurial sutures.

Sufficient relaxation of the tissues to permit tension-free repair can usually be obtained by positioning the nearby joints or by mobilizing and re-routing the nerve. If this does not solve the problem then a primary nerve graft must be considered. A traction lesion – especially of the brachial plexus – may leave a gap too wide to close. These injuries are best dealt with in specialized centres, where primary grafting or nerve transfer can be carried out.

If a tourniquet is used it should be a pneumatic one; it must be released and bleeding stopped before the wound is closed.

The limb is splinted in a position to ensure minimal tension on the nerve; if flexion needs to be excessive, a graft is required. The splint is retained for 3 weeks and thereafter physiotherapy is encouraged.

Delayed repair

Late repair, i.e. weeks or months after the injury, may be indicated because: (1) a closed injury was left alone but shows no sign of recovery at the expected time; (2) the diagnosis was missed and the patient presents late; or (3) primary repair has failed. The options must be carefully weighed: if the patient has adapted to the functional loss, if it is a high lesion and re-innervation is unlikely within the critical 2-year period, or if there is a pure motor loss which can be treated by tendon transfers, it may be best to leave well alone. Excessive scarring and intractable joint stiffness may, likewise, make nerve repair questionable; yet in the hand it is still worthwhile simply to regain protective sensation.

The lesion is exposed, working from normal tissue above and below towards the scarred area. When the nerve is in continuity it is difficult to know whether resection is necessary or not. If the nerve is only slightly thickened and feels soft, or if there is conduction across the lesion, resection is not advised; if the 'neuroma' is hard and there is no conduction on nerve stimulation, it should be resected, paring back the stumps until healthy fascicles are exposed.

How to deal with the gap? The nerve must be sutured without tension. The stumps may be brought together by gently mobilizing the proximal and distal segments, by flexing nearby joints to relax the soft tissues, or (in the case of the ulnar nerve) by transposing the nerve trunk to the flexor aspect of the elbow. In this way, gaps of 2 cm in the median nerve, 4–5 cm in the ulnar nerve and 6–8 cm in the sciatic nerve can usually be closed, the limb being splinted in the 'relaxing' position for 4–6 weeks after the operation. Elsewhere, gaps of more than 1–2 cm usually require grafting.

Nerve guides

It is now apparent that nerve gaps can regenerate through a tube which excludes the surrounding tissue from each end. The tubes can be autogenous vein, freeze-dried muscle, silicone or metal; soluble guides (flexible at body temperature) which dissolve over weeks or months are also used. This technology offers a simple way of avoiding a nerve graft yet achieving results which are at least as good in both digital nerves and probably in main trunks.

Nerve grafting

Free autogenous nerve grafts can be used to bridge gaps too large for direct suture. The sural nerve is most commonly used; up to 40 cm can be obtained from each leg. Because the nerve diameter is small, several strips may be used (cable graft). The graft should be long enough to lie without any tension, and it should be routed through a well-vascularized bed. The graft is attached at each end either by fine sutures or with fibrin glue.

It is crucial that the motor and sensory fascicles are appropriately connected by the graft. There are various techniques which can help. Careful inspection of the fascicular alignment, structure and vascular markings is often helpful. Enzyme-staining techniques can be used.

Vascularized grafts are used in special situations. If the ulnar and median nerves are both damaged (e.g. in Volkmann's ischaemia) a pedicle graft from the ulnar nerve may be used to bridge the gap in the median. It is also possible to use free vascularized grafts for certain brachial plexus lesions.

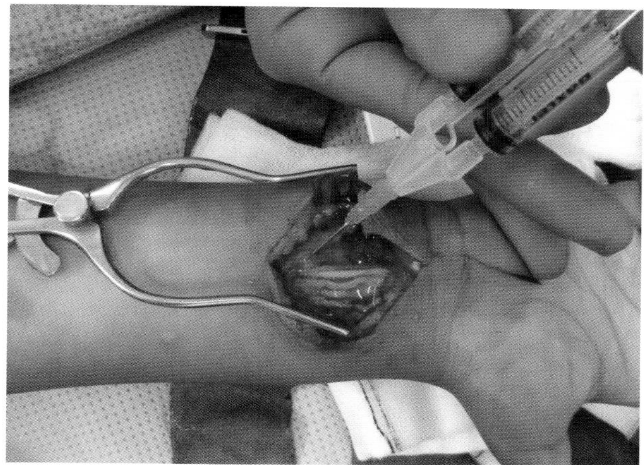

11.8 Nerve graft using fibrin polymer glue

Nerve transfer

In root avulsions of the upper brachial plexus, too proximal for direct repair, nerve transfer can be used. The spinal accessory nerve can be transferred to the suprascapular nerve, and intercostal nerves can be transferred to the musculocutaneous nerve. If biceps has failed because too much time has passed since the injury, an entire muscle (gracilis or latissimus dorsi) can be transferred as a free flap, attached between elbow and shoulder and then innervated by joining

PRINCIPLES OF TENDON TRANSFER

Assess the problem
- Which muscles are missing?
- Which muscles are available?

The donor muscle should be:
- expendable
- powerful enough
- an agonist or synergist

The recipient site should:
- be stable
- have mobile joints and supple tissues

The transferred tendon should be:
- routed subcutaneously
- placed in a straight line of pull
- capable of firm fixation

The patient should be:
- motivated
- able to comprehend and attend hand therapy

intercostal nerves or the spinal accessory nerve to the stump of the original nerve supplying that muscle.

Care of paralysed parts

While recovery is awaited the skin must be protected from friction damage and burns. The joints should be moved through their full range twice daily to prevent stiffness and minimize the work required of muscles when they recover. 'Dynamic' splints may be helpful.

Tendon transfers

Motor recovery may not occur if the axons, regenerating at about 1 mm per day, do not reach the muscle within 18–24 months of injury. This is most likely when there is a proximal injury in a nerve supplying distal muscles. In such circumstances, tendon transfers should be considered. The principles can be summarized in the Box on the previous page.

Recommended transfers are discussed under the individual nerve lesions.

Prognosis

Type of lesion Neurapraxia always recovers fully; axonotmesis may or may not; neurotmesis will not unless the nerve is repaired.

Level of lesion The higher the lesion, the worse the prognosis.

Type of nerve Purely motor or purely sensory nerves recover better than mixed nerves, because there is less likelihood of axonal confusion.

Size of gap Above the critical resection length, suture is not successful.

Age Children do better than adults. Old people do poorly.

Delay in suture This is a most important adverse factor. The best results are obtained with early nerve repair. After a few months, recovery following suture becomes progressively less likely.

Associated lesions Damage to vessels, tendons and other structures makes it more difficult to obtain recovery of a useful limb even if the nerve itself recovers.

Surgical techniques Skill, experience and suitable facilities are needed to treat nerve injuries. If these are lacking, it is wiser to perform the essential wound toilet and then transfer the patient to a specialized centre.

REGIONAL SURVEY OF NERVE INJURIES

BRACHIAL PLEXUS INJURIES

Pathological anatomy

The brachial plexus is formed by the confluence of nerve roots from C5 to T1; the network and its branches are shown diagrammatically in Figure 11.9. The plexus, as it passes from the cervical spine between the muscles of the neck and beneath the clavicle en route to the arm, is vulnerable to injury –

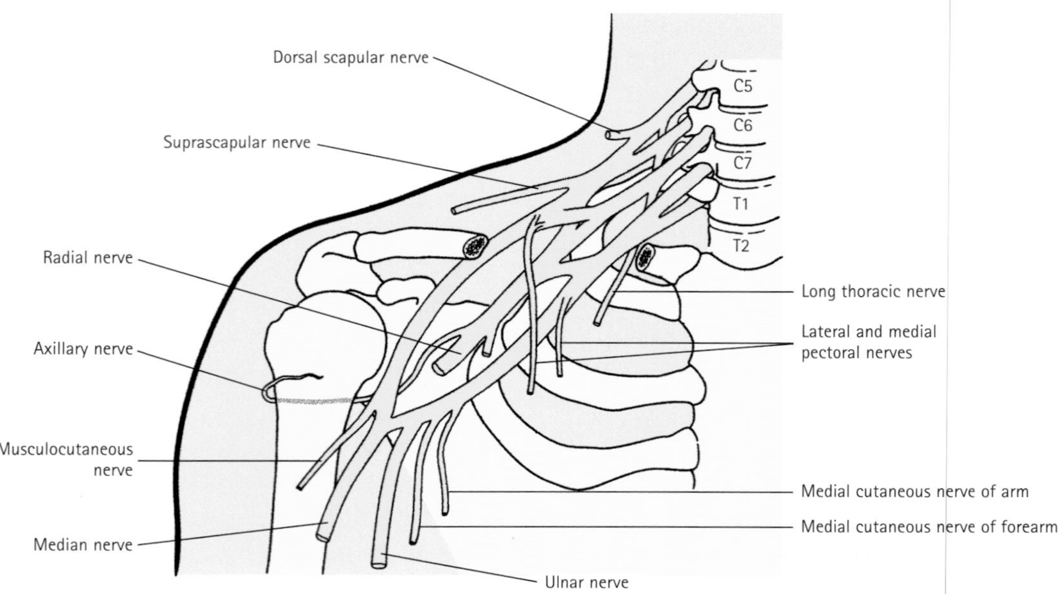

11.9 Brachial plexus Diagram of the brachial plexus and its relationship to the clavicle (some of the less important nerve branches and the posterior attachment of the second rib have been omitted).

either a stab wound or severe traction caused by a fall on the side of the neck or the shoulder.

Traction injuries are generally classed as supraclavicular (65 per cent), infraclavicular (25 per cent) and combined (10 per cent). *Supraclavicular lesions* typically occur in motorcycle accidents: as the cyclist collides with the ground or another vehicle his neck and shoulder are wrenched apart. In the most severe injuries the arm is practically avulsed from the trunk, with rupture of the subclavian artery. *Infraclavicular lesions* are usually associated with fractures or dislocations of the shoulder; in about a quarter of cases the axillary artery also is torn. Fractures of the clavicle rarely damage the plexus and then only if caused by a direct blow.

The injury may affect any level, or several levels within the plexus, often involving a mixture of nerve root(s), trunk(s) and nerve(s). An important distinction is made between preganglionic and postganglionic lesions. Avulsion of a nerve root from the spinal cord is a *preganglionic lesion*, i.e. disruption proximal to the dorsal root ganglion; this cannot recover and it is surgically irreparable. Rupture of a nerve root distal to the ganglion, or of a trunk or peripheral nerve, is a *postganglionic lesion*, which is surgically reparable and potentially capable of recovery. *Lesions in continuity*, from first to fourth degree, generally have a better prognosis than complete ruptures. *Mild lesions (neurapraxia)* are fairly common and may be caused by comparatively trivial trauma such as sudden compression by a tight harness or motor vehicle seatbelt; these recover spontaneously but mild residual symptoms may prove a nuisance for many months.

Clinical features

Brachial plexus injuries are often overshadowed by other, life-threatening trauma which needs immediate attention. Associated injuries, such as rupture of the subclavian or axillary artery, should be sought and attended to, otherwise a poor outcome is inevitable.

Neurological dysfunction soon becomes obvious. Detailed clinical examination is directed at answering specific questions: What is the level of the lesion? Is it preganglionic or postganglionic? If postganglionic, what type of lesion is it?

THE LEVEL OF THE LESION

In upper plexus injuries (C5 and 6) the shoulder abductors and external rotators and the forearm supinators are paralysed. Sensory loss involves the outer aspect of the arm and forearm.

Pure lower plexus injuries are rare. Wrist and finger flexors are weak and the intrinsic hand muscles are paralysed. Sensation is lost in the ulnar forearm and hand.

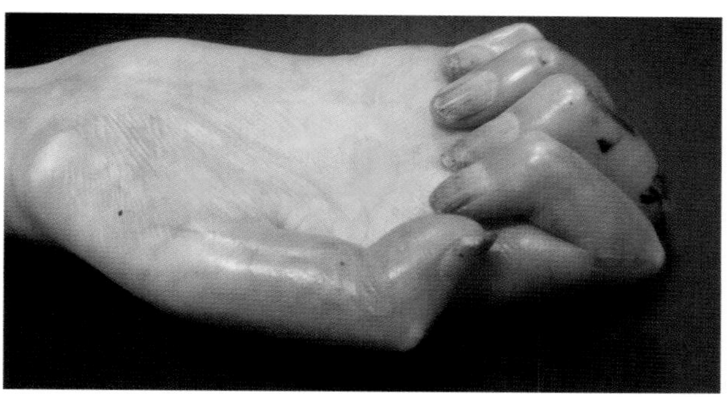

11.10 Brachial plexus injury Ischaemic insensate hand.

If the entire plexus is damaged, the whole limb is paralysed and numb.

Sometimes the scapular muscles and one side of the diaphragm too are involved. By examining systematically for each component of the brachial plexus (roots, trunks, divisions, cords and branches) the exact site of the lesion may be identified. For instance, preservation of the dorsal scapular nerve (rhomboids), long thoracic nerve (serratus anterior) and suprascapular nerve (supraspinatus), but loss of musculocutaneous nerve function (biceps), radial nerve (triceps) and axillary nerve (deltoid) suggest a lateral and posterior cord injury.

PRE- OR POST-GANGLIONIC?

It is crucial to establish how far from the cord the lesion is. Preganglionic lesions (root avulsions) are irreparable; postganglionic lesions may either recover (axonotmesis) or may be amenable to repair. Features suggesting root avulsion are: (1) crushing or burning pain in an anaesthetic hand; (2) paralysis of scapular muscles or diaphragm; (3) Horner's syndrome – ptosis, miosis (small pupil), enophthalmos and anhidrosis; (4) severe vascular injury; (5) associated fractures of the cervical spine; and (6) spinal cord dysfunction (e.g. hyper-reflexia in the lower limbs).

The *histamine test* is intriguing. Intradermal injection of histamine usually causes a triple response in the surrounding skin (central capillary dilatation, a wheal and a surrounding flare). If the flare reaction persists in an anaesthetic area of skin, the lesion must be proximal to the posterior root ganglion, i.e. it is probably a root avulsion. With a postganglionic lesion the test will be negative because nerve continuity between the skin and the dorsal root ganglion is interrupted.

CT myelography or *MRI* may show pseudomeningoceles produced by root avulsion. Note that during the first few days a 'positive' result is unreliable because the dura can be torn without there being root avulsion.

Nerve conduction studies need careful interpretation. If there is sensory conduction from an anaesthetic dermatome, this suggests a preganglionic lesion

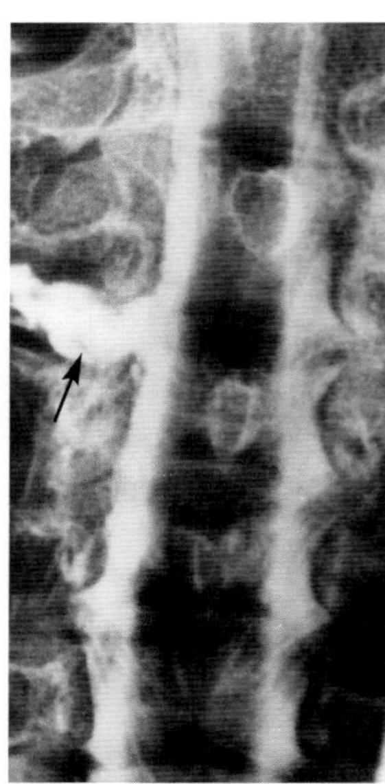

11.11 Brachial plexus The myelogram shows leakage of the contrast medium, indicating root avulsion.

(i.e. the nerve distal to the ganglion is not interrupted). This test becomes reliable only after a few weeks, when wallerian degeneration in a postganglionic lesion will block nerve conduction.

THE TYPE OF LESION

Once a postganglionic lesion has been diagnosed, it becomes important to decide how severely the nerve has been damaged. The history is informative: the mechanism of injury and the impact velocity may suggest either a mild (first or second degree) or a severe (fourth or fifth degree) injury. With the former a period of observation is justified; a first or second degree lesion may show signs of recovery by 6 or 8 weeks. If a neurotmesis seems likely then early operative exploration is called for. Since there may be different degrees of injury within the plexus, some muscles may recover while others fail to do so.

Management

The patient is likely to be admitted to a general unit where fractures and other injuries will be given priority. Emergency surgery is required for brachial plexus lesions associated with penetrating wounds, vascular injury or severe (high energy) soft-tissue damage whether open or closed; clean cut nerves should be repaired or grafted. This is best performed by a team specializing in this field of work.

All other closed injuries are left until detailed examination and special investigations have been completed. Patients with root avulsion or severe, mutilating injuries of the limb will be unsuitable for nerve surgery, at least until the prognosis for limb function becomes clear.

Progress of the neurological features is carefully monitored. As long as recovery proceeds at the expected rate, watchful conservation is the byword. If recovery falters, or if special investigations show that it is more than a second degree lesion, then the patient should be referred to a special centre for surgical exploration of the brachial plexus and nerve repair, grafting or nerve transfer procedures. The sooner this decision is made, the better: during the early days operative exposure is easier and the response to repair more reliable. Repairs performed after 6 months are unlikely to succeed.

THE PATTERN OF INJURY

Surgical exploration reveals three typical patterns of injury:

- *C5,6(7) avulsion* or *rupture with C(7)8, T1 intact*: this group has the most favourable outcome as hand function is preserved and muscles innervated from the upper roots often recover after plexus repair or nerve transfer.
- *C5,6(7) rupture with avulsion of C7,8,T1*: these may recover shoulder and elbow movement after repair and grafting of the upper levels, but hand function is irretrievably lost.
- *C5–T1 avulsion*: these cases have a poor outcome. There are few donor axons available to neurotize the upper levels (shoulder and elbow function) and no recovery will take place in the hand.

The implication is that all efforts for nerve repair or nerve transfer are directed towards lesions involving C5 and 6. The objectives are to regain shoulder abduction, elbow flexion, wrist extension, finger flexion, and sensibility over the lateral (radial) side of the hand.

NERVE GRAFTING AND NERVE TRANSFER

Nerve grafting is often necessary and the results for restoration of shoulder and elbow function are quite good; however, the outcome for lesions affecting the forearm and hand is disappointing .

Nerve transfer is an alternative way of providing functioning axons. If C5 and C6 are avulsed, then the spinal accessory nerve can be transferred to the suprascapular nerve; or two or three intercostal nerves can be transferred to the musculocutaneous nerve.

If one nerve root is available (e.g. C5) then this should be grafted on to the lateral cord which will supply elbow flexion, finger flexion and sensation over the radial side of the hand. If two roots are available (e.g. C5, C6) these can be grafted on to the lateral and posterior cords. These procedures bypass the suprascapular nerve which is joined to the spinal accessory nerve.

With complete preganglionic loss, the contralateral C7 root can be extended across the chest with autologous graft and then used as an axon source into the plexus. There is remarkably little deficit in the donor limb.

Two or three years must pass before the final results of plexus reconstruction are apparent.

LATER RECONSTRUCTION

The best results of plexus reconstruction are obtained after very early operation. If the patient is not seen until very late after injury, or if plexus reconstruction has failed, then there are a number of options:

Tendon transfer to achieve elbow flexion Various muscles can be transferred as elbow flexors: pectoralis major (Clarke's transfer), the common flexor origin (Steindler transfer), latissimus dorsi, or triceps. The nerve supply to these muscles must remain intact, so they are suitable only for certain patterns of injury.

Free muscle transfer Gracilis, rectus femoris or the contralateral latissimus dorsi can be transferred as a free flap and innervated with two or three intercostal nerves or contralateral C7. Elbow flexion and wrist extension can be regained.

Shoulder arthrodesis Arthrodesis is usually reserved for an unstable or painful shoulder, perhaps after failure of re-innervation of the supraspinatus. The position must be tailored to the needs of the particular patient.

OBSTETRICAL BRACHIAL PLEXUS PALSY

Obstetrical palsy is caused by excessive traction on the brachial plexus during childbirth, e.g. by pulling the bay's head away from the shoulder or by exerting traction with the baby's arm in abduction. Three patterns are seen: (1) *upper root injury (Erb's palsy)*, typically in overweight babies with shoulder dystocia at delivery; (2) *lower root injury (Klumpke's palsy)*, usually after breech delivery of smaller babies; and (3) *total plexus injury*.

Clinical features

The diagnosis is usually obvious at birth: after a difficult delivery the baby has a floppy or flail arm. Further examination a day or two later will define the type of brachial plexus injury.

Erb's palsy is caused by injury of C5, C6 and (sometimes) C7. The abductors and external rotators of the shoulder and the supinators are paralysed. The arm is held to the side, internally rotated and pronated. There may also be loss of finger extension. Sensation cannot be tested in a baby.

(a)

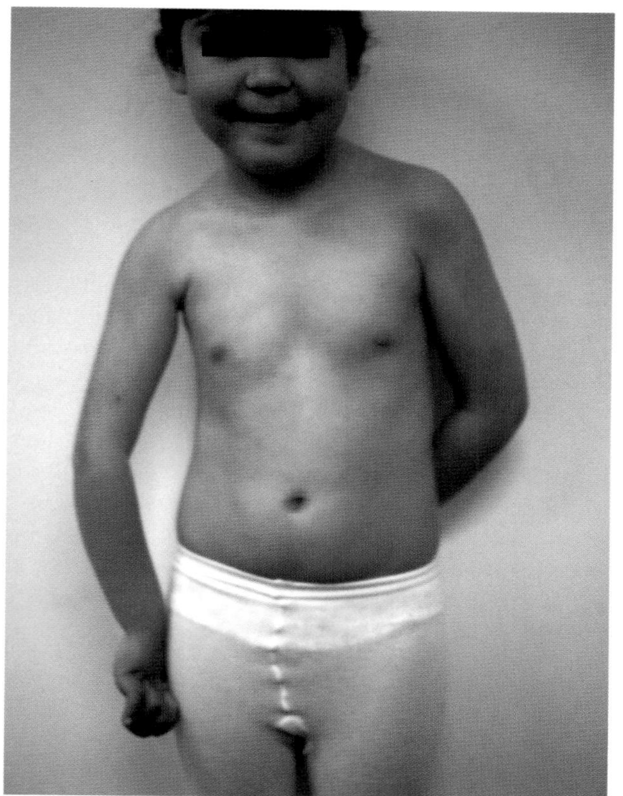

(b)

11.12 Obstetrical brachial plexus palsy (a) Paralysis of the abductors and external rotators of the shoulder, as well as the forearm supinators, results in the typical posture demonstrated in this baby with Erb's palsy of the left arm. (b) Young boy with Klumpke's palsy of the right arm.

Klumpke's palsy is due to injury of C8 and T1. The baby lies with the arm supinated and the elbow flexed; there is loss of intrinsic muscle power in the hand. Reflexes are absent and there may be a unilateral Horner's syndrome.

With a total plexus injury the baby's arm is flail and pale; all finger muscles are parlysed and there may also be vasomotor impairment and a unilateral Horner's syndrome.

X-rays should be obtained to exclude fractures of the shoulder or clavicle (which are not uncommon and which can be mistaken for obstetrical palsy).

Management

Over the next few weeks one of several things may happen.

Paralysis may recover completely Many (perhaps most) of the upper root lesions recover spontaneously. A fairly reliable indicator is return of biceps activity by the third month. However, absence of biceps activity does not completely rule out later recovery.

Paralysis may improve A total lesion may partially resolve, leaving the infant with a partial paralysis.

Paralysis may remain unaltered This is more likely with complete lesions, especially in the presence of a Horner's syndrome.

While waiting for recovery, physiotherapy is applied to keep the joints mobile.

OPERATIVE TREATMENT

If there is no biceps recovery by 3 months, operative intervention should be considered. Unless the roots are avulsed, it may be possible to excise the scar and bridge the gap with free sural nerve grafts; if the roots are avulsed, nerve transfer may give a worthwhile result. This is highly demanding surgery which should be undertaken only in specialized centres.

The shoulder is prone to fixed internal rotation and adduction deformity. If diligent physiotherapy does not prevent this, then a subscapularis release will be needed, sometimes supplemented by a tendon transfer. In older children, the deformity can be treated by rotation osteotomy of the humerus.

LONG THORACIC NERVE

The long thoracic nerve of Bell (C5, 6, 7) may be damaged in shoulder or neck injuries (usually an axonotmesis) or during operations such as first rib resection, transaxillary sympathectomy or radical mastectomy. However, serratus anterior palsy is also seen after comparatively benign events, such as carrying loads on the shoulder, and even viral illnesses or toxoid injections.

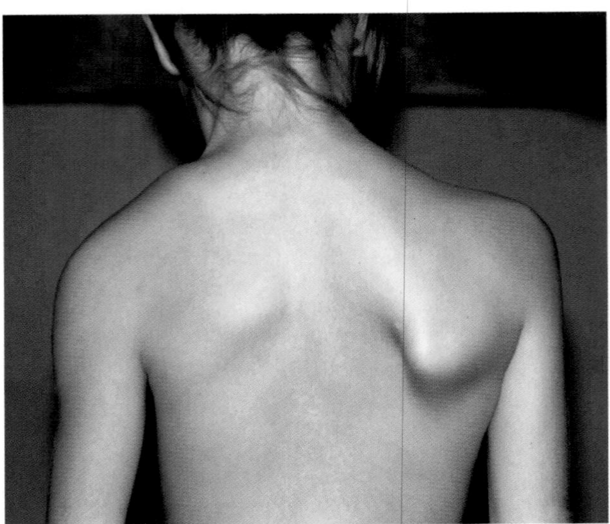

11.13 Long thoracic nerve palsy Winging of the scapula is demonstrated by the patient pushing forwards against the wall. If the serratus anterior is paralysed, the scapula cannot be held firmly against the rib-cage.

Clinical features

Paralysis of serratus anterior is the commonest cause of winging of the scapula. The patient may complain of aching and weakness on lifting the arm. Examination shows little abnormality until the arm is elevated in flexion or abduction. The classic test for winging is to have the patient pushing forwards against the wall or thrusting the shoulder forwards against resistance.

Treatment

Except after direct injury or division, the nerve usually recovers spontaneously, though this may take a year or longer. Persistent winging of the scapula occasionally requires operative stabilization by transferring pectoralis minor or major to the lower part of the scapula.

SPINAL ACCESSORY NERVE

The spinal accessory nerve (C2–6) supplies the sternomastoid muscle and then runs obliquely across the posterior triangle of the neck to innervate the upper half of the trapezius. Contrary to general belief, the nerve appears also to have sensory functions, including pain sensibility. Because of its superficial course, it is easily injured in stab wounds and operations in the posterior triangle of the neck (e.g. lymph node biopsy). It is occasionally injured in whiplash injuries.

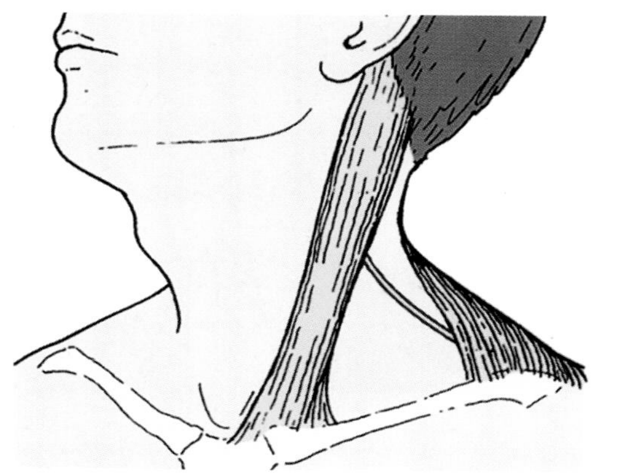

11.14 Accessory nerve The accessory nerve is embedded in the fascia which covers the posterior triangle and is easily damaged during lymph node biopsy or excision (and in stab wounds).

Clinical features

Following an open wound or operation, the patient complains of severe pain and 'stiffness' of the shoulder. Examination reveals asymmetry or drooping of the shoulder, reduced ability to hitch or hunch the shoulder and weakness on abduction of the arm; typically there is mild winging of the scapula on attempting active abduction against resistance; unlike the deformity in serratus anterior palsy, this disappears on flexion or forward thrusting of the shoulder. Often the true nature of the problem is not appreciated and diagnosis is delayed for weeks or months. In late cases there may be wasting of the trapezius.

Treatment

Stab injuries and surgical injuries should be explored immediately and the nerve repaired. If the exact cause of injury is uncertain, it is prudent to wait for about 8 weeks for signs of recovery. If this does not occur, the nerve should be explored: (a) to confirm the diagnosis and (b) to repair the lesion by direct suture or grafting. While waiting for recovery the arm is held in a sling to prevent dragging on the neck muscles. The results of early nerve repair are generally good but some patients continue to complain of shoulder fatigue during lifting and overhead activities.

SUPRASCAPULAR NERVE

The suprascapular nerve, which arises from the upper trunk of the brachial plexus (C5, 6), runs through the suprascapular notch to supply the supra- and infraspinatus muscles. It may be injured in fractures of the scapula, dislocation of the shoulder, by a direct blow or sudden traction, or simply by carrying a heavy load over the shoulder.

Clinical features

There may be a history of injury, but patients sometimes present with unexplained pain in the suprascapular region and weakness of shoulder abduction – symptoms readily mistaken for a rotator cuff syndrome. There is usually wasting of the supraspinatus and infraspinatus, with diminished power of abduction and external rotation. Electromyography may help to establish the diagnosis.

Treatment

This is usually an axonotmesis which clears up spontaneously after 3 months. If no recovery is seen at this stage the nerve should be explored. In the absence of trauma one might suspect a nerve entrapment syndrome, and decompression by division of the suprascapular ligament often brings improvement. The operative approach is through a posterior incision above and parallel to the spine of the scapula.

AXILLARY NERVE

The axillary nerve (C5, 6) arises from the posterior cord of the brachial plexus and runs along subscapularis and across the axilla just inferior to the shoulder joint. It emerges behind the humerus, deep to the deltoid; after supplying the teres minor, it divides into a medial branch which supplies the posterior part of the deltoid and a patch of skin over the muscle and an

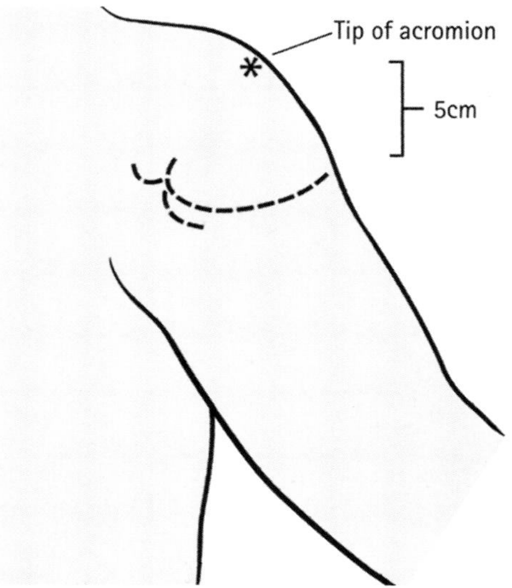

11.15 Axillary nerve Surface marking of the axillary nerve.

anterior branch that curls round the surgical neck of the humerus to innervate the anterior two-thirds of the deltoid. The landmark for this important branch is 5 cm below the tip of the acromion.

The nerve is sometimes ruptured in a brachial plexus injury. More often it is injured during shoulder dislocation or fractures of the humeral neck. Iatrogenic injuries occur in transaxillary operations on the shoulder and with lateral deltoid-splitting incisions. It is sometimes injured at the same time as the suprascapular nerve in shoulder dislocation. Simultaneous rupture of the rotator cuff can add to the diagnostic confusion by causing weak or absent arm abduction after shoulder dislocation.

Clinical features

The patient complains of shoulder 'weakness', and the deltoid is wasted. Although abduction can be initiated (by supraspinatus), it cannot be maintained. Retropulsion (extension of the shoulder with the arm abducted to 90 degrees) is impossible. Careful testing will reveal a small area of numbness over the deltoid (the 'sergeant's patch').

Treatment

Nerve injury associated with fractures or dislocations recovers spontaneously in about 80 per cent of cases. If the deltoid shows no sign of recovery by 8 weeks, EMG should be performed; if the tests suggest denervation then the nerve should be explored through a combined deltopectoral and posterior (quadrilateral space) approach. Excision of the nerve ends and grafting are usually necessary; a good result can be expected if the nerve is explored within 3 months of injury. However, if the operation fails and the shoulder is painfully unstable, then provided that trapezius and serratus anterior are functioning, shoulder arthrodesis can provide both stability and some degree of 'abduction'.

RADIAL NERVE

The radial nerve may be injured at the elbow, in the upper arm or in the axilla.

Clinical features

Low lesions are usually due to fractures or dislocations at the elbow, or to a local wound. Iatrogenic lesions of the posterior interosseous nerve where it winds through the supinator muscle are sometimes seen after operations on the proximal end of the radius. The patient complains of clumsiness and, on testing, cannot extend the metacarpophalangeal joints of the hand. In the thumb there is also weakness of extension and retroposition. Wrist extension is preserved because the branch to the extensor carpi radialis longus arises proximal to the elbow.

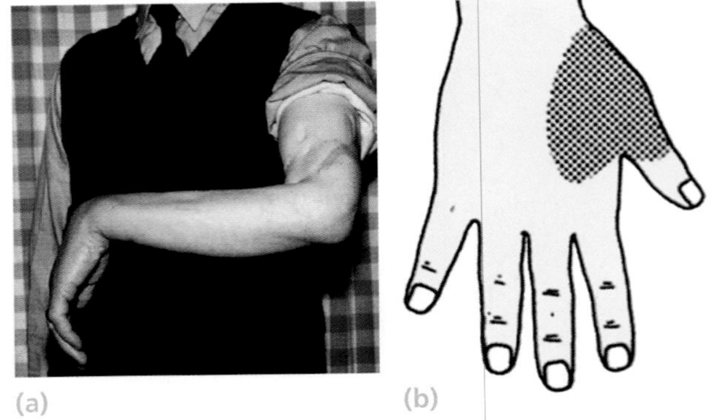

11.16 Radial nerve palsy (a) This man developed a complete drop-wrist palsy following a severe open fracture of the humerus and division of the radial nerve. (b) The typical area of sensory loss.

High lesions occur with fractures of the humerus or after prolonged tourniquet pressure. There is an obvious wrist drop, due to weakness of the radial extensors of the wrist, as well as inability to extend the metacarpophalangeal joints or elevate the thumb. Sensory loss is limited to a small patch on the dorsum around the anatomical snuffbox.

Very high lesions may be caused by trauma or operations around the shoulder. More often, though, they are due to chronic compression in the axilla; this is seen in drink and drug addicts who fall into a stupor with the arm dangling over the back of a chair ('Saturday night palsy') or in thin elderly patients using crutches ('crutch palsy'). In addition to weakness of the wrist and hand, the triceps is paralysed and the triceps reflex is absent.

Treatment

Open injuries should be explored and the nerve repaired or grafted as soon as possible.

Closed injuries are usually first or second degree lesions, and function eventually returns. In patients with fractures of the humerus it is important to examine for a radial nerve injury on admission, before treatment and again after manipulation or internal fixation. If the palsy is present on admission, one can afford to wait for 12 weeks to see if it starts to recover. If it does not, then EMG should be performed; if this shows denervation potentials and no active potentials then a neurapraxia is excluded and the nerve should be explored. The results, even with delayed surgery and quite long grafts, can be gratifying as the radial nerve has a straightforward motor function.

If it is certain that there was no nerve injury on admission, and the signs appear only after manipulation or internal fixation, then the chances of an iatropathic injury are high and the nerve should be explored and – if necessary – repaired or grafted without delay.

While recovery is awaited, the small joints of the hand must be put through a full range of passive movements. The wrist is splinted in extension. 'Lively' hand splints are avoided as they tend to hold the metacarpophalangeal joints in extension with the proximal interphalangeal joints flexed and this will lead to fixed contractures.

If recovery does not occur, the disability can be largely overcome by tendon transfers: pronator teres to the short radial extensor of the wrist, flexor carpi radialis to the long finger extensors and palmaris longus to the long thumb abductor.

ULNAR NERVE

Injuries of the ulnar nerve are usually either near the wrist or near the elbow, although open wounds may damage it at any level.

Clinical features

Low lesions are often caused by cuts on shattered glass. There is numbness of the ulnar one and a half fingers. The hand assumes a typical posture in repose – the claw hand deformity – with hyperextension of the metacarpophalangeal joints of the ring and little fingers, due to weakness of the intrinsic muscles. Hypothenar and interosseous wasting may be obvious by comparison with the normal hand. Finger abduction is weak and this, together with the loss of thumb adduction, makes pinch difficult. The patient is asked to grip a sheet of paper forcefully between thumbs and index fingers while the examiner tries to pull it away; powerful flexion of the thumb interphalangeal joint signals weakness of adductor pollicis and first dorsal interosseous with overcompensation by the flexor pollicis longus (Froment's sign).

Entrapment of the ulnar nerve in the pisohamate tunnel (Guyon's canal) is often seen in long-distance cyclists who lean with the pisiform pressing on the handlebars. Unexplained lesions of the distal (motor) branch of the nerve may be due to compression by a deep carpal ganglion or ulnar artery aneurysm.

High lesions occur with elbow fractures or dislocations. The hand is not markedly deformed because the ulnar half of flexor digitorum profundus is paralysed and the fingers are therefore less 'clawed' (the *'high ulnar paradox'*). Otherwise, motor and sensory loss are the same as in low lesions.

'Ulnar neuritis' may be caused by compression or entrapment of the nerve in the medial epicondylar (cubital) tunnel, especially where there is severe valgus deformity of the elbow or prolonged pressure on the elbows in anaesthetized or bed-ridden patients. It is important to be aware of this condition in patients who start complaining of ulnar nerve symptoms some

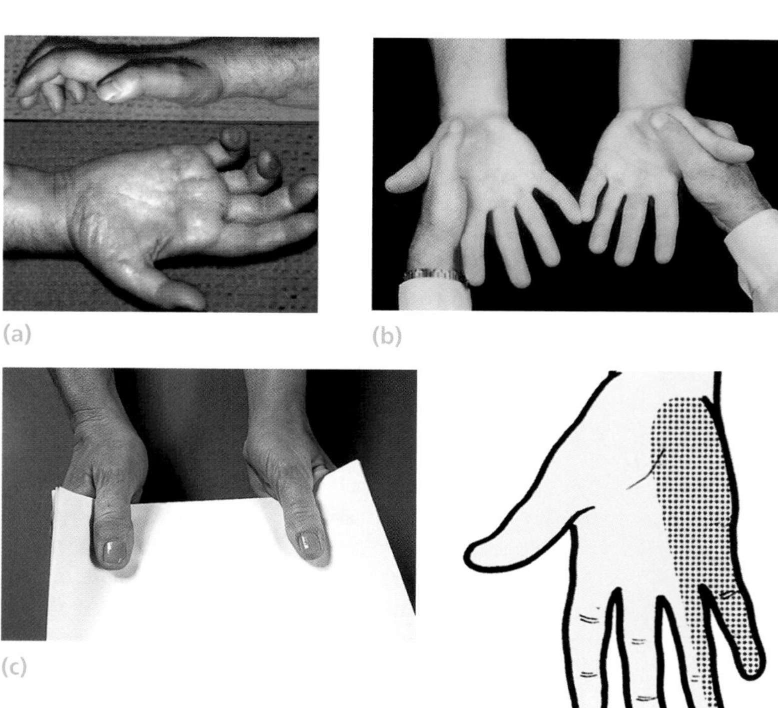

11.17 Ulnar nerve palsy (a) Clawing of the ring and little fingers and wasting of the intrinsic muscles. (b) A good test for interosseous muscle weakness. Ask the patient to spread his fingers (abduct) as strongly as possible and then force his hands together with the little fingers apposed; the weaker side will collapse (the left hand in this case). (c) *Froment's sign*: the patient is asked to grip a card firmly between thumbs and index fingers; normally this is done using the thumb adductors while the interphalangeal joint is held extended. In the right hand, because the adductor pollicis is weak, the patient grips the card only by acutely flexing the interphalangeal joint of the thumb (flexor pollicis longus is supplied by the median nerve). (d) Typical area of sensory loss.

weeks after an upper limb injury; one can easily be misled into thinking that the nerve lesion is due to the original injury!

Treatment

Exploration and suture of a divided nerve are well worthwhile, and anterior transposition at the elbow permits closure of gaps up to 5 cm. While recovery is awaited, the skin should be protected from burns. Hand physiotherapy keeps the hand supple and useful.

If there is no recovery after nerve division, hand function is significantly impaired. Grip strength is diminished because the primary metacarpophalangeal flexors are lost, and pinch is poor because of the weakened thumb adduction and index finger abduction. Fine, coordinated finger movements are also affected.

Metacarpophalangeal flexion can be improved by extensor carpi radialis longus to intrinsic tendon transfers (Brand), or by looping a slip of flexor digitorum superficialis around the opening of the flexor sheath (Zancolli procedure). Index abduction is improved by transferring extensor pollicis brevis or extensor indicis to the interosseous insertion on the radial side of the finger.

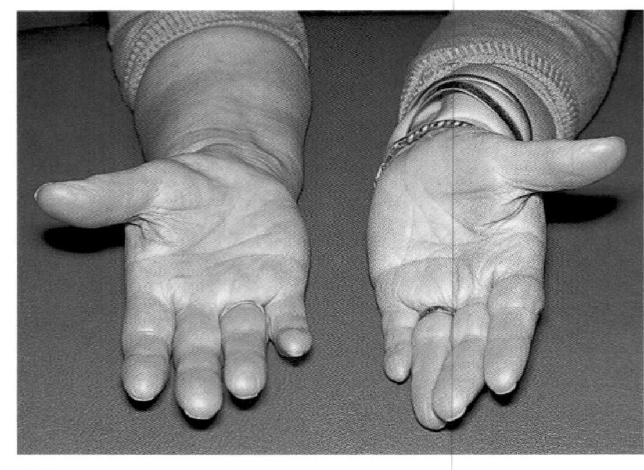

(a)

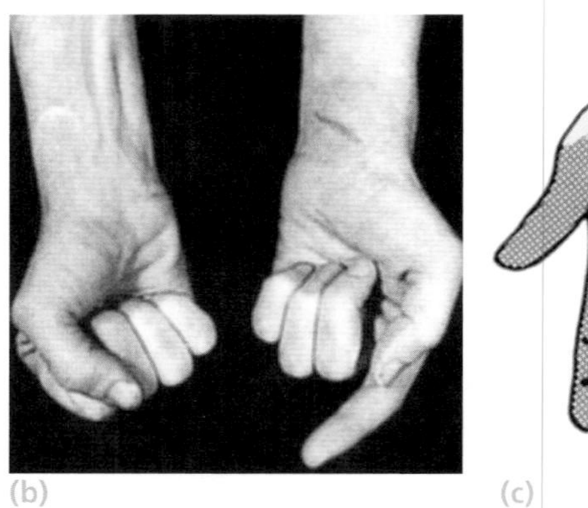

(b) (c)

11.19 Median nerve lesions (a) Wasting of the thenar eminence on the right side. (b) In high median nerve lesions, the long flexors to the thumb and index fingers are also paralysed and the patient shows the 'pointing index sign'. (c) Typical area of sensory loss.

MEDIAN NERVE

The median nerve is most commonly injured near the wrist or high up in the forearm.

Clinical features

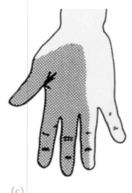

Low lesions may be caused by cuts in front of the wrist or by carpal dislocations. The patient is unable to abduct the thumb, and sensation is lost over the radial three and a half digits. In longstanding cases the thenar eminence is wasted and trophic changes may be seen.

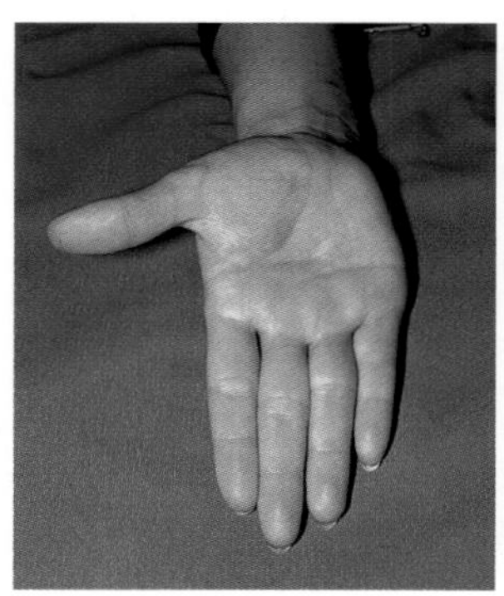

(a)

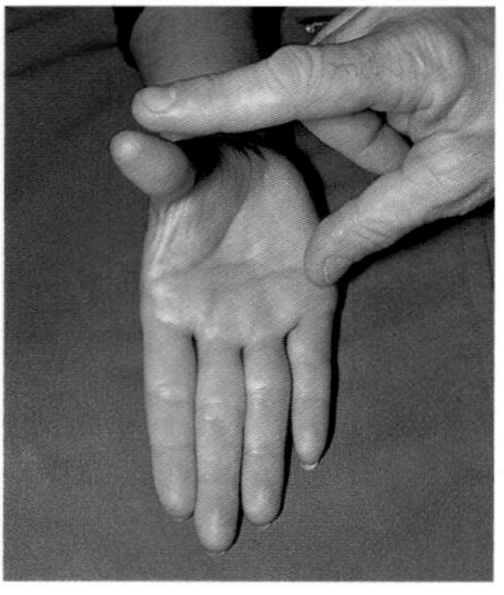

(b)

11.18 Median nerve – testing for abductor power (a) The hand must remain flat, palm upwards. (b) The patient is told to point the thumb towards the ceiling against the examiner's resistance.

High lesions are generally due to forearm fractures or elbow dislocation, but stabs and gunshot wounds may damage the nerve at any level. The signs are the same as those of low lesions but, in addition, the long flexors to the thumb, index and middle fingers, the radial wrist flexors and the forearm pronator muscles are all paralysed. Typically the hand is held with the ulnar fingers flexed and the index straight (the 'pointing sign'). Also, because the thumb and index flexors are deficient, there is a characteristic pinch defect: instead of pinching with the thumb and index fingertips flexed, the patient pinches with the distal joints in full extension.

Isolated anterior interosseous nerve lesions are extremely rare. The signs are similar to those of a high median nerve injury, but without any sensory loss. The usual cause is brachial neuritis (Parsonage–Turner Syndrome) which is associated with shoulder girdle pain after immunization or a viral illness.

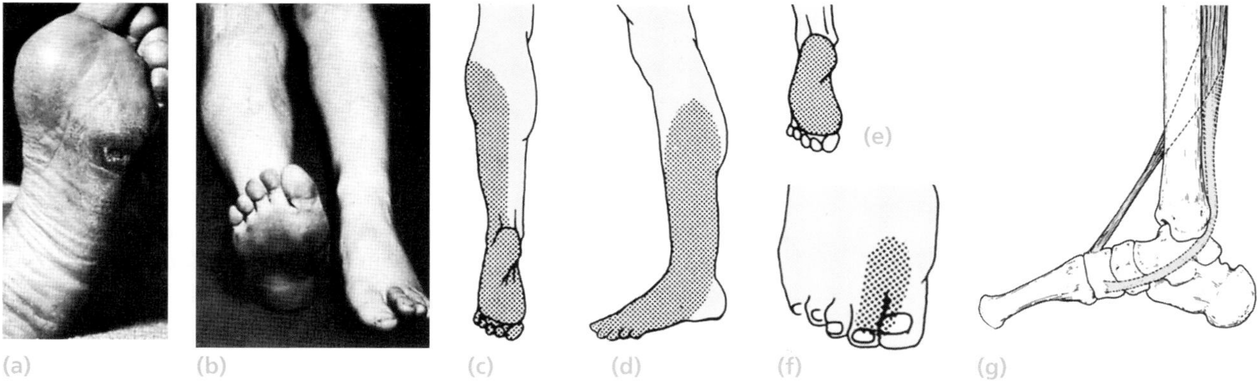

11.20 Two problems in sciatic nerve lesions are (a) trophic ulcers because of sensory loss and (b) foot drop. Sensory loss following division of (c) complete sciatic nerve, (d) common peroneal nerve, (e) posterior tibial nerve and (f) anterior tibial nerve. (g) Drop foot can be treated by rerouting tibialis posterior so that it acts as a dorsiflexor.

Treatment

If the nerve is divided, suture or nerve grafting should always be attempted. Postoperatively the wrist is splinted in flexion to avoid tension; when movements are commenced, wrist extension should be prevented.

Late lesions are sometimes seen. If there has been no recovery, the disability is severe because of sensory loss and deficient opposition. If sensation recovers but not opposition, extensor indicis proprius or, less suitably, abductor digiti minimi can be re-routed to the insertion of abductor pollicis brevis. Extensor carpi radialis longus is available as a transfer for flexor digitorum profundus, brachioradialis for flexor pollicis longus and extensor indicis for abductor pollicis brevis.

LUMBOSACRAL PLEXUS

The plexus may be injured by massive pelvic trauma. These lesions are usually incomplete and often missed; the patient may complain of no more than patchy muscle weakness and some difficulty with micturition. Sensation is diminished in the perineum or in one or more of the lower limb dermatomes. Some patients, however, have significant problems with incontinence, impotence and neurogenic pain. *Plexus injuries should always be sought in patients with fractures of the pelvis.*

Surgery is rarely undertaken.

FEMORAL NERVE

The femoral nerve may be injured by a gunshot wound, by pressure or traction during an operation or by bleeding into the thigh.

Clinical features

Quadriceps action is lacking and the patient is unable to extend the knee actively. There is numbness of the anterior thigh and medial aspect of the leg. The knee reflex is depressed. Severe neurogenic pain is common.

Treatment

This is a fairly disabling lesion and, where possible, counter-measures should be undertaken. A thigh haematoma may need to be evacuated. A clean cut of the nerve may be treated successfully by suturing or grafting but results are disappointing. The alternative would be a caliper to stabilize the knee, or tendon transfers of hamstrings to quadriceps.

SCIATIC NERVE

Division of the main sciatic nerve is rare except in gunshot wounds. Traction lesions may occur with traumatic hip dislocations and with pelvic fractures. Intraneural haemorrhage in patients receiving anticoagulants is a rare cause of intense pain and partial loss of function.

Iatropathic lesions are sometimes discovered after total hip replacement – due either to inadvertent division, compression by bone levers or possibly thermal injury from extruded acrylic cement; in most cases, though, no specific cause can be found and injury is assumed to be due to traction (see below).

Clinical features

In a complete lesion the hamstrings and all muscles below the knee are paralysed; the ankle jerk is absent. Sensation is lost below the knee, except on the medial side of the leg which is supplied by the saphenous branch of the femoral nerve. The patient walks with a drop foot and a high-stepping gait to avoid dragging the insensitive foot on the ground.

Sometimes only the deep part of the nerve is affected, producing what is essentially a common peroneal (lateral popliteal) nerve lesion (see below). This is the usual presentation in patients suffering foot-drop after hip replacement; however, careful examination will often reveal minor abnormalities also in the tibial (medial popliteal) division. Electrodiagnostic studies will help to establish the level of the injury.

If sensory loss extends into the thigh and the gluteal muscles are weak, suspect an associated lumbosacral plexus injury.

In late cases the limb is wasted, with fixed deformities of the foot and trophic ulcers on the sole.

Treatment

If the nerve is known to be divided, suture or nerve grafting should be attempted even though it may take more than a year for leg muscles to be re-innervated. While recovery is awaited, a below-knee drop-foot splint is fitted. Great care is taken to avoid damaging the insensitive skin and to prevent trophic ulcers.

The chances of recovery are generally poor and, at best, will be long delayed and incomplete. Partial lesions, in which there is protective sensation of the sole, can sometimes be managed by transferring tibialis posterior to the front in order to counteract the drop foot. The deformities should be corrected if they threaten to cause pressure sores. If there is no recovery whatever, amputation may be preferable to a flail, deformed, insensitive limb.

Sciatic palsy after total hip replacement

The incidence of overt sciatic nerve dysfunction is reported as 0.5–3 per cent following primary hip replacement and about twice as high after revision. However, subclinical EMG changes are quite common. The vast majority of these resolve fairly quickly and do not manifest as postoperative nerve lesions. The less fortunate patients present soon after operation with weakness of ankle dorsiflexion, or a foot-drop, and abnormal sensibility in the distribution of the common peroneal nerve – a combination which is readily mistaken for a peroneal nerve lesion (wishful thinking in almost every case!). The reason for this is that the 'peroneal' portion of the sciatic nerve lies closest to the acetabulum and is most easily damaged. Careful examination will often show minor abnormalities also in the tibial nerve. If there is any doubt about the level of the lesion, EMG and nerve conduction tests will help.

X-rays may show a bone fragment or extruded cement (with the possibility of thermal damage) in the soft tissues; MRI may be needed to establish its proximity to the sciatic nerve. However, in most cases no cause is identified and one is left guessing whether the nerve was inadvertently injured by a scalpel point, haemostat, electrocautery, suture knot or traction levers. Delayed onset palsy may be due to a haematoma.

In about half the cases the lesion proves to be a first or second degree injury; some of these recover within weeks, others take months and may not recover completely. Unless a definite cause is known or strongly suspected, it is usually worth waiting for 6 weeks to see if the condition improves. During this time the patient is fitted with a drop-foot splint and physiotherapy is begun.

There is no agreement about the indications for immediate operation. Those who argue against it say they are unlikely to find any specific pathology and anyway if they do discover evidence of nerve damage, the chances of functional recovery after nerve repair are probably no better than those of waiting for spontaneous improvement. Our own indications for early operation are: (1) total sciatic palsy; (2) a partial lesion associated with severe burning pain; and (3) strong evidence of a local, and possibly reversible, cause such as a bone fragment, acrylic cement or haematoma near the nerve. If the exploratory operation reveals a local cause, it should be corrected. If the nerve is divided or shows full thickness damage, repair or grafting may be worthwhile. At best, recovery will take several years and will be incomplete. Partial lesions are better left alone and the resulting disability managed by splintage and/or tendon transfers.

PERONEAL NERVES

Injuries may affect either the common peroneal (lateral popliteal) nerve or one of its branches, the deep or superficial peroneal nerves.

Clinical features

The *common peroneal nerve* is often damaged at the level of the fibular neck by severe traction when the knee is forced into varus (e.g. in lateral ligament injuries and fractures around the knee, or during operative correction of gross valgus deformities), or by pressure from a splint or a plaster cast, from lying with the leg externally rotated, by skin traction or by wounds. A ganglion from the superior tibio-fibular joint can also present with this palsy. The patient has a drop foot and can neither dorsiflex nor evert the foot. He or she walks with a high-stepping gait to avoid catching the toes. Sensation is lost over the front and outer half of the leg and the dorsum of the foot. Pain may be significant.

The *deep peroneal nerve* runs between the muscles of the anterior compartment of the leg and emerges at the lower border of the extensor retinaculum of the ankle. It may be threatened in an anterior compartment syndrome, causing pain and weakness of dorsiflexion and sensory loss in a small area of skin between the first and second toes. Sometimes the distal portion is cut during operations on the ankle, resulting in paraesthesia and numbness on the dorsum around the first web space.

The *superficial peroneal nerve* descends along the fibula, innervating the peroneal muscles and emerging through the deep fascia 5–10 cm above the ankle to supply the skin over the dorsum of the foot and the medial four toes. The muscular portion may be involved in a lateral compartment syndrome. The patient complains of pain in the lateral part of the leg and numbness or paraesthesia of the foot; there may be weakness of eversion and sensory loss on the dorsum of the foot. The cutaneous branches alone may be trapped where the nerve emerges from the deep fascia, or stretched by a severe inversion injury of the ankle, causing pain and sensory symptoms without muscle weakness.

Treatment

Direct injuries of the common peroneal nerve and its branches should be explored and repaired or grafted wherever possible. As usual, the earlier the repair, the better the result. While recovery is awaited a splint may be worn to control ankle weakness. Pain may be relieved and drop foot is improved in almost 50 per cent of patients, especially those who are operated on early. If there is no recovery, the disability can be minimized by tibialis posterior tendon transfer or by hind-foot stabilization; the alternative is a permanent splint.

Traction injuries from a knee dislocation may damage the nerve over a large length, needing a graft so long that recovery is hopeless. Splintage and tendon transfers are required.

TIBIAL NERVES

The tibial (medial popliteal) nerve is rarely injured except in open wounds. The distal part (posterior tibial nerve) is sometimes involved in injuries around the ankle.

Clinical features

The *tibial nerve* supplies the flexors of the ankle and toes. With division of the nerve, the patient is unable to plantarflex the ankle or flex the toes; sensation is absent over the sole and part of the calf. Because both the long flexors and the intrinsic muscles are involved, there is not much clawing. With time the calf and foot become atrophic and pressure ulcers may appear on the sole.

The *posterior tibial nerve* runs behind the medial malleolus under the flexor retinaculum, gives off a small calcaneal branch and then divides into *medial* and *lateral plantar nerves* which supply the intrinsic muscles and the skin of the sole. Fractures and dislocations around the ankle may injure any of these branches and the resultant picture depends on the level of the lesion. Thus, posterior tibial nerve lesions cause wide sensory loss and clawing of the toes due to paralysis of the intrinsics with active long flexors; but injury to one of the smaller branches causes only limited sensory loss and less noticeable motor weakness. A compartment syndrome of the foot (e.g. following metatarsal fractures) is easily missed if one fails to test specifically for plantar nerve function.

Treatment

A complete nerve division should be sutured as soon as possible. A peculiarity of the tibial nerve is that injury or repair (especially delayed repair) may be followed by causalgia.

While recovery is awaited, a suitable orthosis is worn (to prevent excessive dorsiflexion) and the sole is protected against pressure ulceration. In suitable cases, weakness of plantar flexion can be treated by hind-foot fusion or transfer of the tibialis anterior to the back of the foot.

NERVE COMPRESSION (ENTRAPMENT) SYNDROMES

Pathophysiology

Wherever peripheral nerves traverse fibro-osseous tunnels they are at risk of entrapment and compression, especially if the soft tissues increase in bulk (as they may in pregnancy, myxoedema or rheumatoid arthritis) or if there is a local obstruction (e.g. a ganglion or osteophytic spur).

Nerve compression impairs epineural blood flow and axonal conduction, giving rise to symptoms such as numbness, paraesthesia and muscle weakness; the relief of ischaemia explains the sudden improvement in symptoms after decompressive surgery. Prolonged or severe compression leads to segmental demyelination, target muscle atrophy and nerve fibrosis; symptoms are then less likely to resolve after decompression.

Peripheral neuropathy associated with generalized disorders such as diabetes or alcoholism may render a nerve more sensitive to the effects of compression. There is evidence, too, that proximal compression (e.g. discogenic root compression) impairs the synthesis and transport of neural substances, so predisposing the nerve to the effects of distal entrapment – the so-called '*double-crush syndrome*'.

Common sites for nerve entrapment are the *carpal tunnel* (median nerve) and the *cubital tunnel* (ulnar nerve); less common sites are the *tarsal tunnel* (posterior tibial nerve), the *inguinal ligament* (lateral cutaneous nerve of the thigh), the *suprascapular notch* (suprascapular nerve), the *neck of the fibula* (common peroneal nerve) and the *fascial tunnel of the superficial peroneal nerve.* A special case is the *thoracic outlet*, where the subclavian vessels and roots of the brachial plexus cross the first rib between the scalenus anterior and medius muscles. In these cases there may be vascular as well as neurological signs.

Clinical features

The patient complains of unpleasant tingling or pain or numbness. Symptoms are usually intermittent and sometimes related to specific postures which compromise the nerve. Thus, in the *carpal tunnel syndrome* they occur at night when the wrist is held still in flexion, and relief is obtained by moving the hand 'to get the circulation going'. In *ulnar neuropathy*, symptoms recur whenever the elbow is held in acute flexion for long periods. In the *thoracic outlet syndrome*, paraesthesia in the distribution of C8 and T1 may be provoked by holding the arms in abduction, extension and external rotation.

Areas of altered sensation and motor weakness are mapped out. In longstanding cases there may be obvious muscle wasting. The likely site of compression should be carefully examined for any local cause.

Electromyography and nerve conduction tests help to confirm the diagnosis, establish the level of compression and estimate the degree of nerve damage. Conduction is slowed across the compressed segment and EMG may show abnormal action potentials in muscles that are not obviously weak or wasted, or fibrillation in cases with severe nerve damage.

Treatment

In early cases splintage may help (e.g. holding the wrist or elbow in extension) and steroid injection into the entrapment area can reduce local tissue swelling. If symptoms persist, operative decompression will usually be successful. However, in longstanding cases with muscle atrophy there may be endoneurial fibrosis, axonal degeneration and end-organ decay; tunnel decompression may then fail to give complete relief.

MEDIAN NERVE COMPRESSION

Three separate syndromes are recognized: (1) carpal tunnel syndrome (far and away the most common); (2) proximal median nerve compression (the 'pronator syndrome'); and (3) anterior interosseous nerve compression.

CARPAL TUNNEL SYNDROME

This is the best known of all the entrapment syndromes. In the normal carpal tunnel there is barely room for all the tendons and the median nerve; consequently, any swelling is likely to result in compression and ischaemia of the nerve. Usually the cause eludes detection; the syndrome is, however, common at the menopause, in rheumatoid arthritis, pregnancy and myxoedema.

Clinical features

The history is most helpful in making the diagnosis. Pain and paraesthesia occur in the distribution of the median nerve in the hand. Night after night the patient is woken with burning pain, tingling and numbness. Hanging the arm over the side of the bed, or shaking the arm, may relieve the symptoms. In advanced cases there may be clumsiness and weakness, particularly with tasks requiring fine manipulation such as fastening buttons.

The condition is far more common in women than in men. The usual age group is 40–50 years; in younger patients it is not uncommon to find related factors such as pregnancy, rheumatoid disease, chronic renal failure or gout.

Sensory symptoms can often be reproduced by percussing over the median nerve (*Tinel's sign*) or by

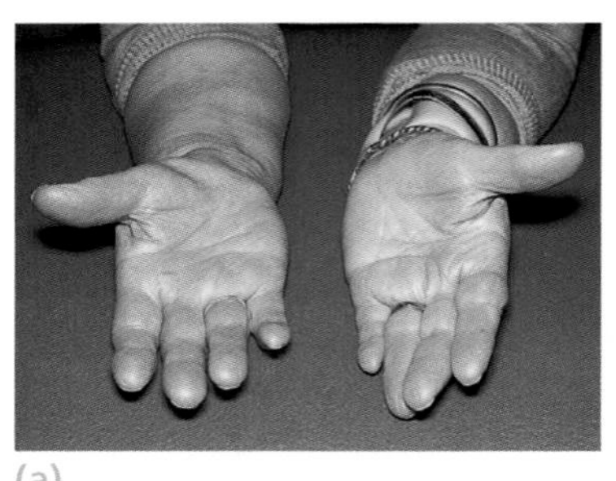

(a)

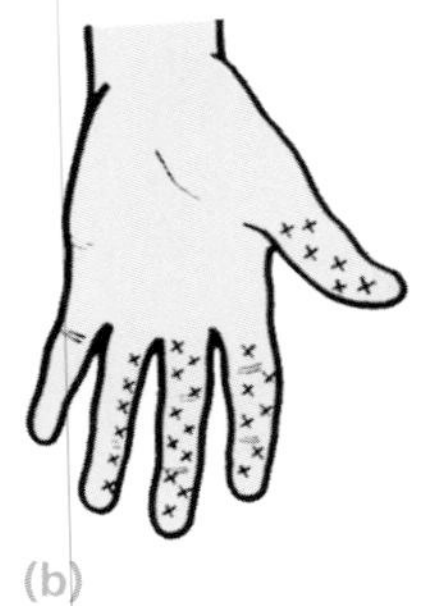

(b)

11.21 Median nerve compression (a) Thenar wasting in the right hand, (b) sensory loss.

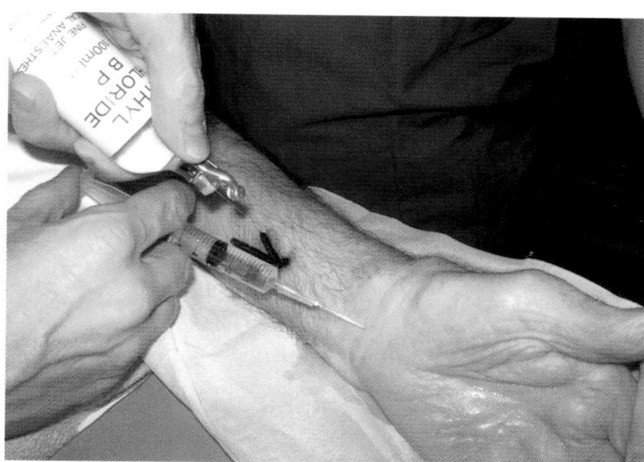

(a)

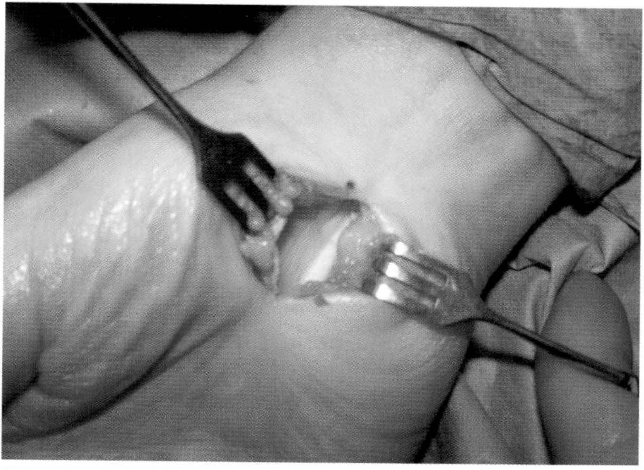

(b)

11.22 Median nerve compression – treatment
(a) Carpal tunnel injection, (b) open carpal tunnel release.

holding the wrist fully flexed for less than 60 seconds (*Phalen's test*). In late cases there is wasting of the thenar muscles, weakness of thumb abduction and sensory dulling in the median nerve territory.

Electrodiagnostic tests, which show slowing of nerve conduction across the wrist, are reserved for those with atypical symptoms. Radicular symptoms of cervical spondylosis may confuse the diagnosis and may coincide with carpal tunnel syndrome.

Treatment

Light splints that prevent wrist flexion can help those with night pain or with pregnancy-related symptoms. Steroid injection into the carpal canal, likewise, provides temporary relief.

Open surgical division of the transverse carpal ligament usually provides a quick and simple cure. The incision should be kept to the ulnar side of the thenar crease so as to avoid accidental injury to the palmar cutaneous (sensory) and thenar motor branches of the median nerve. Internal neurolysis is not recommended. Endoscopic carpal tunnel release offers an alternative with slightly quicker postoperative rehabilitation; however, the complication rate is higher.

Proximal median nerve compression

The median nerve can be (very rarely) compressed beneath one of several structures around the elbow including the ligament of Struthers (a connection between the medial epicondyle and the humerus), the bicipital aponeurosis or the arch-like origins of either pronator teres or flexor digitorum superficialis. This variability is not well conveyed by the more common term *'pronator syndrome'*. Symptoms are similar to those of carpal tunnel syndrome, although night pain is unusual and forearm pain is more common. Phalen's test will obviously be negative; instead, symptoms can be provoked by resisted elbow flexion with the forearm supinated (tightening the bicipital aponeurosis), by resisted forearm pronation with the elbow extended (pronator tension) or by resisted flexion of the middle finger proximal interphalangeal joint (tightening the superficialis arch). Pain may be felt in the forearm and there may be altered sensation in the territory of the palmar cutaneous branch of the median nerve (which originates proximal to the carpal tunnel). Tinel's sign may be positive over the nerve proximally but not at the carpal tunnel. Nerve conduction studies may localize the level of the compression but are often negative, particularly in postural compression. X-ray examination may show a bony spur at the attachment of Struthers' ligament (a very rare association).

Surgical decompression involves division of the bicipital aponeurosis and any other restraining structure (pronator teres, arch of flexor digitorum superficialis); great care is needed in the dissection.

ANTERIOR INTEROSSEOUS NERVE SYNDROME

The anterior interosseous nerve can be selectively compressed at the same sites as the proximal median nerve. However, spontaneous (and usually temporary) physiological failure (Parsonage–Turner syndrome) is a more likely cause. There is motor weakness without sensory symptoms. The patient is unable to make the 'OK sign' – pinching with the thumb and index finger joints flexed, like a ring – because of weakness of the flexor pollicis longus and flexor digitorum profundus. Isolated loss of flexor pollicis longus can occur. Pressure over the belly of this muscle in the forearm will flex the thumb-tip, thus excluding tendon rupture. The condition usually settles spontaneously within a few months. If it does not, surgical exploration and release or tendon transfer may be considered.

ULNAR NERVE COMPRESSION

This occurs most commonly at the elbow and less commonly at the wrist.

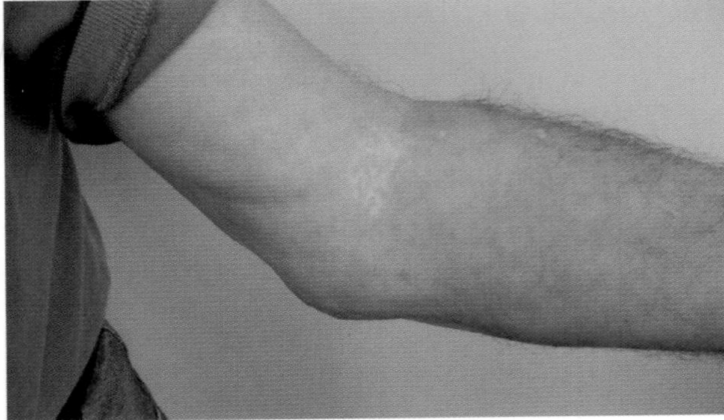

(a)

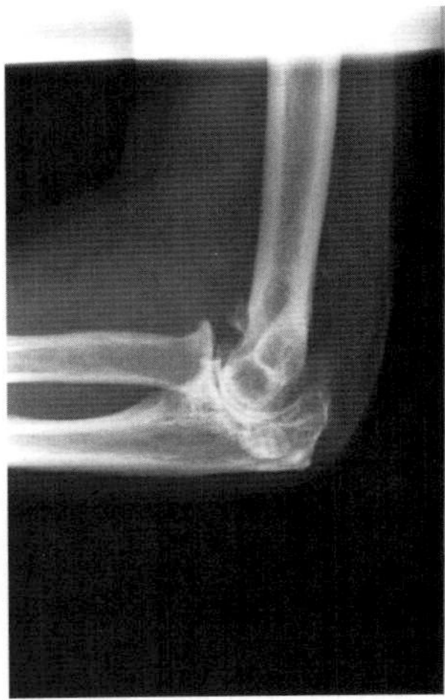

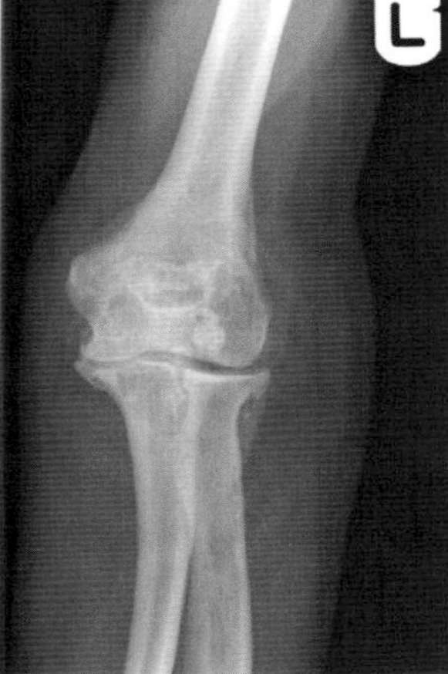

(b)

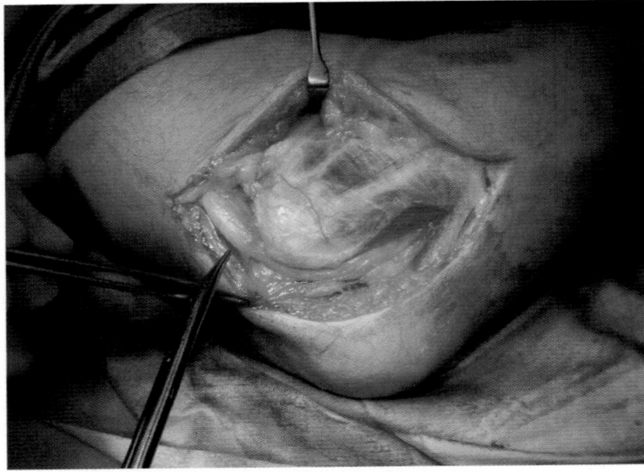

(c)

11.23 Ulnar nerve compression at the elbow The ulnar nerve may be compressed in the cubital tunnel by (a) tension in a valgus elbow or (b) osteoarthritic spurs. (c) Surgical release in situ.

Cubital tunnel syndrome

The ulnar nerve is easily felt behind the medial epicondyle of the humerus (the 'funny bone'). It can be trapped or compressed within the cubital tunnel (by bone abnormalities, ganglia or hypertrophied synovium), proximal to the cubital tunnel (by the fascial arcade of Struthers) or distal to the cubital tunnel as it passes through the two heads of flexor carpi ulnaris to enter the forearm (Osbourne's canal). Sometimes it is 'stretched' by a cubitus valgus deformity or simply by holding the elbow flexed for long periods.

Clinical features

The patient complains of numbness and tingling in the little and the ulnar half of the ring finger; symptoms may be intermittent and related to specific elbow postures (e.g. they may appear only while the patient is lying down with the elbows flexed, or while holding the newspaper – again with the elbows flexed). Initially there is little to see but in late cases there may be weakness of grip, slight clawing, intrinsic muscle wasting and diminished sensibility in the ulnar nerve territory. Froment's sign and weakness of abductor digiti minimi can often be demonstrated.

Bone or soft-tissue abnormalities may be obvious. Tinel's percussion test, tenderness over the nerve behind the medial epicondyle, reproduction of the symptoms with flexion of the elbow, and weakness of flexor carpi ulnaris and the flexor digitorum profundus to the little finger all suggest compression at the elbow rather than at the wrist.

The diagnosis may be confirmed by nerve conduction tests; however, since the symptoms are often postural or activity related, a negative test does not exclude the diagnosis.

Treatment

Conservative measures such as modification of posture and splintage of the elbow in mid-extension at night should be tried.

If symptoms persist, and particularly if there is intrinsic wasting, operative decompression is indicated. Options include simple release of the roof of the cubital tunnel, anterior transposition of the nerve into a subcutaneous or submuscular plane, or medial epicondylectomy. Simple release is preferable as it avoids the potential denervation associated with transposition or the persisting epicondylar pain associated with epicondylectomy. During the surgical approach, great care is taken to avoid damaging the posterior branch of the medial cutaneous nerve of the forearm; otherwise troublesome numbness, if not neurogenic pain or even complex regional pain syndrome, may result.

Compression in Guyon's canal

The ulnar nerve can be compressed as it passes through Guyon's canal at the ulnar border of the wrist. The symptoms can be pure motor, pure sensory or mixed, depending on the precise location of entrapment. A ganglion from the triquetrohamate joint is the most common cause; a fractured hook of hamate and ulnar artery aneurysm (seen with overuse of a hammer) are much rarer causes. Preservation of sensation in the dorsal branch of the ulnar nerve (which leaves the nerve proximal to Guyon's canal) suggests entrapment at the wrist rather than elbow; similarly, power to flexor carpi ulnaris and flexor digitorum profundus to the little finger will be maintained.

After electrophysiological localization of the lesion to the wrist, further investigations should be considered: MRI may demonstrate a ganglion, CT a carpal fracture and Doppler studies an ulnar artery aneurysm. Depending on the results of these investigations, surgery can be planned.

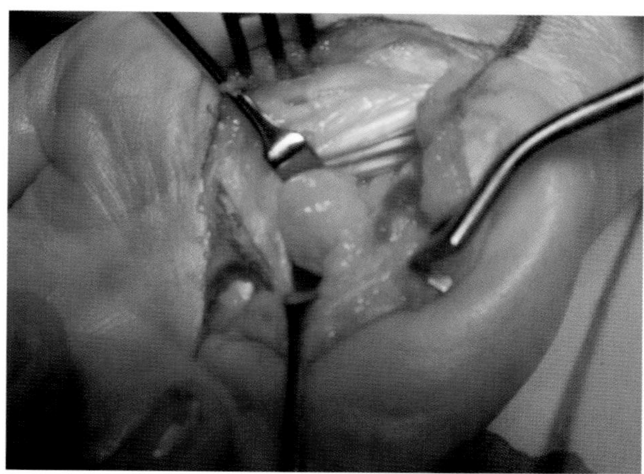

(a)

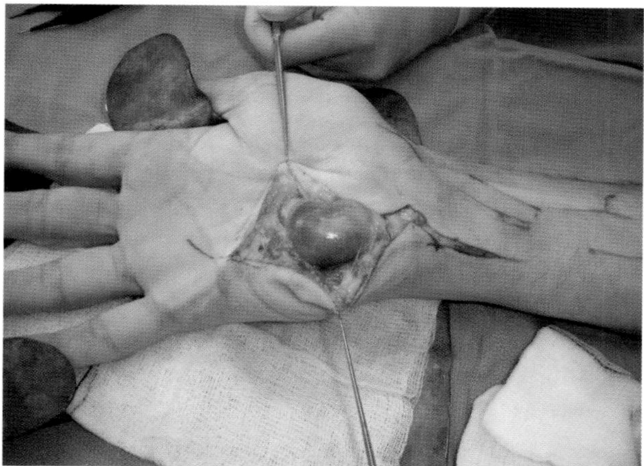

(b)

11.24 Ulnar nerve compression in Guyon's canal (a) Schwannoma pushing on the ulnar nerve. (b) Ulnar artery aneurysm.

Radial (posterior interosseous) nerve compression

The radial nerve itself is rarely the source of 'entrapment' symptoms. Just above the elbow, it divides into a superficial branch (sensory to the skin over the anatomical snuffbox) and the posterior interosseous nerve which dives between the two heads of the supinator muscle before supplying motor branches to extensor carpi ulnaris and the metacarpophalangeal extensors (branches to extensor carpi radialis longus and brevis arise above the elbow).

Posterior interosseous nerve compression may occur at five sites, represented by the mnemonic *FREAS* [*F*ibrous bands around radiocapitellar joint; *R*ecurrent arterial branches; *E*xtensor carpi radialis brevis, *A*rcade of Frohse (a thickening at the proximal edge of supinator); distal edge of *S*upinator]. It may also be caused by a space-occupying lesion pushing on the nerve – a ganglion, a lipoma or severe radio-capitellar synovitis.

Two clinical patterns are encountered: the *posterior interosseous syndrome* and the *radial tunnel syndrome.*

Posterior interosseous syndrome

Clinical features

This is a pure motor disorder and there are no sensory symptoms. Gradually emerging weakness of metacarpophalangeal extension affects first one or two and then all the digits. Wrist extension is preserved (the nerves to extensor carpi radialis longus arise proximal to the supinator) but the wrist veers into radial deviation because of the weak extensor carpi ulnaris. This feature helps to distinguish posterior interosseous nerve entrapment from conditions such as neuralgic amyotrophy, in which the more proximally supplied muscles are often affected.

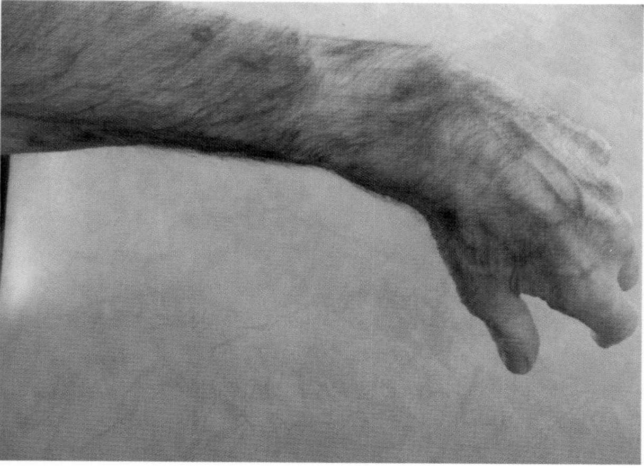

11.25 Posterior interosseous nerve compression Wrist in radial deviation; fingers dropped.

Compression usually occurs within the tunnel (FREAS) but it may also be caused by swellings (a lipoma, a ganglion or synovial proliferation) in or around the radial tunnel. MRI may help to pinpoint the diagnosis.

Treatment

Surgical exploration is warranted if the condition does not resolve spontaneously within three months or earlier if MRI shows a swelling. Recovery after surgery is slow; if there is no improvement by the end of a year, and if muscle weakness is disabling, tendon transfer is needed.

RADIAL TUNNEL SYNDROME

This syndrome is controversial; the symptoms resemble those of 'tennis elbow' and the condition is sometimes labelled *'resistant tennis elbow'*. However a careful history and examination should distinguish between the two.

Although a motor nerve is involved the patient presents with pain, often work-related or at night, just distal to the lateral aspect of the elbow. Resisted wrist extension may precipitate the pain. Unlike posterior interosseous syndrome, there is no weakness and there is not an association with a mass lesion. Electrodiagnostic tests are not helpful.

If the symptoms do not resolve with prolonged non-operative measures (modification of activities and splintage), then surgery is considered. The nerve is freed beneath the extensor carpi radialis brevis and supinator muscle. However, the patient should be warned that surgery often fails to relieve the symptoms.

SUPRASCAPULAR NERVE COMPRESSION

Chronic or repetitive compression of the suprascapular nerve and its branches is much more common than is generally recognized. The peculiar anatomy of the nerve makes it unusually vulnerable to both traction and compression. However, the symptoms of this condition closely mimic those of rotator cuff lesions and cervical radiculopathy; unless the diagnosis is kept in mind in all such cases, it is likely to be missed.

The suprascapular nerve arises from the upper trunk of the brachial plexus in the posterior triangle of the neck and then courses through the suprascapular notch beneath the superior transverse scapular ligament to supply the supraspinatus and infraspinatus muscles. It also sends sensory branches to the posterior part of the glenohumeral joint, the acromioclavicular joint, the subacromial bursa, the ligaments around the shoulder and (in a small proportion of people) the skin on the outer, upper aspect of the arm.

Compression or entrapment occurs at two sites: (a) the suprascapular notch and (b) a fibro-osseous tunnel where the infraspinatus branch curves around the edge of the scapular spine. Causes are continuous pressure or intermittent impact on the supraclavicular muscles (e.g. by carrying loads on the shoulder) or repetitive traction due to forceful shoulder movements (e.g. in games which involve pitching and throwing). In some cases nerve compression may be produced by a soft-tissue mass such as a large 'ganglion' at the back of the shoulder joint.

Clinical features

There may be a history of injury to the pectoral girdle; more often patients present with unexplained pain in the suprascapular region or at the back of the shoulder, and weakness of shoulder and upper arm movements – symptoms readily mistaken for cervical radiculopathy or a rotator cuff disorder. There is usually wasting of the supraspinatus muscle and diminished power of abduction and external rotation. Tensing the nerve by forceful adduction (pulling the arm across the front of the chest) causes increased pain.

Special investigations

Electromyography and measurement of nerve conduction velocity may help to establish the diagnosis. Ultrasonography and MRI are useful in excluding a soft-tissue mass.

Treatment

The first step is to stop any type of activity which might stress the suprascapular nerve; after a few weeks, graded muscle-strengthening exercises can be introduced. If the condition is likely to settle, it will do so within 3–6 months.

If there is no improvement, or if imaging studies reveal a soft-tissue mass, operative decompression is justified. The nerve is approached through a posterior incision above and parallel to the spine of the scapula. Provided the diagnosis was correct, there is a good chance that symptoms will be improved; however, some muscle wasting will probably remain.

THORACIC OUTLET SYNDROME

Neurological and vascular symptoms and signs in the upper limbs may be produced by compression of the lower trunk of the brachial plexus (C8 and T1) and subclavian vessels between the clavicle and the first rib.

The subclavian artery and lower brachial trunk pass through a triangle based on the first rib and bordered by scalenus anterior and medius. These neurovascular structures are made taut when the shoulders are braced back and the arms held tightly to the sides; an extra rib (or its fibrous equivalent extending from a large costal process), or an anomalous scalene muscle, exaggerates this effect by forcing the vessel and nerve upwards.

These anomalies are all congenital, yet symptoms are rare before the age of 30. This is probably because, with increasing age, the shoulders sag, thus putting more traction on the neurovascular bundle; indeed drooping shoulders alone may cause the syndrome and symptoms are characteristically posture-related.

Stretching or compression of the lower nerve trunk produces sensory changes along the ulnar side of the forearm and hand, and weakness of the intrinsic hand muscles. The subclavian artery is rarely compressed but the lumen may contract due to irritation of its sympathetic supply, or else its wall may be damaged leading to the formation of small emboli. Even more unusual are signs of venous compression – oedema, cyanosis or thrombosis.

Clinical features

The patient, typically a woman in her 30s, complains of pain and paraesthesia extending from the shoulder, down the ulnar aspect of the arm and into the medial two fingers. Symptoms tend to be worse at night and are aggravated by bracing the shoulders (wearing a back-pack) or working with the arms above shoulder height. Examination may show mild clawing of the ulnar two fingers with wasting and weakness of the intrinsic muscles. If a female, the patient is often long-necked with sloping shoulders (like a Modigliani painting).

Vascular signs are uncommon, but there may be cyanosis, coldness of the fingers and increased sweating. *Unilateral Raynaud's phenomenon should make one think 'thoracic outlet'.*

Symptoms and signs may be reproduced by various provocative manoeuvres. In *Adson's test* the patient's neck is extended and turned towards the affected side while he or she breathes in deeply; this compresses the interscalene space and may cause paraesthesia and obliteration of the radial pulse. In *Wright's test* the arms are abducted and externally rotated; again the symptoms recur and the pulse disappears on the abnormal side. The examination is continued by asking the patient to hold his or her arms high above their head and then open and close the fingers rapidly; this may cause cramping pain on the affected side (*Roos's test*). Unfortunately these tests are neither sensitive nor specific enough to clinch the diagnosis.

Investigations

X-rays of the neck occasionally demonstrate a cervical rib or an abnormally long C7 cervical process. X-rays should also be obtained of the lungs (is there an apical tumour?) and the shoulders (to exclude any painful local lesion).

Angiography and *venography* are reserved for the few patients with vascular symptoms.

Electrodiagnostic tests are helpful mainly to exclude peripheral nerve lesions such as ulnar or median nerve compression which may confuse the diagnosis.

Diagnosis

In the absence of clear motor signs (which are rare!) the diagnosis of thoracic outlet syndrome is not easy. Some of the symptoms occur as transient phenomena in *normal individuals*, and 'cervical ribs' are sometimes discovered as incidental findings in patients who are x-rayed for other reasons. Postural obliteration of the radial pulse, likewise, may be quite normal; the provocative tests should be interpreted as positive only if they affect the pulse *and* reproduce the sensory symptoms.

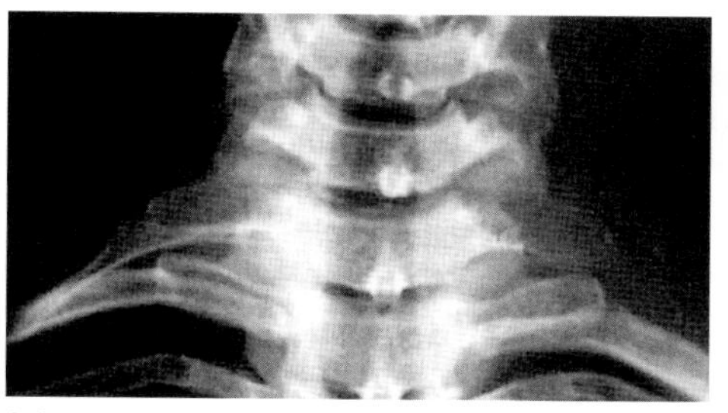
(a)

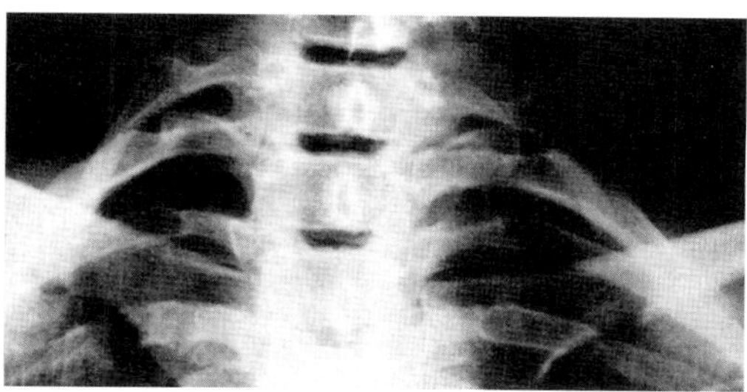
(b)

11.26 Cervical rib (a) Unilateral on right side and (b) bilateral.

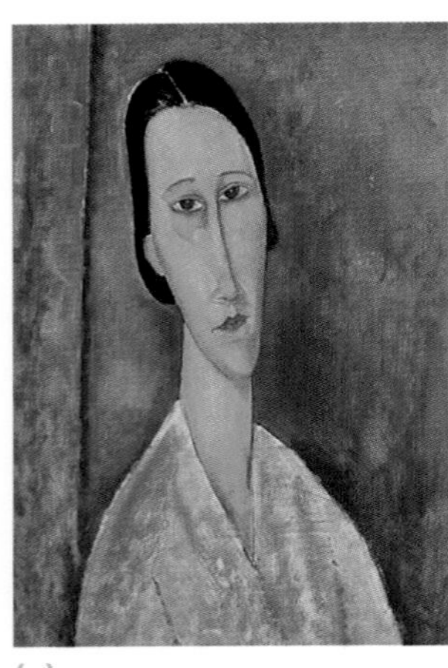

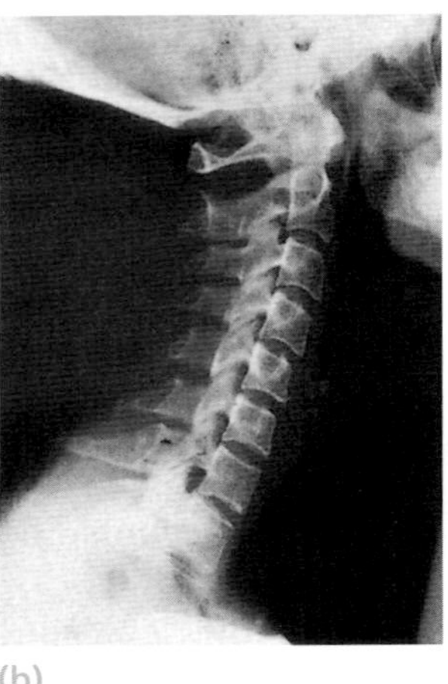

(a) (b)

11.27 Thoracic outlet syndrome (a) Amadeo Modigliani's painting of Madame Zborowska (courtesy of the Tate Gallery, London). (b) X-ray of a long-necked woman: all the vertebrae down to T1 are above the clavicle.

The early symptoms and signs can be mistaken for those of *ulnar nerve compression*. In fact, ulnar neuropathy may accompany thoracic outlet compression as a manifestation of the double-crush syndrome. There is pain and numbness over the medial side of the forearm and hand. In severe cases there will be wasting of all the intrinsic muscles (T1) and weakness of the long flexors (C8).

Cervical spondylosis is sometimes discovered on x-ray. However, this disorder seldom involves the T1 nerve root.

Pancoast's syndrome, due to apical carcinoma of the bronchus with infiltration of the structures at the root of the neck, includes pain, numbness and weakness of the hand. A hard mass may be palpable in the neck and x-ray of the chest shows a characteristic opacity.

Rotator cuff lesions sometimes cause pain radiating down the arm. However, there are no neurological symptoms and shoulder movement is likely to be abnormal.

Treatment

Most patients can be managed by *conservative treatment*: exercises to strengthen the shoulder girdle muscles, postural training and instruction in work practices and ways of preventing shoulder droop and muscle fatigue. Analgesics may be needed for pain.

Operative treatment is indicated if pain is severe, if muscle wasting is obvious or if there are vascular disturbances. The thoracic outlet is decompressed by removing the first rib (or the cervical rib). This is accomplished by either a supraclavicular approach or a transaxillary approach; in the latter, care must be taken to prevent injury to the brachial plexus and subclavian vessels, or perforation of the pleura. Patients with arterial obstruction, distal embolism or a local aneurysm will need vascular reconstruction as well as decompression.

LOWER LIMB COMPRESSION SYNDROMES

COMPRESSION OF LATERAL CUTANEOUS NERVE OF THE THIGH

The lateral cutaneous nerve can be compressed as it runs through the inguinal ligament just medial to the anterior superior iliac spine.

The patient complains of numbness, tingling or burning discomfort over the anterolateral aspect of the thigh (*meralgia paraesthetica*). Testing for sensibility to pinprick will reveal a patch of numbness over the upper outer thigh.

If the symptoms are troublesome the nerve can be released.

Tarsal tunnel syndrome

Pain and sensory disturbance over the plantar surface of the foot may be due to compression of the posterior tibial nerve behind and below the medial malleolus. The pain may be precipitated by prolonged weightbearing. It is often worse at night and the patient may seek relief by walking around or stamping his or her foot. Paraesthesia and numbness should follow the characteristic sensory distribution, but these symptoms are not as well defined as in other entrapment syndromes. Tinel's percussion test may be positive behind the medial malleolus. The diagnosis is difficult to establish but nerve conduction studies may show slowing of motor or sensory conduction.

Treatment

Tarsal tunnel entrapment may be relieved by fitting a medial arch support that holds the foot in slight varus. If this fails, surgical decompression is indicated. The nerve is exposed behind the medial malleolus and followed into the sole; sometimes it is trapped by the belly of abductor hallucis arising more proximally than usual. Unfortunately symptoms are not consistently relieved by this procedure.

DIGITAL NERVE COMPRESSION IN THE FOOT

Compression neuropathy of the digital nerve (Morton's metatarsalgia) is dealt with in Chapter 21.

OTHER PERIPHERAL NERVE DISORDERS

Compartment syndromes

Capillary perfusion of a nerve may be markedly reduced by swelling within an osteofascial compartment. Direct trauma, prolonged compression or arterial injury may result in muscle swelling and a critical rise in compartment pressure; if unrelieved, this causes further impedance of blood flow, more prolonged ischaemia and so on into a vicious circle of events ending in necrosis of nerve and muscle. This may occur after proximal arterial injury, soft-tissue bleeding from fractures or operations, circular compression by tight dressings or plasters, and even direct pressure in a comatose person lying on a hard surface. Lesser, self-relieving effects are sometimes produced by muscle swelling due to strenuous exercise. Common sites are the forearm and leg; less common are the foot, upper arm and thigh.

ACUTE COMPARTMENT SYNDROME

Acute compartment syndrome and its late effects (Volkmann's contracture) are described in Chapter 23.

CHRONIC COMPARTMENT SYNDROME

Long-distance runners sometimes develop pain along the anterolateral aspect of the calf, brought on by muscular exertion. Swelling of the anterior calf muscles contained within the inexpansile deep fascia causes ischaemia of the deep peroneal nerve as it traverses the compartment. The condition is diagnosed from the history and can be confirmed by measuring the compartment pressure before and after exercise. Release of the fascia is curative. The same syndrome is very rarely seen in the forearm muscles.

IATROPATHIC INJURIES

Positioning the patient for diagnostic or operative procedures needs careful attention so as to avoid compression or traction on nerves at vulnerable sites. The brachial plexus, radial nerve, ulnar nerve and common peroneal nerve are particularly at risk. Recovery may take anything from a few minutes to several months; permanent loss of function is unusual.

During operation an important nerve may be injured by accidental scalpel or diathermy wounds, excessive traction, compression by instruments, snaring by sutures or heating and compression by extruded acrylic cement. Nerves most frequently involved are the spinal accessory or the trunks of the brachial plexus (during operations in the posterior triangle of the neck), the axillary and musculocutaneous nerves (during operations for recurrent dislocation of the shoulder), the posterior interosseous branch of the radial nerve (during approaches to the proximal end of the radius), the median nerve at the wrist (in tendon surgery), the palmar cutaneous branch of the median nerve (in carpal tunnel release), the cutaneous branch of the radial nerve (when operating for de Quervain's disease), the digital nerves (in operations for Dupuytren's contracture), the sciatic nerve (in hip arthroplasty), the common peroneal nerve (in operations around the knee) and the sural nerve (in operations on the calcaneum).

Tourniquet pressure is an important cause of nerve injury in orthopaedic operations. Damage is due to direct pressure rather than prolonged ischaemia; injury is therefore more likely with very high cuff pressure (it need never be more than 75 mmHg above systolic pressure), a non-pneumatic tourniquet or a very narrow cuff. However, ischaemic damage may occur at 'acceptable' pressures if the tourniquet is left on for more than 2 hours.

Manipulative pressure or traction – e.g. during reduction of a fracture or dislocation – may injure a nerve coursing close to the bone or across the joint. Shoulder abduction and varus angulation of the knee under anaesthesia are particularly dangerous. Even moderate pressure or traction can be harmful in patients with peripheral neuropathy; this is always a risk in alcoholics and diabetics.

Injections are occasionally misdirected and delivered into a nerve (usually the radial or sciatic during intramuscular injection, the median nerve during non-operative treatment of carpal tunnel syndrome or the brachial plexus during axillary blockade).

Irradiation may cause irreparable nerve damage, a mishap not always avoidable when treating cancer. The effects may not appear until a year or two after exposure.

Diagnosis

Following operations in 'high-risk' areas of the body, local nerve function should always be tested as soon as the patient is awake. Even then it may be difficult to distinguish true weakness or sensory change from the 'normal' postoperative discomfort and unwillingness to move.

Initially it may be impossible to tell whether the lesion is a neurapraxia, axonotmesis or neurotmesis. With closed procedures it is more likely to be a lesser injury, with open ones a greater. If there is no recovery after a few weeks, EMG may be helpful. The demonstration of denervation potentials suggests either axonotmesis or neurotmesis. Surgical exploration at this early stage gives the best chance of a favourable outcome.

Prevention and treatment

Awareness is all. Knowing the situations in which there is a real risk of nerve injury is the best way to prevent the calamity. The operative exposure should be safe and well rehearsed; important nerves should be given a wide berth or otherwise kept under vision and out of harm's way; retraction should be gentle and intermittent; hidden branches (such as the posterior interosseous nerve in the supinator muscle) should be retracted with their muscular covering. It goes without saying that self-retaining retractors should never be used to retract nerves.

If a nerve is seen to be divided during surgery, it should be repaired immediately; if this cannot be done, the wound can be closed, help can be summoned and the nerve can be re-explored as soon as possible.

If the injury is discovered only after the operation, it is best to re-operate as soon as possible, referring the patient to a specialized centre if needed.

If nerve division is thought to be unlikely, then it is wiser to wait for signs that might clarify the diagnosis. If there is marked loss of function and no flicker of recovery by 6 weeks, the nerve should be explored. Even then, fibrosis may make diagnosis difficult; nerve stimulation will show whether there is conduction across the injured segment. Partial lesions or injuries that cause only minor disability are probably best left alone. More serious lesions may need excision and repair or grafting.

LEPROSY

Long-term disabilities in patients with leprosy are due mainly to peripheral nerve abnormalities which result in *loss of sensibility* and *muscle weakness* affecting the hands and feet (see Chapter 2). The former may result in poor wound healing, ulceration and scarring – mainly affecting the hands. The latter may result in deformity and joint instability.

THE HAND

The ulnar nerve is most often affected; combined ulnar and median nerve paralysis is less common and triple nerve (ulnar, median and radial) paralysis is rare. Any other kind of paralysis is extremely rare. The clinical features associated with these conditions are summarized in Table 11.1 and typical deformities are shown in the accompanying figures.

Claw-finger correction

This deformity is improved, and the movements lost due to intrinsic muscle paralysis are restored, by rebalancing muscle pull at the metacarpophalangeal (MCP) or proximal interphalangeal (PIP) joint or at both joints. A number of operations have been employed to achieve this end (Table 11.2). The operation currently favoured by most surgeons is the 'lasso operation' of Zancolli in which one tendon of flexor digitorum superficialis (FDS) is split into four slips and one slip each is looped around the A1 pulley of each affected finger so as to provide an independent flexor to MCP joints.

The thumb in ulnar palsy

The severely unstable thumb due to flexor pollicis brevis (FPB) paresis (Figs 11.30 and 11.31) can be

Table 11.1 Clinical features of paralytic hand deformities in leprosy

Pattern of paralysis	Frequency	Deformity	Consequence	Disability
Isolated (high or low) ulnar nerve paralysis	Most common	Partial claw-hand Ulnar palsy thumb, Z deformity	Intrinsic muscle deficiency Froment's sign	Poor precision handling Weak grip
Combined ulnar and low median nerve paralysis	Less common	Total claw-hand Claw fingers and claw thumb	'Intrinsic zero' hand All intrinsic muscles paralysed Fingers and thumb activated by long muscles only	Only thumb–index (lateral pinch or 'key grip') and hook grips possible. Power grip and precision handing become difficult or impossible
Ulnar, low median and radial nerve paralysis	Rare	Drop-wrist and dropped digits	'Long-flexor driven' hand All intrinsic muscles and long extensors paralysed	Severe loss of function Cannot grasp or hold objects
Combined ulnar and high median nerve paralysis	Very rare	Mild clawing	'Extensor driven' hand All intrinsic muscles and long flexors paralysed	Very severe functional loss Cannot grip
Ulnar, high median and radial nerve paralysis	Very rare	Drop-wrist	Denervated hand All muscles below elbow paralysed	Total loss of function

Table 11.2 Strategies and tactics for claw-finger correction

Strategy	Tactic	Procedure
Restore balance at MCP joint	Reduce extending force Increase flexing forces Increase flexor moment arm	Extensor diversion graft[1] operation Capsulodesis[2] Tenodesis[3,4] Dermodesis[5] Pulley advancement[6]
Restore balance at PIP joint	Reduce flexing force Increase extending force	FDS transfer of Bunnell[7] FDS transfer of Bunnell[7]
Restore balance at both joints	Tendon transfer operations in which the transfer is routed volar to MCP and dorsal to PIP joints	ECRL/ECRB transfers of Brand[8] Palmaris longus transfer of Antia[9] Fowler's digital extensor transfer and other similar procedures

[1]Srinivasan, [2]Zancolli, [3]Parkes, [4]Riordan, [5]Srinivasan, [6]Palande, [7]Bunnell, [8]Brand, [9]Antia, [10]Zancolli.
ECRB, extensor carpi radialis brevis; ECRL, extensor carpi radialis longus; FDS, flexor digitorum superficialis; MCP, metacarpophalangeal; PIP, proximal interphalangeal.

corrected by augmenting flexion at the MCP joint or extension at the interphalangeal joint or both. In one procedure, the radial half of flexor pollicis longus (FPL) tendon is 'dorsalized' by bringing it over the proximal phalanx distal to the MCP joint and fixing it to extensor pollicis longus tendon, turning FPL into an MCP flexor. Alternatively, FPB can be substituted by transferring the radial half of the index flexor superficialis tendon.

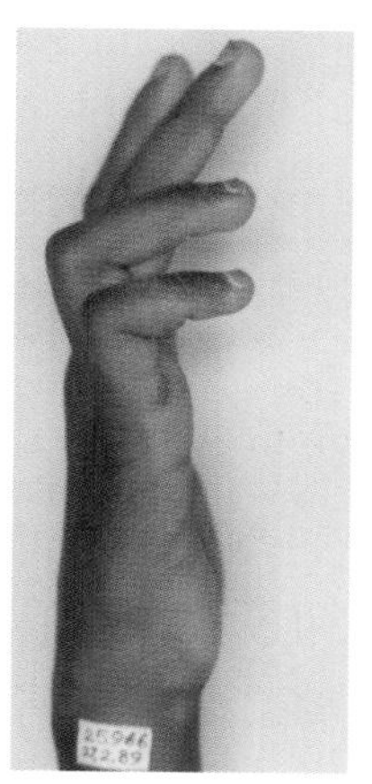

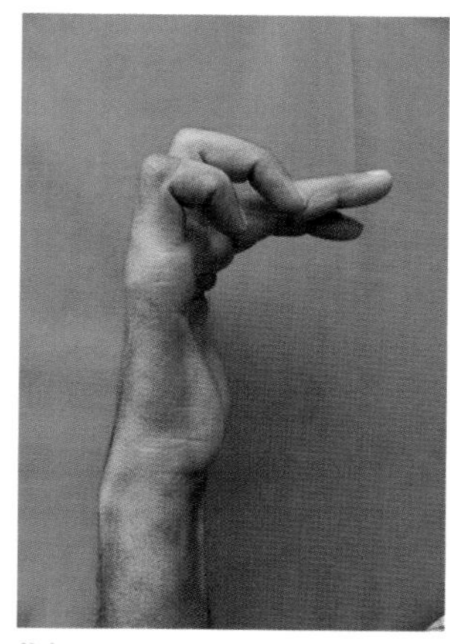

(a) (b)

11.28 Partial claw hand (a) Partial claw-hand deformity in ulnar nerve paralysis: ring and little fingers are clawed more severely than index and middle fingers. The virtually straight terminal phalanges of the clawed ring and little fingers indicate that flexor digitorum profundus going to these two fingers is paralysed, so this must be a case of 'high' ulnar paralysis. (Courtesy of Dr G. N. Malaviya.) (b) 'Intrinsic minus' disability: isolated PIP extension. Keeping the metacarpophalangeal joints in flexion is not possible. (Courtesy of Dr Santosh Rath.)

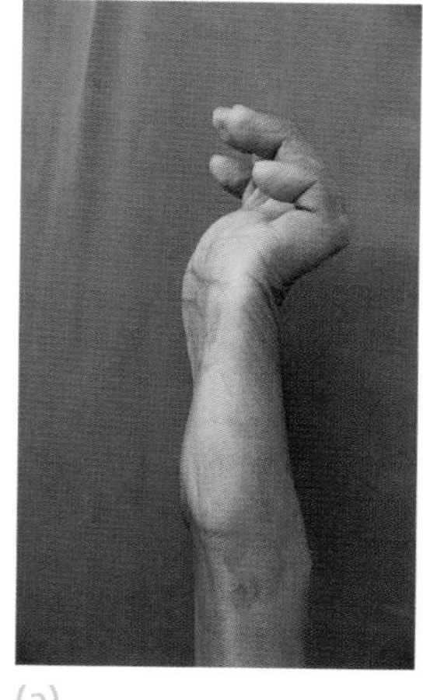

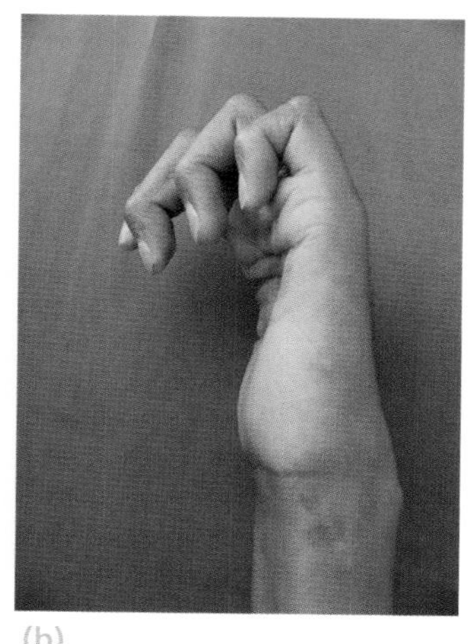

(a) (b)

11.29 Total claw hand (a) Total claw-hand deformity in combined paralysis of ulnar and median nerves. The flexed terminal phalanges of the ring and little fingers indicate that this is a case of 'low' ulnar paralysis, i.e. distal to the elbow beyond the points of origin of the motor branches of flexor digitorum profundus. (b) With intrinsic minus disability, isolated metacarpophalangeal flexion is not possible. (Courtesy of Dr Santosh Rath.)

The thumb in combined ulnar and median nerve paralysis

Complete paralysis of all thenar muscles (the '*intrinsic-zero*' thumb) results in loss of effective power and precision-grip (Fig. 11.30). Correction requires stabilization of the carpometacarpal joint in the 'opponens position' (abduction, flexion and internal rotation) by opponensplasty using flexor superficialis of the middle or ring finger or extensor indicis proprius.

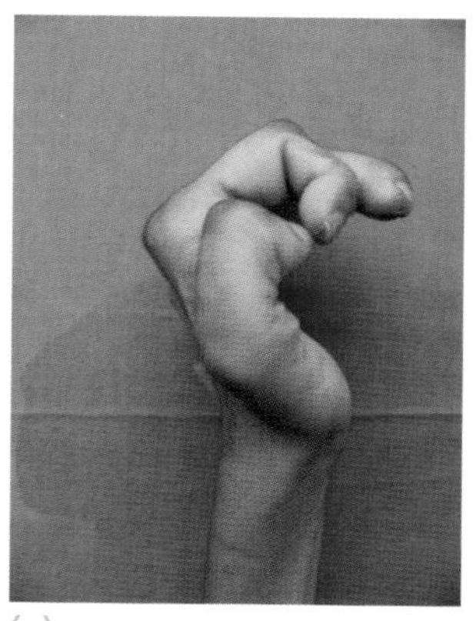

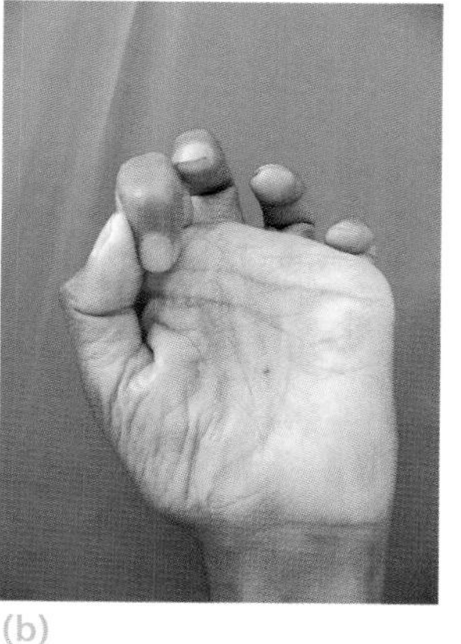

(a) (b)

11.30 Claw thumb (a) 'Claw-thumb' (hyperextended at the basal and flexed at the middle and distal joints) in combined ulnar and median nerve paralysis. Note wasting of the thenar eminence. (b) Illustrating pinch in thenar paralysis. Only the lateral or 'key-pinch' is possible for these hands. (Courtesy of Dr Santosh Rath.)

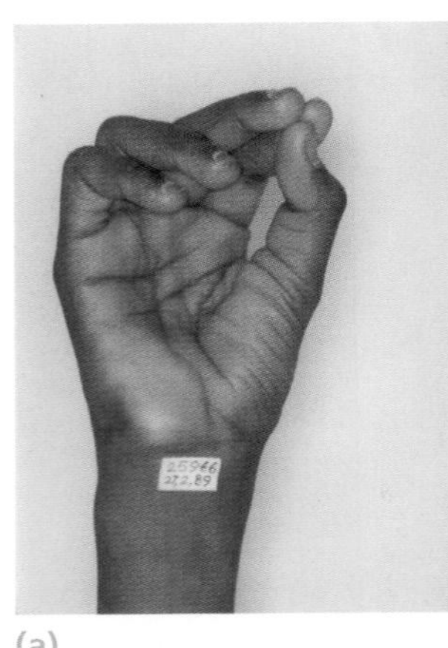

(a)

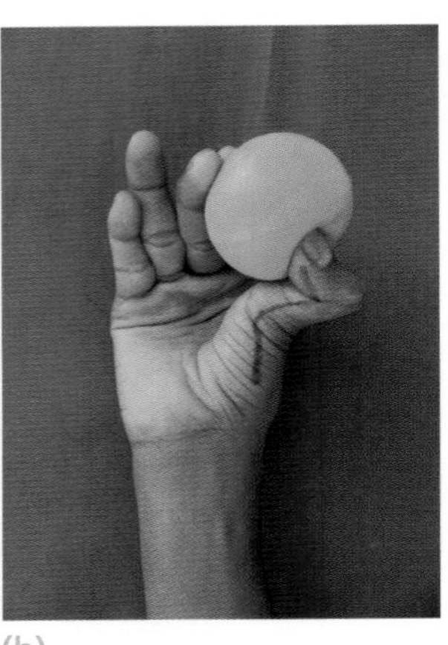

(b)

11.31 Thumb in ulnar palsy with paralysis of flexor pollicis brevis (a) While at rest the proximal phalanx is de-rotated and lies in line with the metacarpal instead of being flexed by about 25 degrees, and the distal phalanx is flexed by about 15 degrees. (Courtesy of Dr G. N. Malaviya.) (b) Acting against resistance, the thumb collapses into hyperextension at the metacarpophalangeal joint and hyperflexion at the interphalangeal joint (Z deformity). (Courtesy of Dr Santosh Rath.)

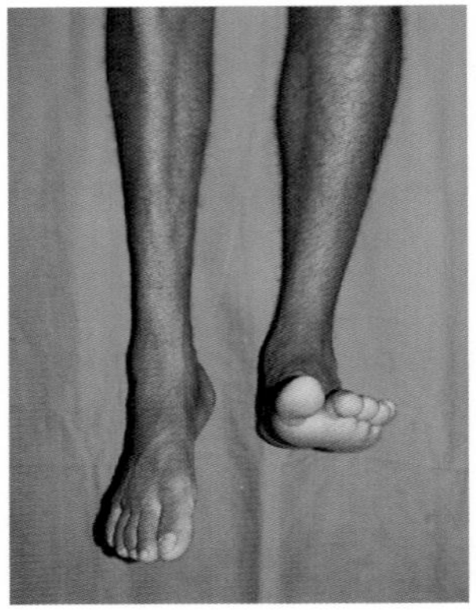

(a)

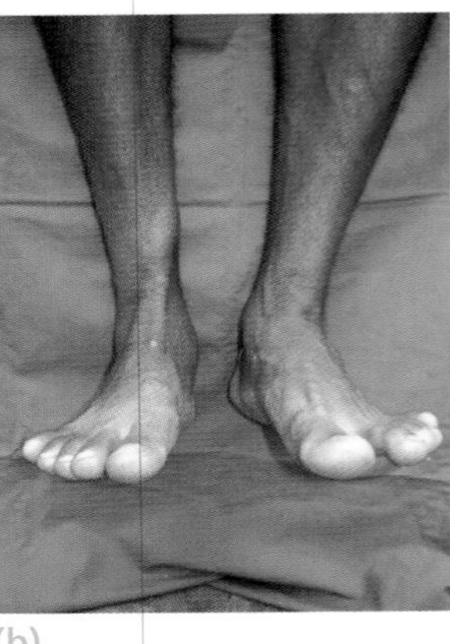

(b)

11.32 Right drop-foot (a) Preoperative deformity. The patient is attempting to lift both feet but can do so only on the left side. (b) Same patient one year after surgical correction by two-tailed circumtibial transfer of tibialis posterior to extensor hallucis longus and extensor digitorum longus tendons over the dorsum of the foot. (Courtesy of Dr Santosh Rath.)

Triple paralysis

Combined loss of ulnar, median and radial nerve function causes very severe disability. The patient has a 'flexor driven' hand as only the long flexors of the fingers and the wrist flexors are active. Multiple tendon transfers to stabilize the wrist, fingers and thumb in extension are needed; the resulting functionally 'intrinsic zero' hand is then corrected.

THE FOOT IN LEPROSY

Feet are involved less often than hands but the consequences are more serious. Problems include drop-foot, claw toes, plantar ulceration and tarsal disorganization.

Drop-foot

'Drop-foot' occurs in 1–2 per cent of leprosy patients, because of paralysis of muscles in the anterior and lateral compartments of the leg consequent to damage to the common peroneal nerve. Sometimes only the dorsiflexors or the evertors of the foot are paralysed.

In *dorsiflexor paralysis* the patient has to lift the leg higher than usual during walking for clearing the ground (high-stepping gait). If the condition is neglected, the foot becomes stiff in equinus with intractable forefoot ulceration.

In *evertor paralysis* the foot remains inverted when striking the ground and during the push-off stage of walking. In the course of time, the foot becomes stiff in varus, the weightbearing lateral part of the foot gets damaged and ulcers develop here. In neglected cases the outer part of the foot is destroyed by repeated ulceration.

A suitable drop-foot orthosis offers a temporary solution, only until corrective surgery is available. The choice of operation depends on whether the deformity is mobile or fixed.

Mobile drop-foot This is corrected by transfer of tibialis posterior tendon, which is almost never paralysed in leprosy. The tendon is re-routed to run in front of the ankle and is fixed in the foot so that the muscle now acts as a dorsiflexor (Fig. 11.32b). Skeletal fixation of the transferred tendon is not advised as that might precipitate tarsal disorganization. Circumtibial, two-tailed tibialis posterior tendon transfer to extensor hallucis and extensor digitorum longus tendons over the dorsum of the foot is most commonly done; it is usually combined with tendo calcaneus lengthening. When only the anterior compartment muscles are paralysed, a similar transfer of peroneus longus is done.

Fixed drop-foot deformity Fixed equinus or equinovarus usually requires triple arthrodesis of the hindfoot (Lambinudi's operation), which should provide the patient with a plantigrade foot.

Claw-toes

This condition, due to plantar intrinsic muscle paralysis, is more common than drop-foot. It increases the risk of plantar ulceration greatly. Treatment depends on the severity of the deformity.

First degree (mild) claw-toes There is no joint stiffness but the tips of the toes become ulcerated. The deformity is corrected by transfer of the long flexor to the extensor expansion of each toe.

Second degree (moderate) claw-toes The interphalangeal joints have fixed flexion but the metatarsophalangeal joints remain mobile. PIP arthrodesis, with or without excision of the distal interphalangeal (DIP) joint, is needed.

Third degree (severe) claw-toes Fixed flexion of the IP joints is associated with dorsal migration of the toes and fixed hyperextension of the metatarsophalangeal (MTP) joints; the metatarsal heads are pushed down towards the sole of the forefoot (plunger effect). Trans-metatarsal amputation is probably the treatment of choice, but patients usually reject this option. A more conservative solution requires open reduction of the MTP joints, proximalization of the long extensor tendons and PIP arthrodesis. Surgical syndactyly helps to fix a 'floating toe'.

Plantar ulceration (trophic ulcers)

Painless chronic ulcers that occur 'spontaneously' are commonly seen in the soles of neurologically compromised feet. They heal with difficulty and recur easily. Loss of sensibility is the main predisposing cause and the risk of ulceration increases greatly when plantar intrinsic muscles are paralysed or when there is some deformity. Plantar ulcers are colonized by 'street bacteria'; they remain chronic because they are not treated properly.

About 80 per cent of the ulcers are located in the ball of the foot (the majority under the first MTP joint), about 8 per cent in the cubo-metatarsal joint region, about 10 per cent in the heel, and about 2 per cent over the tips of the toes.

PATHOGENESIS

During walking the body-load shifts from the heel to the forefoot and from the lateral to the medial side of the forefoot. In this process the subcutaneous tissues suffer significant compression, shear and stretch, which is normally countered by the intrinsic muscles. These stresses are increased momentarily with each step when the intrinsic muscles are paralysed. Even slightly increased stresses, if repetitive, eventually lead to tissue damage. A *necrosis blister* develops and that breaks down to form an ulcer.

Injuries occurring in insensitive feet are often neglected because the patient does not experience pain. Wounds fester and develop into ulcers. Even in the absence of any injury, the lack of sweating in the denervated sole predisposes to the development of cracks and fissures and they easily become infected.

NATURAL HISTORY

The natural history of plantar ulcers is a dismal cycle of: ulceration – infection – tissue loss – healing – breakdown of scar – recurrent ulceration – spread of infection with further tissue loss – healing with deformity – more frequent recurrences, and so on until the forefoot is destroyed, tarsal sepsis supervenes and the foot is lost or removed. Sometimes lethal complications (gas gangrene, septicaemia or malignancy) supervene.

MANAGEMENT

A *necrosis blister* should be treated promptly by compression bandaging, rest and elevation for 3 days, followed by a below-knee walking plaster of Paris cast for 3 weeks. If the blister is likely to burst, it is opened under aseptic conditions and dressed before applying the cast.

Simple ulcers present as chronic, shallow lesions. They remain unhealed because they are subjected to the repetitive trauma of walking. A below-knee walking-cast, which eliminates the forefoot stage of the walking cycle, is applied and kept on for 6 weeks. Split-thickness skin grafting hastens healing of large simple ulcers. Walking is resumed gradually and only with protective footwear.

Acute infected ulcers require bed rest, elevation of the foot, frequent wet dressings and local irrigation. Systemic antibiotics are used if there are symptoms and signs of general infection. Surgery is limited to drainage procedures.

Complicated ulcers are chronic ulcers associated with additional factors such as infection of deeper structures or deformity. The principles of management are ulcer debridement (which may have to be repeated many times) and protected weightbearing; deformity correction and stabilizing operations (like arthrodesis) are performed, if needed, after sound healing has been obtained. Sometimes chronic ulcers present as 'cauliflower growths' which commonly turn out to be pseudo-epitheliomas or less commonly epitheliomas of low grade malignancy. Deep local excision is adequate as treatment and essential for histological confirmation.

Recurrent plantar ulcers occur because the original causes (anaesthesia, muscle paralysis and walking) persist. Additional factors are: poor quality skin, excessive loading of the scar, deep-seated infection and poor blood supply. The risk can be minimized by constant vigilance and attention to hydration of the sole, the use of protective footwear, restricted walking and correction of stress-inducing deformities.

Excessive pressures due to prominent metatarsal heads on the sole of the foot can be treated by: (a) plantar condylectomy and transfer of the long extensor tendons to the metatarsal necks; (b) dorsal displacement metatarsal osteotomies; or (c) excision of an entire ray in the foot.

Intractable ulceration along the lateral border of the foot, due to equinovarus deformity, will need an appropriate triple arthrodesis or a more complicated joint-sparing procedure to render the foot plantigrade.

Heel scars may require plastic surgical flaps combined with 'bumpectomy' to remove bony prominences. Deformities of the calcaneum which produce high-pressure areas should be treated by re-establishing the posterior pillar of the arch of the foot, by doing an appropriately designed calcaneal osteotomy. Sometimes subtotal resection of the calcaneum is needed to get rid of persistent infection; after this type of surgery the inside of the shoe heel will need to be padded.

OTHER OPERATIONS

In suitably selected cases, posterior tibial neurovascular decompression behind and above the ankle improves the blood supply to the sole and helps heal a recurring or non-healing ulcer.

'Flail foot' after loss of the talus is corrected by tibio-calcaneal fusion.

Neuropathic tarsal disorganization

ASEPTIC DISORGANIZATION

Aseptic tarsal disorganization is uncommon. It may follow an inadequately treated fracture of a tarsal bone. In the early stages the patient may have mild pain during walking and on examination there is local swelling, warmth and tenderness. X-rays show the typical features of neuropathic bone necrosis and disorganization (Fig. 11.33)

Treatment consists of complete avoidance of all weightbearing and movement, enforced bed rest and application of a total-contact cast that is renewed periodically until the soft-tissue swelling disappears (usually 8–12 weeks), and then for another 4 weeks. If the foot is then found to be stable, a walking cast is applied for a further 4–6 weeks, to be followed by the use of an appropriate orthosis. If the foot is unstable, operative stabilization will be needed.

SEPTIC TARSAL DISORGANIZATION

Infection may spread from a plantar ulcer to underlying tarsal bones and joints and destroy these structures. Once the infection is controlled, the foot is immobilized in a below-knee cast; the involved bones fuse together and a stable, rigid foot results. An unstable foot will need surgical stabilization after clearing the infection.

Amputations

Occasionally amputation is necessary to keep the patient ambulatory. However, this step should not be taken without careful consideration; amputation merely shifts the problem to a more proximal level where it will be even more difficult to manage because the stump is often insensitive in these patients. Moreover, facilities for prostheses are scarce in many of the areas where leprosy is endemic, and even where they are available, hand deformities or poor vision in affected persons make their use difficult. The guiding principles are: amputate only if you must, amputate conservatively and try to provide an end-bearing stump where possible.

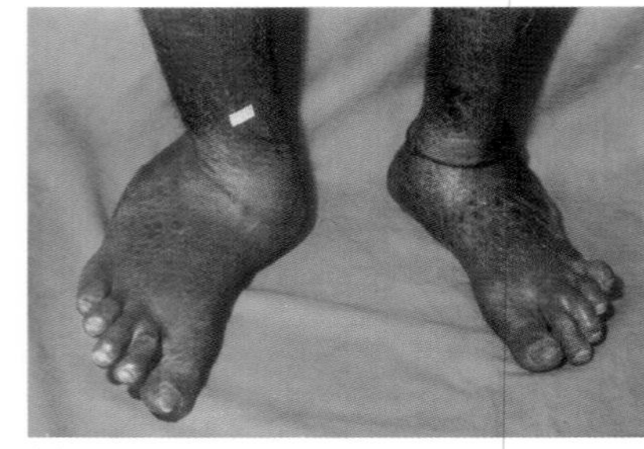

(a)

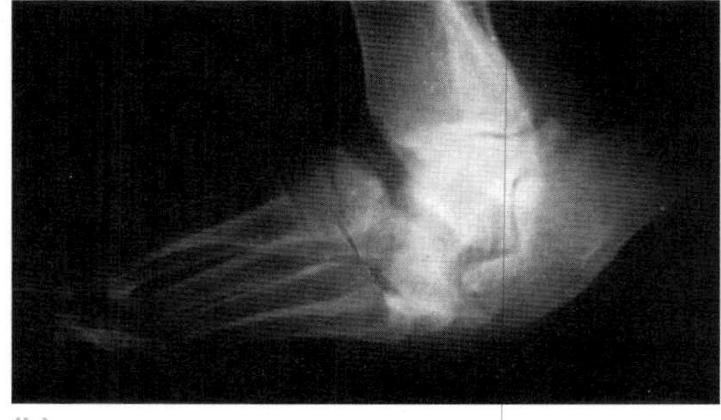

(b)

11.33 The neuropathic foot (a) Neuropathic tarsal disorganization (right foot). (b) Radiograph of the same foot. There is disruption at the mid-tarsal level with separation of the forefoot from the talus and calcaneum. The talo-calcaneal articulation is intact, the talus is plantarflexed and the calcaneum is in equinus. The head of the plantarflexed talus has ploughed through the mid foot and has become directly weightbearing as may be seen from the clinical photograph. Because he could feel no pain in the foot, this patient was able to walk on the foot despite the severe damage. (Courtesy of Dr G. N. Malaviya.)

REFERENCES AND FURTHER READING

Birch R. Brachial plexus injuries. *J Bone Joint Surg*, 1996; **78B:** 986–92.

Birch R, Bonney G, Wyn Parry CB. Surgical Disorders of the Peripheral Nerves. Churchill Livingstone, 1998.

Brand PW. Deformity in leprosy. Ch. XXI in *Leprosy in Theory and Practice*, ed RG Cochrane, Bristol, John Wright, pp 265–319, 1959.

Brand PW. Deformity in leprosy. In *Leprosy in Theory and Practice*, Edn 2, eds RG Cochrane and TF Davy, Bristol, John Wright, pp 447–94, 1964.

Brand PW. Pressure sores – the problem. In *Bed Sore Biomechanics*, ed Kenedi RM, Cowden JM & Scales JT, London, Macmillan, pp 19–23, 1976.

Brandsma W, Schwarz R (eds). *Surgical Reconstruction & Rehabilitation in Leprosy and Other Neuropathies.* Kathmandu (Nepal), Ekta Books, 2004.

Dong Li Wen. *Microscopic surgical techniques in leprosy*, Published by Shanghai Skin Disease & STD Hospital, Shanghai 2001, containing papers reprinted from Indian J Lepr (1999) **71,** pp 285–295, 297–309, 423–436, 437–450, vol. (2000) **72,** pp 227–244, 431–436: and Lepr Rev (1992), **63,** pp 141–144.

Landsmeer JMF. Functional considerations. Ch. 9 in *Atlas of Anatomy of the Hand.* Edinburgh, Churchill Livingstone, pp 315–344, 1976.

Gravem PE. Role of flaps and skin grafts in the management of neuropathic plantar ulcers. Ch. 16 in *Surgical Reconstruction & Rehabilitation in Leprosy and Other Neuropathies*, Kathmandu (Nepal), Ekta Books, pp 227–236, 2004.

McDowell F, Enna CD (eds.). *Surgical Rehabilitation in Leprosy*, Baltimore, Williams Wilkins, 1974.

Mulder JD, Landsmeer JMF. The mechanism of claw finger. *J Bone Joint Surg* 1968; **50B:** 664–8.

Seddon HJ. A classification of nerve injuries. *BMJ*, 1942; **2:** 237–239.

Sunderland S. Nerves and Nerve Injuries, 2nd ed. Edinburgh, Churchill Livingstone, 1978.

Srinivasan H. Disability, deformity and rehabilitation. Ch. 20 in *Leprosy*, 2nd edn. ed. Robert C Hastings, Edinburgh, Churchill Livingstone, pp 411–448, 1994.

Srinivasan H. *Atlas of Corrective Surgical Procedures Commonly Used in Leprosy.* Published by the author, Chennai, India, 2004.

Srinivasan H, Desikan KV. Cauliflower growths in neuropathic plantar ulcers in leprosy patients. *J Bone Joint Surg* 1971; **53A:** 123–32.

Srinivasan H, Palande DD. *Essential Surgery in Leprosy*, Geneva, World Health Organization, 1997.

Srinivasan H, Mukherjee SM, Subramaniam RA. Two-tailed transfer of tibialis posterior for correction of drop-foot in leprosy. *J Bone Joint Surg* 1968; **50B:** 623–8.

Tsuge K, Hashizume C. Reconstruction of opposition in the paralyzed hand. Ch.23 in *Surgical Rehabilitation in Leprosy*, ed. Frank McDowell and Carl D. Enna, Baltimore, Williams & Wilkins, pp 185–198, 1974.

Zancolli EA. *Structural and Dynamic Basis of Hand Surgery.* 4th edn Philadelphia, JB Lippincott, 1979.

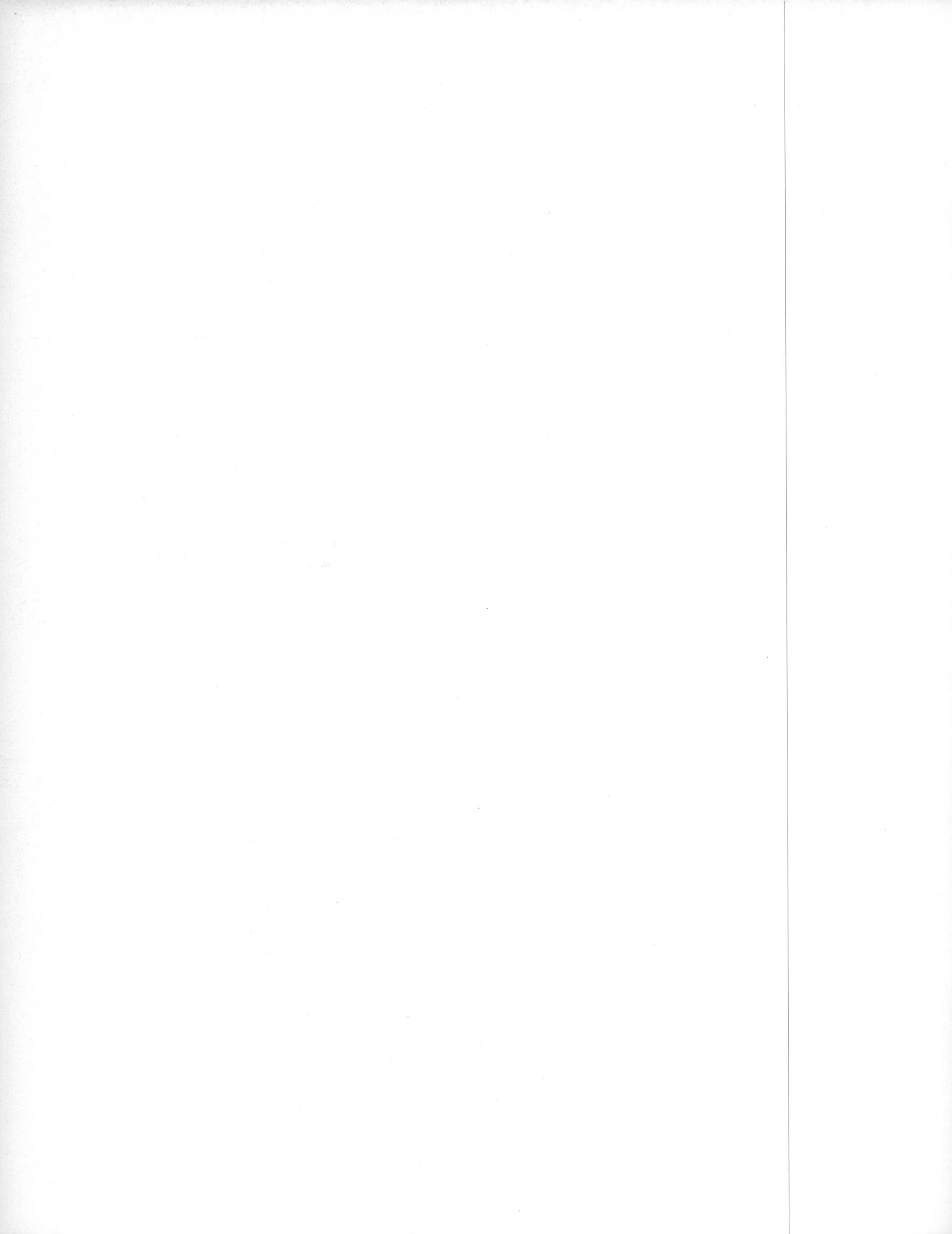

Orthopaedic operations 12

Selvadurai Nayagam, David Warwick

The art and skill of orthopaedic surgery is directed not simply to reshaping or constructing a particular arrangement of parts but to restoring function to the whole.

In this chapter principles applying to orthopaedic operations will be discussed and fundamental techniques of soft-tissue and bone repair will be described. For detailed descriptions of the various operative procedures the reader is referred to standard textbooks on operative orthopaedic surgery and monographs dealing with specific regional subjects.

PREPARATION

PLANNING

Operations upon bone must be carefully planned in advance, when accurate measurements can be made and bones can be compared for symmetry with those of the opposite limb. X-rays, magnetic resonance imaging (MRI) and computed tomography (CT) (if necessary with three-dimensional re-formation) are helpful; transparent templates may be needed to help size and select the most appropriate implant.

Corrective osteotomies and implant positioning can be simulated on x-ray or paper cut-outs before the operation is undertaken. In today's era of digital imaging, these methods have been superseded by image manipulation software, which allows measurement of angles and skeletal axes as well as 'cutting' and 'rearranging' of parts on digital files of x-ray images. Before new or complex reconstructive operations are undertaken they should, ideally, be rehearsed using artificial bones and joints at a workbench. This is a facility that is now widely used in training programmes.

EQUIPMENT

The minimum requirements for orthopaedic operations are drills (for boring holes), osteotomes (for cutting cancellous bone), saws (for cutting cortical bone), chisels (for shaping bone), gouges (for removing bone) and plates, screws and screwdrivers (for fixing bone).

Many operations such as joint replacement, spinal fusion and the various types of internal fixation require special implants and instruments to ensure that the implants are correctly aligned and fixed. Surgeons should familiarize themselves with the implants they plan to use, their advantages and disadvantages and the pitfalls encountered in their use. Most important of all, the surgeon is responsible for ensuring that the necessary instruments and implants (in appropriate sizes!) are available in the operating theatre before starting the operation; the explanation that a particular item 'was not on the instrument table' is no excuse for failure.

INTRAOPERATIVE RADIOGRAPHY

Intraoperative radiography is often helpful and sometimes essential for certain procedures. Fracture reduction, osteotomy alignments and the positioning of implants and fixation devices can be checked before allowing the patient off the operating table. Angiography may be needed to diagnose a vascular injury or demonstrate the success of a vascular repair.

X-ray cassettes must be wrapped in sterile drapes. Portable equipment must be positioned accurately and more time is lost while the plates are developed. However, conventional x-ray films show excellent resolution of bone architecture and provide a permanent record of the procedure. Image intensification and fluoroscopy are more efficient and, although fine features may not be seen in such detail, the resolution is usually adequate. Some fluoroscopy machines are fitted with a printer, so that a permanent copy is available.

X-RAY GUIDANCE SYSTEMS

By using a navigation system based on implanted markers and intraoperative radiography with suitable

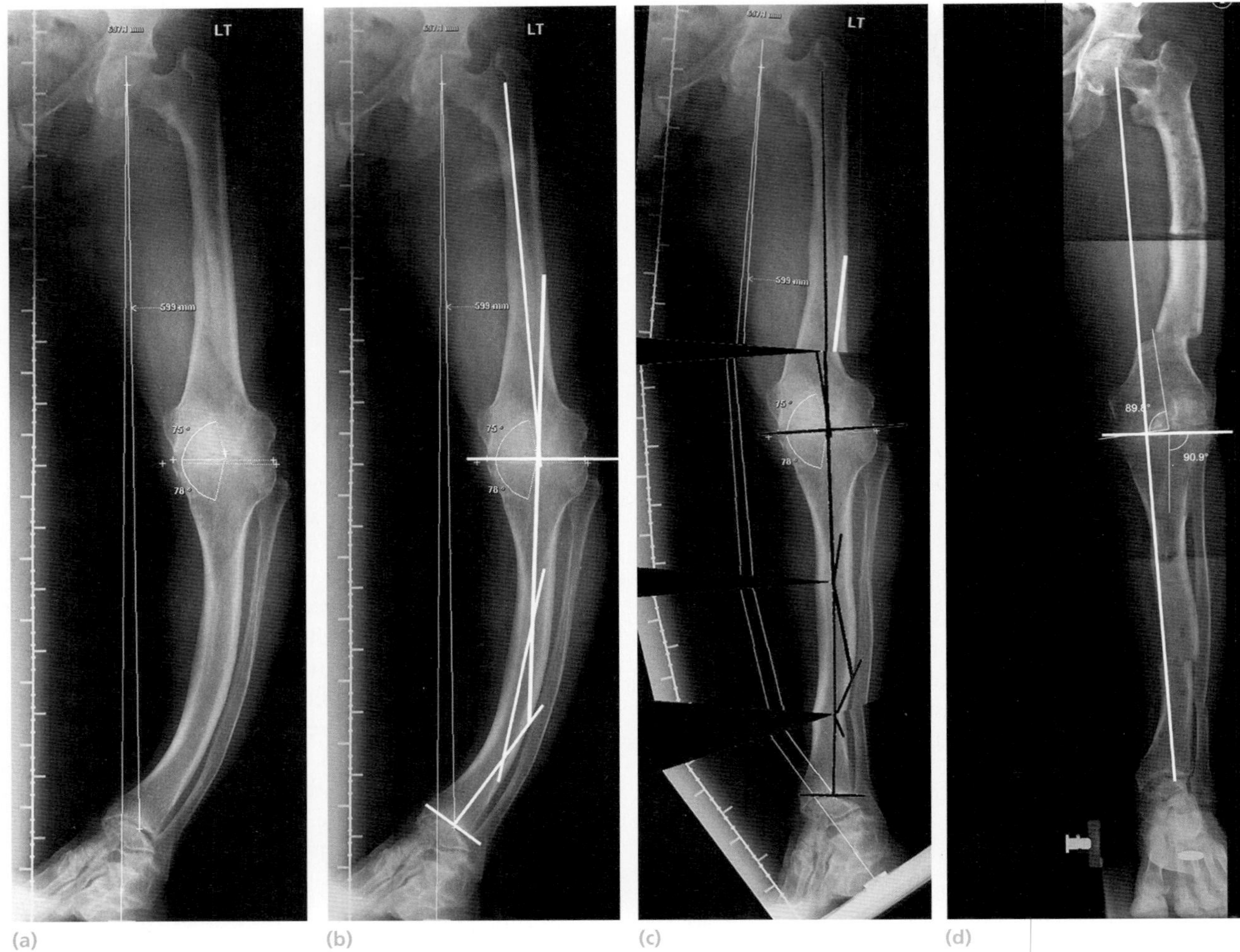

12.1 Preoperative planning on digitized x-ray images The computer software allows the deformity to be analyzed (a,b) and the correction simulated (c). The end result then mimics the simulation (d).

computer software, surgeons are able to improve their accuracy and consistency in placing implants correctly. Examples are insertion of screws into vertebral pedicles and positioning of joint replacement components.

Radiation exposure

Intraoperative radiography involves the risk of exposure to radiation; both the patient and surgeon are affected. The dose limit for the general public is 1 mSv per year, which is the equivalent of 1000 chest x-rays. Each chest x-ray in turn produces the same radiation dose as is endured during a 4-hour airline flight. Fluoroscopic images acquired during operations are usually pulsed exposures rather than continuous screening, so a few minutes of exposure to the patient during a protracted operation would still amount to a negligible additional risk of developing cancer. However, for the surgeon the risk is far greater because of the repeated use of fluoroscopy.

Total exposure varies with the type of procedure performed (operations on limb extremities produce the least, hip operations middling and spine operations the most) as well as the number of procedures needing x-ray assistance and the protective measures used. The latter influence the cumulative exposure significantly and lead aprons are therefore compulsory; further attenuation of radiation exposure is gained through the use of thyroid shields and, if practical, eye goggles. Using a hip procedure as an example, lead aprons will reduce the effective dose received by a factor of 16 for anteroposterior projections and by a factor of 4–10 for lateral projections. Using a thyroid shield decreases the dose by another 2.5 times (Theocharopoulos et al., 2003).

Magnification

Magnification is an integral part of peripheral nerve and hand surgery. The improved view minimizes the trauma of surgery and allows more accurate apposition of tissues during reconstruction.

Operating loupes range in power from 2–6 × magnification. As the magnification increases, the field of view decreases and the interruption by unwanted head movements becomes more apparent. Most surgeons, therefore, choose between 2.5 and 3.5 × magnification.

The operating microscope allows much greater magnification with a stable field of view. It is particularly important when very accurate apposition of tissue is required, for example when aligning nerve fascicles during nerve repair or nerve grafting, when anastomosing small vessels or when operating in a narrow corridor of safety as in microdiscectomy of the spine.

THE 'BLOODLESS FIELD'

Many operations on limbs (and particularly the hand) can be done more rapidly and accurately if bleeding is prevented by the application of a tourniquet (Noordin et al., 2009).

TOURNIQUET CUFF

Only a pneumatic cuff should be used and it should be at least as wide as the diameter of the limb. Wide cuffs reduce the pressure needed for vascular occlusion. A tied rubber bandage is a potentially dangerous substitute and should not be used; the pressure beneath the bandage cannot be controlled and there is a real risk of damage to the underlying nerves and muscle. A layer of wool bandage beneath the pneumatic tourniquet will distribute the pressure and prevent wrinkling of the underlying skin. During skin preparation, it is essential that the sterilizing fluid does not leak beneath the cuff as this can cause a chemical burn. Isolating the tourniquet with a plastic drape prevents this complication.

EXSANGUINATION

Elevation of the lower limb at 60 degrees for 30 seconds will reduce the blood volume by 45 per cent; increasing the elevation time does not alter the percentage significantly. The same pattern is observed in the upper limb (Blond et al., 2002; Blond and Madsen, 2002). This simple manoeuvre will therefore suffice to 'drain' the tissues if a truly bloodless field is not essential, or when surgery is being undertaken for tumour or infection and forceful exsanguination might squeeze pathological tissue into the proximal part of the limb. The 'squeeze' method, in which pressure on the palm or foot is followed by sequential squeezing of the limb in a proximal direction, is also effective. If a clearer field is required then exsanguination can be achieved by pressure using an Esmarch or gauze bandage wrapped from distal to proximal, or a rubber tubular exsanguinator. These methods reduce blood volume by an additional 20 per cent.

TOURNIQUET PRESSURE

A tourniquet pressure of 150 mmHg above systolic is recommended for the lower limb and 80–100 mmHg above systolic for the upper limb. This may need to be increased in hypertensive, obese or very muscular patients. Higher pressures are unnecessary and will increase the risk of damage to underlying muscles and nerves.

Tourniquet time

An absolute maximum tourniquet time of 3 hours is allowed, although it is safer (and more advisable) to keep this under 2 hours; transient nerve-related symptoms may occur with 3-hour tourniquet times but full recovery is usual by the fifth day. Time can be saved by ensuring that the limb is shaved, prepared, draped and marked before inflating the cuff. The time of application of the tourniquet should be recorded and the surgeon should be informed of the elapsed time at regular intervals, particularly as the 2-hour period is approached.

Deflating and re-inflating the tourniquet

This has serious local and systemic effects. Locally deflation is followed by a hyperaemic response that reduces by half in 5, 12 and 25 minutes, respectively after ischaemic times of 1, 2 and 3 hours (Klenerman et al., 1982). This information is useful to the surgeon trying to obtain haemostasis after tourniquet release. There is also a variable amount of swelling, unrelated to the length of the ischaemic period; it would therefore be wise to omit tourniquet use for those limbs where significant swelling is already evident so as not to jeopardize wound healing. At the systemic level, tourniquet deflation induces a free radical-mediated reperfusion syndrome, which adds to any muscle damage already produced by the ischaemic period. 'Breathing periods' (deflation followed after a pause by re-inflation), which were once popular to enable extended tourniquet times, are no longer recommended as the reperfusion effects are cumulative even though the local limb anoxia is relieved at each tourniquet deflation (Bushell et al., 2002). If a prolonged tourniquet time is required, and if this is anticipated due to the complexity of surgery to be undertaken, it is wise to warn the patient of the possibility of transient nerve-related symptoms and to obtain their consent to use the absolute maximum period of 3 hours.

Finger tourniquet

This is suitable for relatively minor hand operations. A sterile rubber glove-finger makes a good cuff; the tip is cut and the margin is then rolled back proximally. This has the combined effect of exsanguinating the finger and acting as a tourniquet. A stretched rubber catheter must not be used as this may damage the underlying structures. *Always check that the finger tourniquet has been removed at the end of the operation.*

Complications

Complications of tourniquet usage usually relate to nerve injury (more often due to compression than duration of ischaemia), skin burns from leakage of alcoholic antiseptic solutions beneath the tourniquet cuff and a failure to diagnose peripheral vascular disease before surgery (Klenerman, 2003). These mishaps can be prevented, or the risk minimized, by always using a wide cuff, sealing the cuff against seeping fluids and avoiding excessive tourniquet pressures. A wise precaution is to not employ a bloodless field at all in patients with impaired peripheral circulation or those with arterial prostheses or stents that may not expand sufficiently after tourniquet deflation to re-establish an adequate blood flow.

MEASURES TO REDUCE RISK OF INFECTION

SKIN PREPARATION AND DRAPING

Hair removal

Shaving the limb is more likely to be harmful than helpful. Shaving before surgery causes superficial skin damage and leads to local bacterial proliferation. Depilatory creams have been shown to remove hair effectively and, if hair removal is deemed necessary, they can be used the day before surgery without an increase in wound problems.

Skin cleaning

The limb may benefit from washing with soap to remove particulate matter and grease. This is particularly useful in managing open fractures and in cases where the limb has been wrapped in a cast or splint for some time. Skin preparation prior to surgery should be carried out with an alcohol-based preparation where safe; alcohol is not to be applied over open wounds, exposed joints or nerve tissue. Iodine or chlorhexidine preparations are available but there is evidence that chlorhexidine is more effective after a single application, having longer residual activity and maintaining efficacy in the presence of blood and serum (Milstone et al., 2008). The use of colouring in the preparation fluid will help to ensure that the limb is fully covered. However, use of red colouring should be avoided if a tourniquet is used since it may make it difficult to determine whether blood flow has returned after releasing the tourniquet.

Drapes

These function to isolate the surgical field from the rest of the patient and reduce contamination from outside. There are disposable and re-usable varieties and, as yet, none has been shown to be superior as long as they have the following qualities: (1) barrier effectiveness throughout the length of the procedure; (2) quality that is maintained if it is re-used (for re-usable varieties); (3) configurability to cover different areas of body or limb; (4) tear-resistance and does not lint; (5) no cause for skin reactions through allergy or abrasiveness; (6) reasonable cost (Rutala and Weber, 2001). Plastic adhesive coverings, some impregnated with iodine, function primarily to secure the drapes, especially if the limb is moved during surgery. This method of skin isolation was thought to reduce wound contact with some of the resident bacteria around the skin incision; however there is no evidence that they reduce surgical site infections and they may even increase them! (Webster and Alghamdi 2007).

SURGICAL ATTIRE

Gowns

Gowns need to share the requisite qualities of drapes but should also be comfortable.

Gloves

Gloves are available in latex and non-latex varieties. The latter are needed if either the surgeon or the patient has a latex hypersensitivity. This could apply to patients who are constantly exposed to latex devices, e.g. urinary catheters. Latex allergy is second only to muscle relaxants for inducing anaphylaxis during surgery (Lieberman, 2002). Double gloving, with a coloured inner glove (so-called indicator glove) reduces the number of inner glove perforations and allows outer glove perforations to be picked up more quickly, but a difference in surgical site infections has yet to be established (Tanner and Parkinson, 2006).

Face mask

This hallmark of the surgeon in theatre has been questioned in its ability to reduce surgical site infections. As studies provide conflicting views (Lipp and Edwards, 2002), for the time being at least, face masks should continue to be used if only for protection of the surgical staff. Modern face masks incorporate visors (eye shields), which substantially reduce the risk of contact with blood.

VACCINATION

There is a risk of transmission of blood-borne infections to orthopaedic surgeons, not least because of the nature of surgery but also due to frequent handling of instruments and bone fragments with sharp edges. Transfer of infectious agents through blood occurs mainly by contact (percutaneous or mucocutaneous) and through aerosols (Wong and Leung, 2004). The face and neck may become contaminated and this may go unnoticed until after the procedure; splashes and aerosol sprays often happen during the use of power tools and irrigation fluids (Quebbeman et al, 1991). Exposure is more likely if the operation continues for over 3 hours or when blood loss is greater than 300 mL (Gerberding et al., 1990). A barrier created by surgeon attire must be coupled to the correct etiquette for handling and passing instruments between staff. This reduces the likelihood of accidental needle-stick injury but will need augmenting by prophylaxis through vaccination.

Hepatitis B

Transmission may occur through inoculation or even from contact with a contaminated surface (the virus is able to survive for a week in dried blood). There is a 30 per cent risk of transmission from a single inoculation of an unvaccinated person (Alter et al., 1976). Vaccination is safe, effective and immunity, for those who respond after a course of injections, indefinite. Those who do not respond to immunization will need post-exposure prophylaxis using a combination of hepatitis B immunoglobulin and the vaccine.

Hepatitis C

The risk of accidental transmission is lower than for hepatitis-B (less than 7 per cent). Unfortunately neither effective vaccines nor post-exposure protection is available.

Human immunodeficiency virus

The risk of human immunodeficiency virus (HIV) infection after accidental injury is very low (less than 0.5 per cent) (Ippolito et al., 1999), although this may vary between individuals. Vaccination is not available but post-exposure treatment with antivirals is essential.

THROMBOPROPHYLAXIS

Venous thromboembolism (VTE) is the commonest complication of lower limb surgery. It comprises three associated disorders: *deep vein thrombosis* (DVT), *pulmonary embolism* (PE) and the later complication of *chronic venous insufficiency*. Approximately one in 30–40 patients operated on for hip fractures or hip and knee replacements will develop a symptomatic thromboembolic complication despite the use of prophylaxis during their hospital stay. The most important risk factors are increasing age, obesity and a history of previous thrombosis.

PATHOPHYSIOLOGY

According to Virchow, thrombosis results from an interaction between vessel wall damage, alterations in blood components and venous stasis. All of these occur in major orthopaedic operations. The surgery is highly thrombogenic. Soft-tissue exposure, bone cutting and reaming induce a systemic hypercoagulable state and fibrinolytic inhibition. Blood flow in the femoral vein is obstructed by the torsion needed to expose the femoral canal and the acetabulum in hip replacements; this damages the endothelium, both in the proximal femoral vein (by torsion) and in the distal veins (by distension). Furthermore, venous obstruction allows a concentration of clotting factors. In knee replacement, the anterior subluxation of the tibia and vibration from the saw may cause local endothelial damage. In addition, the relative immobility that follows lower limb operations induces some degree of venous stasis.

DVT occurs most frequently in the veins of the calf and less often in the proximal veins of the thigh and pelvis. It is from the larger and more proximal thrombi that fragments sometimes get carried to the lungs, where they may give rise to symptomatic pulmonary embolism (PE) and, in a small percentage of cases, fatal pulmonary embolism (FPE).

CLINICAL FEATURES AND DIAGNOSIS

Thromboembolic events can be represented as a pyramid; most of these events are asymptomatic but a

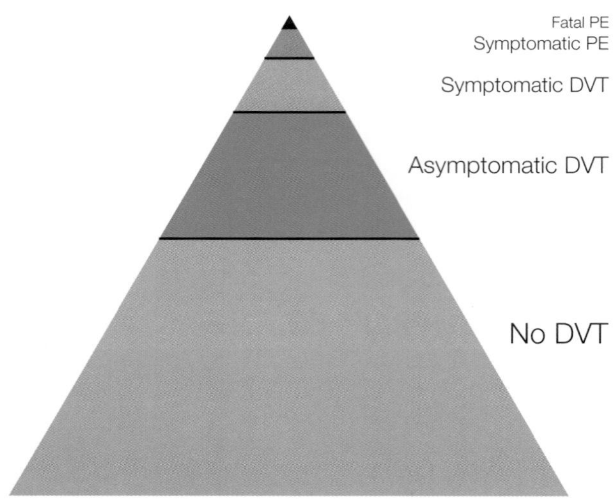

12.2 The thromboembolism pyramid

proportion is revealed clinically (Fig. 12.2). Hence DVT is, in the main, an occult disease and considerably more common than the symptoms and signs suggest.

Deep venous thrombosis

DVT is usually asymptomatic, although some patients present with pain in the calf or thigh. A sudden slight increase in temperature and pulse rate may develop. There are usually no signs but there may be calf swelling and tenderness. Homans' test (increased pain on passive dorsiflexion of the foot), although still frequently employed, is now regarded as unreliable.

Pulmonary embolism (PE)

Patients may develop pleuritic pain in the chest and shortness of breath, but other conditions, such as myocardial infarction or fulminant pneumonia can be mistaken for PE. In most cases PE is completely asymptomatic and fatal PE usually presents as a sudden collapse without prior symptoms in the legs or chest; in such cases the diagnosis is confirmed by post-mortem examination.

Imaging studies help to confirm the diagnosis in patients who have a moderate or high clinical probability of thromboembolism. Ultrasound or venography is important for demonstrating DVT and computer tomographic pulmonary angiography or ventilation-perfusion (VQ) scans are helpful in the diagnosis of PE.

Post-thrombotic syndrome

Post-thrombotic syndrome (PTS) presents with leg discomfort, swelling, skin changes and even ulceration. This is a debilitating condition that directly influences quality of life (Kahn et al., 2008). Approximately one-third of patients with *symptomatic* DVT will develop features of PTS within 2 years but it is not yet established whether the much more frequent *asymptomatic* DVT after joint replacement predis-

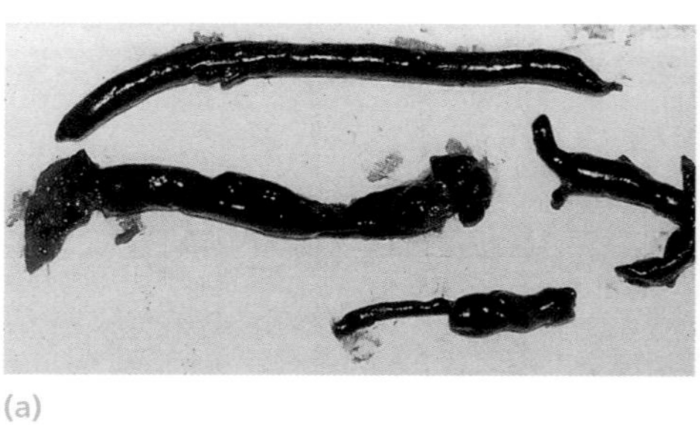

(a)

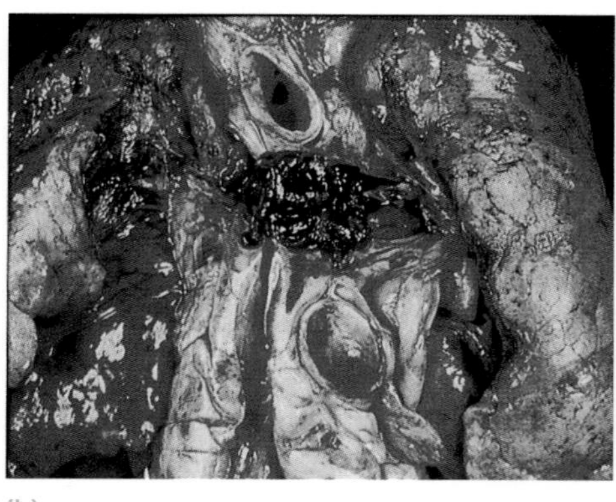

(b)

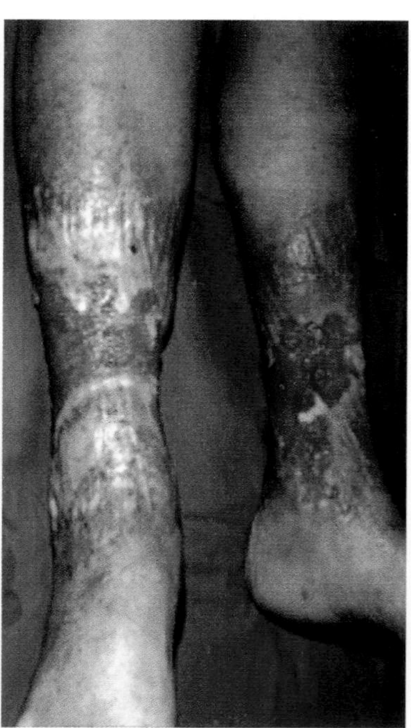

(c)

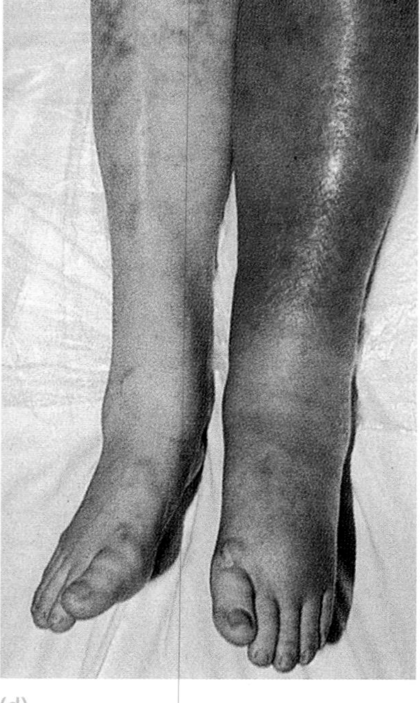

(d)

12.3 Venous thromboembolism (a) Venous thrombosis – embolism from the deep veins of the leg, extracted from the lung at post mortem. (b) Fatal pulmonary embolism at post mortem (c) chronic venous insufficiency (d) acute thrombophlebitis.

Table 12.1 Risk of venous thromboembolism (VTE)

Procedure or condition	Fatal PE	Symptomatic VTE	Asymptomatic DVT
Hip fracture	1 per cent	4 per cent	60 per cent
Hip replacement	0.2–0.4 per cent	3–4 per cent	55 per cent
Knee replacement	0.2 per cent	3–4 per cent	60 per cent
Isolated lower limb trauma	Unknown	0.4–2 per cent	10–35 per cent
Spinal surgery	Unknown	6 per cent	18 per cent
Knee arthroscopy	Unknown	0.2 per cent	7 per cent
Major trauma	Unknown	Unknown	58 per cent
Spinal cord injury	Unknown	13 per cent	35 per cent
Upper limb surgery	Unknown	Vv rare	Vv rare
Minor lower limb surgery	Vv rare	Vv rare	Vv rare

DVT, deep vein thrombosis; PE, pulmonary embolism; VTE, venous thromboembolism. Derived from the International Consensus Statement (Nicolaides et al., 2006) and ACCP Guidelines (Geerts et al., 2008).

poses to this long-term outcome (Pesavento et al., 2006).

Chronic pulmonary hypertension

This is a potential sequel for those who survive a symptomatic PE but the incidence is unknown.

INCIDENCE OF THROMBOEMBOLIC EVENTS

It is generally accepted that the risk of symptomatic thromboembolism and fatal PE is less now than it was 20 or 30 years ago, due to more efficient surgery and anaesthesia as well as earlier mobilization and the widespread use of prophylaxis.

Much of the information used to calculate risk reduction with prophylaxis is derived from studies using a venographic surrogate. Venograms are sensitive and specific in identifying venous thrombi but the relationship between 'venographic DVT' and symptomatic events has not been fully defined. Many asymptomatic venographic thrombi resolve without untoward effects. However, there is reasonable evidence to show that a reduction in venographic DVT would produce a proportionate reduction in symptomatic DVT or even fatal PE, thus shrinking the pyramid of risk (Table 12.1).

PREVENTION

The overall risk of DVT and PE can be reduced by prophylaxis. Patients admitted for surgery, whether electively or in emergency, need a risk assessment, which can be simplified by including an active reminder or checklist prior to surgery. This ensures that safe, effective prophylaxis is routinely given according to a protocol that has been accepted by the surgeons and anaesthetists (Tooher et al., 2005; Warwick et al, 2008).

General measures

- *Neuraxial anaesthesia* – Spinal or epidural anaesthesia reduces mortality, enhances peri-operative analgesia and reduces the risk of VTE by about 50 per cent through enhancing blood flow. It is wise to avoid giving neuraxial anaesthesia and chemical prophylaxis too close together to avoid a spinal haematoma. Local guidelines should be followed.
- *Surgical technique* – Rough surgical technique will potentiate thromboplastin release. Prolonged torsion of a major vein, when maintaining a dislocated hip for purposes of replacement or during aggressive dorsal retraction of the tibia during knee replacement, inhibits venous return and damages the endothelium.
- *Tourniquet* – A tourniquet probably does not change the risk; clotting factors that accumulate whilst the tourniquet is inflated are flushed out by the hyperaemia on tourniquet deflation.
- *Early mobilization* – This is a simple physiological means of improving venous flow.

Physical methods

- *Graduated compression stockings* can halve the incidence of DVT when compared to no prophylaxis; there is a suggestion that below-knee stockings may be just as effective as above-knee types, as long as the stockings are properly woven and well-fitted (Phillips et al., 2008).

- *Intermittent plantar venous compression* takes advantage of the fact that blood from the sole of the foot is normally expressed during weightbearing by intermittent pressure on the venous plexus around the lateral plantar arteries; this, in turn, increases venous blood flow in the leg. A mechanical foot-pump can reproduce this physiological mechanism in patients who are confined to bed. It should not be used in combination with compression stockings as these impair refill of the venous plexus after emptying by the foot pump. There is some evidence that this technique provides effective thromboprophylaxis in hip fracture, hip arthroplasy and knee arthroplasty, especially if combined with a chemical method (Pellegrini et al., 2008).
- *Intermittent pneumatic compression of the leg* has also been shown to reduce the risk of 'radiological DVT' after hip replacements and in trauma. It is, however, impractical for patients undergoing operations at or below the knee.
- *Inferior vena cava filters* resemble an umbrella and are percutaneously passed through the femoral vein and lodged in the inferior vena cava. They merely catch an embolus to prevent it from reaching the lungs. They have a specific role in the occasional case where the risk of embolism is high yet anticoagulation is contra-indicated, e.g. in a patient with a pelvic fracture who has already developed a DVT but needs a major surgical reconstruction. The complication rate, which includes death from proximal coagulation, should restrict use of these devices.

Chemical methods

These are generally safe, effective, easy to administer (tablet or injection) and can be used for extended periods. They are relatively inexpensive compared with the overall cost of surgery. However, all chemical methods incur a risk of bleeding, which is a natural concern for both the orthopaedic surgeon and the anaesthetist. Methods include:

- *Aspirin* – Whilst some authorities still recommend the use of aspirin, others (NICE in the United Kingdom, the American College of Chest Physicians, The International Consensus Statement) advise against its use because of its relatively poor efficacy, the risk of bleeding and the tendency to cause gastrointestinal irritation.
- *Unfractionated heparin* – This carries a risk of increased bleeding after operation and is contraindicated in elderly people.
- *Low molecular weight heparin* (LMWH) – This class of drug has haematological and pharmacokinetic advantages over unfractionated heparin including ready bio-availability and a wide window of safety; therefore monitoring is not required. They are safe if used properly (with an adequate time between administration and surgery or regional anaesthesia, and a reduced dose for those with impaired renal function). They are more effective than placebo or unfractionated heparin and at least as effective as warfarin, compression devices and foot pumps. Randomized studies have shown that it effectively reduces the prevalence of venographic DVT in hip and knee replacement surgery, and the effect may be amplified when coupled to physical methods.
- *Pentasaccharide* – This synthetic injectable antithrombotic drug (fondaparinux) precisely inhibits activated Factor X. It is at least as effective as LMWH but must not be given too close to surgery (it is best given 6–8 hours after surgery) or bleeding may become a significant problem. The drug is excreted by the kidneys rather than metabolized by the liver and so must be used carefully or avoided in those with poor renal function.
- *Direct anti-Xa inhibitors* and *direct thrombin inhibitors* – These drugs are likely to transform thromboprophylaxis. They are given orally and have a broad therapeutic and safety window (so that no monitoring is required). They are given after surgery and should be continued for as long as the patient is at risk of VTE. There is good evidence of equivalence of efficacy with LMWH in hip and knee replacement surgery. They provide a pragmatic solution for after-hospital prophylaxis, requiring neither injections nor complex monitoring. Drug activity is difficult to reverse. Presently, two are available: a direct thrombin inhibitor (dabigatran) and an anti-Xa inhibitor (rivaroxaban).
- *Warfarin* – Warfarin has been used fairly widely, particularly in North America. It reduces the prevalence of DVT after hip and knee replacement and FPE is extremely rare. Drawbacks are the difficulty in establishing appropriate dosage levels and the need for constant monitoring. If it is used at all it must be maintained at an international normalized ratio (INR) level of 2–3.

Timing and duration of prophylaxis

Risk factors for thromboembolism are most pronounced during surgery but, in some patients (particularly those with hip or major long-bone fractures of the lower limb), immobility and a hypercoagulable state may begin before the operation. In general prophylaxis it is given on admission to hospital in this group, particularly if surgery is delayed beyond 24 hours. Chemical prophylaxis should not be given too close to surgery otherwise there is a risk of provoking a bleeding complication. If it is given too long before surgery, metabolism or excretion may reduce its potency; if given too long after surgery, the thrombogenic process will be established and the drug is now therapeutic instead of prophylactic.

The ideal duration of thromboprophylaxis is not known (Warwick et al., 2007). Traditional recommendations suggesting that it should be continued until the patient is fully mobile have been superseded by evidence that the cumulative risk for VTE lasts for up to 1 month after knee replacement surgery and 3 months with hip surgery (Bjornara et al., 2006). Half of the VTE events after knee replacement and two-thirds after hip replacement occur beyond hospital discharge. The duration of risk in other orthopaedic conditions is not known. Therefore, thromboprophylaxis should be prolonged for some time after discharge from hospital.

Randomized clinical trials have shown that the risk of after-discharge symptomatic DVT can be reduced by two-thirds by prolonging thromboprophylaxis. The precise period depends on many factors, including individual patient factors, which are difficult to quantify, but current evidence supports 14 days for knee replacement and 4–5 weeks for hip replacement and hip fracture. Whilst many of the chemical methods may be appropriate, oral agents that do not require monitoring (e.g. anti-Xa and anti-thrombin inhibitors) facilitate effective and practical extended duration prophylaxis (NICE, 2010).

Multimodal prophylaxis

Risk assessment of patients may determine that a combination of physical and chemical prophylaxis is needed. This form of *multimodal prophylaxis* is gaining popularity and some studies point to increased efficacy. For patients at particularly high risk of bleeding, the mechanical method should be used until the bleeding risk has resolved and until the device is no longer tolerated. It is then safely replaced by a chemical product, which is continued for as long as there is a risk of thrombosis. For patients with a particularly high risk of thrombosis, the mechanical device is started immediately after surgery and continued for as long as tolerated; the chemical is started as close to surgery as is safe (e.g. 6 hours postoperatively) and continued for as long as the risk of VTE persists.

OPERATIONS ON BONES

OSTEOTOMY

Osteotomy may be used to correct deformity, to change the shape of the bone, or to redirect load trajectories in a limb so as to influence joint function. Preoperative planning is essential; principles of deformity analysis and osteotomy are well described in the monograph by Paley (2002).

Knowledge of the limb axes and their relation to the joints is the foundation for analyzing skeletal deformity. 'Corrective' surgery is an exercise in balancing the extent of operative interventions needed to produce *anatomical 'normality'* with the *anticipated gain in function*. 'Anatomical' correction, whilst desirable in most cases, is not always necessary. An appropriate example is a skeletal deformity due to a neuromuscular disorder where correction to achieve maximal *functional* gain has to be greater than that for *anatomical* accuracy.

Modern deformity analysis recognizes the three-dimensional basis of most deformities, whether the origin of the problem is within a bone or a joint or a combination of both. Deformity of bone exists as a deviation in the coronal or sagittal plane (or any plane in between) where it can be measured in degrees of angulation or millimetres of translation, or in the axial plane, where it exists as degrees of rotation or millimetres of length abnormality. The lower limb is used to illustrate the principles as applied to the coronal plane.

Limb axes and reference angles

The mechanical axis of a limb is defined by an imaginary line connecting the centre of the most proximal major joint to the centre of the most distal, e.g. in the lower limb from the centre of the hip to the centre of the ankle. In most individuals this line passes close to the centre of the knee joint, usually 8(±7) mm medial to it. If a deformity is present the line may be displaced away from its usual position (Fig. 12.4a). Interestingly, if a deformity should exist at two or more levels in the limb, the resulting displacements may cancel each other out, so that the limb axis ends up in the 'normal' position (Fig. 12.4b). It follows the observed position of the mechanical axis of the lower limb in relation to the knee joint is a 'screening' assessment and does not rule out the presence of deformity. A further step would be to compare reference angles subtended by the mechanical axes of the individual bone segments to joints. It is usual to compare these angles with those of the contralateral 'normal' side but in the event the other is also affected some reference ranges are available (Fig. 12.5):

1. *At the hip* – the angle between the anatomical axis of the femur and the axis of the femoral neck is approximately 128 degrees (±3 degrees).
2. *At the knee* – the angle between the anatomical axis of the femur and a tangent to the joint line of the knee is, on the lateral aspect, approximately 80 degrees (±2 degrees).

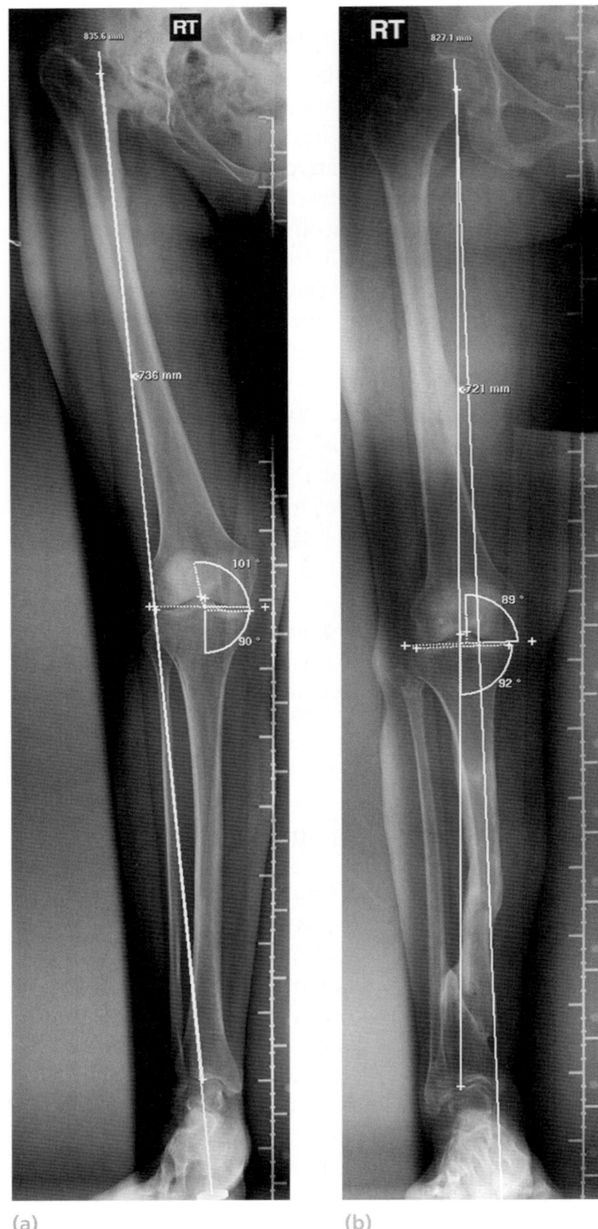

(a) (b)

12.4 (a) Deformity in the lower limb It may be sufficient to alter the mechanical axis of the limb – here it is shifted laterally due to changes at the hip joint. (b) If there are two deformities, the mechanical axis may be normal if the effect of each is to shift the axis in equal and opposite directions – a compensated deformity.

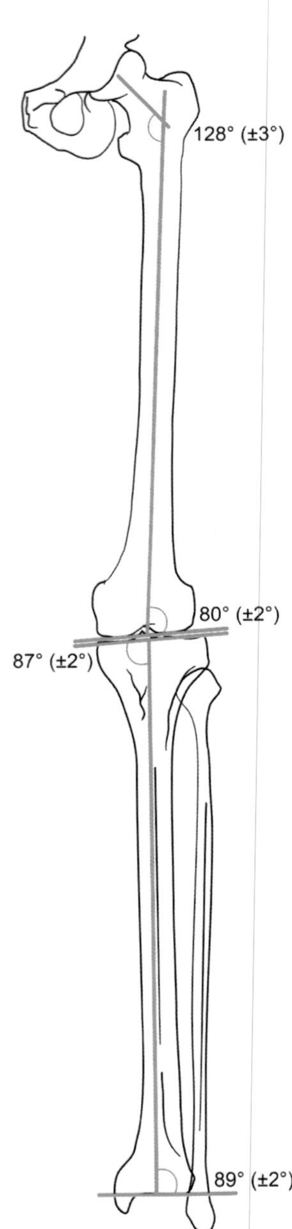

12.5 Analysis of coronal plane deformity This can be based on a contralateral normal limb or use of reference angles in relation to the anatomical (or mechanical) axes (Paley, 2002).

3. *At the knee* – the angle between the anatomical axis of the tibia and a tangent to the joint line of the knee is, on the medial aspect, approximately 87 degrees (±2 degrees).
4. *At the ankle* – the angle between the anatomical axis of the tibia and a tangent to the tibial plafond is, on the lateral aspect, approximately 89 degrees (±2 degrees).

If an abnormal value is encountered, it suggests a deformity is present within that bone. However, when drawing out these reference angles and seeking to identify a source of deformity, it is easy to be carried away by abnormal values that differ from the reference ranges by a few degrees. The clinical significance of these 'abnormalities' must be taken in context; an intrinsic (naturally present) varus angulation of a few degrees at the distal femur matters little if the main source of deformity is a larger varus malunion of a tibial fracture further distally – in which case the correction should be in the tibia.

Rules for osteotomy

Most surgeons are familiar with the simple method of drawing the anatomical axes of the bone segments proximal and distal to a deformity and measuring the size of the deformity (in degrees) at the intersection of these axes. In modern deformity analysis this intersection of anatomical axes is referred to as a *centre of rotation of angulation* (CORA) and can also be determined by noting the intersection of the mechanical axes of the segments proximal and distal to the deformity (Fig. 12.6). The CORA is important for the following reasons:

1. It indicates where an axis of rotation, named angulation correction axis or *ACA* (Paley, 2002), should be placed about which the two intersecting axes of the CORA can be brought in line and hence the deformity corrected. This axis of rotation, which enables appropriate realignment of the intersecting axes, should be positioned on either side of the CORA but along a line termed '*the bisector*'. This is, as is implied in its name, the line that bisects the angle described by the deformity (Fig. 12.7a). The effect of placing the axis of rotation on the convex side of the deformity is to envisage an opening wedge correction, and conversely if it is placed on the concave side – a closing wedge correction. Moving the rotation axis further along the bisector increases or decreases the size of the opening, i.e. achieves simultaneous lengthening or shortening with the angular correction (Fig. 12.7b and c). If the rotation axis is not placed on the bisector, a translation deformity will ensue despite satisfactory correction of angulation.
2. It reveals the presence of translation as well as angulation as components of the deformity and can also indicate the presence of multi-apical deformities.
   (a) When the CORA is identified and is found to lie within the boundaries of the bone involved as well as coinciding in level with the apex of the deformity, this indicates only an angular component to the deformity. The rotation axis to correct the deformity can be sited on the bisector and the osteotomy performed at the same level – this is equivalent to classic correction through opening or closing wedge methods (Fig. 12.7b).
   (b) When the CORA lies within the boundaries of the bone involved but is at a different level to that of the apex of deformity, it indicates the presence of translation and angulation within the deformity (Fig. 12.8a). The rotation axis to enable correction should be maintained on the bisector of the CORA but the osteotomy can be sited at either of the two levels (coincident with the apex of deformity or at the CORA): (1) when positioned on the former, correction of both translation and angulation is simultaneously accomplished at the site of original deformity (Fig. 12.8b); (2)

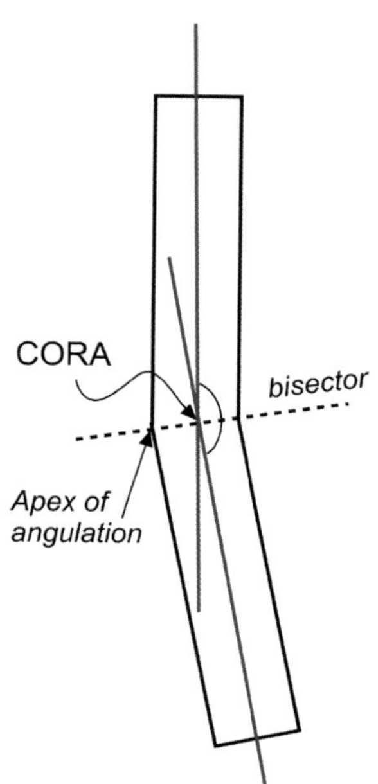

12.6 Location of the CORA It is found at the intersection of the anatomical (or mechanical) axes of the segments proximal and distal to the deformity. The bisector is the line that divides the supplement to the angle of deformity. Whilst the apex of angulation and CORA coincide in this example, that is not always so.

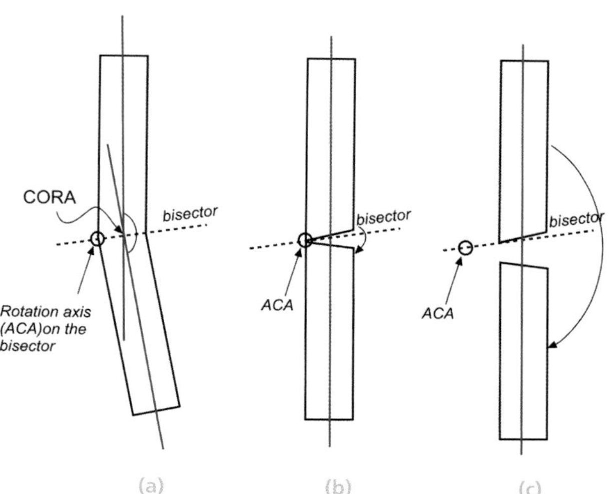

12.7 Axis of rotation It is placed along the bisector of the CORA on the convex side. This achieves an open wedge correction (a,b). If the rotation axis is moved further along the bisector, lengthening – in addition to the open wedge realignment – is obtained (c).

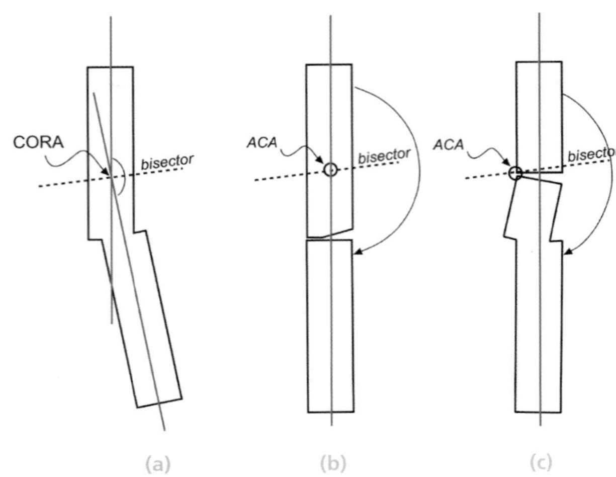

12.8 If the CORA is found to be proximal or distal to the apex of angulation, but within the boundaries of the bone, this suggests the presence of translation as an additional component to the deformity (a). Simultaneous correction can be achieved by placing the axis of rotation on the CORA or its bisector; the osteotomy can be either at the apex of angulation (b) or at the same level as the CORA (c).

when sited on the latter, a new deformity is created which correctly 'balances' the malalignment produced from the original site (Fig. 12.8c).

(c) When the CORA lies outside the boundaries of the involved bone, a multi-apical deformity is likely to be present (and the deformity more akin to a curve). The deformity would need to be resolved through multiple osteotomies.

These features of the CORA are, in essence, the rules of osteotomy as described by Paley (2002). It explains why it is permissible to perform osteotomies away from the apex of the deformity as long as the correction is achieved through a rotation axis placed on the CORA or on its bisector. Many examples in orthopaedics illustrate this principle, e.g. performing an intertrochanteric or subtrochanteric osteotomy to correct malalignment of the femoral neck in a child with a slipped capital femoral epiphysis, or inducing translation in correcting a genu valgum arising from the femoral joint line – both of which are examples of the 2(b) scenario above.

Complications of osteotomy and deformity correction

General As with all bone operations, thrombo-embolism and infection are calculated risks.

Undercorrection and overcorrection Under- and over-correction of the deformity can be avoided by careful preoperative planning. In difficult cases, intra-operative x-ray or fluoroscopy is essential. If the fault is recognized while the patient is still under the anaesthetic, it should be corrected straightaway. If discovered on a postoperative x-ray check, the impact of the mistake will need to be gauged and, if significant, it may still be advisable to re-do the procedure.

Nerve tension Correction of severe deformities may put excessive tension on a nearby nerve. The commonest example is peroneal nerve palsy after corrective osteotomy for a marked valgus deformity of the knee. In general, acute long-bone corrections greater than 20 degrees should be avoided and if there is a known risk of nerve injury it should be limited to 10 degrees. If greater correction is needed it can be done gradually in an appropriate external fixator (see on page 319, under the Ilizarov method).

Compartment syndrome Osteotomy of the tibia or forearm bones is at risk of this rare but potentially limb-threatening complication. The limb should be checked repeatedly for signs and prompt action taken if danger signals appear (see Chapter 23).

Non-union Non-union may occur if fixation is inadequate or if the soft tissues are damaged by excessive stripping during surgical exposure. Gentle handling of tissues and respect for the blood supply to bone together with sound fixation techniques will minimize the risk.

BONE FIXATION

Stabilizing two segments or fragments of bone is usually by internal or external fixation methods. In internal fixation, this may involve screws, wires, plates or intramedullary rods. External fixators come in a variety of types. There are basic rules for choosing and using either method.

Internal fixation by screws

Screws can be used simply by holding two fragments in close proximity or to fix a plate to the bone. They may also be used to compress two fragments together through what is called the 'lag principle'. By over-drilling the near fragment, the threads of the screw only engage the far fragment and, when the screw is tightened, it draws the two parts together in compression. The lag screw works best if passed at right angles to the plane between the bone fragments. If there is a long fracture line, several screws can be inserted at different levels with each screw at right angles to the fracture plane at their respective sites. A similar lag effect is achieved if the screw is threaded only near its tip – a partially threaded screw.

The pull-out strength of a screw fixed in bone depends on factors involving both the screw and the bone: it increases (1) with the size of screw and the length of screw embedded; (2) with the thickness and density of the bone in which it is embedded; (3) if both cortices are engaged by the screw.

Most screws are inserted after drilling a pilot-hole and tapping, although self-drilling and self-tapping varieties are available. In cancellous bone, and particularly if it is osteoporotic, it may be preferable not the tap after pre-drilling; tapping removes additional bone that would help anchor the screw.

INTERNAL FIXATION BY PLATES AND SCREWS

Plates of varying design may be incorporated: (1) simple *straight compression plates*, which will allow compression along the axis of the plate; (2) *contoured plates* to fit specific bones; (3) *low-profile plates* that reduce the 'footprint' on the bone so as to preserve local vascularity; (4) *locked plates* where the screw also engages the plate by a secure mechanism so as to create a stable construct and prevent toggling.

The plate may be applied subperiosteally by a formal exposure of the fracture or osteotomy, or extraperiosteally (in the submuscular plane) so as to span the site. These are internal splints that should not be used as loadbearing devices. The ability to control loads across the bone will depend on the degree of contact

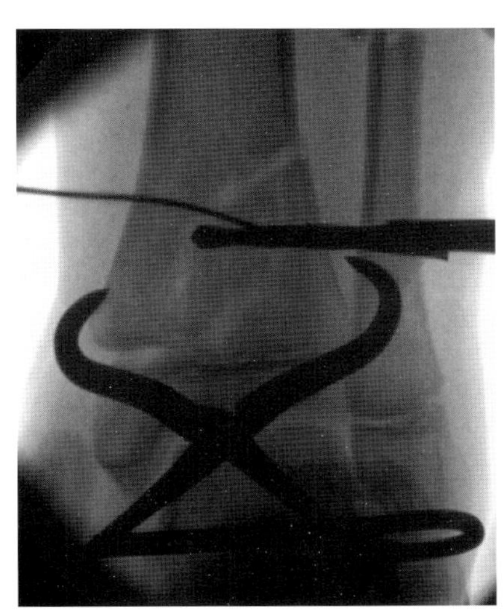

(a)

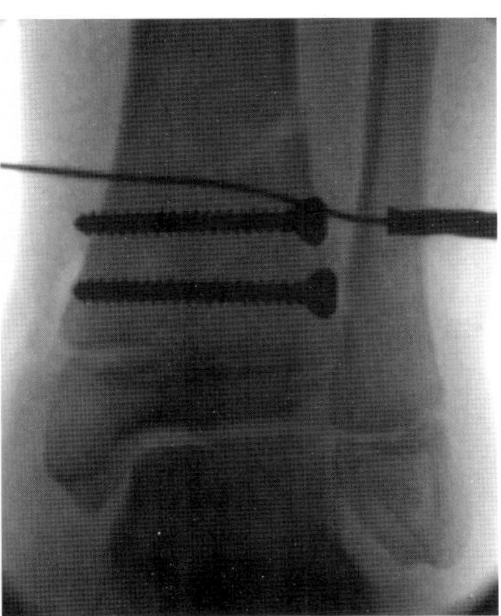

(b)

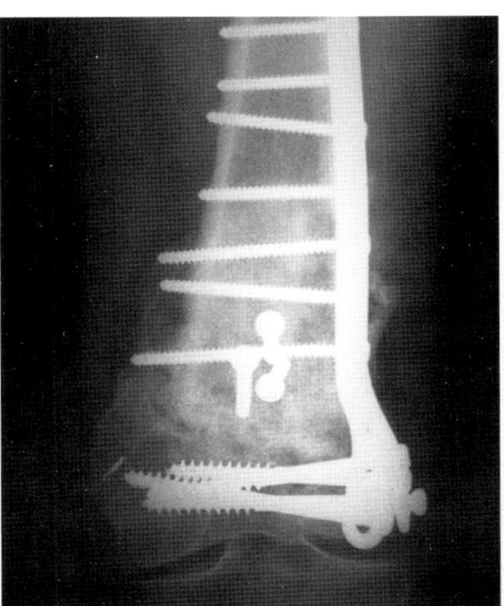

(c)

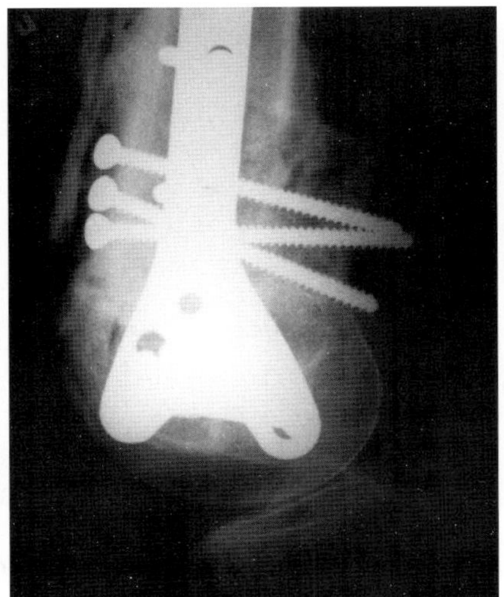

(d)

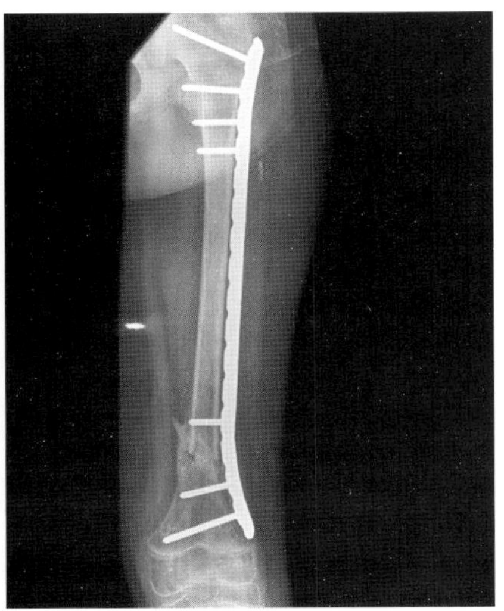

(e)

12.9 Lag screw fixation This is accomplished through design of the screw (being unthreaded for part of the shank) or through overdrilling the near fragment (a,b). Lag screws are thus used individually or in conjunction with a plate (c,d). Plates can be applied to control twisting forces (here they are used in conjunction with lag screws) or simply as long internal splints, as in indirect submuscular plating of fractures (e).

between the bone ends; it is important that this should be accomplished, usually by compression across the bone ends by a lag screw or through the plate itself (Fig. 12.9).

In addition to improving contact between the bone ends, compression through the plate can be utilized as part of the tension-band concept. Curved long bones have a compression side and tension side when axially loaded; plate application on the tension side will convert the loading forces that attempt to separate the fracture ends into compressive ones and thereby maintain bone contact.

INTERNAL FIXATION BY INTRAMEDULLARY DEVICES

Two major design types are used: those with and those without interlocking capabilities. *Interlocking nails* have become a standard fixation method for most shaft fractures of the tibia and femur in adults. Stability from these nails is due to a combination of an interference (frictional) fit within the medullary canal and the capture of bone to nail by means of the interlocking screws. Interlocked intramedullary nails offer better control of length and torsion than the unlocked varieties of this device. Older nail designs had an open cross-section but these are being replaced by closed section devices, which provide greater torsional stiffness.

The medullary canals of the femur and tibia are not simple curves and there are variations between individuals. None of the present-day nail designs are anatomically contoured; therefore intramedullary reaming to a diameter greater than the nail to be used allows unimpeded insertion of the device. Insufficient reaming potentially risks the bone splitting during nail insertion as a result of hoop stresses (expansile forces) generated.

Unlocked intramedullary nails are increasingly used in the treatment of long-bone shaft fractures in children. These flexible rods are inserted so as not to damage the physes at either end of the long bone and function as internal splints until callus formation takes over (Fig. 12.10).

EXTERNAL FIXATION

External fixators are useful for open fractures and for reconstruction of limbs using the Ilizarov method. They can also be used as temporary fracture stabilization devices when the local soft tissue conditions need improving before open surgery, or during emergency fixation of multiple long-bone fractures (Fig. 12.11).

The fixator functions as an exoskeleton through which the patient's own skeleton can be supported and adjusted. The basic components are wires or pins inserted into bone to which rods or rings are attached and interconnected. Pin- or wire-related problems have limited widespread adoption of this method; newer pin designs, and some with hydroxyapatite coating have reduced the frequency of problems. The mechanics of pin-hold in bone is governed by similar factors to that of screws.

External fixators are mainly of the *unilateral-planar* or *circular* types; there are also designs that combine

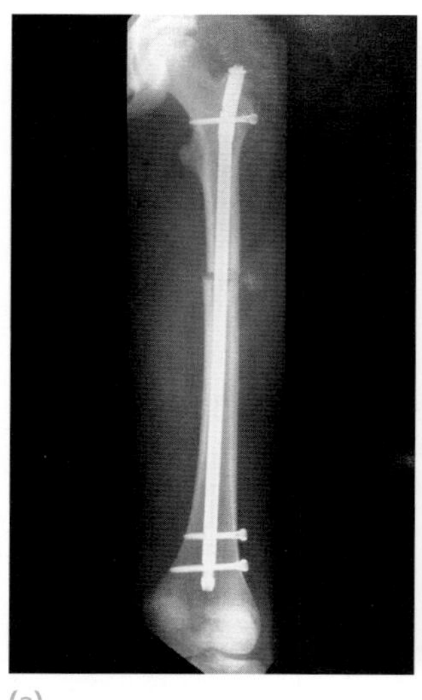
(a)

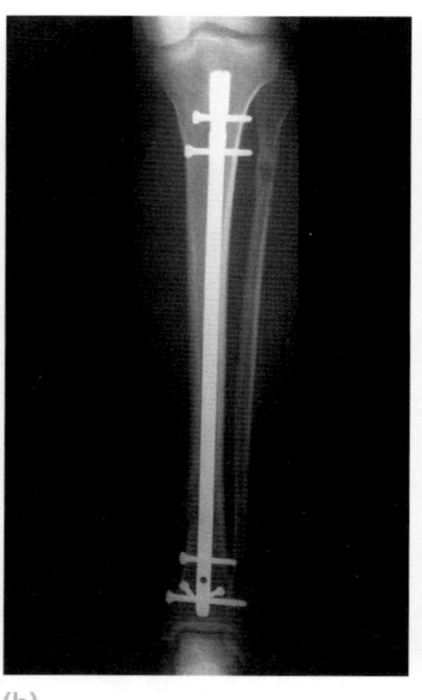
(b)

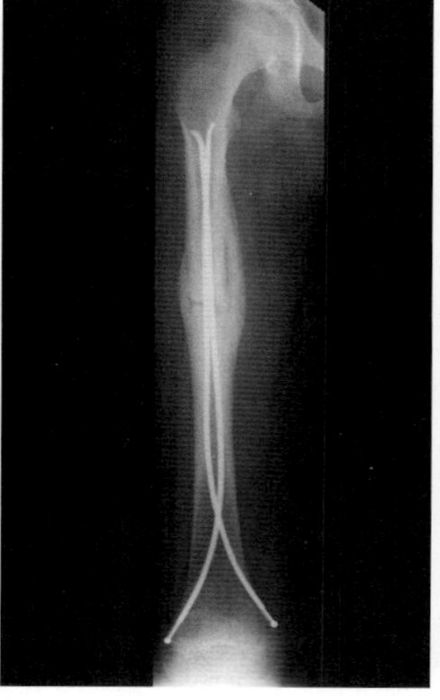
(c)

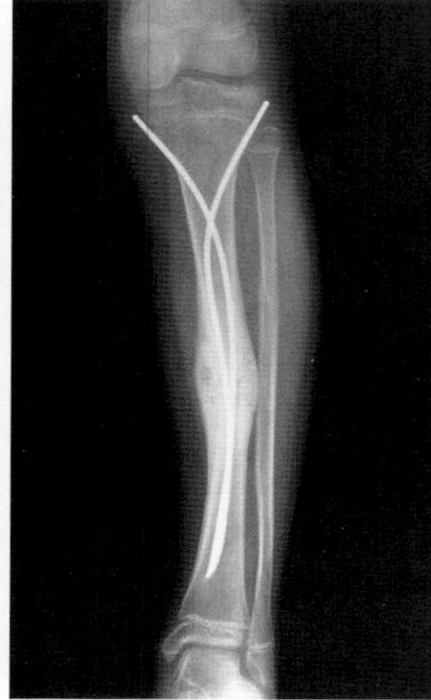
(d)

12.10 Intramedullary nails These are excellent for stabilizing shaft fractures of the major long bones: (a) femur; (b) tibia. Locked nails have the added benefit of controlling length and torsion. Flexible and elastic nails work by three-point fixation and are suitable for paediatric fractures where damage to the physis can be avoided (c, d).

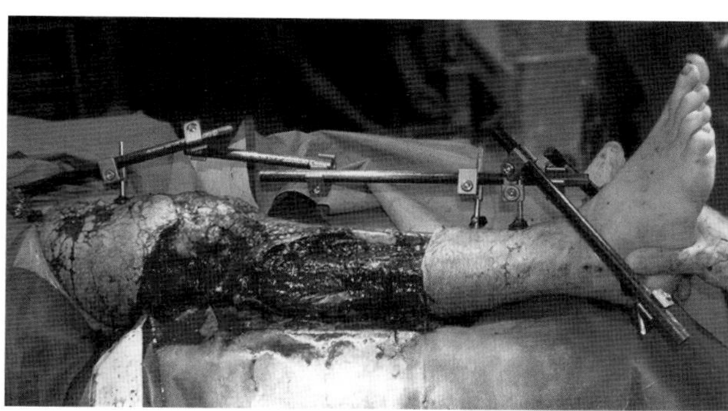

(a)

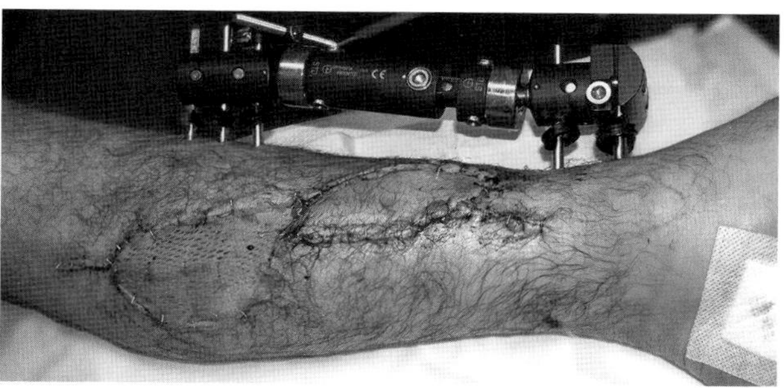

(b)

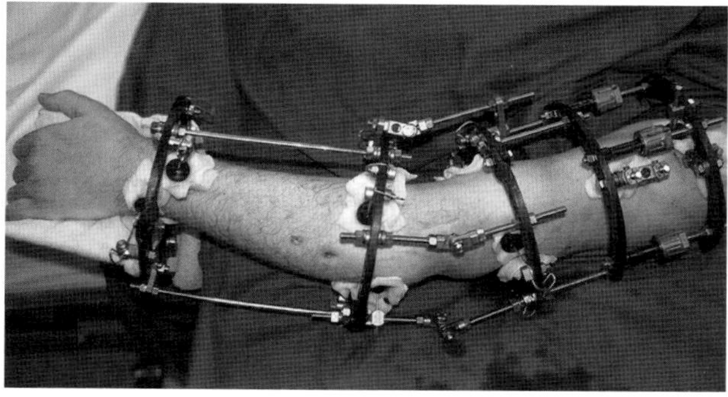

(c)

12.11 External fixators (a) These are useful for provisional fracture control, as in severe open fractures. Fixators are also used for definitive fracture treatment (b) and for Ilizarov limb reconstruction surgery (c).

aspects of both types (*hybrid*). Each possesses specific biomechanical properties with regard to control of movement at the fracture or osteotomy site, especially when the patient loads the limb on walking. The choice of a fixator type will depend on many factors including the intended purpose of its use and the surgeon's familiarity with the device.

BONE GRAFTS AND SUBSTITUTES

Bone grafts are both *osteoinductive* and *osteoconductive*: (1) they are able to stimulate osteogenesis through the differentiation of mesenchymal cells into osteoprogenitor cells; (2) they provide linkage across defects and a scaffold upon which new bone can form. Osteogenesis is brought about partly by the activity of cells surviving on the surface of the graft but mainly by the action of osteoprogenitor cells in the host bed.

Three basic requirements for osteogenesis are the presence of osteoprogenitor cells, a bone matrix and growth factors.

AUTOGRAFTS (AUTOGENOUS GRAFTS)

Bone is transferred from one site to another in the same individual. These are the most commonly used grafts and are satisfactory provided that sufficient bone of the sort required is available and that, at the recipient site, there is a clean vascular bed.

Cancellous autografts

Cancellous bone can be obtained from the thicker portions of the ilium, greater trochanter, proximal metaphysis of the tibia, lower radius, olecranon, or from an excised femoral head. Cortical autografts can be harvested from any convenient long bone or from the iliac crest; they usually need to be fixed with screws, sometimes reinforced by a plate and can be placed on the host bone, or inlaid, or slid along the long axis of the bone. Cancellous grafts are more rapidly incorporated into host bone than cortical grafts, but sometimes the greater strength of cortical bone is needed to provide structural integrity.

The autografts undergo necrosis, though a few surface cells remain viable. The graft stimulates an inflammatory response with the formation of a fibrovascular stroma; through this, blood vessels and osteoprogenitor cells can pass from the recipient bone into the graft. Apart from providing a stimulus for bone growth (osteoinduction), the graft also provides a passive scaffold for new bone growth (osteoconduction). Cancellous grafts become incorporated more quickly and more completely than cortical grafts (Fig. 12.12).

Vascularized grafts

This is theoretically the ideal graft; bone is transferred complete with its blood supply, which is anastomosed to vessels at the recipient site. The technique is difficult and time consuming and requires microsurgical skill. Available donor sites include the iliac crest (complete with one of the circumflex arteries), the fibula (with the peroneal artery) and the radial shaft. Vascularized grafts remain completely viable and become incorporated by a process analogous to fracture healing.

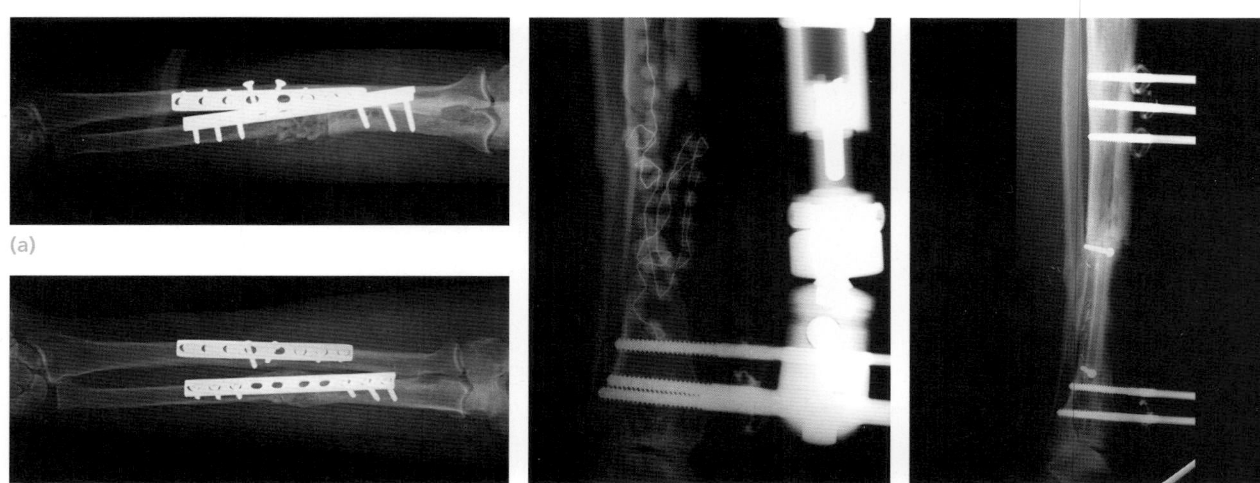

12.12 Autogenous cancellous bone grafts (a) Here autogenous grafts are used to fill a defect of the ulna and they unite with the host bone in 4 months (b). Free vascularized bone transfer (in this case a portion of fibula) is also helpful when larger defects need to be filled (c,d).

Bone marrow aspirates

Bone marrow contains stem cells and osteoprogenitor cells, which are able to transform into osteoblasts in the appropriate environment and with stimulation. The number of these mesenchymal cells in aspirates from the iliac crest decreases with age and more so in females (Muschler et al., 2001). In addition, the aspiration technique from the iliac crest can influence the number of osteoblast progenitors obtained; this may account for the variable results reported in the small clinical series thus far published. The recommended procedure is to take multiple small-volume aspirates (four 1 mL aspirates from separate site punctures). Centrifugation of the aspirate, in order to concentrate the cellular contents, has provided encouraging results in animal experiments; early evidence suggests this also may be the optimal method for using bone marrow aspirates in humans (Hernigou et al., 2005).

Platelet-derived activators

'Activators' are now available through centrifugation of venous blood. These factors activate repair of tissues (not just bone) and may augment healing processes in vivo. Further strong clinical evidence to their efficacy is awaited.

Allografts (homografts)

Allografts consist of bone transferred from one individual (alive or dead) to another of the same species. They can be stored in a bone bank and, as supplies can be plentiful, are particularly useful when large defects have to be filled. However, sterility must be ensured. The potential for transfer of infection is either from contamination at the time of harvesting or from diseases present in the donor. The graft must be harvested under sterile conditions and the donor must be cleared for malignancy, syphilis, cytomegalovirus, hepatitis and HIV; this requires prolonged (several months) testing of the donor before the graft is used. Sterilization of the donor material can be done by exposure to ethylene oxide or by ionizing radiation, but the physical properties and potential for osteoinduction are considerably altered (De Long et al., 2007).

Fresh allografts, though dead, are not immunologically acceptable. They induce an inflammatory response in the host and this may lead to rejection. However, antigenicity can be reduced by freezing (at –70°C), freeze-drying or by ionizing radiation.

Demineralization is another way of reducing antigenicity and it may also enhance the osteoinductive properties of the graft. Acid extraction of allograft bone yields ***demineralized bone matrix***, which contains collagen and growth factors. It is available in a variety of forms (putty, powder, granules) and is sometimes combined with other types of bone substitutes. The osteoinductive capability of demineralized bone matrix is variable; most human studies have not shown the impressive osteoinductive capacity found in animal experiments. One way to supplement the properties of demineralized bone matrix is to use it as an autologous bone graft expander.

Allografts are most often used in reconstructive surgery where pieces are inserted for structural support; an example is revision hip arthroplasty where bone loss from prosthesis loosening is replaced. The process of incorporation of allografts (when it occurs) is similar to that with autografts but slower and less complete.

Bone morphogenetic proteins (BMPs)

These substances were originally extracted from allograft bone but were too difficult to produce in commercially suitable quantities. BMP-2 and BMP-7 are now manufactured using recombinant techniques and are available commercially.

BMPs are osteoinductive. There is evidence to support their use in the treatment of non-union and open tibial fractures where the success rate is equivalent to that of autogenous bone grafts. They are used with a carrier, which may be allograft, demineralized bone matrix, collagen or bioactive bone cement. Currently, the cost of purchase is a barrier to widespread adoption.

Calcium-based synthetic substitutes

Calcium phosphate, hydroxyapatite (a crystalline calcium phosphate) and calcium sulphate are primarily osteoconductive and need a pore size of around 400 μm for osteoprogenitor cells to lay down bone.

The calcium phosphate and hydroxyapatite varieties are usually used to fill metaphyseal defects in fracture surgery, e.g. tibial plateau, distal radius and calcaneal fractures; in this context, several studies have reported good results. Various forms of the material are available, including granules, chips and paste. Despite claims by manufacturers to the contrary, these synthetic substitutes do not possess sufficient compressive strength to withstand high loads and should be used in stabilized fractures and not as a means of contribution to stability. Calcium phosphate materials are usually absorbed completely by 6–9 months, but hydroxyapatite substitutes are still visible on x-ray after several years. This slow resorption has prompted hydroxyapatite and calcium phosphate mixtures to be made available, in the hope that the faster resorption of the latter will enable more rapid bone replacement. Calcium phosphate has also been successfully mixed with autologous bone marrow and bovine collagen to produce results equivalent to those of autogenous bone graft (Chapman et al., 1997).

In contrast, calcium sulphate materials are usually resorbed within 6–9 weeks and are useful, in combination with gentamicin or tobramycin, as a means of local antibiotic delivery in the treatment of cavities or 'dead space' after surgery in chronic osteomyelitis (McKee et al., 2002) (Fig. 12.13).

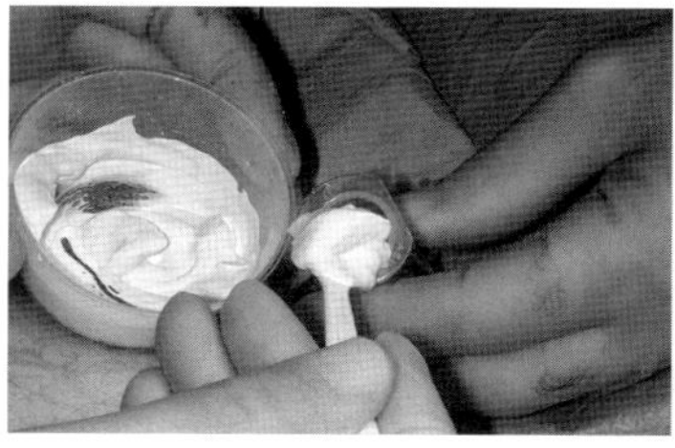

(a)

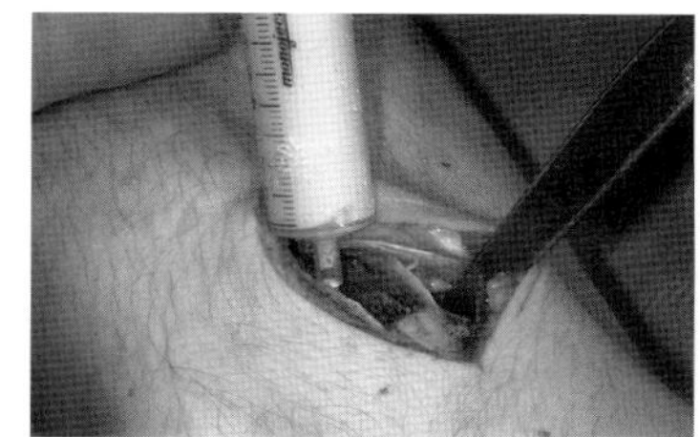

(b)

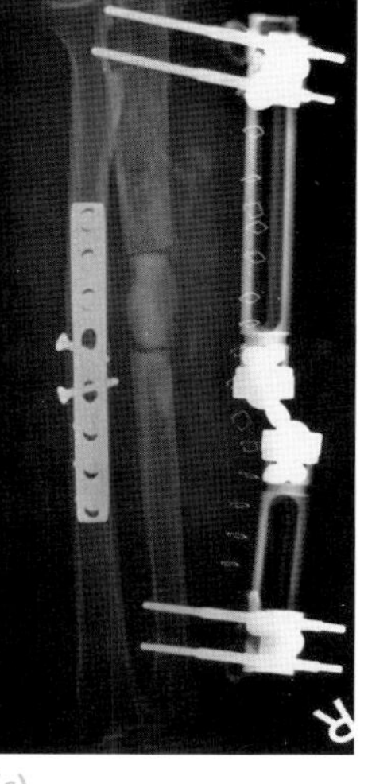

(c)

12.13 Synthetic bone substitutes These are used primarily as osteoconductive agents or as a delivery medium for antibiotics. Several forms are available, including putties and injectable pastes (a,b). They are used to fill small defects or can act as antibiotic-eluting spacers after bone resection in chronic osteomyelitis (c).

DISTRACTION OSTEOGENESIS AND LIMB RECONSTRUCTION – ILIZAROV METHOD

Distraction osteogenesis is a form of tissue engineering founded on the principle of *tension-stress*, which is the generation of new bone in response to gradual increases in tension. Discovered in the 1950s by Gavril Ilizarov in Russia, the application of this principle to orthopaedic conditions represents a significant advance; it has opened opportunities for treatment in conditions that hitherto were poorly treated or even untreatable. The term *'Ilizarov method'* embraces the various applications of this principle, emphasizing minimally invasive surgery (many of the techniques are performed percutaneously) and an early return of function.

Distraction osteogenesis

Callotasis

Callus distraction, or *callotasis*, is perhaps the single most important application of the tension-stress principle. It is used for limb lengthening or filling of large segmental defects in bone, either through bone transport or other strategies. The basis of the technique is to produce a careful fracture of bone, followed by a short wait before the young callus is gradually distracted via a circular or unilateral external fixator. It is worth noting that all tissue types are created during the distraction process and the term *distraction histogenesis* is perhaps more appropriate.

The external fixator is applied using transfixing wires or screws proximal and distal to the proposed osteogenesis site. The surgical fracture to allow distraction osteogenesis to commence is done by several methods. In a *corticotomy*, the bony cortex is partially divided with a sharp osteotome through a small skin incision and the break completed by osteoclasis, leaving the medullary blood supply and endosteum largely intact. Alternatively, the periosteum can be incised and elevated and the bone then drilled several times before using an osteotome to complete the division; the periosteum is then repaired. Both techniques are exacting – simply dividing the bone with a power saw results in nothing being formed in the gap. After an initial wait of 5–10 days, distraction is begun and proceeds at 1 mm a day, with small (usually 0.25 mm) increments spaced out evenly throughout the day. The first callus is usually seen on x-ray after 3–4 weeks; in optimum conditions it appears on x-ray as an even column of partially radio-opaque material in the gap between the bone fragments (this is called the *regenerate*). If the distraction rate is too fast, or the osteotomy performed poorly, the regenerate may be thin with an hourglass appearance; conversely if distraction is too slow, it may appear bulbous or worse still may consolidate prematurely, thereby preventing any further lengthening.

When the desired length is reached, a second wait follows, which allows the regenerate column to consolidate and harden. Weightbearing is permitted throughout this period and it assists the consolidation process. The regenerate column is first seen on x-ray to be divided by an irregular line (the *fibrous interzone*), which gradually disappears when the column of bone completely ossifies. Regular x-rays allow the surgeon to check on the quality of regenerate (Fig. 12.14). When cortices of even thickness are seen in the regenerate on x-ray, the fixator is ready to be removed. Throughout treatment, physiotherapy is important to preserve joint movement and avoid contractures.

CHONDRODIATASIS

Bone lengthening can also be achieved by distracting the growth plate (*chondrodiatasis*). No osteotomy is needed but the distraction rate is slower, usually 0.25 mm twice daily. Although a wide, even column of regenerate is usually seen, the fate of the physis is sealed – the growth plate frequently closes after the process. This technique is best reserved for children close to the end of growth.

BONE TRANSPORT

Distraction osteogenesis is used not only for limb lengthening but also as a means of filling segmental defects in bone. In *bone transport*, the defect (or gap) is filled gradually by creating a 'floating' segment of bone through a corticotomy either proximal or distal to the defect, and this segment is moved slowly across the defect. An external fixator provides stability and the ability to control this segment during the process. As the segment is transported from the corticotomy site to the new docking site, new bone is created in its wake, which effectively fills the defect (Fig. 12.15).

A variant of the bone transport technique is *bifocal*

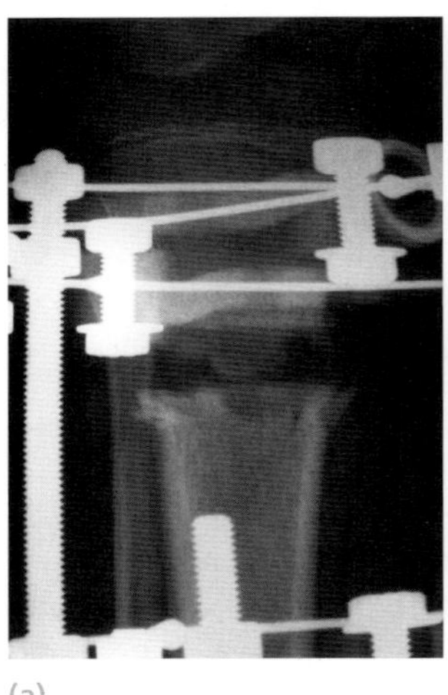
(a)

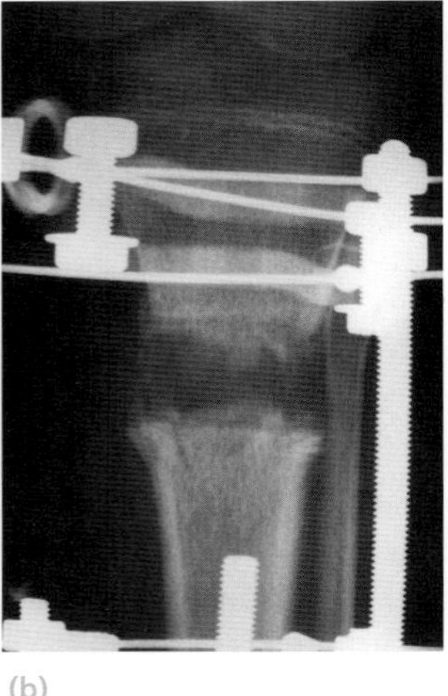
(b)

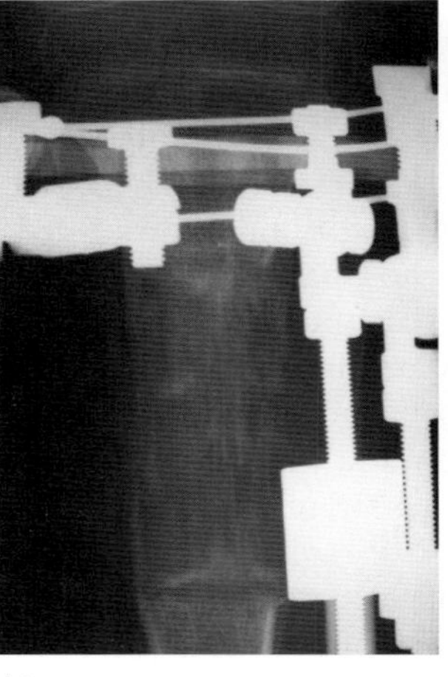
(c)

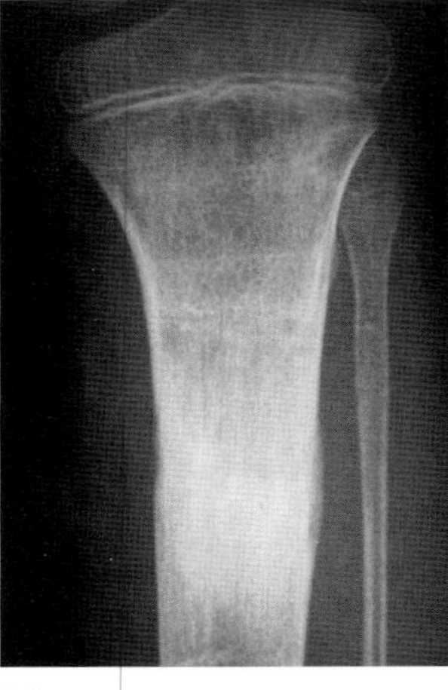
(d)

12.14 Distraction osteogenesis Early on there is little activity in the distracted gap (a). A little later, columns of bone are seen reaching for the centre of the distracted zone, leaving a clear space in between – the fibrous interzone (b). When the columns bridge the gap, the regenerate bone matures and, finally, a medullary cavity is re-established (c,d).

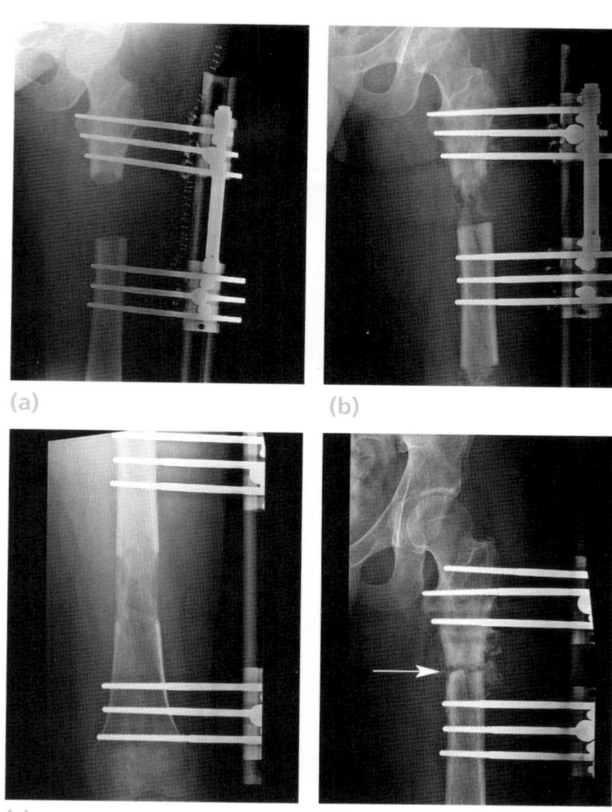

12.15 Bone transport. A segment of bone 'travels' across a defect. The limb length is, therefore, unchanged. (a,b,c) The segment is created by osteotomy and gradual distraction produces new bone. The docking site (arrow) often needs attending to in order to heal (d).

compression-distraction. With this method, the defect is closed by instantly bringing the bone ends together; a corticotomy is then performed at a different level and length is restored by callotasis. In this case the limb is shortened temporarily, whereas in bone transport overall limb length remains unchanged.

Correcting bone deformities and joint contractures

Angular deformities are corrected by carefully planned osteotomies. However, the amount of correction needed may induce, if undertaken acutely, an unwanted sudden tension on soft tissues, particularly nerves. With the Ilizarov method, it is now possible to undertake large corrections with a much lower risk. The correction is performed gradually with the aid of an external fixator; length, rotation and translation deformities can be dealt with simultaneously (Fig. 12.16).

The principle of tension stress can also be applied to correcting soft-tissue contractures. For example, a resistant club-foot deformity is dealt with by applying gradual tension to the contracted soft tissue structures through an external fixator and slowly altering the position of the ankle, subtalar and midtarsal joints until a normal position is achieved. The assembly of the external fixator to accomplish this technique is complex, but the results are often gratifying.

LEG LENGTH EQUALIZATION

Inequality of leg length may result from many causes, including congenital anomalies, malunited fractures, epiphyseal and physeal injuries, infections and paralysis. Marked inequality leads to inefficient walking and a noticeable limp. The longer leg has to be lifted higher to clear the ground during swing-through and the pelvis and shoulders dip noticeably during the stance phase on the shorter side; both of these adjustments increase energy consumption. Pelvic tilt and the associated compensatory scoliosis tend to cause backache, and there is a higher reported incidence of osteoarthritis of the hip on the longer side – possibly because of the 'uncovering' of the femoral head due to pelvic obliquity.

Inequality greater than 2.5 cm needs treatment, which may amount to no more than a shoe-raise, or it may involve an operation to either the shorter or longer leg.

Techniques for correcting leg length

There are four choices:

- shortening the longer leg
- slowing growth in the longer leg
- lengthening the shorter leg
- speeding up growth in the shorter leg.

The problem of leg length inequality often presents in childhood. Several questions need to be answered before a technique appropriate for the particular child is determined:

- What will the discrepancy be when the child is mature?
- What is the expected adult height of the child?
- When will the child reach skeletal maturity?
- Is there a deformity associated with the leg length discrepancy?

Leg length difference at maturity is estimated through charts and tables and by plotting the rate of change in discrepancy over a period. Expected adult height is calculated through formulae – the TW3 method is one (Tanner et al., 2001), and the time of skeletal maturity is obtained by reading the bone age from an x-ray of the non-dominant hand.

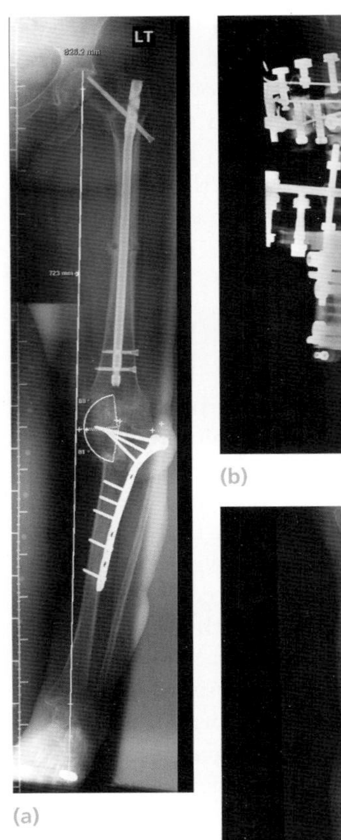
(a)

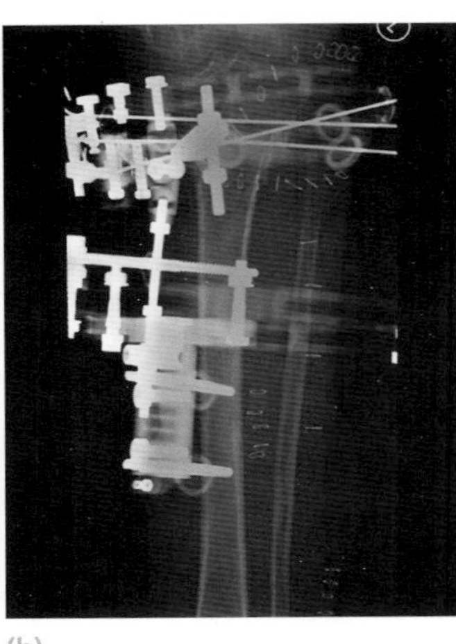
(b)

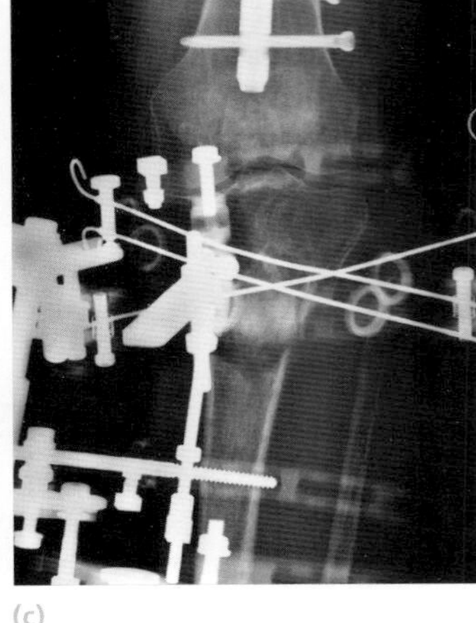
(c)

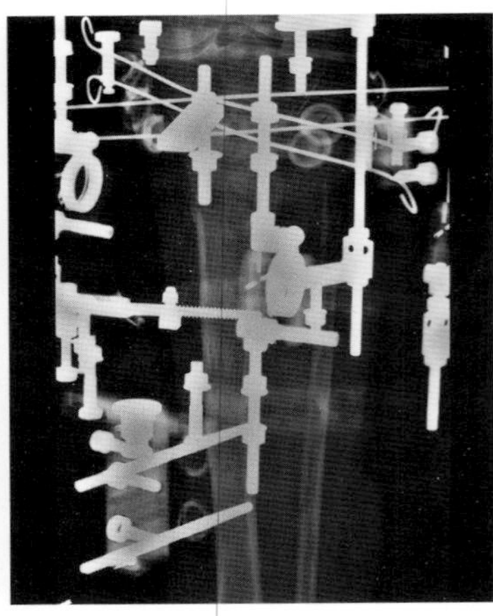
(d)

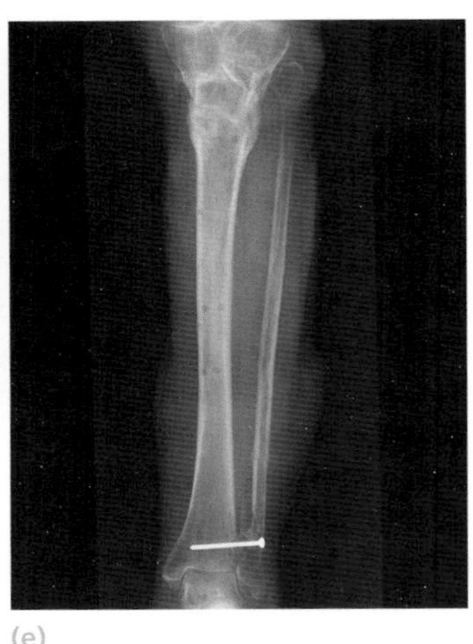
(e)

12.16 Correction of deformity (a) Varus malunion in a fracture of the proximal tibia was corrected by osteotomy and gradual realignment in a circular external fixator (b–d). A cuneiform-shaped mass of bone formed after the axes were aligned (e).

Operations on the longer leg

Physeal arrest

In children, physeal arrest is an effective method of slowing the rate of growth of the longer leg; it can be temporary, using removable staples fixed across the growth plate, or permanent, by drilling across the physis and curetting out the growth plate. Another method is to excise a rectangular block of bone across the physis, rotate the block through 90 degrees and then reinsert it into the original bed. When the physis fuses (epiphyseodesis), longitudinal growth at that site ceases and the overall gain in length of the limb is retarded. In due course the difference in lengths should be reduced.

The timing and technique of epiphyseodesis is important. If it is inaccurately timed, a difference in leg lengths will remain, and if improperly done, deformity may occur. Physeal arrest will create a loss of 10 mm of length a year from the distal femur and 6 mm a year from the proximal tibia. As the physes close naturally at 16 years of age in boys and 14 years in girls, a predicted length discrepancy at maturity of 45 mm can, for example, be addressed by both a distal femoral and proximal tibial physeal arrest performed about 3 years before skeletal maturity.

Epiphyseodesis produces approximate length equalization, often to within 10 mm of estimated length, if performed in a timely fashion. Other methods of predicting the timing of epiphyseodesis are chart based (Moseley, 1977; Eastwood and Cole, 1995) or use a multiplier method (Aguilar et al., 2005).

Bone shortening

Epiphyseodesis is feasible only in a growing child. In adults, it is necessary to excise a segment of bone, preferably from the femur, since tibial shortening is more complicated and is cosmetically unattractive; up to 7.5 cm of femoral shortening can be achieved without permanent loss of function. The safest technique is to excise a segment from between the lesser trochanter and the femoral isthmus, to approximate the cut ends, and to fix them together with a locking intramedullary nail or plate. Open excision of bone segments from the long leg has several disadvantages, among which scarring and poor muscle tone are important. The scarring results from a longitudinal incision being suddenly subjected to a concertina effect, which causes the wound to gape widely. Shorter segments can be removed by 'closed' intramedullary techniques, which rely on an intramedullary saw and bone splitter, and thereby avoid the problem with scars. In general, shortening of the long leg is reserved for situations where the patient is too old for an epiphyseodesis or where lengthening the short leg is deemed too risky, e.g. in the presence of unstable joints or infection.

Shortening should, of course, be applied only if the patient's residual height will still be acceptable. It should also be remembered that the longer leg is usually the normal one and if a serious complication such as non-union ensues, the patient may be worse off than not having an operation in the first place.

Lengthening the shorter leg

Lengthening the short leg is most easily accomplished by wearing a raised shoe, but this is often inadequate or unacceptable – a shoe raise of more than 5 cm can risk injury to the ankle!

Stimulation of the growth plate can be achieved by the technique of periosteal division. A circumferential 5 mm strip is excised from around the distal femoral or proximal tibial physis (Wilde and Baker, 1987). The physis responds with an accelerated growth rate that may last for up to 2 years. However, like epiphyseodesis, poor technique may produce deformity; the method is probably best reserved for young children (younger than 6 years) as the effects on older children are unpredictable.

Limb lengthening by the Ilizarov method is a suitable method for predicted length discrepancies of greater than 5 cm. Distraction osteogenesis has become much safer since it was appreciated that distraction has to be slow if neural or vascular damage is to be avoided (see earlier). Major length corrections can be tackled by staging the treatment process over several years, or by attempting to lengthen at two levels within the same bone (*bifocal lengthening*). The latter method, although attractive, has a higher rate of complications largely from the soft tissues being distracted too quickly.

OPERATIONS TO INCREASE STATURE

Bilateral leg lengthening is a feasible procedure for people with achondroplasia and other individuals of short stature, but detailed consultation is an essential preliminary. The prospective patient must understand that treatment is painful, prolonged, and may be associated with a substantial number of complications such as pin-site sepsis, deformity or fracture. Moreover, gain in height is not the same as 'normality'. Nevertheless, successful treatment is so rewarding ("People no longer look at me in the street; I can now get things off a shelf without having to climb up") that it should not be withheld if the patient is otherwise normal and is psychologically prepared. Referral to a specialized centre is wise.

The techniques of lengthening are as described earlier and two bones can be dealt with simultaneously. It is more usual to lengthen both tibiae at one procedure and both femora at another. Gains in height averaging 20–25 cm have been achieved by combining the bone lengthening with soft-tissue releases (McAndrew and Saleh, 2007).

OPERATIONS ON JOINTS

ARTHROTOMY

Arthrotomy (opening a joint) may be indicated to: (1) inspect the interior or perform a synovial biopsy; (2) drain a haematoma or an abscess; (3) remove a loose body or damaged structure (e.g. a torn meniscus); (4) to excise inflamed synovium. The intra-articular tissues should be handled with great care, and if postoperative bleeding is expected (e.g. after synovectomy) a drain should be inserted – postoperative haemarthrosis predisposes to infection. Following the operation the joint should be rested for a few days, but thereafter movement must be encouraged.

ARTHRODESIS

The most reliable operation for a painful or unstable joint is arthrodesis; where stiffness does not seriously affect function, this is often the treatment of choice. Examples are the spine, tarsus, ankle, wrist and interphalangeal joints. Arthrodesis is also useful for a knee that is already fairly stiff (provided the other knee has good movement) and for a flail shoulder. More controversial is arthrodesis of the hip. Though it is a reasonable alternative to arthroplasty or osteotomy for joint disease in young patients, there is an understandable resistance to sacrificing all movement in such an important joint. It is difficult to convey to the patient that a fused hip can still 'move' by virtue of pelvic tilting and rotation; the best approach is to introduce the patient to someone who has had a successful arthrodesis.

The principles of arthrodesis are straightforward and involve four stages: (1) *exposure* – both joint

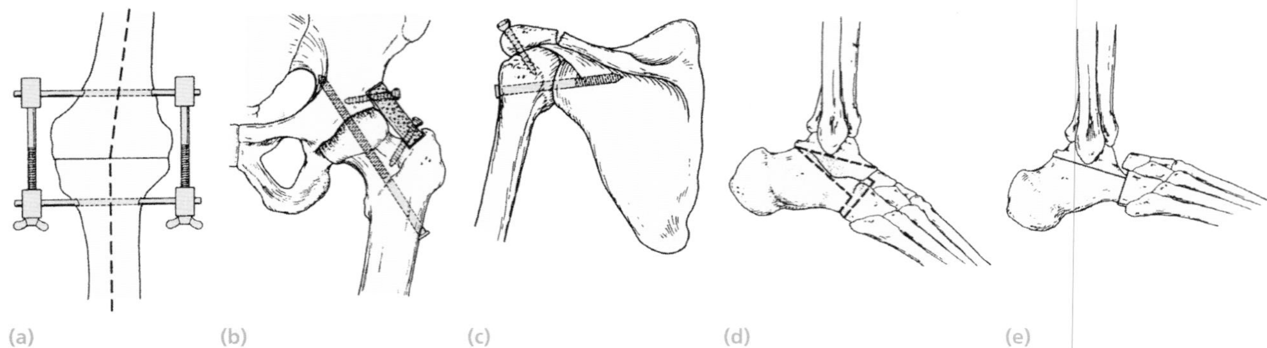

12.17 Arthrodesis (a) Compression arthrodesis; (b) screw plus bone graft; (c) similar technique using the acromion. (d,e) Subtalar mid-tarsal fusion.

surfaces need to be well visualized and often this means an extensile incision, but some smaller joints are now accessible by arthroscopic means; (2) *preparation* – both articular surfaces are denuded of cartilage and sometimes the subchondral bone is 'feathered' to increase the contact area; (3) *coaptation* – the prepared surfaces are apposed in the optimum position, ensuring good contact; (4) *fixation* – the surfaces are held rigidly by internal or external fixation. Sometimes bone grafts are added in the larger joints to promote osseous bridging (Fig. 12.17).

The main *complication* is non-union with the formation of a pseudoarthrosis. Rigid fixation lessens this risk; where feasible (e.g. the knee and ankle), the bony parts are squeezed together by compression-fixation devices.

ARTHROPLASTY

Arthroplasty, the surgical refashioning of a joint, aims to relieve pain and to retain or restore movement. The following are the main varieties (Fig. 12.18):

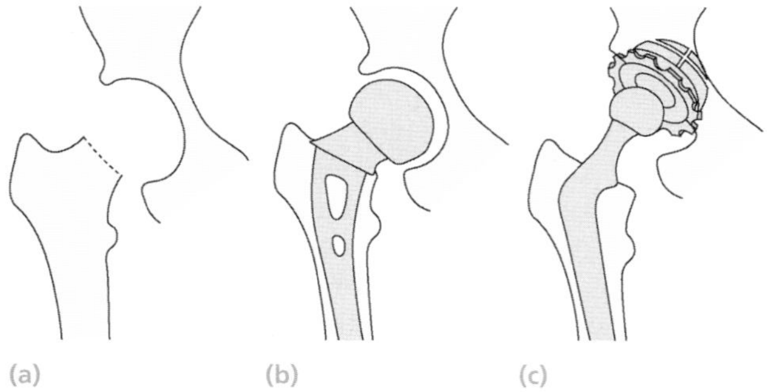

12.18 Arthroplasty The main varieties as applied to the hip joint: (a) excision arthroplasty (Girdlestone); (b) partial replacement – an Austin Moore prosthesis has been inserted after removing the femoral head; (c) total replacement – both articular surfaces are replaced.

- *Excision arthroplasty* – Sufficient bone is excised from the articulating parts of the joint to create a gap at which movement can occur (e.g. Girdlestone's hip arthroplasty). This movement is limited and occurs through intervening fibrous tissue, which forms in the gap. In some situations, e.g. after excising the trapezium, a shaped 'spacer' can be inserted; this is often tendon harvested from nearby.
- *Partial replacement* – One articulating part only is replaced (e.g. a femoral prosthesis for a fractured femoral neck, without an acetabular component); or one compartment of a joint is replaced (e.g. the medial or lateral half of the tibiofemoral joint). The prosthesis is kept in position either by acrylic cement or by a press-fit between implant and bone.
- *Replacement* – Both the articulating parts are replaced by prosthetic implants; for biomechanical reasons, the convex component is usually metal and the concave high-density polyethylene. Metal-on-metal replacements are also becoming more common. Irrespective of type, these components are fixed to the host bone, either with acrylic cement or by a cementless press-fit technique. Using hip replacement as an example, the rationale, indications and complications of total joint replacement are discussed in detail in Chapter 19.

MICROSURGERY AND LIMB REPLANTATION

Microsurgical techniques are used in repairing nerves and vessels, transplanting bone or soft tissue with a vascular pedicle, transferring a less essential digit (e.g. a toe) to replace a lost essential one (e.g. a thumb) and – occasionally – for reattaching a severed limb or digit. Essential prerequisites are an operating microscope, special instruments, microsutures, a chair with

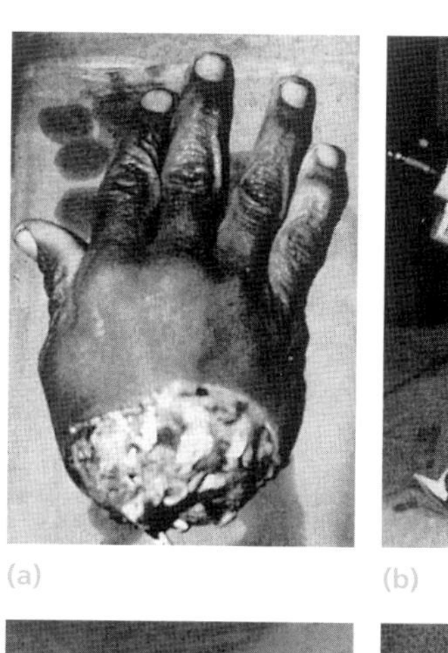
(a)

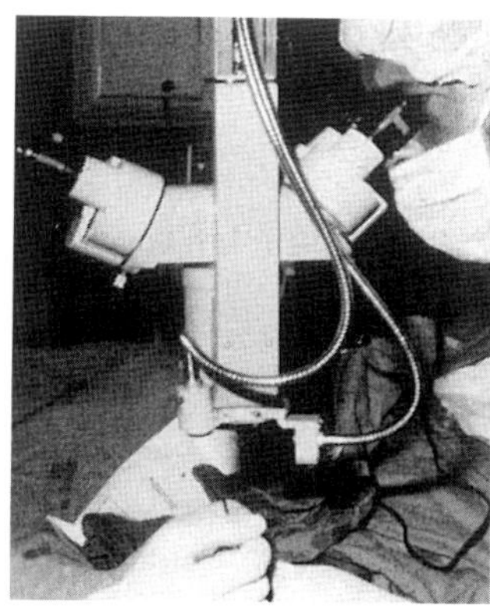
(b)

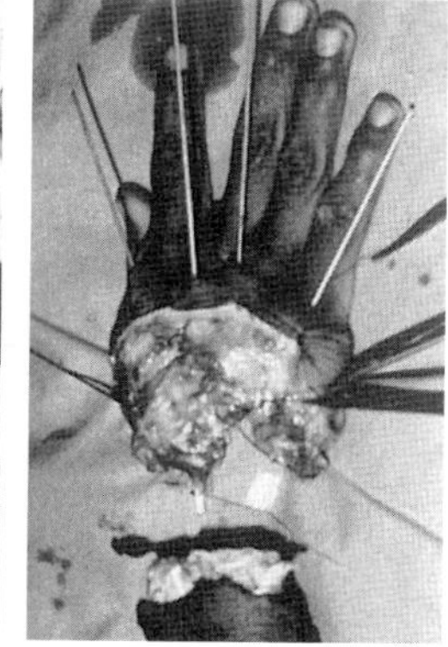
(c)

(d)

(e)

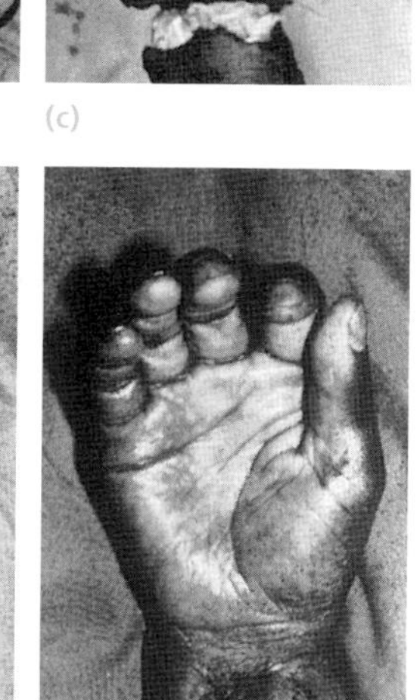
(f)

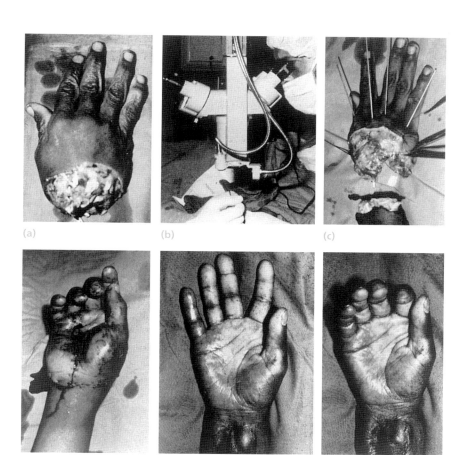

12.19 Microsurgery and limb replantation (a) The problem – a severed hand. (b) The solution – replantation with microsurgical techniques. (c) The bones of the severed hand have been fixed with K-wires as a preliminary to suturing vessels and nerves. (d) The appearance at the end of the operation. (e,f) The limb 1 year later; the fingers extend fully and bend about halfway. But the hand survived, has moderate sensation and the patient was able to return to work (as a guillotine operator in a paper works!)

arm supports and – not least – a surgeon well practised in microsurgical techniques.

For *replantation*, the severed part should be kept cool during transport. The more muscle in the amputated part, the shorter the period it will last; warm ischaemic periods of greater than 6 hours are likely to result in permanent muscle damage and may even produce severe systemic upset in the patient when reperfusion of the muscle occurs. Two teams dissect, identify and mark each artery, nerve and vein of the stump and the limb. Following careful debridement the bones are shortened to reduce tension and are stabilized internally. Next the vessels are sutured – veins first and (if possible) two veins for each artery. Nerves and tendons next need to be sutured. Only healthy ends of approximately equal diameter should be joined; tension, kinking and torsion must be prevented. Decompression of skin and fascia, as well as thrombectomy, may be needed in the postoperative period (Fig. 12.19).

Replantation surgery is time consuming, expensive and often unsuccessful. It should be carried out only in centres specially equipped and by teams specially trained for this work.

AMPUTATIONS

INDICATIONS

Alan Apley, in characteristic style, encapsulated the indications for amputation in the never-to-be-forgotten 'three Ds': (1) *Dead,* (2) *Dangerous* and (3) *Damned nuisance*:

Dead (or dying) Peripheral vascular disease accounts for almost 90 per cent of all amputations. Other causes of limb death are *severe trauma*, *burns* and *frostbite*.

Dangerous 'Dangerous' disorders are *malignant tumours*, *potentially lethal sepsis* and *crush injury*. In crush injury, releasing the compression may result in renal failure (the crush syndrome).

Damned nuisance Retaining the limb may be worse than having no limb at all. This may be because of: (1) pain; (2) gross malformation; (3) recurrent sepsis or (4) severe loss of function. The combination of deformity and loss of sensation is particularly trying, and in the lower limb is likely to result in pressure ulceration.

Varieties

A *provisional amputation* may be necessary because primary healing is unlikely. The limb is amputated as distal as the causal conditions will allow. Skin flaps sufficient to cover the deep tissues are cut and sutured loosely over a pack. Re-amputation is performed when the stump condition is favourable.

A *definitive end-bearing amputation* is performed when pressure or weight is to be borne through the end of a stump. Therefore the scar must not be terminal, and the bone end must be solid, not hollow, which means it must be cut through or near a joint. Examples are through-knee and Syme's amputations.

A *definitive non-end-bearing amputation* is the commonest variety. All upper limb and most lower limb amputations come into this category. Because weight is not to be taken at the end of the stump, the scar can be terminal.

AMPUTATIONS AT SITES OF ELECTION

Most lower limb amputations are for ischaemic disease and are performed through the site of election below the most distal palpable pulse. The selection of amputation level can be aided by Doppler indices; if the ankle/brachial index is greater than 0.5, or if the occlusion pressure at the calf and thigh are greater than 65 mmHg and 50 mmHg respectively, then there is a greater likelihood the below-knee amputation will succeed (Sarin et al., 1991). An alternative means is by using transcutaneous oxygen tension as a guide, but the level that assures wound healing and avoids unnecessary above-knee amputations has not been confidently determined. The knee joint should be preserved if clinical examination and investigations suggest this is at all feasible – energy expenditure for a trans-tibial amputee is 10–30 per cent greater as compared to a 40–67 per cent increase in trans-femoral cases (Czerniecki, 1996; Esquenazi and Meier, 1996; Mattes et al., 2000).

The sites of election are determined also by the demands of prosthetic design and local function. Too short a stump may tend to slip out of the prosthesis. Too long a stump may have inadequate circulation and can become painful, or ulcerate; moreover, it complicates the incorporation of a joint in the prosthesis (Fig. 12.20). For all that, the skill of the modern prosthetist has made it possible to amputate at almost any site.

Principles of technique

A tourniquet is used unless there is arterial insufficiency. Skin flaps are cut so that their combined length equals 1.5 times the width of the limb at the site of amputation. As a rule anterior and posterior flaps of equal length are used for the upper limb and for trans-femoral (above-knee) amputations; below the knee a long posterior flap is usual.

Muscles are divided distal to the proposed site of bone section; subsequently, opposing groups are sutured over the bone end to each other and to the periosteum, thus providing better muscle control as well as better circulation. It is also helpful to pass the sutures that anchor the opposing muscle groups through drill-holes in the bone end, creating an *osteomyodesis*. Nerves are divided proximal to the bone cut to ensure a cut nerve end will not bear weight.

The bone is sawn across at the proposed level. In trans-tibial amputations the front of the tibia is usually bevelled and filed to create a smoothly rounded contour; the fibula is cut 3 cm shorter.

The main vessels are tied, the tourniquet is removed and every bleeding point meticulously ligated. The skin is sutured carefully without tension. Suction drainage is advised and the stump covered without constricting passes of bandage; figure-of-eight passes are better suited and prevent the creation of a venous tourniquet proximal to the stump.

Aftercare

If a haematoma forms, it is evacuated as soon as possible. After satisfactory wound healing, gradual

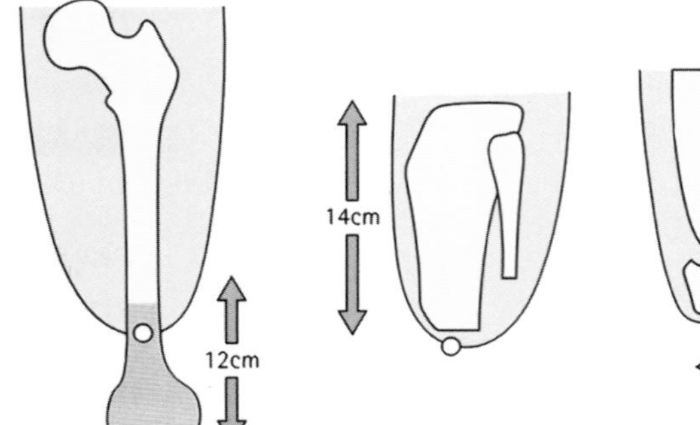

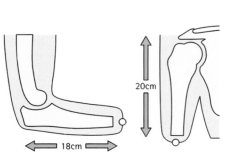

12.20 Amputations The traditional sites of election; the scar is made terminal because these are not end-bearing stumps.

compression stump socks are used to help shrink the stump and produce a conical limb-end. The muscles must be exercised, the joints kept mobile and the patient taught to use his prosthesis.

AMPUTATIONS OTHER THAN AT SITES OF ELECTION

Interscapulo-thoracic (forequarter) amputation) This mutilating operation should be done only for traumatic avulsion of the upper limb (a rare event), when it offers the hope of eradicating a malignant tumour, or as palliation for otherwise intractable sepsis or pain.

Disarticulation at the shoulder This is rarely indicated, and if the head of the humerus can be left, the appearance is much better. If 2.5 cm of humerus can be left below the anterior axillary fold, it is possible to hold the stump in a prosthesis.

Amputation in the forearm The shortest forearm stump that will stay in a prosthesis is 2.5 cm, measured from the front of the flexed elbow. However, an even shorter stump may be useful as a hook to hang things from.

Amputations in the hand These are discussed in Chapter 16.

Hemipelvectomy (hindquarter amputation) This operation is performed only for malignant disease.

Disarticulation through the hip This is rarely indicated and prosthetic fitting is difficult. If the femoral head, neck and trochanters can be left, it is possible to fit a tilting-table prosthesis in which the upper femur sits flexed; if, however, a good prosthetic service is available, a disarticulation and moulding of the torso is preferable.

Transfemoral amputations A longer stump offers the patient better control of the prosthesis and it is usual to leave at least 12 cm below the stump for the knee mechanism. However, recent gait studies suggest some latitude is present as long as the amputated femur is at least 57 per cent of the length of the contralateral femur (Baum et al., 2008).

Around the knee The Stokes–Gritti operation (in which the trimmed patella is apposed to the trimmed femoral condyle) is rarely performed because the bone may not unite securely; the end-bearing stump is rarely satisfactory and there is no room for a sophisticated knee mechanism.

Amputation through the knee is used at times but is often associated with poorer functional and psychological outcomes to above-knee amputees. Fitting a modern knee mechanism is troublesome and the sitting position reveals the knees to be grossly unequal in level. The main indication for this procedure is in children because the lower femoral physis is preserved, effectively permitting a stump length equivalent to an above-knee amputation to be reached when the child is mature.

Transtibial (below-knee) amputations Healthy below-knee stumps can be fitted with excellent prostheses allowing good function and nearly normal gait. Even a 5–6 cm stump may be fitted with a prosthesis in a thin patient; greater length makes fitting easier, but there is no advantage in prolonging the stump beyond the conventional 14 cm.

Above the ankle Syme's amputation This is sometimes very satisfactory, provided the circulation of the limb is good. It gives excellent function in children, and shares the same advantage as a through-knee amputation in that the distal physis is preserved. In adults it is well accepted by men, but women find it cosmetically undesirable. The indications are few and the operation is difficult to do well. Because the stump is designed to be end-bearing, the scar is brought away from the end by cutting a long posterior flap. The flap must contain not only the skin of the heel but the fibrofatty heel pad so as to provide a good surface for weightbearing. The bones are divided just above the malleoli to provide a broad area of cancellous bone, to which the flap should stick firmly; otherwise the soft tissues tend to wobble about.

Pirogoff's amputation Similar in principle to Syme's but this is rarely performed. The back of the os calcis is fixed onto the cut end of the tibia and fibula.

Partial foot amputation The problem here is that the tendo-Achillis tends to pull the foot into equinus; this can be prevented by splintage, tenotomy or tendon transfers. The foot may be amputated at any convenient level; for example, through the mid-tarsal joints (Chopart), through the tarsometatarsal joints (Lisfranc), through the metatarsal bones or through the metatarsophalangeal joints. It is best to disregard the classic descriptions and to leave as long a foot as possible provided it is plantigrade and that an adequate flap of plantar skin can be obtained. The only prosthesis needed is a specially moulded slipper worn inside a normal shoe.

In the foot Where feasible, it is better to amputate through the base of the proximal phalanx rather than through the metatarsophalangeal joint. With diabetic gangrene, septic arthritis of the joint is not uncommon; the entire ray (toe plus metatarsal bone) should be amputated.

PROSTHESES

All prostheses must fit comfortably, should function well and look presentable. The patient accepts and uses a prosthesis much better if it is fitted soon after operation; delay is unjustifiable now that modular components are available and only the socket need be made individually.

In the upper limb, the distal portion of the prosthesis is detachable and can be replaced by a 'dress hand' or by a variety of useful terminal devices. Electrically powered limbs are available for both children and adults.

In the lower limb, weight can be transmitted through the ischial tuberosity, patellar tendon, upper tibia or soft tissues. Combinations are permissible; recent developments in silicon and gel materials provide improved comfort in total-contact self-suspending sockets.

COMPLICATIONS OF AMPUTATION STUMPS

EARLY COMPLICATIONS

In addition to the complications of any operation (especially secondary haemorrhage), there are two special hazards: breakdown of skin flaps and gas gangrene:

Breakdown of skin flaps This may be due to ischaemia, suturing under excess tension or (in below-knee amputations) an unduly long tibia pressing against the flap.

Gas gangrene Clostridia and spores from the perineum may infect a high above-knee amputation (or re-amputation), especially if performed through ischaemic tissue.

LATE COMPLICATIONS

Skin Eczema is common, and tender purulent lumps may develop in the groin. A rest from the prosthesis is indicated.

Ulceration is usually due to poor circulation, and re-amputation at a higher level is then necessary. If, however, the circulation is satisfactory and the skin around an ulcer is healthy, it may be sufficient to excise 2.5 cm of bone and resuture.

Muscle If too much muscle is left at the end of the stump, the resulting unstable 'cushion' induces a feeling of insecurity that may prevent proper use of a prosthesis; if so, the excess soft tissue must be excised.

Blood supply Poor circulation gives a cold, blue stump that is liable to ulcerate. This problem chiefly arises with below-knee amputations and often re-amputation is necessary.

Nerve A cut nerve always forms a neuroma and occasionally this is painful and tender. Excising 3 cm of the nerve above the neuroma sometimes succeeds. Alternatively, the epineural sleeve of the nerve stump is freed from nerve fascicles for 5 mm and then sealed with a synthetic tissue adhesive or buried within muscle or bone away from pressure points.

'Phantom limb' This term is used to describe the feeling that the amputated limb is still present. In contrast, residual limb pain exists in the area of the stump. Both features are prevalent in amputees to a varying extent, and appear to have greater significance in those who also have features of depressive symptoms. The patient should be warned of the possibility; eventually the feeling recedes or disappears but, in some, long-term medication may be needed. A painful phantom limb is very difficult to treat.

Joint The joint above an amputation may be stiff or deformed. A common deformity is fixed flexion and fixed abduction at the hip in above-knee stumps (because the adductors and hamstring muscles have been divided). It should be prevented by exercises. If it becomes established, subtrochanteric osteotomy may be necessary. Fixed flexion at the knee makes it difficult to walk properly and should also be prevented.

Bone A spur often forms at the end of the bone, but is usually painless. If there has been infection, however, the spur may be large and painful and it may be necessary to excise the end of the bone with the spur.

If the bone is transmitting little weight, it becomes osteoporotic and liable to fracture. Such fractures are best treated by internal fixation.

IMPLANT MATERIALS

METAL

Metal used in implants (screws, plates, intramedullary nails and joint replacement prostheses) should be tough, strong, non-corrosive, biologically inert and easy to sterilize. Those commonly used are stainless steel, cobalt–chromium alloys and titanium alloys. No one material is ideal for all purposes.

Stainless steel, because of its relative plasticity, can be cold worked. This is a process in which the metal is reshaped or resized, usually at room temperature, which increases its hardness and strength. The form of stainless steel used in orthopaedic surgery is 316L; in addition to iron, it contains chromium (which forms an oxide layer providing resistance to corrosion), carbon (which adds strength but needs to be in low concentrations – hence the L suffix – or else it offsets corrosion resistance), nickel and molybdenum as the main elements used in the alloy. The tensile plasticity (ductility) of stainless steel makes it possible to bend plates to required shapes during an operation without seriously disturbing their strength.

Cobalt chromium-based alloys are widely used in joint prosthesis manufacture. Chromium is added to cobalt for *passivation*; an adherent oxide layer formed by the chromium provides corrosion resistance, as it does in stainless steel. Other elements are sometimes added, e.g. tungsten and molybdenum, to improve strength and machining ability. These alloys have a long track record of biocompatibility in human tissue and have also, through forging and cold-working, high strength.

Titanium alloys are used in fracture fixation devices and joint prostheses. They usually contain aluminium and vanadium in low concentrations for strength; passivation (and thus corrosion resistance) is obtained by creating a titanium oxide layer. The elastic modulus of the metal is close to that of bone and this reduces the stress concentrations that can occur when stainless steel or cobalt chromium alloys are used. Additionally, the corrosion resistance (which is superior to that of the other two alloys) augments this metal's biocompatibility. A disadvantage of titanium alloy is notch sensitivity; this is when a scratch or sharp angle created in the metal, either at manufacture or during insertion of the implant, can significantly reduce its fatigue life.

Implant failure

Metal implants may fail for a variety of reasons: (1) defects during manufacture; (2) incorrect implant selection for intended purpose; (3) exposure to repeated high stresses from incorrect seating of the implant or from exceeding the fatigue life as when there is delay in a fracture union (Fig. 12.21).

Corrosion

Corrosion is inevitable unless the implanted metal is treated, e.g. by passivation, which creates a protective passive layer; this is usually an oxide layer formed from chemical treatment. In stainless steel and cobalt chromium, it is the chromium component that helps in creating an oxide layer but, in titanium, the element itself forms it. With passivated metal alloys used in orthopaedic surgery, corrosion is rarely a problem except when damage to the passive layer occurs; it may be initiated by abrasive damage or minute surface cracks due to fatigue failure. Even in the absence of these faults, failure can occur through crevice corrosion (where the process is heightened by low oxygen concentrations in crevices – e.g. beneath the heads of screws and plates) or stress corrosion (where repeated low stresses in a corrosive environment cause failure before the fatigue life of the implant is reached). The products of corrosion, metal ions and debris, cause a local inflammatory response that accelerates loosening.

Dissimilar metals

Dissimilar metals immersed in solution in contact with one another may set up galvanic corrosion with accelerated destruction of the more reactive (or 'base') metal. In the early days of implant surgery, when highly corrodible metals were used, the same thing happened in the body. However, the passive alloys now used for implants do not exhibit this phenomenon (titanium being particularly resistant to chemical attack), and the traditional fear of using dissimilar metals in bone implants is probably exaggerated.

Friction and wear

These mechanical concepts are relevant to understanding joint function and prosthesis design. Friction

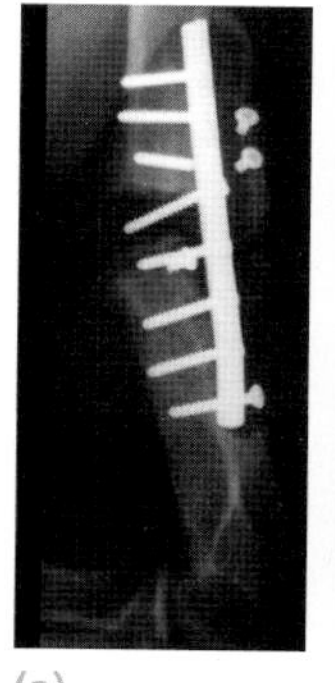
(a)

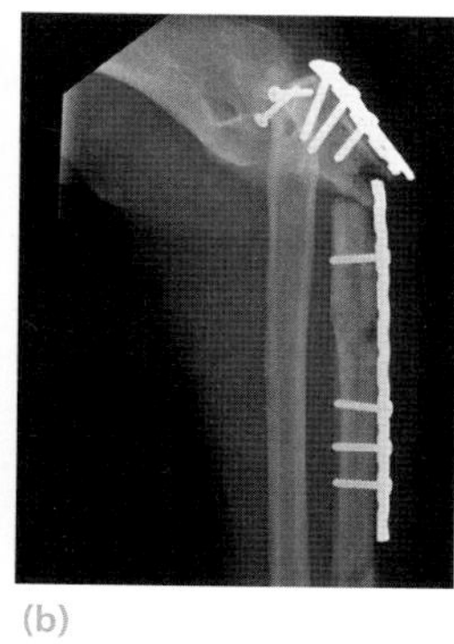
(b)

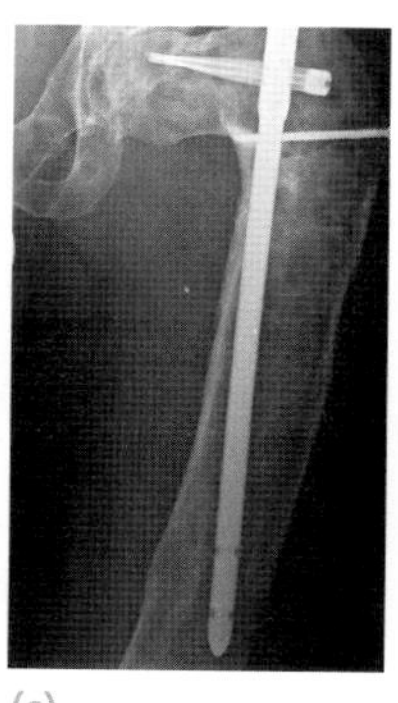
(c)

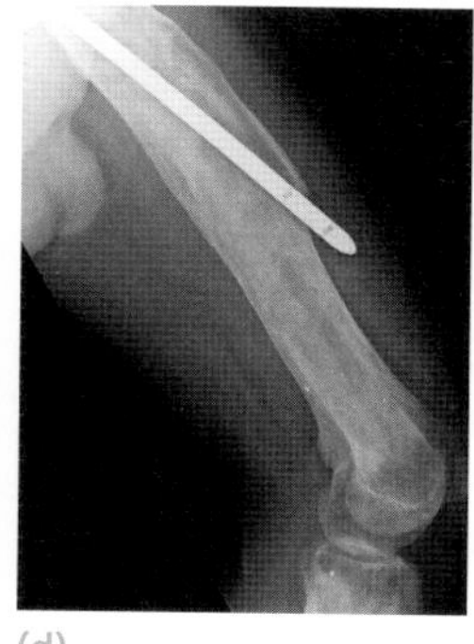
(d)

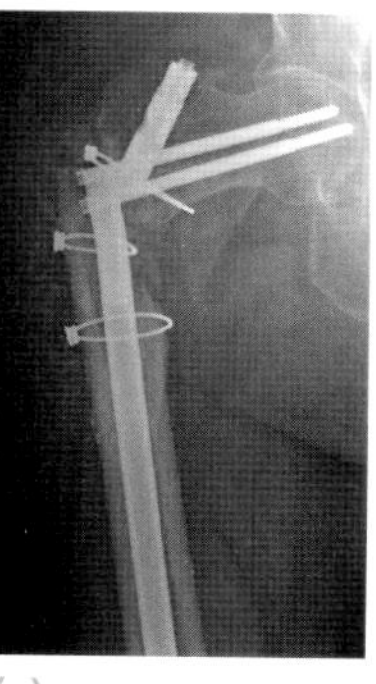
(e)

12.21 Fatigue failure of implants Fatigue failure can be due to (a,b) incorrect implant selection (too small or too weak) or (c,d) incorrect positioning. Other factors are also involved: infection may delay union and lead to eventual implant fracture (e).

between two sliding surfaces will not be affected by the area of contact or the speed of movement but will depend on the applied load. Therefore, any two surfaces can have a coefficient of friction derived to represent this interaction – it is the ratio of the force needed to start a sliding movement to the normal compression force between the surfaces.

Normal human joints possess coefficients of friction that are about ten times lower than those of various combinations of metal-on-metal. Metal-on-ultra high molecular weight polyethylene produces a better (lower) coefficient of friction and this is improved further if the metal is replaced by a ceramic, e.g. alumina or zirconium.

An important modulator of friction characteristics in joints is lubrication. Synovial fluid reduces the coefficient of friction either by forming a layer of fluid that is greater in width than the surface irregularities on normal articular cartilage (fluid film lubrication) or, in the absence of this interposed fluid layer, a molecular-width coating that resists abrasion (boundary lubrication). Both methods may be involved under different joint loading conditions.

Friction and joint lubrication are related to wear – the loss of surface material due to sliding motion under load. Wear is proportional to the load and distance of movement between the two surfaces. Wear between surfaces can be the result of abrasion (a harder surface eroding the surface of the softer material), adhesion (where the two surfaces bond more tightly than particles within one of the surfaces), or from debris that becomes trapped between articulating surfaces and causes abrasion (third-body wear). Metal wear particles may cause local inflammation and scarring, and occasionally a toxic or allergic reaction; most importantly, however, they may cause implant loosening following their uptake by macrophages and subsequent activation of osteoclastic bone resorption. Metal wear particles have also been demonstrated in lymph nodes and other organs far distant from the implant; the significance of this finding is uncertain. Wear of articular cartilage is offset partly by an ability to repair, although this capacity diminishes with age; this mechanism is obviously not possessed by prostheses.

Infection

Metal does not cause infection. Titanium alloys have been shown to be less susceptible to the development of infection when exposed to the same inoculums of bacteria (as compared to stainless steel), but the mechanism of this difference is uncertain. Once infection is established, several mechanisms come into play that encourage its persistence: (1) the metal implant acts as a foreign body that is devoid of blood supply and thereby inaccessible to immune processes; (2) it promotes the formation of biofilms that encase micro-colonies of the bacteria and render them immune to defence mechanisms and antibiotics; (3) the implant impedes drainage.

Malignancy

A few cases of malignancy at the site of metal implants have been reported, but the number is so small in comparison with the number of implants that the risk can probably be discounted.

ULTRA-HIGH MOLECULAR WEIGHT POLYETHYLENE

Ultra-high molecular weight polyethylene (UHMWPE) is an inert thermoplastic polymer. Its density is close to that of the low-density polyethylenes but the very high molecular weight provides increased strength and wear resistance over other types of polyethylene. The material is manufactured for hip (acetabular cup) and knee (tibial tray) prostheses and sterilized by gamma irradiation. The latter process was noted to cause oxidation of the material and detrimentally alter its physical and chemical properties to the extent that a 'shelf life' for the component was created. Consequently, current techniques of sterilization involve gamma irradiation in an oxygen-free environment, e.g. in nitrogen. Although ethylene oxide sterilization is an alternative way, irradiation of UHMWPE enables cross-linking of the polymer, which also improves wear rates.

In contact to polished metal UHMWPE has a low coefficient of friction and it therefore seemed ideal for joint replacement. This has proved to be true in hip reconstruction with a simple ball-and-socket articulation. However, UHMWPE has disadvantages: (1) the cross-linked form may have improved wear properties but poorer yield strength, which may influence crack development and propagation; (2) being a viscoelastic material, it is susceptible to deformity (stretching) and creep; (3) UHMWPE is also easily abraded, a reflection of poor hardness, and chips of bone or acrylic cement trapped on its surface cause it to disintegrate.

SILICON COMPOUNDS

There is a wide variety of silicon polymers, of which silicone rubber (Silastic) is particularly useful. It is firm, tough, flexible and inert, and was used to make hinges for replacing finger and toe joints. However, long-term results are tainted by the material's susceptibility to fracture if the implant surface is nicked or torn by a sharp instrument or piece of bone.

The presence of silicon particles in the body may induce a giant-cell synovitis; sometimes bone erosion and 'cyst' formation are seen at some distance from the actual implant. For these reasons the main use for Silastic is as temporary spacers to lie within tendon pulleys prior to tendon transplants.

CARBON

This eminently biocompatible material is looking for a purpose. As graphite it has wear and lubricant properties that might fit it for joint replacement. As carbon fibre it is sometimes used to replace ligaments; it induces the formation of longitudinally aligned fibrous tissue, which substitutes for the natural ligament. However, the carbon fibres tend to break up and if particles find their way into the synovial cavity they induce a synovitis. Carbon composites are also used to manufacture plates and joint prostheses; these have a lower modulus of elasticity than metal and may therefore be more compatible with the bone to which they are attached. Carbon fibre is also extensively used for the manufacture of external fixation devices, e.g. connecting rods and even circular rings, as the combination of lightweight, rigidity and x-ray lucency is attractive.

ACRYLIC CEMENT

In joint replacement the prostheses are often fixed to the bone with acrylic cement (polymethylmethacrylate – PMMA), which acts as a grouting material. It is usually presented as a liquid (the PMMA monomer) and powder (the PMMA polymer plus copolymers or other additives), which is mixed to set off an exothermic reaction of polymerization. Before the mixture sets, it is applied to the bone in which the prosthesis is embedded. With sufficient pressure the pasty material is forced into the bony interstices and, when fully polymerized, the hard compound prevents all movement between prosthesis and bone. It can withstand large compressive loads but is easily broken by tensile stress.

Cement mixing and cement introduction techniques have been shown to influence the tensile strength. An almost 50 per cent increase in tensile strength can be obtained by vacuum mixing or centrifugation of the mixture prior to application; this reduces the number of voids within the mixture. Additionally, pressurization of the cement within the bone cavity, prior to introduction of the implant, improves the interdigitating lock that is created between cement and interstices of the bone surface.

When the partially polymerized cement is forced into the bone there is often a drop in blood pressure; this is attributed to the uptake of residual monomer, which can cause peripheral vasodilatation, but there may also be fat embolization from the bone marrow. This is seldom a problem in fit patients with osteoarthritis, but in elderly people who are also osteoporotic, monomer and marrow fat may enter the circulation very rapidly when the cement is compressed and the fall in blood pressure can be alarming (and occasionally fatal).

With good cementing technique osseointegration can and does take place on the acrylic surface. However, if the initial cement application is not perfect, a fibrous layer forms at the cement/bone interface, its thickness depending on the degree of cement penetration into the bone crevices. In this flimsy membrane fine granulation tissue and foreign body giant cells can be seen. This relatively quiescent tissue remains unchanged under a wide range of biological and mechanical conditions, but if there is excessive movement at the cement/bone interface, or if polyethylene or metallic wear products track down into the cement/bone interface, an aggressive reaction ensues that produces bone resorption and disintegration of the interlocking surface; occasionally this is severe enough to justify the term 'aggressive granulomatosis' or 'aggressive osteolysis'. Bone resorption and cement loosening may also be associated with low-grade infection, which can manifest for the first time many years after the operation; whether the infection in these cases precedes the loosening or vice versa is still not known.

HYDROXYAPATITE

The mineral phase of bone exists largely in the form of crystalline hydroxyapatite (HA). It is not surprising, therefore, that this material has been used to reproduce the osteoinductive and osteoconductive properties of bone grafts. Porous hydroxyapatite obtained from coral exoskeleton is rapidly incorporated in living bone and synthetic implants consisting of hydroxyapatite and tricalcium phosphate are commercially available as bone graft substitutes (see earlier). HA can also be plasma sprayed onto implants; the HA coating is a highly acceptable substrate for bone cells and promotes rapid osseointegration. This technique has found a place in the use of uncemented hip replacement prostheses and with external fixator pins.

REFERENCES AND FURTHER READING

Aguilar JA, Paley D, Paley J *et al.* Clinical validation of the multiplier method for predicting limb length discrepancy and outcome of epiphysiodesis, part II. *J Pediatr Orthop* 2005; **25:** 192–6.

Alter HJ, Seeff LB, Kaplan PM *et al.* Type B hepatitis: the infectivity of blood positive for e antigen and DNA polymerase after accidental needlestick exposure. *N Engl J Med* 1976; **295:** 909–13.

Baum BS, Schnall BL, Tis JE, Lipton JS. Correlation of residual limb length and gait parameters in amputees. *Injury* 2008; **39:** 728–33.

Bjornara BT, Gudmundsen TE, Dahl OE. Frequency and timing of clinical venous thromboembolism after major joint surgery. *J Bone Joint Surg* 2006; **88B:** 386–91.

Blond L, Kirketerp-Moller K, Sonne-Holm S, Madsen JL. Exsanguination of lower limbs in healthy male subjects. *Acta Orthop Scand* 2002; **73:** 89–92.

Blond L, Madsen JL. Exsanguination of the upper limb in healthy young volunteers. *J Bone Joint Surg* 2002; **84B:** 489–91.

Bushell AJ, Klenerman L, Taylor S *et al.* Ischaemic preconditioning of skeletal muscle: 1. Protection against the structural changes induced by ischaemia/reperfusion injury. *J Bone Joint Surg* 2002; **84B:** 1184–8.

Chapman MW, Bucholz R, Cornell C. Treatment of acute fractures with a collagen-calcium phosphate graft material. A randomized clinical trial. *J Bone Joint Surg* 1997; **79A:** 495–502.

Czerniecki JM. Rehabilitation in limb deficiency. 1. Gait and motion analysis. *Arch Phys Med Rehabil* 1996; **77(Suppl 1):** S3–8.

De Long WG Jr, Einhorn TA, Koval K *et al.* Bone grafts and bone graft substitutes in orthopaedic trauma surgery. A critical analysis. *J Bone Joint Surg* 2007; **89A:** 649–58.

Eastwood DM, Cole WG. A graphic method for timing the correction of leg-length discrepancy. *J Bone Joint Surg* 1995; **77B:** 743–7.

Esquenazi A, Meier RH III. Rehabilitation in limb deficiency. 4. Limb amputation. *Arch Phys Med Rehabil* 1996; **77(Suppl 1):** S18–28.

Geerts WH, Bergqvist D, Pineo GF *et al.* Prevention of venous thromboembolism: American College of Chest Physicians Evidence-Based Clinical Practice Guidelines (8th edition). *Chest* 2008; **133(Suppl):** 381S–453S.

Gerberding JL, Littell C, Tarkington A *et al.* Risk of exposure of surgical personnel to patients' blood during surgery at San Francisco General Hospital. *N Engl J Med* 1990; **322:** 1788–93.

Hernigou P, Poignard A, Beaujean F, Rouard H. Percutaneous autologous bone-marrow grafting for nonunions. Influence of the number and concentration of progenitor cells. *J Bone Joint Surg* 2005; **87A:** 1430–7.

Ippolito G, Puro V, Heptonstall J *et al.* Occupational human immunodeficiency virus infection in health care workers: worldwide cases through September 1997. *Clin Infect Dis* 1999; **28:** 365–83.

Kahn SR, Shbaklo H, Lamptin DL *et al.* Determinants of health-related quality of life during the 2 years following deep vein thrombosis. *J Thromb Haemost* 2008; **6:** 1105–12.

Klenerman L. *The Tourniquet Manual – Principles and Practice.* Springer, London; 2003.

Klenerman L, Crawley J, Lowe A. Hyperaemia and swelling of a limb upon release of a tourniquet. *Acta Orthop Scand* 1982; **53:** 209–13.

Lieberman P. Anaphylactic reactions during surgical and medical procedures. *J Allergy Clin Immunol* 2002; **110(Suppl):** S64–9.

Lipp A, Edwards P. Disposable surgical face masks for preventing surgical wound infection in clean surgery. *Cochrane Database of Systematic Rev* 2002; CD002929.

Mattes SJ, Martin PE, Rover TD. Walking symmetry and energy cost in persons with unilateral transtibial amputations: Matching prosthetic and intact limb inertial properties. *Arch Phys Med Rehabil* 2000; **81:** 561–8.

McAndrew AR, Saleh M. Limb lengthening by the Vilarrubias method: the Sheffield Children's Hospital experience. *J Pediatr Orthop B* 2007; **16:** 233–5.

McKee MD, Wild LM, Schemitsch EH, Waddell JP. The use of an antibiotic-impregnated, osteoconductive, bioabsorbable bone substitute in the treatment of infected long-bone defects: Early results of a prospective trial. *J Orthop Trauma* 2002; **16:** 622–7.

Milstone AM, Passaretti CL, Perl TM. Chlorhexidine: expanding the armamentarium for infection control and prevention. *Clin Infect Dis* 2008; **46:** 274–81.

Moseley CF. A straight-line graph for leg-length discrepancies. *J Bone Joint Surg* 1977; **59A:** 174–9.

Muschler GF, Nitto H, Boehm CA, Easley KA. Age- and gender-related changes in the cellularity of human bone marrow and the prevalence of osteoblastic progenitors. *J Orthop Res* 2001; **19:** 117–25.

NICE. Venous thromboembolism – reducing the risk. www.guidance.nice.org.uk/CG92; 2010.

Nicolaides AF, Kakkar J, Breddin AK *et al.* Prevention and treatment of venous thromboembolism. International Consensus Statement (guidelines according to scientific evidence). *International Angiology* 2006; **25:** 101–61.

Noordin S, McEwen JA, Kragh JF, Eisen A, Masri BA. Surgical Tourniquets in Orthopaedics. *J Bone Joint Surg* 2009; **91A:** 2958–67.

Paley D. *Principles of Deformity Correction.* Springer, Berlin Heidelberg; 2002.

Pellegrini VD Jr, Sharrock NE, Paiement GD, Morris R, Warwick DJ. Venous thromboembolic disease after total hip and knee arthroplasty: current perspectives in a regulated environment. *Instr Course Lect* 2008; **57:** 637–61.

Pesavento R, Bernardi E, Concolato A *et al.* Postthrombotic syndrome. *Semin Thromb Hemost* 2006; **32:** 744–51.

Phillips SM, Gallagher M, Buchan H. Use graduated compression stockings postoperatively to prevent deep vein thrombosis. *BMJ* 2008; **336:** 943–4.

Quebbeman EJ, Telford GL, Hubbard S *et al.* Risk of blood contamination and injury to operating room personnel. *Ann Surg* 1991; **214:** 614–20.

Rutala WA, Weber DJ. A review of single-use and reusable gowns and drapes in health care. *Infect Control Hosp Epidemiol* 2001; **22:** 248–57.

Sarin S, Shami S, Shields DA *et al.* Selection of amputation level: a review. *Eur J Vasc Surg* 1991; **5:** 611–20.

Tanner J, Healy M, Goldstein H, Cameron N. *Assessment of skeletal maturity and prediction of adult height (TW3 method).* WB Saunders, London; 2001.

Tanner J, Parkinson H. Double gloving to reduce surgical cross-infection. *Cochrane Database of Syst Rev* 2006; **3:** CD003087.

Theocharopoulos N, Perisinakis K, Damilakis J *et al.* Occupational exposure from common fluoroscopic projections used in orthopaedic surgery. *J Bone Joint Surg* 2003; **85A:** 1698–1703.

Tooher RP, Middleton P, Pham C *et al.* A systematic review of strategies to improve prophylaxis for venous thromboembolism in hospitals. *Ann Surg* 2005; **241:** 397–415.

Warwick D, Dahl OE, Fisher WD *et al.* Orthopaedic thromboprophylaxis: limitations of current guidelines. *J Bone Joint Surg* 2008; **90B:** 127–32.

Warwick D, Friedman RJ, Agnelli G *et al.* Insufficient duration of venous thromboembolism prophylaxis after total hip or knee replacement when compared with the time course of thromboembolic events. Findings from the Global Orthopaedic Registry. *J Bone Joint Surg* 2007; **89B:** 799–807.

Webster J, Alghamdi AA. Use of plastic adhesive drapes during surgery for preventing surgical site infection. *Cochrane Database Syst Rev* 2007; **4:** CD006353.

Wilde GP, Baker GC. Circumferential periosteal release in the treatment of children with leg-length inequality. *J Bone Joint Surg* 1987; **69B:** 817–21.

Wong KC, Leung KS. Transmission and prevention of occupational infections in orthopaedic surgeons. *J Bone Joint Surg* 2004; **86A:** 1065–76.

Section 2

Regional Orthopaedics

The shoulder and pectoral girdle

13

Andrew Cole, Paul Pavlou

CLINICAL ASSESSMENT

SYMPTOMS

Pain is the commonest symptom. However, 'pain in the shoulder' is not necessarily 'shoulder pain'! If the patient points to the top of the shoulder, think of the acromioclavicular joint, or referred pain from the neck. Pain from the shoulder joint and the rotator cuff is felt, typically, over the front and outer aspect of the joint, often as far down as the middle of the arm. The relationship to posture may be significant: pain which appears when the arm is in the 'window-cleaning' position is characteristic of rotator cuff impingement; pain which comes on suddenly when the arm is held high overhead suggests instability.

Beware the trap of *referred pain*. Mediastinal disorders, including cardiac ischaemia, can present with aching in either shoulder.

Weakness may appear as a true loss of power, suggesting a neurological disorder, or as a sudden and surprising inability to abduct the shoulder – perhaps due to a tendon rupture. Between these extremes there is weakness in performing only certain movements and weakness associated with pain.

Instability symptoms may be gross and alarming ('my shoulder jumps out of its socket when I raise my arm'); more often they are quite subtle: a click or jerk when the arm is held overhead, or the 'dead arm' sensation that overtakes the tennis player as he or she prepares to serve.

Stiffness may be progressive and severe – so much so as to merit the term 'frozen shoulder'.

Swelling may be in the joint, the muscle or the bone; the patient will not know the difference.

Deformity may consist of muscle wasting, prominence of the acromioclavicular joint, winging of the scapula or an abnormal position of the arm.

Loss of function is usually expressed as difficulty with dressing and grooming, or inability to lift objects or work with the arm above shoulder height.

THE PAINFUL SHOULDER	
Referred pain syndromes Cervical spondylosis Mediastinal pathology Cardiac ischaemia	**Rotator cuff disorders** Tendinitis Rupture Frozen shoulder
Joint disorders Glenohumeral arthritis Acromioclavicular arthritis	**Instability** Dislocation Subluxation
Bone lesions Infection Tumours	**Nerve injury** Suprascapular nerve entrapment

SIGNS

The patient should always be examined from in front and from behind. Both upper limbs, the neck, the outline of the scapula and the upper chest must be visible.

Look

Skin Scars or sinuses are noted; do not forget the axilla!

Shape The two sides should be compared. Asymmetry of the shoulders, winging of the scapula, wasting of the deltoid, supraspinatus and infraspinatus muscles and acromioclavicular dislocation are best seen from behind; swelling of the acromioclavicular or sternoclavicular joint or wasting of the pectoral muscles is more obvious from the front. A joint effusion causes swelling anteriorly and occasionally 'points' in the axilla. Wasting of the deltoid suggests a nerve lesion whereas wasting of the supraspinatus may be due to either a full-thickness tear or a suprascapular nerve lesion. The typical 'Popeye' bulge of a ruptured biceps is more easily seen if the elbow is flexed.

Position If the arm is held internally rotated, think of posterior dislocation of the shoulder.

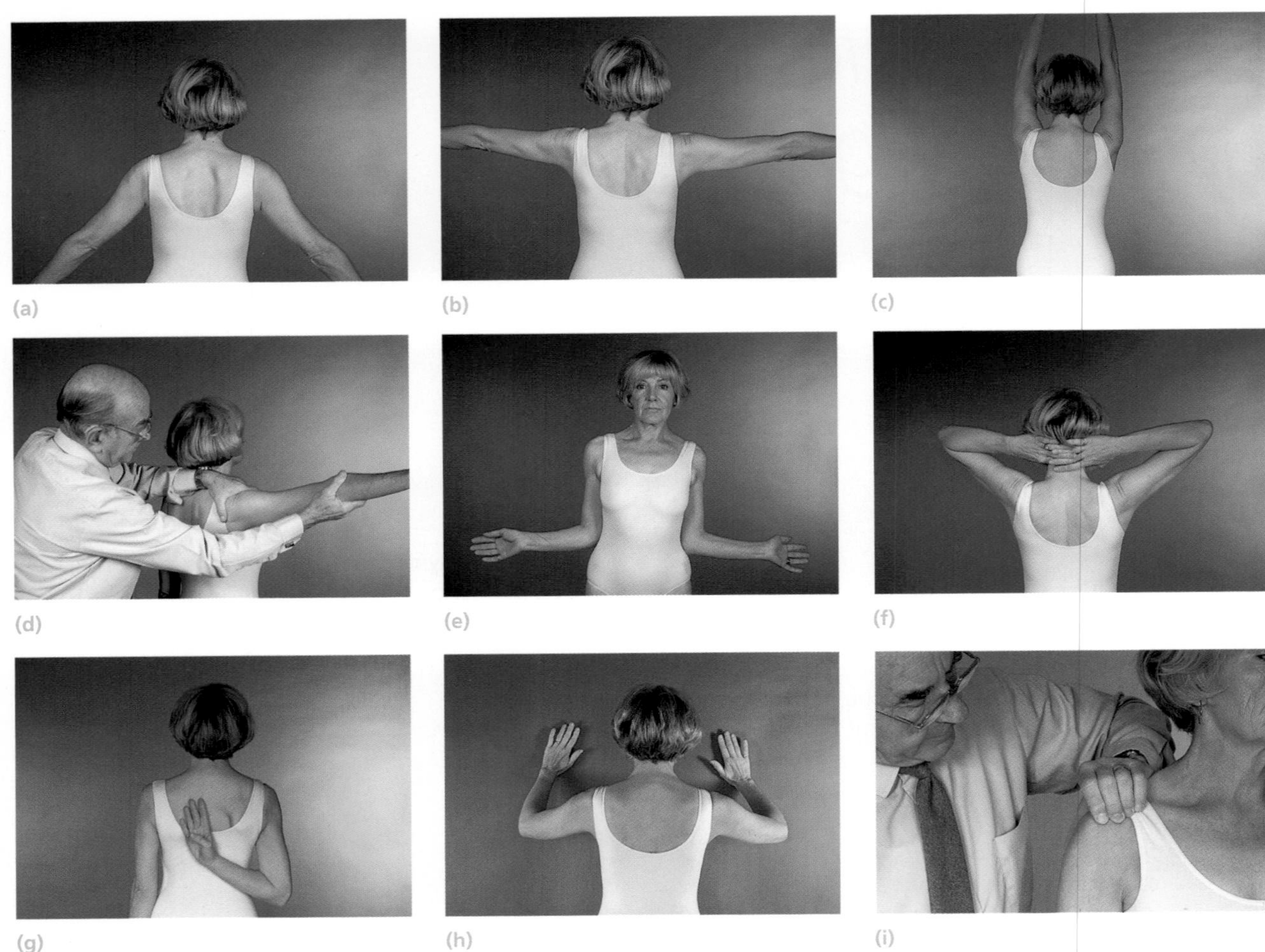

13.1 Examination Active movements are best examined from behind the patient, paying careful attention to symmetry and the coordination between scapulo-thoracic and gleno-humeral movements. (a) Abduction; (b) limit of gleno-humeral abduction; (c) full abduction and elevation, a combination of scapulo-thoracic and gleno-humeral movement. (d) The range of true gleno-humeral movement can be assessed by blocking scapular movement with a hand placed firmly on the top edge of the scapula. (e) External rotation. (f,g) Complex movements involving abduction, rotation and flexion or extension of the shoulder. (h) Testing for serratus anterior weakness. (i) Feeling for supraspinatus tenderness.

Feel

Skin Because the joint is well covered, inflammation rarely influences skin temperature.

Bony points and soft tissues The deeper structures are carefully palpated, following a mental picture of the anatomy. Start with the sternoclavicular joint, then follow the clavicle laterally to the acromioclavicular joint, and so onto the anterior edge of the acromion and around the acromion. The anterior and posterior margins of the glenoid should be palpated. With the shoulder held in extension, the supraspinatus tendon can be pinpointed just under the anterior edge of the acromion; below this, the bony prominence bounding the bicipital groove is easily felt, especially if the arm is gently rotated so that the hard ridge slips medially and laterally under the palpating fingers. Crepitus over the supraspinatus tendon during movement suggests tendinitis or a tear.

Move

Active movements Movements are observed first from in front and then from behind, with the patient either standing or sitting. Sideways elevation of the arms normally occurs in the plane of the scapula, i.e. about 20 degrees anterior to the coronal plane, with the arm rising through an arc of 180 degrees. However, by convention, abduction is performed in the coronal plane and flexion–extension in the sagittal plane.

Abduction starts at 0 degrees; the early phase of movement takes place almost entirely at the gleno-humeral joint, but as the arm rises the scapula begins to rotate on the thorax and in the last 60 degrees of movement is almost entirely scapulo-thoracic (hence sideways movement beyond 90 degrees is sometimes called 'elevation' rather than 'abduction'). The rhythmic transition from gleno-humeral to scapulo-thoracic movement is disturbed by disorders in the joint or by dysfunction of the stabilizing tendons

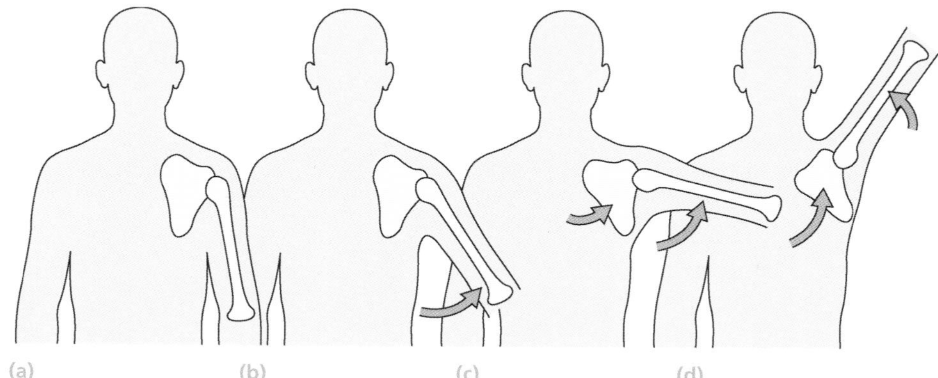

13.2 Scapulo-humeral rhythm (a–c) During the early phase of abduction, most of the movement takes place at the gleno-humeral joint. As the arm rises, the scapula begins to rotate on the thorax (c). In the last phase of abduction, movement is almost entirely scapulo-thoracic (d).

around the joint. Thus, abduction may be (1) difficult to initiate, (2) diminished in range or (3) altered in rhythm, the scapula moving too early and creating a shrugging effect. If movement is painful, the arc of pain must be noted; pain in the mid-range of abduction suggests a minor rotator cuff tear or supraspinatus tendinitis; pain at the end of abduction is often due to acromioclavicular arthritis.

Flexion and extension are examined by asking the patient to raise the arms forwards and then backwards. The normal range is 180 degrees of flexion and 40 degrees of extension.

Rotation is tested in two ways: The arms are held close to the body with the elbows flexed to 90 degrees; the hands are then separated as widely as possible (external rotation) and brought together again across the body (internal rotation). This is a rather unnatural movement and one learns more by simply asking the patient to clasp his (or her) fingers behind his neck (external rotation in abduction) and then to reach up his back with his fingers (internal rotation in adduction); the two sides are compared.

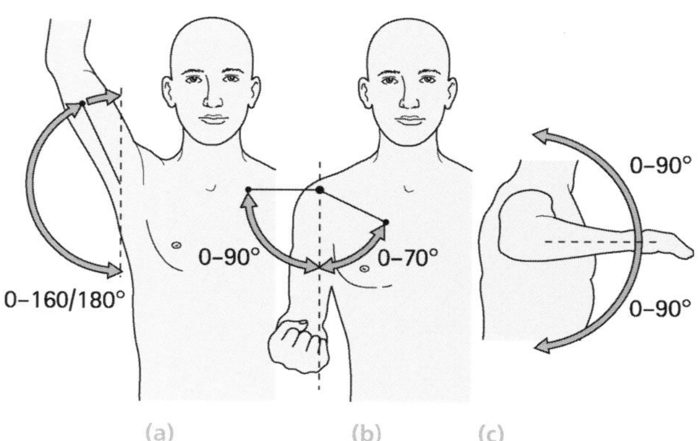

13.3 Normal range of movement (a) Abduction is from 0° to 160° (or even 180°), but only 90° of this takes place at the gleno-humeral joint (in the plane of the scapula, 20° anterior to the coronal place); the remainder is scapular movement. (b) External rotation is usually about 80° but internal is rather less because the trunk gets in the way. (c) With the arm abducted to a right angle, internal rotation can be assessed without the trunk getting in the way.

Passive movements To test the range of gleno-humeral movement (as distinct from combined gleno-humeral and scapular movement) the scapula must first be anchored; this is done by the examiner pressing firmly down on the top of the shoulder with one hand while the other hand moves the patient's arm. Grasping the angle of the scapula as a method of anchorage is less satisfactory.

Power The deltoid is examined for bulk and tautness while the patient abducts against resistance. To test serratus anterior (long thoracic nerve, C5, 6, 7) the patient is asked to push forcefully against a wall with both hands; if the muscle is weak, the scapula is not stabilized on the thorax and stands out prominently (winged scapula). Pectoralis major is tested by having the patient thrust both hands firmly into the waist. Rotator power is tested by asking the patient to stand with his arms tucked into his side and the elbows flexed, then to externally rotate against resistance. Weakness may be associated with a rotator cuff lesion, instability or a neurological disorder.

Other systems Clinical assessment is completed by examining the cervical spine (as a common source of referred pain), testing for generalized joint laxity (a frequent accompaniment of shoulder instability) and performing a focussed neurological examination.

Special clinical tests

Special clinical tests have been developed for localizing more precisely the site of pain and tenderness, the source of muscle weakness and the presence of instability. These are described in the relevant sections that follow.

Examination after local anaesthetic injection

It is sometimes possible to localize the source of shoulder pain by injecting local anaesthetic into the target site (for example the supraspinatus tendon or the acromioclavicular joint) and thus to see whether there is a temporary reduction in pain on movement. Injection into the subacromial space may help to distinguish loss of movement due to pain from that due to a rotator cuff tear.

Diagnostic focus

Important as it is to adopt a systematic approach in the clinical examination, the practical exercise of working towards a diagnosis requires a sensible balance in the focus of attention. A young athletic person who develops pain and weakness on abduction and external rotation of the shoulder is more likely to be suffering from a rotator cuff disorder than an inflammatory arthritis of the shoulder and therefore the full panoply of special tests for localization of pain and weakness would be justified, whereas some of these tests would be quite inappropriate in an elderly person with the longstanding pain and swelling of an arthritic condition.

IMAGING

X-rays At least two x-ray views should be obtained: an anteroposterior in the plane of the shoulder and an axillary projection with the arm in abduction to show the relationship of the humeral head to the glenoid. Look for evidence of subluxation or dislocation, joint space narrowing, bone erosion and calcification in the soft tissues. The acromioclavicular joint is best shown by an anteroposterior projection with the tube tilted upwards 20 degrees (the cephalic tilt view). The subacromial space is viewed by tilting the tube downwards 30 degrees (the caudal tilt view).

Arthrography This is useful for detecting rotator cuff tears and some larger Bankart lesions found with anterior instability. It is now usually combined with CT or MRI.

Computed tomography Particularly when enhanced with intra-articular contrast, CT scans can identify cuff tears and labral detachments.

Ultrasound In experienced hands, ultrasound provides a reliable and simple means of identifying rotator cuff tears, calcific tendinitis and biceps problems. It can also be useful to identify areas of hypervascularity and perform ultrasound-guided injections and barbotage (the practice of inserting a needle into a calcific deposit and aspirating or fragmenting the material).

Magnetic resonance imaging The information which is provided by MRI depends on the quality of the equipment and the imaging sequences which are chosen. For patients with suspected rotator cuff pathology, MRI gives information on the site and size of a tear, as well as the anatomy of the coracoacromial arch and acromioclavicular joint (Recht and Resnick, 1993). For patients with symptoms and signs suggesting instability, it can demonstrate associated anomalies of the capsule, labrum, glenoid and humeral head. MRI is also useful in detecting osteonecrosis of the head of the humerus and in the diagnosis and staging of tumours.

Magnetic resonance arthrography Using MR arthrography, a sensitivity of 91 per cent and a specificity of 93 per cent have been reported in the detection of

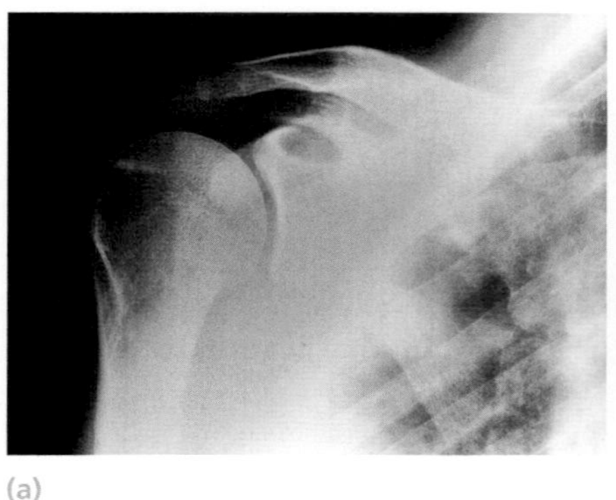
(a)

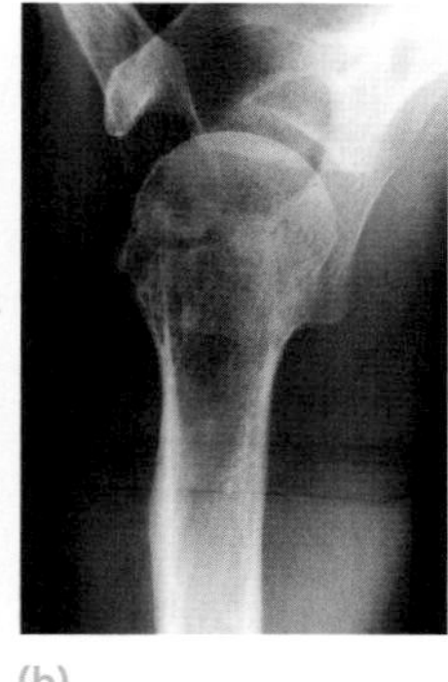
(b)

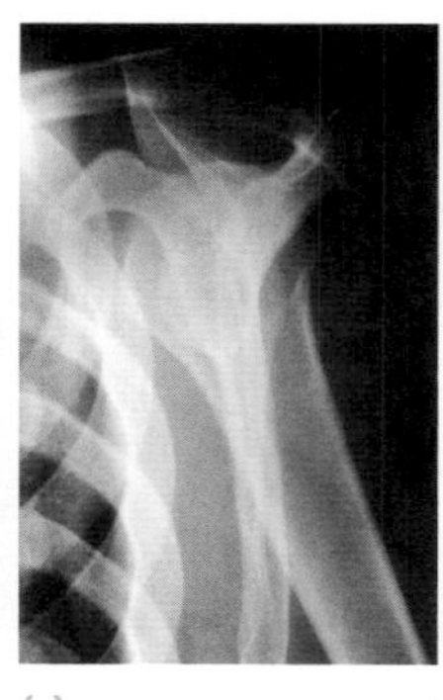
(c)

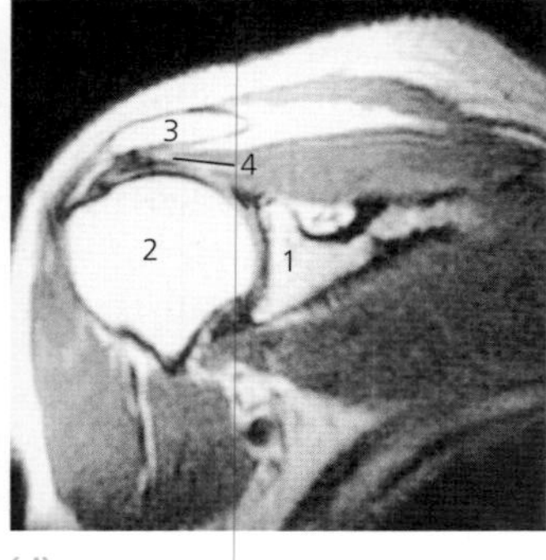

(d)

13.4 Imaging (a) Anteroposterior x-ray. (b) Axillary view showing the humeral head opposite the shallow glenoid fossa, and the coracoid process anteriorly. The acromion process shadow overlaps that of the humeral head. (c) Lateral view; the head of the humerus should lie where the coracoid process, the spine of the scapula and the blade of the scapula meet. (d) MRI. Note (1) the glenoid, (2) the head of the humerus, (3) the acromion process and (4) the supraspinatus (with degeneration of the tendon).

pathological labral conditions (Palmer et al., 1994). For identifying rotator cuff partial undersurface tears, MRA has been shown to be more sensitive and specific than MRI alone (Tirman et al., 1994)

ARTHROSCOPY

Arthroscopy can be useful to diagnose (and treat) intra-articular lesions, detachment of the labrum or capsule and impingement or tears of the rotator cuff. Arthroscopy is said to be the best means by which superior labrum, anterior and posterior (SLAP) tears may be diagnosed.

DISORDERS OF THE ROTATOR CUFF

The rotator cuff is made up of the lateral portions of the infraspinatus, supraspinatus and subscapularis muscles and their conjoint tendon which is inserted into the greater tuberosity of the humerus. The musculotendinous cuff passes beneath the coracoacromial arch, from which it is separated by the subacromial bursa; during abduction of the arm the cuff slides outwards under the arch. The deep surface of the cuff is intimately related to the joint capsule and the tendon of the long head of the biceps.

Although contraction of the individual muscles that make up the rotator cuff exerts a rotational pull on the proximal end of the humerus, the main function of the conjoint structure is to draw the head of the humerus firmly into the glenoid socket and stabilize it there when the deltoid muscle contracts and abducts the arm. Consequently, patients with rotator cuff tendinitis experience pain and weakness on active abduction and those with a severe tear of the cuff are unable to initiate abduction but can hold the arm abducted once it has been raised aloft by the examiner.

The commonest cause of pain around the shoulder is a disorder of the rotator cuff. This is sometimes referred to rather loosely as *'rotator cuff syndrome'*, which comprises at least four conditions with distinct clinical features and natural history:

- supraspinatus impingement syndrome and tendinitis
- tears of the rotator cuff
- acute calcific tendinitis
- biceps tendinitis and/or rupture.

In all these conditions the patient is likely to complain of pain and/or weakness during certain movements of the shoulder. Pain may have started recently, sometimes quite suddenly, after a particular type of exertion; the patient may know precisely which movements now reignite the pain and which to avoid, providing a valuable clue to its origin. 'Rotator cuff' pain typically appears over the front and lateral aspect of the shoulder during activities with the arm abducted and medially rotated, but it may be present even with the arm at rest. Tenderness is felt at the anterior edge of the acromion.

Pain and tenderness directly in front along the delto-pectoral boundary could be associated with the biceps tendon. Localized pain over the top of the shoulder is more likely to be due to acromioclavicular pathology, and pain at the back along the scapular border may come from the cervical spine. All these sites should be inspected for muscle wasting, carefully palpated for local tenderness and constantly compared with the opposite shoulder.

If there is weakness with some movements but not with others, then one must rule out a partial or complete tendon rupture; here again, as with pain, localization to a specific site is the key to diagnosis. In both cases clinical examination should include a number of provocative tests to determine the source of the patient's symptoms. These are described in the relevant sections below.

IMPINGEMENT SYNDROME, SUPRASPINATUS TENDINITIS AND CUFF DISRUPTION

Pathology

Rotator cuff impingement syndrome is a painful disorder which is thought to arise from repetitive compression or rubbing of the tendons (mainly supraspinatus) under the coracoacromial arch. Normally, when the arm is abducted, the conjoint tendon slides under the coracoacromial arch. As abduction approaches 90 degrees, there is a natural tendency to externally rotate the arm, thus allowing the rotator cuff to occupy the widest part of the subacromial space. If the arm is held persistently in abduction and then moved to and fro in internal and external rotation (as in cleaning a window, painting a wall or polishing a flat surface) the rotator cuff may be compressed and irritated as it comes in contact with the anterior edge of the acromion process and the taut coracoacromial ligament. This attitude (abduction, slight flexion and internal rotation) has been called the 'impingement position'. Perhaps significantly, the site of impingement is also the 'critical area' of diminished vascularity in the supraspinatus tendon about 1 cm proximal to its insertion into the greater tuberosity.

Although the concept of 'impingement' as a primary pathogenetic factor has now become

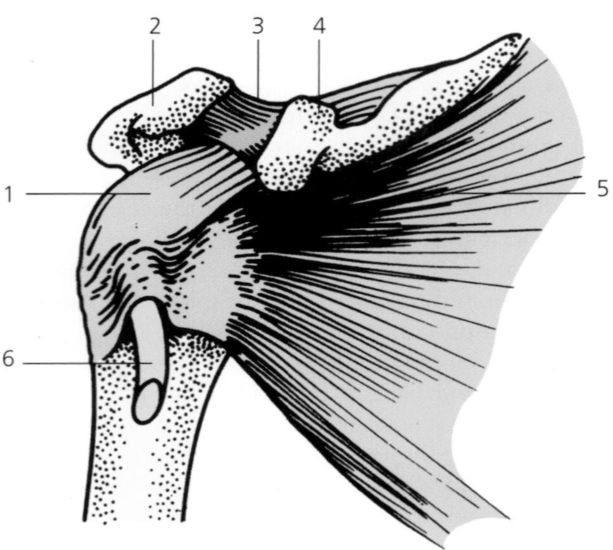

13.5 Anatomy The tough coracoacromial ligament stretches from the coracoid to the underside of the anterior third of the acromion process; the humeral head moves beneath this arch during abduction and the rotator cuff may be irritated or damaged as it glides in this confined space. Key: 1 Rotator cuff; 2 acromion process; 3 coracoacromial ligament; 4 coracoid process; 5 suscapularis; 6 long head of biceps.

entrenched, it should be mentioned that there is still some controversy about whether supraspinatus tendinitis may also occur *ab initio* in response to severe repetitive stress, and the slightly swollen tendon then start impinging on the acromioclavicular arch.

Other factors which may predispose to repetitive impingement are osteoarthritic thickening of the acromioclavicular joint, the formation of bony ridges or 'osteophytes' on the anterior edge of the acromion, and swelling of the cuff or the subacromial bursa in inflammatory disorders such as gout or rheumatoid arthritis. In 1986, Bigliani and Morrison described three variations of acromial morphology. Type I is flat, type II curved and type III the hooked acromion. They suggested that the type III variety was most frequently associated with impingement and rotator cuff tears.

The mildest injury is a type of friction, which may give rise to localized oedema and swelling ('tendinitis'). This is usually self-limiting, but with prolonged or repetitive impingement – and especially in older people – minute tears can develop and these may be followed by scarring, fibrocartilaginous metaplasia or calcification in the tendon. Healing is accompanied by a vascular reaction and local congestion (in itself painful) which may contribute to further impingement in the constricted space under the coraco-acromial arch whenever the arm is elevated.

Sometimes – perhaps where healing is slow or following a sudden strain – the microscopic disruption extends, becoming a partial or full-thickness tear of the cuff; shoulder function is then more seriously compromised and active abduction may be impossible. The tendon of the long head of biceps, lying adjacent to the supraspinatus, also may be involved and is often torn.

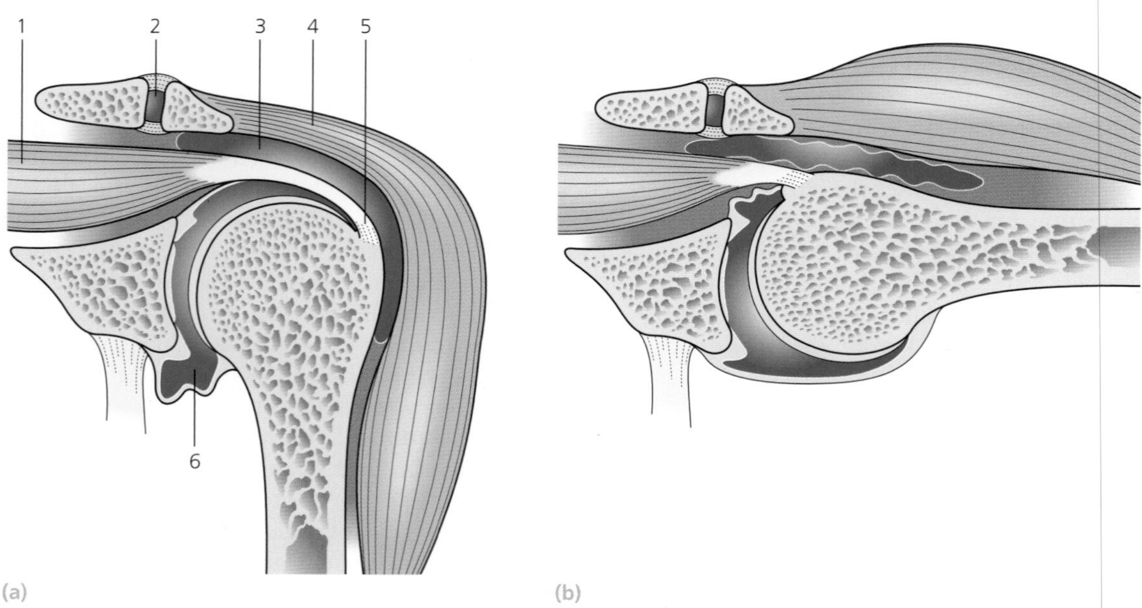

13.6 Rotator cuff impingement Coronal sections through the shoulder to illustrate show how the subdeltoid bursa and supraspinatus tendon can be irritated by repeated impingement under the coracoacromial arch or a rough acromioclavicular joint during abduction. (a) Joint at rest. (b) In abduction. Key: 1 Supraspinatus muscle; 2 acromioclavicular joint; 3 subdeltoid bursa; 4 deltoid muscle; 5 supraspinatus tendon; 6 synovial joint.

Secondary arthropathy Large tears of the cuff eventually lead to serious disturbance of shoulder mechanics. The humeral head migrates upwards, abutting against the acromion process, and passive abduction is severely restricted. Abnormal movement predisposes to osteoarthritis of the gleno-humeral joint. Occasionally this progresses to a rapidly destructive arthropathy – the so-called 'Milwaukee shoulder' (named after the city where it was first described by McCarty).

CLINICAL FEATURES

Early clinical features are typically those of a 'rotator cuff syndrome', as described above. Subsequent progress depends on the stage of the disorder, the age of the patient and the vigour of the healing response. Three patterns are encountered:

- *Subacute tendinitis* – the 'painful arc syndrome', due to vascular congestion, microscopic haemorrhage and oedema.
- *Chronic tendinitis* – recurrent shoulder pain due to tendinitis and fibrosis.
- *Cuff disruption* – recurrent pain, weakness and loss of movement due to tears in the rotator cuff.

Subacute tendinitis (painful arc syndrome)

The patient develops anterior shoulder pain after vigorous or unaccustomed activity, e.g. competitive swimming or a weekend of house decorating. The shoulder looks normal but is acutely tender along the anterior edge of the acromion. Point tenderness is most easily elicited by palpating this spot with the arm held in extension, thus placing the supraspinatus tendon in an exposed position anterior to the acromion process; with the arm held in flexion the tenderness disappears.

TESTS FOR CUFF IMPINGEMENT PAIN

- *The painful arc:* On active abduction scapulo-humeral rhythm is disturbed and pain is aggravated as the arm traverses an arc between 60 and 120 degrees. Repeating the movement with the arm in full external rotation may be much easier for the patient and relatively painless.
- *Neer's impingement sign:* The scapula is stabilized with one hand while with the other hand the examiner raises the affected arm to the full extent in passive flexion, abduction and internal rotation, thus bringing the greater tuberosity directly under the coracoacromial arch. The test is positive when pain, located to the subacromial space or anterior edge of acromion, is elicited by this manoeuvre. The test is over 80 per cent sensitive for subacromial impingement or a rotator cuff tear but it has poor specificity and may be positive also in patients with acromioclavicular osteoarthritis, gleno-humeral instability and SLAP lesions.
- *Neer's test for impingement:* If the previous manoeuvre is positive, it may be repeated after injecting 10 mL of 1 per cent lignocaine into the subacromial space; if the pain is abolished (or significantly reduced), this will help to confirm the diagnosis.
- *Hawkins–Kennedy test* (Hawkins and Kennedy, 1980): The patient's arm is placed in 90 degrees forward flexion with the elbow also flexed to 90 degrees. The examiner then stabilizes the upper arm with one hand while using the other hand to internally rotate the arm fully. Pain around the anterolateral aspect of the shoulder is noted as a positive test. As with the Neer sign, this test is highly sensitive but weakly specific.

Subacute tendinitis is often reversible, settling down gradually once the initiating activity is avoided.

Chronic tendinitis

The patient, usually aged between 40 and 50, gives a history of recurrent attacks of subacute tendinitis, the pain settling down with rest or anti-inflammatory treatment, only to recur when more demanding activities are resumed.

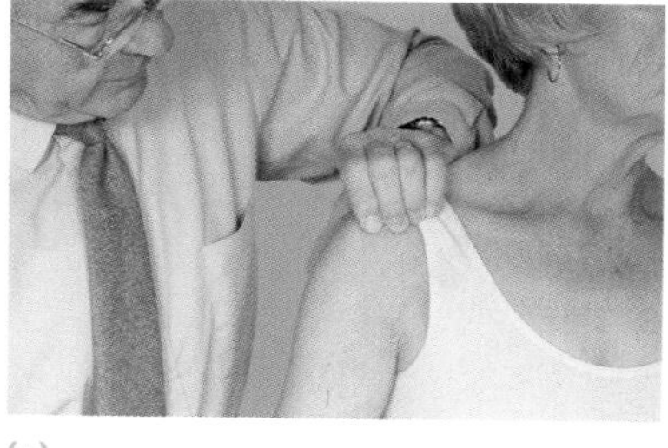
(a)

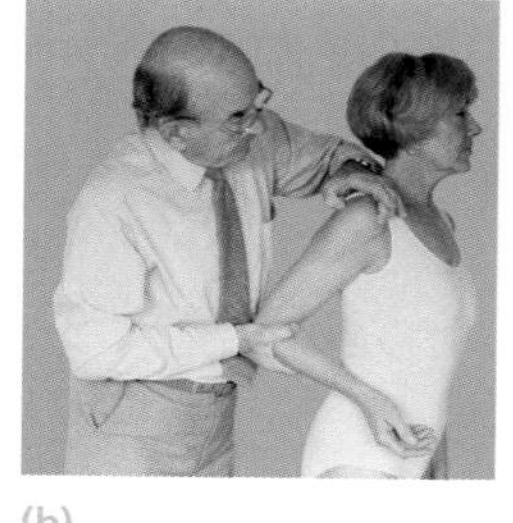
(b)

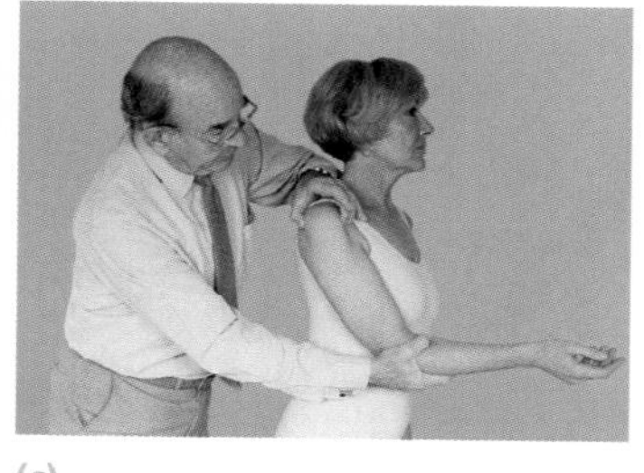
(c)

13.7 Supraspinatus tenderness (a) The tender spot is at the anterior edge of the acromion process. When the shoulder is extended (b) tenderness is more marked; with the shoulder slightly flexed (c) the painful tendon disappears under the acromion process and tenderness disappears.

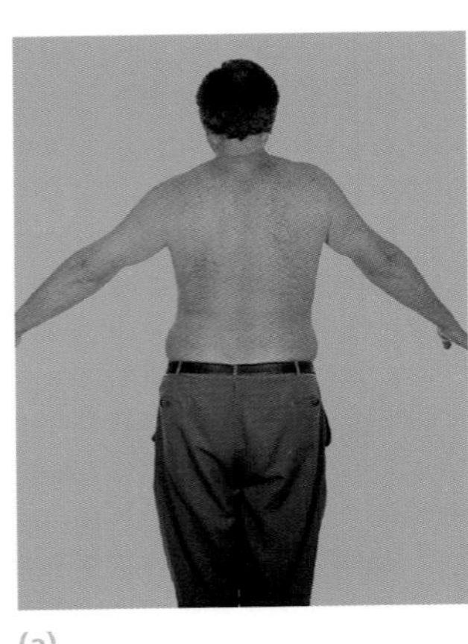
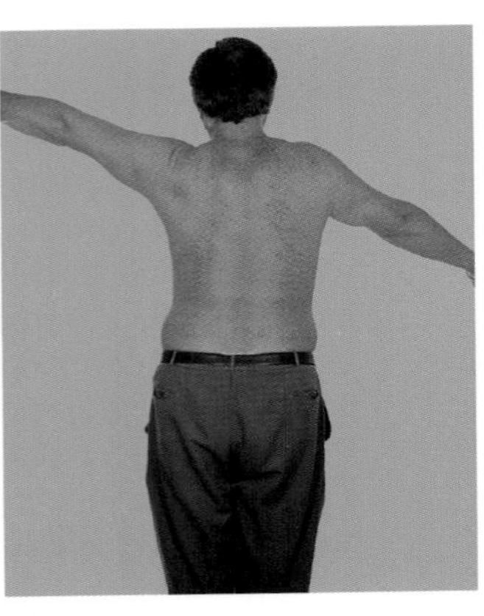
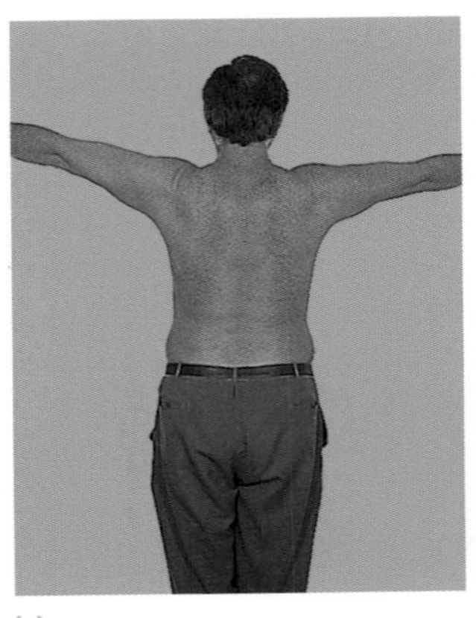
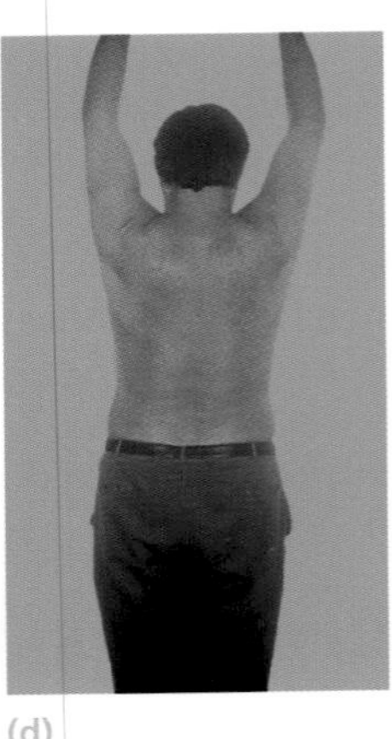

(a) (b) (c) (d)

13.8 The painful arc (a,b) In abduction, scapulo-humeral rhythm is disturbed on the right and the patient starts to experience pain at about 60°. (c,d) As the arm passes beyond 120° the pain eases and the patient is able to abduct and elevate up to the full 180°.

Characteristically pain is worse at night; the patient cannot lie on the affected side and often finds it more comfortable to sit up out of bed. Pain and slight stiffness of the shoulder may restrict even simple activities such as hair grooming or dressing. The physical signs described above should be elicited. In addition there may be signs of bicipital tendinitis: tenderness along the bicipital groove and crepitus on moving the biceps tendon.

A disturbing feature is coarse crepitation or palpable snapping over the rotator cuff when the shoulder is passively rotated; this may signify a partial tear or marked fibrosis of the cuff. Small, unsuspected tears are quite often found during arthroscopy or operation.

Cuff disruption

The most advanced stage of the disorder is progressive fibrosis and disruption of the cuff, resulting in either a partial or full thickness tear. The patient is usually aged over 45 and gives a history of refractory shoulder pain with increasing stiffness and weakness.

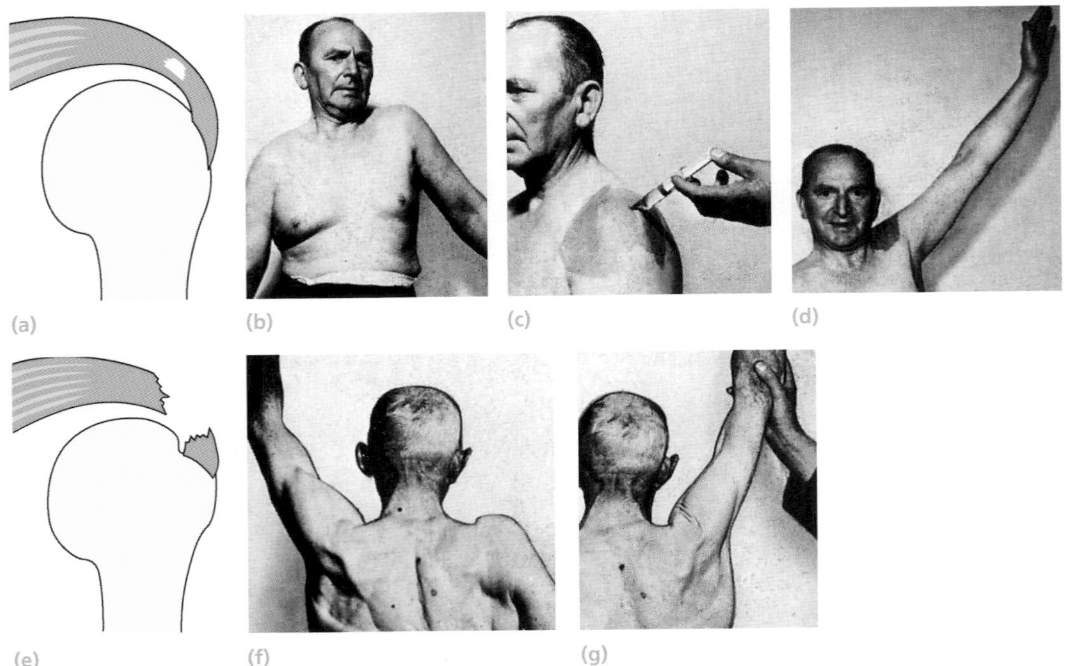

13.9 Torn supraspinatus (a–d) Partial tear of left supraspinatus: the patient can abduct actively once pain has been abolished with local anaesthetic. (e–g) Complete tear of right supraspinatus: active abduction is impossible even when pain subsides (f), or has been abolished by injection; but once the arm is passively abducted, the patient can hold it up with her deltoid muscle (g).

Partial tears may occur within the substance or on the deep surface of the cuff and are not easily detected, even on direct inspection of the cuff. They are deceptive also in that continuity of the remaining cuff fibres permits active abduction with a painful arc, making it difficult to tell whether chronic tendinitis is complicated by a partial tear.

A *full thickness tear* may follow a long period of chronic tendinitis, but occasionally it occurs spontaneously after a sprain or jerking injury of the shoulder. There is sudden pain and the patient is unable to abduct the arm. Passive abduction also may, in the early stages, be limited or prevented by pain. If the diagnosis is in doubt, pain can be eliminated by injecting a local anaesthetic into the subacromial space. If active abduction is now possible the tear must be only partial. If active abduction remains impossible, then a complete tear is likely.

If some weeks have elapsed since the injury the two types are more easily differentiated. With a complete tear, pain has by then subsided and the clinical picture is unmistakable: active abduction is impossible and attempting it produces a characteristic shrug; but passive abduction is full and once the arm has been lifted above a right angle the patient can keep it up by using his deltoid (the 'abduction paradox'); when he lowers it sideways it suddenly drops (the 'drop arm sign').

With time there may be some recovery of active abduction, though power in both abduction and external rotation is weaker than normal. There is usually wasting of the supraspinatus and infraspinatus, and on testing the biceps there may be an old tear of the long head tendon (see Fig. 13.10). There is often tenderness of the acromioclavicular joint.

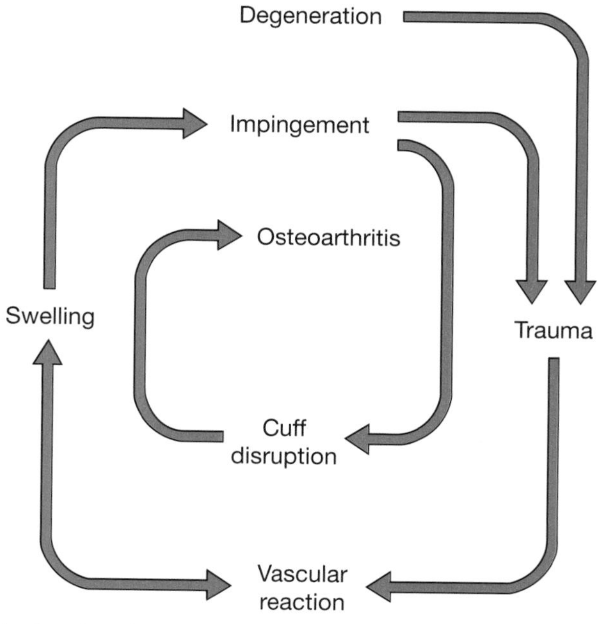

13.10 The vicious spiral of rotator cuff lesions

In longstanding cases of partial or complete rupture, secondary osteoarthritis of the shoulder may supervene and movements are then severely restricted.

TESTS FOR ISOLATED WEAKNESS

The 'abduction paradox' and 'drop arm sign' are helpful in the diagnosis of a complete rupture of the cuff. For partial tears of the cuff, more subtle tests are used to identify weakness in isolated components of the cuff.

- *Supraspinatus – the 'empty can' test* (Jobe and Jobe, 1983): Supraspinatus strength can be tested in isolation as follows. The patient (seated or standing) is asked to raise his or her arms to a position of 90 degrees abduction, 30 degrees of forward flexion and internal rotation (thumbs pointing to the floor, as if emptying an imaginary can). The examiner stands behind the patient and applies downward pressure on both arms, with the patient resisting this force. The result is positive when the affected side is weaker than the unaffected side, suggesting a tear of the supraspinatus tendon.
- *Infraspinatus – resisted external rotation:* The patient stands holding his or her arms close to the body and the elbows flexed to 90 degrees. He or she is instructed to externally rotate both arms while the examiner applies resistance; lack of power on one side signifies weakness of infraspinatus. The test can be repeated, this time with the arm in 90 degrees of forward elevation in the plane of the scapula. The patient is asked to laterally rotate the arm against resistance; the ability to do so despite feeling pain can indicate tendinitis whilst an inability to resist at all suggests a tear of infraspinatus.
- *Infraspinatus* and *posterior cuff* – the *'lag sign'* and the *'drop sign':* For the *external rotation lag sign* the patient's arms are lifted slightly away from the body and placed in maximum external rotation; a positive test is signalled when the patient cannot maintain that position on one side and allows the arm to drift into a more neutral position. This suggests a tear of infraspinatus or supraspinatus. The *drop sign* is similar: here the examiner lifts and places the arm in 90 degrees of abduction, the elbow at a right angle and the arm maximally externally rotated; when the examiner lets go the patient would normally hold that position, but if the arm 'drops' it signals a positive test (Hertel et al., 1996). This is seen in patients with tears of the infraspinatus and posterior part of the rotator cuff.
- *Subscapularis – 'the lift-off' test:* The patient is asked to stand and place one arm behind his or her back with the dorsum of the hand resting against the mid-lumbar spine. The examiner then lifts the patient's hand off the back and the patient is told to hold it there. Inability to do this signifies subscapularis

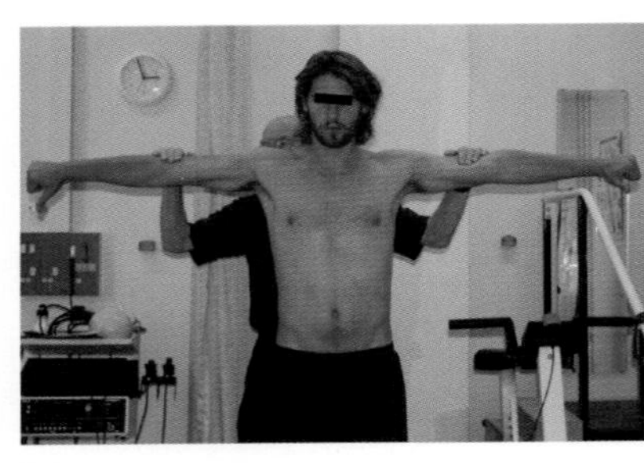
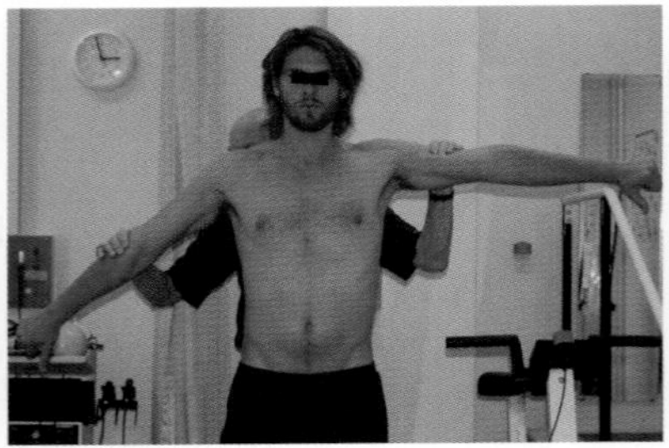
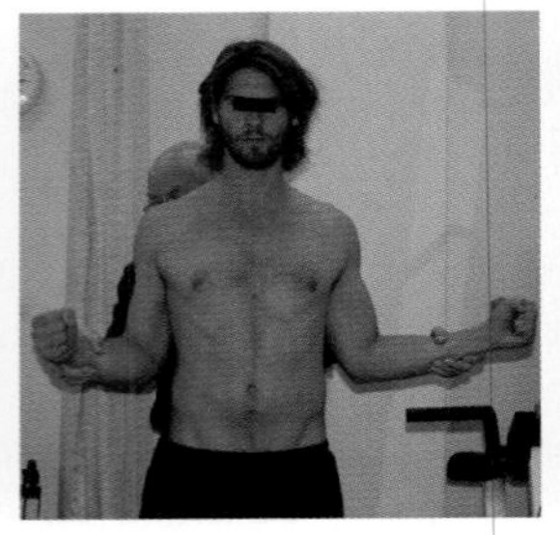
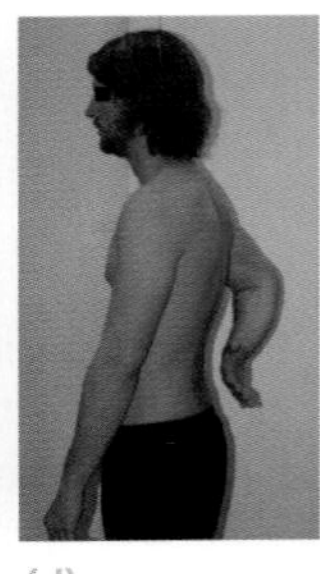

(a) (b) (c) (d)

13.11 Tests for cuff weakness (a) Position for Jobes' test for supraspinatus power. (b) Jobe's test – right side weaker than left. (c) Test for infraspinatus – right side weaker than left. (d) Normal 'lift-off' test for subscapularis.

weakness, possibly due to rupture (Gerber and Krushell, 1991). A drawback is that the test calls for full passive internal rotation, so it cannot be used if internal rotation is painful or restricted.

IMAGING FOR ROTATOR CUFF DISORDERS

X-ray examination X-rays are usually normal in the early stages of the cuff dysfunction, but with chronic tendinitis there may be erosion, sclerosis or cyst formation at the site of cuff insertion on the greater tuberosity. In chronic cases the caudal tilt view may show roughening or overgrowth of the anterior edge of the acromion, thinning of the acromion process and upward displacement of the humeral head. Osteoarthritis of the acromioclavicular joint is common in older patients and in late cases the glenohumeral joint also may show features of osteoarthritis. Sometimes there is calcification of the supraspinatus, but this is usually coincidental and not the cause of pain (see Fig. 13.12).

Magnetic resonance imaging MRI effectively demonstrates the structures around the shoulder and gives valuable ancillary information (regarding lesions of the glenoid labrum, joint capsule or surrounding muscle or bone). However, it should be remembered that up to a third of asymptomatic individuals have abnormalities of the rotator cuff on MRI (Sher et al., 1995). Changes on MRI need to be correlated with the clinical examination.

Ultrasonography Ultrasonography has comparable accuracy with MRI for identifying and measuring the size of full thickness and partial thickness rotator cuff tears (Teefe et al., 2004). It has the disadvantage that it cannot identify the quality of the remaining muscle as well as MRI and cannot always be accurate in predicting the reparability of the tendons.

TREATMENT OF CUFF DISORDERS

Conservative treatment

Uncomplicated impingement syndrome (or tendinitis) is often self-limiting and symptoms settle down once the aggravating activity is eliminated. Patients should be taught ways of avoiding the 'impingement

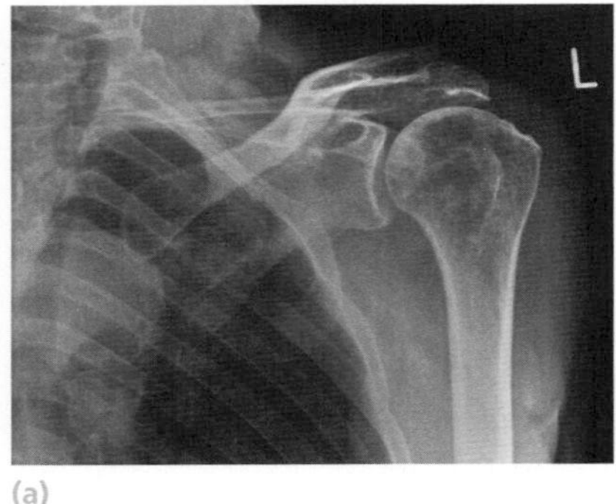

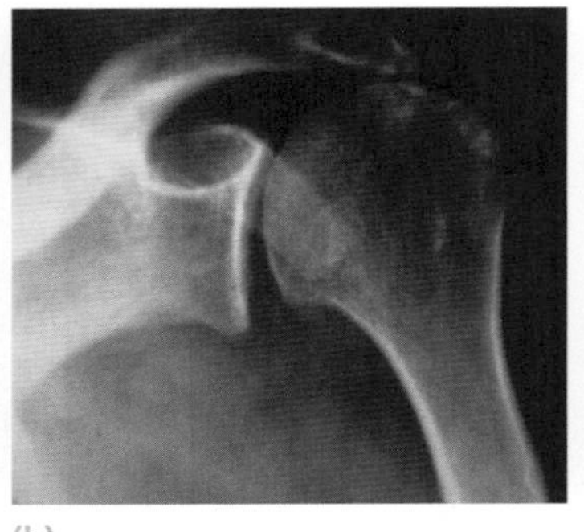
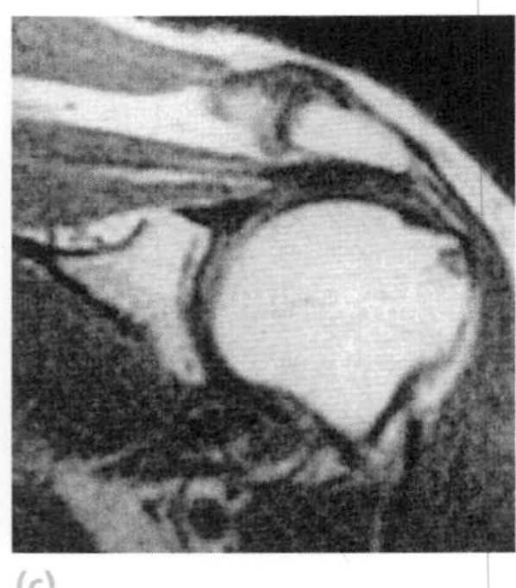

(a) (b) (c)

13.12 Supraspinatus tendinitis – x-rays (a) X-ray of the shoulder showing a typical thin band of sclerosis at the insertion of supraspinatus and narrowing of the subacromial space. The rest of the joint looks normal. (b) X-ray at a later stage showing upward displacement of the humeral head due to a large cuff rupture. There is almost complete loss of the subacromial space, and osteoarthritis of the glenohumeral joint. (c) MRI showing thickening of the supraspinatus and erosion at its insertion; the acromioclavicular joint is swollen and clearly abnormal.

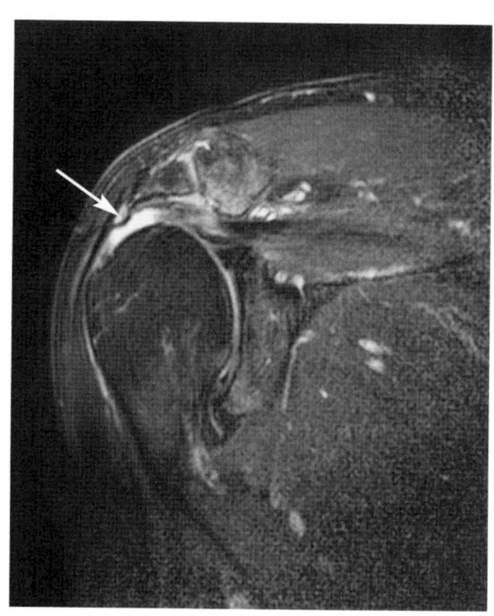

13.13 Rotator cuff tear – MRI High signal on MRI, indicating a full-thickness tear of the rotator cuff.

position'. Physiotherapy, including ultrasound and active exercises in the 'position of freedom', may tide the patient over the painful healing phase. A short course of non-steroidal anti-inflammatory tablets sometimes brings relief. If all these methods fail, and before disability becomes marked, the patient should be given one or two injections of depot corticosteroid into the subacromial space. In most cases this will relieve the pain, and it is then important to persevere with protective modifications of shoulder activity for at least 6 months. Healing is slow, and a hasty return to full activity will often precipitate further attacks of tendinitis.

Surgical treatment

The indications for surgical treatment are essentially clinical; the presence of a cuff tear does not necessarily call for an operation. Provided the patient has a useful range of movement, adequate strength and well-controlled pain, non-operative measures are adequate. If symptoms do not subside after 3 months of conservative treatment, or if they recur persistently after each period of treatment, an operation is advisable. Certainly this is preferable to prolonged and repeated treatment with anti-inflammatory drugs and local corticosteroids. The indication is more pressing if there are signs of a partial rotator cuff tear and in particular if there is good clinical evidence of a full thickness tear in a younger patient. The object is to decompress the rotator cuff by excising the coraco-acromial ligament, undercutting the anterior part of the acromion process and, if necessary, reducing any bony excrescences at the acromioclavicular joint (Rockwood and Lyons, 1993). This can be achieved by open surgery or arthroscopically. The latter is technically more demanding but it can produce results equivalent to those of open surgery (Sachs et al., 1994; Nutton et al., 1997).

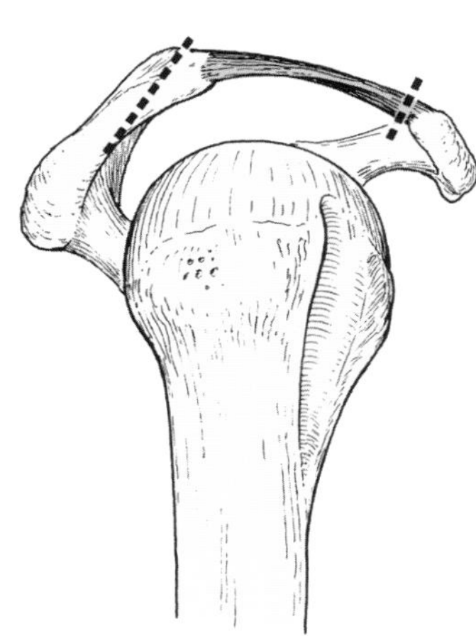

13.14 Impingement syndrome – surgical treatment The coraco-acromial ligament and underside of the anterior third of the acromion are removed to enlarge the space for the rotator cuff. This can be performed by open surgery or arthroscopically.

OPEN ACROMIOPLASTY

Through an anterior incision the deltoid muscle is split and the part arising from the anterior edge of the acromion is dissected free, exposing the coracoacromial ligament, the acromion and the acromioclavicular joint. The coracoacromial ligament is excised and the anteroinferior portion of the acromion is removed by an undercutting osteotomy. The cuff is then inspected: if there is a defect, it is repaired. Excrescences on the undersurface of the acromioclavicular joint are pared down. If the joint is hypertrophic, the outer 1 cm of clavicle is removed; this last step exposes even more of the cuff and permits reconstruction of larger defects. An important step is careful reattachment of the deltoid to the acromion, if necessary by suturing through drill holes in the acromion; failure to obtain secure attachment may lead to postoperative pain and weakness. After the operation, shoulder movements are commenced as soon as pain subsides.

ARTHROSCOPIC ACROMIOPLASTY

Arthroscopic acromioplasty should achieve the same basic objectives as open acromioplasty (Nutton et al., 1997). The underside of the acromion (and, if necessary, the acromioclavicular joint) must be trimmed and the coracoacromial ligament divided or removed. If a cuff tear is encountered, then it may be possible to repair it; otherwise the edges can be debrided or an open repair undertaken (Gartsman, 1997).

This procedure has now become the gold standard and allows earlier rehabilitation than open acromioplasty because detachment of the deltoid is not performed. Arthroscopy allows good visualization inside the gleno-humeral joint and therefore the detection of other abnormalities which may cause pain (present in up to 30 per cent of patients). It allows good visualization of both sides of the rotator cuff and the identification of partial and full thickness tears.

OPEN REPAIR OF THE ROTATOR CUFF

The indications for open repair of the rotator cuff are chronic pain, weakness of the shoulder and significant loss of function. The younger and more active the patient, the greater is the justification for surgery. The operation always includes an acromioplasty as described above. The cuff is mobilized, if necessary by releasing the coraco-humeral ligament and the glenoid attachment of the capsule; this dissection should not stray more than 2 cm medial to the glenoid rim lest the suprascapular nerve is damaged.

It may be possible to approximate the ends of the cuff defect. Larger tears can be dealt with by suturing the cuff tendon directly to a roughened area on the greater tuberosity using drill holes or soft-tissue anchors.

Postoperatively, movements are restricted for 6–8 weeks and then graded exercises are introduced.

The results of open cuff repair are reasonably good, with satisfactory pain relief in about 80 per cent of patients. This alone usually improves function, even if strength and range of movement are still restricted (Ianotti, 1994).

Massive full thickness tears that cannot be reconstructed are treated by subacromial decompression and debridement of degenerate cuff tissue; the relief of pain may allow reasonable abduction of the shoulder by the remaining muscles (Rockwood et al., 1995). Other methods to reconstruct irreparable tears in the younger patient include supraspinatus advancement, latissimus dorsi transfer, rotator cuff transposition, fascia lata autograft and synthetic tendon graft.

Acute rupture of the rotator cuff in patients over 70 years usually becomes painless; although movement is restricted, operation is contraindicated.

ARTHROSCOPIC ROTATOR CUFF REPAIR

Since the 1990s the repair of full thickness tears has undergone a transition from open techniques to arthroscopically assisted (mini open) repairs and now full arthroscopic techniques. The arthroscopic instruments, suture anchors and knot tying techniques have quickly evolved to allow full arthroscopic repairs although most authors describe a steep learning curve. Advantages of the techniques include less soft-tissue damage, faster rehabilitation and a better cosmetic appearance. Double row arthroscopic repair is now producing similar outcomes and results to open repairs (Huijsmans et al., 2007).

CALCIFICATION OF THE ROTATOR CUFF

ACUTE CALCIFIC TENDINITIS

Acute shoulder pain may follow deposition of calcium hydroxyapatite crystals, usually in the 'critical zone' of the supraspinatus tendon slightly medial to its insertion, occasionally elsewhere in the rotator cuff. The condition is not unique to the shoulder, and similar lesions are seen in tendons and ligaments around the ankle, knee, hip and elbow.

The cause is unknown but it is thought that local ischaemia leads to fibrocartilaginous metaplasia and deposition of crystals by the chondrocytes. Calcification alone is probably not painful; symptoms, when they occur, are due to the florid vascular reaction which produces swelling and tension in the tendon. Resorption of the calcific material is rapid and it may soften or disappear entirely within a few weeks.

Clinical features

The condition affects 30–50 year-olds. Aching, sometimes following overuse, develops and increases in severity within hours, rising to an agonizing climax. After a few days, pain subsides and the shoulder gradually returns to normal. In some patients the process is less dramatic and recovery slower. During the acute stage the arm is held immobile; the joint is usually too tender to permit palpation or movement.

X-RAYS

Calcification just above the greater tuberosity is always present. An initially well-demarcated deposit becomes more 'woolly' and then disappears.

Treatment

NON-OPERATIVE TREATMENT

Conservative treatment is successful in up to 90 per cent of patients. The main methods are non-steroidal anti-inflammatory drugs, subacromial injection of corticosteroids, physiotherapy, extracorporeal shockwave therapy, needle aspiration and irrigation.

Non-steroidal anti-inflammatory drugs are the mainstay of non-operative treatment. Although corticosteroid injections are commonly used in the treatment of calcifying tendinitis, there is no conclusive evidence that they promote resorption of the calcium deposit. The efficacy of physiotherapy in the form of therapeutic ultrasound remains uncertain.

Extracorporeal shockwave therapy employs acoustic waves to induce fragmentation of the mechanically hard crystals. Its use as an alternative treatment for calcifying tendinitis has gained increasing popularity in the last few years and its efficacy has been confirmed in several prospective studies which show that the deposit disappears in up to 86 per cent of cases with a significant reduction in pain. However, most of these studies have only a short-term follow-up.

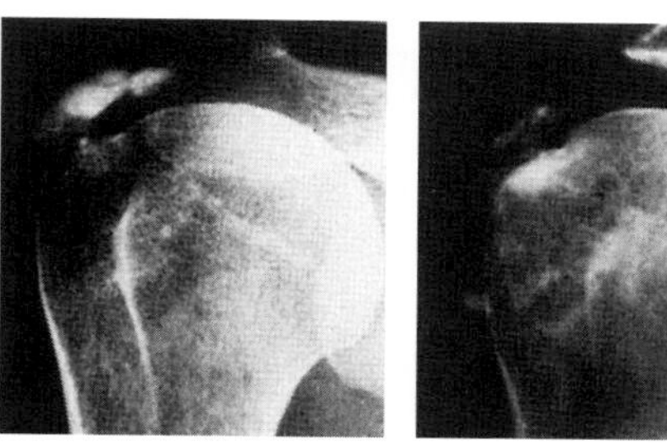
(a)
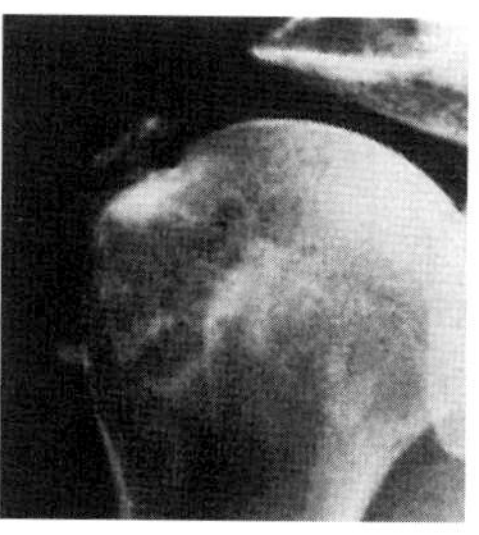
(b)
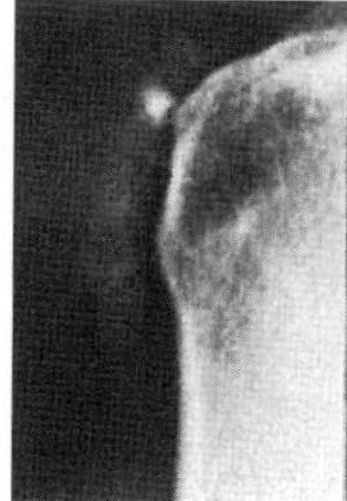
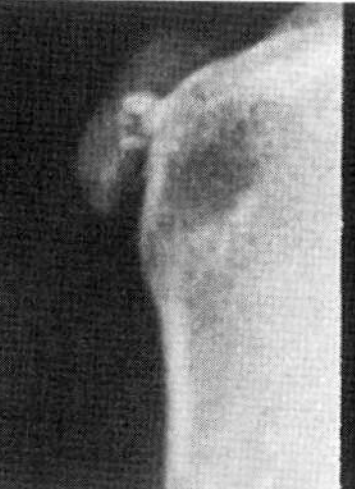
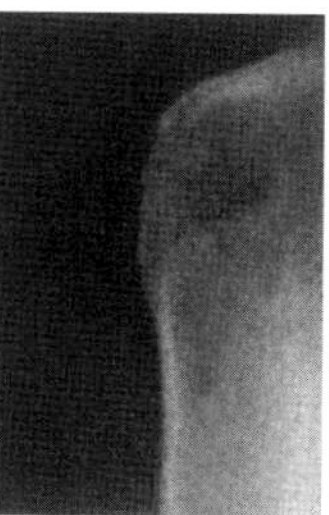
(c)
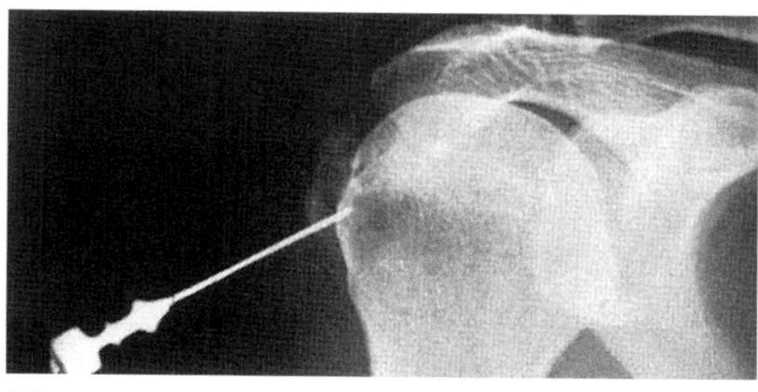
(d)

13.15 Acute calcification of supraspinatus (a) Dense mass in the tendon. (b) Following the 'reaction' some calcium has escaped into the subdeltoid bursa; (c) spontaneous dispersal. (d) An attempt at treatment by aspiration; this procedure is much more likely to succeed if image-intensification and ultrasound control are used.

Needle aspiration and irrigation (barbotage) aims to drain a substantial portion of the calcium deposit, thereby stimulating cell-mediated progressive resorption. Needle aspiration can be readily done under local anaesthesia in the outpatient setting with ultrasound guidance. A combination of local anaesthetic and corticosteroid is used. The best results are obtained in patients with an acutely painful shoulder, typically during the resorption stage in which the calcium is of toothpaste-like consistency.

OPERATIVE TREATMENT

While operative treatment is still a controversial issue, there is wide agreement that surgery is indicated for patients with severe disabling symptoms which have persisted for more than 6 months and are resistant to conservative treatment. The procedure involves a gleno-humeral arthroscopy with special attention to the 'critical zone' of the rotator cuff. Once the calcium deposit is identified, the capsule is carefully incised from the bursal side with a knife in line with fibre orientation of the tendon; a curette is then used to milk out the toothpaste-like deposit. A subacromial decompression is also usually performed.

CHRONIC CALCIFICATION

Asymptomatic calcification of the rotator cuff is common and often appears as an incidental finding in shoulder x-rays. When it is seen in association with the impingement syndrome, it is tempting to attribute the symptoms to the only obvious abnormality – supraspinatus calcification. However, the connection is spurious and treatment should be directed at the impingement lesion rather than the calcification.

LESIONS OF THE BICEPS TENDON

Tendinitis

The long head of biceps is subject to tenosynovitis because of its anatomy; the tendon has a synovial sheath and follows a constrained path in the bicipital groove.

Bicipital tendinitis usually occurs together with rotator cuff impingement; rarely, it presents as an isolated problem in young people after unaccustomed shoulder strain. Tenderness is sharply localized to the bicipital groove. Two manoeuvres that often cause pain are: (1) resisted flexion with the elbow straight and the forearm supinated (Speed's test); and (2) resisted supination of the forearm with the elbow bent (Yergason's test).

Rest, local heat and deep transverse friction usually bring relief. If recovery is delayed, a corticosteroid injection will help. For refractory cases, a number of surgical solutions have been described including arthroscopic decompression, biceps tenotomy and biceps tenodesis.

Rupture

Rupture of the tendon of the long head of biceps usually accompanies rotator cuff disruption, but sometimes the biceps lesion is paramount. The patient is usually aged over 50. While lifting he or she feels something snap in the shoulder and the upper arm becomes painful and bruised. Ask the patient to flex the elbow: the detached belly of the biceps forms a prominent lump in the lower part of the arm.

Isolated tears in elderly patients need no treatment. However, if the rupture is part of a rotator cuff lesion

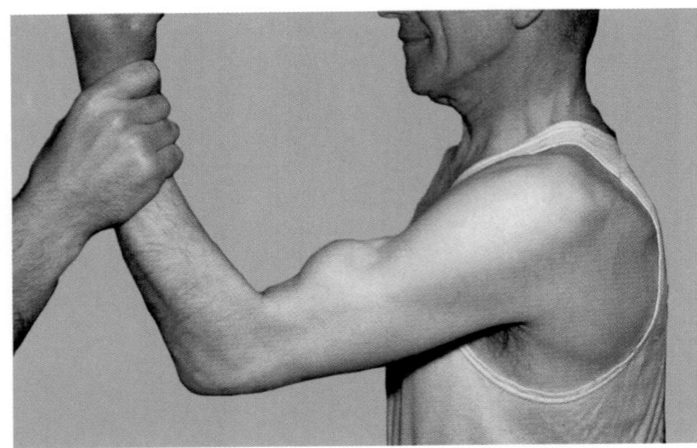

13.16 Ruptured long head of biceps The lump in the front of the arm becomes even more prominent when the patient contracts the biceps against resistance.

– and especially if the patient is young and active – this is an indication for anterior acromioplasty; at the same time the distal tendon stump can be sutured to the bicipital groove (biceps tenodesis). Postoperatively the arm is lightly splinted with the elbow flexed for 4 weeks. (Avulsion of the distal attachment of the biceps is discussed in Chapter 14.)

Hypertrophy and intra-articular entrapment (the hourglass biceps)

The biceps tendon sometimes hypertrophies, e.g. in association with advanced disease of the rotator cuff, and is unable to slide into the bicipital groove. This causes buckling of the tendon on elevation of the shoulder with entrapment of the tendon between the humeral head and glenoid, leading to pain and a block to terminal elevation.

Instability

Both subluxations and dislocations of the long head of biceps have been described. Subluxation is defined as a partial and/or transient loss of contact between the tendon and its groove. Dislocation is the complete and permanent loss of contact between the tendon and the groove; it is usually classified into intra-articular, intra-tendinous and extra-articular subtypes.

Dislocation is nearly always associated with a tear of subscapularis, except in the rare cases of extra-articular dislocation in which the tendon is resting anterior to subscapularis.

SLAP LESIONS

Compressive loading of the shoulder in the flexed abducted position (e.g. in a fall on the outstretched hand) can damage the superior labrum anteriorly and posteriorly (SLAP). The injury of the superior labrum begins posteriorly and extends anteriorly, stopping before or at the mid-glenoid notch and including the 'anchor' of the biceps tendon to the labrum. Four main types are described:

1. non-traumatic superior labral degeneration, usually in older people and often asymptomatic;
2. avulsion of the superior part of the labrum – the commonest type (Fig. 3.17);
3. a 'bucket handle' tear of the superior labrum;
4. as for type 3 with an extension into the tendon of long head of biceps.

Further subtypes that include associated lesions have also been described.

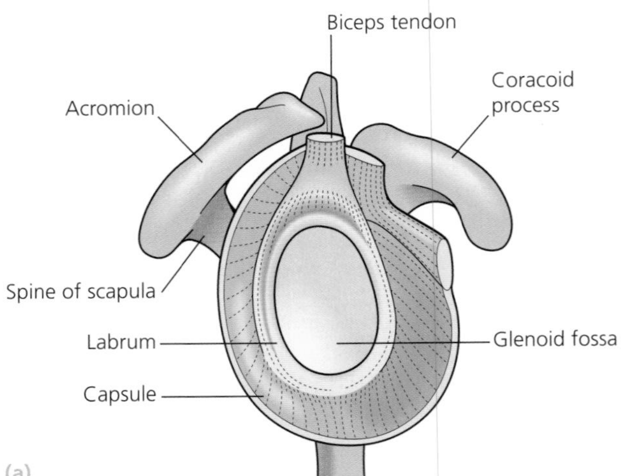

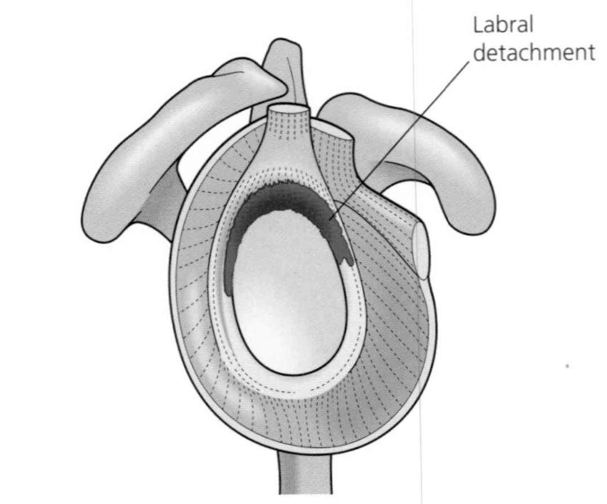

13.17 SLAP lesions (a) Diagram of the normal anatomy, looking into the glenoid fossa. Note that the biceps tendon takes its origin from the superior part of the labrum. (b) The labrum may tear or become detached from the glenoid. This illustration shows a partial tear. Other types are described in the text.

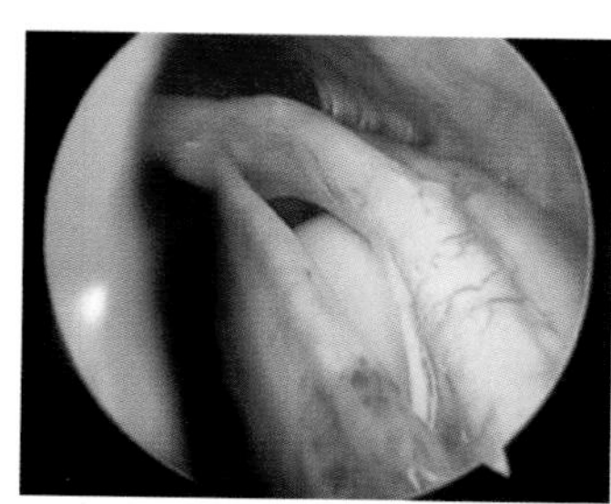

13.18 SLAP lesions
Arthroscopic appearance of a type III SLAP lesion.

Clinical features

There is usually a history of a fall on the arm. As the initial acute symptoms settle, the patient continues to experience a painful 'click' on lifting the arm above shoulder height, together with loss of power when using the arm in that position. He or she may also complain of an inability to throw.

O'Briens test The patient is instructed to flex the arm to 90 degrees with the elbow fully extended and then to adduct the arm 10–15 degrees medial to the sagittal plane. The arm is then maximally internally rotated and the patient resists the examiner's downward force. The procedure is repeated in supination. Pain elicited by the first manoeuvre which is reduced or eliminated by the second signifies a positive test.

Imaging

MRI is the modality of choice though the diagnosis is best confirmed by arthroscopic examination and at the same time the lesion is treated by debridement or repair.

Treatment

Very few patients with SLAP lesion injuries return to full capability without surgical intervention. Arthroscopic repair of an isolated superior labral lesion is successful in the majority (91 per cent) of patients. However, the results in patients who participate in overhead sports are not as satisfactory as those in patients who are not involved in overhead sports (Seung-Ho Kim et al., 2002)

ADHESIVE CAPSULITIS (FROZEN SHOULDER)

The term 'frozen shoulder' should be reserved for a well-defined disorder characterized by progressive pain and stiffness of the shoulder which usually resolves spontaneously after about 18 months. The cause remains unknown. The histological features are reminiscent of Dupuytren's disease, with active fibroblastic proliferation in the rotator interval, anterior capsule and coraco-humeral ligament (Bunker, 1997. The condition is particularly associated with diabetes, Dupuytren's disease, hyperlipidaemia, hyperthyroidism, cardiac disease and hemiplegia. It occasionally appears after recovery from neurosurgery.

Clinical features

The patient, aged 40–60, may give a history of trauma, often trivial, followed by aching in the arm and shoulder. Pain gradually increases in severity and

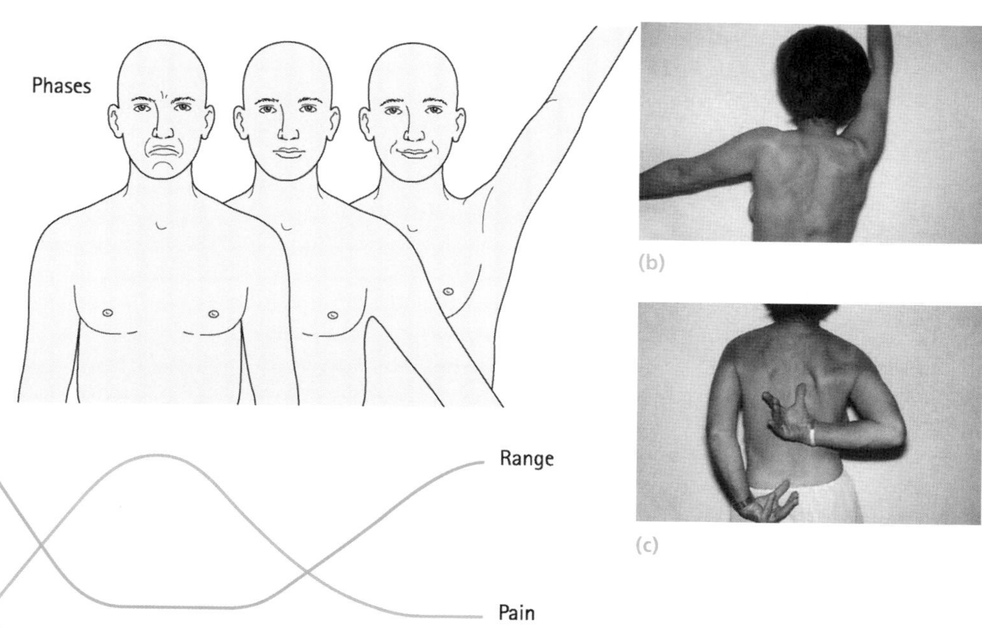

13.19 Frozen shoulder
(a) Natural history of frozen shoulder. The face tells the story. (b,c) This patient has hardly any abduction but manages to lift her arm by moving the scapula. She cannot reach her back with her left hand.

often prevents sleeping on the affected side. After several months it begins to subside, but as it does so stiffness becomes an increasing problem, continuing for another 6–12 months after pain has disappeared. Gradually movement is regained, but it may not return to normal and some pain may persist.

Apart from slight wasting, the shoulder looks quite normal; tenderness is seldom marked. The cardinal feature is a stubborn lack of active and passive movement in all directions.

X-rays are normal unless they show reduced bone density from disuse. Their main value is to exclude other causes of a painful, stiff shoulder.

Diagnosis

Not every stiff or painful shoulder is a frozen shoulder, and indeed there is some controversy over the criteria for diagnosing 'frozen shoulder' (Zuckerman et al., 1994). Stiffness occurs in a variety of conditions – arthritic, rheumatic, post-traumatic and postoperative. The diagnosis of frozen shoulder is clinical, resting on two characteristic features: (1) painful restriction of movement in the presence of normal x-rays; and (2) a natural progression through three successive phases.

When the patient is first seen, a number of conditions should be excluded:

Infection In patients with diabetes, it is particularly important to exclude infection. During the first day or two, signs of inflammation may be absent.

Post-traumatic stiffness After any severe shoulder injury, stiffness may persist for some months. It is maximal at the start and gradually lessens, unlike the pattern of a frozen shoulder.

Diffuse stiffness If the arm is nursed over-cautiously (e.g. following a forearm fracture) the shoulder may stiffen. Again, the characteristic pattern of a frozen shoulder is absent.

Reflex sympathetic dystrophy Shoulder pain and stiffness may follow myocardial infarction or a stroke. The features are similar to those of a frozen shoulder and it has been suggested that the latter is a form of reflex sympathetic dystrophy. In severe cases the whole upper limb is involved, with trophic and vasomotor changes in the hand (the 'shoulder–hand syndrome').

Treatment

CONSERVATIVE TREATMENT

Conservative treatment aims to relieve pain and prevent further stiffening while recovery is awaited. It is important not only to administer analgesics and anti-inflammatory drugs but also to reassure the patient that recovery is certain.

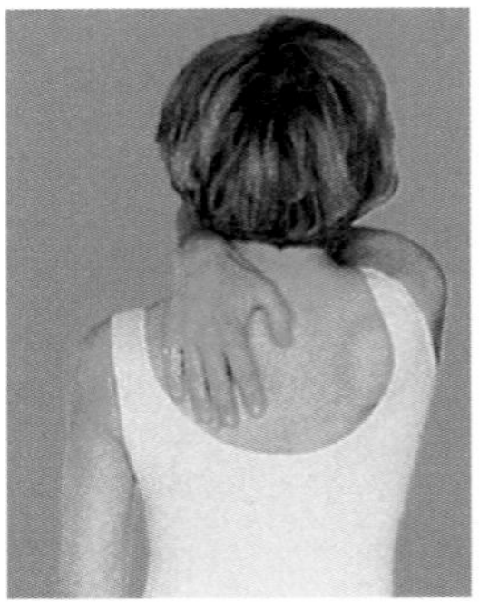

(a)

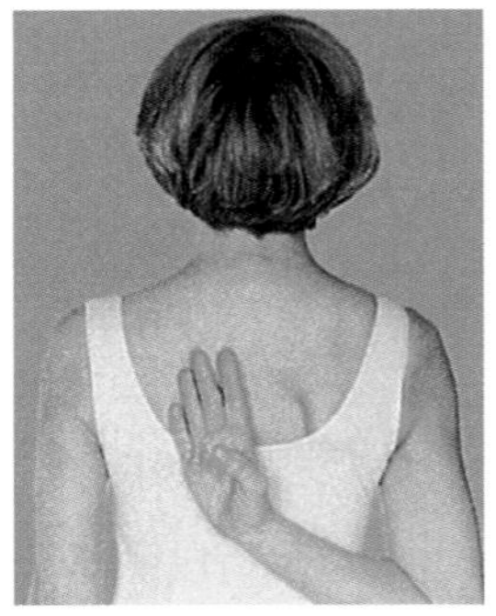

(b)

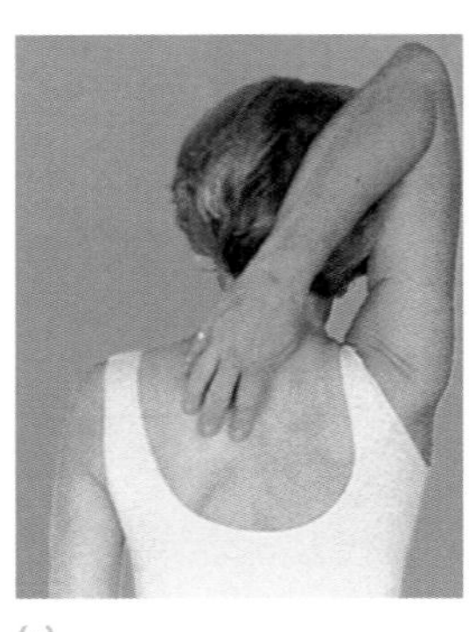

(c)

13.20 Shoulder pain – the scratch test 'Shoulder' pain may be due to disorders of the shoulder joint itself (e.g. gleno-humeral arthritis), the acromioclavicular joint (injury or arthritis) or structures around the joint (e.g. the rotator cuff syndromes). But it could also be referred from more distant lesions (e.g. brachial neuralgia, cervical spondylosis or cardiac ischaemia). If the patient can scratch the opposite scapula in these three ways, the shoulder joint and its tendons are unlikely to be at fault.

Exercises are encouraged, the most valuable being 'pendulum' exercises in which the patient leans forward at the hips and moves his arm as if stirring a giant pudding (this is really a form of assisted active movement, the assistance being supplied by gravity). However, the patient is warned that moderation and regularity will achieve more than sporadic masochism. The role of physiotherapy is unproven and the benefits of steroid injection are debatable.

Manipulation under general anaesthesia may improve the range of movement. The shoulder is moved gently but firmly into external rotation, then abduction and flexion. Special care is needed in elderly, osteoporotic patients as there is a risk of fracturing the neck of the humerus. At the end, the joint is injected with methylprednisolone and lignocaine. An alternative method of treatment is to distend the joint by injecting a large volume (50–200 mL) of sterile

Table 13.1 The painful shoulder

Referred pain syndromes	Rotator cuff disorders
Cervical spondylosis	Tendinitis
Mediastinal pathology	Rupture
Cardiac ischaemia	Frozen shoulder
Joint disorders	**Instability**
Gleno-humeral arthritis	Dislocation
Acromioclavicular arthritis	Subluxation
Bone lesions	**Nerve injury**
Infection	Suprascapular nerve entrapment
Tumours	

saline under pressure. Arthroscopy has shown that both manipulation and distension achieve their effect by rupturing the capsule.

The results of conservative treatment are subjectively good, most patients eventually regaining painless and satisfactory function; however, examination is likely to show some residual restriction of movement (especially external rotation) in over 50 per cent of cases (Shaffer et al., 1992).

Most studies on outcome are small. In the largest of these, Hand et al. (2008) reported on patients who were followed up for a mean of 4.4 years: 59 per cent had normal or near-normal shoulders, and of the remainder 94 per cent had only mild symptoms.

SURGICAL TREATMENT

Surgery does not have a well-defined role. The main indication is prolonged and disabling restriction of movement which fails to respond to conservative treatment.

Arthroscopic capsular release is increasingly employed. New techniques enable the surgeon to release intra-articular, subacromial and subdeltoid adhesions without dividing the subscapularis. Active range of motion can be started immediately (Harryman et al., 1997).

INSTABILITY OF THE SHOULDER

The shoulder achieves its uniquely wide range of movement at the cost of stability. The humeral head is held in the shallow glenoid socket by the glenoid labrum, the gleno-humeral ligaments, the coracohumeral ligament, the overhanging canopy of the coracoacromial arch and the surrounding muscles. Failure of any of these mechanisms may result in instability of the joint.

One must distinguish between *joint laxity* and *joint instability*. Joint laxity implies a degree of translation in the gleno-humeral joint which falls within a physiological range and which is asymptomatic. Joint instability is an abnormal symptomatic motion for that shoulder which results in pain, subluxation or dislocation of the joint.

Dislocation is defined as complete separation of the gleno-humeral surfaces, whereas *subluxation* implies a symptomatic separation of the surfaces without dislocation.

Pathogenetic classification

The aetiology and classification of shoulder instability is complex, although the Stanmore Instability Classification system developed at the Royal National Orthopaedic Hospital in London is now increasingly used. It recognizes that there are two broad reasons why shoulders become unstable: (1) structural changes due to major trauma such as acute dislocation or recurrent micro-trauma; and (2) unbalanced muscle recruitment (as opposed to muscle weakness) resulting in the humeral head being displaced upon the glenoid.

From a clinical and therapeutic point of view, three polar types of disorder can be identified:

Type I Traumatic structural instability.
Type II Atraumatic (or minimally traumatic) structural instability.
Type III Atraumatic non-structural instability (muscular dyskinesia).

The triangular relationship between these conditions allows for the fact there are intermediate types that lie between the 'poles'; the balance of abnormalities can shift and patients may 'move' from one group to another over time or present with a combination of pathologies: for example, a purely structural disorder which, if allowed to persist, becomes associated with abnormal muscle patterning to the extent that *both*

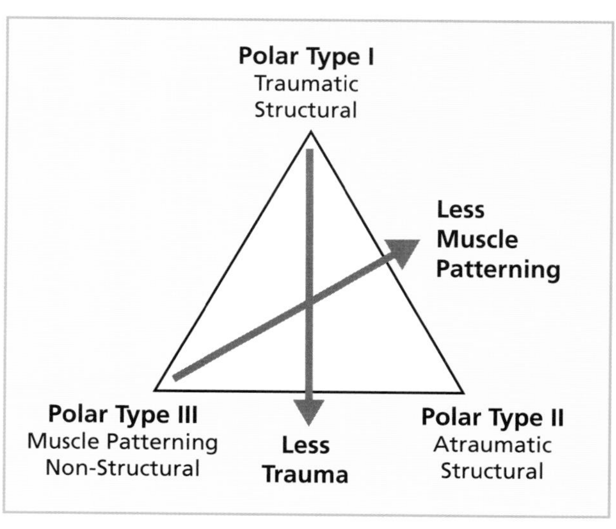

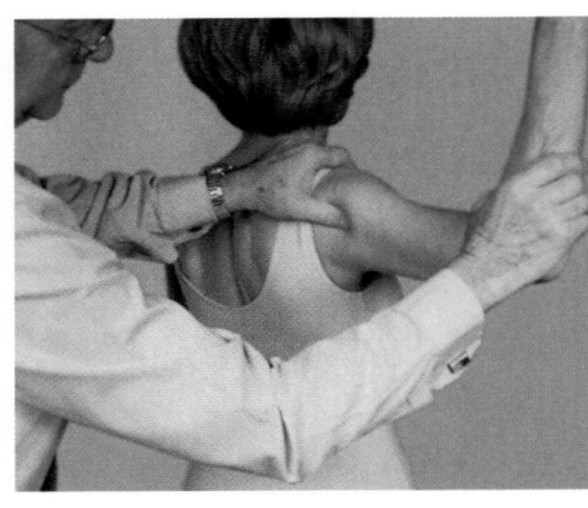
(a)

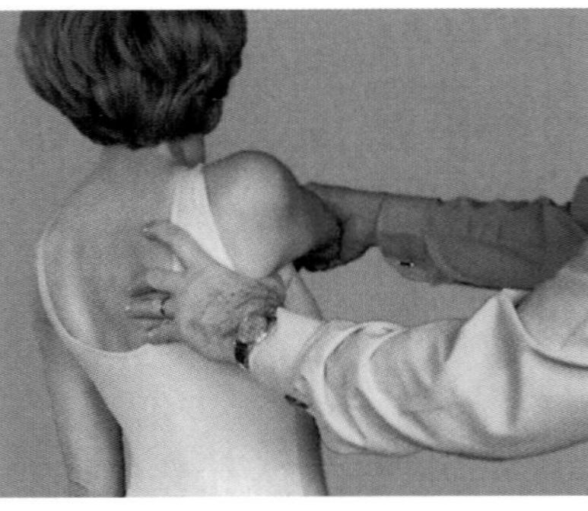
(b)

13.21 Shoulder instability – the apprehension test (a) This is the apprehension test for *anterior subluxation* or *dislocation*. Abduct, externally rotate and extend the patient's shoulder while pushing on the head of the humerus. If the patient feels that the joint is about to dislocate, she will forcibly resist the manoeuvre. (b) *Posterior dislocation* can be tested for in the same way by drawing the arm forward and across the patient's body (adduction and internal rotation).

Table 13.2 Pathological changes in each of the polar types

Pathology	Group I	Group II	Group III
Trauma	Yes	No	No
Articular surface damage	Yes	Yes	No
Capsular problem	Bankart lesion	Dysfunctional	Dysfunctional
Laxity	Unilateral	Uni/bilateral	Often bilateral
Muscle patterning	Normal	Normal	Abnormal

conditions need to be treated and the problems grow in complexity. The system also recognizes that there is a gradation in the opposite direction, from dyskinetic muscle patterning to structural abnormality (Lewis, Kitamura and Bayley, 2004).

TRAUMATIC ANTERIOR INSTABILITY – POLAR TYPE I

PATHOLOGY

This is far and away the commonest type of instability, accounting for over 95 per cent of cases. Traumatic anterior instability usually follows an acute injury in which the arm is forced into abduction, external rotation and extension. In *recurrent dislocation* the labrum and capsule are often detached from the anterior rim of the glenoid (the classic Bankart lesion). In addition there may be an indentation on the posterolateral aspect of the humeral head (the Hill–Sachs lesion), a compression fracture due to the humeral head being forced against the anterior glenoid rim each time it dislocates. In some cases *recurrent subluxation* may alternate with recurrent dislocation. In other cases the shoulder never dislocates completely and in these the labral tear and bone defect may be absent, although the inferior gleno-humeral ligament will be stretched. In patients over the age of 50, dislocation is often associated with tears of the rotator cuff.

Clinical features

The patient is usually a young man or woman who gives a history of the shoulder 'coming out', perhaps during a sporting event. The first episode of *acute dislocation* is a landmark and he or she may be able to describe the mechanism precisely: an applied force with the shoulder in abduction, external rotation and extension. The diagnosis may have been verified by x-ray and the injury treated by closed reduction and 'immobilization' in a bandage or sling for several weeks. This may be the first of many similar episodes: *recurrent dislocation* requiring treatment develops in about one-third of patients under the age of 30 and in about 20 per cent of older patients, with an overall redislocation rate of 48 per cent (Hovelius et al., 1996). Some studies have reported instability rates following acute dislocation between 88 per cent and 95 per cent in patients under the age of 20. A greater proportion have instability without actual dislocation.

Recurrent subluxation Symptoms and signs of recurrent subluxation are less obvious. The patient may describe a 'catching' sensation, followed by 'numbness' or 'weakness' – the so-called 'dead arm syndrome' – whenever the shoulder is used with the arm in the overhead position (e.g. throwing a ball, serving at tennis or swimming). Pain with the arm in abduction may suggest a rotator cuff syndrome; it is as well to remember that recurrent subluxation may actually cause supraspinatus tendinitis.

On examination, between episodes of dislocation, the shoulder looks normal and movements are full. Clinical diagnosis rests on provoking subluxation. In the *apprehension test,* with the patient seated or lying, the examiner cautiously lifts the arm into abduction, external rotation and then extension; at the crucial moment the patient senses that the humeral head is about to slip out anteriorly and his or her body tautens in apprehension. The test should be repeated with the examiner applying pressure to the front of the shoulder; with this manoeuvre, the patient feels more secure and the apprehension sign is negative.

The same effect can be demonstrated by the *fulcrum test*. With the patient lying supine, arm abducted to 90 degrees, the examiner places one hand behind the patient's shoulder to act as a fulcrum over which the humeral head is levered forward by extending and laterally rotating the arm; the patient immediately becomes apprehensive.

If instability is marked the *drawer test* may be positive (see Fig. 13.23). With the patient supine, the scapula is stabilized with one hand while the upper arm is grasped firmly with the other so as to manipulate the head of the humerus forwards and backwards (like a drawer).

Investigations

Most cases can be diagnosed from the history and examination alone. The Hill–Sachs lesion (when it is present) is best shown by an *anteroposterior x-ray* with the shoulder internally rotated, or in the axillary view. Subluxation is seen in the axillary view.

MRI or *MR arthrography* is useful for demonstrating bone lesions and labral tears.

Arthroscopy is sometimes needed to define the labral tear.

Examination under anaesthesia can help to determine the direction of instability. This forms an essential part of assessing instability. Both shoulders need to be examined. Reports have demonstrated sensitivities and specificities of 100 per cent and 93 per cent, respectively.

Treatment

If dislocation recurs at long intervals, the patient may choose to put up with the inconvenience and simply try to avoid vulnerable positions of the shoulder. There is some evidence that dislocation predisposes to osteoarthritis, although it is probably the initial dislocation rather than recurrence that causes this (Hovelius et al., 1996).

OPERATIVE TREATMENT

The indications for operation include frequent dislocation, especially if this is painful, and recurrent subluxation or a fear of dislocation sufficient to prevent participation in everyday activities, including sport. There is growing evidence to support primary surgery in young adults engaged in highly demanding physical activities following first acute traumatic dislocation (Handoll et al., 2004). Two types of operation are employed:

Anatomical repairs These are operations that repair the torn glenoid labrum and capsule, e.g. the Bankart procedure (Bankart, 1939; Gill et al., 1997).

Non-anatomical repairs These procedures are designed to counteract the pathological tendency to joint displacement: (a) operations that shorten the anterior capsule and subscapularis by an overlapping repair (e.g. the Putti–Platt operation); (b) operations that reinforce the anteroinferior capsule by redirecting other muscles across the front of the joint (e.g. the Bristow–Laterjet operation); and (c) a bone operation to correct a reduced retroversion angle of the humeral head by osteotomy (Kronberg and Brostrum, 1995).

The Putti–Platt operation, in which the subscapularis is overlapped and shortened, prevents redislocation but at the cost of significant loss of external

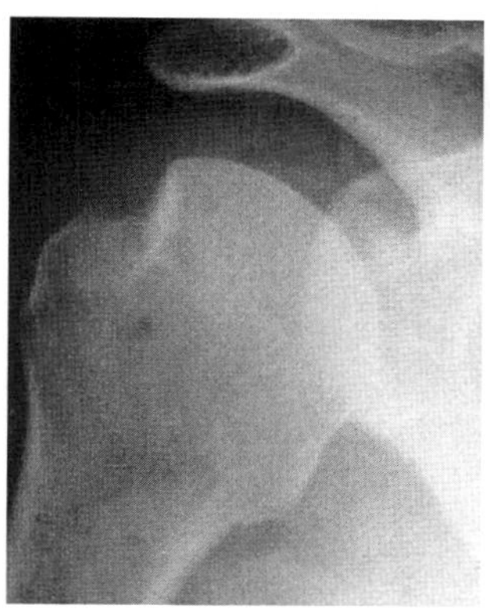
(a)

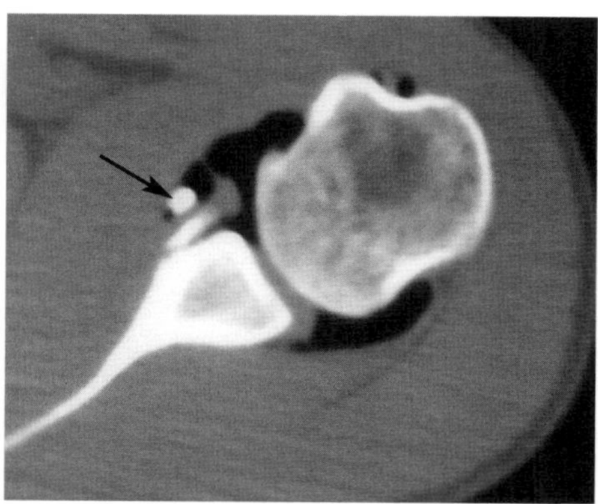
(b)

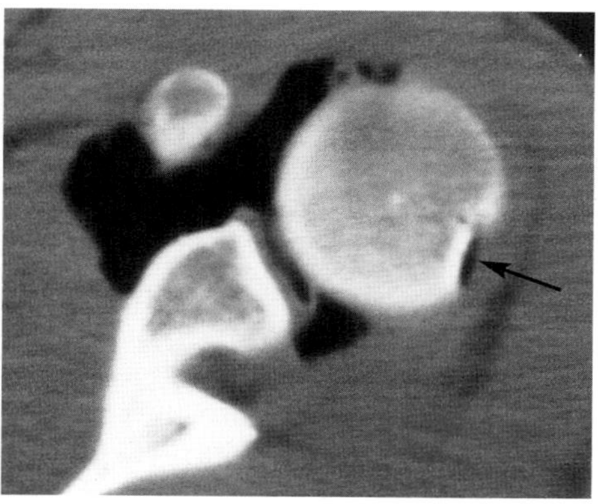
(c)

13.22 Anterior instability – imaging (a) The plain x-ray shows a large depression in the posteriosuperior part of the humeral head (the Hill–Sachs sign). (b,c) MRI shows both a Bankart lesion, with a flake of bone detached from the anterior edge of the glenoid, and the Hill–Sachs lesion (arrows).

rotation. It is now not commonly used. The Bristow–Laterjet operation, in which the coracoid process with its attached muscles is transposed to the front of the neck of the scapula, produces less restriction of external rotation (Singer et al., 1995). In general, non-anatomical operations are now thought to have a limited role in the management of shoulder instability. They do not address the underlying pathological changes and they are often associated with an unacceptable loss of function. Reports of recurrent instability of 20 per cent, loss of external rotation and late-onset degenerative joint disease are common.

If the labrum and anterior capsule are detached, and there is no marked joint laxity, the Bankart operation combined with anterior capsulorrhaphy is the procedure of choice. The labrum is re-attached to the glenoid rim with suture anchors or drill holes and, if necessary, the capsule is tightened by an overlapping tuck without shortening the subscapularis. Bankart initially described this as an open operation through the deltopectoral approach; however, arthroscopic techniques have been developed with advanced anchor materials and the development of specialized arthroscopic instruments. With careful patient selection clinical outcomes and recurrence rates of arthroscopic and open stabilization are now comparable; however, after either type of operation there is still a significant recurrence rate (about 20 per cent), usually following another injury (Cole et al., 2000). If there is bone loss on either the glenoid aspect or the humeral head the outcome following arthroscopic surgery is considerably worse (Boileau et al., 2006).

ATRAUMATIC OR MINIMALLY TRAUMATIC INSTABILITY – POLAR TYPES II AND III

The terminology of these groups is somewhat confusing: *'atraumatic instability'* can include entities such as the 'loose shoulder', multidirectional instability, voluntary dislocation and habitual dislocation. In these cases it is often difficult to decide whether the problem is 'structural' or 'non-structural'.

ATRAUMATIC STRUCTURAL INSTABILITY

This is an acquired multidirectional instability due either to repetitive micro-trauma which has placed undue stress upon the soft tissues or to rapid, forceful movements that contribute to the development of overall laxity of the joint; occasionally a predisposing factor such as glenoid dysplasia is identified.

Atraumatic structural instability is a recognized problem in athletes, particularly swimmers and throwers. They develop symptoms of instability due to overload and fatigue in the stabilizing muscles of the shoulder; dislocation may occur in several different directions. It is doubly important in these cases to rule out the presence of any pathological condition, such as a labral lesion, and to assess whether there is any contributory element of abnormal muscle patterning.

Treatment

REHABILITATIVE MEASURES

Dedicated physiotherapy is focused on strengthening the muscles normally involved in stabilizing the shoulder and restoring muscular coordination and control. Associated problems of muscle patterning are also addressed and patients may need special instruction in the kinematics of shoulder movements and control of stability, as well as advice about modification of physical activities.

SURGICAL TREATMENT

If rehabilitative measures fail to reduce the problem and the patient is genuinely incapacitated operative treatment may be required – usually some type of capsular plication (which can be performed arthroscopically) or a capsular shift (by open operation) (Neer and Foster, 1980).

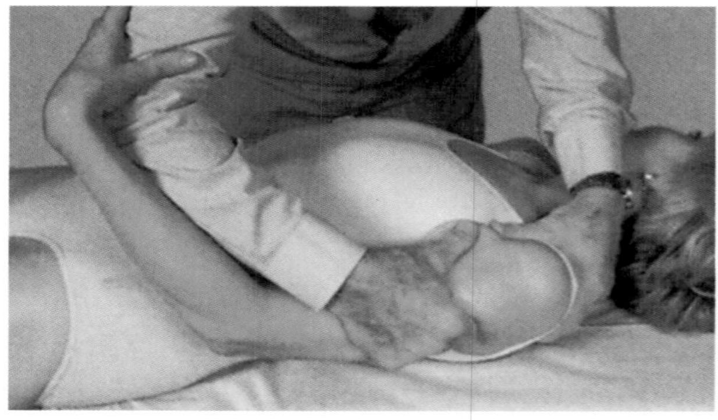

(a)

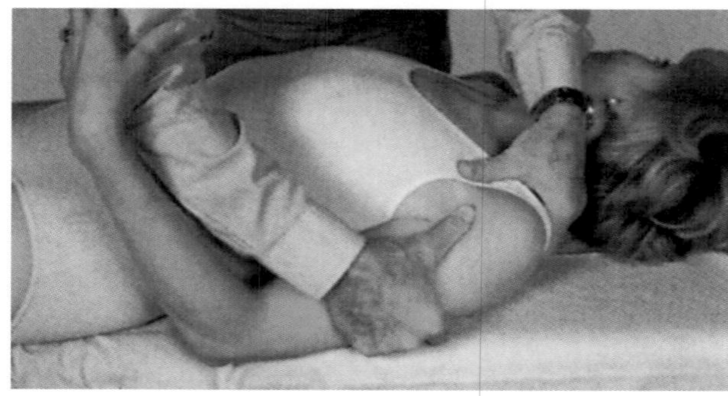

(b)

13.23 Multidirectional instability (a) The anterior and (b) posterior drawer tests are best performed with the patient lying supine. The amount of movement is compared with that on the unaffected side.

Atraumatic non-structural instability (altered muscle patterning)

The stability of the shoulder joint throughout its large range of motion comes partly from precise synchronized muscle contractions and relaxations during movement. Each of the muscles moving and stabilizing the shoulder needs to be activated at a specific time in coordination with other protagonistic and antagonistic muscles. If this pattern is altered instability can occur.

Muscle patterning instability usually occurs in younger patients who can voluntarily slip the shoulder out of joint as a trick movement (habitual), but may then go on to dislocate repeatedly (uncontrolled or involuntary dislocation).

Treatment

The aim is to regain normal neuromuscular control and patterning. This can be difficult, time consuming and require the participation of a full team comprising a specialist shoulder physiotherapist, shoulder surgeon and sometimes an occupational therapist and a psychologist. Treatment follows much the same lines as for atraumatic structural instability but surgery should be avoided if possible.

Inferior subluxation

Some weeks after an injury to the shoulder girdle a patient sometimes develops a feeling of instability in the shoulder, as if it 'slips out of joint', particularly when carrying something heavy with that arm. X-ray examination of the shoulder may show that the head of the humerus has subluxated inferiorly; if this is not immediately apparent, further views with the patient carrying a 10 kg weight in each hand will show the head of the humerus lying below the glenoid socket on the affected side (Fig. 13.25). The condition is due to (temporary) weakness of the shoulder muscles, usually because of prolonged splintage of the arm and lack of exercise.

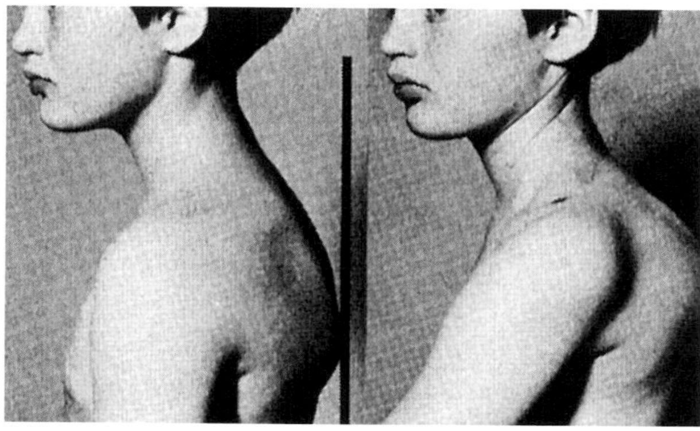

13.24 Habitual subluxation The clue is in the unconcerned expression.

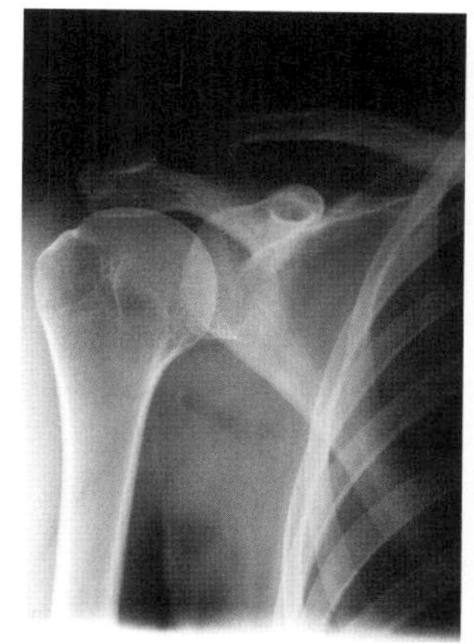

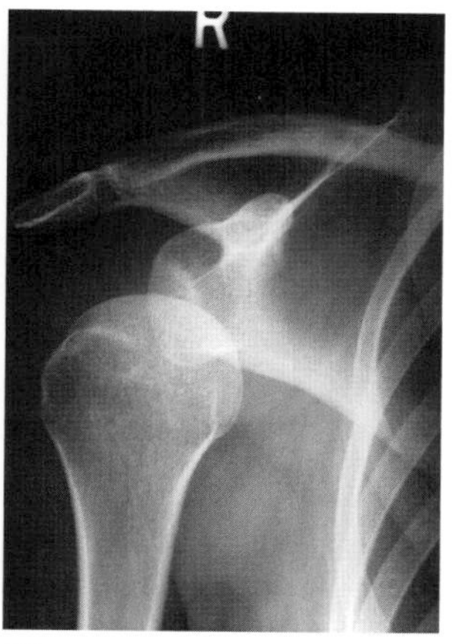

(a) (b)

13.25 Inferior subluxation (a) X-ray of a young woman who developed 'clicking' and instability in the right shoulder after recovering from an injury to the neck and right upper limb. Plain x-ray examination showed no abnormality, but when the anteroposterior view was repeated with the patient carrying 15 kg weights in both hands, subluxation due to laxity of the anteroinferior capsule was demonstrated to the right side (b).

The condition usually corrects itself after a period of normal muscular activity, but physiotherapy will help to speed up the process. In the occasional case, tissue laxity is more persistent and capsular reefing may be advisable.

POSTERIOR INSTABILITY

Pathology

This condition is usually due to a violent jerk in an unusual position or following an epileptic fit or a severe electric shock. Dislocation may be associated with fractures of the proximal humerus, the posterior capsule is stripped from the bone or stretched, and there may be an indentation on the anterior aspect of the humeral head. Recurrent instability is almost always a *posterior subluxation* with the humeral head riding back on the posterior lip of the glenoid.

Clinical features

Acute posterior dislocation is rare, and when it does occur it is often missed. There may be a history of fairly violent injury or an electric shock. On examination the arm is held in internal rotation and attempts

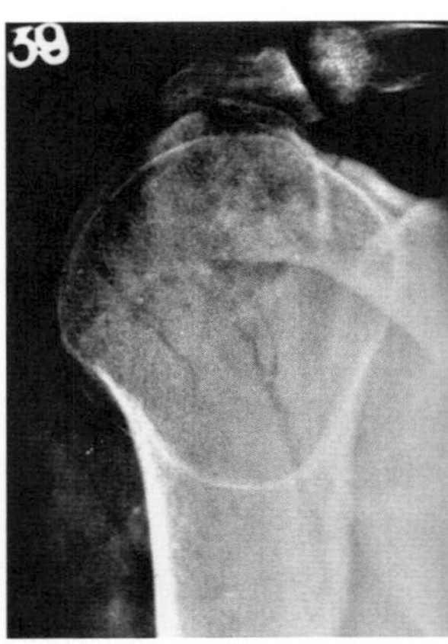

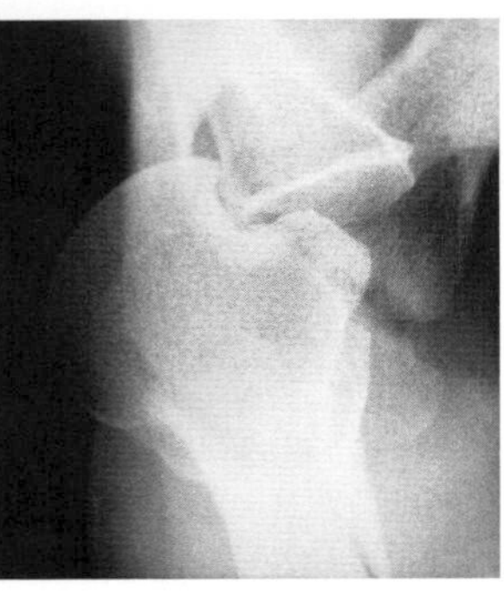

(a) (b)

13.26 Posterior dislocation (a) In the anteroposterior view the humeral head looks globular – the so-called 'light bulb' appearance. (b) In the lateral view one can see the humeral head is lying behind the glenoid fossa, with an impaction fracture on the anterior surface of the head.

at external rotation are resisted. The anteroposterior x-ray may show a typical 'light bulb' appearance of the proximal humerus (the humeral head looks symmetrically bulbous because the shoulder is internally rotated). If the arm can be abducted, an axillary view will show the dislocation quite clearly.

Recurrent posterior instability usually takes the form of subluxation when the arm is used in flexion and internal rotation. On examination, the posterior drawer test (scapular spine and coracoid process in one hand, humeral head pushed backwards with the other) and posterior apprehension test (forward flexion and internal rotation of the shoulder with a posterior force on the elbow) confirm the diagnosis.

TREATMENT

Recurrent posterior instability due to muscle patterning and proprioceptive problems should be treated with physiotherapy. It is essential that this is undertaken by a therapist trained and experienced in dealing with shoulder instability, as the rehabilitation can be long and arduous.

Surgery should be considered only if the primary abnormality is found to be structural (e.g. a Bankart lesion, bony lesion or capsular injury). The particular operation depends on the injuries; it is therefore essential to identify the pathology and treat accordingly. No single operation applies to all patients with posterior instability. Soft-tissue reconstructions are the mainstay of treatment. Rarely there is a bone problem, such as excessive glenoid retroversion (shown on CT scan), in which case glenoid osteotomy should be considered. In extreme cases a bony block to posterior translation of the humeral head is employed though failure rates are reported to be high.

DISORDERS OF THE GLENOHUMERAL JOINT

TUBERCULOSIS (see also Chapter 2)

Tuberculosis of the shoulder is uncommon. It usually starts as an osteitis but is rarely diagnosed until arthritis has supervened. This may proceed to abscess and sinus formation, but in some cases the tendency is to fibrosis and ankylosis. If there is no exudate the term 'caries sicca' is used; however, one suspects that many such cases, formerly diagnosed on the basis of coexisting pulmonary tuberculosis rather than joint biopsy or bacteriological examination, are actually examples of frozen shoulder.

Clinical features

Adults are mainly affected. They complain of a constant ache and stiffness lasting many months or years. The striking feature is wasting of the muscles around the shoulder, especially the deltoid. In neglected cases a sinus may be present over the shoulder or in the axilla. There is diffuse warmth and tenderness and all movements are limited and painful. Axillary lymph nodes may be enlarged.

X-rays show generalized rarefaction, usually with some erosion of the joint surfaces. There may be abscess cavities in the humerus or glenoid, with little or no periosteal reaction.

Treatment

In addition to systemic treatment with antituberculous drugs, the shoulder should be rested until acute

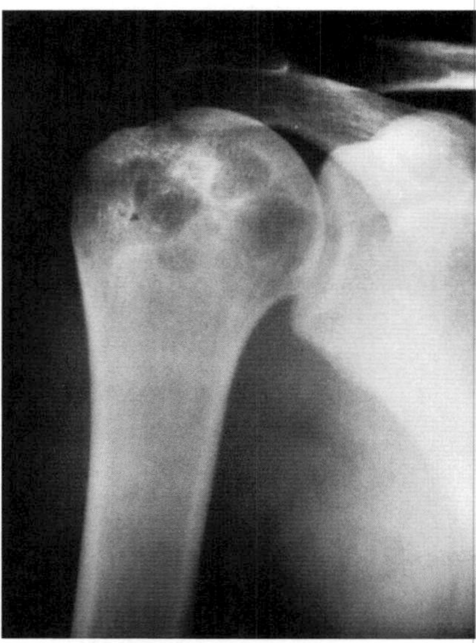

13.27 Tuberculosis X-ray of the shoulder showing tuberculous abscesses in the head of the humerus.

symptoms have settled. Thereafter movement is encouraged and, provided the articular cartilage is not destroyed, the prognosis for painless function is good. If there are repeated flares, or if the articular surfaces are extensively destroyed, the joint should be arthrodesed.

RHEUMATOID ARTHRITIS

(see also Chapter 3)

This is the most common arthropathy to affect the shoulder complex; 90 per cent of patients with rheumatoid arthritis have involvement of the acromioclavicular joint, the shoulder joint and the various synovial pouches around the shoulder.

The *acromioclavicular joint* develops an erosive arthritis which may go on to capsular disruption and instability. This is sometimes the first site to be diagnosed from routine x-rays of the chest.

The *gleno-humeral* joint, with its lax capsule and folds of synovium, shows marked soft-tissue inflammation. Often there is an accumulation of fluid and fibrinoid particles which may rupture the capsule and extrude into the muscle planes. Cartilage destruction and bone erosion are often severe.

The *subacromial bursa* and the *synovial sheath* of the long head of biceps become inflamed and thickened; often this leads to rupture of the rotator cuff and the biceps tendon.

Clinical features

The patient may be known to have generalized rheumatoid arthritis; occasionally, however, acromioclavicular erosion discovered on an x-ray of the chest is the first clue to the diagnosis.

Pain and swelling are the usual presenting symptoms; the patient (usually a woman) has increasing difficulty with simple tasks such as combing her hair or washing her back. Although it may start on one side, the condition usually becomes bilateral.

Synovitis of the *joint* results in swelling and tenderness anteriorly, superiorly or in the axilla. *Tenosynovitis* produces features similar to those of cuff lesions, including tears of supraspinatus or biceps. Joint and tendon lesions usually occur together and conspire to cause the marked weakness and limitation of movement that are features of the disease.

X-rays

Neer described three radiological patterns: *wet* (peri-articular erosions, rapid progress, early cuff rupture), *dry* (subchondral sclerosis, osteophytes, slow progress, cuff intact) and *resorptive* (marked bone loss, few erosions).

Treatment

The general treatment of rheumatoid arthritis is discussed in Chapter 3. In the early stages, local treatment in the form of intra-articular injections of methylprednisolone may be needed.

If synovitis persists, operative synovectomy is carried out; at the same time, cuff tears may be repaired. Excision of the lateral end of the clavicle may relieve acromioclavicular pain.

In advanced cases pain and stiffness can be very disabling. Provided the rotator cuff is not completely destroyed and there is still adequate bone stock, total joint replacement with an unconstrained prosthesis may be carried out. This operation provides good pain relief, moderate shoulder function and reasonable durability (Stewart and Kelly, 1997). Surface replacement arthroplasty has comparable outcomes to total

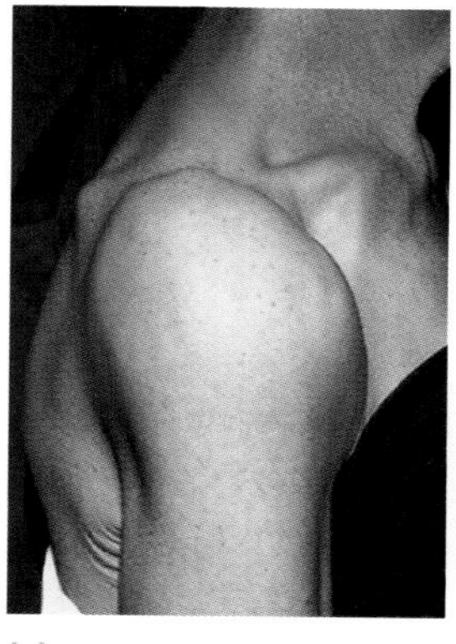
(a)

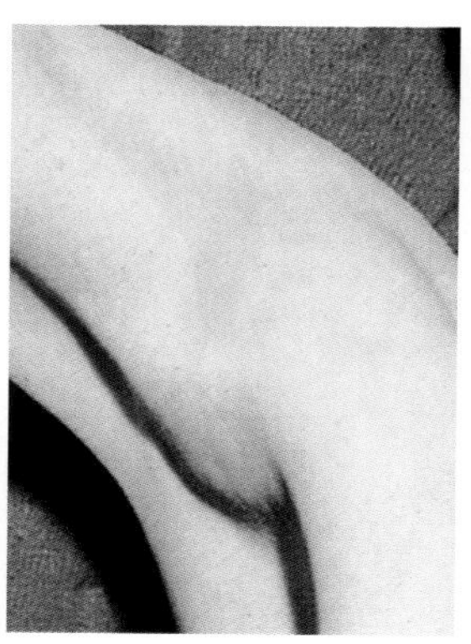
(b)

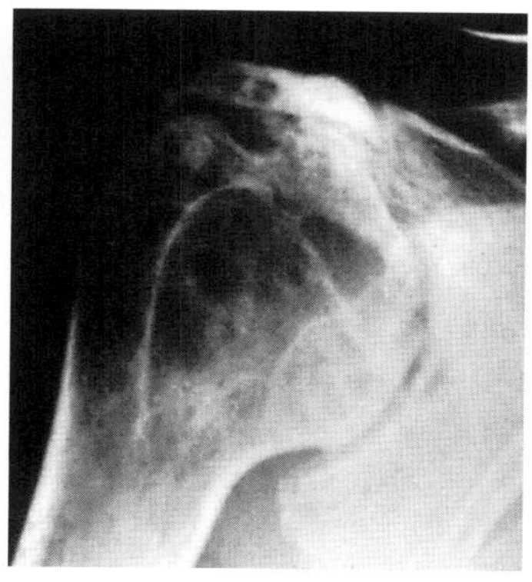
(c)

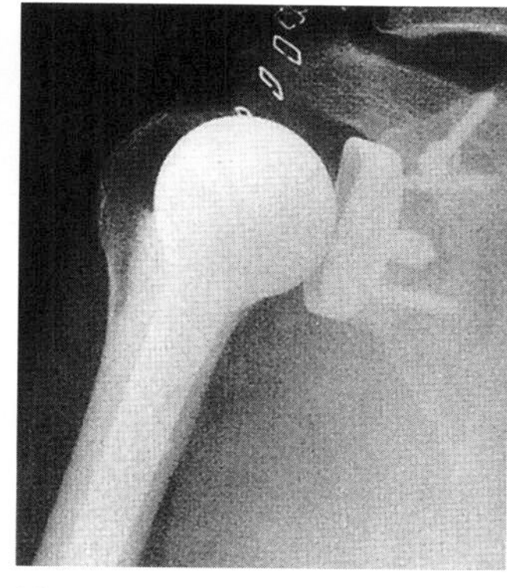
(d)

13.28 Rheumatoid arthritis (a) Large synovial effusions cause easily visible swelling; small ones are likely to be missed, especially if they present in the axilla (b). (c) X-rays show progressive erosion of the joint. (d) X-ray appearance after total joint replacement.

joint replacement but is not suitable for severely damaged joints in which the humeral head is insufficient or too soft (Levy et al., 2004).

If the rotator cuff is destroyed, or bone erosion very advanced, arthrodesis may be preferable; despite its apparent limitations, it gives improved function because scapulo-thoracic movement is usually undisturbed.

OSTEOARTHRITIS

Osteoarthritis of the gleno-humeral joint is more common than is generally recognized. It is usually secondary to local trauma, recurrent subluxation or longstanding rotator cuff lesions. Often chondrocalcinosis is present as well but it is not known whether this predisposes to osteoarthritis or appears as a sequel to joint degradation.

Clinical features

The patient is usually aged 50–60 and may give a history of injury, shoulder dislocation or a previous painful arc syndrome. There is usually little to see but shoulder movements are restricted in all directions.

X-rays show distortion of the joint, bone sclerosis and osteophyte formation; the articular 'space' may be narrowed or may show calcification.

Treatment

Analgesics and anti-inflammatory drugs relieve pain, and exercises may improve mobility. Most patients manage to live with the restrictions imposed by stiffness, provided pain is not severe. However, if both shoulders are involved then the disability can be severe.

In advanced cases, if pain becomes intolerable, shoulder arthroplasty is justified. Arthroplasty is discussed in more detail later in this section. It may not always improve mobility much, but it does relieve pain. The alternative is arthrodesis.

RAPIDLY DESTRUCTIVE ARTHROPATHY (MILWAUKEE SHOULDER)

Occasionally, in the presence of longstanding or massive cuff tears, patients develop a rapidly progressive and destructive form of osteoarthritis in which there is severe erosion of the gleno-humeral joint, the acromion process and the acromioclavicular joint – what Neer and his colleagues (1983) called a *cuff tear arthropathy*. The changes are now attributed to hydroxyapatite crystal shedding from the torn rotator cuff and a synovial reaction involving the release of lysosomal enzymes (including collagenases) which lead to cartilage breakdown (McCarty et al., 1981). A similar condition is seen in other joints such as the hip and knee. The shoulder disorder, however, has come to be known as *Milwaukee shoulder*, after the city from whence McCarty hailed.

Clinical features

The patient is usually aged over 60 and may have suffered with shoulder pain for many years. Over a period of a few months the shoulder becomes swollen and increasingly unstable. On examination there is marked crepitus in the joint and loss of active movements.

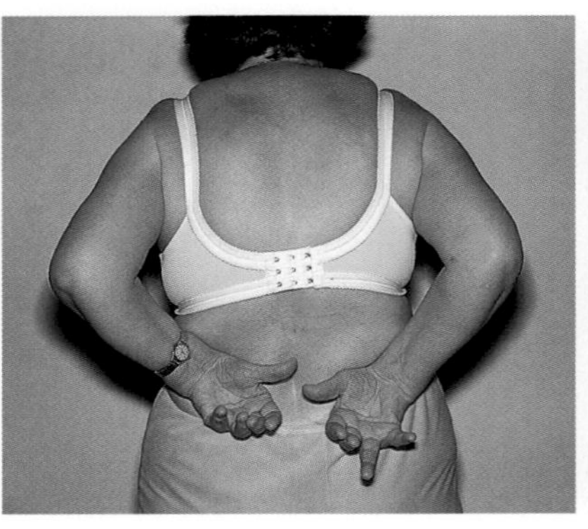
(a)

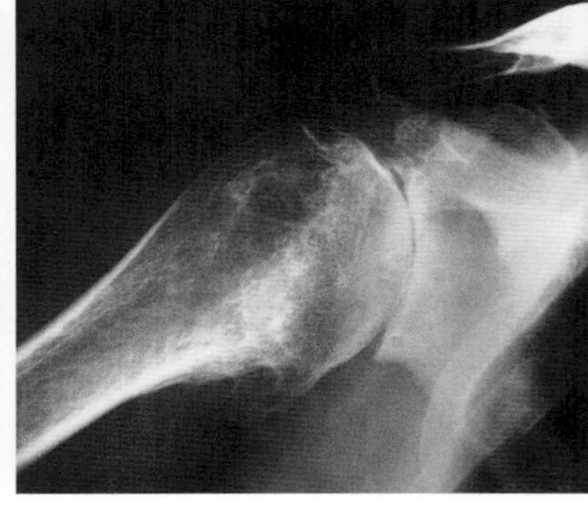
(b)

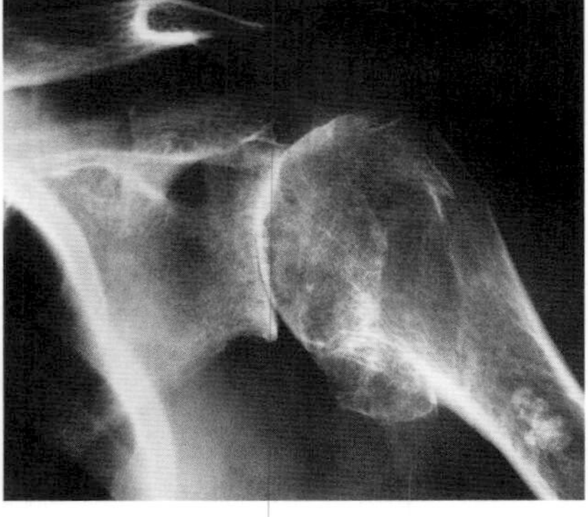
(c)

13.29 Osteoarthritis of the shoulder (a) This woman has advanced osteoarthritis of both shoulders. Movements are so restricted that she has difficulty dressing herself and combing her hair. (b,c) X-rays show the severe degree of articular destruction.

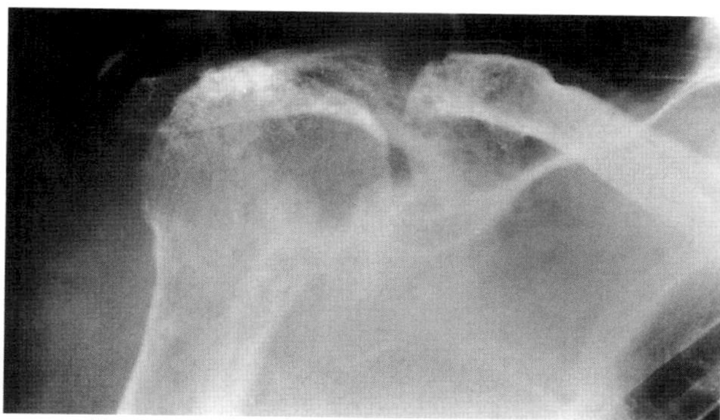

13.30 Milwaukee shoulder X-ray showing a destructive arthropathy with marked swelling and calcification in the soft tissues around the shoulder.

X-rays show severe erosion of the articular surfaces, subluxation of the joint and calcification in the soft tissues.

Treatment

Resurfacing arthroplasty relieves pain and allows good rotations at waist level but will not improve abduction, because the rotator cuff is disrupted and the joint is unstable. It is quick and minimally invasive, retaining bone stock and keeping options open for future revision or arthrodesis.

Reverse shoulder arthroplasty in cuff tear arthropathy allows good elevation in the presence of a well-functioning deltoid as it depends less on the status of the cuff. Problems may occur in the long-term follow-up regarding progressive glenoid loosening due to the so-called 'inferior notching', which is supposed to be a result of an impingement at the inferior glenoid rim followed by increased polyethylene wear and progressive osteolysis. It is thus advisable to avoid reverse shoulder arthroplasty in the younger patient.

OSTEONECROSIS (see also Chapter 6)

The shoulder is the second most common site of steroid-induced osteonecrosis. The condition may also be seen in association with marrow storage disorders, sickle-cell disease and caisson disease, or following irradiation of the axilla.

The clinical features and diagnosis are discussed in Chapter 6. Articular collapse occurs more slowly than in weightbearing joints and operative treatment can usually be delayed for several years. If this should become necessary, joint replacement is the method of choice.

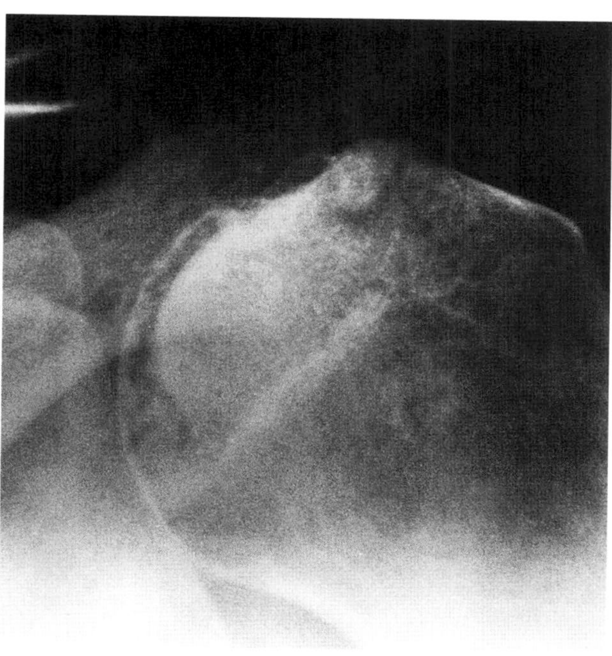

13.31 Osteonecrosis A young woman with systemic lupus erythematosus was treated with large doses of prednisolone. She developed pain in one hip and one shoulder. X-ray of the shoulder shows the classic features of osteonecrosis, including a long subarticular fracture of the humeral head.

DISORDERS OF THE SCAPULA AND CLAVICLE

CONGENITAL ELEVATION OF THE SCAPULA

The scapulae normally complete their descent from the neck by the third month of fetal life; occasionally one or both scapulae remain incompletely descended. Associated abnormalities of the cervical spine are common and sometimes there is a family history of scapular deformity.

CLINICAL FEATURES

Two similar, and possibly related, conditions are encountered.

Sprengel's deformity Deformity is the only symptom and it may be noticed at birth. The shoulder on the affected side is elevated; the scapula looks and feels abnormally high, smaller than usual and somewhat prominent; occasionally both scapulae are affected. The neck appears shorter than usual and there may be kyphosis or scoliosis of the upper thoracic spine. Shoulder movements are painless but abduction and

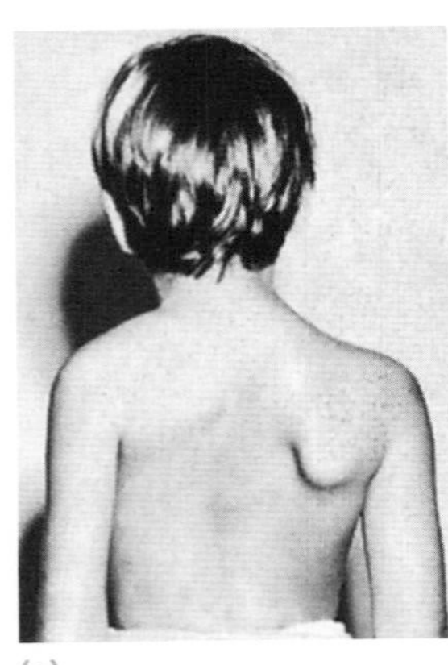

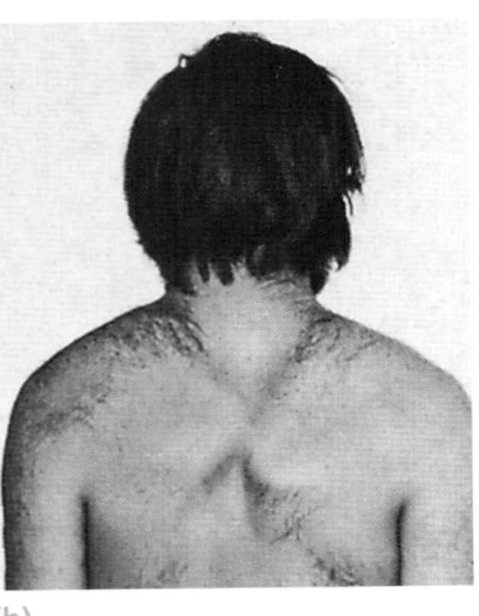

(a) (b)

13.32 Scapular disorders (a) Sprengel shoulder; (b) Klippel–Feil syndrome.

elevation may be limited by fixation of the scapula. *X-rays* will show the elevated scapula and any associated vertebral anomalies; sometimes there is also a bony bridge between the scapula and the cervical spine (the omo-vertebral bar).

Klippel–Feil syndrome This is usually a more widespread disorder. There is bilateral failure of scapular descent associated with marked anomalies of the cervical spine and failure of fusion of the occipital bones. Patients look as if they have no neck; there is a low hairline, bilateral neck webbing and gross limitation of neck movement. This condition should not be confused with *bilateral shortness* of the *sternomastoid muscle* in which the head is poked forward and the chin thrust up; the absence of associated congenital lesions is a further distinguishing feature.

TREATMENT

Mild cases are best left untreated. Surgical treatment aims to decrease deformity and improve shoulder function. In children under 6 years of age, the scapula can be repositioned by releasing the muscles along the vertebral and superior borders of the scapula, excising the supraspinous portion of the scapula and the omovertebral bar, pulling the scapula down, then reattaching the muscles to hold it firmly in its new position. In older children this carries a risk of brachial nerve compression or traction between the clavicle and first rib; here it is safer merely to excise the supraspinous portion of the scapula in order to improve the appearance but without improving movement. Before undertaking any operation the cervical spine should be carefully imaged in order to identify any abnormalities of the odontoid process or base of skull.

CLEIDOCRANIAL DYSOSTOSIS

This is a heritable disorder (autosomal dominant) characterized by hypoplasia or aplasia of the clavicles and flat bones (pelvis, scapulae and skull). Those affected have a typical appearance, with drooping shoulders, an usually narrow chest and the ability to bring the shoulders together across the front of the chest.

X-rays show hypoplasia or complete absence of the clavicles, and sometimes also of the scapulae. Other skeletal defects, which occur in varying degree, are delayed closure of the fontanelles, brachycephaly, underdevelopment of the pelvis, coxa vara and scoliosis.

Treatment is usually unnecessary and, despite the widespread defects, patients enjoy good function.

CONGENITAL PSEUDARTHROSIS OF THE CLAVICLE

The typical clinical picture is that of a child with a painless lump in the mid-shaft of the clavicle. This always occurs on the right side, except in the presence of dextrocardia. X-ray shows the break in the clavicle, which usually heals only after excision of the 'non-union' and bone grafting.

Treatment, if required, is by excision of the pseudarthrosis and bone grafting across the gap.

SCAPULAR INSTABILITY

Winging of the scapula is due to weakness of the serratus anterior muscle. It results in asymmetry of the shoulders but the deformity may not be obvious until the patient tries to contract the serratus anterior against resistance. The typical appearance is shown in Figure 13.33.

There are several causes of weakness or paralysis of the serratus anterior muscle:

- neuralgic amyotrophy (see page 259)
- injury to the brachial plexus (a blow to the top of the shoulder, severe traction on the arm or carrying heavy loads on the shoulder
- direct damage to the long thoracic nerve (e.g. during radical mastectomy)
- fascioscapulohumeral muscular dystrophy.

Disability is usually slight and is best accepted. However, if function is noticeably impaired, it is possible to stabilize the scapula by transferring the sternal

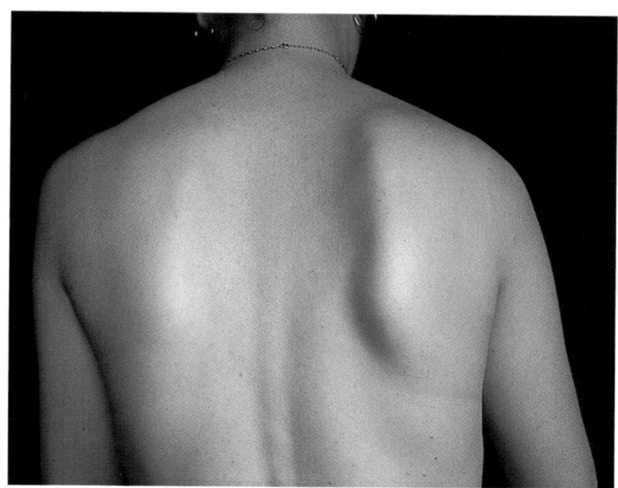

13.33 Winged scapula This young woman's right scapula was somewhat prominent even at rest, but here the 'winging' is enhanced by having her thrust her arms forcibly against the wall.

portion of pectoralis major and attaching it via a fascia lata graft to the lower pole of the scapula; or the scapula can be fixed to the rib-cage to provide the deltoid and the rotator cuff muscles with a stable base from which to control the shoulder.

A less obvious, but sometimes more disabling, form of scapular instability may follow *injury* to the *spinal accessory nerve* (e.g. following operations in the posterior triangle of the neck). The trapezius muscle is an important stabilizer of the shoulder and loss of this function results in weakness and pain on active abduction against resistance. Early recognition may permit nerve repair or grafting.

GRATING SCAPULA

Asymptomatic scapulo-thoracic crepitus is found in about a third of healthy persons. People with symptoms complain of grating or clicking on moving the arm; the condition is often painless but annoying, though it does sometimes become painful. Usually no cause is found, though bony, muscular and bursal abnormalities have been blamed.

Tangential x-ray views of the scapula should be obtained to exclude an osteochondroma on the undersurface of the scapula. A CT scan with three-dimensional reconstruction can be helpful; if an osteochondroma is present, the lesion can be excised. If a bony lesion is not identified conservative treatment is usually adopted.

SEPTIC ARTHRITIS OF THE STERNO-CLAVICULAR JOINT

This condition is rare except in drug abusers following intravenous injections, and as a secondary complication of sterno-clavicular haemarthrosis following trauma. Local signs may be misleadingly mild but persistent pain, swelling and tenderness associated with systemic signs of infection should arouse suspicion.

Imaging *X-rays* are usually normal until fairly late when they may show erosion of the sterno-clavicular joint and the adjacent bone. If infection is suspected then further imaging of the joint will be required, such as *MRI* or *CT*, which will allow the extent of any spread of infection or bony destruction to be identified. *Radioscintigraphy* is able to identify multifocal septic arthritis.

Investigations If infection is suspected then blood cultures and aspiration of the joint will be required. A wide range of organisms have been found to cause infection at this site.

Treatment If frank pus is present in the joint then an arthrotomy with formal washout will be required. If there is delay in diagnosis or institution of the correct treatment, rupture of the joint capsule may occur with tracking of pus into the chest wall, retrosternum or superior mediastinum.

STERNO-CLAVICULAR HYPEROSTOSIS

Several individually uncommon disorders are associated with pain and swelling over the clavicle or the sterno-clavicular joint. They are often confused, though certain characteristic features permit appropriate differentiation in the majority of cases.

Condensing osteitis of the clavicle

This is usually seen in women of 20–40 years who present with pain at the medial end of the clavicle, which is aggravated by abducting the arm. The clavicle may be thickened and tender. X-rays reveal sclerosis and radionuclide scanning shows increased activity in the affected bone (Cone et al., 1983).

The condition may be no more than a reaction to the mechanical stress of excessive lifting activities, and treatment consists simply of avoiding such activities. Of greater importance is the need to distinguish it from the other hyperostotic disorders.

Condensing osteitis shares both morphological and radiological features with osteitis of the ilium and osteitis of the pubis. It has been noted that all of these bones have a fibrocartilaginous covering which may explain the predilection of the condition for those sites.

Sterno-costo-clavicular hyperostosis

This condition in some ways resembles condensing osteitis, but it is seen in slightly older people (both men and women) and is usually bilateral. Patients develop pain, swelling and tenderness over the sterno-clavicular region and x-rays show hyperostosis of the medial ends of the clavicles, the adjacent sternum, the anterior ends of the upper ribs and the soft tissues in between. Vertebrae also may be affected and the ESR may be increased; little wonder that it has been suggested that this is a type of seronegative spondarthropathy. Biopsy is of little help; the histological changes are non-specific and micro-organisms have not been identified. A peculiarity which links this condition with the next is an association with pustular lesions on the palms and soles (palmo-plantar pustulosis) and pustular psoriasis.

Subacute or chronic multifocal osteomyelitis

Multifocal osteomyelitis usually occurs in children and adolescents; the clavicle and lower limb metaphyses are sites of predilection. It may present as a painful, fusiform swelling of the clavicle and x-rays show thickening and sclerosis of the medial third of the bone. Like sterno-costo-clavicular hyperostosis, it is sometimes associated with palmo-plantar pustulosis. The diagnosis is strongly suggested if pustulosis is present, otherwise it usually emerges gradually as other sites become affected over the course of the next year or two and x-rays show the typical lytic areas in the metaphyses and/or epiphyses close to the physis. The full-blown picture is well described in the paper by Carr et al. (1993). There is no effective treatment; the lesions almost invariably heal spontaneously over a period of months or years, the only trace of the condition being the thickened bone ends.

OSTEOARTHRITIS OF THE ACROMIO-CLAVICULAR JOINT

Osteoarthritis of the acromioclavicular joint is common in middle-aged and older people. Predisposing factors are trauma (subluxation of the joint) and occupational stress (habitually carrying weights on the shoulder or working with pneumatic hammers and drills), but the condition also occurs in the absence of any suggestive history. The patient may complain of 'shoulder pain', but if you ask him or her to point, he or she will direct your attention to the prominent bump at the outer end of the clavicle; tenderness is sharply localized to this area. Shoulder movements are usually not restricted (unless the shoulder joint itself is involved) but there may be pain at the extremes of abduction and flexion.

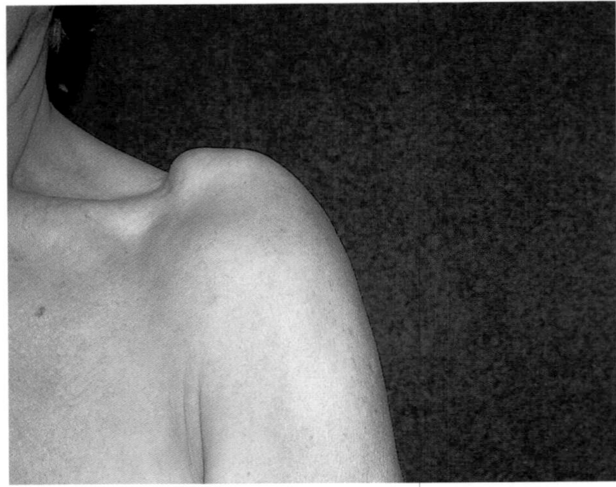

13.34 Osteoarthritis of the acromioclavicular joint Osteophytic thickening of the acromioclavicular joint produced a small (but very tender) bump on top of the left shoulder. Occasionally the joint capsule herniates, producing a large 'cyst' over the acromioclavicular joint.

X-ray shows the characteristic features of osteoarthritis; the changes are often bilateral, even though only one side may be hurting. In some cases the condition is discovered while examining the patient for an impingement syndrome; indeed, acromioclavicular OA may *cause* impingement.

TREATMENT

If analgesics or steroid injections are ineffectual, pain may be relieved by excision of the lateral end of the clavicle. This procedure can now be performed arthroscopically. Trimming of the bony roughness, or excision of the outer end of the clavicle, may also be needed during subacromial decompression for rotator cuff impingement.

OPERATIONS

Rotator cuff surgery and shoulder stabilization are described in the relevant sections.

ARTHROSCOPY

Arthroscopy is a useful technique for the *diagnosis* of peri-articular and intra-articular disorders, such as rotator cuff disruption and instability. At the same time a *biopsy* can be taken which may assist in the diagnosis of synovial disorders such as rheumatoid arthritis or pigmented villonoduar synovitis.

Arthroscopic surgery is now well established. There has been a transition over the last 20 years from its usage in diagnosis to that of repair and reconstructive procedures. It is the first-line surgical option for subacromial decompression, acromioclavicular joint excisions, debridement of rotator cuff tears and release of frozen shoulder. Arthroscopic repair of Bankart lesions produces results comparable to those obtained by open surgery.

ARTHROPLASTY OF THE SHOULDER

Shoulder replacement was initially introduced by Neer in the 1950s for the treatment of proximal humeral fractures. Subsequent modifications and the introduction of glenoid resurfacing broadened the indications to include other disease processes, including end-stage gleno-humeral osteoarthritis and rheumatoid arthritis. If non-operative treatment fails, the two surgical options commonly considered are humeral head replacement (HHR) and total shoulder replacement (TSR). The optimal treatment choice, however, remains controversial.

Indications

The indications for arthroplasty are:

1. osteoarthritis causing pain and loss of movement
2. rheumatoid arthritis
3. complex fractures of the proximal humerus
4. avascular necrosis of the humeral head
5. tumours of the proximal humerus
6. severe arthritis with cuff arthropathy.

The choice of procedure lies between total shoulder replacement, humeral head replacement (hemiarthroplasty) – which can be stemmed or resurfacing – and more constrained shoulder replacements such as the reverse polarity shoulder replacements. The relative merits of total shoulder arthroplasty and hemiarthroplasty are not clear. Glenoid resurfacing is contraindicated if inadequate bone stock or irreparable rotator cuff tears (or both) are present. Hemiarthroplasty affords the benefits of decreased operation time, blood loss and technical difficulty which would otherwise attend glenoid exposure and resurfacing. On the other hand, individual studies have reported less consistent pain relief with isolated humeral head replacement. With isolated humeral head replacement, the glenoid can undergo progressive erosion over time, often leading to deteriorating results.

Relative indications for TSR in patients with gleno-humeral arthritis include loss of articular cartilage or incongruent osseous surfaces, with normal or reparable rotator cuff tendons. TSR requires more operative time and is technically more challenging than hemi-arthroplasty, and the procedure introduces the concern of glenoid loosening, the most common complication. However, proponents of TSR suggest it may yield more consistent pain relief and a better range of motion.

In a systematic review of the literature there is a suggestion that overall TSR may yield superior results; however, it remains unclear if one procedure is significantly better than the other (Radnay et al., 2007).

Complications

The commonest, in order of frequency, are loosening of the components, gleno-humeral instability, rotator cuff failure, peri-prosthetic fracture, infection and implant failure. Glenoid fixation remains a challenge;

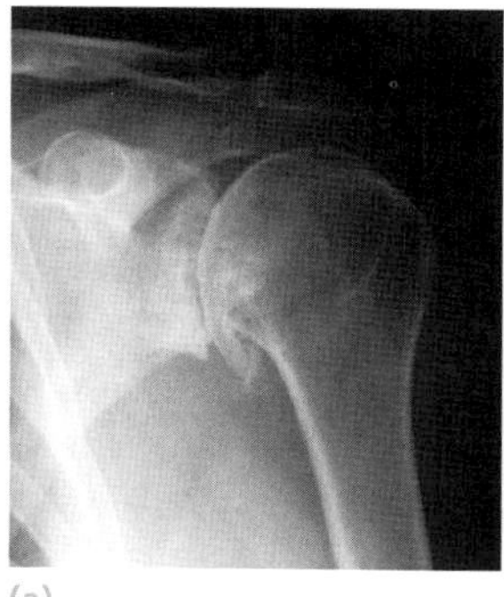
(a)

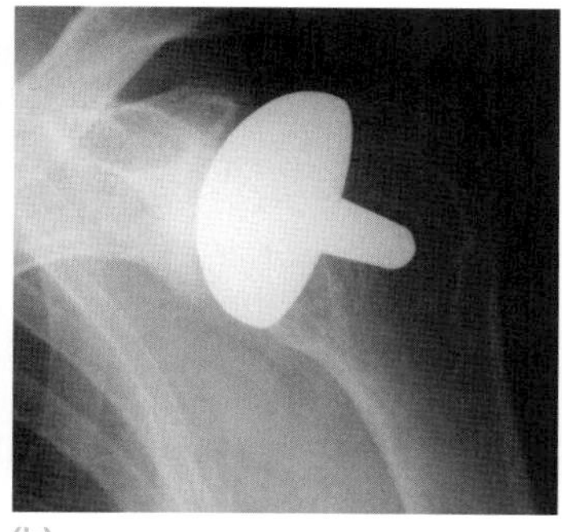
(b)

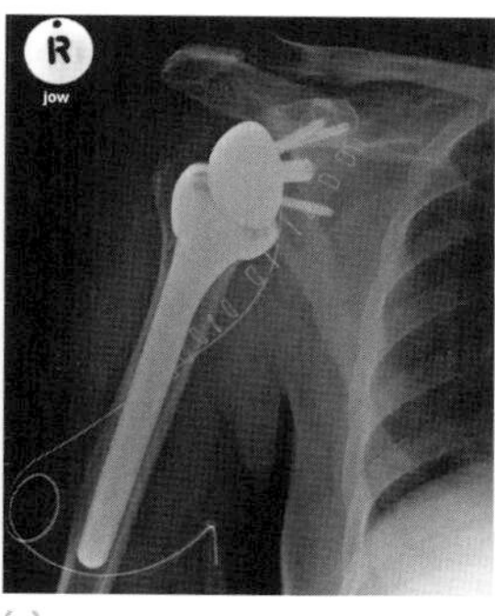

(c)

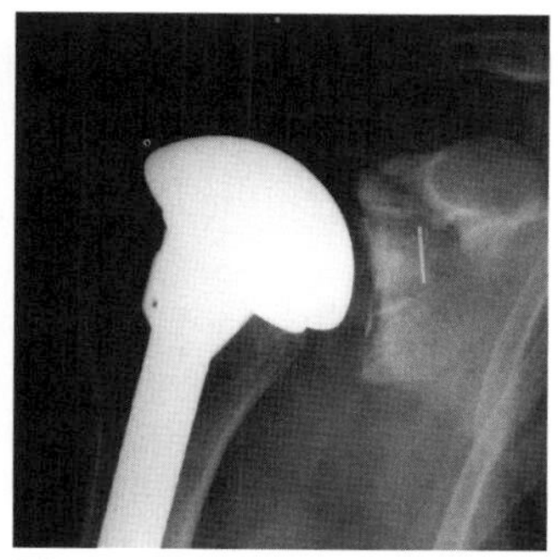
(d)

13.35 Shoulder replacements (a,b) Osteoarthritis and a resurfacing arthroplasty. (c) Early postoperative x-ray of a reverse polarity shoulder replacement. (d) Total shoulder replacement with replacement of the glenoid.

lucent lines around the glenoid component are very common, although not always symptomatic (Wirth and Rockwood, 1996).

Outcome

This depends largely on the indications for surgery. Arthroplasty for fractures, avascular necrosis or proximal humeral tumours gives good pain relief and shoulder movement, although power is always diminished. Where there is more extensive joint destruction and disruption of the soft tissues (e.g. in rheumatoid arthritis), pain relief is still excellent but the range of movement is only moderately improved. The greater the integrity of the surrounding soft tissues (and especially the rotator cuff), the more stable will the new joint be, and thus the better the outcome of the operation. In severe cuff failure, reverse geometry arthroplasty has been used with reasonable success in the short term in elderly patients, though further research is needed to assess longevity and continued functional improvement.

ARTHRODESIS

Arthrodesis of the gleno-humeral joint is now seldom performed, but it is still a useful operation for severe shoulder dysfunction.

Indications

The indications for shoulder arthrodesis are:

1. paralysis of the scapulo-humeral muscles
2. infective disorders of the gleno-humeral joint (including tuberculous arthritis)
3. advanced erosive arthritis with massive disruption of the rotator cuff
4. failed total shoulder arthroplasty
5. uncontrolled instability.

The operation

A prerequisite is stable and powerful scapulo-thoracic movement, because with a fused shoulder 'movement' is achieved entirely by rotation of the scapula on the thorax. A number of techniques have been reported with extra-articular arthrodesis, intra-articular arthrodesis and a combination of both. Internal fixation has been used more frequently in recent years,

Extra-articular arthrodesis is primarily a historic procedure that was used before the antibiotic era to treat tuberculosis.

A variety of methods of internal fixation for intra-articular arthrodesis have been described. It is generally agreed that internal fixation is desirable because it maintains the position of the arthrodesis and can decrease the length of time spent in plaster immobilization.

The optimal position is 30 degrees of flexion, 30 degrees of abduction and 30 degrees of internal rotation. A thermoplastic orthosis needs to be worn for 6 weeks.

Outcome

Despite the restriction of gleno-humeral movement, postoperative function is surprisingly good; and of course the joint is free of pain!

Complications include non-union, infection, malposition often with too much internal rotation, prominence of the internal fixation and fracture of the humerus.

NOTES ON APPLIED ANATOMY

Joints

The anatomy of the shoulder is uniquely adapted to allow freedom of movement and maximum reach for the hand.

Five 'articulations' are involved:

- the gleno-humeral joint
- the pseudojoint between the humerus and the coracoacromial arch
- the sternoclavicular joint
- the acromioclavicular joint
- the scapulothoracic articulation.

Stability

The shallow gleno-humeral articulation has little inherent stability because the glenoid surface area is only one-quarter that of the humeral articular surface. The extent to which the socket is deepened by the labrum may seem trivial, but it must be significant because labral tears are associated with dislocation. Stability depends mainly on the integrity of the ligaments and capsule. The muscles provide kinetic stability: during abduction the rotator cuff muscles draw the head of the humerus firmly into its socket while the deltoid elevates the arm.

Rotator cuff

The rotator cuff is a sheet of conjoint tendons closely applied over the top of the shoulder capsule and inserting into the greater tuberosity of the humerus. It is made up of subscapularis in front, supraspinatus above and infraspinatus and teres minor behind. The 'rotator' muscles have an important function in stabilizing the head of the humerus by pulling it firmly into the glenoid whenever the deltoid lifts the arm forwards or sideways. The rotator interval lies between the supraspinatus and infraspinatus tendons.

Arching over the cuff is a fibro-osseous canopy – the coracoacromial arch – formed by the acromion process posterosuperiorly, the coracoid process anteriorly and the coracoacromial ligament joining them. Separating the tendons from the arch, and allowing them to glide, is the subacromial bursa. Of the four cuff tendons, the supraspinatus is the most exposed; it runs over the top of the shoulder under the anterior edge of the acromion and the adjacent acromio-clavicular joint, with the intra-articular portion of the biceps tendon closely applied to its deep surface.

Movement

Abduction and flexion of the shoulder look simple; in fact they are very complex movements involving all the joints of the shoulder girdle. Imagine what would happen if the deltoid muscle acted alone in abducting the shoulder. Because of the relatively unstable fulcrum, the deltoid would simply shrug the arm upwards at the side of the body. In reality, the rotator cuff muscles, particularly the supraspinatus, draw the head of the humerus firmly into the socket and slightly downwards, thus allowing the deltoid to act as a true abductor.

The first 30 degrees of abduction occurs almost entirely at the gleno-humeral joint with slight movement of the clavicle at the sterno-clavicular joint. From 30 to 90 degrees of abduction the scapula gradually comes into play, with about one-third of the movement coming from the scapula rotating on the thorax. From 90 to 180 degrees, the movement is mainly scapulo-thoracic and for this reason it is termed 'elevation' rather than 'abduction'. As the arm rises above shoulder height, it rolls into external rotation so that the greater tuberosity clears the projecting acromion. The sterno-clavicular joint participates in movements close to the trunk (e.g. shrugging or bracing the shoulders); the acromioclavicular joint moves in the last 60 degrees of abduction.

REFERENCES AND FURTHER READING

Bankart ASB. The pathology and treatment of recurrent dislocation of the shoulder joint. *Brit J Surg* 1939; **26:** 23–9.

Bigliani LV, Levine WN Subacromial impingement syndrome. *J Bone Joint Surg* 1997; **79A:** 1854–68.

Boileau P, Ahrens PM, Hatzidakis AM. Entrapment of the long head of the biceps: the hourglass biceps: a cause of pain and locking of the shoulder. *J Shoulder Elbow Surg* 2004; **13:** 249–57.

Boileau P, Villalba M, Héry JY *et al.* Risk factors for recurrence of shoulder instability after arthroscopic Bankart repair. *J Bone Joint Surg* 2006; **88A:** 1755–1763.

Bunker TD. Frozen shoulder: unravelling the engima. *Ann R Coll Surg Engl* 1997; **79:** 210–13.

Carr AJ, Cole WG, Roberton DM, Chow CW. Chronic multifocal osteomyelitis. *J Bone Joint Surg* 1993; **75B:** 582–91.

Cole BJ, L'Insalata J, Irrgang J, Warner JJ. Comparison of arthroscopic and open anterior shoulder stabilization. A two to six-year follow-up study. *J Bone Joint Surg* 2000; **82A:** 1108–14.

Cone RD, Resnick D, Goergen TG *et al.* Condensing osteitis of the clavicle. *Am J Roentgenol* 1983; **141:** 387–8.

Gartsman GM. Arthroscopic treatment of rotator cuff disease. *J Shoulder Elbow Surg* 1995; **4:** 228–41.

Gartsman GM. Combined arthroscopic and open treatment of tears of the rotator cuff. *J Bone Joint Surg* 1997; **79A:** 776–83.

Gerber C, Krushell RJ. Isolated rupture of the tendon of the subscapularis muscle. Clinical features in 16 cases. *J Bone Joint Surg* 1991; **73B:** 389–94.

Gill TJ, Micheli LJ, Geghard F, Binder C. Bankart repair for anterior instability of the shoulder. *J Bone Joint Surg* 1997; **79A:** 850–57.

Hand C, Clipsham K, Rees JL, Carr AJ. Long-term outcome of frozen shoulder. *J Shoulder Elbow Surg* 2008; **17(2):** 231–6.

Handoll HH, Almaiyah MA, Rangan A. Surgical versus non-surgical treatment for acute anterior shoulder dislocation. *Cochrane Database Syst Rev* 2004.

Harryman DT, Matsen FA, Sidles JA. Arthroscopic management of refractory shoulder stiffness. *Arthroscopy* 1997; **13:** 1–8.

Hawkins, RJ, Kennedy JC. Impingement syndrome in athletes. *Am J Sports Med* 1980; **8:** 151–8.

Hertel R, Ballmer FT, Lambert SM, Gerber C. Lag signs in the diagnosis of rotator cuff rupture. *J Shoulder Elbow Surg*, 1996; **5:** 307–13.

Hertzog R. Magnetic resonance imaging of the shoulder. *J Bone Joint Surg* 1997; **79A:** 934–53.

Hovelius L, Augustini BG, Fredin OH *et al.* Primary anterior dislocation of the shoulder in young patients. *J Bone Joint Surg* 1996; **78A:** 1677–84.

Huijsmans PE, Pritchard MP, Berghs BM *et al.* Arthroscopic rotator cuff repair with double-row fixation. *J Bone Joint Surg* 2007; **89A:** 1248–57.

Ianotti JP. Full thickness rotator cuff tears: factors affecting surgical outcome. *J Am Acad Orthop Surgeons* 1994; **2:** 87–95.

Jobe FW, Jobe CM. Painful athletic injuries of the shoulder. *Clin Orthop Relat Res* 1983; **173:** 117–24.

Jobe FW, Moynes DR. Delineation of diagnostic criteria and a rehabilitation program for rotator cuff injuries. *Am J Sports Med* 1982; **10:** 336–9.

Kronberg M, Brostrum L-A. Rotation osteotomy of the

proximal humerus to stabilise the shoulder. *J Bone Joint Surg* 1995; **77B:** 924–27.

Levy O, Funk L, Sforza G, Copeland SA. Copeland surface replacement arthroplasty of the shoulder in rheumatoid arthritis. *J Bone Joint Surg* 2004; **86A:** 512–8.

Lewis A, Kitamura T, Bayley JIL. The classification of shoulder instability: new light through old windows! *Curr Orthop* 2004; **18(2):** 97–108.

McCarty DJ, Halverson PB, Carrera GF *et al.* Milwaukee shoulder: association of microspheroids containing hydroxyapatite crystals, active collagenase and neutral protease with rotator cuff defects. *Arthritis Rheumat* 1981; **24:** 464–73.

Nam EK, Snyder SJ. The diagnosis and treatment of superior labrum, anterior and posterior (SLAP) lesions. *Am J Sports Med* 2003; **31(5):** 798–810.

Neer CS. Anterior acromioplasty for the chronic impingement syndrome in the shoulder. *J Bone Joint Surg* 1972; **54A:** 41–50.

Neer CS, Foster CR. Inferior capsular shift for involuntary inferior and multidirectional instability of the shoulder. A preliminary report. *J Bone Joint Surg* 1980; **62A:** 897–908.

Neer CS, Welsh RP. The shoulder in sports. *Orthop Clin North Am* 1997; **8:** 583–91.

Neer CS, Craig EV, Fukuda HF. Cuff tear arthropathy. *J Bone Joint Surg* 1983; **65A:** 1232–1244.

Nutton RW, McBirnie JM, Phillips C. Treatment of chronic rotator cuff impingement by arthroscopic subacromial decompression. *J Bone Joint Surg* 1997; **79B:** 73–76.

Palmer WE, Brown JH, Rosenthal DI. Labral-ligamentous complex of the shoulder: evaluation with MR arthrography. *Radiology* 1994; **190:** 645.

Radnay CS, Setter K, Chambers L, Levine W, Bigliani L, Ahmad C. Total shoulder replacement compared with humeral head replacement for the treatment of primary glenohumeral arthritis. A systematic review. *J Shoulder Elbow Surg* 2007; **16(4):** 396–402.

Recht MP, Resnick D. Magnetic resonance-imaging studies of the shoulder. *J Bone Joint Surg* 1993; **75A:** 1244–53.

Rockwood CA, Lyons FR. Shoulder impingement syndrome: diagnosis, radiographic evaluation and treatment with a modified Neer acromioplasty. *J Bone Joint Surg* 1993; **75A:** 409–24.

Rockwood CA, Williams GR, Burkhead WZ. Debridement of degenerative, irreparable lesions of the rotator cuff. *J Bone Joint Surg* 1995; **77A:** 857–66.

Sachs RA, Stone ML, Devine S. Open versus arthroscopic acromioplasty – a prospective randomised study *Arthroscopy* 1994; **10:** 248–54.

Seung-Ho Kim, Kwon-Ick Ha, Sang-Hyun Kim, Hee-Joon Choi. Results of arthroscopic treatment of superior labral lesions. *J Bone Joint Surg* 2002; **84A:** 981–985.

Shaffer B, Tibone JE, Kerlan RK. Frozen shoulder. A long term follow-up. *J Bone Joint Surg* 1992; **74A:** 738–46.

Sher JS, Urbie JW, Posada A, *et al.* Abnormal findings on MRI of asymptomatic shoulders. *J Bone Joint Surg* 1995; **77A:** 10–15.

Singer GC, Kirkland PM, Emery RJH. Coracoid transposition for recurrent anterior dislocation of the shoulder. *J Bone Joint Surg* 1995; **77B:** 73–6.

Snyder SJ, Karzel RP, Del Pizzo W, *et al.* SLAP lesions of the shoulder. *Arthroscopy* 1990; **6(4):** 274–9.

Stewart MPM, Kelly IG. Total shoulder replacement in rheumatoid disease. *J Bone Joint Surg* 1997; **79B:** 68–72.

Teefey SA, Rubin DA, Middleton WD *et al.* Detection and quantification of rotator cuff tears. Comparison of ultrasonographic, magnetic resonance imaging, and arthroscopic findings in seventy-one consecutive cases. *J Bone Joint Surg* 2004; **86A:** 708–16.

Tirman PFJ, Bost FW, Garvin GJ, *et al.* Posterosuperior glenoid impingement of the shoulder: findings at MR imaging and MR arthrography with arthroscopic correlation. *Radiology* 1994; **193:** 431–6.

Warner JJP. Frozen shoulder: diagnosis and management. *J Am Acad Orthop Surgeons* 1997; **5:** 130–40.

Wirth MA, Rockwood CA. Complications of total shoulder replacement arthroplasty *J Bone Joint Surg* 1996; **78A:** 603–16.

Zuckerman JD, Cuomo F, Rokito S. Definition and classification of frozen shoulder – a consensus approach. *J Shoulder Elbow Surg* 1994; **3:** S72.

The elbow and forearm

14

David Warwick

CLINICAL ASSESSMENT

SYMPTOMS

Pain from the elbow is fairly diffuse and may extend into the forearm. Localized pain over the lateral or medial epicondyle of the humerus is usually due to tendinitis. The patient may have noticed that it is triggered, or aggravated, by certain activities. So often is this the case that the symptom has acquired colloquial definitions: 'tennis elbow' for lateral epicondylar pain and 'golfer's elbow' for medial epicondylar pain. Pain over the back of the elbow is often due to an olecranon bursitis. *Remember that 'pain in the elbow' is sometimes referred pain from the cervical spine!*

Stiffness, if it is mild, may hardly be noticed. If it is severe, it can be very disabling; the patient may be unable to reach up to the mouth (loss of flexion) or the perineum (loss of extension); limited supination makes it difficult to carry large objects.

Swelling may be due to injury or inflammation; a soft lump on the back of the elbow suggests an olecranon bursitis.

Deformity is uncommon except in rheumatoid arthritis and after trauma. Always ask about previous injuries.

Instability – the feeling that the elbow 'moves out of joint' – is due either to previous trauma or to destructive joint disease.

Ulnar nerve symptoms (tingling, numbness and weakness of the hand) may occur in elbow disorders because of the nerve's proximity to the joint.

Loss of function is noticed mainly in grooming, carrying and placing activities. However good the hand, if the elbow cannot put it out into the environment and bring it back to the individual, upper limb function is seriously degraded.

SIGNS

Both upper limbs should be completely exposed, and it is essential to look at the back of the elbow as well as the front. Often the neck, shoulders and hands also need to be examined.

Look

Both upper limbs must be completely exposed. The patient holds his or her arms alongside the body, elbows fully extended, with palms forwards. In this position the forearms are normally angled slightly outwards – a valgus or *carrying angle* of 5–15 degrees. 'Varus' or 'valgus' *deformity* is determined by angular deviations medialwards or lateralwards beyond those limits or, in unilateral abnormalities, by comparison with the normal side.

Varus and valgus deformities (*cubitus varus* and *cubitus valgus*) are usually the result of trauma around the elbow. By far the best way to demonstrate a varus deformity is to ask the patient to lift his or her arms sideways to shoulder height; in this position the deformity becomes much more obvious, the arm taking on the appearance of a rifle butt (*gunstock deformity*, shown in Fig. 14.5).

Feel

Start by identifying the most obvious bony landmarks: the olecranon process posteriorly, the medial and lateral epicondyles and the head of the radius just

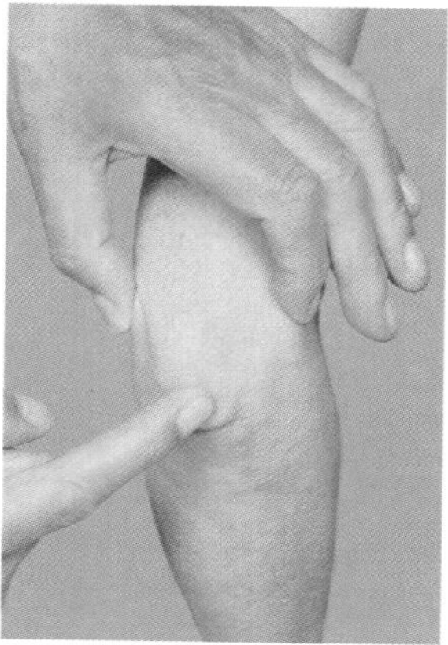

14.1 Examination Feeling begins with the skin. Is there undue warmth? Next, feel the bony landmarks. With the elbow flexed, the tips of the medial and lateral epicondyles and the olecranon process form an isosceles triangle. With the elbow extended, they lie transversely in line with each other. These relationships are disturbed in post-traumatic deformities of the elbow.

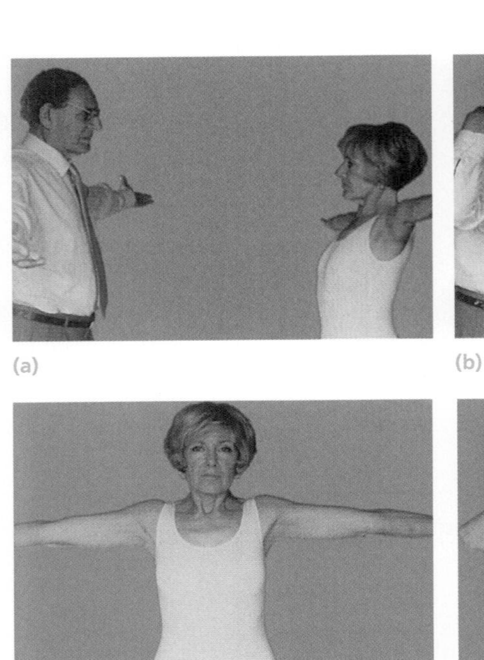
(a)

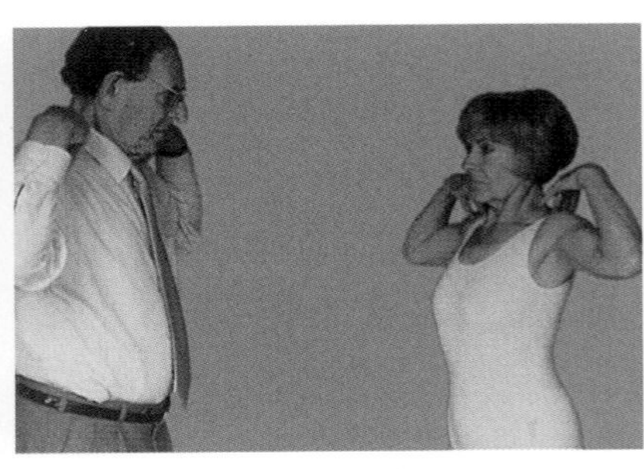
(b)

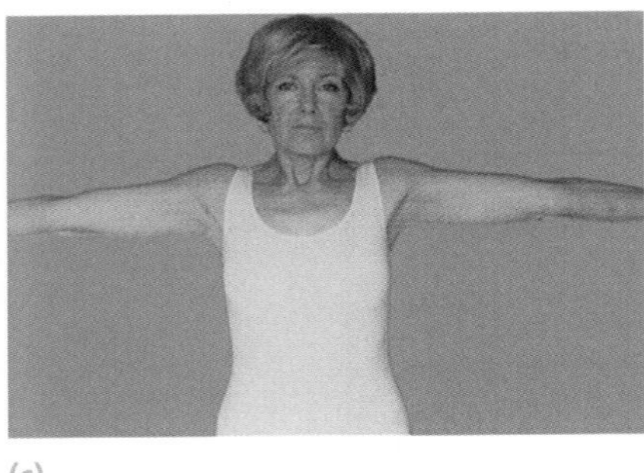
(c)

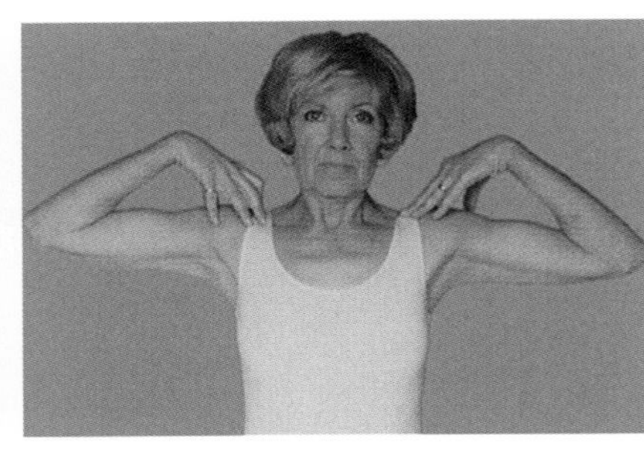
(d)

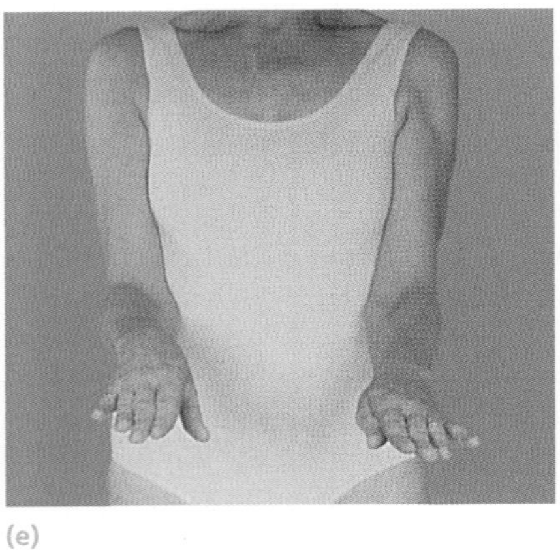
(e)

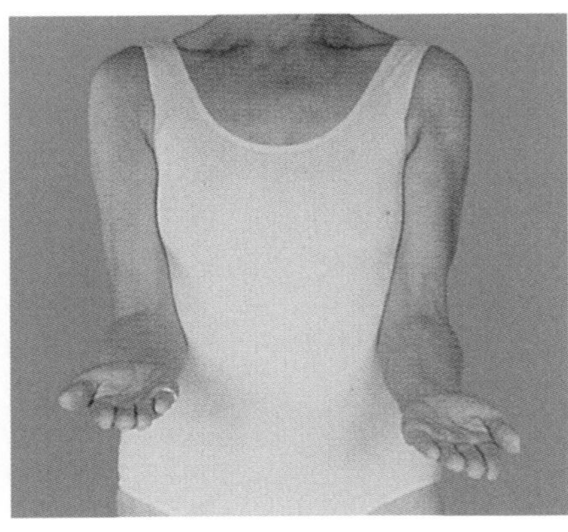
(f)

14.2 (a,b) The best way to examine active movements is to stand in front of the patient and show her what to do. (c,d) The normal range of flexion is from 0° (full extension) to 140° (full flexion). (e,f) To test pronation and supination, ask the patient to tuck her elbows tightly into her body and then turn the hands fully palms down and then palms up. The normal range is 90° in each direction.

distal to the lateral epicondyle; pronating and supinating the forearm makes it easier to find the mobile radial head and the lateral joint line. The ulna can be palpated throughout its length, the radius only at its proximal end and in the distal third of the forearm.

The back of the elbow is palpated for warmth and swelling (signs of an olecranon bursitis) and subcutaneous nodules (a feature of rheumatoid arthritis). Feel more widely for synovial thickening and fluid (fluctuation on each side of the olecranon). The ulnar nerve is very superficial behind the medial condyle and here it can be rolled under the fingers to feel if it is thickened or hypersensitive.

Last of all, feel for tenderness and try to determine which structure is affected.

Move

Active and passive flexion and extension are compared on the two sides. The elbow should be able to extend to the zero position (absolutely straight); people with lax joints can extend even beyond that point. As a rough guide, people are normally able to flex the elbow sufficiently to touch the top of the shoulder with their fingers, but bear in mind that those with bulky upper arm muscles may not be able to do so. Pronation and supination of the forearms are tested with the patient holding the arms tucked into the waist and flexed to a right angle; 80–90 degrees each way is normal. *Stability* must also be tested carefully after trauma. The humerus is stabilized, the elbow is flexed to about 25 degrees to unlock any contribution to stability by the olecranon and the elbow is stressed in torsion and collateral stress.

General examination

Clinical examination should include the neck and shoulder (which are sources of referred pain to the elbow) and the hand (for signs of nerve dysfunction).

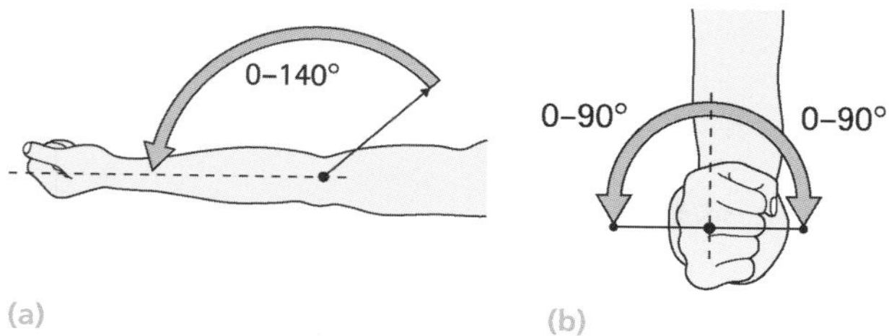

(a) (b)

14.3 Normal range of movement (a) The extended position is recorded as 0° and any hyperextension as a minus quantity; flexion is full when the arm and forearm make contact. (b) From the neutral position the radio-ulnar joint rotates 90° into pronation and 90° into supination.

Imaging

Plain x-ray

The position of each bone is noted, then the joint line and space. Next, the individual bones are inspected for evidence of old injury or bone destruction. There may be some calcification over the epicondyles in cases of tennis or golfer's elbow. Finally, loose bodies are sought.

In children the epiphyses are largely cartilaginous and the articular relations often have to be deduced from the shape and position of the emerging secondary ossific centres. The average ages at which they appear are easily remembered by the mnemonic CRITOE: Capitulum – 2 years; Radial head – 4 years; Internal (medial) epicondyle – 6 years; Trochlea – 8 years; Olecranon – 10 years; External (lateral) epicondyle – 12 years.

Computed tomography

Arthrography with CT imaging is a useful method for defining loose bodies and detailed changes in osteoarthritis.

Magnetic resonance imaging

MRI will be needed to reveal articular changes (such as osteochondritis dissecans) and soft-tissue abnormalities (e.g. ligament injuries).

CONGENITAL DISORDERS

Congenital dislocation of the radial head

This may be anterior or posterior and is usually bilateral. The patient may notice the lump, which is easily palpable and can be felt to move when the forearm is rotated. X-rays show that the dislocated radial head is dome-shaped (due to abnormal modelling).

Function is usually surprisingly good and pain is unusual. Surgery is therefore rarely required; however, if the lump limits elbow flexion it can be excised (beware of the posterior interosseous nerve).

Congenital synostosis

Congenital deficiencies of the forearm bones are occasionally associated with fusion of the humerus to the radius or ulna. This disabling condition is, fortunately, very rare. A more useful angle of forearm rotation can be achieved by osteotomy.

Proximal radio-ulnar synostosis causes loss of rotation, but elbow flexion is retained and the inconvenience is often only moderate. Surgery to regain rotation rarely succeeds. A rotational osteotomy can give a more suitable angle of pronation–supination tailored to the individual patient's needs.

ACQUIRED DEFORMITIES

Cubitus valgus

The normal carrying angle of the elbow is 5–15 degrees of valgus; anything more than this is regarded as a valgus deformity, which is usually quite obvious when the patient stands with arms to the sides and palms facing forwards.

The commonest cause is longstanding non-union of a fractured lateral condyle; the deformity may be associated with marked prominence of the medial condylar outline. The importance of cubitus valgus is the liability to delayed ulnar palsy; years after the causal injury the patient notices weakness of the hand, with numbness and tingling of the ulnar fingers. The deformity itself needs no treatment, but for delayed ulnar palsy the nerve should be transposed to the front of the elbow. Great care is needed in performing the operation. Excessive dissection of the nerve or rough handling can impair nerve function.

Cubitus varus ('gun-stock' deformity)

The deformity is most obvious when the elbow is extended and the arms are elevated. The most common cause is malunion of a supracondylar fracture. The deformity can be corrected by a wedge osteotomy of the lower humerus but this is best left until skeletal maturity.

Subluxation of the radial head

This is commonly associated with bone dysplasias in which the ulna is disproportionately shortened (e.g. hereditary multiple exostosis). It usually causes little

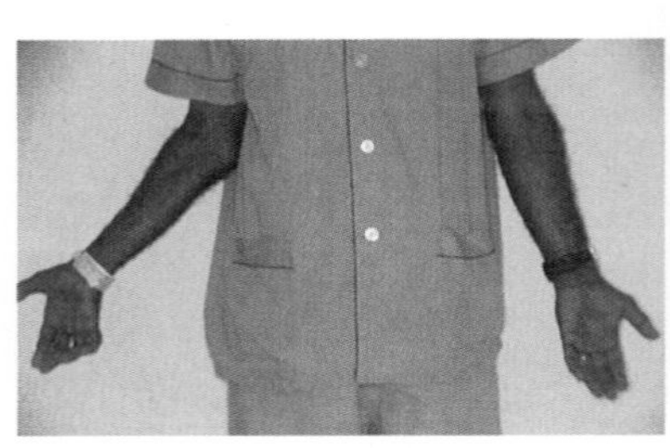

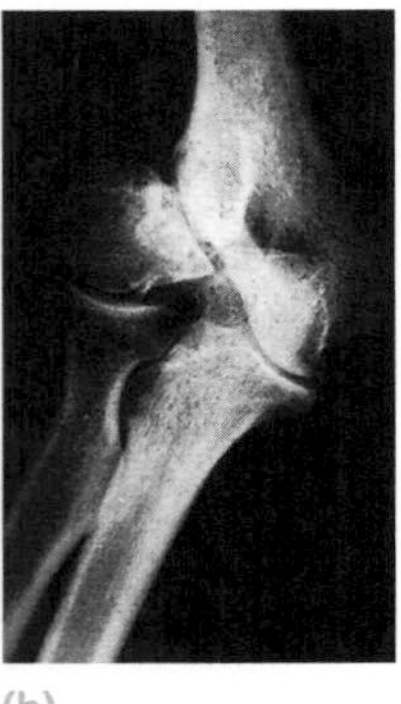

(a) (b)

14.4 Cubitus valgus (a) This man has excessive valgus of the right elbow. But his main complaint was of weakness and deformity in the hand, which was caused by traction on the ulnar nerve secondary to the elbow deformity. (b) Valgus deformity from an un-united fracture of the lateral condyle.

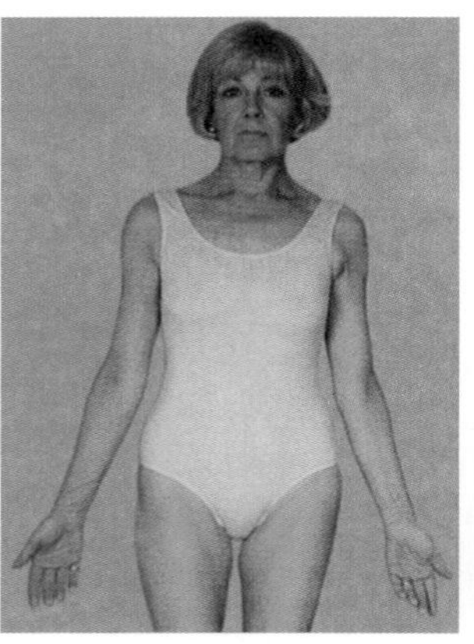

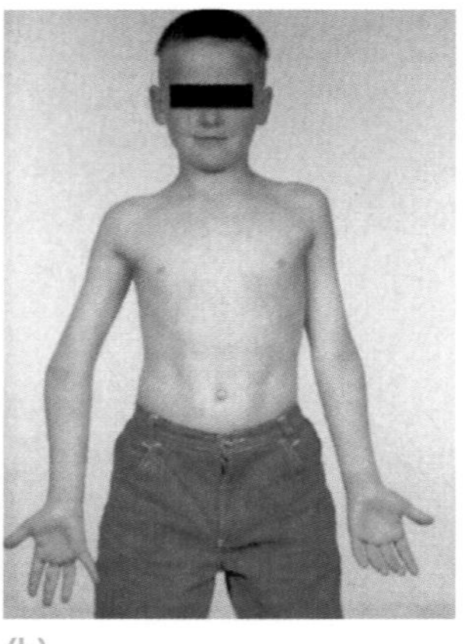

(a) (b)

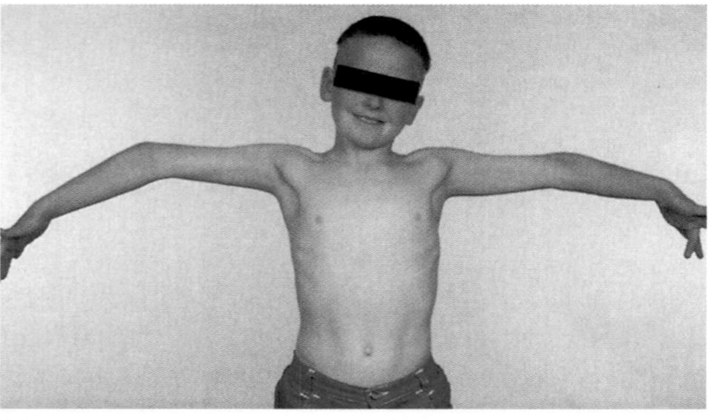

(c)

14.5 Cubitus varus (a) Note that the elbows are normally held in 5–10° of valgus (the carrying angle). (b) This young boy ended up with slight varus angulation after a supracondylar fracture of the distal humerus. The deformity is much more obvious (c) when he raises his arms (gun-stock deformity).

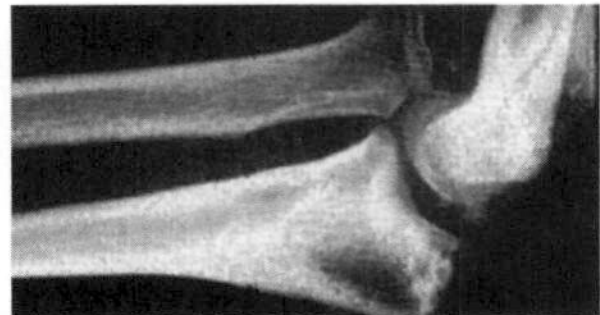

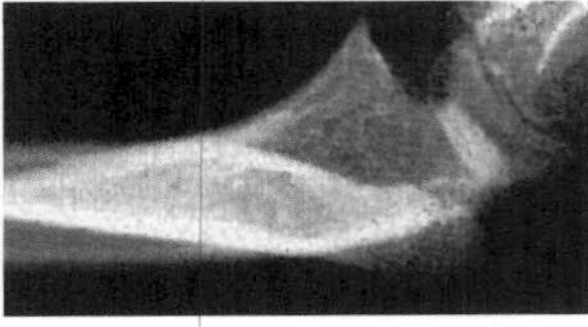

(a) (b)

14.6 Dislocated radial head (a) Anterior dislocation from old Monteggia fracture; (b) posterior dislocation, most likely congenital.

disability, but if it becomes too troublesome the radial head can be excised after all growth has ceased.

UNREDUCED DISLOCATION OF THE HEAD OF RADIUS

An unreduced Montegia fracture-dislocation will leave the radial head permanently dislocated. Open reduction and realignment of the ulna, together with soft-tissue reconstruction, may improve function.

'PULLED ELBOW'

Downward dislocation of the head of the radius from the annular ligament is a fairly common injury in children under the age of 6 years. There may be a history of the child being jerked by the arm and subsequently complaining of pain and inability to use the arm. The limb is held more or less immobile with the elbow fully extended and the forearm pronated; any attempt to supinate the forearm is resisted. The diagnosis is essentially clinical, though x-rays are usually obtained in order to exclude a fracture.

The radial head can be forcibly pulled out of the noose of the annular ligament only when the forearm is pronated; even then the distal attachment of the ligament is sometimes torn.

If the history and clinical picture are suggestive, an attempt should be made to reduce the subluxation or dislocation. While the child's attention is diverted, the elbow is quickly supinated and then slightly flexed; the radial head is relocated with a snap. (This sometimes happens 'spontaneously' while the radiographer is positioning the arm!)

OSTEOCHONDRITIS DISSECANS

(see also Chapter 6)

The capitulum is one of the common sites of osteochondritis dissecans. This may be due to repeated stress following prolonged or unaccustomed activity but can occur spontaneously. The pathological changes are described in Chapter 6.

The patient – usually a young male adolescent –

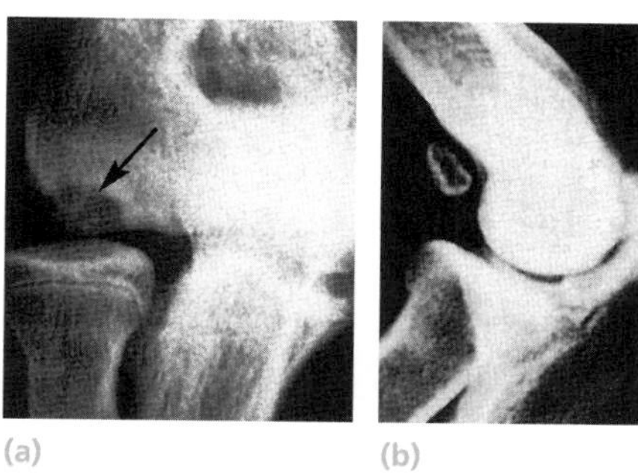

(a) (b)

14.7 Osteochondritis dissecans (a) The capitulum is fragmented and slightly flattened. (b) Sometimes the fragment separates and lies in the joint.

complains of aching which is aggravated by activity and relieved by rest. On examination there may be swelling, signs of an effusion, tenderness over the capitulum and slight limitation of movement. If the fragment has separated, there may be intermittent locking.

X-rays may show fragmentation or, at a much later stage, flattening of the capitulum.

CT and *MRI* are more useful for defining the lesion.

Treatment is usually symptomatic. The lesion can heal and symptoms resolve. Repeated CT or MRI scanning will monitor this. However, if the fragment has separated and is lying free in the joint, it should be removed. A large loose fragment which is often still partly attached can be pinned back. These procedures can be done arthroscopically.

LOOSE BODIES

Loose bodies in the elbow may be due to: (1) acute trauma (an osteocartilaginous fracture); (2) osteochondritis dissecans; (3) synovial chondromatosis (a cluster of mainly cartilaginous 'pebbles'); or (4) osteoarthritis (separation of osteophytes).

The patient may complain of sudden locking and unlocking of the joint. Symptoms of osteoarthritis may coexist.

A loose body is rarely palpable. When degenerative changes have occurred, extremes of movement are limited.

X-rays may reveal the loose body or bodies (see Fig. 14.8); in the special case of osteochondritis dissecans there is a rarefied cystic area in the capitulum and enlargement of the radial head. A CT arthrogram will define the size and the number of loose bodies.

If loose bodies are troublesome, they should be removed by arthroscopic or open means, depending on the size of the loose body and the experience of the surgeon.

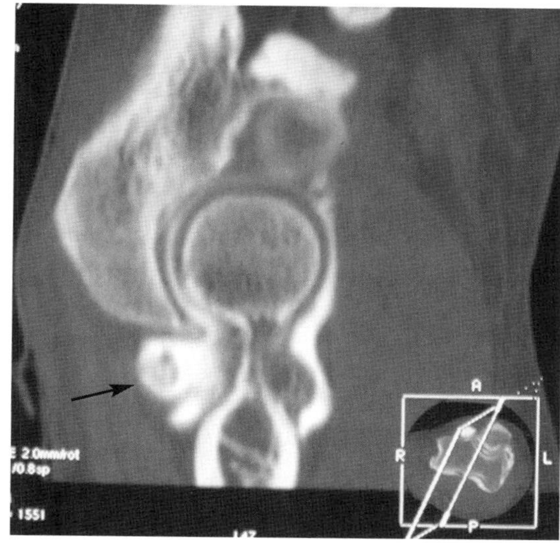

14.8 Loose body CT scan showing a loose body in the back of the elbow joint.

TUBERCULOSIS (see also Chapter 2)

Clinical features

The elbow is affected in about 10 per cent of patients with skeletal tuberculosis. Although the disease begins as synovitis or osteomyelitis, patients are rarely seen until arthritis supervenes. The onset is insidious with a long history of aching and stiffness. The most striking physical sign is the marked wasting. While the disease is active the joint is held flexed, looks swollen, and feels warm and diffusely tender; movement is considerably limited and accompanied by pain and spasm. Always feel for the supratrochlear and axillary lymph nodes; they may be enlarged.

X-rays

The typical features are peri-articular osteoporosis and joint erosion. There may also be subchondral cystic lesions.

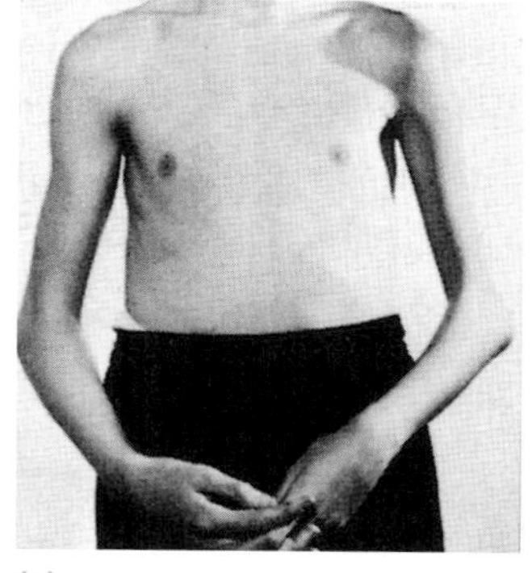

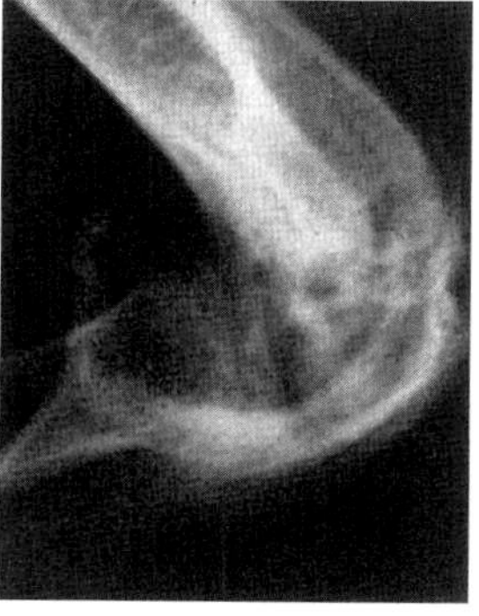

(a) (b)

14.9 Tuberculosis of the elbow Muscle wasting is marked and bone destruction extensive.

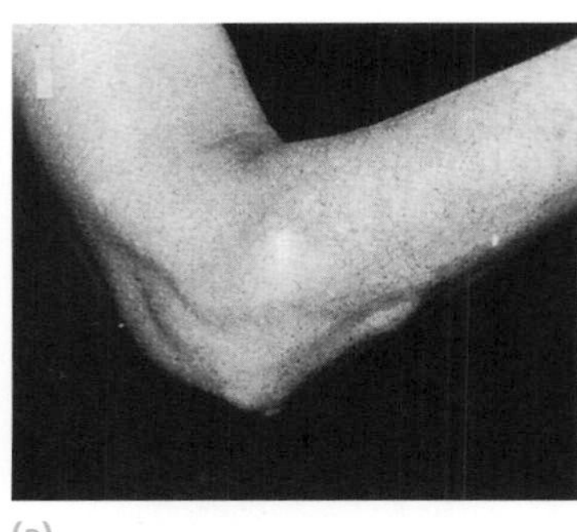

(a)

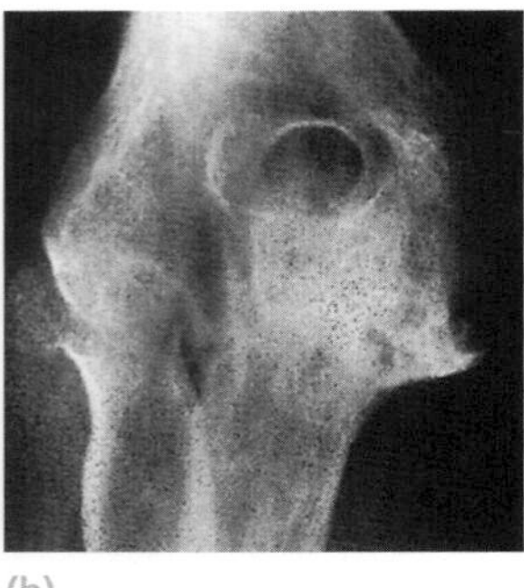

(b)

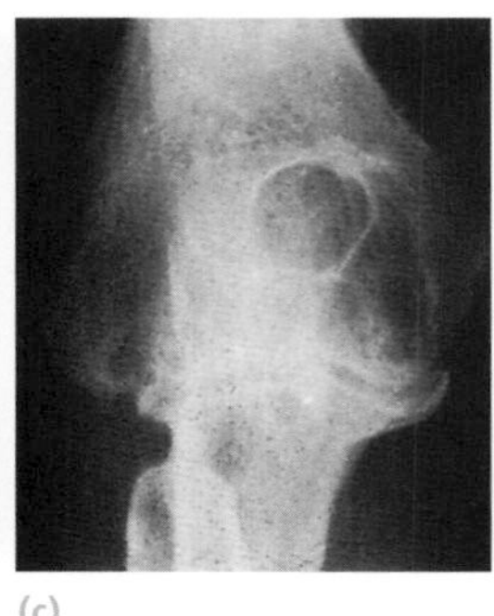

(c)

14.10 Rheumatoid arthritis (a) This rheumatoid patient has nodules over the olecranon and a bulge over the radiohumeral joint; (b) his x-rays show deformity of the radial head and marked erosion of the rest of the elbow. (c) Excision of the radial head combined with synovectomy relieved the pain and improved elbow movement.

Other investigations

Aspiration, synovial biopsy and microbiological investigation will usually confirm the diagnosis.

Treatment

General antituberculous treatment is essential. The elbow is rested until the acute symptoms subside – at first in a splint and positioned at 90 degrees of flexion and mid-rotation, later simply by applying a collar and cuff. As soon as possible, however, movement is encouraged.

Late residual effects – chronic pain, stiffness or deformity – may be troublesome enough to justify excisional or replacement arthroplasty or (rarely) arthrodesis.

RHEUMATOID ARTHRITIS

The elbow is involved in more than 50 per cent of patients with polyarticular rheumatoid arthritis, and in the majority of cases the condition is bilateral.

Clinical features

Ulnar bursitis and rheumatoid nodules are often found on the back of the elbow even if the joint itself is not affected. With true joint involvement, synovitis gives rise to pain and tenderness, especially over the lateral aspect of the radio-humeral joint.

Later the entire elbow may be swollen. Movements are restricted but, if bone destruction is marked, the joint becomes unstable.

Synovial swelling occasionally causes ulnar nerve or posterior interosseous nerve compression, with symptoms and signs in the wrist and hand. It is important to distinguish these features from those of local weakness and tendon rupture due to generalized disease.

X-rays

X-ray examination reveals bone erosion, with gradual destruction of the radial head and widening of the trochlear notch of the ulna. Sometimes large synovial extensions penetrate the articular surface and appear as 'cysts' in the proximal radius or ulna.

Treatment

In addition to general treatment, the elbow should be splinted during periods of active synovitis. Local injections of corticosteroid preparations may reduce pain and swelling – at least for a while.

OPERATIVE TREATMENT

If, despite adequate conservative treatment, synovitis persists – and more particularly if this is associated with erosion of the radial head – synovectomy is worthwhile. This is usually performed through a lateral approach, with excision of the radial head. There are two reasons for this: first, the radio-capitellar surfaces are almost invariably eroded, and second, radial head excision permits wider access to the hypertrophic synovium. The operation relieves pain and may slow the progress of the disease, but after 5–6 years erosion of the humeroulnar joint often causes increasing instability and recurrence of pain. A drawback of radial head excision is that it may jeopardize the result of joint replacement if this should later become necessary.

Progressive bone destruction and instability may call for reconstructive surgery. Arthrodesis is very disabling and is unlikely to be accepted by the patient. Joint replacement is usually successful in relieving pain and maintaining a functional range of movement. Good 10-year results have been reported in about 80 per cent of patients. However, the operation is difficult to perform and prone to complications such as infection, instability and dislocation, ulnar neuropathy and aseptic loosening of the implants.

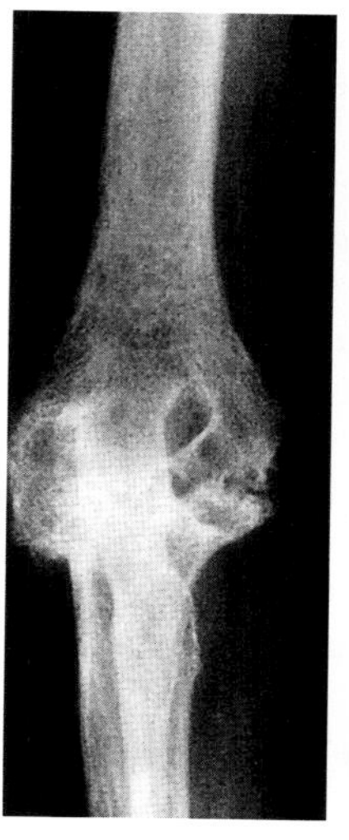

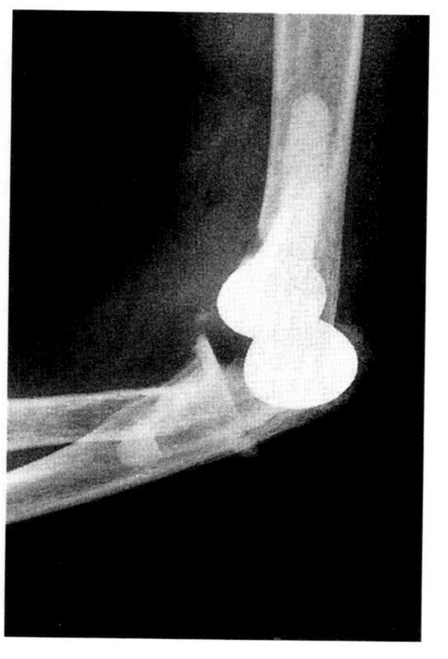

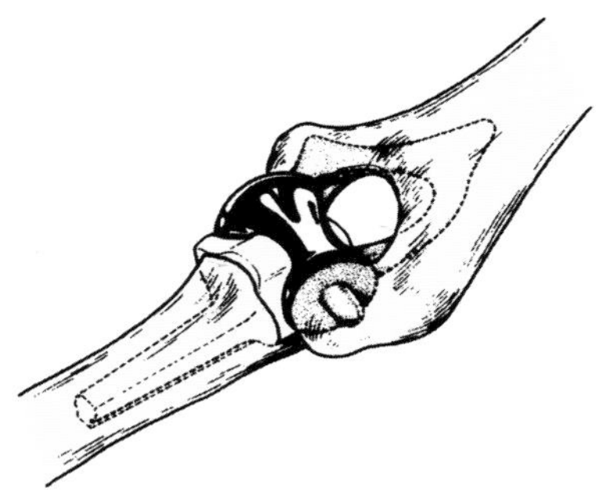

(a) (b) (c)

14.11 Total elbow replacement (a) Severe rheumatoid arthritis of the elbow. (b) X-ray after joint replacement. (c) The Souter arthroplasty; a metal humeral prosthesis and polyethylene ulnar implant.

GOUT AND PSEUDOGOUT

The elbow – or more precisely the olecranon bursa – is a favourite site for gout. In an acute attack the area rapidly becomes painful, swollen and inflamed. The swelling and redness may extend well down the forearm and the condition is easily mistaken for cellulitis or joint infection. The serum uric acid level may be raised and the bursal aspirate will contain urate crystals. Treatment is with high dosage anti-inflammatory preparations.

Similar attacks occur in pseudogout, due to the deposition of CPPD crystals, which can be identified in the aspirate (see Chapter 4).

Chronic calcium pyrophosphate arthropathy This condition should always be suspected when 'osteoarthritic' changes appear spontaneously in an unusual site such as the elbow; x-rays may show, additional features such as chondrocalcinosis and peri-articular calcification. The diagnosis can be confirmed by demonstrating the typical positively birefringent crystals in fluid aspirated from the joint. Treatment is as for osteoarthritis (see below).

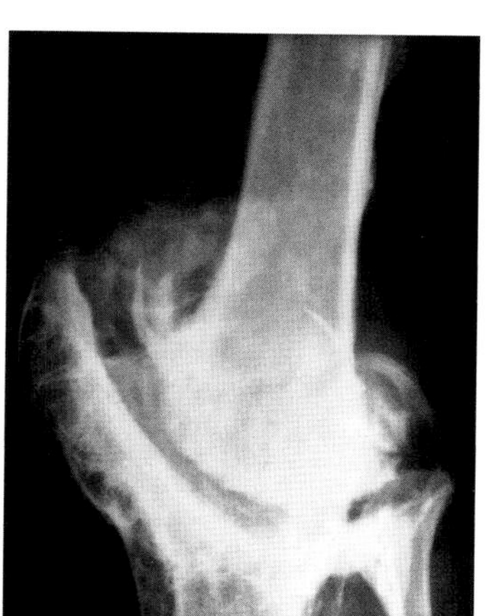

14.12 Pyrophosphate arthropathy Osteoarthritis of the elbow is unusual except after trauma. These x-rays show a destructive arthritis and typical flared osteophytes in a patient with generalized pyrophosphate arthropathy.

OSTEOARTHRITIS (see also Chapter 4)

Osteoarthritis of the elbow is uncommon and usually denotes some recognizable underlying pathology – a previous fracture or ligamentous injury, loose bodies in the joint, longstanding occupational stress, inflammatory arthritis or gout. 'Primary' osteoarthritis – especially when it is part of a polyarticular disorder – suggests calcium pyrophosphate deposition disease (see above).

Clinical features

The patient usually complains of pain and stiffness, especially following periods of inactivity. Examination shows local tenderness, thickening of the joint, crepitus and restriction of movement. Osteophytic hypertrophy may cause ulnar nerve palsy.

X-rays

X-ray examination shows narrowing of the joint space with sclerosis and osteophytes. One or more loose bodies may be seen; chondrocalcinosis and peri-articular calcification are typical of pyrophosphate arthropathy.

Treatment

Treatment is usually limited to pain control and the use of non-steroidal anti-inflammatory preparations.

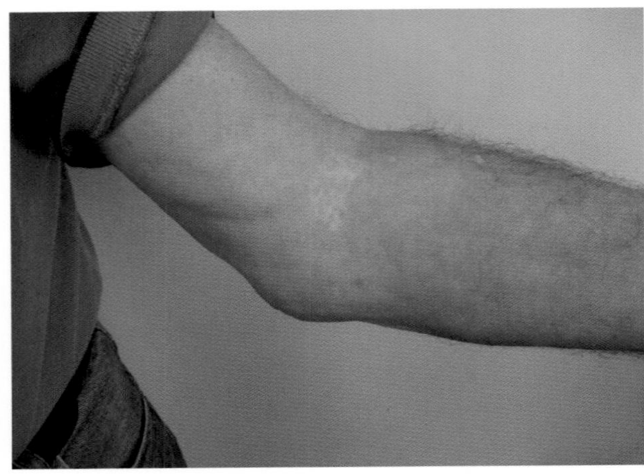

(a)

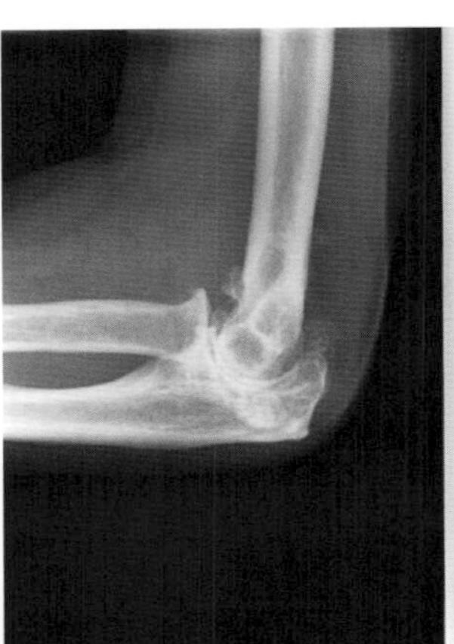

(b)

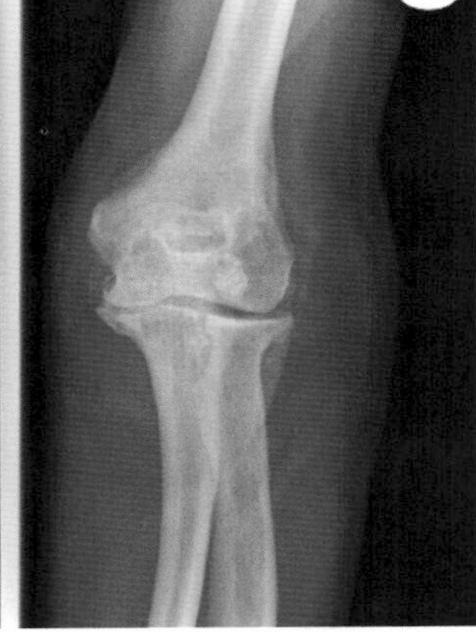

(c)

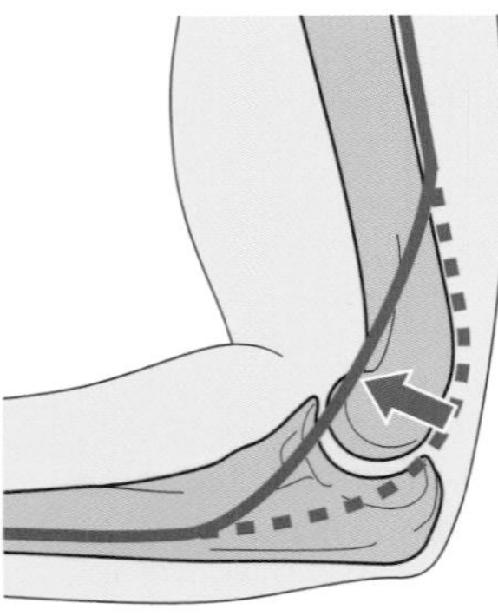

(d)

14.13 Osteoarthritis (a) Valgus elbow; (b,c) x-ray with new bone and loose bodies; (d) transposition of ulnar nerve anteriorly to treat the associated ulnar nerve symptoms.

Loose bodies, if they cause locking, should be removed. If there are signs of ulnar neuropathy, the nerve should be transposed.

Debridement of the joint may be helpful. This can be done arthroscopically with debridement of synovium and loose cartilage, burring of osteophytes, trimming of the olecranon and coronoid fossae and removal of loose cartilage. The debridement can also be performed by an open approach. Through a dorsal incision the posterior compartment is cleared; the thin bone of the olecranon fossa is then removed to expose the anterior compartment (the so-called 'OK procedure'). This will improve movement and impingement pain, often for several years.

An alternative to joint replacement in the younger patient is an interposition *arthroplasty*, in which a layer of fascia, subcutis or tendon is placed into the joint space. A hinged external fixator maintains some distraction yet allows movement and protects the reconstruction.

In advanced cases in older patients, joint replacement can be considered; however, upper limb activities will have to be permanently restricted in order to reduce the risk of implant loosening.

NEUROPATHIC ARTHRITIS

Neuropathic arthritis of the elbow is seen in syringomyelia and diabetes mellitus. Sometimes neurological features predominate and the diagnosis may be known; occasionally the patient presents with progressive instability of the elbow. The joint may be markedly swollen and hypermobile, with coarse crepitation on passive movement, or it may be completely flail.

The condition must be distinguished from other causes of flail elbow, such as advanced rheumatoid arthritis and unreduced (or ununited) fracture-dislocations.

Treatment consists of splintage to maintain stability. Arthrodesis usually fails and is functionally disabling. A semi-constrained arthroplasty is technically difficult and prone to early failure in this setting.

STIFFNESS OF THE ELBOW

Stiffness of the elbow may be due to *congenital abnormalities* (various types of synostosis, or arthrogryposis), *infection, inflammatory arthritis, osteoarthritis* or the late effects of *trauma*. Most of these conditions are dealt with in other chapters. Here consideration will be given to post-traumatic stiffness, which is an important cause of disability.

Post-traumatic stiffness

For reasons that are not entirely clear, the elbow is particularly prone to post-traumatic stiffness. The more obvious causes (as with other joints) are either extrinsic (e.g. soft-tissue contracture or heterotopic bone formation), intrinsic (e.g. intra-articular adhesions and articular incongruity), or a combination of these. Clinical assessment should include examination

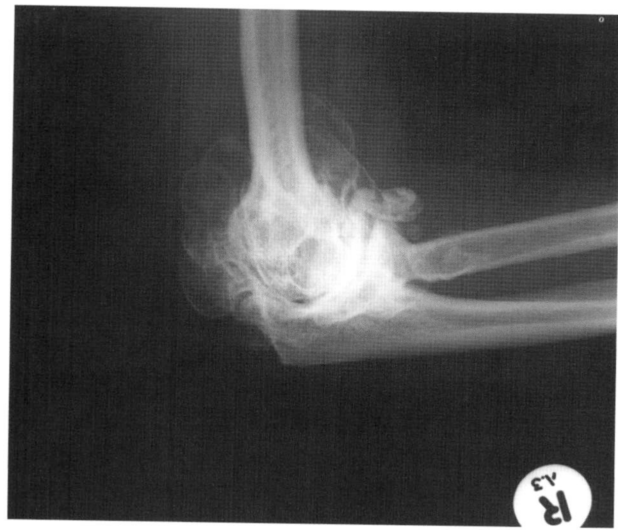

(a)

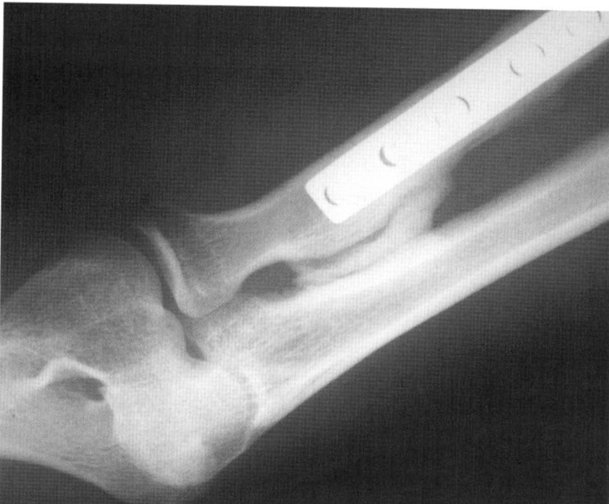

(b)

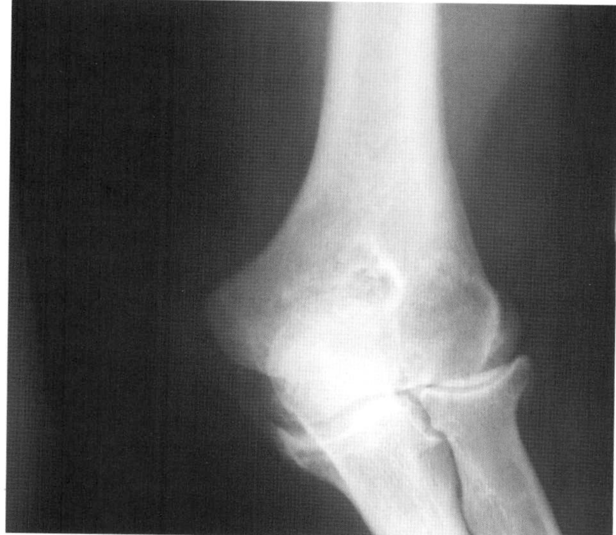

(c)

14.14 Elbow stiffness (a) Osteochondrosis; (b) radio-ulnar synostosis; (c) osteoarthritis.

of all the joints of the upper limb as well as an evaluation of the functional needs of the particular patient. Most of the activities of daily living can be managed with a restricted range of elbow motion: flexion from 30 to 130 degrees and pronation and supination of 50 degrees each. Any greater loss is likely to be disabling.

NON-OPERATIVE TREATMENT

The most effective treatment is prevention, by early active movement through a functional range. If movement is restricted and fails to improve with exercise, serial splintage may help; aggressive passive manipulation may aggravate more than help.

OPERATIVE TREATMENT

The indication for operative treatment is failure to regain a functional range of movement at 12 months after injury. There are a few caveats: the limb as whole should be useful; there should be no over-riding neurological impairment; and the patient should be cooperative and motivated. If there is heterotopic ossification, it is important to wait until the bone is 'mature', i.e. showing clear cortical margins and trabecular markings on x-ray. There is no point in a soft-tissue release if the x-ray or CT shows that bone incongruity is blocking movement.

The objectives are determined by the type of pathology. Heterotopic bone can be excised. Capsular release or capsulectomy (open or arthroscopic) may restore a satisfactory range of movement. Intra-articular procedures include fixing of ununited fractures or correction of malunited fractures.

Post-traumatic radio-ulnar synostosis sometimes follows internal fixation of fractures of the radius and ulna. It is treated by resection when the synostosis has matured (this takes about one year) followed by diligent physiotherapy.

RECURRENT ELBOW INSTABILITY

Following a dislocation or severe sprain, the lateral collateral ligament can be stretched or ruptured. The patient may present with painful clunking and locking. On examination, an apprehension response can be elicited by supinating the forearm while applying a valgus force to the elbow during flexion.

The lateral collateral ligament can be directly repaired or reconstructed with a tendon autograft (e.g. palmaris longus).

Medial instability is less frequent after trauma; a chronic instability can develop in javelin throwers and baseball players. Ligament reconstruction with a tendon graft and careful graduated rehabilitation can give very good results.

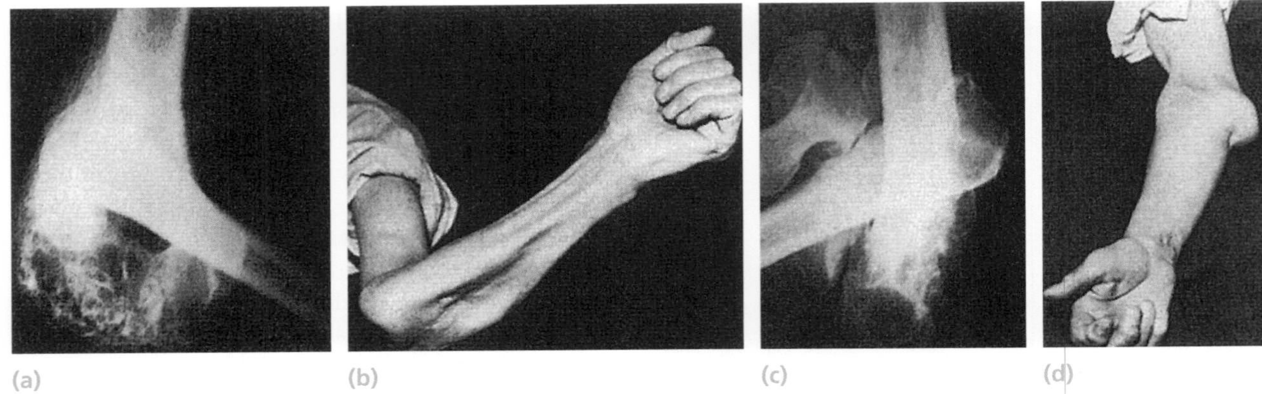

(a) (b) (c) (d)

14.15 Flail elbow (a,b) Following gunshot wound; (c,d) neuropathic arthritis.

EPICONDALGIA

The elbow is prone to painful disorders of the tendon attachment. Sometimes this occurs spontaneously, sometimes after sudden unaccustomed use. These conditions have acquired names derived from the activities in which they were encountered when they were first described.

TENNIS ELBOW (LATERAL EPICONDALGIA)

Pain and tenderness over the lateral epicondyle of the elbow (or, more accurately, the bony insertion of the common extensor tendon) is a common complaint among tennis players – but even more common in non-players who perform similar activities involving forceful repetitive wrist extension. It is the extensor carpi radialis tendon (which automatically extends the wrist when gripping) which is pathological in tennis elbow (Fig. 14.16). Like supraspinatus tendinitis, it may result in small tears, fibrocartilaginous metaplasia, microscopic calcification and a painful vascular reaction in the tendon fibres close to the lateral epicondyle.

Clinical features

The patient is usually an active individual of 30 or 40 years. Pain comes on gradually, often after a period of

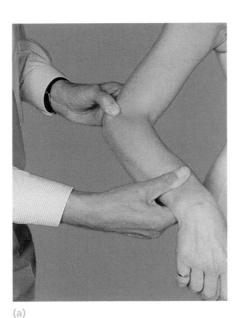

(a)

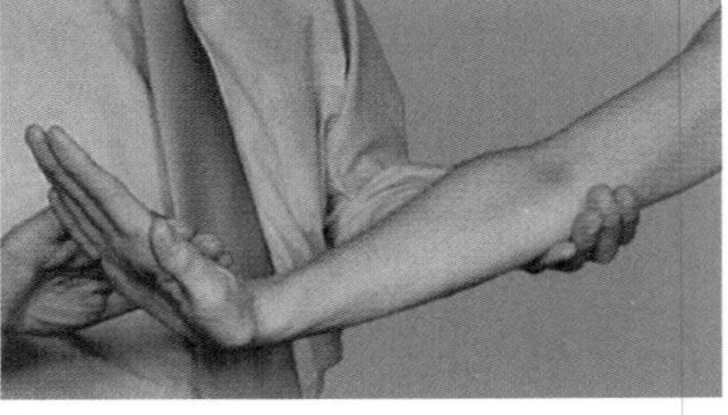

(b)

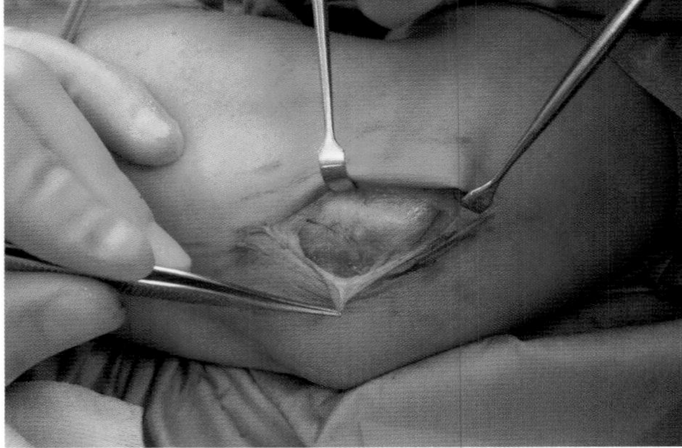

(c)

14.16 Tennis elbow (a) Tenderness over the anterior aspect of the lateral epicondyle; (b) pain provoked by resisted wrist extension; (c) tennis elbow surgery – the abnormal extensor carpi radialis brevis origin is excised.

unaccustomed activity involving forceful gripping and wrist extension. It is usually localized to the lateral epicondyle, but in severe cases it may radiate widely. It is aggravated by movements such as pouring out tea, turning a stiff doorhandle, shaking hands or lifting with the forearm pronated. Among tennis players it is usually blamed on faulty technique.

The elbow looks normal, and flexion and extension are full and painless.

Characteristically there is localized tenderness at or just below the lateral epicondyle; pain can be reproduced by passively stretching the wrist extensors (by the examiner acutely flexing the patient's wrist with the forearm pronated) or actively by having the patient extend the wrist with the elbow straight.

X-ray is usually normal, but occasionally shows calcification at the tendon origin.

Diagnosis

In patients with longstanding symptoms which do not respond to treatment, the possibility of a painful radial nerve entrapment ('radial tunnel syndrome') should be considered (see Chapter 11).

Treatment

Many methods of treatment are available but the benefits of most are unclear; it is well to remember that 90 per cent of 'tennis elbows' will resolve spontaneously within 6–12 months.

The first step is to identify, and then restrict, those activities which cause pain. Modification of sporting style may solve the problem. A tennis elbow clasp is helpful. The role of physiotherapy and manipulation is uncertain. Injection of the tender area with corticosteroid and local anaesthetic relieves pain but is not curative.

OPERATIVE TREATMENT

Some cases are sufficiently persistent or recurrent for operation to be indicated. The origin of the common extensor muscle is detached from the lateral epicondyle. Additional procedures such as division of the orbicular ligament or removal of a 'synovial fringe' are sometimes advocated; they probably make very little difference to the outcome. Surgery is successful in about 85 per cent of cases.

GOLFER'S ELBOW (MEDIAL EPICONDYLITIS)

This is similar to tennis elbow but about three times less common. In this case it is the pronator origin that is affected. Often there is an associated ulnar nerve neuropathy. A medial collateral ligament injury should be excluded.

Treatment is the same as for lateral epicondylitis but the outcome of surgery seems less predictable. The abnormal tissue at the flexor–pronator origin is excised, great care being taken to preserve the medial collateral ligament. The medial antebrachial cutaneous nerve must be respected during the skin incision to avoid a troublesome postoperative neuroma.

BASEBALL PITCHER'S ELBOW

Repetitive, vigorous throwing activities can cause damage to the bones or soft-tissue attachments around the elbow. Professional baseball players may develop hypertrophy of the lower humerus and incongruity of the joint, or loose-body formation and osteoarthritis. The junior equivalent (*'little leaguer's elbow'*) is due to partial avulsion of the medial epicondyle. The only remedy – however grudgingly accepted – is to stay off baseball until the condition clears up completely.

JAVELIN THROWER'S ELBOW

The over-arm action employed by javelin throwers may avulse or cause impingement upon the tip of the olecranon process. However, this sport (like other throwing sports) places huge strain on the medial collateral ligament which can become either acutely injured or chronically attenuated. There may also be symptoms of ulnar nerve impairment. The pain usually settles down after a period of rest and modification of activities. However, an attenuated medial collateral ligament may need reconstruction with a tendon graft.

AVULSION OF THE DISTAL TENDON OF BICEPS

The typical patient is a man of about 45 years who feels sudden pain and weakness at the front of the elbow after strenuous effort. Feel for the distal biceps tendon while the patient flexes the elbow against resistance (ask him to grip the desk or table as if to lift it; normally the biceps tendon stands out as a taut cord across the elbow crease). Loss of supination power with the elbow flexed (negating supinator muscle) is a good physical sign. The tendon may be partially or completely avulsed from its insertion into the bicipital tuberosity of the radius.

The diagnosis is often missed because elbow flexion

and supination, although weaker than normal, are preserved by brachialis and supinator action. MRI helps to confirm the diagnosis but must not delay surgical treatment. Clinical diagnosis should usually suffice.

Treatment

Operative repair is not always necessary; some patients are content to manage with slightly reduced elbow flexion: in time, the other elbow flexors will compensate (brachioradialis, brachialis). However, there will be a very obvious cosmetic defect and greatly reduced power of supination. For these reasons, many patients will choose repair. The best results are achieved by operation within 2 weeks, before the tendon retracts and the interosseous tunnel becomes occluded. A two-incision technique is recommended to avoid nerve damage and heterotopic ossification; tissue anchors or sutures-through-drillholes can be used to attach the tendon to its insertion point. The results of early surgery and careful rehabilitation are usually very good.

BURSITIS

The olecranon bursa sometimes becomes enlarged as a result of *continual pressure* or *friction;* this used to be called 'student's elbow'. If the enlargement is a nuisance the fluid may be aspirated.

The commonest non-traumatic cause is *gout*; there may be a sizeable lump with calcification on x-ray. In *rheumatoid arthritis*, also, the bursa may become enlarged, and sometimes nodules can be felt in the lump or just distal to it over the proximal ulna. In both conditions other joints are likely to be affected as well.

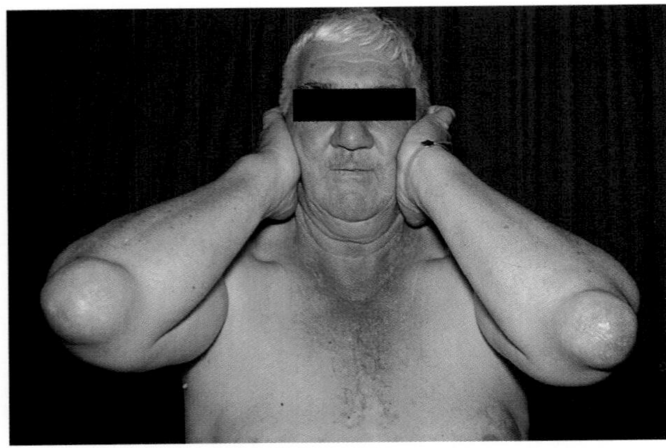

14.17 Olecranon bursitis The enormous red lumps over the points of the elbows are enlarged olecranon bursae; the ruddy complexion completes the typical picture of gout.

A chronically enlarged bursa may prove a severe nuisance and need to be excised. However, wound healing can be a problem.

OPERATIONS

ARTHROSCOPY

Arthroscopy of the elbow is technically demanding; its role for diagnosis and treatment continues to evolve.

Indications

An arthroscopic approach may be employed for intra-articular procedures such as removal of loose bodies, irrigation for infection or trimming of osteophytes. More advanced indications include synovectomy, capsular release, removal of coronoid or olecranon osteophytes and radial head excision.

Technique

The risk of this operation is a devastating injury to the median nerve, ulnar nerve or posterior interosseous nerve, each of which lies less than a centimetre from the joint and very close to the portals used for access. The operation therefore requires special training and a very clear appreciation of the anatomy. Pre-distension of the joint with fluid and the use of blunt trochars help to reduce the risk. Capsulectomy carries a particularly high risk.

ARTHROPLASTY

A complex anatomy and relatively fragile bone structure make it more challenging to repeat the success stories of hip and knee replacement. Nevertheless, in specific circumstances it is better than the alternative of a painful, stiff or unstable joint.

Indications

The most common indication for arthroplasty is rheumatoid arthritis; it is also occasionally suitable for the treatment of osteoarthritis. It has a valuable role in the treatment of comminuted distal humerus fractures in osteopaenic bone for those individuals with lower demands. Elbows which are ankylosed (e.g. due to previous infection) can be successfully salvaged with elbow replacement.

One should think carefully before advocating this operation to patients who intend to return to heavy work or leisure activities or to those with single-joint disease, i.e. without the protective effect against overuse of other involved joints in the same limb.

Design

Earlier *constrained* (single-axis hinge) implants had a high failure rate due to loosening. *Unconstrained* designs are associated with instability and dislocation. However, 90 per cent good results can be achieved in carefully selected patients (those with good bone stock and competent ligaments). *Semi-constrained* implants allow some of the forces to be absorbed by the soft tissues whilst maintaining some intrinsic stability.

Outcome

The majority of patients with an elbow replacement can expect relief of pain and a functional range of movement. Ten-year survival rates as high as 80 per cent have been achieved in patients with rheumatoid arthritis (perhaps the joint is protected because of poor function in the rest of the limb) whereas the survival rate for those with osteoarthritis or distal humeral non-union is less certain. A good outcome can also be achieved in selected trauma patients (older individuals with low demand).

Complications

The operation has a relatively high complication rate, particularly ulnar nerve palsy, wound failure and collateral ligament instability. This is particularly likely in patients with inadequate bone stock due to rheumatoid disease, previous infection or previous operations.

Arthrodesis

Arthrodesis is rarely indicated. It is a technically difficult and very disabling procedure. Even with normal wrist and shoulder function it is not possible to fuse the elbow in a position which would facilitate both feeding (i.e. 100 degrees of flexion) and perineal hygiene (about 45 degrees of flexion). Compression plating is the most straightforward and stable technique.

NOTES ON APPLIED ANATOMY

The elbow needs to be able to convey the hand upwards to the head and mouth, downwards to the perineum and legs, and also to a wide variety of working positions at bench, desk, wall or table. A varied combination of flexion and extension with pronation and supination is clearly needed. Although the normal elbow is capable of full extension, flexion to about 130 degrees and 90 degrees of both pronation and supination, the *functional range of movement* is 30–130 degrees of flexion and 50 degrees both pronation and supination.

The forearm is normally in slight valgus relative to the upper arm, the average carrying angle being about 15 degrees. The complex geometry of the joint allows for the fact that when the elbow is flexed the forearm comes to lie directly upon the upper arm. The carrying angle may be altered by malunion of a fracture or by damage to the physis, resulting in cubitus valgus or cubitus varus.

The joint acts as a 'sloppy hinge', permitting a few degrees of valgus/varus movement and some rotational laxity. Stability is provided by: (1) the relative conformity of the humeral trochlea with the olecranon; (2) the medial collateral ligament (particularly the anterior band); and (3) the lateral collateral ligament (particularly the ulnar part). The radial head is a secondary constraint to valgus instability; it can be excised with relative impunity as long as the medial collateral ligament, humero-ulnar articulation and interosseous membrane are intact. The elbow is not really a 'non-weightbearing' joint – forces of up to three times body weight pass across it with normal use.

Pronation and supination take place mainly at the radio-ulnar joints with a small amount of abduction and adduction between the olecranon and the trochlea. The movement is often supplemented by rotation at the shoulder. The humeroradial joint is held in position by the strong annular (orbicular) and collateral ligament which embraces the head and neck of the radius but is not attached to it. The capsule of the elbow is attached to the annular ligament but is not attached to the radius. The circular and slightly concave upper surface of the radius ensures that in all positions of rotation it retains adequate contact with the hemispheric capitulum.

Nerves

The ulnar nerve passes behind the medial condyle of the humerus; it may be stretched if there is marked cubitus valgus. Distal to the condyle the nerve is closely applied to the elbow capsule, and there also it may be compromised if the joint is osteoarthritic.

On the lateral side of the elbow the radial nerve passes between brachialis and brachioradialis. It then splits to become the superficial radial nerve and the posterior interosseous nerve. The latter passes beneath extensor carpi radialis brevis and then between two parts of the supinator muscle; it is vulnerable to injury during surgical approaches to the proximal part of the radius.

In front of the elbow lie the brachialis muscle and also the median nerve in company with the great vessels; these relationships make an anterior approach to the elbow somewhat challenging.

The wrist 15

David Warwick, Roderick Dunn

The wrist and hand function together, for all practical purposes, as a single articulated unit. The hand would be unable to perform its range of complicated movements without the reciprocal movement, positioning and stabilizing action of the wrist. Loss of movement at the wrist limits the manipulative skill of the fingers and thumb; and pain in the wrist makes it impossible to grip or pinch with full strength. Disorders of the wrist and hand are often interrelated and therefore, in the clinical setting, these two units should be examined and analysed together. However, for the sake of emphasis, they are treated here in two separate chapters.

CLINICAL ASSESSMENT

SYMPTOMS

Pain may be localized to the radial side (especially in de Quervain's disease and thumb base arthritis), to the ulnar side (e.g. in distal radio-ulnar joint arthritis and piso-triquetral arthritis) or to the dorsum (in radio-carpal arthritis, Kienböck's disease and occult dorsal wrist ganglion).

Stiffness is often not noticed until it is severe in the flexion–extension plane; loss of rotation is noticed earlier and can be very disrupting.

Swelling may signify involvement of either the joint or the tendon sheaths or a ganglion.

Deformity is a late symptom except after trauma or radial nerve palsy. Ask if it is localized to a particular site (e.g. an overly-prominent head of ulna, suggesting subluxation of the distal radio-ulnar joint) or involving the posture of the wrist as a whole [progressive radial deviation in advanced rheumatoid arthritis (RA)].

Loss of function refers mainly to the hand, though the patient may be aware that the problem lies in the wrist.

Clicks are common and usually of no relevance; *clunks* with pain or weakness may signify instability.

SIGNS

Examination of the wrist is not complete without also examining the elbow, forearm and hand. Both upper limbs should be completely exposed.

Look

The skin is inspected for scars. Both wrists and forearms are compared to see if there is any deformity. If there is swelling, note whether it is diffuse or localized to one of the tendon sheaths. Look also at the hands and fingers to see if there are any related abnormalities.

The posture of the wrist at rest and during movement varies with different positions of the hand and fingers. This is discussed in the opening sections of Chapter 16.

Feel

Palpation of the wrist will yield valuable information only if the surface anatomy is thoroughly understood

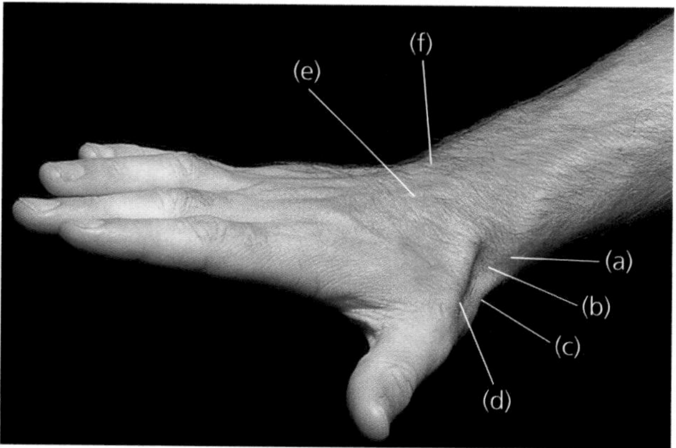

15.1 Tender points at the wrist **(a)** Tip of the radial styloid process; **(b)** anatomical snuffbox, bounded on the radial side by **(c)** the extensor pollicis brevis and on the ulnar side by **(d)** the extensor pollicis longus; **(e)** the extensor tendons of the fingers; and **(f)** the head of the ulna.

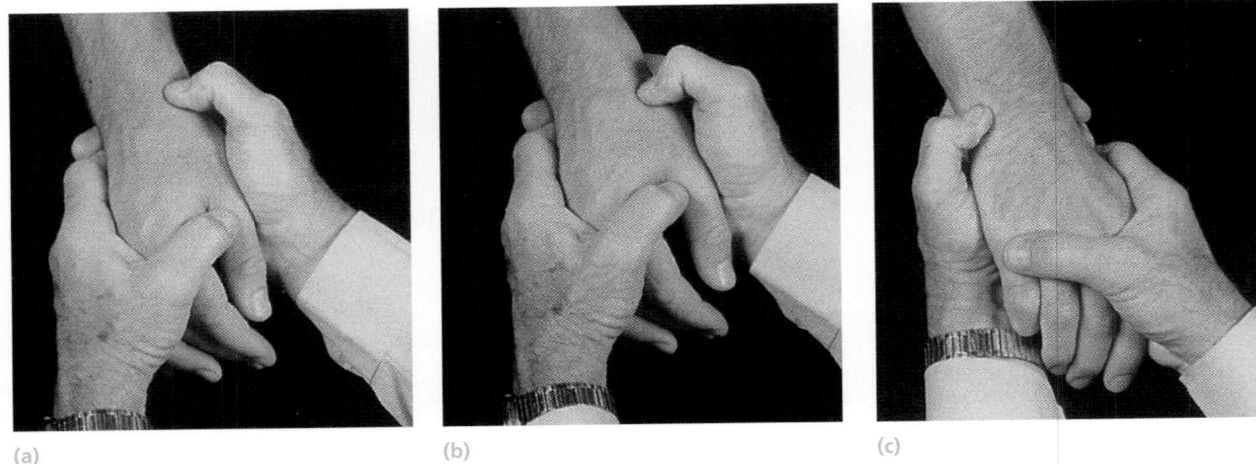

(a) (b) (c)

15.2 (a) Tenderness at the tip of the radial styloid suggests de Quervain's disease (tenovaginitis of the combined sheath for extensor pollicis brevis and abductor pollicis longus). This diagnosis can be confirmed by *Finkelstein's test*. Hold the patient's hand with his thumb tucked firmly unto the palm; then turn the wrist into full ulnar deviation; in a positive test, this will elicit sharp pain in the affected sheath. (b) Tenderness in the anatomical snuffbox is typical of a scaphoid injury (c) Tenderness just distal to the head of the ulna is found in extensor carpi ulnaris tendinitis.

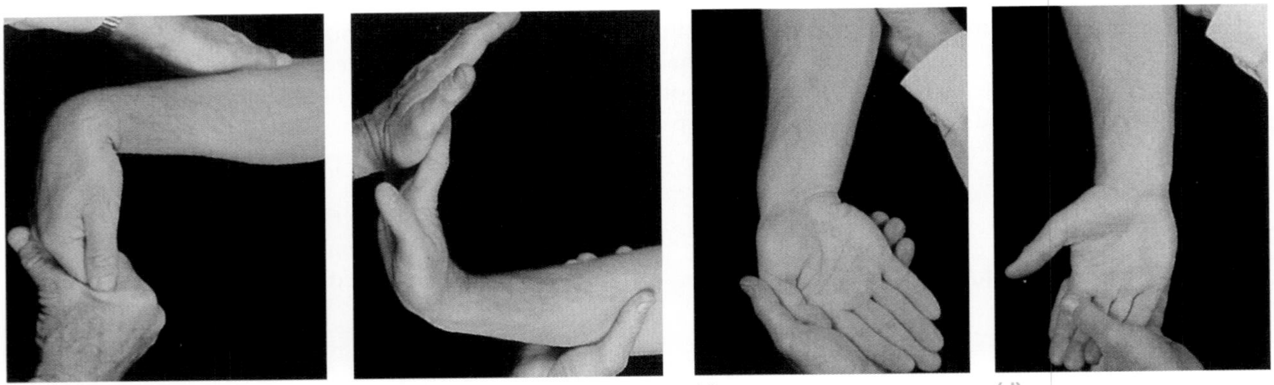

(a) (b) (c) (d)

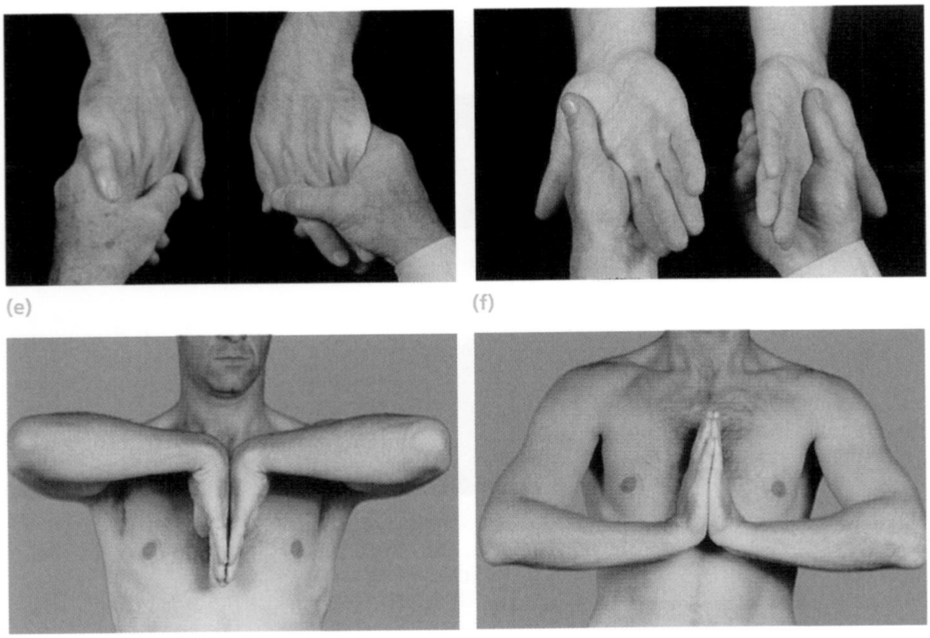

(e) (f)

(g) (h)

15.3 (a-f) Testing for wrist flexion, extension, ulnar deviation, radial deviation, pronation and supination. When testing pronation and supination, the patient must keep his elbows flexed. (g,h) This is a good way to test flexion and extension of the wrists; you can compare the two sides.

(see Figure 15.1). Tender areas must be accurately localized and the various landmarks compared with those of the normal wrist. The site of tenderness may be diagnostic, for example in de Quervain's disease (tip of radial styloid), scaphoid fracture (anatomical snuffbox), carpo-metacarpal osteoarthritis (base of first metacarpal), Kienböck's disease (over the lunate), triangular fibrocartilage complex (just distal to the head of the ulna) and localized tenosynovitis of any of the wrist tendons. At the same time note if the skin feels unduly warm.

If the head of the ulna seems abnormally prominent on the dorsum of the wrist, try to jar the distal radio-ulnar joint by pressing down sharply on the ulnar prominence; if it moves up and down the joint is unstable (this is aptly named the 'piano-key sign').

Move

Passive movements To compare passive dorsiflexion of the wrists the patient places his palms together in the position of prayer, then elevates his elbows. Palmar flexion is examined in a similar way. Radial and ulnar deviation are measured in either the palms-up or the palms-down position. With the elbows at right angles and tucked in to the sides, pronation and supination are assessed.

While testing passive movements, the presence of abnormal 'clunks' should be noted; they may signify one or other form of carpal instability.

Active movements Ask the patient to pull the hand backwards to its limit (*extension*), then forwards as far as possible (*flexion*), and then sideways to right and left (*radial and ulnar deviation*). Active *pronation and supination* should be performed with the patient's elbows tucked tightly into the waist. These movements are then repeated but carried out against resistance, to test for muscle power. Finally, grip strength is measured, preferably using a mechanical dynamometer. Loss of power may be due to pain, tendon rupture or muscle weakness.

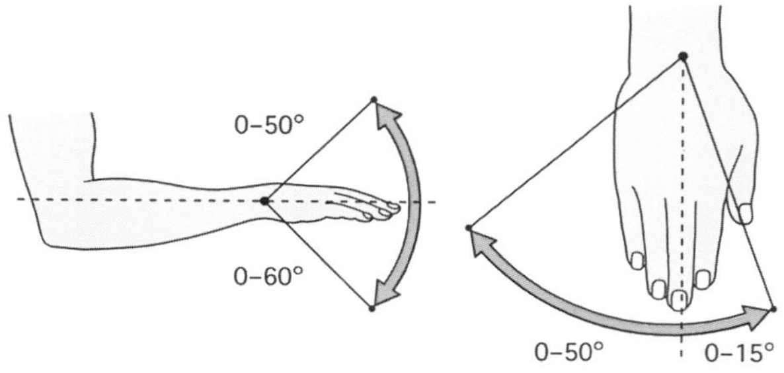

15.4 Normal range of movement From the neutral position dorsiflexion is slightly less than palmarflexion. Most hand functions are performed with the wrist in ulnar deviation; normal radial deviation is only about 15°.

Provocative tests

Special tests are needed to assess stability of the carpal articulations. The *luno-triquetral joint* is tested by gripping or pinching the lunate with one hand, the triquetral-pisiform with the other, and then applying a sheer stress: pain or clicking suggests an incompetent luno-triquetral ligament. The *piso-triquetral joint* is tested by pushing the pisiform radialwards against the triquetrum. Stability of the *scapho-lunate joint* is tested by pressing hard on the palmar aspect of the scaphoid tubercle while moving the wrist alternately in abduction and adduction: pain or clicking on abduction (radial deviation) is abnormal. The *triangular fibrocartilage* is tested by pushing the wrist medially then flexing and extending it. The *distal radio-ulnar joint* is tested for stability by holding the radius and then ballotting the ulnar head up and down. These tests are mentioned again in the section on carpal instability.

IMAGING

X-rays

Anteroposterior and lateral views are obtained routinely. Note the position and shape of the individual carpal bones and whether there are any abnormal spaces between them. Then look for evidence of joint space narrowing, especially at the radio-carpal joint and the carpo-metacarpal joint of the thumb. The wrist x-ray should be taken in a standard position of mid-pronation with the elbow at 90 degrees; often both wrists must be x-rayed for comparison. Special views may be necessary to show a scaphoid fracture or carpal instability. Moving the wrist under image intensification is useful to investigate some cases of carpal instability.

Arthrography

The wrist contains three separate compartments – the radio-carpal joint, the distal radio-ulnar joint and the midcarpal joint. Defects in the triangular fibrocartilage, scapho-lunate ligaments or luno-triquetral ligaments can be identified by arthrography.

Computed tomography

CT is the ideal method for assessing congruity of the distal radio-ulnar joint, fractures of the hook of hamate, and alignment of scaphoid fractures prior to surgery for non-union or malunion.

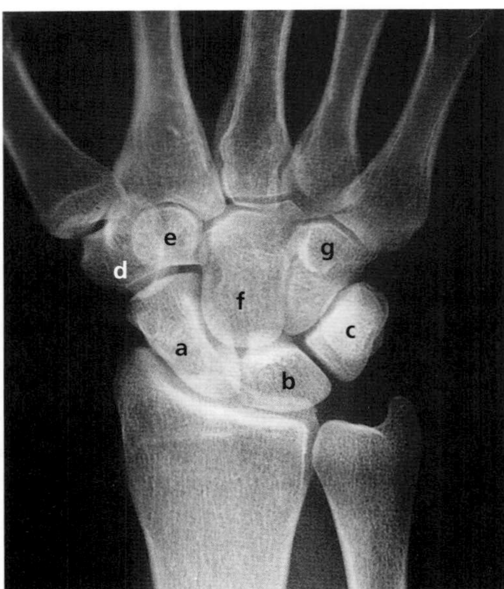

15.5 X-ray Note the shape and position of the bones which make up the normal carpus: **(a)**, scaphoid, **(b)**, lunate, **(c)**, triquetrum overlain by pisiform, **(d)**, trapezium, **(e)**, trapezoid, **(f)**, capitate, **(g)**, hamate.

Magnetic resonance imaging

MRI is particularly useful for detecting changes associated with scaphoid fractures, avascular necrosis of the lunate (Kienböck's disease), occult dorsal ganglia and intra-osseous ganglia. The thickness of the cuts may be too large to detect injury to thin structures such as the luno-triquetral ligament, scapho-lunate ligament or triangular fibrocartilage. MRI arthrography increases the sensitivity.

Radionuclide scan

A localized area of increased activity may reveal an osteoid osteoma, an occult scaphoid fracture or early osteoarthritis.

Fluoroscopy

Fluoroscopic examination may be needed to demonstrate some patterns of carpal instability.

ARTHROSCOPY

The wrist is suspended by finger traps, inflated with saline and inspected through specific portals into the radio-carpal joint, the ulno-carpal joint and the mid-carpal joint. Ligament tears, articular cartilage damage, osteoarthritis, occult ganglia, synovitis and triangular fibrocartilage lesions can be recognized and in some cases treated.

CONGENITAL ANOMALIES OF THE WRIST AND HAND

Abnormalities occurring in the upper limb anlage during the first three months of embryonic life are likely to affect more than one segment (or indeed the whole) of the developing limb; not surprisingly, therefore, congenital anomalies often occur together in the forearm, wrist and hand. For this reason, we have dealt with the subject under a single heading.

The embryonic arm buds appear about 4 weeks after fertilization and from then on the limbs develop progressively from proximal to distal. By 6 weeks the digital rays begin to appear and then develop in concert with the general mesenchymal differentiation that gives rise to the primitive skeleton and muscles. Growth goes hand in hand with genetically programmed cell death that results in modelling of the limbs and the formation of joints and separate digits. The process is more or less complete by the end of the eighth week after fertilization, at which time primary ossification centres begin to appear in the long bones. Ossification centres in the epiphyses and carpal bones do not emerge until after birth, so x-rays in the neonatal period must be interpreted with this in mind.

Malformations may occur during embryonic development because of either defective formation or incomplete separation of mesenchymal components, the former accounting for partial or complete absence of a part and the latter for coalitions between adjacent elements. It must also be remembered that other organs developing during the same period may also be affected; thus musculoskeletal malformations are often associated with other abnormalities.

The overall incidence of congenital upper limb anomalies is estimated to be about 1 in 600 live births, but in only a fraction of those affected are the defects severe enough to require operative treatment. Some of the malformations are caused by heritable genetic mutations or by intrauterine damage from drugs, infection or ionizing radiation; in the majority of cases the cause is unknown.

CLASSIFICATION

The classification of congenital limb malformation adopted by the International Federation of Societies for Surgery of the Hand (IFSSH) lists seven major categories: (1) failure of formation of parts; (2) failure of differentiation of parts; (3) duplication; (4) overgrowth; (5) undergrowth; (6) constriction bands; and (7) generalized skeletal abnormalities. Some conditions do not fit readily into a single category (e.g. thumb hypoplasia, which sits equally well in 'failure of formation' and 'undergrowth').

General considerations

Initial consultation

The parents and child are likely to be anxious, and may have been given conflicting information by non-specialist physicians. There may be issues of maternal guilt, parental anger and resentment, and unrealistic expectations about the outcome and possibilities of surgery. It is important to gain the confidence of the family at the initial consultation; remember that the children are likely to be long-term patients.

They must be given a *diagnosis*, an indication of *prognosis*, *reassurance about the future* and *a long-term plan of treatment*, including a *schedule of surgery*, which may have to be carried out in several stages. Many children manage well into adulthood with untreated congenital anomalies, and the requirement for surgery is not always clear.

Clinical examination

The clinic should be held in a child-friendly setting. Toys should be available to allow children to play in an unrestrained manner, which permits close observation of hand function. It may be easier to examine a child while he or she is sitting on the parent's lap. The diagnosis is not always obvious, though the absence of skin creases suggests some congenital abnormality such as absent joints or joints which do not move.

Remember that many congenital wrist and hand anomalies are part of a larger syndrome. Radial dysplasia, for example, may be associated with vertebral anomalies, anal atresia, cardiovascular anomalies, tracheo-oesophageal fistula, renal anomalies and other limb defects (embodied in the acronym VACTERL). The child should always be investigated fully and, if necessary, referred to other specialists. Genetic counselling should be made available for inherited or unusual conditions, and indeed may be helpful in reaching a diagnosis.

Indications for operative treatment

Whenever the need for operative treatment is considered, four general precepts should be borne in mind:

- *Function:* Consider how important is the affected part to everyday activity, for example when deciding whether to use a normal index finger to reconstruct an absent or defective thumb.
- *Progression of deformity:* Decide whether further growth is likely to increase the deformity or give rise to other deformities. For example, syndactyly involving digits of unequal length – say the ring and little fingers – may cause progressive deviation of the fingers.
- *Appearance:* The hand is second only to the face in self-consciousness of appearance. If it looks normal, a child is more likely to use it normally. If it looks abnormal, the child will hide it away. This concept is known as 'dynamic cosmesis'.
- *Pain:* Although malformations are usually not painful, some may come to need treatment for this reason. An example is a tender fingertip in constriction ring syndrome when there is poor soft-tissue cover over the bone.

Failure of formation

Transverse arrest

This can exist anywhere between the shoulder and the phalanges. The most common levels of absence are at the proximal forearm and mid-carpus, then at the metacarpals and humerus. Associated anomalies are unusual.

Proximal forearm Prosthetic fittings in young children may be desirable for cosmetic reasons. For older children and adolescents, myoelectric prostheses may be considered and can improve function, though many youngsters manage surprisingly well without them.

Transverse arrest of fingers The child with vestigial fingers (*symbrachydactyly*) can be treated by microvascular transfer of a toe if there are proximal enabling structures available (skin, tendons and nerves), or by non-vascularized transfer of a toe phalanx into the existing skin envelope.

Longitudinal arrest

Longitudinal arrest may involve *radial* (pre-axial), *ulnar* (post-axial), *central* (cleft hand) or *intersegmental* (intercalated) structures.

RADIAL DYSPLASIA

This rare condition (incidence 1:50 000 to 1:100 000 live births) may involve any (or all) of the structures from the elbow to the thumb. It usually occurs as an isolated abnormality but is occasionally associated with other skeletal, cardiac, haematological, renal or craniofacial anomalies, which should be sought.

The infant is born with the wrist in marked radial deviation – hence the use of the term *'radial club hand'*; half the patients are affected bilaterally. There is absence of the whole or part of the radius; often the thumb, scaphoid and trapezium fail to develop normally.

Treatment Mild radial dysplasia is treated from birth by gentle stretching and splintage, best done by the parents. More serious cases can be treated by distraction prior to a tension-free soft-tissue correction

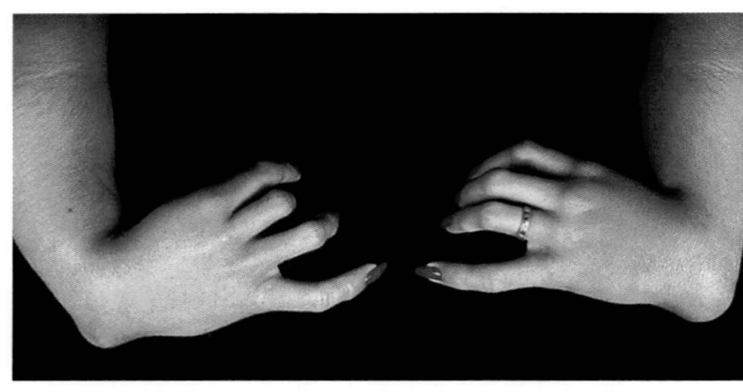

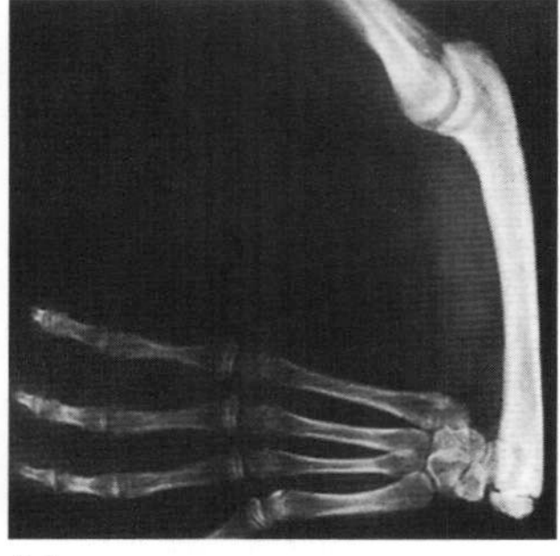

(a) (b)

15.6 Radial dysplasia (a) Bilateral. (b) X-ray showing that the entire radius is absent.

which has less effect on growth of the carpus and distal ulna than the older technique of 'centralizing' the carpus over the remaining forearm structures. Prolonged splintage is still required to avoid recurrence of the deformity. Attention must be paid to the elbow; if the joint is stiff, the radially deviated wrist can actually be advantageous, as the child can then get the hand to his or her mouth (for eating) and the perineum (for toilet care). Surgical correction of the wrist in these cases can result in a functional disaster.

If the *thumb* is affected this can present serious problems in treatment. Hypoplasia may be associated with a tight first web space and instability of the metacarpophalangeal (MCP) joint, requiring advanced reconstructive surgery, tendon transfers and joint stabilization. If the thumb is absent, pollicization of the index finger or microvascular toe transfer may be required. (See also below under Undergrowth.)

ULNAR DYSPLASIA

This is even less common than radial dysplasia. Most cases are sporadic, but the condition may be part of a larger syndrome, together with anomalies in other limbs.

Here the new-born infant presents with ulnar deviation of the wrist (or both wrists), due to partial or complete absence of the ulna; in addition some of the carpal bones may be absent and the ulnar rays of the hand may be missing. With growth the radius elongates disproportionately and becomes bowed; ultimately the radial head may dislocate.

Treatment During the first few months stretching and splinting may be helpful. If wrist deformity and radial bowing are progressive and severe, surgery may be advisable and consists of excision of any tethering ulnar anlage and osteotomy of the radius. If the radial head has dislocated and elbow movement is restricted, the radial head can be excised; if the forearm is unstable, the distal radius can be fused to the proximal ulna (the Straub procedure).

Secondary ulnar dysplasia A similar but milder deformity sometimes occurs in children over the age of about 10 years who were born with hereditary multiple exostoses

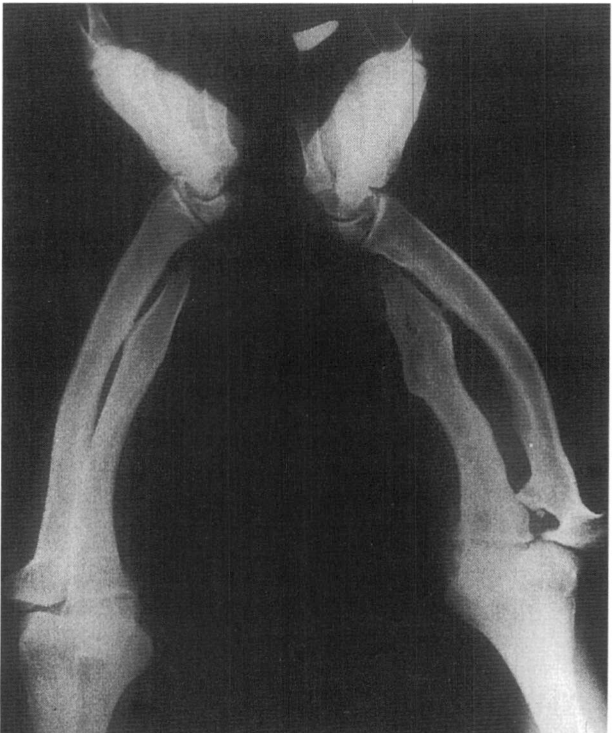

15.7 Distal ulnar deformity The x-ray characteristically shows a tapering, carrot-shaped distal end of ulna. This bilateral case was due to hereditary multiple exostoses; there is bilateral bowing of the radius and on the right side the radial head has subluxated.

or dyschondroplasia. If the distal ulna is affected in these conditions, growth at the distal physis may be retarded; the distal ulna tapers to a carrot shape and is short. If the radius remains unaffected and goes on growing normally, it becomes bowed and the radial head tends to subluxate or dislocate (see page 161). In most cases the elbow and forearm are completely stable and no treatment is needed (except, possibly, for cosmetic reasons).

CENTRAL DYSPLASIA (CLEFT HAND)

True cleft hand presents with a V-shaped cleft in the centre of the hand which may be associated with the absence of one or more digits, transverse bones, syndactyly of digits bordering the cleft, and a tight first web space. It is often familial (dominant inheritance), may be unilateral or bilateral, and can be associated with 'cleft feet'. Other anomalies, such as cleft lip, cleft palate and congenital heart disease may also be present. The condition differs from so-called 'atypical cleft hand' (*symbrachydactyly)*, which is not heritable and not associated with other anomalies.

Surgery is complex, having to deal with closure of the cleft, reconstruction of the first web space and – in some cases – correction of other anomalies in the adjacent digits. Redundant soft tissue from closing the cleft can be used to augment the tight first web space.

INTERCALARY SEGMENTAL DYSPLASIA

Very rarely an intercalary segment in the upper limb fails to develop and the forearm or hand may be attached directly to the trunk, or the hand is attached to the humerus. This condition, also known as *phocomelia*, may affect more than one limb and is sometimes associated with craniofacial deformities.

For the upper limb, there is no satisfactory treatment apart from designing and fitting a cosmetically preferable prosthesis.

Failure of differentiation

Syndactyly

Conjoined digits is the commonest congenital malformation of the hand (incidence about 1:2000 live births). The anomaly may be *simple* (soft tissue only) or *complex* (skin and bone), *complete* (affecting the entire web) or *incomplete* (only part of the web).

Mild, incomplete syndactyly of central digits may need no treatment. Treatment of complete syndactyly involves separation of the conjoined structures and skin grafting. When multiple digits are involved (*achrosyndactyly*), this should be tackled one web space at a time, at separate operations, so as to avoid potential compromise of both digital arteries. If the border digits (thumb and index, ring and little fingers) are affected this can cause progressive deformity with growth and requires early surgical reconstruction.

Synostosis

Failure of embryological separation of skeletal components can result in conjoined normal-looking bones or fused (unseparated) joints. This may occur at any level from the fingers to the humerus and can be longitudinal (e.g. humero-ulnar synostosis) or transverse (e.g. proximal radio-ulnar synostosis or carpal coalitions). The condition may appear in isolation or as part of a wider syndrome.

If there is no significant loss of function then operative treatment is unnecessary. If important movements are affected (e.g. uncompensated loss of forearm rotation in proximal radio-ulnar synostosis, or fusion at the elbow joint), osteotomy and re-positioning of the limb in a more favourable position may be considered. Carpal fusions usually need no treatment.

Camptodactyly

'Bent finger' is a flexion deformity of the proximal interphalangeal joint, usually of the little finger. It may be an isolated condition or part of a syndrome. It may be inherited or sporadic, and two-thirds of cases are bilateral.

The condition presents as two groups: those occurring in infancy and affecting males and females equally, and those presenting in adolescence, mainly affecting females. There is often an abnormal muscle insertion (usually one of the lumbricals), and there may be a characteristic abnormal radiographic appearance of the head of the proximal phalanx.

The mainstay of treatment is splinting. Surgery may be indicated if the deformity is marked or is a severe nuisance. Soft-tissue releases and/or muscle transfers are advocated by some surgeons but the results are disappointing. If there is a bony block to interphalangeal extension, a corrective osteotomy will improve the situation.

Clinodactyly In this condition a digit is bent sideways (radially or ulnarwards), usually due to an abnormally shaped middle phalanx – a so-called 'delta' deformity in which the epiphysis is curved. It usually affects the little finger and is often inherited and bilateral. As it is often part of a more widespread syndrome, the child should be examined for other defects. Severe cases can be treated by corrective osteotomy and bone grafting.

The condition must be distinguished from *Kirner's syndrome,* in which the distal phalanx of the little finger is similarly bent. This usually presents in adolescence and treatment is the same as for clinodactyly.

Duplication

Polydactyly ('extra digits') may occur on the radial (pre-axial), the ulnar (post-axial) or the central part of the hand.

Duplication of the little finger is one of the most common congenital anomalies of the hand. It is often inherited and is much commoner in black people than in whites. The extra digit is often attached only by skin and a neurovascular bundle, and may be removed under local anaesthesia; this is easiest when the child is less than 4 months old. If a phalanx or entire digit is duplicated, removal and soft-tissue reconstruction should be performed a little later under formal operating theatre conditions.

Duplications of the thumb or central digits are extremely rare and require complex reconstructive surgery of the digit, its tendons and the overlying skin. In the thumb, even small 'tags' should be approached with care so as to avoid the risk of damaging tendons that need reconstruction.

Overgrowth

Macrodactyly must be distinguished from other forms of enlarged digits (neurofibromatosis, multiple enchondromatosis, vascular malformations). There are two forms: *static* (present at birth and growing proportionately to other digits) and *progressive* (enlargement of a digit in early childhood, growing faster than other digits with deviation of the digit). The condition is rare, and the majority of cases are unilateral, affecting the index, middle, thumb, ring or little finger, in order of frequency. The median or ulnar nerve is often enlarged, and may become compressed.

Surgical correction is extremely difficult and generally unrewarding. It includes debulking, epiphyseal arrest (when the digit has reached adult size) and nerve excision and grafting. Amputation may be the best option but beware, an adjacent digit may start 'overgrowing'!

Undergrowth

Undergrowth (brachydactyly) is common and may be part of a wider syndrome (e.g. Turner's syndrome). It can affect a single bone, a digit or an entire limb.

Thumb hypoplasia ranges from mild (requiring no treatment) to severe phalangeal or metacarpal hypoplasia with joint instability, or even complete absence of the digit. When the first carpo-metacarpal (CMC) joint is present, reconstruction of the first web space and ulnar collateral ligament as well as an opposition transfer may be necessary. In the absence of the first CMC joint, it is usual to pollicize the index finger to reconstruct the thumb (as long as the index finger is not hypoplastic).

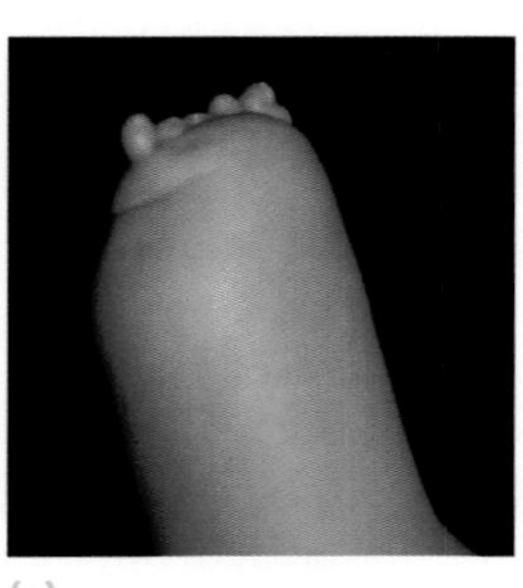

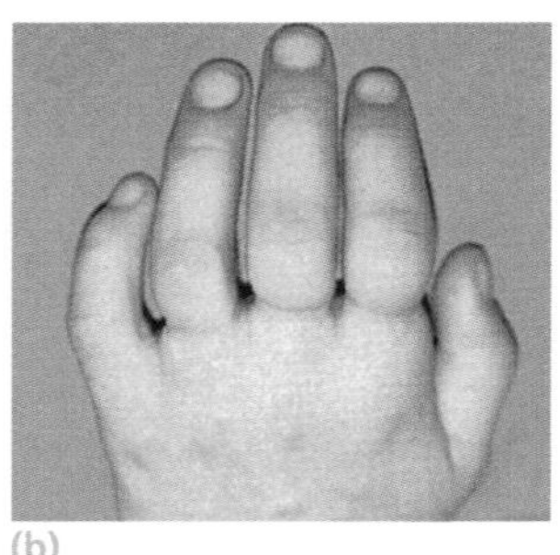

(a) (b)

15.8 Congenital variations (a) Transverse failure of formation; (b) constriction rings.

Constriction ring syndrome

The aetiology of this condition is thought to be early, *in utero,* rupture of the amniotic membrane and the formation of constricting amniotic membrane strands. Associated deformities (e.g. club feet) are common.

The condition presents as a localized 'strangulation', most commonly of the ring finger; the distal part of the finger may be painful, swollen and cyanotic, or sometimes threatened with amputation. Even if the disorder is not that severe, it may compromise growth.

Treatment consists of excision of the constricting band and soft-tissue reconstruction using multiple Z-plasties.

Miscellaneous conditions

Madelung's deformity In this deformity, which may be either congenital or post-traumatic, the lower radius curves forwards (ventrally), carrying with it the carpus and hand but leaving the lower ulna sticking out as a lump on the back of the wrist. The congenital disorder may appear as an isolated entity or as part of a generalized dysplasia; although the abnormality is present at birth, the deformity is rarely seen before the age of 10 years, after which it increases until growth is complete. Function is usually excellent.

If deformity is severe, the lower end of the ulna may be shortened; this is sometimes combined with osteotomy of the radius. Excision of the physeal tether and replacement with a free fat graft is an alternative in certain cases.

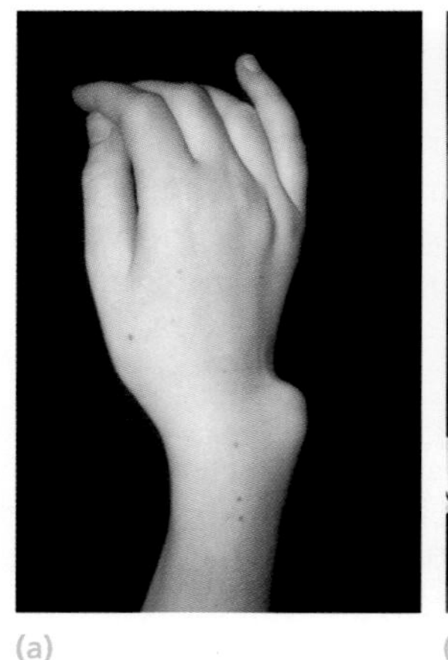

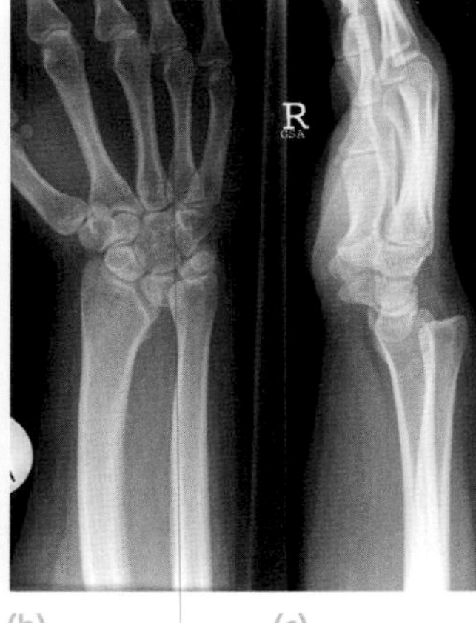

(a) (b) (c)

15.9 Madelung's deformity (a) Note prominent ulnar head and radial tilt; (b) characteristic x-ray showing increased slope of radius and (c) subluxation of ulma.

Congenital clasped thumb Infants with this condition clasp their thumbs persistently under the fingers. The disorder appears to be due to weakness or absence of the extensor tendons, in severe cases aggravated by flexion contractures of the MCP and CMC joints. It may present as an isolated problem or as part of a syndrome. However, the diagnosis should not be made before the third month as it is normal for infants to hold their thumbs in the palm before then.

Treatment is by splintage, but if this fails tendon transfers may be required later.

Congenital trigger thumb Care should be taken to distinguish this condition from the clasped thumb syndrome described above. It is unlikely that it is a truly congenital disorder but it may occur within a few months after birth. It appears to be a form of stenosing tenovaginitis of flexor pollicis longus. Thickening of the tendon, or a small nodule (Notta's node), may be palpable at the base of the thumb.

Triggering often resolves spontaneously, but if the condition is still present at one year it can be treated successfully by surgical division of the A1 pulley of the flexor tendon sheath.

Symphalangism This term describes congenital stiffness of the proximal interphalangeal joints of the fingers. These joints are abnormal and the fingers are underdeveloped. Surgical intervention is usually unrewarding.

Arthrogryposis multiplex congenita (AMC) Arthrogryposis is described in Chapter 10. Part or the whole of the upper limb may be affected, giving rise to muscle weakness and joint contractures. The shoulders are usually adducted, the elbows stiff, the wrists and fingers flexed and the thumbs clasped in adduction and flexion. The overlying skin is smooth and devoid of the normal creases.

Treatment is by early stretching and splinting; later joint releases and tendon transfers may be called for.

Other generalized syndromes Many generalized disorders involve the upper limbs. Examples include Down's syndrome (short little fingers), Marfan's syndrome (long fingers, camptodactyly), neurofibromatosis (macrodactyly) and cerebral palsy. The hand problems will require specialized treatment in their own right, in addition to management of the general disorder.

ACQUIRED DEFORMITIES OF THE WRIST

Physeal injury

Fracture-separation of the distal radial epiphysis may result in partial fusion of the physis, with pain and asymmetrical growth deformity of the wrist. The bony bridge crossing the physis, if it is small, may be excised and replaced by a fat graft.

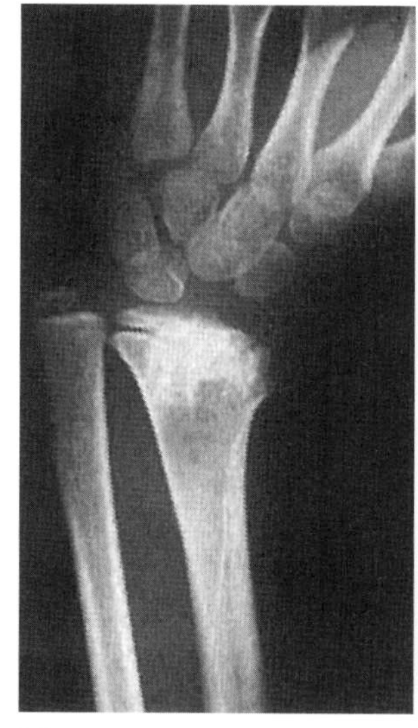

(a)

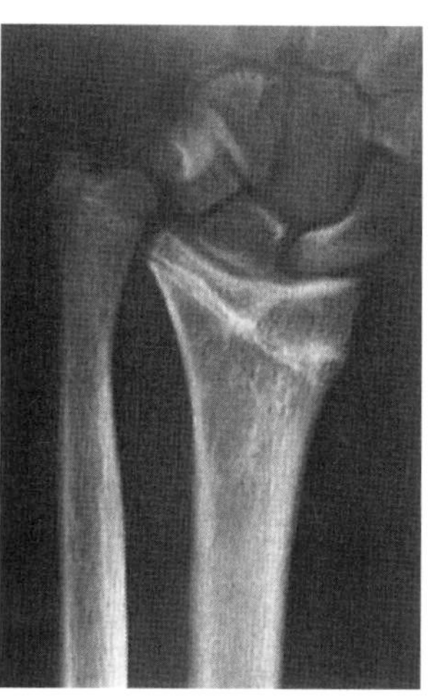

(b)

15.10 Growth plate arrest (a) Impacted physeal fracture; (b) later arrest of radius, relative overgrowth of ulna.

Once growth slows down the deformity can be corrected by a suitable osteotomy, if necessary combined with soft-tissue release; the circular frame apparatus can be used for this.

Forearm fractures

After a Colles' fracture radial deviation, posterior angulation and prominence of the radial head are common. These deformities may be unsightly but cause little disability.

Subluxation of the distal radio-ulnar joint may result in prominence of the ulnar head, painful rotation and loss of pronation or supination. This should be treated by reconstructing the distal radius; *the ulnar head should never be excised.* Abnormal angulation of the radius may lead to midcarpal malalignment with pain and loss of grip strength. A radial osteotomy is then necessary; the bone fragments are fixed with a locking plate and bone grafts are added.

Rheumatoid deformities

The typical rheumatoid deformity is radial deviation of the wrist, swelling of the extensor tendons, dorsal prominence of the ulnar head and sometimes tendon rupture. The carpus falls into flexion and supination as the ulnar side sags forwards away from the prominent ulnar head.

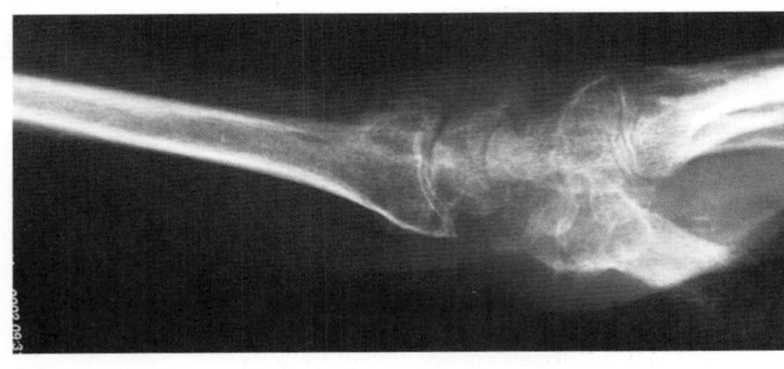

(a)

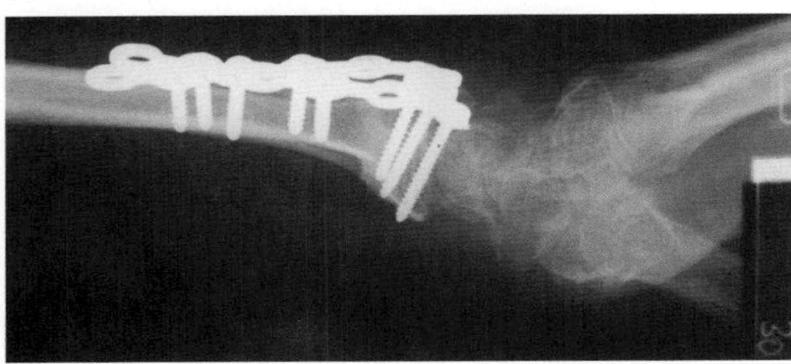

(b)

15.11 Malunion of radius (a) Malunion of Colles' fracture with dorsal tilt of distal radius. (b) Position following corrective osteotomy.

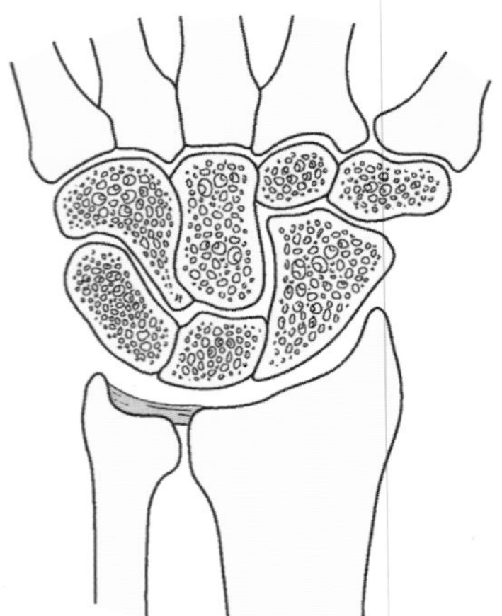

15.12 The carpal joints This schematic section through the wrist shows the radio-carpal joint between the radius and the proximal row of carpal bones and the mid-carpal joint between the proximal and distal rows of carpal bones. The proximal row is an intercalcated segment.

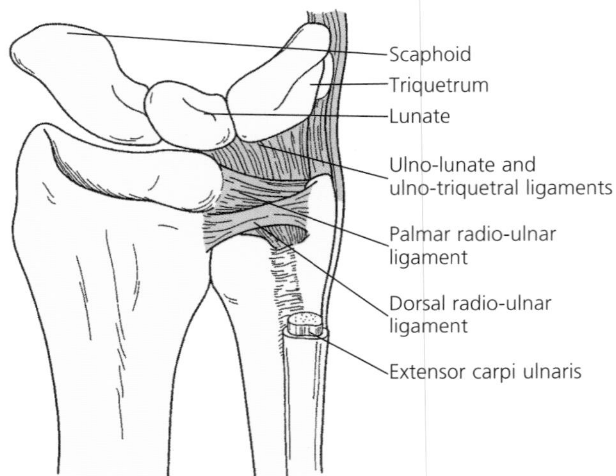

15.13 The distal radio-ulnar joint The joint incorporates the triangular fibrocartilage complex. The fibrocartilaginous plate is connected as its apex to the base of the ulnar styloid process and laterally to the inferomedial ridge of the radius. Its outer fibres blend with those of the ligaments around the ulnar aspect of the wrist.

'Drop-wrist'

Radial nerve palsy causes the wrist to drop into flexion and active extension is lost. With a posterior interosseous nerve palsy, the wrist will extend radialwards because extensor carpi radialis longus function is preserved.

If the nerve does not recover, tendon transfers will greatly improve function (see Chapter 11).

CHRONIC INSTABILITY OF THE WRIST

Movements of the wrist and hand are interdependent, the wrist providing appropriate mobility and stability to position and steady the hand for the remarkable range of actions and tactile sensibility employed in our daily activities. Abnormalities of wrist mechanics are a common source of functional disability; this is seen most often in rheumatoid arthritis, in association with congenital laxity and after local trauma.

Articulations of the wrist

The wrist comprises three movable joints: the *distal radio-ulnar joint,* the *radio-carpal joint* (between the radius and the proximal row of carpal bones) and the *midcarpal joint* (between the proximal and distal rows of carpal bones).

THE DISTAL RADIO-ULNAR JOINT (DRUJ)

The distal radius and ulna are linked to each other by the interosseous membrane, the capsule of the DRUJ and *the triangular fibrocartilage complex (TFCC).* The head of the ulna articulates congruently with the sigmoid notch of the distal radius; movement at the joint occurs by the radius both rotating and sliding in an arc around the head of the ulna during pronation and supination of the forearm. Interposed between the head of the ulna and the carpus is a fibrocartilaginous disc, a fan-shaped structure spreading from an apical attachment at the base of the ulnar styloid process to the rim of the radial sigmoid notch. Its dorsal and volar edges are coextensive with the dorsal and palmar radio-ulnar ligaments; further attachments to the joint capsule, the ulno-triquetral and ulno-lunate ligaments, the ulnar collateral ligament and the sheath of the extensor carpi ulnaris tendon complete the fibrocartilage complex. The peripheral attachments of the TFCC have a good vascular supply and can heal after injury; the central area of the triangular plate is avascular and tears do not heal.

THE RADIO-CARPAL AND MIDCARPAL JOINTS

Movements in the sagittal plane (flexion and extension) occur at both the radio-carpal and midcarpal joints. Movements in the frontal plane (adduction or ulnar deviation and abduction or radial deviation) occur mainly at the radio-carpal joint, but they inevitably involve also the scaphoid which has to flex forwards as the trapezium moves towards the radial styloid during abduction.

The bones of the distal carpal row (hamate, capitate, trapezium and trapezoid) are joined by ligaments to each other and to the bases of the metacarpals. Although there is some movement of the fifth carpometacarpal joint, there is very little movement in the remaining carpo-metacarpal articulations.

The distal row articulates through the midcarpal joint with the bones of the proximal row (triquetrum, lunate and scaphoid), which are likewise held together by stout interosseous ligaments. Because these bones have no muscles attaching to them, their position is determined by the way they all fit together and by the constraints of the interosseous ligaments. The proximal row is, in a sense, 'interposed' between the forearm bones and the hand bones and is called an *intercalated segment*.

The articular surface of the radius slopes obliquely forwards at 11 degrees and ulnarwards at 22 degrees; the radial styloid is about 11 mm distal to the ulnar styloid (the 'rule of elevens').With the wrist in the neutral position, tightening of the long muscles will tend to drag the carpus down the slope, and when the wrist is pulled into abduction this tendency is increased. By contrast, when the wrist is adducted about 30 degrees, muscle pull draws the carpus most securely into the radial 'socket'. This is, in fact, the *'position of function'* (or maximum stability) and there is a natural inclination to adopt this position during power grip. This action is mediated by flexor carpi ulnaris (which is why it is unwise to choose that muscle for a tendon transfer).

The scaphoid is potentially the most unstable of all the carpal bones. As the wrist flexes and extends, so does the scaphoid bone; the lunate and triquetrum follow passively, guided by the interosseous ligaments. With abduction, the space between the trapezium and radial styloid closes down so the scaphoid moves out of the way by flexing palmarwards and sliding ulnarwards. During adduction, the scaphoid tilts dorsally

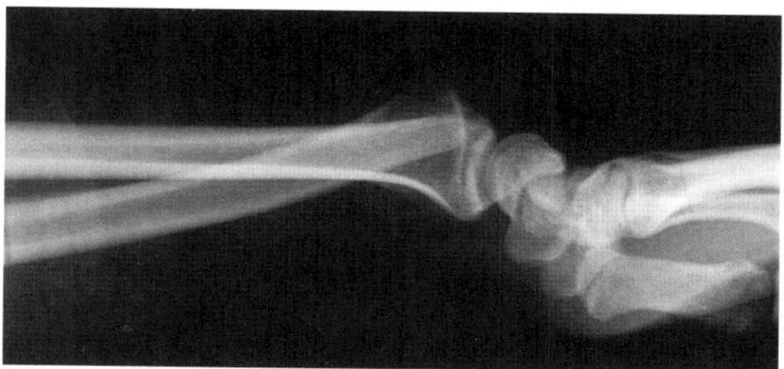

15.14 Ulnar head instability The ulnar head has subluxated dorsally.

and slides radially. As the wrist abducts and adducts, the helical surface of the hamate also causes the triquetrum to move.

INSTABILITY OF THE DISTAL RADIO-ULNAR JOINT

Chronic instability of the distal radio-ulnar joint may result from trauma, rheumatoid arthritis or excision of the distal end of the ulna. The previous history is therefore important. Fracture of the radial shaft is associated with dislocation of the distal radio-ulnar joint (Galeazzi fracture-dislocation); after reduction of the radius, one must be certain that the radio-ulnar joint also is reduced.

The patient complains of painful restriction of pronation and supination, clunking and undue prominence of the ulnar head. There may be tenderness directly over the radio-ulnar joint and grip strength is sometimes reduced. The unstable ulna can be 'balloted' by holding the patient's forearm pronated and pushing sharply upon the prominent head of the ulna (the *piano-key sign*).

Imaging

X-ray examination may show evidence of previous injury, previous surgery or rheumatoid arthritis. However, the most effective way of demonstrating radio-ulnar incongruity or subluxation is by CT.

Treatment

This depends on the cause. If the ulnar head is intact, then the TFCC can be reattached by arthroscopic or open methods. Ulnar shortening osteotomy can tighten the ulnar corner and improve stability; a tendon weave to reproduce the volar and dorsal radio-ulnar ligaments is the most reliable but difficult reconstruction. The ulnar head must never be excised to treat instability; that will only worsen the problem.

If the ulnar head has previously (and usually unwisely) been removed, ulnar head replacement will usually be needed to restore stability. Special implants have been developed for the failed Sauve–Kapandji procedure (fusion of the distal ulna to the radius).

Longitudinal instability of the radius and ulna

Fracture of the radial head is sometimes accompanied by disruption of the interosseous membrane and dislocation of the distal radio-ulnar joint (the Essex-Lopresti lesion). Excision of the radial head can lead to proximal migration of the radius and ulno-carpal impaction (see below); whenever possible the radial head should be preserved or replaced by a metal implant. Chronic longitudinal instability causes ulnar-sided wrist pain and loss of grip strength.

Treatment of the distal radio-ulnar joint symptoms is generally unsatisfactory. A combination of radial head replacement and an ulnar shortening osteotomy sometimes improves symptoms. Radio-ulnar fusion is sometimes employed as the only salvage procedure.

Disorders of the triangular fibrocartilage complex

Clinically significant disorders of the TFCC can be divided into traumatic and degenerative conditions.

Traumatic disruption

There may be a history of a fall on the outstretched hand or a twisting injury of the forearm. The patient complains of pain, and sometimes clicking or even instability in the distal radio-ulnar joint, particularly on twisting the wrist. There is tenderness over the ulno-carpal joint and pain on rotation of the forearm. Symptoms can also be reproduced by holding the wrist in adduction and compressing the ulnar head against the carpus. The distal ulna should be tested for instability. The diagnosis is confirmed by contrast arthrography, MRI or, most sensitively, arthroscopy.

Treatment Peripheral tears can be re-attached by either open or arthroscopic techniques with a reasonable expectation that they will heal. If this fails then a tendon reconstruction is needed. Central tears, in the absence of ulno-carpal impaction (see below), are best managed by arthroscopic debridement.

Ulno-carpal impaction and TFCC degeneration

The TFCC tends to degenerate with age; usually this is asymptomatic. However, progressive degenerative change may be associated with a relatively long ulna, impaction of the ulnar head against the ulnar side of the lunate and ulno-carpal arthritis (the *ulno-carpal impaction syndrome*). X-ray examination (standard views with the shoulder abducted 90 degrees, the elbow flexed 90 degrees and the forearm in mid-pronation-supination) may show a relatively long ulna (*'positive ulnar variance'*) and in late cases there may be arthritic changes in the ulno-lunate articulation.

Treatment Initial treatment is with simple analgesics, splintage and steroid injections. If this is not successful then the long ulna is shortened using a special jig and compression plate. A better alternative for just 2 or 3 mm of positive variance is an arthroscopic excision of the distal dome of the ulnar head. *The ulnar head itself should never be excised for this condition.*

Chronic instability of the radio-carpal and intercarpal joints

Abnormal movement between the carpus and the forearm bones, or between individual carpal bones, results from loss of the bony relationships and/or

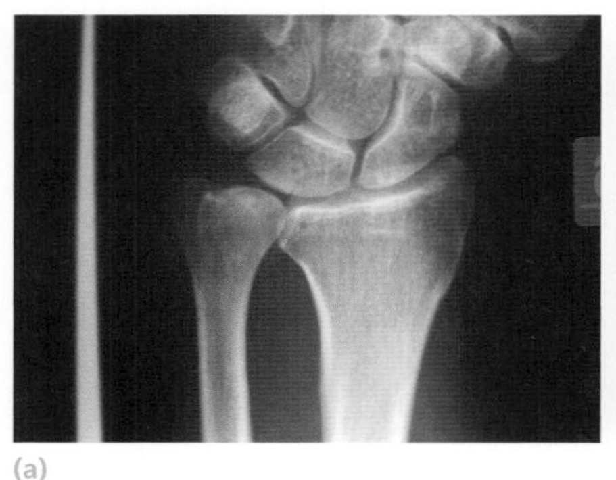

(a)

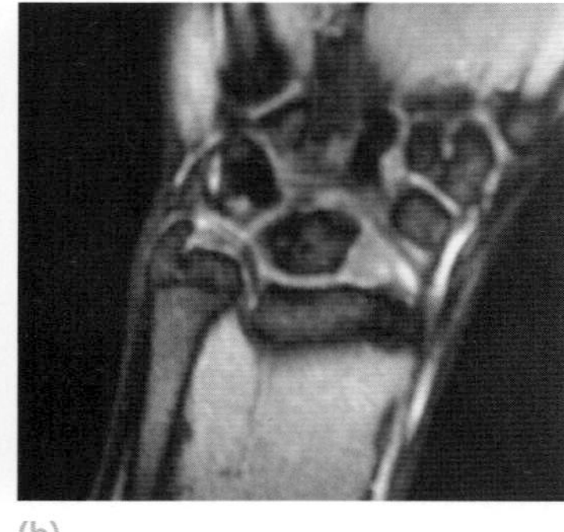

(b)

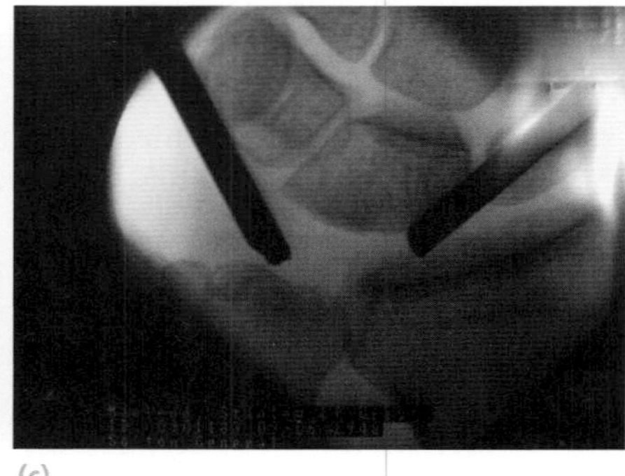

(c)

15.15 Ulno-carpal impaction (a) X-ray; (b) MRI; (c) intra-operative x-ray during arthroscopic removal of the distal dome of the ulna.

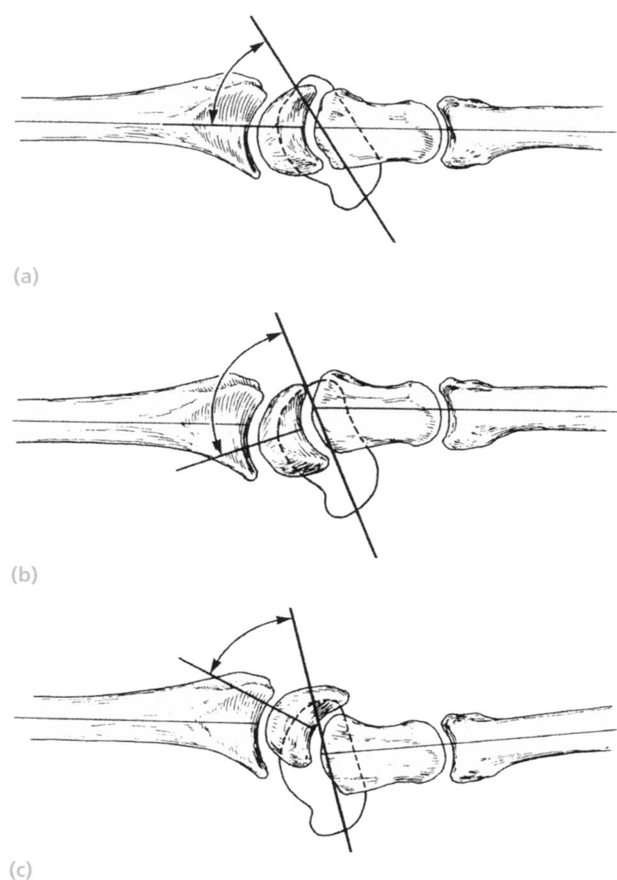

15.16 Carpal instability The relationships of the carpal bones in (a) the normal wrist, (b) DISI and (c) VISI.

ligamentous constraints which normally stabilize the wrist. The initiating cause is usually some type of injury – a wrist sprain with ligament damage, subluxation or dislocation at one of the radio-carpal or intercarpal joints or a fracture of one of the wrist bones – but chronic instability may also arise insidiously in erosive joint disorders such a rheumatoid arthritis.

PATTERNS OF CARPAL INSTABILITY

Acute carpal injuries are dealt with in Chapter 25. Here we shall consider the problems associated with chronic carpal instability. The disorder affects mainly the intercalated segment (proximal carpal row) of the wrist. The common patterns are:

Dorsal intercalated segment instability (DISI) Following a fracture of the scaphoid or rupture of the scapholunate ligament (scapho-lunate dissociation), the lunate no longer passively follows the scaphoid. The scaphoid tends to flex and the lunate assumes its default position of extension (dorsal tilt).

Volar intercalated segment instability (VISI) Less commonly, the luno-triquetral ligament is ruptured. The lunate, unrestrained by the triquetrum, but still controlled by the scaphoid, tends to flex whilst the capitate tends to extend.

Midcarpal instability This usually emerges as a chronic problem, associated with generalized ligamentous laxity. The proximal and distal rows become unstable through the midcarpal joint.

Adaptive midcarpal instability If a distal radius fracture heals with the radial articular surface tilted dorsally, then the proximal carpal row tends also to tilt dorsally and the midcarpal joint flexes to maintain the palm in line with the forearm. This is painful and grip is reduced.

Radio-carpal translocation Chronic synovitis and articular erosion (as in RA) gradually leads to attenuation of the wrist ligaments and subluxation of the entire radio-carpal joint. In advanced RA the carpus usually shifts ulnarwards and simultaneously deviates into abduction and supination.

Clinical features of carpal instability

The patient with scapho-lunate or luno-triquetral incompetence presents with pain and weakness of the wrist, and sometimes also clunking during movement or gripping actions. It is important to enquire about any previous injury, however trivial it may have seemed at the time.

On examination, there may be generalized tenderness over the carpus from synovitis or more localized tenderness, for example at the scapho-lunate junction or over the scaphoid itself. Grip strength is reduced. Provocative tests are useful.

Watson's test for scapho-lunate incompetence Thumb pressure is applied to the volar aspect of the wrist over the distal pole of the scaphoid (this restores the alignment of the volar-tilted scaphoid). While maintaining this position, the wrist is moved alternately into adduction and abduction. A painful 'clunk' occurs as the proximal pole of the scaphoid subluxes dorsally.

Luno-triquetral ballottement With one hand the examiner grasps and stabilizes the lunate between index finger and thumb. With the other thumb he presses on the pisiform/triquetrum to produce a shearing motion between lunate and triquetrum. If there is pain and excessive movement, this suggests incompetence of the luno-triquetral ligament.

Pivot shift test The examiner grasps the patient's forearm with one hand and the patient's hand with the other; he then compresses the wrist axially while moving it from abduction to adduction. A painful 'clunk' suggests mid-carpal instability.

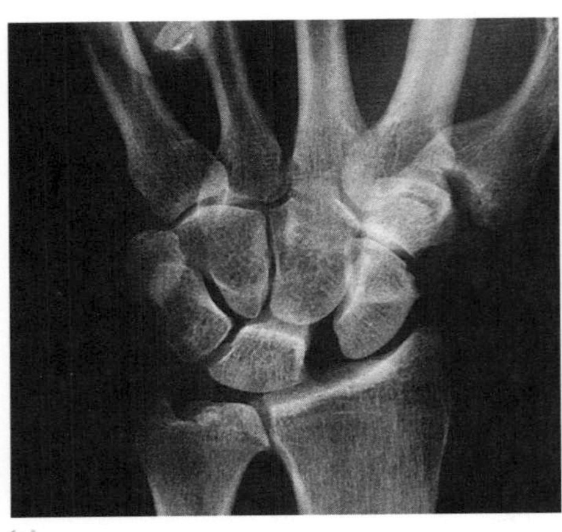
(a)

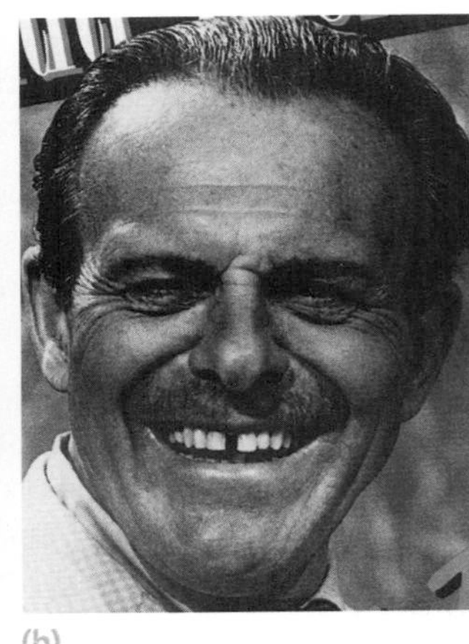
(b)

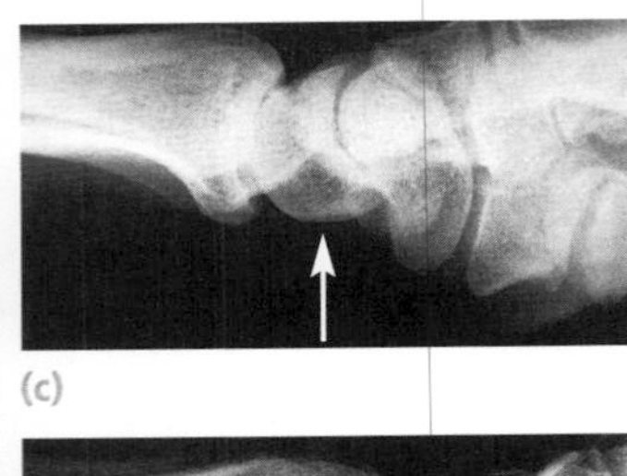
(c)

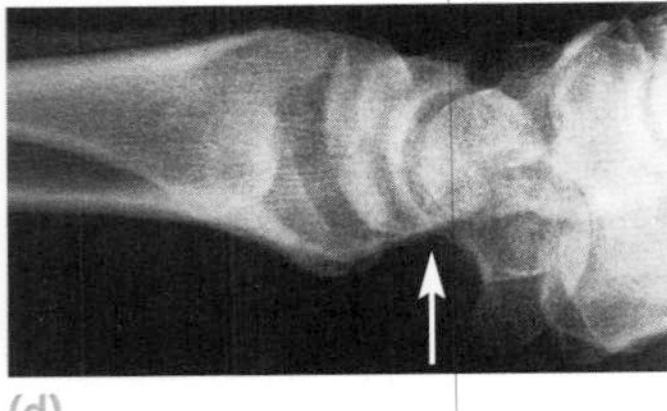
(d)

15.17 Carpal instability **(a)** A year after 'straining' his wrist this patient was still complaining of pain; the x-ray shows a gap between the scaphoid and lunate (the *Terry-Thomas sign*) and rotation of the scaphoid. **(b)** The actor Terry Thomas with the trademark gap between his front teeth (reproduced by permission; © United Artists Inc.). **(c)** In the lateral view the lunate is tilted dorsally and the scaphoid ventrally (DISI); compare this with **(d)**, an example of VISI, showing volar tilt of the lunate.

X-rays

An anteroposterior x-ray may show an old or new scaphoid fracture. There may be widening of the scapho-lunate interval (*the Terry-Thomas sign*); if the scaphoid is flexed, it will look foreshortened and the tubercle may appear as a dense 'ring' in the bone.

A true lateral view is examined to assess the relative alignment of the distal radius, the lunate, capitate and scaphoid. In a normal wrist, the articular surfaces of the radius, lunate and capitate are parallel. In the DISI deformity, the capitate axis is shifted dorsally but it flexes relative to the lunate, the lunate tilts backwards and the scaphoid flexes; the scapho-lunate angle is greater than 70 degrees. In a VISI deformity, the lunate is flexed forwards and the scapho-lunate angle is less than 30 degrees; the capitate tilts dorsally.

In an anteroposterior 'clenched fist view' the scaphoid is seen to flex and a scapho-lunate gap becomes more apparent.

Anteroposterior views with the wrist adducted and abducted emphasize scapho-lunate gaps and abnormal scaphoid flexion (the ring sign), particularly when compared with x-rays of the other side.

Further investigations

Image intensification helps to define the site of instability in difficult cases.

Arthrography shows leakage of contrast through incompetent scapho-lunate or luno-triquetral spaces.

MRI will reveal any associated injuries, such as a scaphoid fracture. The scapho-lunate and luno-triquetral interosseous ligaments are so slim that the resolution of MRI scanning may be inadequate to detect significant injuries.

Arthroscopy of the radio-carpal and midcarpal joints is the best method for demonstrating carpal instability. Ligament tears, certain patterns of instability, synovitis and damaged articular cartilage can be detected.

Treatment

Scapho-lunate and luno-triquetral dissociation The best results are obtained if the ligaments heal in an anatomical position. The diagnosis should, therefore, be made as soon as possible after injury; this requires a high index of suspicion. The surgeon should be alerted by a history of wrist pain following a fall on the outstretched hand and a finding of midcarpal tenderness. Arthrography or arthroscopy may be needed to secure the diagnosis. The ligaments are repaired, the bones stabilized with K-wires and the wrist held in a cast for at least 2 months.

Patients seen more than 3 months after injury will require a more extensive type of carpal reduction and ligament reconstruction. For scapho-lunate incompetence various reconstructions have been described. Perhaps the Brunelli is the most reliable. Half of flexor carpi radialis tendon is passed through a drill hole in the scaphoid and then secured across the back of the carpus. This pulls up the flexed scaphoid from its flexed position and tightens the carpus transversely.

If the displacement cannot be reduced, or if soft-tissue repair fails or if osteoarthritis supervenes, then a salvage operation is needed. The options include a proximal row carpectomy (if the lunate-capitate junction is preserved) or a scaphoid excision with four-corner fusion (if the lunate-capitate joint is arthritic or if the patient needs the strongest wrist especially in torsion).

For *luno-triquetral instability*, tendon reconstruction is not reliable enough. A luno-triquetral fusion is the most suitable treatment.

Symptomatic midcarpal instability Treatment includes proprioceptive training (a gyroscopic device can help). Intractable symptoms may respond to arthroscopic shrinkage of the capsule with a diathermy probe. The alternative of a ligament reconstruction is unreliable, and midcarpal fusion causes very significant loss of movement (about 50 per cent).

Dorsal malunions of the distal radius A dorsal tilt deformity that is symptomatic may be treated by a corrective osteotomy of the distal radius; normal carpal alignment should be restored.

KIENBÖCK'S DISEASE

Robert Kienböck, in 1910, described what he called 'traumatic softening' of the lunate bone. This is a form of ischaemic necrosis, probably due to chronic stress or injury, though one cannot be certain about this. It has been suggested that relative shortening of the ulna ('negative ulnar variance') predisposes to stress overload of the lunate between the distal edge of the radius and the carpus, but this has not been proven convincingly.

Pathology

As in other forms of ischaemic necrosis, the pathological changes proceed in four stages: *stage 1*, ischaemia without naked-eye or radiographic abnormality; *stage 2*, trabecular necrosis with reactive new bone formation and increased radiographic density, but little or no distortion of shape; *stage 3*, collapse of the bone; and *stage 4*, disruption of radio-carpal congruence and secondary osteoarthritis.

Clinical features

The patient, usually a young adult, complains of ache and stiffness; only occasionally is there a history of acute trauma. Tenderness is localized over the lunate

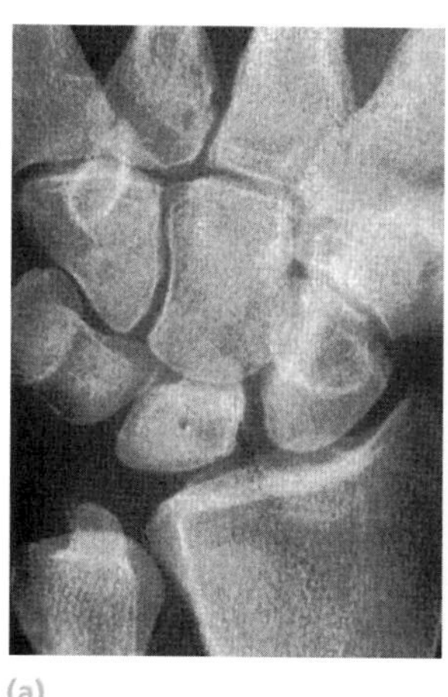
(a)

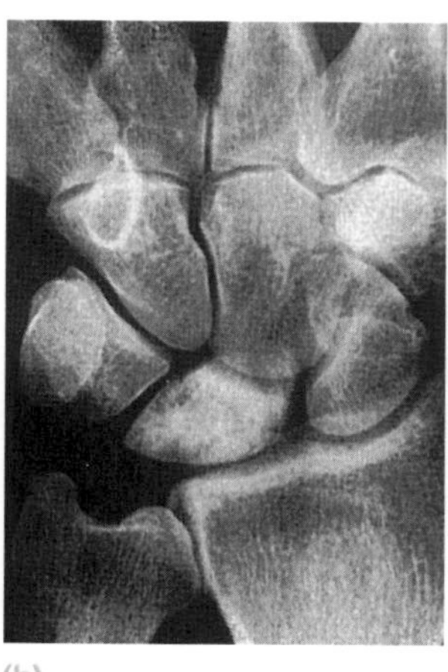
(b)

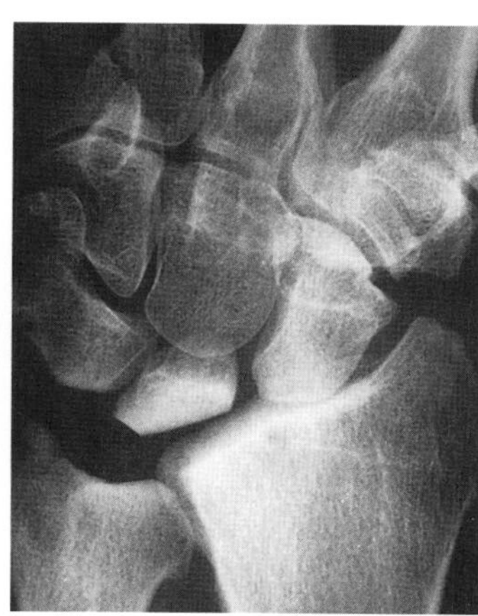
(c)

15.18 Kienböck's disease (a) In stage 2 the bone shows mottled increase of density, but is still normal in shape. (b) In stage 3 density is more marked and the lunate looks slightly squashed. (c) In stage 4 the bone has collapsed and there is radio-carpal osteoarthritis. In all three the ulna looks disproportionately short.

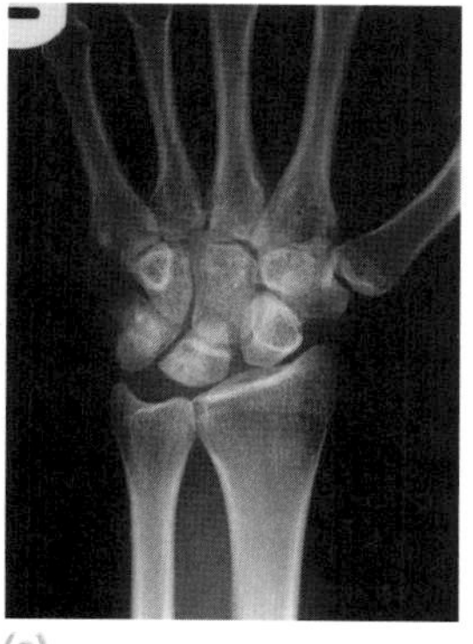
(a)

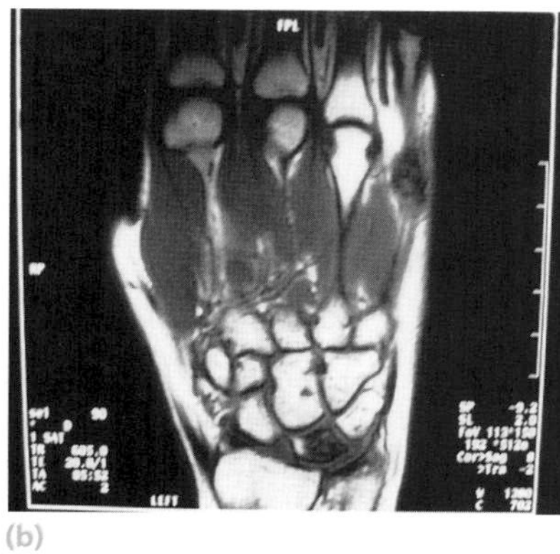

(b)

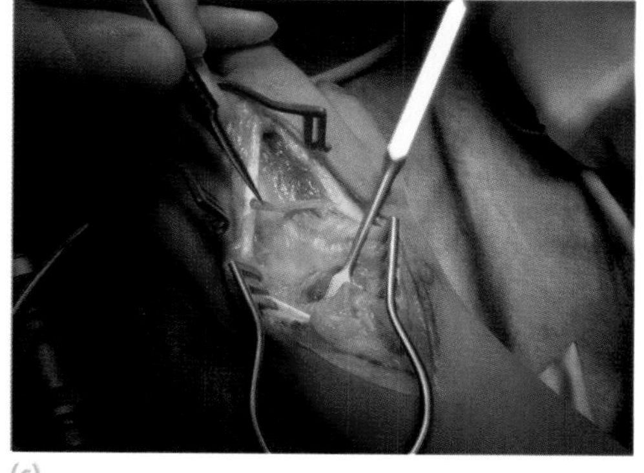
(c)

15.19 Kienböck's disease grade (a) Not seen on x-ray; (b) seen on MRI scan; (c) treated by vascular bundle implantation.

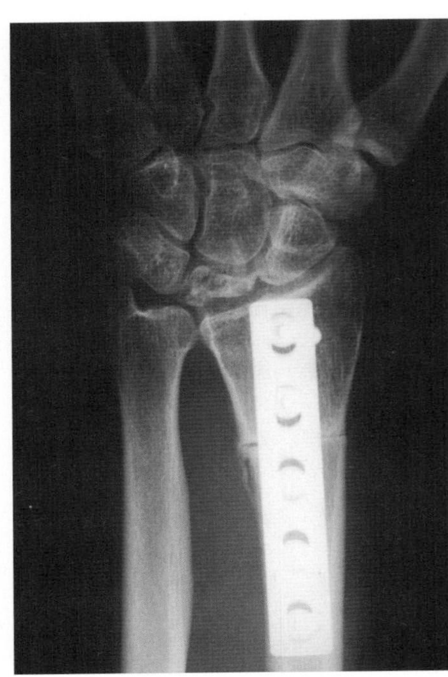

(a)

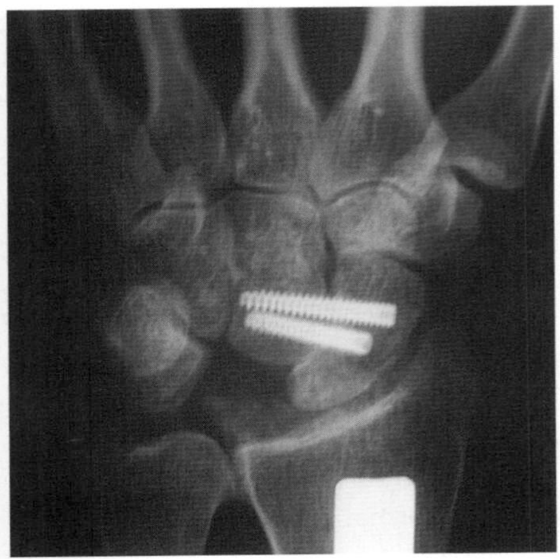

(b)

15.20 Kienböck's disease-treatment (a) Radial shortening; (b) scapho-capitate fusion.

and grip strength is diminished. In the later stages wrist movements are limited and painful.

Imaging

X-rays at first show no abnormality, but radioscintigraphy may reveal increased activity. Later, x-rays may show either mottled or diffuse density of the bone, and later still the bone looks intensely sclerotic and irregular in shape or squashed. The capitate migrates proximally into the space left by the collapsing lunate and the scaphoid flexes forward. Eventually, there are osteoarthritic changes in the wrist. Ulnar variance should be assessed by standardized x-ray examination with the shoulder abducted to 90 degrees, the forearm in neutral rotation and the wrist in neutral flexion-extension. As the lunate collapses, the relative length of the capitate from third metacarpal bone to distal radius increases.

MRI is the most reliable way of detecting the early changes. A gadolinium-enhanced MRI scan will demonstrate the condition even if plain x-rays are normal.

Treatment

NON-OPERATIVE TREATMENT

In early cases, splintage of the wrist for 6–12 weeks relieves pain and possibly reduces mechanical stress. If bone healing catches up with ischaemia, the lunate may remain virtually undistorted; this is more likely in very young patients. However, if pain persists, and even more so if the bone begins to flatten, operative treatment is indicated.

Table 15.1 Stages of Kienböck's Disease

Stage	X-ray, MRI	Treatment
1	Normal x-ray, changes on MRI	Cast for 3 months Vascularized bone graft
2	Lunate sclerosis on plain x-ray, fracture lines sometimes present	Vascularized bone graft If negative ulnar variance: radial shortening If positive ulnar variance: radial dome osteotomy
3a	Fragmentation of lunate; height preserved	Proximal row carpectomy
3b	Collapse of lunate, proximal migration of capitate, fixed scaphoid rotation	Scapho-capitate fusion Scapho-trapezium-trapezoid fusion Proximal row carpectomy
4	Midcarpal or radio-carpal arthritis	Proximal row carpectomy Total wrist fusion Wrist replacement

OPERATIVE TREATMENT

In its earliest stages, before collapse, the bone can be revascularized with a pedicled bone graft or vascular bundle implantation.

While the wrist architecture is only minimally disturbed (i.e. up to early stage 3), it seems rational to aim for a reduction of carpal stress by shortening the radius. The same effect can be achieved by lengthening the ulna, but a bone graft is needed and union is less predictable.

Once the bone has collapsed, the options are limited. A wrist neurectomy is worth trying; this will preserve movement yet reduce pain. Lunate replacement by a silicone prosthesis, once popular, gives poor long-term results and particle shedding is liable to cause synovitis. Other procedures, such as intercarpal fusion or excision of the proximal row of the carpus, may improve function but in the long term may not prevent the occurrence of osteoarthritis.

If pain and restriction of movement become intolerable, *radio-carpal arthrodesis* is the one reliable way of providing a stable, pain-free wrist. Wrist replacement is an alternative in individuals with lesser demands.

PREISER'S DISEASE

This is a very rare condition in which the scaphoid undergoes spontaneous avascular necrosis. Early disease, diagnosed on MRI, can respond to vascularized bone grafting. Later symptomatic disease with advanced destruction of the scaphoid would need joint-preserving surgery (proximal row carpectomy or scaphoidectomy–four-corner fusion).

TUBERCULOSIS (see also Chapter 2)

At the wrist, tuberculosis is rarely seen until it has progressed to a true arthritis. Pain and stiffness come on gradually and the hand feels weak. The forearm looks wasted; the wrist is swollen and feels warm. Involvement of the flexor tendon compartment may give rise to a large fluctuant swelling that crosses the wrist into the palm (compound palmar ganglion). In a neglected case there may be a sinus. Movements are restricted and painful.

X-rays show localized osteoporosis and irregularity of the radio-carpal and intercarpal joints; there may also be bone erosion.

Diagnosis

The condition must be differentiated from rheumatoid arthritis. Bilateral arthritis of the wrist is nearly always rheumatoid in origin, but when only one wrist is affected the signs resemble those of tuberculosis. X-rays and serological tests may establish the diagnosis, but often a biopsy is necessary.

Treatment

Antituberculous drugs are given and the wrist is splinted. If an abscess forms, it must be drained. If the wrist is destroyed, systemic treatment should be continued until the disease is quiescent and the wrist is then arthrodesed.

RHEUMATOID ARTHRITIS
(see also Chapter 3)

After the metacarpo-phalangeal (MCP) joints, the wrists and distal radio-ulnar joints are the most common sites of rheumatoid arthritis. Wrist and hand should always be considered together when dealing with this condition.

Pathology

In the early stages, the characteristic features are synovitis of the joints and tendon sheaths. If the disease

(a)

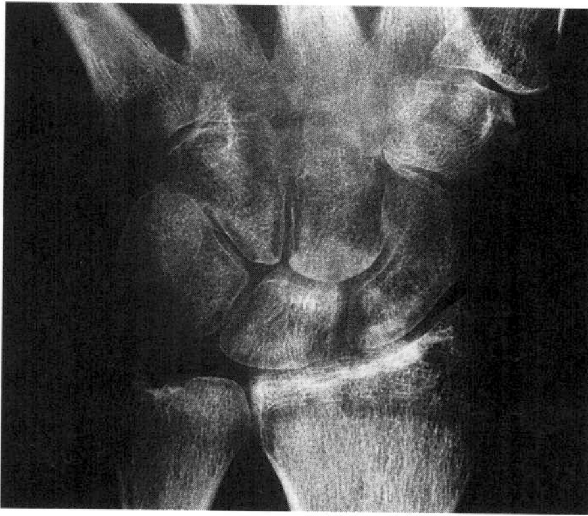

(b)

15.21 Tuberculosis of the wrist (a) Pointing abscess; (b) x-ray showing diffuse osteoporosis.

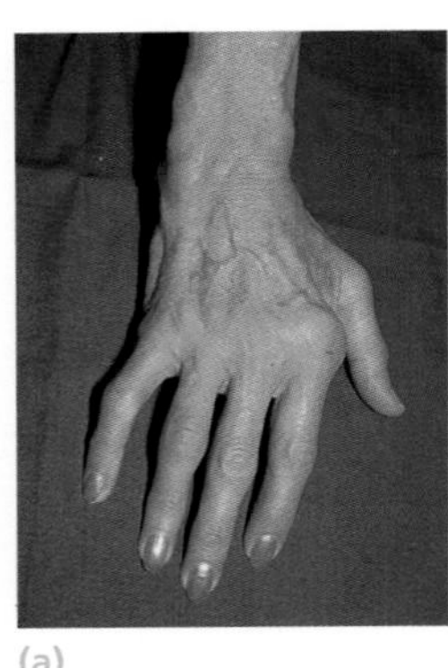

(a)

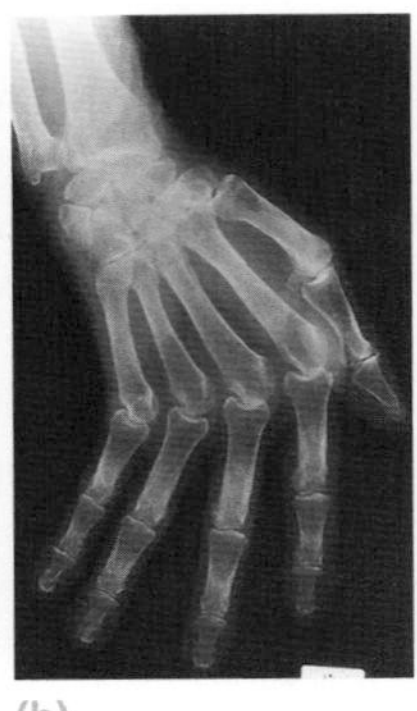

(b)

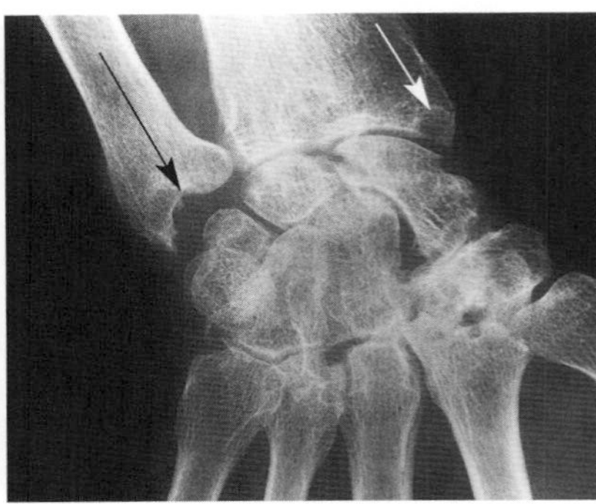

(c)

15.22 Rheumatoid arthritis (a) Typical zig-zag deformity in established rheumatoid arthritis. The wrist is deviated radialwards and the fingers ulnarwards. (b) X-ray of the same patient. (c) Enlarged x-ray view – note the characteristic erosions at the distal ends of the radius and ulna (arrows).

persists, the distal radio-ulnar joint (DRUJ), radio-carpal joint and intercarpal joints become eroded; this, together with attenuation of the ligaments and tendons, leads to instability and progressive deformity of the wrist and hand.

The ulnar side of the carpus gradually shifts towards flexion and volar subluxation, causing the head of the ulna to jut out prominently on the dorsum of the wrist. The proximal carpal row slides ulnarwards and the metacarpal bones deviate radialwards, which mechanically predisposes to a reciprocal ulnar deviation of the fingers – a cardinal feature of the 'rheumatoid hand'. At the same time, the scaphoid falls into marked flexion because of erosion of the interosseous ligaments and loss of carpal height. The combination of instability and erosive tenosynovitis eventually leads to tendon rupture – typically one or more of the long extensor tendons.

An unstable wrist means a weak hand; deformities of the MCP joints are almost invariably associated with complementary deformities of the wrist.

Clinical features

Early symptoms are pain, swelling and stiffness of the wrists. At first the swelling is usually localized to the common extensor tendon sheath or the extensor carpi ulnaris, but as time progresses the joints become thickened and tender. Swelling of the synovium in the carpal tunnel may cause median nerve compression.

Gradually the wrist becomes unstable as the articular surfaces erode and ligaments become attenuated. Early infiltration of tendons may lead to weakness of wrist extension and flexion. Instability of the DRUJ aggravates the dorsal protrusion of the ulnar head, which can often be jogged up and down by pressing upon it with your thumb (the *piano-key sign*).

Tendon lesions are common in the late stage. The first to rupture is usually the extensor digiti minimi, followed by the extensor communis tendons of the little and ring fingers. Extensor pollicis longus tendon is also vulnerable. The flexor tendons also sometimes rupture, either within the digital sheaths or in the cramped confines of the carpal tunnel.

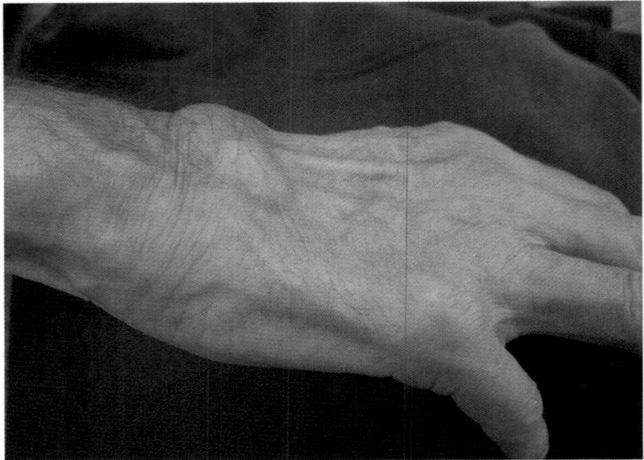

15.23 Rheumatoid arthritis Synovitis around the ulnar head with rupture of extensor digiti minimi.

The proximal joints in both upper limbs should be examined as well. It is important to know whether the arm is able to place the wrist and hand in functional positions.

X-rays

Typical signs are peri-articular osteoporosis and erosion of the ulnar styloid and the radio-carpal and intercarpal joints. In most cases the hands also will be affected, but there is a well-recognized group of patients (mostly elderly men) in whom the wrists carry the brunt of the disease.

Treatment

EARLY STAGE DISEASE

During the early stages of rheumatoid arthritis the objectives of treatment are to relieve pain and counteract synovitis. In addition to systemic treatment, synovitis of the wrist and/or tendons will be helped by intermittent splintage and intrasynovial injections of corticosteroid preparations.

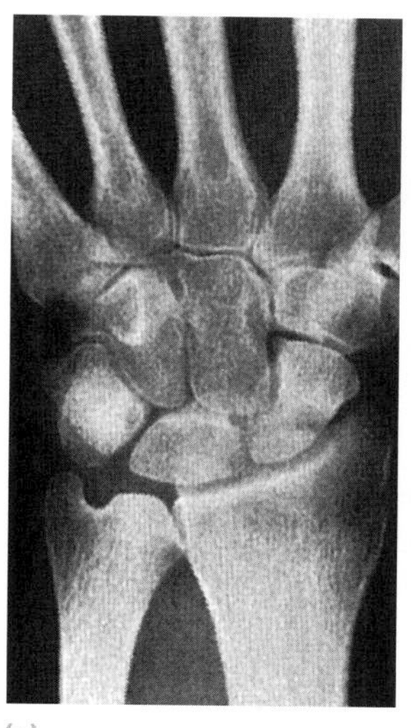
(a)

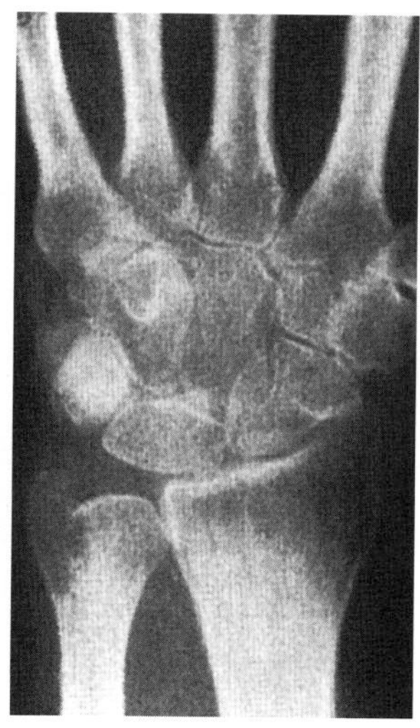
(b)

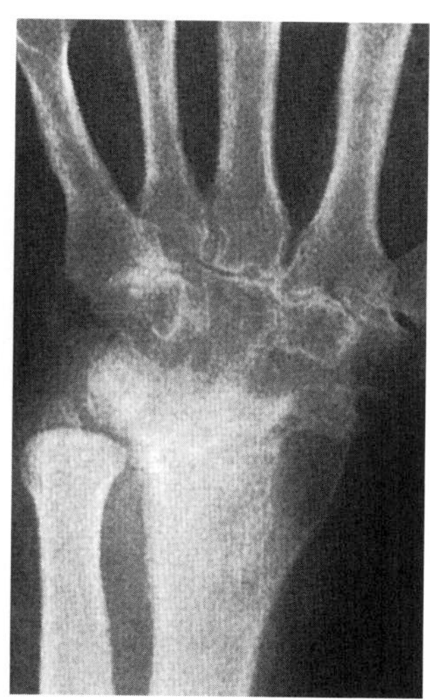
(c)

15.24 Rheumatoid arthritis (a) At first the x-rays show only soft-tissue swelling. (b) Two years later, this patient shows early bone changes – peri-articular osteoporosis and diminution of the joint space. (c) Five years later still, bony erosions and joint destruction are marked.

ESTABLISHED DISEASE

As joint erosion makes its appearance, the focus turns increasingly to the safeguarding of joint stability and the prevention of deformity.

Extensor tenosynovectomy and soft-tissue stabilization of the wrist may forestall further deterioration. Through a dorsal longitudinal incision the extensor retinaculum is exposed and carefully dissected but left attached at the radial side. The thickened synovium around the extensor tendons, as well as any bony protrusions on the back of the wrist, are removed. The preserved extensor retinaculum is then placed beneath the tendons to further reduce the risk of later tendon rupture.

If the *radio-ulnar joint* is involved, synovectomy can be combined with excision of the ulnar head and transposition of the extensor carpi radialis longus to the ulnar side of the wrist (to counteract the tendency to radial deviation). Fusion of the lunate to the radius (Chamay procedure) prevents ulnar slide of the carpus.

Flexor tenosynovitis is not as obvious as extensor tendon involvement. It may present as *carpal tunnel syndrome* – median nerve compression by swollen tendons in the carpal tunnel – which requires open release of the flexor retinaculum and tenosynovectomy. Obvious bony protrusions in the floor of the carpal tunnel (due to carpal collapse) should be removed and the raw area covered with a soft-tissue flap. Bear in mind that median nerve symptoms in patients with rheumatoid arthritis may be caused by pathology in the proximal part of the limb or the cervical spine, so these patients should always undergo nerve conduction studies and electromyography before the carpal tunnel decompression.

LATE DISEASE

In the late stage tendon ruptures at the wrist, joint destruction, instability and deformity may require reconstructive surgery.

Ruptured extensor tendons can seldom be repaired; side-to-side suture of a distal tendon stump to an adjacent tendon, tendon grafting or tendon transfer gives a satisfactory if not perfect result.

Rupture of the flexor pollicis longus tendon in the carpal tunnel may be caused by scuffing of the tendon against the distal pole of the scaphoid or the edge of the trapezium – the so-called *'Mannerfelt lesion'*. Repair or grafting gives disappointing results; the simplest way of dealing with this problem is to fuse the thumb interphalangeal joint and rely on the other motors to manipulate this important digit.

Painful joint destruction, instability and deformity can be dealt with by either joint replacement or arthrodesis. Arthroplasty using a silicone 'spacer' has a high failure rate; silicone synovitis and the difficulty of revision have led to it being abandoned. Total wrist replacement with a metal–polyethylene device is becoming more reliable, but is only suitable for those with well-preserved bone stock.

Arthrodesis is widely considered to be the best option for dealing with painful instability in the radiocarpal joint. If the wrist is already 'fusing' itself spontaneously, simple stabilization with a Steinman pin passed between the second and third metacarpals, across the carpus and into the distal radius is all that is needed. Bone grafts are not necessarily added but can be taken from the ulnar head if it is excised. For patients with better bone stock, pin fixation is inadequate; formal arthrodesis with a wrist fusion plate is preferable. In this group, ulnar head replacement rather than ulnar head excision should be considered.

As a general rule, wrist deformities should be corrected before hand deformities. Furthermore the dominant wrist should, if possible, be fused in slight extension to provide reliable power grip, while the non-dominant wrist is fused in some flexion (or replaced) so as to provide the posture needed for perineal care.

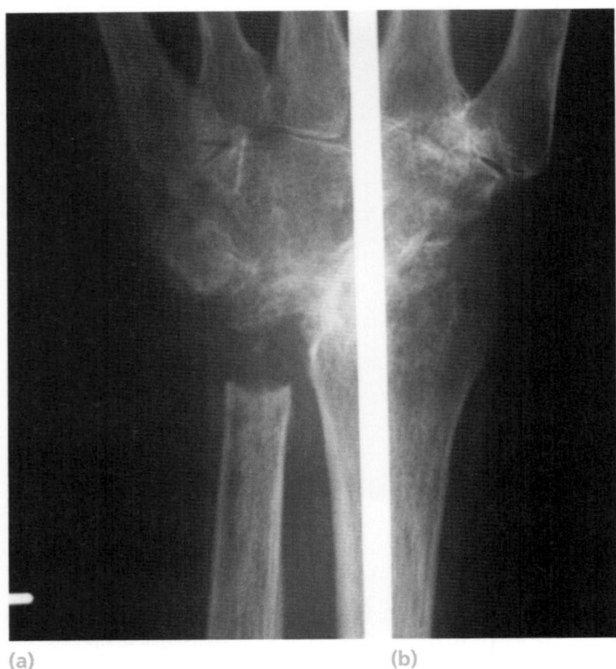

(a) (b)

15.25 Rheumatoid arthritis wrist fusion Surgical fusion using a long intramedullary pin. The ulnar head has been excised.

OSTEOARTHRITIS OF THE WRIST

Osteoarthritis of the wrist appears at three main sites: the radio-carpal joint, the distal radio-ulnar joint and the first carpo-metacarpal joint. Since these usually present as distinct syndromes, they are considered separately.

RADIO-CARPAL OSTEOARTHRITIS

Osteoarthritis of the radio-carpal joint is uncommon and when it does occur it is sometimes a late sequel to an injury such as an intra-articular fracture of the distal radius, an ununited or malunited fracture of the scaphoid, scapholunate ligament rupture or Kienböck's disease; yet it should be borne in mind that, while trauma of all kinds is common, only a fraction of all such injuries lead to arthritis in later life.

Clinical features

The patient may have forgotten the original injury. Years later he or she complains of pain and stiffness. At first these symptoms occur intermittently after use; later they become more constant, with frequent exacerbations or recurrent 'wrist sprains'.

The appearance may be normal but there is often swelling over the back of the wrist and movements are limited and painful.

X-rays

Typical features are narrowing of the radio-carpal joint, subchondral sclerosis and osteophyte formation at the margins of the joint. A predisposing cause, such as an old fracture or Kienböck's disease, may be apparent.

Treatment

CONSERVATIVE MEASURES

Analgesic medication and rest, in a polythene splint, are often sufficient treatment. However, if pain is intolerable or if function is seriously disturbed (e.g. if the patient is unable to grip firmly or lift moderately heavy objects), surgical options have to be considered.

SURGICAL TREATMENT

Partial excision of the radial styloid Osteoarthritis following a scaphoid fracture may be limited to that part of the joint. In that case excision of the tip of the radial styloid process is helpful, but no more than 7 mm must be removed to avoid destabilizing the carpus. This can be done by open or arthroscopic means and at the same time a partial wrist denervation may be performed.

OPERATIONS ON CARPAL BONES

For advanced changes, it may be necessary to operate on the carpus, but wrist movement should be preserved if possible. The entire proximal row of carpal bones can be removed *(proximal row carpectomy);* the head of the capitate then articulates on the lunate fossa of the radius. In some cases *scaphoidectomy and four-corner fusion* may be more appropriate: the lunate–capitate–hamate–triquetrum are fused with wires, a circular plate or buried screws.

TYPICAL SITES OF X-RAY CHANGES

Distal radius: radius-scaphoid degeneration

Scaphoid fracture (SNAC wrist = scaphoid non-union advanced collapse)
- Stage 1: radial styloid and distal scaphoid
- Stage 2: scapho-capitate joint (proximal scaphoid and reciprocal radius spared, cf. scapho-lunate arthritis)
- Stage 3: peri-scaphoid arthritis, lunate-capitate arthritis. Lunate-radius preserved

Scapho-lunate ligament failure (SLAC wrist = scapho-lunate advanced collapse)
- Stage 1: radial styloid and distal scaphoid
- Stage 2: entire radioscaphoid joint
- Stage 3: capitate-lunate joint. Lunate-radius preserved

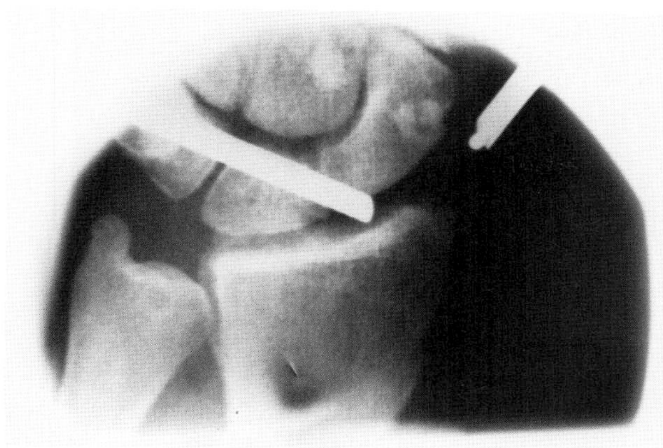

15.26 Radio-carpal arthritis Early stage treated by arthroscopic radial styloidectomy.

The outcome of these procedures is similar (about 60 per cent grip strength, 60 per cent movement). Proximal row carpectomy is easier to perform and risks fewer complications; four-corner fusion gives a more stable grip in torsion.

Total arthrodesis of the wrist This is occasionally necessary. The radio-carpal and intercarpal joints are decorticated, bone graft is impacted and a compression plate is fixed to the third metacarpal and the distal radius. Contouring the plate to 15 degrees of dorsiflexion improves grip strength.

Arthroplasty Wrist replacement with metal or polythene implants is becoming more reliable, although at present this operation is reserved for those with low functional demands. Long-term survivorship studies have yet to show whether replacement arthroplasty will hold up in patients with higher demands.

Distal radio-ulnar arthritis

Progressive destruction of the distal radio-ulnar joint is a characteristic feature of severe rheumatoid arthritis. Lesser degenerative changes are seen in secondary osteoarthritis, possibly following marked and longstanding instability of the joint.

If pain and loss of function cannot be controlled by conservative measures, the patient may benefit from ulnar head replacement. Older operations that involve excision of the ulnar head have been abandoned because of the high risk of causing severe and intractable instability.

Carpo-metacarpal osteoarthritis

Osteoarthritis of the trapezio-metacarpal joint is common in postmenopausal women. It is often accompanied by Heberden's nodes of the finger joints, in which case it is usually bilateral and part of a generalized osteoarthritis.

Clinical features

The patient, usually a middle-aged or older woman, complains of diffuse pain around the base of her thumb. Pinch and grip are weakened. On examination, the joint is swollen and in advanced cases is held in an adducted position, with prominence of the subluxed metacarpal base. With more established fixed adduction of the thumb base, the metacarpophalangeal joint hyperextends to provide a competent thumb–index span. The carpo-metacarpal joint is tender and the 'grind test' (compressing and rotating

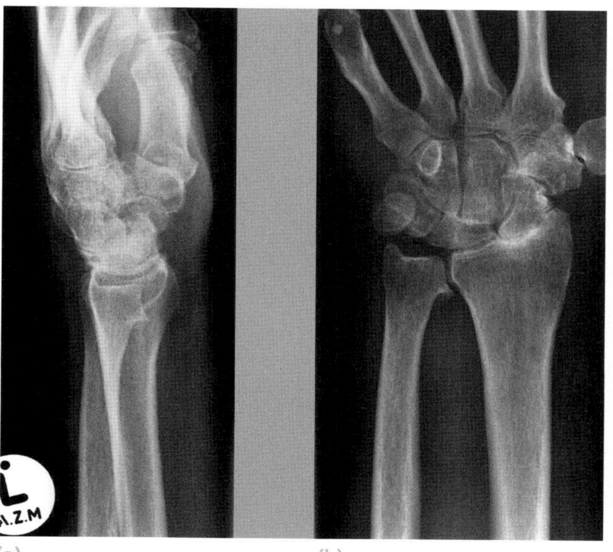

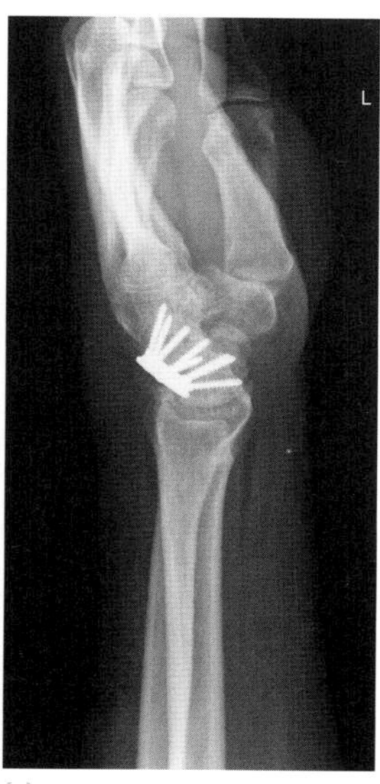

(a) (b) (c)

15.27 Radiocarpal arthritis (a,b) The so-called 'SLAC wrist' – scapho-lunate advanced collapse; (c) treated by scaphoid excision and four-corner fusion.

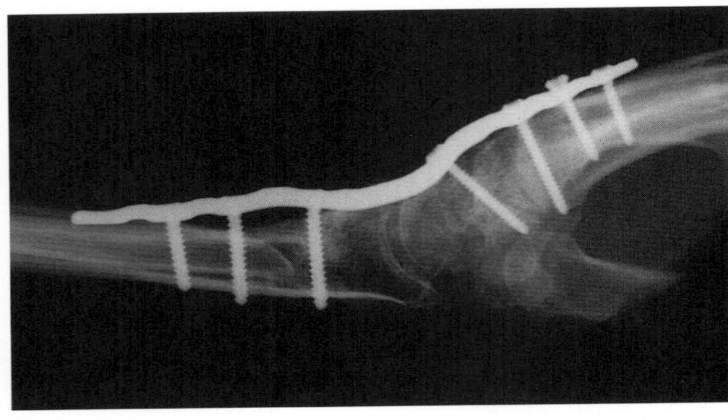

(a)

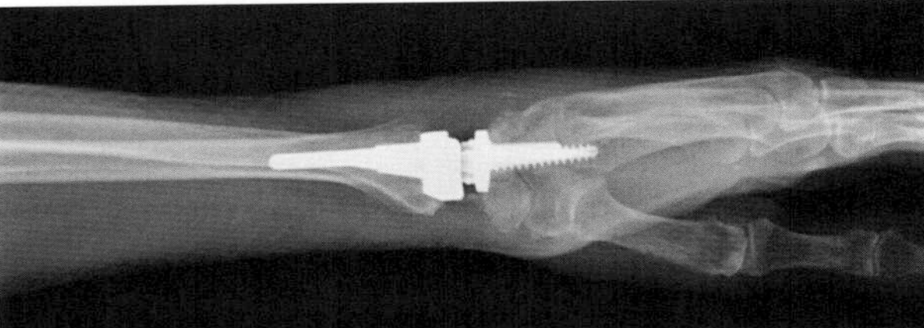

(b)

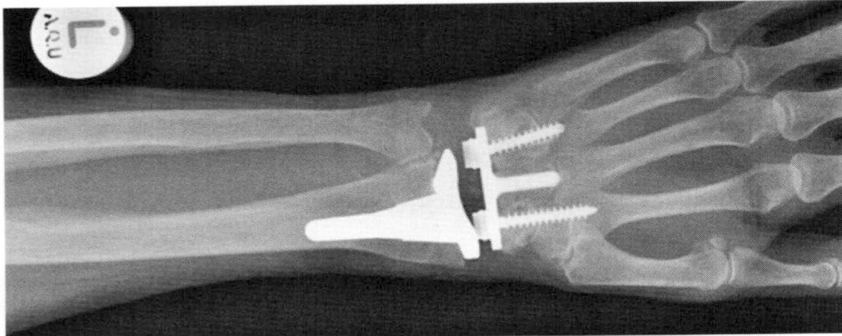

(c)

15.28 Wrist arthritis (a) Total wrist fusion; (b,c) total wrist replacement.

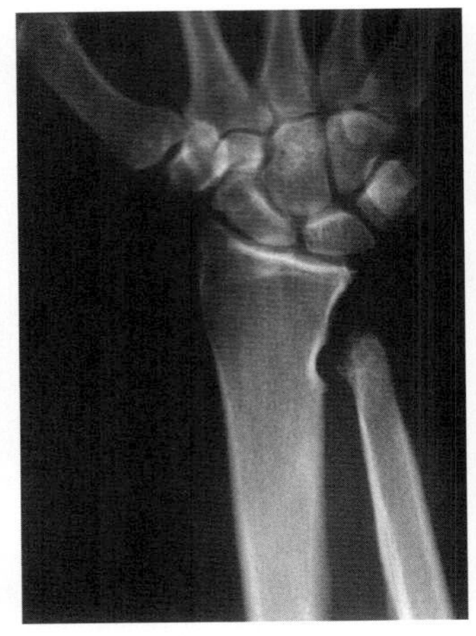

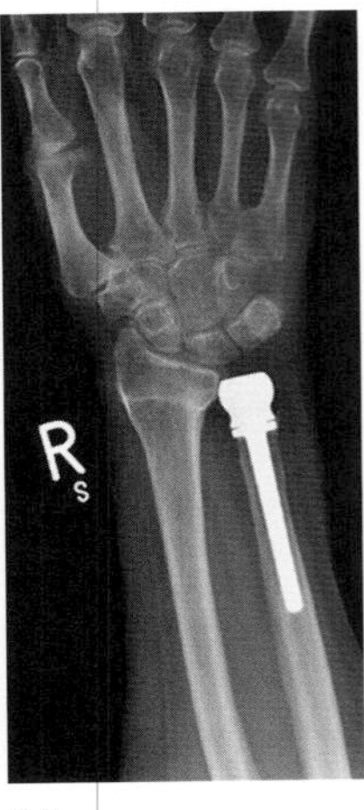

(a) (b)

15.29 Distal radio-ulnar joint arthritis – operative treatment (a) Excising too much of the distal ulna may cause painful radio-ulnar impingement. (b) One alternative is an ulnar head replacement.

the metacarpal longitudinally against the trapezium) is painful.

X-rays show narrowing and then lateral subluxation of the trapezio-metacarpal joint. Radioscintigraphy is useful in early cases when the diagnosis is in doubt; increased activity precedes the more obvious x-ray changes.

Treatment

Most patients can be treated by anti-inflammatory preparations, local corticosteroid injections and temporary splintage. There may be a role for intra-articular hyaluronidase. If these measures fail to control pain, or if instability becomes marked, operative treatment is considered.

SURGICAL TREATMENT

Joint-preserving operations In early cases, joint-preserving operations are helpful in about 70 per cent. The options are either *extension osteotomy* or *ligament reconstruction*. These procedures alter the joint forces and thus improve pain and function.

Excisional arthroplasty Excision of the trapezium gives pain relief and return of function, though thumb pinch is always weak. The bone can be removed through either the palmar approach or the anatomical snuffbox, taking care not to damage the superficial radial nerve, the radial artery or the flexor carpi radialis tendon. Attempts have been made to prevent postoperative collapse of the joint and proximal migration of the metacarpal by re-routing a slip of flexor carpi radialis or abductor pollicis longus tendon and attaching it to a drill hole in the metacarpal base; the benefit of this extra intervention has not been established.

Replacement arthroplasty Replacement arthroplasty using a silicone spacer has a high complication rate and the results are unpredictable. Metal-on-polyethene implants and pyrocarbon implants are also available but longer-term outcome is uncertain.

Arthrodesis Arthrodesis of the trapezio-metacarpal joint relieves pain, but the restriction of movement and high failure rate are distinct drawbacks. The scapho-trapezial joint should be normal.

If the metacarpo-phalangeal joint has been secondarily damaged by hyperextension, then either a sesamoid arthrodesis (which restores flexion but preserves movement) or fusion (at 25 degrees for stable pinch) is indicated.

SCAPHOID-TRAPEZIUM-TRAPEZOID (STT) ARTHRITIS

The joint between the distal end of the scaphoid and the underside of the trapezium and trapezoid ('the triscaphe joint') can develop arthritis either in isola-

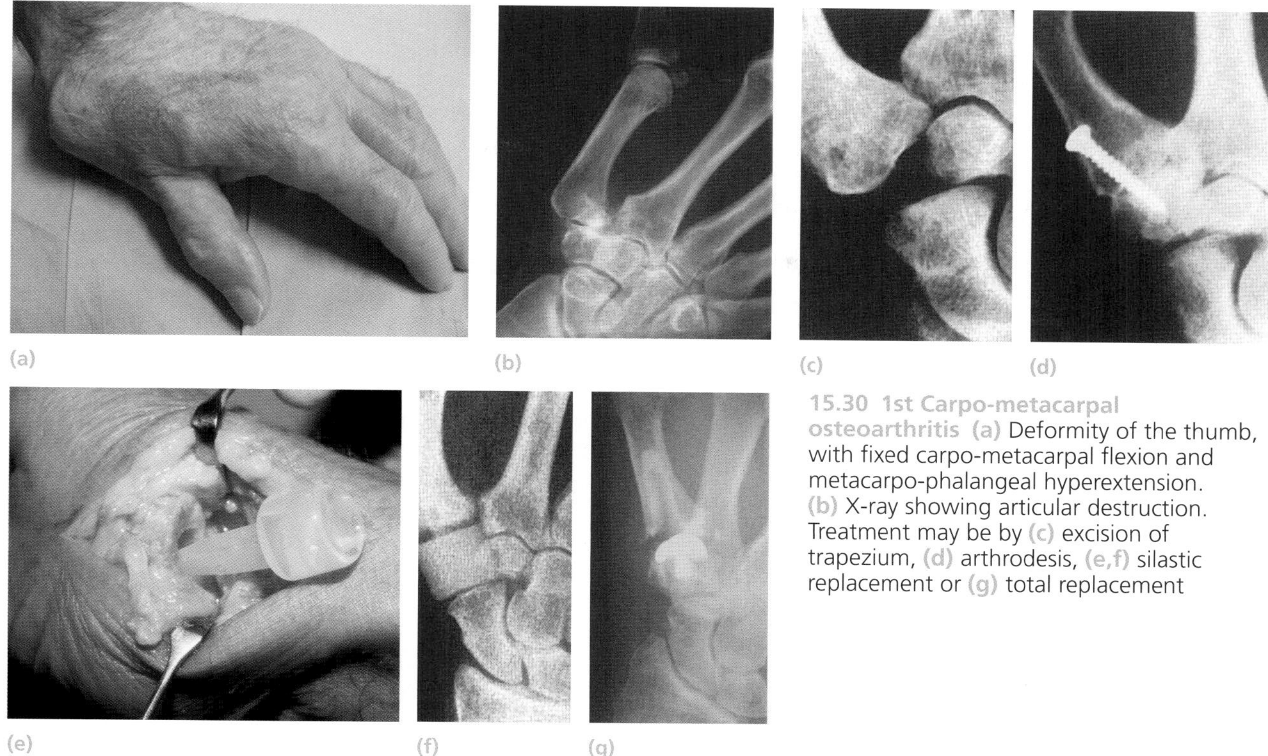

15.30 1st Carpo-metacarpal osteoarthritis (a) Deformity of the thumb, with fixed carpo-metacarpal flexion and metacarpo-phalangeal hyperextension. (b) X-ray showing articular destruction. Treatment may be by (c) excision of trapezium, (d) arthrodesis, (e,f) silastic replacement or (g) total replacement

tion or in association with arthritis of the carpo-metacarpal joint.

Late middle-aged females are most commonly affected. The patient points to the front of the scaphoid tubercle as the source of the pain (whereas in carpo-metacarpal arthritis the patient points to the back of the thumb base).

Treatment

Treatment is initially along standard lines – adaptive measures, anti-inflammatory medication, cortisone injection and splintage.

Patients with severe symptoms may benefit from surgery. However, there is as yet no completely satis-

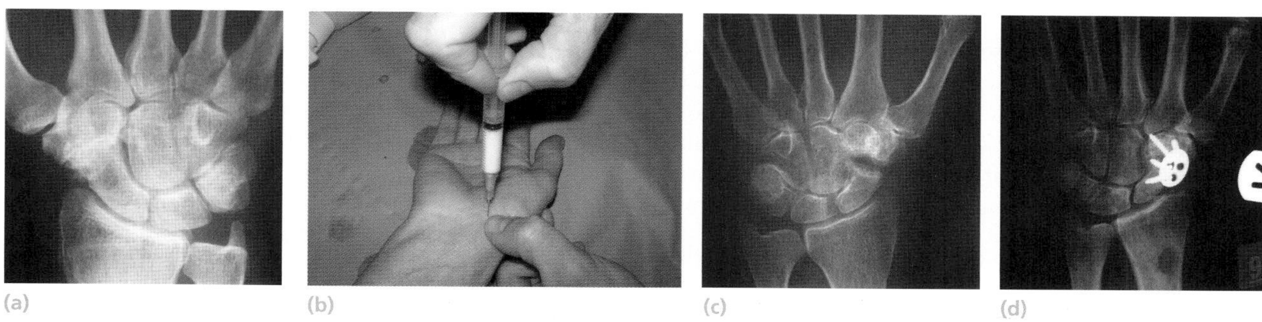

15.31 Scaphoid-trapezium-trapezoid arthritis (a) Changes on x-ray; (b) steroid injection; (c) distal pole of scaphoid excision (do not remove too much!); (d) STT fusion.

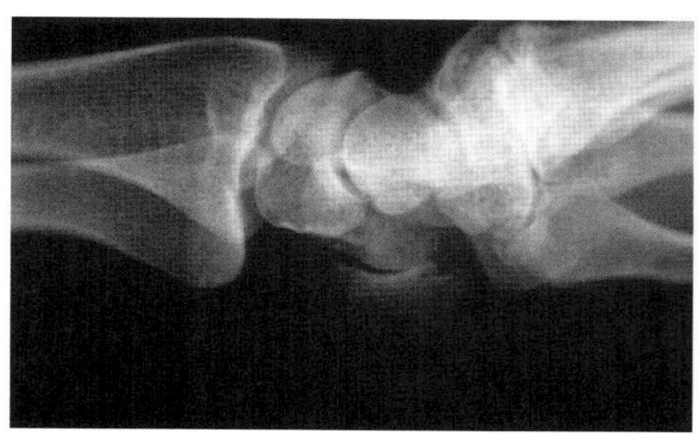

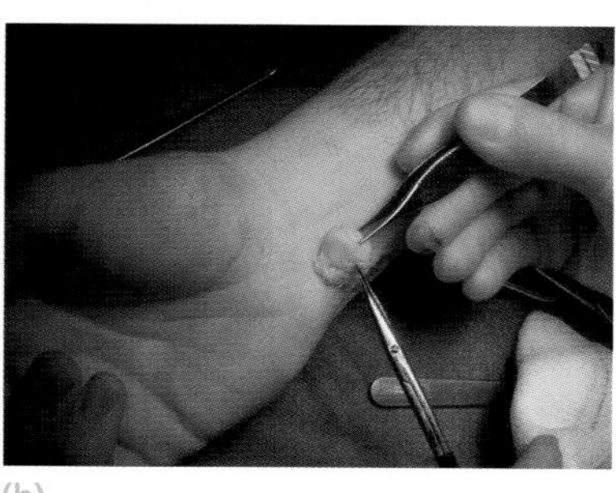

15.32 Piso-triquetral arthritis (a) Shown on 30° supinated view. (b) Pisiform excision gives good results – but beware the ulnar nerve!

factory operation. *STT fusion* removes the painful joint but is technically difficult. *Excision of the distal pole of the scaphoid* is easier but can cause midcarpal collapse. *Trapeziectomy with under-cutting of the trapezoid* is probably the most reliable and straightforward, especially if there is concomitant trapeziometacarpal arthritis. *Pyrocarbon interposition arthroplasty* has also been employed but long-term follow-up data are lacking.

TENOSYNOVITIS AND TENOVAGINITIS

The extensor retinaculum has six compartments which transmit tendons lined with synovium. Tenosynovitis can be caused by unaccustomed overuse but sometimes it occurs spontaneously. The resulting synovial inflammation causes secondary thickening of the sheath and stenosis of the compartment, which further compromises the tendon. Early treatment, including rest, anti-inflammatory medication and injection of corticosteroids, may break this vicious circle.

The first dorsal compartment (abductor pollicis longus and extensor pollicis brevis) and the second dorsal compartment (extensor carpi radialis brevis) are most commonly affected.

The flexor tendons are affected far less frequently.

De Quervain's disease

Pathology

This condition, first described in 1895, is caused by reactive thickening of the sheath around the extensor pollicis brevis and abductor pollicis longus tendons within the first extensor compartment. It may be initiated by overuse but it also occurs spontaneously, particularly in middle-aged women, and sometimes during pregnancy.

Clinical features The patient is usually a woman aged 40–50, who complains of pain on the radial side of the wrist. There may be a history of unaccustomed activity such as pruning roses or wringing out clothes. Sometimes there is a visible swelling over the radial styloid and the tendon sheath feels thick and hard. Tenderness is most acute at the very tip of the radial styloid.

The pathognomonic sign is elicited by *Finkelstein's test*. The examiner places the patient's thumb across the palm in full flexion and then, holding the patient's hand firmly, turns the wrist sharply into adduction. In a positive test this is acutely painful; repeating the movement with the thumb left free is relatively painless. Resisted thumb extension (hitch-hiker's sign) is also painful.

The *differential diagnosis* includes arthritis at the base of the thumb, scaphoid non-union and the intersection syndrome (see below).

Treatment

The early case can be relieved by a corticosteroid injection into the tendon sheath, sometimes combined with hand therapy (ultrasound, frictions, splintage). Resistant cases need an operation, which consists of slitting the thickened tendon sheath. Sometimes there is duplication of tendons and even of the sheath, in which case both sheaths need to be divided. Care should be taken to prevent injury to the dorsal sensory branches of the radial nerve, which may cause intractable dysaesthesia.

Intersection syndrome

This condition, otherwise known as *crossover syndrome* or *peri-tendinitis crepitans*, is characterized by pain, swelling and crepitus over the tendons of extensor pollicis brevis and abductor pollicis longus 4–6 cm proximal to the extensor retinaculum. It is found in weight-lifters, canoeists and rowers. It should be dis-

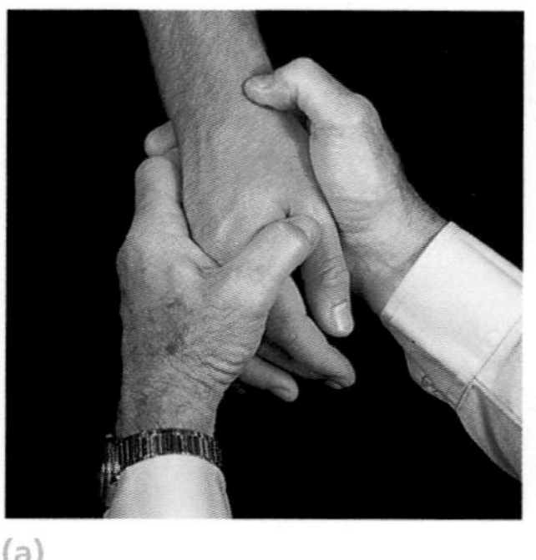
(a)

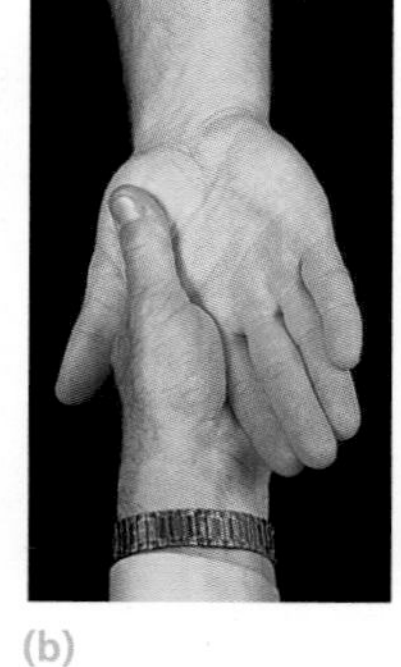
(b)

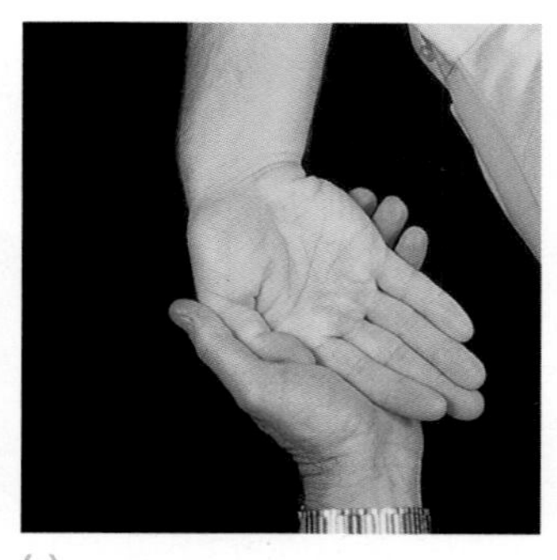
(c)

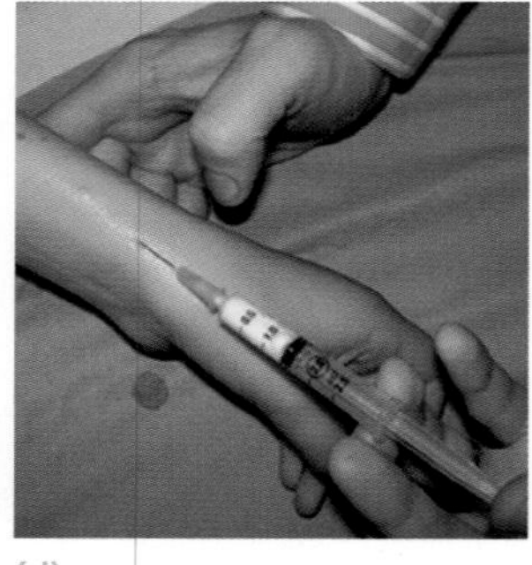
(d)

15.33 De Quervain's disease (a) There is point tenderness at the tip of the radial styloid process. (b,c) Finkelstein's test: Ulnar deviation with the thumb left free is relatively painless (b), but if the movement is repeated with the thumb held close to the palm (c), the pull on the thumb tendons causes intense pain. (d) Injecting the tendon sheath.

tinguished clinically from de Quervain's disease. The condition is generally attributed to friction between these tendons (the so-called 'outcropping tendons') and the underlying longitudinally-aligned extensor tendons, leading to an adventitious bursa or a tenosynovitis. There is usually an associated tenosynovitis within the second extensor compartment containing extensors carpi radialis longus and brevis.

Treatment involves rest, splintage, steroid injection and, in resistant cases, surgical widening of the second compartment and exploration of the intersection.

OTHER SITES OF EXTENSOR TENOSYNOVITIS

Overuse tenosynovitis of *extensor carpi radialis brevis* (the most powerful extensor of the wrist) or *extensor carpi ulnaris* may cause pain and point tenderness just medial to the anatomical snuffbox or immediately distal to the head of the ulna, respectively (see Figure 15.2). Splintage and corticosteroid injections are usually effective.

The common extensor compartment is occasionally irritated by direct trauma. Patients present with pain and crepitus on the dorsum of the wrist; flexing and extending the fingers produces a fine, palpable crepitus over the common extensor compartment. Treatment is by rest and splintage of the wrist.

Extensor tenosynovitis is also a common feature of rheumatoid disease.

FLEXOR TENDINITIS

Except in specific inflammatory disorders such as rheumatoid arthritis, the flexor tendons are rarely affected.

Flexor carpi radialis tendinitis causes pain on the front of the wrist alongside the scaphoid tubercle; symptoms are reproduced by resisted wrist flexion. Tenderness is sharply localized and should be distinguished from that of de Quervain's disease or osteoarthritis of the basal joint of the thumb.

Flexor carpi ulnaris can become inflamed near its insertion into the pisiform. Occasionally x-rays show calcific deposits around the sheath.

Treatment of these conditions is the same as for the other types of tenosynovitis.

OCCUPATIONAL PAIN DISORDERS

Terms such as *repetitive stress injury* and *cumulative trauma disorder* have been used for a controversial syndrome comprising ill-defined and unusually disabling pain around the wrist and forearm (and sometimes the entire limb) which is usually ascribed to a particular work practice. In some cases there is clinical evidence of tenosynovitis, which could have been caused by unaccustomed or prolonged activity of a particular kind. Other defined and treatable conditions such as carpal tunnel syndrome, thumb base arthritis and de Quervain's should be excluded. Epidemiological studies suggest that these conditions are no more common amongst keyboard operators than in the general population. What has fuelled the controversy surrounding the 'occupational' disorders is their apparent severity and intractability compared with other types of overuse syndrome and the potential rewards for successful litigation. There are often social and psychological aspects which confound the picture. The term 'work relevant upper limb disorder' is preferred as it acknowledges that the symptoms are noticed at work but does not imply causation.

SWELLINGS AROUND THE WRIST

GANGLION CYSTS

Pathology

The ganglion cyst is the most common swelling in the wrist. It arises from leakage of synovial fluid from a

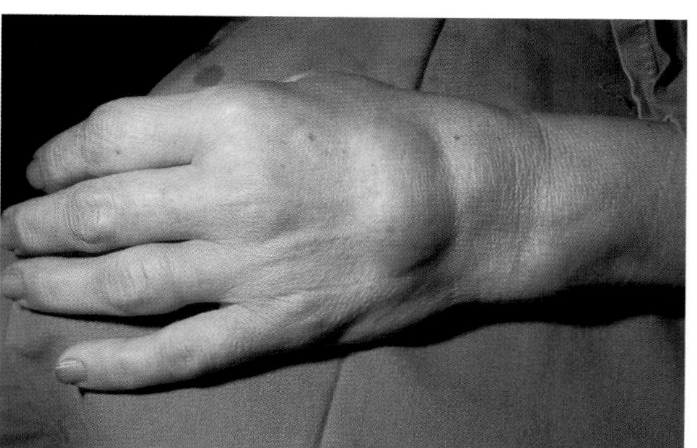
(a)

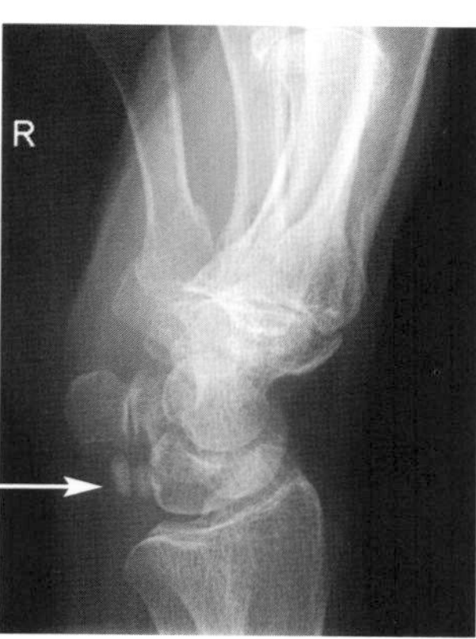

(b)

15.34 Other types of tendinitis (a) Rheumatoid; (b) calcific tendinitis of flexor carpi ulnaris.

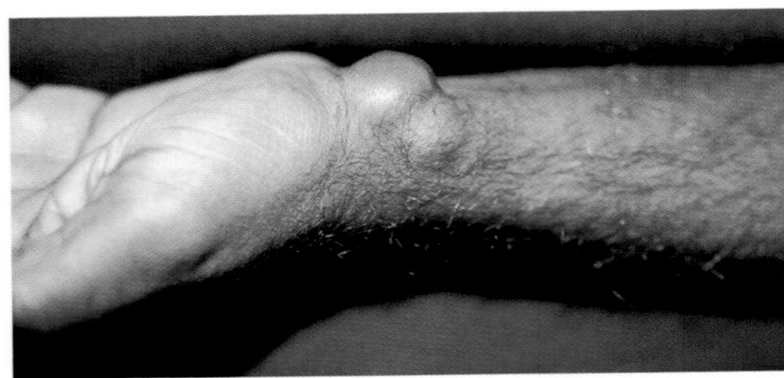

15.35 Volar wrist ganglion

joint or tendon sheath and contains a glairy, viscous fluid. Although it can appear anywhere around the carpus, it usually develops on the dorsal surface of the scapho-lunate ligament. Palmar wrist ganglia usually arise from the scapho-lunate or scapho-trapezio-trapezoid joint.

Clinical features

The patient, often a young adult, presents with a painless lump, though occasionally there is slight ache and weakness. The lump is well defined, cystic and not tender; it can sometimes be transilluminated. It does not move with the tendons. The back of the wrist is the commonest site; less frequently a ganglion emerges alongside the radial artery on the volar aspect. Occasionally a small, hidden ganglion is found to be the cause of compression of the deep (muscular) branch of the ulnar nerve.

Treatment

Treatment is usually unnecessary. The lump can safely be left alone; it often disappears spontaneously. However, it can be aspirated to reassure the patient. If it becomes troublesome – and certainly if there is any pressure on a nerve – operative removal is justified. Even then it may recur with embarrassing persistence; it is not easy to ensure that every shred of abnormal tissue is removed.

Occult ganglion or dorsal synovial impingement

Sometimes patients complain of pain in the back of the wrist, provoked by extending the wrist. On examination there is a discrete tender point over the back of the mid-carpus and the pain is reproduced by full passive wrist extension. Ultrasound, or preferably MRI, will show either a small ganglion or thickening of the synovium at the radio-carpal or midcarpal joint.

Treatment should be initially with a steroid injection; if that fails, then arthroscopic excision may succeed.

Extensor tenosynovitis

Localized swelling of a tendon sheath on the dorsum of the wrist sometimes occurs in rheumatoid disease and can be mistaken for a 'cyst'.

Carpo-metacarpal boss

A firm round swelling over the back of the second and third carpo-metacarpal joint is sometimes seen in a young adult. It is not always tender. It is thought that it may be caused by some instability at the joint.

Treatment involves reassurance; the lump can be excised but if it recurs, the underlying joint should be fused.

'Compound palmar ganglion'

This lesion is neither a ganglion nor compound. Chronic inflammation distends the common sheath of the flexor tendons both above and below the flexor retinaculum. Rheumatoid arthritis and tuberculosis are the commonest causes. The synovial membrane

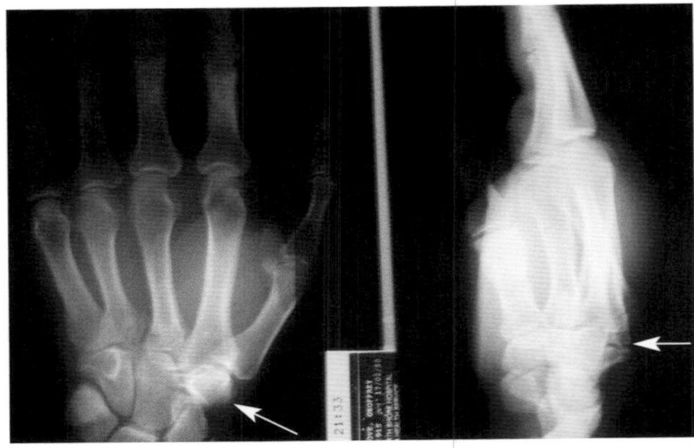

(a)

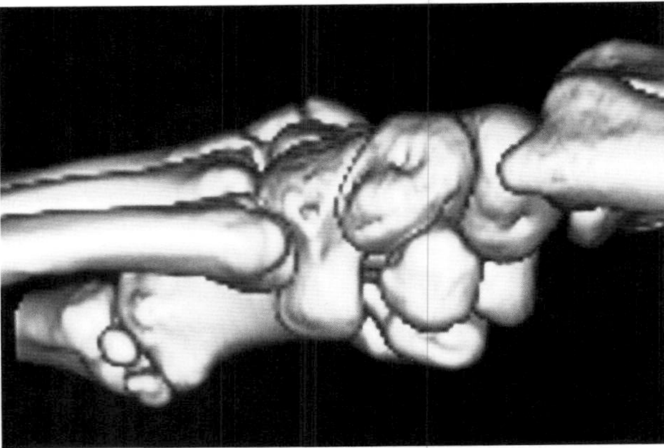

(b)

15.36 Carpo-metacarpal boss (a) X-ray; (b) three-dimensional CT.

becomes thick and villous. The amount of fluid is increased and it may contain fibrin particles moulded by repeated movement to the shape of melon seeds. The tendons may eventually fray and rupture.

Clinical features

Pain is unusual but paraesthesia due to median nerve compression may occur. The swelling is hourglass in shape, bulging above and below the flexor retinaculum; it is not warm or tender; fluid can be pushed from one part to the other (cross-fluctuation).

Treatment

If the condition is tuberculous, general treatment is begun. The contents of the sac are evacuated, streptomycin is instilled and the wrist rested in a splint. If these measures fail, the entire flexor sheath is dissected out. Complete excision is also the best treatment when the cause is rheumatoid disease.

CARPAL TUNNEL SYNDROME

The carpal tunnel syndrome, due to median nerve compression under the flexor retinaculum of the wrist, is described together with other nerve compression disorders in Chapter 11.

NOTES ON APPLIED ANATOMY

In most positions of the forearm the styloid process of the radius is more distal than that of the ulna, but with the forearm supinated the two processes are at approximately the same level. This relationship, known as *ulnar variance*, may be altered as a result of growth abnormalities or injury.

Relative shortness of the ulna appears as an anatomical variant in association with Kienböck's disease. *Relative overlength* is associated with ulna-carpal impaction syndrome (central TFCC perforations and late ulno-carpal arthritis).

Gilula's arcs

These lines are helpful radiographic indicators. They are illustrated in Figure 15.37. The congruent lines between the distal radius/ulna and proximal carpal row, and between the proximal and distal carpal row, are disturbed in midcarpal instability, Kienböck's disease and dislocation of the wrist.

Normal angles: radial tilt 22 degrees, palmar tilt 11 degrees; scapho-lunate angle 30 to 65 degrees.

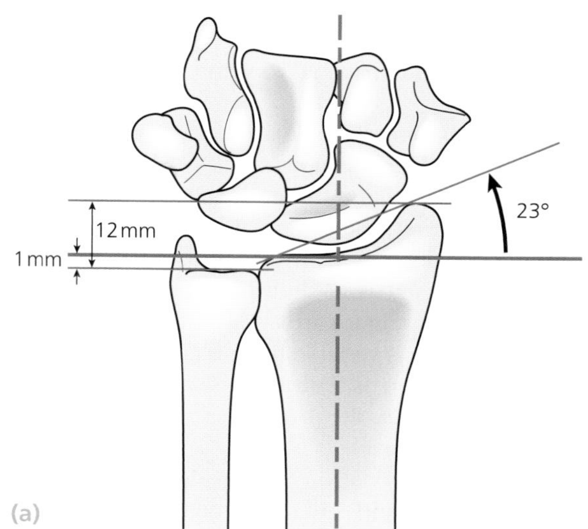

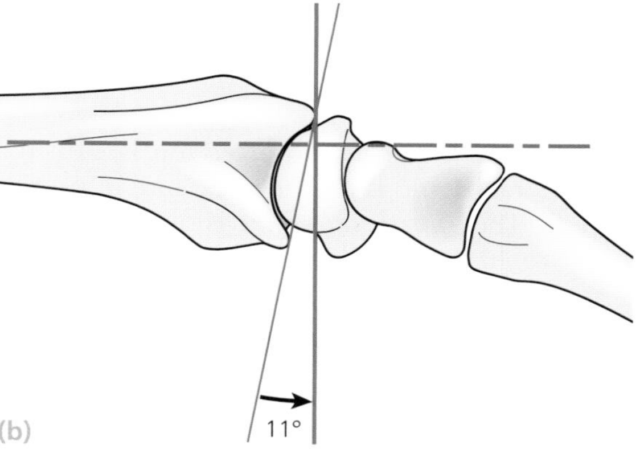

15.37 Angle of the distal radius

Carpal height: the ratio between the distal edge of the capitate and proximal edge of the lunate/third metacarpal is usually 0.54±0.03. The ratio is reduced in carpal collapse (e.g. with Kienböck's disease and scapho-lunate ligament failure).

Just distal to the radial styloid is the scaphoid, immediately beneath the anatomical snuffbox, which is one of the key areas for localizing tenderness. Tenderness at the distal end of the snuffbox may incriminate the carpo-metacarpal joint of the thumb. More proximal tenderness, at the tip of the radial styloid, is characteristic of de Quervain's disease. Dorsal to the snuffbox the oblique course of extensor pollicis longus exposes it to damage by a careless incision.

The carpal bones are arranged in two rows, with the pisiform as the odd man out. The scaphoid crosses both rows. The scaphoid, trapezium and thumb combine to function almost as a separate entity, a 'jointed strut', with independent movement; degenerative arthritis of the wrist occurs most commonly in the joints of this strut.

Kinematics

Wrist flexion: the proximal row and distal row flex and ulnar deviate.

Wrist extension: the proximal row and distal row extend and radially deviate.

Radial deviation: there are two synchronized movements. First, the proximal row flexes (to prevent scaphoid blocking flexion between radial styloid and trapezium); distal row slightly extends. Second, the scaphoid slides ulnarwards, pushing lunate and triquetrum. There is variable flexion and sliding between individuals known as 'column wrist' and 'row wrists'.

Ulnar deviation: the proximal row extends and distal row slightly flexes.

Radial–ulnar deviation is provided 60 per cent by the midcarpal and 40 per cent by the radio-carpal/ulno-carpal joints.

Flexion-extension: this is about 50 per cent mid-carpal and 50 per cent radio-carpal.

Range of movement

Normally the arc of flexion-extension is 110 to 150 degrees; radial tilt is 30 degrees and ulnar tilt 45 degrees. The *functional range* is about 10 degrees flexion to 30 degrees extension.

Surgical anatomy of the nerves

On their volar aspect the carpal bones form a concavity roofed over by the carpal ligament; in the tunnel lie the flexor tendons and the median nerve. The thenar branch of the nerve (supplying the all-important thenar muscles) is in danger if, during a decompression operation, the carpal ligament is divided too far radially. On the dorso-radial side of the wrist, branches of the superficial radial nerve are vulnerable (beware during operations for ganglia, de Quervain's, thumb carpo-metacarpal joint). On the ulnar side, the close relationship of the ulnar nerve to the pisiform and hamate hook must be borne in mind. Operations at the distal end of the ulna threaten the dorsal branch of the ulnar nerve which runs anteriorly about 3 cm proximal to the ulnar styloid.

Ossification of the wrist bones

The ossific centre for the distal radius epiphysis appears at age 2 and fuses at age 16–18. The other bones develop ossification centres in clockwise order (looking at the right hand from behind, fully pronated, i.e. face down). Capitate (1 month), hamate (1 year); triquetrum (2–3 years); lunate (4 years); scaphoid (4–6 years); trapezium (4–6 years); trapezoid (4–6 years); pisiform (8–10 years).

N.B. In an adolescent, the incompletely ossified scaphoid can be mistaken for a scapho-lunate dissociation.

The ligaments of the wrist

The extrinsic ligaments are discrete consolidations of the capsule. The palmar ligaments are stronger than the dorsal (Fig. 15.38).

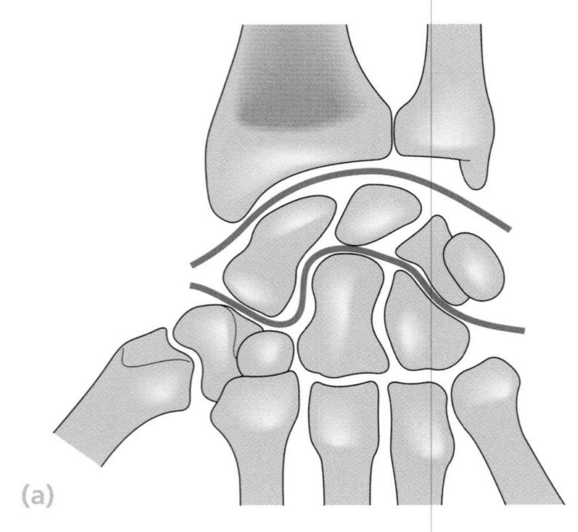

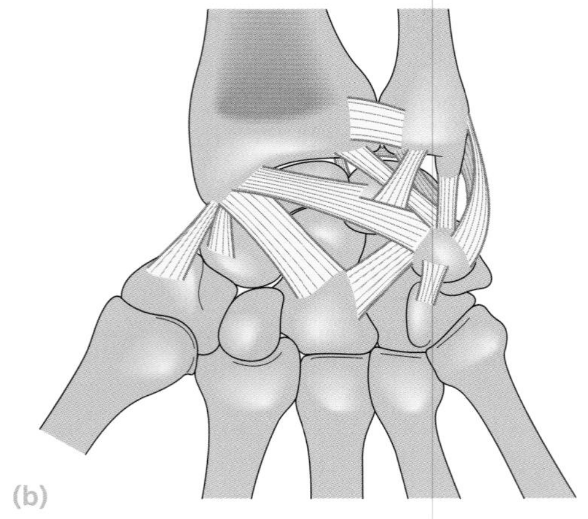

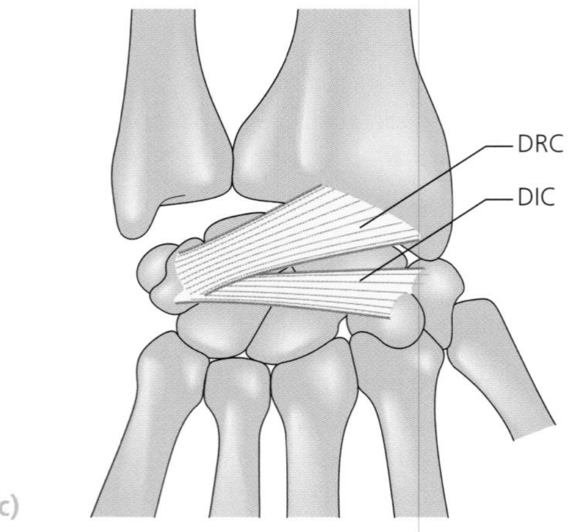

15.38 (a) Gilula's lines; (b) palmar ligaments of the wrist; (c) dorsal ligaments of the wrist. DRC = Dorsal radiocarpal ligament. DIC = Dorsal intercarpal ligament.

EXTRINSIC CARPAL LIGAMENTS (DORSAL)

- *Dorsal radio-carpal ligaments* (radio-scaphoid, radio-triquetral). Rupture contributes to VISI.
- *Dorsal intercarpal ligament* (triquetrum to scaphoid and trapezoid). Available as a donor for tenodesis against palmar rotation of scaphoid.

EXTRINSIC CARPAL LIGAMENTS (PALMAR)

- *Radio-scapho-capitate.* Attaches to palmar edge of radial styloid. Fulcrum for scaphoid flexion. Divided then carefully repaired during palmar approach to scaphoid. Readily seen in arthroscopy. Beware removing attachment by enthusiastic radial styloidectomy.
- *Long radio-lunate ligament.* Restrains lunate from palmar dislocation.
- *Ligament of Testut (radio-scapho-lunate).* Synovial fold, no stabilizing function. Landmark for scapho-lunate ligament in wrist arthroscopy.
- *Short radio-lunate ligament.* From ulnar edge of distal radius to lunate, blends ulnarwards with the ulno-lunate ligament.
- *Ulno-carpal ligament.* Ulno-capitate, ulno-lunate, ulno-triquetral. Blend into volar radio-lunate ligament (i.e. anterior limb of TFCC). Ulno-triquetral ligament blends into sub-sheath of extensor carpi ulnaris (also part of TFCC).

SPACE OF POIRIER

This is the gap between lunate and midcarpal joint through which lunate can dislocate anteriorly.

INTRINSIC (INTEROSSEOUS LIGAMENTS)

- *Scapho-lunate interosseous ligament:* C shaped, thickest dorsally.
- *Luno-triquetral:* C shaped, thickest palmarwards.
- *Capitate-hamate, trapezium-capitate; trapezium-trapezoid.*

Blood supply of the wrist

There are dorsal and palmar arches, supplied by the radial artery, ulnar artery and anterior interosseous artery. These can be used as flaps to vascularize the scaphoid and lunate.

The hand 16

David Warwick, Roderick Dunn

The hand is (in more senses than one) the medium of introduction to the outside world. Its unique repertoire of prehensile movements, grasp, pinch, hook-action and tactile acuity sets us apart from all other species. We can think of the hand as a sophisticated tool, but it is also an organ of communication, used for gesturing and expressing a range of emotions from anxiety and fear to submission and helplessness, scorn and hatred, determination and control, or tenderness and love. We are more aware of our hands than of any other part of the body; when they go wrong we know about it from a very early stage.

CLINICAL ASSESSMENT

SYMPTOMS

Pain may be felt in the palm, the thumb or the finger joints. Remember, though, that a poorly defined pain may be referred from the neck, shoulder or mediastinum.

Deformity may appear suddenly (e.g. due to tendon rupture) or slowly (suggesting bone or joint pathology, a soft-tissue contracture or a postural defect due to a nerve lesion).

Swelling may be localized (and, if associated with throbbing pain, is almost certainly due to infection) or it may be evident in many joints simultaneously. Ask whether the swelling is constant or intermittent, and how long it has been present.

Sensory symptoms and motor weakness provide well-defined clues to neurological disorders. A precise description of the affected area tells us a great deal about the level of the lesion.

Loss of function takes various forms. The patient may have difficulty handling eating utensils, holding a cup or glass, grasping a doorknob (or a crutch), dressing or (most trying of all) attending to personal hygiene. Equally important is loss of function due to sensory change in the fingers.

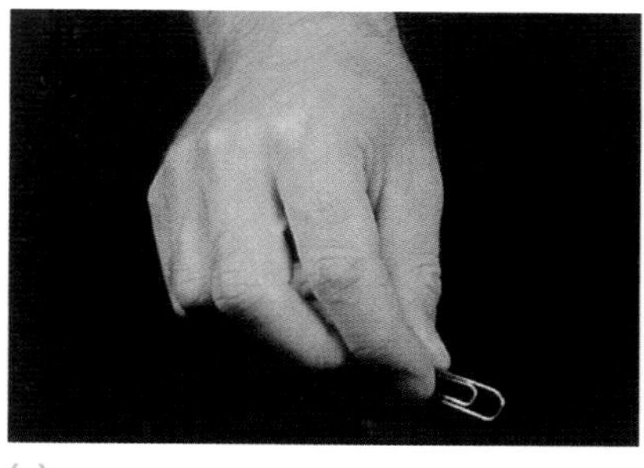

(a)

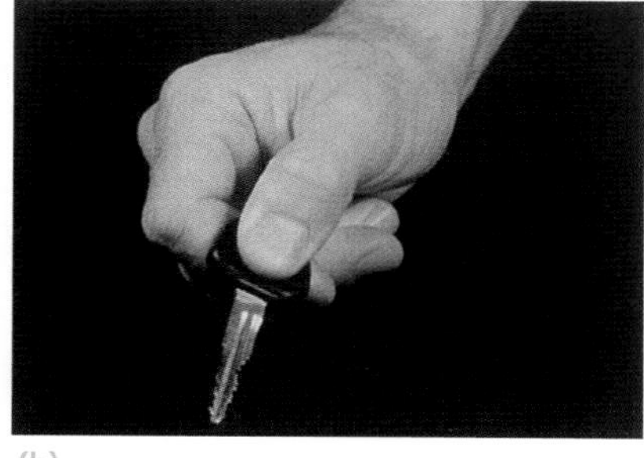

(b)

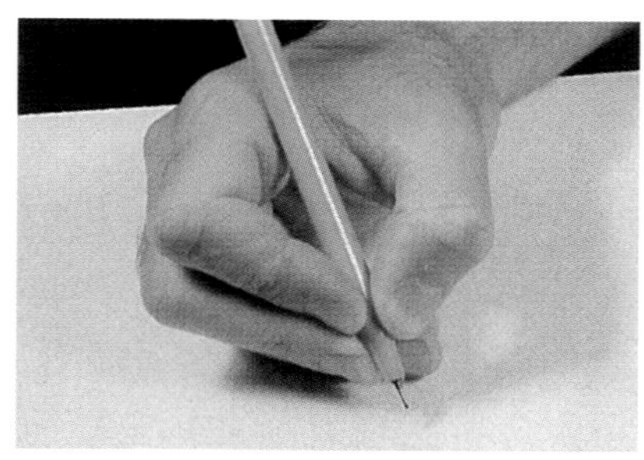

(c)

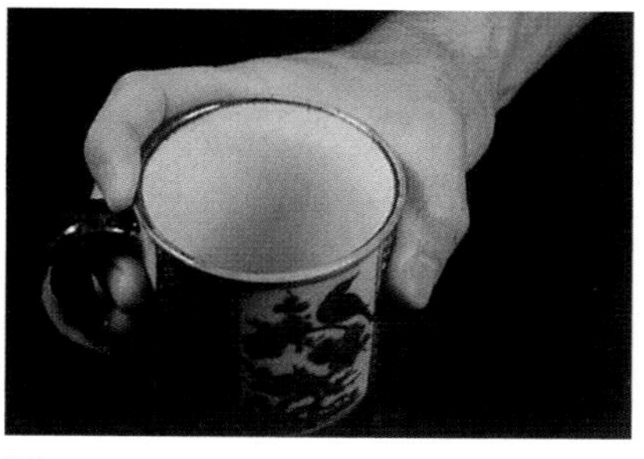

(d)

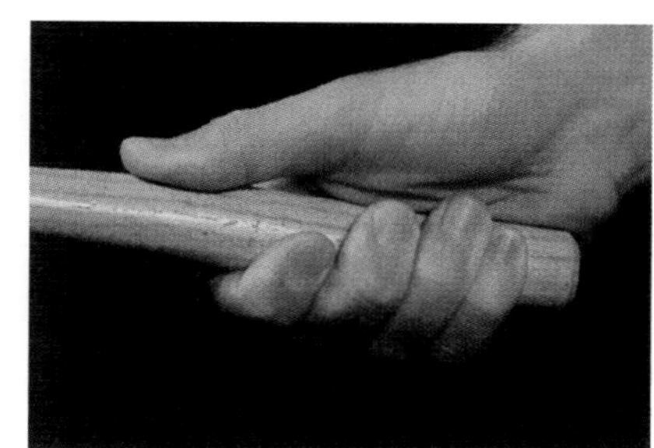

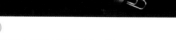

(e)

16.1 Hand function (a) Pinch, (b) key, (c) tripod, (d) grasp and (e) power grip.

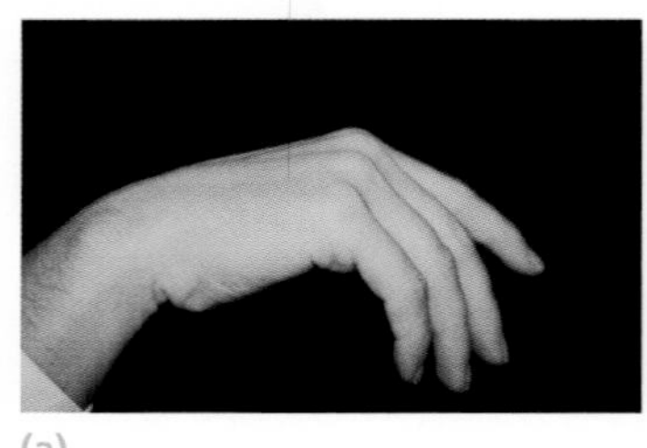

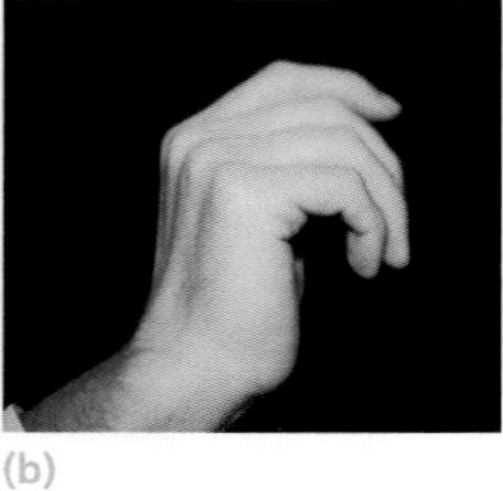

(a) (b)

16.2 Passive tenodesis Note the resting position of the fingers with the wrist (a) flexed, (b) extended.

Signs

Both upper limbs should be bared for comparison. Before focussing on the hands take a quick look at the shoulders and elbows and their range of movement. Also ask which is the dominant hand. A rapid assessment can be carried out in a few minutes. A full examination needs patience and meticulous attention to detail.

Look

Note how the patient holds the hand and uses it during the interview; the resting posture may be suggestive of nerve or tendon damage. Ask the patient to place both hands on the table in front of you, with the palms first upwards and then downwards. The skin may be scarred, altered in colour, dry or moist, and hairy or smooth. Puckering and ridging of the skin in the palm, sometimes extending into one of the fingers, are cardinal signs of Dupuytren's contracture. Deformity of the fingers and the presence of any lumps should be noted. Swelling may arise in the subcutaneous tissues, in a tendon sheath or in a joint. Do not forget to look at the nails; they may show signs of atrophy or disease: e.g. psoriasis, which is sometimes associated with a typical arthropathy, or a 'grooved' nail which is a tell-tale feature of a ganglion cyst at the nail bed.

If multiple joints are involved, take careful note of their distribution. Characteristically, rheumatoid arthritis causes swelling of the proximal joints – metacarpo-phalangeal (MCP) and proximal interphalangeal (PIP) – while osteoarthritis affects mainly the distal interphalangeal (DIP) joints.

Compare the thenar eminences of the two hands and look for wasting on one or other side (a sign of median nerve dysfunction).

Posture in different resting positions While looking at the patient's hands, observe their resting posture in different positions. Normally, with the palm upwards, the fingers fall into a gentle cascade with the MCP joints slightly flexed – about 30 degrees in the index, ranging to 70 degrees in the little. The interphalangeal (IP) joints similarly lie in increasing flexion from index to little. When the hand is turned palm downwards, the fingers straighten out, again in a gentle cascade with greater extension on the index finger than the little finger. If the regular cascade is interrupted, then a tendon is probably either divided or stuck. If the cascade is normal but active movements are not possible, then a nerve injury should be suspected.

Note also that there is a reciprocal relationship between the position of the wrist and the resting position of the fingers (Fig 16.2). Normally as the wrist drops into flexion the fingers automatically tend to straighten, and when the wrist is pulled into extension the fingers flex slightly; contractures of the long flexors will cause the fingers to curl tightly in flexion when the wrist is extended.

Feel

The temperature and texture of the skin are noted and the pulse is felt. Swelling or thickening may be in the subcutaneous tissue, a tendon sheath, a joint or one of the bones. If a nodule is felt, the underlying tendon should be moved (by flexing and extending the relevant finger) to discover if the nodule is attached to the

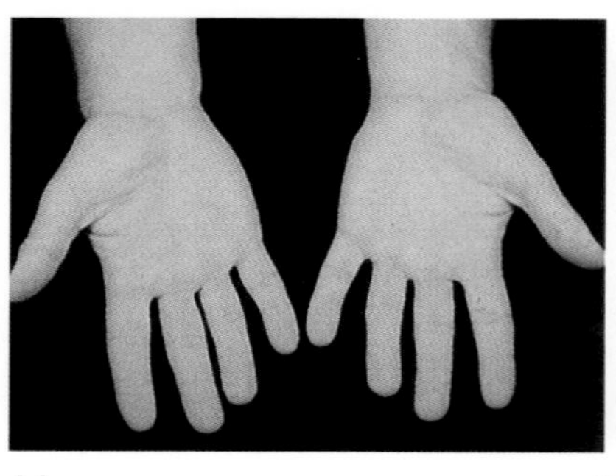

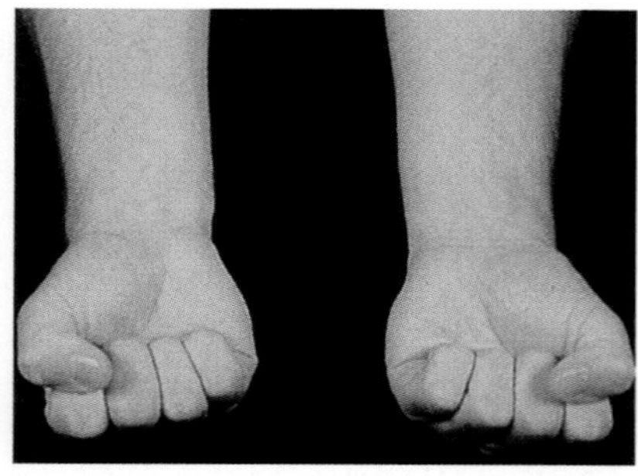

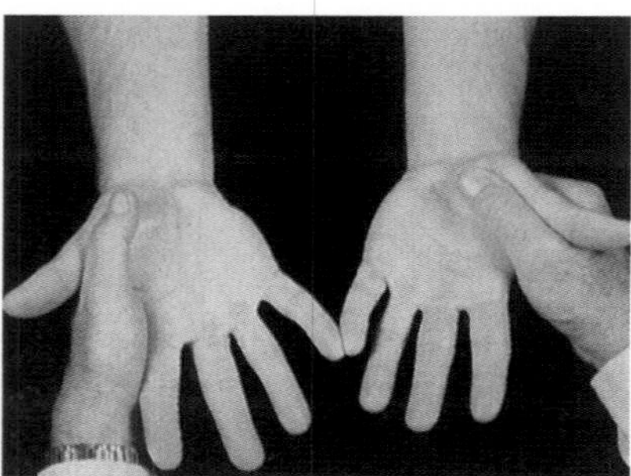

(a) (b) (c)

16.3 Gross active movement (a) Full extension. (b) Full flexion. (c) A good test for abductor power is to have the patient spread his or her fingers as strongly as possible; slowly push the hands together until the tips of the little fingers are forcefully opposing one another; the weaker one will collapse.

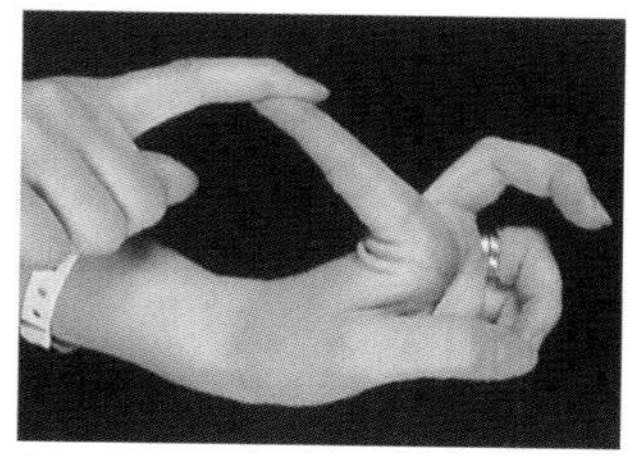
(a)

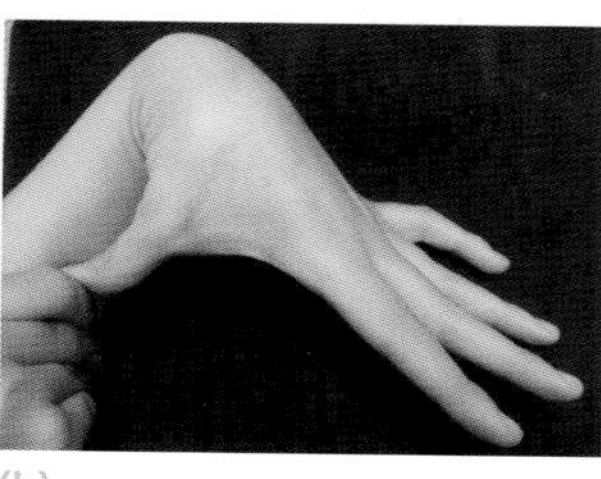
(b)

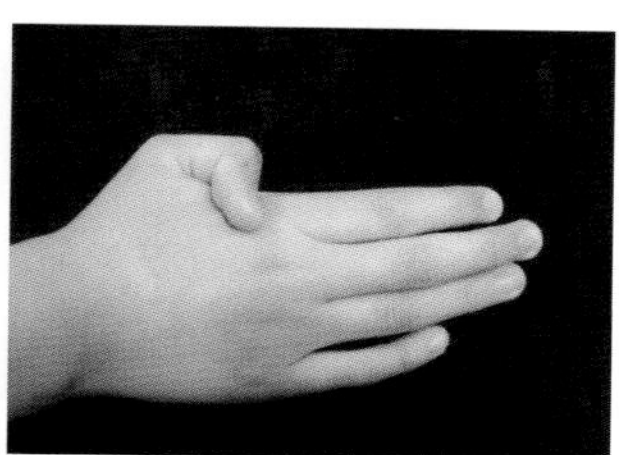
(c)

16.4 Joint laxity (a) in the fingers, (b,c) in the thumb.

tendon or its sheath. This will also reveal whether the tendon glides smoothly or whether it gets stuck momentarily with finger in flexion and then snaps free as the finger is extended (the 'trigger finger' effect). Any point of tenderness should, if possible, be accurately localized to a particular structure.

Move

Passive movements There is a good argument for starting with passive movements, so that you can see whether all the little finger joints are *capable* of moving before testing the *patient's ability* to move them. The thumb and each finger are examined in turn and the range of movement recorded. Note whether the movement causes pain.

Some degree of passive hyperextension at the MCP joints (tested by gently pushing each finger dorsalwards to its limit) is normal but anything more than 90 degrees of (hyper)extension is suggestive of generalized joint laxity; the diagnosis can be confirmed by testing the range of extension in other joints such as the thumbs, elbows and knees.

Active movements Ask the patient to place both hands with the palms facing upwards, to *extend* the fingers and thumbs fully and then to curl them into full *flexion* as if making a gentle fist. A 'lagging finger' is immediately obvious, though it still remains to establish whether this is due to a stiff joint, a defective tendon or loss of motor power. Active movements at each of the MCP, PIP and DIP joints will have to be examined.

Abduction and adduction When the MCP joints are held in extension, they are able to move sideways in the plane of the flattened hand; this is because, in the extended position, the collateral ligaments of the MCP joints are somewhat lax. Spreading the fingers apart is denoted as *abduction* and bringing them back to the neutral position (all the fingers side by side) is *adduction*. Active power can be roughly gauged by having the patient abduct the fingers forcibly and the examiner then pressing against the spread-out index and little fingers, trying to force them back to the neutral position. A better way is to ask the patient to spread the fingers of both hands to the maximum; the examiner then grasps the patient's hands, pushes them towards each other and forces the two little fingers against each other. The weaker (non-dominant) side will normally give way first, but if the difference in one or other hand is very marked it signifies true abductor weakness, a sign of ulnar nerve or T1 root dysfunction.

Thumb movements Movements of the thumb and their nomenclature are unusual, comprising (as they do) the combined mobility of both the first carpometacarpal (CMC) and the first MCP joint. With the hand lying flat, palm upwards, six types of movement are observed:

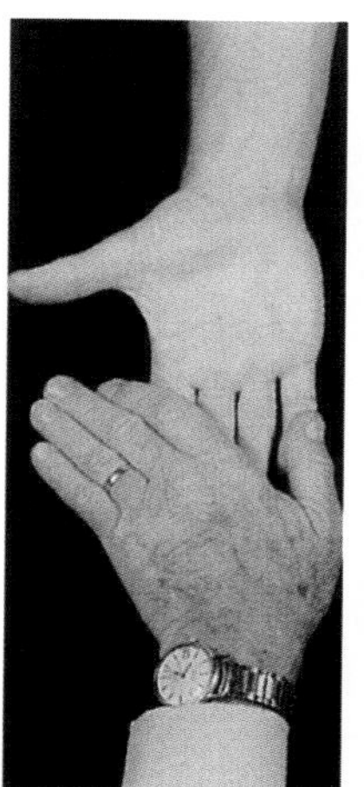
(a)

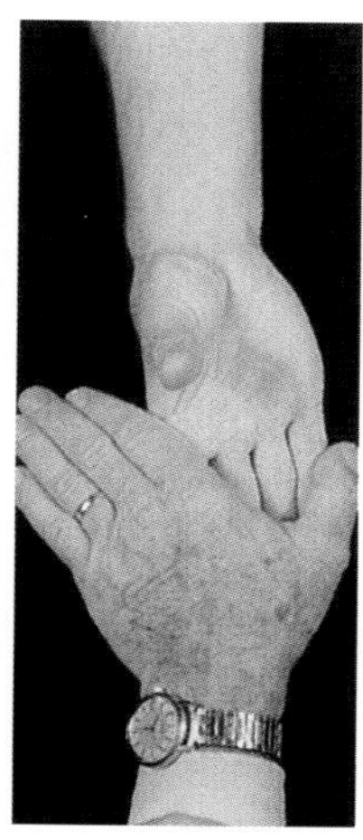
(b)

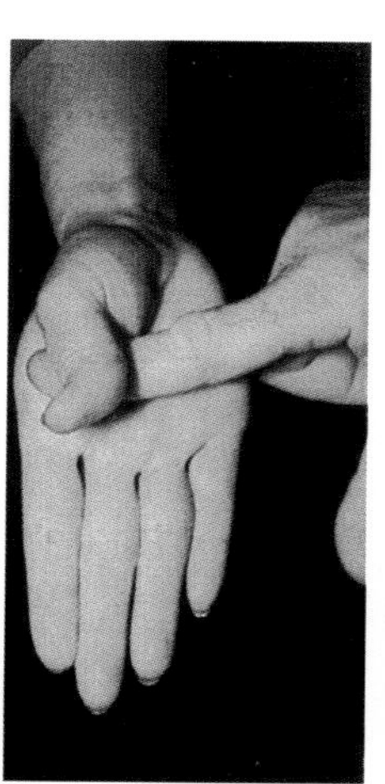
(c)

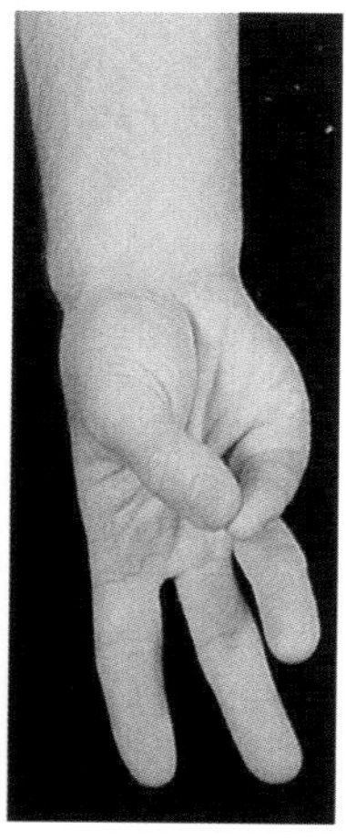
(d)

16.5 Thumb movements You should have no difficulty defining the planes of movement if you follow this routine: (a) hold the patient's hand flat on the table and instruct him or her to 'stretch to the side' (extension), (b) 'point to the ceiling' (abduction), (c) 'pinch my finger' (adduction) and (d) 'touch your little finger' (opposition).

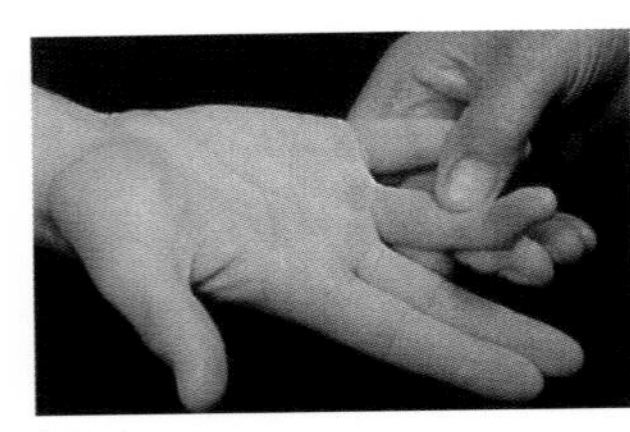
(a)

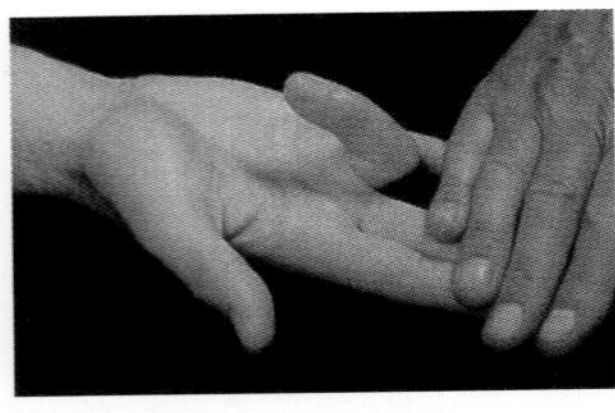
(b)

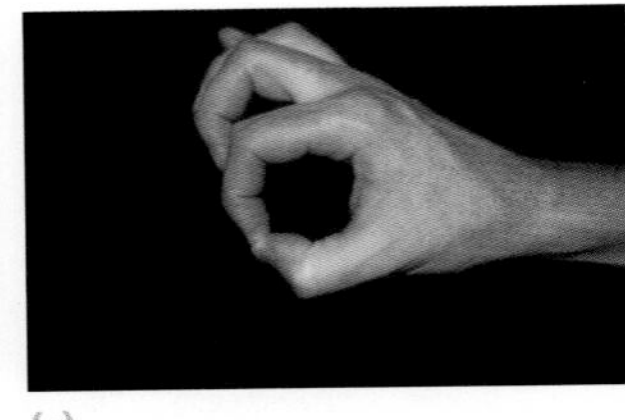
(c)

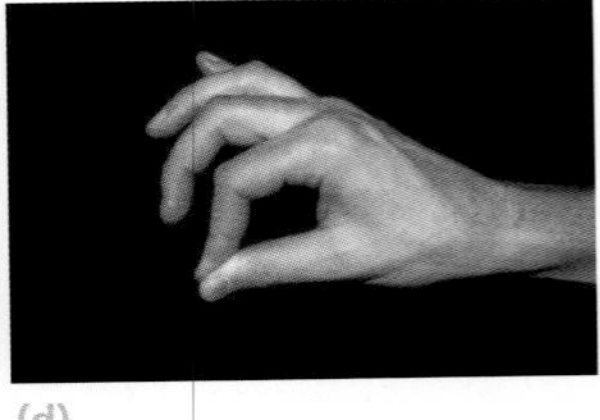
(d)

16.6 Testing for (a) FDP lesser fingers, (b) FDS lesser fingers, (c) FDP index, (d) FDS index.

- *extension* (sideways movement in the plane of the palm)
- *abduction* (upward movement at right angles to the palm)
- *adduction* (pressing against the palm)
- *flexion* (sideways movement across the palm)
- *opposition* (touching the tips of the fingers)
- *retroposition* (lifting the thumbs backwards behind the plane of the hand).

Weakness of abduction (tested simply by pressing against the abducted thumb of each hand) is a cardinal feature of median nerve dysfunction. In advanced cases there will also be obvious wasting of the thenar eminence.

Pain, deformity and loss of motion at the base of the thumb (the first CMC joint) are common symptoms of osteoarthritis.

Testing the muscles and tendons

Flexion of the fingers is motivated mainly by *flexor digitorum profundus* (FDP) and *flexor digitorum superficialis* (FDS); these muscles also assist in flexion of the MCP joints but the main MCP flexors are the *intrinsic muscles.* Active mass flexion can be tested by asking the patient to curl his or her fingers into flexion so as to engage them in the examiner's fingers in a tug of strength. However, the patient's flexors can also be tested independently, as follows.

To test for *flexor digitorum profundus* in an individual finger, the PIP joint is held and immobilized in extension and the patient is then asked to bend the tip of the finger.

To test *flexor digitorum superficialis*, the flexor profundus must first be inactivated, otherwise one cannot tell which tendon is flexing the PIP joint. This is done by grasping all the fingers, except the one being examined, and holding them firmly in full extension; because the profundus tendons share a common muscle belly, this manoeuvre automatically prevents *all* the profundus tendons from participating in finger flexion. The patient is then asked to flex the isolated finger which is being examined; this movement must be activated by flexor digitorum superficialis. There are two exceptions to this rule: First, the little finger sometimes has no independent flexor digitorum superficialis. Second, the index finger often has an entirely separate flexor profundus, which cannot be inactivated by the usual mass action manoeuvre; instead, flexor superficialis is tested by asking the patient to pinch hard with the DIP joint in full extension and the PIP joint in full flexion; this position can be maintained only if the superficialis tendon is active and intact.

Since the thumb has only a single IP joint, the *flexor pollicis longus* is tested by immobilizing the thumb MCP joint and then asking the patient to flex the IP joint.

The *long extensors* are tested by asking the patient to extend the MCP joints. Inability to do this usually signifies either paralysis or tendon rupture; occasionally, a long extensor tendon may simply have slipped off the knuckle into the interdigital gutter (a common occurrence in rheumatoid arthritis).

The *intrinsic muscles (lumbricals and interossei)* can act uniquely to flex the MCP joints with the IP joints held simultaneously in extension (i.e. preventing the long flexors from acting). Ask the patient to extend the fingers with the MCP joints flexed (the 'duckbill' position). The interossei also motivate finger abduction and adduction.

Grip strength

Grip strength is an important indicator of hand and wrist function. A painful wrist will result in a weak hand. Loss of finger function due to pain, stiffness, instability or weakness will also reduce grip. Grip strength should be measured with a mechanical dynamometer; if this is not available, an indication can be derived from having the patient squeeze a partially inflated sphygmomanometer cuff (normally a pressure of 150 mmHg can be achieved easily). Pinch grip also should be measured using a specific pinch gauge.

Neurological assessment

If symptoms such as numbness, tingling or weakness exist – and in all cases of trauma – a full neurological examination of the upper limbs should be carried out, testing power, reflexes and sensation. Further

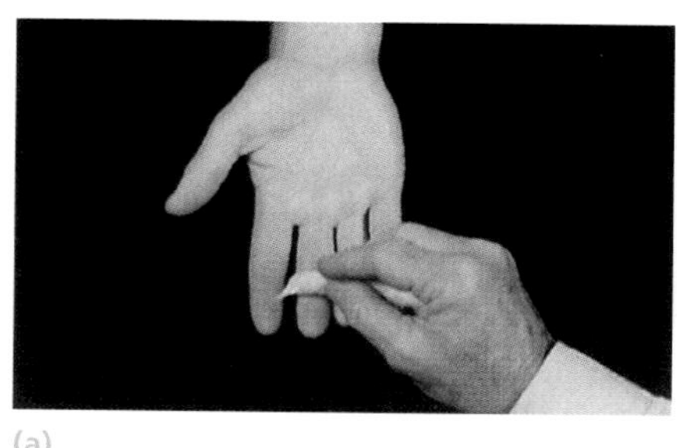
(a)

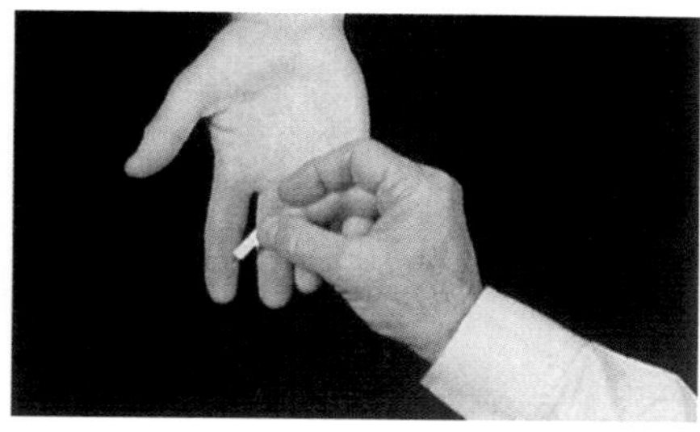
(b)

16.7 Neurological assessment (a) Light touch, (b) pinprick.

refinement is achieved by testing monofilament detection, two-point discrimination, vibration sensibility, proprioception and stereognosis (tactile discrimination).

Functional tests

Ultimately it is function that counts; patients learn to overcome their defects by ingenious modifications and trick movements. Function can be measured subjectively using patient-completed scales, but objective tests are more reliable. There are several types of grip, which can be tested by giving the patient a variety of tasks to perform: picking up a pin (precision grip), holding a sheet of paper (pinch), holding a key (sideways pinch), holding a pen (chuck grip), holding a bag handle (hook grip), holding a glass (span) and gripping a hammer handle (power grip). Stereognosis is evaluated using Moberg's pick-up test (1958). The patient is instructed to pick up a number of small objects and place them in a box; the procedure is timed and efficiency of the affected hand is compared with that of the 'good' hand.

Each finger has its special task: the thumb and index finger are used for pinch. The index finger is also an important sensory organ; slight loss of movement matters little, but if sensation is abnormal the patient probably will not use the finger at all. The middle finger controls the position of objects in the palm. The ring and little fingers are used for power grip; any loss of movement here will affect function markedly.

Stiffness is poorly tolerated in the little finger whereas instability is less worrisome; the opposite is true for the thumb and index finger.

Dexterity is lost in severe carpal tunnel syndrome (median nerve compression) because of the combination of thenar weakness, reduced sensation and diminished stereognosis and proprioception.

CONGENITAL HAND ANOMALIES

The incidence of congenital upper limb abnormalities is estimated to be about 1 in 600 live births. Some are confined to the hand but in most cases the wrist and forearm are involved as well. We have therefore covered congenital anomalies of the wrist and hand as a single subject in Chapter 15.

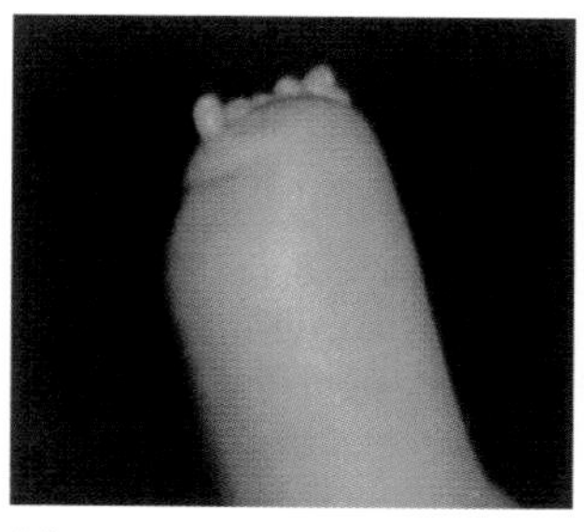
(a)

(b)

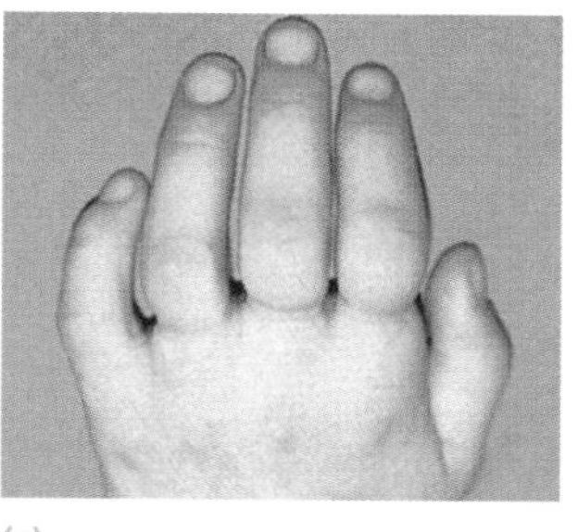
(c)

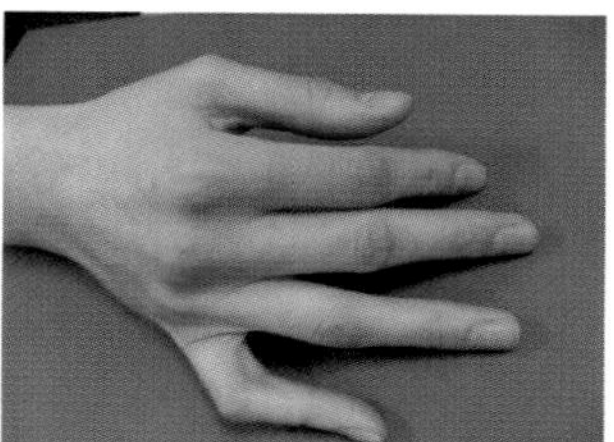
(d)

(e)

16.8 Congenital variations (a) Transverse failure, (b) radial club hand and absent thumb, (c) constriction rings, (d) camptodactyly, (e) clinodactyly.

ACQUIRED DEFORMITIES

Deformity of the hand may result from acquired disorders of the skin, subcutaneous tissues, muscles, tendons, joints, bones or neuromuscular function. Often there is a history of trauma or infection or concomitant disease; at other times the patient is unaware of any cause.

Problems arise for three main reasons: (1) the defect may be unacceptable simply because of its unsightly appearance; (2) function is impaired; and (3) the deformed part becomes a nuisance during daily activities.

Assessment and management of hand deformities demands a detailed knowledge of functional anatomy and, in particular, of the normal mechanisms of balanced movement in the wrist and fingers.

SKIN CONTRACTURE

Cuts and burns of the palmar skin are liable to heal with contracture. *Surgical incisions should never cross skin creases perpendicularly;* they should lie more or less parallel or oblique to them, or in the mid-axial line of the fingers. A useful alternative is a zig-zag incision with the middle part of the Z in the skin crease. Longitudinal wounds can also be closed as Z-plasties.

Established contractures may require excision of the scar, Z-plasty of the remaining skin, skin grafts, a pedicled flap and occasionally a free flap.

SUPERFICIAL PALMAR FASCIA (DUPUYTREN'S) CONTRACTURE

The superficial palmar fascia (palmar aponeurosis) fans out from the wrist towards the fingers, sending extensions across the MCP joints to the fingers. Hypertrophy and contracture of the palmar fascia may lead to puckering of the palmar skin and fixed flexion of the fingers. The condition is dealt with on page 421.

MUSCLE CONTRACTURE

VOLKMANN'S ISCHAEMIC CONTRACTURE

Contracture of the forearm muscles may follow circulatory insufficiency due to injuries at or below the elbow. Shortening of the long flexors causes the fingers to be held in flexion; they can be straightened only when the wrist is flexed so as to relax the long flexors. Sometimes the picture is complicated by associated damage to the ulnar or median nerve (or both). If disability is marked, some improvement may be obtained by lengthening the shortened tendons, or else by excising the fibrosed muscles and restoring finger movement with tendon transfers.

SHORTENING OF THE INTRINSIC MUSCLES

Shortening of the intrinsic muscles in the hand produces a characteristic deformity: flexion at the MCP joints with extension of the IP joints and adduction of the thumb (the so-called *'intrinsic-plus' hand*). Slight degrees of deformity may not be obvious, but can be diagnosed by *Bunnell's 'intrinsic-plus' test*: with the MCP joints pushed passively into hyperextension (thus putting the intrinsics on stretch), it is difficult or impossible to flex the IP joints passively; if the MCP joints are then placed in flexion, the IP joints can be passively flexed.

The causes of intrinsic shortening or contracture are: (1) spasticity (e.g. in cerebral palsy); (2) volar subluxation of the MCP joints (e.g. in rheumatoid arthritis); (3) scarring after trauma or infection; and (4) shrinkage due to ischaemia. Moderate contracture can be treated by resecting a triangular segment of the intrinsic 'aponeurosis' at the base of the proximal phalanx (Littler's operation).

TENDON LESIONS

MALLET FINGER

This results from injury to the extensor tendon of the terminal phalanx. It may be due to direct trauma but more often painlessly follows an innocent event when the finger tip is forcibly bent during active extension, perhaps while tucking the blankets under a mattress or trying to catch a ball. The terminal joint is held flexed and the patient cannot straighten it, but passive movement is normal. With the extensor mechanism unbalanced, the PIP joint may become hyperextended ('swan-neck').

X-rays are taken to show or exclude a fracture. If there is a fracture but minimal subluxation of the joint, it is treated by splintage with the DIP joint in extension for 6 weeks. Operative treatment is considered only if there is a large fragment (>50 per cent) and subluxation of the DIP joint. Otherwise surgery is ill advised, as the complication rate is high and it is unlikely to improve the outcome.

A mallet finger without bone injury is treated with a plastic splint with the DIP joint in extension for 8 weeks, followed by 4 weeks of night splintage. This treatment may still work if presentation is delayed for a few weeks. The great majority do very well. Old lesions need treatment only if the deformity is marked and hand function seriously impaired. The options include fusion for painful arthritic joints or tendon reconstruction.

RUPTURED EXTENSOR POLLICIS LONGUS

The long thumb extensor may rupture after fraying or ischaemia where it crosses the wrist (e.g. after a Colles' fracture, or in rheumatoid arthritis). The distal phalanx drops into flexion; it can be passively extended, and there may still be weak active extension because of thenar muscle insertion into the extensor expansion; however, the thumb cannot be actively elevated backwards above the plane of the hand (retroposition). Direct repair is unsatisfactory and a tendon transfer, using the extensor indicis, is needed. The results are, in over 90 per cent of cases, satisfactory.

DROPPED FINGER

Sudden loss of finger extension at the MCP joint is usually due to tendon rupture at the wrist (e.g. in rheumatoid arthritis). Because direct repair is not usually possible, the distal portion can be attached to an adjacent finger extensor or a tendon transfer performed.

Occasionally the deformity is due to catching of the collateral ligament on a metacarpal osteophyte or rupture of the sagittal band which centralizes the tendon over the back of the knuckle.

BOUTONNIÈRE DEFORMITY

This lesion presents as a flexion deformity of the PIP joint and extension of the DIP joint. It is due to interruption or stretching of the central slip of the extensor tendon where it inserts into the base of the middle phalanx. The lateral slips separate and the head of the proximal phalanx thrusts through the gap like a button through a buttonhole. Ironically while English speakers call it a *'boutonniere'* deformity, the French refer to it as *'le buttonhole'*.The usual causes are direct trauma or rheumatoid disease. Initially the deformity is slight and passively correctable; later the soft tissues contract, resulting in fixed flexion of the proximal and hyperextension of the DIP joint. Early diagnosis is therefore important; an impending deformity should be suspected in anyone with tenderness or a cut over the dorsum of the PIP joint, especially if they cannot actively extend the IP joint with the MCP joints and wrist flexed.

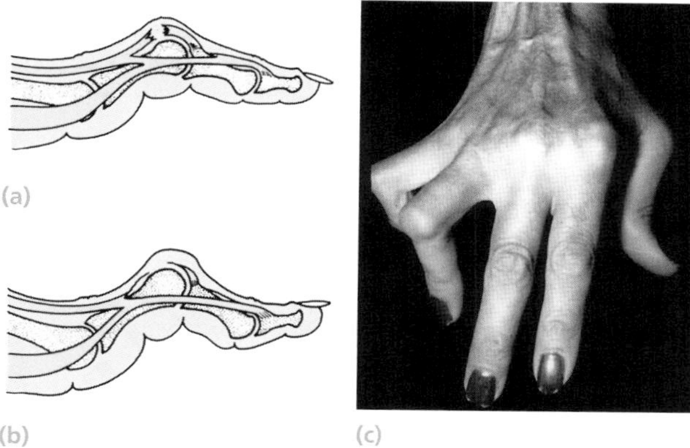

16.9 Boutonnière deformity (a) When the middle slip of the extensor tendon first ruptures there is no more than an inability to extend the PIP joint. (b) Gradually the lateral slips slide volarwards, the knuckle pops through the 'buttonhole' and the DIP joint is pulled into hyperextension. (c) Clinical appearance.

In the early post-traumatic case, splinting the PIP joint in full extension for 6 weeks usually leads to healing; the DIP joint must be moved passively to prevent the lateral bands from sticking. Open injuries of the central slip should be repaired, with the joint protected by a K-wire for 3 weeks.

For later cases where the joint is still passively correctible, several operations have been invented (suggesting that none is too reliable). The easiest and probably most successful procedure is to divide the extensor tendon just proximal to its insertion into the distal phalanx. This allows the extensor mechanism to move proximally, thus enhancing PIP extension and diminishing DIP extension.

Longstanding fixed deformities are extremely difficult to correct and may be better left alone.

SWAN-NECK DEFORMITY

This is the reverse of the boutonnière deformity; the PIP joint is hyperextended and the DIP joint flexed. The deformity can be reproduced voluntarily by lax-jointed individuals. The clinical disorder has many causes, with two things in common: imbalance of extensor versus flexor action at the PIP joint and laxity of the palmar plate. Thus it may occur: (1) if the PIP extensors overact (e.g. due to intrinsic muscle spasm or contracture, after mallet finger, or following volar subluxation of the MCP joint); (2) if the PIP flexors are inadequate (inhibition or division of the flexor superficialis); or (3) if the palmar plate of the PIP joint fails (in rheumatoid arthritis, lax-jointed individuals or trauma). If the deformity is allowed to persist, secondary contracture of the intrinsic muscles, and eventually of the PIP joint itself, makes correction increasingly difficult and ultimately impossible.

Treatment depends on the cause and whether or not the deformity has become fixed. If the deformity corrects passively, then a simple figure-of-eight ring splint to maintain the PIP joint in a few degrees of flexion may be all that is required; if this works but cannot be tolerated, then tenodesis of the PIP joint works well. The options are either to attach one slip of flexor digitorum superficialis to the proximal phalanx, which prevents hyperextension, or to re-route a lateral band anteriorly so it becomes a flexor rather than an extensor of the PIP joint. If the intrinsics are tight they are released.

If the deformity is fixed, then it may respond to gentle manipulation supplemented by temporary K-wire fixation in a few degrees of flexion; if not, then lateral band release from the central slip may be needed. The dorsal skin may not close directly after

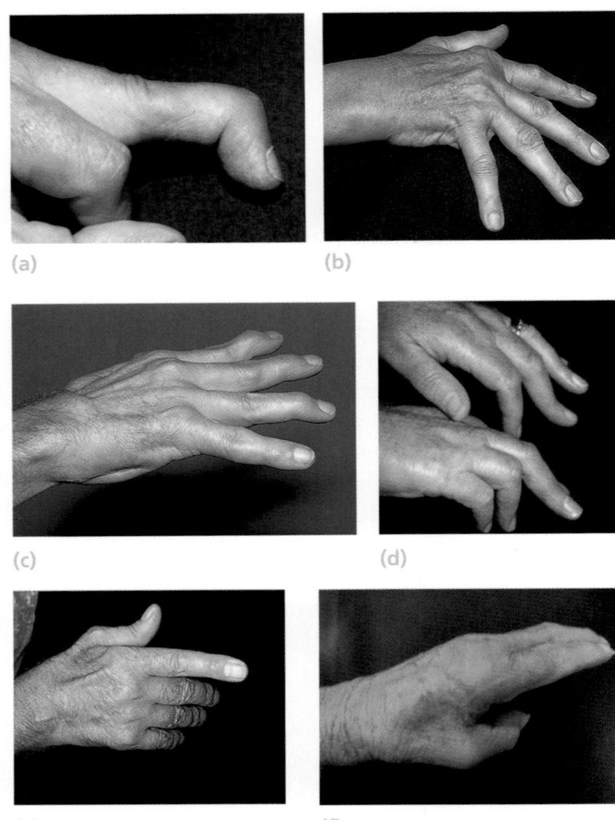

16.10 **Deformities due to tendon lesions** (a) Mallet finger. (b) Dropped fingers due to extensor tendon ruptures at the wrist. (c) Swan-neck deformities. (d) Boutonnière deformities. (e) Rupture of extensor pollicis brevis. (f) Rupture of extensor pollicis longus.

correction. If the swan-neck deformity is secondary to a mallet finger, then the latter should be addressed as described above.

If function is severely impaired and does not respond to one of the above measures, the joint is arthrodesed in a more acceptable position.

Joint disorders

RHEUMATOID ARTHRITIS

Rheumatoid arthritis causes multiple, symmetrical deformities of both hands, typically ulnar deviation of the MCP joints and boutonnière or swan-neck deformities of the proximal finger joints (see page 424).

JUVENILE IDIOPATHIC ARTHRITIS

The pattern of involvement is different from that of adult disease. The wrists tend to develop ulnar (rather than radial) deviation, the MCP joints develop flexion contractures (rather than ulnar drift), and the IP joints also become fixed in flexion (swan-neck deformities are rare). The hands are small because of premature fusion of the physis.

The mainstay of treatment is medical. Long-term splintage of the hand is helpful and synovectomy is sometimes needed. Later, wrist fusion, MCP joint replacement and IP joint fusion also have a role, usually after skeletal maturity.

PSORIATIC ARTHRITIS

Erosive arthropathy of the IP joints leads to profound weakness and instability; the PIP joints may develop fixed flexion deformities. If the disease progresses, psoriatic arthritis can devastate the small joints of the hand ('arthritis mutilans') resulting in severe, and sometimes bizarre, deformities of the IP and MCP joints. The nails are often pitted (onychodystrophy) and skin lesions (a guttate or pustular rash) may be evident. Occasionally joint fusion is needed to relieve pain and to provide stability in a functional position.

SYSTEMIC LUPUS ERYTHEMATOSUS

This autoimmune disease, affecting women five times more frequently than men, causes soft-tissue slackening with extensor tendon dislocation, ulnar deviation at the MCP joints and swan-neck deformities of the fingers. Soft-tissue corrections tend to fail with time and eventually fusions may be needed to maintain function.

SCLERODERMA

Typically the fingers are smooth-skinned and stiff (sclerodactyly), with flexion deformities of the IP joints. Raynaud's phenomenon and painful ulcers may develop. Early on, physiotherapy and splinting help; in the later stages, joint fusion in a functional position and digital sympathectomy to relieve ulcers may be needed. Painful calcific deposits can be excised but wound breakdown is a risk.

OSTEOARTHRITIS

Osteoarthritis, by contrast, affects mainly the DIP joints. It is common in postmenopausal women and may cause deformity. The thumb CMC joint is another common site, and this may result in adduction of the first metacarpal and flexion of the first CMC joint. Treatment is discussed on page 403.

GOUT

Gouty swellings (tophi) and finger deformities are sometimes mistaken for rheumatoid disease. However, the lesions tend to be asymmetrical and the x-ray appearances are distinctive. The diagnosis can be confirmed by identifying urate crystals in the tophaceous material. Curiously, gout and rheumatoid arthritis hardly ever occur in the same patient. In addition to systemic treatment, evacuation of a tophus (or tophi) is sometimes advisable.

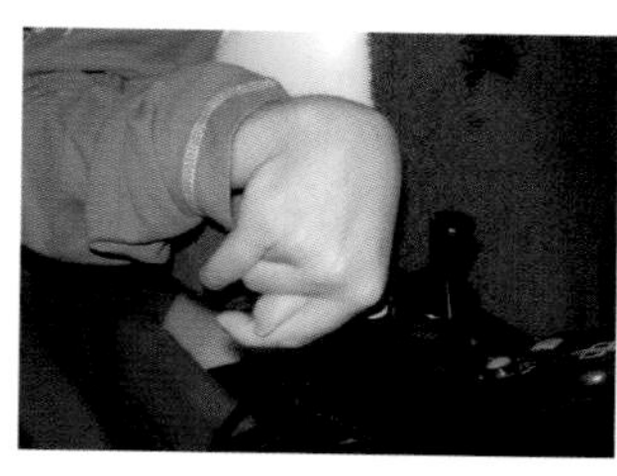
(a)

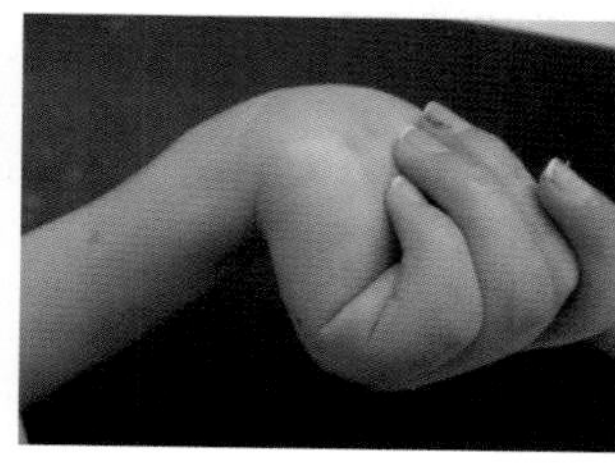
(b)

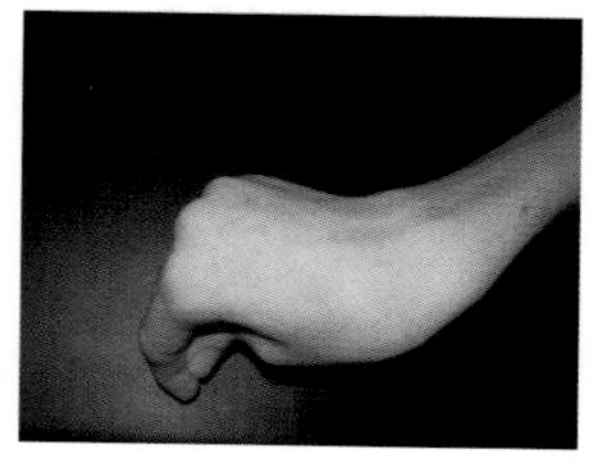
(c)

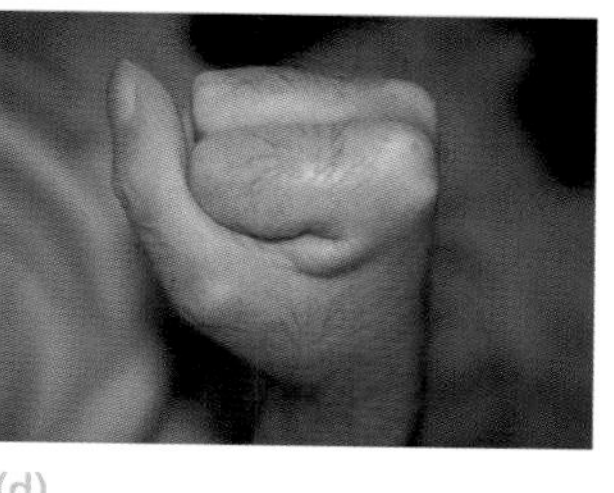
(d)

16.11 Spastic contracture – hand deformities (a,b,c) cerebral palsy, and (d) head injury with brain damage.

TRAUMA

Fractures may go on to malunion and joints may become stiff and swollen. This subject is dealt with in Chapter 26.

BONE LESIONS

A variety of bone lesions (acute infection, tuberculosis, malunited fractures, infantile rickets, tumours) may cause metacarpal or phalangeal deformity. X-rays usually show the abnormality. In addition to treating the pathological lesion, deformity may need correction by osteotomy with internal fixation.

NEUROMUSCULAR DISORDERS

SPASTIC PARESIS

Cerebral palsy, head injury and stroke may result in typical deformities of the hand. The 'intrinsic-plus' posture is easily recognized. Another common disability is 'thumb-in-palm'; the tendency to adduct and flex the thumb into the palm is increased by activity, especially finger flexion. Releasing the adductor pollicis from the third metacarpal may improve the appearance, but normal thumb pinch is rarely restored.

OTHER NEUROLOGICAL DISORDERS

Poliomyelitis, leprosy, syringomyelia and Charcot–Marie–Tooth disease may cause hand deformities. If there is only partial involvement, tendon transfer may be feasible.

PERIPHERAL NERVE LESIONS

The postural deformities are so characteristic that the diagnosis should seldom be in doubt (see Chapter 11). The most common are drop-wrist and drop-fingers (radial nerve palsy), a simian thumb and pointing index finger (median nerve palsy) and partial claw hand (ulnar nerve palsy). The distribution of sensory loss helps to establish the site of the lesion.

THE 'INTRINSIC MINUS' HAND

Among the late neurological defects, *intrinsic paralysis* is particularly disabling. The 'intrinsic minus' hand shows wasting of the small muscles and moderate clawing, with extension of the MCP and partial flexion of the IP joints. If all the intrinsics are affected (e.g. after poliomyelitis or a combined low median and ulnar nerve injury) the thumb lies flat at the side of the hand and cannot be opposed. In ulnar nerve palsy only the ring and little fingers are clawed, because the index and middle lumbricals are supplied by the median nerve; these muscles continue to flex the MCP joints and extend the IP joints. Thumb opposition is retained but thumb pinch is unstable because index-finger abduction (first dorsal interosseous) is weak, and loss of thumb adduction is compensated for by exaggerated IP flexion during strong pinch (Froment's sign).

The objectives of treatment are: (1) stabilization of the MCP joints in flexion – this can be achieved dynamically by a tendon transfer (e.g. flexor superficialis into the intrinsic tendon) or statically by looping a slip of flexor digitorum superficialis around the flexor pulley (Zancolli's operation); (2) restoration of index abduction to provide stable pinch (e.g. by extensor carpi radialis brevis tendon transfer to the first dorsal interosseous); (3) restoration of thumb opposition (if it is lost) by a tendon transfer looped around a fascial or tendon pulley and attached to the radial edge of the proximal phalanx of the thumb. *Before any of these operations, stiff finger joints must be made mobile.*

DUPUYTREN'S CONTRACTURE

This is a nodular hypertrophy and contracture of the superficial palmar fascia (palmar aponeurosis). The condition is inherited as an autosomal dominant trait and is most common in people of European (especially Anglo-Saxon) descent. It is more common in males than females; the prevalence increases with age, but onset at an early stage usually means aggressive disease. There is a high incidence in epileptics receiving phenytoin therapy; associations with diabetes, smoking, alcoholic cirrhosis, AIDS and pulmonary tuberculosis have also been described. There is a contentious and weak association with injury to the hand.

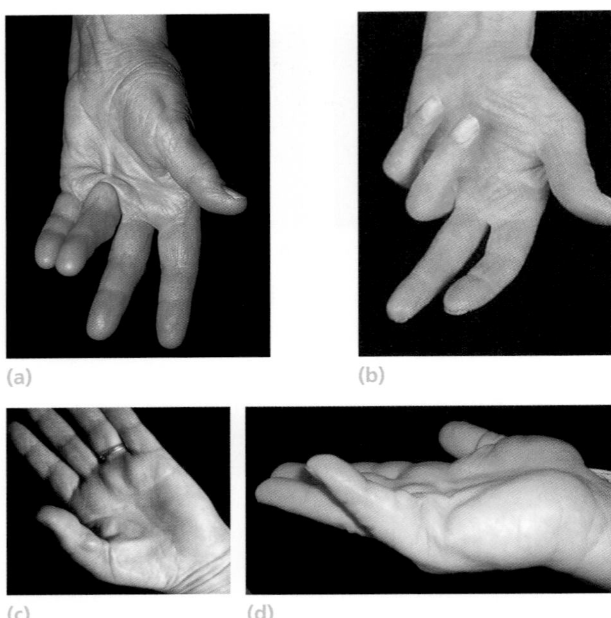

(a) (b) (c) (d)

16.12 Dupuytren's disease Contractures may occur at (a) palmar crease, (b) proximal interphalangeal joint, (c) thumb web, (d) little finger.

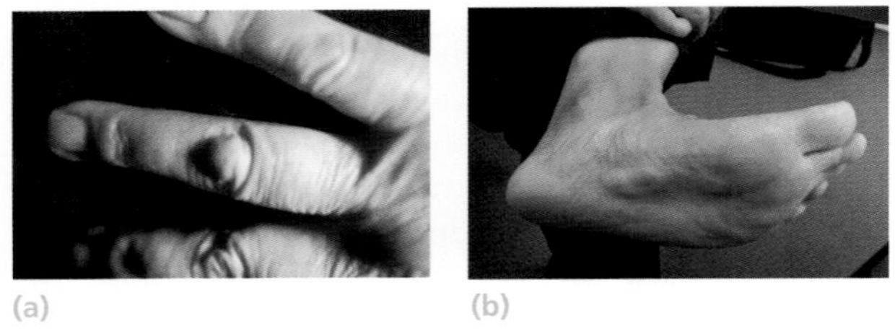

(a) (b)

16.13 Dupuytren's disease – other manifestations (a) Garrod's pads, (b) Ledderhose's nodules.

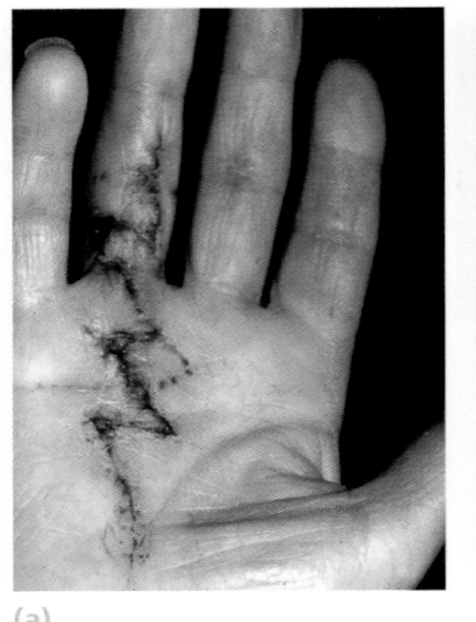

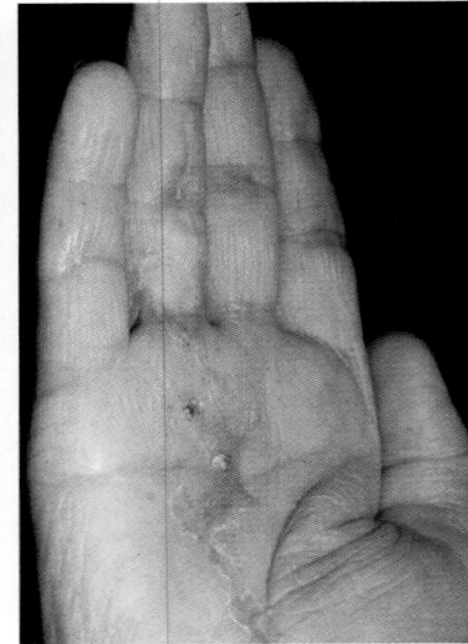

(a)

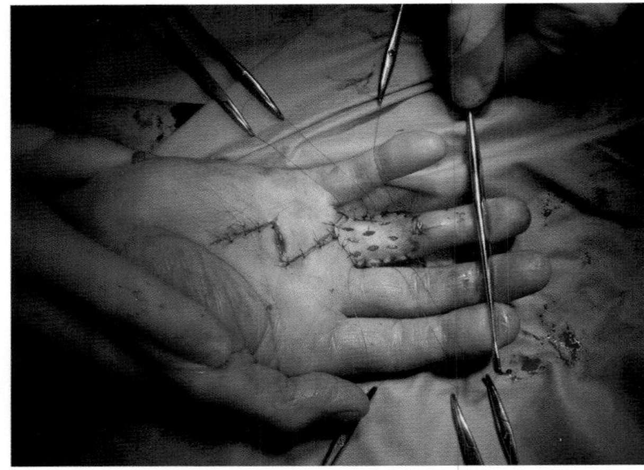

(b)

16.14 Dupuytren's disease – surgery (a) Z-plasty in the hand shortly after operation and two weeks later when healing is almost complete; (b) skin graft in theatre.

PATHOLOGY

The essential problem in Dupuytren's disease is proliferation of myofibroblasts; where they come from and why they proliferate remains unclear. After an initial proliferative phase, fibrous tissue within the palmar fascia and fascial bands within the fingers contracts, causing flexion deformities of the MCP and PIP joints. Fibrous attachments to the skin lead to puckering. The digital nerve is displaced or enveloped, but not invaded, by fibrous tissue. Occasionally the plantar aponeurosis also is affected.

Clinical features

The patient – usually a middle-aged man – complains of a nodular thickening in the palm. Gradually this extends distally to involve the ring or little finger. Pain may occur early on but is seldom a marked feature. Often both hands are involved, one more than the other. The palm is puckered, nodular and thick. If the subcutaneous cords extend into the fingers they may produce flexion deformities at the MCP and PIP joints. Sometimes the dorsal knuckle pads are thickened (Garrod's pads). About 60 per cent of patients give a family history.

Similar nodules may be seen on the soles of the feet (Ledderhose's disease). There is a rare, curious association with fibrosis of the corpus cavernosum (Peyronie's disease).

Diagnosis

Dupuytren's contracture must be distinguished from skin contracture (where the previous laceration is usually obvious), tendon contracture (in which the finger deformity changes with wrist position) and PIP joint contracture (in which there may be a history of clinodactyly or joint injury).

Treatment

Operation is indicated if the deformity is a nuisance or rapidly progressing. In particular, PIP joint contractures can become irreversible. The aim is reasonable, not complete, correction. Surgery does not cure the disease, it only partially corrects the deformity, and recurrence or extension is common. Correction of the MCP joint is more predictable than the PIP joint.

Only the thickened part of the fascia is excised (complete fasciectomy is usually unnecessary). An isolated cord across the front of the MCP joint can be managed by dividing the contracture under local anaesthetic with a bevelled needle ('needle fasciotomy'). If the disease is more extensive, the affected area is approached through a longitudinal or a Z-shaped incision and, after carefully freeing the nerves and blood vessels, the cords are excised. Skin closure may be facilitated by multiple Z-plasties. This has the dual effect of improving the deformity and, if recurrence occurs, preventing a longitudinal wound contracture. The palmar section of the wound can be left open; it will soon heal with dressings. This makes skin closure easier and allows any haematoma (which may predispose to recurrence) to escape. After operative correction a splint is applied, and removed after a few days for active motion exercises. Night splinting for a few months may reduce recurrence.

If there is severe skin involvement (particularly in surgery for recurrent disease), if there is a strong family history, or if the patient is particularly young, then skin grafting should be considered. Amputation or joint fusion is occasionally advisable for severe, recurrent disease in the little finger.

TRIGGER FINGER (DIGITAL TENOVAGINOSIS)

A flexor tendon may become trapped by thickening at the entrance to its sheath; on forced extension it passes the constriction with a snap ('triggering'). A secondary nodule can develop on the tendon. The underlying cause is unknown but the condition is certainly more common in patients with diabetes. People with rheumatoid disease may develop synovial thickening or intratendinous nodules which can also cause triggering. Occupational factors, though sometimes blamed, are unlikely to be causative.

Clinical features

Any digit may be affected, but the thumb, ring and middle fingers most commonly; sometimes several fingers are affected. The patient notices a click as the finger is flexed; when the hand is unclenched, the affected finger initially remains bent at the PIP joint but with further effort it suddenly straightens with a snap. A tender nodule can be felt in front of the MCP joint and the click may be reproduced at this site by alternately flexing and extending the finger.

INFANTILE TRIGGER THUMB

Parents sometimes notice that their baby or infant cannot extend the thumb tip. The diagnosis is often missed, or the condition is wrongly taken for a 'dislocation'. Very occasionally the child grows up with the thumb permanently bent. This condition must be distinguished from the rare *congenitally clasped thumb* in which both the IP joint and the MCP joint are flexed because of congenital insufficiency of the extensor mechanism (see Chapter 15).

Treatment

In adults, early cases may be cured by an injection of corticosteroid carefully placed at the mouth of the tendon sheath. Recurrent triggering up to 6 months later occurs in over 30 per cent of patients – particularly younger patients and those with diabetes, who may then need a second injection. Refractory cases need operation, through an incision over the distal palmar crease, or in the MCP crease of the thumb – the A1 section of the fibrous sheath is incised until the tendon moves freely.

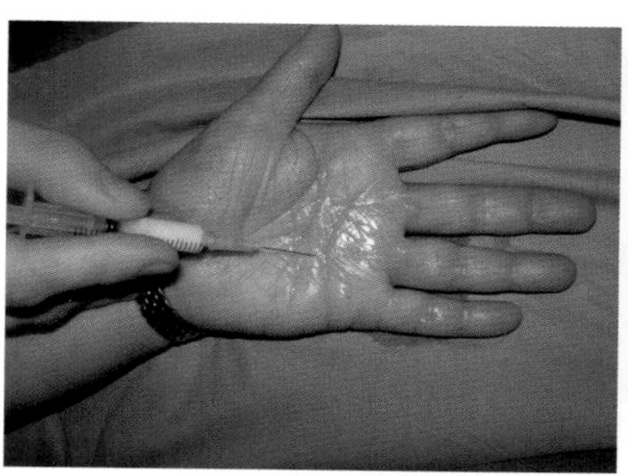
(a)

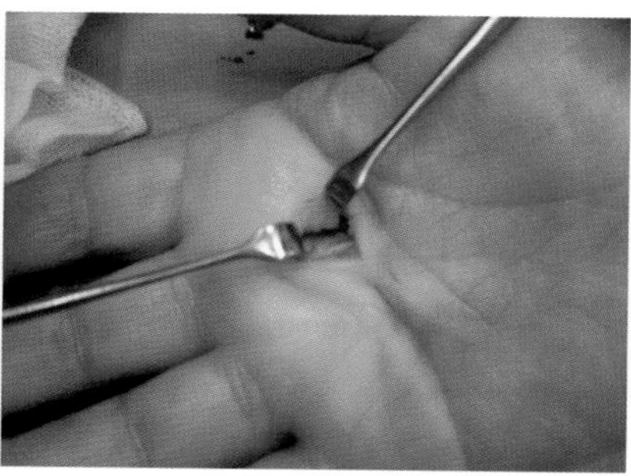
(b)

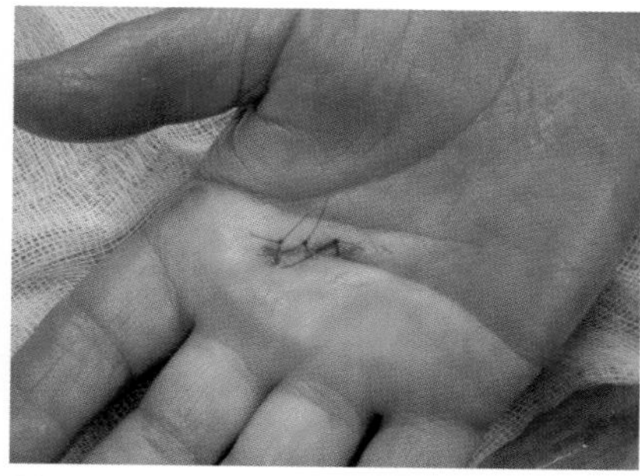
(c)

16.15 Trigger finger (a) Injection of steroid, (b,c) operative treatment.

In babies it is worth waiting until the child is about 3 years old, as spontaneous recovery often occurs. If not, then the pulley is released.

Care should be taken to avoid injury to the digital neurovascular bundles during surgery. The risk is greatest in the thumb (where the nerves are close to the midline) and the index finger (where the radical digital nerve crosses the tendon).

In patients with rheumatoid arthritis the fibrous pulley must be carefully preserved; damage to this structure will predispose to ulnar deviation of the fingers. Flexor synovectomy with excision of one slip of flexor digitorum superficialis is preferred.

RHEUMATOID ARTHRITIS (see also Chapter 3)

The hand, more than any other region, is where rheumatoid arthritis carves its story. The early stage is characterized by synovitis of the joints and tendon sheaths. If the disease progresses, joint and tendon erosions prepare the ground for mechanical derangement. In the late stage, joint destruction, attenuation of the ligaments and tendon ruptures lead to instability and progressive deformity.

With the advent of biological treatment such as anti-TNF agents, the need for surgical treatment has diminished considerably.

Clinical features

Stiffness and swelling of the fingers are early symptoms; the patient may mention that the wrist also is swollen. Sometimes the first symptoms are typical of carpal tunnel compression, caused by flexor tenosynovitis at the wrist.

Examination may reveal swelling of the MCP and PIP joints, giving the fingers a spindle shape; both hands are affected, more or less symmetrically. Swelling of tendon sheaths is usually seen on the dorsum of the wrist and along the ulnar border (extensor carpi ulnaris); thickened flexor tendons may also be felt on the volar aspect of the proximal phalanges. The joints are tender and crepitus may be felt on moving the tendons. Joint mobility and grip strength are diminished.

As the disease progresses, early deformities make their appearance: slight radial deviation of the wrist and ulnar deviation of the fingers, correctable swan-neck deformities of some fingers, an isolated boutonnière or the sudden appearance of a drop-finger or mallet thumb (from extensor tendon rupture).

In the late stage, long after inflammation may have subsided, established deformities are the rule: the carpus settles into radial tilt and volar subluxation; there is marked ulnar drift of the fingers and volar dislocation of the MCP joints, often associated with multiple swan-neck and boutonnière deformities. These 'rheumatoid deformities' are so characteristic that they allow the diagnosis to be made at first glance. When the abnormalities become fixed, functional loss may be so severe that patients can no longer dress or feed themselves.

General features

The hand should not be considered in isolation. Its functional interaction with the wrist and elbow is crucial and, in a generalized disorder such as rheumatoid disease, the condition of all the upper limb joints and the cervical spine should be carefully assessed.

Weakness Rheumatoid hands are weak because of a combination of generalized muscular weakness, pain inhibition, tendon malalignment or rupture, joint stiffness and nerve compression.

Rheumatoid nodules These are associated with aggressive disease in seropositive patients. They tend to

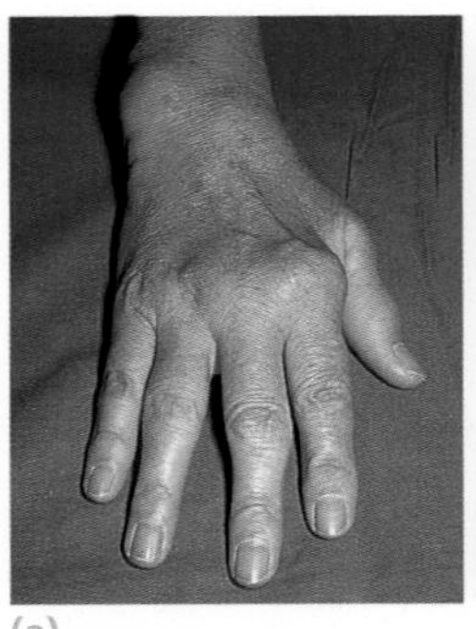
(a)

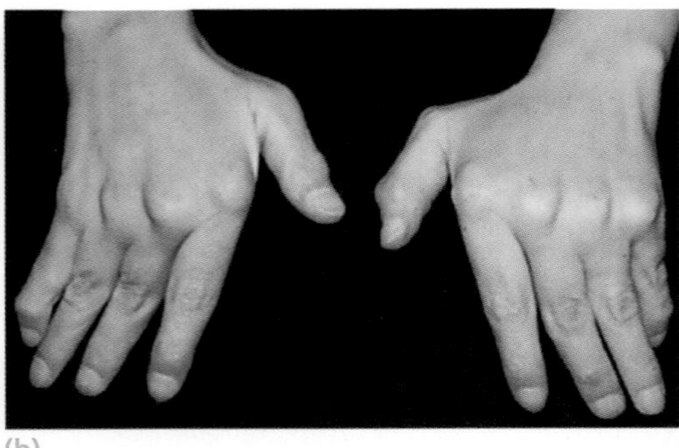
(b)

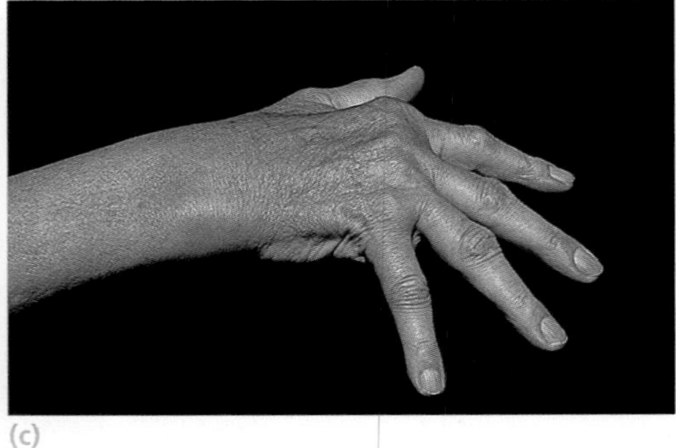
(c)

16.16 Rheumatoid arthritis – clinical features (a) Early case with typical features: radial deviation of the wrist; subluxation of the radio-ulnar joint; swollen MCP joints and ulnar deviation of the fingers. (b) More advanced changes, including subluxation of the MCP joints. (c) Dropped fingers due to rupture of extensor tendons at the wrist.

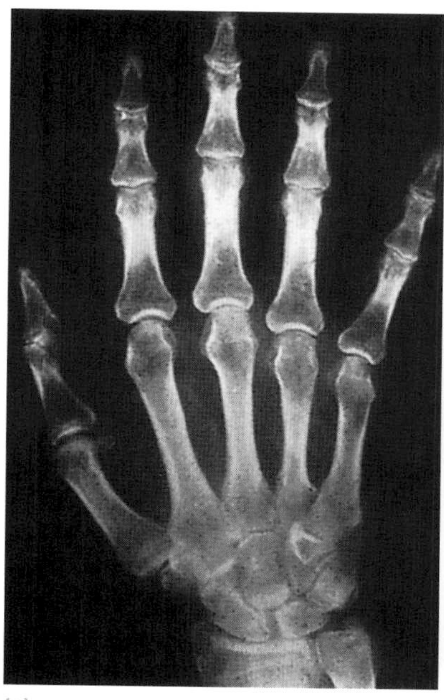
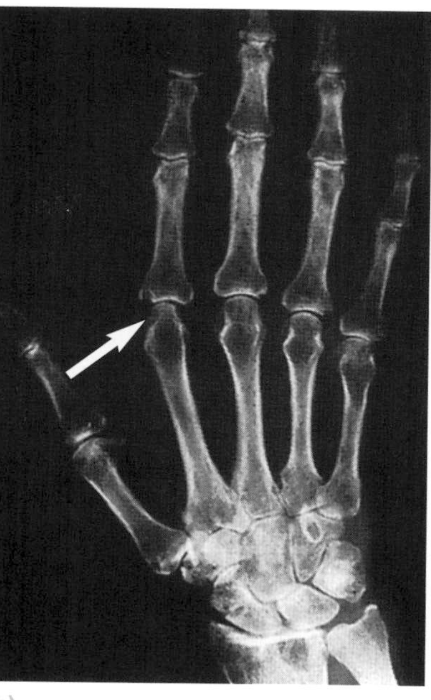
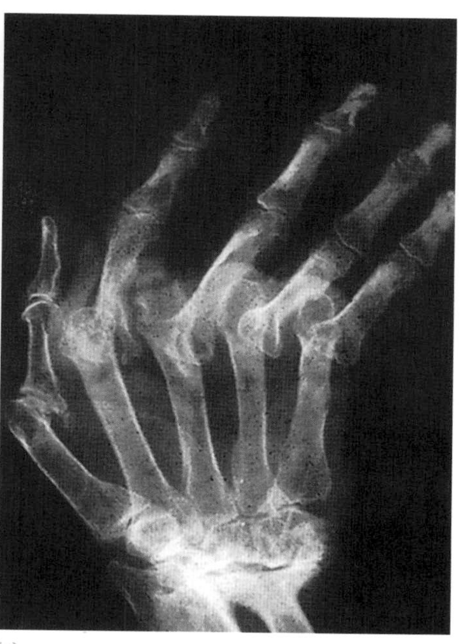

(a) (b) (c)

16.17 Rheumatoid arthritis – x-ray changes (a) Early on, the x-rays may show no more than soft-tissue swelling and juxta-articular osteoporosis. (b) A later stage showing characteristic punched-out juxta-articular erosions at the second and third metacarpo-phalangeal joints. The wrist is now also involved. (c) In the most advanced stage, the metacarpo-phalangeal joints are dislocated and the hand is severely deformed.

occur at pressure areas (e.g. the pulps of the fingers and the radial side of the index finger).

Z-collapse If one of two adjacent joints changes direction, then the overlying long tendons will pull the other joint into the opposite direction. In rheumatoid arthritis, this is typified by radial tilt of the wrist with ulnar drift of the MCP joints, the boutonnière deformity and the swan-neck deformity.

X-rays

During the early stage x-rays show only soft-tissue swelling and osteoporosis around the joints. Later one can usually discern joint 'space' narrowing and small peri-articular erosions; these are commonest at the MCP joints and in the styloid process of the ulna. In advanced cases, articular destruction may be marked, affecting the MCP, PIP and wrist joints almost equally. Joint deformity and dislocation are common.

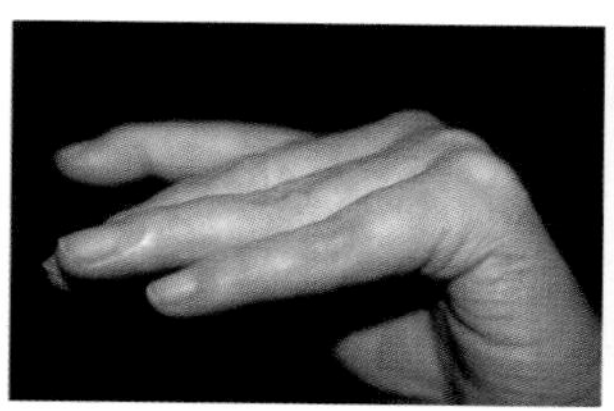
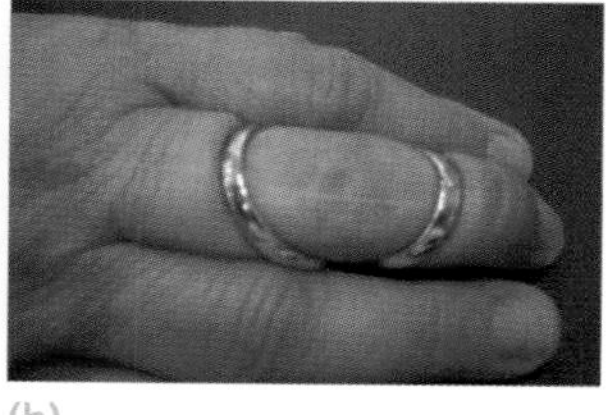

(a) (b)

16.18 Rheumatoid arthritis – treatment (a) Swan-neck deformity; (b) swan-neck 'figure of eight' splint.

Treatment

EARLY STAGE DISEASE

Treatment is directed essentially at controlling the systemic disease and the local synovitis. In addition to general measures, static splints may reduce pain and swelling. These splints are not corrective but are designed to rest inflamed joints and tendons; in mild cases they are worn only at night, in more active cases during the day as well. Persistent synovitis of a few joints or tendon sheaths may benefit from local injections of corticosteroid with local anaesthetic. Only small quantities are injected (e.g. 0.5 mL for an MCP joint or flexor tendon sheath and 1 mL for the wrist). This should not be repeated more than two or three times. A boggy flexor tenosynovitis may not respond to this limited therapeutic assault; operative synovectomy may be needed. If carpal tunnel symptoms are present, the transverse carpal ligament is divided and, if necessary, a flexor synovectomy performed.

Established disease As the disease progresses it becomes increasingly important to prevent deformity. Uncontrolled synovitis of joints or tendons requires operative synovectomy followed by physiotherapy. Excision of the distal end of the ulna, synovectomy of the common extensor sheath and the wrist, and reconstruction of the soft tissues on the ulnar side of the wrist may arrest joint destruction and progressive deformity. Early instability and ulnar drift at the MCP joints can be corrected by

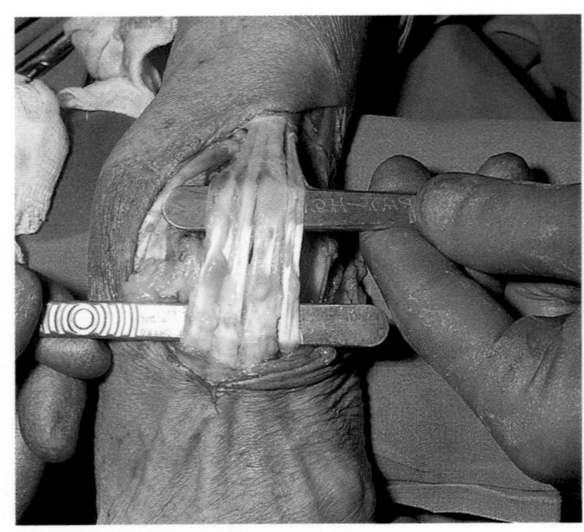

(a)

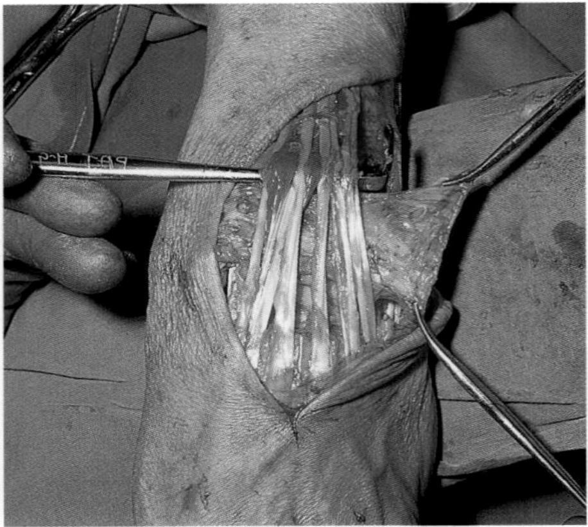

(b)

16.19 Rheumatoid arthritis – synovectomy Synovitis of the common extensor sheath will eventually damage the tendons. (a) Here, after synovectomy, one can see nodules on several tendons. (b) The sheath itself is preserved intact and laid beneath the tendons to cover the back of the joint and provide a bed upon which the tendons can move.

excising the inflamed synovium, tightening the capsular structures and releasing the ulnar pull of the intrinsic tendons. Mobile boutonnière and swan-neck deformities can be treated with splints; if they progress or are fixed, then surgery may be needed. Isolated tendon ruptures are repaired or bypassed by appropriate tendon transfers. These procedures are followed by splintage and hand therapy.

Destruction of the MCP joints without ulnar drift can be treated with surface replacement (chrome–polyethylene or pyrocarbon).

Late disease In late cases deformity is combined with articular destruction; soft-tissue correction alone will not suffice. For the MCP and IP joints of the thumb, arthrodesis gives predictable pain relief, stability and functional improvement. The MCP joints of the fingers can be excised and replaced with Silastic 'spacers', which improve stability and correct deformity. Replacement of IP joints gives less predictable results; if deformity is very disabling (e.g. a fixed swan-neck) it may be better to settle for arthrodesis in a more functional position. At the wrist, painless stability can be regained by fusion of the radio-carpal, midcarpal and CMC joints. Wrist replacement with Silastic or metal–plastic implants, whilst providing some movement, may well fail; the loss of bone stock that accompanies failure means that salvage can be very difficult.

MANAGEMENT OF THUMB DEFORMITIES IN RHEUMATOID ARTHRITIS

Ruptured FPL
- If painless: leave alone
- If painful: tendon graft, flexor digitorum sublimus transfer or IP fusion

Simple boutonnière deformity
- If passively correctible: cortisone injection to MCP joint and splintage
- MCP joint synovectomy and extensor realignment unreliable
- If MCP joint fixed but IP joint passively correctible and CMC joint mobile: fuse MCP joint
- If MCP joint and IP joint fixed: fuse IP joint and either fuse or replace MCP joint

Boutonnière with CMC joint failure
- Trapeziectomy and CMC joint stabilization, with MCP joint and IP joint treated as above

Swan-neck deformity
- CMC joint failure causes adduction contracture of thumb base and MCP joint hyperextension
- If deformity severe: trapeziectomy with soft-tissue reconstruction or fusion of MCP joint

Failure of ulnar collateral ligament (like 'gamekeeper's thumb')
- Synovitis attenuates ulnar collateral ligament. Pinch grip causes increasing deformity
- Ligament reconstruction (if bone and soft-tissue quality allow) or MCP joint fusion

Swan-neck with MCP joint and CMC joint preserved
- Synovitis of MCP joint causes hyperextension with secondary passive flexion of IP joint
- Treat by palmar plate advancement or, if soft tissues tenuous, MCP fusion

Arthritis mutilans
- Arthrodesis with interposition bone graft

The thumb in rheumatoid arthritis

The combination of soft-tissue failure and joint erosion leads to characteristic deformities of the thumb: rupture of flexor pollicis longus tendon, a boutonnière lesion at the MCP joint, CMC instability, swan-neck deformity and ulnar collateral ligament instability.

Depending on the deformity, the patient's demands and the condition of the rest of the hand, treatment may involve various combinations of splintage, tendon repair, joint fusion, excision arthroplasty and joint replacement.

Treatment options are summarized in the accompanying box.

Metacarpo-phalangeal deformities

Chronic synovitis of the MCP joints results in failure of the palmar plate and the collateral ligaments. The powerful flexor tendons drag the proximal phalanx palmarwards, causing subluxation of the joint. The deformity may be aggravated by primary or secondary intrinsic muscle tightness.

The most obvious deformity of the rheumatoid hand is ulnar deviation of the MCP joints. There are several reasons for this: palmar grip and thumb pressure naturally tend to push the index finger ulnarwards; weakening of the collateral ligaments and the first dorsal interosseous muscle reduces the normal resistance to this force; the wrist is usually involved and, as it collapses into radial deviation, the MCP joints automatically veer in the opposite direction (the so-called 'zig-zag mechanism'); once ulnar drift begins, it becomes self-perpetuating due to tightening of the ulnar intrinsic muscles and stretching of the radial intrinsics and the adjacent capsular structures. As the sagittal bands fail, the extensor tendon slips ulnarwards and palmarwards, accentuating the deformity even further.

At an early stage, before joint destruction and soft-tissue instability, synovectomy may relieve pain but the joint usually stiffens somewhat. When ulnar drift has started, splintage may maintain function and retard progression. With marked deformity but little joint damage, a soft-tissue reconstruction (reefing of the radial sagittal bands, tightening of the radial collateral ligament with intrinsic muscle release and transfer) can give a satisfactory and fairly durable correction. Once there is marked damage to the joint surface, replacement with a Silastic spacer, along with the soft-tissue reconstruction, is recommended. There is no point in correcting the MCP joints unless any wrist deformity is also corrected; the tendency to zig-zag deformity will otherwise lead to recurrence of the ulnar drift.

TYPES OF SWAN-NECK DEFORMITY IN RHEUMATOID ARTHRITIS

Type I	PIP joint flexible, independent of MCP position (i.e. Bunnell's test negative). Due to palmar plate failure at PIP joint ± failure of flexor digitorum superficialis
Type II	PIP joint flexibility dependent on MCP position. Intrinsic muscle tightness. Bunnell's test: with MCP joint passively extended, passive PIP joint flexion limited
Type III	PIP joint stiff regardless of MCP position. Due to contracture of joint
Type IV	Destruction of PIP joint

Finger deformities

Boutonnière Synovitis in the proximal IP joint causes elongation or rupture of the central slip which passes over the back of the joint before inserting into the base of the middle phalanx. The lateral bands slip away from the central slip and pass in front of the axis of rotation of the proximal joint but remain behind the axis in the distal joint, to form the characteristic

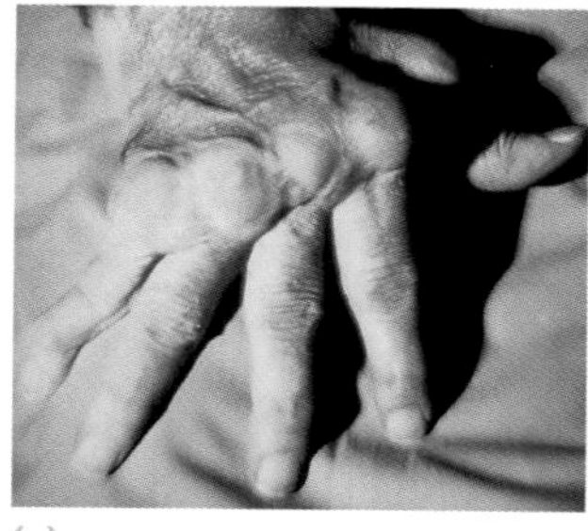
(a)

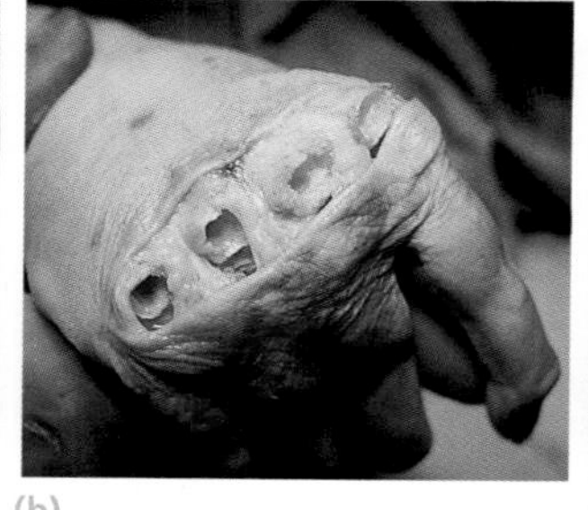
(b)

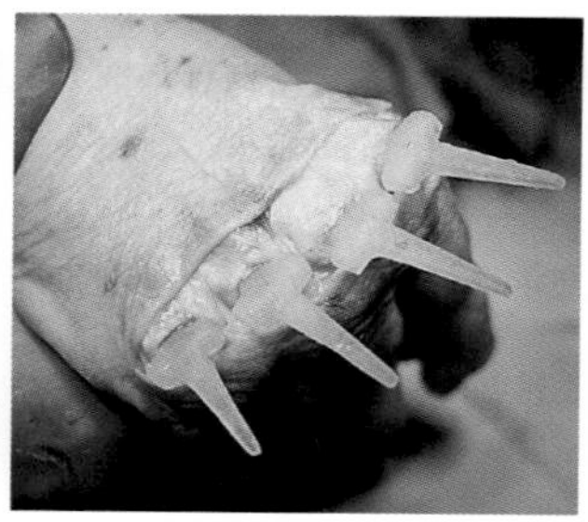
(c)

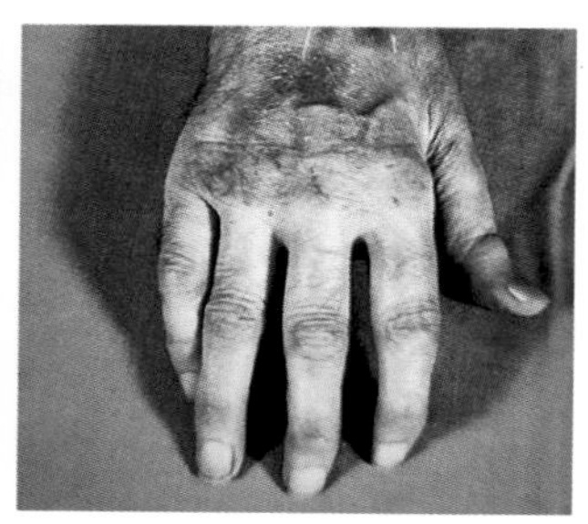
(d)

16.20 Rheumatoid arthritis – joint replacement (a) Before operation. Subluxation and deformity of all the finger MCP joints. (b, c) The eroded metacarpal heads are excised and flexible spacers inserted. (d) Postoperative result.

deformity. Early, correctable deformity responds to splinting and synovectomy; later, central slip reconstruction (an unpredictable procedure) may be required; simple division of the distal insertion is a simpler, and often effective, alternative. In fixed deformities, or those with joint damage, fusion or replacement is considered.

Swan-neck Chronic synovitis may lead to swan-neck deformity by one or more of the following mechanisms: failure of the palmar plate of the PIP joint; rupture of the flexor digitorum superficialis; dislocation or subluxation of the MCP joint and consequent tightening of the intrinsic muscles.

Treatment depends on a careful analysis of the cause and will include figure-of-eight splintage, tendon transfer, intrinsic release and occasionally fusion.

Tenosynovitis and tendon rupture

Extensor tendons Extensor tendon rupture is a common complication of chronic synovitis. Extensor digiti minimi is usually the first to go and predicts rupture of the other tendons. Treatment consists of either suturing the distal tendon stump to an adjacent tendon, inserting a bridge graft (e.g. palmaris longus) or performing a tendon transfer (e.g. extensor indicis proprius). Synovectomy and excision of the distal ulna may also be necessary.

Flexor tendons Flexor tenosynovitis is one of the earliest and most troublesome features of rheumatoid disease. The restriction of finger movement is easily mistaken for arthritis; however, careful palpation of the palm and the nearby joints will quickly show where the swelling and tenderness are located. Secondary problems include carpal tunnel syndrome, triggering of one or more fingers and tendon rupture. Synovitis of the flexor digitorum superficialis also contributes to the swan-neck deformity.

If carpal tunnel release is needed, the operation should include a flexor tenosynovectomy. If the flexor tendons are bulky (best felt over the proximal phalanges) and joint movement is limited, then flexor tenosynovectomy should improve movement and, just as important, should prevent tendon rupture. Triggering, likewise, should be treated by tenosynovectomy rather than simple splitting of the sheath. Rupture of flexor digitorum profundus is best treated by distal IP joint fusion. Rupture of flexor pollicis longus (due to attrition against the underside of the distal radius or flexor synovitis) can be treated either by tendon grafting or by fusion of the thumb IP joint.

OSTEOARTHRITIS

Eighty per cent of people over the age of 65 have radiological signs of osteoarthritis in one or more joints of the hand; fortunately, most of them are asymptomatic.

DISTAL INTERPHALANGEAL JOINTS

Osteoarthritis of the DIP joints is very common in postmenopausal women. It often starts with pain in one or two fingers; the distal joints become swollen and tender, the condition usually spreading to all the fingers of both hands. On examination there is bony thickening around the joints (Heberden's nodes) and some restriction of movement.

Treatment is usually symptomatic. However, if pain and instability are severe, a cortisone injection will give temporary relief. Joint fusion is a good solution. The angle of fusion is debatable. Intramedullary double-pitched screws are effective and avoid the problems of percutaneous wires. However, the final position is one of extension which slightly reduces grip in the little and ring fingers.

Mucous cysts sometimes protrude between the extensor tendon and collateral ligament of an osteoarthritic DIP joint. They press on the germinal matrix of the nail, causing an unsightly groove. They occasionally ulcerate and septic arthritis can develop. If the cyst is too bothersome, excision of the cyst with the underlying osteophyte is effective. With luck, the nail will recover as well.

PROXIMAL INTERPHALANGEAL JOINTS

Not infrequently some of the PIP joints are involved (Bouchard's nodes). These are strongly associated with osteoarthritis elsewhere in the body (polyarticular OA). The joints are swollen and tend to deviate ulnarwards due to mechanical pressure in daily activities.

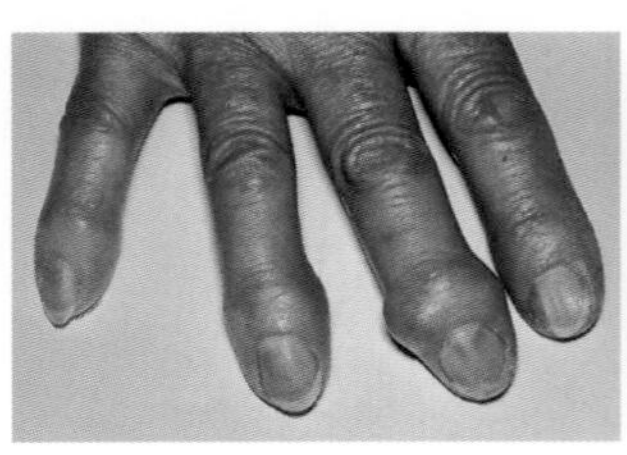
(a)

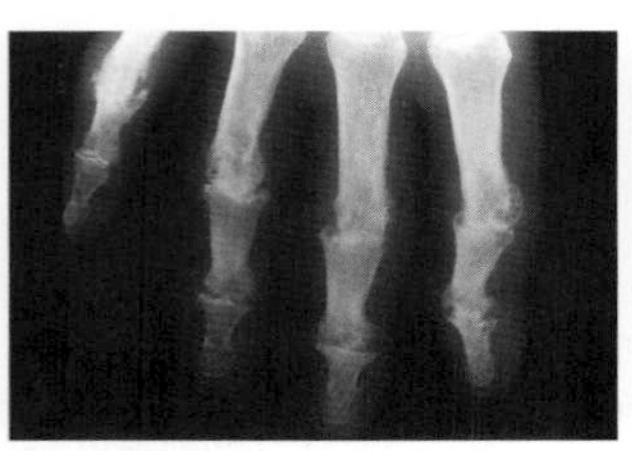
(b)

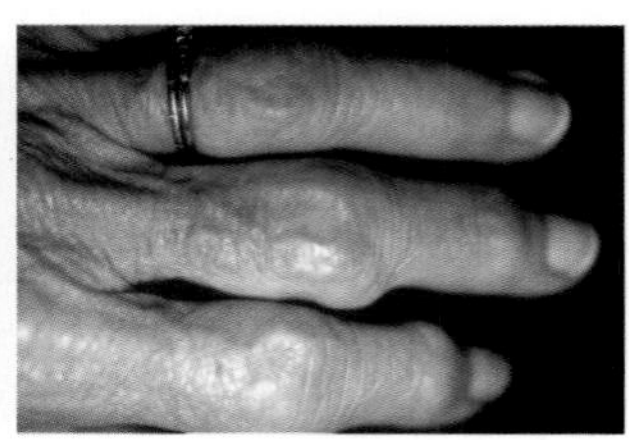
(c)

16.21 Osteoarthritis **(a,b)** The common picture is one of 'knobbly finger-tips' due to involvement of the DIP joints (*Heberden's nodes*). **(c)** In some cases the PIP joints are affected as well (*Bouchard's nodes*).

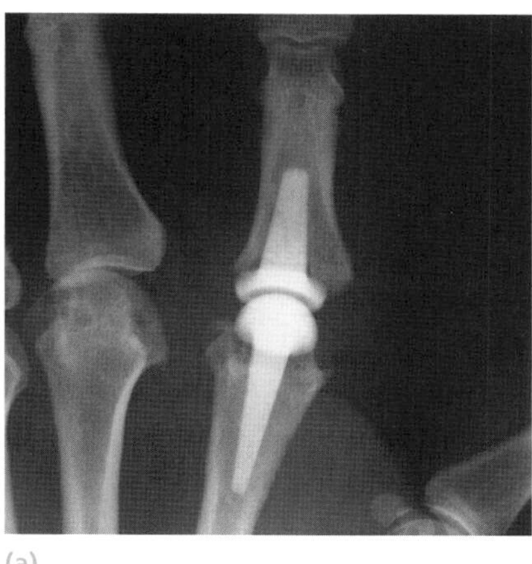
(a)

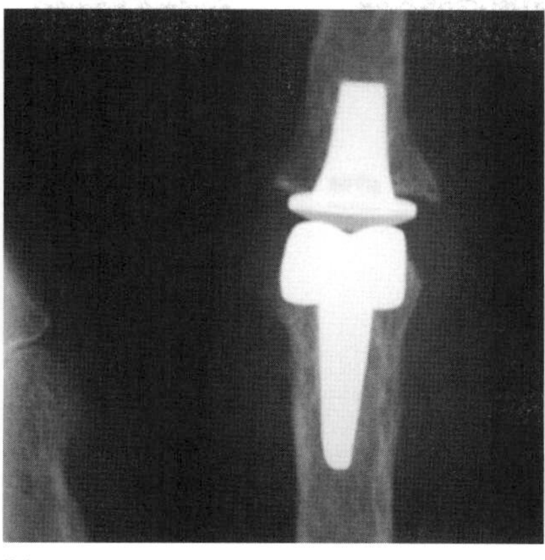
(b)

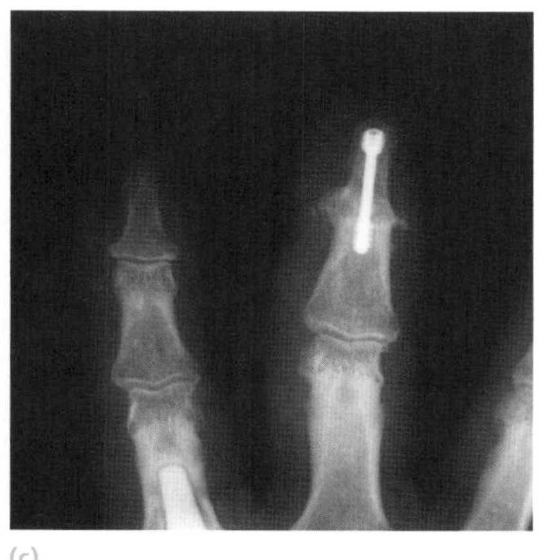
(c)

16.22 Osteoarthritis – operative treatment (a) Pyrocarbon MCP joint replacement. (b) PIP joint replacement. (c) Arthrodesis of the DIP joint.

Treatment is usually non-operative. If the joint is very painful or unstable then surgery is considered. Fusion restores reliable, pain-free pinch in the index and middle finger PIP joints; fusion of the ring and little fingers compromises grip and so joint replacement is usually preferable. Implants made from pyrocarbon, Silastic or metal–polyethylene are available. However, the results are unpredictable: some patients do very well; others have problems with deformity, instability or stiffness.

Metacarpo-phalangeal joints This is an uncommon site for osteoarthritis. When it does occur, a specific cause can usually be identified: previous trauma, infection, gout or haemochromatosis.

Treatment is initially non-operative with the use of analgesics, splints or local injections. Fusion of the thumb MCP gives excellent results; however in the fingers this operation has serious functional consequences and is to be avoided. The MCP joints can be replaced with pyrocarbon or metal–polyethylene implants, with encouraging early and mid-term results.

Carpo-metacarpal joint of the thumb This is discussed on page 403.

Carpo-metacarpal joint of the ring and little fingers These joints can become arthritic, particularly after a fracture-dislocation. Because the fourth and fifth CMC joints normally flex forwards during power grip, pain can be disabling, particularly in patients engaged in heavy manual work. If a steroid injection fails to give improvement, then surgery (usually fusion) is indicated.

ACUTE INFECTIONS OF THE HAND

Infection of the hand is frequently limited to one of several well-defined compartments: under the nail-fold (paronychia); the pulp space (felon) and in the subcutaneous tissues elsewhere; the deep fascial spaces; tendon sheaths; and joints. Usually the cause is a staphylococcus which has been implanted during fairly trivial injury. However, cuts contaminated with unusual organisms account for about 10 per cent of cases.

Pathology

Here, as elsewhere, the response to infection is an acute inflammatory reaction with oedema, suppura-

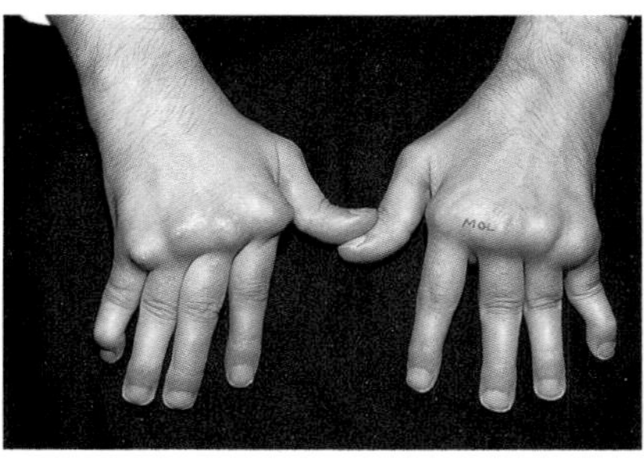
(a)

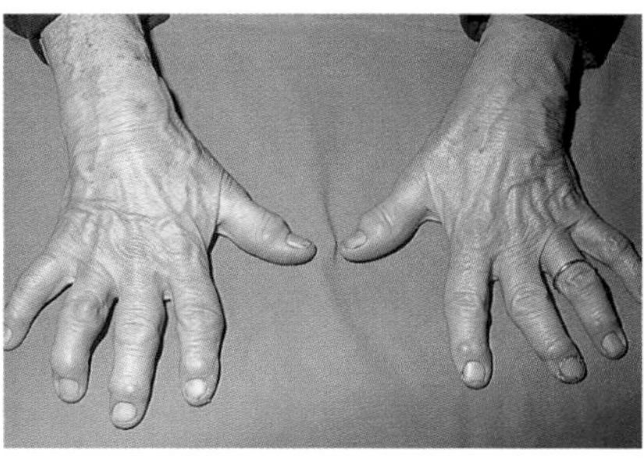
(b)

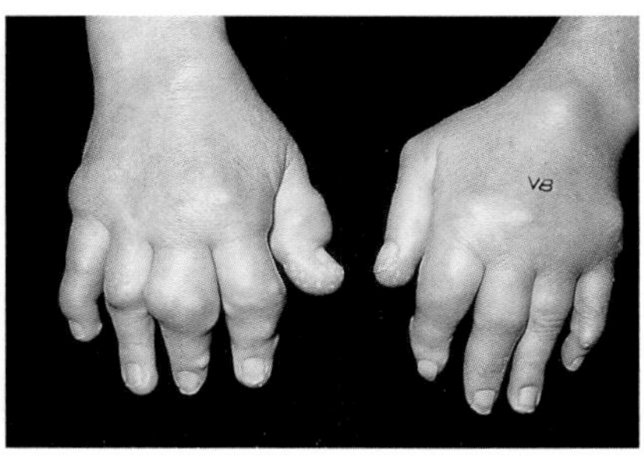
(c)

16.23 Swollen fingers Always be on the alert for 'lookalikes'. The clues (in most cases) are: (a) Proximal joints = rheumatoid arthritis; (b) distal joints = osteoarthritis; asymmetrical joints = gout.

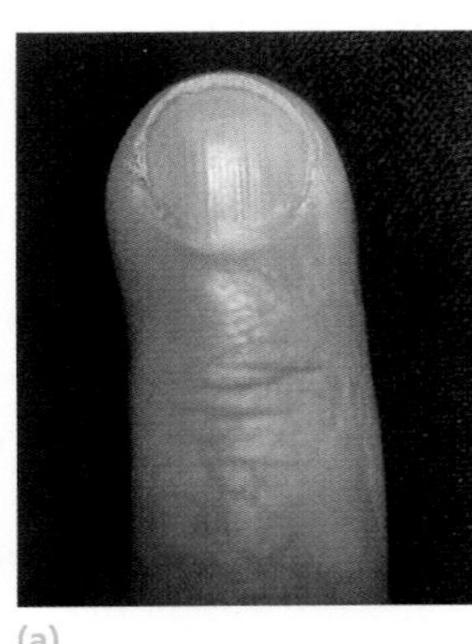

(a)

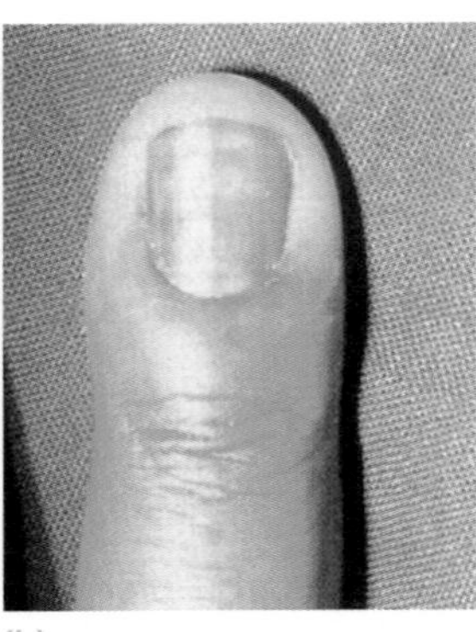

(b)

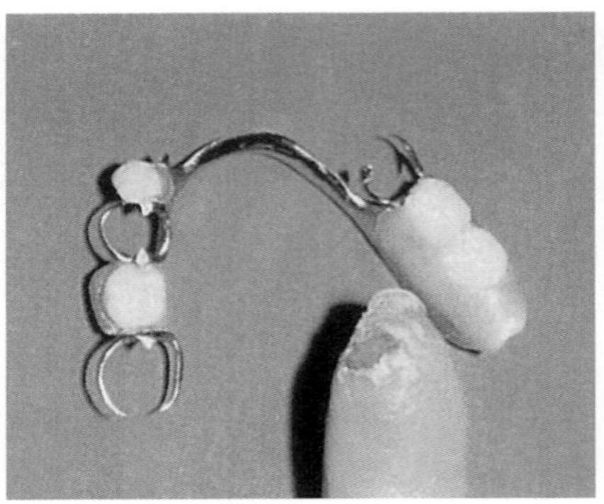

(c)

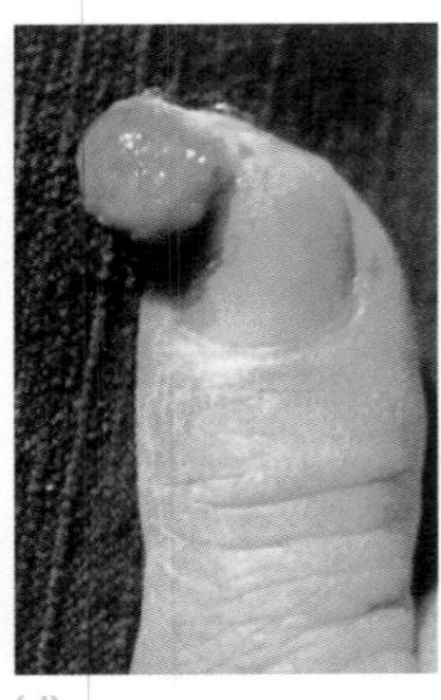

(d)

16.24 Acute infections (1) (a) Acute nail-fold infection (paronychia); and (b) chronic paronychia. (c) Pulp-space infection (felon or whitlow) of the thumb due to a prick-injury on the patient's own denture. (d) Septic granuloma. (Courtesy of Professor S. Biddulph.)

tion and increased tissue tension. In closed tissue compartments (e.g. the pulp space or tendon sheath) pressures may rise to levels where the local blood supply is threatened, with the risk of tissue necrosis. In neglected cases infection can spread from one compartment to another and the end result may be a permanently stiff and useless hand. There is also a danger of lymphatic and haematogenous spread; even apparently trivial infections may give rise to lymphangitis and septicaemia.

Clinical features

Usually there is a history of trauma (a superficial abrasion, laceration or penetrating wound), but this may have been so trivial as to pass unnoticed. A few hours or days later the finger or hand becomes painful and swollen. There may be throbbing and sometimes the patient feels ill and feverish. Ask if he or she can recall any causative incident: a small cut or superficial abrasion, a prick injury (including plant thorns) or a local injection. Also, do not forget to enquire about predisposing conditions such as diabetes mellitus, intravenous drug abuse and immunosuppression.

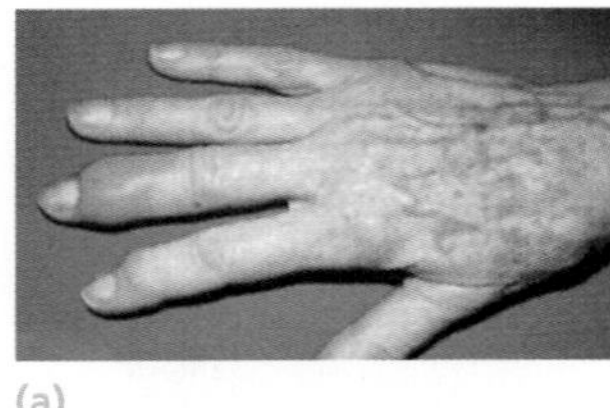

(a)

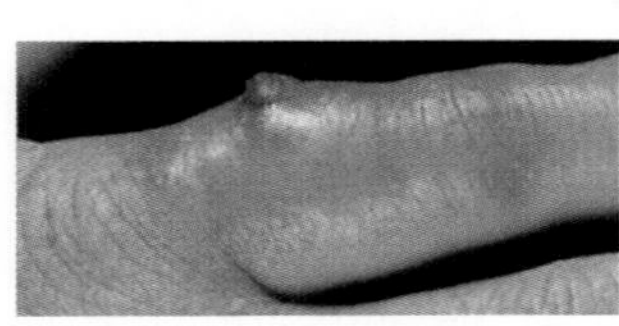

(b)

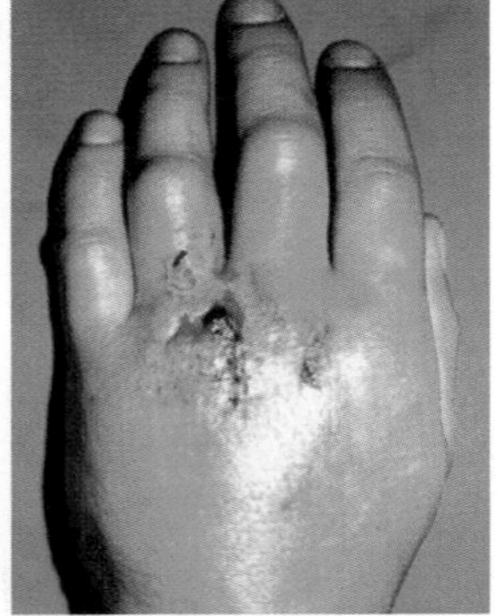

(c)

16.25 Acute infections (2) (a) Septic arthritis of the terminal interphalangeal joint following a cortisone injection. (b) Infected insect 'bite'. (c) Septic human bite resulting in acute infection of the fourth metacarpophalangeal joint. (Courtesy of Professor S. Biddulph.)

On examination the finger or hand is red and swollen, and usually exquisitely tender over the site of tension. However, in immune-compromised patients, in the very elderly and in babies, local signs may be mild. With superficial infection the patient can usually be persuaded to flex an affected finger; with deep infections active flexion is not possible. The arm should be examined for lymphangitis and swollen glands, and the patient more generally for signs of septicaemia.

X-ray examination may disclose a foreign body but is otherwise unhelpful in the early stages of infection. However, a few weeks later there may be features of osteomyelitis or septic arthritis, and later still of bone necrosis.

If pus becomes available, this should be sent for bacteriological examination.

Diagnosis

In making the diagnosis, several conditions must be excluded: an *insect bite or sting* (which can closely mimic a subcutaneous infection), a *thorn prick* (which, itself, can become secondarily infected), acute *tendon rupture* (which may resemble a septic tenosynovitis) and *acute gout* (which is easily mistaken for septic arthritis).

Plant-thorn injuries are extremely common and the distinction between secondary infection and a non-septic reaction to a retained fragment can be difficult. Rose thorn and blackthorn are the usual suspects in the UK, but any plant spine (including cactus needles) can be implicated. The local inflammatory response sometimes leads to recurrent arthritis or tenosynovitis, which is arrested only by removing the retained fragment. If the condition is suspected, the fragment may be revealed by ultrasound scanning or MRI. Secondary infection with unusual soil or plant organisms may occur.

Principles of treatment

Superficial hand infections are common; if their treatment is delayed or inadequate, infection may rapidly extend, with serious consequences. The essentials of treatment are:

- antibiotics
- rest, splintage and elevation
- drainage
- rehabilitation.

Antibiotics As soon as the clinical diagnosis is made, and preferably after a specimen has been taken for Gram stain and culture, antibiotic treatment is started – usually with flucloxacillin or a cephalosporin. If bone infection is suspected, fusidic acid may be added. For bites (which should always be assumed to be infected) a broad-spectrum penicillin is advisable. Agricultural injuries risk infection by anaerobic organisms and it is therefore prudent to add metronidazole. The interim antibiotic may later be changed when the bacterial sensitivity is known.

Rest, splintage and elevation In a mild case the hand is rested in a sling. In a severe case the patient is admitted to hospital; the arm is held elevated in an overhead sling while the patient is kept under observation. Analgesics are given for pain. *The hand must be splinted in the position of safe immobilization* with the wrist slightly extended, the MCP joints in full flexion, the IP joints extended and the thumb in abduction.

Drainage If treated within the first 24–48 hours, many hand infections will respond to antibiotics, rest, elevation and splintage.

If there are signs of an abscess – throbbing pain, marked tenderness and toxaemia – the pus should be drained. A tourniquet and either general or regional block anaesthesia are essential. The hand should be exsanguinated by elevation only; an exsanguinating bandage can spread the sepsis. The incision should be planned to give access to the abscess without causing injury to other structures *but never at right angles across a skin crease.* When pus is encountered it must be carefully wiped away and a search made for deeper pockets of infection. Necrotic tissue should be excised. The area is thoroughly washed out and, in some cases, a catheter may be left in place for further, postoperative, irrigation (e.g. in cases of flexor tenosynovitis). The wound is either left open or lightly sutured, and is then covered with a non-stick dressing and gauze. The pus obtained is sent for culture.

At the end of the operation the hand is splinted in the position of safe immobilization. A removable splint will permit repeated wound dressings and exercises. A sling is used to keep the arm elevated.

The hand should be re-examined within the next

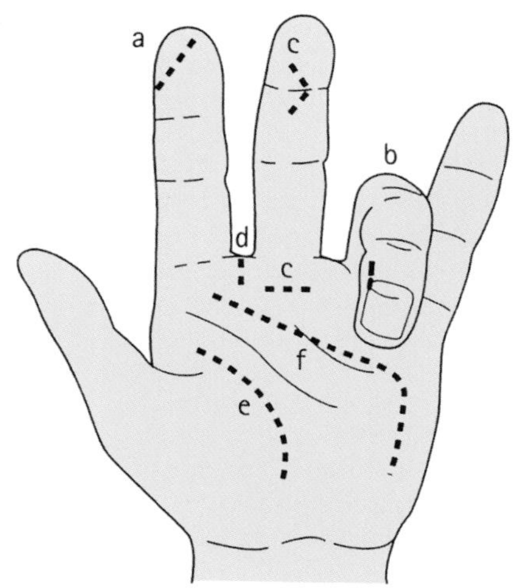

16.27 Infections The incisions for surgical drainage are shown here: **a**, pulp space (directly over the abscess); **b**, nail-fold (it may also be necessary to excise the edge of the nail); **c**, tendon sheath; **d**, web space; **e**, thenar space; **f**, mid-palmar space.

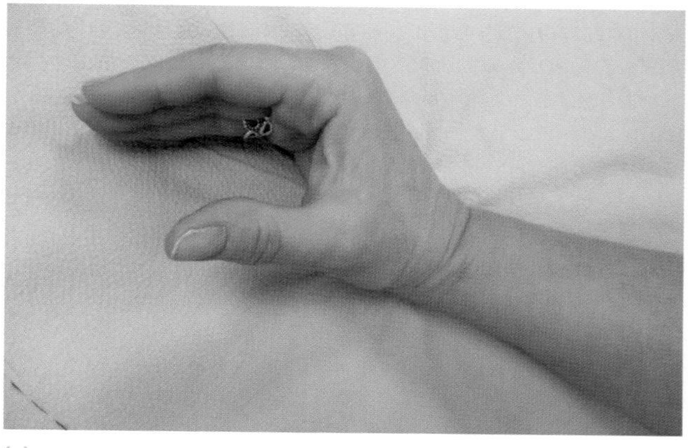

(a)

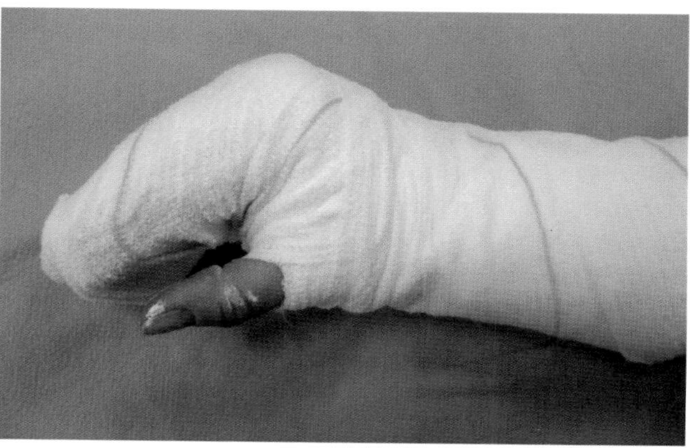

(b)

16.26 The position of safe immobilization The knuckle joints are 90° flexed, the finger joints extended and the thumb abducted. This is the position in which the ligaments are at their longest and splintage is least likely to result in stiffness.

24 hours to ensure that drainage is effective; if it is not, further operative drainage may be needed. Inadequate drainage of acute infection may lead to chronic infection.

Postoperative rehabilitation As soon as the signs of acute inflammation have settled, movements must be started under the guidance of a hand therapist, otherwise the joints are liable to become stiff. For the first few days the resting splint is re-applied between exercise sessions.

Nail-fold infection (paronychia)

Infection under the nail-fold is the commonest hand infection; it is seen most often in children, or in older people after rough nail-trimming. The edge of the nail-fold becomes red and swollen and increasingly tender. A tiny abscess may form in the nail-fold; if this is left untreated, pus can spread under the nail.

At the first sign of infection, treatment with antibiotics alone may be effective. However, if pus is present it must be released by an incision at the corner of the nail-fold in line with the edge of the nail; a pledget of paraffin gauze is used to keep the nail-fold open. If pus has spread under the nail, part or all of the nail may need to be removed.

Chronic paronychia Chronic nail-fold infection may be due to (1) inadequate drainage of an acute infection, or (2) a fungal infection, which requires specific treatment. Topical or oral antifungal agents are used to eradicate fungal infection, but failing this, or for chronic bacterial infection, the nail bed may have to be laid open ('marsupialized'); care should be taken to avoid damaging the germinal nail matrix.

Pulp infection (felon)

The distal finger pad is essentially a closed fascial compartment filled with compact fat and subdivided by radiating fibrous septa. A rise in pressure within the pulp space causes intense pain and, if unrelieved, may threaten the terminal branches of the digital artery which supply most of the terminal phalanx.

Pulp-space infection is usually caused by a prick injury; blackthorn injuries are particularly likely to become infected. The most common organism is *Staphylococcus aureus*. The patient complains of throbbing pain in the finger-tip, which becomes tensely swollen, red and acutely tender.

If the condition is recognized very early, antibiotic treatment and elevation of the hand may suffice. Once an abscess has formed, the pus must be released through a small incision over the site of maximum tenderness. If treatment is delayed, infection may spread to the bone, the joint or the flexor tendon sheath.

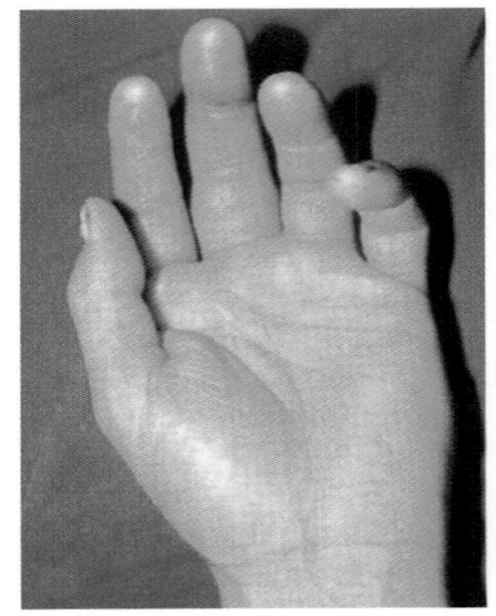

(a)

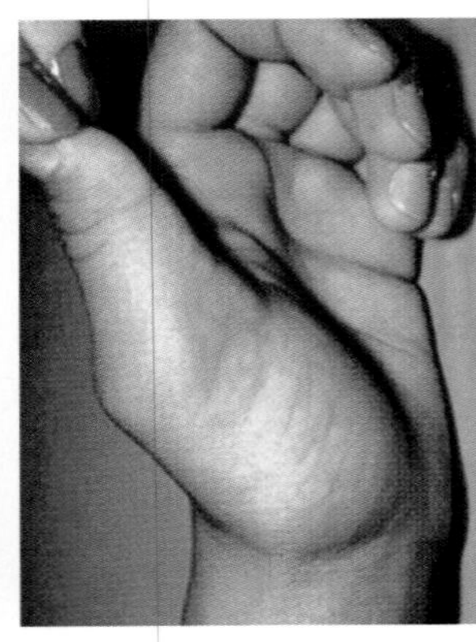

(b)

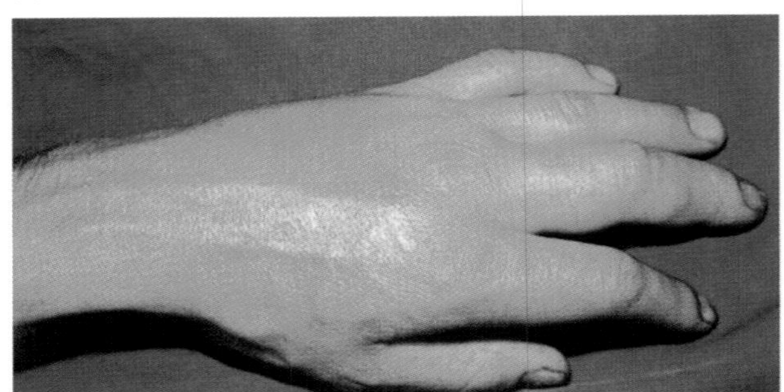

(c)

16.28 Acute infections (a) Flexor tenosynovitis of the middle finger following a cortisone injection. **(b)** Tuberculous synovitis of flexor pollicis longus. **(c)** Diffuse septic extensor tendinitis. (Courtesy of Professor S. Biddulph.)

Postoperatively the finger is dressed with a loose packing of gauze; antibiotic treatment is modified if the results of culture and sensitivity so dictate, and is continued until all signs of infection have cleared. The wound will gradually heal by secondary intention.

Herpetic whitlow The herpes simplex virus may enter the finger-tip, possibly by auto-inoculation from the patient's own mouth or genitalia, or by cross infection during dental surgery. Small vesicles form on the finger-tip, then coalesce and ulcerate. The condition is self-limiting and usually subsides after about 10 days, but may recur from time to time. Herpes whitlow should not be confused with a staphylococcal felon. Surgery is unhelpful and may be harmful, exposing the finger to secondary infection. Aciclovir may be effective in the early stages.

Other subcutaneous infections

Anywhere in the hand a blister, a superficial cut or an insect 'bite' may become infected, causing redness, swelling and tenderness. A local collection of pus should be drained through a small incision over the site of maximal tenderness (but never crossing a skin crease or the web edge); in the finger, a mid-lateral incision is suitable. It is important to exclude a deeper pocket of pus in a nearby tendon sheath or in one of the deep fascial spaces.

Tendon sheath infection (suppurative tenosynovitis)

The tendon sheath is a closed compartment extending from the distal palmar crease to the DIP joint. In the thumb and fifth finger, the sheaths are co-extensive with the radial and ulnar bursae, which envelop the flexor tendons in the proximal part of the palm and across the wrist; these bursae also communicate with Parona's space in the lower forearm.

Pyogenic tenosynovitis is uncommon but dangerous. It usually follows a penetrating injury, the commonest organism being *Staphylococcus aureus*; however, streptococcus and Gram-negative organisms are also encountered.

The affected digit is painful and swollen; it is usually held in slight flexion, is very tender, and the patient will not move it or permit it to be moved. Early diagnosis is based on clinical findings; x-rays are unhelpful but ultrasound scanning may be useful.

Delayed diagnosis results in a progressive rise in pressure within the sheath and a consequent risk of vascular occlusion and tendon necrosis. In neglected cases infection may spread proximally within the radial or ulnar bursa, or from one to the other (*a 'horse-shoe' abscess*); it can also spread proximally to the flexor compartment at the wrist and into Parona's space in the forearm. Occasionally this results in median nerve compression.

KANAVEL'S SIGNS OF FLEXOR SHEATH INFECTION
Flexed posture of digit
Tenderness along the course of the tendon
Pain on passive finger extension
Pain on active flexion

Treatment Treatment must be started as soon as the diagnosis is suspected. The hand is elevated and splinted and antibiotics are administered intravenously – ideally a broad-spectrum penicillin or a systemic cephalosporin. If there is no improvement after 24 hours, surgical drainage is essential. Two incisions are needed, one at the proximal end of the sheath and one at the distal end; using a fine catheter, the sheath is then irrigated (always from proximal to distal) with Ringer's lactate solution. Additional, proximal, incisions may be needed if the synovial bursae are infected.

Postoperatively the hand is swathed in absorbent dressings and splinted in the position of safe immobilization. The dressings should not be too bulky, as this will make it difficult to ensure correct positioning of the joints. The flexor sheath catheter is left in place; using a syringe, the sheath is irrigated with 20 mL of saline three or four times a day for the next 2 days. The catheter and dressings are then removed and finger movements are started.

Stiffness is a very real risk and so early supervised hand therapy must be arranged.

Deep fascial space infection

The large thenar and mid-palmar fascial spaces may be infected directly by penetrating injuries or by secondary spread from a web space or an infected tendon sheath.

Clinical signs can be misleading; the hand is painful but, because of the tight deep fascia, there may be little or no swelling in the palm while the dorsum bulges like an inflated glove. There is extensive tenderness and the patient holds the hand as still as possible.

Treatment As with other infections, splintage and intravenous antibiotics are commenced as soon as the diagnosis is made. For drainage, an incision is made directly over the abscess (being careful not to cross the flexor creases) and sinus forceps inserted; if the web space is infected it, too, should be incised. A *thenar space* abscess can be approached through the first web space (but do not incise in the line of the skin-fold) or through separate dorsal and palmar incisions around the thenar eminence. Great care must be taken to avoid damage to the tendons, nerves and blood vessels. A thorough knowledge of anatomy is essential. The deep *mid-palmar space* (which lies between the flexor tendons and the metacarpals) can be drained through an incision in the web space between the middle and ring fingers, but wider exposure through a transverse or oblique palmar incision is preferable, taking care not to cross the flexor creases directly. Above all, do not be misled by the swelling on the back of the hand into attempting drainage through the dorsal aspect.

Occasionally, deep infection extends proximally across the wrist, causing symptoms of median nerve compression. Pus can be drained by anteromedial or anterolateral approaches; incisions directly over the flexor tendons and median nerve are avoided.

Operation wounds are either loosely stitched or left open. Bulky dressings and saline irrigation are employed, more or less as described for tendon sheath infections.

Septic arthritis

Any of the MCP or finger joints may be infected, either directly by a penetrating injury or intra-articular injection, or indirectly from adjacent structures (and occasionally by haematogenous spread from a distant site). *Staphylococcus* and *Streptococcus* are the usual organisms; *Haemophilus influenzae* is a common pathogen in children. A 'fight-bite' is a common cause of infection of the MCP joints (see Fig. 16.25).

Pain, swelling and redness are localized to a single joint, and all movement is resisted. The presence of lymphangitis and/or systemic features may help to clinch the diagnosis; in their absence, the early symptoms and signs are indistinguishable from those of acute gout. Joint aspiration may give the answer.

Treatment Intravenous antibiotics are administered and the hand is splinted. If the inflammation does not subside within 24 hours, or if there are overt signs of pus, open drainage is needed. Dorso-ulnar or dorsoradial incisons between the collateral ligaments and extensors are recommended for the finger IP joints; for the MCP joints, mid-dorsal incision is needed. The capsule is closed with a soluble suture but the skin wounds are left open, to heal by secondary intention. Copious dressings are applied and the hand is splinted in the 'position of safety' for 48 hours; thereafter, movement is encouraged.

Intravenous antibiotics are continued until all signs of sepsis have disappeared; it is prudent to follow this with another 2-week course of oral antibiotics.

Bites

ANIMAL BITES

Animal bites are usually inflicted by cats, dogs, farm animals or rodents. Many become infected and, although the common pathogens are staphylococci and streptococci, unusual organisms like *Pasteurella multocida* are often reported.

HUMAN BITES

Human bites are generally thought to be even more prone to infection. A wide variety of organisms (including anaerobes) are encountered, the commonest being *Staphylococcus aureus*, *Streptococcus* Group A and *Eikenella corrodens.*

Bites can involve any part of the hand, fingers or thumb; tell-tale signs of a human bite are lacerations on both volar and dorsal surfaces of the finger. Often, though, the 'bite' consists only of a dorsal wound over one of the MCP knuckles, sustained during a fist-fight. *All such wounds should be assumed to be infected.* Moreover, it should be remembered that a laceration of the clenched fist may have penetrated the extensor apparatus and entered the MCP joint; this will not be apparent if the wound is examined with the fingers in extension because the extensor hood and capsule will have retracted proximally.

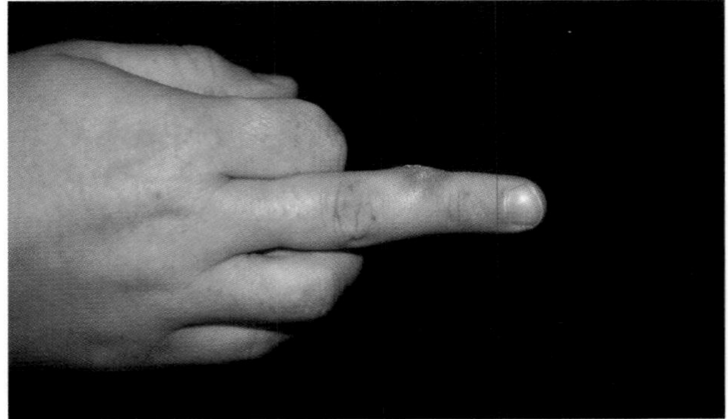

16.29 Mycobacterium marinum Infection in an aquarium keeper.

X-rays should be obtained (to exclude a fracture, tooth fragment or foreign body) and swabs taken for bacterial culture and sensitivity.

Treatment

Fresh wounds should be carefully examined in the operating theatre and, if necessary, extended and debrided. Search for a fragment of tooth or – with a knuckle bite – for a *divot* of articular cartilage from the joint. The hand is splinted and elevated and antibiotics are given prophylactically until the laboratory results are obtained.

Infected bites will need debridement, wash-outs and intravenous antibiotic treatment. The common infecting organisms are all sensitive to broad-spectrum penicillins (e.g. amoxicillin with clavulanic acid) and cephalosporins. With animal bites one should also consider the possibility of rabies.

Postoperative treatment consists, as usual, of copious wound dressings, splintage in the 'safe' position and encouragement of movement once the infection has resolved. Tendon lacerations can be dealt with when the tissues are completely healed.

Mycobacterial infections

Tuberculous tenosynovitis is uncommon even in countries where tuberculosis is still rife. The diagnosis should be considered in patients with chronic synovitis once the alternatives such as rheumatoid disease have been excluded; it can be confirmed by synovial biopsy. Treatment is by synovectomy and then prolonged chemotherapy.

'Fishmonger's infection' is a chronic infection of the hand caused by *Mycobacterium marinum.* The

organism is introduced by prick-injuries from fish spines or hard fins in people working with fish or around fishing boats. It may appear as no more than a superficial granuloma, but deep infection can give rise to an intractable synovitis of tendon or joint. Other causes of chronic synovitis must be excluded; definitive diagnosis usually requires biopsy for histological examination and special culture.

Superficial lesions often heal on their own; if not, they can be excised. Deep lesions usually require surgical synovectomy. Prolonged antibiotic treatment is needed to avoid recurrence; the recommended drug is a broad-spectrum tetracycline such as minocycline, or else chemotherapy with ethambutol and rifampicin.

Fungal infections

Superficial tinea infection of the palm and interdigital clefts (similar to 'athlete's foot') is fairly common and can be controlled by topical preparations. Tinea of the nails can be more difficult to eradicate and may require oral antifungal medication and complete removal of the nail.

Subcutaneous infection by *Sporothrix schenckii* (sporotrichosis) is rarely seen in the UK but is not uncommon in North America, where it is usually caused by a thorn prick. Chronic ulceration at the prick site, unresponsive to antibiotic treatment, may suggest the diagnosis, which can be confirmed by microbiological culture. The recommended treatment is oral potassium iodide.

Deep mycotic infection may involve tendons or joints. The diagnosis should be confirmed by microscopy and microbiological culture. Treatment is by local excision and administration of an intravenous antifungal agent. Resistant cases occasionally require limited amputation.

Opportunistic fungal infections are more likely to occur in debilitated and immunosuppressed patients.

VASCULAR DISORDERS OF THE HAND

Emboli

Arising from the heart or from aneurysms in the arteries of the upper limb, emboli can lodge in distal vessels causing splinter haemorrhages, or in larger, more proximal vessels, causing ischaemia of the arm. A large embolus leads to the classic signs of pain, pulselessness, paraesthesia, pallor and paralysis. Untreated, gangrene or ischaemic contracture ensues.

Raynaud's disease

Raynaud's syndrome is produced by a vasospastic disorder which affects mainly the hands and fingers. Attacks are usually precipitated by cold; the fingers go pale and icy, then dusky blue (or cyanotic) and finally red. Between attacks the hands look normal. The condition is most commonly seen in young women who have no underlying or predisposing disease.

Raynaud's phenomenon is the term applied when these changes are associated with an underlying disease such as scleroderma or arteriosclerosis. Similar, though milder, changes are also seen in thoracic outlet syndrome. The hands must be kept warm. Calcium channel blockade, iloprost infusions or digital sympathectomy (surgical removal of the sympathetic plexus around the digital arteries) may be needed.

Hand–arm vibration syndrome

Excessive and prolonged use of vibrating tools can damage the nerves and vessels in the fingers. The damage is proportional to the duration of exposure and amount of vibration. There are two components: vascular and neurological. The *vascular component* is similar to Raynaud's phenomenon, with the finger-tips turning white in cold weather, then changing through blue and red as the circulation is restored. The *neurological component* involves numbness and tingling in the finger-tips. In advanced cases there can be reduced dexterity. Some patients have clear carpal tunnel syndrome as well.

Treatment is generally unsatisfactory, but includes avoidance of cold weather and smoking as well as, of course, vibrating tools. Carpal tunnel syndrome associated with vibration, in the absence of a more diffuse neuropathy, responds fairly well to standard decompression.

ULNAR ARTERY THROMBOSIS

Repeated blows to the hand, especially using the hypothenar eminence as a hammer, can damage the intima of the ulnar artery, leading to either thrombosis or an aneurysm. The patient presents with cold intolerance in the little finger. Microvascular reconstruction of the ulnar artery is needed.

OTHER GENERAL DISORDERS

A number of generalized disorders should always be borne in mind when considering the diagnosis of any unusual lesion that appears to be confined to the hand. It is beyond the scope of this book to enlarge on these conditions. The few examples shown in Figure 16.30

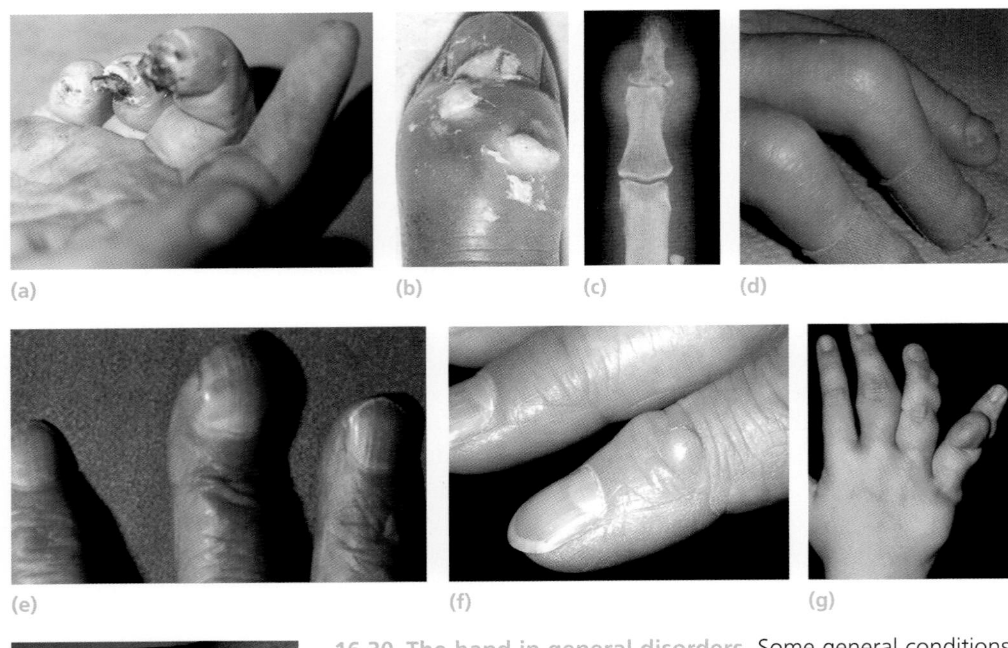

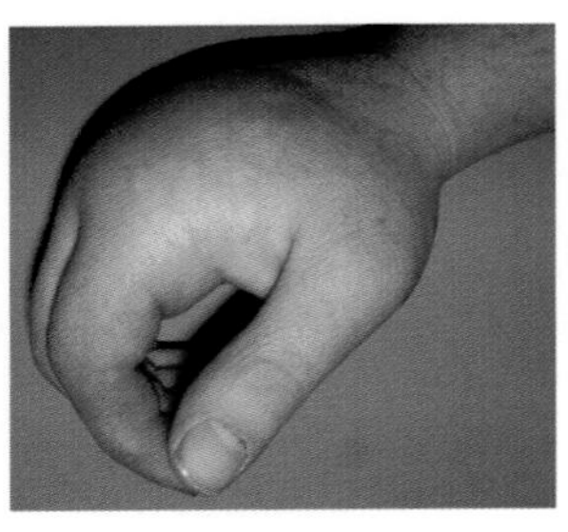

16.30 The hand in general disorders Some general conditions that may manifest with lesions in the hand: (a) scleroderma; (b,c) gouty tophi; (d) psoriasis; (e) implantation dermoid; (f) dermatofibroma; (g) Maffucci's syndrome; (h) Secretan's syndrome (hard odema due to repetitive trauma, often self-inflicted).

serve merely as a reminder that a general history and examination are as important as focussed attention on the hand.

NOTES ON APPLIED ANATOMY

FUNCTION

The hand serves three basic functions: *sensory perception, precise manipulation* and *power grip*. The first two involve the thumb, index and middle fingers; without normal sensation and the ability to oppose these three digits, manipulative precision will be lost. The ring and little fingers provide power grip, for which they need full flexion though sensation is less important.

With the wrist flexed the fingers and thumb fall naturally into extension. With the wrist extended the fingers curl into flexion and the tips of the thumb, index and middle fingers form a functional tripod; this is the *position of function*, because it is best suited to the actions of prehension.

Finger flexion is strongest when the wrist is powerfully extended; normal grasp is possible only with a painless, stable wrist. Spreading the fingers produces abduction to either side of the middle finger; bringing them together, adduction. Abduction and adduction of the thumb occur in a plane at right angles to the palm (i.e. with the hand lying palm upwards, abduction points the thumb to the ceiling). By a combination of movements the thumb can also be opposed to each of the other fingers. Functionally, the thumb is 40 per cent of the hand.

SKIN

The *palmar skin* is relatively tight and inelastic; skin loss can be ill-afforded and wounds sutured under tension are liable to break down. The acute sensibility of the digital palmar skin cannot be achieved by any skin graft. Although the *dorsal skin* seems lax and mobile with the fingers extended, flexion will show that there is very little spare skin. Loss of skin therefore often requires a graft or flap.

Just deep to the palmar skin is the palmar aponeurosis, the embryological remnant of a superficial layer of finger flexors; attachment to the bases of the proximal phalanges explains part of the deformity of Dupuytren's contracture. Incisions on the palmar surface are also liable to contracture unless they are

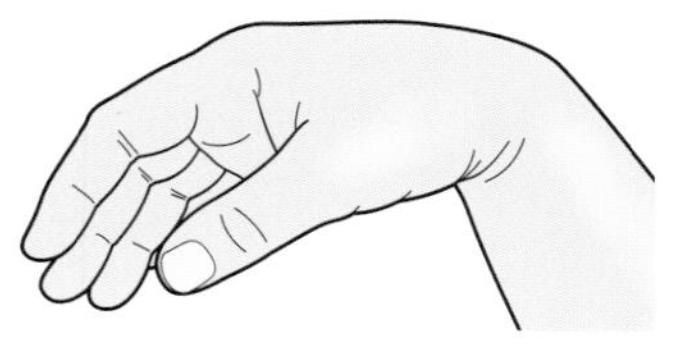
(a)

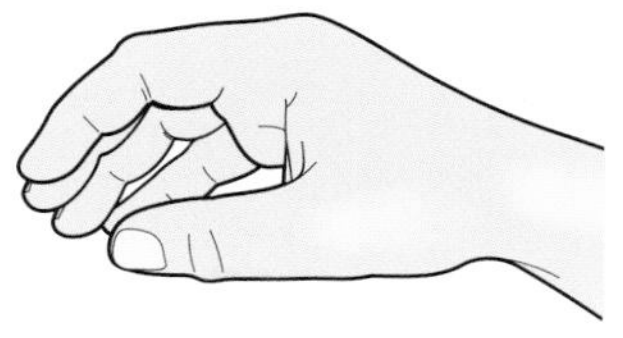
(b)

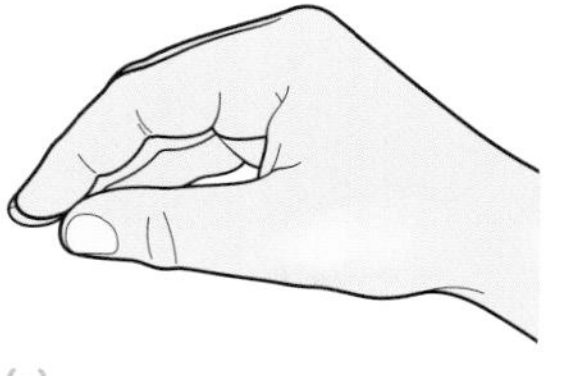
(c)

16.31 Three positions of the hand (a) The position of relaxation, (b) the position of function (ready for action), (c) the position of safe immobilization, with the ligaments taut.

placed in the line of the skin creases, along the midlateral borders of the fingers or obliquely across the creases.

JOINTS

The carpo-metacarpal joints The second and third metacarpals have very little independent movement; the fourth and fifth have more, allowing greater closure of the ulnar part of the hand during power grip. The metacarpal of the thumb is the most mobile and the first CMC joint is a frequent target for degenerative arthritis.

The metacarpo-phalangeal joints These flex to about 90 degrees. The range of extension increases progressively from the index to the little finger. The collateral ligaments are lax in extension (permitting abduction) and tight in flexion (preventing abduction). *If these joints are immobilized they should always be in flexion, so that the ligaments are at full stretch and therefore less likely to shorten if they should fibrose.*

The interphalangeal joints The IP joints are simple hinges, each flexing to about 90 degrees. Their collateral ligaments send attachments to the volar plate and these fibres are tight in extension and lax in flexion; *immobilization of the IP joints, therefore, should always be in extension.*

MUSCLES AND TENDONS

Two sets of muscles control finger movements: the *long extrinsic muscles* (extensors, deep flexors and superficial flexors), and the *short intrinsic muscles* (interossei, lumbricals and the short thenar and hypothenar muscles). The extrinsics extend the MCP joints (long extensors) and flex the IP joints (long flexors). The intrinsics flex the MCP and extend the IP joints; the dorsal interossei also abduct and the palmar interossei adduct the fingers from the axis of the middle finger. Spasm or contracture of the intrinsics causes the *intrinsic-plus* posture – flexion at the MCP joints, extension at the IP joints and adduction of the thumb. Paralysis of the intrinsics produces the *intrinsic-minus* posture – hyperextension of the MCP and flexion of the IP joints ('claw hand').

Tough *fibrous sheaths* enclose the flexor tendons as they traverse the fingers; starting at the MCP joints (level with the distal palmar crease) they extend to the DIP joints. They serve as runners and pulleys, so preventing the tendons from bowstringing during flexion. Scarring within the fibro-osseous tunnel prevents normal excursion.

The long extensor tendons are prevented from bowstringing at the wrist by the extensor retinaculum; here they are liable to frictional trauma. Over the MCP joints each extensor tendon widens into an expansion which inserts into the proximal phalanx and then splits in three; a central slip inserts into the middle phalanx, the two lateral slips continue distally, join and end in the distal phalanx. Division of the middle slip causes a flexion deformity of the PIP joint (boutonnière); rupture of the distal conjoined slip causes flexion deformity of the DIP joint (mallet finger).

NERVES

The median nerve supplies the abductor pollicis brevis, opponens pollicis and lumbricals to the middle and index fingers; it also innervates the palmar skin of the thumb, index and middle fingers and the radial half of the ring finger.

The ulnar nerve supplies the hypothenar muscles, all the interossei, lumbricals to the little and ring fingers, flexor pollicis brevis and adductor pollicis. Sensory branches innervate the palmar and dorsal skin of the little finger and the ulnar half of the ring finger.

The radial nerve supplies skin over the dorsoradial aspect of the hand.

REFERENCES AND FURTHER READING

Warwick D, Dunn R, Melikyan E, Vadher J. *Hand Surgery* 2009: Oxford University Press, Oxford.

Green DP, Hotchkiss RN, Pederson WC, Wolfe SW. *Green's Operative Hand Surgery*, 5th Edition. Elsevier, London.

Mobergh E. Objective methods for determining the functional value of sensitivity in the hand. *Journal of Bone and Joint Surgery* 1958; **40B:** 454–76.

Smith P. *The Hand, Diagnosis and Indications.* 4th Edition. Churchill Livingstone, Edinburgh.

The neck

17

Stephen Eisenstein, Louis Solomon

CLINICAL ASSESSMENT

SYMPTOMS

Pain is felt in the neck itself, but it may also be referred to the shoulders or arms. If it starts suddenly after exertion, and is exaggerated by coughing or straining, think of a disc prolapse. Pain spreading down an arm and forearm with paraesthesiae in the hand will strengthen the likelihood of a disc prolapse with cervical root compression. Chronic or recurrent pain in older people is usually due to chronic disc degeneration and spondylosis. Always enquire if any posture or movement makes it worse; or better.

Stiffness may be either intermittent or continuous. Sometimes it is so severe that the patient can scarcely move the head.

Deformity usually appears as a wry neck; occasionally the neck is fixed in flexion.

Numbness, tingling and weakness in the upper limbs may be due to pressure on a nerve root; weakness in the lower limbs may result from cord compression in the neck.

Headache sometimes emanates from the neck, especially occipital headache, but if this is the only symptom other causes should be suspected.

'Tension' is often mentioned as a cause of neck pain and occipital headache. The neck and back are common 'target zones' for psychosomatic illness.

SIGNS

No examination of the neck is complete without examination of the upper trunk, both upper limbs, and shoulder joints.

Look

Any deformity is noted. Wry neck, due to muscle spasm, may suggest a disc lesion, an inflammatory disorder or cervical spine injury, but it also occurs with intracranial lesions and disorders of the eyes or semicircular canals. Neck stiffness is usually fairly obvious.

Feel

The front of the neck is most easily palpated with the patient seated and the examiner standing behind him or her. The best way to feel the back of the neck is with the patient lying prone and resting his or her head over a pillow; this way he or she can relax and the bony structures are more easily palpated. Feel for tender spots or lumps and note if the paravertebral muscles are in spasm.

Move

Forward flexion, extension, lateral flexion and rotation are tested, and then shoulder movements. Range of motion normally diminishes with age, but even then movement should be smooth and pain-free. While testing for both active and passive movements, ask whether any motion is painful; this could be suggestive of cervical intervertebral disc degeneration. Movement-induced pain or paraesthesia down the arm is particularly noteworthy. In Spurling's test the patient is instructed to rotate the neck to one side with the chin elevated: if ipsilateral upper limb pain and paraesthesiae are reproduced, that would increase the suspicion of a disc prolapse with cervical root compression. Pain may be relieved by having the patient place the arm overhead (the abduction relief sign).

Tests for arterial compression

If the thoracic outlet is tight, the radial pulse may disappear if, when the patient holds a deep breath, the neck is turned towards the affected side and extended (Adson's test), or if the shoulder is elevated and externally rotated (Wright's test).

Neurological examination

Neurological examination of the upper limbs is mandatory in all cases; in some the lower limbs also

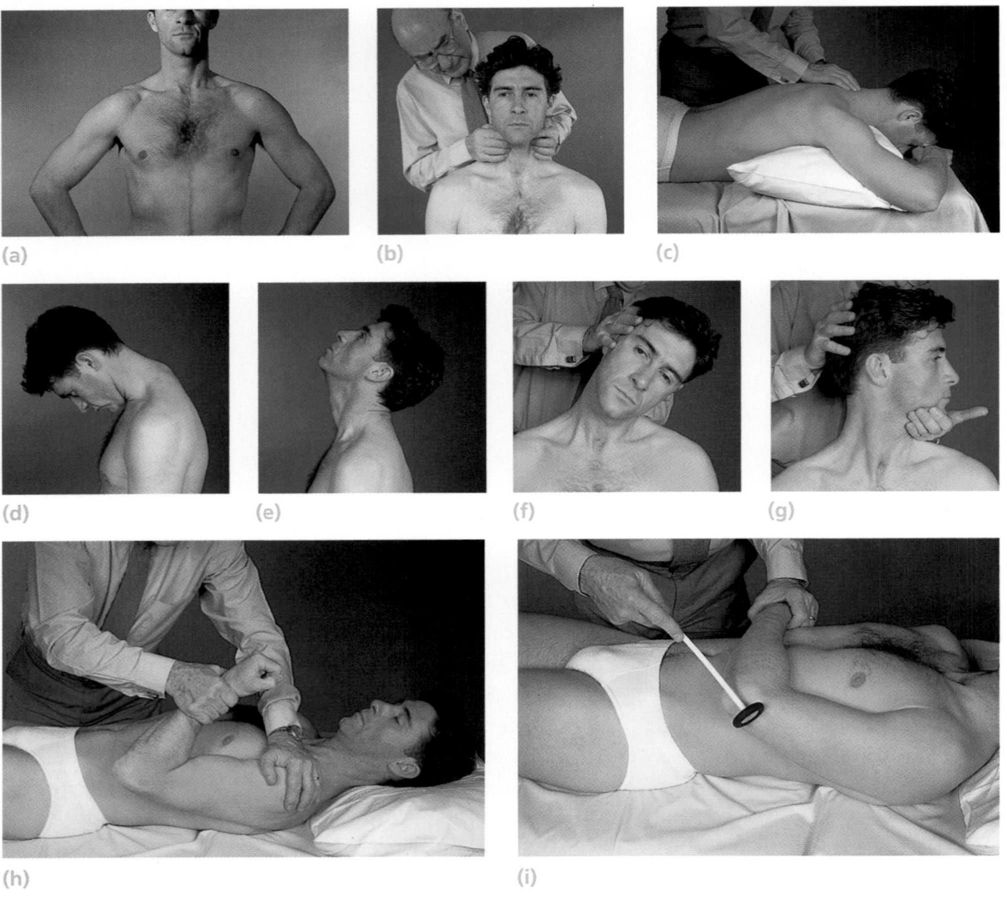

17.1 Examination (a) Look for any deformity or superficial blemish which might suggest a disorder affecting the cervical spine. (b) The front of the neck is felt with the patient seated and the examiner standing behind him. (c) The back of the neck is most easily and reliably felt with the patient lying prone over a pillow; this way muscle spasm is reduced and the neck is relaxed. (d–g) Movement: flexion ('chin on chest'); extension ('look up at the ceiling'); lateral flexion ('tilt your ear towards your shoulder')' and rotation ('look over your shoulder'). (h,i) Neurological examination is mandatory.

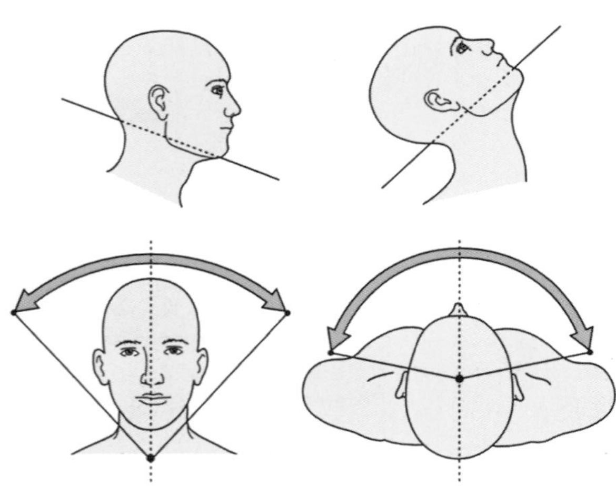

17.2 Normal range of movement Flexion and extension of the neck are best gauged by observing the angle of the occipitomental line – an imaginary line joining the tip of the chin and the occipital protuberance. In full flexion, the chin normally touches the chest; in full extension, the occipitomental line forms an angle of at least 45° with the horizontal, and more than 60° in young people. Lateral flexion is usually achieved up to 45° and rotation to 80° each way.

should be examined. Muscle power, reflexes and sensation should be carefully tested; even small degrees of abnormality may be significant.

IMAGING

X-RAYS

The standard radiographic series for the cervical spine comprises anteroposterior, lateral and open-mouth views. Additional lateral views with the neck in flexion and extension should be obtained provided there is no history of recent neck injury.

The anteroposterior view should show the regular, undulating outline of the lateral masses; their symmetry may be disturbed by destructive lesions or fractures. A projection through the mouth is required to show the upper two vertebrae.

When looking at the lateral view, *make sure that all seven vertebrae can be seen*; patients have been paralysed, and some have lost their lives, because a fracture-dislocation at C6/7 or C7/T1 was missed. The normal cervical lordotic curve shows four parallel lines: one along the anterior surfaces of the vertebral bodies, one along their posterior surfaces, one along the posterior borders of the lateral masses and one along the bases of the spinous processes; any malalignment suggests subluxation. The disc spaces are inspected; loss of disc height and the presence of osteophytic spurs at the margins of adjacent vertebral bodies suggest chronic intervertebral disc degeneration. The posterior interspinous spaces are compared;

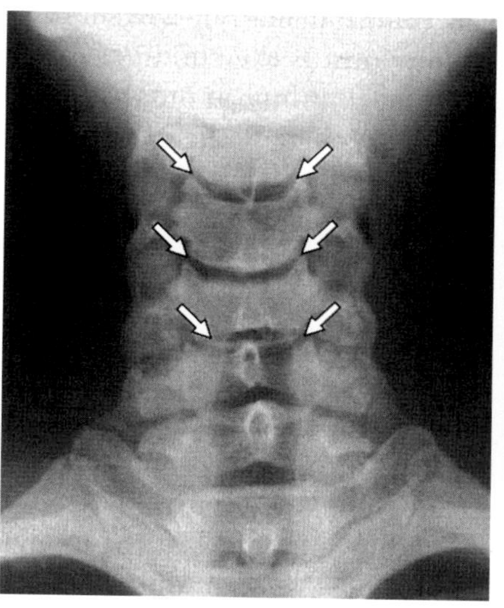

(a)

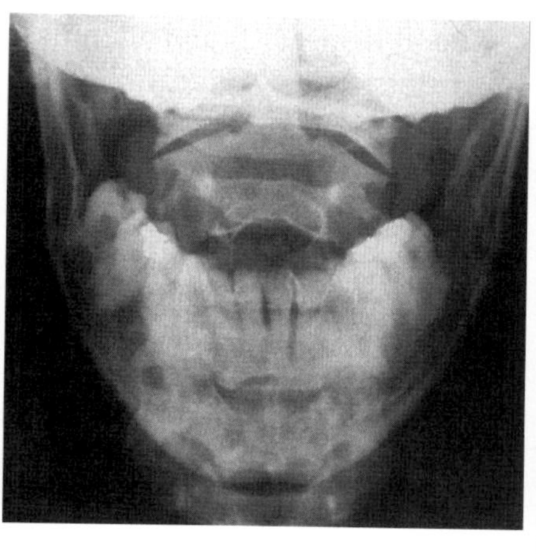

(b)

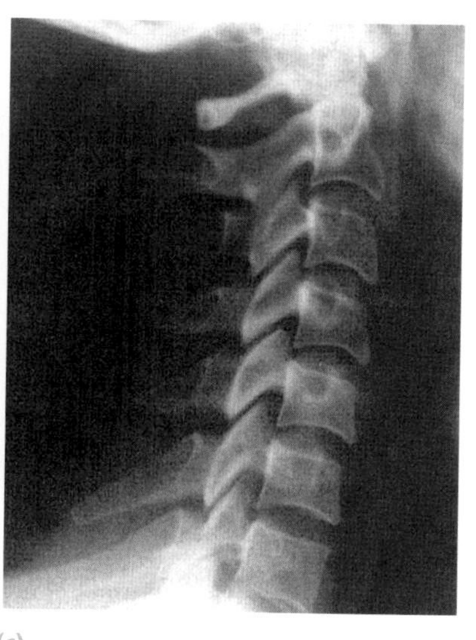

(c)

17.3 Imaging – normal x-rays (a) Anteroposterior view – note the smooth, symmetrical outlines and the clear, wide uncovertebral joints (arrows). (b) Open mouth view – to show the odontoid process and atlanto-axial joints. (c) Lateral view – showing all seven cervical vertebrae.

if one is wider than the rest, this may signify chronic instability of that segment, possibly due to a previously undiagnosed subluxation. Flexion and extension views may be needed to demonstrate instability, though after an acute injury this is best avoided!

Children's x-rays present special problems. Because the ligaments are relatively lax and the bones incompletely ossified, flexion views may show unexpectedly large shifts between adjacent vertebrae; this is sometimes mistaken for abnormal subluxation. Thus, during flexion, the lateral x-ray may show an atlanto-dental interval of 4 or 5 mm (which in an adult would suggest rupture of the transverse ligament), or anterior 'subluxation' at C2/3. Note also that the retropharyngeal space between the cervical spine and pharynx at the level of C3 increases markedly on forced expiration (e.g. when crying) and this can be misinterpreted as a soft-tissue mass. Another error is to mistake the normal synchondrosis between the dens and the body of C2 (which only fuses at about 6 years) for an odontoid fracture. Finally, remember that normal-looking radiographs in children do not exclude the possibility of a spinal cord injury.

CT SCAN

In the cervical spine, CT is particularly helpful for demonstrating the shape and size of the spinal canal and intervertebral foramina, as well as the integrity of the bony structures.

MYELOGRAPHY

Changes in the contour of the contrast-filled thecal sac suggest intradural and extradural compression. However, this is an invasive investigation and fairly non-specific. Its usefulness is enhanced by performing a post-contrast CT scan.

MRI SCAN

This is non-invasive, does not expose the patient to radiation and provides excellent resolution of the intervertebral disc and neural structures. It is the most sensitive method of demonstrating tumours and infection. It provides information on the size of the spinal canal and neural foramina. Its sensitivity can be a drawback: 20 per cent of asymptomatic patients show significant abnormalities and the scans must therefore be interpreted alongside the clinical assessment.

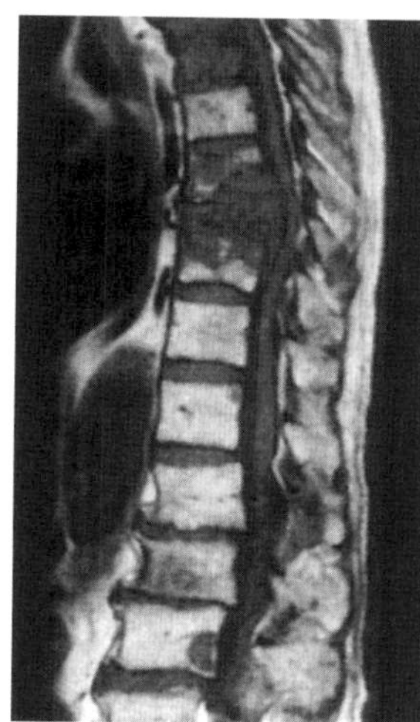

17.4 Magnetic resonance imaging MRI of the lower cervical and upper thoracic spine, showing metastatic deposits (dark grey areas in this Tl-weighted image) in several vertebral bodies. The large tumour deposit at T2/3 is encroaching perilously on the spinal canal.

DEFORMITIES OF THE NECK IN CHILDREN

A variety of deformities are encountered, some reflecting postural adjustments to underlying disorders and others due to developmental anomalies.

TORTICOLLIS

This is a description rather than a diagnosis. The chin is twisted upwards and towards one side. There are many causes. The condition may be either *congenital* or *acquired*.

Infantile (congenital) torticollis

This condition is common. The sternomastoid muscle on one side is fibrous and fails to elongate as the child grows; consequently, progressive deformity develops. The cause is unknown; the muscle may have suffered ischaemia from a distorted position in utero (the association with breech presentation and hip dysplasia is supporting evidence), or it may have been injured at birth.

A history of difficult labour or breech delivery is common. A lump may be noticed in the first few weeks of life; it is well defined and involves one or both heads of the sternomastoid. At this stage there is neither deformity nor obvious limitation of movement and within a few months the lump has disappeared. Deformity does not become apparent until the child is 1–2 years old. The head is tilted to one side, so that the ear approaches the shoulder; the sternomastoid on that side may feel tight and hard. There may also be asymmetrical development of the face (plagiocephaly). These features become increasingly obvious as the child grows.

Other causes of wry neck (bony anomalies, discitis, lymphadenitis) should be excluded. The history and the typical facial appearance are helpful clues. Radiographs must be taken to exclude a bone abnormality or fracture.

Treatment If the diagnosis is made during infancy, daily muscle stretching by the parents may prevent the incipient deformity. Non-operative treatment is successful in most cases. If the condition persists beyond one year, operative correction is required to avoid progressive facial deformity. The contracted muscle is divided (usually at its lower end but sometimes at the upper end or at both ends) and the head is manipulated into the neutral position. After operation, correction must be maintained, with a temporary rigid orthosis followed by stretching exercises.

Secondary torticollis

Childhood torticollis may be secondary to congenital bone anomalies, atlanto-axial rotatory displacement, infection (lymphadenitis, retropharyngeal abscess, tonsillitis, discitis, tuberculosis), trauma, juvenile rheumatoid arthritis, posterior fossa tumours, intraspinal tumours, dystonia (benign paroxysmal torticollis) or ocular dysfunction.

Atlanto-axial rotatory displacement The aetiology of this condition is unclear, but it is thought to be due to muscle spasm resulting from inflammation of the ligaments, capsule and synovium of the atlanto-axial

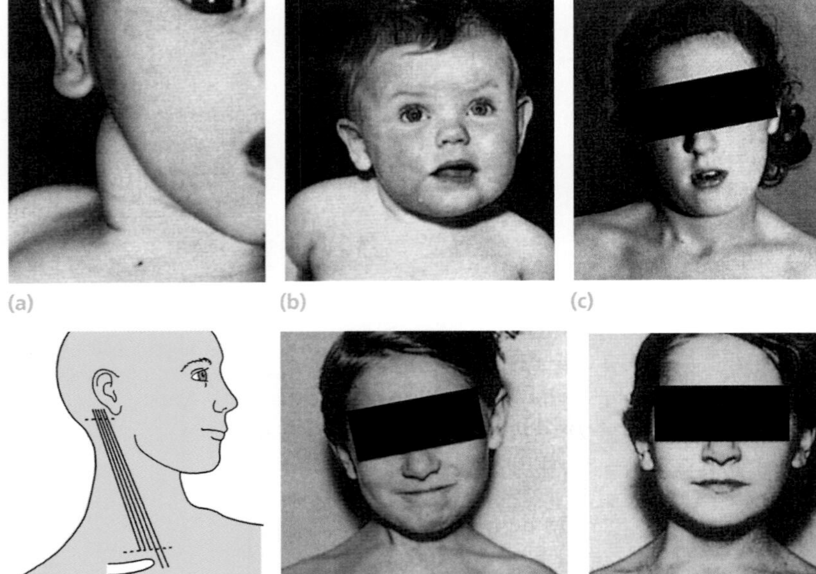

17.5 Torticollis Natural history: (a) sternomastoid tumour in a young baby; (b) early wry neck; (c) deformity with facial hemiatrophy in the adolescent. Surgical treatment: (d) two sites at which the sternomastoid may be divided; (e,f) before and a few months after operation.

region. There may be a history of trauma or upper respiratory tract infection. The child presents with a *painful wry neck*. Plain x-rays are difficult to interpret; a CT scan in both neutral and maximum lateral rotation is the most helpful investigation.

Most cases are mild and can be managed expectantly with a soft collar and analgesics. If there is no resolution after a week, halter traction, bed rest and analgesics should be prescribed. In more resistant cases, halo traction may be required. Occasionally there is anterior displacement of C1 on C2; the articulation may not stabilize following traction and a C1/2 fusion is then indicated.

VERTEBRAL ANOMALIES

There are many vertebral anomalies and most are very rare. Three are described here.

Klippel–Feil Syndrome (cervical-vertebral synostosis)

This developmental disorder represents a failure of segmentation of the cervical somites; it is often associated with abnormalities in the genito-urinary, nervous or cardiovascular systems. Some children have a hearing impediment.

Children with synostosis have a characteristic appearance: the neck is short or non-existent and there may be webbing; the hairline is low; and neck movements are limited. About 1 in 3 children with Klippel–Feil syndrome also has Sprengel's deformity of the scapula. Scoliosis is present in about 60 per cent and rib anomalies in about 30 per cent. Hand deformities such as syndactyly, thumb hypoplasia and extra digits are often present. X-rays reveal fusion of two or more cervical vertebrae.

Symptoms tend to arise in the second or third decades, not from the fused segments but from the adjacent mobile segments. There may be pain due to joint hypermobility, or neurological symptoms from instability.

Children with symptoms may need cervical fusion. For asymptomatic patients, treatment is unnecessary but parents should be warned of the risks of contact sports; sudden catastrophic neurological compromise can occur after minor trauma.

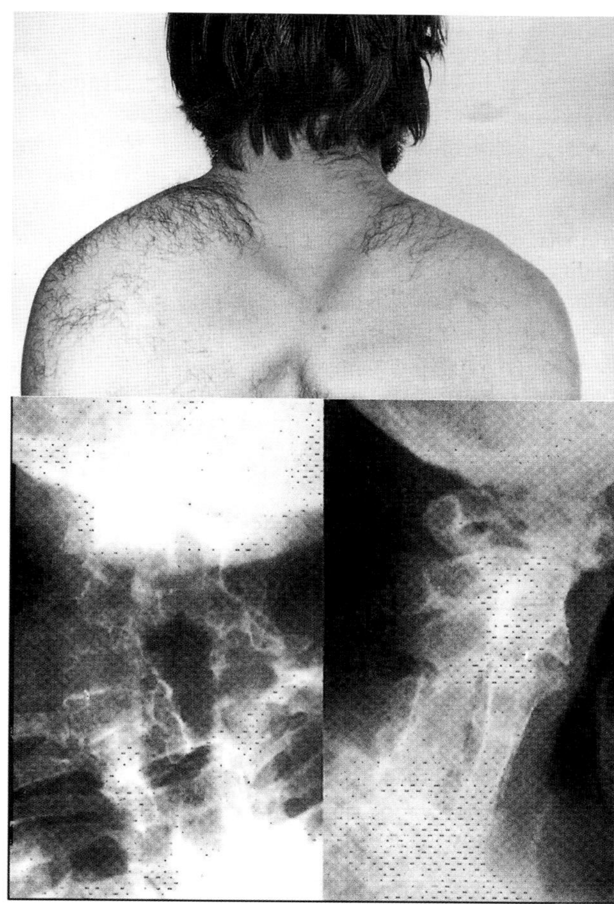

17.6 Klippel–Feil syndrome The short neck and vertebral anomalies in a typical patient.

Basilar impression

In this condition the floor of the skull is indented by the upper cervical spine. The odontoid can impinge upon the brain-stem. The cause is either a primary bone abnormality (associated with other bone defects such as odontoid abnormalities, Morquio syndrome and Klippel–Feil syndrome) or secondary to softening of the bones (osteomalacia, rickets, rheumatoid arthritis, neurofibromatosis, etc.). The relationship between the odontoid process and the foramen magnum can be ascertained on plain radiographs; further information is acquired with CT or MRI. Patients may present – often in the second or third decade – with symptoms of raised intracranial pressure (because the aqueduct of Sylvius becomes blocked), weakness and paraesthesia of the limbs (because of direct compression or ischaemia of the cord). Treatment involves surgical decompression and stabilization.

Odontoid anomalies

The odontoid may be absent or hypoplastic, or there may be a separate ossicle (the os odontoideum). The anomaly should be suspected (and looked for even if the child does not complain) in skeletal dysplasias which involve the spine. This is especially important in patients undergoing operation; the atlanto-axial joint may subluxate under anaesthesia. Some patients present with pain or torticollis, or neurological complications such as transient paralysis, myelopathy with upper motor neuron signs or sphincter disturbances. In the majority of cases the anomaly is discovered by chance in a routine cervical spine x-ray following trauma. Open-mouth radiographs show the abnormality; lateral flexion–extension views may show instability of the C1–C2 articulation.

Patients with symptoms should have surgical stabilization; the prophylactic treatment of asymptomatic patients is controversial.

ACUTE INTERVERTEBRAL DISC PROLAPSE

Acute disc prolapse is not as common in the neck as in the lower back; both segments of the spine are mobile but the mechanical environment in the cervical region is more favourable than that in the lumbosacral region. The pathological features are similar; these are described in some detail in Chapter 18.

The acute prolapse may be precipitated by local strain or injury, especially sudden unguarded flexion and rotation, and usually occurs immediately above or below the sixth cervical vertebra. In many cases (perhaps in all) there is a predisposing abnormality of the disc with increased nuclear tension. Prolapsed material may press on the posterior longitudinal ligament or dura mater, causing neck pain and stiffness as well as pain referred to the upper limb. Pressure on the nerve roots causes paraesthesia, and sometimes weakness, in one or both arms – usually in the distribution of C6 or C7.

Clinical features

The original attack can sometimes be related to a specific strain episode, e.g. acute flexion of the neck during intense physical exertion, or (occasionally) a 'whiplash' injury. Subsequent attacks may be sudden or gradual in onset, and with trivial cause. The patient complains of: (a) pain and stiffness of the neck, the pain often radiating to the scapular region and sometimes to the occiput; and (b) pain and paraesthesia in one upper limb (rarely both), often radiating to the outer elbow, back of the wrist and the index and middle fingers. Weakness is rare. Between attacks the patient feels well, although the neck may feel a bit stiff.

The neck may be held tilted forwards and sideways. The muscles are tender and movements are restricted. The arms should be examined for neurological deficit. The C6 root innervates the biceps reflex, the biceps

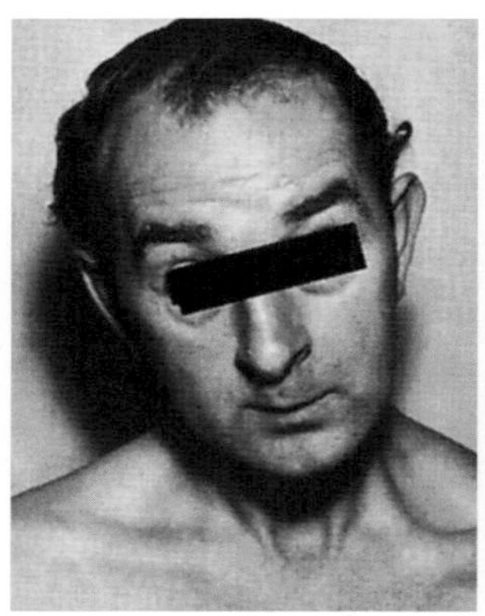

(a)

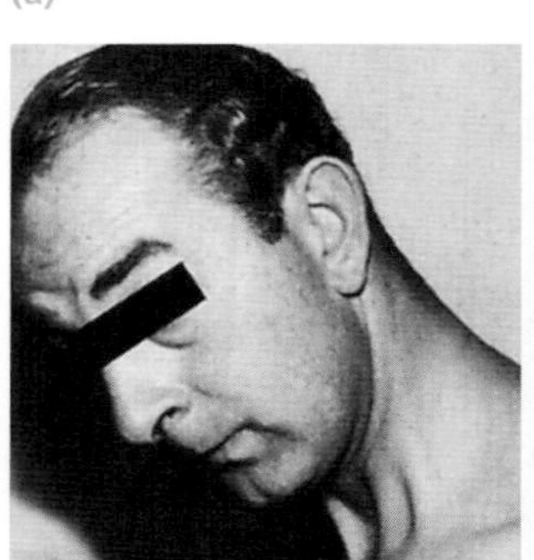

(b)

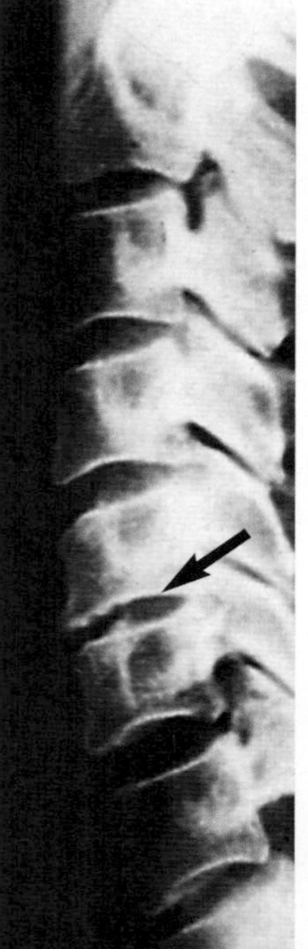

(c)

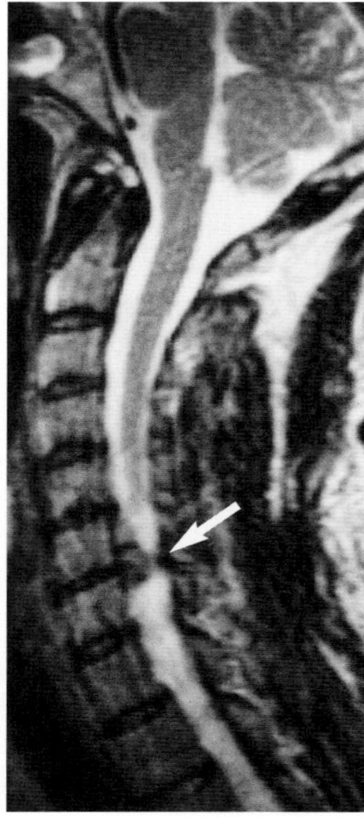

(d)

17.7 Acute disc prolapse (a,b) Acute wry neck due to a prolapsed disc. (c) The intervertebral disc space at C5/6 is reduced. (d) MRI in another case showing a large disc prolapse at C6/7.

muscle and wrist dorsiflexion, and sensation of the lateral forearm, thumb and index finger; C7 innervates the triceps and radial reflexes, the triceps muscle, wrist flexors and finger extensors, and sensation in the middle finger. Rotation and tilting of the neck to the affected side, combined with a Valsalva manoeuvre, may provoke radicular symptoms.

Imaging

X-rays may reveal straightening out of the normal cervical lordosis (due to muscle spasm) and narrowing of the disc space (although this is unlikely during a first attack). The most useful form of imaging is *MRI*, which will show the disc and its relationship to the nerve root in most cases. Even more accurate, but not used routinely because it involves intrathecal injection of contrast medium, is *CT myelography*.

Differential diagnosis

Acute soft-tissue strain Acute strains of the neck are often associated with pain, stiffness and vague 'tingling' in the upper limbs. It is important to bear in mind that pain radiating into the arm is not necessarily due to nerve root pressure.

Neuralgic amyotrophy This condition can closely resemble an acute disc prolapse and should always be thought of if there is no definite history of a strain episode. Pain is sudden and severe, and situated over the shoulder rather than in the neck itself. Careful examination will show that more than one neural level is affected – an extremely rare event in disc prolapse.

Cervical spine infections Pain is unrelenting and local spasm severe. X-rays show erosion of the vertebral end-plates.

Cervical tumours Neurological signs are progressive and x-rays reveal bone destruction.

Rotator cuff lesions Although the distribution of pain may resemble that of a prolapsed cervical disc, tenderness is localized to the rotator cuff and shoulder movements are abnormal.

Treatment

Heat and analgesics are soothing but, as with lumbar disc prolapse, there are only three satisfactory ways of treating the prolapse itself.

Rest A collar will prevent unguarded movement; However, it seldom needs to be worn for more than a week or two.

Reduce Traction may enlarge the disc space, permitting the prolapse to subside. The head of the couch is raised and weights (up to 8 kg) are tied to a harness fitting under the chin and occiput. Traction is applied intermittently for no more than 30 minutes at a time.

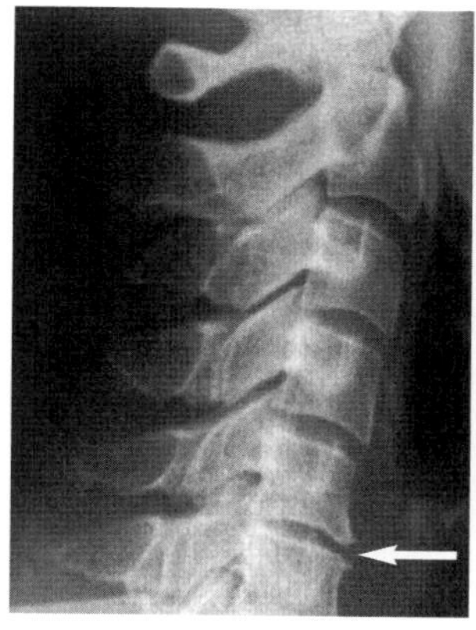

(a)

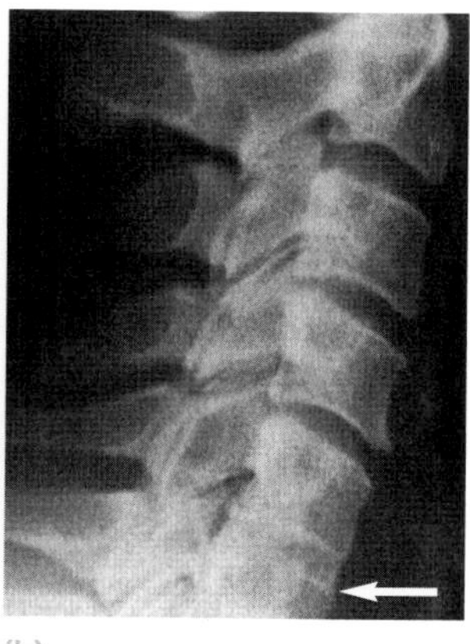

(b)

17.8 Cervical disc prolapse – treatment (a,b) Operative treatment usually consists of anterior disc removal and bone grafting. In this case the intervertebral disc height at C5/6 has been restored but now, some years later, there are signs of disc degeneration above and below the fused segment.

Remove If symptoms are refractory and severe enough, if there is a progressive neurological deficit or if there are signs of an acute myelopathy then surgery is indicated. The disc may be removed through an anterior approach; bone grafts are inserted to fuse the affected segment and to restore the normal intervertebral height. If only one level is affected, and there is no bony encroachment on the intervertebral foramen, anterior decompression can be expected to give good long-term relief from radicular symptoms.

CERVICAL SPONDYLOSIS

This vague term is applied to a cluster of abnormalities arising from chronic intervertebral disc degeneration. Changes are most common in the lower two segments of the cervical spine (C5/6 and C6/7), the area which is prone to intervertebral disc prolapse. The discs degenerate, flatten and become less elastic. The facet joints and the uncovertebral joints are slightly displaced and become arthritic, giving rise to pain and stiffness in the neck. Bony spurs, ridges or bars appear at the anterior and posterior margins of the vertebral bodies; those that develop posteriorly may encroach upon the spinal canal or the intervertebral foramina, causing pressure on the dura (which is pain sensitive) and the neural structures.

Clinical features

The patient, usually aged over 40, complains of *neck pain and stiffness*. The symptoms come on gradually

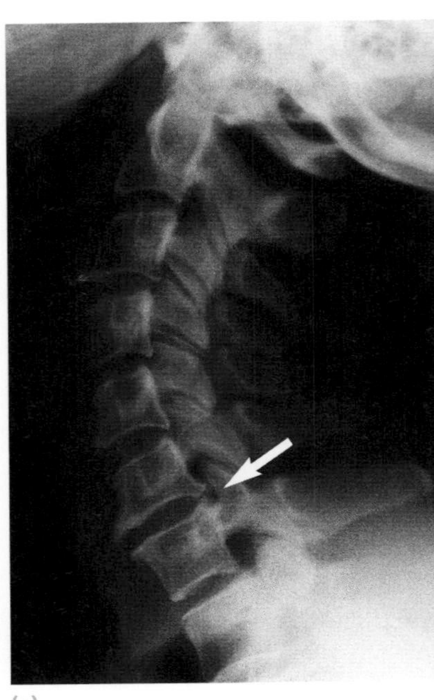

(a)

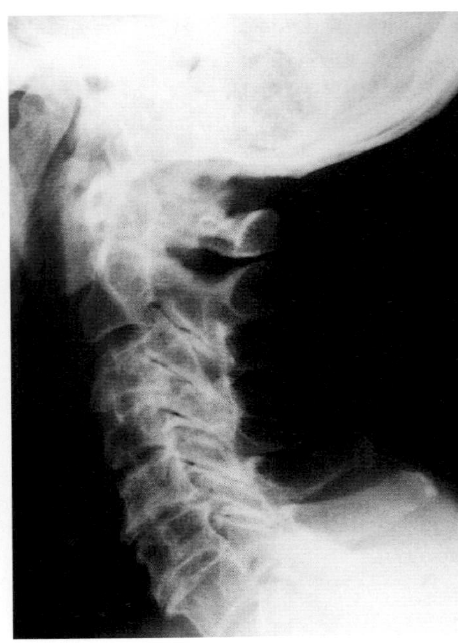

(b)

17.9 Cervical spondylosis – x-rays (a) Degenerative features at one level, C6/7. Note the prominent 'osteophytes' at the anterior and posterior borders of these two vertebral bodies. (b) Marked degenerative changes at multiple levels.

and are often worse on first getting up. The pain may radiate widely: to the occiput, the back of the shoulders and down one or both arms; it is sometimes accompanied by paraesthesia, weakness and clumsiness in the arm and hand. Typically there are exacerbations of more acute discomfort, and long periods of relative quiescence.

The appearance is normal, but the muscles at the back of the neck and across the scapulae are tender. Neck movements are limited and painful.

Sometimes the clinical picture is dominated by features arising from narrowing of the intervertebral foramina and compression of the nerve roots (*radiculopathy*): these include pain referred to the interscapular area and upper limb, numbness and/or paraesthesiae in the upper limb or the side of the face, muscle weakness and depressed reflexes in the arm or hand. In advanced cases there may be narrowing of the spinal canal and changes due to pressure on the cord (*myelopathy* – see below).

Imaging *X-rays* show narrowing of one or more intervertebral spaces, with spur formation (or lipping) at the anterior and posterior margins of the disc. These bony ridges (often referred to as 'osteophytes') may encroach upon the intervertebral foramina. *MRI* is more reliable for showing whether the nerve roots are compressed.

Diagnosis

Other disorders associated with neck and/or arm pain and sensory symptoms must be excluded. Cervical spine 'degenerative changes' are so common after the age of 40 years that they are likely to be seen in most middle-aged and elderly people who complain of pain, and it is easy to persuade oneself that they are the cause of the patient's symptoms.

Nerve entrapment syndromes Median or ulnar nerve entrapment may give rise to intermittent symptoms of pain and paraesthesia in the hand. Characteristically the symptoms are worse at night or are posture related. Careful examination will show that the changes follow a peripheral nerve rather than a root distribution. In doubtful cases, nerve conduction studies and electromyography will help to establish the diagnosis. Remember, though, that the patient may have symptoms from both a peripheral and a central abnormality; indeed, there is some evidence to suggest that longstanding cervical spondylosis may make the patient more vulnerable to the effects of peripheral nerve entrapment.

Rotator cuff lesions Pain may resemble that of cervical spondylosis, but shoulder movements are abnormal and there may be x-ray and MRI features of rotator cuff degeneration.

Cervical tumours Metastatic deposits in the cervical spine can cause misleading symptoms, but sooner or later bone destruction produces diagnostic x-ray changes. With tumours of the spinal cord, nerve roots or lymph nodes, symptoms are usually continuous, and the lesion may appear on imaging.

Thoracic outlet syndrome This condition is described in Chapter 11. Symptoms resemble those of cervical spondylosis; pain and sensory abnormalities appear mainly down the ulnar border of the forearm and may be aggravated by upper limb traction or by elevation and external rotation of the shoulder. Importantly, neck movements are neither painful nor restricted. X-rays may reveal a cervical rib, although the mere presence of this anomaly is not necessarily diagnostic.

Conservative treatment

Analgesics are prescribed when necessary. Heat and massage are often soothing, but restricting neck movements in a collar is the most effective treatment during painful attacks. Physiotherapy is the mainstay of treatment, patients usually being maintained in relative comfort by various measures including exercises, gentle passive manipulation and intermittent traction. Prolonged use of a cervical collar or brace may do more harm than good.

Operative treatment

If conservative measures fail to relieve the patient's symptoms, and particularly if there are neurological symptoms and signs arising from nerve root compression at one or two identifiable levels, surgical treatment may be preferable.

ANTERIOR DISCECTOMY AND FUSION

This operation has a 'track record' of more than 25 years and is particularly suitable if the problem is primarily one of unrelieved neck pain and stiffness, though it is also successful in relieving radicular symptoms (Bohlman et al., 1993). Through the anterior approach the intervertebral disc can be removed without disturbing the posteriorly placed neurological structures. After preparation of the intervertebral space, a suitably shaped bone graft (usually autogenous, taken from the iliac crest) is inserted firmly between the adjacent vertebral bodies. An anterior plate is added if there is uncertainty about stability or if several levels are being fused. Operative complications such as injury to the recurrent laryngeal nerve or (worse) the vertebral artery are unusual if sufficient care is exercised. Postoperative dysphagia and dysphonia (particularly if a plate has been applied) have been reported. Graft dislodgement and failed fusion (with pseudarthrosis) are less likely with intervertebral plating. More worrying is the possibility that fusion at one level may predispose to degeneration at an adjacent level.

FORAMINOTOMY

If the main problems are referred pain in the upper limb and/or neurological symptoms and signs (features of a radiculopathy) and the MRI shows foraminal narrowing and nerve root compression at one or two levels, foraminotomy (through a posterior approach) may be indicated. Only part of the facet joint is removed so this segment should not become unstable. However, patients should be warned that pre-existing *neck pain* may not be eliminated; and, of course, adjacent segments may go on to develop symptomatic disc degeneration in the future, which may then require further surgery.

INTERVERTEBRAL DISC REPLACEMENT

Disc replacement operations have recently been approved in some countries. This has the (theoretical) advantage of removing the offending disc and preserving movement at the affected site. As yet it is too early to assess the long-term outcome of these procedures.

OSSIFICATION OF THE POSTERIOR LONGITUDINAL LIGAMENT

Reports on ossification of the posterior longitudinal ligament (OPLL) have appeared mainly from Japan (Ono et al., 1977; Tsuyama, 1984). However, it is now recognized that this condition is quite common

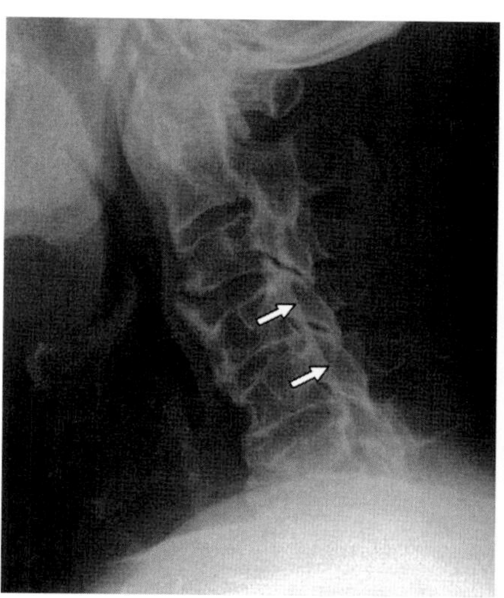

(a)

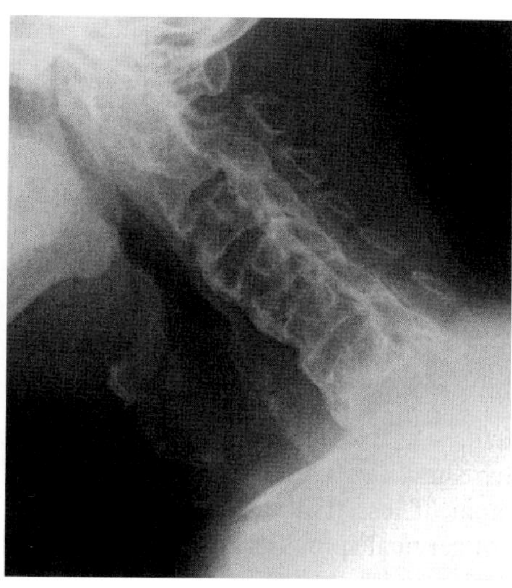

(b)

17.10 Ossification of the posterior longitudinal ligament (a) Lateral x-ray of the cervical spine showing the thin dense band running down the backs of the vertebral bodies (arrows); this appearance is typical of posterior longitudinal ligament ossification, which resulted in cervical spinal stenosis. (b) X-ray taken after posterior spinal decompression (laminoplasty); the spinous processes have been removed, the laminae split on one side of the mid-line and the posterior arch 'jacked' open. The sagittal diameter of the spinal canal is now considerably greater than before. (Courtesy of Mr H. K. Wong, Singapore.)

and widespread. It occurs mainly in the cervical spine and may be associated with bone-forming conditions such as diffuse idiopathic skeletal hyperostosis (DISH) and fluorosis. The cause is unknown. The significance of the disease is that it may give rise to spinal stenosis and cervical myelopathy.

The patient, usually a man between 50 and 70 years of age, may present with any combination of pain in the neck and upper limb(s), sensory symptoms and muscle weakness in the arms and upper motor neuron (cord) symptoms and signs in the lower limbs. The most disturbing features are motor abnormalities such as weakness, incoordination, clumsiness, muscle wasting and incontinence.

X-rays show dense ossification along the back of the vertebral bodies (and sometimes also the ligamentum flavum) in the mid-cervical spine.

Treatment Treatment is not always necessary; indeed people with typical x-ray features may be completely asymptomatic. If the symptoms and signs are disturbing or progressive, operative decompression will be needed. 'Decompression' is performed posteriorly because of the multilevel nature of the condition, and takes the form of one or other type of laminoplasty, leaving the ossified ligament in place.

SPINAL STENOSIS AND CERVICAL MYELOPATHY

The sagittal diameter of the mid-cervical spinal canal (the distance, on plain x-rays, from the posterior surface of the vertebral body to the base of the spinous process) varies considerably from one individual to another; anything less than 11 mm is suggestive of stenosis. Abnormally small canals are seen in rare dysplasias, such as achondroplasia, and may give rise to cord compression. Many asymptomatic, and apparently normal, people also have small canals and they are at risk of developing the clinical symptoms of spinal stenosis if there is any further encroachment due to intervertebral disc degeneration, posterior 'osteophytosis', osteoarthritis of the facet joints, thickening of the ligamentum flavum, ossification of the posterior longitudinal ligament or vertebral displacement. If the changes are severe enough, the patient may develop neurological symptoms and signs (*cervical myelopathy*), which are thought to be due to both direct compression and ischaemia of the cord and nerve roots arising from impaired venous drainage and reduced arterial flow.

Clinical features

Patients usually have neck pain and brachialgia but also complain of paraesthesia, numbness, weakness and clumsiness in the arms and legs. Symptoms may be precipitated by acutely hyperextending the neck, and some patients present for the first time after a hyperextension injury. They may experience involuntary spasms in the legs and, occasionally, episodes of spontaneous clonus. In severe cases there may be urinary and rectal dysfunction or incontinence.

The 'classical' picture of weakness and spasticity in the legs and numbness in the hands is easy to recognize, but the signs are not always as clear-cut as that. However, careful examination should reveal upper motor neuron signs in the lower limbs (increased muscle tone, brisk reflexes and clonus), while sensory signs depend on which part of the cord is compressed: there may be decreased sensibility to pain and temperature (spinothalamic tracts) or diminished vibration and position sense (posterior columns).

The condition is usually slowly progressive, but occasionally a patient with longstanding symptoms starts deteriorating rapidly and treatment becomes urgent.

Imaging A *plain lateral radiograph* which shows an anteroposterior diameter of the spinal canal of less than 11 mm strongly supports the diagnosis of cervical spinal stenosis. A better measure is the Pavlov ratio (the anteroposterior diameter of the canal divided by the diameter of the vertebral body at the same level) because this is not affected by magnification error. A ratio of less than 0.8 is abnormal.

MRI demonstrates the spinal cord and soft-tissue structures, and helps to exclude other causes of similar neurological dysfunction. *CT myelography* is superior to MRI in demonstrating osseous detail.

DIFFERENTIAL DIAGNOSIS

Full neurological investigation is required to eliminate other diagnoses such as multiple sclerosis (episodic symptoms), amyotrophic lateral sclerosis (purely motor dysfunction), syringomyelia and spinal cord tumours.

Treatment

Most patients can be treated conservatively with analgesics, a collar, isometric exercises and gait training. Manipulation and traction should be avoided.

Patients with progressive myelopathy or rapid deterioration should be considered for surgery. Acute, severe myelopathy is a surgical emergency, requiring immediate decompression.

PYOGENIC INFECTION

Pyogenic infection of the cervical spine is uncommon, and therefore often misdiagnosed in the early stages when antibiotic treatment is most effective.

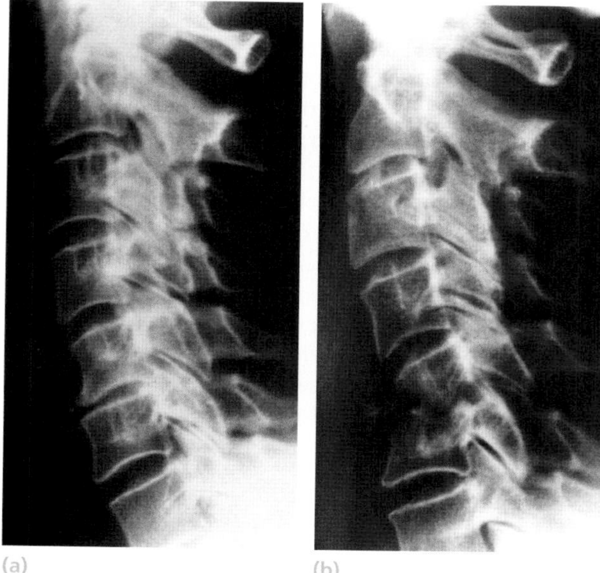

17.11 Pyogenic infection (a) The first x-ray, taken soon after the onset of symptoms, shows narrowing of the C5/6 disc space but no other abnormality. (b) Three weeks later there is dramatic destruction and collapse; the speed at which these have occurred distinguishes pyogenic from tuberculous infection.

The organism – usually a staphylococcus – reaches the spine via the blood stream. Initially, destructive changes are limited to the intervertebral disc space and the adjacent parts of the vertebral bodies. Later, abscess formation occurs and pus may extend into the spinal canal or into the soft-tissue planes of the neck.

Clinical features

Vertebral infection may occur at any age. The patient complains of pain in the neck, often severe and associated with muscle spasm and marked stiffness. However, systemic symptoms are often mild. On examination, neck movements are severely restricted. *Blood tests* may show a leucocytosis and an increased ESR.

X-rays at first show either no abnormality or only slight narrowing of the disc space; later there may be more obvious signs of bone destruction.

Treatment

Treatment is by antibiotics and rest. The cervical spine is 'immobilized' by traction; once the acute phase subsides, a collar may suffice. Operation is seldom necessary; as the infection subsides the intervertebral space is obliterated and the adjacent vertebrae fuse. If there is frank abscess formation, this will require drainage.

TUBERCULOSIS

Cervical spine tuberculosis is rare. As with other types of infection, the organism is blood-borne and the infection localizes in the intervertebral disc and the anterior parts of the adjacent vertebral bodies. As the bone crumbles, the cervical spine collapses into kyphosis. A retropharyngeal abscess forms and points behind the sternomastoid muscle at the side of the neck. In late cases cord damage may cause neurological signs varying from mild weakness to tetraplegia.

Clinical features

The patient – usually a child – complains of neck pain and stiffness. In neglected cases a retropharyngeal abscess may cause difficulty in swallowing or swelling at the side of the neck. On examination the neck is extremely tender and all movements are restricted. In late cases there may be obvious kyphosis, a fluctuant abscess in the neck or a retropharyngeal swelling. The limbs should be examined for neurological defects.

X-rays show narrowing of the disc space and erosion of the adjacent vertebral bodies.

Treatment

Treatment is initially by antituberculous drugs and 'immobilization' of the neck in a cervical brace or plaster cast for 6–18 months.

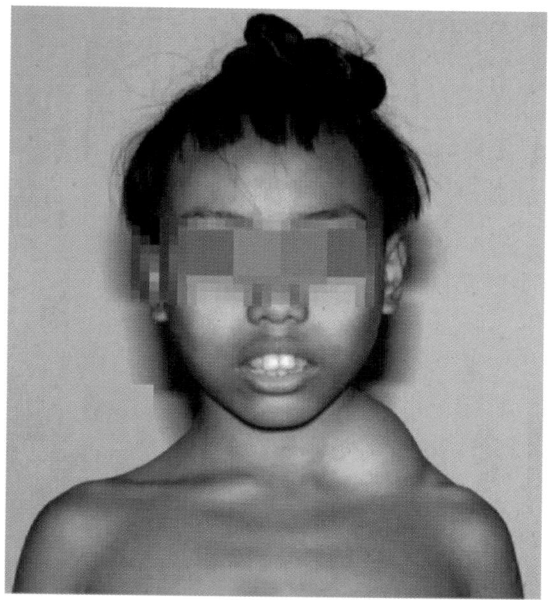

17.12 Tuberculosis This child had been complaining of neck pain and stiffness for several months. Eventually she was brought to the clinic with a lump at the side of her neck – a typical tuberculous abscess.

Operative treatment Debridement of necrotic bone and anterior cervical vertebral fusion with bone grafts may be offered as an alternative to prolonged immobilization in a brace or cast. More urgent indications for operation are (1) to drain a retropharyngeal abscess, (2) to decompress a threatened spinal cord, or (3) to fuse an unstable spine.

RHEUMATOID ARTHRITIS

The cervical spine is severely affected in 30 per cent of patients with rheumatoid arthritis. Three types of lesion are common: (1) erosion of the atlanto-axial joints and the transverse ligament, with resulting instability; (2) erosion of the atlanto-occipital articulations, allowing the odontoid peg to ride up into the foramen magnum (cranial sinkage); and (3) erosion of the facet joints in the mid-cervical region, sometimes ending in fusion but more often leading to subluxation. In addition, vertebral osteoporosis is common, due either to the disease or to the effect of corticosteroid therapy, or both.

Considering the amount of atlanto-axial displacement that occurs (often greater than 1 cm), neurological complications are uncommon. However, they do occur – especially in longstanding cases – and are produced by mechanical compression of the cord, by local granulation tissue formation or (very rarely) by thrombosis of the vertebral arteries.

Clinical features

The patient is usually a woman with advanced rheumatoid arthritis. She has neck pain, and movements are markedly restricted. Symptoms and signs of root compression may be present in the upper limbs; less often there is lower limb weakness and upper motor neuron signs due to cord compression. There may be symptoms of vertebro-basilar insufficiency, such as vertigo, tinnitus and visual disturbance. Some patients, though completely unaware of any neurological deficit, are found on careful examination to have mild sensory disturbance or pyramidal tract signs (e.g. abnormally brisk reflexes).

General debility and peripheral joint involvement can mask the signs of myelopathy. Lhermitte's sign – electric shock sensation down the spine on flexing the neck – may be present. Sudden death from catastrophic neurological compression is rare.

X-rays X-rays show the features of an erosive arthritis, usually at several levels. *Atlanto-axial instability* is visible in lateral films taken in flexion and extension; in flexion the anterior arch of the atlas rides forwards, leaving a gap of 5 mm or more between the back of the anterior arch and the odontoid process; on extension the subluxation is reduced. *Atlanto-occipital erosion* is more difficult to see, but a lateral tomograph shows the relationship of the odontoid to the foramen magnum. Normally the odontoid tip is less than 5 mm above McGregor's line (a line from the posterior edge of the hard palate to the lowest point on the occiput); in erosive arthritis the odontoid tip may be 10–12 mm above this line. Flexion views may also show *anterior subluxation in the mid-cervical region.*

CT and MRI These methods are useful for imaging 'difficult' areas such as the atlanto-axial and atlanto-occipital articulations, and for viewing the soft-tissue structures (especially the cord).

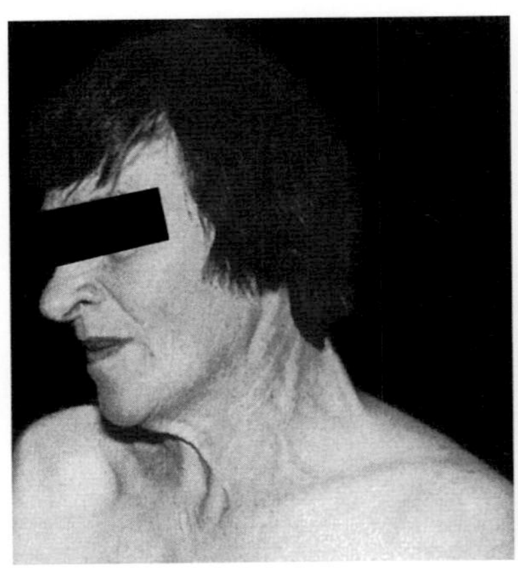
(a)

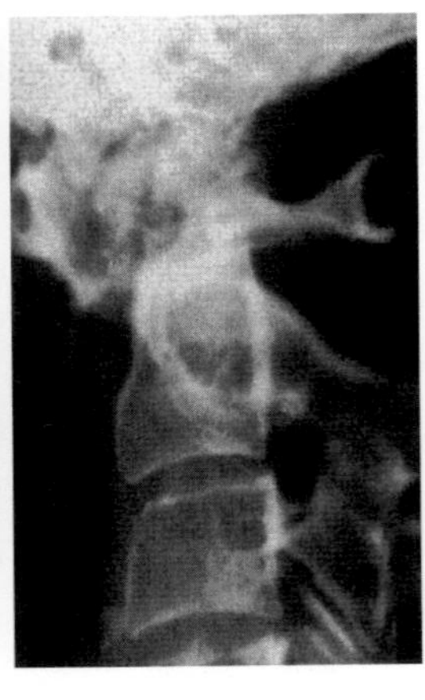
(b)

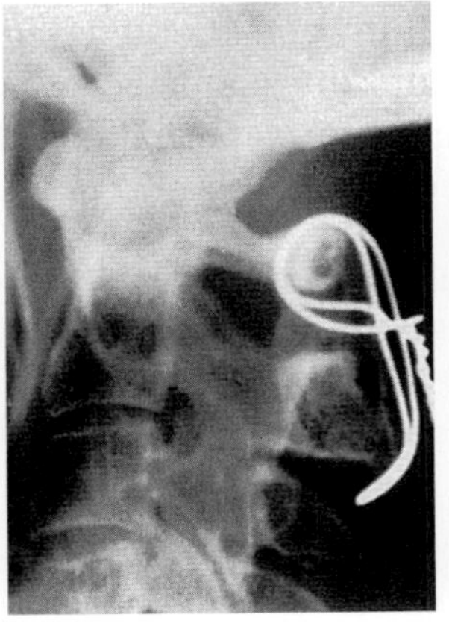
(c)

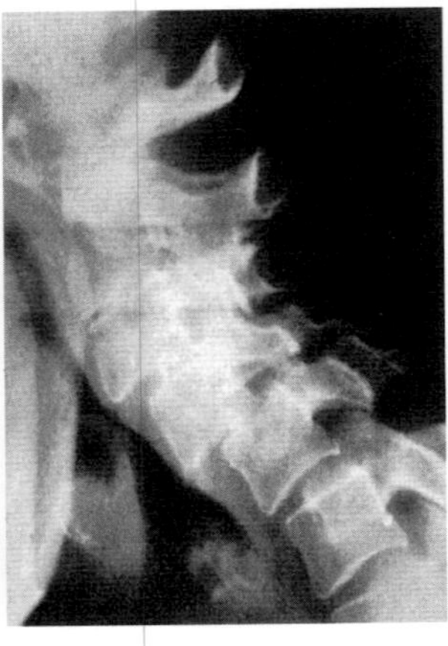
(d)

17.13 Rheumatoid arthritis (a) Movement is severely restricted; attempted rotation causes pain and muscle spasm. (b) Atlanto-axial subluxation is common; erosion of the joints and the transverse ligament has allowed the atlas to slip forward about 2 cm; (c) reduction and posterior fusion with wire fixation. (d) This patient has subluxation, not only at the atlanto-axial joint but also at two levels in the mid-cervical region.

Treatment

Despite the startling x-ray appearances, serious neurological complications are uncommon. Pain can usually be relieved by wearing a collar.

The indications for operative stabilization of the cervical spine are (1) severe and unremitting pain, and (2) neurological signs of root or cord compression. Arthrodesis (usually posterior) is by bone grafting followed by a halo body cast, or by internal fixation (posterior wiring or a rectangular fixator) and bone grafting. Postoperatively a cervical brace is worn for 3 months; however, if instability is marked and operative fixation insecure, a halo jacket may be necessary. In patients with very advanced disease and severe erosive changes, postoperative morbidity and mortality are high. This is an argument for operating at an earlier stage for 'impending neurological deficit', as diagnosed from x-ray signs of severe atlanto-axial subluxation, upward migration of the odontoid or subaxial vertebral subluxation together with CT, myelographic or MR images of cord or brain-stem compression.

ANKYLOSING SPONDYLITIS

Ankylosing spondylitis is the most common seronegative spondyloarthropathy to affect the cervical spine. Neck pain and stiffness tend to occur some years after the onset of backache. The neck becomes progressively stiff and kyphotic although some movement is usually preserved at the atlanto-occipital and atlanto-axial joints.

An unacceptable 'chin-on-chest' deformity, or inability to lift the head high enough to see more than ten paces ahead, are indications for cervical spine osteotomy.

The ankylosed spine is osteoporotic and prone to fracture. A patient with ankylosing spondylitis and an increase in neck pain must be assumed to have a fracture until proven otherwise (by bone scan or MRI if plain radiographs are normal). Neurological compromise is common. A displaced fracture needs careful closed reduction with halo traction then halo vest immobilization. Surgery carries a high complication rate.

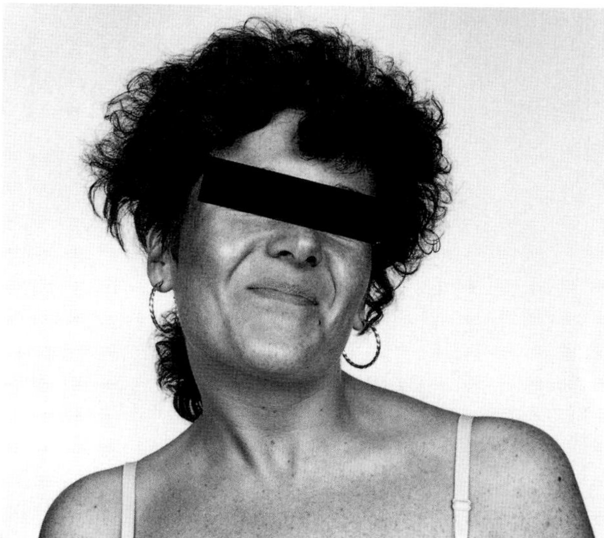

17.14 Spasmodic torticollis Attempted correction was forcibly resisted. The deformity can be very distressing.

SPASMODIC TORTICOLLIS

This, the most common form of focal dystonia, is characterized by involuntary twisting or clonic movements of the neck. Spasms are sometimes triggered by emotional disturbance or attempts at correction. Even at rest the neck assumes an abnormal posture, the chin usually twisted to one side and upwards; the shoulder on that side may be elevated. In some cases involuntary muscle contractions spread to other areas and the condition is revealed as a more generalized form of dystonia.

The exact cause is unknown, but some cases are associated with lesions of the basal ganglia. Correction is extremely difficult; various drugs, including anticholinergics, have been used, though with little success. Some patients respond to local injections of botulinum toxin into the sternomastoid muscle.

NOTES ON APPLIED ANATOMY

In the upright posture the neck has a gentle anterior convexity; this natural lordosis may straighten but is never quite reversed, even in flexion, unless it is abnormal.

Eight pairs of nerve roots from the cervical cord pass through the relatively narrow intervertebral foramina, the first between the occiput and C1, and the eighth between C7 and the first thoracic (T1) vertebra; thus each segmental root from the first to the seventh lies above the vertebra of the same number. Thus a lesion between C5 and C6 might compress the sixth root.

The intervertebral discs lie close to the nerve roots as they emerge through the foramina; even a small herniation often causes root symptoms (shoulder girdle and upper limb pain and paraesthesiae) rather than neck pain. Moreover, disc degeneration is associated with spur formation on both the posterior aspect of the vertebral body and the associated facet joints; the resulting encroachment on the intervertebral foramen traps the nerve root. It is important to remember, however, that 'root pain' alone (i.e. pain in the shoulder and arm) does not necessarily signify nerve-root irritation; it may be referred from the facet joint or the soft structures around it. Only paraesthesiae and sensory or motor loss are unequivocal evidence of nerve root compression.

At the atlanto-occipital joint, the movements that occur are nodding and tilting (lateral flexion); there is no rotation, and when this movement takes place (at the atlanto-axial joint) the atlas and the skull move as one. In the rest of the cervical spine, movements that occur are flexion, extension and tilting to either side; the facets permit subluxation or dislocation to occur without fracture, a displacement that the strong posterior ligaments normally prevent.

REFERENCES AND FURTHER READING

Agarwal AK, Peppelman WC, Kraus DR, Eisenbeis CH. The cervical spine in rheumatoid arthritis. *BMJ 1993;* **306:** 79–80.

Bohlman HH, Emery SE,Goodfellow DB, Jones PK. Robinson anterior cervical discectomy and arthrodesis for cervical radiculopathy: Long-term follow-up of one hundred and twenty patients. *J Bone Joint Surg* 1993; **75A:** 1298–1307.

Copley LA, Dormans JP. Cervical spine disorders in infants and children. *J Am Acad Orthop Surg* 1998; **6:** 204–14.

Garfin SR, Herkowitz HN. (Guest Editors). The degenerative neck. *Orthop Clinics of North America* 1992; **23(3)**.

Hensinger RN. Congenital anomalies of the cervical spine. *Clin Orthop Relat Res* 1991; **264:** 16–38.

Law MD, Bernhardt M, White AA. Evaluation and management of cervical spondylotic myelopathy. *J Bone Joint Surg* 1994; **76A:** 1420–33.

Levine MJ, Albert TJ, Smith MD. Cervical radiculopathy. *J Am Acad Orthop Surg* 1996; **4:** 305–316.

Ono K, Ota H, Tada K, *et al*. Ossified posterior longitudinal ligament. *Spine* 1977; **2:** 126.

Tsuyama N. Ossification of the posterior longitudinal ligament of the spine. *Clin Orthop* 1984; **184:** 71–84.

The back

18

Stephen Eisenstein, Surendar Tuli, Shunmugam Govender

CLINICAL ASSESSMENT

SYMPTOMS

The usual symptoms of back disorders are pain, stiffness and deformity in the back, and pain, paraesthesia or weakness in the lower limbs. The mode of onset is very important: did it start suddenly, perhaps after a lifting strain; or gradually without any antecedent event? Are the symptoms constant, or are there periods of remission? Are they related to any particular posture? Has there been any associated illness or malaise?

Pain, either sharp and localized or chronic and diffuse, is the commonest presenting symptom. Backache is usually felt low down and on either side of the midline, often extending into the upper part of the buttock and even into the lower limbs. Back pain made worse by rest would suggest pain arising from the facet joints. Pain made worse by activity probably comes from any of the soft-tissue supports of the spine (muscles and ligaments) including the annulus of the intervertebral disc.

Sciatica is the term originally used to describe intense pain radiating from the buttock into the thigh and calf – more or less following the distribution of the sciatic nerve and therefore suggestive of nerve root compression or irritation. However Kellgren (1977), in a classic experiment, showed that almost any structure in a spinal segment can, if irritated sufficiently, give rise to *referred pain* radiating into the lower limbs. Unfortunately, with the passage of time, many clinicians have taken to describing all types of pain extending from the lumbar region into the lower limb as 'sciatica'. This is at best confusing and at worst a preparation for misdiagnosis! True *sciatica*, most commonly due to a prolapsed intervertebral disc pressing on a nerve root, is characteristically more intense than referred low back pain, is aggravated by coughing and straining and is often accompanied by symptoms of root pressure such as numbness and paraesthesiae, especially in the foot.

Stiffness may be sudden in onset and almost complete (in a 'locked back' attack, or after a disc prolapse) or continuous and predictably worse in the mornings (suggesting arthritis or ankylosing spondylitis).

Deformity is usually noticed by others, but the patient may become aware of shoulder asymmetry or of clothes not fitting well.

Numbness or *paraesthesia* is felt anywhere in the lower limb, but can usually be mapped fairly accurately over one of the dermatomes. It is important to ask if it is aggravated by standing or walking and relieved by sitting down – the classic symptom of spinal stenosis.

Urinary retention or *incontinence* can be due to pressure on the cauda equina.

Faecal incontinence or urgency, and *impotence*, may also occur.

Other symptoms important in back disorders are: (1) urethral discharge; (2) diarrhoea; (3) sore eyes – classical features of Reiter's disease.

SIGNS WITH THE PATIENT STANDING

Adequate exposure is essential; patients should strip to their underclothes.

Look

Start by examining the skin. Scars (previous surgery or injury), pigmentation (neurofibromatosis?) or abnormal tufts of hair (spina bifida?) are important clues to underlying spinal disorders.

Look carefully at the patient's shape and posture, both from the front and behind. Asymmetry of the chest, trunk or pelvis may be obvious, or may appear only when the patient bends forward. Lateral deviation of the spinal column is described as a *list* to one or other side; lateral curvature is *scoliosis.*

Seen from the side, the back normally has a slight forward curve, or *kyphosis*, in the thoracic region and a shorter backward curve, or *lordosis*, in the lumbar segment (the 'hollow' of the back). Excessive thoracic

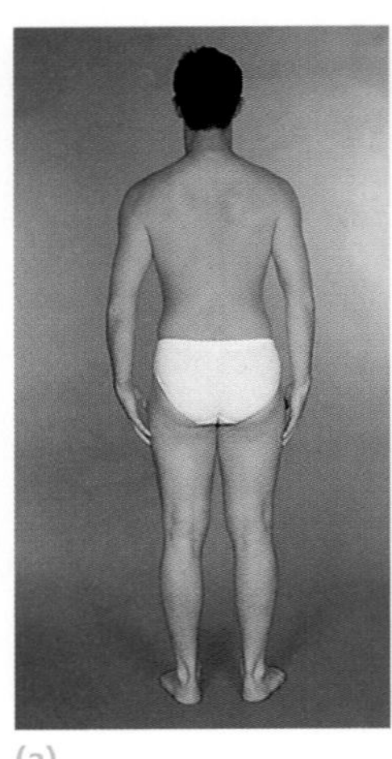
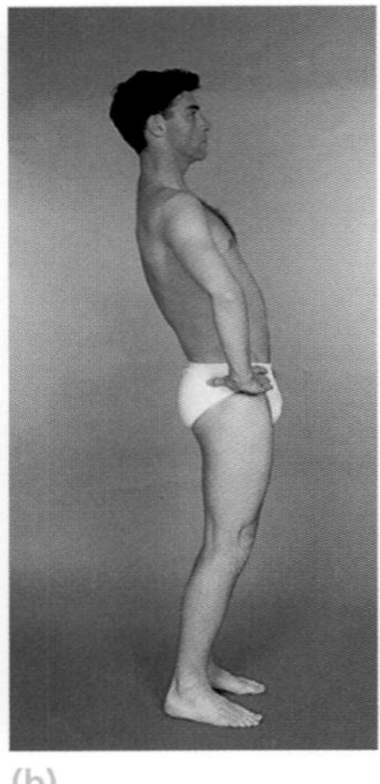
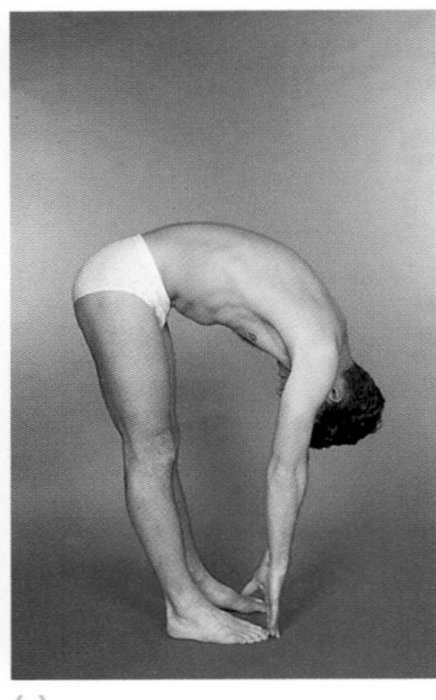
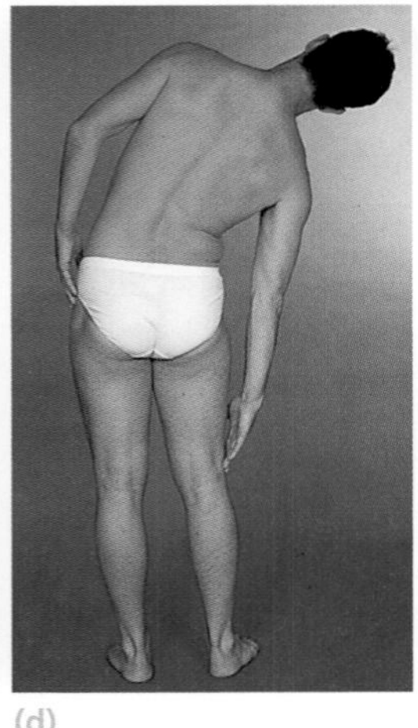
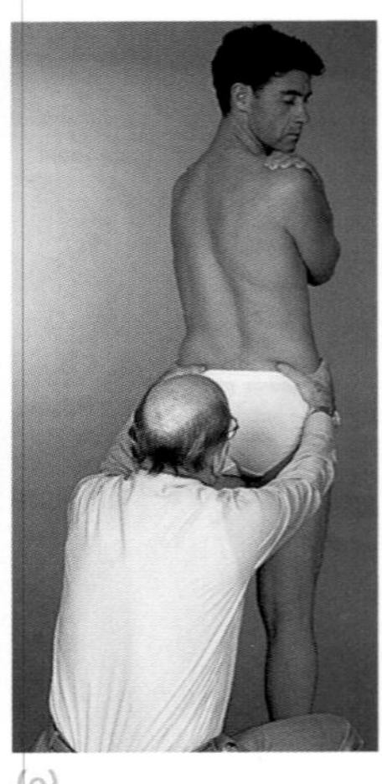

(a) (b) (c) (d) (e)

18.1 Examination With the patient standing upright (a), look at his general posture and note particularly the presence of any asymmetry or frank deformity of the spine. Then ask him to lean backwards (extension) (b), forwards to touch his toes (flexion) (c) and then sideways as far as possible (d), comparing his level of reach on the two sides. Finally, hold the pelvis stable and ask the patient to twist first to one side and then to the other (rotation). Note that rotation occurs almost entirely in the thoracic spine (e) and not in the lumbar spine.

kyphosis is sometimes called *hyperkyphosis*, to distinguish it from the normal; if the spine is sharply angulated the prominence is called a *kyphos* or *gibbus*. The lumbar spine may be excessively lordosed (hyperlordosis) or unusually flat (effectively a lumbar kyphosis).

Undue or asymmetrical prominence of the paravertebral muscles may be due to spasm, an important sign in acute back disorders.

If the patient consistently stands with one knee bent (even though his legs are equal in length) this suggests nerve root tension on that side; flexing the knee relaxes the sciatic nerve and reduces the pull on the nerve root.

Feel

Feel for the spinous processes and the interspinous ligaments, noting any unusual prominence or a 'step'. Tenderness should be localized to: (1) bony structures; (2) intervertebral tissues; (3) paravertebral muscles and ligaments, especially where they insert into the iliac crest.

Move

Flexion is tested by asking the patient to try to touch his toes. Even with a stiff back he may be able to do

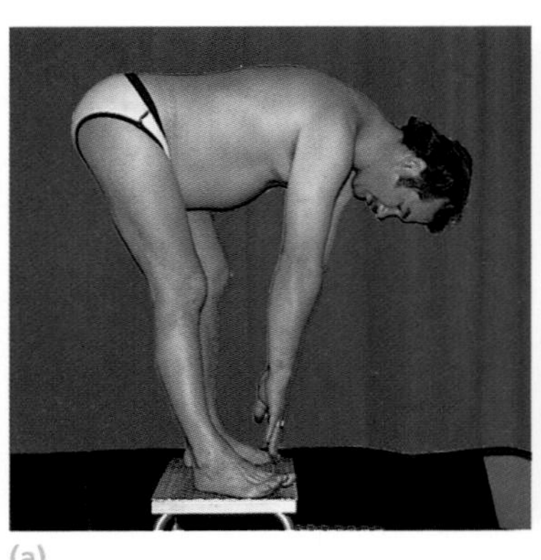
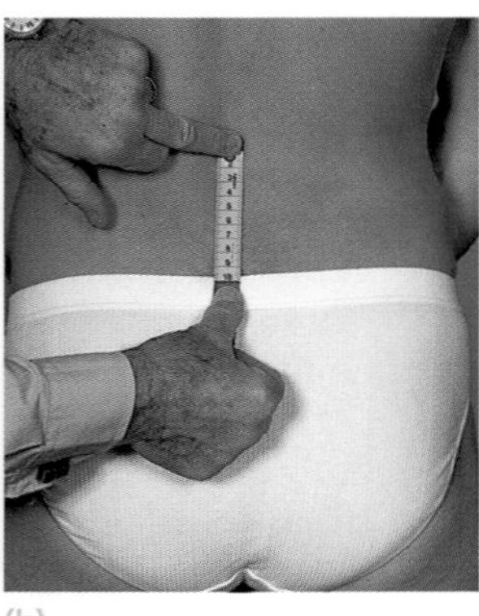
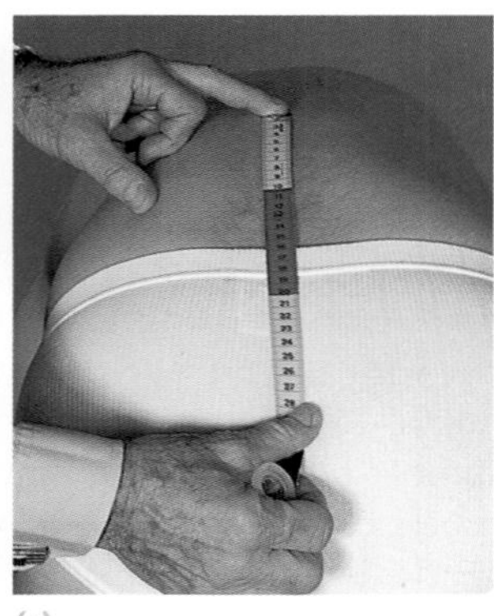

(a) (b) (c)

18.2 Measuring the range of flexion Bending down and touching the toes may look like lumbar flexion but this is not always the case. The patient in (a) has anklyosing spondylitis and a rigid lumbar spine, but he is able to reach his toes because he has good flexibility at the hips. Compare his flat back with the rounded back of the model in Figure 18.1c. You can measure the lumbar excursion. With the patient upright, select two bony points 10 cm apart and mark the skin (b); as the patient bends forward, the two points should separate by at least a further 5 cm (c).

this by flexing the hips; so watch the lumbar spine to see if it really moves, or, better still, measure the spinal excursion. *The mode of flexion* (whether it is smooth or hesitant) and the way in which the patient comes back to the upright position are also important. In clinical lumbar instability the patient tends to regain the upright position by pushing on the front of his thighs. To test *extension*, ask the patient to lean backwards, but see that he doesn't cheat by bending his knees. A patient with good forward bending but much pain on extension probably has painful facet joints.

The '*wall test*' will unmask a minor flexion deformity (kyphosis, as in ankylosing spondylitis or Scheuermann's osteochondrosis); standing with the back flush against a wall, the heels, buttocks, shoulders and occiput should all make contact with the vertical surface.

Lateral flexion is tested by asking the patient to bend sideways, sliding his hand down the outer side of his leg; the two sides are compared. *Rotation* is examined by asking him to twist the trunk to each side in turn while the pelvis is anchored by the examiner's hands; this is essentially a thoracic movement and is not limited in lumbosacral disease.

Rib-cage excursion is assessed by measuring the *chest circumference* in full expiration and then in full inspiration; the normal difference is about 7 cm. A reduced excursion may be the earliest sign of ankylosing spondylitis.

While the patient is standing, you can test *muscle power* in the legs by asking him to stand up on his toes (plantarflexion) and then to rock back on his heels (dorsiflexion); small differences between the two sides are easily spotted.

SIGNS WITH THE PATIENT LYING PRONE

Make sure that the patient is lying comfortably on the examination couch, and remove the pillow so that he is not forced to arch his back (or smother himself). Again, look for localized deformities and muscle spasm, and examine the buttocks for *gluteal wasting*.

Feel the *bony outlines* (is there an unexpected 'step' or prominence?) and check for consistently localized lumbosacral *tenderness* or soft-tissue 'trigger' points.

The popliteal and posterior tibial *pulses* are felt, hamstring *power* is tested and *sensation* on the back of the limbs assessed.

The *femoral nerve stretch test* (for lumbar 3rd or 4th nerve root sensitivity) is carried out by gently flexing the patient's knee or by lifting the hip into extension (or both in one movement); pain may be felt in the front of the thigh.

SIGNS WITH THE PATIENT LYING SUPINE

The patient is observed as he turns – is there pain or stiffness? A rapid appraisal of the thyroid, chest (and breasts), and abdomen (and scrotum) is advisable, and essential if there is even a hint of generalized disease. Hip and knee mobility are assessed before testing for spinal cord or root involvement.

The *straight-leg raising test* discloses lumbosacral root tension. Ask the patient to hold his or her knee absolutely straight, then lift the patient's leg slowly until he or she experiences pain – not merely in the lower back (which is common and not significant) but also in the buttock, thigh and calf (Lasègue's test, but attribution is controversial); the angle at which this occurs is noted. Normally it should be possible to raise the limb to 80–90 degrees; people with lax ligaments can go even further. In a full-blown disc prolapse with nerve root compression, straight-leg raising may be restricted to less than 30 degrees because of severe pain in the sciatic distribution, not back pain. At the point where the patient experiences discomfort, passive dorsiflexion of the foot may cause an additional stab of sciatic pain. A gentler (and some would say more meaningful) way of testing straight-leg raising is to ask the *patient* to raise the leg with the knee straight and rigid – and to stop when he or she feels pain.

The '*bowstring' sign* is even more specific. Raise the

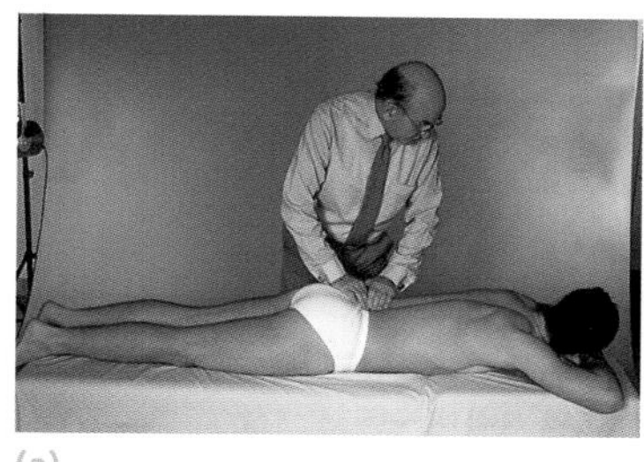
(a)

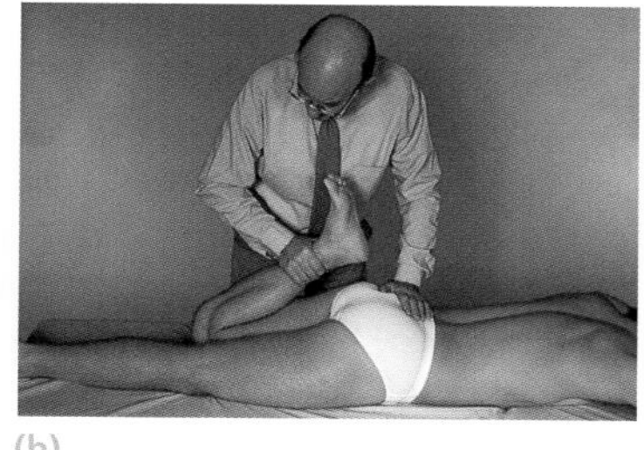
(b)

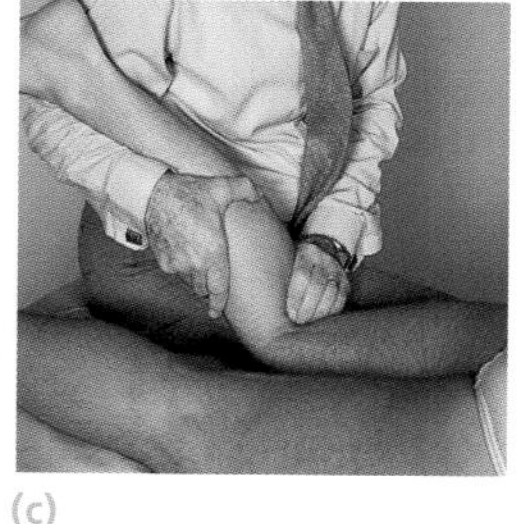
(c)

18.3 Examination with the patient prone (a) Feel for tenderness, watching the patient's face for any reaction. (b) Performing the femoral stretch test. You can test for lumbar root sensitivity either by hyperextending the hip or by acutely flexing the knee with the patient lying prone. Note the point at which the patient feels pain and compare the two sides. (c) While the patient is lying prone, take the opportunity to feel the pulses. The popliteal pulse is easily felt if the tissues at the back of the knee are relaxed by slightly flexing the knee.

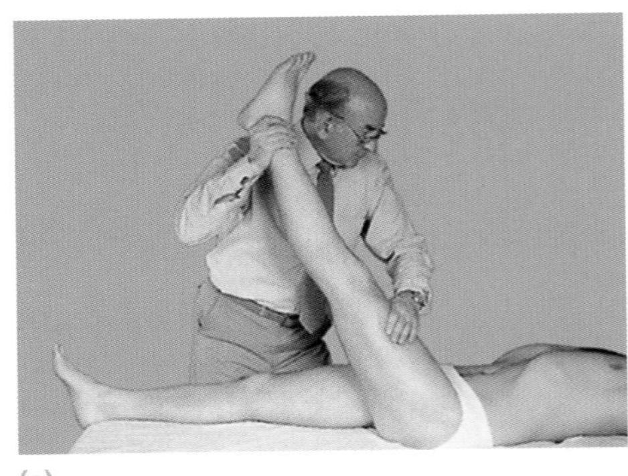

(a)

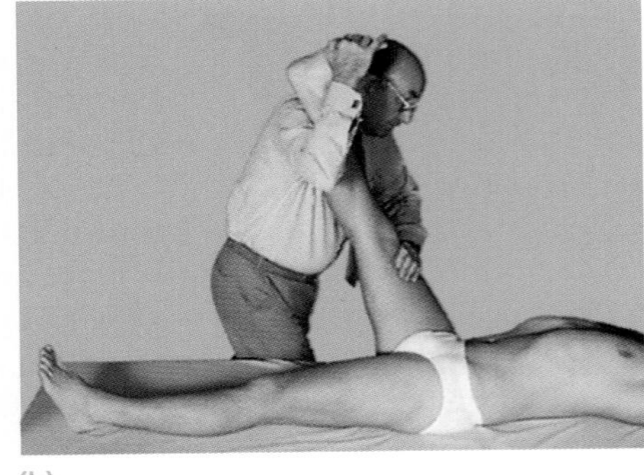

(b)

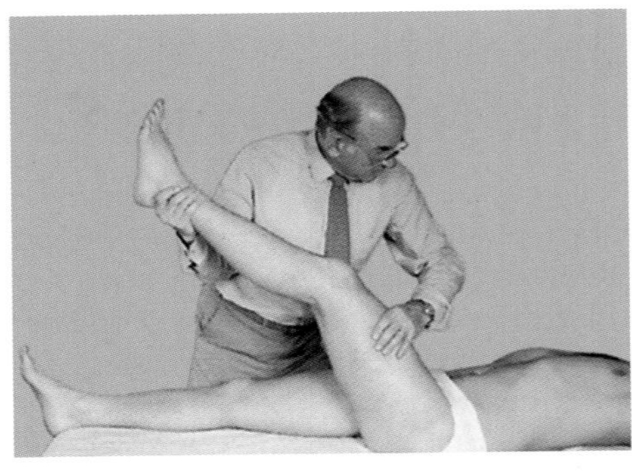

(c)

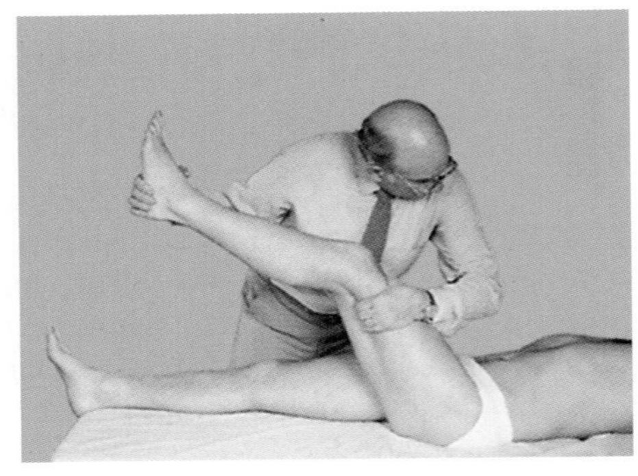

(d)

18.4 Sciatic stretch tests (a) Straight-leg raising. The knee is kept absolutely straight while the leg is slowly lifted (or raised by the patient himself); note where the patient complains of tightness and pain in the buttock – this normally occurs around 80 or 90°. (b) At that point a more acute stretch can be applied by passively dorsiflexing the foot – this may cause an added stab of pain. (c) The 'bowstring sign' is a confirmatory test for sciatic tension. At the point where the patient experiences pain, relax the tension by bending the knee slightly; the pain should disappear. Then apply firm pressure behind the lateral hamstrings to tighten the common peroneal nerve (d); the pain recurs with renewed intensity.

patient's leg gently to the point where he or she experiences sciatic pain; now, without reducing the amount of lift, bend the knee so as to relax the sciatic nerve. Buttock pain is immediately relieved; pain may then be re-induced without extending the knee by simply pressing on the lateral popliteal nerve behind the lateral tibial condyle, to tighten it like a bowstring.

Sometimes straight-leg raising on the unaffected side produces pain on the affected side. This *crossed sciatic tension* is indicative of severe root compression, usually due to a large central disc prolapse, and warns of the risk to the sacral nerve roots that control bladder function (the cauda equina syndrome – one of very few surgical emergencies in spinal disorders).

A *full neurological examination* of the lower limbs is then carried out. An absent ankle jerk on the side of sciatica, combined with paraesthesiae along the lateral border of the foot, suggests compression of the S1 nerve root; normal reflexes combined with paraesthesiae on the dorsum of the foot, suggests compression of the L5 nerve root. Check for clonus and a positive Babinski sign; if present there should be some alarm regarding possible spinal cord compression.

Ankle clonus with a positive Babinski sign suggests brain or spinal cord pathology until proved otherwise.

The lower limbs should be carefully examined for *length discrepancy and trophic changes*; the *pulses* are felt in the groin, the popliteal fossa and around the ankle.

Unless the signs point unequivocally to a spinal disorder, *rectal* and *vaginal examination* may also be necessary.

IMAGING

Plain x-rays

Begin with anteroposterior and lateral views of the spine; for the lumbar region, oblique views of the spine, an anteroposterior x-ray of the pelvis and a postero-anterior view of the sacroiliac joints may also be needed.

In the anteroposterior view the spine should look perfectly straight and the soft-tissue shadows should outline the normal muscle planes. Curvature (scoliosis) is obvious, and best shown in erect views. Bulging of the psoas muscle or loss of the psoas shadow may indicate a paravertebral abscess. Individual vertebrae may show alterations in structure, e.g. asymmetry or collapse. Check the outlines of the pedicles, which normally look like oval footprints near the lateral edges of each rectangular vertebral body: a missing or misshapen pedicle could be due to erosion by infection, a neurofibroma or metastatic disease.

In the lateral view the normal thoracic kyphosis (up to 40 degrees) and lumbar lordosis should be regular and uninterrupted. Anterior shift of an upper segment upon a lower (spondylolisthesis) may be associated with defects of the posterior arch, which show best in oblique views. Vertebral bodies, which should be rectangular, may be wedged or biconcave, deformities typical of osteoporosis or old injury. Bone density and trabecular markings also are best seen in lateral films. Lateral views in flexion and extension may reveal

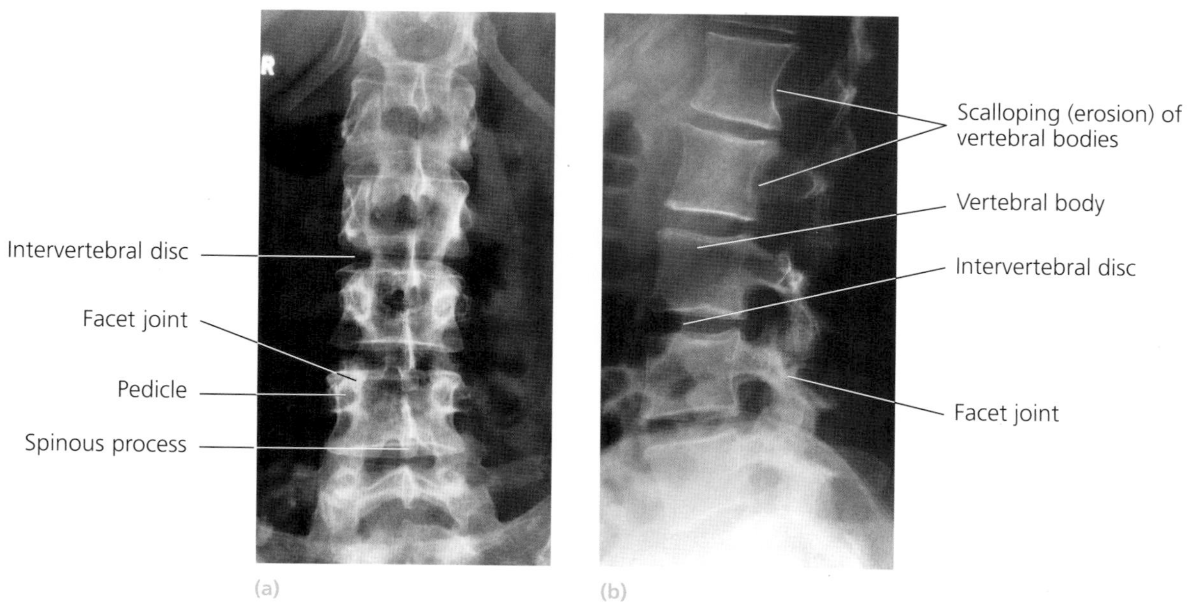

18.5 Lumbar spine x-rays (a,b) The most important normal features are demonstrated in the lower lumbar spine. In this particular case there are also signs of marked posterior vertebral body and facet joint erosions at L1 and L2, features that are strongly suggestive of an expanding neurofibroma.

excessive intervertebral movement, a possible cause of back pain.

The intervertebral spaces may be edged by bony spurs (suggesting longstanding disc degeneration) or bridged by fine bony syndesmophytes (a cardinal feature of ankylosing spondylitis).

The sacroiliac joints may show erosion or ankylosis, as in tuberculosis (TB) or ankylosing spondylitis, and the hip joints may show arthrosis, not to be missed in the older patient with backache.

Radioisotope scanning

Isotope scans may pick up areas of increased activity, suggesting a fracture, a local inflammatory lesion or a 'silent' metastasis.

Computed tomography

Computed tomography (CT) is helpful in the diagnosis of structural bone changes (e.g. vertebral fracture) and intervertebral disc prolapse. When combined with *myelography* it gives valuable information about the contents of the spinal canal.

Discography and facet joint arthrography

These are sometimes performed in the investigation of chronic back pain. Remember, though, that disc degeneration and facet joint arthritis are common in older people and are not necessarily the cause of the patient's symptoms. These are painful investigations, no longer easily justified where MRI is available.

Magnetic resonance imaging

MRI has virtually done away with the need for myelography, discography, facet arthrography, and much of CT scanning. The spinal canal and disc spaces are clearly outlined in various planes. Scans can reveal the physiological state of the disc as regards dehydration, as well as the effect of disc degeneration on bone marrow in adjacent vertebral bodies.

SPINAL DEFORMITIES

'Spinal deformity' (as opposed to deformities of individual vertebrae) affects the entire shape of the back and manifests as abnormal curvature, in either the coronal plane (scoliosis) or the sagittal plane (hyperkyphosis and hyperlordosis).

Variations and abnormalities of segmentation are common; they include anomalies such as lumbarization of the first sacral segment, 'sacralization' of one or both transverse processes of the fifth lumbar vertebra and asymmetry of the apophyseal joints, all of which are harmless, as well as such conditions as hemivertebra, which may give rise to severe spinal deformity (see later).

The most serious type of *congenital defect* is spina bifida.

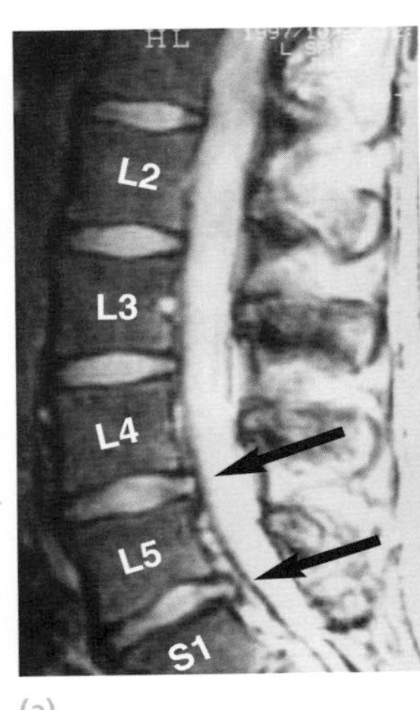

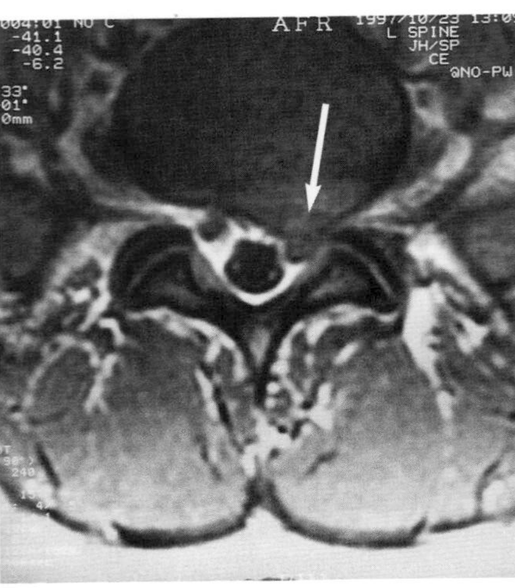

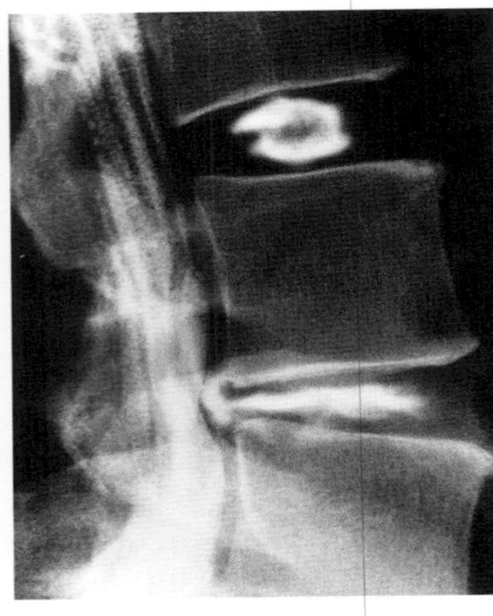

(a) (b) (c)

18.6 MRI and discography (a) The lateral T_2-weighted MRI shows a small posterior disc bulge at L4/5 and a larger protrusion at L5/S1. (b) The axial MRI shows the disc prolapse encroaching on the intervertebral canal and the nerve root on the left side. (c) Discography, showing normal appearance at the upper level and a degenerate disc with prolapse at the level below.

SCOLIOSIS

Scoliosis is an apparent lateral (sideways) curvature of the spine. 'Apparent' because, although lateral curvature does occur, the commonest form of scoliosis is actually a triplanar deformity with lateral, anteroposterior and rotational components (Dickson et al., 1984). Two broad types of deformity are defined: *postural* and *structural.*

Postural Scoliosis

In postural scoliosis the deformity is secondary or compensatory to some condition outside the spine, such as a short leg, or pelvic tilt due to contracture of the hip. When the patient sits (thereby cancelling leg length asymmetry) the curve disappears. Local muscle spasm associated with a prolapsed lumbar disc may cause a skew back; although sometimes called 'sciatic scoliosis' this, too, is a spurious deformity.

Structural scoliosis

In structural scoliosis there is a non-correctable deformity of the affected spinal segment, an essential component of which is vertebral rotation. The spinous processes swing round towards the concavity of the curve and the transverse processes on the convexity rotate posteriorly. In the thoracic region the ribs on the convex side stand out prominently, producing the rib hump, which is a characteristic part of the overall deformity. Dickson and co-workers (1984) have pointed out that this is really a lordoscoliosis associated with rotational buckling of the spine. The initial

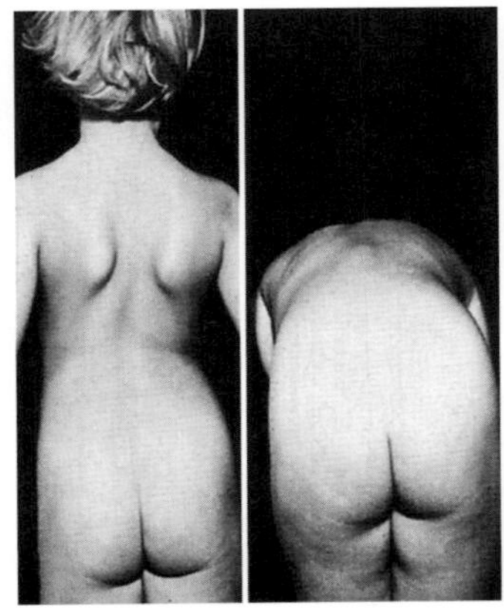

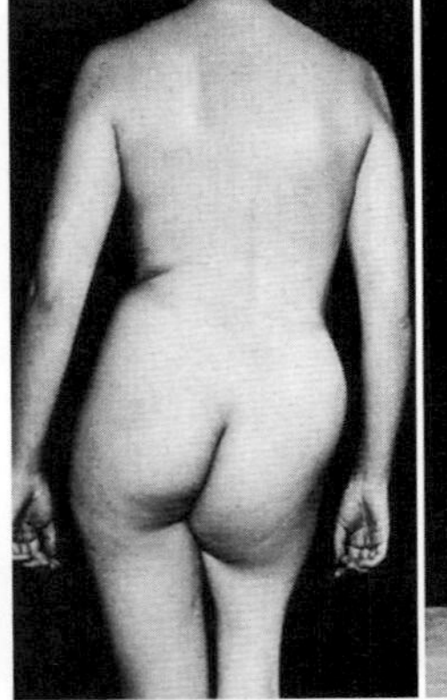

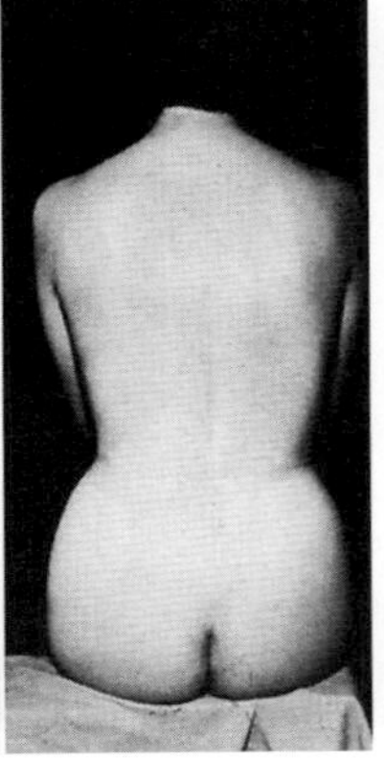

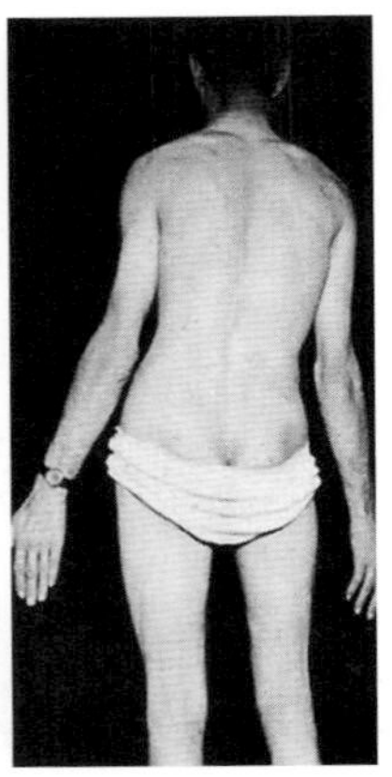

(a) (b) (c)

18.7 Postural scoliosis (a) This young girl presented with thoracolumbar 'curvature'. When she bends forwards, the deformity disappears; this is typical of a postural or mobile scoliosis. (b) Short-leg scoliosis disappears when the patient sits. (c) Sciatic scoliosis disappears when the prolapsed disc settles down or is removed.

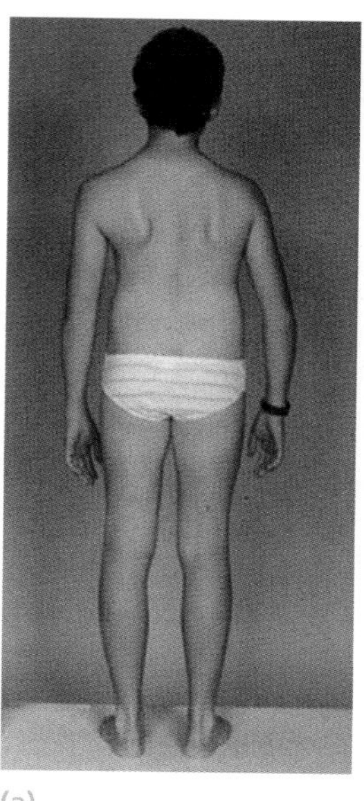
(a)

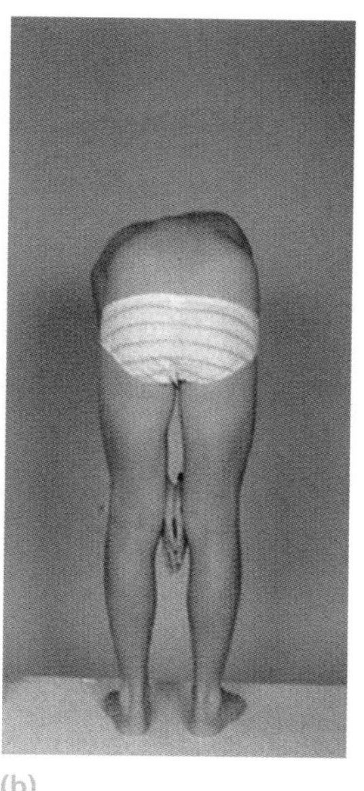
(b)

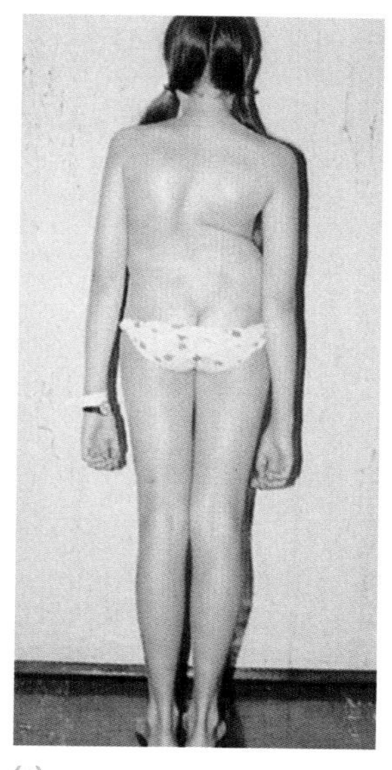
(c)

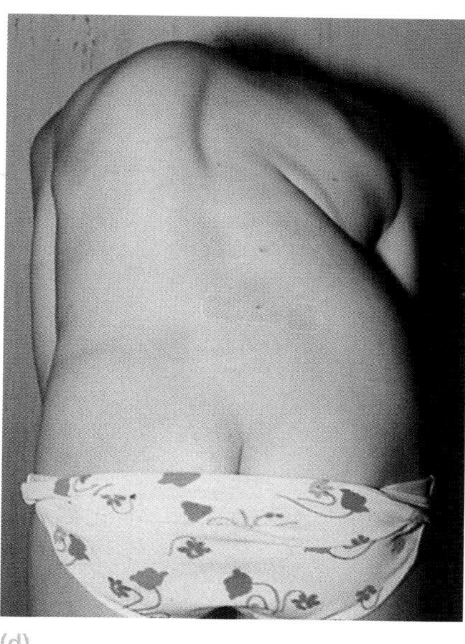
(d)

18.8 Structural scoliosis (a) Slight curves are often missed on casual inspection but the deformity becomes apparent when the spine is flexed (b). The young girl in (c) has a much more obvious scoliosis and asymmetry of the hips but what really worries her is the prominent rib hump, seen best when she bends over (d).

deformity is probably correctable, but once it exceeds a certain point of mechanical stability the spine buckles and rotates into a fixed deformity that does not disappear with changes in posture. Secondary (compensatory) curves nearly always develop to counterbalance the primary deformity; they are usually less marked and more easily correctable, but with time they, too, become fixed.

Once fully established, the deformity is liable to increase throughout the growth period. Thereafter, further deterioration is slight, though curves greater than 50 degrees may go on increasing by 1 degree per year. With very severe curves, chest deformity is marked and cardiopulmonary function is usually affected.

Most cases have no obvious cause (*idiopathic scoliosis*); other varieties are *congenital* or *osteopathic* (due to bony anomalies), *neuropathic, myopathic* (associated with some muscle dystrophies) and a miscellaneous group of connective-tissue disorders.

Clinical features

Deformity is usually the presenting symptom: an obvious skew back or a rib hump in thoracic curves, and asymmetrical prominence of one hip in thoracolumbar curves. Balanced curves sometimes pass unnoticed until an adult presents with backache. Where school screening programmes are conducted, children will be referred with very minor deformities.

Pain is a rare complaint and should alert the clinician to the possibility of a neural tumour and the need for MRI. Scoliosis in children is a painless deformity. Scoliosis with pain suggests a spinal tumour until proved otherwise.

There may be a *family history* of scoliosis or a record of some abnormality *during pregnancy* or *childbirth*; the *early developmental milestones* should be noted.

The trunk should be completely exposed and the patient examined from in front, from the back and from the side. *Skin* pigmentation and congenital anomalies such as sacral dimples or hair tufts are sought.

The *spine* may be obviously deviated from the midline, or this may become apparent only when the patient bends forward (the Adams test). The level and direction of the major curve convexity are noted (e.g. 'right thoracic' means a curve in the thoracic spine and convex to the right). The hip (pelvis) sticks out on the concave side and the scapula on the convex. The breasts and shoulders also may be asymmetrical. With thoracic scoliosis, rotation causes the rib angles to protrude, thus producing an asymmetrical rib hump on the convex side of the curve. In balanced deformities the occiput is over the midline; in unbalanced (or decompensated) curves it is not. This can be determined more accurately by dropping a plumbline from the prominent spinous process of C7 and noting whether it falls along the gluteal cleft.

The diagnostic feature of fixed (as distinct from postural or mobile) scoliosis is that forward bending makes the curve more obvious. Spinal mobility should be assessed and the effect of lateral bending on the curve noted; is there some flexibility in the curve and can it be passively corrected?

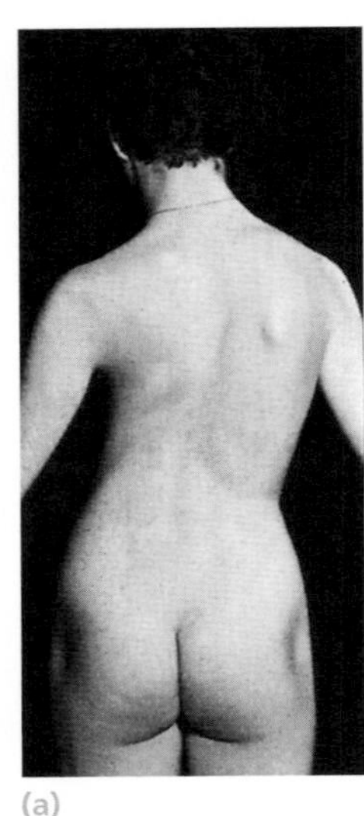

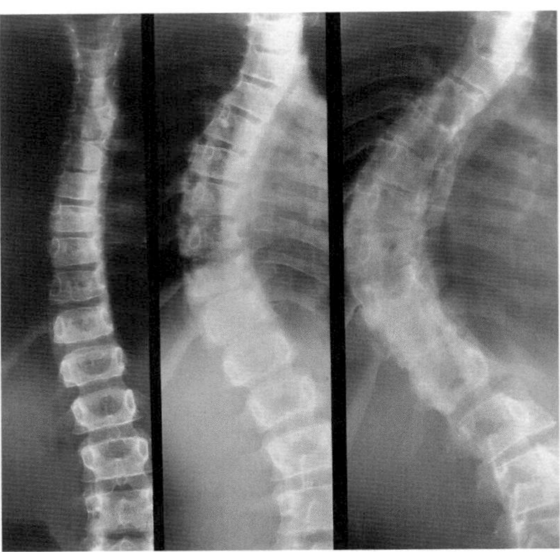

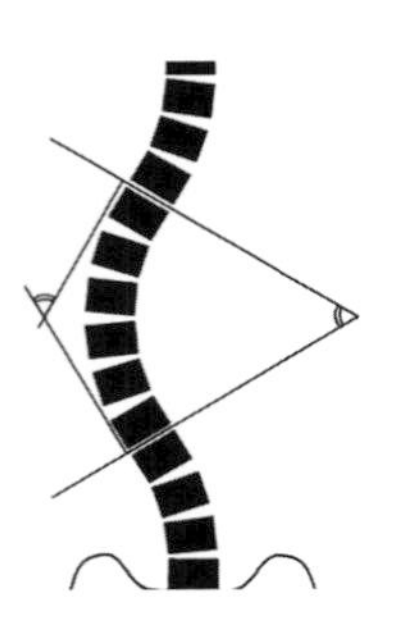

(a) (b) (c)

18.9 Adolescent idiopathic scoliosis (a) Typical thoracic deformity. (b) Serial x-rays show how this curve increased over a period of 4 years. (c) The angle of curvature is measured on the x-ray by Cobb's method: Lines projected from the top of the uppermost and the bottom of the lowermost vertebral bodies in the primary curve define Cobb's angle.

Side-on posture should also be observed. There may appear to be excessive kyphosis or lordosis.

Neurological examination is important. Any abnormality suggesting a spinal cord lesion calls for CT and/or MRI.

Leg length is measured. If one side is short, the pelvis is levelled by standing the patient on wooden blocks and the spine is re-examined.

General examination includes a search for the possible cause and an assessment of cardiopulmonary function (which is reduced in severe curves).

Imaging

PLAIN X-RAYS

Full-length posteroanterior (PA) and lateral x-rays of the spine and iliac crests must be taken with the patient erect. Structural curves show vertebral rotation: in the PA x-ray, vertebrae towards the apex of the curve appear to be asymmetrical and the spinous processes are deviated towards the concavity. Remember that PA in relation to the patient is not PA in relation to the rotated vertebrae!

The upper and lower ends of the curve are identified as the levels where vertebrae start to angle away from the curve. The degree of curvature is measured by drawing lines on the x-ray at the upper border of the uppermost vertebra and the lower border of the lowermost vertebra of the curve; the angle subtended by these lines is the *angle of curvature* (Cobb's angle).

The site of the curve apex should be noted. Right thoracic curves are the commonest, the great majority in girls in adolescent idiopathic scoliosis. Left thoracic curves are so unusual that if seen they should be further investigated by MRI to exclude spinal tumours. The primary structural curve is usually balanced by compensatory curves above and below, or by a second 'primary' curve also with vertebral rotation (sometimes there are multiple 'primary' curves).

What is not readily appreciated from these films is the degree of lordosis in the primary curve(s) and kyphosis in the compensatory curves (Archer and Dickson, 1989); indeed it is postulated that flattening or reversal of the normal thoracic kyphosis superimposed on coronal plane asymmetry leads, with growth, to progressive idiopathic scoliosis. Lateral bending views are taken to assess the degree of curve correctability.

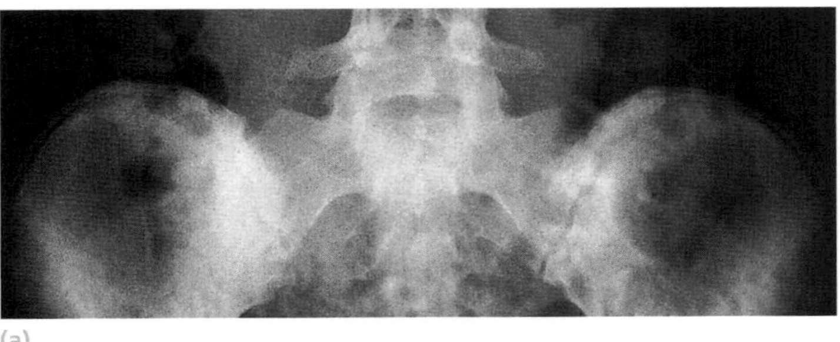

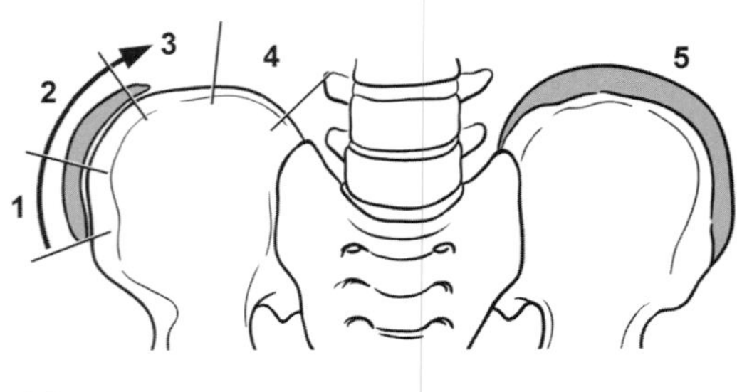

(a) (b)

18.10 Risser's sign The iliac apophyses normally appear progressively from lateral to medial (stages 1–4). When fusion is complete, spinal maturity has been reached and further increase of curvature is negligible (stage 5).

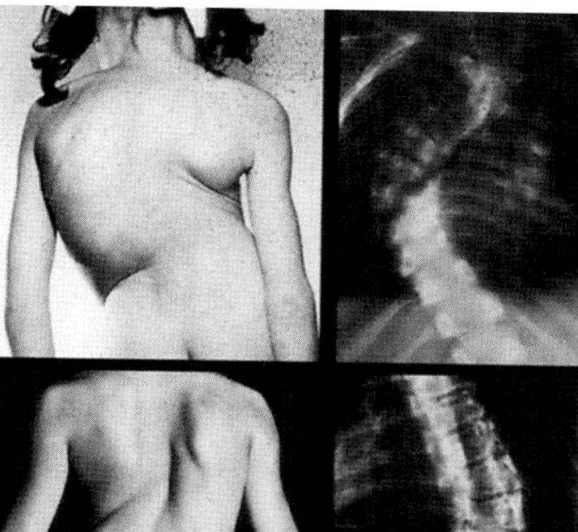

Infantile thoracic
60 per cent male
90 per cent convex to left.
Associated with ipsilateral plagiocephaly
May be resolving or progressive.
Progressive variety becomes severe.
Adolescent thoracic
90 per cent female
90 per cent convex to right.
Rib rotation exaggerates the deformity.
50 per cent develop curves of greater than 70°.

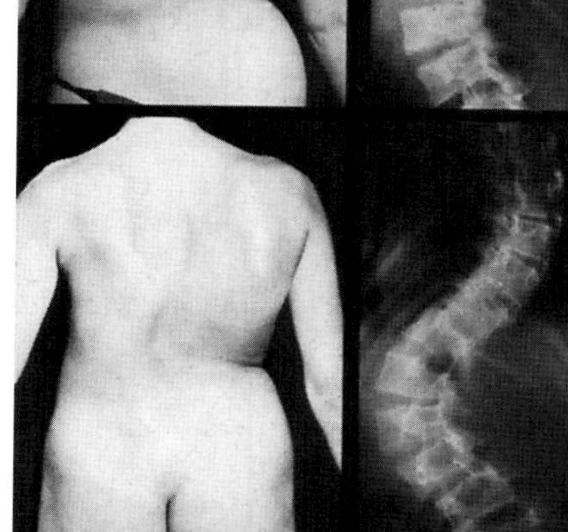

Thoracolumbar
Slightly more common in females.
Slightly more common to right.
Features mid-way between adolescent thoracic and lumbar.
Lumbar
More common in females.
80 per cent convex to left.
One hip prominent but no ribs to accentuate deformity.
Therefore not noticed early, but backache in adult life.
Combined
Two primary curves, one in each direction.
Even when radiologically severe, clinical deformity relatively slight because always well balanced.

18.11 Patterns of idiopathic scoliosis Bracing is used far less than previously because of serious doubts as to its effectiveness beyond natural history.

SKELETAL MATURITY – RISSER'S SIGN

This is assessed in several ways (this is important because the curve often progresses most during the period of rapid skeletal growth and maturation). The iliac apophyses start ossifying shortly after puberty; ossification extends medially and, once the iliac crests are completely ossified, further progression of the scoliosis is minimal (Risser's sign). This stage of development usually coincides with fusion of the vertebral ring apophyses. 'Skeletal age' may also be estimated from x-rays of the wrist and hand.

SPECIAL IMAGING

CT and MRI may be necessary to define a vertebral abnormality or cord compression.

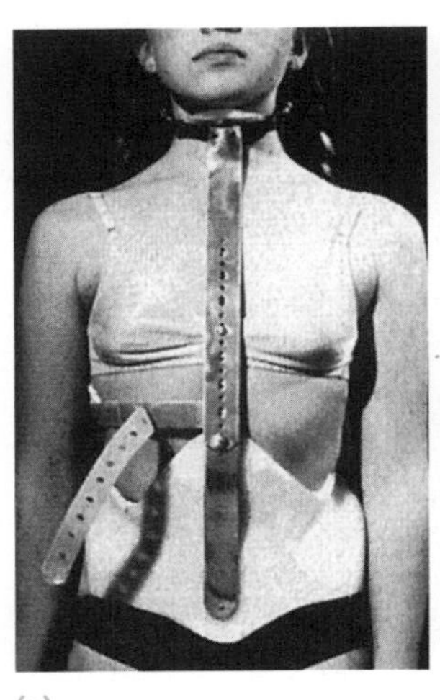
(a)

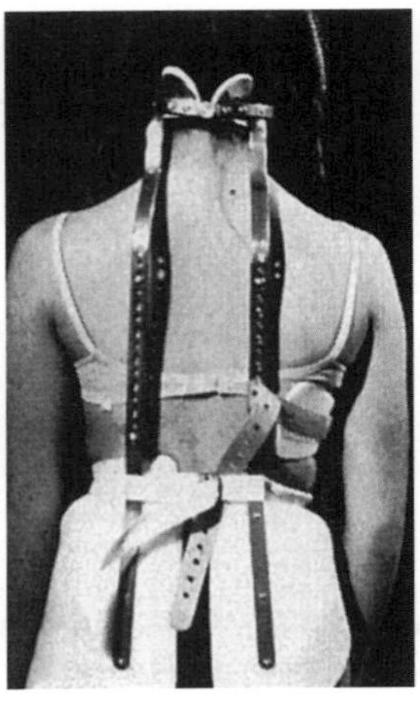
(b)

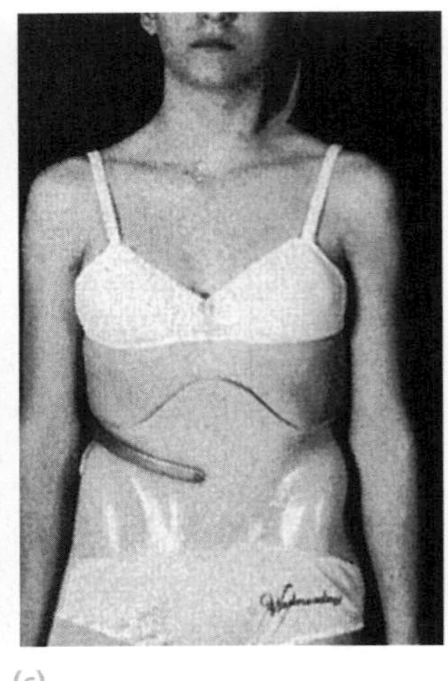
(c)

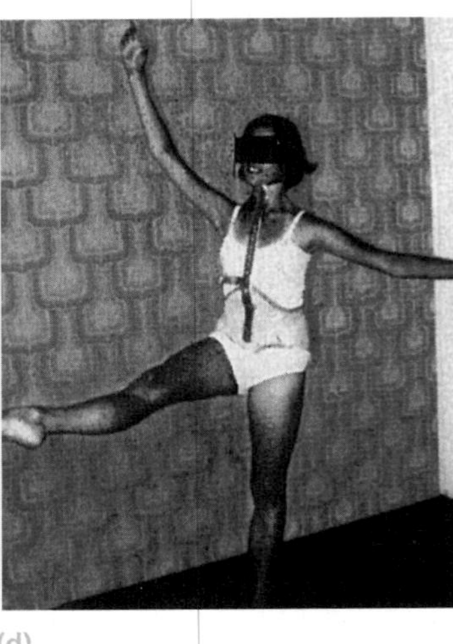
(d)

18.12 Structural scoliosis – bracing (a,b) The Milwaukee brace fits snugly over the pelvis below; chin and head pads promote active postural correction and a thoracic pad presses on the ribs at the apex of the curve. (c) The Boston brace is used for low curves. All braces are cumbersome, but (d) if well made they need not interfere much with activity. Nowadays bracing is used far less often than before because of doubts about its ability to alter the natural progress of structural scoliosis.

Special investigations

Pulmonary function tests are performed in all cases of severe chest deformity. A marked reduction in vital capacity is associated with diminished life expectancy and carries obvious risks for surgery.

Patients with muscular dystrophies or connective tissue disorders require full *biochemical* and *neuromuscular* investigation of the underlying condition.

Prognosis and treatment

Prognosis is the key to treatment: the aim is to prevent severe deformity. Generally speaking, the younger the child and the higher the curve the worse is the prognosis. Management differs for the different types of scoliosis, which are considered later.

IDIOPATHIC SCOLIOSIS

This group constitutes about 80 per cent of all cases of scoliosis. The deformity is often familial and the population incidence of serious curves (over 30 degrees and therefore needing treatment) is three per 1000; trivial curves are very much more common. The age at onset has been used to define three groups: *adolescent*, *juvenile* and *infantile*. A simpler division now in general use is *early-onset* (before puberty) and *late-onset scoliosis* (after puberty).

LATE-ONSET (ADOLESCENT) IDIOPATHIC SCOLIOSIS (AGED 10 OR OVER)

This is the commonest type, occurring in 90 per cent of cases, mostly in girls. Primary thoracic curves are usually convex to the right, lumbar curves to the left; intermediate (thoracolumbar) and combined (double primary) curves also occur. Progression is not inevitable; indeed, most curves less than 20 degrees either resolve spontaneously or remain unchanged. However, once a curve starts to progress, it usually goes on doing so throughout the remaining growth period (and, to a much lesser degree, beyond that). Reliable predictors of progression are: (1) a very young age; (2) marked curvature; (3) an incomplete Risser sign at presentation (Lonstein and Carlson, 1984). In prepubertal children, rapid progression is liable to occur during the growth spurt.

Treatment

The aims of treatment are: (1) to prevent a mild deformity from becoming severe; (2) to correct an existing deformity that is unacceptable to the patient. A period of preliminary observation may be needed before deciding between conservative and operative treatment. At 4–9-monthly intervals the patient is examined, photographed and x-rayed so that curves can be measured and checked for progression.

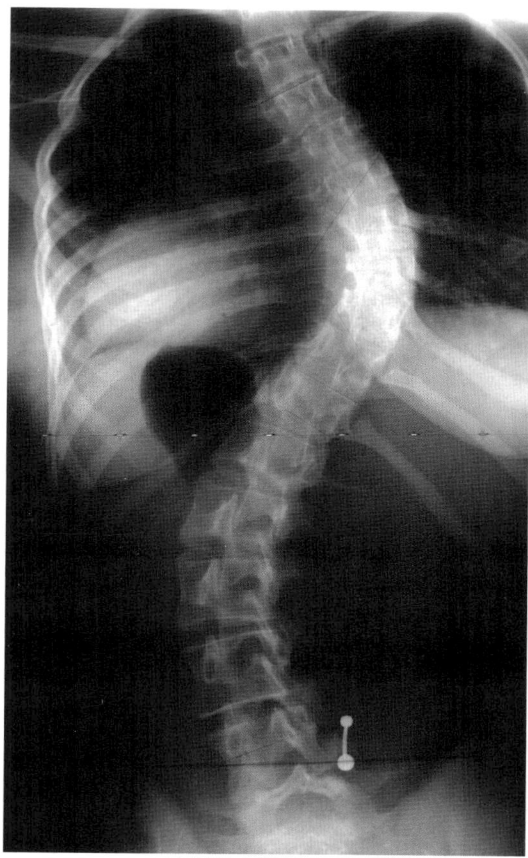
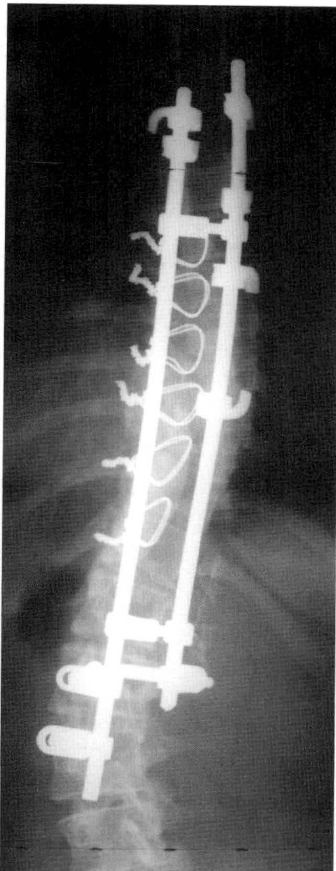
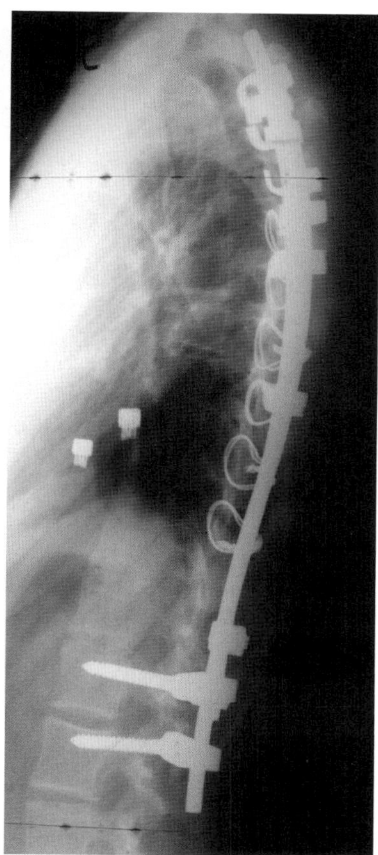

18.13 Scoliosis – posterior instrumentation Idiopathic scoliosis treated by posterior double-rod fixation.

NON-OPERATIVE TREATMENT

If the patient is approaching skeletal maturity and the deformity is acceptable (which usually means it is less than 30 degrees and well balanced), treatment is probably unnecessary unless sequential x-rays show definite progression.

Exercises are often prescribed; they have no effect on the curve but they do maintain muscle tone and may inspire confidence in a favourable outcome.

Bracing has been used for many years in the treatment of progressive scoliotic curves between 20 and 30 degrees. The *Milwaukee brace* is principally a thoracic support consisting of a pelvic corset connected by adjustable steel supports to a cervical ring carrying occipital and chin pads; its purpose is to reduce the lumbar lordosis and encourage active stretching and straightening of the thoracic spine. The *Boston brace* is a snug-fitting underarm brace that provides lumbar or low thoracolumbar support. Corrective pads may be added to these devices to apply pressure at a particular site. A well-made brace can be worn 23 hours out of 24 and does not preclude full daily activities, including sport and exercises.

It has long been recognized that bracing will not improve the curve – at best it will merely stop it from getting worse. Many orthopaedic surgeons no longer employ this method of treatment, arguing that there is insufficient evidence of its benefits. Their preference now is to wait for the curve to progress to the stage when corrective surgery would be justified.

OPERATIVE TREATMENT

Surgery is indicated: (1) for curves of more than 30 degrees that are cosmetically unacceptable, especially in pre-pubertal children who are liable to develop marked progression during the growth spurt; (2) for milder deformity that is deteriorating rapidly. Balanced, double primary curves require operation only if they are greater than 40 degrees and progressing.

The objectives are: (1) to halt progression of the deformity; (2) to straighten the curve (including the rotational component) by some form of instrumentation; (3) to arthrodese the entire primary curve by bone grafting. Surgical options include:

Harrington system In the original system a rod was applied posteriorly along the concave side of the curve; attached to the rod were movable hooks that were engaged in the uppermost and lowermost vertebrae so as to distract the curve. If the curve is flexible, it will

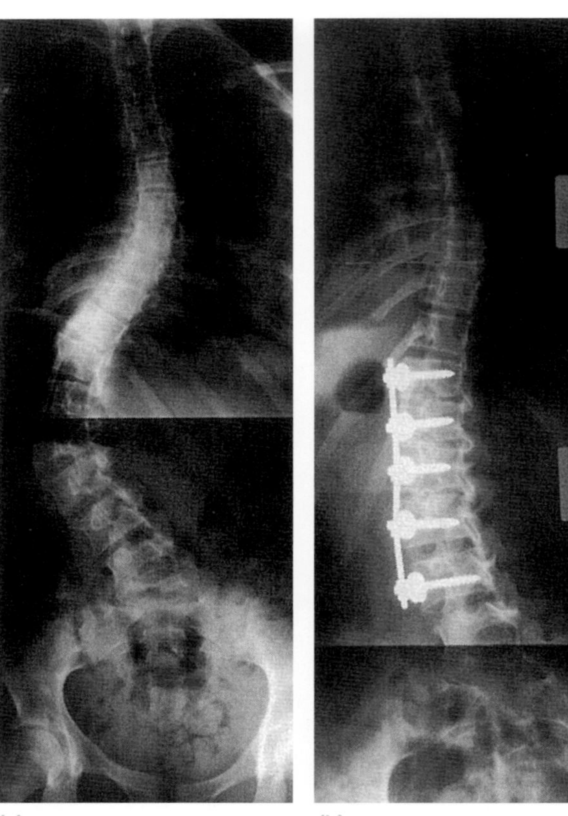

(a) (b)

18.14 Scoliosis – anterior instrumentation (a) This 14-year-old girl had a very stiff lumbar curve. It was planned to correct this by two-stage anterior and posterior release and fusion. (b) X-ray taken after the Zielke anterior instrumentation.

passively correct and bone grafts are then applied to obtain fusion over the length of the curve. A major drawback of the original distraction instrumentation is that it does not correct the rotational deformity at the apex of the curve and thus the rib prominence remains virtually unchanged.

Rod and sublaminar wiring (Luque) This is a modification of the Harrington system. Wires are passed under the vertebral laminae at multiple levels and fixed to the rod on the concave side of the curve, thus providing a more controlled and secure fixation. By bending the rod and arranging the mechanism so that the wires pull backwards rather than merely sideways, the rotational component of the deformity can also be substantially improved. However, the sublaminar wires are dangerously close to the dura and the risk of neurological damage is increased.

Cotrel-Dubousset system This mechanism combines a pedicle screw 'box' foundation at the caudal end of the deformity, with multiple hooks which can be placed at various levels to produce either distraction or compression. With double rods one can distract on the concave and compress on the convex side of the curve; by appropriate manipulation of the implants one can obtain correction also in the sagittal plane. It has been claimed that this system can correct the rotational deformity. It is also sufficiently rigid to make postoperative bracing unnecessary.

Anterior instrumentation (Dwyer; Zielke; Kaneda) Rigid curves and thoracolumbar curves associated with lumbar lordosis can be corrected by approaching the spine from the front, removing the discs throughout the curve and then applying a compression device (either a braided cable or a rod linking transverse vertebral body screws) along the convex side of the curve. Bone grafts are added to achieve fusion. In some cases combined anterior and posterior instrumentation is necessary

Advantages of this system are: (1) that it provides strong fixation with fewer vertebral segments having to be fused; (2) that overall shortening of the deformed section (by disc excision and vertebral compression) lessens the risk of cord injury due to spinal distraction. In some centres, transthoracic scoliosis surgery is now performed endoscopically through several ports, in order to reduce the morbidity associated with open thoracic surgery and rib resection.

Warning Whatever method is used, spinal cord function should be monitored during the operation. Ideally this is done by measuring somatosensory and motor evoked potentials during spinal correction. If these facilities are not available, the 'wake-up test' is used: anaesthesia is reduced to bring the patient to a semi-awake state and he or she is then instructed to move their feet. If there are signs of cord compromise, the instrumentation is relaxed or removed and re-applied with a lesser degree of correction. Patients have no memory of the wake-up procedure.

Rib hump The best of the instrumentation systems cannot completely eliminate the rib hump – and it is often this that troubles the patient most of all. If the deformity is marked, it can be reduced significantly by performing a costoplasty, where short sections of rib are excised at multiple levels on the rib hump (convex) side, close to the vertebral articulation.

Complications of surgery

Neurological compromise With modern techniques the incidence of permanent paralysis has been reduced to less than 1 per cent. From the patient's point of view this is small comfort. Every effort should be made to provide adequate safeguards.

Spinal decompensation Overcorrection may produce an unbalanced spine. This should be avoided by careful preoperative planning and selection of the appropriate levels of fusion.

Pseudarthrosis – Incomplete fusion occurs in about 2 per cent of cases and may require further operation and grafting.

Implant failure – Hooks may cut out and rods may break. If this is associated with a symptomatic pseudarthrosis, revision fusion/fixation will be needed.

EARLY-ONSET (JUVENILE) IDIOPATHIC SCOLIOSIS

Presenting in children aged 4–9, this type is uncommon. The characteristics of this group are similar to those of the adolescent group, but the prognosis is worse and surgical correction may be necessary before puberty. However, if the child is very young, a brace may hold the curve stationary until the age of 10 years, when fusion is more likely to succeed.

EARLY-ONSET (INFANTILE) IDIOPATHIC SCOLIOSIS

This variety, which presents in children aged 3 or under, is rare in North America and is becoming uncommon elsewhere, perhaps because most babies nowadays are allowed to sleep prone. Boys predominate and most curves are thoracic with convexity to the left. Although 90 per cent of infantile curves resolve spontaneously, progressive curves can become very severe; those in which the rib-vertebra angle at the apex of the curve differs on the two sides by more than 20 degrees are likely to deteriorate (Mehta, 1972). Because this also influences the development of the lungs, there is a high incidence of cardiopulmonary dysfunction.

Curves assessed as being potentially progressive should be treated by applying serial elongation-derotation-flexion (EDF) plaster casts under general anaesthesia, until the deformity resolves or until the child is big enough to manage in a brace. From about the age of 4 years onwards curve progression slows down or ceases and the child may not need further treatment. If the deformity continues to deteriorate, surgical correction may be required. This takes the form of anterior disc excision and fusion to control the apex of the curve, combined with posterior fusion to prevent posterior overgrowth.

OSTEOPATHIC (CONGENITAL) SCOLIOSIS

Although fractures and bone softening (as in rickets or osteogenesis imperfecta) may lead to scoliosis, the commonest bony cause is some type of vertebral anomaly – *hemivertebra, wedged vertebra* (failure of formation), and *fused vertebrae* – sometimes combined with *absent* or *fused ribs* (failure of segmentation). Overlying tissues often show angiomas, naevi,

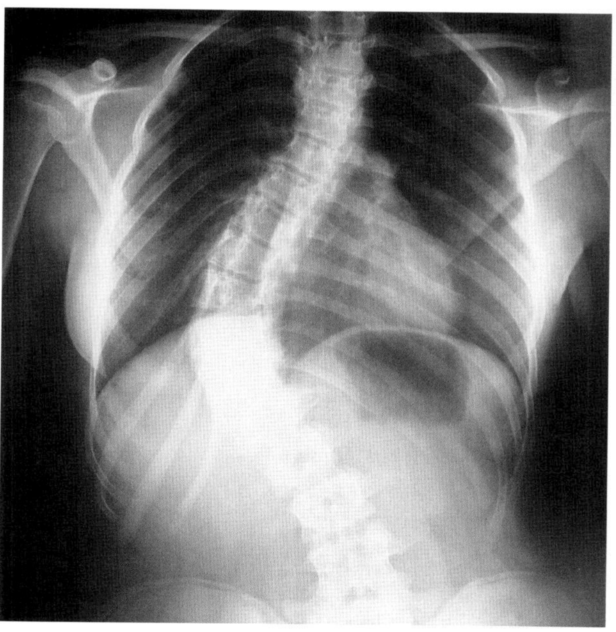

18.15 Early onset scoliosis 'Idiopathic' curves in young children usually resolve, but some increase progressively and become very severe. Measurement of the rib-vertebra angles at the curve apex in the early stages of the deformity is a good prognostic indicator (Mehta, 1972).

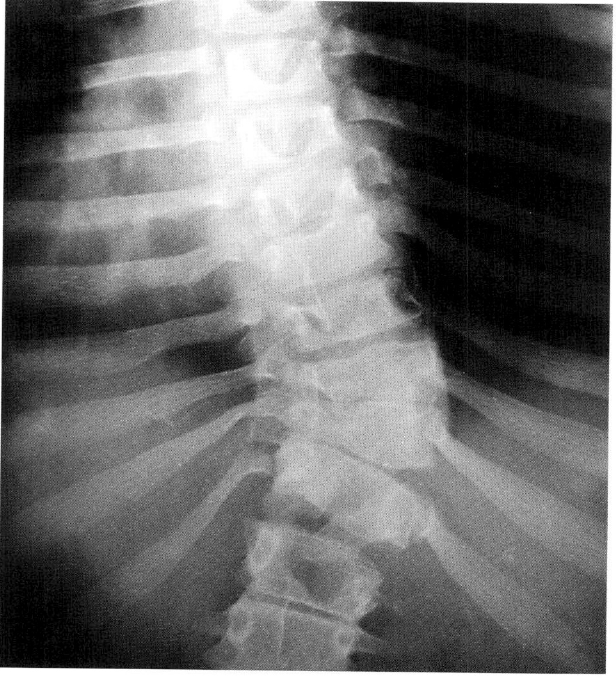

18.16 Congenital scoliosis Failure of segmentation and formation of the vertebrae at T10, 11 and 12 has resulted in a localized scoliosis.

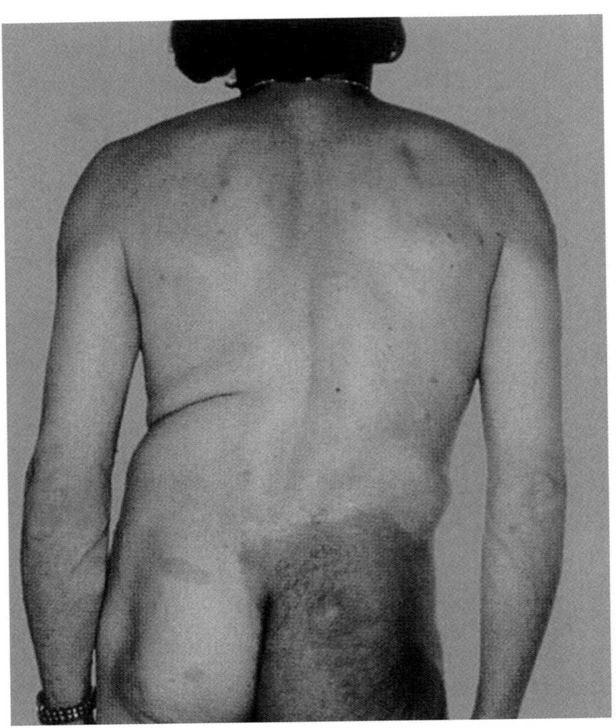

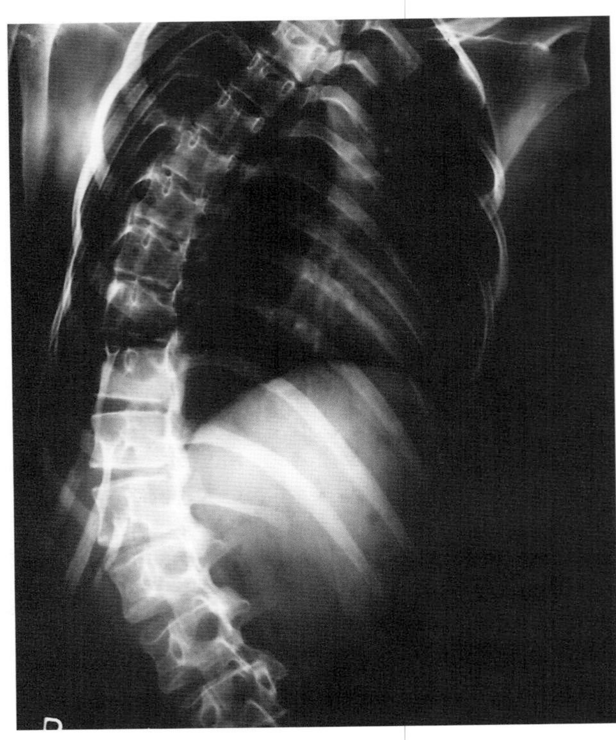

(a) (b)

18.17 Other types of scoliosis (a) This patient has a short structural curve plus multiple skin lesions – features suggesting neurofibromatosis. (b) By contrast, the typical post-poliomyelitis 'paralytic' scoliosis shown in this x-ray is characterised by a long C-shaped curve.

excess hair, dimples or a pad of fat. Spina bifida may be associated and visceral anomalies are common, especially in the heart and kidneys. These children require painstaking clinical investigation and imaging (1) in order to discover any other congenital anomalies; (2) to assess the risk of spinal cord damage.

While congenital scoliosis is often mild, some cases progress to severe deformity, particularly those with unilateral fusion of vertebrae (unilateral unsegmented bar). There must be a management assumption that the deformity will get worse, until proved otherwise. Before any operation is undertaken, advanced imaging is needed to exclude an associated dysraphism, particularly diastematomyelia and cord tethering, which must be dealt with prior to curve correction.

Treatment

Treatment is more difficult and specialized than that of idiopathic infantile scoliosis. Progressive deformities (usually involving rigid curves) will not respond to bracing alone, and surgical correction carries a significant risk of cord injury. These children should be treated in special units: the approach is to undertake staged resection of the curve apex, followed by instrumentation and spinal fusion. If multiple segments of the spine are involved, surgery may be too hazardous and should probably be withheld.

Neuropathic and myopathic scoliosis

Neuromuscular conditions associated with scoliosis include poliomyelitis, cerebral palsy, syringomyelia, Friedreich's ataxia and the rarer lower motor neuron disorders and muscle dystrophies; the curve may take some years to develop. The typical paralytic curve is long, convex towards the side with weaker muscles (spinal, abdominal or intercostal), and at first is mobile. In severe cases the greatest problem is loss of stability and balance, which may make even sitting difficult or impossible. Additional problems are generalized muscle weakness and (in some cases) loss of sensibility with the attendant risk of pressure ulceration.

X-ray with traction applied shows the extent to which the deformity is correctable.

Treatment

Treatment depends upon the degree of functional disability. Mild curves may require no treatment at all. Moderate curves with spinal stability are managed as for idiopathic scoliosis. Severe curves, associated with pelvic obliquity and loss of sitting balance, can often be managed by fitting a suitable sitting support. If this does not suffice, operative treatment may be indicated. This involves stabilization of the entire paralyzed segment by combined anterior and posterior instrumentation and fusion.

Scoliosis and neurofibromatosis

About one-third of patients with neurofibromatosis develop spinal deformity, the severity of which varies from very mild (and not requiring any form of treatment) to the most marked manifestations accompanied by skin lesions, multiple neurofibromata and bony dystrophy affecting the vertebrae and ribs. The scoliotic curve is typically 'short and sharp'. Other clues to the diagnosis lie in the appearance of the skin lesions and any associated skeletal abnormalities.

Mild cases are treated as for idiopathic scoliosis. More severe deformities will usually need combined anterior and posterior instrumentation and fusion. As with other forms of skeletal neurofibromatosis, graft dissolution and pseudarthrosis are not uncommon.

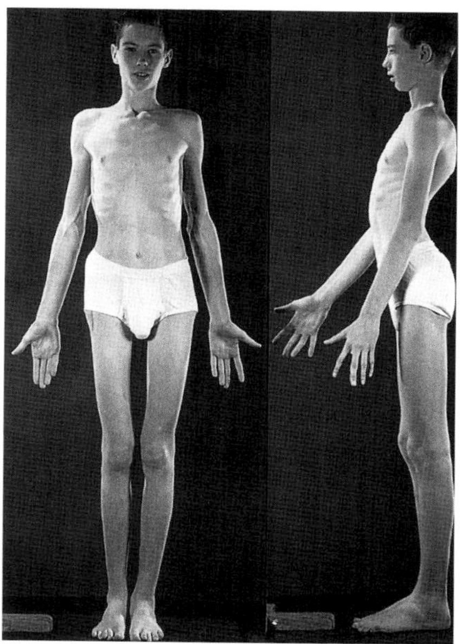

18.18 Postural kyphosis This tall teenager has Marfans' disease and ligamentous laxity. He has also developed a postural thoracic hyperkyphosis and lumbar hyperlordosis.

KYPHOSIS

Rather confusingly, the term 'kyphosis' is used to describe both the normal (gentle rounding of the thoracic spine) and the abnormal (excessive thoracic curvature or straightening out of the cervical or lumbar lordotic curves). Excessive thoracic curvature might be better described as 'hyperkyphosis'. *Kyphos*, or gibbus, is a sharp posterior angulation due to localized collapse or wedging of one or more vertebrae. This may be the result of a congenital defect, a fracture (sometimes pathological) or spinal tuberculosis (see Fig. 18.24).

Postural Kyphosis

Postural kyphosis is usually associated with other postural defects such as flat feet. It is voluntarily correctable. If treatment is needed, this consists of posture training and exercises.

Compensatory kyphosis is secondary to some other deformity, usually increased lumbosacral lordosis. This deformity, too, is correctable.

Structural kyphosis

Structural kyphosis is fixed and associated with changes in the shape of the vertebrae. In *children* this may be due to congenital vertebral defects; it is also seen in skeletal dysplasias such as achondroplasia and in osteogenesis imperfecta. Older children may develop severe deformity secondary to tuberculous spondylitis.

In *adolescence* the commonest cause is Scheuermann's disease (see later). In *adults* kyphosis could be due to an old childhood disorder; tuberculous spondylitis, ankylosing spondylitis or spinal trauma. In *elderly people*, osteoporosis may result in vertebral compression and an increase in a previously mild, asymptomatic deformity.

CONGENITAL KYPHOSIS

Vertebral anomalies leading to kyphosis may be due to failure of formation (type I), failure of segmentation (type II) or a combination of these:

Type I (failure of formation) This is the commonest (and the worst) type. If the anterior part of the vertebral body fails to develop, progressive kyphosis and posterior displacement of the hemivertebra may lead to cord compression. In children younger than 6 years with curves of less than 40 degrees, posterior spinal fusion alone may prevent further progression. Older children or more severe curves may need combined anterior and posterior fusion, and those with neurological complications will require cord decompression as well as fusion.

Type II (failure of segmentation) Type II usually takes the form of an anterior intervertebral bar; as the posterior elements continue to grow, that segment of the spine gradually becomes kyphotic. The risk of neurological compression is much less, but if the curve is progressive a posterior fusion will be needed.

ADOLESCENT KYPHOSIS (JUVENILE OSTEOCHONDROSIS; SCHEUERMANN'S DISEASE)

Scheuermann, in 1920, described a condition that he called 'juvenile dorsal kyphosis', distinguishing it from the more common postural (correctable) kyphosis. The characteristic feature was a fixed round-back deformity associated with wedging of several thoracic vertebrae. The term 'vertebral osteochondritis' was adopted because the primary defect appeared to be in the ossification of the ring epiphyses that define the peripheral rims on the upper and lower surfaces of each vertebral body. The true nature of the disorder is still not known; the cartilaginous end-plates may be weaker than normal (perhaps due to a collagen defect) and are then damaged by pressure of the adjacent intervertebral discs during strenuous activity. The normal curve of the thoracic spine ensures that the anterior edges of the vertebrae are subjected to the greatest stress and this is where the damage is greatest. Similar changes may occur in the lumbar spine, but here wedging is unusual.

Clinical features

The condition starts at puberty and affects boys more often than girls. The parents notice that the child, an otherwise fit teenager, is becoming increasingly round-shouldered. The patient may complain of backache and fatigue; this sometimes increases after the end of growth and may become severe.

A smooth thoracic kyphosis is seen; it may produce a marked hump. Below it is a compensatory lumbar lordosis. The deformity cannot be corrected by changes in posture. Movements are normal but tight hamstrings often limit straight leg raising. A mild scoliosis is not uncommon. Rare complications are spastic paresis of the lower limbs and – with severe deformity of the thorax – cardiopulmonary dysfunction.

In later life patients with thoracic kyphosis may develop lumbar backache. This has been attributed to chronic low back strain or facet joint dysfunction due to compensatory hyperextension of the lumbar spine. In some cases, however, lumbar Scheuermann's disease itself may cause pain (see later).

X-ray

In lateral radiographs of the spine the vertebral end-plates of several adjacent vertebrae (usually T6–10) appear irregular or fragmented. The changes are more marked anteriorly and one or more vertebral bodies may become wedge shaped. There may also be small radiolucent defects in the subchondral bone (Schmorl's nodes), which are thought to be due to central (axial) disc protrusions.

The angle of deformity is measured in the same way as for scoliosis, except that here the lateral x-ray is used and the lines mark the uppermost and lowermost affected vertebrae. Wedging of more than 5 degrees in three adjacent vertebrae and an overall kyphosis angle of more than 40 degrees are abnormal. Mild scoliosis is not uncommon.

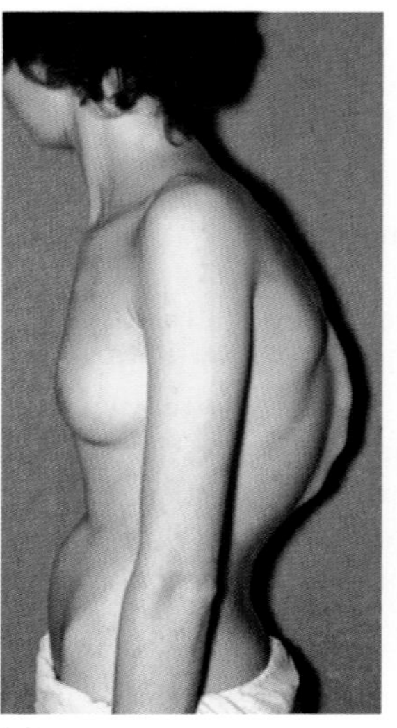
(a)

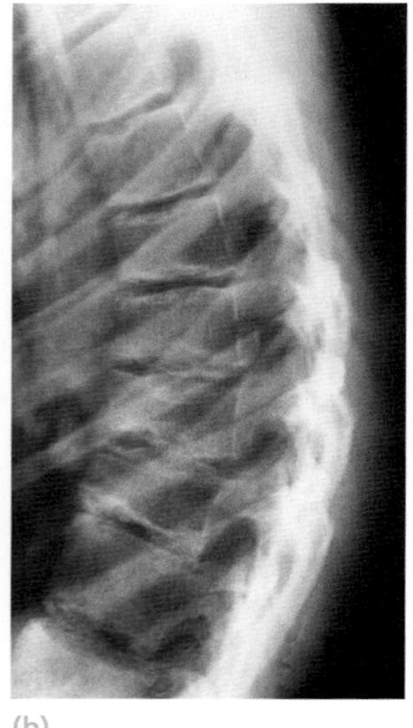
(b)

18.19 Scheuermanns disease (a) A young girl with marked exaggeration of the usual thoracic kyphosis. (b) X-ray examination showed the typical indentations in the vertebral end-plates and wedging of vertebral bodies.

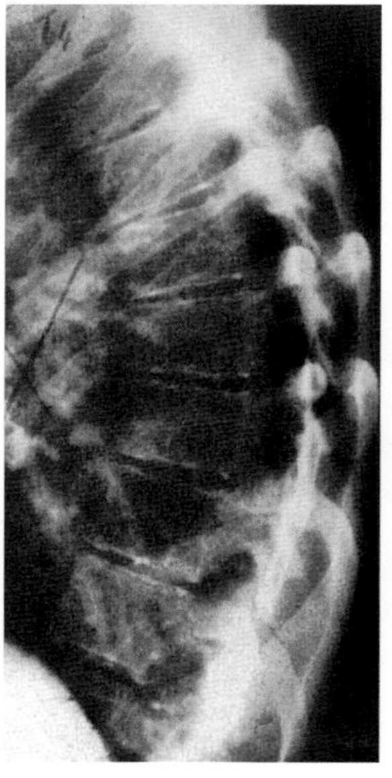
(a)

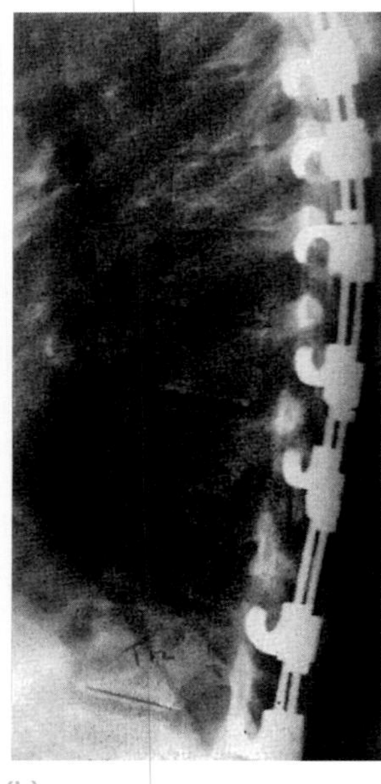
(b)

18.20 Scheuermann's disease – operative treatment A severe curve may need operation especially if, as in this girl (a), it is associated with chronic pain. (b) The same girl after operative correction and fixation with Wisconsin rods; bone grafts were added and can be expected to produce fusion after a year or two.

Differential diagnosis

Postural kyphosis Postural 'round back' is common in adolescence. It is painless, and the patient can correct the deformity voluntarily. The curve is a long one and other postural defects are common. The x-ray appearance is normal.

Discitis, osteomyelitis and tuberculous spondylitis If the changes are restricted to one intervertebral level, they can be mistaken for an infective lesion. However, infection causes more severe pain, may be associated with systemic symptoms and signs and produces more marked x-ray changes, including signs of bone erosion and paravertebral soft-tissue swelling.

Spondyloepiphyseal dysplasia In mild cases this can produce changes at multiple levels resembling those of Scheuermann's disease. Look for the characteristic defects in other joints.

Outcome

The condition is often quite painful during adolescence, but (except in the most severe cases) symptoms subside after a few years. There may be a recurrence of backache in later life, though overall disability is seldom marked (Murray et al, 1993).

Treatment

Curves of 40 degrees or less require only back-strengthening exercises and postural training. More severe curvature in a child who still has some years of growth ahead responds well to a period of 12–24 months in a brace that holds the lumbar spine flat and the thoracic spine in 'extension' (decreased kyphosis). Check the position by x-ray to ensure that the brace is effective.

The older adolescent or young adult with a rigid curve of more than 60 degrees may need operative correction and fusion using a hook-rod system (modified Harrington or Cotrel-Dubousset). In severe cases (kyphosis of greater than 75 degrees), an anterior release operation and fusion should precede the posterior fusion. Even then, the deformity is usually only partially corrected.

Thoraco-lumbar Scheuermann's disease

Vertebral end-plate defects are sometimes limited to the lower thoracic and/or the lumbar spine. In mild cases the condition is usually asymptomatic and discovered only incidentally when x-rays are obtained for other reasons (see Fig. 18.21). In some cases, however, the patient (usually a teenager at the end of growth or a young adult) complains of back pain and

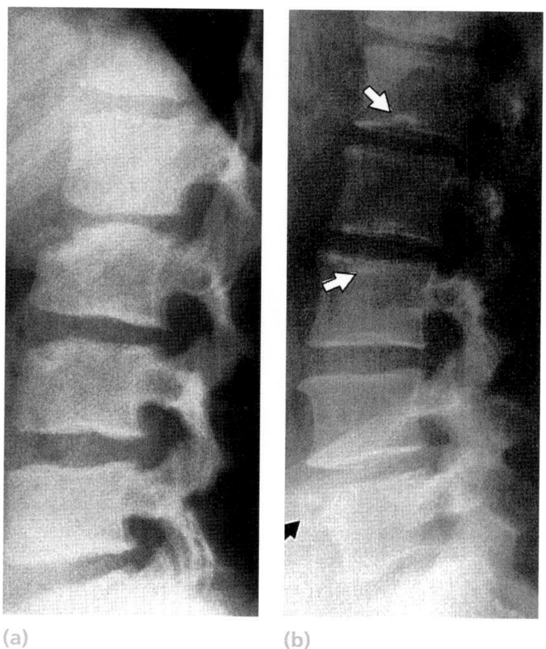

18.21 Lumbar Scheuermann's disease (a) The x-ray appearances of lumbar Scheuermann's disease are often mistaken for a fracture (or worse). The 'fragmentation' anteriorly is due to abnormal ossification of the ring epiphysis. (b) Schmorl's nodes (arrows) may also be seen.

inability to undertake sustained bending, lifting and carrying activities. There is nothing striking to see on clinical examination and it may be difficult to determine whether the backache is due to the Scheuermann disorder or to some other condition such as spondylolysis or facet joint dysfunction.

TREATMENT

Treatment consists of muscle strengthening exercises and avoidance of excessive bending and lifting.

KYPHOSIS IN THE ELDERLY

Degeneration of intervertebral discs probably produces the gradually increasing stoop characteristic of the aged. The disc spaces become narrowed and the vertebrae slightly wedged. There is little pain unless osteoarthritis of the facet joints is also present.

Osteoporotic kyphosis

Postmenopausal osteoporosis may result in one or more compression fractures of the thoracic spine. Patients are usually in their 60s or 70s and may complain of pain. Kyphosis is seldom marked. Often the main complaint is of lumbosacral pain, which results from the compensatory lumbar lordosis in an ageing,

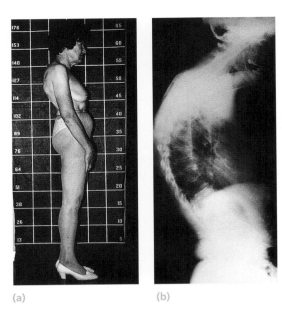

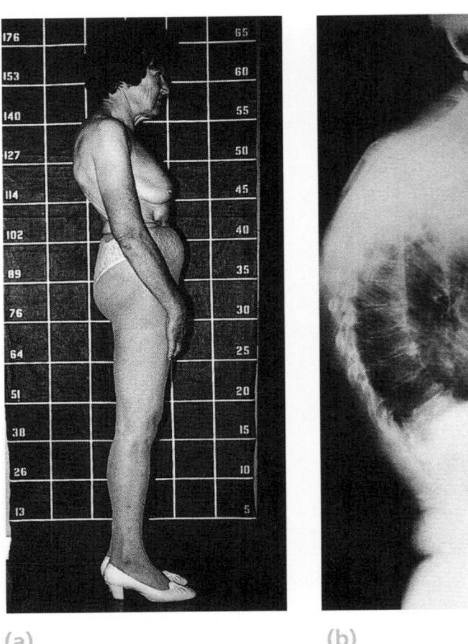

(a) (b)

18.22 Osteoporotic kyphosis (a,b) Postmenopausal osteoporosis often results in compressive wedging of the thoracic vertebral bodies and a gradual increase in the natural thoracic kyphosis.

osteoarthritic spine. Treatment is directed at the underlying condition and may include hormone and bone mineral replacement therapy.

Senile osteoporosis affects both men and women. Patients are usually over 75 years of age, often incapacitated by some other illness, and lacking exercise. They complain of back pain, and spinal deformity may be marked. X-rays reveal multiple vertebral fractures. It is important to exclude other conditions such as *metastatic disease* or *myelomatosis*.

TREATMENT

Treatment is symptomatic. Bed rest and spinal bracing merely aggravate the osteoporosis. More recently, fresh compression fractures are being treated by the transpedicular injection of methacrylate or bone graft substitute paste in order to stop further deformity and control pain ('vertebroplasty') or to correct the wedge deformity and maintain correction ('kyphoplasty'). The authors believe it is too early to recommend this treatment as the long-term outcome and potential complications have yet to be fully assessed.

SPINAL INFECTION

The axial skeleton accounts for 2–7 per cent of all cases of osteomyelitis. Predisposing factors include diabetes mellitus, malnutrition, substance abuse, human immunodeficiency virus (HIV) infection, malignancy, long-term use of steroids, renal failure and septicaemia.

PYOGENIC OSTEOMYELITIS

Acute pyogenic infection of the spine is uncommon and diagnosis and treatment are often unnecessarily delayed. The elderly, chronically ill and immunodeficient patients are at greatest risk.

Pathology

Staphylococcus aureus is responsible in 50–60 per cent of all cases, but in immunosuppressed patients Gram-

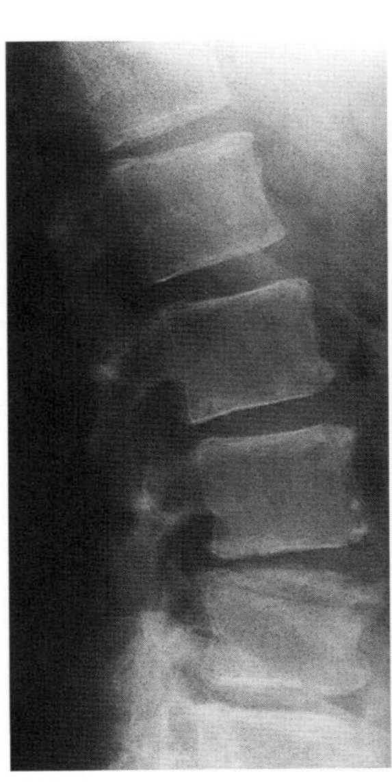

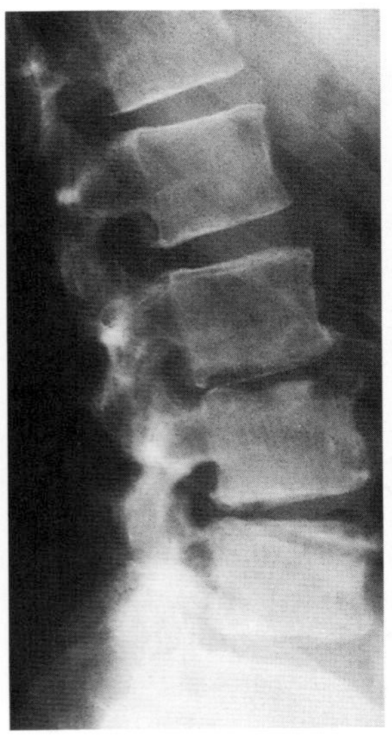

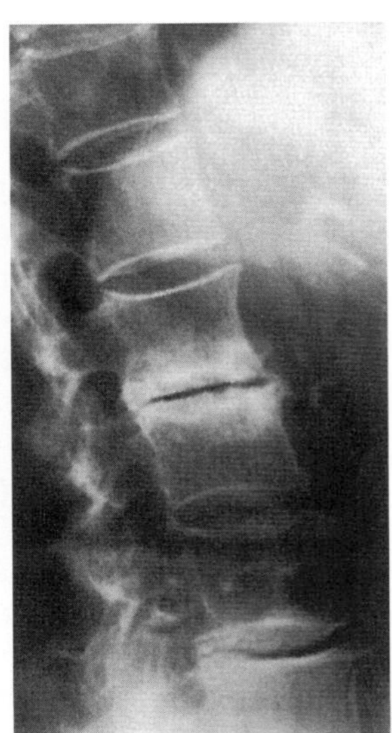

(a) (b) (c)

18.23 Pyogenic osteomyelitis and discitis Typical x-ray features are loss of disc height, irregularity of the disc 'space', end-plate erosion and reactive sclerosis. Progressive changes are shown in (a) and (b). Reactive bone changes, shown in (c), may end with fusion at the affected level. In many cases it is impossible to tell whether the infection began in the disc or in the adjacent bone.

negative organisms such as *Escherichia coli* and *Pseudomonas* are the most common. The usual sources of infection are: (1) haematogenous spread from a distant focus of infection or (2) inoculation during invasive procedures (spinal injections and disc operations).

The infection usually begins in the vertebral end-plates with secondary spread to the disc and adjacent vertebra. It may also spread along the anterior longitudinal ligament to an adjacent vertebra, or outwards into the paravertebral soft tissues: from the thoracic spine along the psoas to the groin; from the lumbar region to the buttock, the sacroiliac joint or the hip.

The spinal canal is rarely involved but when it is, in the form of an epidural abscess, that is a surgical emergency! Despite rapid surgical decompression, the patient is often left with some degree of permanent paralysis.

Clinical features

Localized pain – the cardinal symptom – is often intense, unremitting and associated with muscle spasm and restricted movement. There may also be point tenderness over the affected vertebra. Intercostal neuralgia is a frequent symptom with thoracic spine involvement.

The patient may give a history of some invasive spinal procedure or a distant infection during the preceding few weeks. A careful history and general examination are essential to exclude a focus of infection (skin, ENT, chest, pelvis).

Systemic signs such as pyrexia and tachycardia are often present but not particularly marked. In children the diagnosis can be particularly difficult; often they have an awkward gait with a stiff spine, or if the lumbar spine is involved they can present with abdominal symptoms and signs.

Imaging

X-rays may show no change for several weeks; if the diagnosis is delayed, the examination should be repeated. Early signs are loss of disc height, irregularity of the disc space, erosion of the vertebral end-plate and reactive new bone formation. Soft-tissue swelling may be visible. The early loss of disc height distinguishes vertebral osteomyelitis from metastatic disease, where the disc can remain intact despite advanced bony destruction.

Radionuclide scanning will show increased activity at the site but this is non-specific.

MRI may show characteristic changes in the vertebral end-plates, intervertebral disc and paravertebral tissues; this investigation is highly sensitive but not specific.

Similar features may be seen in discitis. *Needle biopsy* may help with diagnosis, but often no organism is found.

Other investigations

The white cell count, C-reactive protein (CRP) level and erythrocyte sedimentation rate (ESR) are usually elevated, and antistaphylococcal antibodies may be present in high titres. Agglutination tests for *Salmonella* and *Brucella* should be performed, especially in endemic regions and in patients who have recently visited these areas. Blood culture is essential in patients who are febrile though it is often negative in the early stages of infection.

Treatment

If the blood culture is negative a closed needle biopsy is performed for bacteriological culture and tests for antibiotic sensitivity. Treatment is started on the basis of a clinical diagnosis of infection and includes bed rest, pain relief and intravenous antibiotic administration using a 'best guess' preparation that can be changed once the laboratory results and sensitivities are known. As methicillin-resistant *Staphylococcus aureus* (MRSA) has become a common infecting agent, vancomycin or linezolid may be required.

Intravenous antibiotics are continued for 4–6 weeks; if there is a good response (clinical improvement, a falling CRP and ESR. and a normal white cell count), oral antibiotics are then used for a further 6–8 weeks and the patient is mobilized in a spinal brace. The duration of antibiotic treatment depends on the clinical, haematological and radiological findings. During this period nutritional support and management of co-morbidities are essential in ensuring a successful outcome.

Operative treatment is seldom needed. The indications for an open biopsy and decompression are: (1) failure to obtain a positive yield from a closed needle biopsy and a poor response to conservative treatment; (2) the presence of neurological signs; (3) the need to drain a soft-tissue abscess. An anterior approach is preferred; necrotic and infected material is removed and, if necessary, the cord is decompressed. The anterior column defect is reconstructed with rib or iliac grafts. If the spine is unstable, posterior fixation may be necessary. Postoperatively the spine is supported in a brace until healing occurs. In the elderly and in immunocompromised patients a posterolateral extraplueral/retroperitoneal decompression and instrumentation is effective. For a primary epidural abscess, laminectomy is indicated.

The outcome (with prompt and effective treatment) is usually favourable. Spontaneous fusion of infected vertebrae is a common radiological feature of healed staphylococcal osteomyelitis.

DISCITIS

Infection limited to the intervertebral disc is rare and when it does occur it is usually due to direct inoculation following discography, chemonucleolysis or discectomy. The vertebral end-plates are rapidly attacked and the infection then spreads into the vertebral body.

Clinical features and investigations

With direct infection there is always a history of some invasive procedure. Acute back pain and muscle spasm following an injection into the disc should never be attributed merely to the irritant effect of the injection. Systemic features are usually mild, but the ESR is elevated.

In children the infection is assumed to be blood-borne. There may be a history of a flu-like illness followed by back pain, muscle spasm and severe limitation of movement. X-rays, radioscintigraphy and MRI show the same features as in pyogenic spondylitis.

Treatment

Prevention is always better than cure. Following an injection into the disc, a broad-spectrum antibiotic should be administered intravenously. Non-iatrogenic discitis is usually self-limiting. During the acute stage bed rest and analgesics are essential. If symptoms do not resolve rapidly, a needle biopsy is advisable. Only if there are signs of abscess formation or cord or nerve root pressure is surgical evacuation or decompression indicated. This is rarely necessary.

TUBERCULOSIS

The spine is the most common site of skeletal tuberculosis (TB), and accounts for 50 per cent of all musculoskeletal TB. It is thought that there are approximately 2 million people with spinal tuberculosis worldwide.

Pathology

Blood-borne infection usually settles in a vertebral body adjacent to the intervertebral disc. Bone destruction and caseation follow, with infection spreading to the disc space and the adjacent vertebrae. A paravertebral abscess may form, and then track along muscle planes to involve the sacro-iliac or hip joint, or along the psoas muscle to the thigh. As the vertebral bodies collapse into each other, a sharp angulation (gibbus or kyphos) develops. There is a major risk of cord damage due to pressure by the abscess, granulation tissue, sequestra or displaced bone, or (occasionally) ischaemia from spinal artery thrombosis.

With healing, the vertebrae recalcify and bony fusion may occur between them. Nevertheless, if there has been much angulation, the spine is usually 'unsound', and flares are common, resulting in further illness and further vertebral collapse. With progressive kyphosis there is again a risk of cord compression.

Clinical features

There is usually a long history of ill-health and backache; in late cases a gibbus deformity is the dominant feature. Concurrent pulmonary TB is a feature in

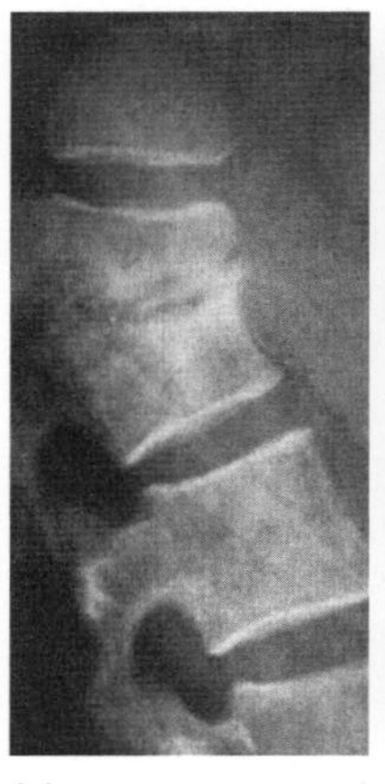
(a)

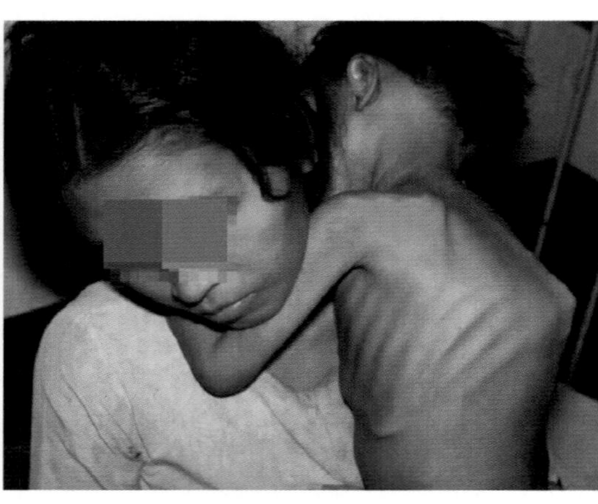
(b)

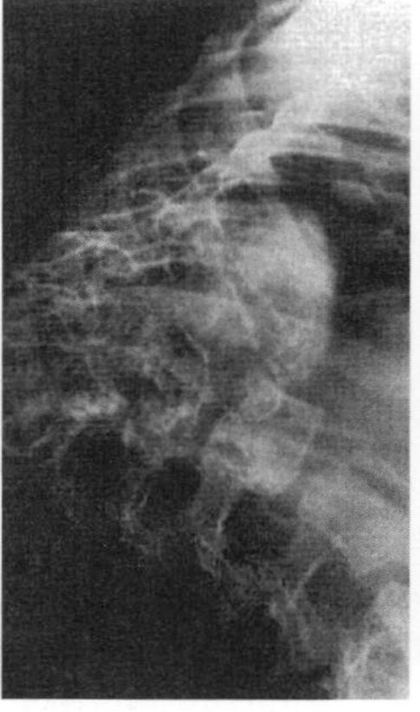
(c)

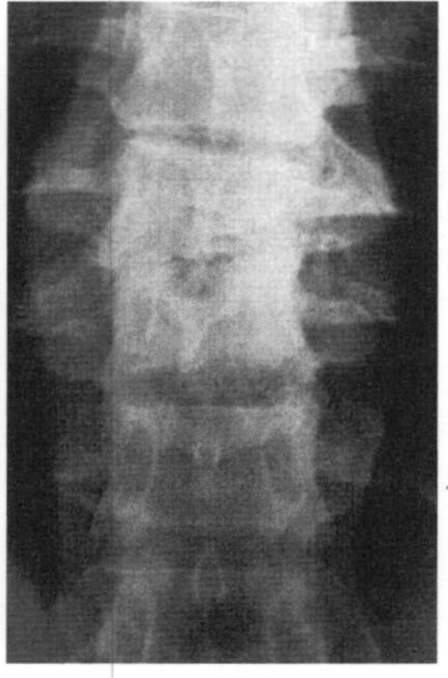
(d)

18.24 Tuberculosis of the spine (a) Early x-ray changes with loss of disc space. (b) Young patient with advanced tuberculous deformity. (c) X-ray showing vertebral collapse and severe kyphosis. (d) X-ray appearance of a psoas abscess in the paravertebral tissues.

most children under 10 years with thoracic spine involvement. Occasionally the patient may present with a cold abscess pointing in the groin, or with paraesthesiae and weakness of the legs. There is local tenderness in the back and spinal movements are restricted.

In cervical spine disease dyspnoea and dysphagia are features of advanced infection, especially in children; these patients present with a stiff painful neck. Children under 10 years of age with thoracic spine TB usually develop a *pectus carinatum* ('pigeon chest') deformity.

Neurological examination may show motor and/or sensory changes in the lower limbs. As spinal tuberculosis is found mostly in the thoracic spine, spastic paraparesis is a common presentation in adults.

ATYPICAL FEATURES

Even in areas where tuberculosis is no longer as common as it was in the past, it is important to be alert to the possibility of this diagnosis. The task is made harder when the patient presents with atypical features:

- Lack of deformity, e.g. a patient with a primary epidural abscess
- Involvement of only the posterior vertebral elements
- Infection confined to a single vertebral body
- Involvement of multiple vertebral bodies and posterior elements (especially in HIV-positive patients) resulting in a kyphoscoliosis.

POTT'S PARAPLEGIA

Paraplegia is the most feared complication of spinal tuberculosis. *Early-onset paresis* (usually within 2 years of disease onset) is due to pressure by inflammatory oedema, an abscess, caseous material, granulation tissue or sequestra. The patient presents with lower limb weakness, upper motor neuron signs, sensory dysfunction and incontinence. CT and MRI may reveal cord compression. In these cases the prognosis for neurological recovery following surgery is good. *Late-onset paresis* is due to direct cord compression from increasing deformity, or (occasionally) vascular insufficiency of the cord; recovery following decompression is poor.

Imaging

The entire spine should be x-rayed, because vertebrae distant from the obvious site may also be affected without any obvious deformity. The earliest signs of infection are local osteoporosis of two adjacent vertebrae and narrowing of the intervertebral disc space, with fuzziness of the end-plates. Progressive disease is associated with signs of bone destruction and collapse of adjacent vertebral bodies into each other. Paraspinal soft-tissue shadows may be due either to oedema, swelling or a paravertebral abscess. The radiological picture may mimic those of other infections including fungal infections and parasitic infestations. A chest x-ray is essential.

With healing, bone density increases, the ragged appearance disappears and paravertebral abscesses may undergo resolution or fibrosis or calcification.

MRI and *CT scans* are invaluable in the investigation of hidden lesions, involvement of posterior vertebral elements, paravertebral abscesses, an epidural abscess and cord compression. Myelography is appropriate when these facilities are not available.

Special investigations

The Mantoux test may be positive and in the acute stage the ESR is raised. In patients with no neurological signs a needle biopsy is recommended to confirm the diagnosis by histological and microbiological investigations. If this does not provide a firm diagnosis, tissue should be obtained by open operation. If there are signs of neurological involvement, operative debridement and decompression of the spinal cord will be required.

Patients with HIV infection (usually showing generalized lymphadenopathy, skin and mucocutaneous lesions and marked weight loss) should be referred for voluntary counselling and testing (VCT). If positive, the CD4/CD8 count should be monitored with TB and antiretroviral therapy.

Differential diagnosis

Spinal tuberculosis must be distinguished from other causes of vertebral pathology, particularly pyogenic and fungal infections, malignant disease and parasitic infestations such as hydatid disease. Disc space collapse is typical of infection; disc preservation is typical of metastatic disease. Metastases may cause vertebral body collapse similar to that seen in TB but, in contrast to tuberculous spondylitis, the disc space is usually preserved.

Treatment

The objectives are to: (1) eradicate or at least arrest the disease; (2) prevent or correct deformity; (3) prevent or treat the major complication – paraplegia.

Antituberculous chemotherapy (rifampicin 600 mg daily plus isoniazid 300 mg daily plus pyrazinamide 2 g daily) is as effective as any other method (including surgical debridement) in stemming the disease. These drugs must be given in combination for 6 months, dropping the pyrazinamide after the first 2 months. The dosages listed are for adults of average weight. Because so much of current tuberculosis is a complication of acquired immune deficiency syn-

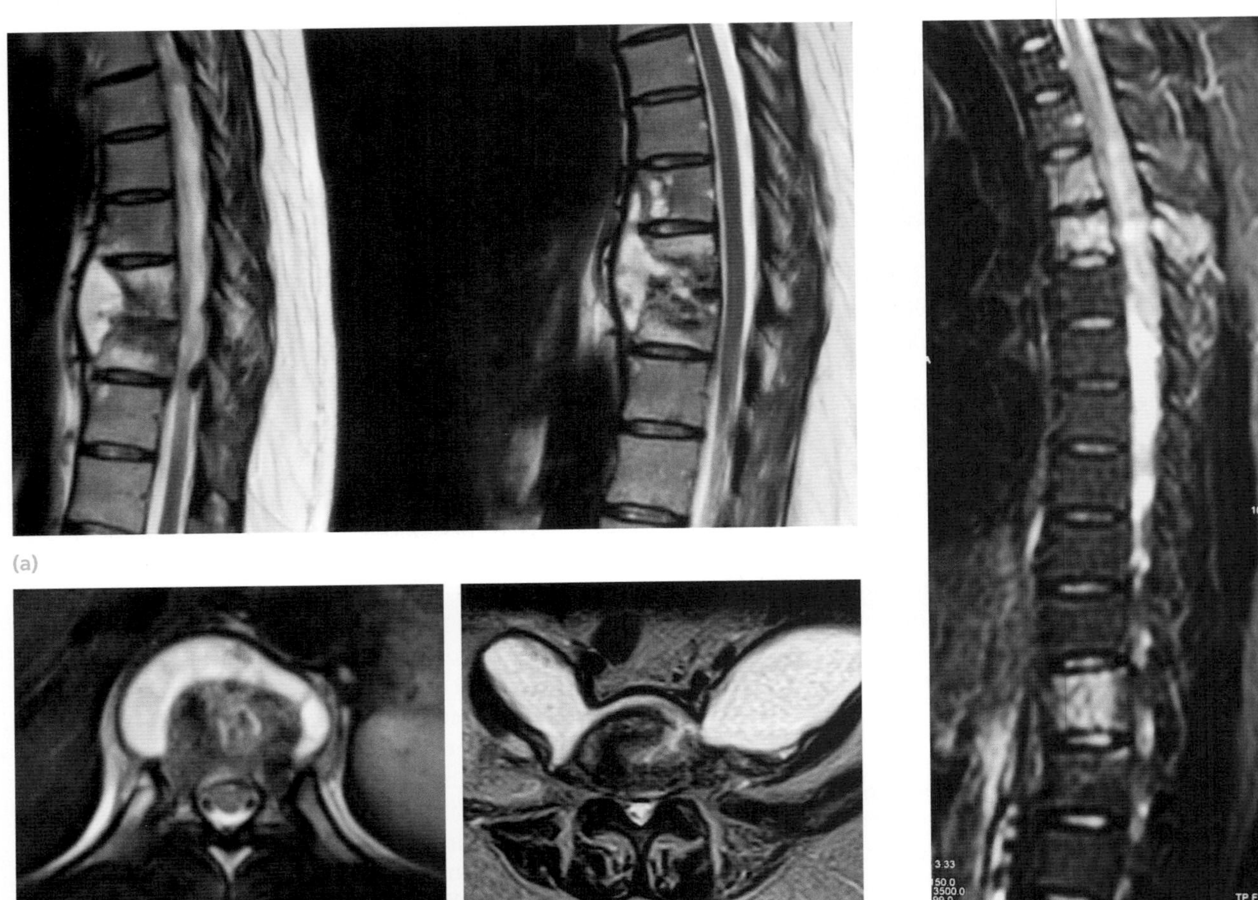

18.25 Spinal tuberculosis – MRI features Scanning in several planes shows details that cannot be seen in plain x-rays. (a) Sagittal MR images of advanced tuberculous infection with abscess formation beneath the anterior longitudinal ligament. (b,c) Axial images showing psoas abscesses communicating across the front of the spine. (d) In countries where TB is endemic, additional active lesions can be detected by MRI in almost 40 per cent of patients presenting with 'local' lesions.

drome (AIDS), resistant mycobacteria are an increasing problem. Ethionamide and streptomycin may have to be substituted for isoniazid.

However, conservative treatment alone carries the risk of progressive kyphosis if the infection is not quickly eradicated. Anterior resection of diseased tissue and anterior spinal fusion with a strut graft offers the double advantage of early and complete eradication of the infection and prevention of spinal deformity (Figure 18.26). After weighing up the pros and cons, the following approach is advocated:

- *Ambulant chemotherapy alone* – is suitable for early or limited disease with no abscess formation or neurological deficit. Treatment is continued for 6–12 months, or until the x-ray shows resolution of the bone changes. Therapeutic compliance is sometimes a problem.
- *Continuous bed rest* and *chemotherapy* – may be used for more advanced disease when the necessary skills and facilities for radical anterior spinal surgery are not available, or where the technical problems are too daunting (e.g. in lumbosacral tuberculosis) – provided there is no abscess that needs to be drained.
- *Operative treatment* – is indicated: (1) when there is an abscess that can readily be drained; (2) for advanced disease with marked bone destruction and threatened or actual severe kyphosis; (3) neurological deficit including paraparesis that has not responded to drug therapy.

Through an anterior approach, all infected and necrotic material is evacuated or excised and the gap is filled with iliac crest or rib grafts that act as a strut. If several levels are involved, anterior or posterior fixation and fusion may be needed for additional stability. Children who are growing and are seen to be at risk of developing severe kyphosis may need fusion of the posterior elements to minimize the expected deformity. Antituberculous chemotherapy is still necessary, of course.

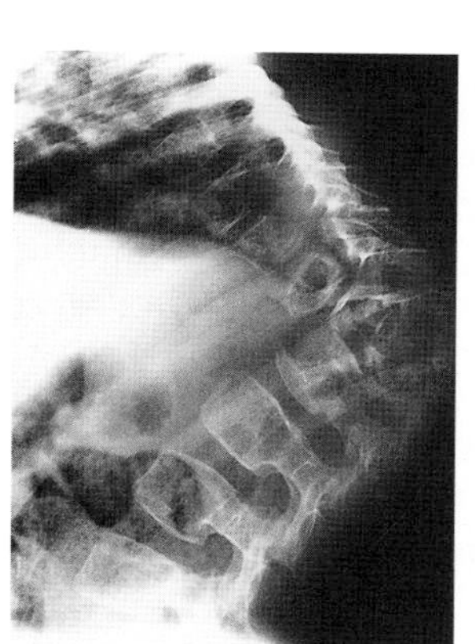
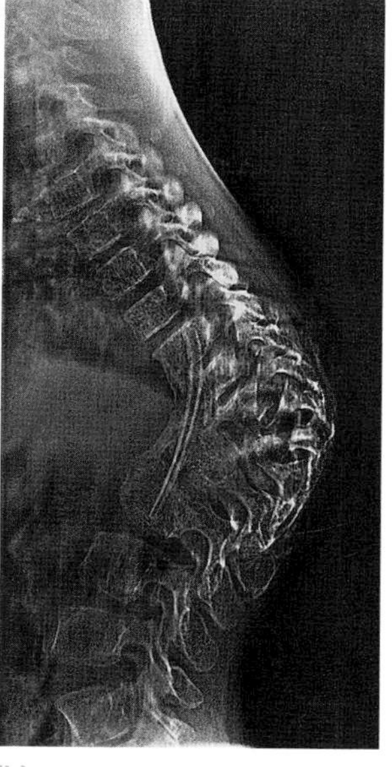

(a) (b)

18.26 Spinal tuberculosis – operative treatment (a) Marked bone collapse and kyphosis, threatening neurological complications. (b) After debridement and spinal fusion with a rib strut graft.

Human immunodeficiency virus and spinal tuberculosis

One of the main reasons for the resurgence of TB, especially in the developing world, is the spread of HIV. Spinal TB, which is an extrapulmonary focus, is AIDS defining.

These patients are prone to developing opportunistic infections and atypical mycobacterial infections (*Mycobacterium intracellulare*, *M. avium*, *M. fortuitum)*. The tuberculous infection usually involves multiple vertebrae and results in severe deformity. A primary epidural abscess is not uncommon.

Decompression and stabilization for neurological deficit are performed through an extrapleural posterolateral approach with instrumentation to minimize pulmonary complications. A primary epidural abscess is drained through a laminectomy.

Postoperatively antituberculous therapy and antiretroviral treatment are commenced. Compliance with treatment and regular monitoring of viral loads and CD4/CD8 counts are essential to ensure a successful outcome.

FUNGAL INFECTION

These are opportunistic infections occurring in an immunocompromised host (e.g. due to HIV, malignancy, steroid therapy or chronic granulomatous disease) and a patient with extensive burns; however, they may also affect a normal host. *Aspergillosis* and *Cryptococcus* are airborne fungi that initially affect the lungs; the spine is involved by haematogenous spread.

In children with chronic granulomatous disease, thoracic spine involvement is due to contiguous spread from the lungs. The presentation, clinical findings and radiographic features may mimic those of TB. The chest X-ray may show a fungal ball or pneumonia. The diagnosis is made by sputum examination and bronchoscopy. The immunodiffusion test is specific for *Aspergillosis* and the latex agglutination test for *Cryptococcus.* A biopsy is performed to confirm the diagnosis.

Treatment

Neurological deficit is an indication for operative decompression. Specific treatment includes 5-flucytosine and amphotericin B, which act synergistically. Synthetic oral antifungals (ketoconazole, fluconazole, itraconazole) are well absorbed and the serum and cerebrospinal fluid (CSF) concentrations are high. Concurrent treatment of the underlying immunocomprised state is essential.

PARASITIC INFESTATION

The commonest parasitic infestation affecting the spine is due to the cestode worm *Echinococcus granulosis*, which causes hydatid disease. It is encountered mainly in areas where sheep are raised: Australasia, South America, parts of Africa, Wales and Iceland. The definitive host is the dog and as well as other canine animals.

The sheep is the intermediate host and humans are affected by the ingestion of ova that are usually carried in the dog's excreta or fur. The embryo worm enters the human host by being either ingested through faecal contamination or by inhalation of dessicated particles in dust. In that way the embryos come to lodge in the liver and the lungs, but in about 10 per cent of cases there is dissemination to other sites, including the bones (mainly the spine, skull and long bones) where hydatid cysts develop in about 1 per cent of cases.

Hydatid disease is usually picked up in childhood but it may be many years before the diagnosis is made. The presentation and clinical features are similar to those of other forms of spondylitis. X-rays may reveal a translucent area with a sclerotic margin in the affected vertebral body. In untreated cases this can lead to bone destruction. Neurological deficit, the difficulty in eradicating the disease and the tendency to recurrence make for significant morbidity and mortality.

Systemic treatment is with albendazole, which is active against the larvae and the cysts; three cycles of 25 days each is the usual recommendation. Operative treatment to achieve spinal decompression may be called for; spillage of cyst contents must be avoided.

The prognosis is generally poor when the liver and lungs are affected.

NON-INFECTIVE INFLAMMATORY DISEASE

Ankylosing spondylitis and seronegative spondyloarthropathies are dealt with in Chapter 3.

DEGENERATIVE DISORDERS OF THE SPINE

INTERVERTEBRAL DISC DEGENERATION

Lumbar backache is one of the most common causes of chronic disability in western societies, and in the majority of cases the backache is associated with degeneration of the intervertebral discs in the lower lumbar spine. This is an age-related phenomenon that occurs in over 80 per cent of people who live for more than 50 years and in most cases it is asymptomatic.

Pathology

With normal ageing the disc gradually dries out: the nucleus pulposus changes from a turgid, gelatinous bulb to a brownish, desiccated structure. The annulus fibrosus develops fissures parallel to the vertebral end-plates running mainly posteriorly, and small herniations of nuclear material squeeze into and through the annulus. Disc cells proliferate and collect into clusters, then die at an increased rate. Glycosaminoglycans production is diminished, leading to poor water retention and gradual 'drying out' of the disc (Roberts et al., 2006). This process begins surprisingly early in life and increases gradually with age. The discs flatten down and bulge slightly beyond the margins of the vertebral bodies. Where they protrude against the ligaments,

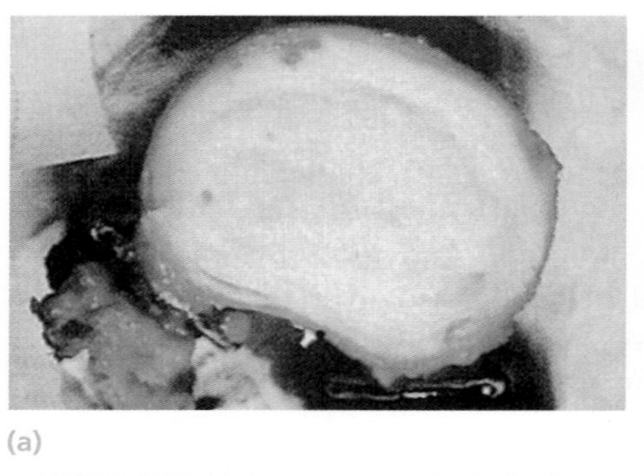

(a)

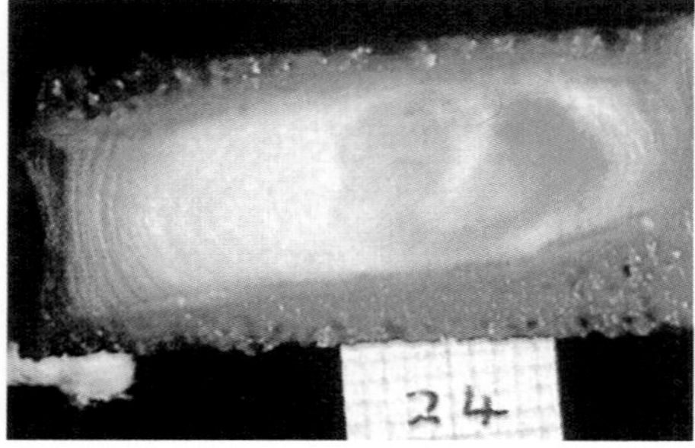

(b)

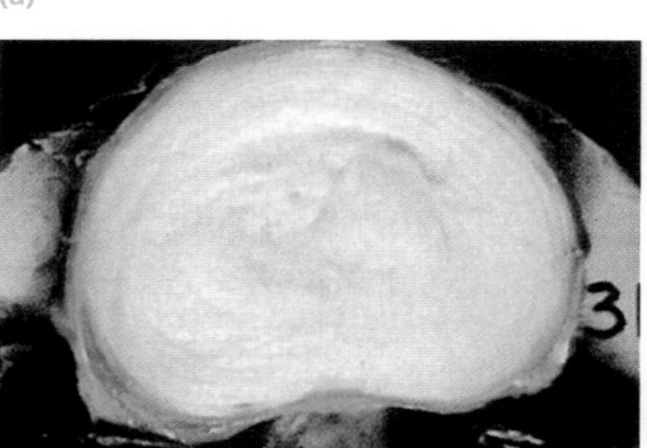

(c)

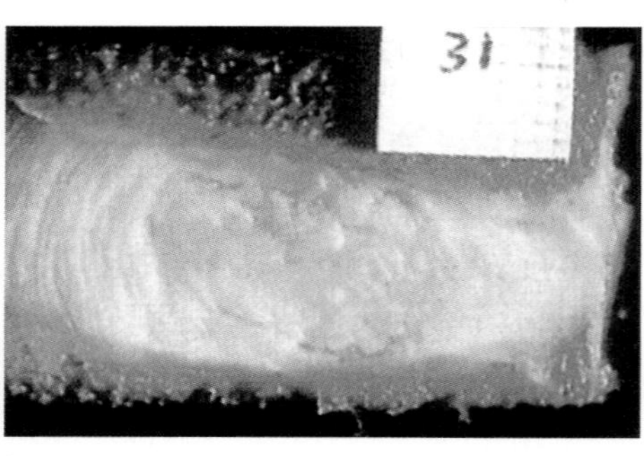

(d)

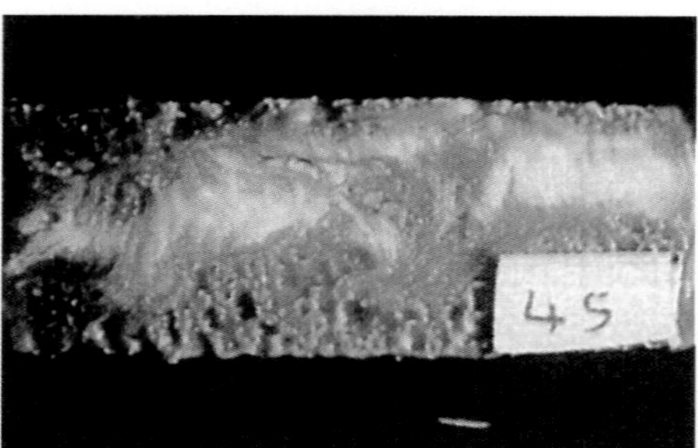

(e)

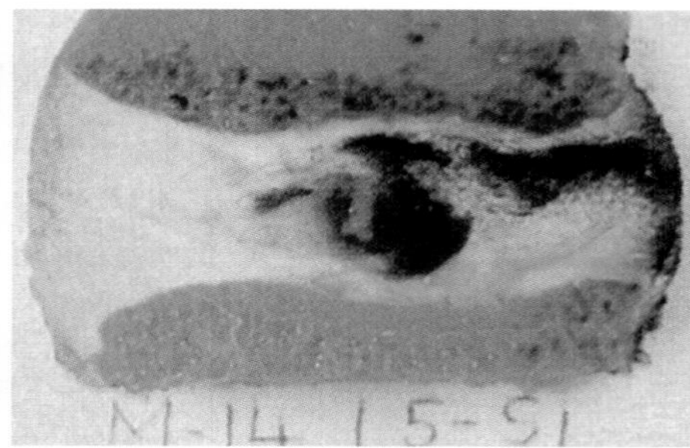

(f)

18.27 Disc lesions – pathology (a,b) Transverse and sagittal sections through a young (teenage) intervertebral disc. The nucleus is soft, homogeneous and almost translucent. The annulus is composed of regular lamellae of fibrocartilage. (c,d) Mature (50-year-old) normal disc. The nucleus is more fibrous and less homogeneous. The annulus is thickened and the vertebral body and end-plates are intact. (e) Degenerating disc, which is markedly flattened with break-up of the nucleus and disruption of the vertebral body end-plates. (f) Young disc stained with analine blue dye to demonstrate a fissure extending posteriorly through the annulus fibrosis.

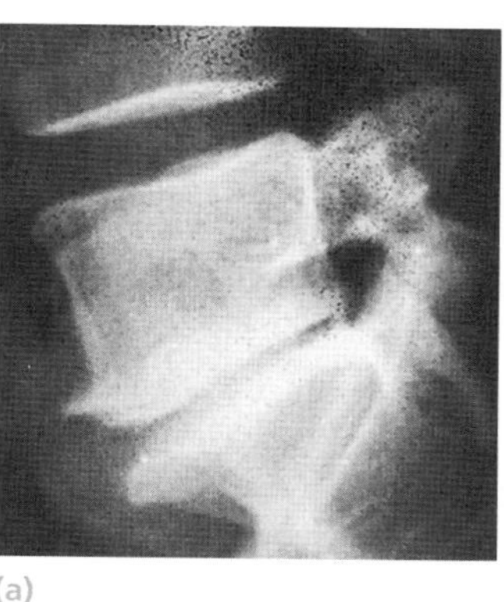
(a)

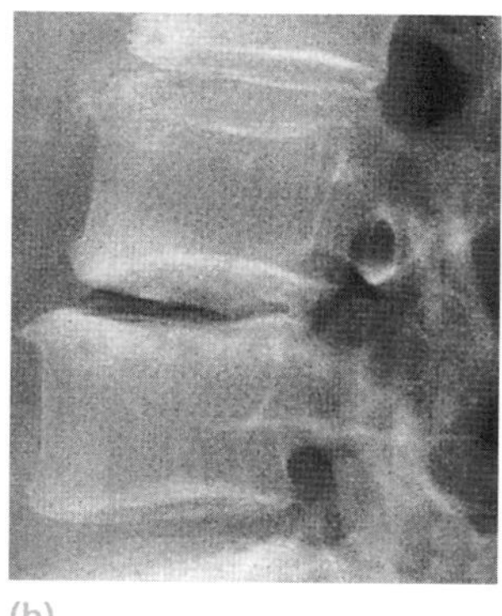
(b)

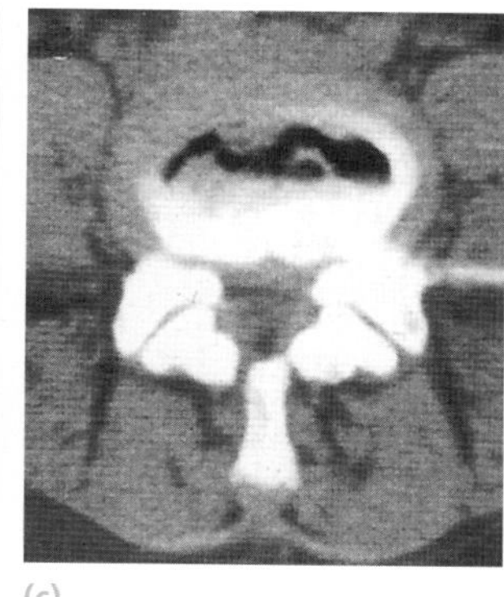
(c)

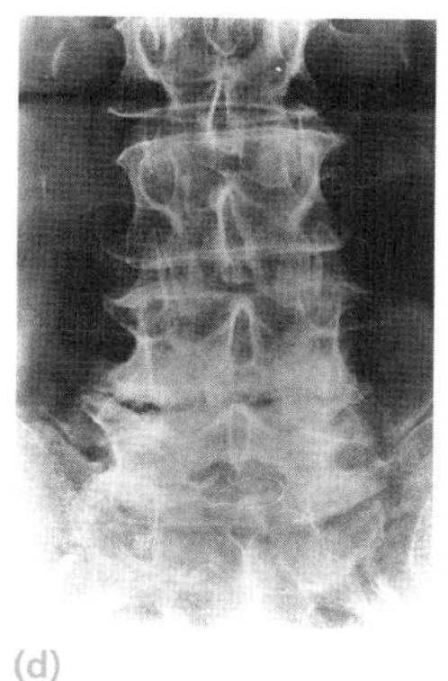
(d)

18.28 Spondylosis and osteoarthritis Typical x-ray features are (a) narrowing of the intervertebral space and anterior 'osteophytes'. (b) Other features are slight retrolisthesis and a dark (vacant) area in the disc space – the 'vacuum sign' – better demonstrated in the axial CT (c), which also shows the hypertrophic osteoarthritis of the facet joints. (d) In advanced cases there are well marked signs of osteoarthritis.

reactive new bone formation produces bony ridges (erroneously called 'osteophytes', because in two-dimensional x-ray images they do indeed look like osteophytic projections). In the adjacent vertebrae the end plates ossify and become sclerotic; fatty change occurs in the subchondral bone marrow. The picture as a whole is referred to as *spondylosis*. A classification of the age-related changes in lumbar discs appears in the paper by Boos et al. (2002).

Secondary effects

Once the degenerative process gets going, secondary changes ensue. *Displacement of the facet joints* and forward or backward *shifts of adjacent vertebral bodies* (as shown in x-ray images) are often interpreted as signs of 'segmental instability'. This, combined with increased stress in the facet joints, may ultimately lead to *osteoarthritis* of these small synovial joints. If the changes are marked, new bone formation may narrow the lateral recesses of the spinal canal and the intervertebral foramina causing *root canal stenosis* and, in some cases, *spinal stenosis. Thickening of the ligamentum flavum* and bulging of the disc annulus contribute further to the circumferential nature of acquired stenosis.

Clinical features

As noted earlier, disc degeneration of itself is usually asymptomatic. When symptoms such as chronic backache or low-back pain on strenuous effort do appear they may well be due to the secondary effects of disc collapse rather than the disc degeneration *per se*. These are described later.

X-Rays

Radiographic features of intervertebral disc degeneration – typically flattening of the disc 'space' and marginal 'osteophyte' formation – appear relatively late. Other secondary changes such as vertebral displacement and facet joint osteoarthritis may also become apparent, making it increasingly difficult to ascribe the patient's symptoms to any particular abnormality. Indeed, even if there are no overt signs apart from the primary discogenic changes, it cannot be determined for certain that the disc pathology is the cause of a patient's backache, because disc degeneration and non-specific low-back pain are both extremely common in older people. It is also not possible to prognosticate about whether an asymptomatic individual with clear x-ray signs of disc degeneration will in the future develop disabling backache.

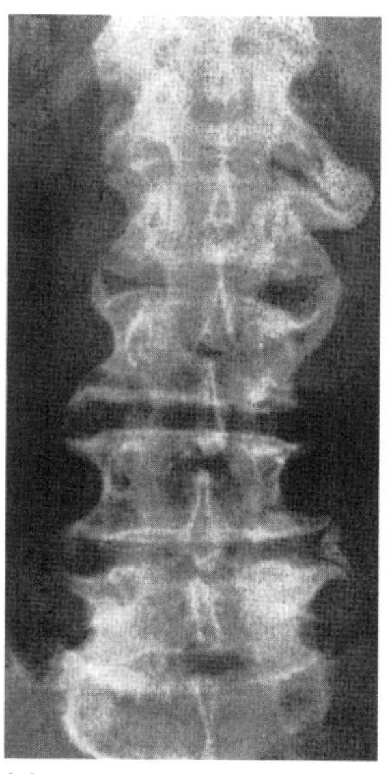
(a)

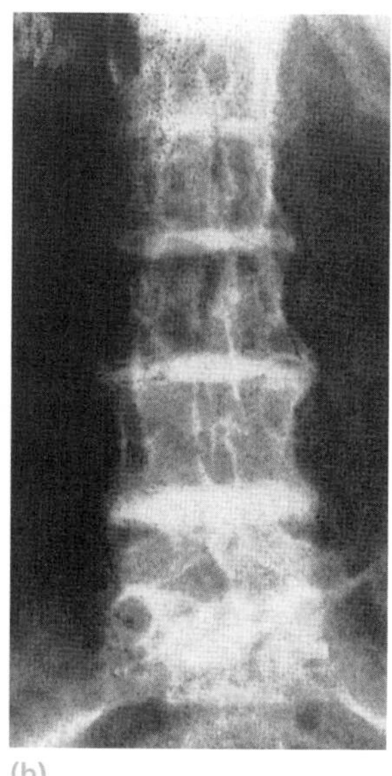
(b)

18.29 Conditions resembling spondylosis
(a) *Forestier's disease*: at first sight this looks like osteoarthritic spondylosis; there are large spurs at multiple levels, but the disc spaces are usually preserved.
(b) *Ochronosis*: intervertebral calcification is characteristic.

For the early features of disc degeneration, including those that can be demonstrated in asymptomatic individuals, more advanced imaging techniques must be considered (Boos et al., 2002).

MRI

The most obvious change on MRI is bulging of the annulus fibrosus in both sagittal and axial projections. However, subtle changes such as diminished thickness and reduced signal intensity of the degenerating disc, or small tears and fissures can also be distinguished and counted. These appearances have been used to produce a classification through grades I to V of increasing severity (Pfirrmann et al., 2001), yet even that method has been found to be wanting on the grounds that it provides a discontinuous scale of progressive degeneration (Haughton, 2006).

A significant secondary change, evidently arising from altered loading characteristics of the degenerating disc, was described by Modic et al. (1989). Oedema, fatty infiltration of the marrow and fibrosis in the subchondral bone adjacent to the vertebral end-plates produce varying imaging characteristics that now form the basis of the Modic classification (Figure 18.30). Although these changes are rarely encountered in asymptomatic individuals, it is also true that most patients with proven disc pathology do not show Modic changes; i.e. as diagnostic markers the Modic signs have relatively low sensitivity.

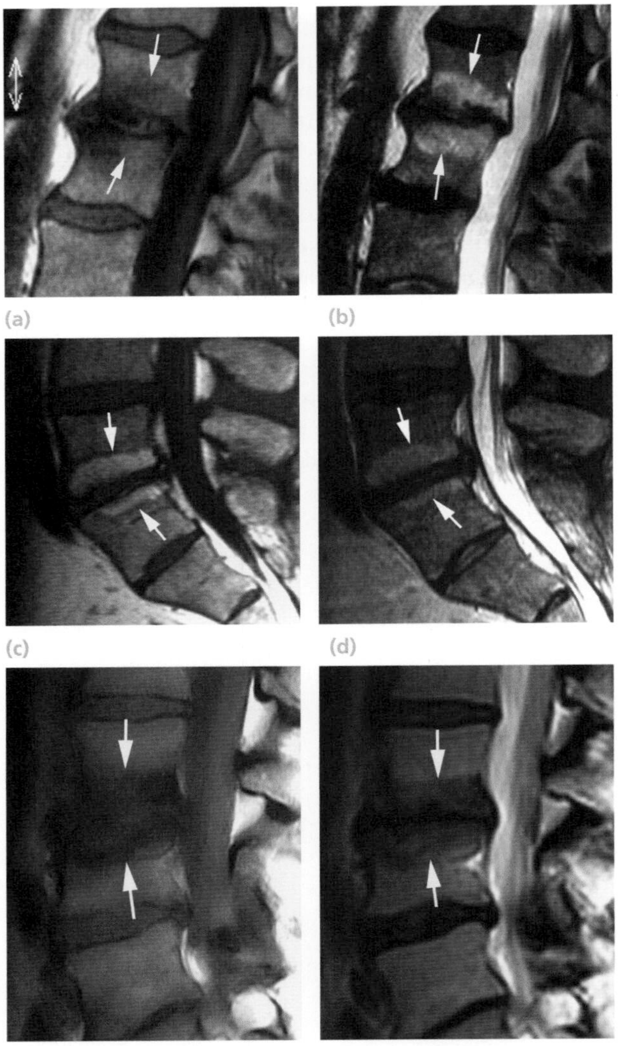

(a) (b) (c) (d) (e) (f)

18.30 MRI – Modic types of vertebral change Sagittal T_1 and T_2 weighted images of (a,b) *Type 1*, (c,d) *Type 2* and (e,f) *Type 3* Modic changes in lumbar vertebral end-plates. *Type 1* suggests oedema, but this may also occur in infection and metastatic disease. Type 2 suggests fatty change; *Type 3* is due to bony sclerosis.

Treatment

Asymptomatic lumbar disc degeneration (often discovered incidentally during x-ray examination for other conditions) does not necessarily presage the future onset of symptoms and does not need any treatment. The management of patients with chronic 'non-specific' low-back pain, with or without obvious signs of disc degeneration, is discussed on page 487. Secondary features of disc degeneration, such as vertebral displacement and facet joint osteoarthritis may need focussed management, sometimes including operative treatment.

ACUTE INTERVERTEBRAL DISC PROLAPSE

Acute disc herniation (prolapse, rupture) is much less common but considerably more dramatic than chronic degeneration. Physical stress (a combination of flexion and compression) is the proximate cause but, even at L4/5 or L5/S1 (where stress is most severe) it seems unlikely that a disc would rupture unless there was also some disturbance of the hydrophilic properties of the nucleus. A *'protrusion'* is a posteriorly bulging disc with some outer annulus intact. When *rupture* does occur, fibrocartilaginous disc material is extruded posteriorly (*'extrusion'*) and usually bulges to one or other side of the posterior longitudinal ligament. With a complete rupture, part of the nucleus may sequestrate and lie free in the spinal canal or work its way into the intervertebral foramen (*sequestration*).

A large central rupture may cause compression of the cauda equina. A posterolateral rupture presses on the nerve root proximal to its point of exit through

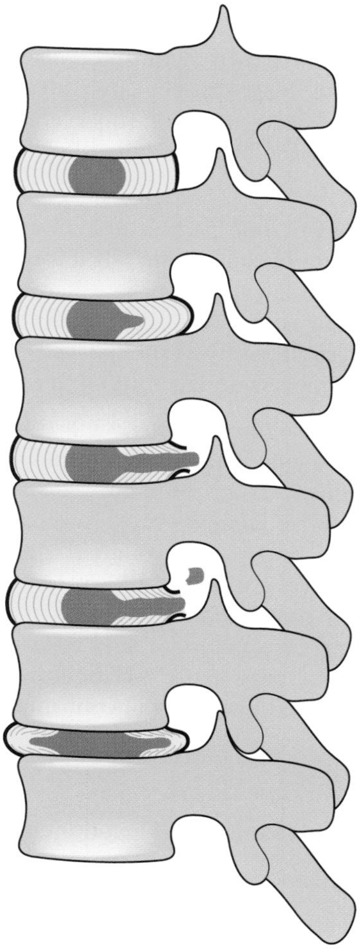

Normal disc

Protrusion
Increased nuclear pressure causing bulging

Extrusion
Ruptured annulus and ligament

Sequestration

Degeneration and joint displacement

18.31 Disc lesions – pathology From above, downwards: an abnormal increase in pressure within the nucleus causes splitting and bulging of the annulus; the posterior segment may rupture, allowing disc material to extrude into the spinal canal; with chronic degeneration (lowest level) the disc space narrows and the posterior facet joints are displaced, giving rise to osteoarthritis.

the intervertebral foramen; thus a herniation at L4/5 will compress the fifth lumbar nerve root, and a herniation at L5/S1, the first sacral root. Sometimes a local inflammatory response with oedema aggravates the symptoms.

Acute back pain at the onset of disc herniation probably arises from disruption of the outermost layers of the annulus fibrosus and stretching or tearing of the posterior longitudinal ligament. If the disc protrudes to one side, it may irritate the dural covering of the adjacent nerve root causing pain in the buttock, posterior thigh and calf (*sciatica*). Pressure on the nerve root itself causes *paraesthesia* and/or *numbness* in the corresponding dermatome, as well as *weakness* and *depressed reflexes* in the muscles supplied by that nerve root.

Clinical features

Acute disc prolapse may occur at any age, but is uncommon in the very young and the very old. The patient is usually a fit adult aged 20–45 years. Typically, while lifting or stooping he has severe back pain and is unable to straighten up. Either then or a day or two later pain is felt in the buttock and lower limb (sciatica). Both backache and sciatica are made worse by coughing or straining. Later there may be paraesthesia or numbness in the leg or foot, and occasionally muscle weakness. Cauda equina compression is rare but may cause urinary retention and perineal numbness.

The patient usually stands with a slight list to one side ('sciatic scoliosis'). Sometimes the knee on the painful side is held slightly flexed to relax tension on the sciatic nerve; straightening the knee makes the skew back more obvious. All back movements are restricted, and during forward flexion the list may increase.

There is often tenderness in the midline of the low back, and paravertebral muscle spasm. Straight leg raising is restricted and painful on the affected side; dorsiflexion of the foot and bowstringing of the lateral popliteal nerve may accentuate the pain. Sometimes raising the unaffected leg causes acute sciatic tension on the painful side ('crossed sciatic tension'). With a high or mid-lumbar prolapse the femoral stretch test may be positive.

Neurological examination may show muscle weakness (and, later, wasting), diminished reflexes and sensory loss corresponding to the affected level. L5 impairment causes weakness of knee flexion and big toe extension as well as sensory loss on the outer side of the leg and the dorsum of the foot. Normal reflexes at the knee and ankle are characteristic of L5 root compression. Paradoxically, the knee reflex may appear to be *increased*, because of weakness of the antagonists (which are supplied by L5). S1 impairment causes weak plantar-flexion and eversion of the foot, a depressed ankle jerk and sensory loss along the lateral border of the foot. Occasionally an L4/5 disc prolapse compresses both L5 and S1. Cauda equina compression causes urinary retention and sensory loss over the sacrum.

Imaging

X-rays are helpful, not to show an abnormal disc space but to exclude bone disease. After several attacks the disc space may be narrowed and small osteophytes appear.

Myelography (radiculography) using iopamidol (Niopam) is a fairly reliable method of confirming the nerve root distortion resulting from a disc protrusion, localizing it and excluding intrathecal tumours; however, it carries a significant risk of unpleasant side

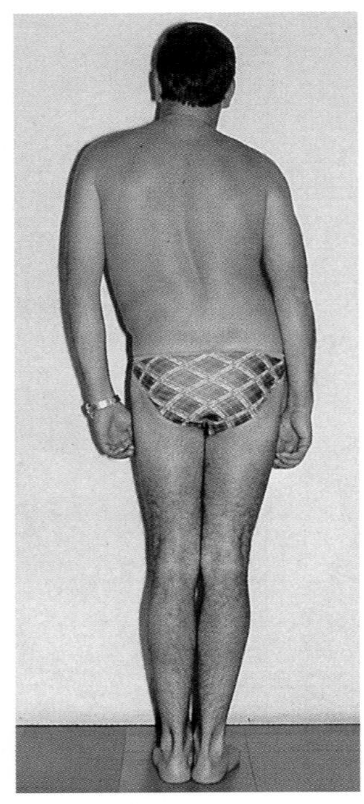

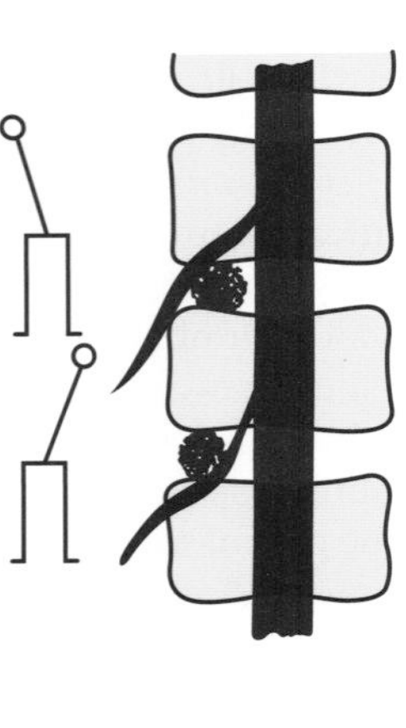

(a) (b)

18.32 Lumbar disc – signs (a) The patient has a sideways list or tilt. (b) If the disc protrudes medial to the nerve root the tilt is towards the painful side (to relieve pressure on the root); with a far lateral prolapse (lower level) the tilt is away from the painful side.

effects, such as headache (in over 30 per cent), nausea and dizziness. Myelography is unsuitable for diagnosing a far lateral disc protrusion (lateral to the intervertebral foramen); if this is suspected CT or MRI is essential.

CT and *MRI* are more reliable than myelography and have none of its disadvantages. These are now the preferred methods of spinal imaging.

Differential diagnosis

The full-blown syndrome is unlikely to be misdiagnosed, but with repeated attacks and with lumbar spondylosis gradually supervening (see later), the features often become atypical. There are two diagnostic aphorisms:

- *Lower limb pain* is not always the sciatica of root compression; frequently it is referred pain from backache and can occur in other lumbar spine disorders.
- *Disc rupture* affects at most two neurological levels; if multiple levels are involved, suspect a cauda equina compression (see box) or a neurological disorder.

Inflammatory disorders such as infection or ankylosing spondylitis, cause severe stiffness, a raised ESR and erosive changes on x-ray.

Vertebral tumours cause severe pain, marked muscle spasm and pain through the night. With metastases the patient is ill, the ESR is raised and the x-rays show bone destruction or sclerosis.

Nerve tumours such as a neurofibroma of the cauda equina, may cause 'sciatica' but pain is continuous. Advanced imaging will confirm the diagnosis.

FEATURES OF CAUDA EQUINA SYNDROME

Bladder and bowel incontinence

Perineal numbness

Bilateral sciatica

Lower limb weakness

Crossed straight-leg raising sign

Note: Scan urgently and operate urgently if a large central disc is revealed.

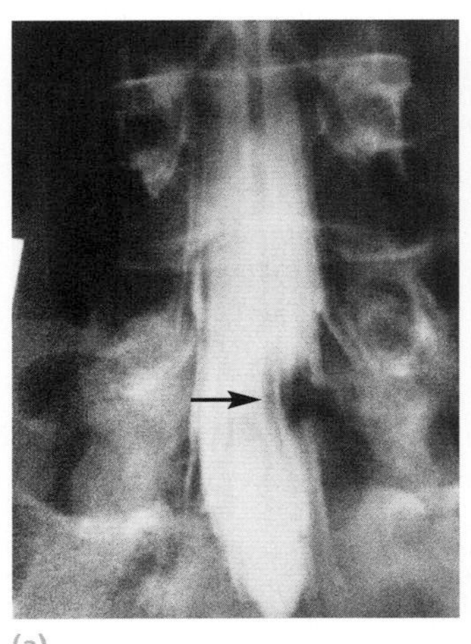

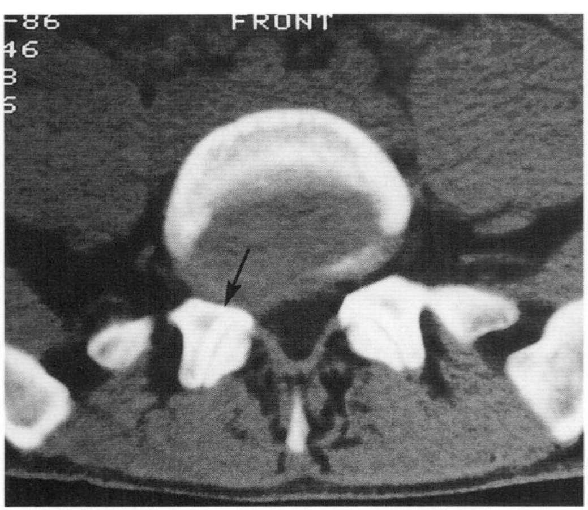

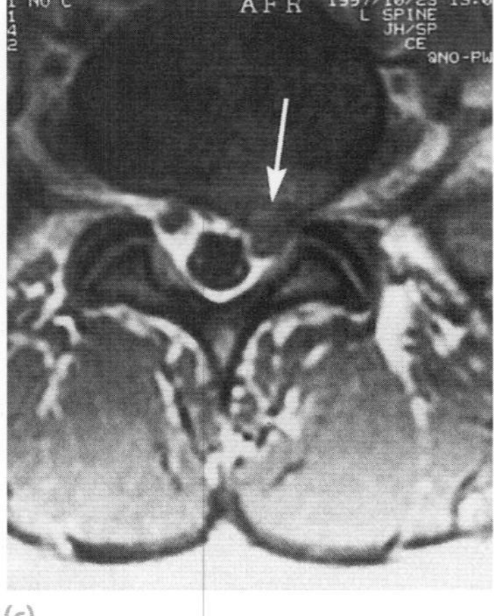

(a) (b) (c)

18.33 Disc prolapse – imaging (a) Radiculogram in which the gap in the contrast medium (arrow) shows where a disc has protruded. (b) CT scan showing how disc protrusion can obstruct the intervertebral foramen. (c) MRI, axial view, showing the relationship of the disc protrusion to the dural sac and intervertebral foramen.

Treatment

Heat and analgesics soothe, and exercises strengthen muscles, but there are only three ways of treating the prolapse itself – *rest, reduction* or *removal,* followed by *rehabilitation*:

Rest With an acute attack the patient should be kept in bed, with hips and knees slightly flexed. A non-steroidal anti-inflammatory drug is useful.

Reduction Continuous bed rest and traction for 2 weeks may reduce the herniation. If the symptoms and signs do not improve during that period, an epidural injection of corticosteroid and local anaesthetic may help.

Chemonucleolysis dissolution of the nucleus pulposus by percutaneous injection of a proteolytic enzyme (chymopapain) – is in theory an excellent way of reducing a disc prolapse. However, controlled studies have shown that it is less effective (and potentially more dangerous) than surgical removal of the disc material (Ejeskär et al., 1982).

Removal The indications for operative removal of a prolapse are: (1) a cauda equina compression syndrome – this is an emergency; (2) neurological deterioration while under conservative treatment; (3) persistent pain and signs of sciatic tension (especially crossed sciatic tension) after 2–3 weeks of conservative treatment. The presence of a prolapsed disc, and the level, must be confirmed by CT, MRI or myelography before operating. Surgery in the absence of a clear preoperative diagnosis is usually unrewarding. The two operations most widely performed are *laminotomy* and *microdiscectomy.*

Laminotomy is nowadays preferred to the older, more destructive type of laminectomy. Ligamentum flavum on the relevant side and at the relevant level is removed, if necessary with some margin of the bordering laminae and medial third of the facet joint. The dura and nerve root are then gently retracted towards the midline and the pea-like disc bulge or extrusion/sequestration is displayed. If the outer layer of the annulus is seen still to be intact, it is incised and the mushy disc material plucked out piecemeal with pituitary forceps. The nerve is traced to its point of exit in order to exclude other pathology.

A far lateral disc protrusion is very difficult to expose by the standard interlaminar approach without damaging the facet joint. An intertransverse approach may be more suitable for these cases.

The main intraoperative complication is bleeding from epidural veins. This is less likely to occur if the patient is placed on his side or in the kneeling position, thus minimizing pressure on the abdomen and a rise in venous pressure. The major postoperative complication is disc space infection, but fortunately this is rare. Recurrent prolapse with sciatica is more common and may require revision decompression surgery.

Microdiscectomy is essentially similar to the standard posterior operation, except that the exposure is very limited and the procedure is carried out with the aid of an operating microscope. Morbidity and length of hospitalization are certainly less than with conventional surgery, but there are drawbacks: careful x-ray control is needed to ensure that the correct level is entered; intraoperative bleeding may be difficult to control; there is a considerable 'learning curve' and the inexperienced operator risks injuring the dura or a stretched nerve root, or missing essential pathology; there is a slightly increased risk of disc space infection, and prophylactic antibiotics are advisable.

Rehabilitation After recovery from an acute disc rupture, or disc removal, the patient is taught isometric exercises and how to lie, sit, bend and lift with the least strain. Ideally this should be done as part of an education programme in a 'back school' (Zachrisson, 1981).

PERSISTENT POSTOPERATIVE BACKACHE AND SCIATICA

Persistent symptoms after operation may be due to: (1) residual disc material in the spinal canal; (2) disc prolapse at another level; (3) nerve root pressure by a hypertrophic facet joint or a narrow lateral recess ('root canal stenosis'). After careful investigation, any of these may call for re-operation; but second procedures do not have a high success rate – third and fourth procedures still less.

ARACHNOIDITIS

Diffuse back pain and vague lower limb symptoms such as 'cramps', 'burning' or 'irritability' sometimes appear after myelography, epidural injections or disc operations. This diagnosis is now rarely made and is believed to have been a complication of oil-based contrast media used in myelography 30 years ago. There may also be sphincter dysfunction and male impotence. Patients complain bitterly and many are labelled neurotic. However, in some cases there are electromyographic abnormalities, and dural scarring with obliteration of the subarachnoid space can be demonstrated by MRI or at operation.

Treatment is generally unrewarding. Corticosteroid injections at best give only temporary relief, and surgical 'neurolysis' may actually make matters worse. Sympathetic management in a pain clinic, psychological support and a graduated activity programme are the best that can be offered.

FACET JOINT DYSFUNCTION

Facet joint abnormalities that have been demonstrated at operation or necropsy are: (1) anatomical variations that limit articular movement; (2) anatomical variations that permit excessive movement; (3) malapposition of the articular surfaces secondary to loss of disc height; (4) softening and fibrillation of the facet articular cartilage; (5) loose bodies in the facet joint; (6) synovial thickening; (7) classical changes of osteoarthritis, progressing from fibrillation to complete loss of articular cartilage and osteophytic thickening of the facets.

Some of these abnormalities are associated with radiologically demonstrable vertebral shift; in others the abnormal movement is considered to be more subtle and it is not surprising that this has given rise to semantic arguments about the concept (and indeed the very existence) of a condition called 'segmental instability', which could give rise to otherwise inexplicable low-back pain.

The concept of 'segmental instability' was elaborated on more than 25 years ago (Kirkaldy-Willis and Farfan, 1982) in an attempt to explain the back pain on the basis of disordered biomechanics of the spine (or a spinal segment). It was widely recognized that patients with chronic backache may develop intermittent episodes of severe pain with radiation into the buttock and thighs in the absence of any sign of intervertebral disc prolapse. These attacks are usually triggered by fairly modest lifting strains, but they can also occur 'spontaneously'. Kirkaldy-Willis suggested that the symptoms are due to abnormal movement and mechanical stress at the posterior facet joints, arising from local injury or non-specific 'dysfunction' of the lower lumbar vertebral segments. The theory is controversial, partly because of differences about the meaning of the word 'instability' in this context and partly because some patients with demonstrably abnormal vertebral motion have no symptoms at all. Radiological images that are interpreted as showing instability may or may not be accepted by a bioengineer as proof of instability in mechanical terms.

Clinical features

Whatever the doubts about aetiology, the clinical appearances of this syndrome are easily recognizable. The patient, usually a young adult engaged in bending and/or lifting activities, experiences mild backache from time to time. Typically this culminates in a particular episode of more severe back pain, possibly accompanied by pain in the buttock or the back of the thighs, but no true neurological symptoms. Pain is usually relieved by rest, mobilization exercises or chiropractic manipulation, only to recur a few weeks or months later after a similar episode of physical stress.

In the established case, the patient gives a history of intermittent backache related to spells of hard work, standing, bending, or walking a lot, or sometimes after sitting in one position during a long journey.

Most patients find relief by lying down, or sitting and resting when backache appears during strenuous activity. A suspicion of 'instability' is favoured inasmuch as the patient achieves relief through recumbency. However, a large minority of patients describe a contrasting pattern: pain aggravated by rest and recumbency and partially relieved by movement; they usually manage full forward bending without discomfort but backward bending (which stresses the facet joints more) is dramatically halted by pain. This is reminiscent of 'arthritic' pain in other synovial joints and could signify the onset of osteoarthritis (OA) in the facet joints. Interestingly, pathological features of OA have been described in specimens excised at surgery during operations for intractable back pain of this pattern (Eisenstein and Parry, 1987).

With time, pain becomes more constant and can sometimes be temporarily relieved only by manipulation, local warmth and anti-inflammatory drugs; at that stage there are likely to be x-ray signs of osteoarthritis in the facet joints.

Examination during a painful episode may reveal muscle spasm, local tenderness and restriction of back movements, but little else. Occasionally the patient presents with a *'locked back'*, which is dramatically relieved by skilful manipulation.

Between acute attacks, physical signs are less obvious and often unconvincing. The *range* of movement may not be much restricted, but the *pattern of movement* is often recognizable: characteristically the patient bends forward quite easily but when asked to return to the upright position he or she does so with a noticeable 'heave' or 'catch', sometimes seeking support by pressing upon the thighs.

Straight-leg raising may be slightly restricted (in this case only because of back pain), but neurological examination is normal.

Imaging

X-RAY

X-rays may look completely normal. However, in many cases there are mild to moderately severe features of intervertebral disc degeneration, mainly flattening of the 'disc space' and marginal osteophytes. A singular feature, which is held to be characteristic of 'segmental instability', is the appearance of a 'traction spur', a bony projection anteriorly a little distance from the upper or lower rim of the vertebral body. In the lateral view, there may be slight displacement of one vertebra upon another, either forwards (spondylolisthesis) or backwards (retrolisthesis); this may become apparent only during flexion or extension.

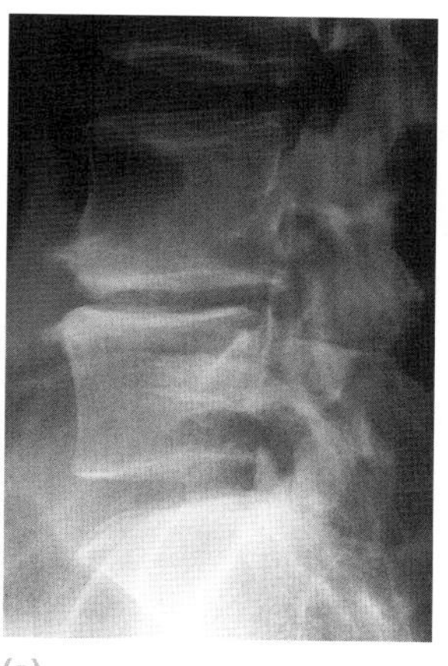

(a)

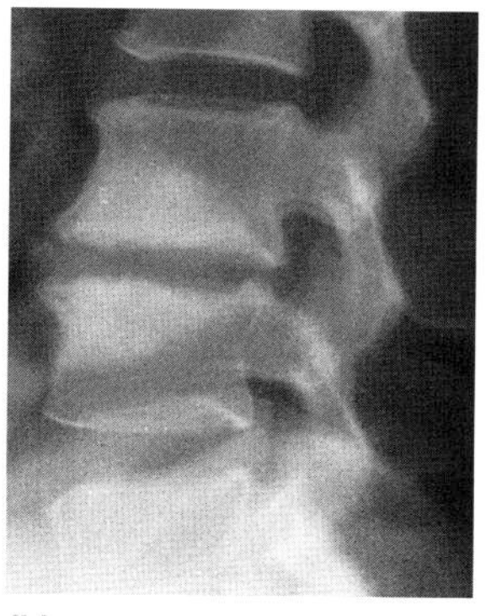

(b)

18.34 Facet joint dysfunction X-ray features of spondylosis and facet joint dysfunction: (a) Narrowing of the disc space and slight retrolisthesis at L4/5, with two small traction spurs at the anterior borders of the adjacent vertebrae. (b) Narrowing of the disc space at L3/4 and areas of subchondral sclerosis in the adjacent vertebral bodies (reminiscent of the Modic type 3 MRI changes shown in Fig.18.30).

Discography and facetography may reveal disc abnormalities, but these investigations are not routinely available and in any case there is some controversy about their reliability.

CT AND MRI

These investigations may reveal signs of disc degeneration as well as early features of OA in the facet joints (loss of articular cartilage space and curling over of the joint surfaces). 'Modic' changes are worth noting (see Fig. 18.30).

Diagnosis

Recurrent backache is often attributed to one particular abnormal feature, such as 'disc degeneration' or 'an annular tear'. It is difficult to prove a causative association of this kind. The discovery of one abnormality should, however, prompt the clinician to look for others; it is the *set* of clinical and imaging features rather than any single sign that elucidates the diagnosis.

Treatment

Whatever pattern the back pain may present, the pain may be sufficiently distressing or disabling to justify treatment in increasing degrees of invasiveness.

CONSERVATIVE MEASURES

Initially the symptoms are neither severe nor disabling; conservative measures should be encouraged for as long as possible:

General care and attention Poor understanding has led to the condition being neglected and, unless there is a very obvious abnormality that is amenable to surgery, patients soon come to feel that the doctor has lost interest in their complaints; little wonder that many of them turn for help to 'alternative' practitioners. They should be given a clear explanation of the likely cause of their symptoms and an outline of the proposed treatment. In more enlightened (and better supported) centres patients are enrolled in a 'back school'.

Physical therapy Conventional physiotherapy, including spinal 'mobilization', often relieves pain dramatically – at least for a while. In the longer term, weight control and strengthening of the vertebral and abdominal muscles will make for fewer recurrences. There is also no reason why orthopaedic surgeons and chiropractors or osteopaths should not be able to collaborate in designing treatment programmes.

Drug treatment Mild analgesics may be needed for pain control. Long term non-steroidal anti-inflammatory drug (NSAID) medication is still preferable to the drastic remedy of spinal fusion surgery, but should be combined with an appropriate gut protector such as omeprazole. However, beware the patient who becomes dependent on increasing doses of medication.

Spinal support A soft lumbar support may give relief in some cases; obese patients benefit from having their centre of gravity pulled in close to the spine.

Modification of activities One of the most important aspects of treatment is modification of daily activities (bending, lifting, climbing, etc.) and specific activities relating to work. The patient may need retraining for a different job. The co-operation of employers is essential.

Psychological support Chronic back pain can be psychologically as well as physically debilitating. Counselling and support are often welcomed by the patient. Perhaps the most successful treatment is the reassurance that the surgeon can provide for the vast majority of patients, to the effect that the patient has no serious spinal disease.

Trigger point and facet joint injection If clinical and x-ray signs point consistently to one or two facet levels, injection of local anaesthetic and corticosteroids may be carried out under fluoroscopic control. Most patients can be expected to obtain short-term benefit and some are relieved of symptoms for periods of more than a year. Lumbosacral trigger points (Travell, 1983) in the midline or along the iliac crests, are a common finding in chronic low back pain. If they are focal and consistent they may respond dramatically, if only temporarily, to deep soft tissue local infiltration without the need for fluoroscopic control.

SURGERY

Only after all of the above measures have been tried and found to be ineffectual should a spinal fusion be considered. Even then very strict guidelines should be followed if embarking on a road already crowded with patients labelled 'failed back surgery' is to be avoided:

1. Repeated examination should ensure that there is no other treatable pathology.
2. There should have been at least some response to conservative treatment; patients who 'benefit from nothing' will not benefit from spinal fusion either.
3. There should be unequivocal evidence of facet joint instability or osteoarthritis at a specific level.
4. The patient should be emotionally stable and should not exaggerate his symptoms nor display inappropriate physical signs (see later).
5. The patient should be warned that: (1) a 'fusion' doesn't always fuse (there is a 10–20 per cent failure rate); (2) a fusion at one level does not preclude further pathology developing at another level; Lehmann et al (1987), in a long-term follow-up of patients who had undergone spinal fusion, found that after 10 years 40 per cent had developed signs of instability elsewhere.

Whether the surgery is performed anteriorly or posteriorly, or from both approaches combined, or whether implants of one kind or another are employed, seems not to affect the final result materially. The surgeon must be allowed to perform the procedure in which he/she has the most confidence. There is no doubt however, that the more extensive and more complex procedures carry a higher complication rate.

SPONDYLOLISTHESIS

'Spondylolisthesis' means forward translation of one segment of the spine upon another. The shift is nearly always between L4 and L5, or between L5 and the sacrum. Normal discs, laminae and facets constitute a locking mechanism that prevents each vertebra from moving forwards on the one below. Forward shift (or slip) occurs only when this mechanism has failed.

Classification

Various classifications have been suggested. Basically there are six types of spondylolisthesis:

Dysplastic (20 per cent) The superior sacral facets are congenitally defective; slow but inexorable forward slip leads to severe displacement. Associated anomalies (usually spina bifida occulta) are common.

Lytic or isthmic (50 per cent) In this, the commonest variety, there are defects in the pars interarticularis (spondylolysis), or repeated breaking and healing may lead to elongation of the pars. The defect (which occurs in about 5 per cent of people) is usually present by the age of 7, but the slip may appear only some years later (Eisenstein, 1978; Fredrickson et al., 1984). It is difficult to exclude a genetic factor because spondylolisthesis often runs in families, and is more common in certain races, notably Eskimos; but the incidence increases with age up to the late teenage years, although clinical presentation with pain can continue into late middle age. An acquired factor probably supervenes to produce what is essentially an ununited stress fracture. The condition is more common than usual in those whose spines are subjected to extraordinary stresses (e.g. competitive gymnasts and weight-lifters).

Degenerative (25 per cent) Degenerative changes in the facet joints and the discs permit forward slip (nearly always at L4/5 and mainly in women of middle age) despite intact laminae. Many of these patients have generalized osteoarthritis and pyrophosphate crystal arthropathy.

Post-traumatic Unusual fractures may result in destabilization of the lumbar spine.

Pathological Bone destruction (e.g. due to tuberculosis or neoplasm) may lead to vertebral slipping.

Postoperative (iatropathic) Occasionally, excessive operative removal of bone in decompression operations results in progressive spondylolisthesis.

Pathology

In the common lytic type of spondylolisthesis the pars interarticularis on both sides is disrupted, as in an ununited fracture (*spondylolysis*), leaving the posterior neural arch separated from the vertebral body anteriorly; the gap is occupied by fibrous tissue. With stress, the vertebral body and superior facets in front of the gap may subluxate or dislocate forwards, carrying the superimposed vertebral column with it (*spondylolisthesis*); the isolated segment of neural arch maintains its normal relationship to the sacral facets. When there is no gap, the pars interarticularis is elongated or the facets are defective.

The degree of slip is measured by the amount of overlap of adjacent vertebral bodies and is usually expressed as a percentage.

With forward slipping there may be pressure on the dura mater and cauda equina, or on the emerging nerve roots; these roots may also be compressed in the narrowed intervertebral foramina. Disc prolapse is liable to occur.

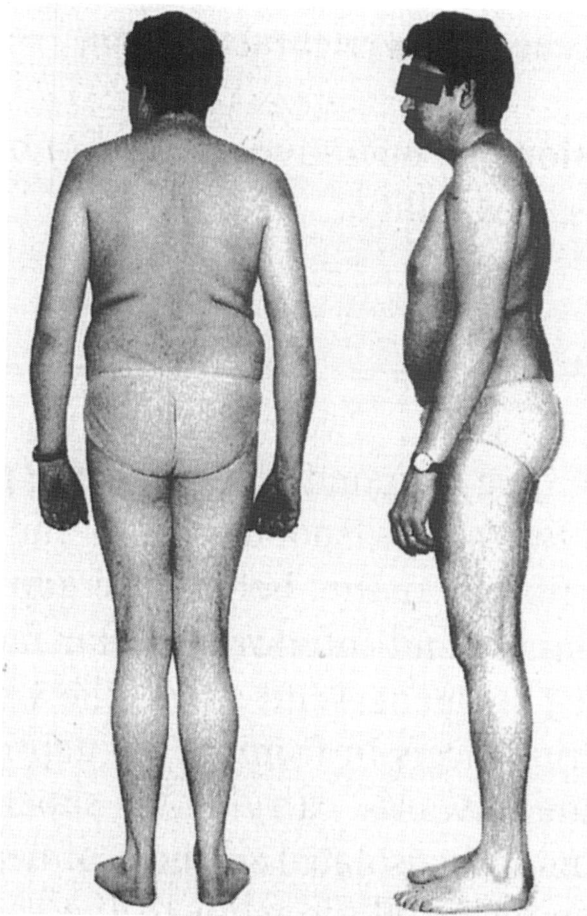

18.35 Spondylolisthesis – clinical appearance The transverse loin creases, forwards tilting of the pelvis and flattening of the lumbar spine are characteristic.

Clinical features

Spondylolysis, and even a well-marked spondylolisthesis, may be discovered incidentally during routine x-ray examination.

In *children* the condition is usually painless but the mother may notice the unduly protruding abdomen and peculiar stance. In *adolescents* and *adults* backache is the usual presenting symptom; it is often intermittent, coming on after exercise or strain. Sciatica may occur in one or both legs. *Patients aged over 50* are usually women with degenerative spondylolisthesis. They always have backache, some have sciatica and some present because of claudication due to spinal stenosis.

On examination the buttocks look curiously flat, the sacrum appears to extend to the waist and transverse loin creases are seen. The lumbar spine is on a plane in front of the sacrum and looks too short. Sometimes there is a scoliosis.

A 'step' can often be felt when the fingers are run down the spine. Movements are usually normal in the younger patients but there may be 'hamstring tightness'; in the degenerative group the spine is often stiff.

X-RAYS

Lateral views show the forward shift of the upper part of the spinal column on the stable vertebra below; elongation of the arch or defective facets may be seen. The gap in the pars interarticularis is best seen in the oblique views. In doubtful cases, reversed gantry CT may be helpful.

Prognosis

Dysplastic spondylolisthesis appears at an early age, often goes on to a severe slip and carries a significant risk of neurological complications.

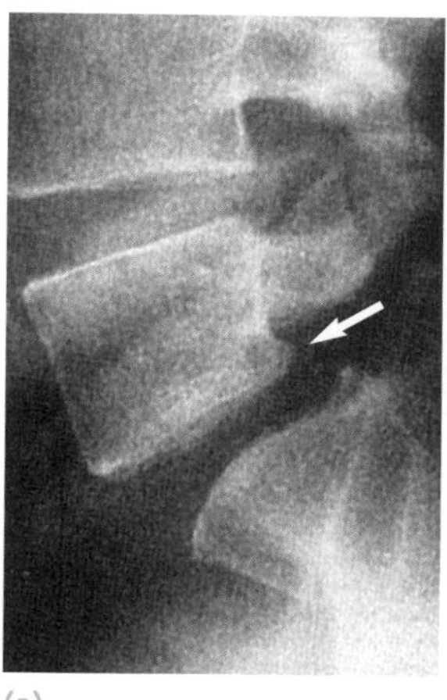

(a)

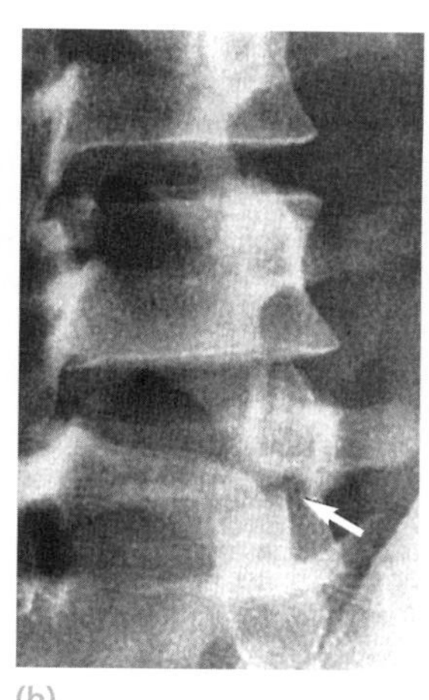

(b)

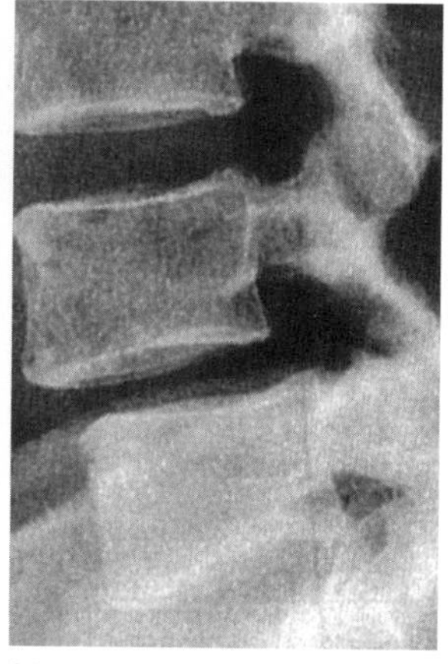

(c)

18.36 Spondylolisthesis – x-rays (a) There is a break in the pars interarticularis of L5, allowing the anterior part of the vertebra to slip forwards. In this case the gap is easily seen in the lateral x-ray, but usually it is better seen in the oblique view (b). In degenerative spondylolisthesis there is no break in the pars – the degenerate disc and eroded facet joints permit one vertebra to slide forwards on the other (c). There is no pars defect; the dehydrated disc permits slipping, usually at L4/5.

Lytic (isthmic) spondylolisthesis with less than 10 per cent displacement does not progress after adulthood, but may predispose the patient to later back problems. It is not a contraindication to strenuous work unless severe pain supervenes (Wiltse et al., 1990). With slips of more than 25 per cent there is an increased risk of backache in later life.

Degenerative spondylolisthesis is rare before the age of 50, progresses slowly and seldom exceeds 30 per cent.

Treatment

Conservative treatment, similar to that for other types of back pain, is suitable for most patients.

Operative treatment is indicated: (1) if the symptoms are disabling and interfere significantly with work and recreational activities; (2) if the slip is more than 50 per cent and progressing; (3) if neurological compression is significant.

For children, posterior intertransverse fusion in situ is almost always successful; if neurological signs appear, decompression can be carried out later. For adults, either posterior or anterior fusion is suitable. However, in the 'degenerative' group, where neurological symptoms predominate, decompression without fusion may suffice.

Note on post-traumatic spondylolisthesis The patient found to have spondylolysis or spondylolisthesis after recent back injury (usually hyperextension) may have fractured the pars, or merely strained the fibrous tissue of a pre-existing lesion. If doubt exists (and it usually does) a plaster jacket should be worn for 3 months; the recent fracture may join spontaneously. If union does not occur the assumption is that spondylolisthesis was present before injury and treatment is along the lines already indicated.

A detailed discussion of surgical options appears in a review paper by Jones and Raj (2009).

SPINAL STENOSIS

The lumbar spinal canal is normally round or oval in cross-section; in a minority of cases the L5 canal is trefoil-shaped and the lateral recesses are narrower than usual, yet still wide enough to allow free passage of the nerve roots through the intervertebral foramina (Eisenstein, 1980). The term *spinal stenosis* is used to describe abnormal narrowing of the central canal, the lateral recesses or the intervertebral foramina to the point where the neural elements are compromised. When this occurs the patient develops neurological symptoms and signs in the lower limbs.

The causes of spinal stenosis are: (1) congenital vertebral dysplasia (e.g. in achondroplasia or hypochondroplasia); (2) chronic disc protrusion and peri-discal fibrosis or ossification; (3) displacement and hypertrophy, or osteoarthritis, of the apophyseal (facet) joints; (4) hypertrophy, folding, or ossification of the ligamentum flavum; (5) bone thickening due to Paget's disease; (6) spondylolisthesis. Unilateral narrowing of the intervertebral foramen (*root canal stenosis*) may result from an unresolved lateral disc herniation, post-discectomy fibrosis or unilateral facet joint ost.

What constitutes abnormal narrowing, or stenosis? Two measurements are used: the mid-sagittal (anteroposterior) diameter and the interpedicular (transverse)

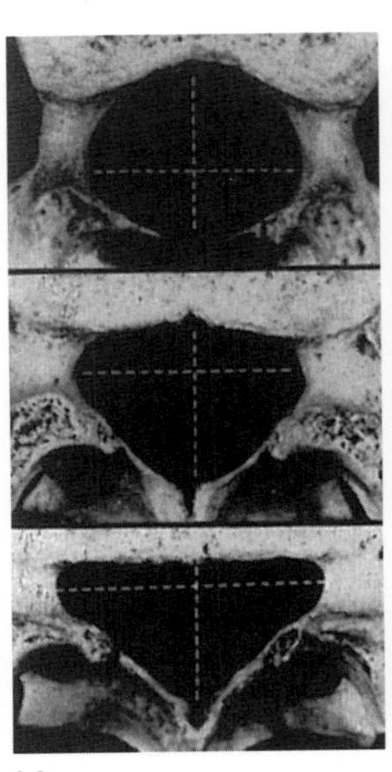
(a)

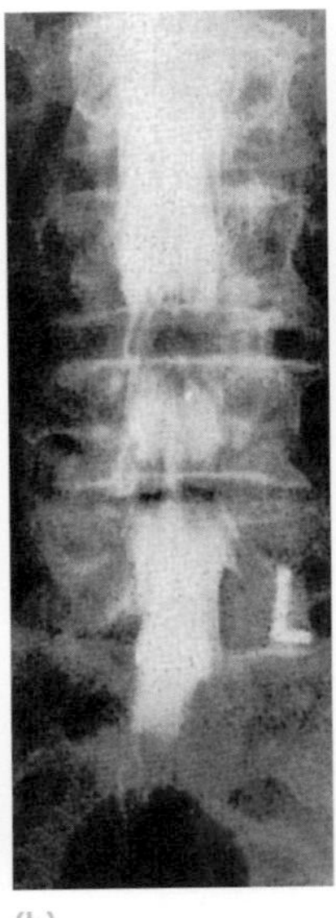
(b)

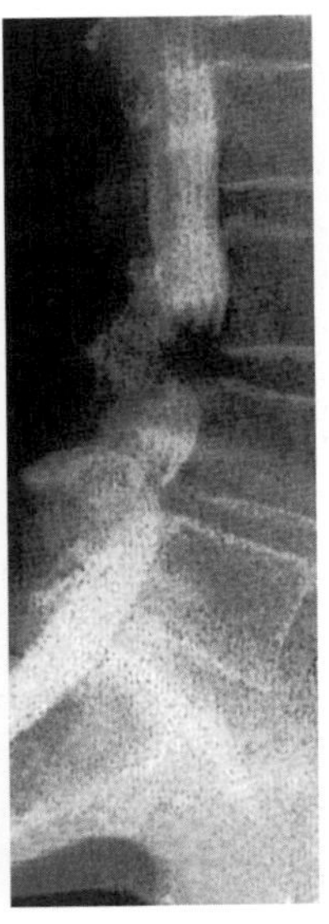
(c)

18.37 Spinal stenosis (a) The shape of the lumbar spinal canal varies from oval (with a large capacity) to trefoil (with narrow lateral recesses); further encroachment on an already narrow canal can cause an ischaemic neuropathy and 'spinal claudication'. **(b,c)** Myelogram showing marked narrowing of the radio-opaque column at the level of stenosis.

diameter of the spinal canal. On plain x-rays the lower limits of normal for the lumbar vertebrae are usually taken as 15 mm for the anteroposterior and 20 mm for the transverse diameters (Eisenstein, 1977; 1983). However, the boundaries of the canal are sometimes difficult to define and more accurate measurements can be obtained from CT; anything less than 11 mm for the anteroposterior diameter and 16 mm for the transverse diameter is considered abnormal.

Clinical features

The patient, usually a man aged over 50, complains of aching, heaviness, numbness and paraesthesia in the thighs and legs; it comes on after standing upright or walking for 5–10 minutes, and is consistently relieved by sitting, squatting or leaning against a wall to flex the spine (hence the term 'spinal claudication'). The patient may prefer walking uphill, which flexes the spine (and maximizes the spinal canal capacity), to downhill, which extends it. With root canal stenosis the symptoms may be unilateral. The patient sometimes has a previous history of disc prolapse, chronic backache or spinal operation.

Examination, especially after getting the patient to reproduce the symptoms by walking, may (rarely) show neurological deficit in the lower limbs. Intact pedal pulses would confirm the claudication as spinal rather than arterial, but beware of the older patient who could have both spinal and arterial claudication.

Imaging

X-rays will usually show features of disc degeneration and proliferative osteoarthritis or degenerative spondylolisthesis. Measurement of the spinal canal can be carried out on plain films, but more reliable information is obtained from myelography, CT and MRI.

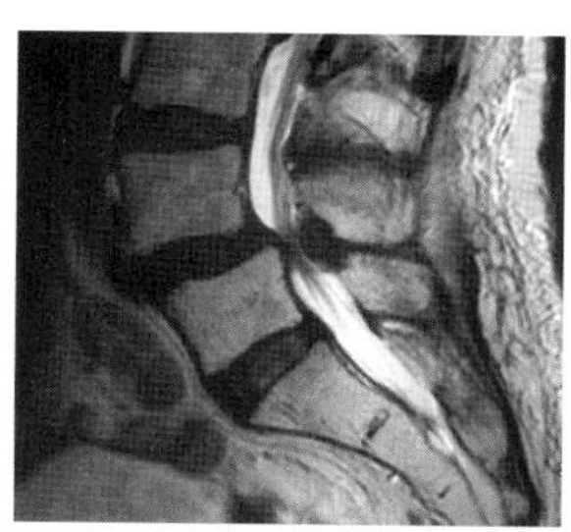

(a)

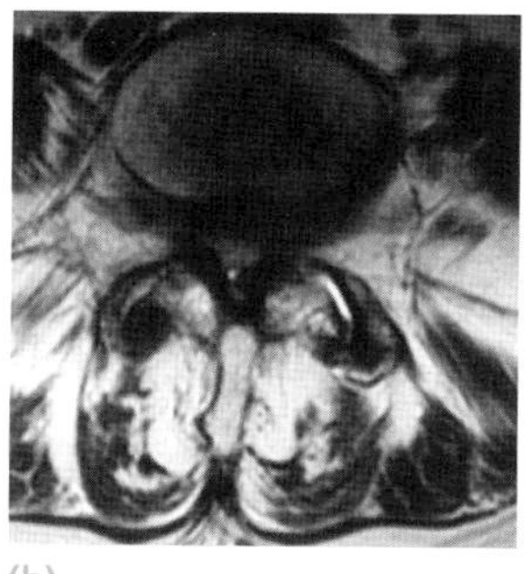

(b)

18.38 Spinal stenosis – MRI T_2-weighted sagittal and axial images showing circumferential spinal stenosis at L4/5 in a middle-aged woman with marked osteoarthritis of the facet joints.

Treatment

Conservative measures, including instruction in spinal posture, may suffice. Most patients are prepared to put up with their symptoms and simply avoid uncomfortable postures. If discomfort is marked and activities such as standing and walking are severely restricted, operative decompression is almost always successful. A large laminotomy with flavectomy, medial facetectomy and discectomy is performed at every relevant level and on every relevant side, if necessary extending over several levels and laterally to clear the nerve root canals. This relieves the leg pain, but not the back pain, and occasionally the surgery actually increases spondylolisthesis and back pain; consequently in patients under 60 the operation is sometimes combined with spinal fusion (Eisenstein, 2002).

APPROACH TO DIAGNOSIS IN PATIENTS WITH LOW BACK PAIN

Chronic backache is such a frequent cause of disability in the community that it has become almost a disease in itself. The following is a suggested approach to more specific diagnosis.

Careful history taking and examination will uncover one of five pain patterns:

1. *Transient backache following muscular activity* This suggests a simple back strain that will respond to a short period of rest followed by gradually increasing exercise. People with thoracic kyphosis (of whatever origin), or fixed flexion of the hip, are particularly prone to back strain because they tend to compensate for the deformity by holding the lumbosacral spine in hyperlordosis.

2. *Sudden, acute pain and sciatica* In young people (those under the age of 20) it is important to exclude *infection* and *spondylolisthesis*; both produce recognizable x-ray changes. Patients aged 20–40 years are more likely to have an acute disc prolapse: diagnostic features are: (1) a history of a lifting strain, (2) unequivocal sciatic tension; (3) neurological symptoms and signs. Elderly patients may have osteoporotic *compression fractures*, but *metastatic disease* and *myeloma* must be excluded.

3. *Intermittent low back pain after exertion* Patients of almost any age may complain of recurrent backache following exertion or lifting activities and this is relieved by rest. Features of disc prolapse are absent but there may be a history of acute sciatica in the past. In early cases x-rays usually show no abnormality; later there may be signs of *lumbar spondylosis* in those over

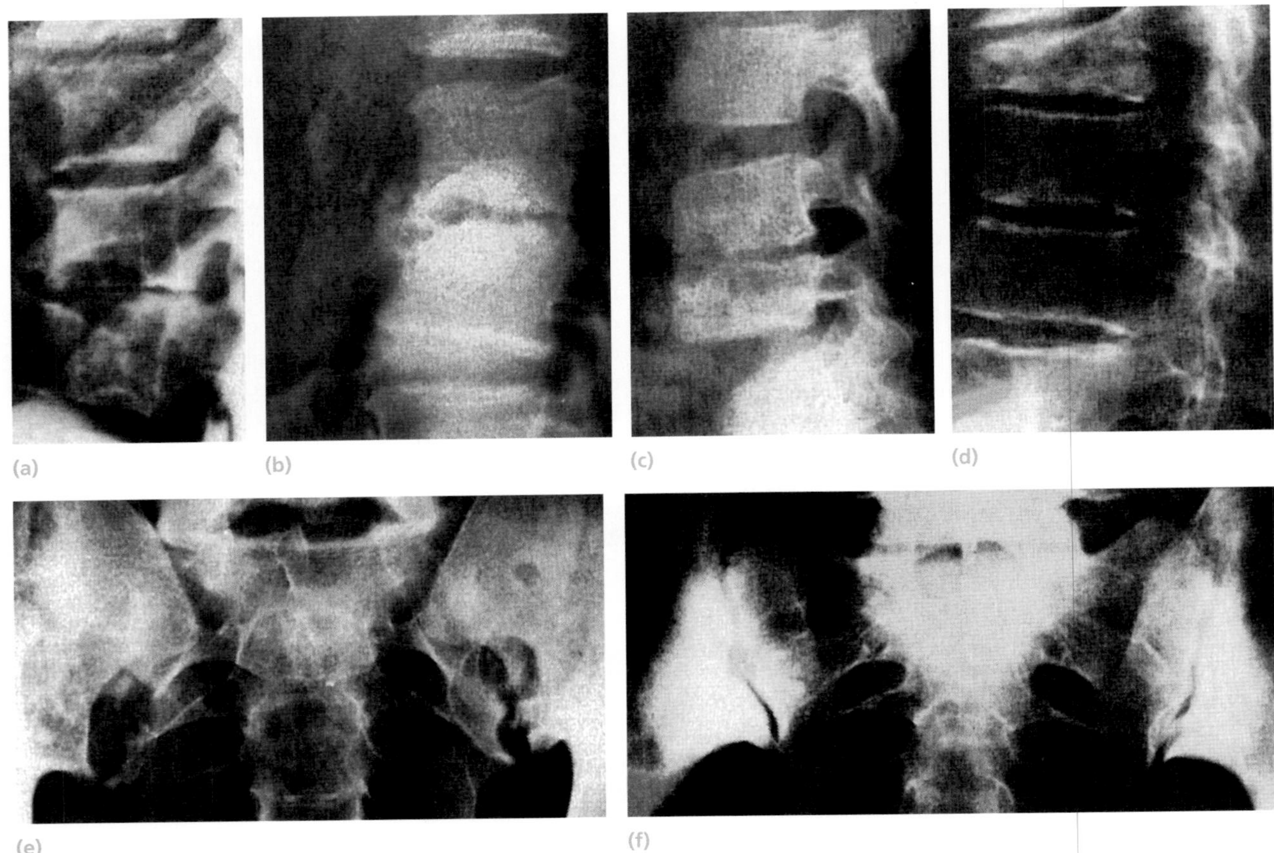

18.39 Some causes of chronic back pain (a) Tuberculosis; (b) acute osteomyelitis – note the sclerosis that developed within a few weeks; (c) discitis; (d) metastatic disease; (e) bilateral sacroiliac tuberculosis; (f) osteitis condensans ilii, which is probably not the cause of the backache.

50 years and *osteoarthritis* of the facet joints is common. These patients need painstaking examination to: (1) uncover any features of radiological segmental instability or facet joint osteoarthritis; (2) determine whether those features are incidental or are likely to account for the patient's symptoms. In the process, disorders such as ankylosing *spondylitis*, *chronic infection*, *myelomatosis* and other *bone diseases* must be excluded by appropriate imaging and blood investigations.

4. Back pain plus pseudoclaudication These patients are usually aged over 50 and may give a history of previous, longstanding back trouble. The diagnosis of *spinal stenosis* should be confirmed by CT and/or MRI.

5. Severe and constant pain localized to a particular site This suggests local bone pathology, such as a compression fracture, Paget's disease, a tumour or infection. Spinal osteoporosis in middle-aged men is pathological and calls for a full battery of tests to exclude primary disorders such as *myelomatosis*, *carcinomatosis*, *hyperthyroidism*, *gonadal insufficiency*, *alcoholism* or *corticosteroid usage*.

CHRONIC BACK PAIN SYNDROME

Patients with chronic backache may despair of finding a cure for their trouble (or, indeed, even a diagnosis that everyone agrees on), and they often develop affective and psychosomatic ailments that subsequently become the chief focus of attention. This 'illness behaviour' is both self-perpetuating and self-justifying. It is usually accompanied by *'non-organic' (inappropriate) physical signs* (Waddell et al., 1980; 1984), such as: (1) pain and tenderness of bizarre degree or distribution; (2) pain on performing impressive but non-stressful manoeuvres such as pressing vertically on the spine or passively rotating the entire trunk; (3) variations in response to tests such as straight leg raising while distracting the patient's attention; (4) sensory and/or motor abnormalities that do not fit the known anatomical and physiological patterns; (5) overdetermined behaviour during physical examination (trembling, sweating, hyperventilating, inability to move, a tendency to fall and exaggerated withdrawal) – usually accompanied by loud groaning and exclamations of discomfort. Patients with these features are unlikely to respond to surgery and they may require prolonged support and management in a special pain clinic – but only after every effort has been made to exclude organic pathology.

NOTES ON APPLIED ANATOMY

THE SPINE AS A WHOLE

The spine has to move, to transmit weight and to protect the spinal cord. In upright man the lumbar segment is lordotic and the column acts like a crane; the paravertebral muscles are the cables that counterbalance any weight carried anteriorly. The resultant force, which passes through the nucleus pulposus of the lowest lumbar disc, is therefore much greater than if the column were loaded directly over its centre; even at rest, tonic contraction of the posterior muscles balances the trunk, so the lumbar spine is always loaded. Nachemson and Morris (1964) measured the intradiscal pressure in volunteers during various activities and found it as high as 10–15 kg/cm^2 while sitting, about 30 per cent less on standing upright and 50 per cent less on lying down. Leaning forward or carrying a weight produces much higher pressures, though when a heavy weight is lifted breathing stops and the abdominal muscles contract, turning the trunk into a tightly inflated bag that cushions the force anteriorly against the pelvis. (Could it be that champion weight-lifters benefit in this way from having voluminous bodies?)

Seen from the side, the dorsal spine is convex backwards (kyphosis); the cervical and lumbar regions are convex forwards (lordosis). In forward flexion the lordotic curves straighten out. Lying supine with the legs straight tilts the pelvic brim forwards; the lumbar spine compensates by increasing its lordosis. If the hips are unable to extend fully (fixed flexion deformity), the lumbar lordosis increases still more until the lower limbs lie flat and the flexion deformity is masked.

VERTEBRAL COMPONENTS

Each segment of the vertebral column transmits weight through the vertebral body anteriorly and the facet joints posteriorly. Between adjacent bodies (and firmly attached to them) lie the intervertebral discs. These compressible 'cushions', and the surrounding ligaments and muscles, act as shock-absorbers; if they are degenerate or weak their ability to absorb some of the force is diminished and the bones and joints suffer the consequences.

The vertebral body is cancellous, but the upper and lower surfaces are condensed to form sclerotic end-plates. In childhood these are covered by cartilage, which contributes to vertebral growth. Later the peripheral rim ossifies and fuses with the body, but the central area remains as a thin layer of cartilage adherent to the intervertebral disc. The epiphyseal end-plates may be damaged by disc pressure during childhood, giving rise to irregular ossification and abnormal vertebral growth (Scheuermann's disease).

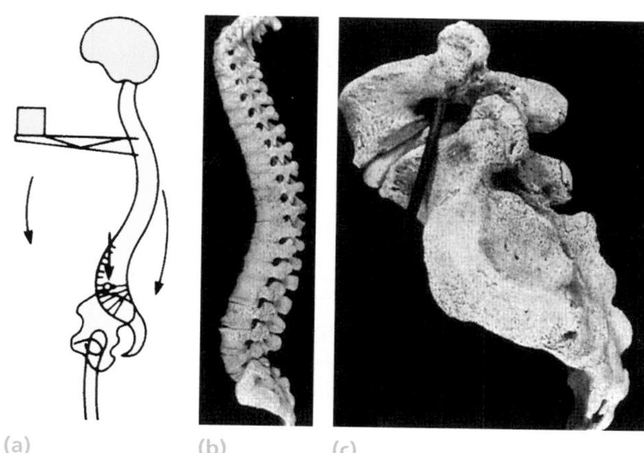

(a) (b) (c)

18.40 Anatomy (a,b) The vertebral column has a series of gentle curves that produce lordosis in the cervical and lumbar regions and kyphosis in the dorsal segment. The column functions like a crane, the weight in front of the spine being counterbalanced by contraction of the posterior muscles. (c) Relationship of nerve root to disc and facet joint.

INTERVERTEBRAL DISC

The disc consists of a central *avascular nucleus pulposus* – a hydrophilic gel made of protein-polysaccharide, collagen fibres, sparse chondroid cells and water (88 per cent), surrounded by concentric layers of fibrous tissue – the *annulus fibrosus.* If the physicochemical state of the nucleus pulposus is normal, the disc can withstand almost any load that the muscles can support; if it is abnormal, even small increases in force can produce sufficient stress to rupture the annulus.

MOVEMENTS

The axis of movements in the thoracolumbar spine is the nucleus pulposus; the disposition of the facet joints determine which movements occur. In the lumbar spine these joints are in the anteroposterior plane, so flexion, extension and sideways tilting are free but there is virtually no rotation. In the thoracic spine the facet joints face backwards and laterally, so rotation is relatively free; flexion, extension and tilting are possible but are grossly restricted by the ribs. The costovertebral joints are involved in respiration and their limitation is an early feature of ankylosing spondylitis.

The spinal canal

The shape of the canal changes from ovoid in the upper part of the lumbar spine to triangular in the lower. Variations are common and include the trefoil canal, whose shape is mainly due to thickening of the laminae (Eisenstein, 1980). This shape is harmless in itself, but further encroachment on the canal (e.g. by a bulging disc or hypertrophic facet joints) may cause compression of the spinal contents (spinal stenosis).

Spinal cord

The spinal cord ends at about L1 in the conus medullaris, but lumbosacral nerve roots continue in the spinal canal as the cauda equina and leave at appropriate levels lower down. The dural sac continues as far as S2, and whenever a nerve root leaves the spine it takes with it a dural sleeve as far as the exit from the intervertebral foramen. These dural sleeves can be outlined by contrast medium radiography (radiculography).

Intervertebral foramina and nerve roots

Each intervertebral foramen is bounded anteriorly by the disc and adjoining vertebral bodies, posteriorly by the facet joint, and superiorly and inferiorly by the pedicles of adjacent vertebrae. It can therefore be narrowed by a bulging disc or by joint osteophytes. The segmental nerve roots leave the spinal canal through the intervertebral foramina, each pair below the vertebra of the same number (thus, the fourth lumbar root runs between L4 and L5). The segmental blood vessels to and from the cord also pass through the intervertebral foramen. Occlusion of this little passage may occasionally compress the nerve root directly or may cause nerve root ischaemia (especially when the spine is held in extension).

Nerve supply of the spine

The spine and its contents (including the dural sleeves of the nerve roots themselves) are supplied by small branches from the anterior and posterior primary rami of the segmental nerve roots. Lesions of different structures (e.g. the posterior longitudinal ligament, the dural sleeve or the facet joint) may therefore cause pain of similar distribution. Pain down the thigh and leg ('sciatica') does not necessarily signify root pressure; it may equally well be referred from a facet joint or any painful spinal tissue.

Blood supply

In addition to the spinal arteries, which run the length of the cord, segmental arteries from the aorta send branches through the intervertebral foramina at each level. Accompanying veins drain into the azygos system and inferior vena cava, and anastomose profusely with the extradural plexus, which extends throughout the length of the spinal canal (Batson's plexus).

REFERENCES AND FURTHER READING

Archer IA, Dickson RA. Spinal deformities. 1. Basic principles. *Curr Orthop* 1989; **3:** 72–6.

Boos N, Weissbach S, Rohrbach H *et al*. Classification of age-related changes in lumbar intervertebral discs. *Spine* 2002; **27:** 2631–44.

Carroll L. (Macmillan, 1865). Alice Through the Looking Glass. Quoted from reprinted edition, Peebles Press International Inc, New York, (undated), p. 205.

Cotrel Y, Dubousset J, Guillamet M. New universal instrumentation in spinal surgery. *Clin Orthop Relat Res* 1988; **227:** 10–23.

Dickson RA. Idiopathic spinal deformities. *Curr Orthop* 1989; **3:** 77–85.

Dickson RA, Lawton JD, Archer IA, Butt WP. The pathogenesis of idiopathic scoliosis. *J Bone Joint Surg* 1984; **66B:** 8–15.

Eisenstein S. Morphometry and pathological anatomy of the lumbar spine in South African Caucasions and Negroes with special reference to spinal stenosis. *J Bone Joint Surg* 1977; **59B:** 173–80.

Eisenstein S. Spondylolysis: a skeletal investigation of two population groups. *J Bone Joint Surg* 1978; **60B:** 488–94.

Eisentein S. The trefoil configuration of the lumbar vertebral canal. *J Bone Joint Surg* 1980; **63B:** 73–7.

Eisenstein S. Lumbar vertebral canal morphometry for computerised tomography in spinal stenosis. *Spine* 1983; **8:** 187–91.

Eisenstein S, Parry CR. The lumbar facet arthrosis syndrome. Clinical presentation and articular surface changes. *J Bone Joint Surg* 1987; **69B:** 3–7.

Eisenstein S. 'Instability' and low back pain. A way out of the semantic maze. In: Szpalski M, Gunzburg R, Pope M (Eds) *Lumbar Segmental Stability*. Lippincott Williams & Wilkins, Philadelphia, 1999, pp 39–44.

Eisenstein S. Fusion for spinal stenosis: a personal view. *J Bone Joint Surg* 2002; **84B:** 9–10.

Ejeskär A, Nachemson A, Herberts P *et al*. Surgery versus chemonucleolysis for herniated lumbar discs. *Clin Orthop Relat Res* 1982; **171:** 252–9.

Fredrickson BE, Baker DR, McHolick WJ *et al*. The natural history of spondylolysis and spondylolisthesis. *J Bone Joint Surg* 1984; **66A:** 699–700.

Haughton V. Imaging intervertebral disc degeneration. *J Bone Joint Surg* 2006; **88A(Suppl 2):** 15–20.

Jones TR, Rao RD. Adult isthmic spondylolisthesis. *J Am Acad Orth Surg* 2009; **17:** 609–17.

Kellgren JH. The anatomical source of back pain. *Rheumatol Rehab* 1977; **16:** 3–14.

Kirkaldy-Willis WH, Farfan HF. Instability of the lumbar spine. *Clin Orthop Relat Res* 1982; **165:** 110–23.

Kostuik JP. Operative treatment of idiopathic scoliosis. *J Bone Joint Surg* 1990; **72A:** 1108–13.

Lehmann TR, Spratt KF, Tozzi JE *et al*. Long-term follow-up of lower lumbar fusion patients. *Spine* 1987; **12:** 97–104.

Leong JCY. Spinal infections. Pyogenic and tuberculous infections. In: Weinstein JN, Wiesel SW (Eds) *The Lumbar Spine*. WB Saunders, Philadelphia, 1990, pp 699–723.

Lonstein JE, Carlson JM. The prediction of curve progression in untreated idiopathic scoliosis during growth. *J Bone Joint Surg* 1984; **6A:** 1061–71.

McCulloch JA. Chemonucleolysis: experience with 2000 cases. *Clin Orthop Relat Res* 1980; **146:** 128–35.

Mehta MH. The rib-vertebra angle in the early diagnosis between resolving and progressive infantile scoliosis. *J Bone Joint Surg* 1972; **54B:** 230–43.

Modic MT, Ross JS, Masaryk TJ. Imaging of degenerative disease of the cervical spine. *Clin Orthop Relat Res* 1989; **239:** 109–20.

Murray PM, Weinstein SL, Spratt KF. The natural history and long-term follow-up of Scheuermann kyphosis. *J Bone Joint Surg* 1993; **75A:** 236–48.

Nachemson A, Morris JM. In vivo measurements of intradiscal pressure. *J Bone Joint Surg* 1964; **46A:** 1077–92.

Pfirrmann CW, Metzdorf A, Zanetti M *et al*. Magnetic resonance classification of lumbar intervertebral disc degeneration. *Spine* 2001; **26:** 1873–8.

Roberts S, Evans H, Trivedi J, Menage J. Histology and pathology of the human intervertebral disc. *J Bone Joint Surg* 2006; **88A(Suppl 2):** 10–14.

Travell JG, Simons DG. Myofascial Pain and Dysfunction. Williams & Wilkins, Baltimore, 1983, 1992.

Waddell G, McCulloch JA, Kummel E, Venner RM. Nonorganic physical signs in low-back pain. *Spine* 1980; **5:** 117–25.

Waddell G, Bircher M, Finlayson D, Main CJ. Symptoms and signs: physical disease or illness behaviour. *BMJ* 1984; **289:** 739–41.

Wiltse LL, Rothman SLG, Wilanowska K *et al*. Lumbar and lumbosacral spondylolisthesis. In: Weinstein JN, Weisell WB (Eds) *The Lumbar Spine* WB Saunders, Philadelphia, 1990, pp 471–545.

Zachrisson M. The back school. *Spine* 1981; **6:** 104–6.

The hip

19

Louis Solomon, Reinhold Ganz, Michael Leunig, Fergal Monsell, Ian Learmonth

CLINICAL ASSESSMENT

SYMPTOMS

Pain arising in the hip joint is felt in the groin, down the front of the thigh and, sometimes, in the knee; occasionally knee pain is the only symptom! Pain at the back of the hip is seldom from the joint; it usually derives from the lumbar spine.

Limp is the next most common symptom. It may simply be a way of coping with pain, or it may be due to a change in limb length, weakness of the hip abductors or joint instability.

Snapping or *clicking* in the hip suggests a number of causes: slipping of the gluteus maximus tendon over the greater trochanter, detachment of the acetabular labrum or psoas bursitis.

Stiffness and *deformity* are late symptoms, and tend to be well compensated for by pelvic mobility.

Walking distance may be curtailed; or, reluctantly, the patient starts using a walking stick.

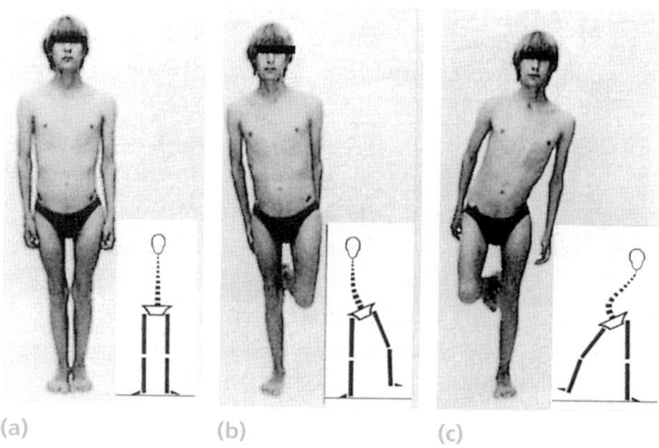

19.1 Trendelenburg's sign (a) Standing normally on two legs. (b) Standing on the right leg which has a normal hip whose abductor muscles ensure correct weight transference. (c) Standing on the left leg whose hip is faulty, and so abduction cannot be achieved; the pelvis drops on the unsupported side and the shoulder swings over to the left.

SIGNS WITH THE PATIENT UPRIGHT

Start by standing face to face with the patient and note his or her general build and the symmetry of the lower limbs. First impressions are important and can be put to the test as the examination proceeds. The patient in Figure 19.1, for example, seems to have unusually short lower limbs in comparison to his trunk length. Is it a mild type of bone dysplasia, or are the hips dislocated?

Trendelenburg's sign

This is a test for postural stability when the patient stands on one leg. In normal two-legged stance the body's centre of gravity is placed midway between the two feet. Normally, in one-legged stance, the pelvis is pulled up on the unsupported side and the centre of gravity is placed directly over the standing foot. If the weightbearing hip is unstable, the pelvis *drops* on the unsupported side; to avoid falling, the person has to throw his body towards the loaded side so that the centre of gravity is again over that foot.

If the difference between the two hips is marked you can detect it by simply looking at the patient's stance. However, small differences are not so obvious. In the classical Trendelenburg test the examiner stands behind the patient and looks at the buttock-folds. Normally in one-legged stance the buttock on the opposite side rises as the person lifts that leg; in a positive (abnormal) test the opposite buttock-fold drops (Fig. 19.2).

The causes of a positive Trendelenburg sign are: (1) pain on weightbearing; (2) weakness of the hip abductors; (3) shortening of the femoral neck; and (4) dislocation or subluxation of the hip.

Gait

Now ask the patient to walk, and observe each phase of the gait. The commonest abnormalities are a *short-leg limp* (a regular, even dip on the short side), an *antalgic gait* (an irregular limp, with the patient

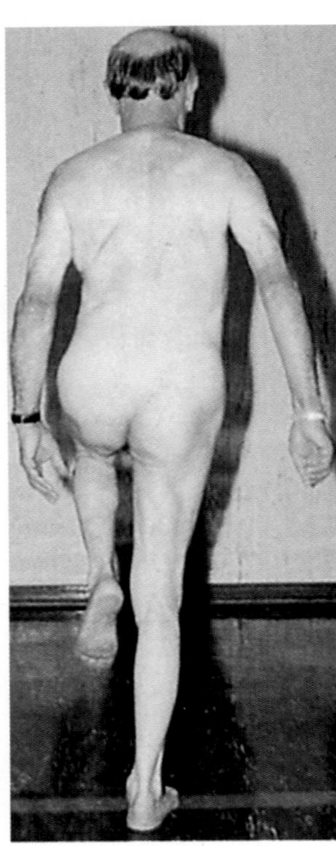

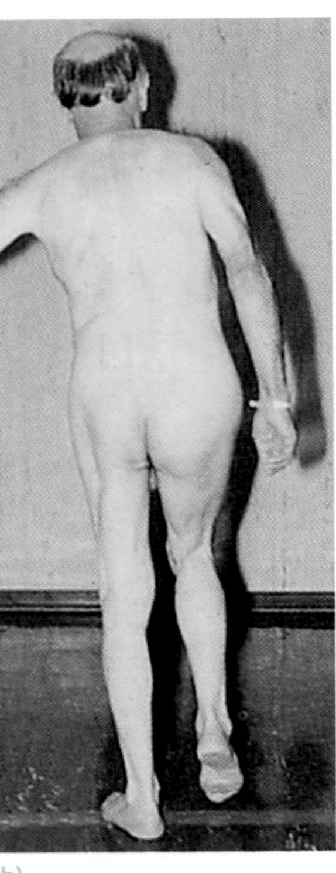

(a) (b)

19.2 Trendelenburg's test This man has a positive Trendelenburg sign on the left due to osteoarthritis of the hip. (a) He can steady himself perfectly well when balancing on the right hip; (b) when he attempts to stand on the left hip, his pelvis dips and the right buttock drops.

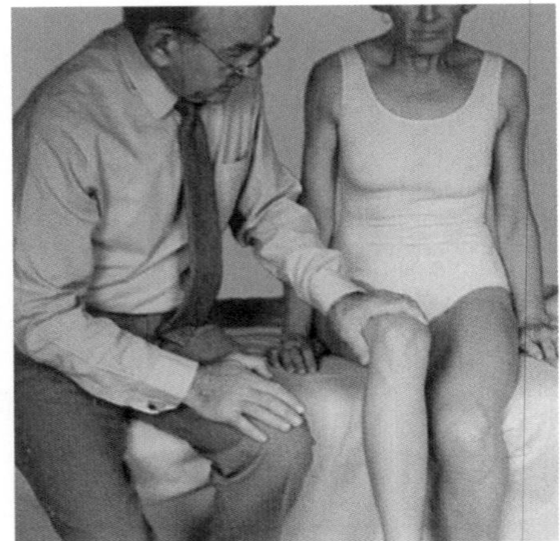

19.3 Testing iliopsoas function This is best done with the patient sitting. Ask him or her to lift the thigh (flex the hip) against resistance. In this position the psoas is acting while the other hip flexors are relaxed. Pain or weakness suggests a local disorder such as a psoas bursitis.

moving more quickly off the painful side) and a *Trendelenburg lurch* (a variant of Trendelenburg's sign).

While the patient is upright, take the opportunity to examine the spine for deformity or limitation of movement.

Signs with the patient sitting

This is the best way to test for iliopsoas function. The patient should be sitting on the edge of the examination couch. Place a hand firmly on his thigh and ask him to lift the thigh (flex the hip) against resistance. This is a predominantly psoas action; pain or weakness suggests a local disorder such as tendinitis or psoas bursitis.

Signs with the patient lying

Look

Scars or sinuses may be seen (or they may be at the back of the hip). Compare the two sides for signs of muscle wasting or swelling.

Check that the pelvis is horizontal (both anterior superior iliac spines at the same level) and the legs placed symmetrically. Limb length can be gauged by looking at the ankles and heels, but measurement is more accurate. With the two legs in identical positions, measure the distance from the anterior superior iliac spine to the medial malleolus on each side. The limb may lie in an abnormal position; excessive rotation is easy to detect but other deformities are often masked by tilting of the pelvis.

Sometimes the *real length*, as determined by measuring between two bony points, is quite different from the *apparent length* with the patient lying in repose. This happens when the pelvis is tilted and one limb is hitched upwards. Almost invariably this is due to an uncorrectable deformity at the hip: with fixed adduction on one side, the limbs would tend to be crossed; when the legs are placed side by side the pelvis has to tilt upwards on the affected side, giving the impression of a shortened limb. The exact opposite occurs when there is fixed abduction, and the limb seems to be longer on the affected side.

If real shortening is present it is usually possible to establish where the fault lies. With the knees flexed and the heels together, it can be seen whether the discrepancy is below or above the knee. If it is above, the next question is whether the abnormality lies above the greater trochanter. The thumbs are pressed firmly against the anterior superior iliac spines and the middle fingers grope for the tops of the greater trochanters; any elevation of the trochanter on one side is readily appreciated.

Feel

Skin temperature and *soft-tissue* contours can be felt, but are unhelpful unless the patient is very thin.

Bone contours are felt when levelling the pelvis and

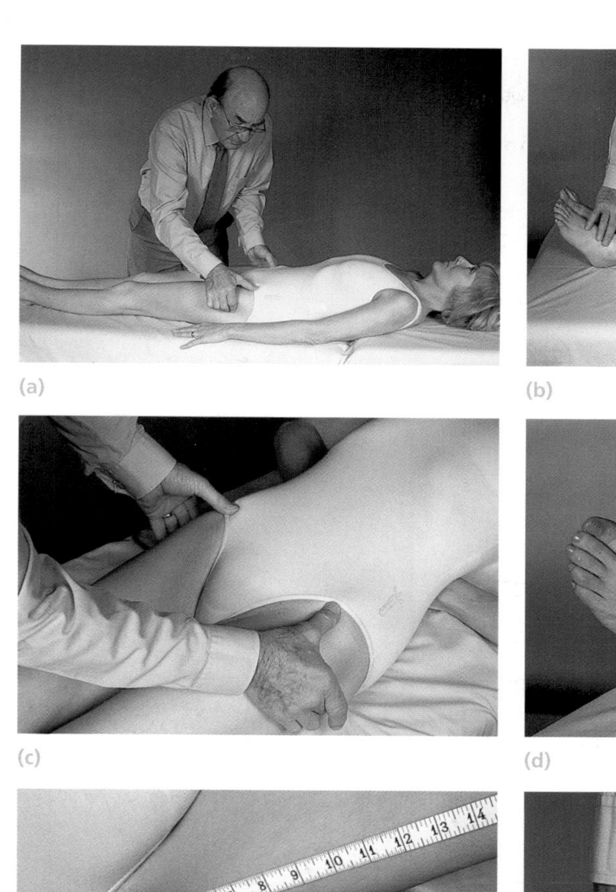

(a)

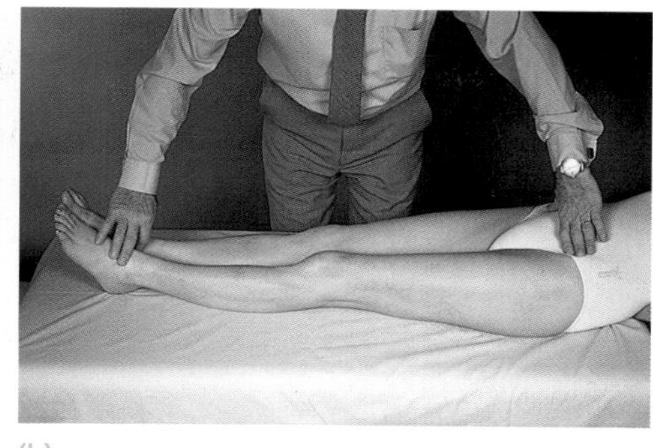

(b)

(c)

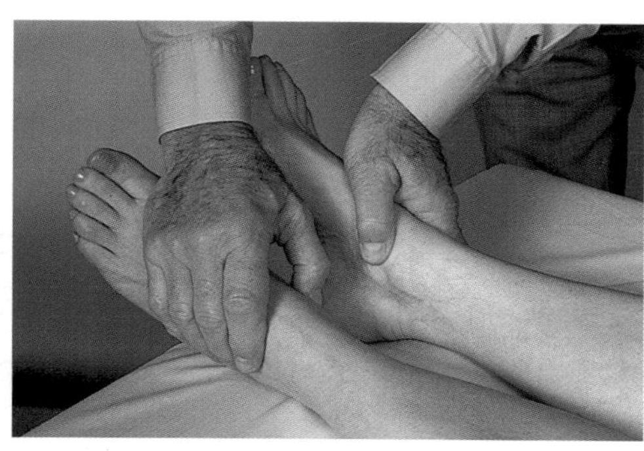

(d)

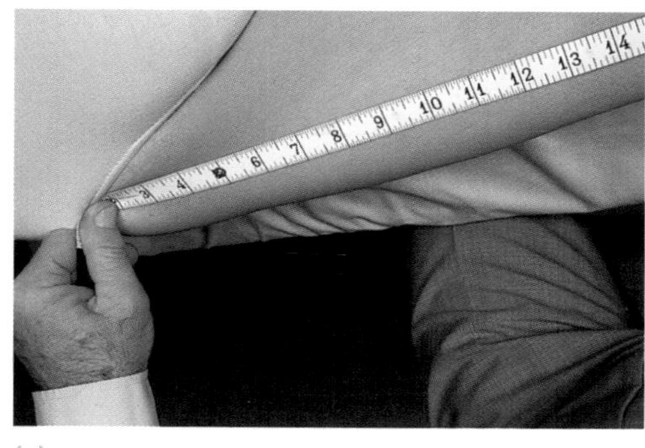

(e)

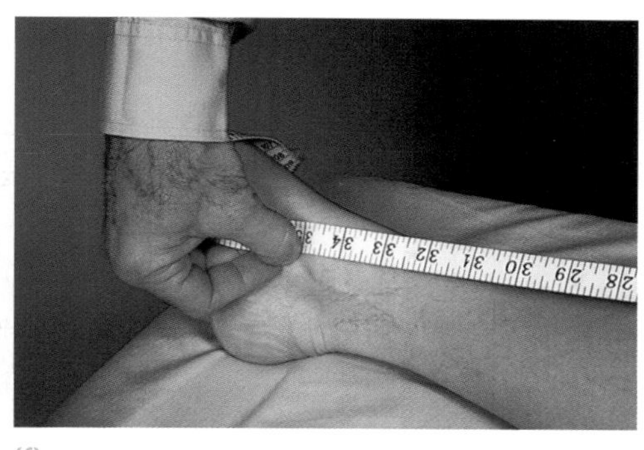

(f)

19.4 Measurement (a,b) Make sure the patient is lying straight on the examination couch and that the pelvis is absolutely level – the anterior superior iliac spines at the same level in relation to the longitudinal axis of the body (c). Then check the medial malleoli (d); discrepancy in leg length will usually be obvious. (e,f) Leg length is most accurately assessed by measuring from the anterior superior iliac spine to the tip of the medial malleolus on each side.

judging the height of the greater trochanters. *Tenderness* may be elicited in and around the joint.

Move

The assessment of hip movements is difficult because any limitation can easily be obscured by movement of the pelvis. Thus, even a gross limitation of extension, causing a *fixed flexion deformity,* can be completely masked simply by arching the back into excessive lordosis. Fortunately it can be just as easily unmasked by performing *Thomas' test* (Fig. 19.5): both hips are flexed simultaneously to their limit, thus completely obliterating the lumbar lordosis; holding the 'sound' hip firmly in position (and thus keeping the pelvis still), the other limb is lowered gently; with any flexion deformity the knee will not rest on the couch. Meanwhile the full range of *flexion* will also have been noted; the normal range is about 130 degrees.

Similarly, when testing *abduction* the pelvis must be prevented from tilting sideways. This is achieved by placing the 'sound' hip (the hip opposite to the one being examined) in full abduction and keeping it there. A hand is placed on one iliac crest to detect the slightest movement of the pelvis. Then, after checking that the anterior superior iliac spines are level, the affected joint is moved gently into abduction. The normal range is about 40 degrees.

Adduction is tested by crossing one limb over the other; the pelvis must be watched and felt to determine the point at which it starts to tilt. The normal range of adduction is about 30 degrees.

To test *rotation* both legs, lifted by the ankles, are rotated first internally (medially) and then externally (laterally); the patellae are watched to estimate the amount of rotation. Rotation in flexion is tested with the hip and knee each flexed 90 degrees.

If internal rotation is full with the hip extended, but

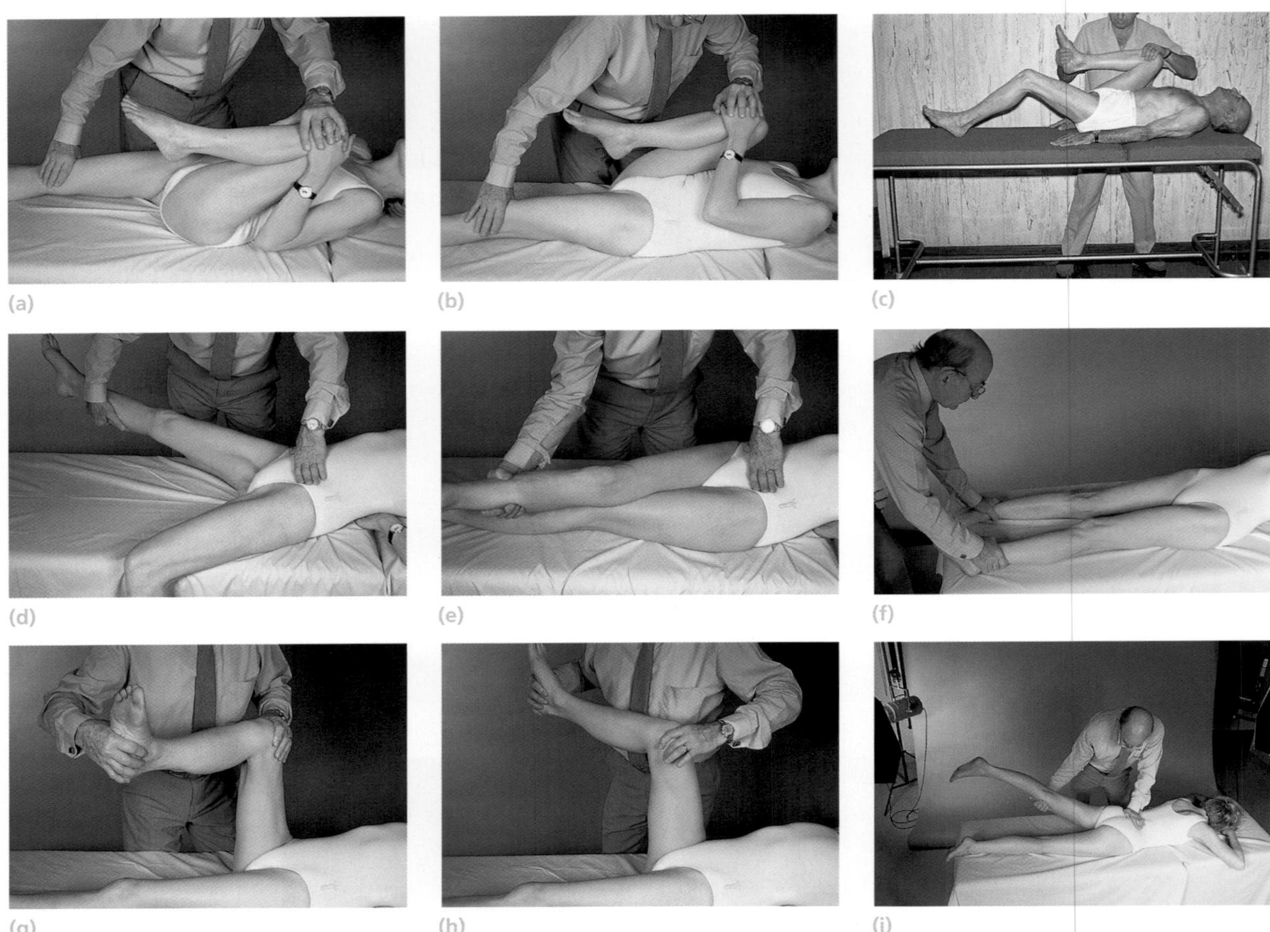

19.5 Movement (a) Forcing one hip into full flexion will straighten out the lumbar spine; the other hip should still be capable of full extension in this position. (b) Now the position is reversed; the right hip is held in full flexion. (c) If the hip cannot straighten out completely, this is referred to as a *fixed flexion deformity*. (d) Testing for abduction. The pelvis is kept level by placing the opposite leg over the edge of the examination couch with that hip also in abduction (the examiner's left hand checks the position of the anterior spines) before abducting the target hip. (e) Testing for adduction. (f–h) External and internal rotation are assessed (f) first with the hips in full extension and then (g,h) in 90° of flexion. (i) Testing for extension.

restricted in flexion, this suggests pathology in the anterosuperior portion of the femoral head, probably avascular necrosis (the so-called 'sectoral sign'). However, in a young person, pain on internal rotation with the hip flexed may indicate a torn acetabular labrum.

Abnormal movement is rarely elicited. Telescoping (excessive movement when the limb is alternately pulled and pushed in its long axis) is a sign of gross instability.

Do not forget the back of the hip. Ask the patient to roll over into the prone position. Check for scars and sinuses. Feel for tenderness and test the range of hip extension. Rotation can also be assessed by flexing both knees and moving the legs, first away from each other (producing internal rotation at the hips) and then towards or crossing each other (external rotation).

IMAGING

Plain x-rays The minimum required is an anteroposterior x-ray of the pelvis showing both hips and a lateral view of each hip separately. The two sides can be compared: any difference in the size, shape or position of the femoral heads is important. With a normal hip Shenton's line, which continues from the inferior border of the femoral neck to the inferior border of the pubic ramus, looks continuous; any interruption in the line suggests an abnormal position of the femoral head. Narrowing of the joint 'space' is a sign of articular cartilage loss, a feature of both inflammatory and non-inflammatory arthritis.

A lateral view is obligatory for assessing the shape, position and architecture of the femoral head; for

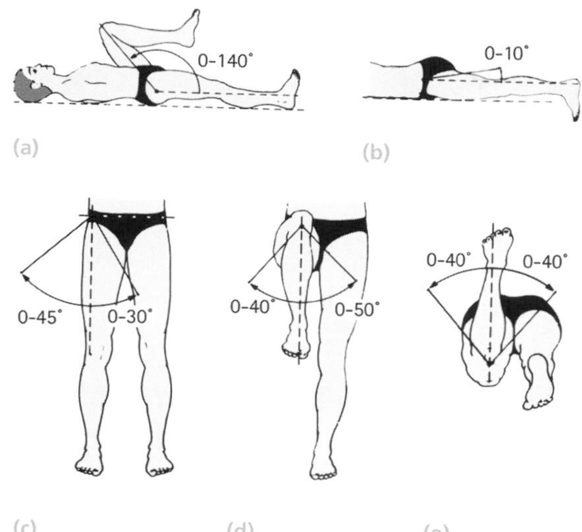

19.6 Normal range of movements (a) The hip should flex until the thigh meets the abdomen, but (b) extends only a few degrees. (c) Abduction is usually greater than adduction. The relative amounts of internal and external rotation may vary according to whether the hip is in (d) flexion or (e) extension.

example, when a slipped epiphysis or avascular necrosis is suspected.

Special tangential views are helpful when assessing congruency between the acetabular socket and the femoral head.

Ultrasonography Ultrasound scans are useful for demonstrating intra-articular effusions. This is also the ideal method of imaging in the early diagnosis of neonatal hip dysplasia, when the joint is entirely cartilaginous.

Arthrography Arthrography may be used to show the outline of the cartilaginous femoral head in young children. It may also reveal loose bodies, a loose flap of articular cartilage or a tear of the acetabular labrum.

Computed tomography CT is ideal for demonstrating structural abnormalities of the joint, e.g. in the assessment of fracture-dislocations of the hip.

Radioscintigraphy Radioisotope scans are helpful in investigating the blood supply of the femoral head or cellular activity in the subchondral bone (new bone formation or an inflammatory 'hot spot').

Magnetic resonance imaging This is ideal for detecting changes in the marrow and is the only certain way of diagnosing early avascular necrosis, in which the changes are confined to the marrow.

ARTHROSCOPY

Arthroscopy has come much later to the hip than to other joints such as the knee and shoulder. The indications for its use are still being defined. In a review of 328 patients presenting with pain in the hip and subsequently undergoing arthroscopy, it was reported that in over half the cases the procedure contributed to the diagnosis beyond the information derived from clinical and imaging studies. In 172 cases some type of operation was performed as well, usually debridement

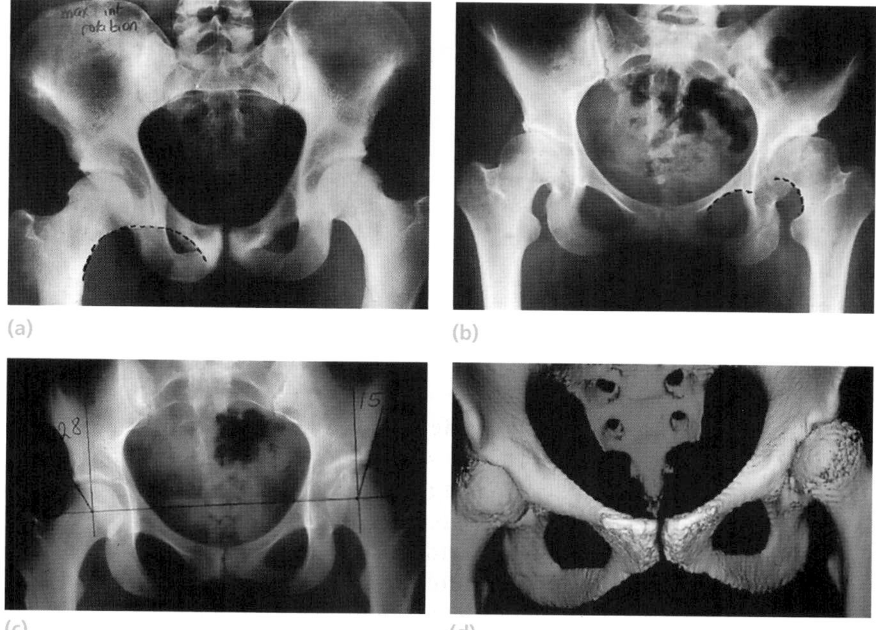

19.7 Imaging (a) Anteroposterior x-ray of normal hips, showing Shenton's line. (b) X-ray of a patient with secondary osteoarthritis of the left hip due to congenital subluxation. The joint 'space' is narrowed and Shenton's line is broken. (c,d) X-ray and three-dimensional CT showing how shallow the acetabula are, and how much of the femoral head is uncovered, especially in this dysplastic left hip. (Courtesy of Professor Kjeld Søballe. Århus Universitetshopital.)

Table 19.1 The diagnostic calendar: age of onset can be a guide to probable diagnosis

Age of onset (years)	Probable diagnosis
0 (birth)	Developmental dysplasia
0–5	Infections
5–10	Perthes' disease
10–20	Slipped epiphysis
Adults	Arthritis

of osteoarthritic tissue, extraction of loose bodies, debridement of labral tears and biopsies (Baber et al., 1999). Arthroscopy is now considered to be more reliable than MRI for the diagnosis of non-osseous loose bodies, labral tears and cartilage surface damage.

THE DIAGNOSTIC CALENDAR

Hip disorders are characteristically seen in certain well-defined age groups. While there are exceptions to this rule, it is sufficiently true to allow the age at onset to serve as a guide to the probable diagnosis (see Table 19.1).

DEVELOPMENTAL DYSPLASIA OF THE HIP

The terminology used to describe abnormalities of the paediatric hip is imprecise and confusing. The term 'congenital dislocation of the hip' (CDH) has been largely superseded by *developmental dysplasia of the hip (DDH)* in an attempt to describe the range and evolution of abnormalities that occur in this condition. This comprises a spectrum of disorders including acetabular dysplasia without displacement, subluxation and dislocation. Teratological forms of malarticulation leading to dislocation are also included.

Normal hip development depends on proportionate growth of the acetabular triradiate cartilages and the presence of a concentrically located femoral head. Whether the instability comes first and then affects acetabular development because of imperfect seating of the femoral head, or is a result of a primary acetabular dysplasia, is still uncertain. Both mechanisms might be important.

The reported incidence of neonatal hip instability in northern Europe is approximately 1 per 1000 live births, but this is dependent on the definition of 'instability'. Barlow (1962) described an incidence of 1:60; however 60 per cent stabilized by one week and 88 per cent by 8 weeks. The incidence is considerably higher in some ethnic groups – 25–50 cases per 1000 live births in Lapps and Native Americans!

Girls are much more commonly affected than boys, the ratio being about 7:1. The left hip is more often affected than the right; in 1 in 5 cases the condition is bilateral.

Aetiology and pathogenesis

Genetic factors must play a part in the aetiology, for DDH tends to run in families and even in entire populations (e.g. in countries along the northern and eastern Mediterranean seaboard). Wynne-Davies (1970) identified two heritable features which could predispose to hip instability: generalized joint laxity (a dominant trait), and shallow acetabula (a polygenic trait which is seen mainly in girls and their mothers). However, this cannot be the whole story because in 4 out of 5 cases only one hip is dislocated.

Hormonal factors (e.g. high levels of maternal oestrogen, progesterone and relaxin in the last few weeks of pregnancy) may aggravate ligamentous laxity in the infant. This could account for the rarity of instability in premature babies, born before the hormones reach their peak.

Intrauterine malposition (especially a breech position with extended legs) favours dislocation; this so-called 'packaging disorder' is linked with the higher incidence in first-born babies, among whom spontaneous version is less likely. Unilateral dislocation usually affects the left hip; this fits with the usual vertex presentation (left occiput anterior) in which the left hip is adjacent to the mother's sacrum, placing it in an adducted position. Other manifestations of intrauterine crowding, including plagiocephaly, congenital torticollis and postural foot deformities, are also associated with a higher than usual incidence of DDH.

Postnatal factors may contribute to persistence of neonatal instability and acetabular maldevelopment. Dislocation is very common in Lapps and North American Indians who swaddle their babies and carry them with legs together, hips and knees fully extended, and is rare in southern Chinese and African Negroes who carry their babies astride their backs with legs widely abducted. There is also experimental evidence that simultaneous hip and knee extension leads to hip dislocation during early development (Yamamuro and Ishida, 1984).

Pathology

At birth the hip, though unstable, is probably normal in shape but the capsule is often stretched and redundant.

During infancy a number of changes develop, some

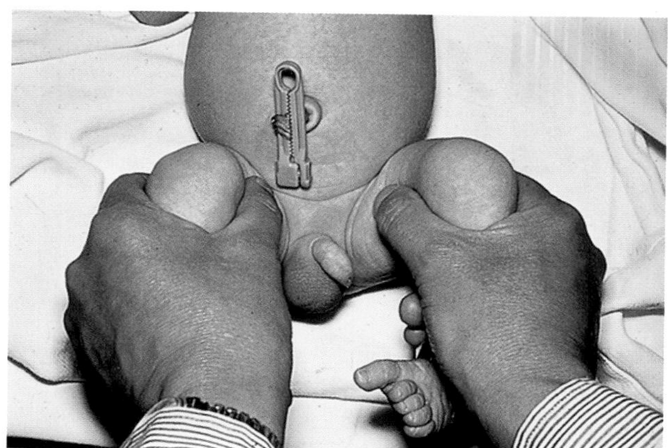

19.8 Developmental dysplasia of the hip (DDH) – early signs Position of the hands for performing Ortolani's test.

of them perhaps reflecting a primary dysplasia of the acetabulum and/or the proximal femur, but most of them from adaptation to persistent instability and abnormal joint loading.

The femoral head dislocates posteriorly but, with extension of the hips, it comes to lie first posterolateral and then superolateral to the acetabulum. The cartilaginous socket is shallow and anteverted. The cartilaginous femoral head is normal in size but the bony nucleus appears late and its ossification is delayed throughout infancy.

The capsule is stretched and the ligamentum teres becomes elongated and hypertrophied. Superiorly the acetabular labrum and its capsular edge may be pushed into the socket by the dislocated femoral head; this fibrocartilaginous limbus may obstruct any attempt at closed reduction of the femoral head.

After weightbearing commences, these changes are intensified. Both the acetabulum and the femoral neck remain anteverted and the pressure of the femoral head induces a false socket to form above the shallow acetabulum. The capsule, squeezed between the edge of the acetabulum and the psoas muscle, develops an hourglass appearance. In time the surrounding muscles become adaptively shortened.

Clinical features

The ideal, still unrealized, is to diagnose every case at birth. For this reason, every newborn child should be examined for signs of hip instability. Where there is a family history of congenital instability, and with breech presentations or signs of other congenital abnormalities, extra care is taken and the infant may have to be examined more than once. Even then some cases are missed.

In the neonate There are several ways of testing for instability. In *Ortolani's test*, the baby's thighs are held with the thumbs medially and the fingers resting on the greater trochanters; the hips are flexed to 90 degrees and gently abducted. Normally there is smooth abduction to almost 90 degrees. In congenital dislocation the movement is usually impeded, but if pressure is applied to the greater trochanter there is a soft 'clunk' as the dislocation reduces, and then the hip abducts fully (the 'jerk of entry'). If abduction stops halfway and there is no jerk of entry, there may be an irreducible dislocation.

Barlow's test is performed in a similar manner, but here the examiner's thumb is placed in the groin and, by grasping the upper thigh, an attempt is made to lever the femoral head in and out of the acetabulum during abduction and adduction. If the femoral head is normally in the reduced position, but can be made to slip out of the socket and back in again, the hip is classed as 'dislocatable' (i.e. unstable).

Every hip with signs of instability – however slight – should be examined by *ultrasonography.* This shows the shape of the cartilaginous socket and the position of the femoral head. If there is any abnormality, the infant is placed in a splint with the hips flexed and abducted (see under Management) and is recalled for re-examination – in the splint – at 2 weeks and at 6 weeks. By then it should be possible to assess whether the hip is reduced and stable, reduced but unstable (dislocatable by Barlow's test), subluxated or dislocated.

Late features An observant mother may spot asymmetry, a clicking hip, or difficulty in applying the napkin (diaper) because of limited abduction.

With unilateral dislocation the skin creases look asymmetrical and the leg is slightly short (Galeazzi's sign) and externally rotated; a thumb in the groin may feel that the femoral head is missing. With bilateral dislocation there is an abnormally wide perineal gap. Abduction is decreased.

Contrary to popular belief, late walking is not a marked feature; nevertheless, in children who do not walk by 18 months dislocation must be excluded. Likewise, a limp or Trendelenburg gait, or a waddling gait could be a sign of missed dislocation.

Imaging

Ultrasonography Ultrasound scanning has replaced radiography for imaging hips in the newborn. The radiographically 'invisible' acetabulum and femoral head can, with practice, be displayed with static and dynamic ultrasound. Sequential assessment is straightforward and allows monitoring of the hip during a period of splintage.

Plain x-rays X-rays of infants are difficult to interpret and in the newborn they can be frankly misleading. This is because the acetabulum and femoral head are

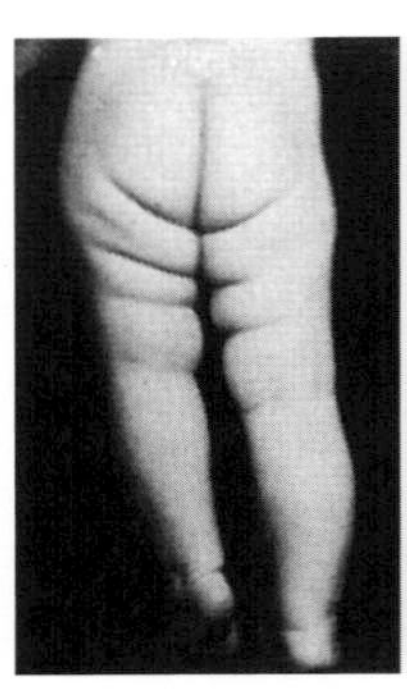

(a)

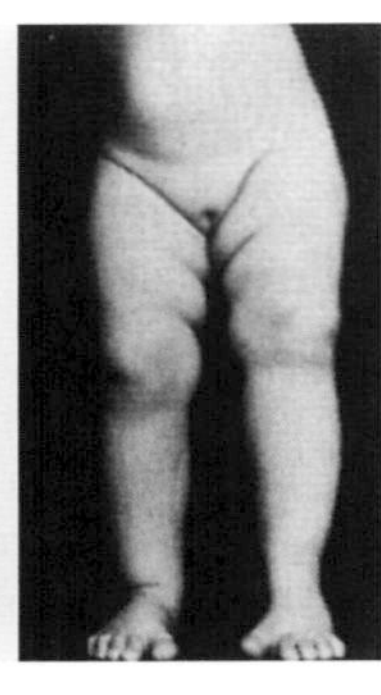

(b)

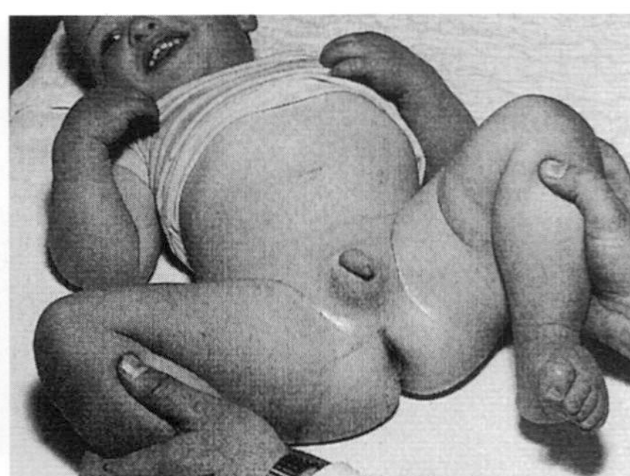

(c)

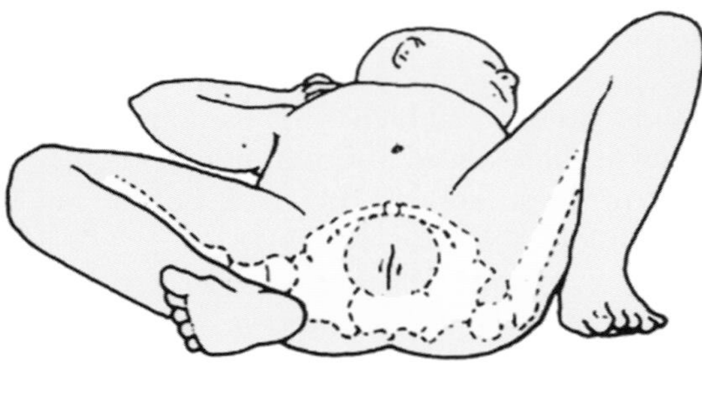

(d)

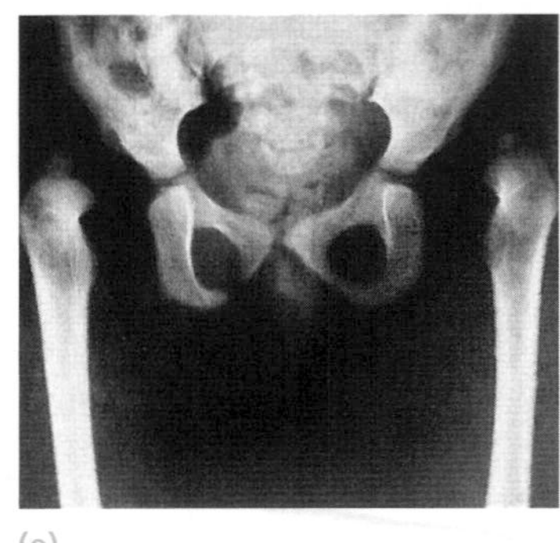

(e)

19.9 DDH – late signs (a,b) Unilateral dislocation of the left hip. (c) The left hip does not abduct more than half way, and (d) the drawing shows why – the femoral head is caught up on the rim of the acetabulum. (e) X-ray showing bilateral displacement of the hip.

largely (or entirely) cartilaginous and therefore not visible on x-ray. X-ray examination is more useful after the first 6 months, and assessment is helped by drawing lines on the x-ray plate to define three geometric indices (Fig. 19.10).

Screening

Neonatal screening in dedicated centres has led to a marked reduction in missed cases of DDH. *Risk factors* such as family history, breech presentation, oligohydramnios and the presence of other congenital abnormalities are taken into account in selecting newborn infants for special examination and ultrasonography. Ideally all neonates should be examined, but if the programme is to be effective those doing the examining should receive special training (Harcke and Kumar, 1991; Jones, 1994).

Management

THE FIRST 3–6 MONTHS

Where facilities for ultrasound scanning are available, all newborn infants with a high-risk background or a suggestion of hip instability are examined by ultrasonography. If this shows that the hip is reduced and has a normal cartilaginous outline, no treatment is required but the child is kept under observation for 3–6 months. In the presence of acetabular dysplasia or hip instability, the hip is splinted in a position of flexion and abduction (see below) and ultrasound scanning is repeated at intervals until stability and normal anatomy are restored or a decision is made to abandon splintage in favour of more aggressive treatment.

If ultrasound is not available, the simplest policy is to regard all infants with a high-risk background or a positive Ortolani or Barlow test, as 'suspect' and to nurse them in double napkins or an abduction pillow for the first 6 weeks. At that stage they are re-examined: those with stable hips are left free but kept under observation for at least 6 months; those with persistent instability are treated by more formal abduction splintage (see below) until the hip is stable and x-ray shows that the acetabular roof is developing satisfactorily (usually 3–6 months)

There are two drawbacks to this approach: (1) the sensitivity of the clinical tests is not high enough to ensure that all cases will be spotted (Jones, 1994); and (2) of those hips that are unstable at birth, 80–90 per cent will stabilize spontaneously in 2–3 weeks. It therefore seems more sensible not to start splintage immediately unless the hip is already dislocated. This reduces the small (but significant) risk of epiphyseal necrosis that attends any form of restrictive splintage in the neonate. Thus: if a hip is dislocatable but not habitually dislocated, the baby is left untreated but re-examined weekly; if at 3 weeks the hip is still unstable, abduction splintage is applied (see below). If the hip is already dislocated at the first examination, it is gently placed in the reduced position and abduction splintage is applied from the outset. Reduction is maintained until the hip is stable; this may take only a

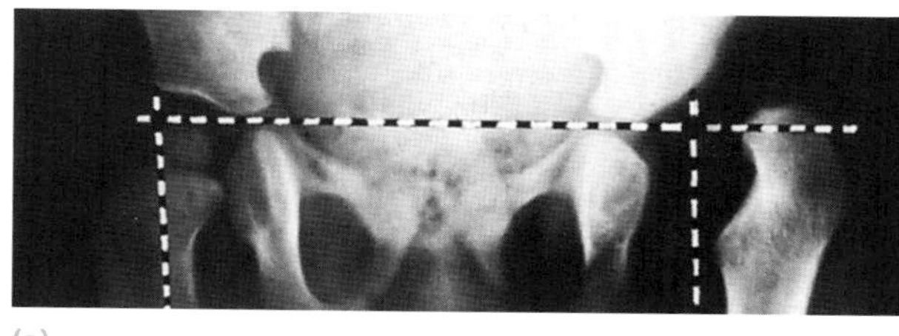

(a)

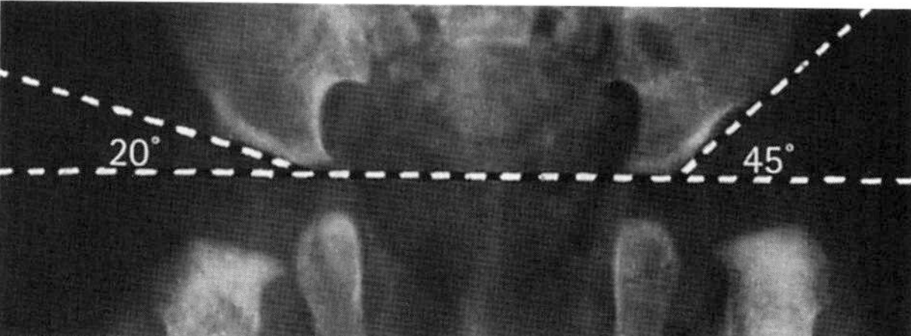

(b)

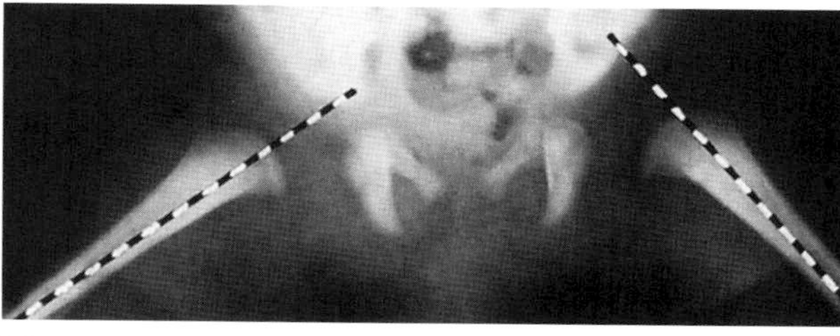

(c)

19.10 DDH – X-rays (a) The left hip is dislocated, the femoral head is underdeveloped and the acetabular roof slopes upwards much more steeply than on the right side. In this case the features are very obvious but lesser changes can be gauged by geometrical tests. The epiphysis should lie medial to a vertical line which defines the outer edge of the acetabulum (Perkins' line) and below a horizontal line which passes through the triradiate cartilages (Hilgenreiner's line). (b) The acetabular roof angle should not exceed 30°. (c) Von Rosen's lines: with the hips abducted 45° the femoral shafts should point into the acetabula. In each case the left side is shown to be abnormal.

few weeks, but the safest policy is to retain some sort of splintage until x-ray shows a good acetabular roof.

Splintage The object of splintage is to hold the hips somewhat flexed and abducted; extreme positions are avoided and the joints should be allowed some movement in the splint. Von Rosen's splint is an H-shaped malleable splint that has the merit of being easy to apply (and the demerit of being equally easy to take off!). The Pavlik harness is more difficult to apply but gives the child more freedom while still maintaining position. The three golden rules of splintage are: (1) the hip must be properly reduced before it is splinted; (2) extreme positions must be avoided; (3) the hips should be able to move. If the hip is splinted in a subluxed/dislocated position, the posterior wall of the acetabulum is at risk of growth disturbance, leading to considerable difficulties with later reconstruction. This situation must be avoided; if the hip fails to locate, splintage should be abandoned in favour of closed or operative reduction at a later date.

Follow-up Whatever policy is adopted, follow-up is continued until the child is walking. Sometimes, even with the most careful treatment, the hip may later show some degree of acetabular dysplasia.

PERSISTENT DISLOCATION: 6–18 MONTHS

If, after early treatment, the hip is still incompletely reduced, or if the child presents late with a 'missed' dislocation, the hip must be reduced – preferably by closed methods but if necessary by operation – and held reduced until acetabular development is satisfactory.

Closed reduction Closed reduction is suitable after the age of 3 months and is performed under general anaesthesia with an arthrogram to confirm a concentric reduction. To minimize the risk of avascular necrosis, reduction must be gentle and may be preceded by gradual traction to both legs.

Failure to achieve concentric reduction should lead to abandoning this method in favour of an operative approach at approximately 1 year of age. The hips should be stable in a safe zone of abduction, which may be increased with a closed adductor tenotomy.

Splintage The concentrically reduced hip is held in a plaster spica at 60 degrees of flexion, 40 degrees of abduction and 20 degrees of internal rotation. After 6 weeks the spica is changed and the stability of the hips

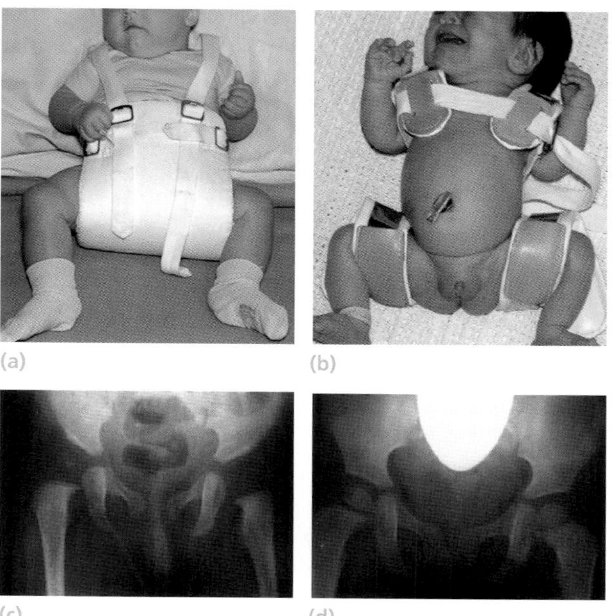

(a) (b) (c) (d)

19.11 DDH – early treatment (a,b) Various types of abduction splint. (c,d) X-rays showing result of splintage for DDH of the right hip at 3 months and 18 months.

assessed under anaesthesia. Provided the position and stability are satisfactory the spica is retained for a further 6 weeks. Following plaster removal the hip is either left unsplinted or managed in a removable abduction splint which is retained for up to 6 months depending on radiological evidence of satisfactory acetabular development.

Operation If, at any stage, concentric reduction has not been achieved, open operation is needed. The psoas tendon is divided; obstructing tissues (redundant capsule and thickened ligamentum teres) are removed and the hip is reduced. It is usually stable in 60 degrees of flexion, 40 degrees of abduction and 20 degrees of internal rotation. A spica is applied and the hip is splinted as described above.

If stability can be achieved only by markedly internally rotating the hip, a corrective subtrochanteric osteotomy of the femur is carried out, either at the time of open reduction or 6 weeks later. In young children this usually gives a good result (Fig. 19.12a, b).

PERSISTENT DISLOCATION: 18 MONTHS – 4 YEARS

In the older child, closed reduction is less likely to succeed; many surgeons would proceed straight to arthrography and open reduction.

Traction Even if closed reduction is unsuccessful, a period of traction (if necessary combined with psoas and adductor tenotomy) may help to loosen the tissues and bring the femoral head down opposite the acetabulum.

Arthrography An arthrogram at this stage will clarify the anatomy of the hip and show whether there is an inturned limbus or any marked degree of acetabular dysplasia.

Operation The joint capsule is opened anteriorly, any redundant capsule is removed along with any other blocks to reduction including the hypertrophied ligamentum teres and transverse acetabular ligament and the femoral head is seated in the acetabulum. Usually a derotation femoral osteotomy held by a plate and screws will be required. At the same time a 1 cm segment can be removed from the proximal femur to reduce pressure on the hip (Klisic and Jankovic, 1976). If there is marked acetabular dysplasia, some form of acetabuloplasty will also be needed – either a pericapsular reconstruction of the acetabular roof (Pemberton's operation) or an innominate (Salter) osteotomy which repositions the entire innominate bone and acetabulum (Fig. 19.12).

Splintage After operation, the hip is held in a plaster spica for 3 months and then left unsupported to allow recovery of movement. The child is kept under intermittent clinical and radiological surveillance until skeletal maturity.

DISLOCATION IN CHILDREN OVER 4 YEARS

Reduction and stabilization become increasingly difficult with advancing age. Nevertheless, in children between 4 and 8 years – especially if the dislocation is unilateral – it is still worth attempting, bearing in mind that the risk of avascular necrosis and hip stiffness is reported as being in excess of 25 per cent. The principles of treatment are as described immediately above.

Unilateral dislocation in the child over 8 years often leaves the child with a mobile hip and little pain. This is the justification for non-intervention, though in that case the child must accept the fact that gait is distinctly abnormal. If reduction is attempted it will require an open operation and acetabular reconstruc-

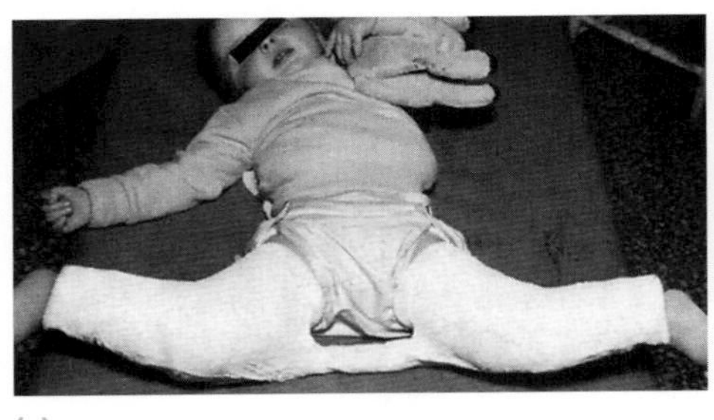
(a)

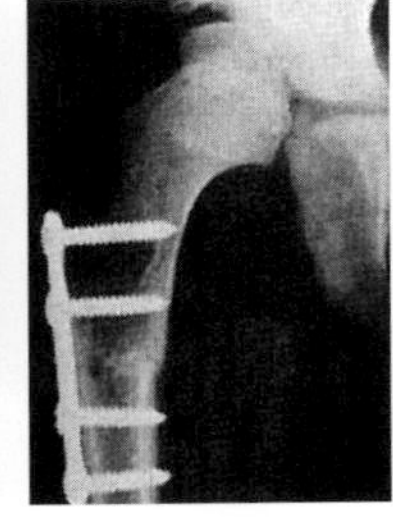
(b)

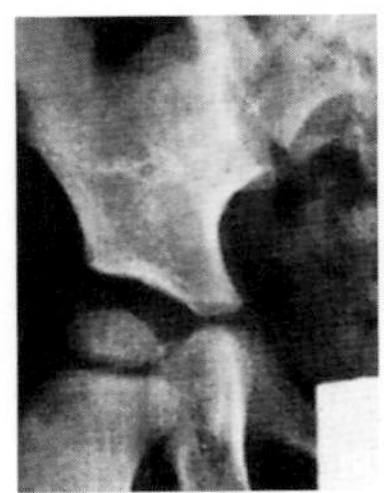
(c)

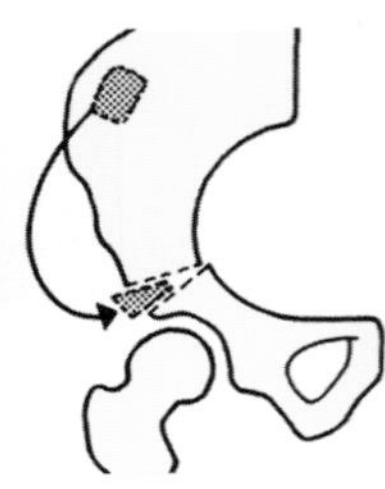
(d)

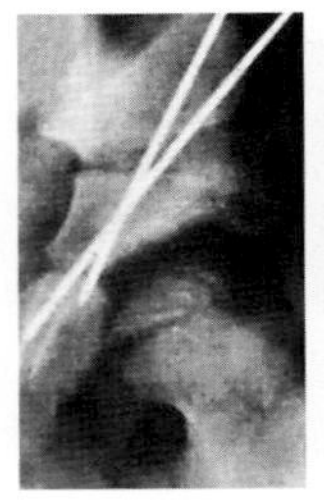
(e)

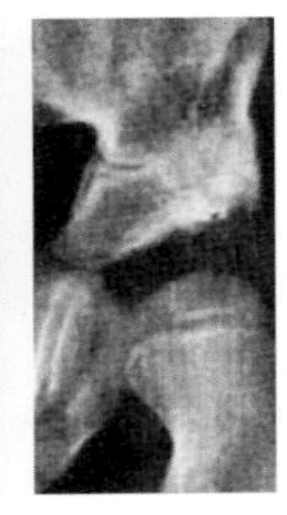
(f)

19.12 Congenital hip dislocation – operative treatment (a) Reduced open, but stable only in medial rotation – 6 weeks later; (b) derotation osteotomy. (c) Reduced open, but head poorly covered; (d) innominate osteotomy. (e,f) X-rays after Salter innominate osteotomy of the left hip.

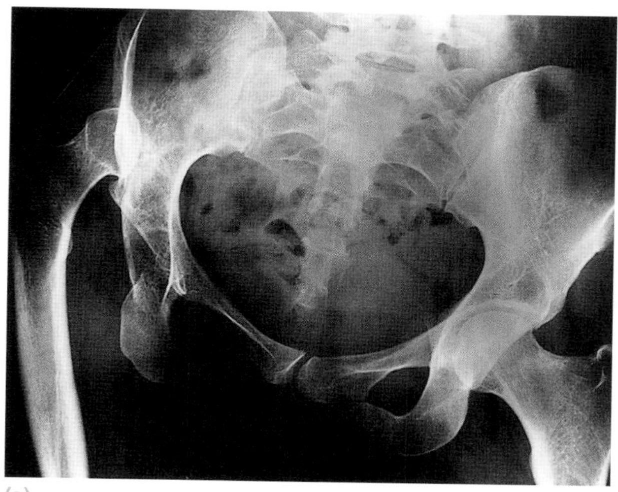

(a)

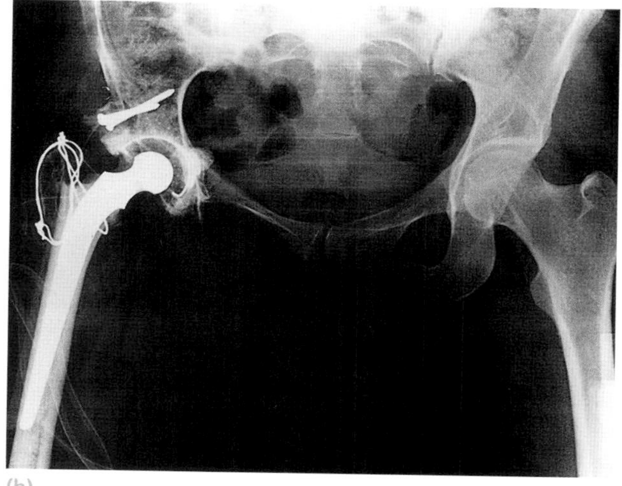

(b)

19.13 Untreated DDH (a) This patient, aged 35 years, had a short leg, a severe limp and back pain. (b) Hip replacement restored her to near normality.

tion. These procedures are best undertaken in centres specializing in this area.

With *bilateral dislocation* the deformity – and the waddling gait – is symmetrical and therefore not so noticeable; the risk of operative intervention is also greater because failure on one or other side turns this into an asymmetrical deformity. Therefore, in these cases, most surgeons avoid operation above the age of 6 years unless the hip is painful or deformity unusually severe. The untreated patient walks with a waddle but may be surprisingly uncomplaining.

Complications

Failed reduction Multiple attempts at treatment, with failure to achieve concentric reduction, may be worse than no treatment. The acetabulum remains undeveloped, the femoral head may be deformed, the neck is usually anteverted and the capsule is thickened and adherent. It is important to enquire also *why* reduction failed: is the dislocation part of a generalized condition, or a neuromuscular disorder associated with muscle imbalance? The principles of treatment for children over 8 years are the same as those discussed above.

Avascular necrosis A much-feared complication of treatment is ischaemia of the immature femoral head. It may occur at any age and any stage of treatment and is probably due to vascular injury or obstruction resulting from forceful reduction and hip splintage in abduction. The effects vary considerably: in the mildest cases the changes are confined to the ossific nucleus, which appears to be slightly distorted and irregular on x-ray. The cartilaginous epiphysis retains the shape and physical growth is normal. After 12–24 months the appearances return to normal. In more severe cases the epiphyseal and physeal growth plates also suffer; the ossific nucleus looks fragmented, the epiphysis is distorted to greater or lesser extent and metaphyseal changes lead to shortening and deformity of the femoral neck.

Prevention is the best cure: forced manipulative reduction should not be allowed; traction should be gentle and in the neutral position; positions of extreme abduction must be avoided; soft-tissue release (adductor tenotomy) should precede closed reduction; and if difficulty is anticipated open reduction is preferable.

Once the condition is established, there is no effective treatment except to avoid manipulation and weightbearing until the epiphysis has healed. In the mildest cases there will be no residual deformity, or at worst a femoral neck deformity which can be corrected by osteotomy. In severe cases the outcome may be flattening and mushrooming of the femoral head, shortening of the neck (with or without coxa vara), acetabular dysplasia and incongruency of the hip. Surgical correction of the proximal femur and pelvic osteotomy to reposition or deepen the acetabulum may be needed.

Persistent dislocation in adults

Adults who appear to have managed quite well for many years may present in their thirties or forties with increasing discomfort due to an unreduced congenital dislocation. Walking becomes more and more tiring and backache is common. With bilateral dislocation, the loss of abduction may hamper sexual intercourse in women.

Disability may be severe enough to justify *total joint replacement*. The operation is difficult and should be

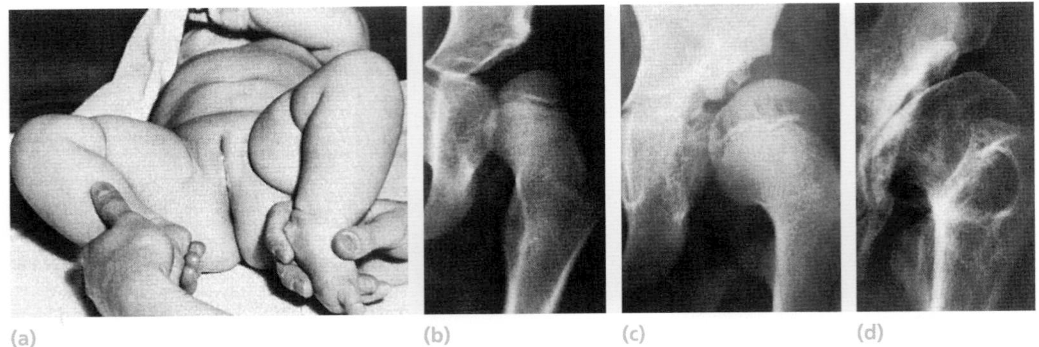

(a) (b) (c) (d)

19.14 Congenital subluxation (a) The cardinal physical sign, restricted abduction; (b) X-ray in childhood; (c) in adolescence; (d) degeneration in early adult life.

undertaken only by those with experience of hip reconstructive surgery. The femoral head is seated above the acetabulum, which is shallow or completely obliterated. A new socket should be fashioned at the normal anatomical site; however, the pelvic wall is usually thin and it may be necessary to build up the roof of the socket with bone grafts. It is then difficult to bring the femoral head down to the level of the socket without risking damage to the sciatic nerve; if necessary, an osteotomy should be performed and a small segment of femoral bone removed to allow a safe fit. The proximal femur is usually very narrow and the neck may be markedly anteverted; this also may need correction when the osteotomy is performed, and special implants are available to fit the small medullary canal.

ACETABULAR DYSPLASIA AND SUBLUXATION OF THE HIP

Acetabular dysplasia may be genetically determined or may follow incomplete reduction of a congenital dislocation, damage to the lateral acetabular epiphysis or maldevelopment of the femoral head (either congenital or, for example, after Perthes' disease). The socket is unusually shallow, the roof is sloping and there is deficient coverage of the femoral head superolaterally and anteriorly; in some cases the hip subluxates. Faulty load transmission in the lateral part of the joint may lead to secondary osteoarthritis (OA).

Clinical features

During infancy, dysplasia may be clinically silent and only apparent on ultrasound examination. If there is associated instability, Barlow's test may be positive, but other clinical indicators including loss of abduction may be absent.

In children the condition is usually asymptomatic and discovered only when the pelvis is x-rayed for some other reason. Sometimes, however, the hip is painful – especially after strenuous activity – and the child may develop a limp. If there is subluxation the Trendelenburg sign is positive, leg length may be asymmetrical and the femoral head may be felt as a

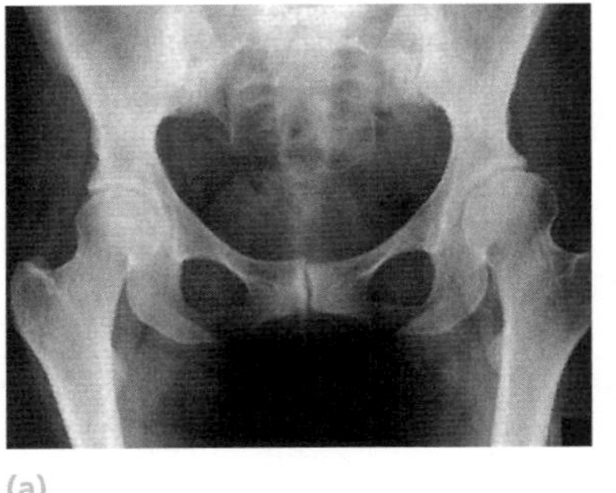

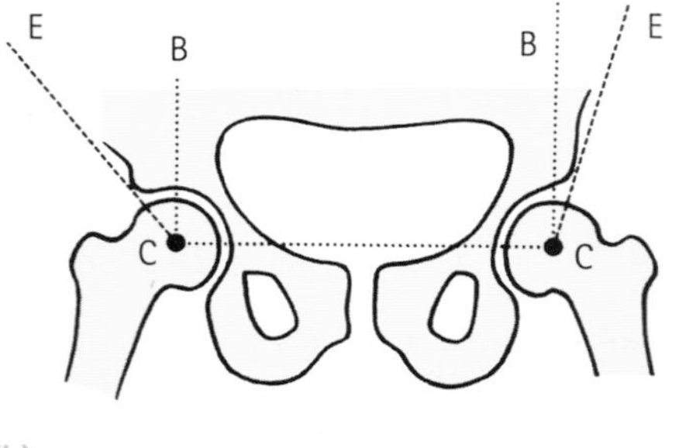

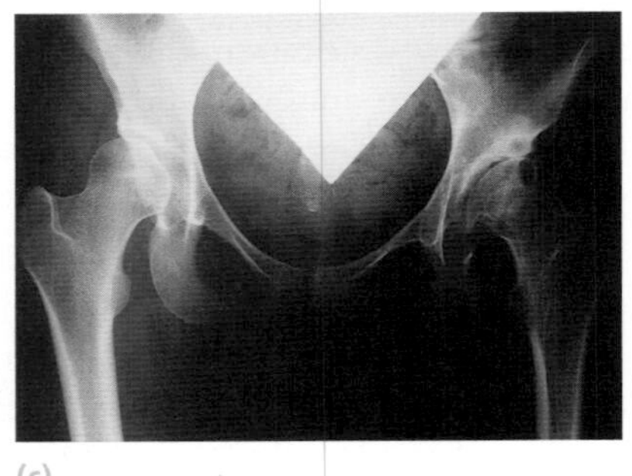

(a) (b) (c)

19.15 Acetabular dysplasia (a) X-ray showing a dysplastic left acetabulum. The socket is shallow and the roof sloping, leaving much of the femoral head uncovered. Note that the femoral neck–shaft angle is somewhat valgus on both sides. (b) Measuring Wiberg's centre–edge (CE) angle; the line C–C joins the centre of each femoral head; C–B is perpendicular to this and C–E cuts the superior edge of the acetabulum. The angle BCE should not be less than 30°; in this case the left hip is abnormal. (c) X-ray of another patient showing acetabular dysplasia on the right side and secondary osteoarthritis in an untreated dysplastic left hip.

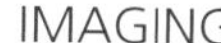

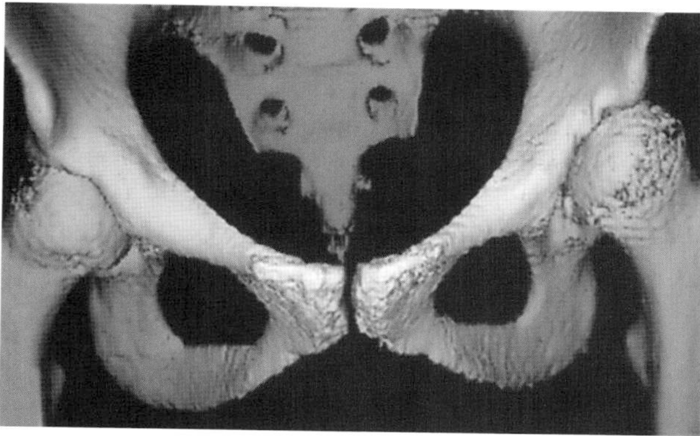

19.16 Acetabular dysplasia – three-dimensional CT Three-dimensional CT shows the full extent of the hip dysplasia in several planes, which is ideal for planning reconstructive surgery.

lump in the groin; movement – particularly abduction in flexion – is restricted.

Older adolescents and *young adults* may complain of pain over the lateral side of the hip, probably due to muscle fatigue and/or segmental overload towards the edge of the acetabulum. Some experience episodes of sharp pain in the groin, possibly the result of a labral tear or detachment.

Older adults (predominantly in their thirties and forties) usually present with features of secondary OA. Indeed, in southern Europe dysplasia of the hip is the commonest cause of symptomatic OA.

NOTE: It is worth emphasizing that most people with mild acetabular dysplasia go through life without knowing that they are in any way abnormal and the condition exists only as a 'x-ray diagnosis'.

IMAGING

X-rays should be taken lying and standing (the latter may show minor degrees of incongruity). In the supine anteroposterior radiograph, the acetabulum looks shallow, the roof is sloping and the femoral head is uncovered. Subtle abnormalities are revealed by measuring the depth of the socket and the relationship between the centre of the femoral head and the edge of the acetabulum – Wiberg's centre–edge (CE) angle. With subluxation, Shenton's line is broken. The *faux profil* (oblique view) of the hip in the standing position will demonstrate acetabular dysplasia and incipient OA in the young adult. Congruity and stability of the hip may be best assessed by examination and dynamic arthrography under anaesthesia (Catterall, 1992).

CT and *MRI* are helpful in those who are considered for operative treatment. Three-dimensional CT reconstruction is particularly useful in providing an accurate picture of the anatomy.

Diagnosis

It is often difficult to be sure that the patient's symptoms are due to the dysplastic acetabulum; other conditions causing pain and limp must be excluded (see Box on page 514).

Bilateral dysplasia is a feature of developmental disorders, such as multiple epiphyseal dysplasia.

Treatment

Infants with subluxation are treated as for dislocation: the hip is splinted in abduction until the acetabular roof looks normal.

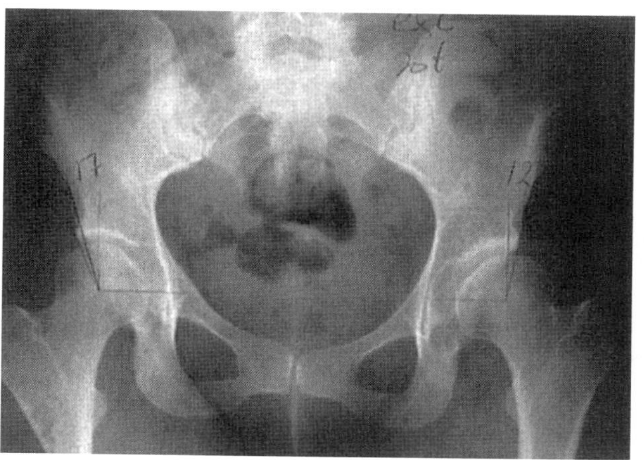

(a)

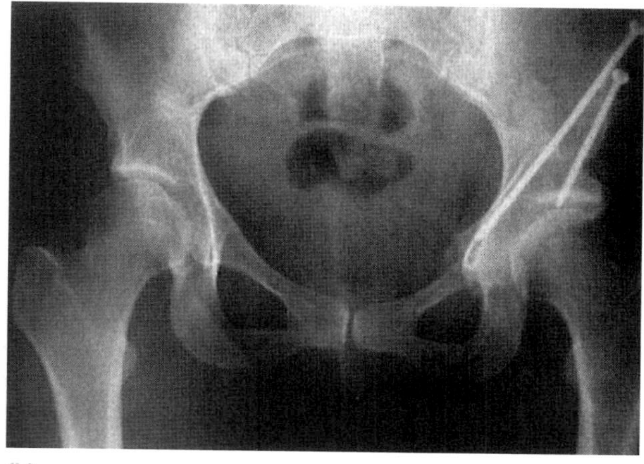

(b)

19.17 Acetabular dysplasia – peri-acetabular osteotomy (a) Bilateral acetabular dysplasia, symptomatic on the left. (b) X-ray after peri-acetabular osteotomy. Cuts were made through the innominate, the ischium and the lateral part of the superior pubic ramus; the entire segment containing the acetabulum was then rotated so as to cover the load-bearing part of the femoral head superolaterally and anteriorly. (Courtesy of Professor Kjeld Søballe. Århus Universitetshopital.)

Young children (4–10) are treated with a Salter innominate osteotomy, provided the dysplastic acetabulum remains congruent. It is often difficult to recommend surgery for an asymptomatic condition, but significant persistent dysplasia, without improvement of the acetabular index, in a child over 5 years old merits serious discussion.

Older children and *young adolescents*, provided the hip is reducible and congruent, often manage with no more than muscle-strengthening exercises. If symptoms persist, they may need an operation to augment the acetabular roof, either a lateral shelf procedure or a limited pelvic osteotomy such as the Chiari operation, either of which may be combined with a varus osteotomy of the proximal femur.

Older adolescents and *young adults* with pain, weakness, instability and subluxation of the hip are candidates for peri-acetabular osteotomy and three-dimensional re-orientation of the entire hip (Ganz et al., 1998).

Patients with *secondary OA* may need intertrochanteric osteotomy or total hip replacement.

ACQUIRED DISLOCATION OF THE HIP

Dislocation occurring after the first year of life is usually due to one of three causes: *pyogenic arthritis*, *muscle imbalance* or *trauma*. Rare causes of acquired dislocation include tuberculosis and Charcot's disease.

Dislocation following sepsis

Septic arthritis of the hip in early childhood, whether from direct infection of the joint or via spread from metaphyseal osteomyelitis, may result in partial or complete destruction of the largely cartilaginous femoral head and pathological dislocation of the hip (see Chapter 2). *On x-ray* the femoral head appears to be completely absent; however, some part of it often survives, although it is too osteoporotic to be seen.

Although the infection may be overcome and some measure of bone regeneration later appears, the dislocation persists and the child presents with signs resembling those of DDH – plus the telltale scars of old sinuses or an operation. Total destruction of the femoral head often results in a completely unstable joint (*Tom Smith's arthritis*).

Treatment of the acute infection is discussed in Chapter 2. If there is a threat of joint instability, a hip spica should be applied until the soft-tissue infection has settled completely. In the absence of a femoral head, the greater trochanter can be placed in the acetabulum or stability can be restored by performing a valgus (Shanz) osteotomy with limb lengthening to equality. In later life the patient will require further reconstructive surgery or total joint replacement.

Dislocation due to muscle imbalance

Unbalanced paralysis in childhood may result in the hip abductors being weaker than the adductors. This is seen in *cerebral palsy*, in *myelomeningocele* and after *poliomyelitis* (see Chapter 10). The foetal anteversion of the femoral neck persists, the greater trochanter fails to develop properly, the femoral neck becomes valgus and the hip may subluxate or dislocate.

Treatment is similar to that of congenital dislocation, but in addition some muscle-rebalancing operation is essential.

Persistent traumatic dislocation

Occasionally dislocation of the hip is missed while attention is focussed on some more distal (and more obvious) injury. Reduction is essential, if necessary by open operation; even if avascular necrosis or hip stiffness supervenes, a hip in the anatomical position presents an easier prospect for reconstructive surgery than one that remains persistently dislocated.

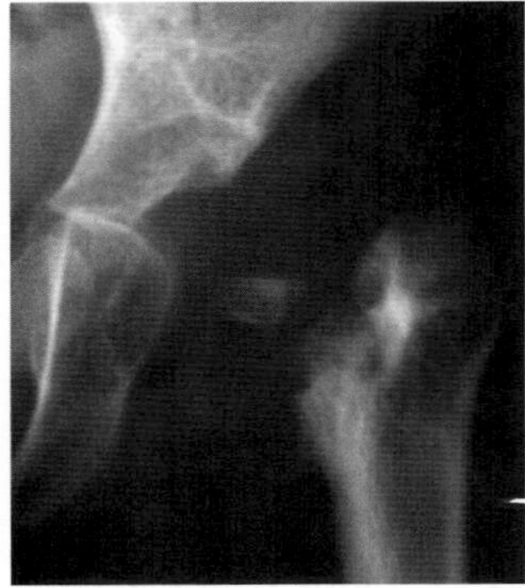

(a)

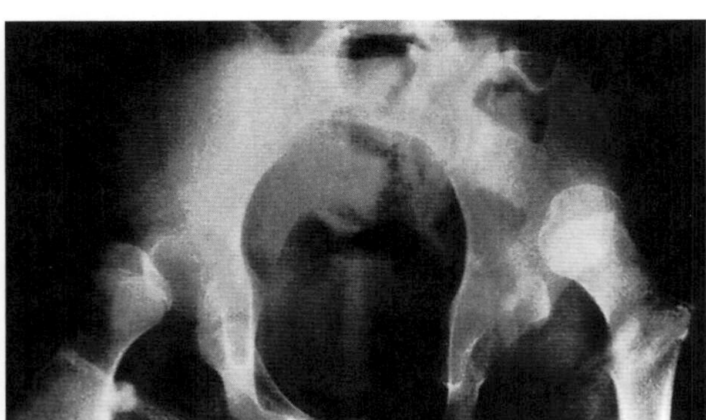

(b)

19.18 Acquired dislocation in children (a) Almost complete destruction of the femoral head following neglected septic arthritis. (b) Bilateral dislocation in a child with muscle imbalance due to spina bifida.

FEMORAL ANTEVERSION AND RETROVERSION ('IN-TOEING' AND 'OUT-TOEING')

Children with in-toeing (and less commonly out-toeing) are often 'taken to the doctor' because of an awkward gait. Usually this is no more than one extreme of the normal developmental spectrum.

The in-toeing child tends to trip over his or her feet when running. The cause is rarely serious but a paternalistic assurance that the child 'will grow out of it' may fail to convince the parents and certainly will not satisfy the grandparents.

Internal rotation of the tibia is common at birth and is usually associated with an equivalent degree of genu varum. This may produce in-toeing in the toddler, which gradually resolves over a period of 2–3 years. External tibial torsion, producing out-toeing, is less common.

In children between 3 and 10 years, the cause of in-toeing is usually femoral anteversion. ('Version' in this context describes the angle in the axial plane subtended by the femoral neck and the femoral shaft, with 'anteversion' being an anterior tilt and 'retroversion' a posterior tilt of the femoral neck and head.) In the young child anteversion may be as much as 40 degrees, thus requiring the rest of the leg to turn inwards in order to keep the femoral head within the acetabulum. Femoral neck anteversion decreases to approximately 20 degrees by the age of 10 years, and this is associated with a gradual loss of in-toeing (Engel and Staheli, 1974; Kling and Hensinger, 1983).

The gait may look clumsy but that is no bar to athletic prowess and usually improves with growth. These children often sit on the floor in the 'television position' with the knees facing each other. With the child standing, the patellae are turned inwards ('squinting patellae') and there may be compensatory external torsion of the tibiae.

The arc of rotatory movement of the hip is assessed with the child prone and knees flexed. An in-toeing gait is associated with greater medial rotation of the hip than lateral, but is considered to be within the normal range as long as there is 20 degrees of lateral rotation. Similarly, an out-toeing child has a normal range if there is at least 20 degrees of internal rotation.

The alignment of the sole of the foot to the thigh is known as the *thigh–foot angle* and combines the effect of any foot deformity as well as tibial torsion. Palpation of the positions of the malleoli demonstrates the presence of tibial torsion.

Rotational profiles in the normal child are variable and charts documenting normal values are available. A rotational profile which lies outside two standard deviations of the mean is considered abnormal and a pathological cause should be considered (Staheli et al, 1985).

Femoral neck anteversion can also be assessed by ultrasonography or by obtaining axial CT scans across the hips and the knees and measuring the angle between the axis of the femoral neck and the transverse axis across the femoral condyles.

Physiological rotational abnormalities have not been shown to have any long-term consequences and parental reassurance is the cornerstone of treatment. Shoe modifications and orthotics are unnecessary (Kling and Hensinger, 1983; Staheli, 1994).

PROTRUSIO ACETABULI (OTTO PELVIS)

In this condition the socket is too deep and bulges into the cavity of the pelvis. The *'primary'* form shows a slight familial tendency. It affects females much more often than males and develops soon after puberty; at this stage there are usually no symptoms

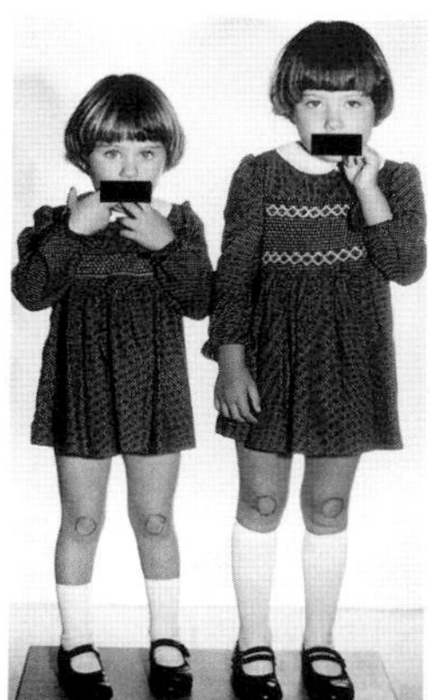

(a)

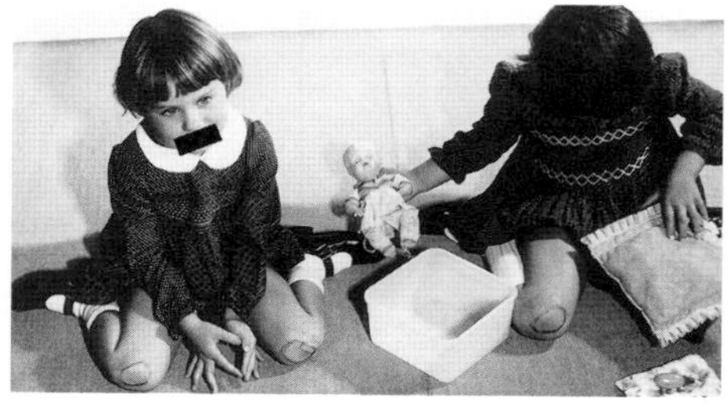

(b)

19.19 In-toe gait (a) These two sisters have excessive anteversion with an in-toe gait. (b) This explains their sitting posture when playing or watching television.

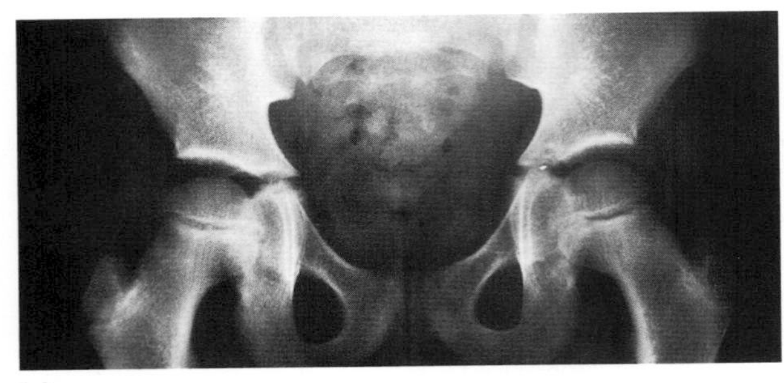

(a)

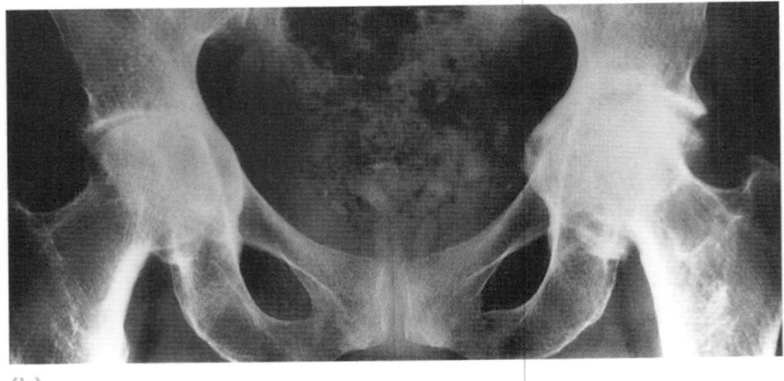

(b)

19.20 Protrusio acetabuli (a) The early stage in a child. (b) In this adult with protrusio, degenerative changes have developed in both hips.

although movements are limited. *X-rays* show the sunken acetabulum, with the inner wall bulging beyond the ilio-pectineal line. Secondary OA may develop in later life, but until then the condition does not require treatment.

Protrusio may occur in later life secondary to bone 'softening' disorders, such as *osteomalacia* or *Paget's disease*, and in longstanding cases of *rheumatoid arthritis*. If pain is severe, or movements are markedly restricted, joint replacement is indicated.

COXA VARA

The normal femoral neck–shaft angle is 160 degrees at birth, decreasing to 125 degrees in adult life. An angle of less than 120 degrees is called coxa vara. The deformity may be either congenital or acquired.

Congenital coxa vara

This is a rare developmental disorder of infancy and early childhood. It is due to a defect of endochondral ossification in the medial part of the femoral neck. When the child starts to crawl or stand, the femoral neck bends or develops a stress fracture, and with continued weightbearing it collapses increasingly into varus and retroversion. Sometimes there is also shortening or bowing of the femoral shaft. As the child grows, the proximal femur keeps elongating but the neck–shaft angle goes into increasing varus. The condition is bilateral in about one-third of cases.

Clinical features

The condition is usually diagnosed when the child starts to walk. The leg is short and the thigh may be bowed. X-rays show that the femoral neck is in varus and abnormally short. Often there is a separate fragment of bone in a triangular notch on the inferomedial surface of the femoral neck. Because of the distorted anatomy, it is difficult to measure the neck–shaft angle. A helpful alternative is to measure *Hilgenreiner's epiphyseal angle* – the angle subtended by a horizontal line joining the centre (triradiate cartilage) of each hip and another parallel to the physeal line; the normal angle is about 30 degrees (Fig. 19.21a) while the angle on the abnormal side is much larger (Fig. 19.21c). At maturity the deformity may be quite bizarre. With bilateral coxa vara the patient may not be seen until he or she presents as a young adult with OA.

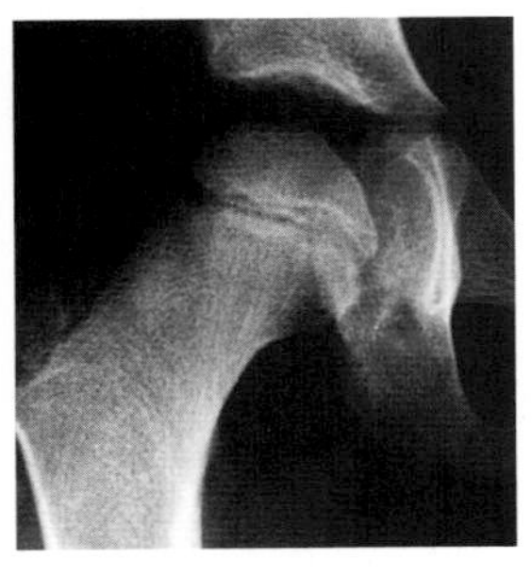

(a)

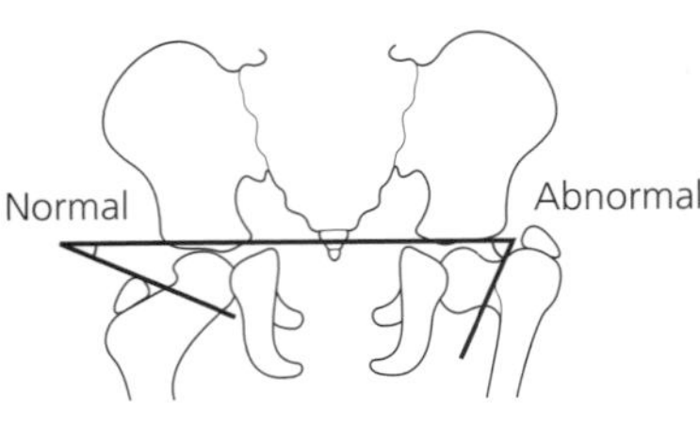

(b)

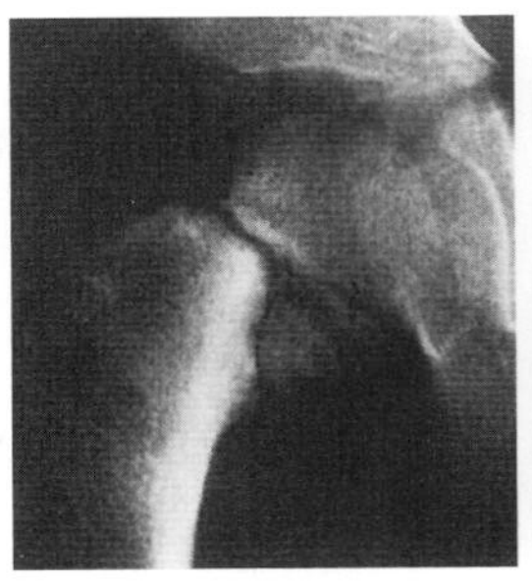

(c)

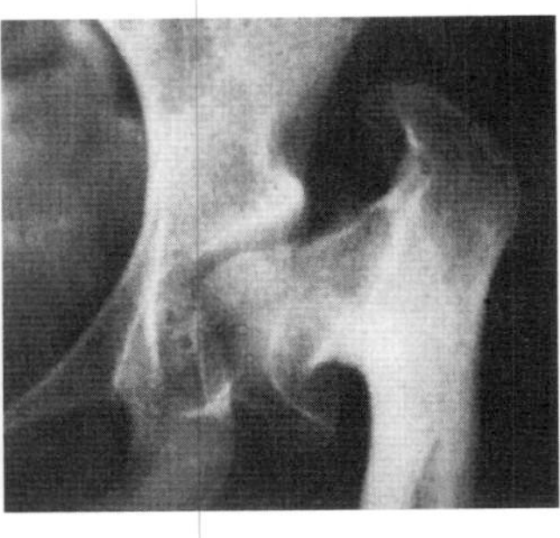

(d)

19.21 Infantile coxa vara In the normal hip (a) Hilgenreiner's epiphyseal angle is well within the normal range of 30–40°. The measurements are shown in (b). On the opposite side (c) the physis is too vertical: 45–60° calls for careful follow-up and review, and more than 60° is an indication for Pauwels' valgus osteotomy. In a neglected case (d) the trochanteric physis allows further growth but the femoral neck may remain fixed in marked varus.

Treatment

If the epiphyseal angle is more than 40 but less than 60 degrees, the child should be kept under observation and re-examined at intervals for signs of progression. If it is more than 60 degrees, or if shortening is progressive, the deformity should be corrected by a subtrochanteric or intertrochanteric valgus osteotomy.

Pauwels demonstrated that permanent correction was possible if the plane of the physeal plate was restored to normal and the characteristic triangular metaphyseal fragment and protruding femoral head were supported on the femoral neck. These objectives are possible with a Y-shaped intertrochanteric osteotomy of the proximal femur (Fig. 19.22). Cordes et al. (1991) evaluated 14 hips at a mean follow-up of 11 years and reported good/excellent function in 78 per cent. Patients with the three hips rated 'poor' had a persistent Trendelenburg gait and fatigue pain.

Acquired coxa vara

Coxa vara can develop if the femoral neck bends or if it breaks. A 'mechanical' coxa vara sometimes results from severe shortening of the femoral neck and relative overgrowth of the greater trochanter; during weightbearing the abductor muscles are at a mechanical disadvantage and the patient walks with a severe Trendelenburg gait.

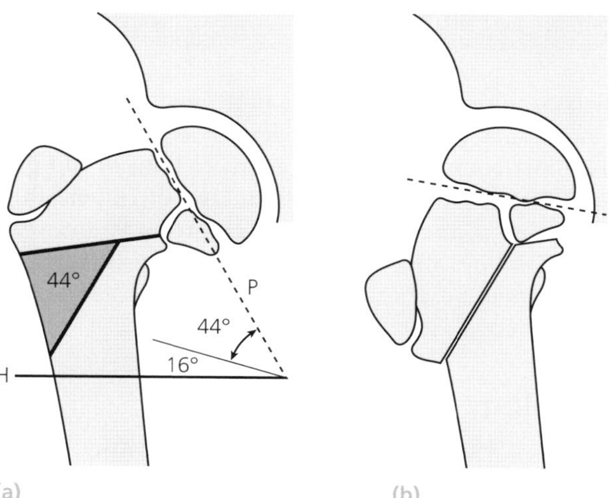

19.22 Pauwels' valgus osteotomy (a) Preoperative planning on a tracing of the preoperative radiograph. P = the plane of the physis. H is a horizontal line drawn well below the lesser trochanter. In this case a 44° closing wedge osteotomy is required to correct the inclination of the physis to 16°. (b) After the osteotomy and removal of the 44° wedge from the lateral side of the proximal femur, the femoral head and adjacent neck are supported by the calcar femorale. (From Cordes et al., 1991. With permission from the *Journal of Bone and Joint Surgery*.)

During childhood, coxa vara is seen in rickets and bone dystrophies, and sometimes after Perthes' disease. Deformity presenting *in adolescence* is more likely to be due to epiphysiolysis.

At any age bone 'softening' may result in coxa vara; causes include osteomalacia, fibrous dysplasia, pathological fracture or the aftermath of infection. Other causes of deformity are malunited fractures and Paget's disease.

Treatment in the form of a corrective (valgus) osteotomy is needed only if there is marked shortening or intolerable discomfort. If the problem is due to a disproportionately high greater trochanter, distal transposition of the trochanter may suffice.

PROXIMAL FEMORAL FOCAL DEFICIENCY

Proximal focal femoral deficiency (PFFD) or congenital femoral deficiency (CFD) is a rare (possibly teratogenic) anomaly with a spectrum of presentation between femoral hypoplasia and virtual absence of the femur. The condition is easily recognized: the affected limb is abnormally short, sometimes bizarre in appearance with the foot on that side lying at the same level as the knee on the opposite limb; the hip is usually held flexed, abducted and externally rotated; in many cases there are also other anomalies, such as fibular deficiency.

CLASSIFICATION AND MANAGEMENT

The most useful anatomical classification is that of Aitken.

- In *type A* there appears to be a gap in the femoral neck or subtrochanteric region, which is in fact a segment of unossified cartilage. This does eventually ossify, but by then the proximal femur has developed a varus deformity and shortening. The femoral head and acetabulum are present.
- In *type B* the 'gap' persists, the femoral head and acetabulum are dysplastic, the upper end of the femur lies above the acetabulum and there is significant shortening.
- In *type C* the femoral head is missing and the acetabulum is undeveloped.
- In *type D* there is agenesis of the entire proximal femur and acetabulum. Both hips may be affected and in half the cases there are also distal anomalies.

The classification suggested by Gillespie (1998) is probably more useful for planning treatment.

- Patients in Group A have short femurs but stable hips, functional knees and the foot below the level of the middle of the opposite tibia. These can be considered for limb reconstruction and lengthen-

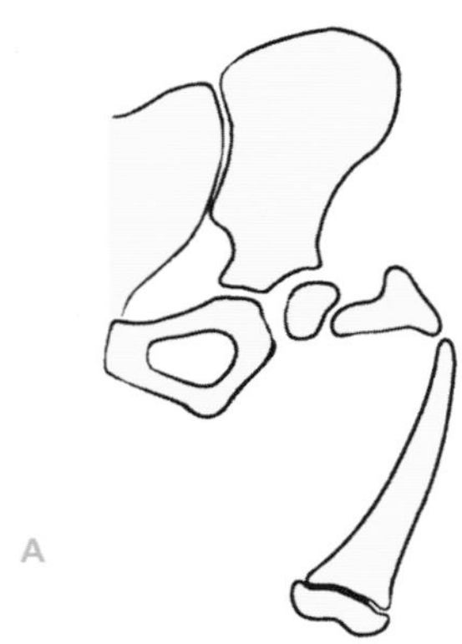

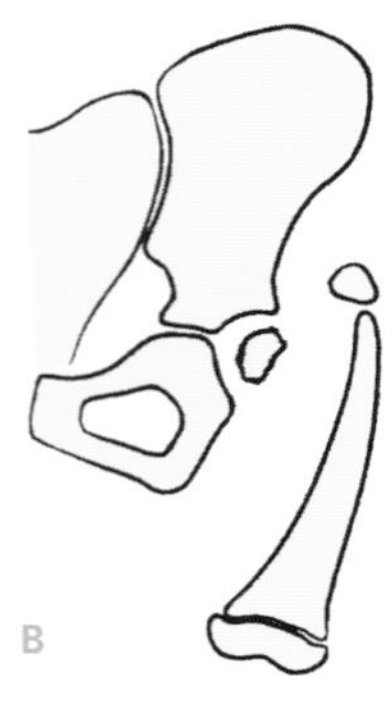

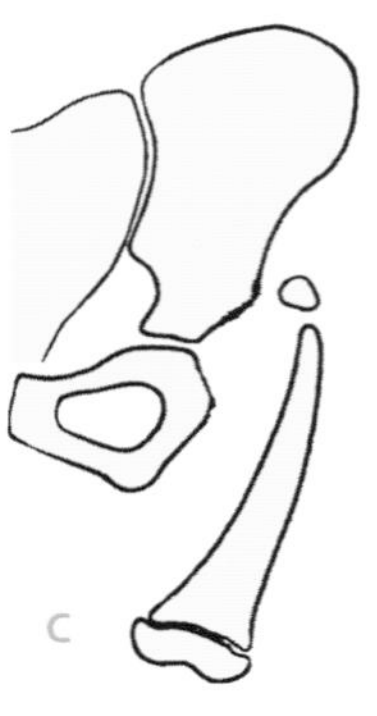

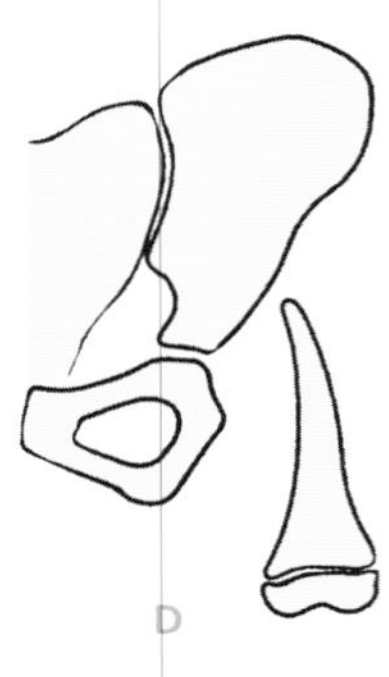

19.23 Proximal femoral focal deficiency – Aitken's classification In types A and B the femoral head and acetabulum are present, though showing varying degrees of dysplasia. Coxa vara may be marked and shortening is significant. In types C and D there is no effective hip joint, shortening is severe and distal deficiencies may be present.

ing. Abnormalities of the knee and foot may have to be addressed as well.

- Patients in group B correspond more or less to those in Aitken's types B and C; most of them can be treated by rotationplasty and a prosthesis or knee fusion combined with ankle disarticulation and a prosthesis.
- Those in Group C correspond to Aitken's type D. They have total (or near-total) absence of the femur, sometimes associated with dysplasia of the hemipelvis and absence of any acetabular development. These patients require a prosthesis and in the most deficient cases retaining the foot may actually be beneficial to the prosthetist.

Patients with bilateral symmetrical anomalies are functionally better than those with unilateral deformity; were it not for the cosmetic problem, they are probably best left alone.

On a personal note: '*Rotationplasty*' (an operation to turn the foot around so that the ankle acts like a knee) sounds better than it turns out to be in real life. The operation is difficult and fraught with complications; patients often end up needing multiple procedures; the limb without a prosthesis is cosmetically questionable; and patients have been known to suffer severe psychological trauma with a foot facing backwards (Fixen, 1983).

(a)

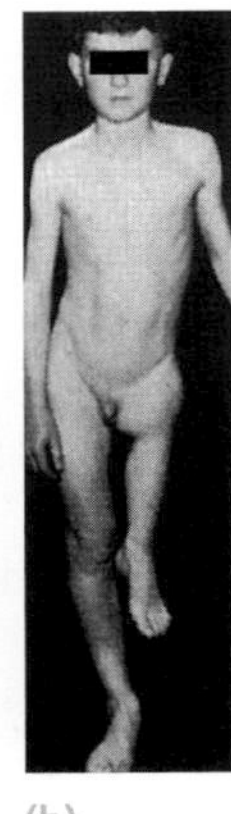

(b)

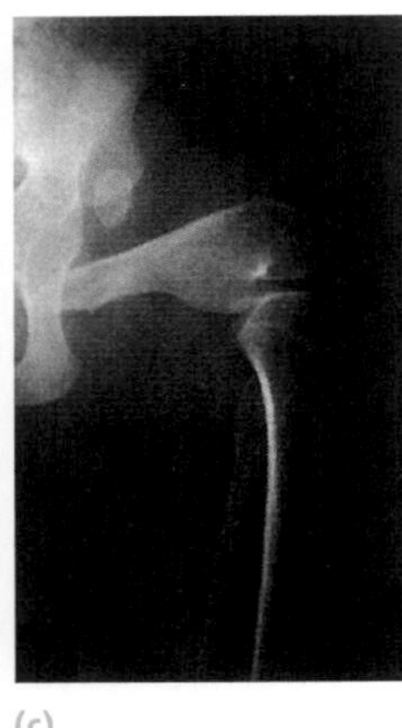

(c)

19.24 Proximal femoral dysplasia **(a)** This man was born with transverse deficiency of the right arm and bilateral proximal femoral focal deficiency. Although unhappy with his appearance, because the lower limb defects were symmetrical he was able to get about remarkably well. **(b)** By contrast, this young man with similar but unilateral dysplasia was severely disabled. **(c)** X-ray showing the proximal femoral deficiency.

THE IRRITABLE HIP (TRANSIENT SYNOVITIS)

This condition is defined as a non-specific, short-lived synovitis, resulting in an effusion of the hip joint. It is the most common cause of an acute limp or hip pain in children, with a reported frequency of 14 per 1000. The most commonly affected age group is 3–8-year-olds with boys affected twice as often as girls. It affects both hips in 5 per cent of cases, although this is rarely simultaneous.

Aetiology

While viral infections, trauma and allergy have been suggested, the exact aetiology remains unclear. The pathological process involves a synovial effusion resulting in an increased intra-articular pressure.

Clinical features

The typical patient presents with pain and a limp, often intermittent and following activity. Pain is felt in the groin or front of the thigh, sometimes reaching as far as the knee. Slight wasting may be detectable but the cardinal sign is restriction of all movements with pain at the extremes of the range in all directions. The diagnosis is based primarily on the clinical features. Standard laboratory investigations including white cell count, erythrocyte sedimentation rate (ESR) and C-reactive protein concentration are usually within normal limits. X-rays do not demonstrate any bony defects, but occasionally there may be a subtle widening of the medial joint space (1–2 mm) when compared with the unaffected side. This is caused by the effusion which allows the femoral head to sublux slightly; it may be confirmed by ultrasonography.

Characteristically, symptoms last for 1–2 weeks and then subside spontaneously; hence the synonym 'transient synovitis'. The child may experience more than one episode, with an interval of months between attacks of pain.

Differential diagnosis

The condition is important largely because it resembles a number of serious disorders which have to be excluded.

Perthes' disease is the main worry. Acute symptoms usually last longer than 2 weeks and x-rays may show an increased 'joint space'. Later, of course, the x-ray features are unmistakable.

Slipped epiphysis may present as an 'irritable hip'. Initially the x-ray looks normal and this may lead to complacency. If the age and general build are suggestive, or if the symptoms persist, the x-ray should be repeated.

Tuberculous synovitis produces a raised ESR and the Heaf test is positive.

Juvenile chronic arthritis and *ankylosing spondylitis* may start with synovitis of one hip and it may take months before other joints are affected. Look for systemic features and a raised ESR. In doubtful cases, synovial biopsy may be helpful.

Septic arthritis should always be borne in mind. The early symptoms and signs are sometimes misleading, especially if someone has already prescribed antibiotics 'just in case!'

Treatment

Treatment involves bed rest, reduced activity and observation, which may be supervised at home or in hospital. Most children recover within a few days and any deterioration in signs or symptoms requires urgent reassessment. Traction, although popular in the past, is not currently recommended as it may increase the intra-articular pressure. Joint aspiration is ineffective; any relief in symptoms tends to be short-lived as the effusion rapidly recurs.

Ultrasonography is repeated at intervals and weightbearing is allowed only when the symptoms disappear and the effusion resolves.

Although this condition carries a good prognosis, recurrence rates of up to 10 per cent have been reported. A causal relationship with Perthes' disease has been suspected but remains unproven.

PERTHES' DISEASE

Perthes' disease – or rather Legg–Calvé–Perthes disease, for in 1910 the condition was described independently by three different people – is a painful disorder of childhood characterized by avascular necrosis of the femoral head. It is uncommon in any community – the quoted incidence is about 1 in 10 000 – with a higher incidence in Japanese, Inuits and central Europeans and a lower incidence in native Australians, native Americans, Polynesians and blacks. Patients are usually 4–10 years old and boys are affected four times as often as girls.

The condition may be part of a general disorder of growth. Epidemiological studies in the UK have shown that there is a higher than usual incidence in underprivileged communities. Affected children and their siblings have slightly retarded growth of the trunk and limbs.

As in other forms of non-traumatic osteonecrosis, inherited thrombophilia has been postulated as a contributory cause and antithrombotic factor deficiencies and hypofibrinolysis have been reported in children with Perthes' disease (Glueck et al., 1996). This hypothesis has been questioned by others (Editorial by R. J. Liesner, 1999).

Pathogenesis

The precipitating cause of Perthes' disease is unknown but the cardinal step in the pathogenesis is ischaemia of the femoral head. Up to the age of 4 months, the femoral head is supplied by (1) metaphyseal vessels which penetrate the growth disc, (2) lateral epiphyseal vessels running in the retinacula and (3) scanty vessels in the ligamentum teres. The metaphyseal supply gradually declines until, by the age of 4 years, it has virtually disappeared; by the age of 7, however, the vessels in the ligamentum teres have developed. Between 4 and 7 years of age the femoral head may depend for its blood supply and venous drainage almost entirely on the lateral epiphyseal vessels whose situation in the retinacula makes them susceptible to stretching and to pressure from an effusion. Although such pressure may be insufficient to block off the arterial flow, it could easily cause venous stasis resulting in a rise in intraosseous pressure and consequent ischaemia (Lin and Ho, 1991). This may be enough to tip the balance towards infarction and necrosis in children who are constitutionally predisposed.

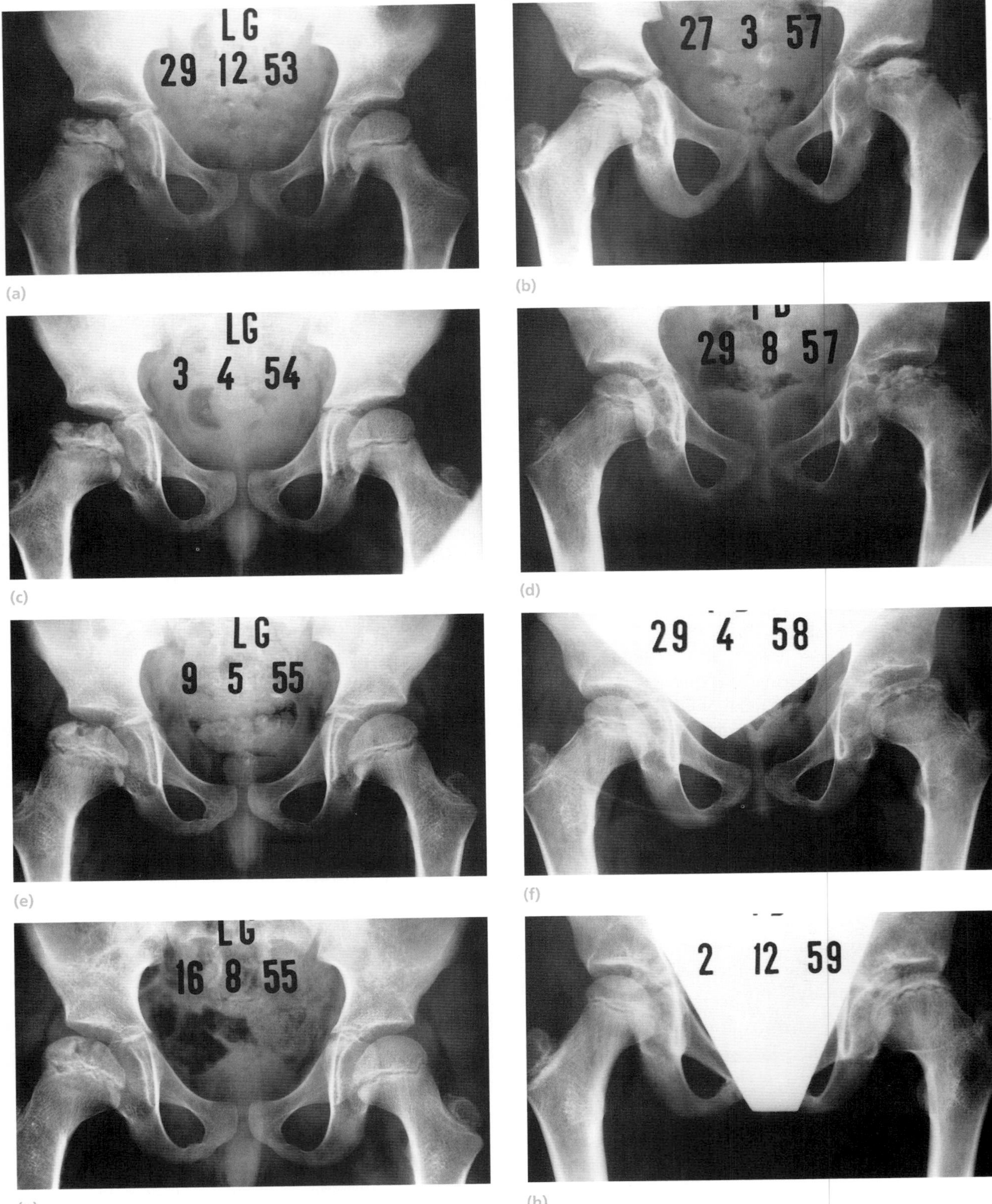

(a) (b) (c) (d) (e) (f) (g) (h)

19.25 Perthes' disease – Herring classification The Herring classification is based on the severity of structural disintegration of the lateral pillar of the femoral epiphysis. Column 1 shows the changes in a boy with moderately severe Perthes' disease of the right hip. Although the central part of the epiphyseal ossific centre seems to be 'fragmented', the lateral part remains intact throughout the progress of the disease. This is a favourable feature and serial x-rays show how the femoral head has gradually re-formed. Column 2 shows progressive changes in another boy with severe Perthes' disease of the left hip. The epiphysis is widely involved from the outset, 'fragmentation' extends to the most lateral portion of the epiphysis and there is progressive flattening of the epiphysis resulting in permanent distortion of the femoral head.

The immediate cause of capsular tamponade may be an effusion following trauma (of which there is a history in over half the cases) or a non-specific synovitis. Two or more such incidents may be needed to produce the typical bone changes.

Pathology

The pathological process goes through several stages which in total may last up to 3 or 4 years.

Stage 1: Ischaemia and bone death All or part of the bony nucleus of the femoral head is dead; it still looks normal on plain x-ray but stops enlarging. The cartilaginous part of the femoral head, being nourished by synovial fluid, remains viable and becomes thicker than normal. There may also be thickening and oedema of the synovium and capsule.

Stage 2: Revascularization and repair Within weeks (possibly even days) of infarction, a number of changes begin to appear. Dead marrow is replaced by granulation tissue, which sometimes calcifies. The bone is revascularized and new lamellae are laid down on the dead trabeculae, producing the appearance of increased density on x-ray. Some of the dead trabecular fragments are resorbed and replaced by fibrous tissue; when this happens, the alternating areas of sclerosis and fibrosis appear on the x-ray as *'fragmentation'* of the epiphysis. The metaphysis may become hyperaemic and on x-ray looks rarefied or cystic. In older children, and more severe cases, morphological changes may also appear in the acetabulum.

Stage 3: Distortion and remodelling If the repair process is rapid and complete, the bony architecture may be restored before the femoral head loses its shape. If it is tardy, the bony epiphysis may collapse and subsequent growth of the femoral head and neck will be distorted: the head becomes oval or flattened – like the head of a mushroom – and enlarged laterally, while the neck is often short and broad. Slowly the femoral head is displaced laterally in relation to the acetabulum. Any residual deformity is likely to be permanent.

Clinical features

The patient – typically a boy of 4–8 years – complains of pain and starts limping. Symptoms continue for weeks on end or may recur intermittently. The child appears to be well, though often somewhat undersized. In 4 per cent there is an associated urogenital anomaly.

The hip looks deceptively normal, though there may be a little wasting. Early on, the joint is irritable so that all movements are diminished and their extremes painful. Often the child is not seen till later, when most movements are full; but abduction (especially in flexion) is nearly always limited and usually internal rotation also.

X-rays

Although the condition may be suspected from the clinical appearances, diagnosis hinges on the x-ray changes.

At first the x-rays may seem normal, though subtle changes such as widening of the 'joint space' and slight asymmetry of the ossific centres are usually present. Radionuclide scanning may show a 'void' in the anterolateral part of the femoral head.

The classic feature of increased density of the ossific nucleus occurs somewhat later. This is often referred to as the '*necrotic phase*', though the radiographically dense areas must surely be due to the new bone formation that always follows bone necrosis. This progresses to the phase of radiographic '*fragmentation*' – alternating patches of density and lucency, or sometimes a crescentic subarticular fracture often best seen in the lateral view. Epiphyseal density increases (the phase of *re-ossification*) and scintigraphy shows increased activity. With *healing* the femoral head may regain its normal (or near-normal) shape; however, in less fortunate cases the femoral head becomes mushroom-shaped, larger than normal and laterally displaced in a dysplastic acetabular socket.

The Catterall classification The radiographic picture varies with the age of the child, the stage of the disease and the amount of head that is necrotic. Catterall (1982) described four groups, based on the appearances in both anteroposterior and lateral x-rays. *In group 1* the epiphysis has retained its height and less than half the nucleus is sclerotic. *In group 2* up to half the nucleus is sclerotic and there may be some collapse of the central portion. *In group 3* most of the nucleus is involved, with sclerosis, fragmentation and collapse of the head. Metaphyseal resorption may be present. *Group 4* is the worst: the whole head is involved, the ossific nucleus is flat and dense and metaphyseal resorption is marked.

The Herring classification This classification embodies a greater degree of predictive value for the outcome of the Perthes changes and is therefore preferred by many orthopaedic surgeons. The features are described below and illustrated in Figure 19.25.

Prognostic features

The outlook for children with Perthes' disease, as a group, is well summarized by Herring (1994): 'A small percentage of patients have a very difficult course, with recurrent loss of motion, pain, and an eventual poor outcome. However, most children have moderate problems in the active phase of the disease and then improve steadily, eventually having a satisfactory outcome.'

This does not, of course, absolve one from undertaking careful analysis and planning in dealing with the individual case. *Age* is the most important prognostic factor: in children under 6 years the outlook is almost always excellent; thereafter, the older the child the less good is the prognosis. There is a poorer prognosis, too, for *girls* than for boys.

A widely used radiographic guide is the *Catterall classification* (see above). The greater the degree of femoral head involvement, the worse the outcome. This is recognized in the simpler *classification of Salter and Thompson*, into those with more and those with less than half the head involved (Simmons et al., 1990). There is also the concept of the *head at risk* – radiographic signs which presage increasing deformity and displacement of the femoral head: (1) progressive uncovering of the epiphysis; (2) calcification in the cartilage lateral to the ossific nucleus; (3) a radiolucent area at the lateral edge of the bony epiphysis (Gage's sign); and (4) severe metaphyseal resorption.

Common to all these predictive systems is the importance of the structural integrity of the superolateral (principal load-bearing) part of the femoral head. This is reflected in Herring's *lateral pillar classification*. In the anteroposterior x-ray, the femoral head is divided into three 'pillars' by lines at the medial and lateral edges of the central 'sequestrum'. Group A are those with normal height of the lateral pillar. Group B are patients with partial collapse (but still more than 50 per cent height) of the lateral pillar; those under 9 years of age usually have a good outcome but older children are likely to develop flattening of the femoral head. Group C cases show more severe collapse of the lateral pillar (less than 50 per cent of normal height); these take longer to heal and usually end up with significant distortion of the femoral head.

Differential diagnosis

The irritable hip of early Perthes' disease must be differentiated from other causes of irritability; the child's fitness, the increased joint space and the patchy bone density are characteristic. In transient synovitis the x-ray is normal.

Morquio's disease, cretinism, multiple epiphyseal dysplasia, sickle-cell disease and Gaucher's disease may resemble Perthes' disease radiologically, especially if they are bilateral; however, in bilateral Perthes' disease the two sides are likely to be at different stages. Moreover, in the other conditions general diagnostic features are usually apparent.

'Old Perthes deformities' in adults, in the 10 per cent of cases with bilateral involvement, may resemble those of certain bone dysplasias, especially multiple epiphyseal dysplasia. Look for changes in other epiphyses.

Management

The initial management of the child with Perthes' disease is determined by the severity of symptoms.

APPROACH TO THE LIMPING CHILD

1. Measure limb length
2. Check the foot
   Splinter? Injury?
   Swollen ankle: Infection? Arthritis?
3. Examine the knee
   Swelling: Infection? Arthritis? Tumour?
4. Examine the hip
   Septic arthritis?
   Dislocation? Subluxation? Coxa vara? Transient synovitis?
   Perthes' disease? Arthritis? Tumour?
5 General assessment
   Exclude non-accidental injury

Analgesia and modification of activities are often sufficient, but hospitalization for bed rest and short periods of traction are sometimes necessary. Wheelchair use and crutch walking should be discouraged in order to avoid unnecessary joint stiffness and contracture. Once joint irritability has subsided, which usually takes about 3 weeks, movement is encouraged, particularly cycling and swimming. Preservation of abduction is also important, with formal stretching used in some children.

The clinical and radiographic features are then reassessed and the bone age is determined from x-rays of the wrist. The choice of further management is between (a) symptomatic treatment and (b) containment.

Symptomatic treatment means pain control (if necessary by further spells of traction), gentle exercise to maintain movement and regular reassessment. During asymptomatic periods the child is allowed out and about but sport and strenuous activities are avoided.

Containment means taking active steps to seat the femoral head congruently and as fully as possible in the acetabular socket, so that it may retain its sphericity and not become displaced during the period of healing and remodelling. This is achieved (a) by holding the hips widely abducted, in plaster or in a removable brace (ambulation, though awkward, is just possible, but the position must be maintained for at least a year); or (b) by operation, either a varus osteotomy of the femur or an innominate osteotomy of the pelvis, or both.

In earlier years there was a good deal of support for non-operative containment, and this is still applicable where specialized surgical facilities are unavailable. However, this has been questioned by more recent outcome studies and the preferred approach is to achieve containment by operative methods (Martinez, 1992; Meehan 1992).

Operative reconstruction provides the advantages of improved containment and early mobilization. Short-term studies also suggest an improvement in the

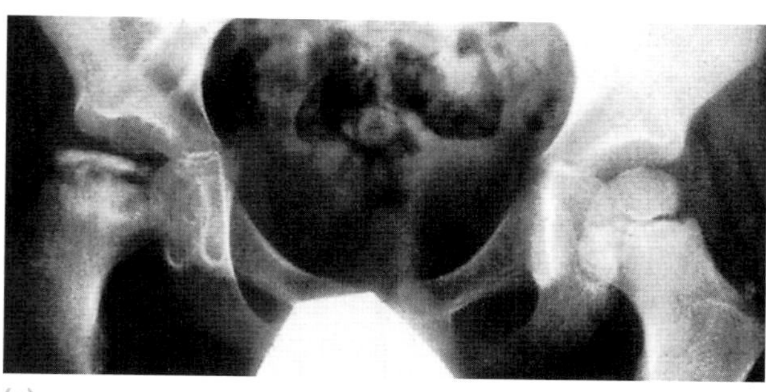

(a)

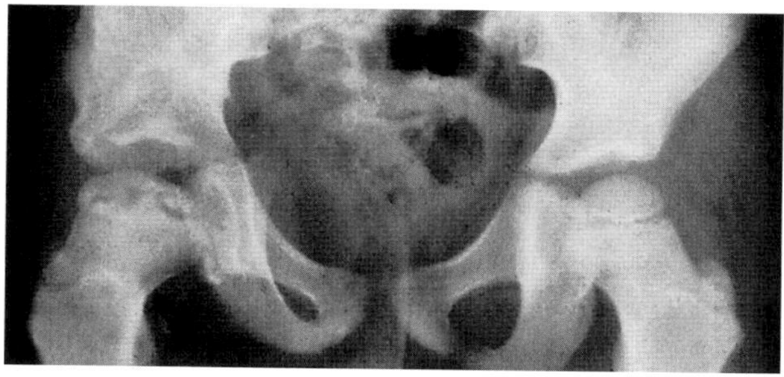

(b)

19.26 Perthes' disease – operative treatment (a) The x-ray shows advanced Perthes changes and lateral displacement of the right femoral head. (b) Following an innominate osteotomy, the femoral head is much better 'contained' and, although not normal, is developing reasonably well.

anatomy of the hip, but there is no convincing evidence of any alteration in the natural history of the disorder or (in particular) the likelihood of needing an arthroplasty in later life.

GUIDELINES TO TREATMENT

There is no general agreement on the 'correct' course of treatment for all cases. Decisions are based on an assessment of the stage of the disease, the prognostic x-ray classifications, the age of the patient and the clinical features, particularly range of abduction and extension. The following guidelines are derived from the review by Herring (1994).

Children under 6 years No specific form of treatment has much influence on the outcome. Symptomatic treatment, including activity modification, is appropriate.

Children aged 6–8 years In this group the bone age is more important than the chronological age.

Bone age at or below 6 years

Lateral pillar group A and B (or Catterall stage I and II) – symptomatic treatment.

Lateral pillar group C (or Catterall stage III and IV) – abduction brace.

Bone age over 6 years

Lateral pillar group A and B (Catterall stage I and II) – abduction brace or osteotomy.

Lateral pillar group C (Catterall stage III and IV) – outcome probably unaffected by treatment, but some would operate.

Children 9 years and older Except in very mild cases (which is rare), operative containment is the treatment of choice.

SLIPPED CAPITAL FEMORAL EPIPHYSIS

Displacement of the proximal femoral epiphysis – also known as femoral capital epiphysiolysis or slipped capital femoral epiphysis (SCFE) – is uncommon (1–3 per 100 000) and virtually confined to children going through the pubertal growth spurt. Boys (usually between 14 and 16 years old) are affected more often than girls (who are, on average, 2–3 years younger). The left hip is affected more commonly than the right and if one side slips there is a 25–40 per cent risk of the other side also slipping.

Aetiology

The slip occurs through the hypertrophic zone of the cartilaginous growth plate. Why should the physis give way during a period of accelerated growth? Many of the patients are either fat and sexually immature or excessively tall and thin. It is tempting to formulate a theory of *hormonal imbalance* as the underlying cause of physeal disruption. Normally, pituitary hormone activity, which stimulates rapid growth and increased physeal hypertrophy during puberty, is balanced by increasing gonadal hormone activity, which promotes physeal maturation and epiphyseal fusion. A disparity between these two processes may result in the physis being unable to resist the shearing stresses imposed by the increase in body weight. This occurs most obviously in the hypogonadal 'Frohlich type' of child, and it may be a factor in cases associated with juvenile hypothyroidism. There are also instances of epiphysiolysis occurring in children with craniopharyngioma after successful treatment and sudden reactivation of pituitary activity. Oestrogens produce a decrease in physeal width and increased physeal strength, which may partly explain the lower incidence in girls and rare occurrence after menarche.

Other factors may also play a part. The perichondrial ring (the retaining 'collar' around the physis) is relatively thinned in this age group and provides less support for the increased load transmitted through the physis during the growth spurt. Most patients with SCFE have a greater than average body mass index. Adolescents with SCFE also have either relative or absolute femoral neck retroversion and the physis

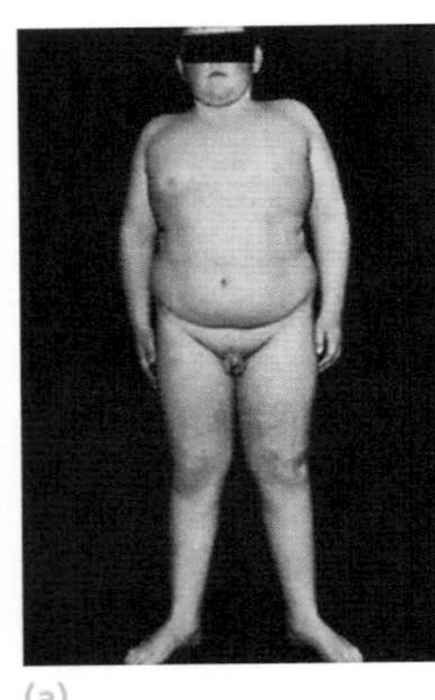
(a)

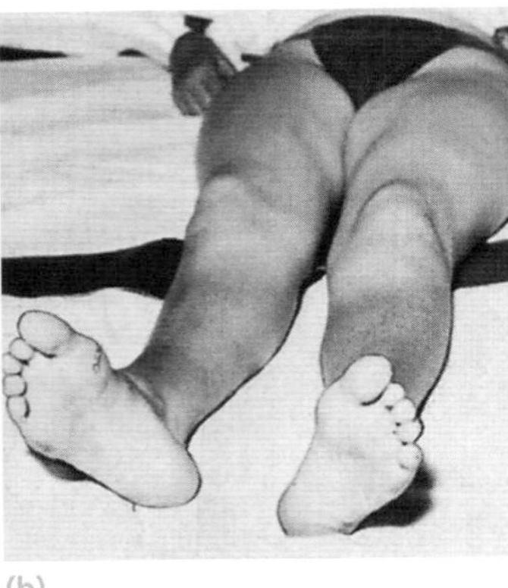
(b)

19.27 Slipped epiphysis – clinical features (a) This boy complained only of pain in his right knee. His build is unmistakable and the resting posture of his right lower limb tends towards external rotation. (b) On examination, abduction and medial rotation were restricted.

has an increased obliquity – on average 11 degrees more vertical than in children who do not develop SCFE (Galbraith et al., 1987).

Trauma plays a part, especially in the 30 per cent of cases with an 'acute' slip. In the other 70 per cent there is a slow, progressive displacement – or a series of slight displacements – sometimes culminating in a major slip after relatively mild mechanical stress (the 'acute-on-chronic' slip).

Pathology

In slipped epiphysis the femoral shaft rolls into external rotation and the femoral neck is displaced forwards while the epiphysis remains seated in the acetabulum. Disruption occurs through the hypertrophic zone of the physis and, relatively speaking, the epiphysis slips posteriorly on the femoral neck. If the slip is severe, the anterior retinacular vessels are torn. At the back of the femoral neck the periosteum is lifted from the bone with the vessels intact; this may be the main – or the only – source of blood supply to the femoral head, and damage to these vessels by manipulation or operation may result in avascular necrosis.

Physeal disruption leads to premature fusion of the epiphysis – usually within 2 years of the onset of symptoms. This is accompanied by considerable bone modelling and, although there may be a permanent external rotation deformity and apparent coxa vara, adaptive changes often ensure good joint function even without treatment.

Clinical features

Slipping usually occurs as a series of minor episodes rather than a sudden, acute event; or there may be a protracted history leading to a severe climax – the 'acute-on-chronic' slip. An initial acute slip occurs in only 15 per cent of cases. In over 50 per cent of cases there is a history of injury. In sequential bilateral slips, the second slip is diagnosed within 18 months of the first slip in 82 per cent of cases (Loder et al., 1993).

The patient is usually a child around puberty, typically overweight or very tall and thin. The presenting symptom is almost invariably pain, sometimes in the groin, but often only in the thigh or knee – which can be very misleading. It may be called a 'sprain'; often, and unfortunately, it is disregarded. It soon disappears only to recur with further exercise. Limp also occurs early and is more constant. Sometimes the child becomes aware that the leg is 'turning out'.

On examination the leg is externally rotated and is 1–2 cm short. Characteristically there is limitation of flexion, abduction and medial rotation. A classic sign is the tendency to increasing external rotation as the hip is flexed.

Following an acute slip, the hip is irritable and all movements are accompanied by pain.

Imaging

X-rays In very early cases the x-ray may be reported as 'normal'; changes can be extremely subtle. This should not be taken as a signal to forego further examination if symptoms persist! In most cases, even trivial slipping can be diagnosed. In the anteroposterior view the epiphyseal plate seems to be too wide and too 'woolly'. A line drawn along the superior surface of the femoral neck should normally intersect the epiphysis. In an early slip the epiphysis may be flush with or even below this line (Trethowan's sign). The metaphyseal blanch sign of Steel is a 'double-density' seen at the level of the metaphysis on an AP x-ray. It reflects the posterior cortical lip of the epiphysis as it is beginning to slip posteriorly and becomes superimposed on the metaphysis.

Capener's sign describes loss of the intracapsular area at the medial aspect of the femoral neck, which normally overlaps the posterior wall of the acetabulum creating a dense triangular shadow.

Decreased epiphyseal height, physeal widening, lesser trochanter prominence due to increased external rotation of the femur and new bone formation in the posterior femoral metaphysis, with anterior-remodelling, are also useful signs in diagnosis.

In the lateral view the femoral epiphysis is tilted backwards; this is the most reliable x-ray sign and minor abnormalities can be detected by measuring the angle subtended by the epiphyseal base and the femoral neck; this is normally a right angle and anything less than 87 degrees means that the epiphysis is tilted posteriorly.

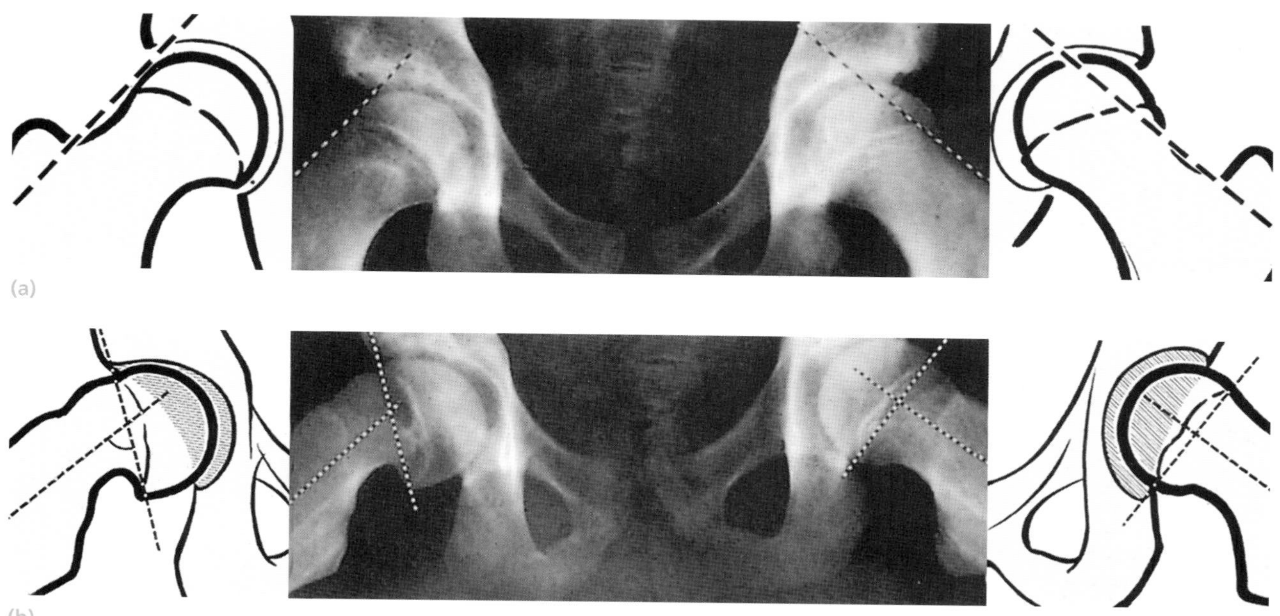

19.28 Slipped epiphysis – x-rays (a) Anteroposterior and (b) lateral views of early slipped epiphysis of the right hip. The upper diagrams show Trethowan's line passing just above the head on the affected side, but cutting through it on the normal side. The lateral view is diagnostically more reliable; even minor degrees of slip can be shown by drawing lines through the base of the epiphysis and up the middle of the femoral neck – if the angle indicated is less than 90°, the epiphysis has slipped posteriorly.

Ultrasonography Ultrasonography may detect a hip effusion associated with an acute event, and may also show metaphyseal remodelling in a chronic slip.

Magnetic resonance imaging MRI has been used to detect and stage avascular necrosis (AVN) of the femoral head.

Computed tomography Three-dimensional CT scanning has proved useful in the preoperative planning of realignment procedures for complex proximal femoral deformities.

Grading

Slipped capital femoral epiphysis can be graded by the clinical presentation and/or radiographic appearance. The simplest classification is based on the timing of onset: *pre-slip*, *acute*, *chronic* or *acute-on-chronic*.

- Pre-slip: The child complains of groin or knee pain, particularly on exertion, and there may be a limp. Examination is often normal, but may demonstrate reduced internal rotation. The x-ray may show widening or irregularity of the physis.
- Acute slip: Symptoms present for less than 3 weeks; painful hip movements with an external rotation deformity, shortening and marked limitation of rotation (the greater the limitation of motion, the greater the degree of slip). Symptoms last for less than 3 months.
- Chronic slip: The child has pain in the groin, thigh or knee lasting more than 3 weeks; episodes of deterioration and remission; loss of internal rotation, abduction and flexion of the hip and limb shortening.
- Acute-on-chronic slip: Long prodromal history and an acute, severe exacerbation.

While this temporal classification is commonly used, it does not correlate to the risk of avascular necrosis or predict the outcome in the longer term.

Loder et al. (1993) described a classification that discriminated between the stable slipped epiphysis when the child walked with or without crutches and the unstable, when walking was not possible. This distinction is clinically useful as it correlates with the risk of avascular necrosis, which occurs in 0 per cent of stable slips and 47 per cent of unstable slips.

Radiological grading is based on measurement of the magnitude of the slip relative to the width of the femoral neck, or the angle of the arc of the slip. The prognosis of a slip is associated with both the distance of slippage and the degree of angulation.

On a 'frog lateral' x-ray the slip is divided into three stages according to the percentage slip of the epiphysis in relation to the femoral neck.

- Mild: Displacement is less than one-third of the width of the femoral neck.
- Moderate: Displacement is between one-third and a half.
- Severe: Displacement is greater than half of the femoral neck width.

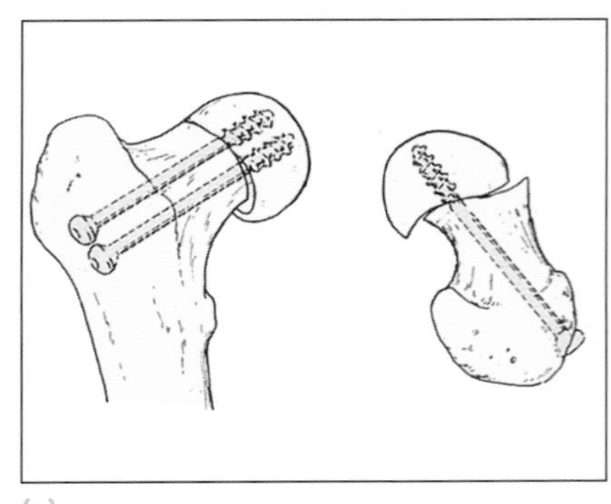
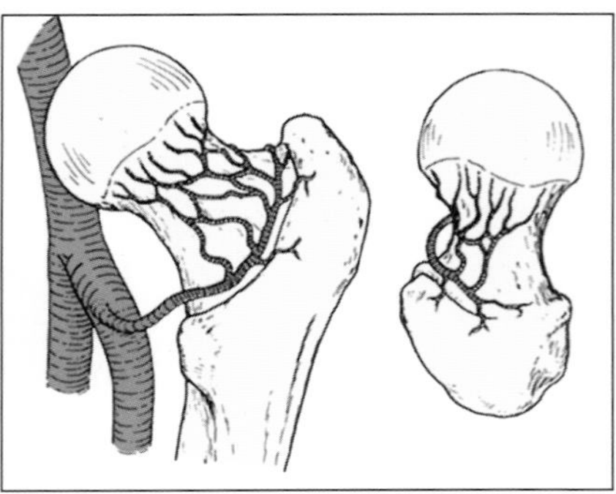
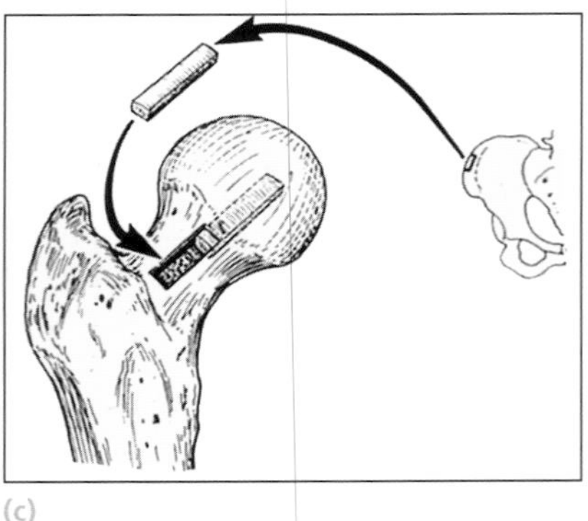

(a) (b) (c)

19.29 Moderate slip – treatment (a) A moderate slip can be accepted and fixed internally; it is essential that the threaded pins or screws enter the femur anteriorly so as not to risk damaging the retinacular vessels on the back of the femoral neck. (b) The femoral neck seen from behind and from above, showing the position of the vessels posterosuperiorly. (c) An alternative method of fixation – the Heyman and Herndon epiphyseodesis.

Jerre and Billing (1994) described a classification based on the magnitude of the epiphyseal–femoral shaft angle seen on the 'frog lateral' view. This requires precise placement of the limb in 90 degrees of external rotation with neutral rotation of the hip and the thigh elevated 25 degrees from the table. *This position is often painful and caution is advised in unstable slips, which may displace further.*

- Mild: Angle less than 30 degrees.
- Moderate: Angle 31–50 degrees.
- Severe: Angle more than 50 degrees.

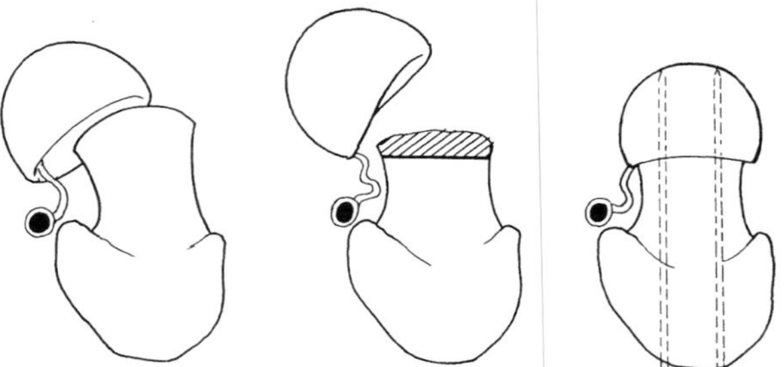

19.30 Severe slip – open reduction Dunn's operation for a severe slip. A small segment of the femoral neck is removed so that the epiphysis can be reduced and pinned without placing tension on the posterior vessels.

Treatment

The aims of treatment are (1) to preserve the epiphyseal blood supply, (2) to stabilize the physis and (3) to correct any residual deformity. Manipulative reduction of the slip carries a high risk of avascular necrosis and should be avoided. The choice of treatment depends on the degree of slip.

Minor slips (less than one-third of the width of the epiphysis on the AP x-ray and less than 20 degrees tilt in the lateral view). Deformity is minimal and needs no correction. The position is accepted and the physis is stabilized by inserting one or two screws or threaded pins along the femoral neck and into the epiphysis, under fluoroscopic control.

Moderate slips (between one-third and two-thirds of the width of the epiphysis on the AP x-ray and 20–40 degrees of tilt in the lateral view). Deformity resulting from this degree of slip, though noticeable, is often tempered by gradual bone modelling and may in the end cause little disability. One can therefore accept the position, fix the epiphysis in situ and then wait: if, after a year or two, there is a noticeable deformity, a corrective osteotomy is performed below the femoral neck (see below). This approach is safe, but 'fixing' the epiphysis is easier said than done: because the head is tilted backwards, pins driven up in the axis of the femoral neck will either enter the most anterior segment of the epiphysis (and be very insecure) or will penetrate the posterior cortex of the femoral neck and damage the retinacular vessels. Therefore, short threaded pins are inserted on the anterior femoral neck and directed posteromedially into the centre of the epiphysis. Alternatively – and probably with less risk of complications – fusion can be achieved by bone graft epiphyseodesis. At the same time any protruding bump on the anterosuperior metaphysis can be trimmed to prevent impingement on the lip of the acetabulum.

Severe slips (more than two-thirds of the width of the epiphysis on the AP x-ray and 40 degrees of tilt in the lateral view). This, the *'unacceptable slip'*, causes marked deformity which, untreated, will predispose to secondary OA. *Closed reduction by manipulation is dangerous and should not be attempted.*

Open reduction by Dunn's method (Dunn and Angel, 1978) gives good results, but should be

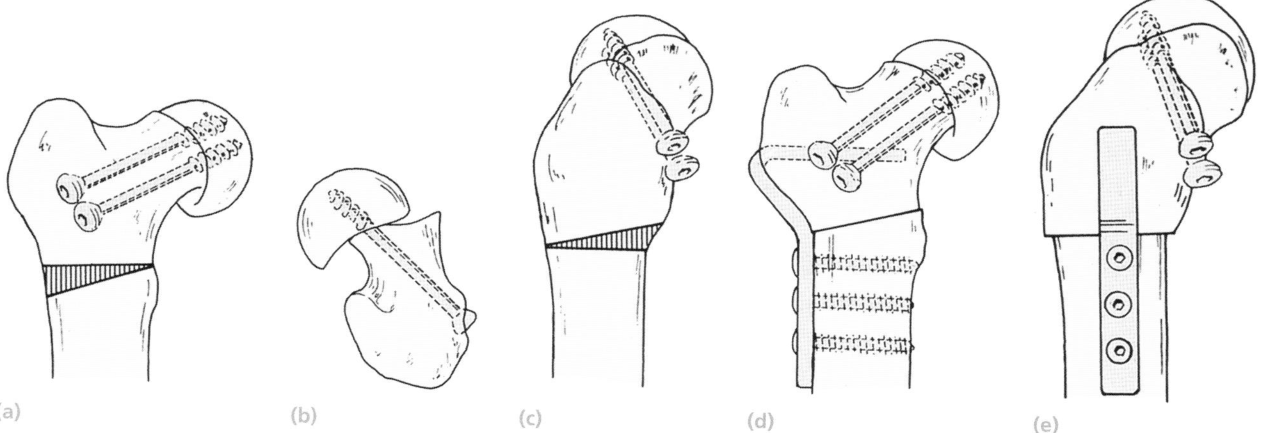

19.31 Severe slip – fixation and osteotomy (a–c) A severe slip can be treated by fixing it and then performing a compensatory osteotomy. Wedges are cut based laterally and anteriorly so as to permit valgus, flexion and rotation at the osteotomy. (d,e) The position after osteotomy and internal fixation.

reserved for the specialist. The greater trochanter is elevated and the femoral neck exposed. By gentle subperiosteal dissection, the posterior retinacular vessels are preserved while mobilizing the epiphysis (which is usually stuck down by young callus). A small segment of the femoral neck is then removed, so that the epiphysis can be repositioned without tension on the posterior structures; once reduced, it is held by two or three pins. In all but the most experienced hands, this still carries a 5–10 per cent risk of avascular necrosis or chondrolysis.

The alternative – and the method recommended for the less experienced surgeon – is to fix the epiphysis as for a 'moderate slip' and then, as soon as fusion is complete, to perform a compensatory intertrochanteric osteotomy: the easiest is a triplane osteotomy with simultaneous repositioning of the proximal femur in valgus, flexion and medial rotation; more anatomical is the geometric flexion osteotomy described by Griffith (1976). However, the patient should be told that this may result in 2–3 cm of shortening.

General note: Most of the complications of slipped epiphysis are related to treatment – injudicious attempts at manipulative reduction of the slip, or failure to recognize the hazards of internal fixation (Riley et al., 1990). The first rule of surgical treatment is 'thou shalt do no harm'!

Complications

Slipping at the opposite hip In at least 20 per cent of cases slipping occurs at the other hip – sometimes while the patient is still in bed. Forewarned is forearmed: the asymptomatic hip should be checked by x-ray and at the least sign of abnormality the epiphysis should be pinned.

Avascular necrosis Death of the epiphysis used to be common. It is now recognized that it hardly ever occurs in the absence of treatment. This iatrogenic complication is minimized by avoiding forceful manipulation and operations which might damage the posterior retinacular vessels.

Articular chondrolysis Cartilage necrosis probably results from vascular damage (often iatrogenic), but in these cases bone changes are minimal. There is progressive narrowing of the joint space and the hip becomes stiff.

This is a recognized complication in SCFE, and does not appear to be related to the method of treatment. In some cases, the condition improves spontaneously while in others it leads to loss of mobility and OA.

Coxa vara A slipped epiphysis that goes unnoticed – or is inadequately treated – may result in coxa vara. Except in the most severe cases, this is more apparent than real; the head slips backwards rather than downwards and the deformity is essentially one of *femoral neck retroversion*. Secondary effects are *external rotation deformity* of the hip, possibly *shortening* of the femur and (still a point of contention) *secondary OA*.

Slipped epiphysis in adults

Epiphysiolysis is occasionally seen in young adults with endocrine disorders (hypogonadism, hypopituitarism or hypothyroidism). This is a risk to be borne in mind in all patients with open physes in the proximal femur, and especially those who are then treated with growth hormone and suddenly increase in stature before the physes stabilize. Treatment is the same as in children.

PYOGENIC ARTHRITIS
(see also Chapter 2)

Pyogenic arthritis of the hip is usually seen in children under 2 years of age. The organism (usually a staphylococcus) reaches the joint either directly from a distant focus or by local spread from osteomyelitis of the femur. Unless the infection is rapidly aborted, the femoral head, which is largely cartilaginous at this age, is liable to be destroyed by the proteolytic enzymes of bacteria and pus.

Adults, also, may develop pyogenic hip infection, either as a primary event in states of debilitation or (more often) secondary to invasive procedures around the hip.

Clinical features

The child is ill and in pain, but it is often difficult to tell exactly where the pain is! The affected limb may be held absolutely still and all attempts at moving the hip are resisted. With care and patience it may be possible to localize a point of maximum tenderness over the hip; the diagnosis is confirmed by aspirating pus or fluid from the joint and submitting it for laboratory examination and bacteriological culture.

In the acute stage x-rays are of little value but sometimes they show soft-tissue swelling, displacement of the femoral head and a vacuum sign in the joint. Ultrasonography will reveal the joint effusion.

Diagnosis can be difficult, especially in neonates who may be almost asymptomatic. If the baby looks ill and no cause is apparent, think of *deep sepsis* and look for a possible source (e.g. an intravascular line). A high index of suspicion is the best aid.

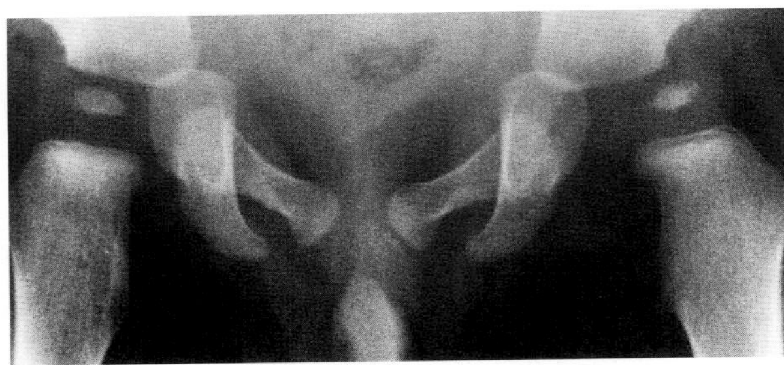

(a)

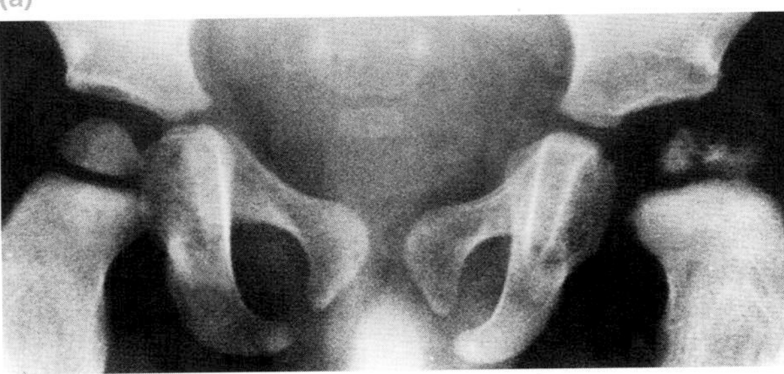

(b)

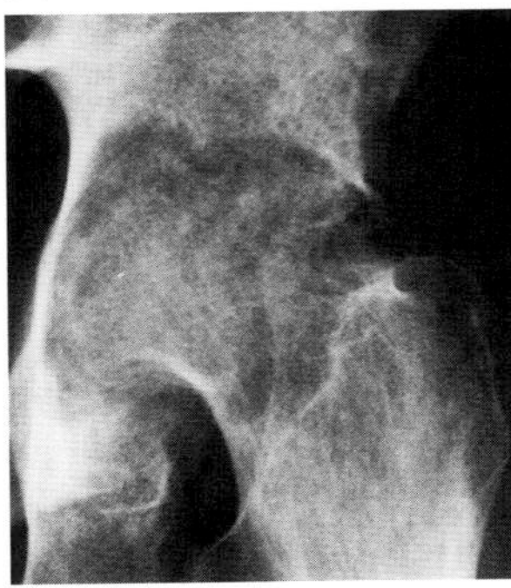

(c)

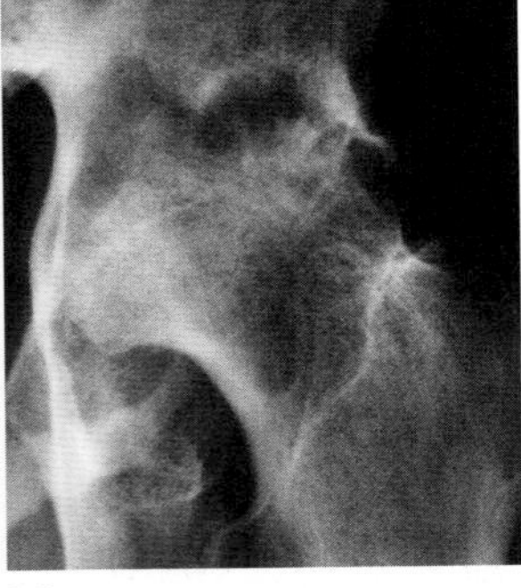

(d)

19.32 Pyogenic arthritis (a,b) *In an infant:* the left hip is distended and the head is drifting out of the socket. Six months later the epiphysis appears to be necrotic. (c,d) *In an adult:* rapid bone destruction over a period of 3 weeks!

Treatment

Intravenous antibiotics should be given as soon as the diagnosis is reasonably certain. The joint is aspirated under general anaesthesia and, if pus is withdrawn, anterior arthrotomy is performed; antibiotics are instilled locally and the wound is closed without drainage. Systemic antibiotics are essential, and the hip is kept on traction or splinted in abduction until all evidence of disease activity has disappeared.

Complications

If the infection is unchecked the head and neck of the femur may be destroyed and a pathological dislocation result. The pus may escape and, when the child recovers, the sinus heals. The hip signs then resemble those of a congenital dislocation, but the telltale scar remains and on x-ray the femoral head is completely absent.

TUBERCULOSIS
(see also Chapter 2)

The disease may start as a synovitis, or as an osteomyelitis in one of the adjacent bones. Once arthritis develops, destruction is rapid and may result in pathological dislocation. Healing usually leaves a fibrous ankylosis with considerable limb shortening and deformity.

Clinical features

The condition starts insidiously with aching in the groin and thigh, and a slight limp; later, pain is more severe and may wake the patient from sleep.

With early disease (synovitis or osteomyelitis) the joint is held slightly flexed and abducted, and extremes of movement are restricted and painful, but

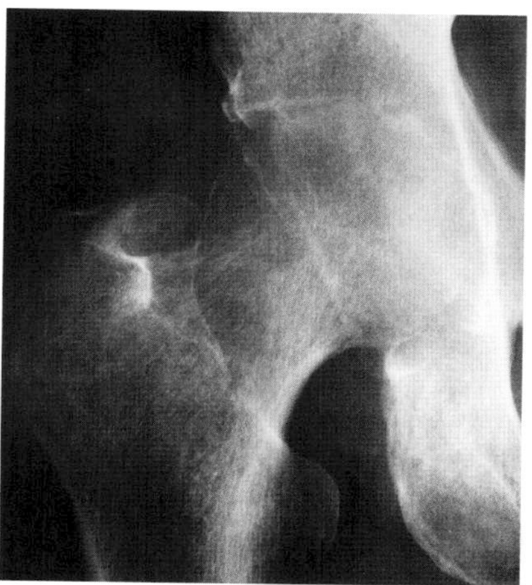
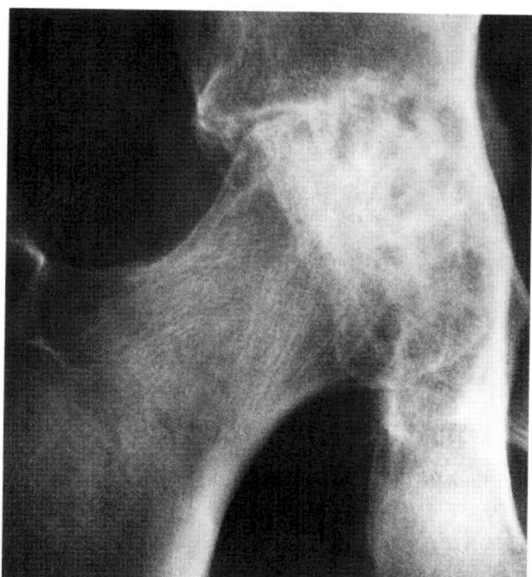
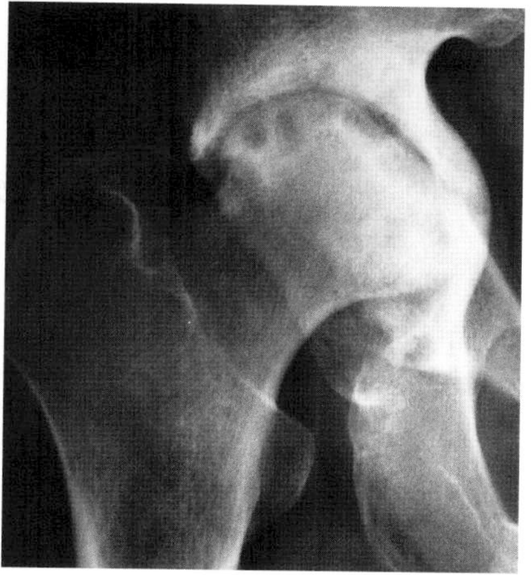

19.33 Hip tuberculosis – drug treatment In this patient, antituberculous drugs alone resulted in healing – though hip movements were still restricted.

until x-ray changes appear the hip is merely 'irritable' and diagnosis is difficult. If arthritis supervenes the hip becomes flexed, adducted and medially rotated, muscle wasting becomes obvious, and all movements are grossly limited by pain and spasm.

X-ray The earliest change is general rarefaction but with a normal joint space and line; the femoral epiphysis may be enlarged or a bone abscess visible; with arthritis, in addition to the general rarefaction, there is destruction of the acetabular roof (wandering acetabulum) or the femoral head, usually both; the joint may be subluxed or even dislocated. With healing the bones re-calcify.

Outcome

Early disease, if properly treated, may heal leaving a normal or almost normal hip, but once the articular surface is destroyed the usual result is an unsound fibrous joint. In untreated cases, the leg becomes scarred and thin; shortening is often severe because of bone destruction, adduction and flexion deformity of the hip and (in children) damage to the upper femoral epiphysis and occasionally premature fusion of the lower femoral epiphysis (especially if the child has been in a spica for too long).

Treatment

Antituberculous drugs are essential, and these alone may result in healing. Skin traction is applied and, for a child, an abduction frame may be used. An abscess in the femoral neck is best evacuated; if the arthritis does not settle, joint 'debridement' is performed. As the disease subsides, traction is discontinued and movement is encouraged.

If the joint has been destroyed, arthrodesis may be necessary once all signs of activity have disappeared, but usually not before the age of 14.

In older patients with residual pain and deformity, if the disease has clearly been inactive for a considerable time, total joint replacement is feasible and often successful; with antituberculous drugs, which are essential, the chances of recurrence are not great.

Girdlestone's excisional arthroplasty is occasionally the only option.

RHEUMATOID ARTHRITIS

(see also Chapter 3)

The hip joint is frequently affected in rheumatoid arthritis; occasionally the disease remains monarticular for several years, but eventually other sites are affected. Persistent synovitis in a weightbearing joint soon leads to the destruction of cartilage and bone; the acetabulum is eroded and eventually the femoral head may per-

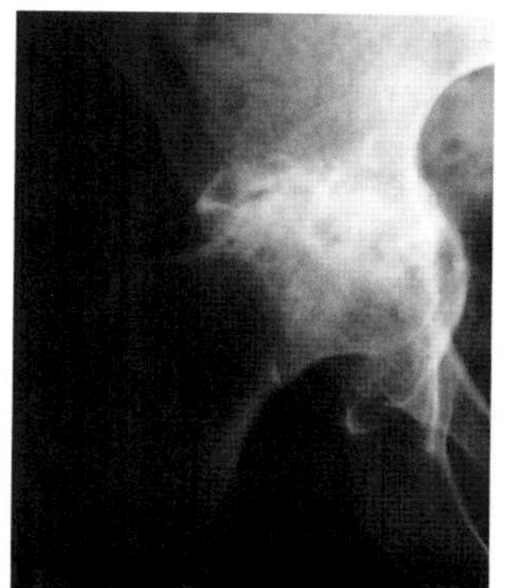
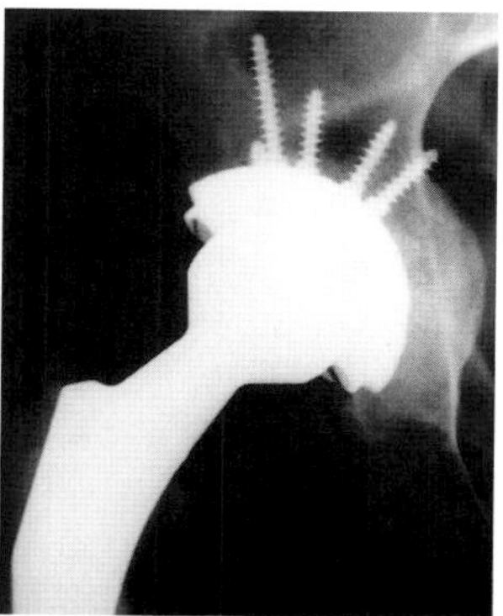

19.34 Rheumatoid arthritis – treatment Severe erosive arthritis treated by hip replacement with an uncemented socket and bone grafting of the acetabulum.

forate its floor. The hallmark of the disease is progressive bone destruction on both sides of the joint without any reactive osteophyte formation.

Clinical features

Usually the patient already has rheumatoid disease affecting many joints. Pain in the groin comes on insidiously; limp, though common, may be ascribed to pre-existing arthritis of the foot or knee. With advancing disease the patient has difficulty getting into or out of a chair, and even movements in bed may be painful. Occasionally the slow symptomatic progression is punctuated by acute flares with intense pain in the hip.

Wasting of the buttock and thigh is often marked, and the limb is usually held in external rotation and fixed flexion. All movements are restricted and painful.

X-rays During the early stages there is osteoporosis and diminution of the joint space; later, the acetabulum and femoral head are eroded. Protrusio acetabuli is common. In the worst cases (and especially in patients on corticosteroids) there is gross bone destruction and the floor of the acetabulum may be perforated.

Treatment

If the disease can be arrested by general treatment, hip deterioration may be slowed down. However, once cartilage and bone are eroded, no treatment will influence the progression to joint destruction. Total joint replacement is then the best answer. It relieves pain and restores a useful range of movement. It is advocated even in younger patients, because the polyarthritis so limits activity that the implants are not unduly stressed.

Care should be taken during operation to prevent fracture or perforation of the osteoporotic bone. If the acetabular floor is deficient, a supportive cage and bone grafting will be needed.

Children with juvenile chronic arthritis may need custom-made prostheses for their small and often delicate bones.

Postoperative infection poses a greater risk in rheumatoid patients than in others – more particularly if the patient is on corticosteroid therapy. Prophylaxis is even more important than usual.

OSTEOARTHRITIS
(see also Chapter 5)

The hip joint is one of the commonest sites of OA, though in some populations (e.g. African Negroes and southern Chinese) this joint seems peculiarly immune to the disease. This may simply be because certain predisposing conditions (acetabular dysplasia, Perthes' disease, slipped epiphysis) show a similar differential incidence in these populations.

Table 19.2 Causes of osteoarthritis of the hip

Abnormal stress	Defective cartilage	Abnormal bone
Subluxation	Infection	Fracture
Coxa magna	Rheumatoid	Necrosis
Coxa vara	Calcinosis	Paget's
Minor deformities		Other causes of scelorosis
Protrusio		

Where there is an obvious underlying cause the term '*secondary osteoarthritis*' is applied (Table 19.2); these patients are often in their third or fourth decade and the appearance of the joint reflects the preceding abnormality. Thus in regions where congenital dislocation and acetabular dysplasia are common (e.g. in southern Europe), women are more often affected than men, the hips may be the only joints affected and lateral subluxation is common.

When no underlying cause is apparent, the term '*primary osteoarthritis*' is used. It is now believed that even in these cases there is some preceding disorder that leads to articular cartilage damage and subtle abnormalities are being sought in patients who would otherwise fall into the 'primary' category. In the case of the hip particular attention has been given to anatomical and mechanical factors that affect joint congruency and predispose to femoro-acetabular impingement and erosion of the articular surface. This comparatively new field of enquiry is explored on page 524.

Pathology

The articular cartilage becomes soft and fibrillated while the underlying bone shows cyst formation and sclerosis. These changes are most marked in the area of maximal loading (chiefly the top of the joint); at the margins of the joint there are the characteristic osteophytes. Synovial hypertrophy is common and capsular fibrosis may account for joint stiffness. The pathology of OA is discussed in greater detail in Chapter 5.

Sometimes articular destruction progresses very rapidly, with erosion of the femoral head or acetabulum (or both), occasionally going on to perforation of the pelvis. This could be due to basic calcium crystal deposition in the joint (see Chapter 4).

Clinical features

Pain is felt in the groin but may radiate to the knee. Typically it occurs after periods of activity but later it

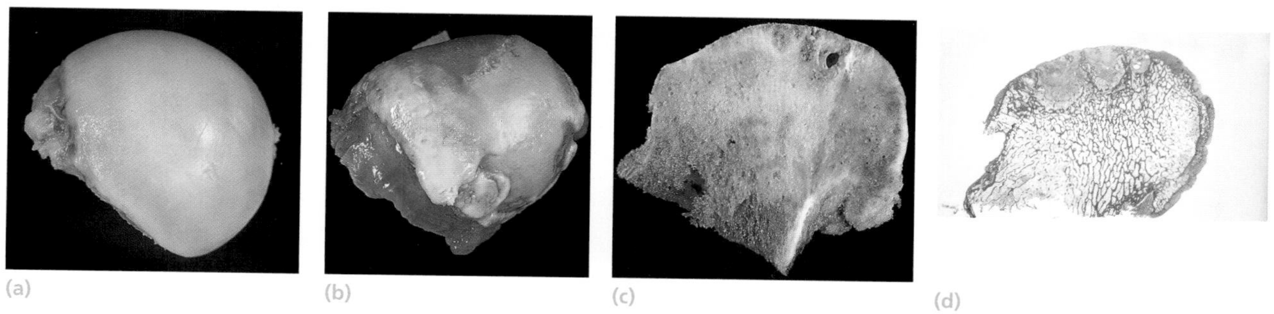

19.35 Osteoarthritis – pathology (a) Normal ageing causes slight degeneration of the articular surface but the general structure is well preserved. (b) By contrast, in progressive osteoarthritis the load-bearing area suffers increasing damage: in this case the superior surface of the femoral head is completely denuded of cartilage and there are large osteophytes around the periphery. In the coronal section (c,d) subarticular cysts are clearly revealed.

is more constant and sometimes disturbs sleep. Stiffness at first is noticed chiefly after rest; later it increases progressively until putting on socks and shoes becomes difficult. Limp is often noticed early and the patient may think the leg is getting shorter.

The patient is usually fit and over 50, but secondary OA can occur at 30 or even 20 years of age. There may be an obvious limp and, except in early cases, a positive Trendelenburg sign. The affected leg usually lies in external rotation and adduction, so it appears short; there is nearly always some fixed flexion, although this may only be revealed by Thomas' test. Muscle wasting is detectable but rarely severe. Deep pressure may elicit tenderness, and the greater trochanter is somewhat high and posterior. Movements, though often painless within a limited range, are restricted; internal rotation, abduction and extension are usually affected first and most severely.

X-ray The earliest sign is a decreased joint space, usually maximal in the superior weightbearing region but sometimes affecting the entire joint. Later signs are subarticular sclerosis, cyst formation and osteophytes. The shape of the femoral head or acetabulum may give a clue to an underlying condition (e.g. old Perthes' disease or a previous inflammatory arthritis). Bilateral cases occasionally show features of a generalized dysplasia.

Treatment

Analgesics and anti-inflammatory drugs may be helpful, and warmth is soothing. The patient is encour-

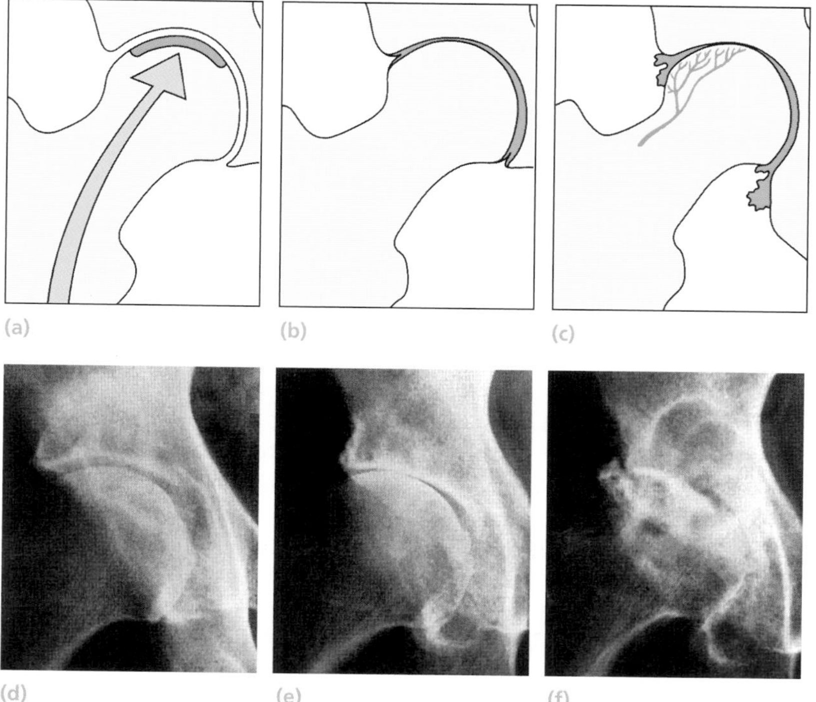

19.36 Osteoarthritis – x-ray (a–c) Cartilage softening and thinning are greatest in the zone of maximal stress. There is a vascular reaction and new-bone formation in the subchondral bone as well as osteophytic growth at the margins of the joint. These changes, as well as subchondral cyst formation, are reflected in the sequential x-ray appearances (d–f).

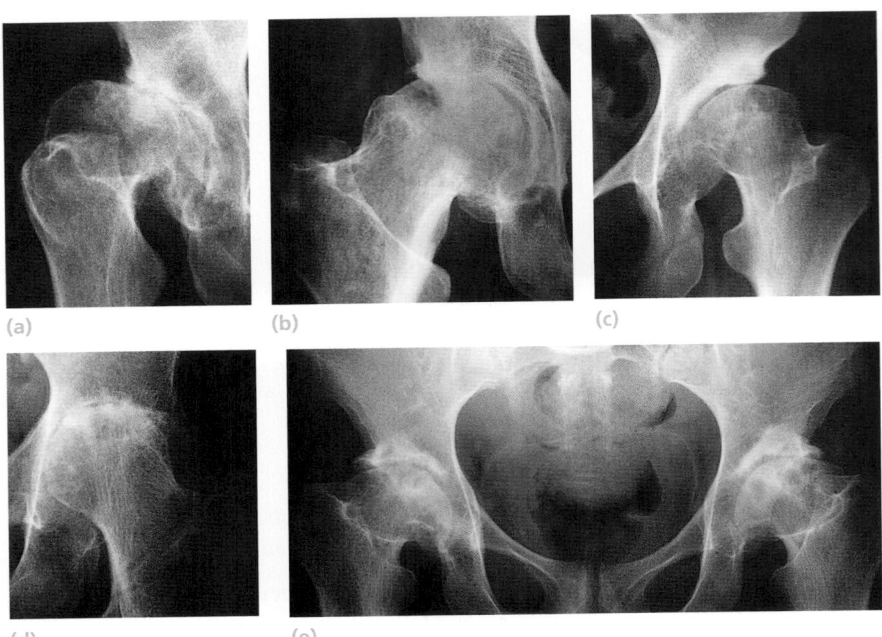

19.37 Secondary osteoarthritis (a) After Perthes' disease. (b) After slipped upper femoral epiphysis. (c) After congenital subluxation. (d) After rheumatoid disease. (e) Bilateral in a patient with multiple epiphyseal dysplasia.

aged to use a walking stick and to try to preserve movement and stability by non-weightbearing exercises. In early cases physiotherapy (including manipulation) may relieve pain for long periods. Activities are adjusted so as to reduce stress on the hip.

Operative treatment The indications for operation are (1) progressive increase in pain, (2) severe restriction of activities, (3) marked deformity and (4) progressive loss of movement (especially abduction), together with (5) x-ray signs of joint destruction.

In the usual case – a patient aged over 60 years with a long history of pain and increasing disability – the preferred operation is *total joint replacement* (see below). In those between 40 and 60 years this may still be the best operation if joint destruction is severe.

In younger patients, particularly those with some preservation of articular cartilage, an *intertrochanteric realignment osteotomy* may be considered. If performed early, it can arrest or delay further cartilage destruction, and if the operation is well planned it does not preclude later replacement arthroplasty.

In recent years *osteochondroplasty* has gained attention following the realization that 'primary' or 'idiopathic' OA of the hip is often associated with malposition or malcongruency of this ball-and-socket joint. This is discussed in the next section.

Arthrodesis of the hip is a practical solution for young adults with marked destruction of a single joint, and particularly when the conditions for advanced reconstructive surgery are less than ideal. If well executed, the operation guarantees freedom from pain and permanent stability, though it has the disadvantages of restricted mobility and a significant incidence of later backache, as well as deformity and discomfort in other nearby joints (Solomon, 1998).

FEMORO-ACETABULAR IMPINGEMENT AND OSTEOARTHRITIS

Reinhold Ganz and Michael Leunig

Although morphological abnormalities of the femoral head and acetabulum have long been recognized in patients with 'secondary' OA of the hip, the concept of femoro-acetabular impingement as a potent cause of 'primary' OA is comparatively new and its pathogenesis has been elaborated only in the last decade.

The human hip is a ball-and-socket joint in which the load-transmitting surfaces are covered by hyaline cartilage, thus offering minimal gliding resistance even during peak loading while permitting sufficient motion to serve the normal activities of daily living.

The range of motion of the hip joint is determined to a large extent by the head–neck ratio and the head size. Other influences include the spatial orientation of the acetabular socket and the proximal end of the femur as well as the femoral neck offset. A certain amount of anteversion of the socket and the femoral neck is necessary for the optimal amount of flexion and internal rotation of the hip. This combination of flexion and internal rotation represents the most important type of motion for optimal bipedal function. It is now known that if the combined angle of anteversion is less than 40 degrees, flexion–internal

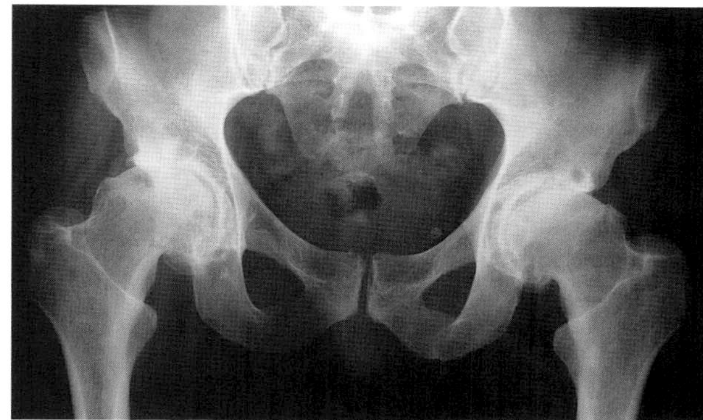

19.38 The 'pistol-grip' deformity X-ray of the pelvis in a man of 59 years who complained of pain in both hips. There is a loss of sphericity of the femoral heads, and unusual bony prominence of the uppermost outline at the head–neck junction in both hips, producing an appearance reminiscent of an old-fashioned pistol grip.

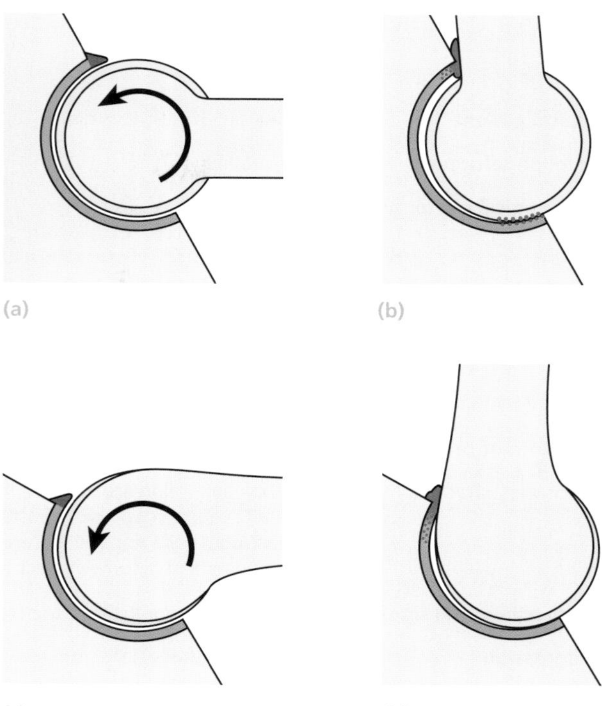

19.39 The two types of FAI *Pincer type of impingement*: (a) Hip in neutral position. Femoral head 'overcovered' by acetabular rim prominence. Arrow indicates intended motion. (b) During internal rotation the femoral neck abuts against the rim prominence; high shearing force posteriorly. *Cam type of impingement*: (c) Bony prominence at anterior head–neck junction. During flexion, internal rotation and adduction (d) the abnormally prominent head/neck abuts against the acetabular rim; the head is jammed in the acetabular cavity producing outside-in avulsion or abrasion of the cartilage from the labrum.

rotation is limited and may be painful, and that this condition is often associated with early OA of the hip (Tönnis and Heinecke, 1999).

Almost 100 years ago, Preisser recognized that limited internal rotation could be a precursor to OA of the hip. During the 1960s–1980s Murray (1965), Solomon (1976), Harris et al. (1986) and Stuhlberg et al. (1975) noted a significant association between early hip OA and subtle morphological abnormalities of the proximal femur, such as retroversion and the so-called 'pistol-grip' deformity of the femoral head (Fig. 19.38). Tönnis and Heinecke (1999) explored the relationship between acetabular and femoral anteversion and OA and gave a detailed description of how to measure these parameters.

These observations led to the theory that most, if not all, cases of so-called 'primary' OA of the hip are secondary to minimal deformities previously unnoticed or ignored, and that the initial cartilage damage is caused by femoro-acetabular impingement (FAI) (Ganz et al., 2003; Beck et al., 2005; Ganz et al., 2008).

Pathomechanics of femoro-acetabular impingement

There are two main subtypes of FAI: *pincer* and *cam*.

In the pincer mechanism there is either global overcoverage of the femoral head (circumferentially as in coxa profunda or protrusio) or local overcoverage of the femoral head by the anterior part of the acetabular rim if the acetabular opening is retroverted. As a consequence a bony ridge (or osteophyte) abuts against the front of the femoral neck during joint motion. This results in fatiguing and degeneration of the anterior part of the acetabular labrum along with a small zone of the adjacent articular cartilage (Fig. 19.39). There may also be an increased shearing force, mostly in the posterior part of the joint during medial rotation of the hip.

In the cam mechanism bony thickening at the femoral head–neck junction (i.e. a low head:neck ratio) causes jamming of the femoral neck against the front of the acetabulum and abrasion or delamination of the acetabular cartilage. During the early phase of cam FAI the acetabular labrum is normal in size and structure, but it may degenerate over time.

The pattern of cartilage damage differs in these two types of FAI; however the majority of FAI hips show a mixed type of impingement with predominance of the cam type. The peripheral anterosuperior part of the joint is severely involved and the central portion of the joint is not involved until there is progression of more advanced OA. However, in the pincer FAI pathology the postero-inferior joint cartilage may develop damage rather early; this could represent a *contre-coup* lesion.

Table 19.3 Characteristics of two types of femoro-acetabular impingement (FAI)

FAI type	Pincer	Cam
Typical patient	Female, 30–40 years old	Male, 20–30 years old, high activity
Level of deformity	Acetabulum	Proximal femur
Pathological anatomy	Deep socket Maloriented socket (idiopathic, iatrogenic)	Non-spherical extension femoral head Prominent metaphysis, retrotilted head Low anteversion femoral neck/low CCD angle (idiopathic, iatrogenic)
Associated disorders	Coxa profunda/ protrusio Acetabular retroversion (idiopathic, proximal focal femoral deficiency, post-traumatic dysplasia, iatrogenic)	Idiopathic, Perthes' disease, avascular necrosis, slipped capital femoral epiphysis, retrotilt after neck fracture, iatrogenic
Structure of primary damage	Labrum	Acetabular cartilage with outside-in abrasion/delamination
Secondary changes	Bone apposition acetabular rim, (double line), *contre-coup* lesion, postero-inferior cartilage, bone apposition, femoral neck, impingement cyst, head–neck junction	Labral degeneration
First radiological signs	Postero-inferior joint space narrowing	Anterolateral migration femoral head
Progression	Slow – rather painful	Rapid, although only mildly symptomatic

Aetiology of femoro-acetabular impingement

Slipped capital femoral epiphysis (SCFE), Perthes' disease and post-traumatic dysplasia are all associated with a high incidence of pincer and cam types of FAI (Ganz et al., 1991; Dora et al., 2000; Leunig et al., 2000) (see Fig.19.39), but the aetiology of most cases of 'idiopathic' FAI remains unknown.

Retroversion of the acetabulum has been associated with hip pain and OA (Reynolds et al., 1999; Giori and Trousdale, 2003). This common deformity is a type of spatial malorientation, not just a deficiency in the posterior wall, and a focal *pincer type FAI* is created by excessive anterior coverage of the femoral head. Iatropathic retroversion has been reported following pelvic osteotomy (Dora et al., 2002), but the aetiology in most cases has not been identified.

Femoral malformation following undiagnosed SCFE was initially thought to be the main cause of *cam type FAI*, but MRI has shown that most of the hips with cam FAI do not manifest the other typical physeal abnormalities associated with SCFE (Siebenrock et al., 2004).

It has also been suggested that rigorous physical activity during skeletal development (causing increased physeal stresses) may play a part in the development of proximal femoral abnormalities.

Clinical features of femoro-acetabular impingement

Groin pain and limited motion are the usual presenting symptoms. During the initial stages of the disease, groin pain may be exacerbated by excessive demand on the hip or may present after sitting for a prolonged period. Examination reveals a restriction of internal rotation in flexion. This test indicates the presence of abnormal morphology of the femoral neck and acetabular rim with recreation of pain, particularly once there is a chondral or labral lesion. Occasionally pain is elicited with flexion–abduction and/or with hyperextension and external rotation pointing towards an impingement in these areas.

The typical patient with predominantly pincer FAI is a woman of 30–40 years. The pain is generated from the injured labrum when there is direct contact between the femoral neck and the sensitive pain fibres of the labrum. Pain can be quite marked although the cartilage damage may be moderate.

The typical patient with predominantly cam FAI is a man, rather muscular and athletic, and about 10 years younger. Pain in this case is less dramatic, probably because FAI is more a jamming of the non-spherical portion of the head into the cavity of the socket. Despite the lesser degree of pain, cartilage destruction is often substantial (Table 19.3).

Standard methods of scoring hip function used for total hip replacement patients are not suitable for young FAI patients with high athletic demands. New outcome scores have been developed and validated for their potential use in hip disorders of the younger patient but so far they have not been widely adopted.

Imaging

An orthograde anteroposterior radiograph of the pelvis and a lateral radiograph of the hip are needed for patients with suspected FAI. The pelvis should be pictured with the coccyx pointing towards the symphysis and a distance of 1–2 cm between them. Besides demonstrating the 'pistol-grip' deformity of the proximal femur, this projection is essential for assessing acetabular version. The quality must be sufficient to allow visualization of the anterior and posterior rims of the acetabulum and to define the double contours of the rim; in a retroverted acetabulum the line of the anterior rim sweeps lateral to the line of the posterior rim (Ganz et al., 2003; Jamali et al., 2007), a feature associated with FAI (Fig. 19.40).

The best lateral view is a 'cross-table lateral', allowing one to detect anterolateral abnormalities of the head/neck contour (Fig. 19.41). MR arthrograms of the hip, including radial cuts, are used to visualize the labrum and cartilage as well as the femoral head/neck morphology.

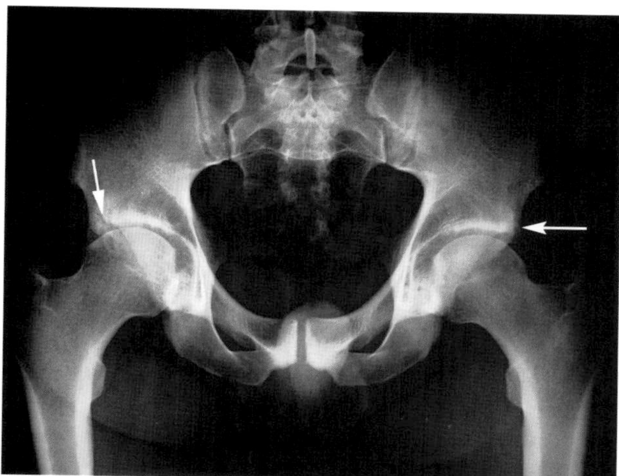

19.40 X-ray – Pincer FAI Anteroposterior radiograph of a 23-year-old man with bilateral retroversion. One can see that in each hip the anterior rim of the acetabulum projects lateral to the posterior rim (arrow, left hip), a sign suggesting retroversion of the hip. At the right hip there is a fatigue fracture of part of the anterior rim of the acetabulum (arrow, right hip).

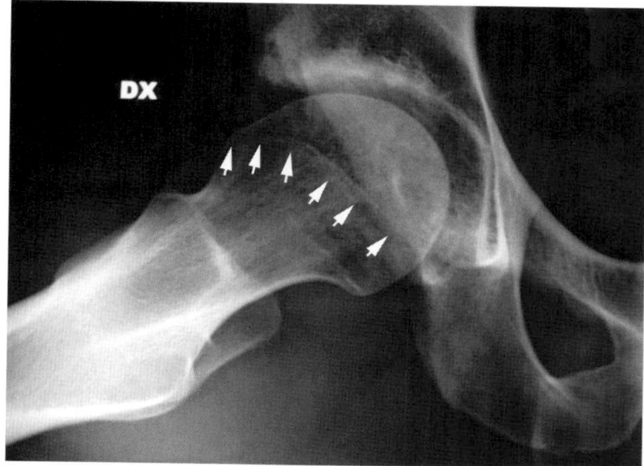

19.41 X-ray – same case as in Figure 19.40 Lateral projection of the right proximal femur. Note the non-spherical expansion of the anterolateral contour of the femoral epiphysis (arrows point to the curved line of the former growth plate).

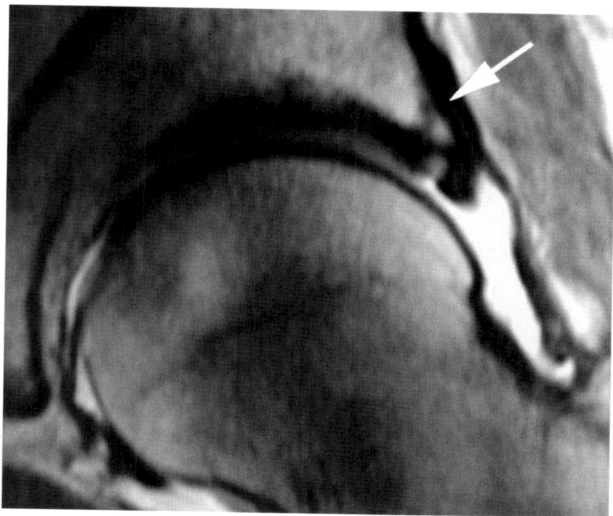

19.42 MR arthrography Section of the lateral joint space of a retroverted left hip, showing the bony projection at the acetabular rim (arrow), a slight signal alteration of the rounded labrum and some irregularity of the adjacent cartilage.

MR arthrograms of the hip are used routinely to visualize the labrum and articular cartilage. These are capable of detecting abnormal sphericity of the femoral head, low offset of the neck, impingement cysts and bone appositions of the rim, all related to FAI. MR arthrography is sensitive and specific for detecting labral and chondral lesions; however, there are limitations in detecting undisplaced delaminations of the acetabular cartilage.

New advanced imaging techniques such as the 3-Tesla system and delayed gadolinium-enhanced MRI of cartilage (dGEMRIC) may in the future be able to detect early cartilage lesions and capsular adhesions.

Treatment

Non-operative The benefits of non-surgical treatment such as physical or anti-inflammatory therapy in FAI are questionable. Restriction of athletic activities may occasionally reduce symptoms; however, a delay in the surgical correction of symptomatic bone dysmorphism may permit progression of articular cartilage destruction, leading to the premature onset of osteoarthritis.

Operative *Arthroscopic procedures* are suitable only for minor and localized structural abnormalities (Fig. 19.43). Isolated treatment of labral lesions without correcting the underlying bony pathology is a major cause of failure.

Open operation with dislocation of the hip is the pre-

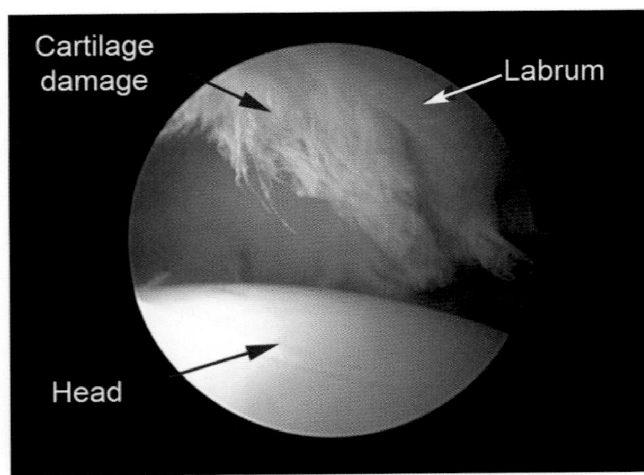

19.43 FAI – arthroscopy Arthroscopic view showing frayed acetabular articular cartilage

ferred approach for treating FAI, offering the advantages of unrestricted access, a precise correction, anatomical labral refixation and the possibility of dynamic control of the correction (Fig 19.44). Osteochondroplasty calls for debridement of damaged cartilage and/or resection of the bony impediments that are responsible for the malarticulation. For cam-type impingement the bony excrescence on the anterior femoral neck needs to be resected; for pincer-type impingement the abnormal overgrowth at the anterior rim of the acetabulum must be removed. In some cases corrective osteotomy of the proximal femur or acetabulum may also be needed (Fig. 19.45).

The morbidity of the procedure is low and the short- to mid-term results are good to excellent (Beck et al., 2004; Murphy et al., 2004; Espinosa et al., 2006; Beaulé et al., 2007).

OSTEONECROSIS

(see also Chapter 6)

The femoral head is the commonest site of symptomatic osteonecrosis, mainly because of its peculiar blood supply which renders it vulnerable to ischaemia from arterial cut-off, venous stasis, intravascular thrombosis, intraosseous sinusoidal compression, or a combination of several of these. The pathogenesis and pathological anatomy of the condition are discussed in Chapter 6.

Post-traumatic osteonecrosis usually follows a displaced fracture of the femoral neck or dislocation of the hip. The main cause is interruption of the arterial blood supply, but contributory factors are venous stasis and thrombosis of intramedullary arterioles and capillaries.

Non-traumatic osteonecrosis is seen in association with infiltrative disorders of the marrow, Gaucher's disease, sickle-cell disease, coagulopathies, caisson disease, systemic lupus erythematosus and – commonest of all – high-dosage corticosteroid administration and alcohol abuse. Perthes' disease is a special example which is dealt with elsewhere in this chapter.

The pathogenesis and pathological anatomy of the bone changes are discussed in Chapter 6.

Clinical features

Post-traumatic osteonecrosis develops soon after injury to the hip, but symptoms and signs may take months to appear.

Non-traumatic osteonecrosis is more insidious. Children are affected in conditions such as Perthes'

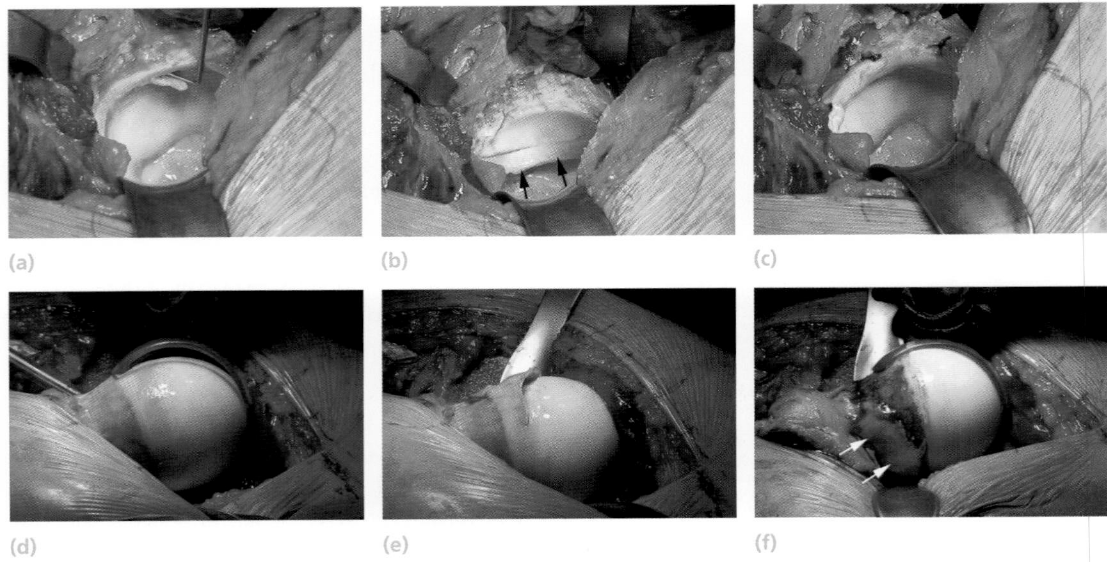

19.44 FAI – open osteochondroplasty Series showing open surgical treatment of FAI. (a–c) Torn acetabular labrum re-fixed and (d–f) non-spherical contour of the femoral head trimmed back.

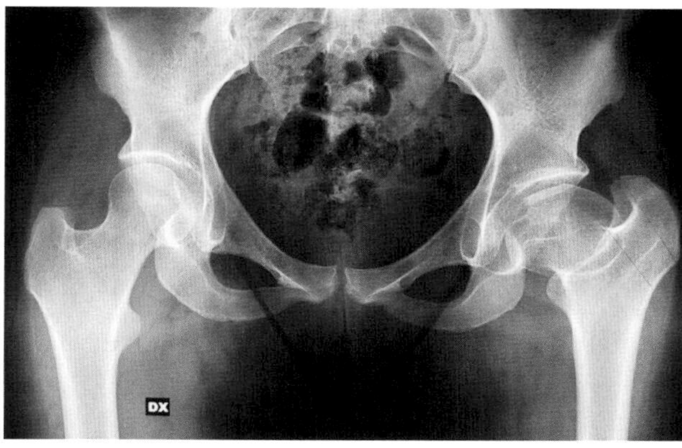

(a)

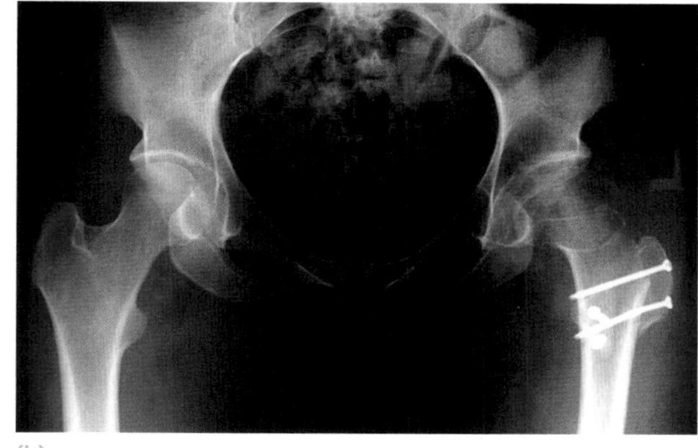

(b)

19.45 FAI – bony correction Bone deformities due to acetabular dysplasia, old Perthes' disease or SCFE may need corrective osteotomy as well. This 19-year-old female had an old Perthes deformity (a) a high-riding greater trochanter with short neck producing extra-articular impingement against the posterosuperior acetabular wall. The prominent anterior border of the femoral head (producing a 'sagging rope sign' on x-ray) led to intra-articular FAI. (b) Correction of the complex impingement was achieved by trimming the femoral head contour and 'lengthening' the femoral neck, together with advancement of both the greater and the lesser trochanter.

disease, sickle-cell disease and Gaucher's disease. Adult patients come from both sexes and all ages.

The presenting complaint is usually pain in the hip (or, in over 50 per cent of cases, both hips), which progresses over a period of 2–3 years to become quite severe. However, in over 10 per cent of cases the condition is asymptomatic and discovered incidentally after x-ray or MRI during investigation of a systemic disorder or longstanding symptoms in the other hip.

On examination, the patient walks with a limp and may have a positive Trendelenburg sign. The thigh is wasted and the limb may be 1 or 2 cm short. Movements are restricted, particularly abduction and internal rotation. A characteristic sign is a tendency for the hip to twist into external rotation during passive flexion; this corresponds to the 'sectoral sign' in which, with the hip extended, internal rotation is almost full, but with the hip flexed it is grossly restricted.

There may be symptoms or signs of an associated, causative disorder or a history of having been treated with corticosteroids – remember that even a short course of high-dosage corticosteroids can result in osteonecrosis and the hip is the commonest target. Another risk factor is high usage of alcohol.

(a)

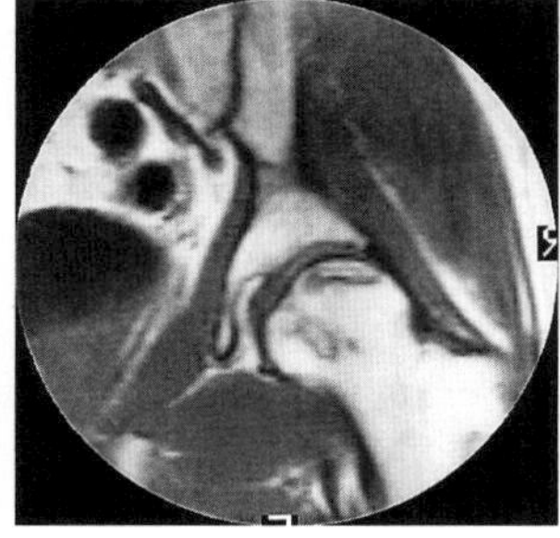

(b)

19.46 Osteonecrosis – imaging, early stage (a) This patient had few symptoms and x-rays that were, at most, equivocal. However, even at that early stage the MRI (b) showed a clear-cut segment of osteonecrosis at the dome of the femoral head.

Imaging

X-rays During the early stages of osteonecrosis plain x-rays are normal. The first signs appear only 6–9 months after the occurrence of bone death and are due mainly to reactive changes in the surrounding (live) bone. Thus, the classic feature of increased density (interpreted as sclerosis) is a sign of repair rather than necrosis. With time, destructive changes do appear in the necrotic segment: a thin subchondral fracture line (the 'crescent sign'), slight flattening of the weightbearing zone and then increasing distortion, with eventual collapse, of the articular surface of the femoral head.

MRI MRI shows characteristic changes in the marrow long before the appearance of x-ray signs – a mean of 3.6 months after the initiation of steroid treatment in one published study (Sakamoto et al., 1997). The diagnostic feature is a band of altered signal intensity running through the femoral head (diminished intensity in the T1 weighted SE image and increased intensity in the STIR image). This 'band' represents the reactive zone between living and dead bone and thus demarcates the ischaemic segment, the extent and location of which are important in staging the lesion.

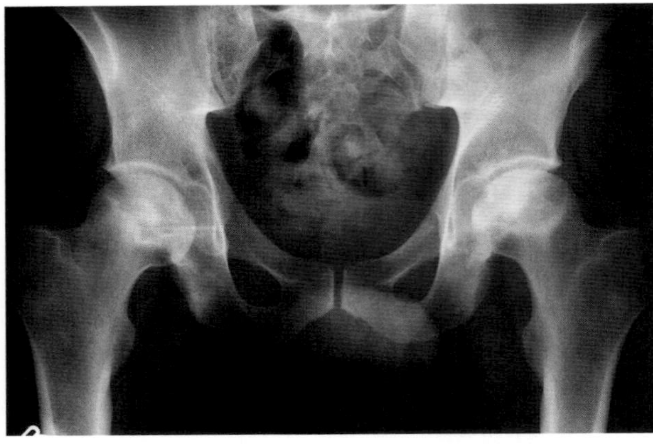

(a)

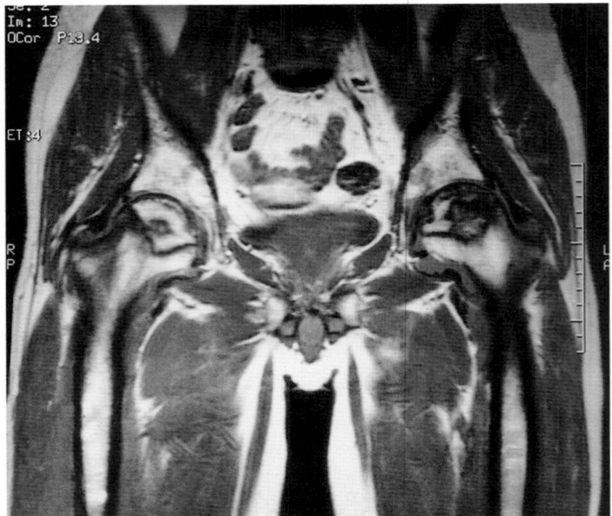

(b)

19.47 Osteonecrosis – imaging, late stage (a) Plain x-ray showing the typical features of bilateral corticosteroid-induced osteonecrosis of the femoral heads. The dense bands define the boundary between dead bone and new-bone formation. (b) The corresponding MRI in the same patient.

Diagnosis

X-ray features of destructive or sclerotic forms of *osteoarthritis* are sometimes mistaken for those of advanced osteonecrosis. There may, indeed, be elements of bone necrosis in some types of OA, but there is an important point of distinction between these two conditions: in OA the articular 'space' diminishes before the bone breaks up, whereas in osteonecrosis the articular 'space' is preserved to the last (because it is not primarily a disease of articular cartilage).

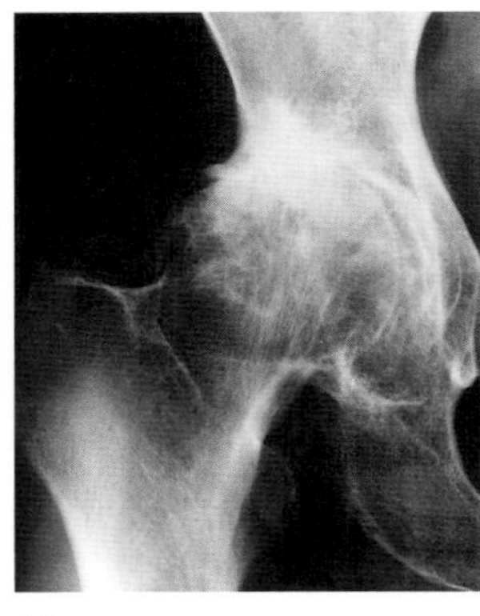

(a)

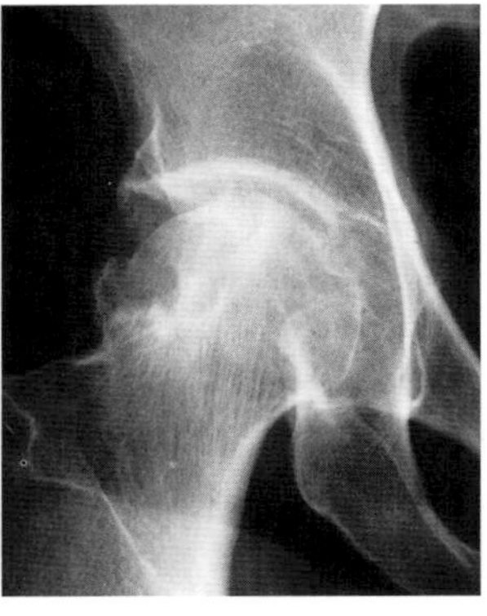

(b)

19.48 Diagnosis (a) Osteoarthritis sometimes shows marked segmental sclerosis on x-ray. These features are often mistaken for those of osteonecrosis. The clue lies in the absent joint 'space', a cardinal sign in osteoarthritis. Compare this with (b), an x-ray of severe osteonecrosis in which the joint 'space' is preserved in the face of bone collapse.

Transient osteoporosis of the hip is sometimes confused with avascular necrosis. The condition is described below.

The causative disorder Diagnosis should include elucidation of the causative disorder. There may be a history of trauma, a familial condition such as sickle-cell disease or Gaucher's disease, an occupational background suggesting dysbaric ischaemia, an underlying disease such as systemic lupus erythematosus, or a known background of corticosteroid administration or alcohol abuse. If there is no such history, the patient should be fully investigated for these associated conditions (see Chapter 6).

It is important to recognize that pathogenic factors are cumulative, so a patient with systemic lupus or a moderately severe alcohol habit may develop osteonecrosis following comparatively low doses of cortisone, and occasionally even after prolonged or excessive use of topical corticosteroids (Solomon and Pearse, 1994).

STAGING (see Chapter 6)

In the past, Ficat and Arlet's radiographic staging of femoral head necrosis was widely used. In *Stage 1* the patient has little or no pain and the plain x-ray shows no abnormality. However, there are typical changes on MRI (see Fig. 19.46). In *Stage 2* there are early x-ray signs but no distortion of the femoral head. *Stage 3 is* more advanced, with increasing signs of bone destruction and femoral head distortion. *Stage 4* is characterized by collapse of the articular surface and joint disorganization. This is a useful descriptive classification of the current state

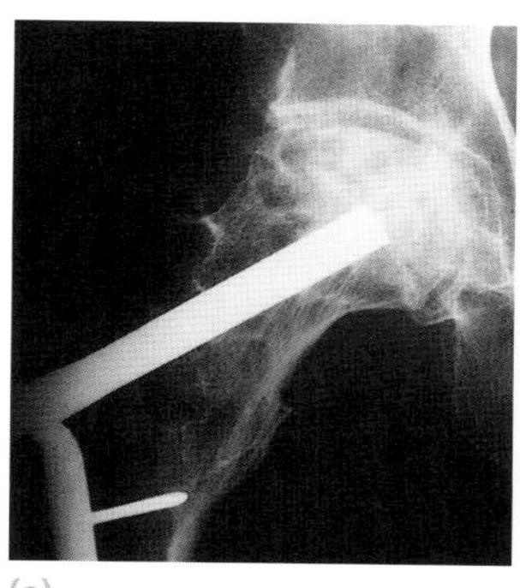

(a)

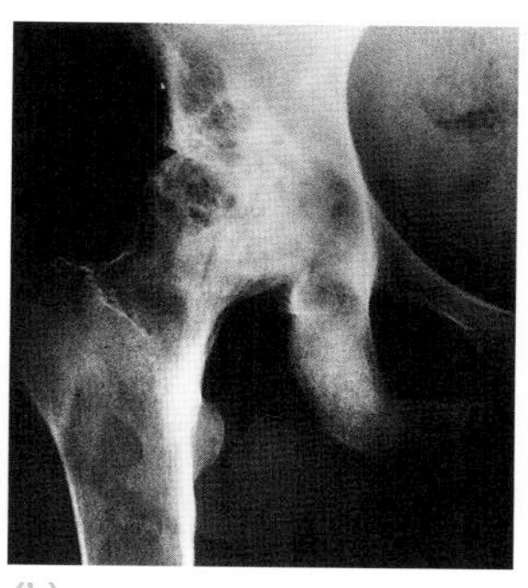

(b)

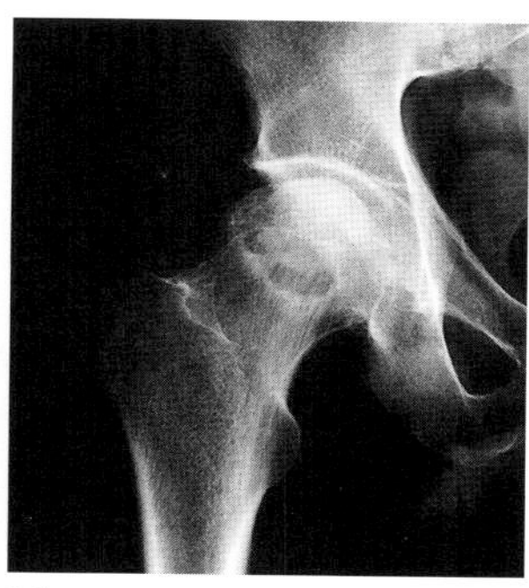

(c)

19.49 Osteonecrosis Femoral head necrosis due to (a) femoral neck fracture, (b) Gaucher's disease and (c) chronic alcohol abuse.

of affairs but it does not provide a guide to prognosis (and therefore treatment) in the early stages of the condition.

Shimizu et al. (1994) proposed a classification based on MR images which defines the extent, location and intensity of the abnormal segment in the femoral head. The risk of femoral head collapse (at least over a period of 2–3 years) was related mainly to the *extent* (the area of the coronal femoral head image involved) and *location* (the portion of the weightbearing surface) in the initial MRI. In general terms, their findings suggested that: (1) the extent of the ischaemic segment is determined at the outset and does not increase over time; (2) lesions occupying less than one-quarter of the femoral head coronal diameter and involving only the medial third of the weightbearing surface rarely go on to collapse; (3) lesions occupying up to one-half of the femoral head diameter and involving between one-third and two-thirds of the weightbearing surface are likely to collapse in about 30 per cent of cases; and (4) lesions occupying more than one-quarter of the femoral head diameter and involving more than two-thirds of the weightbearing surface will collapse within 3 years in over 70 per cent of cases. When discussing treatment, we shall refer to these three degrees of severity as *Grade I*, *Grade II* and *Grade III*.

Note that although this classification is useful for predicting outcome and planning treatment, *extent* (in this context) is not synonymous with *volume*; the true volume of the necrotic segment is very difficult to determine (Kim et al., 1998).

For purposes of comparing data from different sources before and after treatment, the recommended classification is the one proposed by the International Association of Bone Circulation and Bone Necrosis *(Association Research Circulation Osseous – ARCO)* (Table 19.4).

Location / Extent			
	–	+	++
	+	++	+++
	++	+++	++++

19.50 Predictive staging The likelihood of progression to collapse depends on the location and extent of the boundary changes on MRI. In this figure the risk of progression is represented by + signs. The general scheme is based on findings published by Shimuzu et al. (1994).

Treatment of post-traumatic osteonecrosis

Femoral head necrosis following fracture or dislocation of the hip usually ends in collapse of the femoral head. Very young patients (those under 40 years), in whom one is reluctant to perform hip replacement, can be treated by realignment osteotomy, with or without bone grafting of the necrotic segment. They will probably require hip replacement at a later stage.

Older patients will almost invariably opt for partial or total joint replacement.

Treatment of non-traumatic osteonecrosis

Early *Shimuzu Grade I lesions* (those restricted to the medial part of the femoral head) progress very slowly

Table 19.4 ARCO staging of osteonecrosis

Stage 0	Patient asymptomatic and all clinical investigations 'normal' Biopsy shows osteonecrosis
Stage 1	X-rays normal. MRI or radionuclide scan shows osteonecrosis
Stage 2	X-rays and/or MRI show early signs of osteonecrosis but no distortion of bone shape or subchondral 'crescent sign'. Subclassification by area of articular surface involved: A = less than 15 per cent B = 15–30 per cent C = more than 30 per cent
Stage 3	X-ray shows 'crescent sign' but femoral head still spherical Subclassification by length of 'crescent'/articular surface: A = less than 15 per cent B = 15–30 per cent C = more than 30 per cent
Stage 4	Signs of flattening or collapse of femoral head A = less than 15 per cent of articular surface B = 15–30 per cent of articular surface C = more than 30 per cent of articular surface
Stage 5	Changes as above plus loss of 'joint space' (secondary OA)
Stage 6	Changes as above plus marked destruction of articular surfaces

ARCO, Association Research Circulation Osseous; OA, osteoarthritis.

or not at all. Almost any treatment for this group is therefore liable to be assessed as 'beneficial'. All that is needed is symptomatic treatment and reassurance, but it is wise to observe the patient over several years in case there should be a change.

Grade II lesions (those occupying up to one-half of the femoral head and between one and two-thirds of the weightbearing surface) are liable to progress. If they are seen before there is any distortion of the femoral head, it would therefore be justifiable to advise conservative surgery (core decompression or decompression and bone grafting of the femoral head). Coring of the femoral head was introduced by Ficat (1985) as a means of reducing the intraosseous pressure in patients with early non-traumatic osteonecrosis. The intraosseous pressure is measured and, if it is raised, a 7 mm core of bone is removed by drilling up the femoral neck under image intensification fluoroscopy. It is impossible to say which cases will respond favourably, but the attempt is worthwhile and sustained symptomatic improvement is seen in 30–50 per cent of patients. The alternative is realignment osteotomy in younger patients and partial or total hip replacement in patients over 45 years old with increasing symptoms.

Grade III lesions (those occupying a large part of the femoral head and more than two-thirds of the weightbearing surface) have a poor prognosis. Decompression is unlikely to have a lasting effect. For younger patients, therefore, realignment osteotomy is the treatment of choice. X-rays and CT will show exactly where the necrotic segment is and the angulation osteotomy can be planned so as to displace the necrotic segment away from the maximal load-bearing trajectory. A flexion osteotomy will be needed for most cases. The more radical transtrochanteric rotational osteotomy of Sugioka (Sugioka and Mohtai, 1998) is difficult to perform and the results in most hands are no better than those of the more conventional osteotomies. Older patients with intrusive symptoms will be better served by partial or total joint replacement.

Late Patients with advanced osteonecrosis and bone collapse (Ficat stage 3 or 4) will need reconstructive surgery: osteotomy, with or without bone grafting, or joint replacement.

There is a limited place for arthrodesis in young men who are willing to accept the limitations of a 'stiff' hip in return for pain relief (Solomon, 1998).

TRANSIENT OSTEOPOROSIS OF THE HIP (MARROW OEDEMA SYNDROME)

This is a well-recognized, though uncommon, syndrome characterized by pain and rapidly emerging osteoporosis of the femoral head and adjacent pelvis. Radionuclide scanning shows increased activity on both sides of the hip but not in the soft tissues. The condition was originally described in women in the last trimester of pregnancy, but it is now seen in patients of both sexes and all ages from early adulthood onwards. Typically the changes last for 6–12 months, after which the symptoms subside and x-ray gradually returns to normal.

The cause is unknown, but *MRI features* are characteristic of marrow oedema. It has been suggested that the condition is a precursor (or *forme fruste*) of avascular necrosis, but there is little evidence to support this (see Chapter 6).

Treatment The condition almost always resolves spontaneously and most patients require no more than symptomatic treatment. However, pain can be rapidly abolished by operative decompression of the femoral head (drilling up the femoral neck), and some would prefer this to the long wait for a natural 'cure'. If there is any doubt about whether the MRI changes are due to osteonecrosis or marrow oedema, operative decompression is recommended.

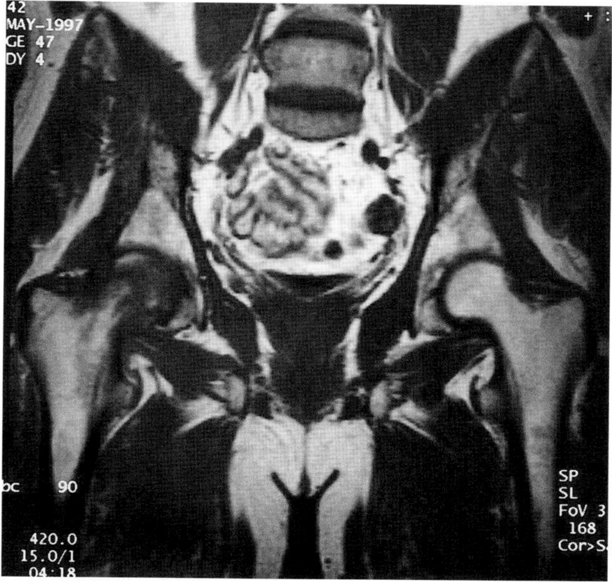

19.51 Marrow oedema syndrome This patient complained of pain in the right hip. X-ray showed no obvious abnormality, although the area around the hip looked somewhat osteoporotic. MRI disclosed the typical picture of diffuse signal reduction (in the right femoral head) in the T1 weighted scans. This contrasts sharply with the localized bands which are characteristic of osteonecrosis.

BURSITIS AND TENDINITIS AROUND THE HIP

Trochanteric bursitis

Pain over the lateral aspect of the hip and thigh may be due to local trauma or overuse, resulting in inflammation of the trochanteric bursa which lies deep to the tensor fasciae latae. There is local tenderness and sometimes crepitus on flexing and extending the hip. Swelling is unusual but post-traumatic bleeding can produce a bursal haematoma.

X-rays may show evidence of a previous fracture, or a protruding metal implant or trochanteric wires dating from some former operation. There may also be calcification or shadows suggesting swelling of the soft tissues. It is important to exclude underlying disorders such as gout, rheumatoid disease and infection (including tuberculosis).

Other causes of pain and tenderness over the greater trochanter are stress fractures (in athletes and elderly patients), slipped epiphysis (in adolescents) and bone infection (in children). The commonest cause of misdiagnosis is referred pain from the lumbar spine.

The usual treatment of trochanteric bursitis is rest, administration of non-steroidal anti-inflammatory drugs and (provided infection is excluded) injection of local anaesthetic and corticosteroid. If a haematoma is present it should be aspirated.

Gluteus medius tendinitis

Acute tendinitis may cause pain and localized tenderness just behind the greater trochanter. This is seen particularly in dancers and athletes. The clinical and x-ray features are similar to those of trochanteric bursitis, and the differential diagnosis is the same. Treatment is by rest and injection of local anaesthetic and corticosteroid.

Adductor longus strain or tendinitis

This overuse injury is often seen in footballers and athletes. The patient complains of pain in the groin and tenderness can be to the adductor longus origin close to the pubis. Swelling below this site may signify an adductor longus tear.

Acute strains are treated by rest and heat. Chronic strains may need prolonged physiotherapy.

Iliopsoas bursitis

Pain in the groin and anterior thigh may be due to an iliopsoas bursitis. The site of tenderness is difficult to define and there may be guarding of the muscles overlying the lesser trochanter. Hip movements are sometimes restricted; indeed, the condition may arise from synovitis of the hip since there is often a potential communication between the bursa and the joint. The most typical feature is a sharp increase in pain on adduction and internal rotation of the hip. Pain can also be elicited by testing psoas contraction against resistance (see Fig. 19.3).

The differential diagnosis of anterior hip pain includes inguinal lymphadenopathy, hernia, a psoas abscess, fracture of the lesser trochanter, slipped epiphysis, local infection and arthritis.

Treatment is by non-steroidal anti-inflammatory drugs and injection of local anaesthetic and steroid; the injection is best performed under fluoroscopic control.

Snapping hip

'Snapping hip' is a disorder in which the patient (usually a young woman) complains of the hip 'jumping out of place, or 'catching', during walking. The snapping is caused by a thickened band in the gluteus maximus aponeurosis flipping over the greater trochanter. In the swing phase of walking the band moves anteriorly; then, in the stance phase, as the gluteus maximus contracts and pulls the hip into extension, the band flips back across the trochanter, causing an audible 'snap'. This is usually painless but it can be quite dis-

PAIN AROUND THE HIP

Anteriorly (groin)
Synovitis and arthritis
Perthes' disease
Labral tear or detachment
Loose bodies in the joint
Stress fracture
Osteitis pubis
Other bone lesions
Inguinal hernia
Inguinal lymphadenopathy
Iliopsoas tendinitis or bursitis
Iliopsoas abscess
Adductor longus strain or tendinitis

Laterally
Referred from spine
Slipped epiphysis
Trochanteric bursitis
Stress fracture
Trochanteric tuberculosis

Posteriorly
Referred from spine
Gluteus medius tendinitis

tressing, especially if the hip gives way. Sometimes there is tenderness around the hip, and it may be possible to reproduce the peculiar sensation by flexing and extending the hip while abducted.

The condition must be distinguished from other causes of painful clicking, particularly a *tear of the acetabular labrum* or an *osteocartilaginous flap* on the femoral head (similar to osteochondritis dissecans). Contrast arthrography, or arthroscopy if this is available, will exclude these entities.

Treatment of the snapping tendon is usually unnecessary; the patient merely needs an explanation and reassurance. Occasionally, though, if discomfort is marked the band can be either divided or lengthened by a Z-plasty.

PRINCIPLES OF HIP OPERATIONS

Exposure of the hip

Operative approaches to the hip can be broadly divided into anterior, anterolateral, lateral and posterior.

The anterior (Smith-Petersen) approach starts in the plane between sartorius and rectus femoris medially and tensor fasciae femoris laterally and remains anterior to the gluteus medius. The hip capsule is exposed by detaching the origins of rectus femoris. This provides adequate exposure for many operations, including open reduction of the dislocated hip in infants and the various types of pelvic osteotomy. However, it is not ideal for major reconstructive surgery in adults.

The anterolateral (Watson-Jones) approach is also anterior to the gluteus medius, but behind the tensor fasciae femoris. It provides reasonable exposure of the hip joint, with minimal detachment of muscles, but the gluteus medius is in the way and this makes hip replacement difficult.

Lateral approaches suffer from the fact that the gluteus medius and minimus obstruct the view of the acetabulum. The abductors are dealt with by (1) retracting them posterosuperiorly (a limited solution), or (2) splitting them and raising the anterior portion intact from the greater trochanter (Hardinge's direct lateral approach), or (3) osteotomizing the greater trochanter and retracting it upwards with the attached abductors (as in the Charnley approach for total joint replacement). This provides excellent exposure; however, there may be problems with reattachment of the trochanteric fragment.

The posterior approach is the most direct. By splitting the anterior part of gluteus maximus, the rotators at the back of the hip are exposed and the sciatic nerve is retracted safely beneath the bulk of the posterior portion of gluteus maximus. Once the short rotators are detached, the hip is entered directly. Many surgeons prefer this approach for joint replacement. It has two minor disadvantages: orientation is more difficult, especially for placing the acetabular cup; and it is associated with an increased incidence of postoperative dislocation.

PLANNING

Reconstructive surgery of the hip needs careful preoperative planning. Tracings of plain x-rays are useful for taking measurements and working out repositioning angles. For the most difficult cases, three-dimensional imaging studies should be obtained.

Osteochondroplasty

Osteochondroplasty for early OA associated with femoro-acetabular impingement (FAI) is dealt with on page 528.

Intertrochanteric osteotomy

Rationale Intertrochanteric osteotomy has three objectives: (1) to change the orientation of the femoral head in the socket so as to reduce mechanical stress in a damaged segment; (2) realigning the proximal femur, to improve joint congruity; and (3) transecting the bone, to reduce intraosseous hypertension and relieve pain. An unintentional, and poorly under-

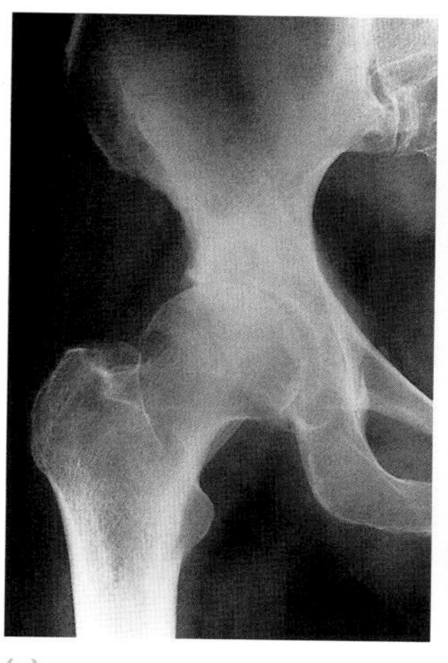
(a)

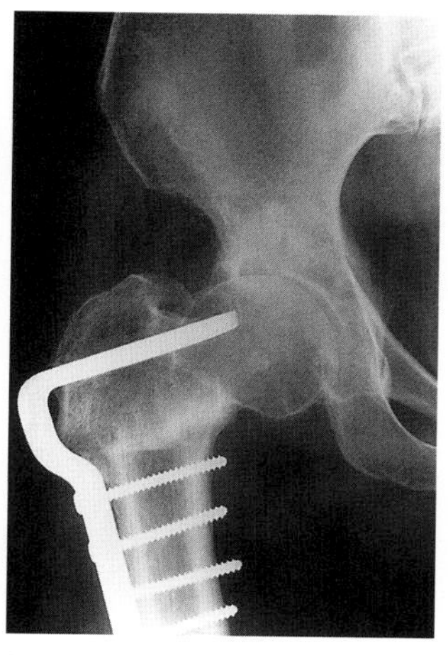
(b)

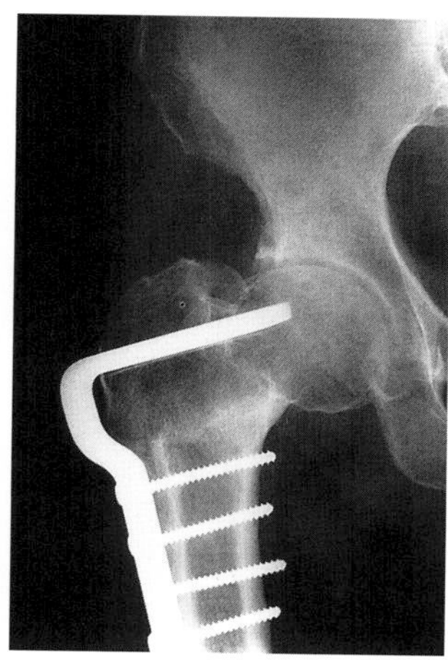
(c)

19.52 Osteoarthritis – treatment by osteotomy Following a varus type of osteotomy this patient lost most of her pain, and the x-rays suggest articular cartilage regeneration.

stood, consequence is (4) fibrocartilaginous repair of the articular surface.

Indications In children osteotomy is used to correct angular or rotational deformities of the proximal femur (e.g. in congenital dislocation, coxa vara or severe slips of the capital epiphysis), or to produce 'containment' of the femoral head in Perthes' disease.

In adults, the main indication is osteoarthritis associated with joint dysplasia, particularly in patients who are younger than 50 years. Pain is often relieved immediately (probably due to reduced vascular congestion) and sometimes the articular space is gradually restored. The other prime indication is in localized avascular necrosis of the femoral head; if only a small segment is involved, realignment can rotate this segment out of the path of maximum stress.

Contraindications Osteotomy is unsuitable in elderly patients and in those with severe stiffness; movement may be even further decreased afterwards. It is also contraindicated in rheumatoid arthritis, and even in OA if there is widespread loss of articular substance; reposition is useless if other parts of the femoral head are equally damaged.

Technical considerations The osteotomy allows repositioning of the femoral head in valgus, varus or different degrees of rotation. Exact placement and angulation can be ensured only by meticulous preoperative planning and painstaking execution of the bone cuts. The fragments are fixed with suitably angled plates and screws. Postoperatively the patient is permitted only partial weightbearing for 3–6 months. About 15 per cent of patients will require some assistance (a walking stick) for the rest of their lives.

Sugioka (Sugioka and Mohtai, 1998) devised a transtrochanteric rotational osteotomy for dealing with anterosuperior segmental destructive lesions of the femoral head, such as localized osteonecrosis. This allows the femoral neck to be rotated on its long axis, thus turning the femoral head through an arc of 90 degrees or more.

Complications The main complication is malposition of the bone. Only careful planning can prevent this. Non-union of the osteotomy is rare.

Results Provided the indications are strictly observed, the results are moderately good. In a series of 368 osteotomies, survivorship analysis showed that 10 years after osteotomy 47 per cent of patients had required no further surgery (Werners et al., 1990).

The operation has not been widely adopted, partly because of its technical complexity, partly because of the risk of complications and partly because of doubts about its long-term effectiveness – particularly in comparison to the outcome of modern methods of total hip replacement.

ARTHRODESIS

Rationale Fusion of the hip is guaranteed to relieve pain and provide stability for a lifetime. But at what cost? Surprisingly, although the joint is fused, the patient retains a great deal of 'mobility' because lumbosacral tilting and rotation are preserved and often increased. Nevertheless, there are restrictions: for sitting comfortably the hip needs 60 degrees of flexion; for climbing stairs, 45 degrees; and for walking, 20 degrees. In the stance phase of walking the normal hip is in slight abduction, but in the swing phase it is carried in slight adduction. No position of fusion can satisfy all these demands, so one aims at a compromise. And sometimes it is wrong, with the result that function is seriously impaired.

Indications Arthrodesis should be considered for any destructive condition of the hip when there are serious contraindications to osteotomy or arthroplasty: for example, a patient who is too young, a hip that is already stiff but painful, and previous infection. Young patients adapt well; those aged over 30–40 years respond unpredictably.

Contraindications Elderly patients, and any patient with a good range of movement, will resent a 'stiff hip'. Other contraindications are lack of bone stock and abnormalities in the 'compensating joints' (lumbar spine, knees and opposite hip).

Technical considerations The recommended position for arthrodesis is 20–30 degrees of flexion, 0–10 degrees of adduction (unless the leg is short) and about 5 degrees of external rotation. However, in young people there is a tendency for the 'joint' to drift into further flexion and by the age of 40 this may be as much as 40 degrees. Some form of internal fixation is used to secure the bones in the desired position. It is important to ensure that these implants do not destroy the abductors; though they are not needed while the hip is arthrodesed, they will be essential if ever the fusion is converted to an arthroplasty.

Complications The major complications are (1) failure to fuse and (2) malposition, which hampers function and puts unwanted strain on other joints. Late complications are (3) compensatory deformities in other joints (knees and opposite hip) and (4) low backache, which occurs in over 60 per cent of patients 20 years after fusion. Women may complain of (5) difficulty with sexual intercourse, and (6) squatting is, of course, impossible. However, it should be remembered that total replacement is still possible after a hip has been arthrodesed.

Results Provided the 'compensating joints' (lumbar spine, knee and opposite hip) are completely normal, young patients in particular may derive benefit from arthrodesis, with many years of reasonable comfort, a well-disguised limp and the ability to walk long distances and play games. Older patients fare less well: they find walking more difficult, tend to develop backache and seem more prone to degenerative changes in other joints.

In countries where advanced facilities and expertise are available, modern techniques of total hip replacement – providing results as high as 90–100 per cent survival rate with excellent function at 10 years postoperatively – have rendered arthrodesis more or less obsolete. This attitude prevails ever more strongly as each new generation of orthopaedic surgeons lacks any sustained training in 'old' types of surgery such as this.

TOTAL HIP REPLACEMENT – GENERAL PRINCIPLES

Rationale Total replacement of the articular surfaces seems the ideal way of treating any disorder causing joint destruction. However, there are several problems to be overcome: (1) the prosthetic implants must be durable; (2) they must permit extraordinary low-friction movement at the articulation; (3) they must be firmly fixed to the skeleton; and (4) they must be inert and not provoke any unwanted reaction in the tissues. The usual combination is a metal femoral component (stainless steel, titanium or cobalt–chrome alloy) articulating with a polyethylene socket. Ceramic components have better frictional characteristics but are more easily broken. Fixation is either by embedding the implant in methylmethacrylate cement, which acts as a grouting material filling the interstices, or by fitting the implant closely to the bone bed without cement. The 'bond' between bone and the implant surface, or cement, is never perfect. The best that can be hoped for is ingrowth of trabecular bone on the implant or cement (osseointegration). There are various ways of enhancing this process: (1) if acrylic cement is used, it is applied under pressure and allowed to cure without movement or extrusion after the implant has been inserted; (2) Ling and his co-workers have shown that a smooth, tapered and collarless femoral prosthesis will continue settling within the cement mantle even after polymerization, thereby maintaining expansile pressure between cement and bone (Fowler et al., 1988); (3) uncemented implants may be covered with a mesh or porous coating that encourages bone ingrowth (Engh et al., 1987); (4) the implant may be coated with hydroxyapatite, an excellent substrate for osteoblastic new-bone formation and osseointegration (Geesink, 1990).

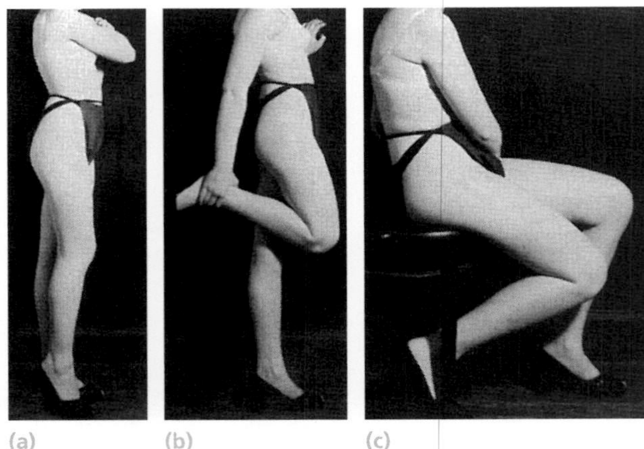

(a) (b) (c)

19.53 Arthrodesis Stiffness of the hip is largely disguised by mobility of the spine and knee.

Indications Because of the tendency for implants to loosen with time, joint replacement was customarily reserved for patients over 60 years. However, with improved cementing techniques and rapid advances in

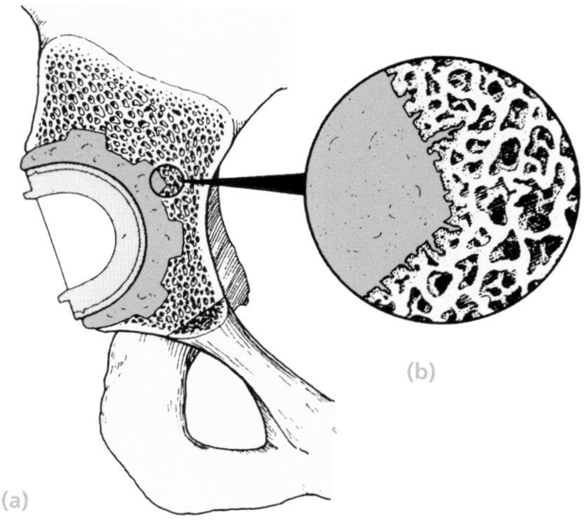

19.54 Prosthetic fixation Fixation between cement and bone is by (a) interlock (interdigitation of large irregularities in cement and bone) and, more completely, by (b) osseointegration (intimate penetration of cement between endosteal trabeculae).

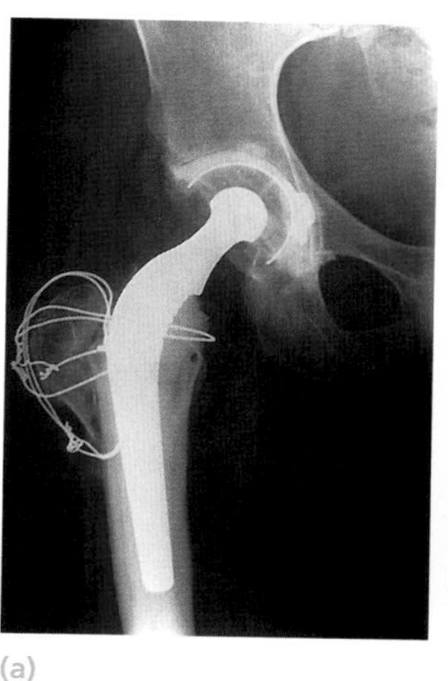

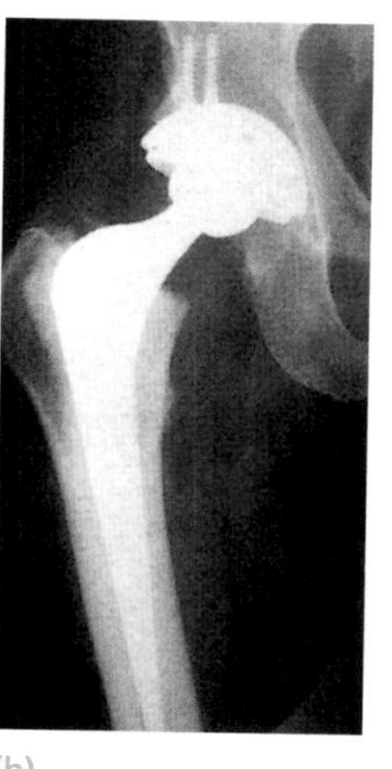

19.55 Total hip replacement (a) X-ray of a Charnley hip replacement system, forerunner of all the modern methods of total hip replacement. This comprises a collared femoral prosthesis with a fairly wide stem and a polyethelene acetabular cup, both implants fixed with acrylic cement. (b) X-ray of a cemented Ling femoral prosthesis – collarless with a tapered stem – and an uncemented acetabular cup.

the design of uncemented prostheses, the operation is being offered to younger patients with destructive hip disorders, and occasionally even to children severely crippled with rheumatoid disease.

Contraindications Overt or latent sepsis is the chief contraindication to joint replacement. An infected arthroplasty spells disaster. Patients under 60 years of age are considered only if other operations are unsuitable.

Technical considerations The fear of infection dictates a host of prophylactic measures, including the use of special ultraclean-air operating theatres, occlusive theatre clothing and perioperative antibiotic cover (Lidwell et al., 1984; Marotte et al., 1987). In addition, some surgeons routinely use antibiotic-laden cement.

The choice of implant should depend on sound biomechanical and biological testing. The array of over 300 different mechanisms currently on the market represents the triumph of hope over reason. The argument of 'cemented versus cementless' goes on. Sound technique is probably more important than anything else.

Postoperatively the implant should be protected from full loading until osseointegration is advanced; 6 weeks on crutches is not unreasonable.

Complications Hip replacements are often performed on patients who are somewhat elderly; some have rheumatoid disease and may be having steroid therapy. Consequently the general complication rate is by no means trivial; deep vein thrombosis is more common than with other elective operations.

Factors that may contribute to the development of complications include previous hip operations, severe deformity, lack of preoperative planning, inadequate 'bone stock', an insufficiently sterile operating environment and lack of experience or expertise on the part of the surgical team.

Intraoperative complications include perforation or even fracture of the femur or acetabulum. Special care should be taken in patients who are very old or osteoporotic and in those who have had previous hip operations.

Sciatic nerve palsy (usually due to traction but occasionally caused by direct injury) may occur with any type of arthroplasty but is more common with a posterior approach. Most cases recover spontaneously but if there is reason to suspect nerve damage the area should be explored.

Postoperative dislocation is rare if the prosthetic components are correctly placed. Reduction is easy and traction in abduction usually allows the hip to stabilize. If malposition of the femoral or acetabular component is severe, revision may be needed, or possibly augmentation of the socket.

Heterotopic bone formation around the hip is seen in about 20 per cent of patients 5 years after joint replacement. The cause is unknown, but patients with skeletal hyperostosis and ankylosing spondylitis are particularly at risk. In severe cases this is associated with pain and stiffness. Ossification can be prevented in high-risk patients by giving either a course of nonsteroidal anti-inflammatory drugs for 3–6 weeks postoperatively or a single dose of irradiation to the hip.

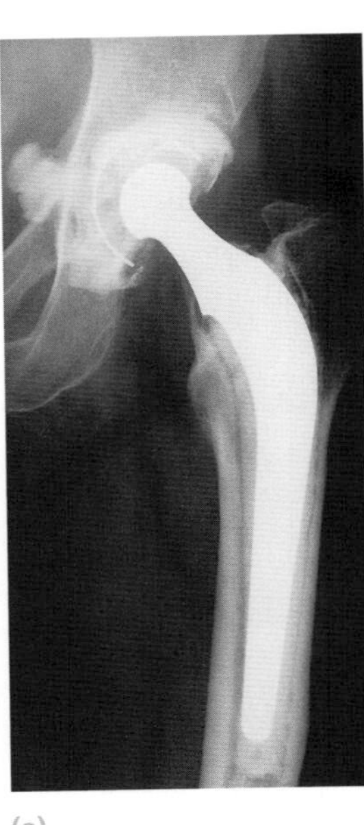

(a)

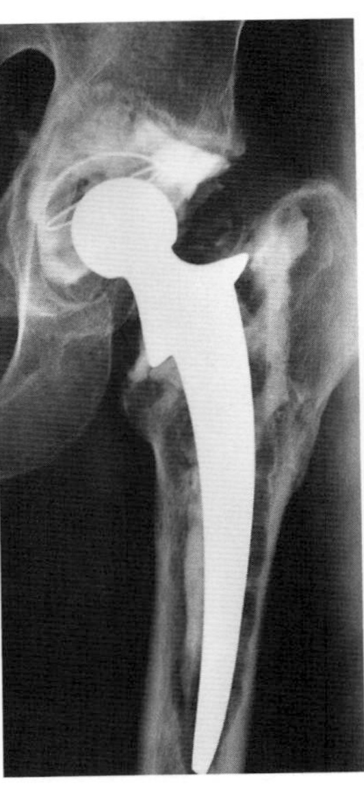

(b)

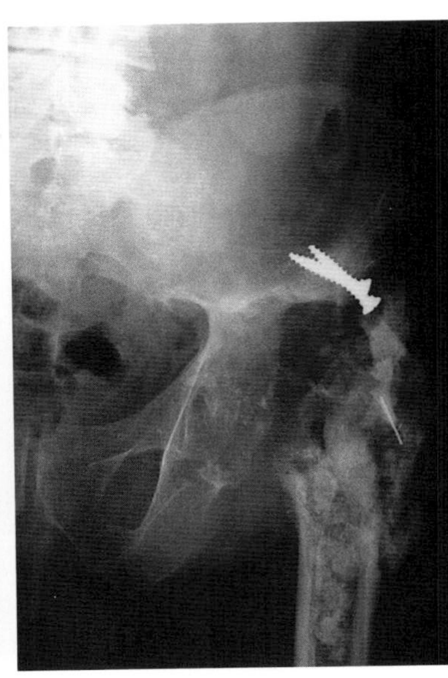

(c)

19.56 Hip replacement – aseptic loosening (a) Ten years after a hip replacement there is a distinct radiolucent line around this femoral implant as well as resorption of the calcar. (b) A further stage shown in another patient. Aggressive osteolysis. (c) The end of the line. This patient, after four 'revisions', ended up with fragmentation of the proximal femur, massive resorption of the acetabulum and fragments of bone and acrylic cement in the soft tissues. Happily, cases such as this are, nowadays, few and far between but the risk is always there.

Aseptic loosening of either the acetabular socket or the femoral stem is the commonest cause of long-term failure. Figures for its incidence vary widely, depending on the criteria used. With modern methods of implant fixation, there is likely to be radiographic evidence of loosening in less than 10 per cent of patients 15 years after operation; at microscopic level many stable implants show cellular reaction and membrane formation at the bone–cement interface (Linder and Carlsson, 1986). Fortunately, only a fraction of these are symptomatic. Pain may be a feature, especially when first taking weight on the leg after sitting or lying, but the diagnosis usually rests on x-ray signs of progressively increasing radiolucency around the implant, fracturing of cement, movement of the implant or bone resorption (Gruen et al., 1979). Radionuclide scanning shows increased activity, and it is claimed that the pattern of ^{99}Tc-HDP and ^{67}Ga uptake can differentiate between aseptic loosening and infection (Taylor et al., 1989). If symptoms are marked, and particularly if there is evidence of progressive bone resorption, the implant and cement should be painstakingly removed and a new prosthesis inserted. Revision arthroplasty can be either cemented or uncemented, depending on the condition of the bone.

Aggressive osteolysis, with or without implant loosening, is sometimes seen. It is associated with granuloma formation at the interface between cement (or implant) and bone. This may be due to a severe histiocyte reaction stimulated by cement, polyethylene or metal particles that find their way into the boundary zone. Revision is usually necessary and this may have to be accompanied by impaction grafting with morsellized bone.

Infection is the most serious postoperative complication. With adequate prophylaxis the risk should be less than 1 per cent, but it is higher in the very old, in patients with rheumatoid disease or psoriasis, and in those on immunosuppressive therapy (including corticosteroids).

The large bulk of foreign material restricts the access of the body's normal defence mechanism; consequently, even slight wound contamination may be serious. Organisms may multiply in the postoperative haematoma to cause early infection, and, even many years later, haematogenous spread from a distant site may cause late infection.

Early wound infection sometimes responds to antibiotics. Later infection does so less often and may need operative 'debridement' followed by irrigation with antibiotic solution for 3–4 weeks. Once the infection has cleared, a new prosthesis can be inserted, preferably without cement. An alternative, more applicable to 'mild' or 'dubious' infection, is a one-stage exchange arthroplasty using gentamicin-impregnated cement. The results of revision arthroplasty for infection are only moderately good. If all else fails the prosthesis and cement may have to be removed, leaving an excisional (Girdlestone) arthroplasty.

Results The success rate of primary total hip replacement is now so high that only with a prolonged follow-up of a large number of cases can we evaluate the relative merits of different models. It is important to compare like with like; present-day cementing (and non-cementing) techniques are far superior to those of only a decade ago and implant survival rates of more than 95 per cent at 15 years are being reported.

TOTAL HIP REPLACEMENT – PRESENT-DAY PERSPECTIVE

Total hip replacement is the second most commonly performed elective surgical procedure in the UK; over 60 000 were performed in 2006.

Charnley (1979) revolutionized the management of the arthritic hip with the development of low-friction arthroplasty. His three major contributions to the evolution of hip replacement were: (1) the concept of *low-friction torque* arthroplasty; (2) the use of *acrylic cement* to fix the components; and (3) the introduction of *high-density polyethylene* as a bearing material. Using this implant, several authors have reported survivorship in the region of 80 per cent at a follow-up of 25 years. Total hip replacement reproducibly alleviates pain and restores mobility while providing joint stability. It has been described as 'the operation of the century'. There has been rapid progress in the technology relating to joint replacement over the last 50 years.

INDICATIONS

The indications for hip replacement include pain, loss of movement and associated disability in the presence of radiographic evidence of joint destruction. Formerly patients had to earn their total hip replacement with severe pain – usually with sleep disturbance – and marked loss of function, with the patient often finally presenting on two crutches. The procedure was largely restricted to the elderly and the infirm. The success of the early implants and vastly improved access to information have persuaded patients that an unacceptable compromise in the quality of life represents a valid indication for joint replacement. These patients expect to return to a full profile of professional and recreational activities. Given their increased expectations it is important that the risks and benefits of total hip replacement be fully discussed with them. Orthopaedic surgeons should avoid promoting unrealistic expectations as this leads to dissatisfaction with the outcome if they are not achieved.

IMPLANT SELECTION

Technological advances have resulted in some of today's implants being very costly. It is essential that the implant selected is effective – that it will function satisfactorily for the individual patient. The objectives are to obtain durable fixation of both components with good orientation and to avoid instability. Care must be taken to reproduce the centre of rotation of the acetabulum, restore the offset and ensure that the limb lengths end up equal. Health economics dictate that the operation should also be cost-effective – the lowest-cost implant that will do the job should be used.

Cemented implants Cemented stems embrace two broad concepts: a taper-slip or force-closed design, and a composite beam or shape-closed design.

The taper slip is a highly polished tapered stem designed to settle within the cement mantle and re-engage the taper. This connects shear stresses to radial hoop stresses, thus optimizing the load distribution to the surrounding bone and cement. Taper slip stems, such as the Exeter prosthesis, have gained increasing popularity among cemented implants. A 100 per cent implant survivorship has been reported at 10-year follow-up with aseptic loosening as the endpoint, and good results have also been noted in younger patients (Yates et al., 2008).

Cement is a grout, not a glue, and fixation is achieved by a mechanical interlock in the bony interstices. Many surgeons today routinely use antibiotic-loaded cement. The antibiotic elutes out of the cement and produces high local concentrations in the early weeks following the operation, thus reducing the incidence of infection. Early methods of cementation entailed little preparation of the bone bed: the cement was introduced antegrade and no real attempt was made at pressurization beyond finger-packing. Contemporary cementing techniques include clearing of the endosteal bone with pulsed lavage, retrograde insertion of cement and sustained pressurization to resist back-bleeding and enhance the mechanical interlock. The Swedish Hip Registry demonstrates the benefits of modern cementation techniques. Cemented total hip replacement is technique-dependent, as the surgeon mixes the bone–cement–implant composite at the time of surgery.

The design of cemented cups has not changed much over the years. The cement is pressurized into an acetabulum that has been cleaned and dried. Cemented cups still have the best results of the designs recorded in the Norwegian Hip Registry.

Cemented total hip replacements are indicated for older, less active patients, although very good results have also been reported in the younger patient.

Uncemented implants The use of uncemented implants has become increasingly popular over the past two decades, particularly in North America. The surface of these implants was often textured (with porous beads or titanium mesh) to enhance bone fixation by osseointegration. It is important to have initial press-fit stability to allow bone on- or ingrowth into the textured surface. More recently bioactive surface coatings – such as hydroxyapatite – have been applied to accelerate bone ongrowth and improve the extent of the osseointegration. Well-fixed uncemented hips provide a durable biological fixation which is cyclically renewed with time.

In the femur the most predictable geometry and good quality bone were available in the diaphysis.

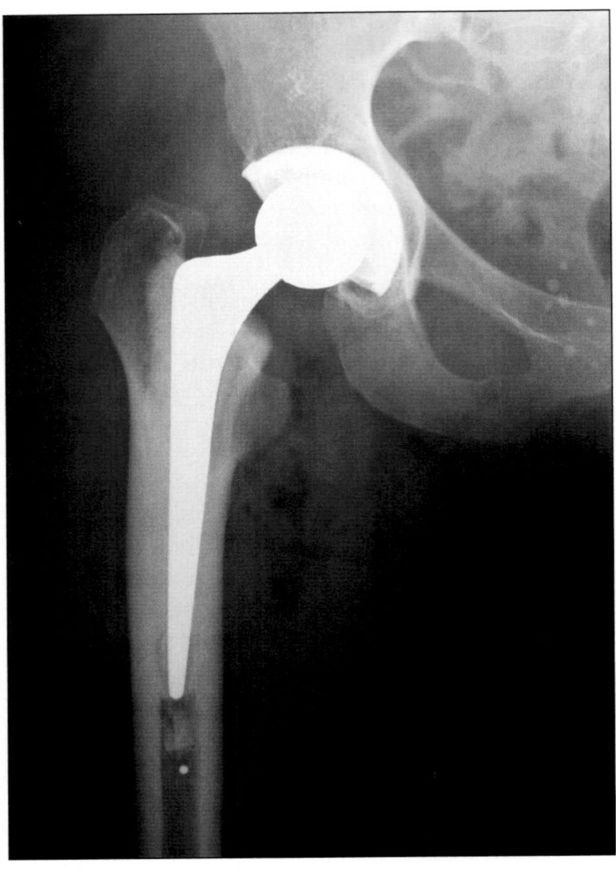

(a)

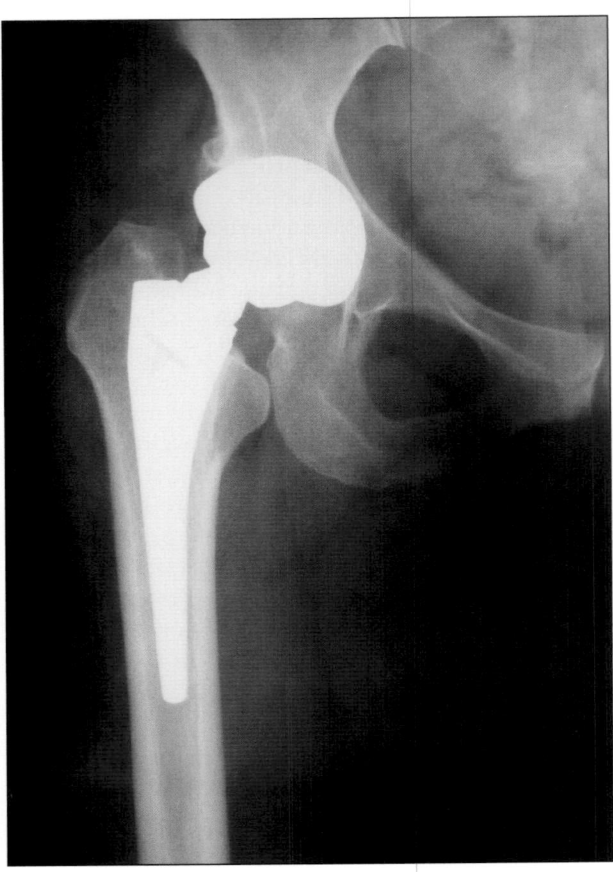

(b)

19.57 Total hip replacement X-rays showing two modern types of total hip replacement: (a) a cemented collarless tapered femoral prosthesis with an uncemented press-fit metal-backed acetabular implant; and (b) modular uncemented implants. Some modular fittings allow a choice of femoral neck angles to overcome problems of severe anteversion or retroversion of the femoral neck,.

Early uncemented implants – which were often extensively textured – were cylindrical distally and gained fixation in the diaphysis. As these stems were often large, this led to thigh pain in up to 40 per cent of patients and stress protection in the proximal femur with associated loss of bone. Subsequently tapered stems were designed in which the surface texturing was limited to the metaphyseal region to promote proximal cancellous bone ingrowth. Three-point stem fixation provided immediate stability. Ten-year survivorship of 100 per cent has been reported with these tapered stems.

Uncemented acetabular components were introduced to address the failure of fixation of cemented polyethylene cups, particularly in the younger patient. Most of these components are hemispherical and initial stability and fixation is achieved by press-fitting the cup into a slightly under-reamed acetabular socket. Excellent survival of fixation has been reported. Failures of these implants were often attributable to malfunction of the locking mechanism of the polyethylene liner and to accelerated wear of the thinner polyethylene liner. This problem has been addressed by improving the locking mechanism and the bearing surfaces. A combination of a cemented stem and an uncemented cup – the so-called 'hybrid hip' – has proved popular for use in the middle-aged patient.

BONE-CONSERVING FEMORAL ARTHROPLASTY

Resurfacing arthroplasty Resurfacing arthroplasty was popular in the 1970s. A large diameter head articulated with a very thin polyethylene cup which was cemented. Catastrophic wear of the plastic occurred, and implant failure of up to 33 per cent was reported in the short- to mid-term. Exploiting the evolving technology of metal-on-metal bearings, McMinn demonstrated that very acceptable mid-term results could be achieved with metal-on-metal resurfacing and hybrid fixation. Concerns remain about fracture of the femoral neck – which occurs in 1–2 per cent of all major series – and remodelling with narrowing of the femoral neck. Resurfacing is not suitable for all hips, and indications and limitations need to be recognized to reduce the number of technique-related failures. The ideal indication is probably the need for hip replacement in males younger than 60 years who have OA.

Short-stemmed implants Patients are now presenting for total hip replacement at an increasingly younger age than in the past. These patients are likely to need at least one revision operation during their lifespan, and one of the major challenges facing the surgeon will be loss of bone stock beneath the cup. Conservative, short-stemmed prostheses have been developed which preserve bone. They are easily inserted through a minimally invasive approach, entail a smaller loss of bone at the time of surgery and conserve bone with more physiological loading of the proximal femur. While excellent mid-term results have been reported with some of these implants, the concept should not be widely embraced until longer-term follow-up has shown results similar to those of conventional stemmed implants.

APPROACHES

As noted earlier in this section, total hip replacement can be carried out through the standard approaches to the hip. The anterolateral and posterolateral approaches remain the most popular. The former is associated with an increased incidence of abductor dysfunction, while the latter is associated with an increased risk of dislocation.

Minimally invasive surgery (MIS) Minimally invasive surgery was initially advocated using the two-incision technique – one anterior and one posterior – but this has been shown to be associated with an unacceptably high incidence of complications including fractures, component malposition and dislocation. It has now largely fallen into disuse.

Single-incision surgery, carried out through a skin incision of less than 10 cm, is reported to reduce pain, blood loss, rehabilitation time and length of hospital stay. An anterior or posterior approach is usually employed. The length of skin incision is a poor determinant of minimally invasive surgery, and will make little difference to the morbidity and speed of rehabilitation if exactly the same soft-tissue dissection is carried out deep to the skin as would have been done with a conventional incision. It is perhaps better to talk about 'soft-tissue sparing surgery'; certainly this raised awareness of minimizing soft-tissue damage has resulted in all incisions becoming very much smaller. Long-term follow-up is needed to show that the proven durability of total hip replacement is not being lost by compromised exposure and malpositioning of the implants.

BEARING SURFACES

The issue of osteolysis had not been resolved by the implantation of uncemented implants. Lytic lesions have been reported with both stable and loose uncemented prostheses, and micron or submicron particles of polyethylene have been identified as the main contributing factors. Indeed this has been recognized as the major limiting factor of conventional total hip replacement and has led to the development of alternative bearing surfaces including highly cross-linked polyethylene and hard-on-hard couples.

Highly cross-linked polyethylene (XLPE) Gamma irradiation of polyethylene causes cross-linking, which greatly improves the wear resistance compared to conventional polyethylene. However, this comes at a price, as the dose of irradiation is inversely proportional to the fracture toughness. Encouraging clinical results with markedly reduced wear have been reported with XLPE. It should be noted that none of the commercially available XLPEs are the same – and the clinical performance is therefore likely to differ.

Ceramic-on-ceramic Alumina ceramics were introduced as a bearing material in the 1970s. They are 'wettable', have very low wear rates, are scratch-resistant and their particulate debris is not biologically very active. However, ceramics are brittle and are susceptible to fractures. Modern ceramics have been strengthened and have much improved fracture toughness. Excellent results have been reported with ceramic–ceramic couples; however, because of their brittle nature it is still not possible to make safe ceramic liners with an inner diameter greater than 86 mm.

Metal-on-metal Metal bearing surfaces have very low wear rates and are self-polishing, which allows for self-healing of surface scratches. Metal is not brittle, unlike ceramic, and components therefore do not have to be as thick as their ceramic counterparts. Thus large head diameters can be combined with monolithic cups. This gives a greater range of motion to impingement, and thus greater mobility and greater stability. The wear of these larger heads is dictated by the lubrication regimen, which is favourably influenced by increasing the head size (thus increasing the entrainment velocity of the lubricating fluid), and optimizing the diametrical clearance and the sphericity of the head. These durable couples allow patients to return to vigorous recreational activities, and are known as 'high performance bearings'.

Although these metal-on-metal couples have very low volumetric wear, they still generate twice the number of particles as metal-on-polyethylene bearings. These particles are very small – in the nano range – but do elicit a biological reaction. This is discussed under Complications.

There are hundreds of different implants and bearing options available on the market. This is not a reflection of the requirement but rather of commercial competition – yet another case of the tail wagging the dog.

Rehabilitation The length of inpatient stay has been reduced to 4–6 days in most hospitals. Patients are well mobilized on crutches or sticks before discharge, and will have negotiated stairs independently. Progress to full weightbearing without support will usually take 6–8 weeks at the patient's own pace.

NOTES ON APPLIED ANATOMY

The ball-and-socket arrangement of the hip combines stability for weightbearing with freedom of movement for locomotion. A deeper acetabulum would confer greater stability but would limit the range of movement. Even with the fibrocartilaginous labrum the socket is not deep enough to accommodate the whole of the femoral head, whose articular surface extends considerably beyond a hemisphere.

The opening of the acetabulum faces downwards and forwards (about 30 degrees in each direction); the neck of the femur points upwards and forwards. Consequently, in the neutral position, the anterior portion of the head is not 'contained'. The amount of forward inclination of the neck relative to the shaft (the angle of anteversion) varies from 10 to 30 degrees in the adult. The upward inclination of the neck is such that the neck–shaft angle is 125 degrees.

A neck–shaft angle of less than 125 degrees is referred to as 'coxa vara' because, were the neck normally aligned relative to the pelvis, the limb would be deviated towards the midline of the body – in varus; a neck–shaft angle greater than 125 degrees (i.e. with the neck unduly vertical) is coxa valga. The angle is mechanically important because the further away the abductor muscles are from the hip, the greater is their leverage and their efficiency.

During standing and walking, the femoral neck acts as a cantilever; the line of body weight passes medial to the hip joint and is balanced laterally by the abductors (especially gluteus medius). The combination of body weight, leverage effect and muscle action means that the resultant force transmitted through the femoral head can be very great – about five times the body weight when walking slowly and much more when running or jumping. It is easy to see why the hip is so liable to suffer from cartilage failure – the essential feature of osteoarthritis.

The ligaments of the hip, though very strong in front, are weak posteriorly; consequently, posterior dislocation is much more common than anterior. When the hip is adducted and medially rotated it is particularly vulnerable, and when this position results from unbalanced paralysis the hip can slip unobtrusively out of position.

During the swing phase of walking not only does the hip flex, it also rotates; this is because the pelvis swivels forwards. As weight comes onto the leg, the abductor muscles contract, causing the pelvis to tilt downwards on the weightbearing side; it is failure of this abductor mechanism which causes the Trendelenburg lurch.

The femoral head receives its arterial blood supply from three sources: (1) intraosseous vessels running up the neck, which are inevitably damaged with a displaced cervical fracture; (2) vessels in the retinacula reflected from capsule to neck, which may be damaged in a fracture or compressed by an effusion; and (3) vessels in the ligamentum teres, which are undeveloped in the early years of life and even later convey only a meagre blood supply. The relative importance of these vessels varies with age, but at all ages avascular necrosis is a potential hazard.

The nerve supply of the hip, unlike the blood supply, is plentiful. Sensory fibres, conveying proprioception as well as pain, abound in the capsule and ligaments. The venous sinusoids of the bones also are supplied with sensory fibres; a rise in the intraosseous venous pressure accounts for some of the pain in osteoarthritis, and a reduction of this pressure for some of the relief which may follow osteotomy.

The tensor fasciae femoris, though a relatively small muscle, has, through its action in tightening the ili-

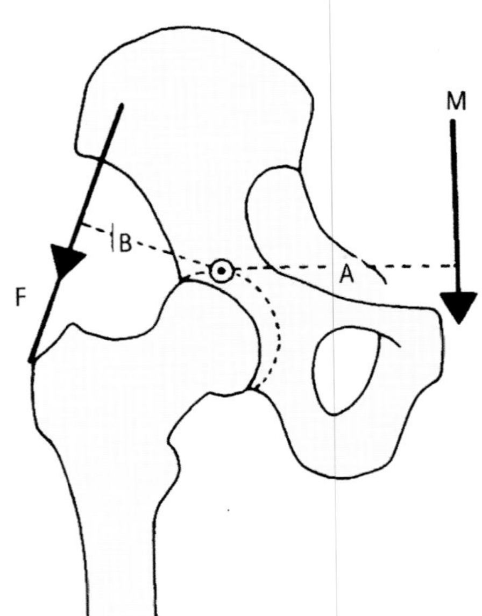

19.58 Forces around the hip When standing on one leg the pelvis is balanced on the femoral head. The vertical force due to the body weight (M) is counterbalanced by contraction of the lateral muscles (F). The force borne by the femoral head is produced by the combined moments M x A and F x B.

otibial tract, a surprisingly large range of functions. This tract is anterior to the axis of knee flexion when the knee is straight, so its tension helps to hold the knee slightly hyperextended while standing. It is also important in getting up from the sitting position, as well as during the phases of walking and running when weight is being taken on the slightly flexed knee.

REFERENCES AND FURTHER READING

Baber YF, Robinson AHN, Villar RN. Is diagnostic arthroscopy of the hip worthwhile? *J Bone Joint Surg* 1999; **81B:** 600–3.

Barlow TG. Early diagnosis and treatment of congenital dislocation of the hip. *J Bone Joint Surg* 1962; **44B:** 292–301.

Beaulé PE, Le Duff MJ, Zaragoza E. Quality of life following femoral head-neck osteochondroplasty for femoroacetabular impingement. *J Bone Joint Surg* 2007; **89A:** 773–9.

Beck M, Leunig M, Parvizi J, Boutier V, Wyss D, Ganz R. Anterior femoroacetabular impingement: part II. midterm results of surgical treatment. *Clin Orthop Relat Res* 2004; **418:** 67–73.

Beck M, Kalhor M, Leunig M, Ganz R. Hip morphology influences the pattern of damage to the acetabular cartilage. Femoroacetabular impingement as a cause of early osteoarthritis of the hip. *J Bone Joint Surg* 2005; **87B:** 1012–8.

Catterall A. *Legg–Calve–Perthes Disease*, Churchill Livingstone, Edinburgh, 1982.

Catterall A. Assessment of adolescent acetabular dysplasia. In Recent Advances in Orthopaedics – 6 (ed. A. Catterall), Churchill Livingstone, Edinburgh, 1992.

Charnley Sir J. *Low Friction Arthroplasty of the Hip*, Springer, Berlin, 1979.

Cohen MS, Griffin PP. Obesity and decreased femoral anteversion in adolescence. *J. Orthop Res.* 1987; (5) 523–528.

Cordes S, Dickens DR, Cole WG. Correction of coxa vara in childhood. The use of Pauwels' Y-shaped osteotomy. *J Bone Joint Surg* 1991: **73B:** 3–6.

Dora C, Zurbach J, Hersche O, Ganz R. Pathomorphological characteristics of posttraumatic acetabular dysplasia. *J Orthop Trauma* 2000; **14:** 483–9.

Dora C, Mascard E, Mladenov K, Seringe R. Retroversion of the acetabular dome after Salter and triple osteotomy for congenital dislocation of the hip. *Pediatr Orthop* 2002; **B11:** 34–40, 2002.

Dunn DM, Angel JC. Replacement of the femoral head by open operation in severe adolescent slipping of the upper femoral epiphysis. *J Bone Joint Surg* 1978; **60B:** 394–403.

Eng CA, Bobyn JD, Glassman AH. Porous-coated hip replacement: the factors governing bone ingrowth, stress shielding and clinical results. *J Bone Joint Surg* 1987; **69B:** 45–55.

Espinosa N, Rothenfluh DA, Beck M, Ganz R, Leunig M. Treatment of femoroacetabular impingement: preliminary results of labral refixation. *J Bone Joint Surg* 2006; **88A:** 925–35.

Ficat RP. Idiopathic bone necrosis of the femoral head: early diagnosis and treatment. *J Bone Joint Surg* 1985; **67B:** 3–9.

Fish J. Cuneiform osteotomy of the femoral neck in the treatment of slipped capital femoral epiphysis. A follow up note. *J Bone Joint Surg* 1994; **76A:** 46–59.

Fishkin Z, Armstrong DG, Shah H *et al.* Proximal femoral physis shear in slipped capital femoral epiphysis – a finite element study. *J Pediatr Orthop.* 2006; **26(3):** 291–4.

Fixen JA. Rotation-plasty. *J Bone Joint Surg* 1983; **65B:** 529–530.

Fixen JA, Lloyd-Roberts GC. The natural history and early treatment of proximal femoral dysplasia. *J Bone Joint Surg* 1974; **56B:** 86–95.

Fowler JL, Gie GA, Lee AJC, Ling RSM. Experience with the Exeter Total Hip since 1970. *Orthopedic Clinics of North America* 1988; **19:** 477–89.

Galbraith RT, Gelberman RH, Hajek PC *et al.* Obesity and decreased femoral anteversion in adolescence. *J Orthop Res* 1987; **5(4):** 523–8.

Ganz R, Bamert P, Hausner P, Isler B, Vrevc F. Cervicoacetabular impingement after femoral neck fracture. *Unfallchirurg* 1991; **94:** 172–5.

Ganz R, Klaue K, Mast J *et al.* Periacetabular osteotomy. In *Hip Surgery – Materials and Developments*, eds. Sedel, L. and Cabanela, M.E. Martin Dunitz, London, 1998.

Ganz R, Parvizi J, Beck M, Leunig M, Nötzli H, Siebenrock KA. Femoroacetabular impingement: a cause for osteoarthritis of the hip. *Clin Orthop Relat Res* 2003; **417:** 112–20.

Ganz R, Leunig M, Leunig-Ganz K, Harris WH. The etiology of osteoarthritis of the hip: an integrated mechanical concept. *Clin Orthop Relat Res* 2008; **466:** 264–72.

Geesink RGT. Hydroxy-apatite-coated total hip prostheses. *Clin Orthop Relat Res* 1990; **261:** 39–58.

Gillespie R. Classification of congenital abnormalities of the femur in: Herring JA, Birch JG (Ed). The Child with a Limb Deficiency. Published by *The Am Acad of Orthop Surg*, Rosemount USA 1998 13–132.

Gillespie R, Torode IP. Classification and management of congenital abnormalities of the femur. *J Bone Joint Surg* 1983; **65B:** 557–68.

Giori NJ, Trousdale RT. Acetabular retroversion is associated with osteoarthritis of the hip. *Clin Orthop Relat Res* 2003; **417:** 263–9.

Glueck CJ, Crawford A, Roy D *et al.* Association by antithrombotic factor deficiencies and hypofibrinolysis with Legg–Perthes disease. *J Bone Joint Surg* 1996; **78A:** 3–13.

Goddard NJ, Hashemi-Nejad A, Fixsen JA. The natural history and treatment of instability of the hip in proximal femoral focal deficiency. *J Pediatr Orthop B* 1995; **4(2):** 145–149.

Griffith MJ. Slipping of the capital femoral epiphysis. *Ann R Coll Surg Engl* 1976; **58:** 34–42.

Gruen TA, McNeice GM, Amstutz HC. 'Modes of failure' of cemented stem-type femoral components. *Clin Orthop Relat Res* 1979; **141:** 17–27.

Harcke T, Kumar J. The role of ultrasound in the diagnosis and management of congenital dislocation and dysplasia of the hip. *J Bone Joint Surg* 1991; **73A:** 622–8.

Harris W. The endocrine basis for slipping of the upper femoral epiphysis: an experimental study. *J Bone Joint Surg*. 1950; **32B(1):** 5–11.

Harris WH. Primary osteoarthritis of the hip: a vanishing diagnosis. *J Rheumatol Suppl* 1983; **9:** 64.

Harris WH. Etiology of osteoarthritis of the hip. *Clin Orthop Relat Res* 1986; **213:** 20–33.

Herring JA. (1994) The treatment of Legg–Calvé–Perthes' disease. *J Bone Joint Surg* 1994; **76A:** 448–8.

Herring JA, Birch JG (eds.) The Child with a Limb Deficiency. *Am Acad Orthop Surg*, Rosemont USA, 1998; pp 63–72.

Jamali AA, Mladenov K, Meyer DC *et al.* Anteroposterior pelvic radiographs to assess acetabular retroversion: High validity of the cross-over sign. *J Orthop Res* 2007; **25:** 758–65.

Jerre R, Billing L, Hansson G *et al.* The contralateral hip in patients primarily treated for unilateral SUFE: long term follow up of 61 hips. *J Bone Joint Surg* 1994; **76B(4):** 563–7.

Jones DA. Principles of screening and congenital dislocation of the hip. *Ann R Coll Surg Engl* 1994; **76:** 245–50.

Kalberer F, Sierra RJ, Madan SS, Ganz R, Leunig M. Ischial spine projection into the pelvis: a new sign for acetabular retroversion. *Clin Orthop Relat Res* 2008; **466:** 677–83.

Kim Y-M, Ahn JH, Kang HS *et al.* Estimation of the extent of osteonecrosis of the femoral head using MRI. *J Bone Joint Surg* 1998; **80B:** 954–8.

King RE. Some concepts of proximal femoral focal deficiency, In Aitken GT (ed) Proximal femoral focal deficiency: a congenital anomaly. Washington DC National Academy of Sciences; 1969; 23–49.

Klisic P, Jankovic L. Combined procedure of open reduction and shortening of the femur in treatment of congenital dislocation of the hip in older children. *Clin Orthop Relat Res* 1976; **119:** 60–9.

Kordelle J, Millis M, Jolesz FA, Kikinis R, Richolt JA. Three-dimensional analysis of the proximal femur in patients with slipped capital femoral epiphysis based on computed tomography. *J Pediatr Orthop* 2001; **21(2):** 179–82.

Leunig M, Werlen S, Ungersböck A, Ito K, Ganz R. Evaluation of acetabular labrum by MR arthrography. *J Bone Joint Surg* 1997; **79B:** 230–4.

Leunig M, Casillas MM, Hamlet M *et al.* Slipped capital femoral epiphysis: early mechanical damage to the acetabular cartilage by the prominent femoral metaphysis. *Acta Orthop Scand* 2000; **71:** 370–5.

Leunig M, Beck M, Kalhor M, Kim YJ, Werlen S, Ganz R. Fibrocystic changes at anteroposterior femoral neck: Prevalence in hips with femoroacetabular impingement. *Radiology* 2005; **236:** 237–46.

Lidwell OM, Lowbury EJL, Whyte W *et al.* Infection and sepsis after operations for total hip or knee joint replacement: influence of ultraclean air, prophylactic antibiotics and other factors. *J Hygiene* (Camb) 1984; **83:** 505–29.

Liesner RJ. Editorial: Does thrombophilia cause Perthes' disease in children? *J Bone Joint Surg* 1999; **81B:** 565–6.

Lin S-L, Ho T-C. The role of venous hypertension in the pathogenesis of Legg–Perthes disease. *J Bone Joint Surg* 1991; **73A:** 194–200.

Linder L, Carlsson AS. The bone–cement interface in hip arthroplasty: a histologic and enzyme study of stable components. *Acta Orthop Scand* 1986; **57:** 495–500.

Loder R. The demographics of slipped capital femoral epiphysis. An international multicenter study. *Clin Orthop Relat Res* 1996; **322:** 8–27.

Loder R, Aronson D, Greenfield L. The epidemiology of SCFE: a study of children in Michigan. *J Bone Joint Surg* 1993; **75A:** 1141.

Loder R, Wiltenberg B, De Silva G. SCFE associated with endocrine disorder. *J Paediatr Orthop* 1995; **15:** 349.

Marotte JH, Lord GA, Blanchard JP *et al.* (1987) Infection rate in total hip arthroplasty as a function of air cleanliness and antibiotic prophylaxis. *JArthroplasty* 2087; **2:** 77–82.

Martinez AG, Weinstein SL, Dietz FR. The weight-bearing abduction brace for the treatment of Legg-Perthes disease. *J Bone Joint Surg* 1992; **74A:** 12–21.

Meehan PL, Angel D, Nelson JM. The Scottish Rite abduction orthosis for the treatment of Legg Perthes disease. *J Bone Joint Surg* 1992; **74A:** 2–12.

Meyer DC, Beck M, Ellit T, Ganz R, Leunig M. Comparison of six radiographic projections to assess femoral head-neck asphericity. *Clin Orthop Relat Res* 2006; **445:** 181–5.

Murphy S, Tannast M, Kim YJ, Buly R, Millis MB. Debridement of the adult hip for femoroacetabular impingement: indications and preliminary clinical results. *Clin Orthop Relat Res* 2004; **429:** 178–81.

Murray RO. The etiology of primary osteoarthritis of the hip. *Br J Radiol* 1965; **38:** 810–24.

Paley D. Lengthening reconstruction surgery for congenital femoral deficiency in: Herring JA, Birch JG (Eds). The Child with a Limb Deficiency. *Am Acad Orthop Surg*, Rosemount USA 1998 113–132.

Preiser G. Statische Gelenkerkrankungen. Ferdinand Enke Verlag, Stuttgart, 1911, p 78

Reynolds D, Lucas J, Klaue K. Retroversion of the acetabulum: A cause of hip pain. *J Bone Joint Surg* 1999; **81B:** 281–8.

Riley PM, Weiner DS, Akron RG. Hazards of internal fixation in the treatment of slipped capital femoral epiphysis. *J Bone Joint Surg* 1990; **72A:** 1500–9.

Sakamoto M, Shimuzu K, Iida S *et al.* Osteonecrosis of the femoral head. A prospective study with MRI. *J Bone Joint Surg* 1997; **79B:** 213–9.

Shimuzu K, Moriya H, Akita T *et al*. Prediction of collapse with magnetic resonance imaging of avascular necrosis of the femoral head. *J Bone Joint Surg* 1994; **76A:** 215–23.

Siebenrock KA, Wahab KH, Werlen S, Kalhor M, Leunig M, Ganz R. Abnormal extension of the femoral head epiphysis as a cause of cam impingement. *Clin Orthop Relat Res* 2004; **418:** 54–60.

Simmons ED, Graham HK, Szalai JP. Interobserver variability in grading Perthes' disease. *J Bone Joint Surg* 1990; **72B:** 202–4.

Solomon L. Geographical and anatomical patterns of osteoarthritis of the hip. *Br J Rheumatol* 1984; **23:** 177–80.

Solomon L. Patterns of osteoarthritis of the hip. *J Bone Joint Surg* 1976; **58B:** 176–83.

Solomon L. Arthrodesis – is there still an indication? In *Hip Surgery – Materials and Developments*, eds. Sedel, L. and Cabanela, M.E. Martin Dunitz, London, 1998.

Solomon L, Beighton P. Osteoarthrosis of the hip and its relationship to preexisting deformity in an African population. *J Bone Joint Surg* 1973; **55B:** 216–7.

Solomon L, Pearse MF. Osteonecrosis following low-dose short-course corticosteroids. *J Orthop Rheumatol* 1994; **7:** 203–5.

Sorensen KH. Slipped upper femoral epiphysis. Clinical study on aetiology. *Acta Orthop Scand* 1968; **39:** 499–517.

Steel HH. Iliofemoral fusion for proximal femoral focal deficiency. In Herring JA, Birch JG (Eds). The Child with a Limb Deficiency. *Am Acad Orthop Surg*, Rosemount USA 1998.

Steel HH, Lyn PS, Betz RR, Kalamchi A, Clancy M. Iliofemoral fusion for proximal femoral focal deficiency. *J Bone Joint Surg* 1987; **69A:** 837–43.

Stuhlberg SD, Cordell LD, Harris WH, Ramsey PL, MacEwen GD. Unrecognized childhood hip disease: a major cause of idiopathic osteoarthritis of the hip. In: Cordell LD, Harris WH, Ramsey PL, MacEwen GD, (Eds) The Hip: Proceedings of the Third Open Scientific Meeting of the Hip Society. St Louis, MO: CV Mosby; 212–28, 1975.

Sugioka Y, Mohtai M. Osteonecrosis of the femoral head: a conservative surgical solution. In *Hip Surgery – Materials and Developments*, (Eds). Sedel, L. and Cabanela, M.E. Martin Dunitz, London, 1998.

Taylor DN, Maughan J, Patel MP, Clegg J. A simple method of identifying loosening or infection of hip prostheses in nuclear medicine. *Nucl Med Commun* 1989; **10:** 551–6.

Tönnis D, Heinicke A. Acetabular and femoral anteversion: Relationship with osteoarthritis of the hip. *J Bone Joint Surg* 1999; **81A:** 1747–70.

Tooke SMT, Amstutz HC, Hedley AK. Results of transtrochanteric rotational osteotomy for femoral head osteonecrosis. *Clin Orthop Relat Res* 1987; **224:** 50–157.

Werners R, Vincent B, Bulstrode C. Osteotomy for osteoarthritis of the hip. *J Bone Joint Surg* 1990; **72B:** 1010–3.

Wynne-Davies R. Acetabular dysplasia and familial joint laxity: two aetiological factors in congenital dislocation of the hip. *J Bone Joint Surg* 1970; **52B:** 704–16.

Yamamuro T, Ishida K. Recent advances in the prevention, early diagnosis and treatment of congenital dislocation of the hip in Japan. *Clin Orthop Relat Res* 1984; **184:** 34–40.

Yates PJ, Burston BJ, Whitley E, Bannister GC. Collarless polished tapered stem. Clinical and radiological results at a minimum of 10 years' follow-up. *J Bone Joint Surg* 2008; **90B:** 16–22.

The knee

20

Louis Solomon, Theo Karachalios

CLINICAL ASSESSMENT

Symptoms

Pain, either insidious in onset or more acute, is the most common knee symptom. With inflammatory or degenerative disorders it is usually diffuse, but with mechanical disorders (and especially after injury) it is often localized – the patient can, and should, point to the painful spot.

If the patient can describe the mechanism of the injury, this is extremely useful: a direct blow to the front of the knee may damage the patello-femoral joint; a blow to the side may rupture the collateral ligament; twisting injuries are more likely to cause a torn meniscus or a cruciate ligament rupture.

Swelling may be diffuse or localized. If there was an injury, it is important to ask whether the swelling appeared immediately (suggesting a haemarthrosis) or only after some hours (typical of a torn meniscus). A complaint of recurrent swelling, with more or less normal periods in between, suggests a longstanding internal derangement – possibly an old meniscal tear, degeneration of the meniscus, a small osteoarticular fracture or loose bodies in the joint. Chronic swelling is typical of synovitis or arthritis.

A small, localized swelling on the anteromedial or anterolateral side of the joint makes one think of a cyst of the meniscus (always on the medial side) or a floating loose body. Swelling over the front of the knee could be due to a prepatellar bursitis; a localized bulge in the popliteal fossa can also be caused by a bursal swelling, but is more often due to ballooning of the synovial membrane and capsule at the back of the joint.

'Stiffness' is a common complaint, but it must be distinguished from inhibition of movement due to pain, or simple weakness of the extensor apparatus. Particularly characteristic is stiffness that appears regularly after periods of rest – so-called 'post-inactivity stiffness' – which suggests some type of chronic arthritis.

Locking is different from stiffness. The knee, quite suddenly, cannot be straightened fully, although flexion is still possible. This happens when a torn meniscus or loose body is caught between the articular surfaces. By wiggling the knee around, the patient may be able to 'unlock' it; sudden *unlocking* is the most reliable evidence that something mobile had previously obstructed full extension. Do not be misled by 'pseudo-locking', when movement is suddenly stopped by pain or the fear of impending pain.

Deformity is seldom a leading symptom; patients are not keen to admit to having 'knock knees' or 'bandy legs'. However, a unilateral deformity, especially if it is progressive, will be more worrying.

Giving way, a feeling of instability, or a lack of trust in the knee suggests a mechanical disorder caused by ligamentous, meniscal or capsular injury, or simple muscle weakness. Giving way, particularly if it occurs when climbing up or down stairs, may also be due to patello-femoral pain or instability. Excessive use of an unstable knee produces post-exercise swelling (effusion or haemarthrosis) and diffuse pain within the joint.

Limp may be due to either pain or instability.

Loss of function manifests as a progressively diminishing walking distance, inability to run and difficulty going up and down steps. Squatting or kneeling may be painful, either because of pressure on the patello-femoral joint or because the knee cannot flex fully.

Signs with the patient upright

For the examination, both lower limbs must be exposed from groin to toe; a mere hitching up of the skirt or rolling back of a trouser leg is not good enough.

Deformity (valgus or varus or hyperextension) is best seen with the patient standing and bearing weight, lower limbs together (if possible!) and feet pointing forward. Normally the knees and ankles can touch in the midline; this means that the knees must be in slight valgus (about 7 degrees in women and

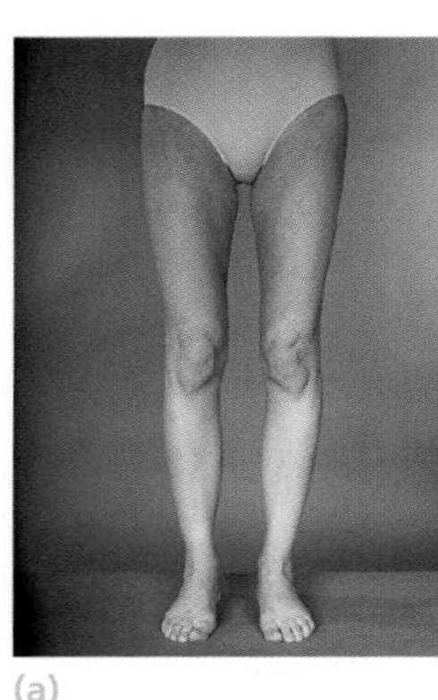
(a)

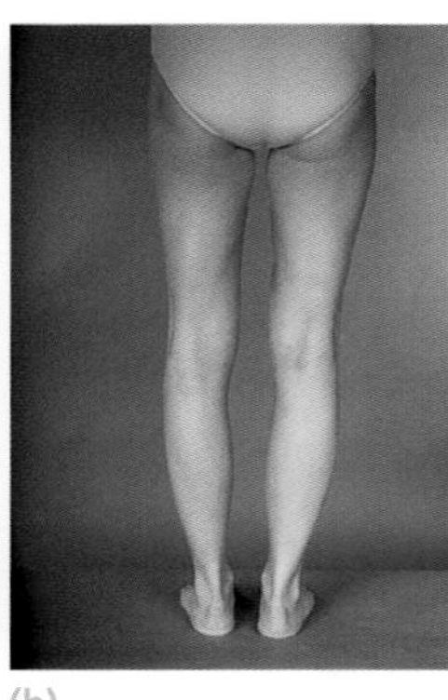
(b)

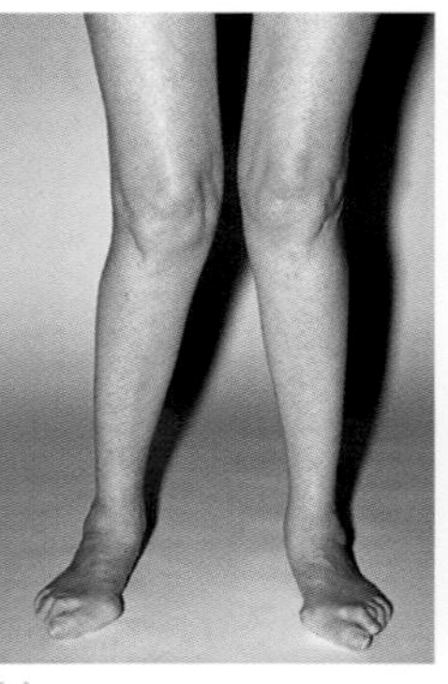
(c)

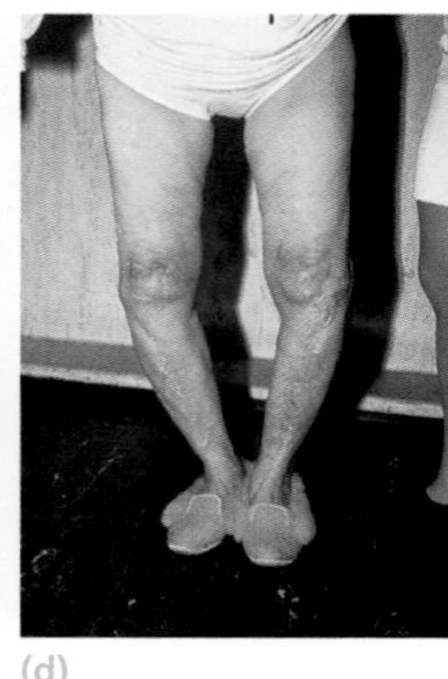
(d)

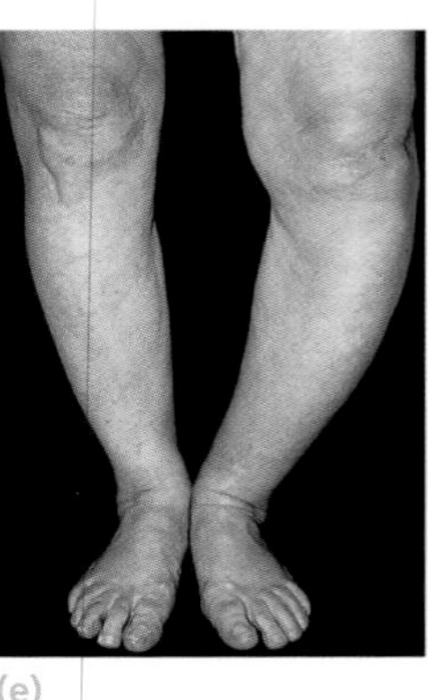
(e)

20.1 Examination standing (a,b) Look at the general shape and posture, first from in front and then from behind. Normally the knees are in slight valgus. Look for swelling of the joint or wasting of the thigh muscles; quadriceps wasting occurs very quickly. (c) This patient has rheumatoid arthritis and bilateral valgus deformities; in contrast, osteoarthritis is likely to lead to varus deformities (d). Unilateral deformity is easier to notice and almost always pathological – this man has Paget's disease of the tibia (e).

5 degrees in men), because the hips are wider than the knees. *Genu valgum* and *genu varum* are determined in relation to this normal anatomical alignment. But look carefully to see whether the deformity is really in the knee (often a sign of arthritis) and not in the lower end of the femur (a bone tumour?) or the upper end of the tibia (e.g. a malunited fracture, or maybe Paget's disease (see Fig. 20.1e)).

Alignment of the extensor mechanism (quadriceps, patella and patellar ligament) can also be measured with the patient standing but is probably more conveniently done with the patient seated (see below).

Gait is important; the patient should also be observed walking with and without any support such as a stick or crutch. In the *stance phase* note whether the knee extends fully (is there a fixed flexion deformity or a hyperextension deformity?) and see if there is any lateral or medial thrust signifying instability. In the *swing phase* note whether the knee moves freely or is held in one position – usually because the joint is painful but perhaps because it really is ankylosed! When the patient walks, is there any sign of a limp? And if so, does it stem from the knee? Or perhaps the hip, or the foot?

Signs with the patient sitting

With the patient sitting sideways on the examination couch, the outlines of the patellae and patellar ligaments, as well as the general shape and symmetry of the two knees and the tibial tubercles, can be made out quite easily. With the knees dangling at 90 degrees of flexion, the patellae should be facing straight forwards; note if they appear to be seated higher than usual (*patella alta*) or lower than usual (*patella baja*). Patella alta is believed to be associated with a higher than normal incidence of chondromalacia patellae.

Next, ask the patient to straighten each knee in turn and observe how the patella moves upwards. Does it remain centred over the femoral condyles or does it veer off towards one side in the early phase of knee extension and then slide back to the centre with full extension – suggesting a tendency to subluxation?

Patellar alignment can also be assessed by measuring the *Q-angle* (quadriceps angle). This is the angle subtended by a line drawn from the anterior superior iliac spine to the centre of the patella and another from the centre of the patella to the tibial tubercle (Fig. 20.2c); it normally averages about 14 degrees in men and 17 degrees in women. An increased Q-angle is regarded as a predisposing factor in the development of chondromalacia; however, small variations from the norm are not a reliable indicator of future pathology.

Signs with the patient lying supine

The knees are the most visible and accessible of all the large joints; with the legs lying side by side, features on one side can be constantly compared with those on the other.

Look

The first things that strike one are the *position of the knee*. Is it symmetrical with the normal side? Is it held in valgus or varus, incompletely extended, or hyperextended? Note also the presence of *swelling*, either of the joint as a whole or as *lumps or bumps* in localized areas.

Wasting of the quadriceps is a sure sign of joint disorder. The visual impression can be checked by *measuring* the girth of the thigh at the same level (e.g. a fixed distance above the joint line or a hand's breadth above the patella) in each limb.

Look more closely for signs of *bruising*, and for *old scars or sinuses*, signifying previous infection or operations.

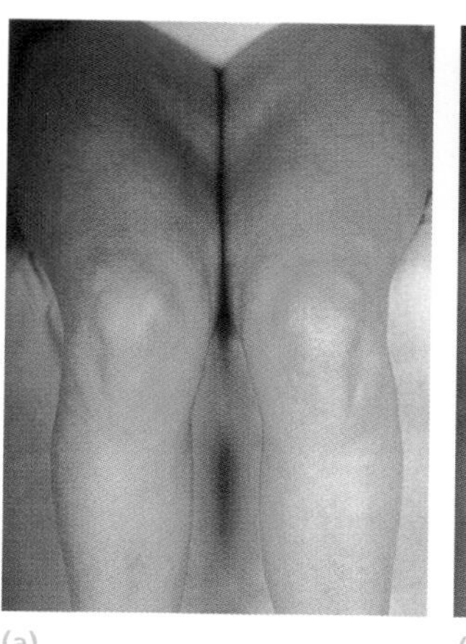
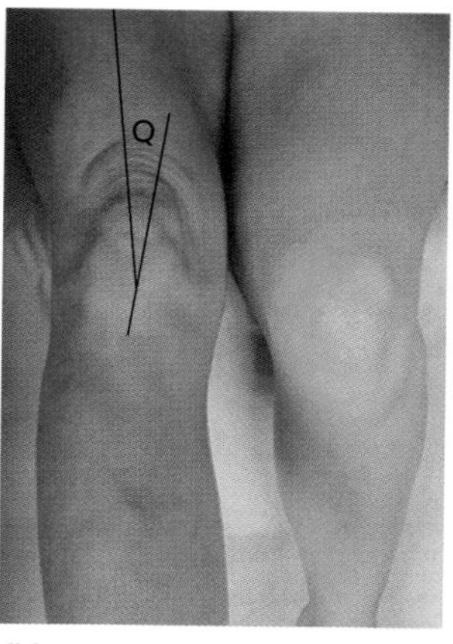

(a) (b)

20.2 Examination with the patient sitting The two knees are compared for shape and symmetry. Note the position of the patellae (a) in relaxation, (b) in full extension and by measuring the Q-angle.

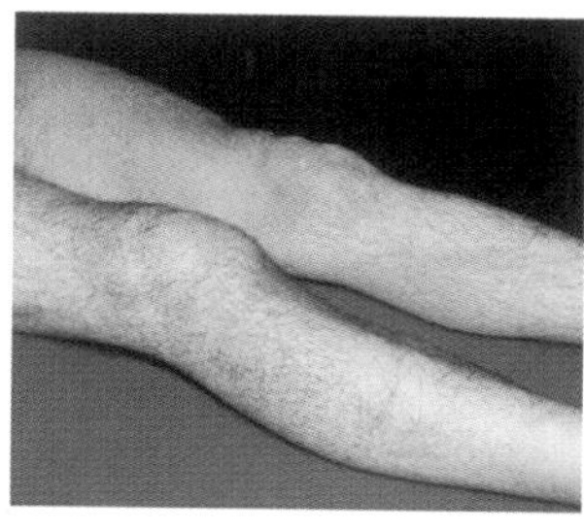
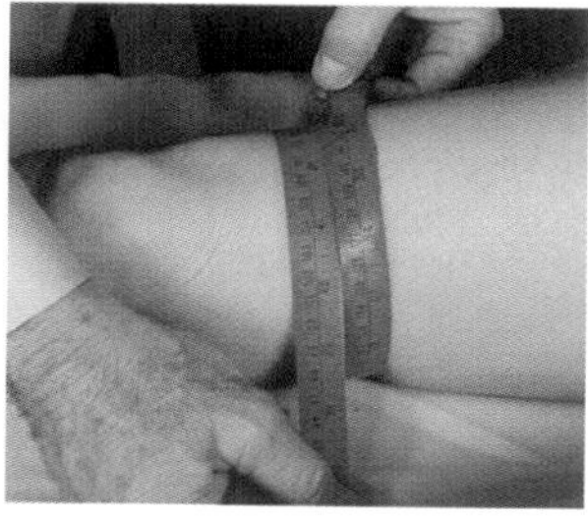

(a) (b)

20.3 Examination with the patient supine (a) Wasting of the quadriceps occurs rapidly after any internal derangement of the knee. (b) The girth is measured at the same level in both limbs, about a hand's breadth above the patella.

Take note of the *shape and position of the patella*, both with the knee at rest and during movement. Always compare the symptomatic with the normal side.

Feel

As with all joints, palpation of the knee – if it is to be rewarding – demands a sound knowledge of the local anatomy.

Start by running your hand down the length of the limb, feeling for changes in *skin temperature* and comparing the symptomatic with the normal side. There is normally a gradual decrease in skin temperature from proximal to distal. Increased warmth over the knee signifies increased vascularity, usually due to inflammation.

The *soft tissues and bony outlines* are then palpated systematically, feeling for abnormal outlines and localized tenderness. This is easier if the joint is flexed and the examiner sits on the edge of the couch facing the knee. By placing both hands over the front of the knee, the outlines of the joint margins, the patellar ligament, the collateral ligaments, the iliotibial band and the pes anserinus are then easily traced with the fingers. The point of maximum tenderness will suggest at least the anatomical site of pathology if not the precise diagnosis.

Synovial thickening is best appreciated as follows: placing the knee in extension, the examiner grasps the edges of the patella in a pincer made of the thumb and middle finger, and tries to lift the patella forwards; normally the bone can be grasped quite firmly, but if the synovium is thickened the fingers simply slip off the edges of the patella.

Move

Passive extension can be tested by the examiner simply holding both legs by the ankles and lifting them off the couch; the knees should straighten fully (or even into a few degrees of hyperextension) and symmetrically. *Active extension* can be roughly tested by the examiner slipping a hand under each knee and then asking the patient to force the knees into the surface of the couch; it is usually easy to feel whether the hands are trapped equally strongly on the two sides. Another way is to have the patient sitting on the edge of the couch with his or her legs hanging over the side and then asking them to extend each knee as far as possible; the test can be repeated with the patient extending the knees against resistance.

Passive and *active flexion* are tested with the patient lying supine. Normally the heel can be pulled up close to the buttock, with the knee moving through a range of 0–150 degrees. The 'heel-to-buttock' distance is compared on the two sides.

Internal and *external rotation*, though normally no more than about 10 degrees, should also be assessed. The patient's hip and knee are flexed to 90 degrees; one hand steadies and feels the knee, the other rotates the foot.

Crepitus during movement may be felt with a hand placed on the front of the knee. It usually signifies patello-femoral roughness.

Movement with compartmental loading is a useful test for localizing the site of joint pain; the medial or lateral compartment of the knee can be loaded separately by applying varus or valgus stress during flexion and noting which manoeuvre is more painful.

Tests for intra-articular fluid

Cross fluctuation This test is applicable only if there is a large effusion. The left hand compresses and empties the suprapatellar pouch while the right hand straddles the front of the joint below the patella; by squeezing with each hand alternately, a fluid impulse is transmitted across the joint.

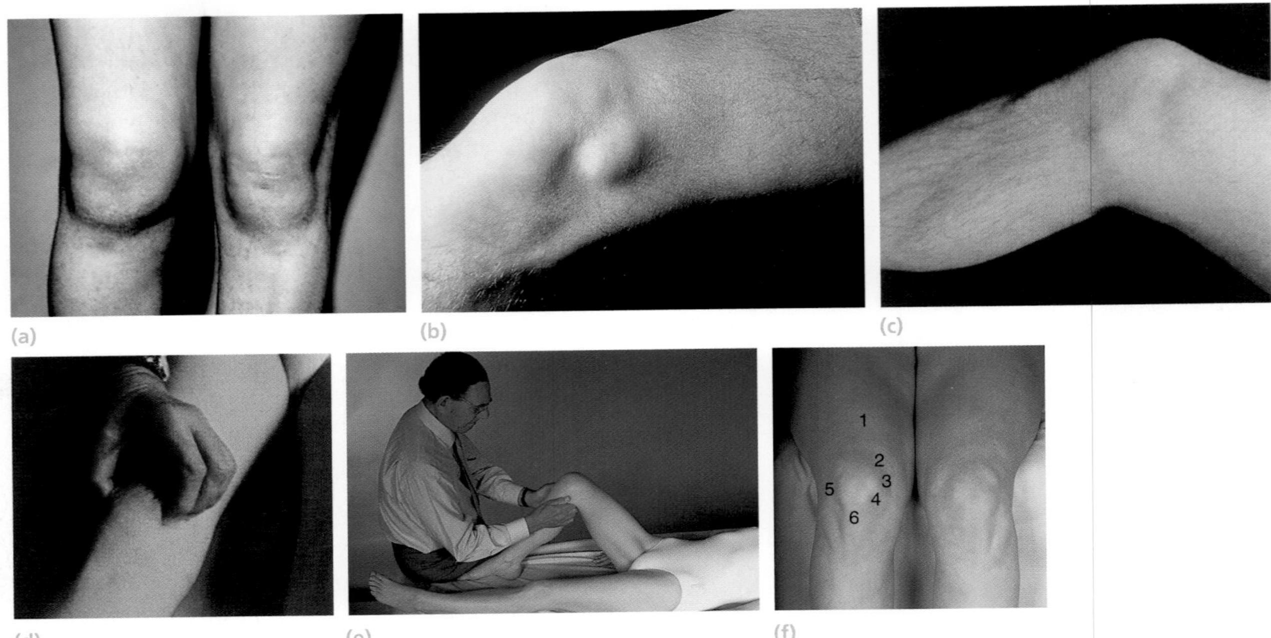

20.4 Examination with the patient supine Swelling may involve either the whole joint, as in this patient (a) with acute synovitis, or may be due to some localized lesion as in patient (b) with a large loose body in the joint and patient (c) with a small meniscal cyst protruding at the medial joint line. (d) Feeling for synovial swelling: try to 'lift' the patella – if the synovium is thickened your fingers will slip off the edges. (e) Feeling for tenderness: sit facing the patient's knee and try to identify the exact site of pain/tenderness. A superficial 'map' is shown in (f): 1, quadriceps tendon; 2, edge of patella; 3, medial collateral ligament; 4, joint line; 5, lateral collateral ligament; 6, patellar ligament.

The patellar tap Again the suprapatellar pouch is compressed with the left hand to squeeze any fluid from the pouch into the joint. With the other hand the patella is then tapped sharply backwards onto the femoral condyles. In a positive test the patella can be felt striking the femur and bouncing off again (a type of ballottement).

The bulge test This is a useful method of testing when there is very little fluid in the joint, though it takes some practice to get it right! After squeezing any fluid out of the suprapatellar pouch, the medial compartment is emptied by pressing on the inner aspect of the joint; that hand is then lifted away and the lateral side is sharply compressed – a distinct ripple is seen on the flattened medial surface as fluid is shunted across.

The juxta-patellar hollow test Normally, when the knee is flexed, a hollow appears lateral to the patellar ligament and disappears with further flexion; if there is excess fluid, the hollow fills and disappears at a lesser angle of flexion (Mann et al., 1991). Compare this in the two knees.

The patello-femoral joint

The *size, shape and position* of the patella are noted. The bone is felt, first on its anterior surface and then

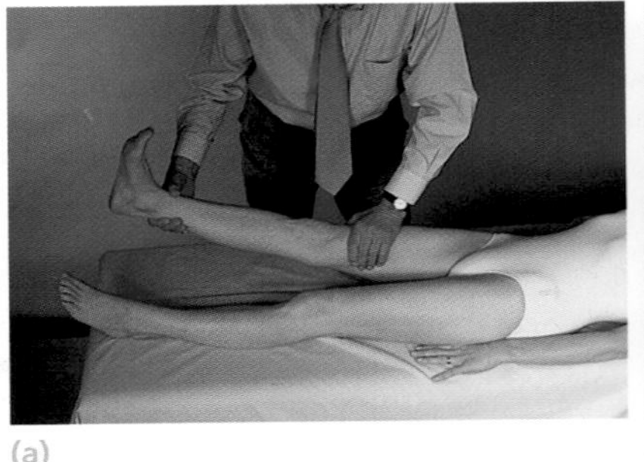
(a)

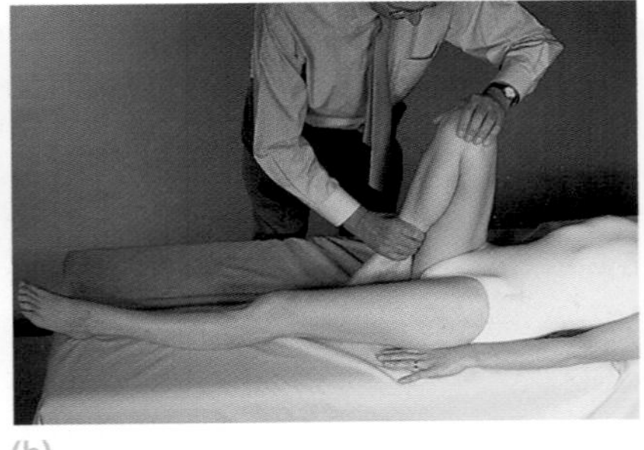
(b)

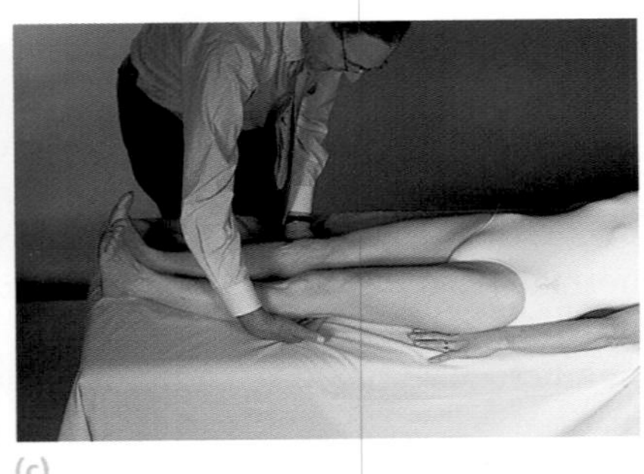
(c)

20.5 Movement The knee should move from full extension (a) through a range of 150 degrees to full flexion (b). Small degrees of flexion deformity (loss of full extension) can be detected by placing the hands under the knees while the patient forces the legs down on the couch (c); if your hand can be extracted more easily on one side than the other, this indicates loss of the final few degrees of complete extension.

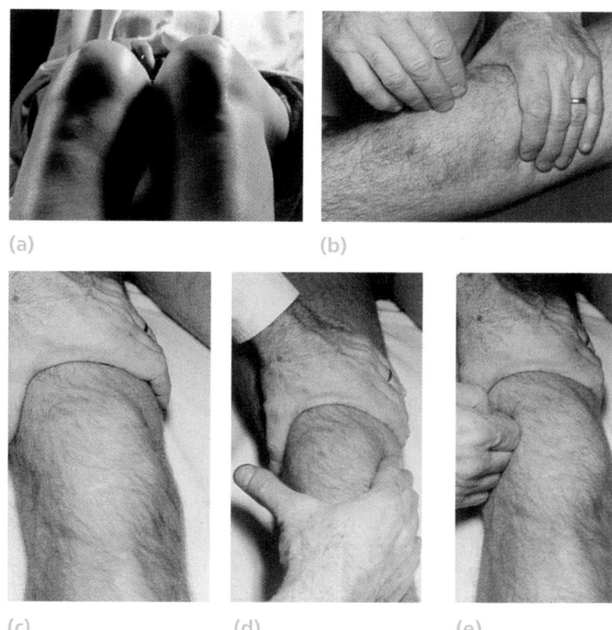

(a) (b) (c) (d) (e)

20.6 Testing for intra-articular fluid (a) The juxta-patellar hollow, which disappears in flexion if there is fluid in the knee. (b) Patellar tap test. (c,d,e) Doing the bulge test: compress the suprapatellar pouch (c), empty the medial compartment (d), push fluid back from the lateral compartment and watch for the bulge on the medial side (e).

along its edges and at the attachments of the quadriceps tendon and the patellar ligament. Much of the posterior surface, too, is accessible to palpation if the patella is pushed first to one side and then to the other; tenderness suggests synovial irritation or articular cartilage softening.

Moving the patella up and down while pressing it lightly against the femur (*the 'friction test'*) causes painful grating if the central portion of the articular cartilage is damaged.

Pressing the patella laterally with the thumb while flexing the knee slowly may induce anxiety and sharp resistance to further movement; this, the *'apprehension test'*, is diagnostic of recurrent patellar subluxation or dislocation.

Tests for stability

Collateral ligaments The medial and lateral ligaments are tested by stressing the knee into valgus and varus: this is best done by tucking the patient's foot under your arm and holding the extended knee firmly with one hand on each side of the joint; the leg is then angulated alternately towards abduction and adduction. The test is performed at full extension and again at 30 degrees of flexion. There is normally some medio-lateral movement at 30 degrees, but if this is excessive (compared to the normal side) it suggests a torn or stretched collateral ligament. Sideways movement in full extension is always abnormal; it may be due to either torn or stretched ligaments and capsule or loss of articular cartilage or bone, which allows the affected compartment to collapse.

Cruciate ligaments Routine tests for cruciate ligament stability are based on examining for abnormal gliding movements in the sagittal plane. With both knees flexed 90 degrees and the feet resting on the couch, the upper tibia is inspected from the side; if its upper end has dropped back, or can be gently pushed back, this indicates a tear of the posterior cruciate ligament (the 'sag sign'). With the knee in the same position, the foot is anchored by the examiner sitting on it (provided this is not painful); then, using both hands, the upper end of the tibia is grasped firmly and rocked backwards and forwards to see if there is any anteroposterior glide (the '*drawer test*'). Excessive anterior movement (a positive anterior drawer sign) denotes anterior cruciate laxity; excessive posterior movement (a positive posterior drawer sign) signifies posterior cruciate laxity.

More sensitive is the *Lachman test*, but this is difficult if the patient has big thighs (or the examiner has small hands). The patient's knee is flexed 20 degrees; with one hand grasping the lower thigh and the other the upper part of the leg, the joint surfaces are shifted backwards and forwards upon each other. If the knee is stable, there should be no gliding. In both the drawer test and Lachman test, note whether the endpoint of abnormal movement is 'soft' or 'hard'.

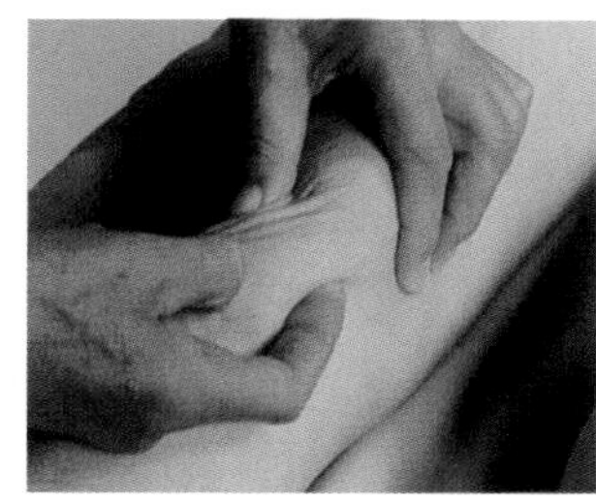

(a)

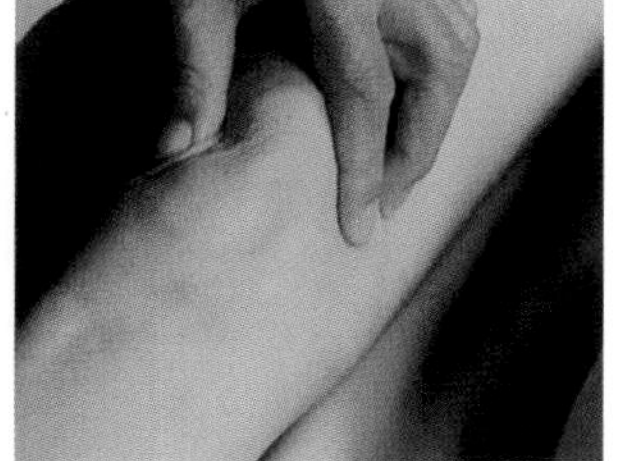

(b)

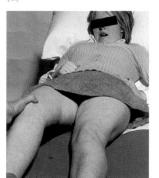

(c)

20.7 Patello-femoral joint (a) Feeling under the edge of the patella. (b) Testing for patello-femoral tenderness. (c) The patellar apprehension test.

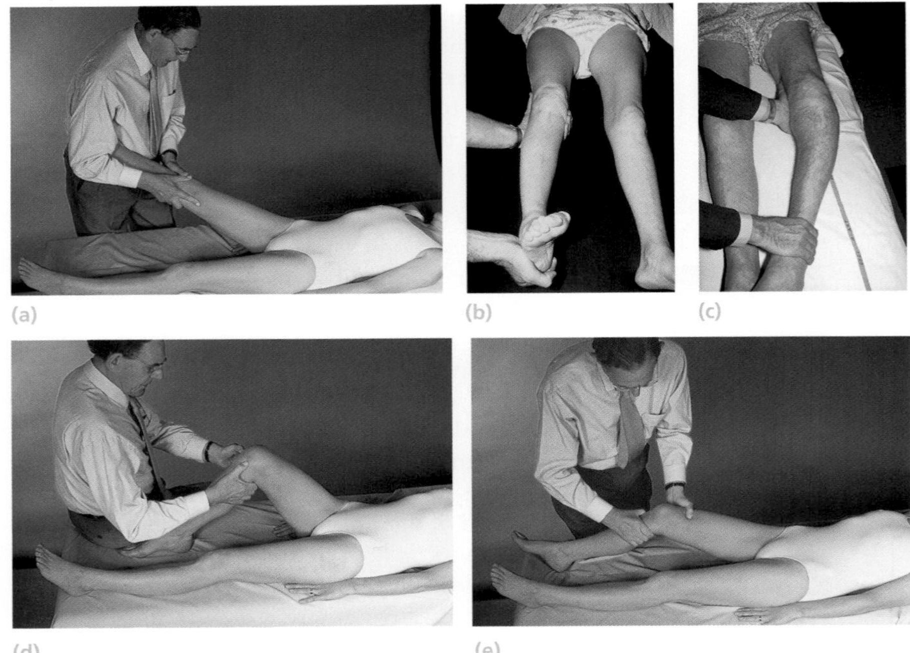

(a) (b) (c) (d) (e)

20.8 Testing for instability There are two ways of testing the collateral ligaments (side-to-side stability): (a) by gripping the foot close to your body and guiding the knee alternately towards valgus and varus; (b) by gripping the femoral condyles (provided your hand is big enough) and then forcing the leg alternately into valgus and varus. (c) In this case there was gross instability on the lateral side, allowing the knee to be pulled into marked varus. Cruciate ligament instability can be assessed by either the drawer test (d) or the Lachman test (e), as described in the text.

Complex ligament injuries When only a collateral or cruciate ligament is damaged the diagnosis is relatively easy: the direction of unstable movement is either sideways or front-to-back. With combined injuries the direction of instability may be oblique or rotational. Special clinical tests have been developed to detect these abnormalities (see Chapter 30); the best known is the *pivot shift test*. The patient lies supine with the lower limb completely relaxed. The examiner lifts the leg with the knee held in full extension and the tibia internally rotated (the position of slight rotational subluxation). A valgus force is then applied to the lateral side of the joint as the knee is flexed; a sudden posterior movement of the tibia is seen and felt as the joint is fully re-located. The test is sometimes quite painful.

Tests for meniscal injuries

McMurray's test This classic test for a torn meniscus is seldom used now that the diagnosis can easily be made by MRI. However, advanced imaging is not always available and the clinical test has not been altogether discarded.

The test is based on the fact that the loose meniscal tag can sometimes be trapped between the articular surfaces and then induced to snap free with a palpable and audible click. The knee is flexed as far as possible; one hand steadies the joint and the other rotates the leg medially and laterally while the knee is slowly extended. The test is repeated several times, with the knee stressed in valgus or varus, feeling and listening for the click.

A positive test is helpful but not pathognomonic; a negative test does not exclude a tear.

Thessaly test This test is based on a dynamic reproduction of load transmission in the knee joint under normal or trauma conditions. With the affected knee flexed to 20 degrees and the foot placed flat on the ground, the patient takes his or her full weight on that leg while being supported (for balance) by the examiner (Fig. 20.9). The patient is then instructed to twist his or her body to one side and then to the other three times (thus, with each turn, exerting a rotational force in the knee) while keeping the knee flexed at 20 degrees. Patients with meniscal tears experience medial or lateral joint line pain and may have a sense of locking. The test has shown a high diagnostic accuracy rate at the level of 95 per cent in detecting meniscal tears, with a low number of false positive and negative recordings (Karachalios et al., 2005).

Signs with the patient lying prone

Scars or lumps in the popliteal fossa are noted. If there is a swelling, is it in the midline (most likely a bulging capsule) or to one side (possibly a bursa)? A semimembranous bursa is usually just above the joint line, a Baker's cyst below it.

The popliteal fossa is carefully palpated. If there is a lump, where does it originate? Does it pulsate? Can it be emptied into the joint?

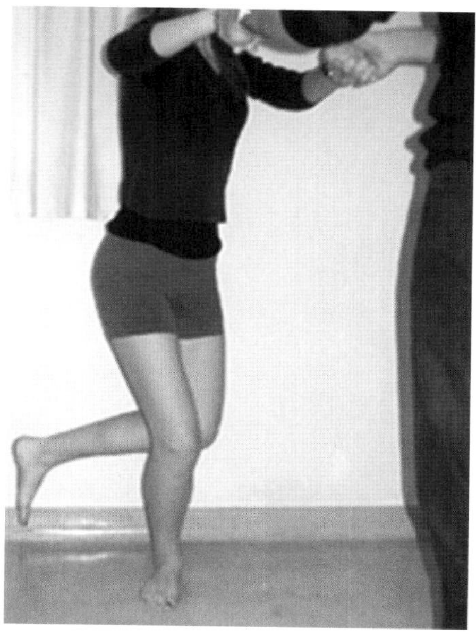

20.9 Meniscal injury – Thessaly test Picture showing how the patient is positioned during the Thessaly test.

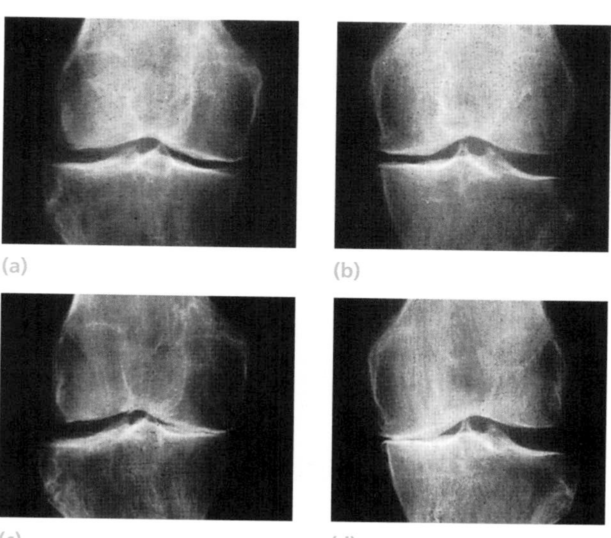

20.10 X-rays Anteroposterior views should always be taken with the patient standing. (a,b) X-rays with the patient lying down show only slight narrowing of the medial joint space on each side; but with weightbearing (c,d) it is clear that these changes are much more marked.

Apley's test With the patient prone the knee is flexed to 90 degrees and rotated while a compression force is applied; this, the *grinding test*, reproduces symptoms if a meniscus is torn. Rotation is then repeated while the leg is pulled upwards with the surgeon's knee holding the thigh down; this, the *distraction test*, produces increased pain only if there is ligament damage.

Lachman's test The Lachman test can be readily performed with the patient prone.

IMAGING

X-RAYS

Anteroposterior and lateral views are routine; it is often useful also to obtain tangential ('skyline') patello-femoral views and intercondylar (or tunnel) views. *The anteroposterior view should always be taken with the patient standing*; unless the femoro-tibial compartment is loaded, narrowing of the articular space may be missed. Both knees should be x-rayed, so as to compare the abnormal with the normal side.

Tibio-femoral alignment can be measured on full-length standing views. Normal indices have also been established for patellar height and patello-femoral congruence. These features are discussed in the relevant sections of the chapter.

OTHER FORMS OF IMAGING

Radioscintigraphy may show increased activity in the subarticular bone in early osteoarthritis. It is also helpful in showing 'hot spots' due to infection after joint replacement.

CT is useful for showing patello-femoral congruence at various angles of flexion.

MRI provides a reliable means of diagnosing lateral and medial meniscal tears and cruciate ligament injuries (Oei et al., 2003). It is also helpful in identifying the early stages of osteoarticular lesions and osteonecrosis of the femoral or tibial condyles.

ARTHROSCOPY

Arthroscopy is useful: (1) to establish or refine the accuracy of diagnosis; (2) to help in deciding whether to operate, or to plan the operative approach with more precision; (3) to record the progress of a knee disorder; and (4) to perform certain operative procedures. Arthroscopy is not a substitute for clinical examination; a detailed history and meticulous assessment of the physical signs are indispensable preliminaries and remain the sheet anchor of diagnosis. However, arthroscopy is especially helpful in diagnosing meniscal injuries – and dealing with them at the same time. *Full asepsis is essential.*

THE DIAGNOSTIC CALENDAR

While most disorders of the knee can occur at any age, certain conditions are more commonly encountered during specific periods of life.

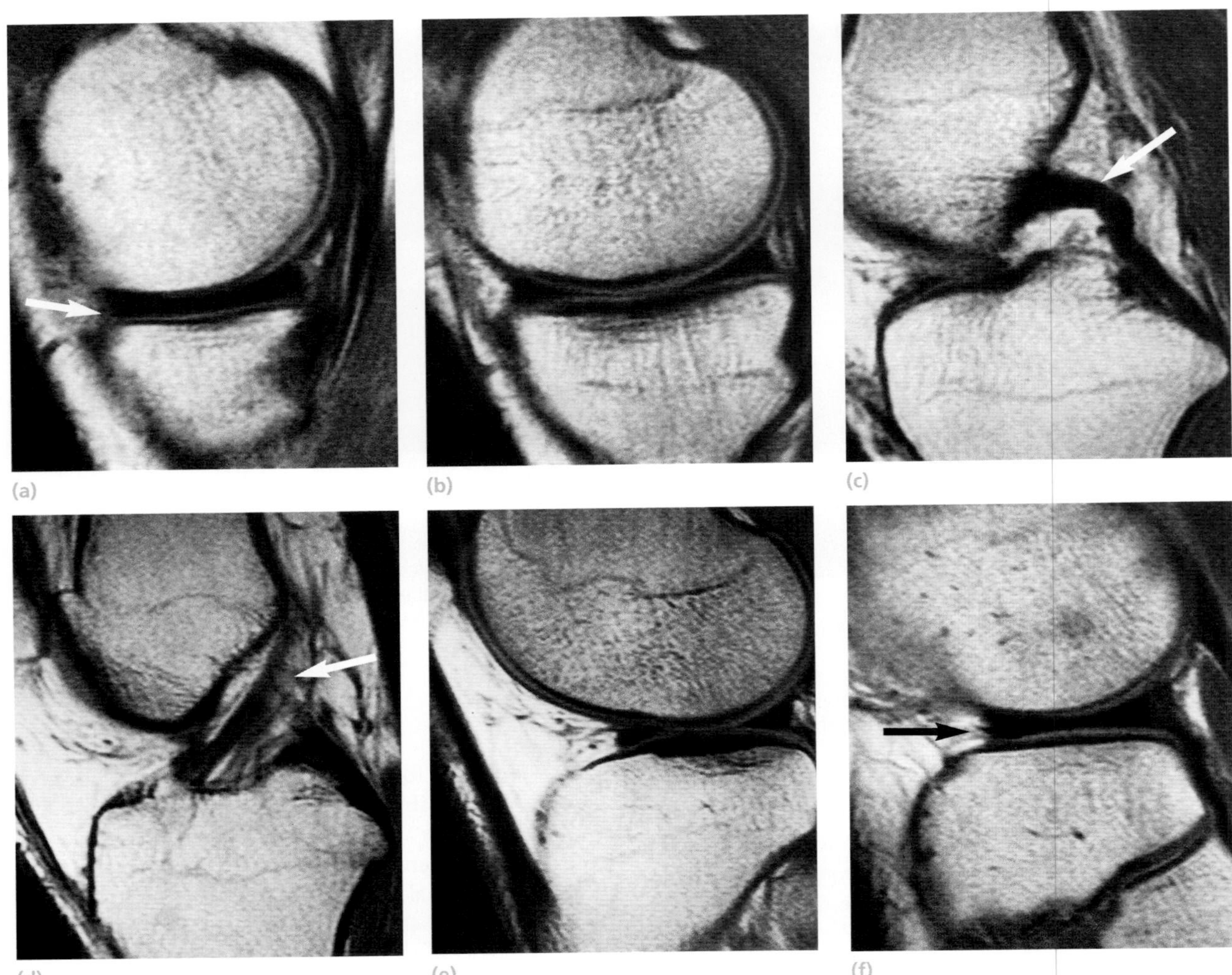

20.11 MRI A series of sagittal T1 weighted images proceeding from medial to lateral show the normal appearances of (a,b) the medial meniscus, (c) the posterior cruciate ligament, (d) the somewhat fan-shaped anterior cruciate ligament and (e,f) the lateral meniscus.

Congenital knee disorders may be present at birth or may become apparent only during the first or second decade of life.

Adolescents with anterior knee pain are usually found to have chondromalacia patellae, patellar instability, osteochondritis or a plica syndrome. But remember – knee pain may be referred from the hip!

Young adults engaged in sports are the most frequent victims of meniscal tears and ligament injuries. Examination should include a variety of tests for ligamentous instability that would be quite inappropriate in elderly patients.

Patients above middle age with chronic pain and stiffness probably have osteoarthritis. With primary osteoarthritis of the knees, other joints also are often affected; polyarthritis does not necessarily (nor even most commonly) mean rheumatoid arthritis.

DEFORMITIES OF THE KNEE

By the end of growth the knees are normally in 5–7 degrees of valgus. Any deviation from this may be regarded as 'deformity', though often it bothers no one – least of all the possessor of the knees. The three common deformities are bow leg (genu varum), knock knee (genu valgum) and hyperextension (genu recurvatum).

BOW LEGS AND KNOCK KNEES IN CHILDREN

Deformity is usually gauged from simple observation. Bilateral bow leg can be recorded by measuring the

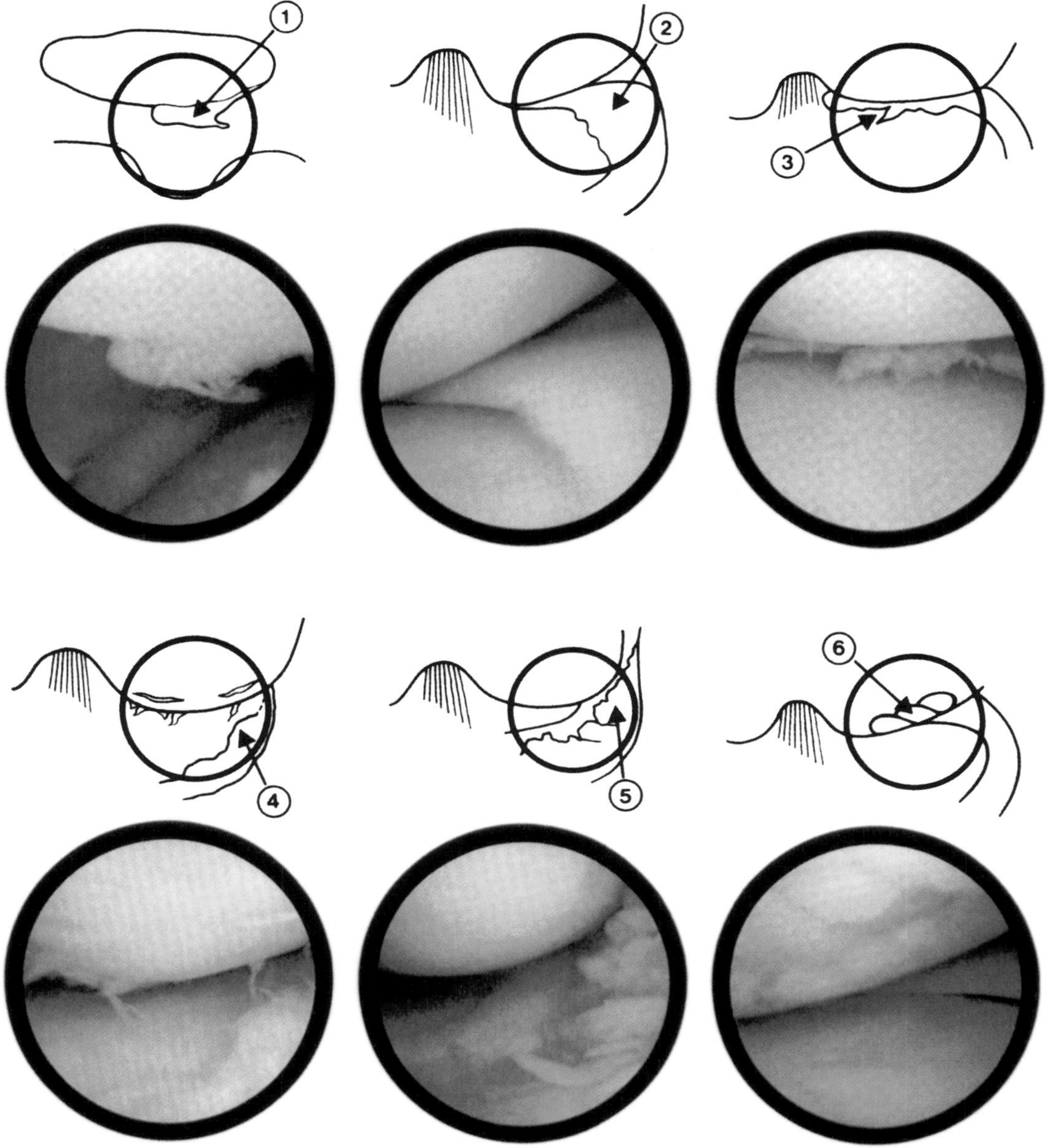

20.12 Arthroscopy Arthroscopic images of the interior of the right knee from the lateral side, showing (1) chrondomalacia patellae; (2) normal medial meniscus; (3) torn medial meniscus; (4) degenerate medial meniscus and osteoarthritic femoral condyle; (5) rheumatoid synovium; (6) osteochondritis dissecans of medial femoral condyle.

distance between the knees with the child standing and the heels touching; it should be less than 6 cm. Similarly, knock knee can be estimated by measuring the distance between the medial malleoli when the knees are touching with the patellae facing forwards; it is usually less than 8 cm.

Physiological bow legs and knock knees

Bow legs in babies and knock knees in 4-year-olds are so common that they are considered to be *normal stages of development*. Other postural abnormalities such as 'pigeon toes' and flat feet may coexist but these children are normal in all other respects; the parents should be reassured and the child should be seen at intervals of 6 months to record progress.

In the occasional case where, by the age of 10, the deformity is still marked (i.e. the intercondylar distance is more than 6 cm or the intermalleolar distance more than 8 cm), operative correction should be advised.

Stapling of the physes on one or other side of the knee can be done to restrict growth on that side and allow correction of the deformity (the staples are removed once the knee has over-corrected slightly); there is a risk, however, that normal growth will not resume when the staples are removed.

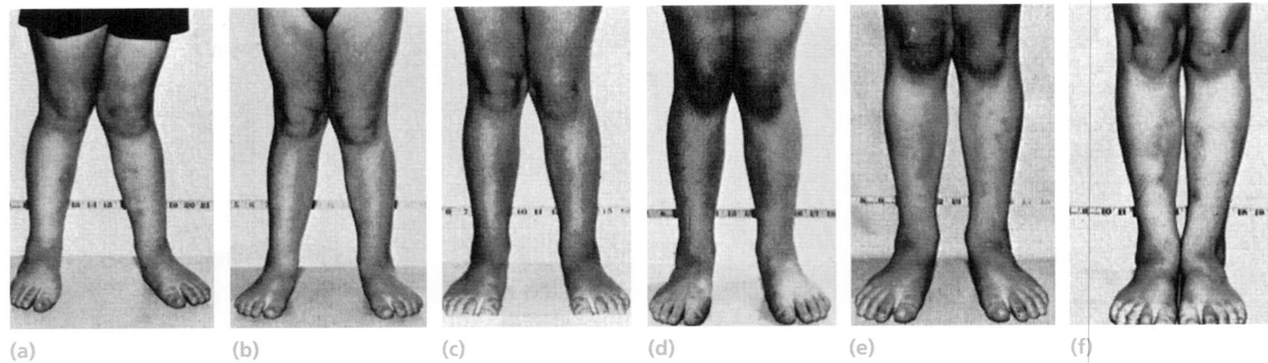

20.13 Physiological genu valgum 'Knock-knees' in young children usually correct spontaneously. These pictures of the same child were obtained at various ages between 3 and 7 years.

Hemi-epiphysodesis (fusion of one-half of the growth plate) on the 'convex' side of the deformity will achieve similar correction; this requires careful timing guided by charting the child's bone age and estimating the corrective effect of arresting further growth on one side of the bone.

Corrective osteotomy (supracondylar osteotomy for valgus knees and high tibial osteotomy for varus knees) may sound sensible; however, the child (and the parents) will have to put up with the 'deformity' until growth is complete before undergoing the operation, otherwise there is a risk of the deformity recurring while the child is still growing.

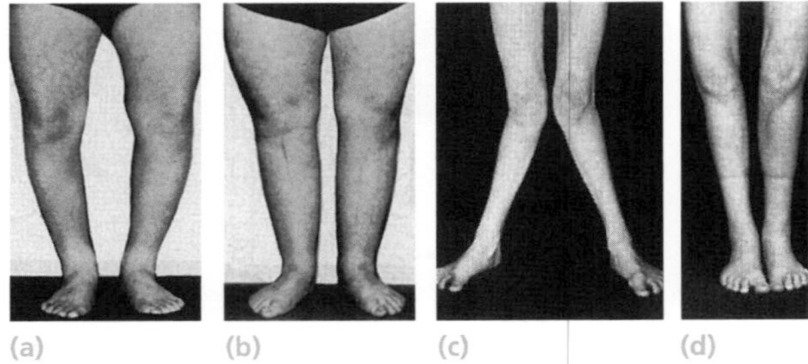

20.14 Persistent deformities (a,b) Persistent genu varum before and after corrective osteotomy. (c,d) Before and after osteotomy for severe genu valgum.

Compensatory deformities

Varus, valgus and rotational deformities of the proximal femur may give rise to complex compensatory deformities of the knees and legs once the child starts to walk. Thus, persistent anteversion of the femoral neck may come to be associated with 'squinting knees' (the patellae face inwards when the hips are fully located), genu valgum, tibial torsion and valgus heels. It is essential to analyse all components of these deformities before focussing on the knees. Often they correct spontaneously by the end of growth, or if some elements persist, they cause little or no problem; only in severe cases – and after the most meticulous preoperative planning – are osteotomies undertaken.

Pathological bow leg and knock knee

Disorders which cause distorted epiphyseal and/or physeal growth may give rise to bow leg or knock knee; these include some of the skeletal dysplasias and the various types of rickets, as well as injuries of the epiphyseal and physeal growth cartilage. A unilateral deformity is likely to be pathological, but it is essential in all cases to look for signs of injury or generalized skeletal disorder. If angulation is severe, operative correction will be necessary, but it should be deferred until near the end of growth lest the deformity recur with further growth.

Blount's disease

This is a progressive bow-leg deformity associated with abnormal growth of the posteromedial part of the proximal tibia. The children are usually overweight and start walking early; the condition is

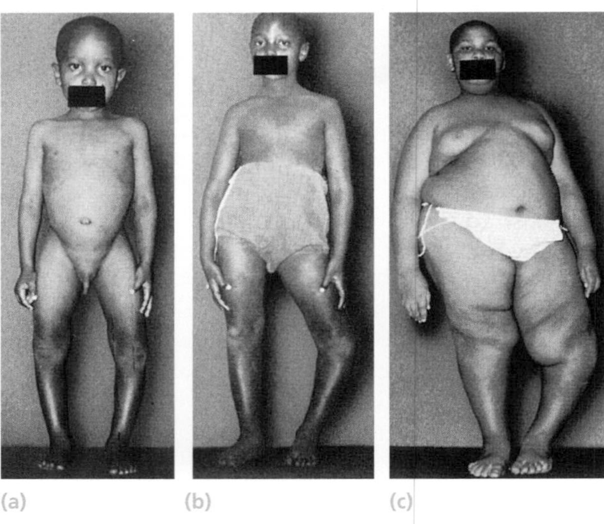

20.15 Pathological bow legs (a) Child with healed rickets. (b) Growth deformity following a fracture involving the proximal tibial physis. (c) The deformity here was due to a 'slipped' proximal tibial epiphysis in a child with an endocrine disorder.

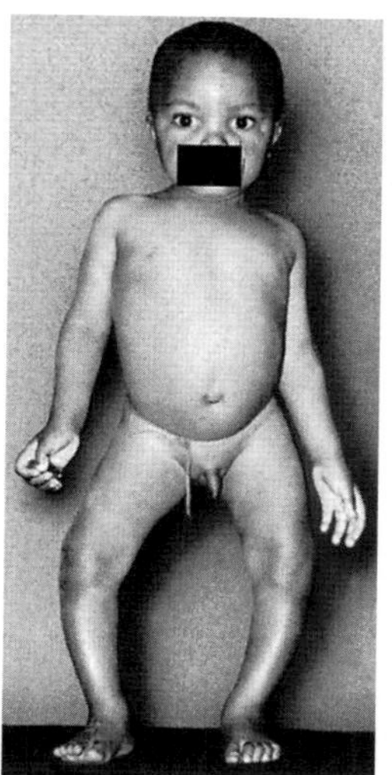

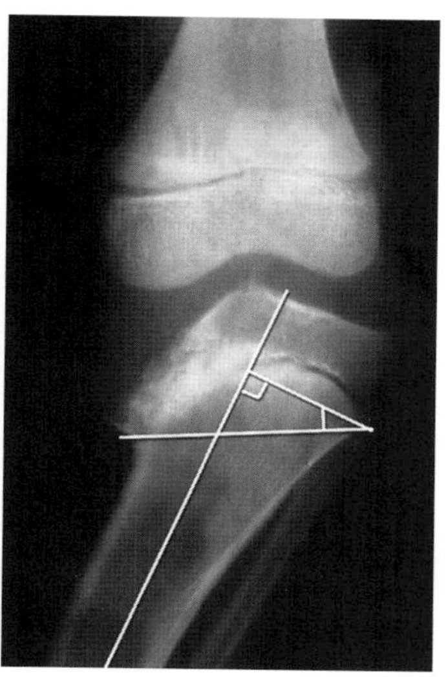

20.16 Blount's disease In contrast to the children in Fig. 20.15, this young boy developed progressive bow-legged deformities from the time he started walking. X-rays showed the typical features of Blount's disease: marked distortion of the tibial epiphysis, as if one half of the growth plate (physis) had fused and stopped growing. Changes can be accurately assessed by measuring the *metaphyseo-diaphyseal angle*: a line is drawn perpendicular to the long axis of the tibia and another across the metaphyseal flare as shown on the x-ray; the acute angle formed by these two lines should normally not exceed 11°.

bilateral in 80 per cent of cases. Children of negroid descent appear to be affected more frequently than others. Deformity is noticeably worse than in physiological bow legs and may include internal rotation of the tibia. The child walks with an outward thrust of the knee; in the worst cases there may be lateral subluxation of the tibia.

X-ray The proximal tibial epiphysis is flattened medially and the adjacent metaphysis is beak-shaped. The medial cortex of the proximal tibia appears thickened; this is an illusory effect produced by internal rotation of the tibia. The tibial epiphysis sometimes looks 'fragmented'; occasionally the femoral epiphysis also is affected. In the late stages a bony bar forms across the medial half of the tibial physis, preventing further growth on that side. The degree of proximal tibia vara can be quantified by measuring the metaphyseo-diaphyseal angle (see Fig. 20.16).

In contrast to physiological bowing, abnormal alignment occurs in the proximal tibia and not in the joint.

Treatment Spontaneous resolution is rare and, once it is clear that the deformity is progressing, a corrective osteotomy should be performed, addressing both the varus and the rotational components. A preoperative (or peroperative) arthrogram, to outline the misshapen epiphysis, will help in planning the operation. Slight over-correction should be aimed for as some recurrence is inevitable. In severe cases it may be necessary also to elevate the depressed medial tibial plateau using a wedge of bone taken from the femur. If a bony bar has formed, it can be excised and replaced by a free fat graft. In older children it may be easier to perform a surgical correction and then (if necessary) lengthen the tibia by the Ilizarov method. All these procedures should be accompanied by fasciotomy to reduce the risk of a postoperative compartment syndrome.

DEFORMITIES OF THE KNEE IN ADULTS

GENU VARUM AND GENU VALGUM

Angular deformities are common in adults (usually bow legs in men and knock knees in women). They may be the *sequel to childhood deformity* and if so usually cause no problems. However, if the deformity is associated with joint instability, this can lead to osteoarthritis – of the medial compartment in varus knees and the lateral compartment in valgus knees. Genu valgum may also cause abnormal tracking of the patella and predispose to patello-femoral osteoarthritis. Even in the absence of overt osteoarthritis, if the patient complains of severe pain, or if there are clinical or radiological signs of joint damage, a 'prophylactic' osteotomy can be performed – above the knee for valgus deformity and below the knee for varus. Preoperative planning should include radiographic measurements to determine the mechanical and anatomical axes of both bones and the lower limb, as well as estimation of the centre of rotation of angulation.

Deformity may be *secondary to arthritis* – usually varus in osteoarthritis and valgus in rheumatoid arthritis. In these cases the joint is often unstable and corrective osteotomy less predictable in its effect. Stress x-rays are essential in the assessment of these cases.

Other causes of varus or valgus deformity are *ligament injuries, malunited fractures* and *Paget's disease.* Where possible, the underlying disorder should be dealt with; provided the joint is stable, corrective osteotomy may be all that is necessary.

GENU RECURVATUM (HYPEREXTENSION OF THE KNEE)

Congenital recurvatum This may be due to abnormal intra-uterine posture; it usually recovers spontaneously. Rarely, gross hyperextension is the precursor of true congenital dislocation of the knee.

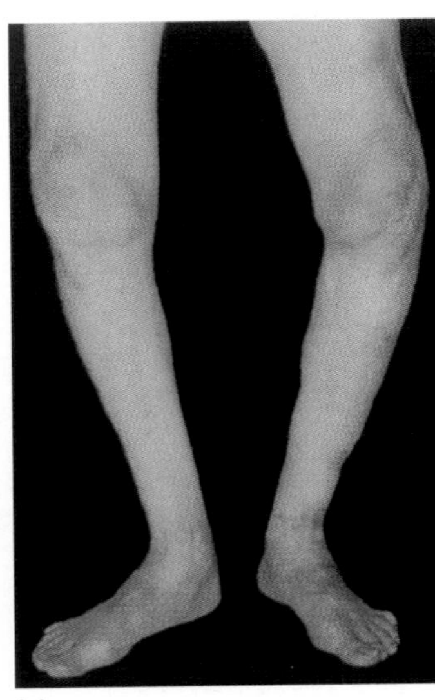

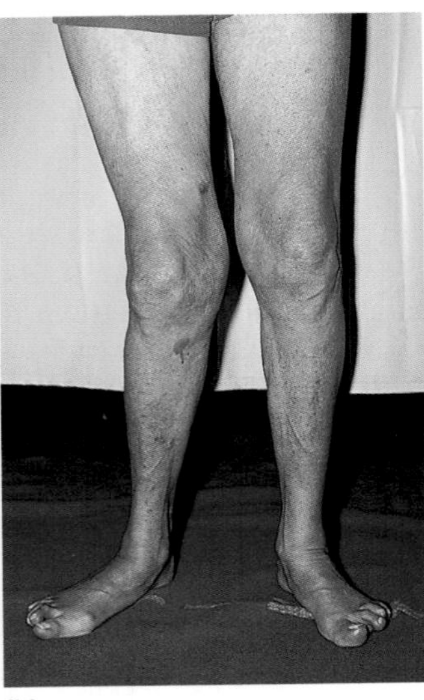

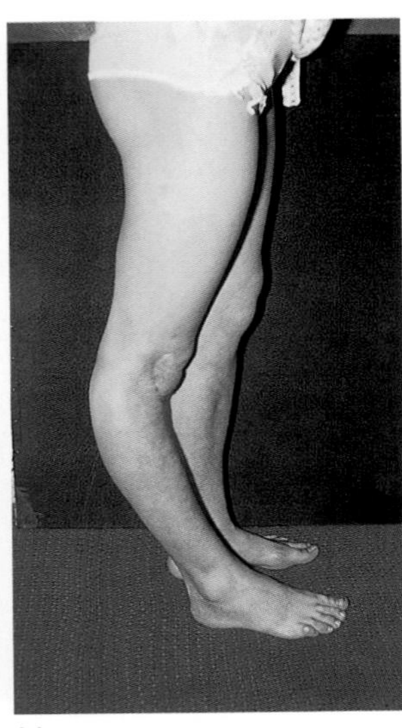

(a) (b) (c)

20.17 Knee deformities in adults Genu varum is usually associated with osteoarthritis (a); genu valgum with rheumatoid arthritis (b); and genu recurvatum (c) with severe destructive arthritis (e.g. Charcot's disease) or a flail joint (e.g. post-poliomyelitis).

Lax ligaments Normal people with generalized joint laxity tend to stand with their knees back-set. Prolonged traction, especially on a frame, or holding the knee hyperextended in plaster, may overstretch ligaments, leading to permanent hyperextension deformity. Ligaments may also become overstretched following chronic or recurrent synovitis (especially in rheumatoid arthritis), the hypotonia of rickets, the flailness of poliomyelitis or the insensitivity of Charcot's disease.

In paralytic conditions such as poliomyelitis, recurvatum is often seen in association with fixed equinus of the ankle: in order to set the foot flat on the ground, the knee is forced into hyperextension. In moderate degrees, this may actually be helpful (e.g. in stabilizing a knee with weak extensors). However, if excessive and prolonged, it may give rise to a permanent deformity. If bony correction is undertaken, the knee should be left with some hyperextension to preserve the stabilizing mechanism. If quadriceps power is poor, the patient may need a caliper. Severe paralytic hyperextension can be treated by fixing the patella into the tibial plateau, where it acts as a bone block (Men et al., 1991).

Miscellaneous Other causes of recurvatum are *growth plate injuries* and *malunited fractures*. These can be safely corrected by osteotomy.

LESIONS OF THE MENISCI

The menisci have an important role in (1) improving articular congruency and increasing the stability of the knee, (2) controlling the complex rolling and gliding actions of the joint and (3) distributing load during movement. During weightbearing, at least 50 per cent of the contact stresses are taken by the menisci when the knee is loaded in extension, rising to almost 90 per cent with the knee in flexion. If the menisci are removed, articular stresses are markedly increased; even a partial meniscectomy of one-third of the width of the meniscus will produce a threefold increase in contact stress in that area.

The medial meniscus is much less mobile than the lateral, and it cannot as easily accommodate to abnormal stresses. This may be why meniscal lesions are more common on the medial side than on the lateral.

Even in the absence of injury, there is gradual stiffening and degeneration of the menisci with age, so splits and tears are more likely in later life – particularly if there is any associated arthritis or chondrocalcinosis. In young people, meniscal tears are usually the result of trauma.

TEARS OF THE MENISCUS

The meniscus consists mainly of circumferential fibres held by a few radial strands. It is, therefore, more likely to tear along its length than across its width. The split is usually initiated by a rotational grinding force, which occurs (for example) when the knee is flexed and twisted while taking weight; hence the frequency in footballers. In middle life, when fibrosis has restricted mobility of the meniscus, tears occur with relatively little force.

Pathology

The medial meniscus is affected far more frequently than the lateral, partly because its attachments to the capsule make it less mobile. Tears of both menisci may occur with severe ligament injuries.

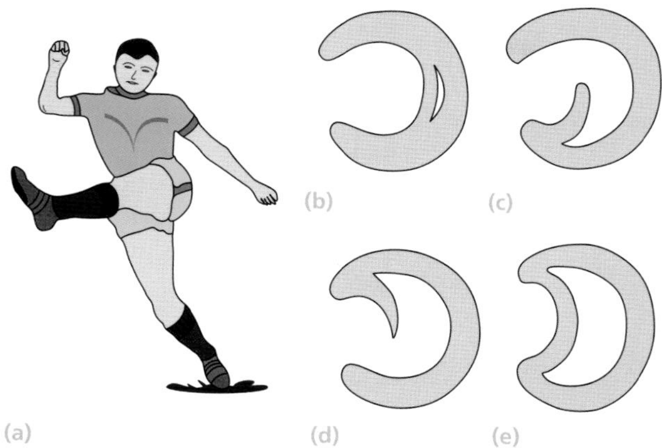

20.18 Torn medial meniscus (a) The meniscus is usually torn by a twisting force with the knee bent and taking weight; the initial split (b) may extend anteriorly (c), posteriorly (d) or both ways to create a 'bucket-handle' tear (e).

In 75 per cent of cases the split *is vertical* in the length of the meniscus. If the separated fragment remains attached front and back, the lesion is called a *bucket-handle tear*. The torn portion sometimes displaces towards the centre of the joint and becomes jammed between femur and tibia, causing a block to extension ('locking'). If the tear emerges at the free edge of the meniscus, it leaves a tongue based anteriorly (an *anterior horn tear)* or posteriorly (a *posterior horn tear*).

Horizontal tears are usually 'degenerative' or due to repetitive minor trauma. Some are associated with meniscal cysts (see below).

Most of the meniscus is avascular and spontaneous repair does not occur unless the tear is in the outer third, which is vascularized from the attached synovium and capsule. The loose tag acts as a mechanical irritant, giving rise to recurrent synovial effusion and, in some cases, secondary osteoarthritis.

Clinical features

The patient is usually a young person who sustains a twisting injury to the knee on the sports field. Pain (usually on the medial side) is often severe and further activity is avoided; occasionally the knee is 'locked' in partial flexion. Almost invariably, swelling appears some hours later, or perhaps the following day.

With rest the initial symptoms subside, only to recur periodically after trivial twists or strains. Sometimes the knee gives way spontaneously and this is again followed by pain and swelling.

It is important to remember that in patients aged over 40 the initial injury may be unremarkable and the main complaint is of recurrent 'giving way' or 'locking'.

'Locking' – that is, the sudden inability to extend the knee fully – suggests a bucket-handle tear. The patient sometimes learns to 'unlock' the knee by bending it fully or by twisting it from side to side.

On examination the joint may be held slightly flexed and there is often an effusion. In longstanding cases the quadriceps will be wasted. Tenderness is localized to the joint line, in the vast majority of cases on the medial side. Flexion is usually full but extension is often slightly limited.

Between attacks of pain and effusion there is a

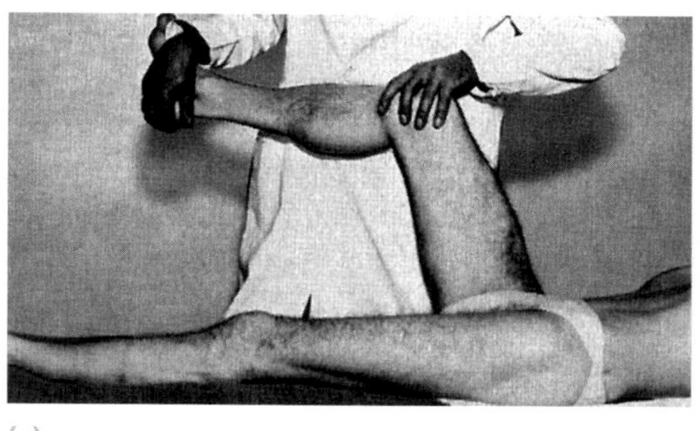

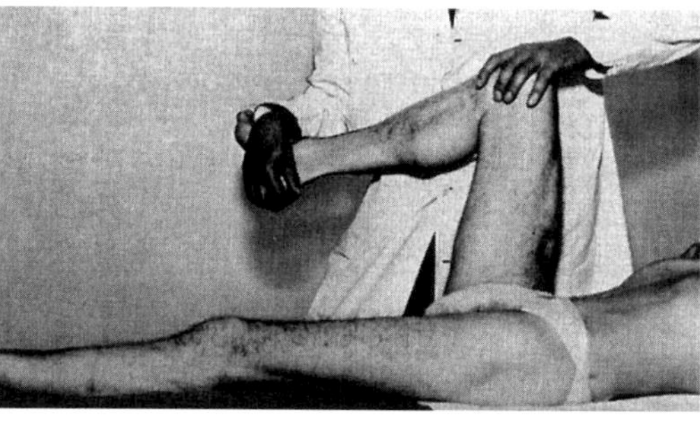

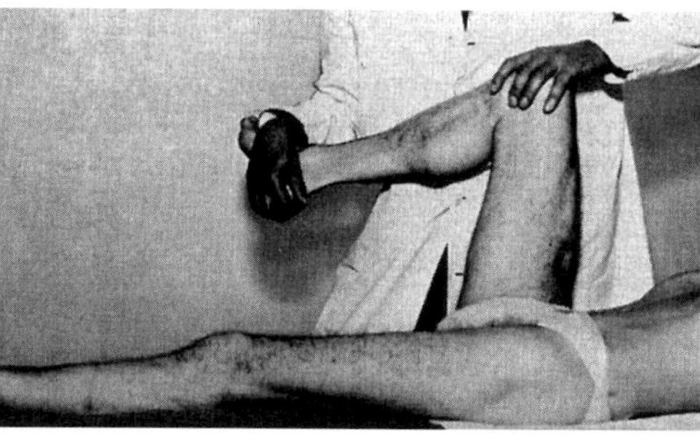

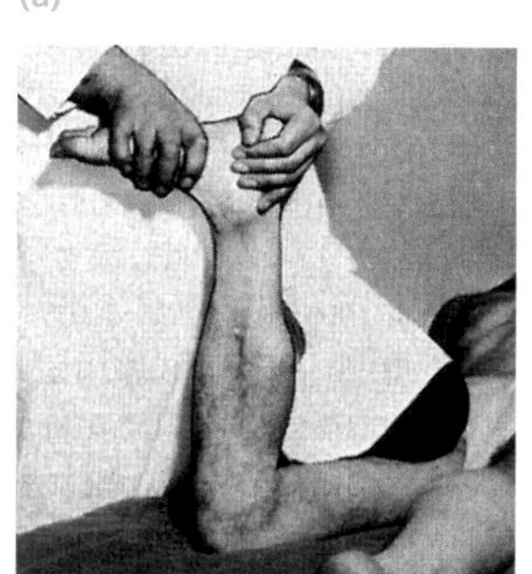

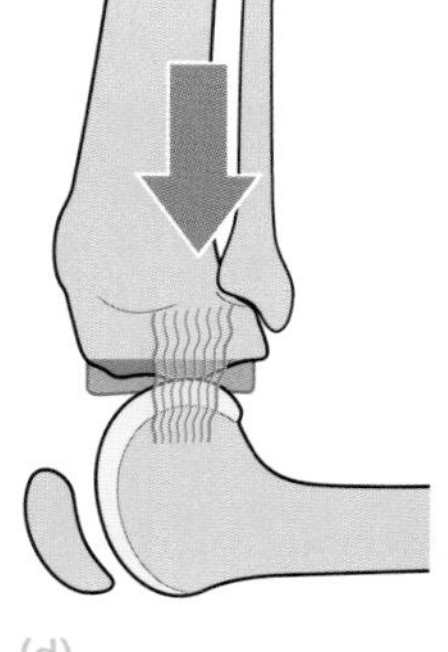

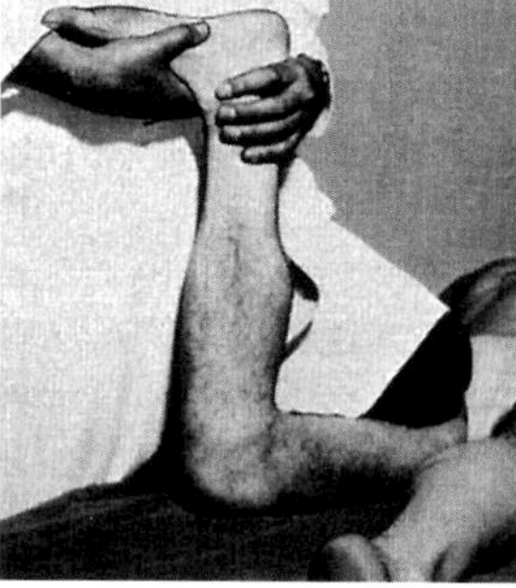

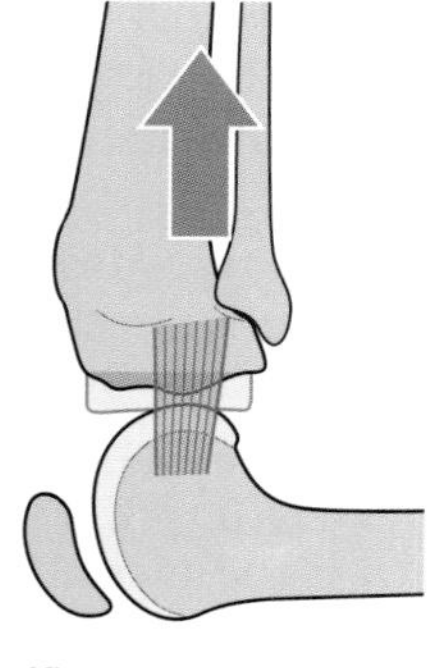

(a) (b) (c) (d) (e) (f)

20.19 Torn medial meniscus – tests (a,b) McMurray's test is performed at varying angles of flexion. (c,d) The grinding test relaxes the ligaments but compresses the meniscus – it causes pain with meniscus lesions. (e,f) The distraction test releases the meniscus but stretches the ligaments and causes pain if these are injured.

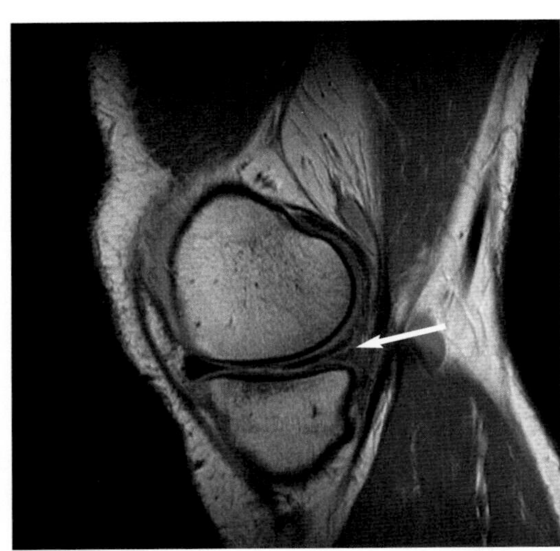

20.20 Torn meniscus – MRI Sagittal MRI showing a tear in the medial meniscus.

disconcerting paucity of signs. The history is helpful, and McMurray's test, Apley's grinding test or the Thessaly test may be positive.

Investigations

Plain x-rays are usually normal, but *MRI* is a reliable method of confirming the clinical diagnosis, and may even reveal tears that are missed by arthroscopy.

Arthroscopy has the advantage that, if a lesion is identified, it can be treated at the same time.

Differential diagnosis

Loose bodies in the joint may cause true locking. The history is much more insidious than with meniscal tears and the attacks are variable in character and intensity. A loose body may be palpable and is often visible on x-ray.

Recurrent dislocation of the patella causes the knee to give way; typically the patient is caught unawares and collapses to the ground. Tenderness is localized to the medial edge of the patella and the apprehension test is positive.

Fracture of the tibial spine follows an acute injury and may cause a block to full extension. However, swelling is immediate and the fluid is blood-stained. X-ray may show the fracture.

A partial tear of the medial collateral ligament may heal with adhesions where it is attached to the medial meniscus, so that the meniscus loses mobility. The patient complains of recurrent attacks of pain and giving way, followed by tenderness on the medial side. Sleep may be disturbed if the medial side rests upon the other knee or the bed. As with a meniscus injury, rotation is painful; but unlike a meniscus lesion, the grinding test gives less pain and the distraction test more pain.

A torn anterior cruciate ligament can cause chronic instability, with a sense of the knee 'giving way' or buckling when the patient turns sharply towards the side of the affected knee. Careful examination should reveal signs of rotational instability, a positive Lachman test or a positive anterior drawer sign. MRI or arthroscopy will settle any doubts.

Treatment

Dealing with the locked knee Usually the knee 'unlocks' spontaneously; if not, gentle passive flexion and rotation may do the trick. Forceful manipulation is unwise (it may do more damage) and is usually unnecessary; after a few days' rest the knee may well unlock itself. However, if the knee does not unlock, or if attempts to unlock it cause severe pain, arthroscopy is indicated. If symptoms are not marked, it may be better to wait a week or two and let the synovitis settle down, thus making the operation easier; if the tear is confirmed, the offending fragment is removed.

Conservative treatment If the joint is not locked, it is reasonable to hope that the tear is peripheral and can therefore heal spontaneously. After an acute episode, the joint is held straight in a plaster backslab for 3–4 weeks; the patient uses crutches and quadriceps exercises are encouraged. Operation can be put off as long as attacks are infrequent and not disabling and the patient is willing to abandon those activities that provoke them. MRI will show if the meniscus has healed.

Operative treatment Surgery is indicated (1) if the joint cannot be unlocked and (2) if symptoms are recurrent. For practical purposes, the lesion is often dealt with as part of the 'diagnostic' arthroscopy. Tears close to the periphery, which have the capacity to heal, can be sutured; at least one edge of the tear should be red (i.e. vascularized). In appropriate cases the success rate for both open and arthroscopic repair is almost 90 per cent.

Tears other than those in the peripheral third are dealt with by excising the torn portion (or the bucket handle). Total meniscectomy is thought to cause more instability and so predispose to late secondary osteoarthritis; certainly in the short term it causes greater morbidity than partial meniscectomy and has no obvious advantages.

Arthroscopic meniscectomy has distinct advantages over open meniscectomy: shorter hospital stay, lower costs and more rapid return to function. However, it is by no means free of complications (Sherman et al., 1986).

Postoperative pain and stiffness are reduced by prophylactic non-steroidal anti-inflammatory drugs. Quadriceps-strengthening exercises are important.

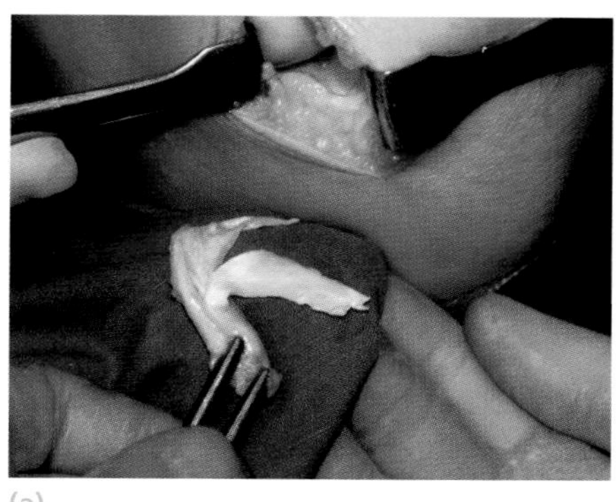
(a)

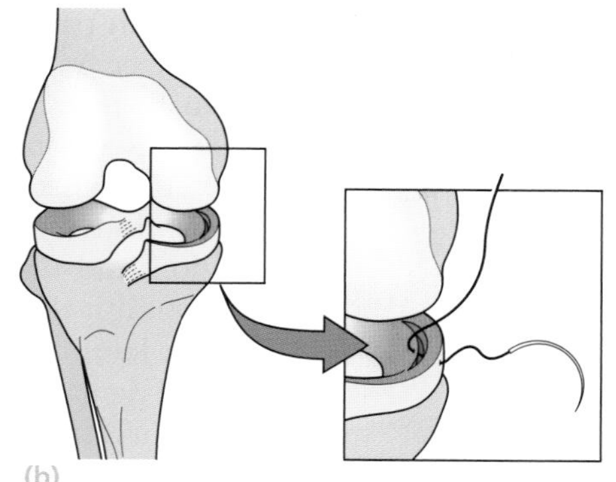
(b)

20.21 Torn meniscus – operation (a) Removal of a torn medial meniscus. (b) Repair is appropriate if at least one edge of the tear is vascularized. This can be done arthroscopically.

Outcome

Neither a meniscal tear by itself nor removal of the meniscus necessarily leads to secondary osteoarthritis. However, the likelihood is increased if the patient has (a) a pre-existing varus deformity of the knee, (b) signs of cruciate ligament insufficiency or (c) features elsewhere of a generalized osteoarthritis.

Meniscal degeneration

Patients over 45 years old may present with symptoms and signs of a meniscal tear. Often, though, they can recall no preceding injury. At arthroscopy there may be a horizontal cleavage in the medial meniscus – the characteristic 'degenerative' lesion – or detachment of the anterior or posterior horn without an obvious tear. Associated osteoarthritis or chrondrocalcinosis is common.

A detached anterior or posterior horn can be sutured firmly in place. Meniscectomy is indicated only if symptoms are marked or if, at arthroscopy, there is a major tear causing mechanical block.

Discoid lateral meniscus

In the fetus the meniscus is not semilunar but disc-like; if this shape persists, symptoms are likely. A young patient complains that, without any history of injury, the knee gives way and 'thuds' loudly. A characteristic clunk may be felt at 110 degrees as the knee is bent and at 10 degrees as it is being straightened. The diagnosis is easily confirmed by MRI.

If there is only a clunk, treatment is not essential. If pain is disturbing, the meniscus may be excised, though a more attractive procedure is arthroscopic partial excision leaving a normally shaped meniscus (Dimakopoulos and Patel, 1990).

Meniscal cysts

Cysts of the menisci are probably traumatic in origin, arising from either a small horizontal cleavage tear or repeated squashing of the peripheral part of the meniscus. It is also suggested that synovial cells infiltrate into the vascular area between meniscus and capsule and there multiply. The multilocular cyst contains gelatinous fluid and is surrounded by thick fibrous tissue.

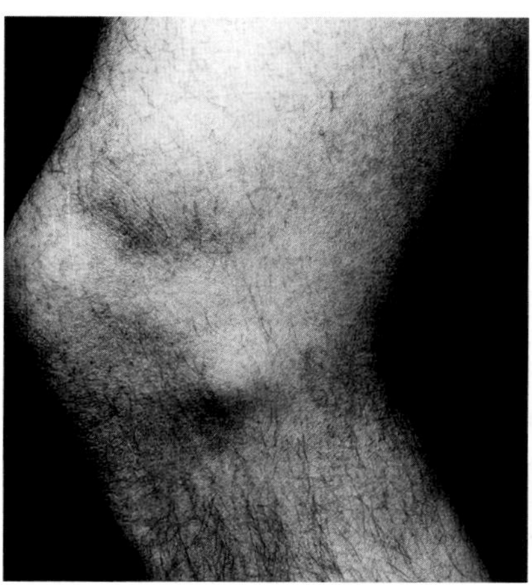
(a)

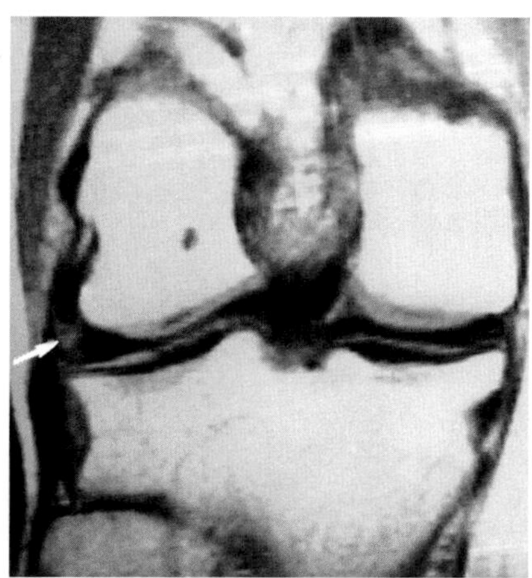
(b)

20.22 Meniscal cyst (a) Typical appearance of a small, firm swelling at or just below the joint line. (b) MRI showing the cyst arising from the edge of the meniscus (arrow).

Clinical features

The lateral meniscus is affected much more frequently than the medial. The patient complains of an ache or a small lump at the side of the joint. Symptoms may be intermittent, or worse after activity.

On examination the lump is situated at or slightly below the joint line, usually anterior to the collateral ligament. It is seen most easily with the knee slightly flexed; in some positions it may disappear altogether. Lateral cysts are often so firm that they are mistaken for a solid swelling. Medial cysts are usually larger and softer.

Differential diagnosis

Apart from cysts, various conditions may present with a small lump along the joint line.

A *ganglion* is quite superficial, usually not as 'hard' as a cyst, and unconnected with the joint.

Calcific deposits in the collateral ligament usually appear on the medial side, are intensely painful and tender, and often show on the x-ray.

A prolapsed, torn meniscus occasionally presents as a rubbery, irregular lump at the joint line. In some cases the distinction from a 'cyst' is largely academic.

Various tumours, both of soft tissue (lipoma, fibroma) and of bone (osteochondroma), may produce a medial or lateral joint lump. Careful examination will show that the lump does not arise from the joint itself.

Treatment

If the symptoms warrant operation, the cyst may be removed. In the past this was usually combined with total meniscectomy, in order to prevent an inevitable recurrence of the cyst. However, it is quite feasible to examine the meniscus by arthroscopy, remove only the torn or damaged portion and then decompress the cyst from within the joint. The recurrence rate following such arthroscopic surgery is negligible (Parisien, 1990).

CHRONIC LIGAMENTOUS INSTABILITY

The knee is a complex hinge which depends heavily on its ligaments for medio-lateral, anteroposterior and rotational stability. Ligament injuries, from minor strains through partial ruptures to complete tears, are common in sportsmen, athletes and dancers. Whatever the nature of the acute injury, the victim may be left with chronic instability of the knee – a sense of the joint wanting to give way, or actually giving way, during unguarded activity. Sometimes this is accompanied by pain and recurrent episodes of swelling. There may be a meniscal tear, but meniscectomy is likely to make matters worse; sometimes patients present with meniscectomy scars on both sides of the knee!

Examination should include special tests for ligamentous instability as well as radiological investigation and arthroscopy. It is important not only to establish the nature of the lesion but also to measure the level of functional impairment against the needs and demands of the individual patient before advocating treatment.

The subject is dealt with in detail in Chapter 30.

RECURRENT DISLOCATION OF THE PATELLA

Acute dislocation of the patella is dealt with in Chapter 30. In 15–20 per cent of cases (mostly children) the first episode is followed by recurrent dislocation or subluxation after minimal stress. This is due, in some measure, to disruption or stretching of the ligamentous structures which normally stabilize the extensor mechanism. However, in a significant proportion of cases there is no history of an acute strain and the initial episode is thought to have occurred 'spontaneously'. It is now recognized that in all cases of recurrent dislocation, but particularly in the latter group, one or more *predisposing factors* are often present: (1) generalized ligamentous laxity; (2) underdevelopment of the lateral femoral condyle and flattening of the intercondylar groove; (3) maldevelopment of the patella, which may be too high or too small; (4) valgus deformity of the knee; (5) external tibial torsion; or (6) a primary muscle defect.

Repeated dislocation damages the contiguous articular surfaces of the patella and femoral condyle; this may result in further flattening of the condyle, so facilitating further dislocations.

Dislocation is almost always towards the lateral side; medial dislocation is seen only in rare iatrogenic cases following overzealous lateral release or medial transposition of the patellar tendon.

Clinical features

Girls are affected more commonly than boys and the condition may be bilateral. Dislocation occurs unexpectedly when the quadriceps muscle is contracted with the knee in flexion. There is acute pain, the knee is stuck in flexion and the patient may fall to the ground.

Although the patella always dislocates laterally, the patient may think it has displaced medially because the uncovered medial femoral condyle stands out prominently. If the knee is seen while the patella is dislocated, the diagnosis is obvious. There is a lump on the

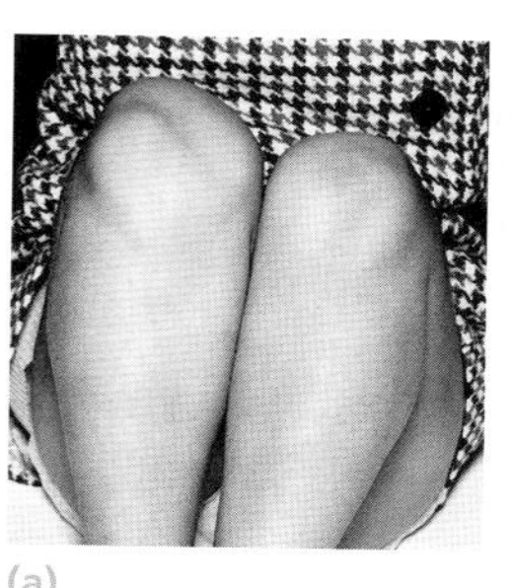
(a)

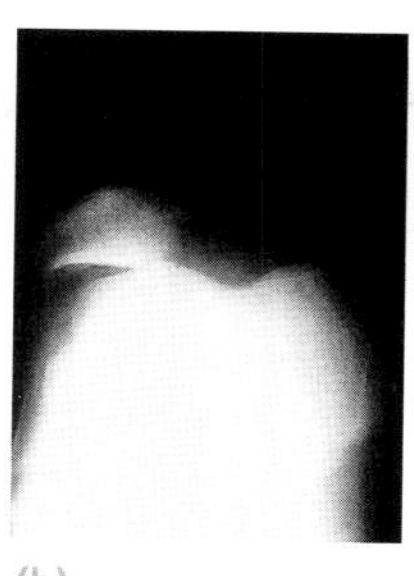
(b)

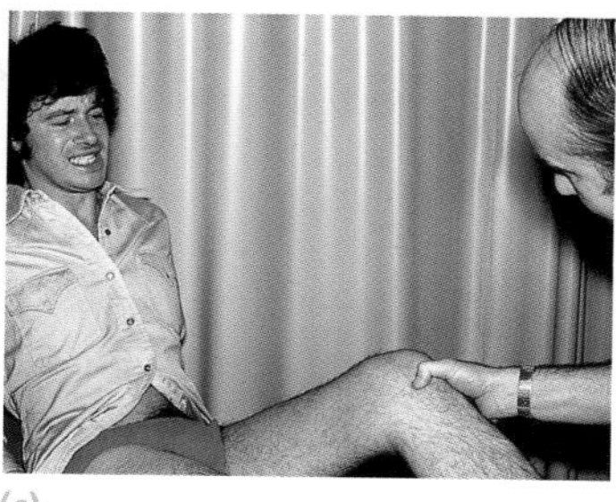
(c)

20.23 Patello-femoral instability (a,b) This young girl presented with recurrent subluxation of the right patella. The knee looks abnormal and the x-ray shows the patella riding on top of the lateral femoral condyle. (c) *The apprehension test*: Watch the patient's face!

lateral side, while the front of the knee (where the patella ought to be) is flat. The tissues on the medial side are tender, the joint may be swollen and aspiration may reveal a blood-stained effusion.

More often the patella has reduced by the time the patient is seen. Tenderness and swelling may still be present and *the apprehension test* is positive: if the patella is pushed laterally with the knee slightly flexed, the patient resists and becomes anxious, fearing another dislocation. The patient will normally volunteer a history of previous dislocation.

Between attacks the patient should be carefully examined for features that are known to predispose to patellar instability (see above).

Imaging

X-rays may reveal loose bodies in the knee, derived from old osteochondral fragments. A lateral view with the knee in slight flexion may show a high-riding patella and tangential views can be used to measure the sulcus angle and the congruence angle.

MRI is helpful and may show signs of the previous patello-femoral soft-tissue disruption.

Treatment

If the patella is still dislocated, it is pushed back into place while the knee is gently extended. The only indications for immediate surgery are (1) inability to reduce the patella (e.g. with a rare 'intra-articular' dislocation), and (2) the presence of a large, displaced osteochondral fragment.

A plaster cylinder or splint is applied and retained for 2–3 weeks; isometric quadriceps-strengthening exercises are encouraged and the patient is allowed to walk with the aid of crutches.

Exercises should be continued for at least 3 months, concentrating on strengthening the vastus medialis muscle. If recurrences are few and far between, conservative treatment may suffice; as the child grows older the patellar mechanism tends to stabilize. However, about 15 per cent of children with patellar instability suffer repeated and distressing episodes of dislocation and for these patients surgical reconstruction is indicated.

OPERATIVE TREATMENT

The principles of operative treatment are (a) to repair or strengthen the medial patello-femoral ligaments, and (b) to realign the extensor mechanism so as to produce a mechanically more favourable angle of pull. This can be achieved in several ways (see Fig. 20.24).

Direct medial patello-femoral ligament repair Occasionally it is possible to perform a direct repair of an attenuated medial patello-femoral ligament.

Suprapatellar realignment (Insall) The lateral retinaculum and capsule are divided. The quadriceps tendon adjacent to the vastus medialis is split longitudinally to the level of the tibial tubercle; the free edge is then sutured over the middle of the patella, thus bringing vastus medialis distally and closer to the midline.

Infrapatellar soft-tissue realignment (Goldthwait) The lateral half of the patellar ligament is detached, threaded under the medial half and reattached more medially and distally. This operation is seldom used by itself but may be combined with suprapatellar realignment.

Infrapatellar bony realignment (Elmslie–Trillat) The tibial tubercle is osteotomized and moved medially, thus improving the angle of pull on the patella. This procedure is only appropriate after closure of the proximal tibial physis; if growth is incomplete, damage to the physis may result in a progressive recurvatum deformity.

NOTE: All these procedures can be combined with repair or tightening of the medial patello-femoral ligament. At the end of the operation it is essential to check that the patella moves smoothly to at least 60 degrees of knee flexion; excessive tightening or uneven tension may cause maltracking (and, occasionally, even medial subluxation!) of the patella.

Patellectomy Occasionally the patello-femoral cartilage is so damaged that patellectomy is indicated, but this operation should be avoided if possible. There is a small risk that after patellectomy the patellar tendon may continue to dislocate and require realignment by the tibial tubercle transfer.

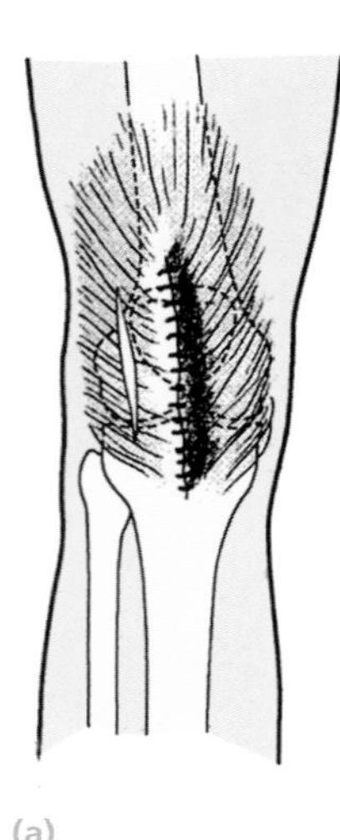
(a)

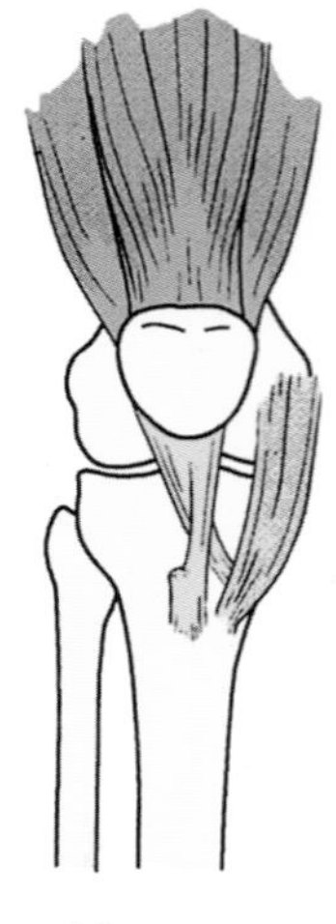
(b)

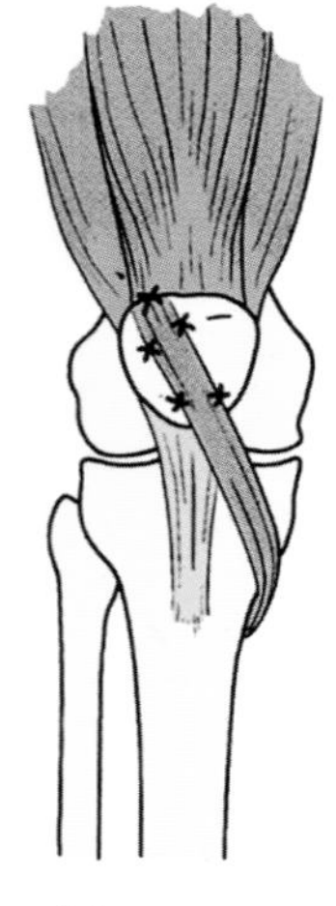
(c)

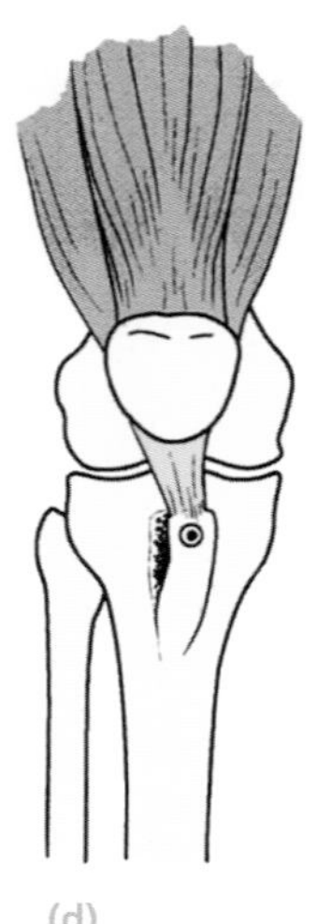
(d)

20.24 Realignment for recurrent patellar dislocation There are several methods popularly used. Most involve a lateral release of the capsule and some form of 'tether' medially. This check-rein may be created from (a) vastus medialis (*Insall*), (b) transposing the lateral half of the patellar ligament medially (*Roux–Goldthwait*) or by (c) the semitendinosus tendon (*Galleazzi*). (d) In adults, bony operations which shift the position of the patellar tubercle may be tried (*Elmslie–Trillat*).

Recurrent subluxation

Patellar dislocation is sometimes followed by recurrent subluxation rather than further episodes of complete displacement. This is the borderline between frank instability and maltracking of the patella (see below).

Other types of non-traumatic dislocation

Congenital dislocation, in which the patella is permanently displaced, is fortunately very rare. Reconstructive procedures, such as semitendinosus tenodesis, have been tried but the results are unpredictable.

Habitual dislocation differs from recurrent dislocation in that the patella dislocates every time the knee is bent and reduces each time it is straightened. In longstanding cases the patella may be permanently dislocated.

The probable cause is *contracture of the quadriceps,* which may be congenital or may result from repeated injections (usually antibiotics) into the muscle.

Treatment requires lengthening of the quadriceps. Additionally a lateral capsular release and medial plication may be needed to hold the patella in the intercondylar groove.

PATELLO-FEMORAL PAIN SYNDROME (CHONDROMALACIA OF THE PATELLA; PATELLO-FEMORAL OVERLOAD SYNDROME)

There is no clear consensus concerning the terminology, aetiology and treatment of pain and tenderness in the anterior part of the knee. This syndrome is common among active adolescents and young adults. It is often (but not invariably) associated with softening and fibrillation of the articular surface of the patella – *chondromalacia patellae.* Having no other pathological label, orthopaedic surgeons have tended to regard chondromalacia as the cause (rather than one of the effects) of the disorder. Against this are the facts that (1) chondromalacia is commonly found at arthroscopy in young adults who have no anterior knee pain, and (2) some patients with the typical clinical syndrome have no cartilage softening.

Pathogenesis and pathology

Pain over the anterior aspect of the knee occurs as one of the symptoms in a number of well-recognized disorders, the commonest of which are bursitis, Osgood–Schlatter disease, a neuroma, plica syndromes, patello-femoral arthritis and tendinitis affecting either the insertion of the quadriceps tendon or the patellar ligament – Sinding-Larsen's disease. When these are excluded and no other cause can be found, one is left with a clinically recognizable syndrome that has earned the unsatisfactory label of 'anterior knee pain' or 'patello-femoral pain syndrome'.

The basic disorder is probably mechanical overload of the patello-femoral joint. Rarely, a single injury (sudden impact on the front of the knee) may damage the articular surfaces. Much more common is repetitive overload due to either (1) *malcongruence* of the patello-femoral surfaces because of some abnormal shape of the patella or intercondylar groove, (2) *malalignment of the lower extremity and/or the patella,* (3) *muscular imbalance of the lower extremity* with decreased strength due to atrophy or inhibition, or relative weakness of the vastus medialis, which causes the patella to tilt, or subluxate, or bear more heavily on one facet than the other during flexion and

Table 20.1 Causes of anterior knee pain

1. Referred from hip
2. Patellofemoral disorders Patellar instability Patello-femoral overload Osteochondral injury Patello-femoral osteoarthritis
3. Knee joint disorders Osteochondritis dissecans Loose body in the joint Synovial chondromatosis Plica syndrome
4. Peri-articular disorders Patellar tendinitis Patellar ligament strain Bursitis Osgood–Schlatter disease

extension, and (4) *overactivity*. 'Overload', as used here, means either direct stress on a load-bearing facet or sheer stresses in the depths of the articular cartilage at the boundary between high-contact and low-contact areas (Goodfellow et al., 1976). Personality and chronic pain response issues must also be considered (Thomee et al., 1999).

Patello-femoral overload leads to changes in both the articular cartilage and the subchondral bone, not necessarily of parallel degree. Thus, the cartilage may look normal and show only biochemical changes such as overhydration or loss of proteoglycans, while the underlying bone shows reactive vascular congestion (a potent cause of pain). Or there may be obvious cartilage softening and fibrillation, with or without subarticular intraosseous hypertension. This would account for the variable relationship between (1) malalignment syndrome, (2) cartilage softening, (3) subchondral vascular congestion and (4) anterior knee pain.

Cartilage fibrillation usually occurs on the medial patellar facet or the median ridge, remains confined to the superficial zones and generally heals spontaneously (Bentley, 1985). It is not a precursor of progressive osteoarthritis in later life. Occasionally the lateral facet is involved – Ficat's 'hyperpression zone' syndrome – and this may well be progressive (Ficat and Hungerford, 1977).

Clinical features

The patient, often a teenage girl or an athletic young adult, complains of pain over the front of the knee or 'underneath the knee-cap'. Occasionally there is a history of injury or recurrent displacement. Symptoms are aggravated by activity or climbing stairs, or when standing up after prolonged sitting. The knee may give way and occasionally swells. It sometimes 'catches' but this is not true locking. Often both knees are affected.

At first sight the knee looks normal but careful examination may reveal malalignment or tilting of the patellae. Other signs include quadriceps wasting, fluid in the knee, tenderness under the edge of the patella and crepitus on moving the knee.

Patello-femoral pain is elicited by pressing the patella against the femur and asking the patient to contract the quadriceps – first with central pressure, then compressing the medial facet and then the lateral. If, in addition, the apprehension test is positive, this suggests previous subluxation or dislocation.

Patellar tracking can be observed with the patient seated on the edge of the couch, flexing and extending the knee against resistance; in some cases subluxation is obvious.

With the patient sitting or lying supine, patellar alignment can be gauged by measuring the quadriceps angle, or Q-angle – the angle subtended by the line of quadriceps pull (a line running from the anterior superior iliac spine to the middle of the patella) and the line of the patellar ligament. It normally averages 14–17 degrees and an angle of more than 20 degrees is regarded as a predisposing factor in the develop-

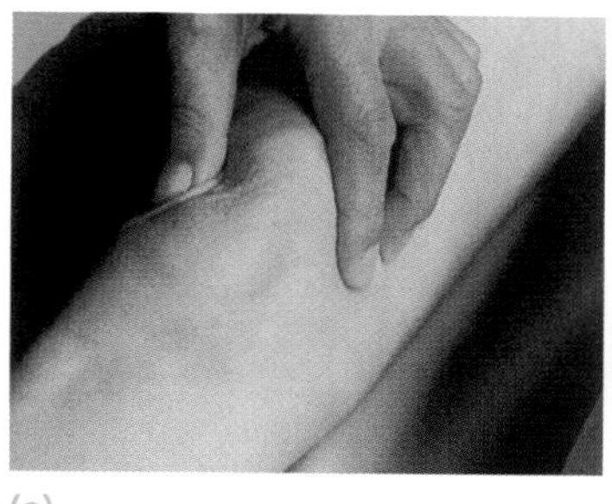
(a)

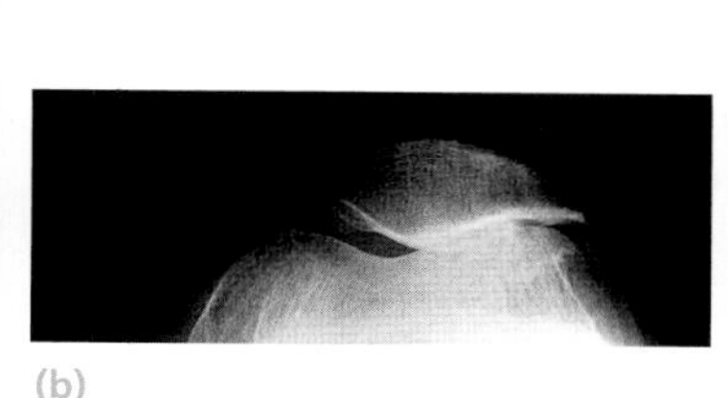
(b)

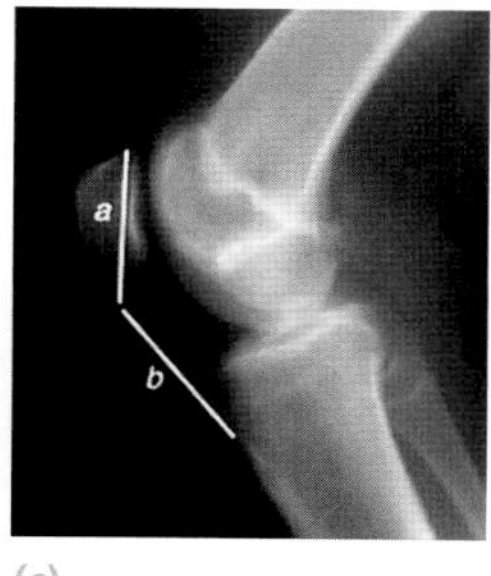

(c)

20.25 Chondromalacia of the patella There is no pathognomonic feature on which to base the diagnosis of chondromalacia, but several signs are suggestive. (a) Hold the patella against the femoral condyles and ask the patient to tighten the thigh muscles; even in normal people this may be uncomfortable, but patients with chondromalacia experience sudden acute pain in the patello-femoral joint. (b) A 'skyline' x-ray with the knee in partial flexion may show obvious tilting of the patella. (c) In the lateral x-ray, with the knee flexed to 45°, the lengths of the patella and the patellar ligament are normally about equal (a ratio of 1:1); in *patella alta* the ratio is less than 1:1.

ment of anterior knee pain. Another predisposing factor is a high-riding patella (*patella alta*); compressive force on the patellar articular surface during flexion and extension is likely to be greater than normal. Patella alta is best measured on the lateral x-ray).

Lastly, the structures around the knee should be carefully examined for other sources of pain, and the hip is examined to exclude referred pain.

Imaging

X-ray examination should include skyline views of the patella, which may show abnormal tilting or subluxation, and a lateral view with the knee half-flexed to see if the patella is high or small.

The most accurate way of showing and measuring patello-femoral malposition is by *CT or MRI* with the knees in full extension and varying degrees of flexion.

Arthroscopy

Cartilage softening is common in asymptomatic knees, and painful knees may show no abnormality. However, arthroscopy is useful in excluding other causes of anterior knee pain; it can also serve to gauge patello-femoral congruence, alignment and tracking.

Differential diagnosis

Other causes of anterior knee pain must be excluded before finally accepting the diagnosis of patello-femoral pain syndrome (see Table 20.1). Even then, the exact cause of the syndrome must be established before treatment: e.g. is it abnormal posture, overuse, patellar malalignment, subluxation or some abnormality in the shape of the bones?

Treatment

CONSERVATIVE MANAGEMENT

In the vast majority of cases the patient will be helped by adjustment of stressful activities and physiotherapy, combined with reassurance that most patients eventually recover without physiotherapy. Exercises are directed specifically at strengthening the medial quadriceps so as to counterbalance the tendency to lateral tilting or subluxation of the patella. Some patients respond to simple measures such as providing support for a valgus foot. Aspirin does no more than reduce pain, and corticosteroid injections should be avoided.

OPERATIVE TREATMENT

Surgery should be considered only if (1) there is a demonstrable abnormality that is correctable by operation, or (2) conservative treatment has been tried for at least 6 months and (3) the patient is genuinely incapacitated. Operation is intended to improve patellar alignment and patello-femoral congruence and to reduce patello-femoral pressure. Various measures are employed: lateral release, with or without one of the realignment procedures illustrated in Figure 20.24, may be needed if there is any sign of patellar instability; other operations are the patellar ligament elevation procedure of Maquet and – as a last resort – patellectomy.

Lateral release The lateral knee capsule and extensor retinaculum are divided longitudinally, either open or arthroscopically. This sometimes succeeds on its own (particularly if significant patellar tilting can be demonstrated on x-ray or MRI), but more often patello-femoral realignment will be needed as well.

Proximal realignment This is achieved by a combined open release of the lateral retinaculum and reefing of the oblique part of the vastus medialis.

Distal realignment The distal soft-tissue and bony realignment procedures are described on page 563. They will improve the tracking angle but run the risk of increasing patello-femoral contact pressures and thus aggravating the patient's symptoms.

Distal elevation of the patellar ligament In Maquet's (1976) tibial tubercle advancement operation the tubercle, with the attached patellar ligament, is hinged forwards and held there with a bone-block. This has the effect of reducing patello-femoral contact pressures. Some patients resent the bump on the front part of the tibia and the operation may substitute a new set of complaints for the old. Alternatively, the Fulkerson anteromedial tibial tubercle transfer and elevation can be used with satisfactory mid-term results.

Chondroplasty Shaving of the patellar articular surface is usually performed arthroscopically using a power tool. Soft and fibrillated cartilage is removed, in severe cases down to the level of subchondral bone; the hope is that it will be replaced by fibrocartilage. The operation should be followed by lavage and can be combined with any of the realignment procedures.

Patellectomy This is a last resort, but patients with severe discomfort are grateful for the relief it brings after other operations have failed.

OSTEOCHONDRITIS DISSECANS

The prevalence of osteochondritis dissecans is between 15 and 30 per 100 000 with males being affected more often than females (ratio 5:3). An increase in its incidence has been observed in recent years, probably due to the growing participation of young children of both genders in competitive sports.

A small, well-demarcated, avascular fragment of

bone and overlying cartilage sometimes separates from one of the femoral condyles and appears as a loose body in the joint. The most likely cause is trauma, either a single impact with the edge of the patella or repeated microtrauma from contact with an adjacent tibial ridge. The fact that over 80 per cent of lesions occur on the lateral part of the medial femoral condyle, exactly where the patella makes contact in full flexion, supports the first of these. There may also be some general predisposing factor, because several joints can be affected, or several members of one family. Lesions are bilateral in 25 per cent of cases.

Pathology

The lower, lateral surface of the medial femoral condyle is usually affected, rarely the lateral condyle, and still more rarely the patella. An area of subchondral bone becomes avascular and within this area an ovoid osteocartilaginous segment is demarcated from the surrounding bone. At first the overlying cartilage is intact and the fragment is stable; over a period of months the fragment separates but remains in position; finally the fragment breaks free to become a loose body in the joint. The small crater is slowly filled with fibrocartilage, leaving a depression on the articular surface.

Classification

Osteochondritis dissecans of the knee is classified according to anatomical location, arthroscopic appearance, scintigraphic or MRI findings and chronological age. For prognostic and treatment purposes it is divided into juvenile and adult forms, either stable or unstable (Kocher et al., 2006).

Clinical features

The patient, usually a male aged 15–20 years, presents with intermittent ache or swelling. Later, there are attacks of giving way such that the knee feels unreliable; 'locking' sometimes occurs.

The quadriceps muscle is wasted and there may be a small effusion. Soon after an attack there are two signs that are almost diagnostic: (1) tenderness localized to one femoral condyle; and (2) Wilson's sign: if the knee is flexed to 90 degrees, rotated medially and then gradually straightened, pain is felt; repeating the test with the knee rotated laterally is painless.

Imaging

Plain x-rays may show a line of demarcation around a lesion in situ, usually in the lateral part of the medial femoral condyle. This site is best displayed in special intercondylar (tunnel) views, but even then a small lesion or one situated far back may be missed. Once the fragment has become detached, the empty hollow may be seen – and possibly a loose body elsewhere in the joint.

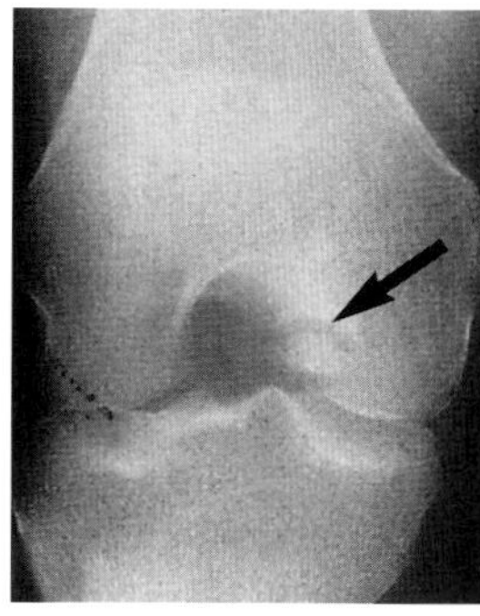

(a)

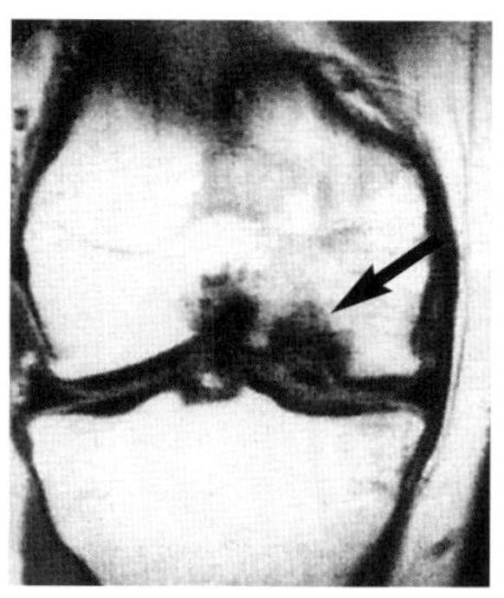

(b)

20.26 Osteochondritis dissecans – imaging The lesion is often missed in the standard anteroposterior x-ray and is better seen in the 'tunnel view', usually along the lateral side of the medial femoral condyle (a). Here the osteochondral fragment has remained in place but sometimes it appears as a separate body elsewhere in the joint. (b) MRI provides confirmatory evidence and shows a much wider area of involvement than is apparent in the plain x-ray.

Radionuclide scans show increased activity around the lesion, and *MRI* consistently shows an area of low signal intensity in the T_1 weighted images; the adjacent bone may also appear abnormal, probably due to oedema. These investigations usually indicate whether the fragment is 'stable' or 'loose'. MRI may also allow early prediction of whether the lesion will heal or not.

Arthroscopy

With early lesions the articular surface looks intact, but probing may reveal that the cartilage is soft. Loose segments are easily visualized.

Differential diagnosis

Avascular necrosis of the femoral condyle – usually associated with corticosteroid therapy or alcohol abuse – may result in separation of a localized osteocartilaginous fragment. However, it is seen in an older age group and on x-ray the lesion is always on the dome of the femoral condyle, and this distinguishes it from osteochondritis dissecans.

Treatment

For the purposes of management, it is useful to 'stage' the lesion; hence the importance of radionuclide scanning, MRI and arthroscopy. Lesions in adults have a greater propensity to instability whereas juvenile osteochondritis is typically stable. Those lesions with an intact articular surface have the greatest potential

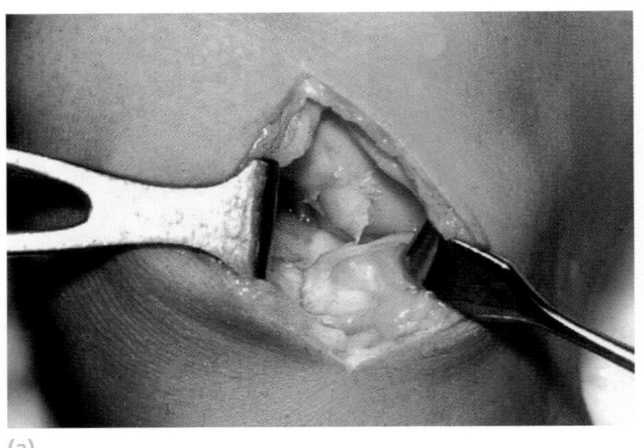
(a)

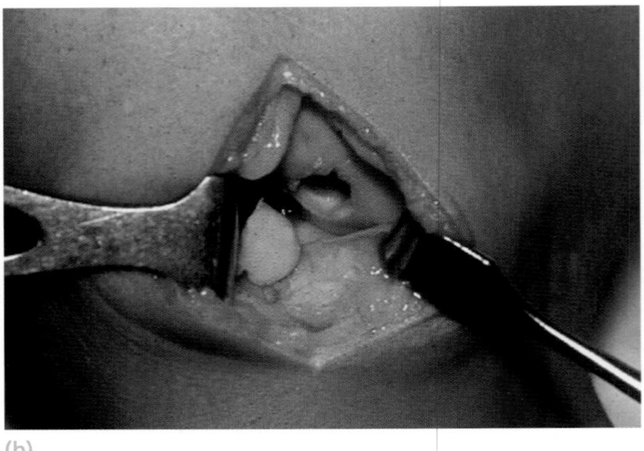
(b)

20.27 Osteochondritis dissecans Intraoperative pictures showing the articular lesion (a) and the defect left after removal of the osteochondral fragment (b).

to heal with non-operative treatment if repetitive impact loading is avoided.

In the earliest stage, when the cartilage is intact and the lesion is 'stable', no treatment is needed but activities are curtailed for 6–12 months. Small lesions often heal spontaneously.

If the fragment is 'unstable', i.e. surrounded by a clear boundary with radiographic 'sclerosis' of the underlying bone, or showing MRI features of separation, treatment will depend on the size of the lesion. A small fragment should be removed by arthroscopy and the base drilled; the bed will eventually be covered by fibrocartilage, leaving only a small defect. A large fragment (say more than 1 cm in diameter) should be fixed in situ with pins or Herbert screws. In addition, it may help to drill the underlying sclerotic bone to promote union of the necrotic fragment. For drilling, the area is approached from a point some distance away, beyond the articular cartilage.

If the fragment is completely detached but in one piece and shown to fit nicely in its bed, the crater is cleaned and the floor drilled before replacing the loose fragment and fixing it with Herbert screws. If the fragment is in pieces or ill-shaped, it is best discarded; the crater is drilled and allowed to fill with fibrocartilage.

In recent years attempts have been made to fill the residual defects by articular cartilage transplantation: either the insertion of osteochondral plugs harvested from another part of the knee or the application of sheets of cultured chondrocytes. This approach should still be regarded as in the 'experimental' stage.

After any of the above operations the knee is held in a cast for 6 weeks; thereafter movement is encouraged but weightbearing is deferred until x-rays show signs of healing.

LOOSE BODIES

The knee – relatively capacious, with large synovial folds – is a common haven for loose bodies. These may be produced by: (1) injury (a chip of bone or

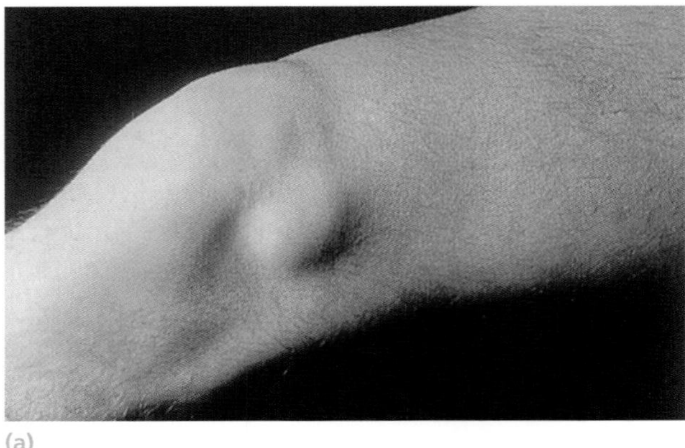
(a)

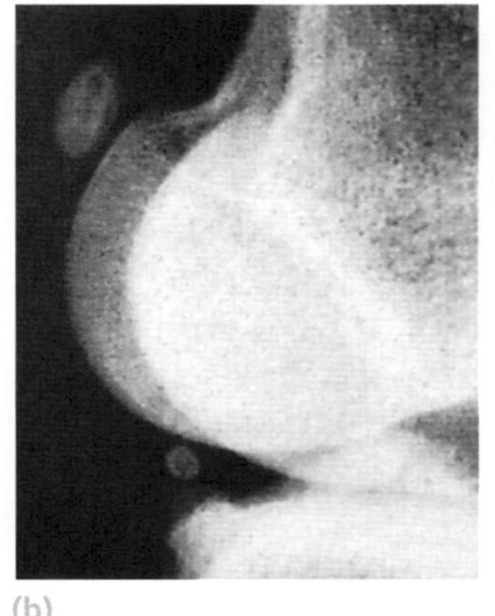
(b)

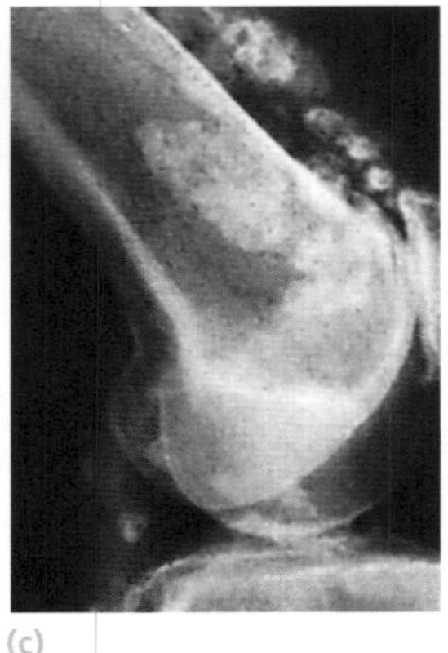
(c)

20.28 Loose bodies (a) This loose body slipped away from the fingers when touched; the term 'joint mouse' seems appropriate. (b) Which is the loose body here? Not the large one (which is a normal fabella), but the small lower one opposite the joint line. (c) Multiple loose bodies are seen in synovial chondromatosis, a rare disorder of cartilage metaplasia in the synovium.

cartilage); (2) osteochondritis dissecans (which may produce one or two fragments); (3) osteoarthritis (pieces of cartilage or osteophyte); (4) Charcot's disease (large osteocartilaginous bodies); and (5) synovial chondromatosis (cartilage metaplasia in the synovium, sometimes producing hundreds of loose bodies).

Clinical features

Loose bodies may be symptomless. The usual complaint is attacks of sudden locking without injury. The joint gets stuck in a position which varies from one attack to another. Sometimes the locking is only momentary and usually the patient can wriggle the knee until it suddenly unlocks. The patient may be aware of something 'popping in and out of the joint'.

In adolescents, a loose body is usually due to osteochondritis dissecans, rarely to injury. In adults osteoarthritis is the most frequent cause.

Only rarely is the patient seen with the knee still locked. Sometimes, especially after the first attack, there is synovitis or there may be evidence of the underlying cause. A pedunculated loose body may be felt; one that is truly loose tends to slip away during palpation (the well-named 'joint mouse').

X-ray Most loose bodies are radio-opaque. The films also show an underlying joint abnormality.

Treatment

A loose body causing symptoms should be removed unless the joint is severely osteoarthritic. This can usually be done through the arthroscope, but finding the loose body may be difficult; it may be concealed in a synovial pouch or sulcus and a small body may even slip under the edge of one of the menisci.

SYNOVIAL CHONDROMATOSIS

This is a rare disorder in which the joint comes to contain multiple loose bodies, often in pearly clumps resembling sago ('snowstorm knee'). The usual explanation is that myriad tiny fronds undergo cartilage metaplasia at their tips; these tips break free and may ossify. It has, however, been suggested that chondrocytes may be cultured in the synovial fluid and that some of the products are then deposited onto previously normal synovium, so producing the familiar appearance (Kay et al., 1989). X-rays reveal multiple loose bodies; on arthrography they show as negative defects.

Treatment The loose bodies should be removed arthroscopically. At the same time an attempt should be made to remove all abnormal synovium.

THE PLICA SYNDROME

A plica is the remnant of an embryonic synovial partition which persists into adult life. During development of the embryo, the knee is divided into three cavities – a large suprapatellar pouch and beneath this the medial and lateral compartments – separated from each other by membranous septa. Later these partitions disappear, leaving a single cavity, but part of a septum may persist as a synovial pleat or plica (from the Latin *plicare* = fold). This is found in over 20 per cent of people, usually as a *median infrapatellar fold* (the ligamentum mucosum), less often as a *suprapatellar curtain* draped across the opening of the suprapatellar pouch or a *mediopatellar plica* sweeping down the medial wall of the joint.

Pathology

The plica in itself is not pathological. But if acute trauma, repetitive strain or some underlying disorder (e.g. a meniscal tear) causes inflammation, the plica may become oedematous, thickened and eventually fibrosed; it then acts as a tight bowstring impinging on other structures in the joint and causing further synovial irritation.

Clinical features

An adolescent or young adult complains of an ache in the front of the knee (occasionally both knees), with intermittent episodes of clicking or 'giving way'. There may be a history of trauma or markedly increased activity. Symptoms are aggravated by exercise or climbing stairs, especially if this follows a long period of sitting.

On examination there may be muscle wasting and a small effusion. The most characteristic feature is tenderness near the upper pole of the patella and over the femoral condyle. Occasionally the thickened band can be felt. Movement of the knee may cause catching or snapping.

Diagnosis

There is still controversy as to whether 'plica syndrome' constitutes a real and distinct clinical entity. In some quarters, however, it is regarded as a significant cause of anterior knee pain. It may closely resemble other conditions such as patellar overload or subluxation; indeed, the plica may become troublesome only when those other conditions are present. The diagnosis is often not made until arthroscopy is undertaken. The presence of a chondral lesion on the femoral condyle secondary to plica impingement confirms the diagnosis.

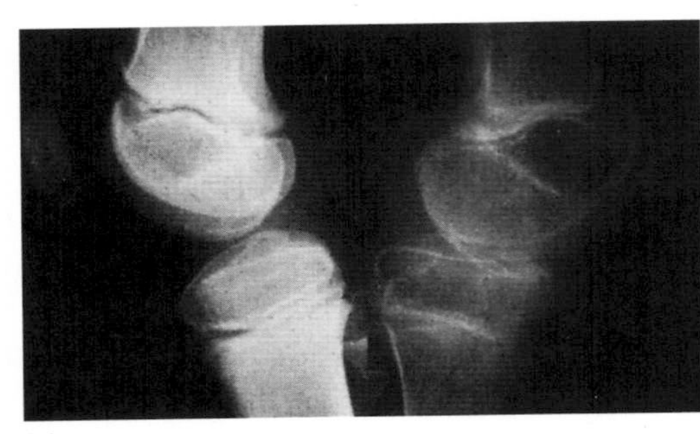

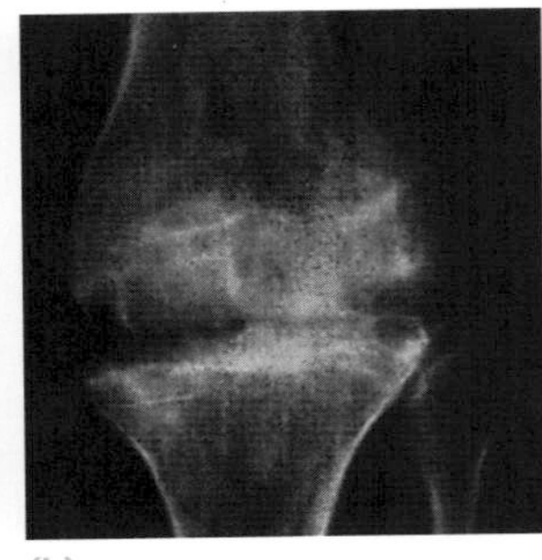

(a) (b)

20.29 Tuberculosis (a) Lateral views of the two knees. On one side the bones are porotic and the epiphyses enlarged, features suggestive of a severe inflammatory synovitis. (b) Later the articular surfaces are eroded.

Treatment

The first line of treatment is rest, anti-inflammatory drugs and adjustment of activities. If symptoms persist, the plica can be divided or excised by arthroscopy.

TUBERCULOSIS

Tuberculosis of the knee may appear at any age, but it is more common in children than in adults.

Clinical features

Early presentation Pain and limp are early symptoms; or the child may present with a swollen joint and a low-grade fever. The thigh muscles are wasted, thus accentuating the joint swelling. The knee feels warm and there is synovial thickening. Movements are restricted and often painful. The Mantoux test is positive and the erythrocyte sedimentation rate (ESR) may be increased.

X-rays show marked osteoporosis and, in children, enlargement of the bony epiphyses. Unlike pyogenic arthritis, joint space narrowing is a late sign; this is because cartilage lysis is prevented by the presence of a plasmin inhibitor in the synovial exudate.

Late features If the disease is allowed to persist the joint surfaces will gradually be eroded and the knee joint will become deformed. The classical picture in neglected cases is a composite deformity: posterior and lateral subluxation or dislocation, external rotation and fixed flexion.

Diagnosis

Monarticular rheumatoid synovitis, or juvenile chronic arthritis, may closely resemble tuberculosis. A synovial biopsy may be necessary to establish the diagnosis.

Treatment

General antituberculous chemotherapy should be given for 12–18 months (see page 49).

In the active stage the knee is rested in a bed splint. The synovitis usually subsides, but if it does not do so after a few weeks' treatment, then surgical debridement will be needed. All obviously diseased and necrotic tissue is removed and bone abscesses are evacuated.

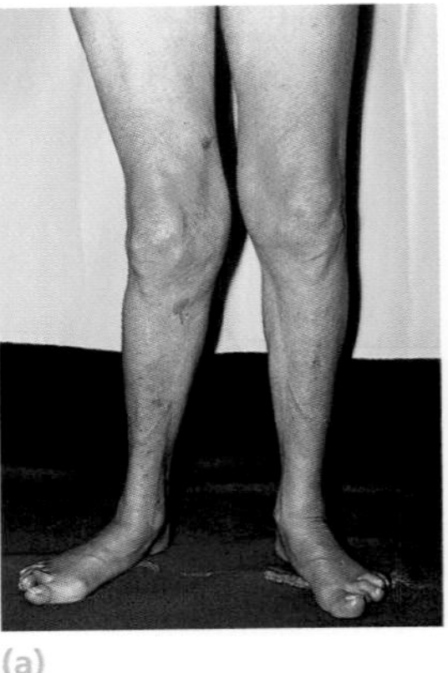

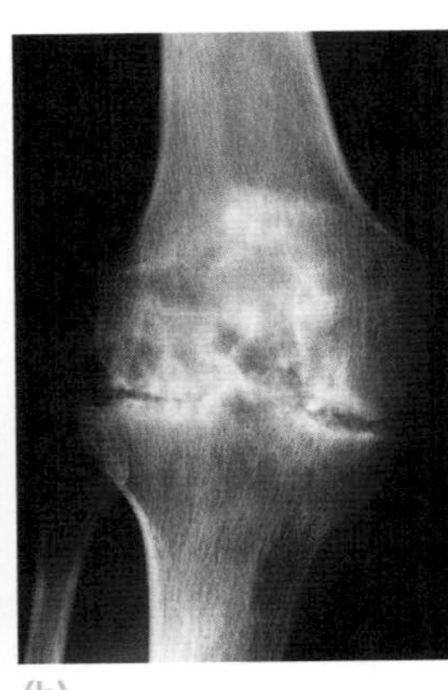

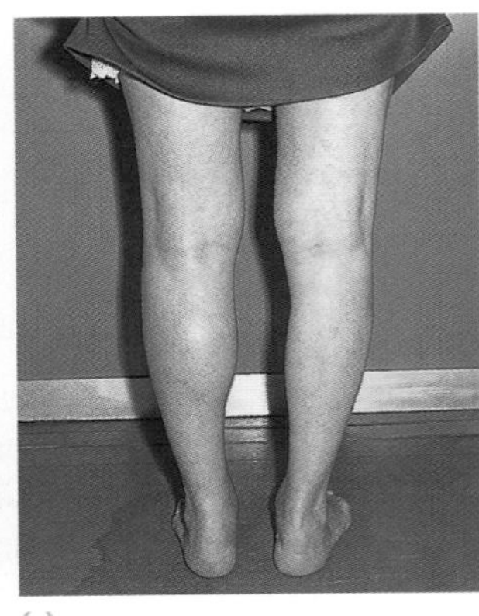

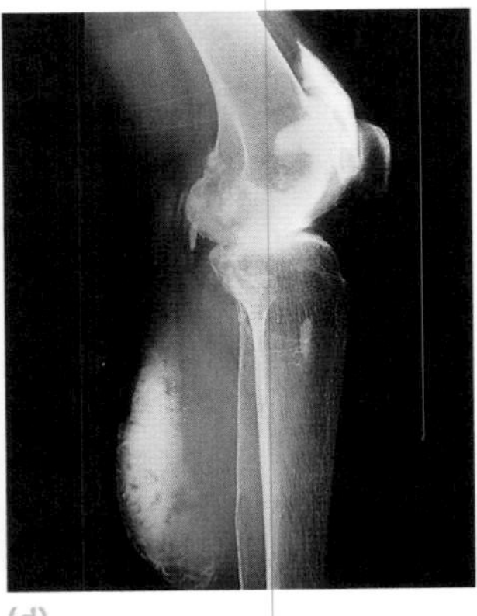

(a) (b) (c) (d)

20.30 Rheumatoid arthritis (a) Patient with rheumatoid arthritis showing the typical valgus deformity of the right knee; the feet and toes also are affected. (b) X-ray showing marked erosive arthritis resulting in joint deformity. (c) This patient presented with a painful swelling of the left calf. She was thought at first to have developed deep vein thrombosis – until we examined her knee and recognized this as a posterior synovial rupture, later confirmed by arthrography (d).

In the healing stage the patient is allowed up wearing a weight-relieving caliper. Gradually this is left off, but the patient is kept under observation for any sign of recurrent inflammation. If the articular cartilage has been spared, movement can be encouraged and weightbearing is slowly resumed. However, if the articular surface is destroyed, immobilization is continued until the joint stiffens.

In the aftermath the joint may be painful; it is then best arthrodesed, but in children this is usually postponed until growth is almost completed. The ideal position for fusion is 10–15 degrees of flexion, 7 degrees of valgus and 5 degrees of external rotation.

In some cases, once it is certain that the disease is quiescent, joint replacement may be feasible.

RHEUMATOID ARTHRITIS

Occasionally, rheumatoid arthritis starts in the knee as a chronic monarticular synovitis. Sooner or later, however, other joints become involved.

Clinical features

The general features of rheumatoid disease are described in Chapter 3.

The early stage is characterized by synovitis; rheumatoid disease occasionally starts with involvement of a single joint. The patient complains of pain and chronic swelling of the knee; there is usually an effusion and the thigh muscles may be wasted. The thickened synovium is often palpable.

Unless there are obvious signs of an inflammatory polyarthritis, the condition has to be distinguished from other types of inflammatory monarthritis, such as gout, Reiter's disease and tuberculosis; biopsy and microbiological investigations may be needed.

During this early stage, while the joint is still stable and the muscles are reasonably strong, there is a danger of rupturing the posterior capsule; the joint contents are extruded into a large posterior bursa or between the muscle planes of the calf, causing sudden pain and swelling which closely mimic the features of calf vein thrombosis.

As the disease progresses the knee becomes increasingly unstable, muscle wasting is marked and there is some loss of flexion and extension.

X-rays may show diminution of the joint space, osteopaenia and marginal erosions. The picture is easily distinguishable from that of osteoarthritis by the complete absence of osteophytes.

In the late stage pain and disability are usually severe. In some patients stiffness is so marked that the patient has to be helped to stand and the joint has only a jog of painful movement. In others, cartilage and bone destruction predominate and the joint becomes increasingly unstable and deformed, usually in fixed flexion and valgus. X-rays reveal the bone destruction characteristic of advanced disease.

Treatment

The majority of patients can be managed by conservative measures. In addition to general treatment with anti-inflammatory and disease-modifying drugs, local splintage and injection of triamcinolone usually help to reduce the synovitis. A more prolonged effect may be obtained by injecting radiocolloids such as yttrium-90 (^{90}Y).

OPERATIVE TREATMENT

Synovectomy and debridement Only if other measures fail to control the synovitis (which nowadays is rare) is synovectomy indicated. This can be done very effectively by arthroscopy. Articular pannus and cartilage tags are removed at the same time. Postoperatively, any haematoma must be drained and movements are commenced as soon as pain has subsided.

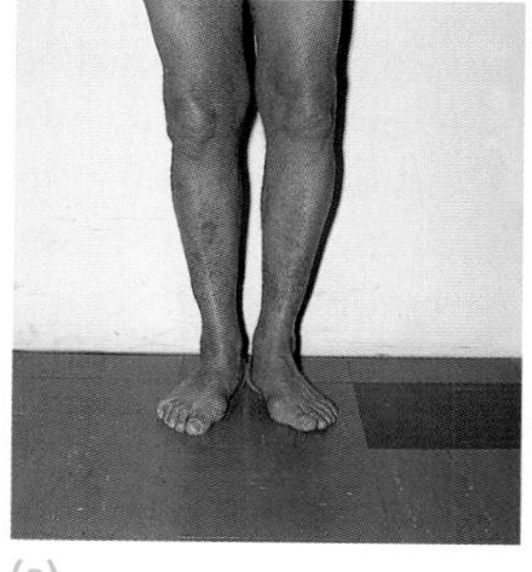
(a)

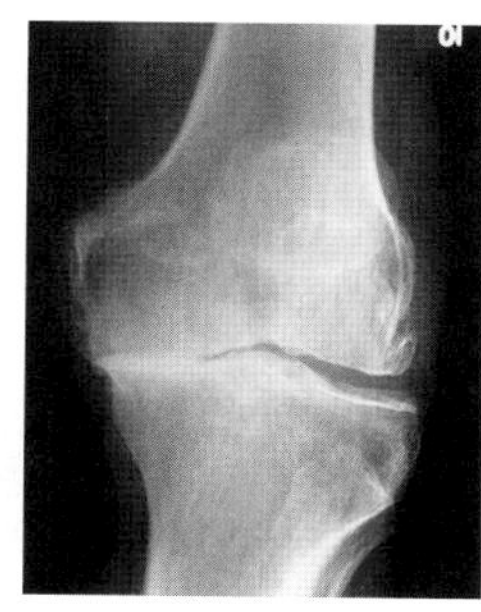
(b)

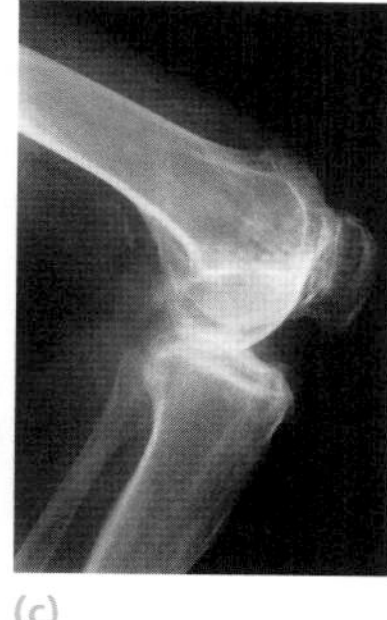
(c)

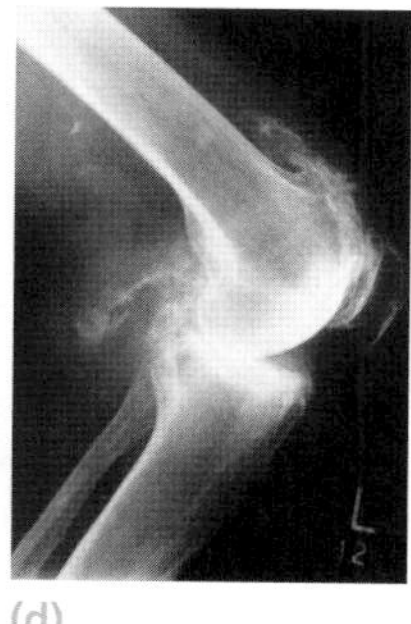
(d)

20.31 Osteoarthritis (a,b) Varus deformity of the left knee suggesting loss of cartilage thickness in the medial compartment. X-ray shows diminished joint space and peripheral osteophytes on the medial side of the knee. (c) Sometimes it is the patello-femoral joint that is mainly affected. (d) Patello-femoral osteoarthritis with long trailing osteophytes is typical of calcium pyrophosphate arthropathy.

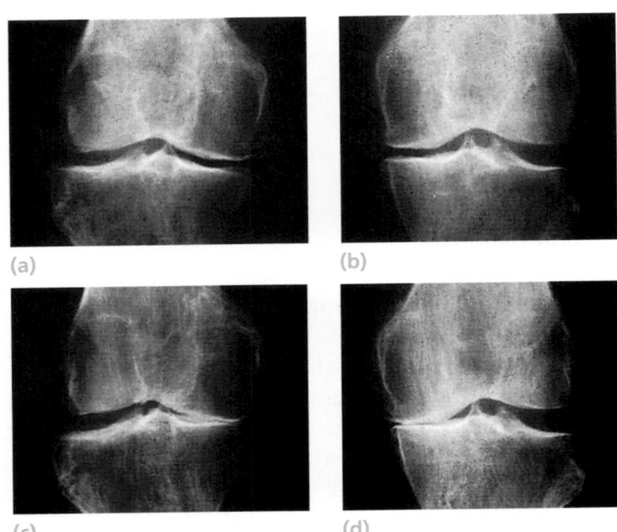

20.32 Osteoarthritis – x-rays Always obtain weightbearing views of the knees. X-rays taken with the patient lying down (a,b) suggest only minor cartilage loss on the medial side of each knee. (c,d) Weightbearing views show the true position: there is severe loss of articular cartilage.

Supracondylar osteotomy Realignment osteotomy is unlikely to have any protective effect in a disease which is marked by generalized cartilage erosion. However, if the knee is stable and pain-free but troublesome because of valgus and flexion deformity, a corrective supracondylar osteotomy is useful.

Arthroplasty Total joint replacement is useful when joint destruction is advanced. However, it is less successful if the knee has been allowed to become very unstable or very stiff; timing of the operation is important.

OSTEOARTHRITIS

The knee is the commonest of the large joints to be affected by osteoarthritis (see Chapter 5). Often there is a predisposing factor: injury to the articular surface, a torn meniscus, ligamentous instability or pre-existing deformity of the hip or knee, to mention a few. However, in many cases no obvious cause can be found. Underlying all of these, there may also be a genetic component. Curiously, while the male:female distribution is more or less equal in white (Caucasian) peoples, black African women are affected far more frequently than their male counterparts.

Osteoarthritis is often bilateral and in these cases there is a strong association with Heberden's nodes and generalized osteoarthritis.

Pathology

Cartilage breakdown usually starts in an area of excessive loading. Thus, with longstanding varus the changes are most marked in the medial compartment. The characteristic features of cartilage fibrillation, sclerosis of the subchondral bone and peripheral osteophyte formation are usually present; in advanced cases the articular surface may be denuded of cartilage and underlying bone may eventually crumble.

Chondrocalcinosis is common, but whether this is cause or effect – or quite unrelated – remains unknown.

Clinical features

Patients are usually over 50 years old; they tend to be overweight and may have longstanding bow-leg deformity.

Pain is the leading symptom, worse after use, or (if the patello-femoral joint is affected) on stairs. After rest, the joint feels stiff and it hurts to 'get going' after sitting for any length of time. Swelling is common, and giving way or locking may occur.

On examination there may be an obvious deformity (usually varus) or the scar of a previous operation. The quadriceps muscle is usually wasted.

Except during an exacerbation, there is little fluid and no warmth; nor is the synovial membrane thickened. Movement is somewhat limited and is often accompanied by patello-femoral crepitus.

It is useful to test movement applying first a varus and then a valgus force to the knee; pain indicates which tibio-femoral compartment is involved. Pressure on the patella may elicit pain.

The natural history of osteoarthritis is one of alternating 'bad spells' and 'good spells'. Patients may experience long periods of lesser discomfort and only moderate loss of function, followed by exacerbations of pain and stiffness (perhaps after unaccustomed activity).

X-ray

The anteroposterior x-ray *must* be obtained with the patient standing and bearing weight; only in this way can small degrees of articular cartilage thinning be revealed. The tibio-femoral joint space is diminished (often only in one compartment) and there is subchondral sclerosis. Osteophytes and subchondral cysts are usually present and sometimes there is soft-tissue calcification in the suprapatellar region or in the joint itself (chondrocalcinosis).

If only the patello-femoral joint is affected, suspect a pyrophosphate arthropathy.

Treatment

If symptoms are not severe, treatment is conservative. Joint loading is lessened by using a walking stick. Quadriceps exercises are important. Analgesics are prescribed for pain, and warmth (e.g. radiant heat or shortwave diathermy) is soothing. A simple elastic support may do wonders, probably by improving proprioception in an unstable knee.

Intra-articular corticosteroid injections will often relieve pain, but this is a stopgap, and not a very good one, because repeated injections may permit (or even predispose to) progressive cartilage and bone destruction.

New forms of medication have been introduced in recent years, particularly the oral administration of glucosamine and intra-articular injection of hyalourans. There is, as yet, no agreement about the long-term efficacy of these products.

OPERATIVE TREATMENT

Persistent pain unresponsive to conservative treatment, progressive deformity and instability are the usual indications for operative treatment.

Arthroscopic washouts, with trimming of degenerate meniscal tissue and osteophytes, may give temporary relief; this is a useful measure when there are contraindications to reconstructive surgery.

Patellectomy is indicated only in those rare cases where osteoarthritis is strictly confined to the patellofemoral joint. However, bear in mind that extensor power will be reduced and if a total joint replacement is later needed pain relief will be less predictable than usual (Paletta and Laskin, 1995).

Realignment osteotomy is often successful in relieving symptoms and staving off the need for 'end-stage' surgery. The ideal indication is a 'young' patient (under 50 years) with a varus knee and osteoarthritis confined to the medial compartment: a high tibial valgus osteotomy will redistribute weight to the lateral side of the joint. The degree and accuracy of angular correction are the most important determinants of mid- and long-term clinical outcome.

Replacement arthroplasty is indicated in older patients with progressive joint destruction. This is usually a 'resurfacing' procedure, with a metal femoral condylar component and a metal-backed polyethylene table on the tibial side. If the disease is largely confined to one compartment, a unicompartmental replacement can be done as an alternative to osteotomy. With modern techniques, and meticulous attention to anatomical alignment of the knee, the results of replacement arthroplasty are excellent.

Arthrodesis is indicated only if there is a strong contraindication to arthroplasty (e.g. previous infection) or to salvage a failed arthroplasty.

OSTEONECROSIS

Osteonecrosis of the knee, though not as common as femoral head necrosis, has the same aetiological and pathogenetic background (see Chapter 6). The usual site is the dome of one of the femoral condyles, but occasionally the medial tibial condyle is affected. Two main categories are identified: (1) *osteonecrosis associated with a definite background disorder* [e.g. corticosteroid therapy, alcohol abuse, sickle-cell disease, hyperbaric decompression sickness, systemic lupus erythematosus (SLE) or Gaucher's disease], and (2) *'spontaneous' osteonecrosis* of the knee, popularly known by the acronym SONK, which is due to a small insufficiency fracture of a prominent part of the osteoarticular surface in osteoporotic bone; the vascular supply to the free fragment is compromised (Yamamoto and Bullough, 2000).

A third type, *postmeniscectomy osteonecrosis,* has been reported; its prevalence and pathophysiology are still unclear (Patel et al., 1998).

Clinical features

Patients are usually over 60 years old and women are affected three times more often than men. Typically they give a history of sudden, acute pain on the medial side of the joint. Pain at rest also is common.

On examination there is usually a small effusion, but the classic feature is tenderness on pressure upon the medial femoral or tibial condyle rather than along the joint line proper.

The patient may offer a history of similar symptoms in the hip or the shoulder. Whether or not this is the case, those joints should be examined as well.

Imaging

X-ray The x-ray appearances are often unimpressive at the beginning, but a radionuclide scan may show increased activity on the medial side of the joint. Later the classic radiographic features of osteonecrosis appear (see Chapter 6). On the femoral side, it is always the *dome* of the condyle that is affected, unlike the picture in osteochondritis dissecans.

Magnetic resonance imaging MRI enhances the ability to visualize bone marrow and to separate necrotic from viable areas with a high level of specificity. It shows the area of reactive bone surrounding the osteonecrotic lesion and can demonstrate the integrity of the overlying cortical shell of bone and articular cartilage. It is also helpful in determining prognosis concerning the natural course of the condition.

Special investigations

Once the diagnosis is confirmed, investigations should be carried out to exclude generalized disorders known to be associated with osteonecrosis (see Chapter 6).

Differential diagnosis

Osteonecrosis of the knee should be distinguished from osteochondritis dissecans, though in truth the two conditions are closely related; however, the age group, aetiology, site of the lesion and prognosis are different and these factors may influence treatment. Other conditions that have a sudden, painful onset and tenderness at the joint line are fracture of an osteoarthritic osteophyte, disruption of a degenerative meniscus, a stress fracture, pes anserinus bursitis and a local tendonitis.

Prognosis

Symptoms and signs may stabilize and the patient be left with no more than slight distortion of the articular surface; or one of the condyles may collapse, leading to osteoarthritis of the affected compartment. The clinical progress depends on the radiographic size of the lesion, the ratio of size of the lesion to the size of the condyle (>40 per cent carries a worse prognosis) and the stage of the lesion (Patel et al., 1998).

Treatment

Treatment is conservative in the first instance and consists of measures to reduce loading of the joint and analgesics for pain. If symptoms or signs increase, operative treatment may be considered.

Surgical options include arthroscopic debridement, drilling with or without bone grafting, core decompression of the femoral condyle at a distance from the lesion, and (for patients with persistent symptoms and well-marked articular surface damage) a valgus osteotomy or unicompartmental arthroplasty. Resurfacing with osteochondral allografts has also been employed, with variable results.

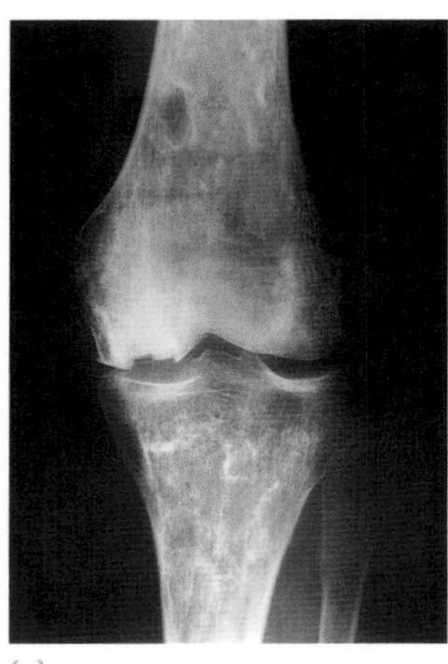

(a)

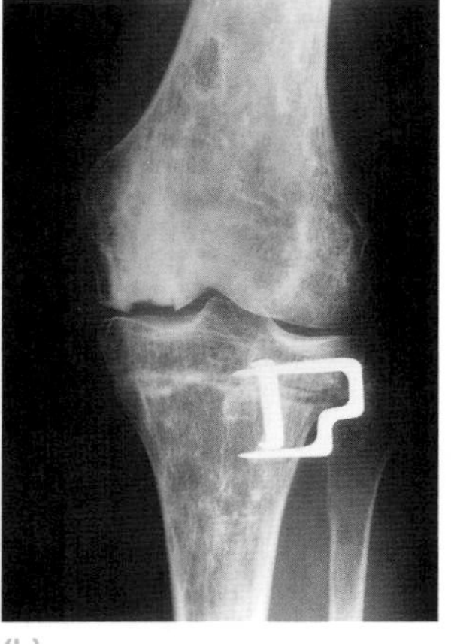

(b)

20.33 Osteonecrosis (a) X-ray showing the typical features of subarticular bone fragmentation and surrounding sclerosis situated in the highest part (the dome) of the medial femoral condyle. (In osteochondritis dissecans, the necrotic segment is almost always on the lateral surface of the medial femoral condyle.) (b) In this case the medial compartment was 'unloaded' by performing a high tibial valgus osteotomy. The patient remained pain-free for 6 years before dying of leukaemia.

CHARCOT'S DISEASE

Charcot's disease (neuropathic arthritis) is a rare cause of joint destruction. Because of loss of pain sensibility and proprioception, the articular surface breaks down and the underlying bone crumbles. Fragments of bone and cartilage are deposited in the hypertrophic synovium and may grow into large masses. The capsule is stretched and lax, and the joint becomes progressively unstable.

Clinical features

The patient chiefly complains of instability; pain (other than tabetic lightning pains) is unusual. The joint is swollen and often grossly deformed. It feels like a bag of bones and fluid but is neither warm nor tender. Movements beyond the normal limits, without pain, are a notable feature. Radiologically the joint is subluxated, bone destruction is obvious and irregular calcified masses can be seen.

Treatment

Patients often seem to manage quite well despite the bizarre appearances. However, marked instability may demand treatment – usually a moulded splint or caliper will do – and occasionally pain becomes intolerable. Arthrodesis is feasible but fixation is difficult and fusion is very slow. Replacement arthroplasty is not indicated.

HAEMOPHILIC ARTHRITIS

The knee is the joint most commonly involved in bleeding disorders. Repeated haemorrhage leads to chronic synovitis and articular cartilage erosion. Movement is progressively restricted and the joint may end up deformed and stiff.

Clinical features

Fresh bleeds cause pain and swelling of the knee, with the typical clinical signs of a haemarthrosis (see Chapter 5). Between episodes of bleeding the knee often

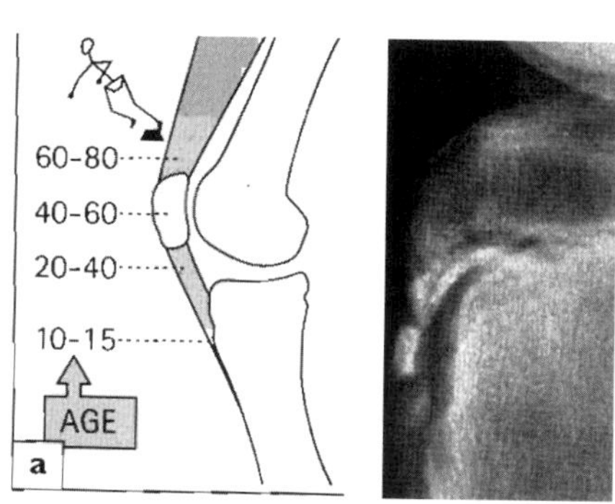

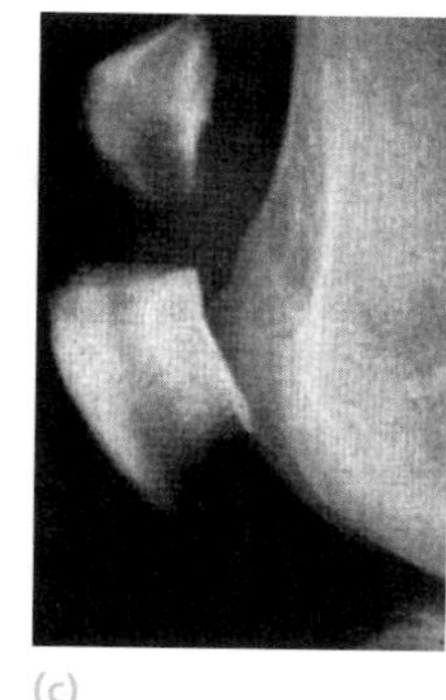

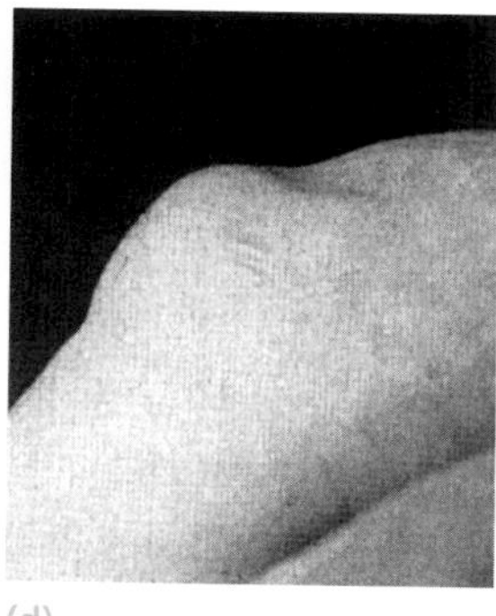

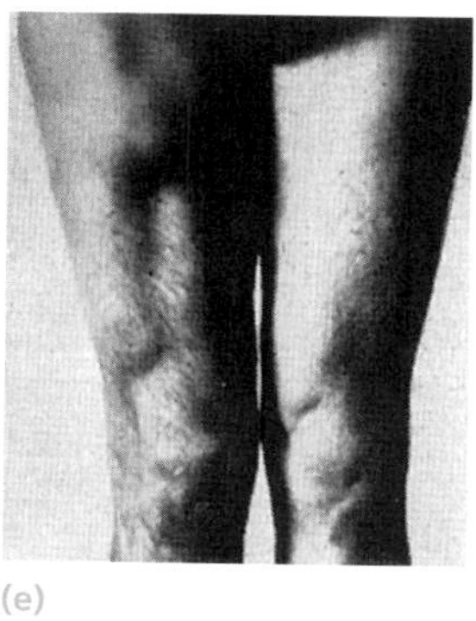

(a) (b) (c) (d) (e)

20.34 Extensor mechanism lesions These follow resisted action of the quadriceps; they usually occur at a progressively higher level with increasing age (a). (b) Osgood-Schlatter's disease – the only one that usually does not follow a definite accident; (c) gap fracture of patella; (d) ruptured quadriceps tendon (note the suprapatellar depression); (e) ruptured rectus femoris causing a lump with a hollow below.

continues to be painful and somewhat swollen, with restricted mobility. There is a tendency to hold the knee in flexion and this may become a fixed deformity.

X-rays Radiographic examination may show little abnormality, apart from local osteoporosis. In more advanced cases the joint space is narrowed and large 'cysts' or erosions may appear in the subchondral bone.

Treatment

Both the haematologist and the orthopaedic surgeon should participate in treatment. The acute bleed may need aspiration, but only if this can be 'covered' by giving the appropriate clotting factor; otherwise it is better treated by splintage until the acute symptoms settle down.

Flexion deformity must be prevented by gentle physiotherapy and intermittent splintage. If the joint is painful and eroded, operative treatment may be considered. However, although replacement arthroplasty is feasible, this should be done only after the most searching discussion with the patient, where all the risks are considered, and only if a full haematological service is available.

RUPTURES OF THE EXTENSOR APPARATUS

Resisted extension of the knee may tear the extensor mechanism. The patient stumbles on a stair, catches his or her foot while walking or running, or may only be kicking a muddy football. In all these incidents, active knee extension is prevented by an obstacle. The precise location of the lesion varies with the patient's age. In the elderly the injury is usually above the patella; in middle life the patella fractures; in young adults the patellar ligament can rupture. In adolescents the upper tibial apophysis is occasionally avulsed; much more often it is merely 'strained'.

Tendon rupture sometimes occurs with minimal strain; this is seen in patients with connective tissue disorders (e.g. SLE) and advanced rheumatoid disease, especially if they are also being treated with corticosteroids.

Rupture above the patella

Rupture may occur in the belly of the rectus femoris. The patient is usually elderly, or on long-term corticosteroid treatment. The torn muscle retracts and forms a characteristic lump in the thigh. Function is usually good, so no treatment is required.

Avulsion of the quadriceps tendon from the upper pole of the patella is seen in the same group of people. Sometimes it is bilateral. Operative repair is essential.

Rupture below the patella

This occurs mainly in young people. The ligament may rupture or may be avulsed from the lower pole of the patella. Operative repair is necessary. Pain and tenderness in the middle portion of the patellar ligament may occur in athletes; CT or ultrasonography will reveal an abnormal area. If rest fails to provide relief the paratenon should be stripped (King et al., 1990).

Partial rupture or avulsion sometimes leads to a traction tendinitis and calcification in the patellar ligament – the *Sinding–Larsen Johansson syndrome* (see below).

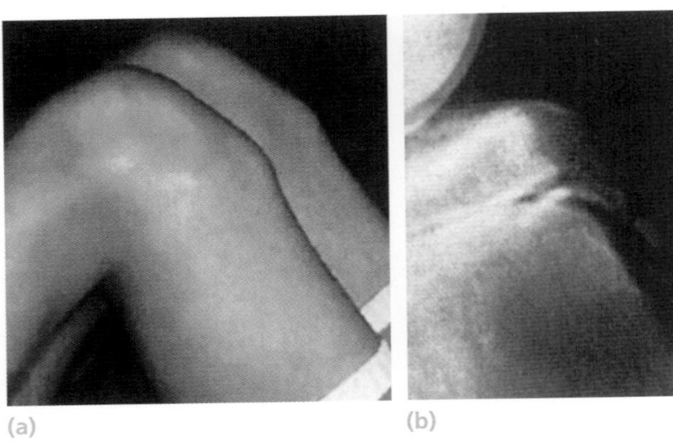

(a) (b)

20.35 Osgood–Schlatter's disease This boy complained of a painful bump below the knee. X-ray shows the traction injury of the tibial apophysis.

Osgood–Schlatter disease ('apophysitis' of the tibial tubercle)

In this common disorder of adolescence the tibial tubercle becomes painful and 'swollen'. Although often called osteochondritis or apophysitis, it is nothing more than a traction injury of the apophysis into which part of the patellar tendon is inserted (the remainder is inserted on each side of the apophysis and prevents complete separation).

There is no history of injury and sometimes the condition is bilateral. A young adolescent complains of pain after activity, and of a lump. The lump is tender and its situation over the tibial tuberosity is diagnostic. Sometimes active extension of the knee against resistance is painful and x-rays may reveal fragmentation of the apophysis.

Spontaneous recovery is usual but takes time, and it is wise to restrict such activities as cycling, jumping and soccer. Occasionally, symptoms persist and, if patience or wearing a back-splint during the day are unavailing, a separate ossicle in the tendon is usually responsible; its removal is then worthwhile.

TENDINITIS AND CALCIFICATION AROUND THE KNEE

Calcification in the medial ligament

Acute pain in the medial collateral ligament may be due to a soft calcific deposit among the fibres of the ligament. There may be a small, exquisitely tender lump in the line of the ligament. Pain is dramatically relieved by operative evacuation of the deposit.

Pellegrini–Stieda disease

X-rays sometimes show a plaque of bone lying next to the femoral condyle under the medial collateral ligament. Occasionally this is a source of pain. It is generally ascribed to ossification of a haematoma following a tear of the medial ligament, though a history of injury is not always forthcoming. Treatment is rarely needed.

Patellar 'tendinopathy' (Sinding–Larsen Johansson syndrome).

This condition was described independently by Sinding-Larsen in 1921 and Johansson in 1922. Following a strain or partial rupture of the patellar ligament the patient (usually a young athletic individual) develops a traction 'tendinitis' characterised by pain and point tenderness at the lower pole of the patella. Sometimes, if the condition does not settle, calcification appears in the ligament (Medlar and Lyne, 1978). CT or ultrasonography may reveal the abnormal area in the ligament. A similar disorder has been described at the proximal pole of the patella.

The condition is comparable to Osgood-Schlatter's disease and usually recovers spontaneously. If rest fails to provide relief, the abnormal area is removed and the paratenon stripped (King et al., 1990; Khan et al., 1998).

SWELLINGS OF THE KNEE

The knee is prone to a number of disorders which present essentially as 'swelling'; and, because it is such a large joint with a number of synovial recesses, the swelling is often painless until the tissues become tense. Conditions to be considered can be divided into four groups: *swelling of the entire joint; swellings in front of the joint; swellings behind the joint;* and *bony swellings.*

Acute swelling of the entire joint

POST-TRAUMATIC HAEMARTHROSIS

Swelling immediately after injury means blood in the joint. The knee is very painful and it feels warm, tense and tender. Later there may be a 'doughy' feel. Movements are restricted. X-rays are essential to see if there is a fracture; if there is not, then suspect a tear of the anterior cruciate ligament.

The joint should be aspirated under aseptic conditions. If a ligament injury is suspected, examination under anaesthesia is helpful and may indicate the need for operation; otherwise a crepe bandage is applied and the leg cradled in a back-splint. Quadriceps exercises are practised from the start. The patient may get up when comfortable, retaining the back-splint until muscle control returns.

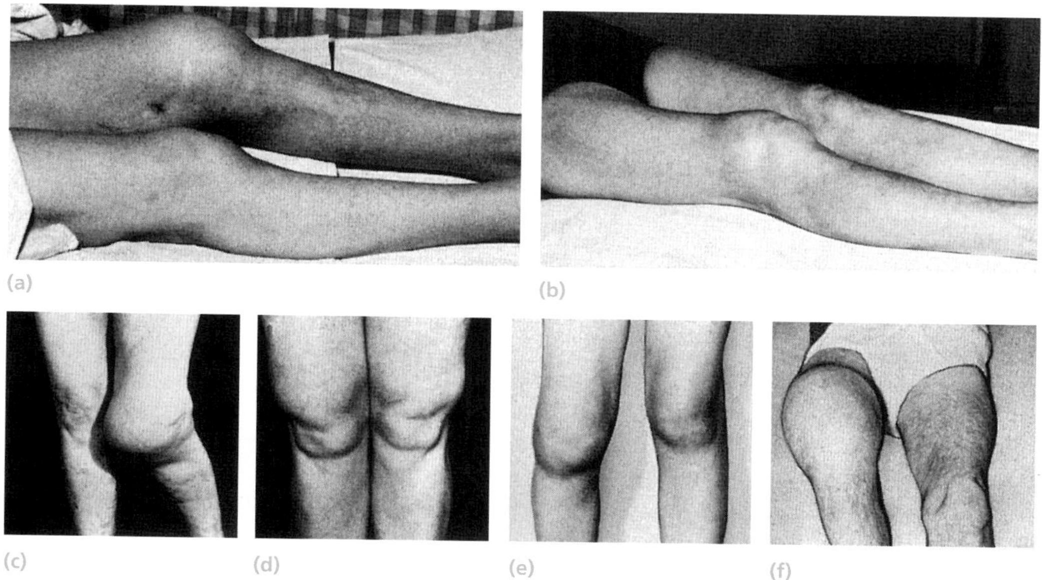

20.36 Swollen knees Some causes of chronic swelling in the absence of trauma: (a) tuberculous arthritis; (b) rheumatoid arthritis; (c) Charcot's disease; (d) villous synovitis; (e) haemophilia; (f) malignant synovioma.

BLEEDING DISORDERS

In patients with clotting disorders, the knee is the most common site for acute bleeds. If the appropriate clotting factor is available, the joint should be aspirated and treated as for a traumatic haemarthrosis. If the factor is not available, aspiration is best avoided; the knee is splinted in slight flexion until the swelling subsides.

ACUTE SEPTIC ARTHRITIS

Acute pyogenic infection of the knee is not uncommon. The organism is usually *Staphylococcus aureus*, but in adults gonococcal infection is almost as common.

The joint is swollen, painful and inflamed; the white cell count and ESR are elevated. Aspiration reveals pus in the joint; fluid should be sent for bacteriological investigation, including anaerobic culture.

Treatment consists of systemic antibiotics and drainage of the joint – ideally by arthroscopy, with irrigation and complete synovectomy; if fluid reaccumulates, it can be aspirated through a wide-bore needle. As the inflammation subsides, movement is begun, but weightbearing is deferred for 4–6 weeks.

TRAUMATIC SYNOVITIS

Injury stimulates a reactive synovitis; typically the swelling appears only after some hours, and subsides spontaneously over a period of days. There is inhibition of quadriceps action and the thigh wastes. The knee may need to be splinted for several days but movement should be encouraged and quadriceps exercise is essential. If the amount of fluid is considerable, its aspiration hastens muscle recovery. In addition, any internal injury will need treatment.

ASEPTIC NON-TRAUMATIC SYNOVITIS

Acute swelling, without a history of trauma or signs of infection, suggests *gout* or *pseudogout*. Aspiration will provide fluid which may look turbid, resembling pus, but it is sterile and microscopy (using polarized light) reveals the crystals. Treatment with anti-inflammatory drugs is usually effective.

CHRONIC SWELLING OF THE JOINT

The diagnosis can usually be made on clinical and x-ray examination. The more elusive disorders should be fully investigated by joint aspiration, synovial fluid examination, arthroscopy and synovial biopsy.

ARTHRITIS

The commonest causes of chronic swelling are *osteoarthritis* and *rheumatoid arthritis*. Other signs, such as deformity, loss of movement or instability, may be present and x-ray examination will usually show characteristic features.

SYNOVIAL DISORDERS

Chronic swelling and synovial effusion without articular destruction should suggest conditions such as *synovial chondromatosis* and *pigmented villonodular synovitis*. The diagnosis will usually be obvious on arthroscopy and can be confirmed by synovial biopsy.

The most important condition to exclude is *tuberculosis*. There has been a resurgence of cases during the last ten years and the condition should be seriously

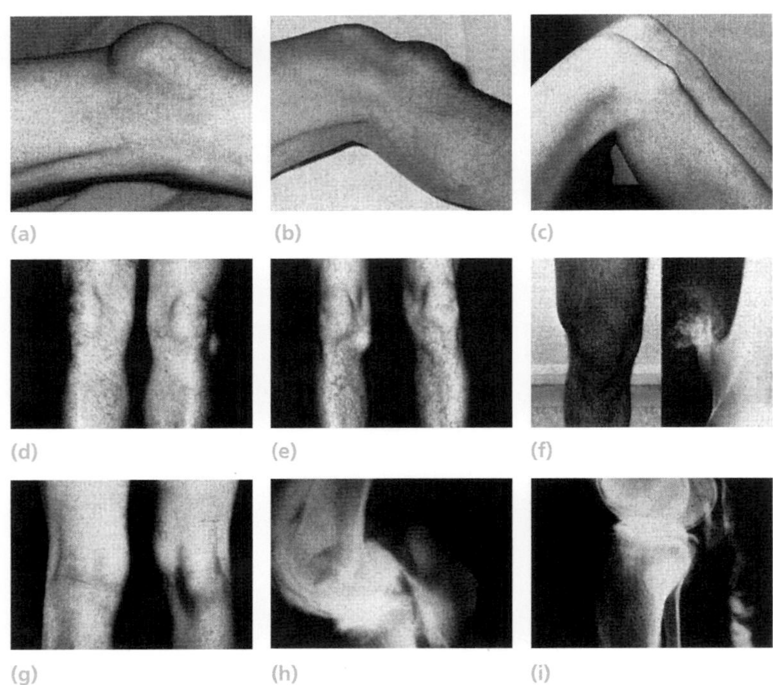

20.37 Lumps around the knee In front: (a) prepatellar bursa; (b) infrapatellar bursa; (c) Osgood–Schlatter disease.

On either side: (d) cyst of lateral meniscus; (e) cyst of medial meniscus; (f) cartilage-capped exostosis.

Behind: (g) semimembranosus bursa; (h) arthrogram of popliteal cyst; (i) leaking cyst.

considered whenever there is no obvious alternative diagnosis. Investigations should include Mantoux testing and synovial biopsy. The ideal is to start antituberculous chemotherapy before joint destruction occurs.

Swellings in front of the joint

PREPATELLAR BURSITIS ('HOUSEMAID'S KNEE')

The fluctuant swelling is confined to the front of the patella and the joint itself is normal. This is an uninfected bursitis due not to pressure but to constant friction between skin and bone. It is seen mainly in carpet layers, paving workers, floor cleaners and miners who do not use protective knee pads. Treatment consists of firm bandaging, and kneeling is avoided; occasionally aspiration is needed. In chronic cases the lump is best excised.

Infection (possibly due to foreign body implantation) results in a warm, tender swelling. Treatment is by rest, antibiotics and, if necessary, aspiration or excision.

INFRAPATELLAR BURSITIS ('CLERGYMAN'S KNEE')

The swelling is below the patella and superficial to the patellar ligament, being more distally placed than prepatellar bursitis; it used to be said that one who prays kneels more uprightly than one who scrubs! Treatment is similar to that for prepatellar bursitis. Occasionally the bursa is affected in gout.

OTHER BURSAE

Occasionally a bursa deep to the patellar tendon or the pes anserinus becomes inflamed and painful. Treatment is non-operative.

Swellings at the back of the knee

SEMIMEMBRANOSUS BURSA

The bursa between the semimembranosus and the medial head of gastrocnemius may become enlarged in children or adults. It presents usually as a painless lump behind the knee, slightly to the medial side of the midline and most conspicuous with the knee straight. The lump is fluctuant but the fluid cannot be pushed into the joint, presumably because the muscles compress and obstruct the normal communication. The knee joint is normal. Occasionally the lump aches, and if so it may be excised through a transverse incision. However, recurrence is common and, as the bursa normally disappears in time, a waiting policy is perhaps wiser.

POPLITEAL 'CYST'

Bulging of the posterior capsule and synovial herniation may produce a swelling in the popliteal fossa. The lump, which is usually seen in older people, is in the midline of the limb and at or below the level of the joint. It fluctuates but is not tender. Injection of radio-opaque medium into the joint, and x-ray, will show that the 'cyst' communicates with the joint.

The condition was originally described by Baker, whose patients were probably suffering from tuberculous synovitis. Nowadays it is more likely to be caused by rheumatoid or osteoarthritis, but it is still often called a 'Baker's cyst'. Occasionally the 'cyst' ruptures and the synovial contents spill into the muscle planes causing pain and swelling in the calf – a combination which can easily be mistaken for deep vein thrombosis.

The swelling may diminish following aspiration and injection of hydrocortisone; excision is not advised, because recurrence is common unless the underlying condition is treated.

POPLITEAL ANEURYSM

This is the commonest limb aneurysm and is sometimes bilateral. Pain and stiffness of the knee may precede the symptoms of peripheral arterial disease, so it is essential to examine any lump behind the knee for pulsation. A thrombosed popliteal aneurysm does not pulsate, but it feels almost solid.

BONY SWELLINGS AROUND THE KNEE

Because the knee is a relatively superficial joint, bony swellings of the distal femur and proximal tibia are often visible and almost always palpable. Common examples are cartilage-capped exostoses (osteochondromata) and the characteristic painful swelling of Osgood–Schlatter disease of the tibial tubercle (see below).

PRINCIPLES OF KNEE OPERATIONS

ARTHROSCOPY

Arthroscopy is useful: (1) to establish or refine the accuracy of diagnosis; (2) to help in deciding whether to operate, and (3) to perform certain operative procedures. Arthroscopy is not a substitute for clinical examination; a detailed history and meticulous assessment of the physical signs are indispensable preliminaries and remain the sheet anchor of diagnosis.

TECHNIQUE

Full asepsis in an operating theatre is essential. The patient is anaesthetized (though local anaesthesia may suffice for short procedures) and a thigh tourniquet applied. Through a tiny incision, a trocar and cannula is introduced; sometimes, saline is injected to distend the joint before it is punctured. Entry into the joint is confirmed when saline flows easily into the joint or, if the joint was distended previously, by the outflow when the trocar is withdrawn. A fibreoptic viewer, light source and irrigation system are attached; a small television camera and monitor make it much easier for the operator to concentrate on manipulating the instruments with both hands ('triangulation'). All compartments of the joint are now systematically inspected; with special instruments and, if necessary, through multiple portals, biopsy, partial meniscectomy, patellar shaving, removal of loose bodies, synovectomy, ligament replacement and many other procedures are possible. Before withdrawing the instrument, saline is squeezed out. A firm bandage is applied; the arthroscopic portals are often small enough not to require sutures. Postoperative recovery is remarkably rapid.

COMPLICATIONS

Intra-articular effusions and small haemarthroses are fairly common but seldom troublesome.

Reflex sympathetic dystrophy (which may resemble a low-grade infection during the weeks following arthroscopy) is sometimes troublesome. It usually settles down with physiotherapy and treatment with non-steroidal anti-inflammatory drugs; occasionally it requires more radical treatment (see pages 261 and 723).

LIGAMENT RECONSTRUCTION

The collateral and cruciate ligaments and the knee capsule are important constraints which allow normal knee function; laxity or rupture of these structures, either singly or in combination, is often the source of recurrent episodes of 'giving way'. Although a significant proportion of such injuries are treated non-operatively, complete ruptures may require surgery in 'high-demand' individuals.

Surgery for ligament reconstruction includes:

1. *Repair*, usually for collateral ligament midsubstance ruptures when they are found in combination with cruciate ligament injuries. This repair can be a simple end-to-end suture.
2. *Substitution*, usually for anterior cruciate ruptures: the semitendinosus and gracilis, either one or two bundle technique, can be carefully anchored to the femur and tibia ensuring that stability is restored without loss of knee movement. Another method is to use an autologous graft from the patellar tendon.
3. *Tenodesis*, using a variety of tendons which are passed either through bony or soft-tissue tunnels to 'check' the abnormal movement resulting from ligament rupture.

OSTEOTOMY

Osteotomy above or below the joint used to be a popular method of treating arthritis of the knee, especially when articular destruction was more or less limited to one compartment and the knee had developed a varus or valgus deformity. With the development of joint replacement techniques, the operation gradually fell into disuse, or at best was seen as a temporizing measure to buy time for patients who would ultimately undergo some form of arthroplasty. However, improvements in technique and the introduction of operations for meniscal and articular cartilage repair have led to renewed interest in this procedure.

The rationale for osteotomy is based on both biomechanical and physiological principles. Malalignment of the limb results in excessive loading and stress in part of the joint and consequently increased damage to the articular cartilage in that area – the medial compartment if the knee is in varus and the lateral compartment in a valgus knee. As the articular surface is destroyed, the deformity progressively increases. Osteotomy and repositioning of the bone fragments, by correcting the deformity, will improve the loadbearing mechanics of the joint. Furthermore, it will reduce the intraosseous venous congestion, and this may relieve some of the patient's pain.

INDICATIONS

Deformity of the knee Severe varus or valgus deformity (e.g. due to a growth defect, epiphyseal injury or a malunited fracture) may of itself call for a corrective osteotomy, and the operation may also prevent or delay the development of osteoarthritis.

Localized articular surface destruction Patients with unicompartmental osteoarthritis or advanced localized osteonecrosis, particularly when this is associated with deformity in the coronal plane, may benefit from an osteotomy which offloads the affected area. Provided the joint is stable and has retained a reasonable range of movement, this offers an acceptable alternative to a unicompartmental arthroplasty. Usually it is the medial compartment that is affected and the knee exhibits a varus deformity. By realigning the joint, load is transferred from the medial compartment to the centre or a little towards the lateral side. Slight over-correction may further offload the medial compartment but marked valgus should be avoided as this will rapidly lead to cartilage loss in the lateral compartment.

Published results suggest that the operation provides substantial improvements in pain and function over a 7–10-year period (Dowd et al., 2006).

Intra-articular reconstructions The introduction of meniscal and articular cartilage reconstruction techniques has led to considerable interest in applying the favourable biomechanical effects of osteotomy to the younger patient who has a full-thickness chondral lesion or an absent meniscus. Similarly, osteotomy in conjunction with either simultaneous or staged cruciate ligament reconstruction appears to be beneficial in patients who have a combination of instability and pain from limb malalignment (Giffin and Fintan, 2007).

TECHNIQUE

For sound biomechanical reasons, a varus deformity is best corrected by a *valgus osteotomy* at the proximal end of the tibia, whereas a valgus deformity should be corrected by a *varus osteotomy* at the femoral supracondylar level.

Angles must be accurately measured and the position of correction carefully mapped out on x-rays before starting the operation.

A high tibial valgus osteotomy can be performed either by removing a pre-determined wedge of bone based laterally and then closing the gap (*closing wedge technique)* or by opening a wedge-shaped gap on the medial side *(opening wedge technique)*.

In the lateral closing wedge method the fibula must first be released either by dividing it lower down or by disrupting the proximal tibio-fibular joint. The tibia is divided just above the insertion of the patellar ligament. Two transverse cuts are made, one parallel to the joint surface and another just below that, angled to create the desired laterally based wedge. The wedge of bone is removed and the fragments are then approximated and fixed in the corrected position either with staples or with compression pins. The limb is immobilized in a cast for 4–6 weeks, by which time the osteotomy should have started to unite.

An opening wedge valgus osteotomy on the medial side offers some advantages: the ability to adjust the degree of correction intra-operatively and the option to correct deformities in the sagittal plane as well as the coronal plane; it also makes it unnecessary to disrupt the tibio-fibular joint. However, there are also disadvantages: the newly-created gap must be filled with a bone graft and a long period of restricted weightbearing is needed after the procedure; there is also a higher rate of non-union or delayed union. These drawbacks can be mitigated by stabilizing the fragments with an external fixator applied to the medial side, waiting for about 5 days and then opening the gap very gradually, allowing it to fill with callus (*hemicallotasis*). Cast immobilization is unnecessary. The external fixator usually remains in place for 10–12 weeks.

If a varus osteotomy is required – usually for active patients with isolated lateral compartment disease and valgus deformity of the knee – this is performed at the supracondylar level of the femur. The method most commonly employed is a medial closing wedge osteotomy, designed to place the mechanical axis at zero. The fragments should be firmly fixed with a blade-plate; in many cases postoperative cast immobilization will also be needed.

RESULTS

High tibial valgus osteotomy, when done for osteoarthritis, gives good results provided (1) the disease is confined to the medial compartment, and (2) the knee has a good range of movement and is stable. Relief of pain is good in 85 per cent of cases in the first year but drops to approximately 60 per cent after 5 years. A recent review has shown that modern medial opening wedge osteotomy techniques can achieve satisfactory postoperative alignment in 93 per cent of patients and survivorship rates of 94 per cent at 5-year, 85 per cent at 10-year, and 68 per cent at 15-year follow-up, with conversion to total knee arthroplasty as the end point (Brower et al., 2007; Virolainen and Aro, 2004).

The clinical results of distal femoral varus osteotomy have been good in selected patients. Substantial improvements in pain and function can be expected in approximately 90 per cent of patients (Preston et al., 2005).

COMPLICATIONS

Compartment syndrome in the leg This is the most important early complication of tibial osteotomy. Careful and repeated checks should be carried out during the early postoperative period to ensure that there are no symptoms or signs of impending ischaemia. Early features of compartment compression in the leg are sometimes mistaken for those of a deep vein thrombosis; this mistake should be avoided at all costs because the consequent delay in starting treatment could make the difference between complete recovery and permanent loss of function.

Peroneal nerve palsy Overzealous attempts at correcting a longstanding valgus deformity can stretch and damage the peroneal nerve. Poor cast techniques may do the same, which is a good reason why postoperative cast application should not be left to an unsupervised junior assistant.

Failure to correct the deformity Under- or overcorrection of the deformity are really failures in technique. With medial compartment osteoarthritis, unless a slight valgus position is obtained, the result is liable to be unsatisfactory. However, marked overcorrection is not only mechanically unsound but the cosmetic defect is liable to be bitterly resented by the patient.

Delayed union and non-union These complications can be avoided by ensuring that fixation of the bone fragments is stable and secure.

ARTHRODESIS

Arthrodesis of the knee has long been considered a demanding procedure that is subject to a variety of postoperative complications and often results in marginal or unacceptable outcomes. A stiff knee is a considerable disability; it makes climbing difficult and sitting in crowded areas distinctly awkward. Consequently, it is not often performed. For these reasons, arthrodesis has typically been held in reserve as a final salvage procedure for patients with irretrievably failed total knee arthroplasties and other comparable conditions.

INDICATIONS

In the past – and even today in some parts of the world – the main indications for arthrodesis of the knee were (and are) *irremediable instability* due to the late effects of poliomyelitis and *painful loss of mobility* due to tuberculosis or chronic pyogenic infection.

In countries with advanced medical facilities the commonest indication is *failed total knee replacement* (either septic or aseptic).

CONTRAINDICATIONS

Contraindications include *severe general disability* because of age or multiple joint disease, especially if associated with problems in the ipsilateral hip or ankle; *amputation* or *knee fusion* of the opposite limb; and *persistent non-union* of a peri-articular fracture or *massive peri-articular bone loss.* Finally, *patient reluctance* may be an important factor. A short period in a plaster cylinder before operation may convince the patient that a rigidly stiff leg is better than a painful and unstable knee.

TECHNIQUE

A vertical midline incision is used. If the operation is for tuberculosis the diseased synovium is excised; otherwise it is disregarded. The posterior vessels and nerves are protected and the ends of the tibia and femur removed by means of straight saw cuts, aiming to end with 15 degrees of flexion and 7 degrees of valgus as the position of fusion. Charnley's method, using thick Steinman pins inserted parallel through the distal femur and proximal tibia, and connecting these with compression clamps, was for many years the standard method. Nowadays, multiplanar external fixation is used, or if the joint is not infected, a long intramedullary nail which may be unlocked or locked.

KNEE REPLACEMENT

INDICATIONS

The main indication for knee replacement is pain, especially when this is combined with deformity and instability. Most replacements are performed for rheumatoid arthritis or osteoarthritis.

TYPES OF OPERATION

Partial replacement The role of unicompartmental replacement has yet to be firmly established. Early results for medial compartment osteoarthritis were promising but longer-term studies have highlighted the need for meticulous and exacting surgical technique to avoid high revision rates. Following a successful operation, relief of pain and restoration of function can be impressive, but for the present it is reserved for older patients; tibial and femoral osteotomies are used in the younger population.

Patellar resurfacing, a kind of partial replacement, is rarely performed alone; usually it is combined with surface replacement of the condyles.

Minimally constrained total replacement The term 'minimally constrained' is used for prostheses where some of the stability after replacement is provided by the prosthesis and some through preservation of the knee ligaments. Most modern minimally constrained designs allow sacrifice of the anterior cruciate ligament; some even allow both cruciates to be removed without detriment to the long-term survival of the prosthesis. 'Totally unconstrained' devices, where both cruciates are preserved, are rarely used because results are poor compared to the minimally constrained group.

At operation all the articular surfaces are replaced – with metal on the femoral side, polyethylene on a metal tray on the tibial side and polyethylene alone on the patella. It is important to ensure correct placement of the implants so as to reproduce the normal mechanics of the knee as closely as possible.

The tibial and patellar components are fixed with cement, whereas the femoral component may be press-fitted. Bone defects may be filled either with bone graft, metal augmentation wedges or cement. The development of suitable prostheses and instrumentation in recent years has led to vast improvements in technique, so the results are now similar to those of hip replacement.

Constrained joints Artificial joints with fixed hinges are used when there is marked bone loss and severe instability. Their main value nowadays is to provide a mobile joint following resection of tumours at the bone ends. The lack of rotation in these implants places severe stresses on the bone/implant interfaces and they are liable to loosen, to break or to erode the tibial or femoral shafts unless physical activity is severely restricted. Moreover, a considerable amount of bone has to be removed, and this makes a subsequent arthrodesis difficult.

Minimally invasive total knee replacement This is in its early stage of development and is not yet widely used. Early results suggest that it provides some benefits over conventional total joint replacement: less pain, faster recovery, better quadriceps strength and a better range of movement.

TECHNIQUE

It is important: (1) to overcome deformity (the knee should finally be about 7 degrees valgus); (2) to promote stability (by tailoring the bone cuts so that the collateral ligaments are equally tense in both flexion and extension); and (3) to permit rotation (otherwise cemented prostheses are liable to loosen).

COMPLICATIONS

General As with all knee operations (except arthroscopy) in which a tourniquet is used, there is a high incidence of deep vein thrombosis. Prophylaxis, either pharmacological (anticoagulants) or mechanical (foot pumps, compression stockings), is recommended.

Infection The methods of preventing and treating infection are similar to those used in hip replacement. For established and intractable infection, treatment by debridement and antibiotics, or by exchange replacement in one or two stages, are obvious possibilities, though probably the safest salvage operation is arthrodesis; this is especially applicable in immunosuppressed patients and in those with resistant bacteria.

Loosening Covert infection is only one cause of implant loosening. Aseptic loosening results from faulty prosthetic design, inaccurate bone shaping, incorrect placement of the implants or a combination of these factors. Revision surgery for loose prostheses must deal with the cause, be it malposition of the prosthesis, accumulation of wear debris or infection. A loose prosthesis can be re-cemented, but unless the cause is dealt with, loosening will recur.

Patellar problems Although relatively uncommon, these can be very disabling. They include: (1) recurrent patellar subluxation or dislocation, which may need realignment; and (2) complications associated with patellar resurfacing, such as loosening of the prosthetic component, fracture of the remaining bony patella, and catching of soft tissues between the patella and the femur.

Patellar tracking as assessed on the operating table after implantation of the prosthesis is important. Any tendency to sublux must be corrected: common causes are unequal soft-tissue tension (for which a lateral release will be needed), a tibial component placed in internal rotation and/or a femoral component placed in internal rotation.

The risk of patellar fracture postoperatively can also be lessened if care is taken not to divide the geniculate vessels when performing a lateral release.

NOTES ON APPLIED ANATOMY

The knee joint combines two articulations – tibiofemoral and patello-femoral. The bones of the tibiofemoral joint have little or no inherent stability; this depends largely upon strong static and dynamic stabilizers such as ligaments and muscles. The patellofemoral joint is so shaped that the patella moves in a shallow path (or track) between the femoral condyles; if this track is too shallow the patella readily dislocates, and if its line is faulty the patellar articular cartilage is subject to excessive wear. One important function of the patella is to increase the power of extension; it lifts the quadriceps forwards, thereby increasing its moment arm.

The patellar tendon is inserted into the upper pole of the patella. It is in line with the shaft of the femur, whereas the patellar ligament is in line with the shaft of the tibia. Because of the angle between them (the Q-angle) quadriceps contraction would pull the patella laterally were it not for the fibres of vastus medialis, which are transverse. This muscle is therefore important and it is essential to try to prevent the otherwise rapid wasting that is liable to follow any effusion.

The shaft of the femur is inclined medially, while the tibia is vertical; thus the normal knee is slightly valgus (average 7 degrees). This amount is physiological and the term 'genu valgum' is used only when the angle exceeds 7 degrees; significantly less than this amount is genu varum.

During walking, weight is necessarily taken alternately on each leg. The line of body weight falls medial to the knee and must be counterbalanced by muscle action lateral to the joint (chiefly the tensor fascia femoris). To calculate the force transmitted across the knee, that due to muscle action must be added to that imposed by gravity; moreover, since with each step the knee is braced by the quadriceps, the force that this imposes also must be added.

Clearly the stresses on the articular cartilage are (as they also are at the hip) much greater than consideration only of body weight would lead one to suppose. It is also obvious that a varus deformity can easily overload the medial compartment, leading to cartilage breakdown; similarly, a valgus deformity may overload the lateral compartment.

For several decades, the prevailing opinion was that the movements of the knee are guided by the cruciate ligaments functioning as a crossed four-bar link. For a knee guided by a four-bar link, this implies that the axis of rotation of the tibia relative to the femur must be at the crossing point of the cruciate ligaments. An important kinematic consequence of the four-bar link is the phenomenon known as 'roll-back'. Roll-back is a progressive movement of the femur backward on the tibia with flexion. The opposite – roll-forward – would then occur during knee extension.

However, recent published work on normal knee kinematics has shown that the knee does not work as a crossed four-bar link. Modern knee kinematics are better understood by dividing the flexion arc into three parts (Freeman and Pinskerova, 2005). From full extension to 20 to 30 degrees of flexion, tibial internal rotation is coupled with flexion and on the lateral side a counter-translation nearing full extension is observed. Knee activities take place mainly between 20 degrees and 120 degrees. Over this arc, the articulating surfaces of the femoral condyles are circular in sagittal section and rotate around a centre. The medial condyle does not move anteroposteriorly (roll-back does not occur medially) but remains stable concerning spinning kinematics, while the contact area transfers from an anterior pair of tibio-femoral surfaces at 10 degrees to a posterior part at about 30 degrees.

Thus, because of the shapes of the bones, the medial contact area moves backwards with flexion to 30 degrees but the condyle does not. On the lateral side a variable spinning motion in mid-flexion (60 degrees) and a rolling motion up to 120 degrees of flexion are observed. Laterally, the femoral condyle and the contact area move posteriorly but to a variable extent in the mid-flexion (roll-back) causing tibial internal rotation to occur with flexion around a medial axis. Flexion beyond 120 degrees can only be achieved passively. Medially, the femur rolls back onto the posterior horn. Laterally, the femur and the posterior horn drop over the posterior tibia. New knee prostheses have been designed to reflect contemporary data regarding knee kinematics.

Situated as they are between these complexly moving surfaces, the fibrocartilaginous menisci are prone to injury, particularly during unguarded movements of extension and rotation on the weightbearing leg. The medial meniscus is especially vulnerable because, in addition to its loose attachments via the coronary ligaments, it is firmly attached at three widely separated points: the anterior horn, the posterior horn and to the medial collateral ligament. The lateral meniscus more readily escapes damage because it is attached only at its anterior and posterior horns and these are close to each other.

The function of the menisci is not known for certain, but they certainly increase the contact area between femur and tibia. They play a significant part in weight transmission and this applies at all angles of flexion and extension; as the knee bends they glide backwards, and as it straightens they are pushed forwards.

The deep portion of the medial collateral ligament, to which the meniscus is attached, is fan-shaped and blends with the posteromedial capsule. It is, therefore, not surprising that medial ligament tears are often associated with tears of the medial meniscus and of the posteromedial capsule. The lateral collateral ligament is situated more posteriorly and does not blend with the capsule; nor is it attached to the meniscus, from which it is separated by the tendon of popliteus.

The two collateral ligaments resist sideways tilting of the extended knee. In addition, the medial ligament prevents the medial tibial condyle from subluxating forwards. Forward subluxation of the lateral tibial condyle, however, is prevented, not by the lateral collateral ligament but by the anterior cruciate. Only when the medial ligament and the anterior cruciate are both torn can the whole tibia subluxate forwards (giving a marked positive anterior drawer sign). Backward subluxation of the tibia is prevented by the powerful posterior cruciate ligament in combination with the arcuate ligament on its lateral side and the posterior oblique ligament on its medial side.

The cruciate ligaments are crucial, in the sense that they are essential for stability of the knee. The anterior cruciate ligament prevents forward displacement of the tibia on the femur and, in particular, it prevents forward subluxation of the lateral tibial condyle, a movement that tends to occur if a person who is running twists suddenly. The posterior cruciate ligament prevents backward displacement of the tibia on the femur and its integrity is therefore important when progressing downhill.

REFERENCES AND FURTHER READING

Apley AG. The diagnosis of meniscus injuries: some new clinical methods. *J Bone Joint Surg* 1947; **29:** 78–84.

Bentley G. Articular cartilage changes in chondromalacia patellae. *J Bone Joint Surg* 1985; **67B:** 769–774.

Bowen JR, Leahy JL, Zhang Z, MacEwen GD. Partial epiphyseodesis at the knee to correct angular deformity. *Clin Orthop* 1985; **198:** 184–90.

Brower RW, van Raaij TM, Bierma-Zeinstra SM *et al.* Osteotomy for treating knee osteoarhtritis. *Cochrane Database Syst Rev* 2007; **18(3)**: CD004019.

Coventry MB. Upper tibial osteotomy for osteoarthritis. *J Bone Joint Surg* 1985; **67A:** 1136–40.

Crotty JM, Monu JU, Pope TL Jr. Magnetic resonance imaging of the musculoskeletal system. Part 4. The knee. *Clin Orthop Relat Res* 1996; **330:** 288–303.

Dandy DJ. Chronic patellofemoral instability. *J Bone Joint Surg* 1995; **78B:** 328–35.

Dimakopoulos P, Patel D. Partial excision of discoid meniscus. *Acta Orthop Scand* 1990; **61:** 1–40.

Dowd GS, Somayaji HS, Uthukuri M. High tibial osteotomy for medial compartment osteoarthritis. *Knee* 2006; **13**: 87–92

Ficat RP, Hungerford DS. Disorders of the Patello-femoral Joint, Williams & Wilkins, Baltimore, 1977.

Freeman MA, Pinskerova V. The movement of the normal tibiofemoral joint. *J Biomech* 2005; **38:** 197–208.

Giffin R, Fintan S. The role of the high tibial osteotomy in the unstable knee**.** *Sports Med Arthrosc* 2007; **15:** 23–31

Goodfellow J, Hungerford DS, Zindel M. Patello-femoral joint mechanics and pathology. 1. Functional anatomy of the patello-femoral joint. *J Bone Joint Surg* 1976; **58B:** 287–90.

Goodfellow J, Hungerford DS, Woods C. Patellofemoral joint mechanics and pathology. 2. Chondromalacia patellae. *J Bone Joint Surg* 1976; **58B:** 291–9.

Goodfellow JW, Kershaw CJ, Benson MKD'A, O'Connor JJ. The Oxford knee for unicompartmental osteoarthritis. *J Bone Joint Surg* 1988; **70B:** 692–701.

Grelsamer RP. Unicompartmental osteoarthrosis of the knee. *J Bone Joint Surg* 1995; **77A:** 278–92

Inone M, Shino K, Hirose H *et al.* Subluxation of the patella. Computed tomography analysis of patellofemoral congruence. *J Bone Joint Surg* 1988; **70A:** 1331–7.

Insall JN, Salvati E. Patella position in the normal knee joint. *Radiology* 1971; **101:** 101.

Karachalios T, Hantes M, Zibis AH *et al.* Diagnostic accuracy of a new clinical test (the Thessaly test) for early detection of meniscal tears. *J Bone Joint Surg* 2005; **87A:** 955–62.

Kay PR, Freemont AJ, Davies DRA. The aetiology of multiple loose bodies. *J Bone Joint Surg* 1989; **71B:** 501–4.

Khan KM, Maffulli N, Coleman BD *et al.* Patellar tendinopathy: some aspects of basic science and clinical management. *Br J Sports Med* 1998; **32:** 346–55.

King JB, Perry DJ, Mourad K, Kumar SJ. Lesions of the patellar ligament. *J Bone Joint Surg* 1990; **72B:** 46–48.

Kocher MS, Tucker R, Ganley TJ, Flynn JM. Management of osteochondritis dissecans of the knee. Current concepts review. *Am J Sports Med* 2006; **34:** 1181–91.

Liu SH, Mirzayan R. Current review. Functional knee bracing. *Clin Orthop Res* 1995; **317:** 273–81.

Mann G, Finsterbush A, Franfkl U *et al.* A method of diagnosing small amounts of fluid in the knee. *J Bone Joint Surg* 1991; **73B:** 346–7.

Maquet PGJ. Biomechanics of the Knee. Springer, Berlin, 1976.

Medlar RC, Lyne ED. Sinding-Larsen Johansson disease. *J Bone Joint Surg* 1978; **60A:** 1113–6.

Men HX, Bian CH, Yang CD *et al.* Surgical treatment of the flail knee after poliomyelitis. *J Bone Joint Surg* 1991; **73B:** 195–8.

Merchant AC, Mercer RL, Jacobsen RH, Cool CR. Roentgenographic analysis of patellofemoral congruence. *J Bone Joint Surg* 1974; **56A:** 1391–6.

Oei EHG, Nikken JJ, Verstijen ACM *et al.* MR Imaging of the menisci and cruciate ligaments: A systematic review. *Radiology* 2003; **226**: 837–48.

Paletta GA Jr, Laskin RS. Total knee arthroplasty after a previous patellectomy. *J Bone Joint Surg* 1995; **77A:** 1708–12.

Parisien JS. Arthroscopic treatment of cysts of the menisci. *Clin Orthop Related Res* 1990; **257:** 154–8.

Patel DV, Breazeale NM, Behr CT *et al.* Osteonecrosis of the knee: current clinical concepts. *Knee Surg Sports Traumatol Arthrosc* 1998; **6**: 2–11.

Preston CF, Fulkerson EW, Meislin R, Di Cesare PE. Osteotomy about the knee: applications, techniques and results. *J Knee Surg* 2005; **18(4)**: 258–72

Salenius P, Vankka E. The development of the tibiofemoral angle in children. *J Bone Joint Surg* 1975; **57A:** 259–61.

Schenck RC Jr, Goodnight JM. Osteochondritis dissecans. *J Bone Joint Surg* 1996; **78A:** 439–56.

Sherman OH, Fox JM, Snyder SJ, *et al.* Arthroscopy – 'No Problem Surgery': An analysis of complications in two thousand six hundred and forty cases. *J Bone Joint Surg* 1986; **68A**: 256–65.

Thomee R, Augustsson J, Karlsson J. Patellofemoral pain syndrome: A review of current issues. *Sport Medicine* 1999; **28:** 245–62.

Virolainen P, Aro HT. High tibial osteotomy for the treatment of osteoarthritis of the knee of the knee: a review of the literature and meta-analysis of follow up studies. *Arch Orthop Trauma Surg* 2004; **124(4)**: 258–61.

Yamamoto T, Bullough PG. Spontaneous osteonecrosis of the knee: the result of subchondral insufficiency fracture. *J Bone Joint Surg* 2000; **82A:** 858–66.

The ankle and foot

21

Gavin Bowyer

CLINICAL ASSESSMENT

SYMPTOMS

Adults with foot and ankle problems often present complaining of pain, swelling, deformity and impaired function including difficulties with work, social and domestic activities. Questions should include those that flag up the possibility of neoplastic or generalized inflammatory disease and diabetes.

Pain over a bony prominence or a joint is probably due to some local disorder; ask the patient to point to the painful spot. Symptoms tend to be well localized to the structures involved, but vague pain across the forefoot (*metatarsalgia*) is less specific and is often associated with uneven loading and muscle fatigue. Often the main complaint is of shoe pressure on a tender corn over a toe joint or a callosity on the sole. Osteoarthritic pain at the first metatarsophalangeal (MTP) joint is often better in firm-soled shoes; hallux valgus/bunions will be exacerbated by close-fitting shoes; a functionally or mechanically unstable ankle often feels better in boots; metatarsalgia is worse in shoes with a higher heel. Morton's neuroma or a prominent metatarsal head feels like a marble or pebble in the shoe.

Deformity is sometimes the main complaint; the patient may abhor a 'crooked toe' or a 'twisted foot', even if it is not painful, and parents often worry about their children who are 'flat-footed' or 'pigeon-toed'. Elderly patients may complain chiefly of having difficulty fitting shoes.

Swelling is common, even in normal people, but it gains more significance if it is unilateral or strictly localized.

Instability of the ankle or subtalar joint produces repeated episodes of the joint 'giving way'. Ask about any previous injury (a 'twisted ankle').

Numbness and *paraesthesia* may be felt in all the toes or in a circumscribed field served by a single nerve or one of the nerve roots from the spine.

General questions that help in reaching a diagnosis, assessing the impact of the condition on function and deciding on treatment in foot and ankle problems are: Have you any pain or stiffness in your muscles, joints or back? Can you dress yourself completely without any difficulty? Can you walk up and down stairs without any difficulty?

SIGNS WITH PATIENT UPRIGHT

It is important to see the patient stand, as deformities will often be much better shown once the patient is weightbearing. The patient, whose lower limbs should be exposed from the knees down, stands first facing the surgeon, then with his or her back to the surgeon. Ask the patient to rise up on tiptoes and then settle back on the heels. Note the posture of the feet throughout this movement. Normally the heels are in slight valgus while standing and inverted on tiptoes; the degree of inversion should be equal on the two sides, showing that the subtalar joint is mobile and the tibialis posterior functioning. Viewed from behind, if there is excessive eversion of one foot, the lateral toes are more easily visible on that side (the '*too-many-toes*' sign).

Gait Observing the gait also helps to identify dynamic problems and pathology on other lower limb joints. The patient is asked to walk normally. Note whether the gait is smooth or halting and whether the feet are well balanced. Gait is easier to analyze if concentrating on the sequence of movements that make up the walking cycle. It begins with heel-strike, then moves into stance, then push-off and finally swing-through before making the next heel-strike. The stance phase itself can be further divided into three intervals: (1) from heel-strike to flat foot; (2) progressive ankle dorsiflexion as the body passes over the foot; (3) ankle plantarflexion leading to toe-off.

Gait may be disturbed by pain, muscle weakness, deformity or stiffness. The position and mobility of each ankle is of prime importance. A fixed equinus deformity results in the heel failing to strike the

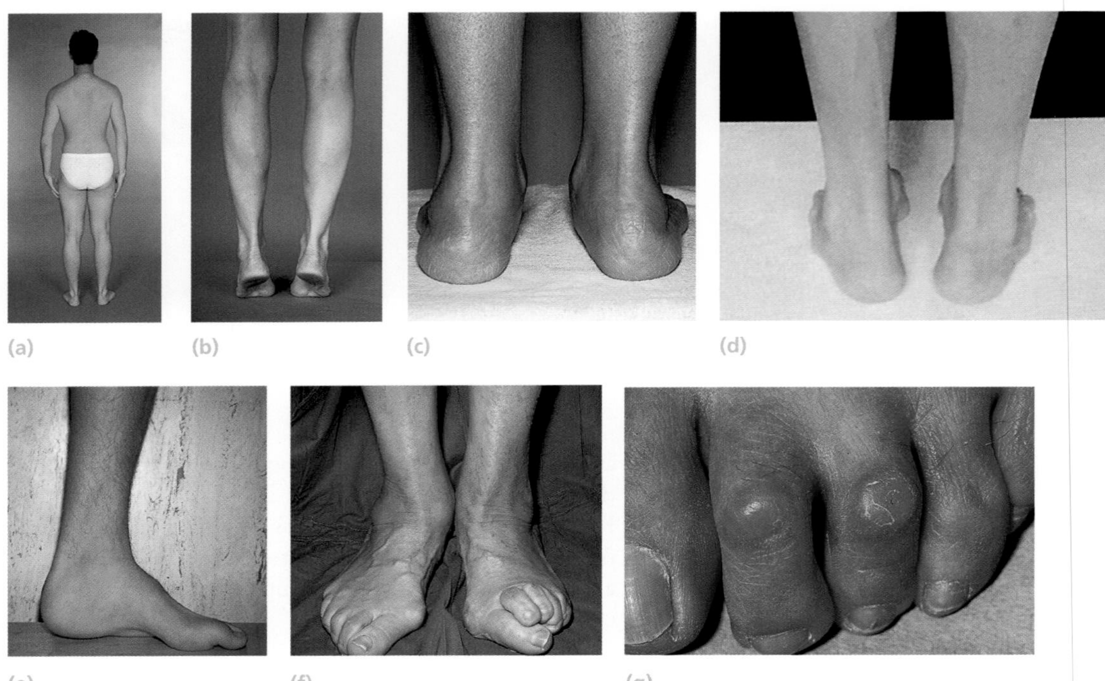

21.1 Examination with patient standing Look at the patient as a whole, first from in front and from behind. (a,b) The heels are normally in slight valgus and should invert equally when a patient stands on his/her toes. (c) This patient has flat feet (pes planus), while the patient in (d) has the opposite deformity, varus heels and an abnormally high longitudinal arch – pes cavus (e). From the front you can again notice (f) the dropped longitudinal arch in the patient with pes planus, as well as the typical deformities of bilateral hallux valgus and overriding toes. (g) Corns on the top of the toes are common.

ground at the beginning of the walking cycle; sometimes the patient forces heel contact by hyperextending the knee.

If the ankle dorsiflexors are weak, the forefoot may hit the ground prematurely, causing a 'slap'; this is referred to as foot-drop (or drop-foot). During swing-through the leg is lifted higher than usual so that the foot can clear the ground (a high-stepping gait).

21.2 Gait – the three rockers of ankle-stance phase The first rocker begins with heel-strike – if the anterior compartment muscles are weak, a 'foot-slap' is noticeable; or if the ankle is in fixed equinus, this rocker may be absent altogether. In mid-stance, the centre of gravity of the body (and ground reaction force) moves from a position posterior to the ankle joint to anterior (second rocker). The third rocker produces an acceleration force that shifts the fulcrum of the pivot forwards to the metatarsal heads, just prior to toe-off (Gage, 1991).

Hindfoot and midfoot deformities may interfere with level ground-contact in the second interval of stance; the patient walks on the inner or outer border of the foot.

Toe contact, especially of the great toe, is also important; pain or stiffness in the first MTP joint may prevent normal push-off.

Signs with patient sitting or lying

A systematic approach to examination, following the 'look, feel, move' steps, will lead to a diagnosis in the majority of cases.

Next the patient is examined lying on a couch, or it may be more convenient if he or she sits opposite the examiner and places each foot in turn on the examiner's lap.

Look

The heel is held square so that any foot deformity can be assessed. The toes and sole should be inspected for *skin changes.* The foot shows areas of overload by producing callosities, and there are often corresponding areas of wear and signs of overload on the footwear. Thickening and keratosis may be seen over the proximal toe joints or on the soles. Atrophic changes in the

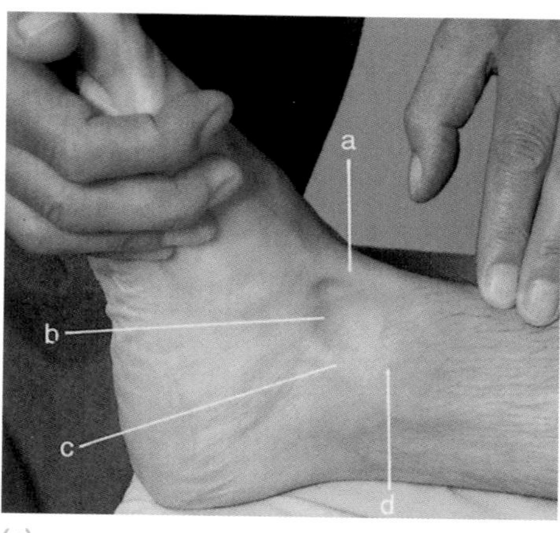

(a)

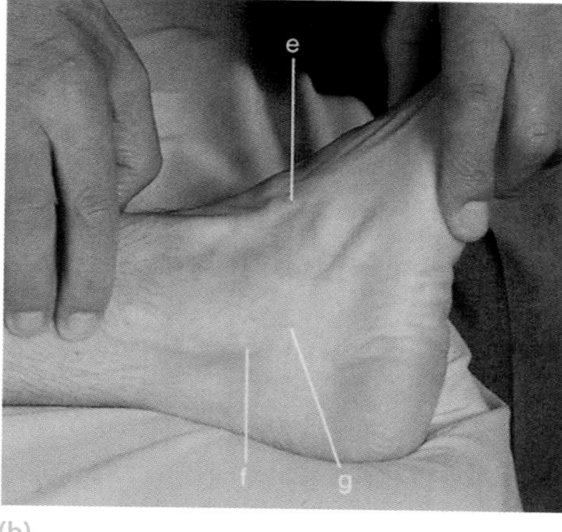

(b)

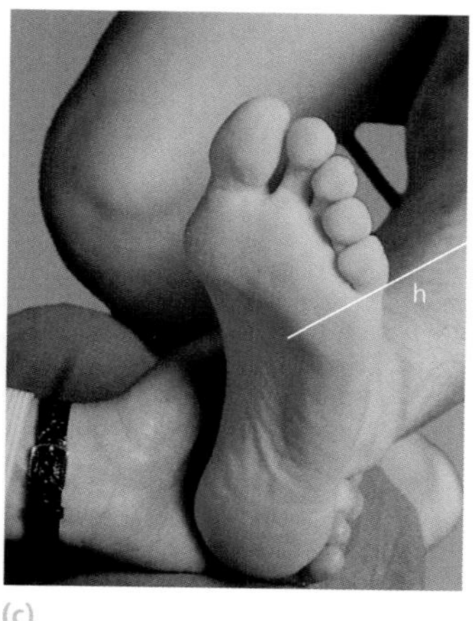

(c)

21.3 Foot – surface anatomy Medial aspect: **a**, tendon of tibialis anterior; **b**, medial malleolus; **c**, tendon of tibialis posterior; **d**, sulcus behind medial malleolus; **e**, extensor tendons of toes; **f**, lateral malleolus; **g**, peroneal tendons curving behind the lateral malleolus; **h**, anterior metatarsal arch.

skin and toe-nails are suggestive of a neurological or vascular disorder.

Deformity may be in the ankle, the foot or toes. A foot that is set flat on the ground at a right angle to the tibia is described as *plantigrade*; if it is set in fixed plantarflexion (pointing downwards) it is said to be in *equinus*; a dorsiflexed position is called *calcaneus*. Common defects are a 'flat-footed' stance (*pes valgus*); an abnormally high instep (*pes cavus*); a downward-arched forefoot (*pes plantaris*); lateral deviation of the great toe (*hallux valgus*); fixed flexion of a single interphalangeal (IP) joint (*hammer toe*) or of all the toes (*claw toes*).

Swelling may be diffuse and bilateral, or localized; unilateral swelling nearly always has a surgical cause and bilateral swelling is more often 'medical' in origin. Swelling over the medial side of the first metatarsal head (a *bunion*) is common in older women.

Corns are usually obvious; *callosities* must be looked for on the soles of the feet.

Feel

Pain and tenderness in the foot and ankle localize very well to the affected structures – the patient really does show us where the problem is. The skin temperature is assessed and the pulses are felt. Remember that one in every six normal people does not have a dorsalis pedis artery. If all the foot pulses are absent, feel for the popliteal and femoral pulses; the patient may need further evaluation by Doppler ultrasound.

If there is tenderness in the foot it must be precisely localized, for its site is often diagnostic. Any swelling, oedema or lumps must be examined.

Sensation may be abnormal; the precise distribution of any change is important. If a neuropathy is suspected (e.g. in a diabetic patient) test also for vibration sense, protective sensation and sense of position in the toes.

Move

The foot comprises a series of joints that should be examined methodically:

- *Ankle joint* – With the heel grasped in the left hand and the midfoot in the right, the ranges of plantarflexion (flexion) and dorsiflexion (extension) are estimated. Beware not to let the foot go into valgus during passive dorsiflexion as this will give an erroneous idea of the range of movement.
- *Subtalar joint* – It is important to 'lock' the ankle joint when assessing subtalar inversion and eversion. This is done simply by ensuring that the ankle is plantigrade when the heel is moved. It is often easier to record the amount of subtalar movement if the patient is examined prone. Inversion is normally greater than eversion.
- *Midtarsal joint* – One hand grips the heel firmly to stabilize the hindfoot while the other hand moves the forefoot up and down and from side to side.
- *Toes* – The MTP and IP joints are tested separately. Extension (dorsiflexion) of the great toe at the MTP joint should normally exceed 70 degrees and flexion 10 degrees.

Stability

Stability is assessed by moving the joints across the normal physiological planes and noting any abnormal 'clunks'. Ankle stability should be tested in both coronal and sagittal planes, always comparing the two joints. Patients with recent ligament injury may have to be examined under anaesthesia.

WHERE DOES IT HURT; WHERE IS IT TENDER?
Anterior ankle joint line – impingement from osteophytes in OA
Anterolateral angle of ankle joint – lateral gutter impingement in post-traumatic ankle with soft tissue problems
Bony tip/lateral malleolus – ankle fracture (Ottawa guidelines)
Posterior/inferior to lateral malleolus – peroneal tenosynovitis or tear
Posterior to medial malleolus/line of tibialis posterior – tibialis posterior tendinitis or tear, and in plano-valgus collapse of hindfoot
Base of fifth metatarsal – fracture/insertional problem with peroneus brevis
Achilles tendon – Achilles tendinitis/paratendinitis
Achilles insertion – insertional tendinitis
Retrocalcaneal bursa – bursitis
Plantar fascia – plantar fasciitis
Medial to first MTP joint – bunion
Dorsal to first MTP joint – OA, hallux limitus/rigidus
Beneath first MTP joint – sesamoiditis
Beneath metatarsal heads – 'metatarsalgia'
In third interspace – Morton's neuroma

Medial and *lateral stability* are checked by stressing the ankle first in valgus and then in varus. *Anteroposterior stability* is assessed by performing an anterior 'drawer test': the patient lies on the examination couch with hips and knees flexed and the feet resting on the couch surface; the examiner grasps the distal tibia with both hands and pushes firmly backwards, feeling for abnormal translation of the tibia upon the talus. Another way of doing this is to stabilize the distal tibia with one hand while the other grasps the heel and tries to shift the hindfoot forwards and backwards.

The same tests can be performed under x-ray and the positions of the two ankles measured and compared.

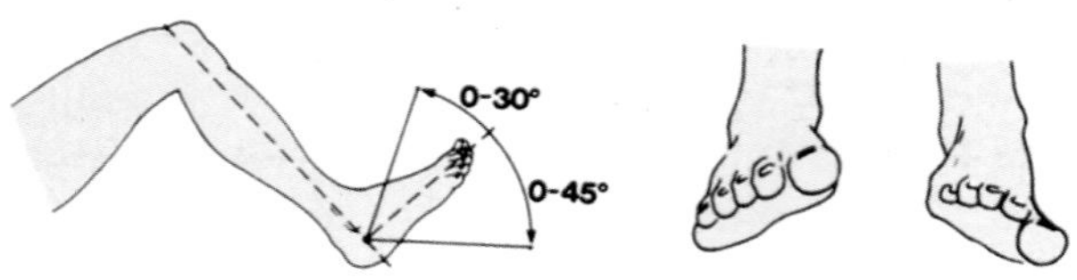

21.4 Normal range of movement All movements are measured from zero with the foot in the 'neutral' or 'anatomical' position: thus, dorsiflexion is 0–15 degrees and plantarfexion 0–40 degrees. Inversion is about 30 degrees and eversion 15 degrees.

Muscle power

Power is tested by resisting active movement in each direction. The patient will be more cooperative if the movement required is demonstrated precisely. While the movement is held, feel the muscle belly and tendon to establish whether they are intact and functioning.

Shoes

Footwear often adds additional clues when examining the foot and ankle, providing valuable information about faulty stance or gait.

General examination

If there are any symptoms or signs of vascular or neurological impairment, or if multiple joints are affected, a more general examination is essential.

Imaging

There are practical problems with imaging in children, and babies in particular because: (1) babies tend not to keep still during examination; (2) their bones are not completely ossified and their shape and position may be hard to define.

X-rays In the adult, the standard views of the ankle are anteroposterior (AP), mortise (an AP view with the ankle internally rotated 15–20 degrees) and lateral. Although the subtalar joint can be seen in a lateral view of the foot, medial and lateral oblique projections allow better assessment of the joint. These views are often used to check articular congruity after treatment of calcaneal fractures. The calcaneum itself is usually x-rayed in axial and lateral views, but a weightbearing view is helpful in defining its relationship to the talus and tibia. The foot, toes and intertarsal joints are well displayed in standing anteroposterior and medial oblique views, but occasionally a true lateral view is needed.

Stress x-rays These complement the clinical tests for ankle stability. The patient should be completely relaxed; if the ankle is too painful, stress x-rays can be performed under regional or general anaesthesia. Both ankles should be examined, for comparison.

CT scan CT provides excellent coronal views and is important in assessing fractures and congenital bony coalitions.

Radioscintigraphy Radioisotope scanning, though non-specific, is excellent for localizing areas of abnormal blood flow or bone remodelling activity; it is useful in the diagnosis of covert infection.

MRI and ultrasound These methods are used to demonstrate soft tissue problems, such as tendon and ligament injuries.

Pedobarography

A record of pressures beneath the foot can be obtained by having the patient stand or walk over a force plate; sensors in the plate produce a dynamic map of the peak pressures and the time over which these are recorded can be obtained. Although this is sometimes helpful in clinical decision making, or for comparing pre- and postoperative function, the investigation is used mainly as a research tool.

CONGENITAL DEFORMITIES

Congenital deformities of the foot are common. Many appear as part of a more widespread genetic disorder; only those in which the foot is the main (or only) problem are considered in this section. Isolated abnormalities of the toes are also dealt with elsewhere.

Talipes equinovarus (idiopathic club-foot)

The term '*talipes*' is derived from *talus* (Latin = ankle bone) and *pes* (Latin = foot). Equinovarus is one of several different talipes deformities; others are talipes calcaneus and talipes valgus.

In the full-blown equinovarus deformity the heel is in equinus, the entire hindfoot in varus and the mid- and forefoot adducted and supinated. The abnormality is relatively common, the incidence ranging from 1–2 per thousand births; boys are affected twice as often as girls and the condition is bilateral in one-third of cases.

The exact cause is not known, although the resemblance to other disorders suggests several possible mechanisms. It could be a germ defect, or a form of

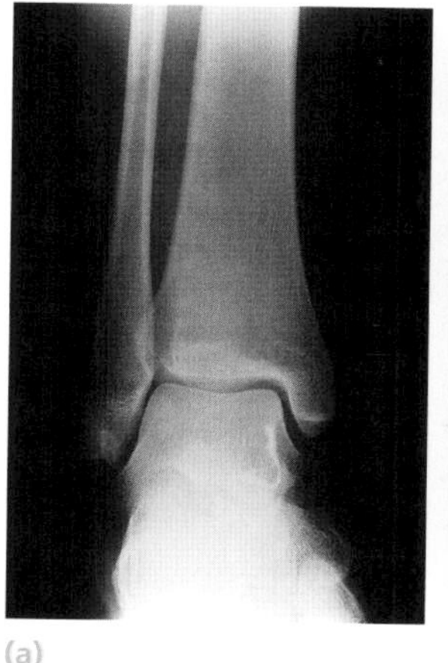
(a)

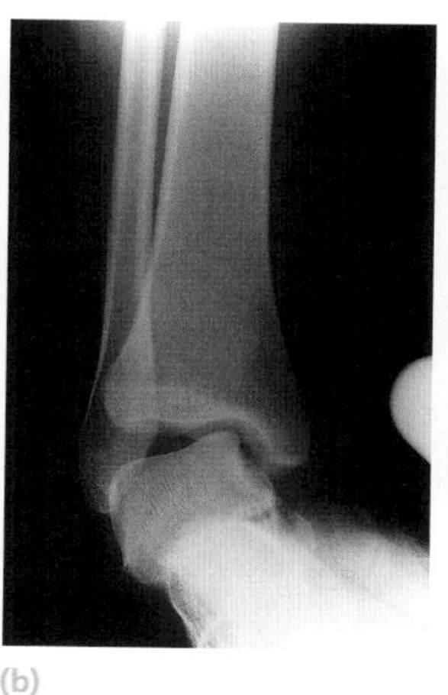
(b)

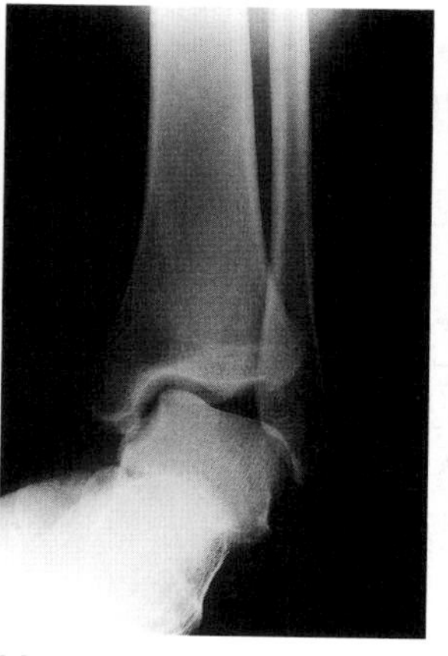
(c)

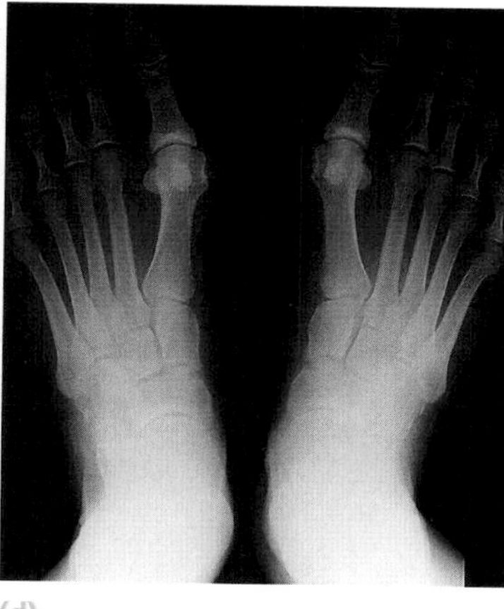
(d)

21.5 X-rays (a) AP view of the ankle in a young woman who complained that after twisting her right ankle it kept giving way in high-heeled shoes. The x-ray looks normal; the articular cartilage width (the 'joint space') is the same at all aspects of the joint. The inversion stress view (b) shows that the talus tilts excessively; always x-ray both ankles for comparison and in this case the left ankle (c) does the same. She has generalized joint hypermobility, not a torn lateral ligament. (d) X-rays of the feet should be taken with the feet flat on the ground.

arrested development. Its occurrence in neurological disorders and neural tube defects (e.g. myelomeningocele and spinal dysraphism) points to a neuromuscular disorder. Severe examples of club-foot are seen in association with arthrogryposis, tibial deficiency and constriction rings. In some cases it is no more than a postural deformity caused by tight packing in an overcrowded uterus.

Pathological anatomy

The neck of the talus points downwards and deviates medially, whereas the body is rotated slightly outwards in relation to both the calcaneum and the ankle mortise (Herzenberg et al., 1988). The posterior part of the calcaneum is held close to the fibula by a tight calcaneo-fibular ligament, and is tilted into equinus and varus; it is also rotated medially beneath the ankle. The navicular and entire forefoot are shifted medially and rotated into supination (the composite varus deformity).

The skin and soft tissues of the calf and the medial side of the foot are short and underdeveloped. If the condition is not corrected early, secondary growth changes occur in the bones; these are permanent. Even with treatment the foot is liable to be short and the calf may remain thin.

Clinical features

The deformity is usually obvious at birth; the foot is both turned and twisted inwards so that the sole faces posteromedially. More precisely, the ankle is in equinus, the heel is inverted and the forefoot is adducted and supinated; sometimes the foot also has a high medial arch (cavus), and the talus may protrude on the dorsolateral surface of the foot. The heel is usually small and high, and deep creases appear posteriorly and medially; some of these creases are incomplete constriction bands. In some cases the calf is abnormally thin.

In a normal baby the foot can be dorsiflexed and everted until the toes touch the front of the leg. In club-foot this manoeuvre meets with varying degrees of resistance and in severe cases the deformity is fixed.

The infant must always be examined for associated disorders such as congenital hip dislocation and spina bifida. The absence of creases suggests arthrogryposis; look to see if other joints are affected.

X-rays

X-rays are used mainly to assess progress after treatment. The *anteroposterior film* is taken with the foot 30 degrees plantarflexed and the tube likewise angled 30 degrees perpendicular. Lines can be drawn through the long axis of the talus parallel to its medial border and through that of the calcaneum parallel to its lateral border; they normally cross at an angle of 20–40 degrees (Kite's angle) but in club-foot the two lines may be almost parallel. Incomplete ossification makes it difficult to decide exactly where to draw these lines and this means that there is a considerable degree of interobserver variation.

The *lateral film* is taken with the foot in forced dorsiflexion. Lines drawn through the midlongitudinal axis of the talus and the lower border of the calcaneum should meet at an angle of about 40 degrees. Anything less than 20 degrees shows that the calcaneum cannot be tilted up into true dorsiflexion; the foot may seem to be dorsiflexed but it may actually have 'broken' at the midtarsal level, producing the so-called *rocker-bottom deformity*.

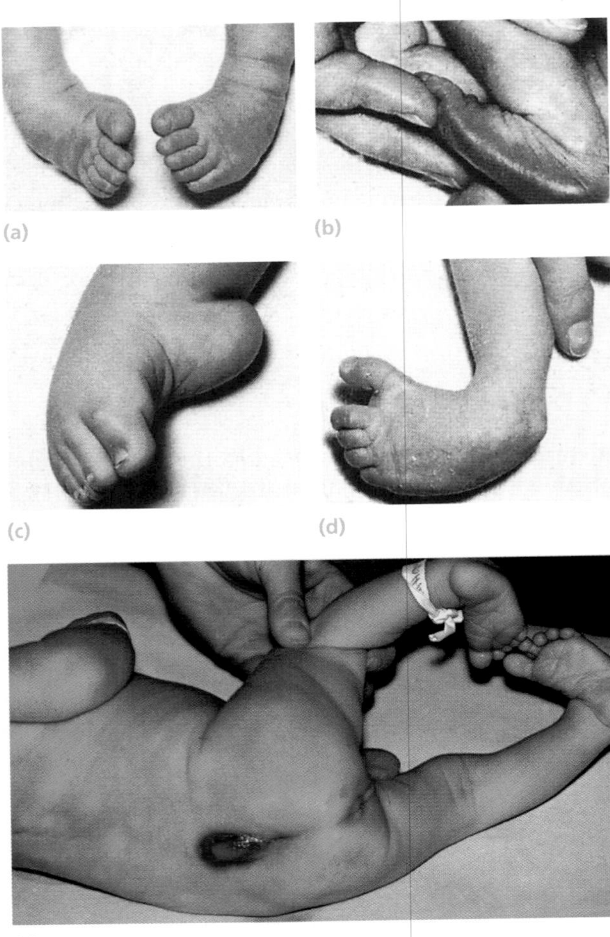

21.6 Talipes equinovarus (club-foot) (a) True club-foot is a fixed deformity, unlike (b) postural talipes, which is easily correctable by gentle passive movement. (c,d) With true club-foot, the poorly developed heel is higher than the forefoot, which points downwards and inwards (varus). (e) Always examine the hips for congenital dislocation and the back for spina bifida (as in the case shown here).

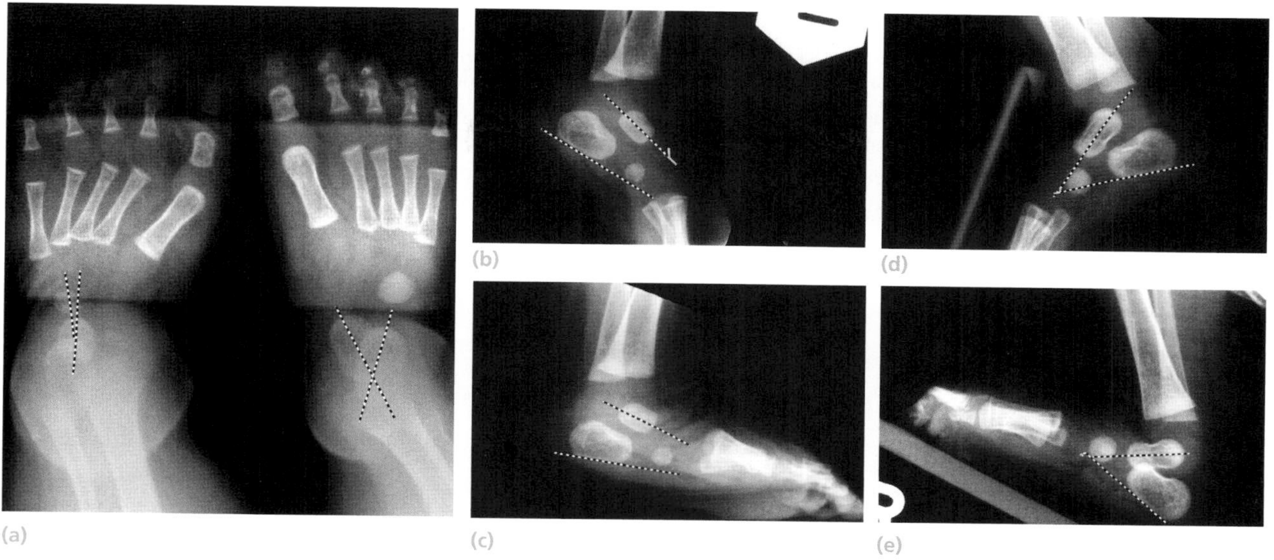

21.7 Talipes equinovarus – x-rays The left foot is abnormal. In the anteroposterior view (a) the talocalcaneal angle is 5 degrees, compared to 42 degrees on the right. In the lateral views, the left talocalcaneal angle is 10 degrees in plantarflexion (b) and 15 degrees in dorsiflexion (c). In the normal foot the angle is unchanged at 44 degrees, whatever the position of the foot (d,e).

Treatment

The aim of treatment is to produce and maintain a plantigrade, supple foot that will function well. There are several methods of treatment but relapse is common, especially in babies with associated neuromuscular disorders.

CONSERVATIVE TREATMENT

Treatment should begin early, preferably within a day or two of birth. This consists of repeated manipulation and adhesive strapping that maintains the correction; the manipulations are taught to the child's mother, who is then able to carry out gentle stretches on a regular basis with the strapping still in place. Treatment is supervised by a physiotherapist, who alters the strapping as correction is gradually obtained. If this level of care is not available, it may be better to hold position by applying a light plaster cast (over a protective layer of strapping), which is soaked off and changed every week.

The three main components of the deformity are always corrected in the following order. First the forefoot must be brought into rotational alignment with the hindfoot; paradoxically this is done by increasing the supination deformity of the forefoot so that it corresponds with the relatively more supinated hindfoot. Next, both hindfoot and forefoot are together gradually brought out of varus and supination; correction is assisted by keeping the fulcrum on the lateral side of the head of the talus. Finally, equinus is corrected by bringing the heel down and dorsiflexing the foot. It may be necessary, en route, to perform percutaneous tendo Achillis lengthening in order to overcome the equinus (Ponsetti, 1992).

The objective (ideally) is to achieve not only correction but *overcorrection*. The position should be checked by x-ray in order to ensure that there is no rocker-bottom defect; attempts to overcome equinus before the other deformities are corrected may 'break' the foot in the midtarsal region.

Resistant cases will usually declare themselves after 8–12 weeks of serial manipulations and strapping. The surgeon then faces a choice of early surgery or continued conservative treatment. The results of early operation, in particular neonatal surgery, have not been shown to be better than those of late surgery. Delaying surgery until the child is near walking age has the advantages of operating on a larger foot (making surgery easier) and using the forces in normal walking to help maintain the correction obtained at surgery.

This delayed operative approach is suitable for severe, rigid deformities; however, for less severe cases it may be preferable to operate at around 6 months of age, but manipulation and splintage must still be continued until the child is walking.

OPERATIVE TREATMENT

The objectives of club-foot surgery are: (1) the complete release of joint 'tethers' (capsular and ligamentous contractures and fibrotic bands); (2) lengthening of tendons so that the foot can be positioned normally without undue tension. A detailed knowledge of the pathological anatomy is a *sine qua non*.

Access to the involved structures is through either an extended posteromedial incision (Turco, 1971), a posterior curved transverse incision extended anteriorly on both medial and lateral sides ('Cincinatti' – Crawford et al., 1982), or a posterolateral incision combined with a separate curved medial incision (Caroll, 1994). The tendo Achillis and tibialis posterior tendons are lengthened through Z-divisions; the posterior capsules of the ankle and subtalar joints often have to be divided to allow adequate correction of hindfoot equinus. Sometimes flexor digitorum longus and flexor hallucis longus also require attention. The calcaneo-fibular ligament, a key structure in keeping the calcaneum malrotated, is then released. A complete subtalar release is performed to allow the hindfoot to be corrected. The superficial deltoid ligament is freed on the medial side but the deep part is preserved to prevent ankle instability.

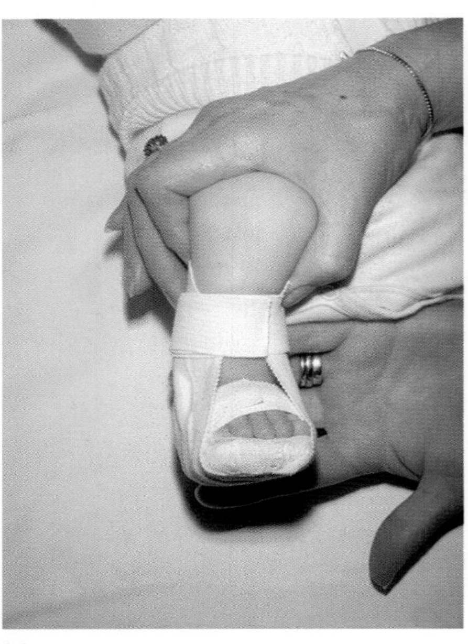
(a)

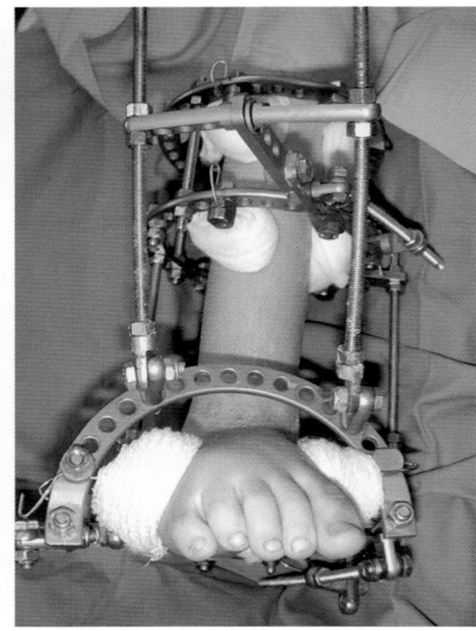
(d)

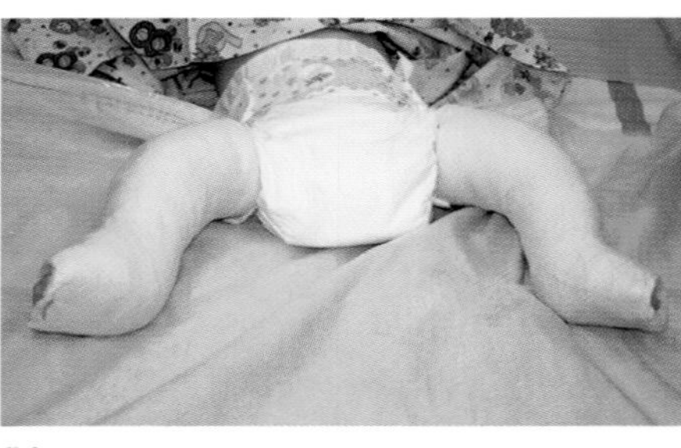
(b)

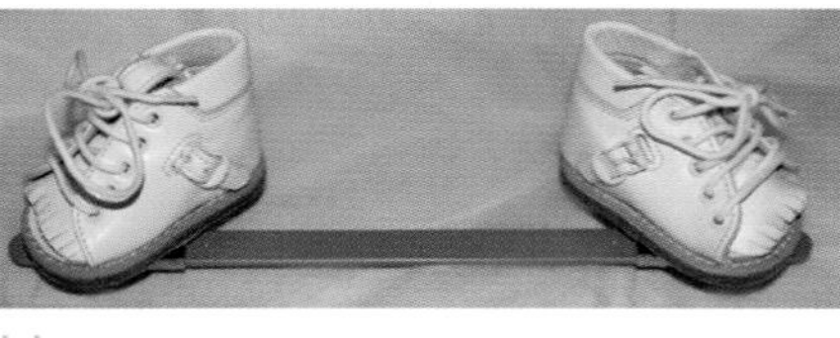
(e)

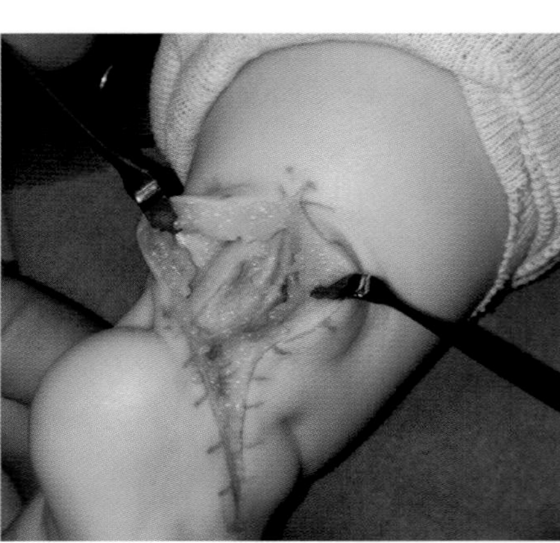
(c)

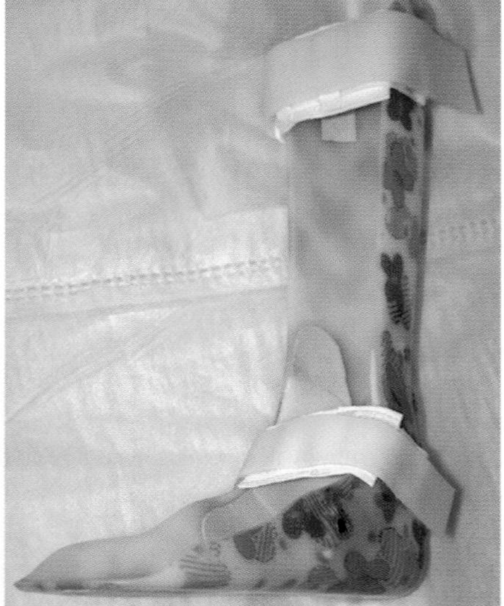
(f)

21.8 Congenital talipes equinovarus – treatment First-line treatment is non-operative. This may be by manipulation and strapping (a) or serial casting (b). If insufficient correction is achieved, a formal open release may be needed (c). Severe relapses need more radical forms of treatment such as the Ilizarov fixator (d). After successful correction of deformity, relapses may be prevented by using Dennis Browne boots in infants (e) or moulded ankle–foot orthoses (f) in older children.

Correction of the forefoot deformity is carried out by releasing the contractures around the talonavicular and calcaneocuboid joints. The interosseous ligament in the sinus canal should be preserved, especially in children with ligamentous laxity, as division may lead to overcorrection. Finally, the origin of the intrinsic muscles and plantar fascia from the calcaneum may need to be divided to reduce any cavus or plantaris deformity.

The foot, in its corrected position, is immobilized in a plaster cast. K-wires are sometimes inserted across the talonavicular and subtalar joints to augment the hold. The wires and cast are removed at 6–8 weeks, after which hobble boots or a custom-made ankle–foot orthosis is used, depending on whether the child has started walking. Stretching exercises that were performed prior to surgery are continued. The period of splintage varies: some surgeons wait until active dorsiflexion and eversion are established whereas others recommend some form of splintage until skeletal maturity.

LATE OR RELAPSED CLUB-FOOT

Late presenters often have severe deformities with secondary bony changes, and the relapsed club-foot is complicated by scarring from previous surgery. If the child is young (aged 4–7), a revision of the soft tissue releases may be considered together with a shortening of the lateral side of the foot by calcaneo-cuboid fusion or cuboid enucleation (The Dilwyn–Evans operation – Evans, 1961). Calcaneal osteotomies, in the form of lateral closing wedges or lateral translations, improve heel varus. Tendon transfers, once popular, now have a more limited role; a split tibialis anterior tendon transfer to the dorsum of the base of the fourth metatarsal may help balance weak evertors, whereas a transfer of tibialis posterior through the interosseous membrane to the dorsum will act as a dorsiflexor in neurological cases. Tendon transfers work well only if the joints are mobile, and this is seldom the case in these patients.

Gradual correction by means of a circular external fixator (the Ilizarov method) has gained popularity in treating difficult relapsed cases and severe deformities; the early results are encouraging. Full corrections can be achieved even in feet severely scarred from previous surgery, and there is often an increase in the size of the foot, which is thought to be due to an increase in the blood supply during distraction. The procedure can be painful and long and for the time being it is best reserved for these very difficult cases.

Despite initially successful surgery, deformities do still recur. A deformed, stiff and painful foot in an adolescent is best salvaged by corrective osteotomies and fusions. The distorted anatomy makes triple arthrodesis a real challenge but it is possible to end up with a plantigrade, stable and pain-free foot.

METATARSUS ADDUCTUS

Metatarsus adductus varies from a slightly curved forefoot to something resembling a mild club-foot. The majority (90 per cent) either improve spontaneously or can be managed non-operatively using serial corrective casts followed by straight-last shoes. The more severe examples need operation. Extensive capsulectomies of the tarso-metatarsal joints followed by prolonged splintage have fallen out of favour because of the risk of early degenerative arthritis in the repositioned joints. Variations of the Dilwyn Evans procedure (which aims to balance the lengths of the medial and lateral columns of the foot), often in combination with basal metatarsal osteotomies, are suitable for the small percentage of children who require surgical treatment.

TALIPES CALCANEOVALGUS

Calcaneovalgus is a common deformity that presents in the newborn as an acutely dorsiflexed foot. There is a deep crease (or several wrinkles) on the front of the ankle, and the calcaneum juts out posteriorly. Unlike congenital vertical talus (which also presents as an acutely dorsiflexed foot) this deformity is flexible. In addition, the anterior creases in congenital vertical talus are located over the midfoot.

Calcaneovalgus is usually bilateral. There is an association with hip dysplasia, especially if it presents on one side only; examination of the hips followed by ultrasound or x-ray examination is therefore recommended.

This is a postural deformity, probably due to abnormal intrauterine positioning, and it often corrects spontaneously in the neonatal period. Severe deformities occasionally require serial casts for correction.

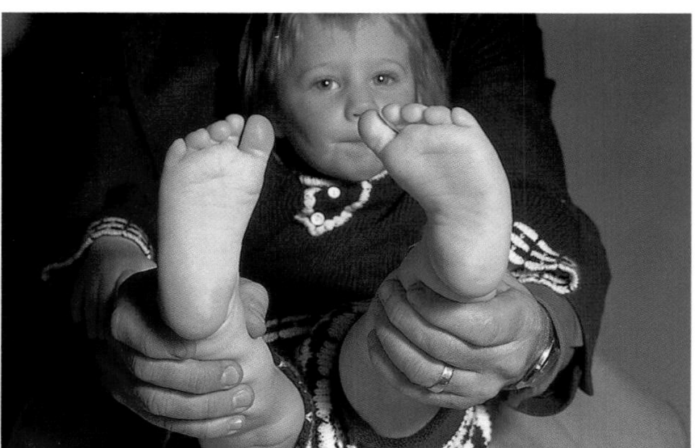

21.9 Metatarsus adductus In contrast to club-foot, the deformity here is limited to the forefoot.

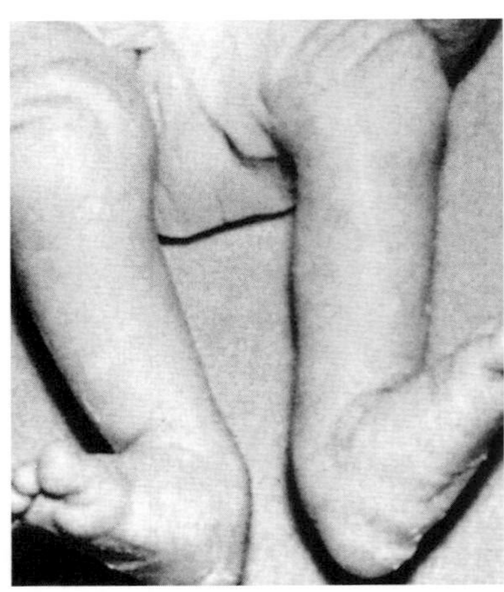

21.10 Talipes calcaneovalgus Bilateral calcaneovalgus. This benign 'deformity' can be easily corrected without hurting the baby. Over time it usually corrects spontaneously.

Congenital convex pes valgus (congenital vertical talus)

This rare condition is seen in infants, usually affecting both feet. Superficially it resembles other types of valgus foot, but the deformity is more severe; the medial arch is not only flat, it is the most prominent part of the sole, producing the appearance of a rocker-bottom foot. The hindfoot is in equinus and valgus and the talus points almost vertically towards the sole; the forefoot is abducted, pronated and dorsiflexed, with subluxation of the talonavicular joint. Passive correction is impossible; by the time the child is seen, the tendons and ligaments on the dorsolateral side of the foot are usually shortened.

X-ray features The calcaneum is in equinus and the talus points into the sole of the foot, with the navicular dislocated dorsally onto the neck of the talus. It is important to repeat the lateral x-ray with the foot maximally plantarflexed; in congenital vertical talus the appearance will be unchanged, whereas in flexible flat-foot the dorsally subluxated navicular returns to the normal position.

Treatment The only effective treatment is by operation, ideally before the age of 2 years. Correction is done in one stage through separate incisions. The tendo Achillis is lengthened, with capsulotomies of the ankle and subtalar joints; via a medial approach the talonavicular joint is reduced and the tibialis anterior tendon is transferred to the neck of the talus; if necessary, the lateral structures are lengthened or released. The reduced position is held with a K-wire transfixing the talonavicular joint and plaster immobilization for 8–12 weeks (the wire can be removed at 6 weeks). Reasonably good results have been reported with this method (Duncan and Fixsen, 1999).

PES PLANUS AND PES VALGUS ('FLAT-FOOT')

"Our feet are no more alike than our faces." This truism from a *British Medical Journal* editorial sums up the problem of 'normally abnormal' feet. The medial arch may be normally high or normally low. The term 'flat-foot' applies when the apex of the arch has collapsed and the medial border of the foot is in contact (or nearly in contact) with the ground; the heel becomes valgus and the foot pronates at the subtalar-midtarsal complex. The problems associated with flat-foot differ in babies, children and adults and these three categories will therefore be considered separately.

Flat-foot in children and adolescents

Flat-foot is a common complaint among children. Or rather their parents, grandparents, and assistants in the shoe-shop – the children themselves usually don't seem to notice it!

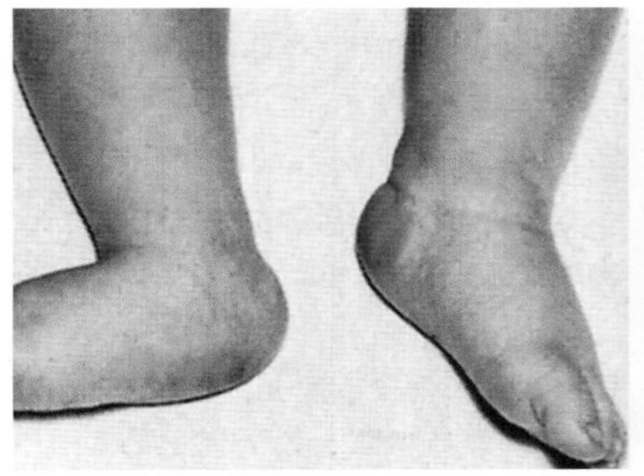

(a)

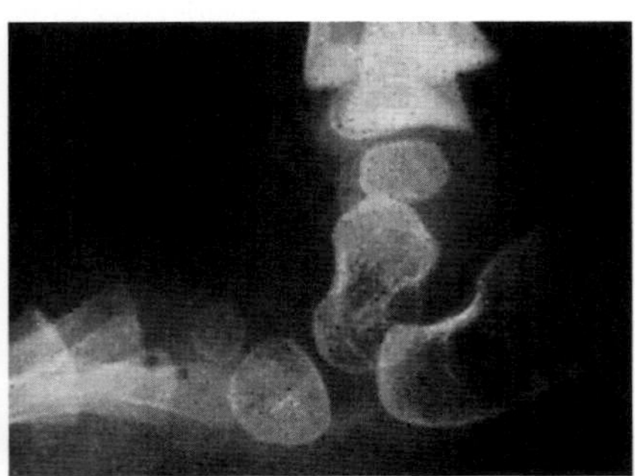

(b)

21.11 Congenital vertical talus (a) The infant's foot is in marked valgus and has a rocker-bottom shape. The deformity is rigid and cannot be corrected. (b) X-ray shows the vertical talus pointing downwards towards the sole and the other tarsal bones rotated around the head of the talus.

Flexible flat-foot Flexible pes valgus appears in toddlers as a normal stage in development, and it usually disappears after a few years, when medial arch development is complete; occasionally, though, it persists into adult life. The arch can often be restored by simply dorsiflexing the great toe (*Jack's test*), and during this manoeuvre the tibia rotates externally (Rose et al., 1985). Many of these children have ligamentous laxity and there may be a family history of both flat feet and joint hypermobility.

Stiff (or 'rigid') flat-foot A deformity that cannot be corrected passively should alert the examiner to an underlying abnormality. *Congenital vertical talus* is dealt with earlier. In older children, conditions to be considered are: (1) *tarsal coalition*; (2) *an inflammatory joint disorder*; (3) a *neurological disorder*.

Compensatory flat-foot This is a spurious deformity that occurs in order to accommodate some other postural defect. For example, a tight tendo Achillis (or a mild fixed equinus) may be accommodated by everting the foot; or if the lower limbs are externally rotated the body weight falls anteromedial to the ankle and the feet go into valgus – the Charlie Chaplin look.

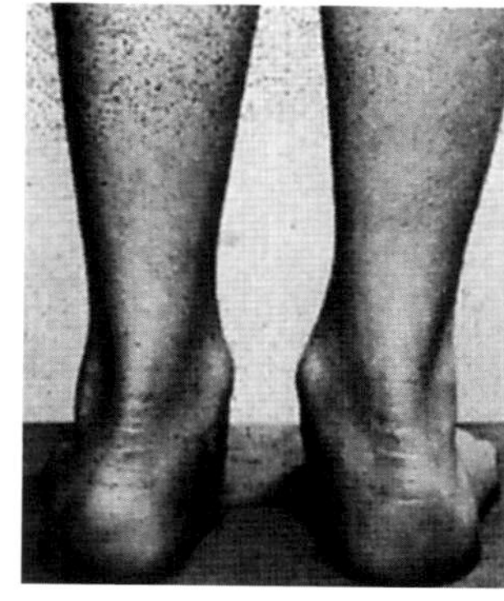

(a)

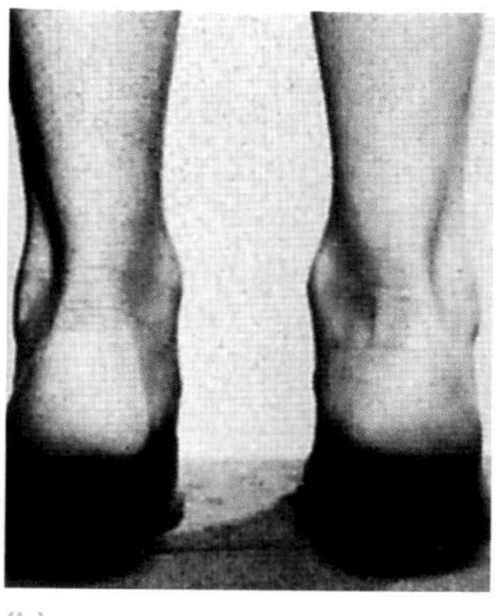

(b)

21.12 Mobile flat feet (a) Standing with the feet flat on the floor, the medial arches appear to have dropped and the heels are in valgus. (b) When the patient goes up on his toes, the medial arches are restored, indicating that these are 'mobile' flat feet. If this does not occur, look carefully for a tarsal coalition.

Clinical assessment

Although there is usually nothing to worry about, the parents' concerns should not be dismissed without a proper assessment of the child. Enquire about neonatal problems and a family history.

Watch the child stand and note the position of the heels from behind. Are they in neutral or valgus, and do they invert when the child stands on tiptoe? The tiptoe test will confirm a mobile subtalar joint and functioning tibialis posterior tendon. Let the child walk: is the gait normal for the child's age? Are the heels set flat during the stance phase, or does the child have tight Achilles tendons?

Examine the foot and note its shape. In the neonate, the rare congenital vertical talus presents as a stiff, acutely dorsiflexed and very flat (almost rocker-bottom) foot. Palpate for tenderness: are there signs of arthritis or infection? Test the movements in the ankle as well as the subtalar and midtarsal joints: a tight Achilles tendon may be 'constitutional' or part of a neuromuscular problem.

Try to correct the flat-foot by gentle passive manipulation. Perform Jack's test (see earlier) to distinguish between a flexible and a stiff ('rigid') deformity.

The spine, hips and knees also should be examined. The clinical assessment is completed by a swift general examination for joint hypermobility and signs of neuromuscular abnormalities.

PERONEAL SPASTIC FLAT-FOOT (TARSAL COALITION)

Older children and teenagers sometimes present with a painful, rigid flat-foot in which the peroneal and extensor tendons are in spasm. X-rays and computed tomography (CT) may show one or several of a variety of unions or partial unions between adjacent tarsal bones; the commonest are talocalcaneal, calcaneonavicular and talonavicular coalitions. The anomaly is inherited as an autosomal dominant condition and is present at birth but it becomes symptomatic only when the abnormal fibrous syndesmosis matures into a stiffer, cartilaginous synchondrosis that later ossifies to become a rigid bar.

The child, usually at puberty or during early adolescence, develops an increasingly stiff flat-foot deformity. Pain may be due to abnormal tarsal stress or even fracture of an ossified bar. The picture differs from that of the more common 'idiopathic' flat-foot in that the deformity is more or less rigid, with spasm of the peroneal muscles. The diagnosis is confirmed by x-ray and/or CT, but other causes of rigid flat-foot must be excluded (e.g. inflammatory arthritis and infection of the hind- or midfoot).

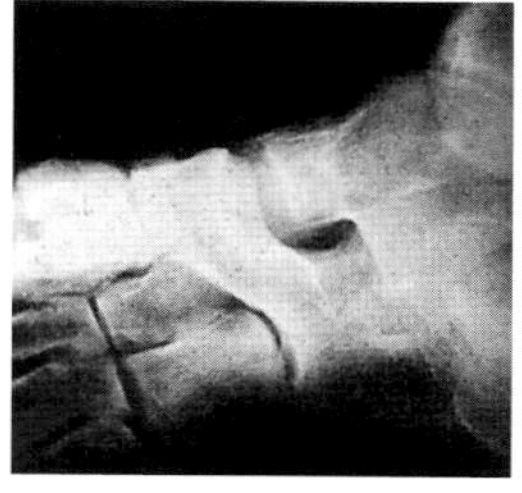

(a)

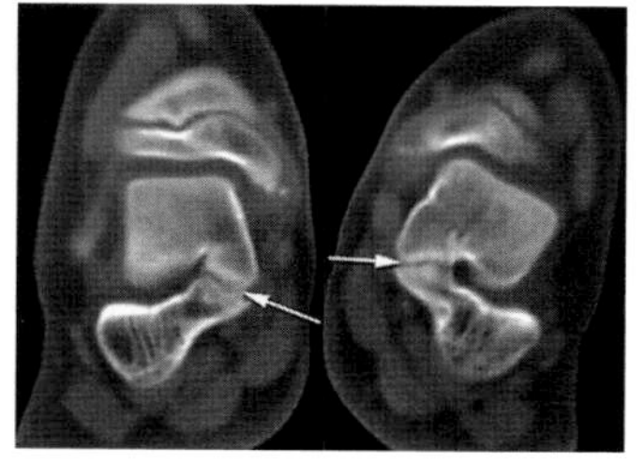

(b)

21.13 Tarsal coalition (a) X-ray appearance of a calcaneonavicular bar. (b) CT image showing incompletely ossified talocalcaneal bars bilaterally (arrows).

Imaging

X-rays are unnecessary for asymptomatic, flexible flat feet. For pathological flat feet (which are usually painful or stiff) standing anteroposterior, lateral and oblique views may help to identify underlying disorders. On the lateral view, 'beaking' of the head of the talus suggests the presence of a tarsal coalition. Narrowing of the talocalcaneal joint, which is sometimes seen in talocalcaneal coalition, is easily mistaken for 'arthritis'. Calcaneonavicular bars, if ossified, can be seen in oblique views of the foot.

CT scanning is the most reliable way of demonstrating tarsal coalitions.

Radioscintigraphy is occasionally used if a covert infection or osteoid osteoma is suspected. It may also help to identify a 'hot' accessory navicular before advocating its removal.

Treatment

Physiological flat-foot Young children with flexible flat feet require no treatment. Parents need to be reassured and told that the 'deformity' will probably correct itself in time; even if it does not fully correct, function is unlikely to be impaired. Some parents will cite examples of other children who were helped by insoles or moulded heel-cups. These appliances serve mainly to alter the pattern of weightbearing and hence that of shoe wear; simply put, they are more effective in treating the shoes than the feet.

Tight tendo Achillis Flat-foot associated with a tight tendo Achillis and restricted dorsiflexion at the ankle may benefit from tendon-stretching exercises.

Accessory navicular Sometimes the main complaint (with a flexible flat-foot) is tenderness over an unusually prominent navicular on the medial border of the midfoot. X-rays may show an extra ossicle at this site – the accessory navicular. Symptoms are due to pressure (and possibly a 'bursitis') over the bony prominence, or repetitive strain at the synchondrosis between the accessory ossicle and the navicular proper. If symptoms warrant it, the accessory bone can be shelled out from within the tibialis posterior tendon. If the medial arch has 'dropped' significantly, the tibialis posterior tendon can be used as a 'hitch' by re-inserting it through a hole drilled in the navicular and suturing the loop with the foot held in maximum inversion (Kidner's operation).

Rigid flat-foot (tarsal coalition) One of the problems with treatment of this condition is that the presence of a tarsal coalition is not necessarily the cause of the patient's symptoms; the anomaly is sometimes discovered as an incidental finding in asymptomatic feet. For this reason the initial treatment should always be conservative. A walking plaster is applied with the foot plantigrade and is retained for 6 weeks; splintage with an outside iron and inside T-strap may have to be continued for another 3–6 months. Obviously if an inflammatory joint disorder is discovered, this will have to be treated. If symptoms do not settle, operative treatment is needed. A calcaneonavicular bar can be resected without much difficulty through a lateral approach, and the operation may be performed before puberty; a portion of the bar is removed and the gap filled with fat or a piece of muscle (e.g. extensor digitorum brevis) to prevent recurrence. Talocalcaneal coalitions are more difficult to deal with and it may be wiser to wait until after the patient reaches puberty and then perform a triple arthrodesis.

FLAT-FOOT IN ADULTS

As in children, the usual picture is of a flexible flat-foot with no obvious cause. However, underlying disorders are common enough to always warrant a careful search for abnormal ligamentous laxity, tarsal coalitions, disorders of the tibialis posterior tendon, post-traumatic deformity, degenerative arthritis, neuropathy and conditions resulting in muscular imbalance.

Painful acquired flat-foot often results from tibialis posterior dysfunction. Tibialis posterior tendon dysfunction affects predominantly women in later midlife. It is usually of insidious onset, affecting one foot much more than the other, and with identifiable systemic factors such as obesity, diabetes, steroids or surgery. There may be recollection of a minor episode of trauma, such as a twisting injury to the foot. The patient experiences aching discomfort in the line of the tibialis posterior tendon, often radiating up the inner aspect of the lower leg. The foot often feels 'tired'. As the tendon stretches out the foot drifts into plano-valgus, producing the typical acquired flat-foot deformity. As the tendon ruptures the ache or pain will often improve, temporarily, but as the foot deformity then worsens the plantar fascia becomes painful and there may be lateral hindfoot pain as the fibula starts to impinge against the calcaneum.

Pathology

The tibialis posterior is a powerful muscle, with a short excursion of its tendon and a strong mechanical advantage as a foot inverter acting to help maintain the medial longitudinal arch of the foot. This tendon is probably inflamed more commonly and ruptures more frequently than the Achilles tendon. There is usually an initial tenosynovitis. Tendon elongation and rupture are probably related to an area of hypovascularity in the tendon. Once the tendon elongates

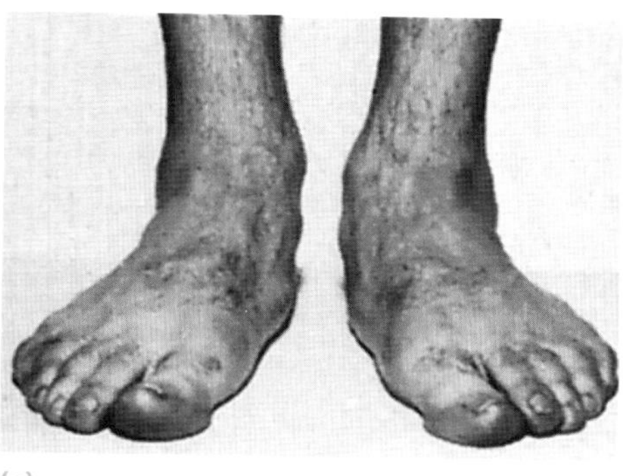

(a)

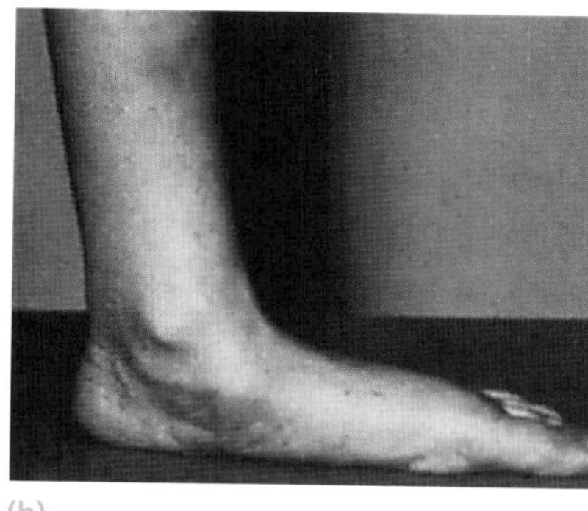

(b)

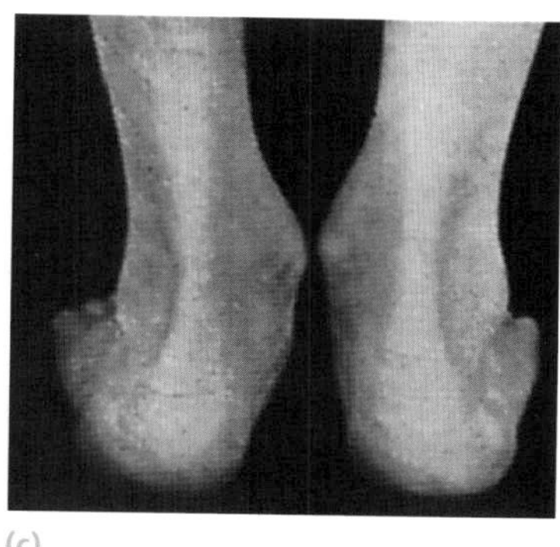

(c)

21.14 Flat-foot in adults – clinical features (a) The medial arches have dropped and the feet appear to be pronated. (b) The medial border of the foot is flat and the tuberosity of the navicular looks prominent. (c) The heels are in valgus and the toes are visible lateral to the outer edge of the heel on the left side (the 'too-many-toes' sign).

the pathology is then related to the loss of powerful hindfoot inversion, probably confounded by associated stretching of the related ligaments, in particular the spring ligament and the plantar fascia.

Examination

There is usually swelling and tenderness in the line of tibialis posterior, at and distal to the medial malleolus. The hindfoot collapse is best appreciated by viewing the patient from behind, when the valgus deformity of the heel is appreciated, and the forefoot abduction leads to 'too many toes' being seen from this position, compared to the contralateral foot. It is difficult for the patient to do a single leg heel raise, as the tibialis posterior cannot stabilize and invert the heel, impairing the heel-raise action of the Achilles tendon.

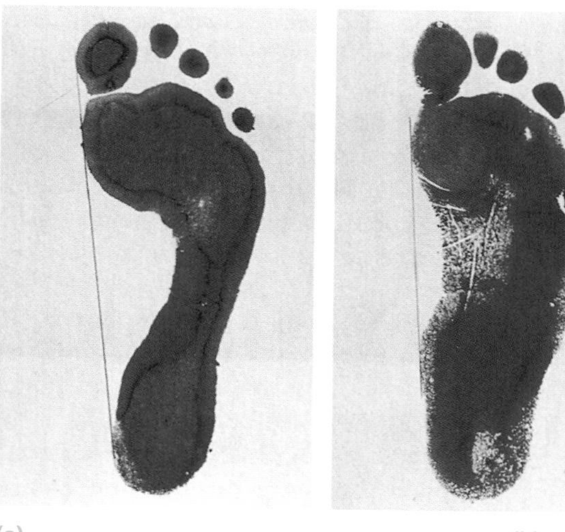

(a) (b)

21.15 Footprints Footprints made with the aid of an ink pad show the difference between normal sole contact and flat-footed contact. (a) Normal footprint, showing the main contact areas across the anterior metatarsal arch, the lateral border of the foot and the heel, with a 'hollow' corresponding to the medial arch. (b) Flat-footed contact, across the sole to the medial side of the foot.

Imaging

Weightbearing x-rays show the altered foot axes. The tendon can be assessed with ultrasound or magnetic resonance imaging (MRI) scan.

Treatment

The key point is to recognize the condition. If it is in the early stages then relative rest (sticks or crutches), support with a temporary insole, elasticated foot/ankle support and oral non-steroidal anti-inflammatory drugs (NSAIDs) may be effective. Whether or not to inject the tendon *sheath* with corticosteroid is contentious; but to inject the tendon itself is just plain wrong! These temporary measures may offer the opportunity to institute more permanent solutions, such as modification of weight and activity, and assessment for definitive orthotics.

ORTHOSES

Functional foot orthoses (FFOs) have a role to play in the adult flexible but symptomatic flat-foot. These appliances (usually called *orthotics*) are used to correct abnormal foot function or biomechanics and, in so doing, they also correct for abnormal lower extremity function; they are very much more than an 'arch support'.

Orthotics are useful in the treatment of a range of painful conditions of the foot and lower extremities, in particular first MTP joint arthritis, metatarsalgia, arch and instep pain, ankle pain and heel pain.

Since abnormal foot function may cause abnormal leg, knee and hip function, orthotics can be used to treat painful tendinitis and bursitis conditions in the ankle, knee and hip, as well as exercise-induced leg pain ('shin splints'). Some types of FFOs are also designed to accommodate painful areas on the soles of the feet (like accommodative foot orthoses).

Orthoses may be made of flexible, semi-rigid or rigid plastic or graphite materials. They are relatively thin and fit easily into several types of shoe. They are fabricated from a three-dimensional model of the foot or scanning the foot with a mechanical or optical scanner.

Assessment for orthotics can be performed by a podiatrist, who can also advise on whether the usual/intended footwear will accommodate such a device and offer the support needed for it to be effective.

'Off-the-shelf' insoles are cheaper, but there are several advantages to prescription foot orthoses. They are custom-made to precisely fit each foot, and are made in relatively rigid, durable materials with a minimal chance of discomfort or irritation to the foot and a greater potential to relieve pain.

PHYSIOTHERAPY

Local treatment of the associated inflammation with physiotherapy might be of benefit. Assessment of the hindfoot biomechanics by a podiatrist might help to prevent progression, and could offer protection to the contralateral side, which is often much less severely affected.

SURGERY

If the condition does not improve with a few weeks of conservative treatment, or the patient presents several months after onset of the symptoms, then surgical intervention should be considered. Options include surgical decompression and tenosynovestomy, or reconstruction of the tendon. The latter is often combined with a calcaneal osteotomy to help to protect the tendon and improve the axis. If there is already degeneration in the hindfoot joints then triple arthrodesis might be indicated (fusing the subtalar, calcaneo-cuboid and talonavicular joints – the ankle joint is not arthrodesed in this procedure, so foot plantarflexion and dorsiflexion are maintained).

PES CAVUS (HIGH-ARCHED FEET)

In pes cavus the arch is higher than normal, and often there is also clawing of the toes. The close resemblance to deformities seen in neurological disorders where the intrinsic muscles are weak or paralyzed suggests that all forms of pes cavus are due to some type of muscle imbalance. There are rare congenital causes, such as arthrogryposis, but in the majority of cases pes cavus results from an acquired neuromuscular disorder see Box opposite. A specific abnormality can often be identified; hereditary motor and sensory neuropathies and spinal cord abnormalities (tethered cord syndrome, diastematomyelia) are the commonest in Western countries but poliomyelitis is the most common cause worldwide. Occasionally the deformity follows trauma – burns or a compartment syndrome resulting in Volkmann's contracture of the sole.

NEUROMUSCULAR CAUSES OF PES CAVUS

Muscular dystrophies	Duchenne, Becker
Neuropathies	HMSN I and II
Cord lesions	Poliomyelitis, syringomyelia, diastomatomyelia, tethered cord
Cerebral disorders	Cerebral palsy, Friedreich's ataxia

Pathology

The toes are drawn up into a 'clawed' position, the metatarsal heads are forced down into the sole and the arch at the midfoot is accentuated. Often the heel is inverted and the soft tissues in the sole are tight. Under the prominent metatarsal heads callosities may form.

Clinical features

Patients usually present at the age of 8–10 years. Deformity may be noticed by the parents or the school doctor before there are any symptoms. There may be a past history of a spinal disorder, or a family history of neuromuscular defects. As a rule both feet are affected.

Pain may be felt under the metatarsal heads or over the toes where shoe pressure is most marked. Callosities appear at the same sites and walking tolerance is reduced. Enquire about symptoms of neurological disorders, such as muscle weakness and joint instability.

The overall cavus deformity is usually obvious; in addition the toes are often clawed and the heel may be varus. Closer inspection will show the components of the high arch; this is important because it leads to an understanding of the responsible deforming forces. Rang (1993) presented a tripod analogy that simplifies the problem. The foot is likened to a tripod of which the calcaneus, fifth metatarsal and first metatarsal form the legs. Combinations of deformities affecting one or more of these 'legs' produce the common types of high arch, namely plantaris, cavovarus, calcaneus and calcaneo-cavus (Fig. 21.17).

The toes are held cocked up, with hyperextension at the MTP joints and flexion at the IP joints. There may

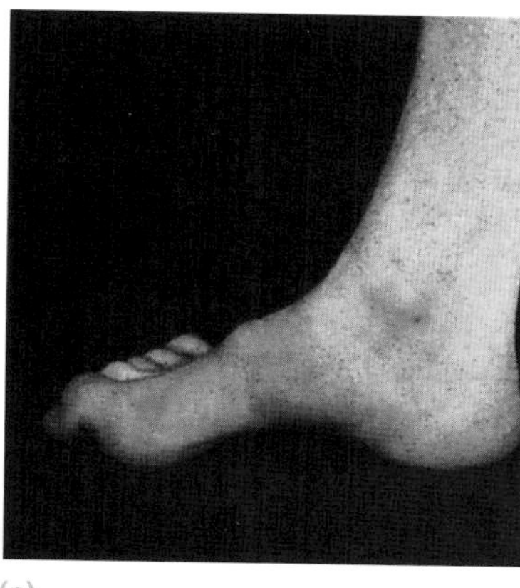
(a)

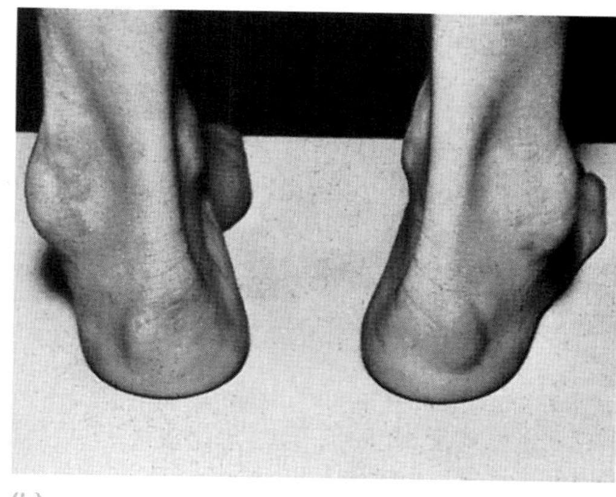
(b)

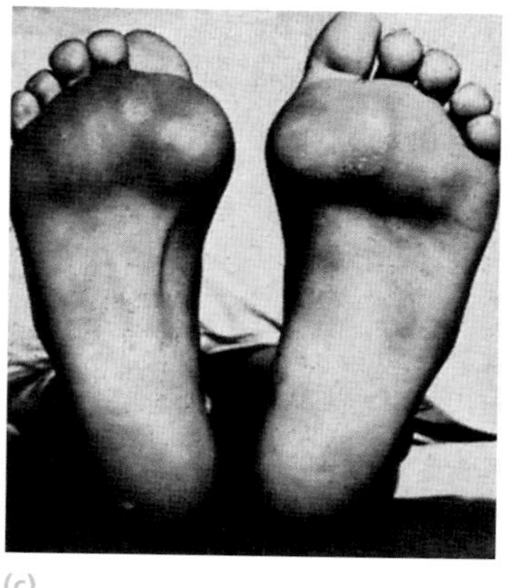
(c)

21.16 Pes cavus and claw-toes (a) Typical appearance of 'idiopathic' pes cavus. Note the high arch and claw-toes. (b) This is associated with varus heels. (c) Look for callosities under the metatarsal heads.

be callosities under the metatarsal heads and corns on the toes. Early on the toe deformities are 'mobile' and can be corrected passively by pressure under the metatarsal heads; as the forefoot lifts, the toes flatten out automatically. Later the deformities become fixed, with the MTP joints permanently dislocated.

Mobility in the ankle and foot joints is important. In the cavo-varus foot, the heel is inverted. The block test (Coleman et al., 1984) is useful to check if the deformity is reversible (Fig. 21.18); if it is, this signifies that the subtalar joint is mobile. If the cavus deformity has been present for a long time, then movements of the ankle, subtalar and midtarsal joints are usually limited.

A neurological examination is important to try to identify a reason for the deformity. Disorders such as hereditary sensory and motor neuropathy and Friedreich's ataxia must always be excluded, and the spine should be examined for signs of dysraphism.

Imaging

Weightbearing x-rays of the foot contribute further to the assessment of the deformity and the state of the individual joints. On the lateral view, measurement of the *calcaneal pitch* and *Meary's angle* help to determine the components of the high arch (Fig. 21.19). In a normal foot the calcaneal pitch is between 10 and 30 degrees, whereas Meary's angle, formed by the axes of the talus and first metatarsal, is zero, i.e. these axes are parallel. In a calcaneus deformity, the calcaneal pitch is increased; in a plantaris deformity, Meary's lines meet at an angle.

MRI scans of the spine will exclude a structural disorder, especially if this is more common than polio as a cause of high-arched feet in the region.

Treatment

Often no treatment is required; apart from the difficulty of fitting shoes, the patient has no complaints.

Foot deformity In general, patients need treatment only if they have symptoms. However, the problem with high-arched feet is that it is often a progressive disorder that becomes more difficult to treat when the deformities are fixed; therefore treatment should start before the feet become stiff. Non-operative treatment

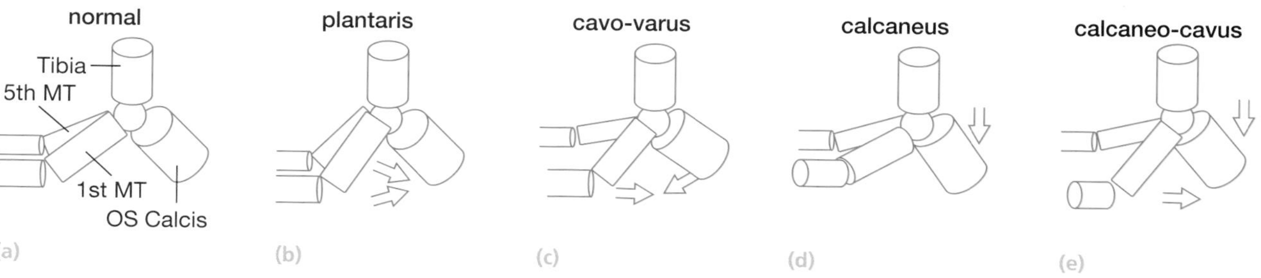

21.17 The tripod analogy for high-arched feet This simplifies understanding of the various types of pes cavus. (a) The calcaneum, first and fifth metatarsals of the foot are likened to the spokes of a tripod. (b) When the first and fifth rays are drawn closer to the heel, a plantaris deformity is present. In a cavo-varus deformity (c), the first ray alone is drawn towards the heel, which itself is in varus. In calcaneus (d), the heel is pushed plantarwards. Finally, a calcaneo-cavus deformity is present (e) when the heel is in calcaneus and the first ray is drawn in.

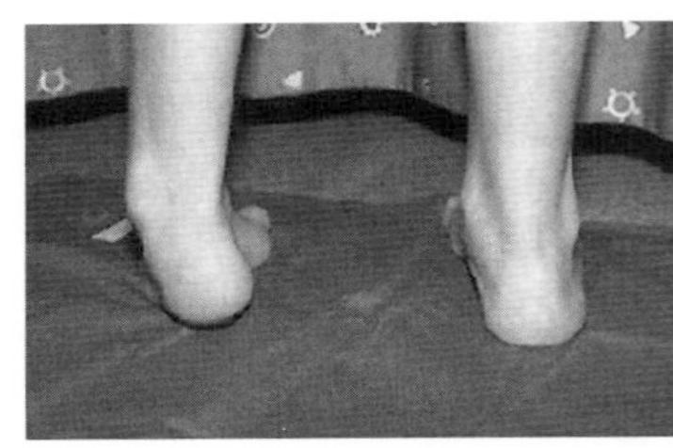

(a)

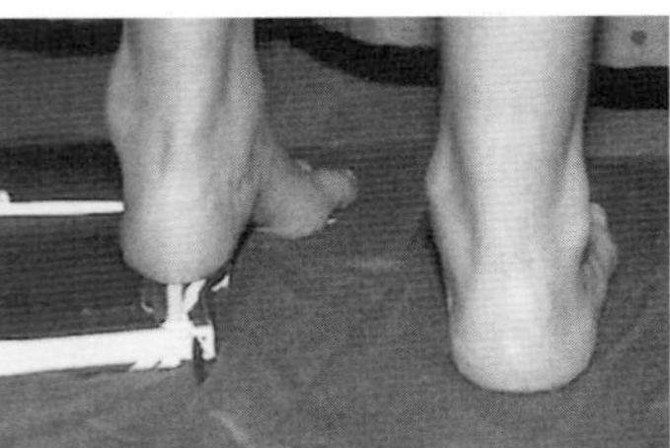

(b)

21.18 Coleman's block test This simple test is used on a high-arched foot to see if the heel is flexible. (a) Normal stance showing the varus position of the heel. (b) With the patient standing on a low block to permit the depressed first metatarsal to hang free, the heel varus is automatically corrected if the subtalar joint is mobile.

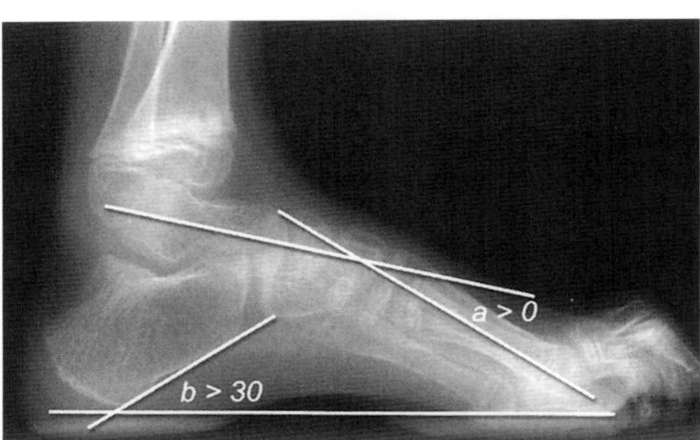

21.19 Weightbearing x-rays in foot deformities Non-weightbearing films are notorious for 'hiding' the true components of foot deformities. In standing lateral views, some measurements are useful in describing the type of high-arched foot: (*a*) the axes of the talus and first metatarsal are parallel in normal feet but cross each other in a plantaris deformity (Meary's angle); (*b*) the calcaneal pitch is greater than 30 degrees in calcaneus deformities.

in the form of custom-made shoes with moulded inserts may provide some relief but does not alter the deformity or influence its progression. Surgery is often needed and the type of procedure will depend on the child's age, underlying cause, site and flexibility of the individual deformities and type of muscle imbalance.

The aim of surgery is to provide a pain-free, plantigrade, supple but stable foot. The methods available are soft tissue releases, osteotomies and tendon transfers. However, the deformity first needs to be corrected before a tendon transfer is considered; additionally, the transfer only works if the joints are mobile.

An equinus contracture is dealt with by lengthening of the tendo Achillis and posterior capsulotomies of the ankle and subtalar joints. The varus hindfoot, if shown to be reversible by Coleman's block test, may benefit from a release of the plantar fascia (the tight fascia acts as a contracted windlass on weightbearing, accentuating the deformity). However, if the subtalar joint is stiff, then calcaneal osteotomy will be needed; two types are commonly used: (1) the lateral closing wedge (an opening wedge on the medial side is a comparable operation but is fraught with wound problems); (2) a lateral translation osteotomy.

Treatment of a calcaneo-cavus deformity (which is the least common type of high arch) differs according to the age of the child. In young children (who usually have a neurological problem) tendon transfers, e.g. transferring the tibialis anterior through the interosseous membrane to the calcaneum, may be combined with tenodesis of the ankle using the tendo Achillis (Banta et al., 1981). Older children may need crescentic calcaneal osteotomies, which will correct both varus and calcaneus deformities (Samilson, 1976) or variations of a triple arthrodesis (Cholmeley, 1953).

Midfoot deformities are usually cavus (plantarflexed first metatarsal) or plantaris (plantarflexed first and fifth metatarsals). The Jones tendon transfer helps elevate the depressed first metatarsal by using the extensor hallucis longus tendon as a sling through the neck of the first metatarsal. Often the peroneus longus is overactive and is partly responsible for pulling the first metatarsal down; some balance is restored by dividing this tendon on the lateral side of the foot and attaching the proximal end to the peroneus brevis, thereby

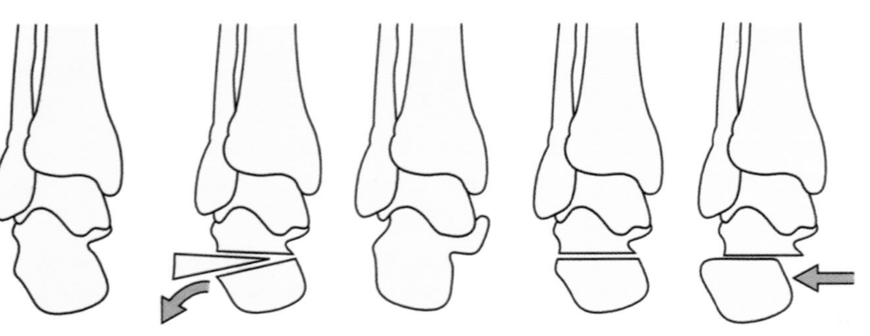

21.20 Treatment of pes cavus 1 In a normal foot (a), the point of contact of the heel is slightly lateral to the centre of the ankle, producing an eversion lever when weight is borne. In a varus heel (b) excising a wedge of bone from the lateral side, or (c) performing a lateral translation osteotomy.

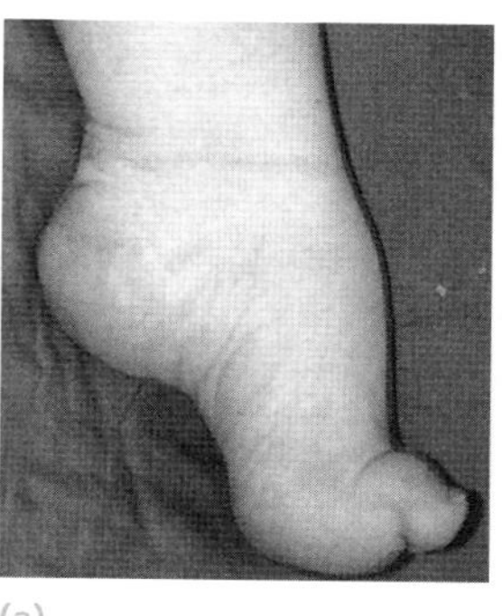
(a)

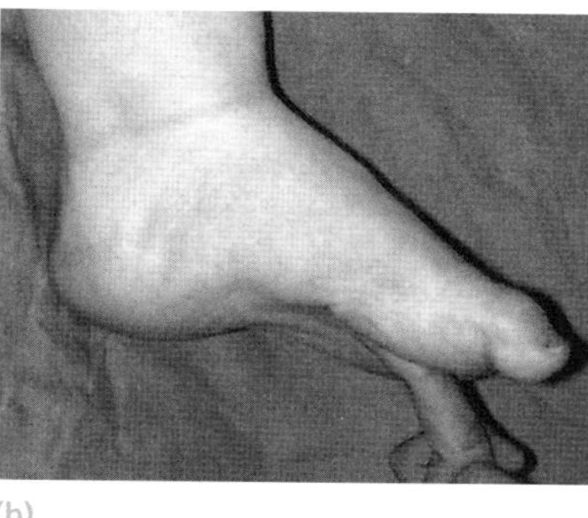
(b)

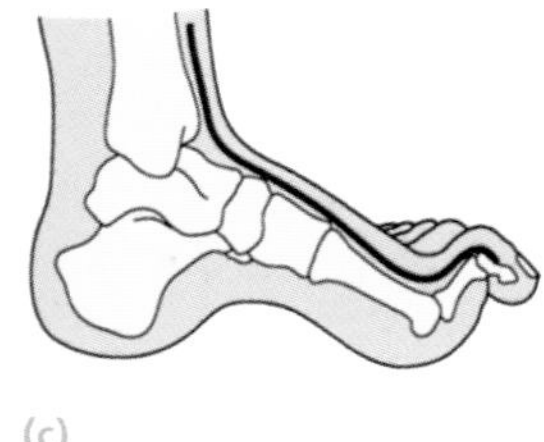
(c)

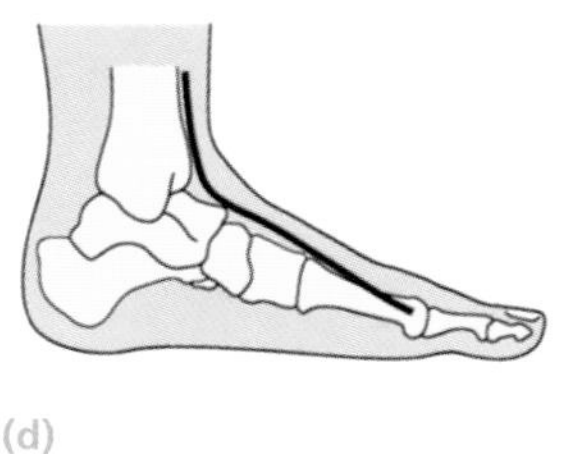
(d)

21.21 Treatment of pes cavus 2 (a,b) If the great toe is clawed and the first metatarsal depressed, reducing the subluxation at the metatarsophalangeal joint by simply elevating the neck of the metatarsal often reduces the severity of the cavus deformity. The surgical equivalent of this effect is (c,d) the Robert Jones tendon transfer: the extensor hallucis longus tendon is detached distally and transferred to the neck of the first metatarsal; the interphalangeal joint is then either fused or tenodesed.

removing the deforming force and improving the power of eversion simultaneously. Occasionally the deformity affecting the first metatarsal is fixed, in which case a dorsal closing wedge osteotomy at the base of the metatarsal is needed. A plantaris deformity is treated along similar lines for the first ray, and combined with a plantar fascia release if the deformity is mobile, but basal metatarsal osteotomies or even a wedge resection and arthrodesis across the midfoot are needed for rigid deformities.

In severe examples and in those who have either relapsed or who have responded poorly with soft tissue releases and osteotomies, salvage surgery in the form of a triple arthrodesis is recommended; it produces a stiff but plantigrade and pain-free foot.

Clawed toes Correction of a clawed first toe is by the Jones tendon transfer, which involves either a tenodesis or fusion of the IP joint. Clawing of the lesser toes is treated with a flexor tendon transfer to the extensor hood of each toe, and MTP joint capsulotomies if the toes are still passively correctable; however, if the deformities are fixed, proximal IP fusion is needed.

HALLUX VALGUS

Hallux valgus is the commonest of the foot deformities (and probably of all musculoskeletal deformities). In people who have never worn shoes the big toe is in line with the first metatarsal, retaining the slightly fan-shaped appearance of the forefoot. In people who habitually wear shoes the hallux assumes a valgus position; but only if the angulation is excessive is it referred to as 'hallux valgus'.

Splaying of the forefoot, with varus angulation of the first metatarsal, predisposes to lateral angulation of the big toe in people wearing shoes – and most of all in those who wear high-heeled shoes. *Metatarsus primus varus* may be congenital, or it may result from loss of muscle tone in the forefoot in elderly people. Hallux valgus is also common in rheumatoid arthritis, probably due to weakness of the joint capsule and ligaments. Heredity plays an important part; a positive family history is obtained in over 60 per cent of cases.

Pathological anatomy

The elements of the deformity are lateral deviation and rotation of the hallux, together with a prominence of the medial side of the head of the first metatarsal (a bunion). Lateral deviation of the hallux may lead to overcrowding and deformity of the other toes and sometimes overriding of adjacent toes. When the valgus deformity exceeds 30 or 40 degrees, the great toe rotates into pronation so that the nail faces medially and the sessamoid bones of flexor hallucis brevis are displaced laterally; in severe deformities the tendons of flexor and extensor hallucis longus bowstring on the lateral side, thus adding to the deforming forces. The contracted adductor hallucis and lateral capsule contribute further to the fixed valgus deformity.

Prominence of the first metatarsal head is due to subluxation of the MTP joint; increasing shoe pressure on the medial side leads to the development of an overlying bursa and thickened soft tissues, additional changes that combine to form the defining 'bunion' that eventually accompanies the great-toe deformity. When exposed at operation, the medial prominence looks like an exostosis (because of a deep sagittal sulcus on the head of the metatarsal) but there is no true exostosis.

In longstanding cases the MTP joint becomes osteoarthritic and osteophytes may then add to the prominence of the metatarsal head.

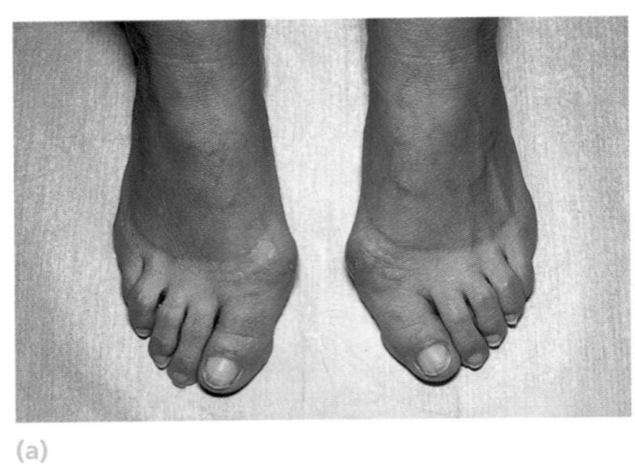
(a)

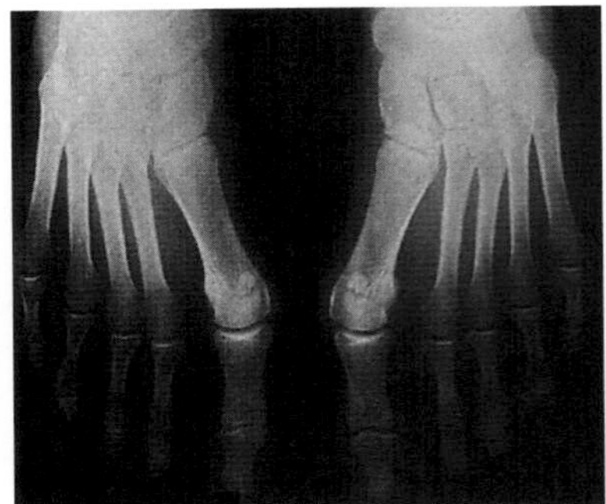
(b)

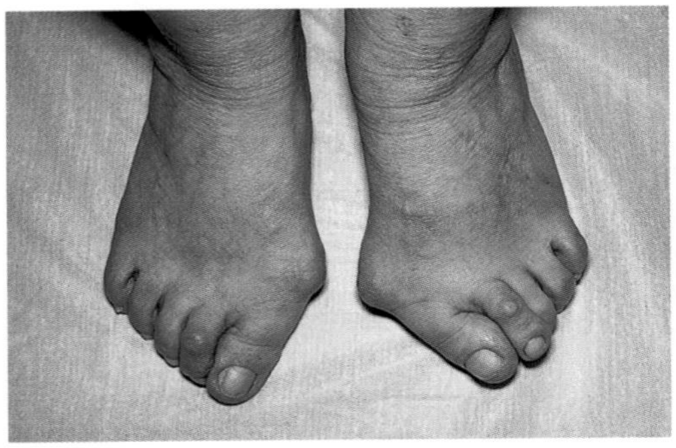
(c)

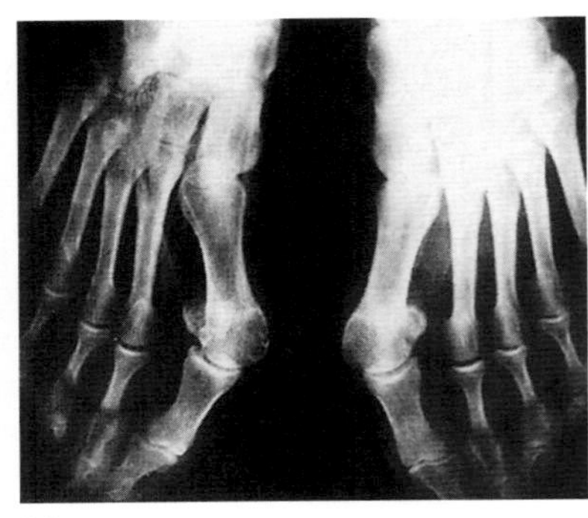
(d)

21.22 Hallux valgus (a,b) This girl's feet are well on the way to becoming as deformed as those of her mother (c,d). Hallux valgus is not uncommonly familial. X-rays should be taken with the patient standing to show the true metatarsal and digital angulation.

Clinical features

The commonest complaints are pain over the bunion, worries about cosmesis and difficulty fitting shoes. Often there is also deformity of the lesser toes and pain in the forefoot. With the patient standing, planovalgus hindfoot collapse may become apparent.

The great toe is in valgus and the bunion varies in appearance from a slight prominence over the medial side of the first metatarsal head to a red and angry-looking bulge that is tender. The MTP joint often retains a good range of movement, but in longstanding cases it may be osteoarthritic.

Always check the circulation and sensation.

X-rays

Standing views will show the degree of metatarsal and hallux angulation. Lines are drawn along the middle of the first and second metatarsals and the proximal phalanx of the great toe; normally the intermetatarsal angle is less than 9 degrees and the valgus angle at the MTP joint less than 15 degrees. Any greater degree of angulation should be regarded as 'hallux valgus'.

Not all types of valgus deformity are equally progressive and troublesome. Based on the x-ray appearances, patients with hallux valgus can be divided into three types (Piggott, 1960): (1) those in whom the MTP joint is normally centred but the articular surfaces, though congruent, are tilted towards valgus; (2) those in whom the articular surfaces are not congruent, the phalangeal surface being tilted towards valgus; (3) those in whom the joint is both incongruent and slightly subluxated (Fig. 21.23). Type 1 is a stable joint and any deformity is likely to progress very slowly or not at all. Type 2 is somewhat unstable and likely to progress. Type 3 is even more unstable and almost certain to progress.

Treatment

ADOLESCENTS

Many young patients are asymptomatic, but worry over the shape of the toe and an anxious mother keen not to let the condition become as severe as her own will bring the patient to the clinic. It is wise to try conservative measures first, mainly because surgical correction in this age group carries a 20–40 per cent recurrence rate. This consists essentially of encouraging the patient to wear shoes with wide and deep toe-boxes, soft uppers and low heels – 'trainers' are a good choice. If x-rays show a type 1 (congruous) deformity, the patient can be reassured that it will progress very slowly, if at all. If there is an incongruous deformity, surgical correction will sooner or later be required.

There are a number of non-operative strategies that may be adopted to deal with the deformity and the resulting limitations, but none that will get rid of the bunion itself. Accommodating, comfortable shoes can help, but are not acceptable for some patients (or

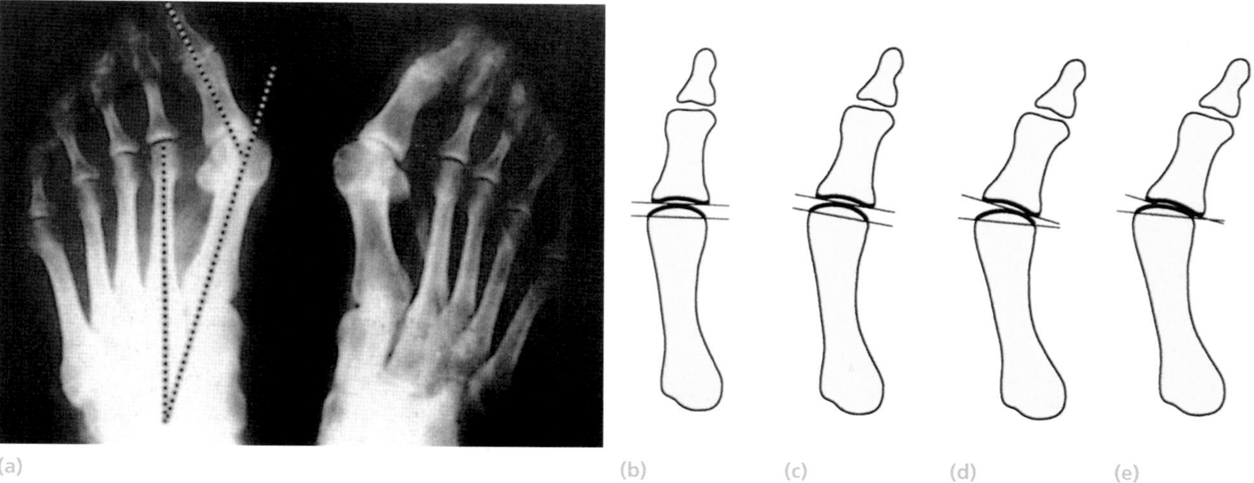

(a) (b) (c) (d) (e)

21.23 X-rays (a) The intermetatarsal angle (between the first and second metatarsals) as well as the metatarsophalangeal angle of the hallux are recorded. Piggott (1960) defined three types of hallux valgus, based on the position and tilt of the first MTP articular surfaces: In *normal feet* (b) the articular surfaces are parallel and centred upon each other. In *congruent hallux valgus* (c) the lines across the articular surfaces are still parallel and the joint is centred, but the articular surfaces are set more obliquely to the long axes of their respective bones. In (d) the *deviated type of hallux valgus*, the lines are not parallel and the articular surfaces are not congruent. In *the subluxated type* (e) the surfaces are neither parallel nor centred.

professions). Lace-up or Velcro-fastening shoes are better than slip-ons, and flat shoes are probably better than those with a raised heel.

Bunion pads (like a Polo/doughnut shape) can help to offload the tender bunion, but strapping and overnight splints are probably a waste of money with no quality research to support their use.

Chiropody can help by taking care of the callosities and skin compromise.

Podiatrists may help to correct the foot biomechanics, but there is no good evidence that anti-pronatory orthoses are effective in the longer term management of the bunion. Diabetic services often provide specialized foot-care.

Operative treatment In the adolescent with mild deformities, where the hallux valgus angle is less than 25 degrees, correction can be obtained by either a soft-tissue rebalancing operation (see later) or by a metatarsal osteotomy. If the x-ray shows a congruent articulation, the deformity is largely bony and therefore amenable to correction by a distal osteotomy.

If the MTP articulation is incongruent the deformity is in the joint and soft-tissue realignment is indicated. The tight structures on the lateral side (adductor hallucis, transverse metatarsal ligament, and lateral joint capsule) are released; the prominent bone on the medial side of the metatarsal head is pared down and the capsule on the medial side is reefed.

In moderate and *severe deformities* the hallux valgus angle may be greater than 30 degrees and inter-metatarsal angle wider than 15 degrees. If the MTP joint is congruent, a distal osteotomy combined with a corrective osteotomy of the base of the proximal phalanx (Aikin's osteotomy) is recommended. For greater deformities, if the joint is subluxed, a soft-tissue adjustment is needed as well as a proximal metatarsal osteotomy. This basal osteotomy is carried

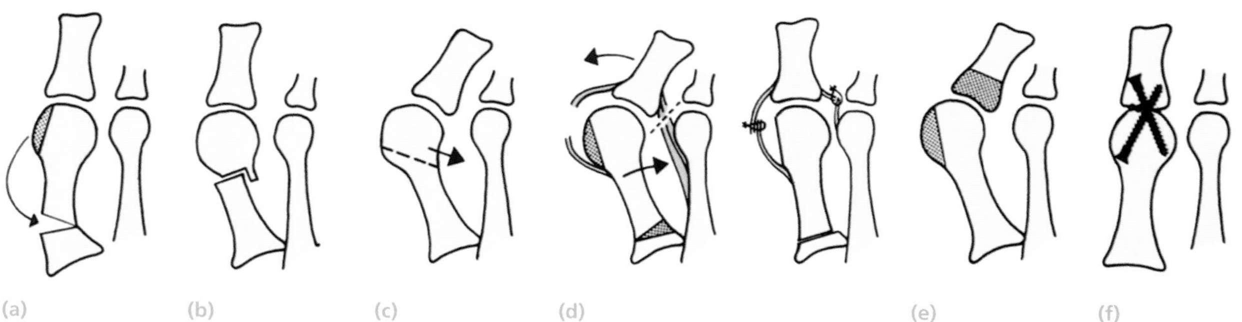

(a) (b) (c) (d) (e) (f)

21.24 Hallux valgus – treatment (a) Basal osteotomy with bone graft inserted. (b) Mitchell's osteotomy. (c) Wilson's osteotomy. (d) Before and after basal osteotomy and capsulorrhaphy. (e) Keller's operation. (f) Arthrodesis.

out to reduce a wide intermetatarsal angle; care is needed not to injure an open physis or else growth of the metatarsal will be stunted.

ADULTS

In the adult, when self-care is insufficient and the bunion is causing pain and difficulty with footwear, surgical options are appropriate. Recurrent infection or ulceration are also indications for operative treatment.

The type of surgery proposed will depend on the level and extent of the deformity. This will usually comprise: (1) an osteotomy to re-align the first metatarsal; (2) soft tissue procedures to rebalance the joint.

A number of different osteotomy patterns have been described and named after their 'inventors' or the pattern of bone cut (chevron, scarf etc.), or the part of the metatarsal that is osteotomized (distal usually if there is less deformity, proximal or basal for greater deformity). These procedures are reviewed in a paper by Robinson and Limbers (2005).

There is convincing evidence to show that a distal osteotomy is associated with reduced pain and increased ability to work in the medium to long term; the safety profile is good, with a less than 10 per cent complication rate and with many procedures being performed as day-case operations and without plaster immobilization in the postoperative period. Patient satisfaction with bunion surgery is generally good, with 75 per cent being satisfied with the outcome.

ELDERLY PATIENTS

Hallux valgus in the elderly is best treated by shoe modifications; where this fails, and in those whose functional demands are low, treatment by excision arthroplasty is usually successful. In the classic *Keller's operation*, the proximal third of the proximal phalanx, as well as the bunion prominence, are removed. This used to be the most common operation for hallux valgus but it has fallen into disuse because of the high rate of recurrent deformity and complications such as loss of control over great toe movement, overload of the other metatarsals, metatarsalgia and dubious cosmetic improvement.

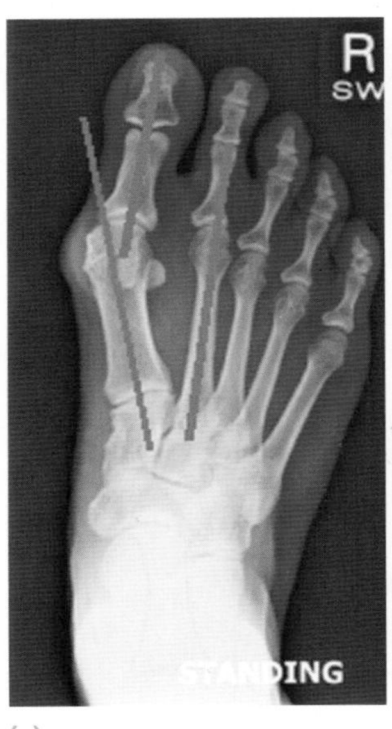

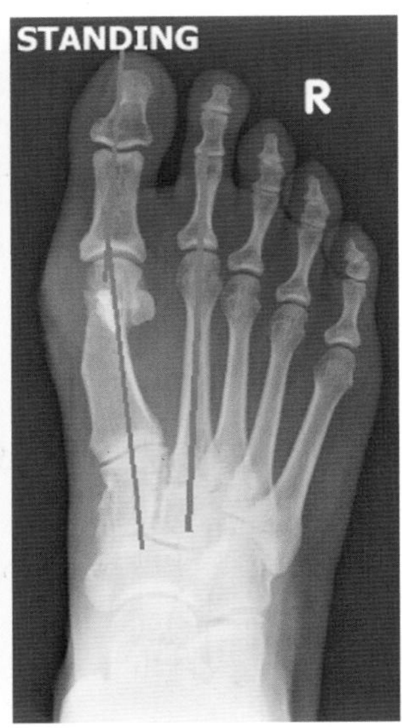

(a) (b)

21.25 Hallux valgus – treatment (a) X-ray before operation. (b) X-ray after distal osteotomy.

Complications

Recurrent infection and *ulceration* are particular problems in the diabetic foot and are an indication for surgery, rather than a contraindication.

Transfer metatarsalgia may occur if the realignment or shortening of the first ray does not take account of the relative lengths of the lesser metatarsals, which then become prominent and overloaded; a metatarsal stress fracture sometimes occurs. Forefoot corrective surgery should strive to produce a balanced forefoot with appropriately distributed weightbearing.

Complex regional pain syndrome is a potential complication of all foot operations.

HALLUX RIGIDUS

'Rigidity' (or stiffness) of the first MTP joint occurs at almost any age from adolescence onwards. In young people it may be due to local trauma or osteochondritis dissecans of the first metatarsal head. In older people it is usually caused by longstanding joint disorders such as gout, pseudogout or osteoarthritis (OA), and is very often bilateral. In contrast to hallux valgus, men and women are affected with equal frequency. A family history is common.

Clinical features

Pain on walking, especially on slopes or rough ground, is the predominant symptom. The patient eventually develops an altered gait, trying to offload the first MTP joint by transferring weight across to the lesser toes; there is also impaired power in toe-off during the gait cycle. The great toe is straight and often has a callosity under the medial side of the distal phalanx. The MTP joint feels knobbly; a tender dorsal 'bunion' (actually a large osteophyte) is diagnostic. Dorsiflexion is restricted and painful, and there may be compensatory hyperextension at the interphalangeal joint. The outer side of the sole of the shoe may be unduly worn – the result of rolling the foot outwards to avoid pressing on the big toe.

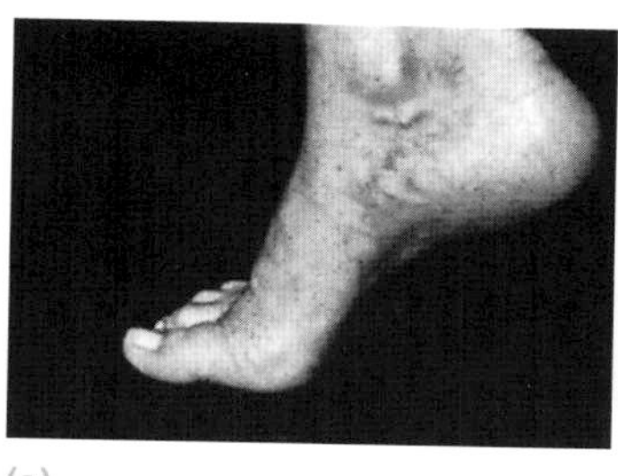
(a)

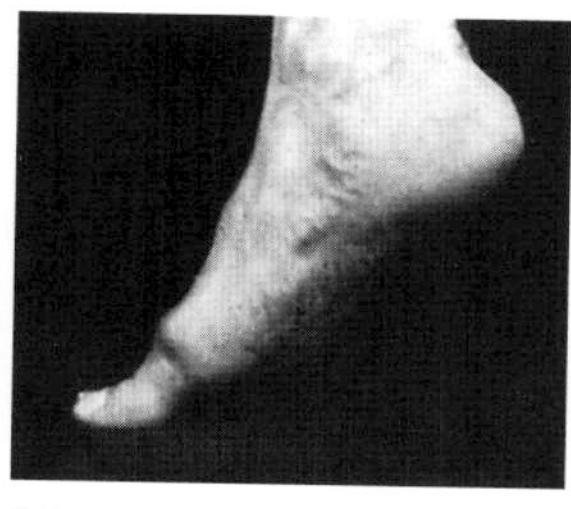
(b)

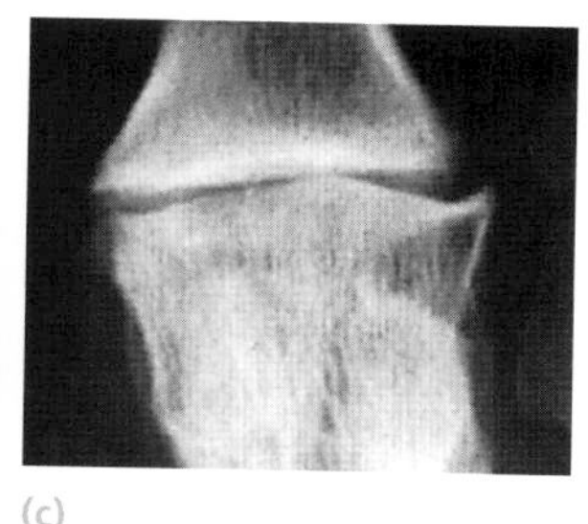
(c)

21.26 Hallux rigidus (a) In normal walking, the big toe dorsiflexes (extends) considerably. With rigidus (b), dorsiflexion is limited. (c) The usual cause is OA of the first MTP joint.

It is important to check the state of the other joints in the foot in order to rule out a polyarthropathy.

X-rays The features are essentially those of OA: narrowing of the joint space, subchondral sclerosis and marginal osteophytes. There may be signs of recent or old osteochondritis ('squaring' of the metatarsal head).

Treatment

If the condition is not interfering with activity then it can be left alone and the patient reassured. Intermittent attacks of pain can be relieved by an intra-articular injection of corticosteroid and local anaesthetic. If, however, the condition is painful and restricting of activity then the risks of long-term NSAIDs must be balanced against those of surgical intervention.

Some orthotic devices will offload or reduce movement at the first MTP joint, but these are usually full-length insoles and relatively bulky – they may not fit in a smart shoe (at least not when the foot is in it as well!) A rocker-soled shoe can abolish pain by allowing the foot to 'roll' without the necessity for dorsiflexion at the MTP joint; many people are unwilling to wear such shoes.

OPERATIVE TREATMENT

Pain at the first MTP joint that is intrusive or limits activity should be an indication for referral. In limited arthritic disease, simply removing the dorsal osteophyte (*cheilectomy*) might be effective, and may be coupled with an extension osteotomy in the proximal phalanx, to alter the loadbearing region of the articulation.

If the joint is more arthritic then a fusion or *arthrodesis* offers a good chance of returning the patient to function, walking comfortably without a limp. The joint should be fused in 10 degrees of valgus and 10–15 degrees of dorsiflexion in relation to the sole of the foot, or with about 5–10 mm clearance between the line of the sole of the foot and the pulp of the great toe. Too little dorsiflexion will cause pain during toe-off and too much will result in the toe

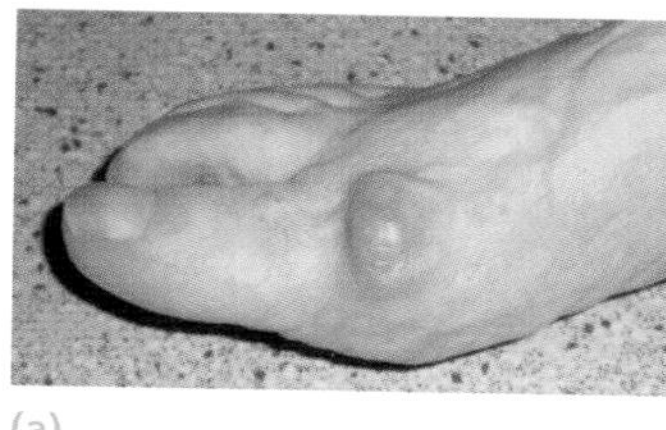
(a)

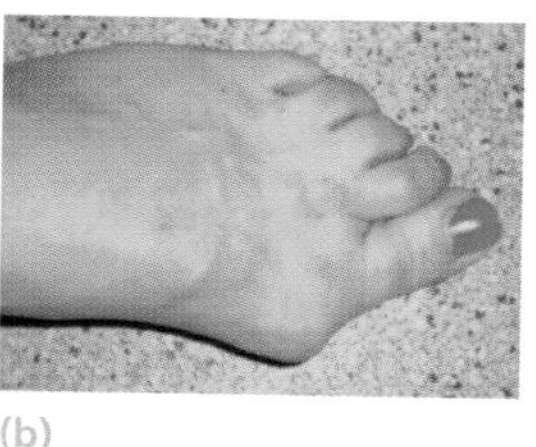
(b)

21.27 'Bunions' Compare the two types of bunion: (a) Dorsal bunion in hallux rigidus and (b) medial bunion in hallux valgus.

pressing against the shoe upper. Female patients may be concerned that they will be unable to wear shoes with a higher heel if the toe is fused, but in fact the majority are able to wear footwear that can include moderate heels.

Arthroplasty is more controversial. Keller's operation (an *excisional arthroplasty*), carries a high risk of complications and seldom brings improvement in function; the procedure is no longer recommended. *Interposition arthroplasty* has from time to time been popular and can provide excellent pain relief, especially in patients with advanced OA. A simple capsular arthroplasty is probably the safest. Silicone implants were often used in the past, but silicone-related complications were common and the operation is no longer recommended for hallux rigidus. Metallic implants have fared better (in experienced hands) but these also produce variable long-term results.

DEFORMITIES OF LESSER TOES

The commonest deformities of the lesser toes are 'claw', 'hammer' and 'mallet'. These terms are often used interchangeably, leading to confusion.

Claw toe is characterized by hyperextension at the MTP joint and flexion at both IP joints.

Hammer toe is an acute flexion deformity of the proximal IP joint only; in severe examples there may be some extension at the MTP joint. The distal IP joint is either straight or hyperextended.

Mallet toe is a flexion deformity of the distal IP joint.

CLAW TOES

The IP joints are flexed and the MTP joints hyperextended. This is an 'intrinsic-minus' deformity that is seen in neurological disorders (e.g. peroneal muscular atrophy, poliomyelitis and peripheral neuropathies) and in rheumatoid arthritis. Usually, however, no cause is found. The condition may also be associated with pes cavus.

Clinical features

The patient complains of pain in the forefoot and under the metatarsal heads. Usually the condition is bilateral and walking may be severely restricted. At first the joints are mobile and can be passively corrected; later the deformities become fixed and the MTP joints subluxed or dislocated. Painful corns may develop on the dorsum of the toes and callosities under the metatarsal heads. In the most severe cases the skin ulcerates at the pressure sites.

Treatment

FLEXIBLE DEFORMITY

So long as the toes can be passively straightened the patient may obtain relief by wearing a metatarsal support or by having a transverse metatarsal bar fitted to the shoe. A daily programme of intrinsic muscle exercises is important. If these measures fail to relieve discomfort, an operation is indicated. 'Dynamic' correction is achieved by transferring the long toe flexors to the extensors. The operation at one stroke removes a powerful IP flexor and converts it to a MTP flexor and IP extensor.

FIXED DEFORMITY

When the deformity is fixed, it may either be accepted and accommodated by special footwear or treated by one of the following operations:

1. *Interphalangeal arthrodesis* – If there is no joint disease, proximal IP arthrodesis and dorsal capsulotomy of the MTP joints permits active flexion of the MTP joints by the long flexors. This is sometimes combined with transfer of the extensor hallucis longus to the first metatarsal, thus removing a deforming force while retaining the muscle as a forefoot stabilizer.
2. *Joint excision* – Fixed claw deformities, usually associated with destruction of the MTP joints (e.g. in rheumatoid arthritis), can be dealt with by excision arthroplasties of the MTP joints – preferably removal of only the bases of the proximal phalanges and trimming of the metatarsal heads. This can usually be achieved through two longitudinal incisions on the dorsum of the foot. If the great toe is affected, a modified Keller's operation is performed. The base of the proximal phalanx is excised and the plantar pad (which is often displaced in these deformities) is returned to its normal position beneath the metatarsal head; the space between the metatarsal and phalanx is then filled by suturing the long extensor tendon to the flexor.
3. *Amputation* – Toes that are severely contracted, dislocated and ulcerated are worse than none. If the circulation is satisfactory and the patient is willing to accept the appearance, amputation of all ten toes is a useful palliative operation.

HAMMER TOE

The proximal IP joint is fixed in flexion, while the distal joint and the MTP joint are extended. The second toe of one or both feet is commonly affected, and

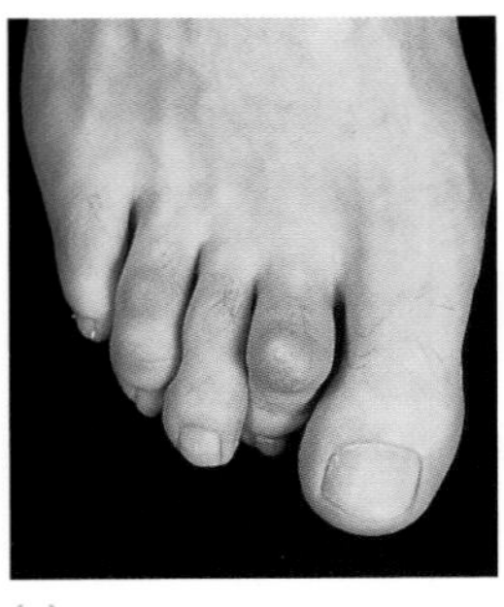
(a)

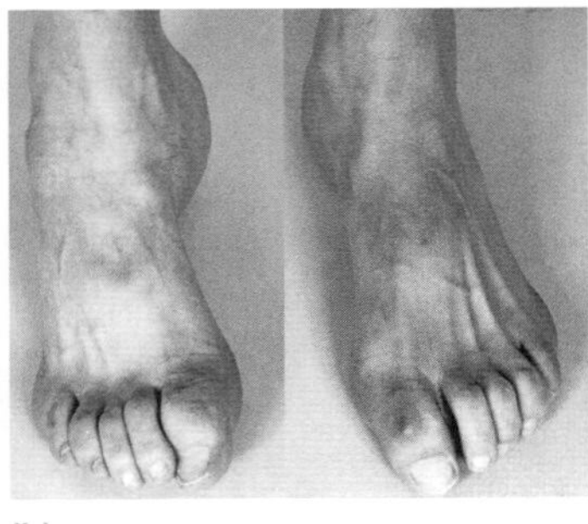
(b)

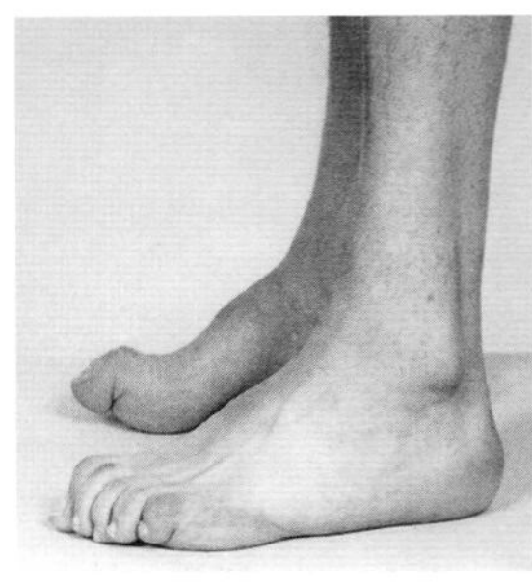
(c)

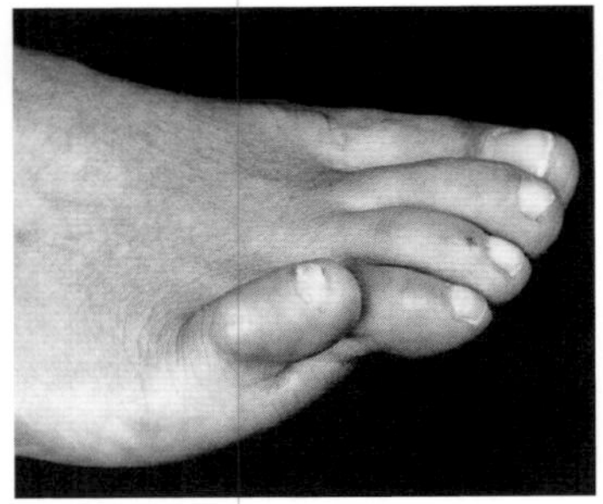
(d)

21.28 Disorders of the lesser toes (a) Hammer-toe deformity. (b,c) Claw toes. This patient suffered from peroneal muscular atrophy, a neurological disorder causing weakness of the intrinsic muscles and cavus feet. (d) Overlapping fifth toe.

hyperextension of the MTP joint may go on to dorsal dislocation. Shoe pressure may produce painful corns or callosities on the dorsum of the toe and under the prominent metatarsal head.

The cause is obscure: the similarity to boutonnière deformity of a finger suggests an extensor dysfunction, a view supported by the frequent association with a dropped metatarsal head, flat anterior arch and hallux valgus. A simpler explanation is that the toe was too long or the shoe too short.

Treatment

Operative correction is indicated for pain or for difficulty with shoes. The toe is shortened and straightened by excising the joint. An ellipse of tissue (including the corn and the underlying extensor tendon) is removed and the proximal IP joint is entered; the articular surfaces are nibbled away and the raw ends of the proximal and middle phalanges are brought together with the toe almost straight. The position is held by a longitudinally placed K-wire, which is retained for 6 weeks. An alternative (and some would say preferable) operation is simple excision of the head of the proximal phalanx, or excision of both articular surfaces, without formal arthrodesis; the toe is splinted for 3 weeks to allow healing in the corrected position.

If the MTP joint is dislocated, a dorsal capsulotomy and elongation of the extensor tendon may be necessary; the toe is held in position by driving the K-wire more proximally, or by inserting a second wire.

MALLET TOE

In mallet toe it is the distal IP joint that is flexed. The toe-nail or the tip of the toe presses into the shoe, resulting in a painful callosity.

If conservative treatment (chiropody and padding) does not help, operation is indicated. The distal IP joint is exposed, the articular surfaces excised and the toe straightened; flexor tenotomy may be needed. A thin K-wire is inserted across the joint and left in position for 6 weeks.

FIFTH TOE DEFORMITIES

OVERLAPPING FIFTH TOE

This is a common congenital anomaly (Fig. 21.28d). If symptoms warrant, the toe may be straightened by a dorsal V/Y-plasty, reinforced by transferring the flexor to the extensor tendon. Tight dorsal and medial structures may have to be released. The toe is held in the overcorrected position with tape or K-wire for 6 weeks. Severe deformities or relapses may need a transfer of the long extensor tendon beneath the proximal phalanx to the abductor digiti minimi (Lapidus, 1942).

COCK-UP DEFORMITY

The MTP joint is dislocated and the little toe sits on the dorsum of the metatarsal head. Operative treatment is usually successful: through a longitudinal plantar incision, the proximal phalanx is winkled out and removed; the wound is closed transversely, thus pulling the toe out of the hyperextended position.

TAILOR'S BUNION

An irritating or painful bunionette may form over an abnormally prominent fifth metatarsal head. If the shoe cannot be adjusted to fit the bump, the bony prominence can be trimmed, taking care not to sever the tendon of the fifth toe abductor. If the metatarsal shaft is bowed laterally (as is often the case), it can be straightened by performing either a distal osteotomy or a varus correction at the base of the metatarsal.

TUBERCULOUS ARTHRITIS

(see also Chapter 2)

Tuberculous infection of the ankle joint begins as a synovitis or as an osteomyelitis and, because walking is painful, may present before true arthritis supervenes. The ankle is swollen and the calf markedly wasted; the skin feels warm and movements are restricted. Sinus formation occurs early.

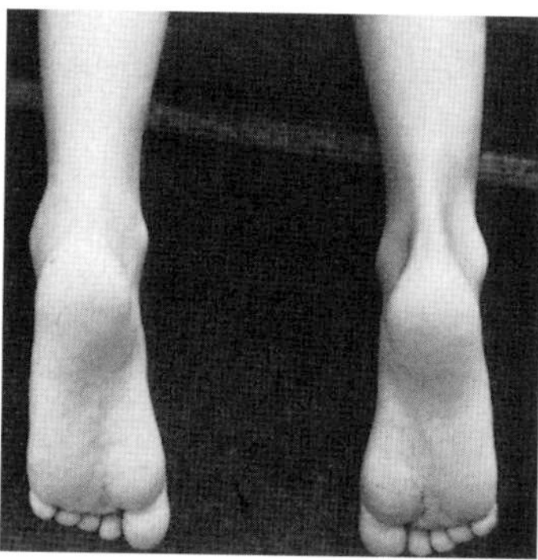

(a)

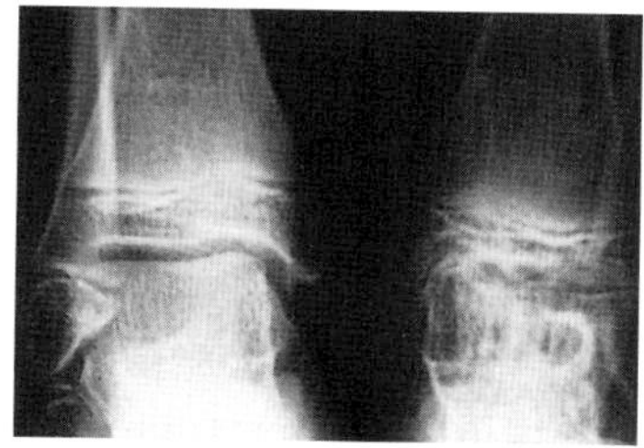

(b)

21.29 Tuberculous arthritis of the ankle (a) The swelling of the left ankle is best seen from behind; (b) shows regional osteoporosis and joint destruction.

X-rays show regional osteoporosis, sometimes a bone abscess and, with late disease, narrowing and irregularity of the joint space.

Treatment

In addition to general treatment (Chapter 2) a removable splint is used to rest the foot in neutral position. If the disease is arrested early, the patient is allowed up non-weightbearing in a calliper; gradually taking more weight and then discarding the calliper altogether. Following arthritis, weightbearing is harmless, but stiffness is inevitable and usually arthrodesis is the best treatment.

RHEUMATOID ARTHRITIS

(see also Chapter 3)

The ankle and foot are affected almost as often as the wrist and hand. Early on there is synovitis of the MTP, intertarsal and ankle joints, as well as of the sheathed tendons (usually the peronei and tibialis posterior). As the disease progresses, joint erosion and tendon dysfunction prepare the ground for increasingly severe deformities.

Forefoot

Pain and swelling of the MTP joints are among the earliest features of rheumatoid arthritis. Shoes feel uncomfortable and the patient walks less and less. Tenderness is at first localized to the MTP joints; later the entire forefoot is painful on pressing or squeezing. With increasing weakness of the intrinsic muscles and joint destruction, the characteristic deformities appear: a flattened anterior arch, hallux valgus, claw toes and prominence of the metatarsal heads in the sole (patients say it feels like walking on pebbles). Subcutaneous nodules are common and may ulcerate. Dorsal corns and plantar callosities also may break down and become infected. In the worst cases the toes are dislocated, inflamed, ulcerated and useless.

X-rays show osteoporosis and peri-articular erosion at the MTP joints. Curiously – in contrast to the situation in the hand – the smaller digits (fourth and fifth toes) are affected first.

Treatment

During the stage of synovitis, corticosteroid injections and attention to footwear may relieve symptoms; operative synovectomy is occasionally needed. Once deformity is advanced, treatment is that of the claw toes and hallux valgus. Sometimes specially made shoes will accommodate the toes in relative comfort. If this does not help, the most effective operation is excision arthroplasty in order to relieve pressure in the sole and to correct the toe deformities. For the hallux, an alternative is MTP fusion.

Forefoot surgery is more likely to succeed if the hindfoot is held in the anatomical position. It is important, therefore, to treat the foot as a whole and attend also to the proximal joints.

Ankle and hindfoot

The earliest symptoms are pain and swelling around the ankle. Walking becomes increasingly difficult and, later, deformities appear. On examination, swelling and tenderness are usually localized to the back of the medial malleolus (tenosynovitis of tibialis posterior) or the lateral malleolus (tenosynovitis of the peronei). Less often the ankle swells (joint synovitis) and its movements are restricted. Inversion and eversion may be painful and limited; subtalar erosion is common. In the late stages the tibialis posterior may rupture (all too often this is missed), or become ineffectual with progressive erosion of the tarsal joints, and the foot gradually drifts into severe valgus deformity. X-rays show osteoporosis and, later, erosion of the tarsal and ankle joints. Soft tissue swelling may be marked.

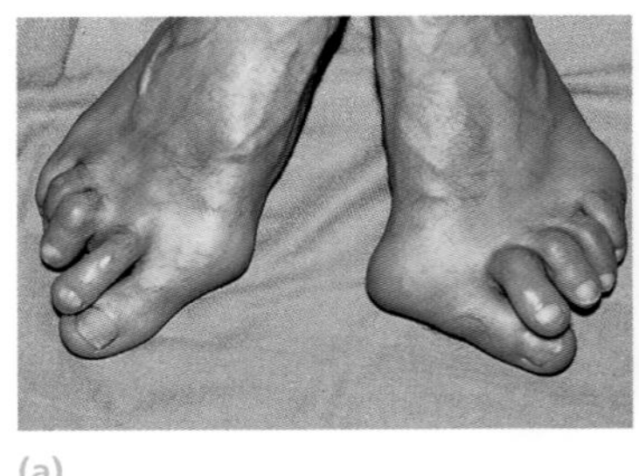
(a)

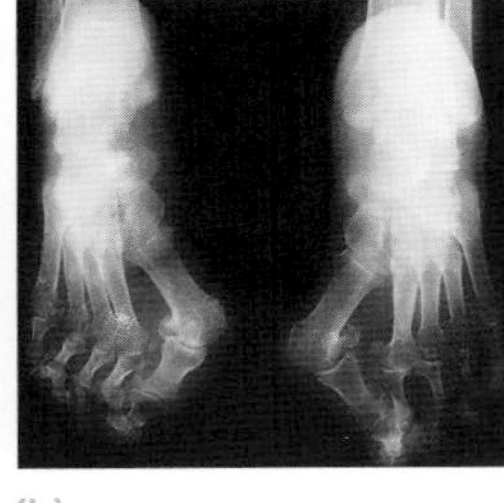
(b)

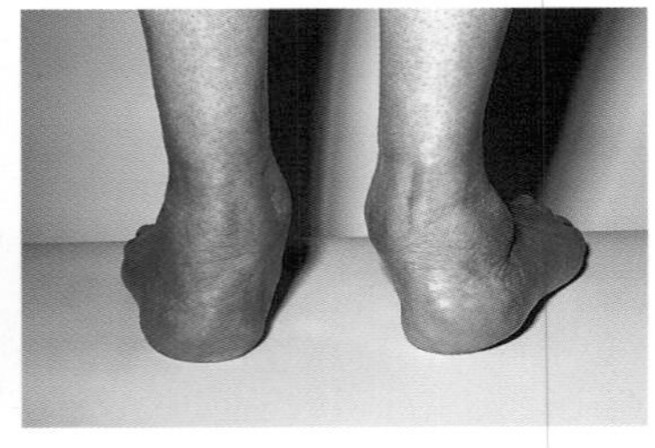
(c)

21.30 Rheumatoid arthritis (a,b) Forefoot deformities are similar to those in non-rheumatoid feet but more severe. They are due to a combination of joint erosion and tendon attrition. (c) Swelling and deformity of the hindfoot due to a combination of arthritis and tenosynovitis. In this case, both the ankle and the subtalar joints are affected.

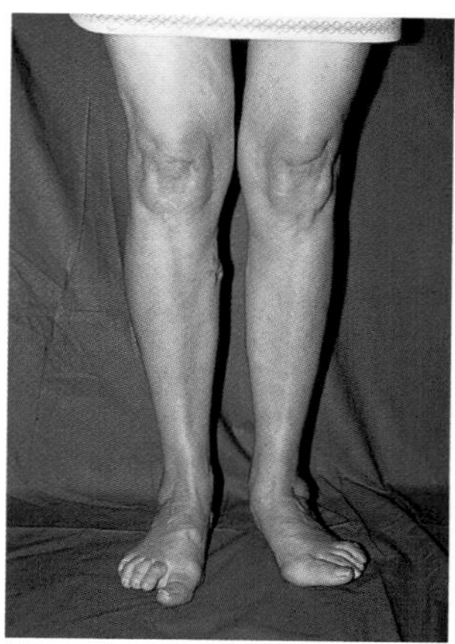

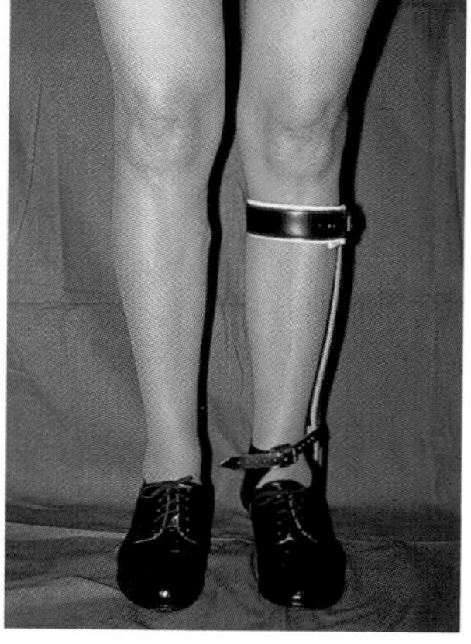

(a) (b)

21.31 Rupture of tibialis posterior tendon (a) This patient with rheumatoid arthritis suddenly developed a painful valgus foot on the left. (b) The deformity was well controlled by a lightweight orthosis, and operative repair was unnecessary.

Treatment

In the stage of synovitis, splintage is helpful (to allow inflammation to subside and to prevent deformity) while waiting for systemic treatment to control the disease. Initially, tendon sheaths and joints may be injected with methylprednisolone, but this should not be repeated more than two or three times because of the risk of tendon rupture. A lightweight below-knee calliper with an inside supporting strap restores stability and may be worn almost indefinitely.

If the synovitis does not subside, operative synovectomy is advisable. Frayed tendons cannot be repaired and, although tendon replacement is technically feasible, progressive erosion of the hindfoot joints will countervail any improvement this might achieve.

In the very late stage, arthrodesis of the ankle and tarsal joints can still restore modest function and abolish pain. The place of arthroplasty is not yet firmly established.

SERONEGATIVE ARTHROPATHIES

The seronegative arthropathies are dealt with in Chapter 3. These conditions are similar to rheumatoid arthritis, but there are differences in the pattern of joint involvement, the severity of the changes and the soft tissue features.

The clinical features are often asymmetrical and the ankle and hindfoot tend to be more severely affected than the forefoot. However, in psoriatic arthritis the toe joints are sometimes completely destroyed.

An inflammatory reaction around the insertions of tendons and ligaments is a feature of the spondyloarthropathies. This appears in the foot as plantar fasciitis and Achilles tendinitis. Splintage and local injection of triamcinolone are helpful.

GOUT (see also Chapter 4)

Swelling, redness, heat and exquisite tenderness of the MTP joint of the great toe ('podagra') is the epitome of gout. The ankle joint, or one of the toes, may be similarly affected – especially following a minor injury. The condition may closely resemble septic arthritis, but the systemic features of infection are absent. The serum uric acid level may be raised.

Treatment with anti-inflammatory drugs will abort the acute attack of gout; until the pain subsides the foot should be rested and protected from injury.

Chronic tophaceous gout Tophi may appear around any of the joints. The diagnosis is suggested by the characteristic x-ray features and confirmed by identifying the typical crystals in the tophus. Treatment may require local curettage of the bone lesions.

Plantar fasciitis Pain under the heel due to plantar fasciitis is another manifestation of gout, though the association may be hard to prove in any particular case.

OSTEOCHONDRITIS DISSECANS OF THE TALUS

Unexplained pain and slight limitation of movement in the ankle of a young person may be due to a small osteochondral fracture of the upper surface of the talus, though the injury may have been forgotten.

X-rays taken at appropriate angles to produce tangential views of the talar surface show the small bony separation (no more than a few millimetres in diameter) at either the anteromedial or posterolateral part of the superior surface of the talus. MRI is also helpful and the lesion may be visualized directly by arthroscopy.

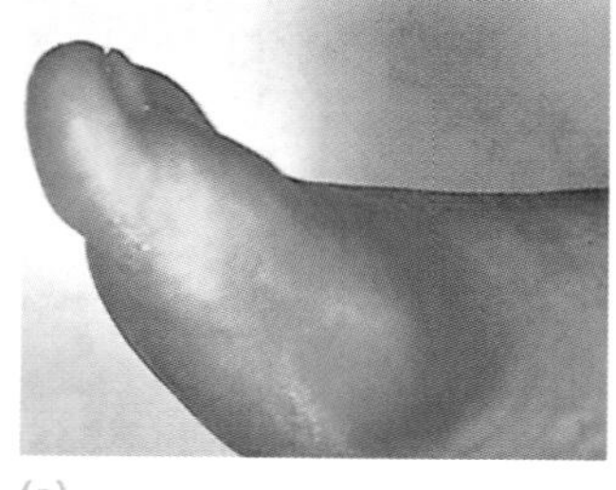

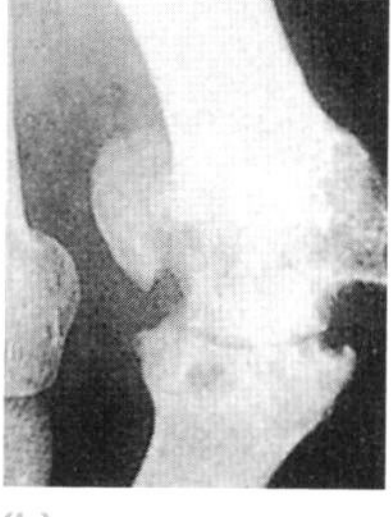

(a) (b)

21.32 Gout (a) The classical image of gout in the big toe. An inflamed 1st MTP joint. (b) X-ray showing large erosions due to tophi at the first metatarsal head.

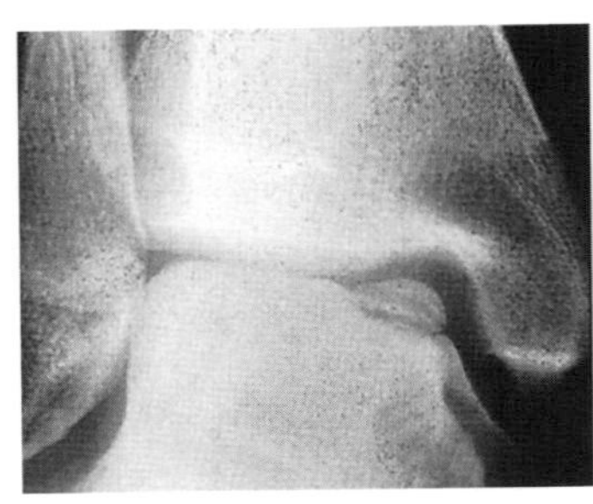

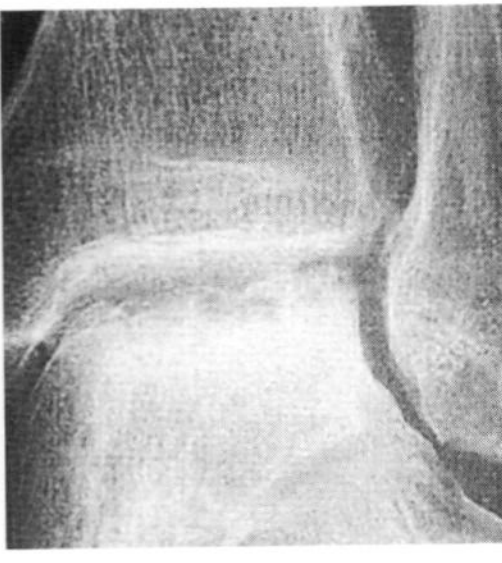

(a) (b)

21.33 Osteochondritis dissecans (a) Osteochondritis dissecans at the common site, the anteromedial part of the articular surface of the talus. (b) More extensive lesions can lead to secondary OA of the ankle.

Treatment depends on the degree of cartilage damage. As long as the articular cartilage is intact, it is sufficient to restrict activities. Once it is softened, arthroscopic drilling may be helpful. A loose fragment may need to be removed, but often the symptoms are insufficient to warrant intervention.

ATRAUMATIC OSTEONECROSIS OF THE TALUS (see also Chapter 6)

Osteonecrosis of the talus is a well-recognized complication of trauma (dislocation or fracture of the neck of the talus). Atraumatic osteonecrosis, though less common than its counterpart in the femoral head, is associated with the same group of systemic disorders as the latter (hypercortisonism, alcoholism, systemic lupus erythematosus, Gaucher's disease, sickle-cell disease etc.) and is often one of multiple sites affected.

Patients complain of pain, which is often aggravated by weightbearing, and gradually increasing restriction of movement. X-rays and MRI show the typical features of osteonecrosis, almost always involving the posterolateral part of the talar dome. Lesions can be staged according to Ficat's radiographic classification (see Chapter 6). For purposes of treatment, it is important to distinguish between 'pre-collapse' and 'collapse' of the talar dome.

Conservative treatment is sometimes effective; the ankle is more forgiving than the hip and patients may cope for some years on simple analgesics and restricted weightbearing. If symptoms persist and interfere significantly with function, *operative treatment* may be needed. During the pre-collapse phase, core decompression is worth trying as a first approach. If this fails, ankle arthrodesis is indicated (Delanois et al., 1998).

ANKLE OSTEOARTHRITIS
(see also Chapter 5)

OA of the ankle is far less common than OA of the hip or knee; when it does occur it is almost always secondary to some underlying disorder: a malunited fracture, recurrent instability, osteochondritis dissecans of the talus, avascular necrosis of the talus or repeated bleeding with haemophilia. Sometimes, however, the ankle is involved in generalized OA and crystal arthropathy (See Chapter 4).

Clinical features

The presentation is usually with pain and stiffness localized to the ankle, particularly noticed at 'start up', when first standing up from rest. Patients often indicate the site of pain as being transversely across the front of the ankle. The ankle is usually swollen, with palpable anterior osteophytes and tenderness along the anterior joint line. Dorsiflexion (extension) and plantarflexion at the ankle are often restricted. If heel inversion and eversion movements are restricted then suspect subtalar joint involvement. Gait is often anatalgic, offloading the affected leg; the foot is often turned outwards as the patient walks through on the affected ankle, to compensate for the loss of ankle movement.

X-rays show the typical features of OA; the predisposing disorder is almost always easily detected.

Treatment

When the condition flares up, minor, generally nonintrusive symptoms can be managed with analgesia or NSAIDs. Relative rest of the joint might be achieved with the use of a walking stick; weight loss might be appropriate. Activity such as walking, cycling and swimming can be encouraged.

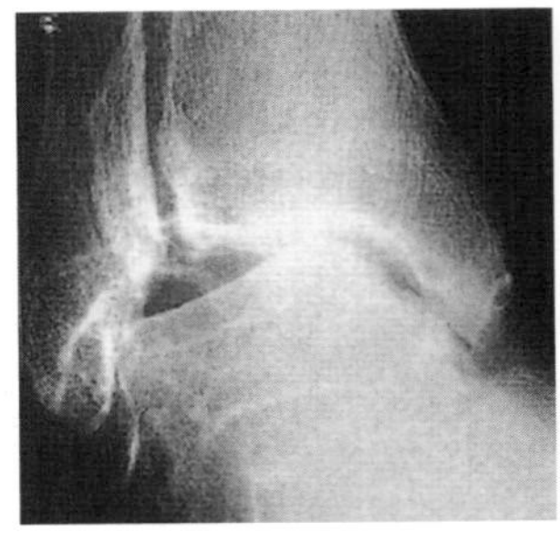

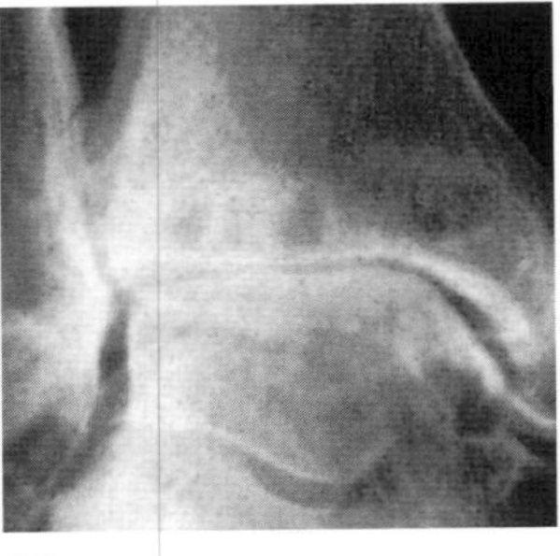

(a) (b)

21.34 OA (a) The obvious malalignment that followed an old injury has led to OA. (b) In this ankle the narrowed joint space and subarticular cysts are characteristic of OA; the cause is not clear, though it may have been trauma.

Physiotherapy can be helpful in improving the range of movement, correcting gait and ensuring correct use of walking aids. An ankle support or brace may help.

OPERATIVE TREATMENT

Ankle arthritis that is interfering with the activities of daily living and limiting work, social or domestic function warrants consideration for operative treatment. Depending on the severity of the condition, ankle surgery such as arthroscopic or open removal of anterior osteophytes (cheilectomy) might be offered, and consideration may be given to ankle arthrodesis; the ideal position for fusion is at zero in the sagittal plane (the foot therefore plantigrade) and 5 degrees of valgus.

Total ankle arthroplasty is not as well established as hip and knee arthroplasty, but encouraging results are being reported.

DIABETIC FOOT

The complications of longstanding diabetes mellitus often appear in the foot, causing chronic disability. More than 30 per cent of patients attending diabetic clinics have evidence of peripheral neuropathy or vascular disease and about 40 per cent of non-trauma-related amputations in British hospitals are for complications of diabetes.

Factors affecting the foot are: (1) a predisposition to peripheral vascular disease; (2) damage to peripheral nerves; (3) reduced resistance to infection; (4) osteoporosis.

Peripheral vascular disease Atherosclerosis affects mainly the medium-sized vessels below the knee. The patient may complain of claudication or ischaemic changes and ulceration in the foot. The skin feels smooth and cold, the nails show trophic changes and the pulses are weak or absent. Doppler studies should corroborate the clinical findings. Superficial ulceration occurs on the toes, deep ulceration typically under the heel; unlike neuropathic ulcers, these are painful and tender. Digital vessel occlusion may cause dry gangrene of one or more toes; proximal vascular occlusion is less common but more serious, sometimes resulting in extensive wet gangrene.

Peripheral neuropathy Early on, patients are usually unaware of the abnormality but clinical tests will discover loss of vibration and joint position sense and diminished temperature discrimination in the feet. Symptoms, when they occur, are mainly due to sensory impairment: symmetrical numbness and paraesthesia, dryness and blistering of the skin, superficial burns and skin cracks or ulceration due to shoe scuffing or localized pressure. Motor loss usually manifests as claw toes with high arches and this, in turn, may predispose to plantar ulceration.

Neuropathic joint disease 'Charcot joints' occur in less than 1 per cent of diabetic patients, yet diabetes is the commonest cause of a neuropathic joint in Europe and America (leprosy and tertiary syphilis being the other common causes worldwide). The mid-tarsal joints are the most commonly affected, followed by the MTP and ankle joints. There is usually a provocative incident, such as a twisting injury or a fracture, following which the joint collapses relatively painlessly. X-rays show marked and fairly rapid destruction of the articular surfaces. These changes are easily mistaken for infection but the simultaneous involvement of several small joints and the lack of systemic signs point to a neuropathic disorder. Joint aspiration and microbiological investigation will also help to exclude infection.

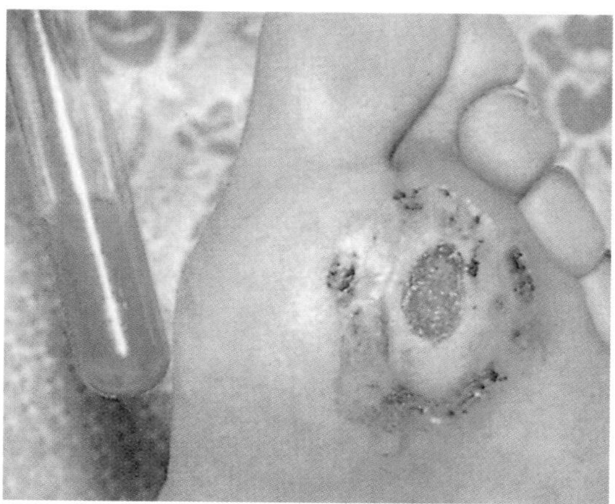
(a)

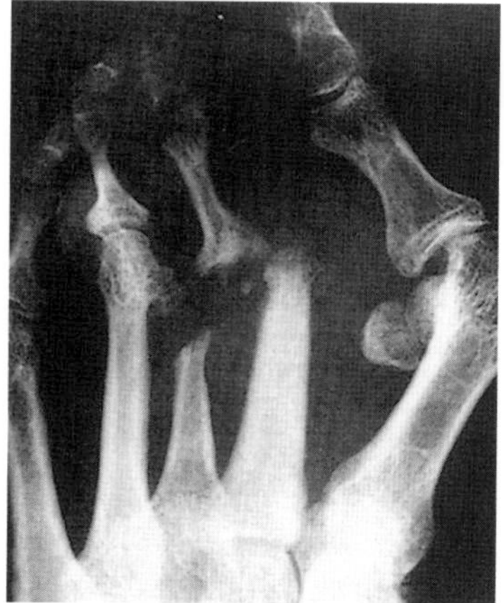
(b)

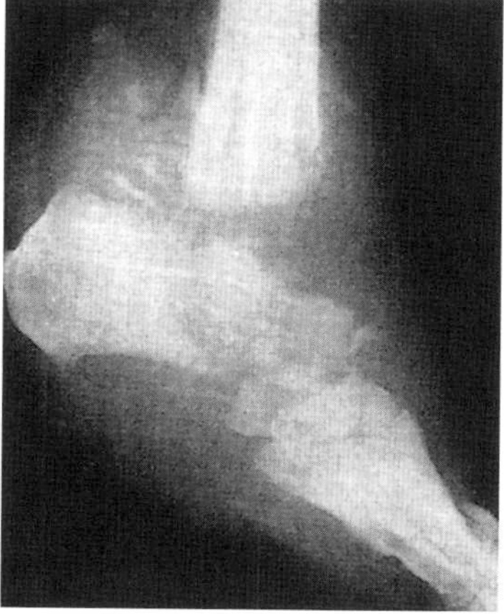
(c)

21.35 The diabetic foot 1 (a) Ulceration in a patient with poorly controlled diabetes. (b,c) Despite the severe changes in these two patients with diabetic neuropathy, the feet were relatively painless.

In late cases there may be severe deformity and loss of function. A rocker-bottom deformity from collapse of the midfoot is diagnostic.

Osteoporosis There is a generalized loss of bone density in diabetes. In the foot the changes may be severe enough to result in insufficiency fractures around the ankle or in the metatarsals.

Infection Diabetes, if not controlled, is known to have a deleterious effect on white cell function. This, combined with local ischaemia, insensitivity to skin injury and localized pressure due to deformity, makes sepsis an ever-recurring hazard.

Management

The orthopaedic surgeon will usually be one member of a multidisciplinary team comprising a physician (or endocrinologist), surgeon, chiropodist and orthotist. The best way of preventing complications is to insist on regular attendance at a diabetic clinic, full compliance with medication, examination for early signs of vascular or neurological abnormality, advice on foot care and footwear and a high level of skin hygiene.

Examination for early signs of neuropathy should include the use of Semmes–Weinstein hairs (for testing skin sensibility) and a biothesiometer (for testing vibration sense). Peripheral vascular examination is enhanced by using a Doppler ultrasound probe. Ulcers must be swabbed for infecting organisms; frequently, multiple bacterial types are isolated (anaerobes make a regular appearance). X-ray examination may reveal periosteal reactions, osteoporosis, cortical defects near the articular margins and osteolysis – often collectively described as 'diabetic osteopathy'.

Great care is needed with nail trimming; skin cracks should be kept clean and covered and ulcers should be treated with local dressings and antibiotics if necessary. Occasionally, septicaemia calls for admission to hospital and treatment with intravenous antibiotics.

Ischaemic changes need the attention of a vascular surgeon who can advise on ways of improving the local blood supply. Arteriography may show that bypass surgery is feasible. Dry gangrene of the toe can be allowed to demarcate before local amputation; severe occlusive disease with wet gangrene may call for immediate amputation.

Indolent neuropathic ulcers require patient dressing and, if infected, antibiotic treatment. Total contact casts may avoid the need for prolonged inpatient stays or bed rest (Coleman et al., 1984). If a bony 'high spot' is identified, it should be trimmed or excised. Custom-made shoes with total contact insoles must follow the successful healing of these ulcers to avoid recurrence.

Insufficiency fractures should be treated, if possible, without immobilizing the limb; or, if a cast is essential, it should be retained for the shortest possible period.

Neuropathic joint disease is a major challenge. Arthrodesis is fraught with difficulty, not least a very poor union rate, and sometimes is simply not feasible. 'Containment' of the problem in a weight-relieving orthosis may be the best option.

Bone or joint infection is an ever-present risk and should be borne in mind in the differential diagnosis of insufficiency fractures and neuropathic joint erosion. This will require urgent treatment.

DISORDERS OF THE TENDO ACHILLIS

ACHILLES TENDINITIS

Athletes, joggers and hikers often develop pain and swelling around the tendo Achillis, due to local irritation of the tendon sheath or the paratenon.

Pathology

The condition usually affects the 'watershed' area about 4 cm above the insertion of the tendon, an area where the blood supply to the tendon is poorer than elsewhere. The tendon sheath or the flimsy tissue around it may become inflamed. In a minority of cases the changes appear at the tendon insertion, or there may be inflammation of the retrocalcaneal bursa just above the calcaneum and deep to the tendon; anatomical deformity of the posterior part of the calcaneum may contribute to the pathogenesis.

Clinical features

The condition may come on gradually, or rapidly following a change in sporting activity (or a change of sports footwear). Less commonly there is a history of direct trauma to the Achilles tendon. The area above the heel may look inflamed and function is inhibited because of pain in the heel-cord, especially at push-off. The tendon feels thickened in the watershed area about 4 cm above its insertion. In chronic cases an ultrasound scan may be helpful in confirming the diagnosis.

If the onset is very sudden, suspect tendon rupture (see later).

Treatment

If the condition starts acutely, it will often settle within about 6 weeks if treated appropriately. Referral for early physiotherapy is important. In the interim, advice on rest, ice, compression and elevation (RICE) and the use of an NSAID (oral or topical) are helpful.

When the symptoms improve, stretching exercises, followed by a muscle strengthening programme, should be advised. The use of a removeable in-shoe heel-raise might be helpful. If there is a plano-valgus hindfoot, correction with orthotics will often bring about improvement and reduce the risk of recurrence.

When the onset is insidious and treatment is started late, symptoms will be prolonged and may last for 9 months or longer.

Operative treatment is seldom necessary but if symptoms fail to settle with physiotherapy then surgery may be appropriate – even more so if there is suspicion of an acute (or missed) tendon rupture. This will involve some type of 'decompressive' operation.

Treatments such as radiofrequency coblation or extracorporeal shockwave lithotripsy are now showing some promise.

Potential pitfalls

Injection with corticosteroids should be avoided. Tendon rupture is a real risk and could well give rise to litigation.

Do not diagnose 'partial rupture' of the Achilles tendon; this should only be entertained if there is clearly some discontinuity of the tendon on ultrasound scan.

ACHILLES TENDON RUPTURE

A ripping or popping sensation is felt, and often heard, at the back of the heel. This most commonly occurs in sports requiring an explosive push-off: squash, badminton, football, tennis, netball. The patient will often report having looked round to see who had hit them over the back of the heel, the pain and collapse are so sudden.

The typical site for rupture is at the vascular watershed about 4 cm above the tendon insertion onto the calcaneum. The condition is often associated with poor muscle strength and flexibility, failure to warm up and stretch before sport, previous injury or tendinitis and corticosteroid injection.

Examination

Plantarflexion of the foot is usually inhibited and weak (although it may be possible, as the long flexors of the toes are also ankle flexors). There is often a palpable gap at the site of rupture; bruising comes out a day or two later. The calf squeeze test (Thompson's or Simmond's test) is diagnostic of Achilles tendon rupture: normally, with the patient prone, if the calf is squeezed the foot will plantarflex involuntarily; if the tendon is ruptured the foot remains still.

Clinical assessment is often sufficient. *Ultrasound scans* must be used to confirm or refute the diagnosis.

Differential diagnosis

Incomplete tear A complete rupture is often mistaken for a partial tear (which is rare). The mistake arises because, if a complete rupture is not seen within 24 hours, the gap is difficult to feel; moreover, the patient may by then be able to stand on tiptoe (just), by using his or her long toe flexors.

Tear of soleus muscle A tear at the musculotendinous junction causes pain and tenderness halfway up the calf. This recovers with the aid of physiotherapy and raising the heel of the shoe.

Treatment

If the patient is seen early, the ends of the tendon may approximate when the foot is passively plantarflexed. If so, a plaster cast or special boot is applied with the foot in equinus; rehabilitation and physiotherapy regimes vary, but it is probably safe, and may be better for eventual tendon strength, to commence physiotherapy within 4–6 weeks. A shoe with a raised heel should be worn for a further 6–8 weeks. The 're-rupture rate' is about 10 per cent.

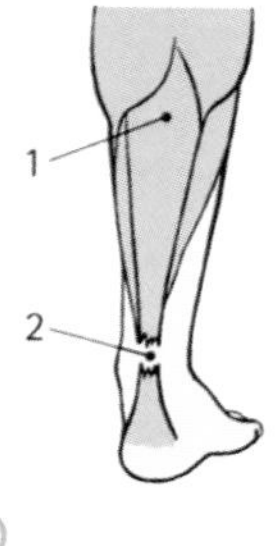

(a)

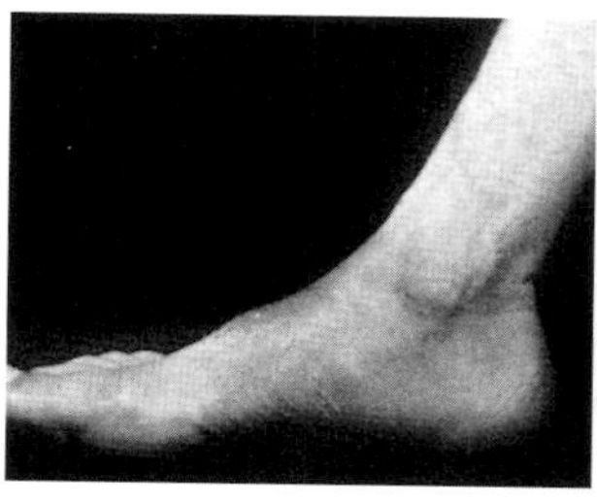

(b)

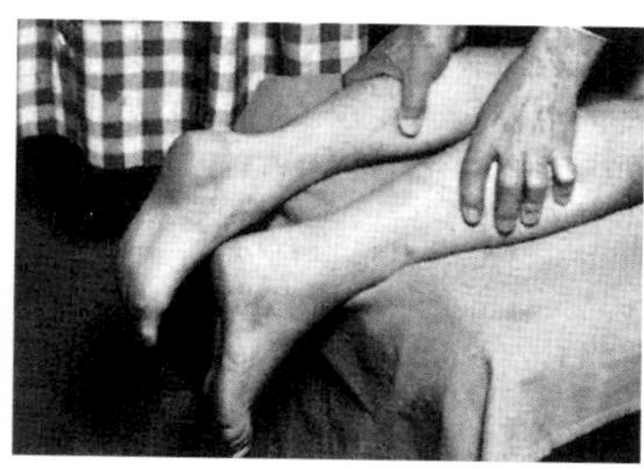

(c)

21.36 Tendo Achillis (a) The soleus may tear at its musculotendinous junction (1), but the tendo Achillis itself ruptures about 5 cm above its insertion (2). (b) The depression seen in this picture at the site of rupture later fills with blood. (c) Simmonds' test: both calves are being squeezed but only the left foot plantarflexes – the right tendon is ruptured.

Operative repair is associated with an earlier return to function, better tendon and calf muscle strength and a lower re-rupture rate. Supported rehabilitation and physiotherapy are commenced early (within a week or two of repair) There are, however, risks associated with operative tendon repair, including wound healing problems and sural nerve neuroma.

For ruptures that present late, reconstruction using local tendon substitutes (e.g. flexor hallucis longus tendon) or strips of fascia lata is still possible.

PARALYZED FOOT

Weakness or paralysis of the foot may be symptomless, or may present in one of three characteristic ways: the patient may: (1) complain of difficulty in walking; (2) 'catch his toe' on climbing stairs (due to weak dorsiflexion); (3) stumble and fall (due to instability).

Clinical features

Upper motor neuron lesions Spastic paralysis may occur in children with cerebral palsy or in adults following a stroke. Muscle imbalance usually leads to equinus or equinovarus deformity. The reflexes are brisk but sensation is normal. The entire limb (or both lower limbs) is usually abnormal.

Lower motor neuron lesions Poliomyelitis was (and in some parts of the world still is) a common cause of foot paralysis. If all muscle groups are affected, the foot is flail and dangles from the ankle; if knee extension is also weak, the patient cannot walk without a calliper. With unbalanced weakness, the foot develops fixed deformity; it may also be smaller and colder than normal, but sensation is normal. Other lower motor neuron disorders such as spinal cord tumours, peroneal muscular atrophy and severe nerve root compression are rare causes of foot weakness or deformity.

Peripheral nerve injuries The sciatic, lateral popliteal or peroneal nerve may be affected. The commonest abnormalities are drop-foot and weakness of peroneal action. Postoperative or postimmobilization drop-foot may be due to pressure on the lateral popiteal or on the peroneal nerve as the leg rolls into external rotation. In addition to motor weakness there is an area of sensory loss. Unless the nerve is divided, recovery is possible but may take many months.

'Peroneal nerve lesion' is sometimes diagnosed after a hip operation. Beware! This is more often due to injury of the peroneal portion of the *sciatic nerve*.

Treatment

The weakness may need no treatment at all, or only a drop-foot splint.

Drop-foot due to nerve palsy can be treated by transferring the tibialis posterior through the interosseous membrane to the midtarsal region.

Spastic paralysis is treated by tendon release and transfer, but great care is needed to prevent overaction in the new direction. Thus, a spastic equinovarus deformity may be converted to a severe valgus deformity by transferring the tibialis anterior to the lateral side; this is avoided if only half the tendon is transferred.

Fixed deformities must be corrected first before doing tendon transfers. If no adequate tendon is available to permit dynamic correction, the joint may be reshaped and arthrodesed; at the same time muscle rebalancing (even of weak muscles) is necessary, otherwise the deformity will recur.

PAINFUL ANKLE

Except after trauma or in rheumatoid arthritis, persistent pain around the ankle usually originates in one of the peri-articular structures or the talus rather than the joint itself. Conditions to be looked for are chronic ligamentous instability, tenosynovitis of the tibialis posterior or peroneal tendons, rupture of the tibialis posterior tendon, osteochondritis dissecans of the dome of the talus or avascular necrosis of the talus.

Tenosynovitis Tenderness and swelling are localized to the affected tendon, and pain is aggravated by active movement – inversion or eversion against resistance. Local injection of corticosteroid usually helps.

Rupture of tibialis posterior tendon Pain starts quite suddenly and sometimes the patient gives a history of having felt the tendon snap. The heel is in valgus during weightbearing; the area around the medial malleolus is tender and active inversion of the ankle is both painful and weak. In physically active patients, operative repair or tendon transfer using the tendon of flexor digitorum longus is worthwhile. For poorly mobile patients, or indeed anyone who is prepared to put up with the inconvenience of an orthosis, splintage may be adequate (see Fig. 21.31).

Osteochondritis dissecans of the talus Unexplained pain and slight limitation of movement in the ankle of a young person may be due to a small osteochondral fracture of the dome of the talus. Tangential x-rays will usually show the tiny fragment. MRI is also helpful and the lesion may be visualized directly by arthroscopy. If the articular surface is intact, it is sufficient to simply

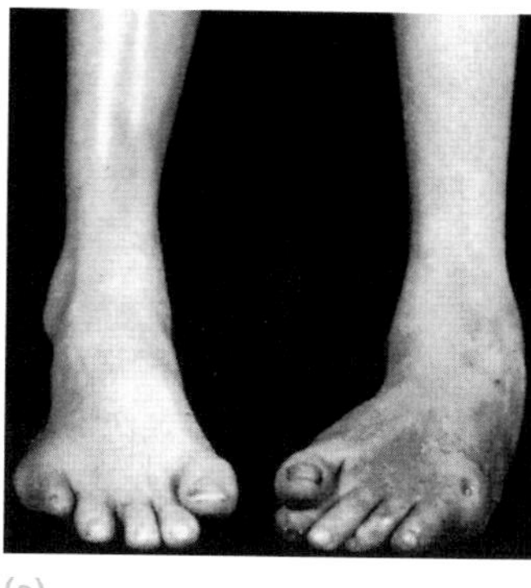
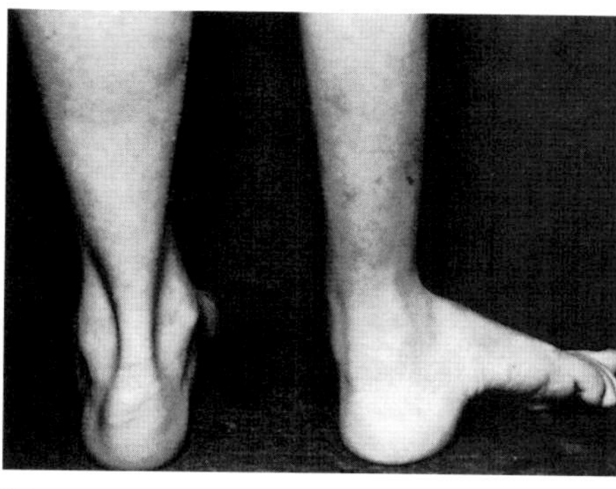
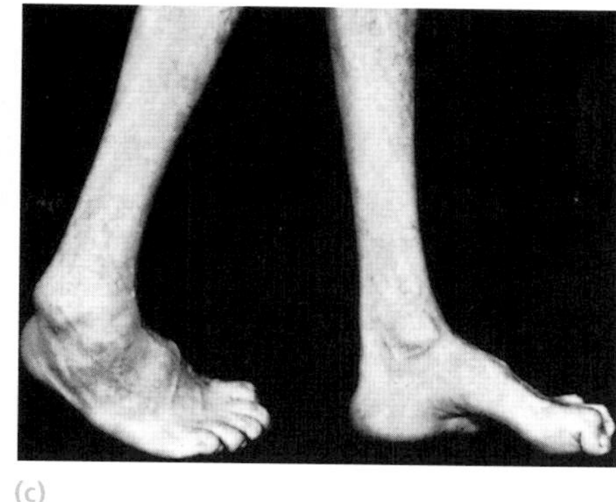

(a) (b) (c)

21.37 The paralyzed foot (a) In spina bifida – the small ulcer is an indication of insensitive skin. (b) Poliomyelitis and (c) peroneal muscular atrophy, in both of which sensation is normal.

restrict activities. If the fragment has separated, it may have to be removed.

Avascular necrosis of the talus The talus is one of the preferred sites of 'idiopathic' necrosis. The causes are the same as for necrosis at other more common sites such as the femoral head. If pain is marked, arthrodesis of the ankle may be needed.

Chronic instability of the ankle This subject is dealt with in Chapter 3.

PAINFUL FEET

"My feet are killing me!" This complaint is common but the cause is often elusive. Pain may be due to: (1) mechanical pressure (which is more likely if the foot is deformed or the patient obese); (2) joint inflammation or stiffness; (3) a localized bone lesion; (4) peripheral ischaemia; (5) muscular strain – usually secondary to some other abnormality. Remember, too, that local disorders may be part of a generalized disease (e.g. diabetes or rheumatoid arthritis), so examination of the entire patient may be indicated.

Specific foot disorders that cause pain are considered later.

POSTERIOR HEEL PAIN

Two common causes of heel pain are traction 'apophysitis' and calcaneal bursitis:

Traction 'apophysitis' (Sever's disease) This condition usually occurs in boys aged about 10 years. It is not a 'disease' but a mild traction injury. Pain and tenderness are localized to the tendo Achillis insertion. The x-ray report usually refers to increased density and fragmentation of the apophysis, but often the painless heel looks similar. The heel of the shoe should be raised a little and strenuous activities restricted for a few weeks.

Calcaneal bursitis Older girls and young women often complain of painful bumps on the backs of their heels. The posterolateral portion of the calcaneum is prominent and shoe friction causes retrocalcaneal bursitis. Symptoms are worse in cold weather and when wearing high-heeled shoes (hence the use of colloquial labels such as 'winter heels' and 'pump-bumps').

Treatment should be conservative – attention to footwear (open-back shoes are best) and padding of the heel. Operative treatment – removal of the bump

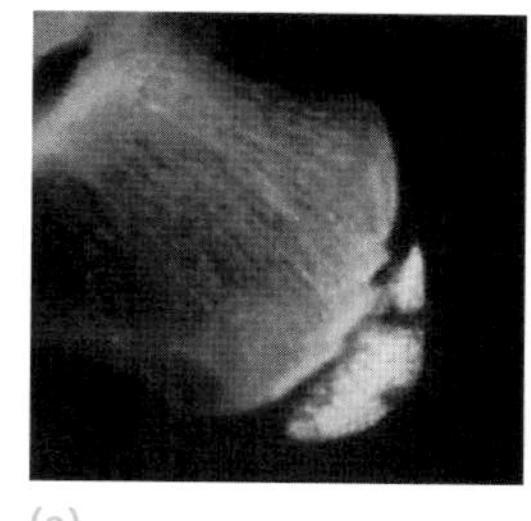
(a)
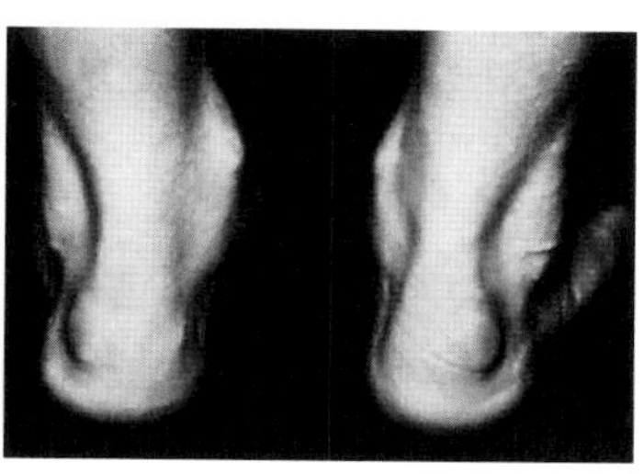
(b)
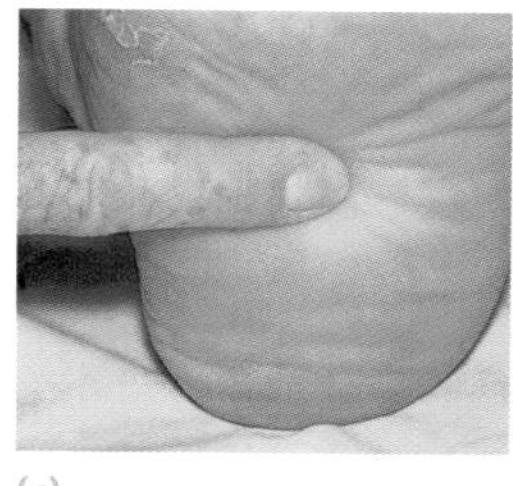
(c)
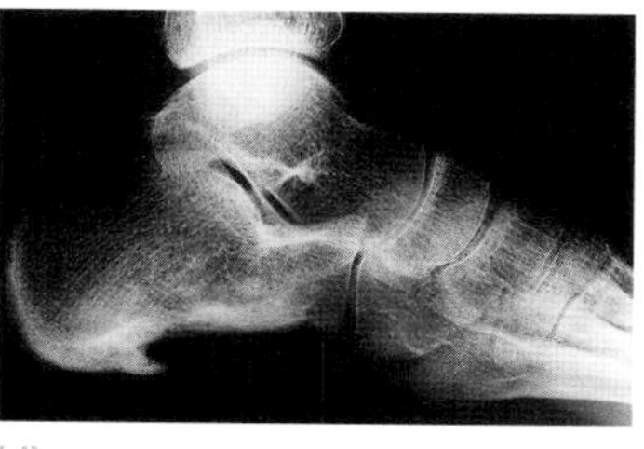
(d)

21.38 Painful heel (a) Sever's disease – the apophysis is dense and fragmented. (b) Bilateral 'heel bumps'. (c) The usual site of tenderness in plantar fasciitis. (d) X-ray in patients with plantar fasciitis often shows what looks like a spur on the undersurface of the calcaneum. In reality this is a two-dimensional view of a small ridge corresponding to the attachment of the plantar fascia. It is doubtful whether the 'spur' is responsible for the pain and local tenderness.

or dorsal wedge osteotomy of the calcaneum – is feasible but the results are unpredictable; despite the reduction in the size of the bumps, patients often continue to experience discomfort, potentially added to by an operation scar.

INFERIOR HEEL PAIN

Calcaneal bone lesions Any bone disorder in the calcaneum can present as heel pain: a stress fracture, osteomyelitis, osteoid osteoma, cyst-like lesions and Paget's disease are the most likely. X-rays usually provide the diagnosis.

PLANTAR FASCIITIS

This is an annoying and painful condition that limits function. There is pain and tenderness in the sole of the foot, mostly under the heel, with standing or walking. The condition usually comes on gradually, without any clear incident or injury but sometimes there is a history of sudden increase in sporting activity, or a change of footwear, sports shoes or running surface. There may be an associated tightness of the Achilles tendon. The pain is often worse when first getting up in the morning, with typical hobbling downstairs, or when first getting up from a period of sitting – the typical start-up pain and stiffness. The pain can at times be very sharp, or it may change to a persistent background ache as the patient walks about.

The condition can take 18–36 months or longer to resolve, but is generally self-limiting, given time.

Pathology

The plantar fascia or aponeurosis is a dense fibrous structure that originates from the calcaneum, deep to the heel fat pad, and runs distally to the ball of the foot, with slips to each toe. The plantar fascia stiffens and becomes less pliable with age. The fascia is probably not actually inflamed in this condition, at least not beyond the first week or two of onset. There may be micro-tears in the fascia, and the fascia thickens.

The term 'plantar fasciitis' is apt in some cases, as the condition is sometimes associated with inflammatory disorders such as gout, ankylosing spondylitis and Reiter's disease, in which enthesopathy is one of the defining pathological lesions.

Clinical features

There is localized tenderness, usually at the medial aspect beneath the heel and sometimes in the midfoot. This is essentially a clinical diagnosis. If there are features suggesting an inflammatory disease (seronegative arthropathy) then blood tests may be indicated. An ultrasound scan shows the thickening and sometimes the Doppler test shows increased local blood flow and neovascularization, but this investigation is not indicated in every case.

A plain lateral x-ray can help to exclude a stress fracture, and will often show what looks like a bony spur on the undersurface of the calcaneum. The 'spur' is, in fact, a bony ridge that looks sharp and localized in the two-dimensional x-ray image; it is an associated, not a causative, feature in plantar fasciitis. Patients, and sometimes doctors, can become fixated on the idea of a spur of bone causing the symptoms by digging into the plantar fascia, and cannot conceive of how the condition could possibly resolve whilst the spur remains – but it can and does get better.

MRI can be helpful in excluding a calcaneal stress fracture, which is an important differential diagnosis.

Treatment

Relative rest and NSAIDs can be helpful in settling the condition in the early stages, with NSAIDs either orally or topically. An analysis of causative factors (footwear, sports and exercise factors) can help the patient to overcome the condition. There is an important role for the patient in managing the condition, with stretching exercises and massage; self-help advice sheets are available.

Patients might expect (or dread!) an injection into the plantar fascia, and they are right to be apprehensive. There is no convincing research to support this, and there is evidence to show that it can lead to rupture of the plantar fascia (which will often immediately ease the symptoms, but leads to a painful flatfoot and impairs sporting function).

A physiotherapist can help to educate the patient about the condition and its likely progress, and can emphasize the need for a regular stretching regime for 8–12 weeks, supplemented with local massage (for instance with a foot roller, golf ball, frozen water bottle). Local manual treatments from the physiotherapist can help, as can the use of taping and a cushioned heel pad.

Night splints have been tried, to keep the foot up in a plantigrade position overnight, preventing stiffening in the Achilles and plantar fascia; there is logic in this, but no clear evidence for its efficacy, and trials have been hampered by poor compliance.

Podiatric assessment of the hindfoot biomechanics may identify predisposing factors such as plano-valgus hindfoot alignment, which can be corrected with orthotics.

OPERATIVE TREATMENT

Patients may lose heart and demand that something be done. However, there is no reliable surgical procedure for this condition. Limited fasciotomy to release part of the plantar fascia can help in some cases, but there is a significant risk of complications including worsening of the condition.

Promising new interventions include shockwave lithotripsy and localized radiofrequency (coblation) therapy, but these have yet to be fully tested in rigorous and large-scale studies.

Potential pitfalls

It is important not to miss a manifestation of a systemic disease such as an inflammatory arthropathy (often seronegative), a peripheral neuropathy (usually diabetic) or a stress fracture.

If a corticosteroid steroid injection is used it should be done cautiously with a small dose into a limited area, and after appropriate warnings to the patient.

Excising a 'spur' is usually a vain endeavour.

Differential diagnosis

Painful fat pad Chronic pain and tenderness directly over the fat pad under the heel sometimes follows a direct blow to the area, e.g. in a fall from a height. The condition is also seen in athletes and has been attributed variously to separation of the fat pad from the bone, loss of its normal shock-absorbing effect and atrophy. Non-specific 'inflammation' has also been blamed. Treatment is palliative: wearing soft-soled shoes or shock-absorbing heel cups, foot baths and anti-inflammatory agents.

Nerve entrapment Entrapment of the first branch of the lateral plantar nerve has been reported as a cause of heel pain. The commonest complaint is pain after sporting activities. Characteristically, tenderness is maximal on the medial aspect of the heel, where the small nerve branch is compressed between the deep fascia of abductor hallucis and the edge of the quadratus plantae muscle. Diagnosis is not easy, because the symptoms and signs may mimic those of plantar fasciitis.

Treatment, in the first instance, is conservative: a long trial (6–8 months) of shock-absorbing orthoses, foot baths, anti-inflammatory preparations and one or two corticosteriod injections. Only if these measures fail to give relief should surgical decompression of the nerve be considered.

Pain over the midfoot

In children, pain in the midtarsal region is rare: one cause is *Kohler's disease* (osteochondritis of the navicular). The bony nucleus of the navicular becomes dense and fragmented. The child, under the age of 5,

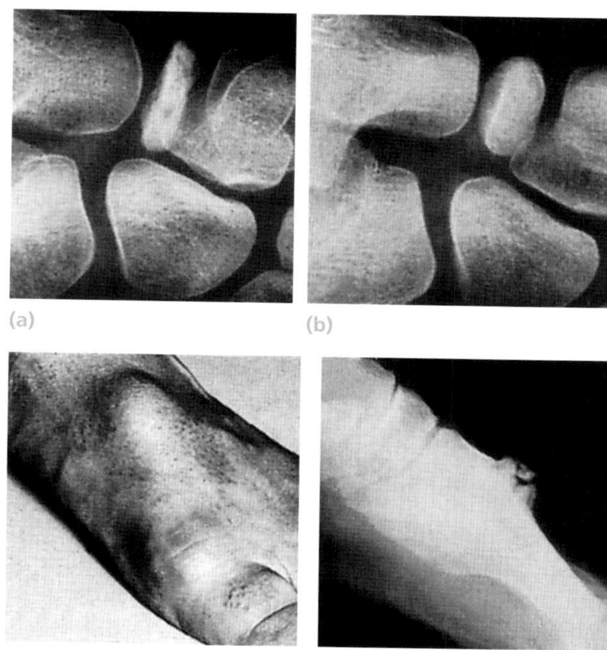

21.39 Pain over the midfoot (a) Köhler's disease compared with (b) the normal foot. (c,d) The bump on the dorsum of the foot due to OA of the first cuneiform-metatarsal joint.

has a painful limp and a tender warm thickening over the navicular. Usually no treatment is needed as the condition resolves spontaneously. If symptoms are severe, a short period in a below-knee plaster helps.

A comparable condition occasionally affects middle-aged women (*Brailsford's disease*); the navicular becomes dense, then altered in shape, and later the midtarsal joint may degenerate.

In adults, especially if the arch is high, a ridge of bone sometimes develops on the adjacent dorsal surfaces of the medial cuneiform and the first metatarsal (the '*overbone*'). A lump can be seen, which feels bony and may become bigger and tender if the shoe presses on it. If shoe adjustment fails to provide relief the lump may be bevelled off.

Generalized pain in the forefoot

Metatarsalgia Generalized ache in the forefoot is a common expression of foot strain, which may be due to a variety of conditions that give rise to faulty weight distribution (e.g. flattening of the metatarsal arch, or undue shortening of the first metatarsal), or merely the result of prolonged or unaccustomed walking, marching, climbing or standing. These conditions have this in common: they give rise to a mismatch between the loads applied to the foot, the structure on which those loads are acting, and the muscular effort required to maintain the structure so that it can support those loads.

Aching is felt across the forefoot and the anterior metatarsal arch may have flattened out. There may even be callosities under the metatarsal heads.

Treatment involves: (1) dealing with the mechanical disorder (correcting a deformity if it is correctable, supplying an orthosis that will redistribute the load, fitting a shoe that will accommodate the foot); and (2) performing regular muscle strengthening exercises, especially for the intrinsic muscles that maintain the anterior (metatarsal) arch of the foot. A good 'do-it-yourself' exercise is for the patient to stand barefoot on the floor, feet together, and then drag their body forwards by repeatedly crimping the toes to produce traction upon the floor. Ten minutes a day should suffice.

Pain in metatarsophalangeal joints Inflammatory arthritis (e.g. rheumatoid disease) may start in the foot with synovitis of the MTP joints. Pain in these cases is associated with swelling and tenderness of the forefoot joints and the features are almost always bilateral and symmetrical.

LOCALIZED PAIN IN THE FOREFOOT

Whereas metatarsalgia involves the entire forefoot, localized pain and tenderness is related to a specific anatomical site in the forefoot and could be due to a variety of bone or soft tissue disorders: 'sesamoiditis', osteochondritis of a metatarsal head (Freiberg's disease), a metatarsal stress fracture or digital nerve entrapment (Morton's disease).

Sesamoiditis

Pain and tenderness directly under the first metatarsal head, typically aggravated by walking or passive dorsiflexion of the great toe, may be due to sesamoiditis. This term is a misnomer: symptoms usually arise from irritation or inflammation of the peritendinous tissues around the sesamoids – more often the medial (tibial) sesamoid, which is subjected to most stress during weightbearing on the ball of the foot.

Acute sesamoiditis may be initiated by direct trauma (e.g. jumping from a height) or unaccustomed stress (e.g. in new athletes and dancers). *Chronic sesamoid pain* and *tenderness* should signal the possibility of sesamoid displacement, local infection (particularly in a diabetic patient) or avascular necrosis.

Sesamoid chondromalacia is a term coined by Apley (1966) to explain changes such as fragmentation and cartilage fibrillation of the medial sesamoid. X-rays in these cases may show a bipartite or multipartite medial sesamoid, which is often mistaken for a fracture.

Treatment, in the usual case, consists of reduced weightbearing and a pressure pad in the shoe. In resistant cases, a local injection of methylprednisolone and local anaesthetic often helps; otherwise the sesamoid should be shaved down or removed, taking great care not to completely interrupt the flexor hallucis brevis tendon.

Freiberg's disease (osteochondritis; osteochondrosis)

Osteochondritis (or osteochondrosis) of a metatarsal head is probably a type of traumatic osteonecrosis of the subarticular bone in a bulbous epiphysis (akin to osteochondritis dissecans of the knee). It usually affects the second metatarsal head (rarely the third) in young adults, mostly women.

The patient complains of pain at the MTP joint. A bony lump (the enlarged head) is palpable and tender and the MTP joint is irritable. X-rays show the head

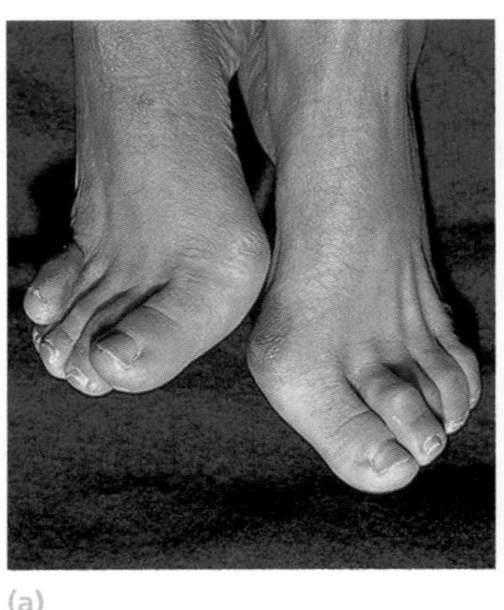

(a)

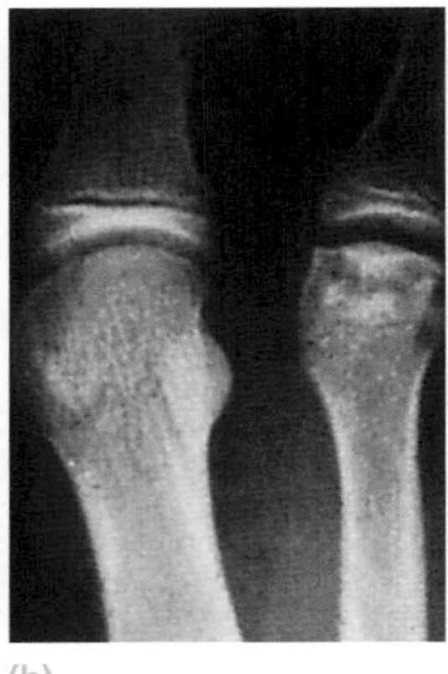

(b)

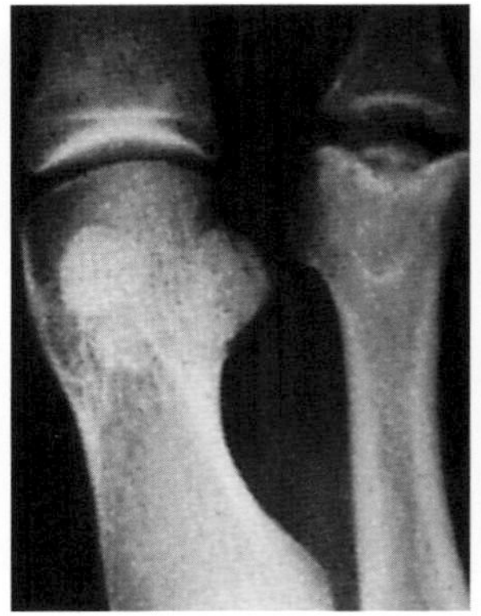

(c)

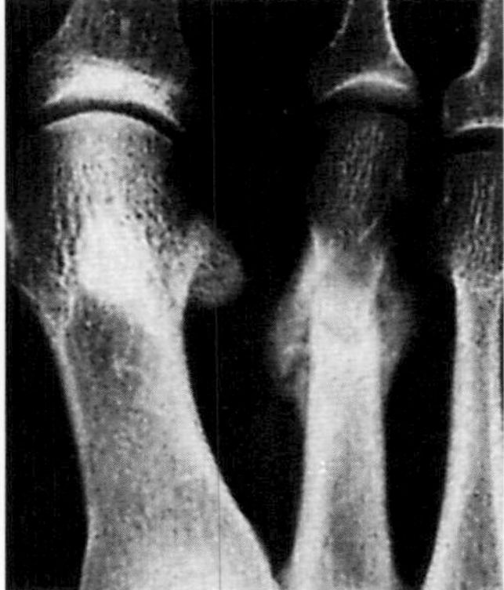

(d)

21.40 Pain in the forefoot (a) Long-standing deformities such as dropped anterior arches, hallux valgus, hammer-toe, curly toes and overlapping toes (all of which are present in this patient) can cause metatarsalgia. Localized pain and tenderness suggest a more specific cause. (b,c) Stages in the development of Freiberg's disease. (d) Periosteal new-bone formation along the shaft of the second metatarsal, the classic sign of a healing stress fracture.

to be flattened and wide, the neck thick and the joint space apparently increased.

If discomfort is marked, a walking plaster or moulded sandal will help to reduce pressure on the metatarsal head. If pain and stiffness persist, operative synovectomy, debridement and trimming of the metatarsal head should be considered. Pain relief is usually good and the range of dorsiflexion is improved.

Stress fracture

Stress fracture, usually of the second or third metatarsal, occurs in young adults after unaccustomed activity or in women with postmenopausal osteoporosis. The dorsum of the foot may be slightly oedematous and the affected shaft feels thick and tender. The x-ray appearance is at first normal, but later shows fusiform callus around a fine transverse fracture. Long before x-ray signs appear, a radioisotope scan will show increased activity. Treatment is either unnecessary or consists simply of rest and reassurance.

Interdigital nerve compression (Morton's metatarsalgia)

Morton's metatarsalgia is a common problem, with neuralgia affecting a single distal metatarsal interspace, usually the third (affecting the third and fourth toes), sometimes the second (affecting the second and third toes), rarely others. The patient typically complains of pain on walking, with the sensation of walking on a pebble in the shoe, or of the sock being rucked-up under the ball of the foot. The pain is worse in tight footwear and often has to be relieved by removing the footwear and massaging the foot. Activities that load the forefoot (running, jumping, dancing) exacerbate the condition, which often consists of severe forefoot pain and then a reluctance to weightbear. In Morton's metatarsalgia the pain is typically reproduced by laterally compressing the forefoot whilst also compressing the affected interspace – this produces the pathognomic Mulder's click as the 'neuroma' displaces between the metatarsal heads.

This is essentially an entrapment or compression syndrome affecting one of the digital nerves, but secondary thickening of the nerve creates the impression of a 'neuroma'. The lesion, and an associated bursa, occupy a restricted space between the distal metatarsals, and are pinched, especially if footwear also laterally compresses the available space.

Treatment A step-wise treatment programme is advisable. Simple offloading of the metatarsal heads by using a metatarsal dome insole and wider fitting shoes may help. If symptoms do not improve with these measures then a steroid injection into the interspace will bring about lasting relief in about 50 per cent of cases.

Surgical intervention is often successful; the nerve should be released by dividing the tight transverse intermetatarsal ligament; this can be done through either a dorsal longitudinal or a plantar incision; most surgeons will also excise the thickened portion of the nerve. This is successful in about 90 per cent of patients; the remaining 10 per cent will continue to experience varying degrees of discomfort.

TARSAL TUNNEL SYNDROME

Pain and sensory disturbance in the medial part of the forefoot, unrelated to weightbearing, may be due to compression of the posterior tibial nerve behind and below the medial malleolus. Sometimes this is due to a space-occupying lesion, e.g. a ganglion, haemangioma or varicosity. The pain is often worse at night and the patient may seek relief by walking around or stamping the foot. Paraesthesia and numbness may follow the characteristic sensory distribution, but these symptoms are not as well defined as in other entrapment syndromes. The diagnosis is difficult to establish but nerve conduction studies may show slowing of motor or sensory conduction.

Treatment To decompress the nerve it is exposed behind the medial malleolus and followed into the sole; sometimes it is trapped by the belly of adductor hallucis arising more proximally than usual.

SKIN DISORDERS

Painful skin lesions are important for two reasons: (1) they demand attention in their own right; (2) postural adjustments to relieve pressure may give rise to secondary problems and metatarsalgia.

Corns and calluses

These are hyperkeratotic lesions that develop as a reaction to localized pressure or friction. Corns are fairly small and situated at 'high spots' in contact with the shoe upper: the dorsal knuckle of a claw toe or hammer toe, or the tip of the toe if it impinges against the shoe. Soft corns also appear on adjacent surfaces of toes that rub against each other. Treatment consists of paring the hyperkeratotic skin, applying felt pads that will prevent shoe or toe pressure, correcting any significant deformity (if necessary by operation) and attending to footwear.

Calluses are more diffuse keratotic plaques on the soles – either under prominent metatarsal heads or under the heel. They are seen mainly in people with 'dropped' metatarsal arches and claw toes, or varus or

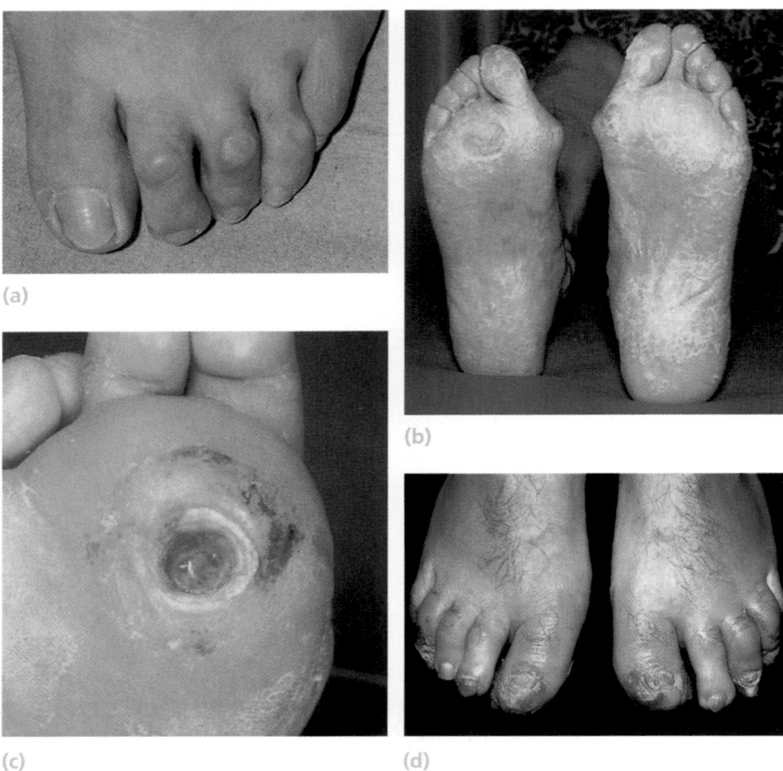

21.41 Skin lesions (a) Corns. (b) Callosities in a patient with claw toes and a 'dropped' anterior metatarsal arch. (c) A typical pressure ulcer in a patient with longstanding diabetic neuropathy. (d) Keratoderma blenorrhagica, a complication of Reiter's disease.

valgus heels. Treatment is much the same as for corns; it is important to redistribute foot pressure by altering the shoes, fitting pressure-relieving orthoses and ensuring that the shoes can accommodate the malshaped feet. Surgical treatment for claw toes may be needed.

Plantar warts

Plantar warts resemble calluses but they tend to be more painful and tender, especially if squeezed. They can be distinguished from calluses by paring down the hyperkeratotic skin to expose the characteristic papillomatous 'core', which is seen to be dotted with fine blood vessels. These are viral lesions but it is usually local pressure that renders them painful.

Treatment is frustrating as they are difficult to eradicate. Salicylic acid plasters are applied at regular intervals, and smaller lesions may respond to cryosurgery. Surgical excision is avoided as this usually leaves a painful scar at the pressure site.

Foreign body 'granuloma'

The sole is particularly at risk of penetration by small foreign bodies (usually a thorn, a splinter or a piece of glass), which may give rise to a painful lump resembling a wart or callus. This diagnosis should always be considered if the 'callosity' is situated in a non-pressure area. X-rays may help to detect the foreign body. Treatment consists of removing the object; the reactive lesion heals quickly.

TOE-NAIL DISORDERS

The toe-nail of the hallux may be ingrown, overgrown or undergrown.

Ingrown toe-nails The nail burrows into the nail groove; this ulcerates and its wall grows over the nail, so the term 'embedded toe-nail' would be better. The patient is taught to cut the nail square, to insert pledgets of wool under the ingrowing edges and to keep the feet clean and dry at all times.

If these measures fail, the portion of germinal matrix that is responsible for the 'ingrow' should be ablated, either by operative excision or by chemical ablation with phenol. The phenol is applied to the exposed matrix with a cotton bud for 3 minutes and then washed off with alcohol, which neutralizes the caustic effect. Rarely is it necessary to remove the entire nail or completely ablate the nail bed.

Overgrown toe-nails (onychogryposis) The nail is hard, thick and curved. A chiropodist can usually make the patient comfortable, but occasionally the nail may need excision.

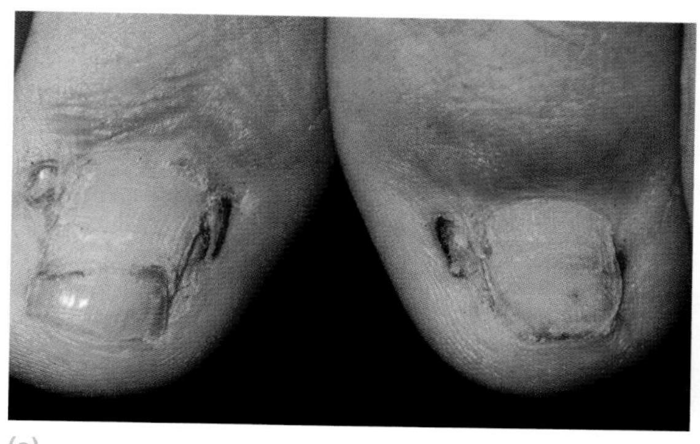
(a)

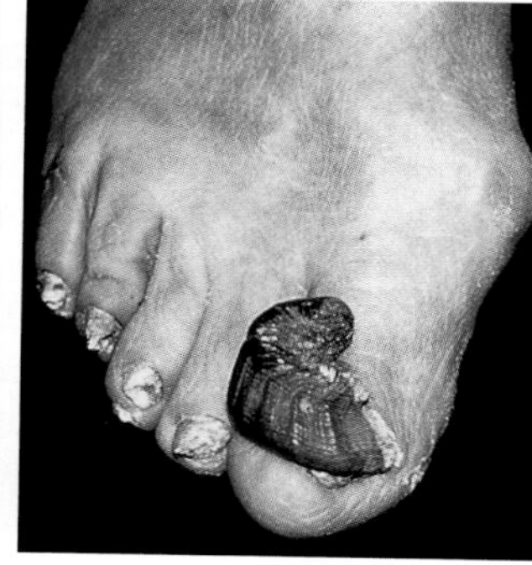
(b)

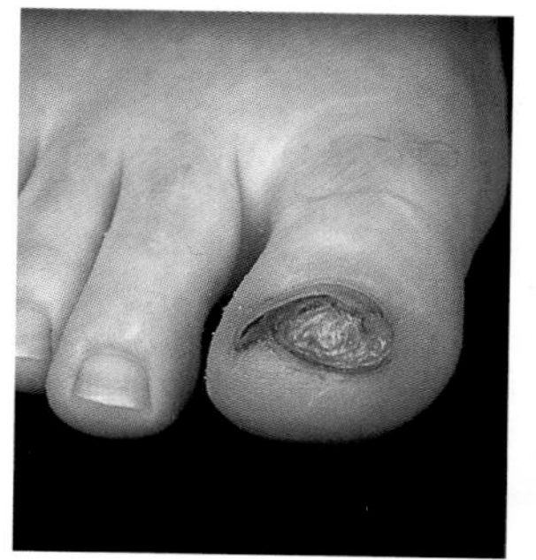
(c)

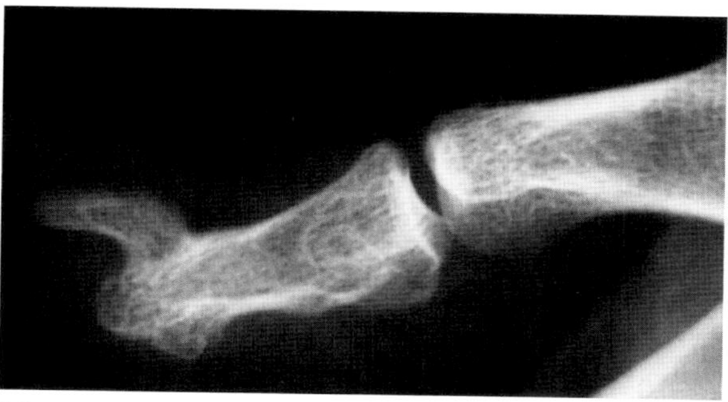
(d)

21.42 Toe-nail disorders (a) Ingrown toe-nails. (b) Overgrown toe-nail (onychogryposis). (c,d) Exostosis from the distal phalanx, pushing the toe-nail up.

Undergrown toe-nails A subungual exostosis grows on the dorsum of the terminal phalanx and pushes the nail upwards. The exostosis should be removed.

NOTES ON APPLIED ANATOMY

The ankle and foot function as an integrated unit, and together provide stable support, proprioception, balance and mobility.

Ankle

The ankle fits together like a tenon and mortise; the tibial and fibular parts of the mortise are bound together by the inferior tibiofibular ligament, and stability is augmented by the collateral ligaments. The medial ligament fans out from the tibial malleolus to the talus, the superficial fibres forming the deltoid ligament. The lateral ligament has three thickened bands: the anterior and posterior talofibular ligaments and, between them, the calcaneofibular ligament. Tears of these ligaments may cause tilting of the talus in its mortise. Forced abduction or adduction may disrupt the mortise altogether by (1) forcing the tibia and fibula apart (diastasis of the tibiofibular joint); (2) tearing the collateral ligaments; (3) fracturing the malleoli.

Foot

The footprint gives some idea of the arched structure of the foot. This derives from the tripodial bony framework between the calcaneum posteriorly and the first and fifth metatarsal heads. The medial arch is high, with the navicular as its keystone; the lateral arch is flatter. The anterior arch formed by the metatarsal bones thrusts maximally upon the first and fifth metatarsal heads and flattens out (spreading the foot) during weightbearing; it can be pulled up by contraction of the intrinsic muscles, which flex the MTP joints.

Movements

The ankle allows movement in the sagittal plane only (plantarflexion and dorsiflexion). Adduction and abduction (turning the toes towards or away from the midline) are produced by rotation of the entire leg below the knee; if either is forced at the ankle, the mortise fractures. Pronation and supination occur at the intertarsal and tarsometatarsal joints; the foot rotates about an axis running through the second metatarsal, the sole turning laterally (pronation) or medially (supination) – movements analogous to those of the forearm. The combination of plantarflexion, adduction and supination is called inversion; the opposite movement of dorsiflexion, abduction and pronation is eversion.

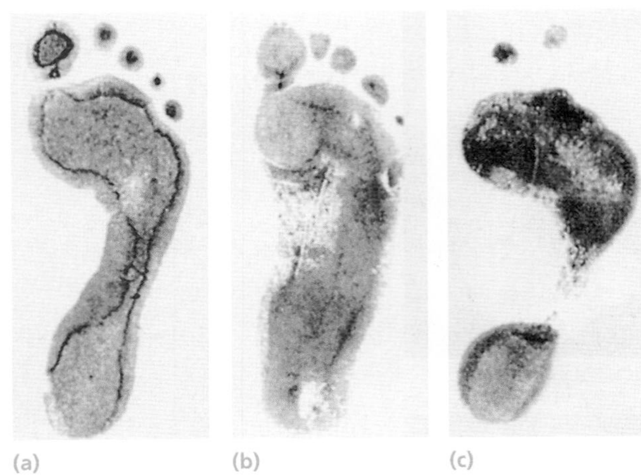

(a) (b) (c)

21.43 Footprints (a) The normal foot, (b) flat-foot (the medial arch touches the ground), and (c) cavus foot (even the lateral arch barely makes contact).

Inversion and eversion are necessary for walking on rough ground or across a slope. If the joints at which they occur are arthrodesed in childhood, a compensatory change may occur at the ankle so that it becomes a ball-and-socket joint.

FOOT POSITIONS AND DEFORMITIES

A downward-pointing foot is said to be in equinus; the opposite is calcaneus. If only the forefoot points downwards the term 'plantaris' is used. Supination with adduction produces a varus deformity; pronation with abduction causes pes valgus. An unusually high arch is called pes cavus. Many of these terms are used as if they were definitive diagnoses when, in fact, they are nothing more than Latin translations of descriptive anatomy.

REFERENCES AND FURTHER READING

Apley AG. Open sessamoid. *Proc R Soc Med* 1966; **59:** 120.

Banta J, Sutherland DH, Wyatt M. Anterior tibialis transfer to os calcis with Achilles tenodesis for calcaneal deformity in myelomeningocoele. *J Paediatr Orthop* 1981; **1:** 125–30.

Caroll NC. Technique of plantar fascia release and calcaneocuboid joint release in clubfoot surgery. In: Simons GW (Ed.) *The Clubfoot.* Springer-Verlag, New York, 1994, pp 246–52.

Cholmeley JA. Elmslie's operation for the calcaneus foot. *J Bone Joint Surg* 1953; **35B:** 46–9.

Coleman WC, Brand PW, Birke JA. The total contact cast. A therapy for plantar ulceration on insensitive feet. *J Am Podiatry Med Assoc* 1984; **74:** 548–52.

Coughlin MJ, Shurnas PS. Hallux rigidus: demographics, etiology, and radiographic assessment. *Foot Ankle Int* 2003; **24:** 731–43.

Crawford A, Marxen J, Osterfeld D. The Cincinatti incision: A comprehensive approach for surgical procedures of the foot and ankle in childhood. *J Bone Joint Surg* 1982; **64A:** 1355–8.

Delanois RE, Mont MA, Yoon TR *et al.* Atraumatic osteonecrosis of the talus. *J Bone Joint Surg* 1998; **80A:** 529–36.

Duncan RD, Fixsen JA. Congenital convex pes valgus. *J Bone Joint Surg* 1999; **81B:** 250–4.

Evans D. Relapsed clubfoot. *J Bone Joint Surg* 1961; **43B:** 722–33.

Gage JR. *Gait Analysis in Cerebral Palsy.* MacKeith Press, New York, 1991.

Herzenberg JE, Carroll NC, Christofersen MR, Lee EH, White S, Munroe R. Clubfoot analysis with three-dimensional computer modeling. *J Paediatr Orthop* 1988; **8:** 257–62.

Lapidus PW. Transplantation of the extensor tendon for correction of the overlapping fifth toe. *J Bone Joint Surg* 1942; **24:** 555–9.

Piggott H. The natural history of hallux valgus in adolescence and early adult life. *J Bone Joint Surg* 1960; **42B:** 749–60.

Ponsetti IV. Treatment of congenital club foot. *J Bone Joint Surg* 1992; **74A:** 448–54.

Rang M. High arches. In: Wenger DR, Rang M (Eds) *The Art and Practice of Children's Orthopaedics.* Raven Press, New York, 1993, pp 168–79.

Robinson AHN, Limbers JP. Modern concepts in the treatment of hallux valgus. *J Bone Joint Surg* 2005; **87B:** 1038–45.

Rose GK, Welton EA, Marshall T. The diagnosis of flat foot in the child. *J Bone Joint Surg* 1985; **67B:** 71–8.

Samilson RL. Proscentic osteotomy of the os calcis for calcaneocavus feet. In: Bateman JE (Ed.) *Foot Science.* WB Saunders, Philadelphia, 1976, p. 18.

Turco V. Surgical correction of the resistant clubfoot. One stage posteromedial release with internal fixation; a preliminary report. *J Bone Joint Surg* 1971; **53A:** 477–97.

Section 3

Fractures and Joint Injuries

The management of major injuries

22

David Sutton, Max Jonas

INTRODUCTION

Aetiology of major trauma

Trauma is the commonest cause of death in people from 1–44 years of age throughout the developed world. The largest proportion of deaths (1.2 million per year) result from road accidents. The World Health Organization (WHO) predicts that by 2020 road traffic injuries will rank third in the causes of premature death and loss of health from disability (Peden et al., 2004). In the UK vehicular accidents causing death or serious injury are usually car related (Figs 22.1 and 22.2).

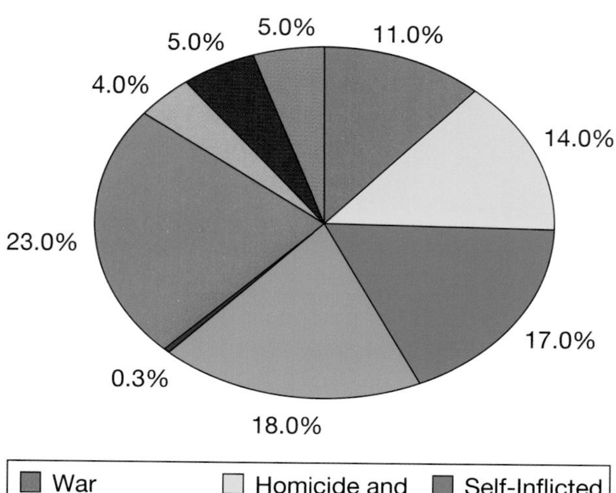

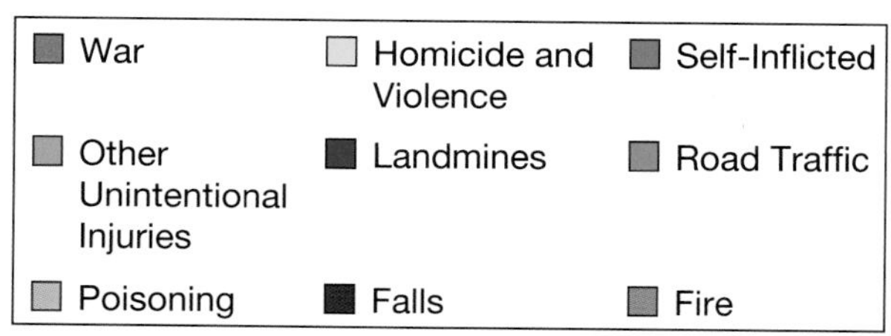

Source: WHO

22.1 Global percentage of deaths due to injury (1999) (World Health Organization, Department of Violence and Injury Prevention).

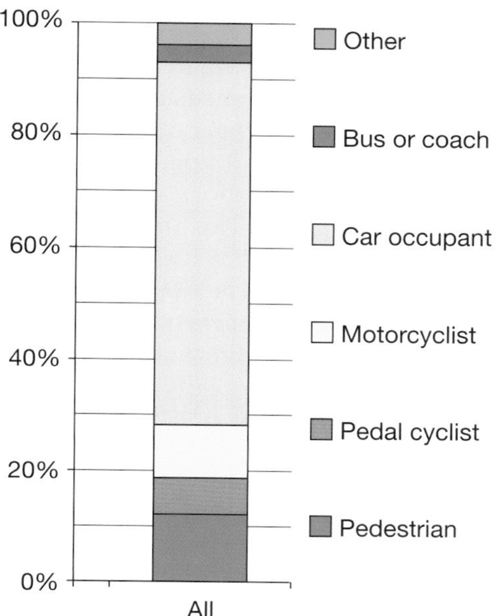

22.2 Proportion of casualties by road user type (UK 2007 Department of Transport data).

For every death from trauma, three victims suffer permanent disability. As well as causing personal tragedy, this represents an enormous drain on a nation's healthcare economy; timely and effective management of major injuries can reduce both morbidity and mortality.

Mode of death

Mortality subsequent to major trauma is dependent on a number of factors, of which the economic level of a nation is a major determinant. The 2004 WHO report (Mock et al., 2004) cites mortality rates for seriously injured adults, i.e. those with an *injury severity score* (ISS) of 9 or higher. ISS will be described in greater detail in a subsequent section. The overall mortality rate, including pre-hospital and in-hospital deaths, is 35 per cent in high-income nations, but rises to 55 per cent in middle-income economies and

63 per cent in low-income economies. More seriously injured patients (ISS 15–24) reaching hospital show a six-fold increase in mortality in low-income economies.

Road traffic deaths and serious injuries show a peak incidence in young people between the ages of 17 (age of learning to drive) and 23.

There is a stark contrast between major trauma mortality in a high-income country hospital (6 per cent) and in a rural area of a low-income country (36 per cent). These statistics demonstrate the impact that a high-income economy with a developed emergency medical system can have on the outcomes of major trauma.

Deaths as a result of trauma classically follow a tri-modal pattern, with three waves following the injury. Some 50 per cent of fatally injured casualties die from non-survivable injuries immediately, or within minutes after the accidents; 30 per cent survive the initial trauma, but die within 1–3 hours; the remaining 20 per cent die from complications at a late stage during the 6 weeks after injury. This trimodality represents civilian trauma deaths; combat deaths in a war fit a bimodal distribution, with merging of the second and third peaks due to the penetrative nature of the injuries and the extended timelines of advanced medical care (Clasper and Rew, 2003).

The initial mortality peak is usually due to non-survivable central nervous system or cardiovascular disruption. The severe nature of the injuries, the immediate nature of the deaths and the usual location in the pre-hospital environment means that very few of these casualties can be saved. However, a small proportion die as a result of early airway obstruction and external haemorrhage, and these deaths can be prevented by immediate first-aid measures. A significant proportion of head-injured casualties who die on the scene succumb not to the primary brain injury but to secondary brain injury caused by the hypoxia and hypercarbia associated with airway obstruction and respiratory dysfunction.

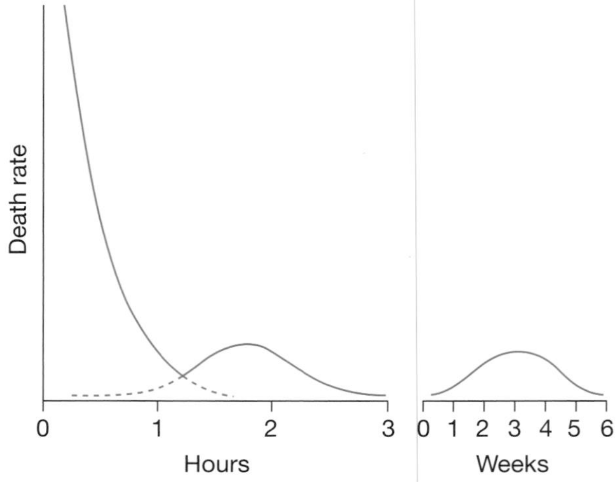

22.4 Death following trauma The trimodal pattern of mortality following severe trauma.

The second peak of deaths during the first few hours after injury is most often due to hypoxia and hypovolaemic shock. A significant proportion of these deaths can be avoided with an effective emergency medical service (EMS); hence, this period has been called 'the golden hour'. One-third of all deaths occurring after major injury may be preventable in hospitals with appropriate resources (Commission on the Provision of Surgical Services, 1988).

The third peak in the cumulative mortality rate within the 6 weeks following injury is largely due to multisystem failure and sepsis. These complications of trauma need a high level of intensive care, but can be reduced by early and effective treatment during the preceding phases of casualty management.

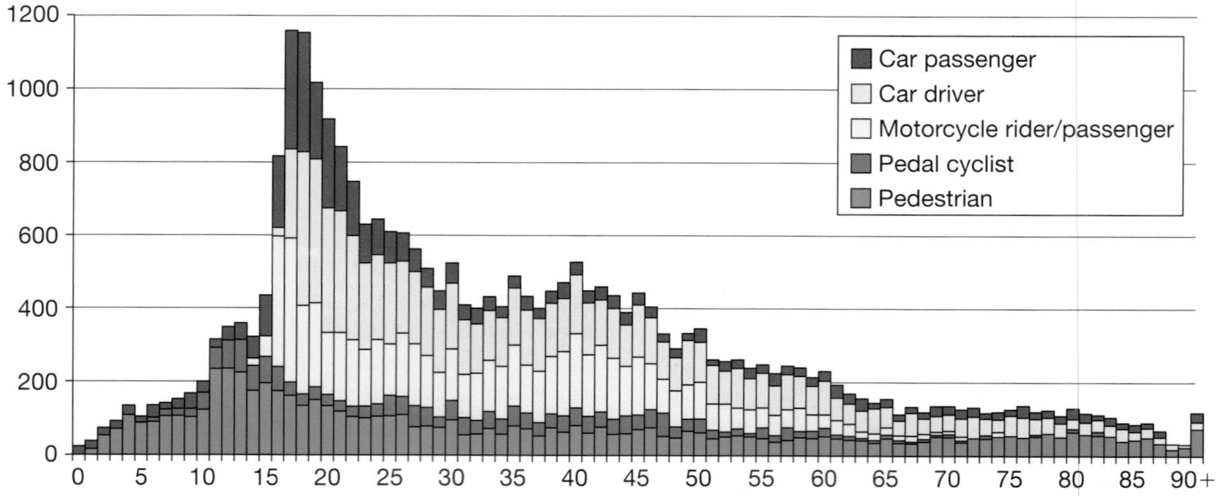

22.3 Deaths and serious injuries by road user type and age (UK 2007 Department of Transport data).

Sequence of management

In developed healthcare systems, an effective EMS is available to initiate management at the scene of the injury and transfer the casualty rapidly to hospital. Immediate first-aid manoeuvres such as opening the airway and controlling external haemorrhage with direct pressure are life-saving interventions that require minimal equipment and training.

More complex treatment requires specialist equipment and expert training not always available at the scene, and rapid transfer to a medical centre is mandatory. However, medical teams can deliver advanced management to entrapped casualties. Such treatment is difficult to deliver in vehicles and aircraft, and a balance has to be drawn between delaying to give treatment on scene and transferring an unstable casualty.

In sophisticated healthcare systems, casualties are taken to the nearest hospital offering comprehensive Emergency Department management. Treatment is centred on *evaluation*, *resuscitation* and *stabilization*. This phase merges into definitive care in the operating theatre, with control of airway, ventilation and surgical management of haemorrhage. Musculoskeletal injuries are initially stabilized, followed by definitive treatment.

Level 2 or 3 critical care may be required to minimize complications and prevent third-phase deaths, and prolonged rehabilitation may be necessary to address the needs of casualties with brain injuries and complex musculoskeletal damage.

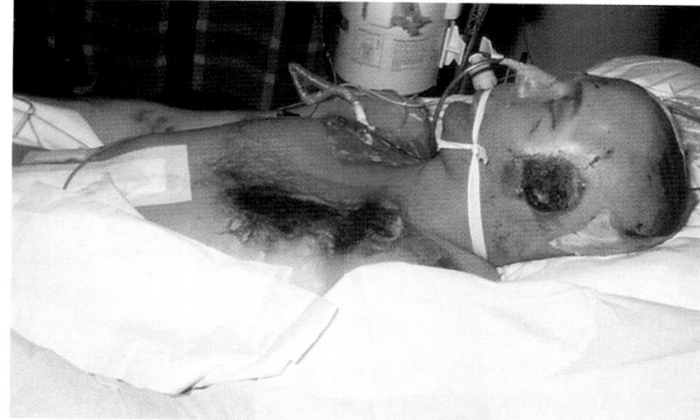

22.5 Acid burns Patient with acid burns to his ear and chest from spilt battery acid during a car accident.

The most integrated system is probably the French Services de l'Aide Medical Urgente (SAMU): all emergencies are triaged by a control room team, which includes a doctor, and an appropriate response is mounted. For major cases, intervention is provided by Services Mobile d'Urgence et de Reanimation (SMUR) teams – hospital-based medical teams with sophisticated equipment and access to a range of transport including helicopters. SMUR teams can deliver an advanced level of care on scene with rapid transfer to an appropriate hospital, and European experience (Frankema et al., 2004) is that a doctor-led pre-hospital service leads to a 2.8-fold improvement in mortality for seriously injured patents. However, the service is very expensive and demands a high number of experienced medical staff (Earlam, 1997).

PRE-HOSPITAL MANAGEMENT

Essential elements include:

1. Organization.
2. Safety on scene.
3. Immediate actions and triage.
4. Assessment and initial management.
5. Extrication and immobilization.
6. Transfer to hospital.
7. Air ambulances.

Organization

Provision of a pre-hospital EMS depends on economic resources, and varies from no provision in rural, low-income countries to sophisticated services linked to hospital care in developed economies. The EMS in most countries is based on ambulances crewed by medical technicians or paramedics. Medical support is variable, ranging from volunteer doctors in the UK by the British Association for Immediate Care (BASICS) to hospital-based teams in North America.

Safety on scene and personal protective equipment

Hospital doctors in acute specialties may be required to form part of a medical team to manage trauma cases on scene. Although surgery on entrapped

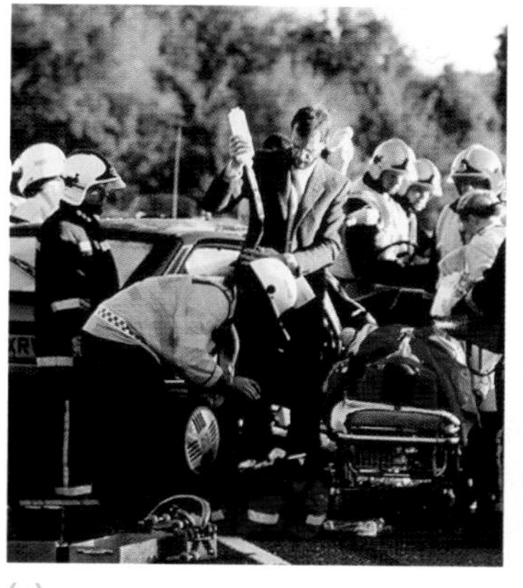

(a)

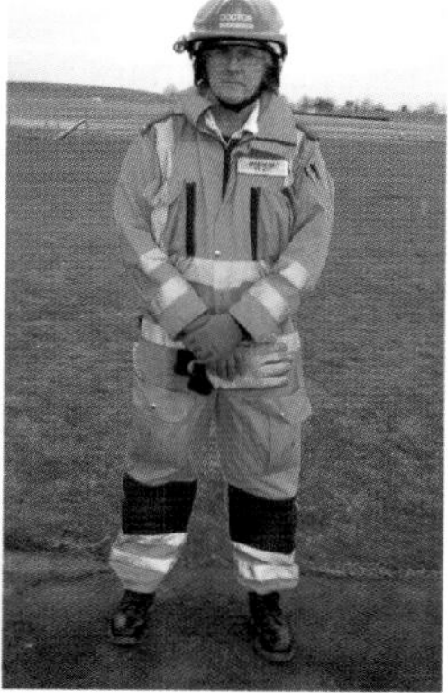

(b)

22.6 Medical personal protective equipment (PPE) (a) Inadequate PPE. (b) Correct PPE.

casualties is a rare event, surgeons may be sent out for serious or major incidents, and so some knowledge of pre-hospital care is important.

The scene of a traumatic incident is invariably hazardous, and the immediate priority for a doctor on scene is personal safety; if this is neglected, the doctor can become a casualty rather than a rescuer. Some hazards are obvious, such as unstable wreckage, jagged metal debris and fire. However, there are concealed hazards that can injure the unwary. Undeployed airbags can be triggered, and a variety of toxic chemicals can be released, such as battery acid.

All members of pre-hospital medical teams should therefore be equipped with personal protective equipment (PPE) and clothing appropriate to the incident, and this should be deployed before the scene is entered (Calland, 2000). The safety of the immediate scene will normally be the responsibility of the fire service, with police controlling the incident overall. Nations' differing EMS will have their own specific regulations covering the specification of PPE for doctors working in the pre-hospital environment. As a rule, PPE must protect the head, eyes, hands, feet, limbs and body to an appropriate extent against physical, chemical, thermal and acoustic risks. Full chemical, biological, radiological and nuclear protection is a specialist requirement rarely applicable to doctors outside a military setting.

Immediate actions and triage

The initial action of a doctor arriving on scene is to establish safety – personal safety, scene safety and casualty safety. Contact should be made with the officers commanding medical, fire and police emergency services for a situation report and direction to casualties on a priority basis. Communications should be established. In the event of multiple casualties, priorities are established by triage.

Triage is a system of medical sorting originating from the Napoleonic battlefields to identify casualties in an order of priority for evacuation and treatment. In trauma management, triage is used when the number of casualties is greater than can be managed simultaneously by the medical personnel available. There are two stages applicable in the pre-hospital environment: a *triage sieve* and a *triage sort* (Hodgetts and Porter, 2002).

The triage sieve is a quick and uncomplicated system based on simple clinical observation of a casualty's ability to walk, breathe and maintain a pulse. It can be performed by trained but non-clinical personnel. The triage sort requires a degree of clinical training and uses physiological measurements to score casualties and place them into priority groups. Both triage systems place casualties into four colour-coded, priority categories:

Priority 1	Immediate
Priority 2	Urgent
Priority 3	Delayed
Priority 4	Dead

In the event of an overwhelming number of casualties, an expectant category can be used. This identifies casualties whose injuries suggest that survival is unlikely, enabling medical resources to be deployed to those more likely to survive. In the event of improved resources, expectant casualties are re-categorized as *Priority 1.*

The category of a casualty does not necessarily dictate the order of evacuation or treatment; for example, the 'walking wounded' and uninjured (*Priority 3*) may be evacuated first ('reverse triage').

Assessment and initial management

Once safety, command, communications and priorities have been established, patients can be given individual attention. This calls for an organized approach involving a*wareness, recognition* and *management* (ARM).

AWARENESS

Awareness of the environment, pattern of damage to a vehicle and the nature of the incident can help the attending doctor predict the likely injuries and facilitate their early recognition. For example, ejection from a vehicle or death of an occupant increases the likelihood of serious injury. Particular impaction patterns and intrusion of wreckage into the passenger compartment can suggest specific injuries; a bulls-eye fracture of a windscreen from inside a car indicates impaction of the passenger's head against the windscreen and likely head, maxillofacial and neck injuries. Entrapment in a fire is associated with smoke inhalation and possible inhalational burns.

RECOGNITION

Recognition of injuries is based on a rapid and systematic questioning and examination of the casualty. An immediate assessment is made of the airway, breathing and circulation – the 'ABC' of trauma assessment. An instant assessment can be made by questioning the patient and eliciting a verbal response; the ability to speak means that the brain is being perfused with oxygenated blood and hence the patient has a patent airway, is breathing and has an adequate circulation. Head injury leading to loss of consciousness is the most common cause of airway obstruction and consequent hypoxia and hypercarbia; lack of response to command or painful stimulus indicates a significant level of coma. Access to an entrapped casualty may be extremely limited, but an assessment can usually be made of the airway and breathing, presence of peripheral pulses and peripheral perfusion, head, chest, abdomen, pelvis and limbs. This initial assessment guides immediate management and the urgency of extrication and transfer to hospital.

MANAGEMENT

Management of injuries is prioritized on treating the most immediately life-threatening injuries first, traditionally following the ABCDE sequence. The exception to this is the casualty suffering external, peripheral haemorrhage. Military experience has shown that bleeding from limb wounds is a leading cause of combat casualty deaths, a significant proportion of which are avoidable. This has led to the development of a CABC sequence, where C stands for catastrophic haemorrhage (Hodgetts et al., 2006). Life-threatening, external bleeding is controlled, and then the usual ABC sequence is followed.

As casualties with airway obstruction succumb within minutes, securing a patent airway is always a priority. Once the airway is open, the casualty must be oxygenated and ventilated if breathing is not adequate. Further circulatory compromise is addressed primarily by control of external haemorrhage; an intravenous cannula should be placed, but fluids must be administered cautiously (see later).

During this immediate management phase, the assumption is always made that damage to the cervical and thoraco-lumbar spine may have occurred. The stability of the cervical spine must be protected at all times until the neck can be cleared from the risk of injury. Stabilization is achieved by two methods: manual immobilization, or securement with head blocks, head straps and a rigid cervical collar. The thoraco-lumbar spine is protected by immobilization with straps on a long spinal board or other extrication device.

Airway The airway is opened initially with the 'bare hands' manoeuvres of chin lift and jaw thrust; the head should not be extended and should be kept in a neutral position. If blood, saliva or vomit are present in the airway, suction should be used. If 'bare hands' techniques are not adequate, an oropharyngeal airway or nasopharyngeal (NP) airway should be carefully placed to prevent the posterior aspect of the tongue obstructing the pharynx. NP airways are particularly useful in casualties with obstructing airways who have retained enough of a gag reflex to resist oropharyngeal airways, however they should be used cautiously in casualties with clinically apparent basal skull fractures. If these manoeuvres are unsuccessful, there is a range of supraglottic devices such as the laryngeal mask airway (LMA), which can be inserted in difficult situations.

Definitive airway securement with intubation or cricothyroidotomy is very difficult in entrapped casualties. Without the use of anaesthetic drugs and muscle relaxants, casualties can only be intubated when jaw tone and protective reflexes have disappeared immediately prior to cardiac arrest. The survival rates of intubation in this situation are, not surprisingly, very poor, however intubation with a rapid sequence of anaesthetic induction remains the gold standard of airway securement for trauma casualties, as it offers reliable protection from airway leaks and aspiration. Prolonged attempts at intubation should not be made without effective oxygenation and ventilation; casualties do not die from not being intubated, they die from hypoxia and hypercarbia. Accumulating evidence suggests that only practitioners with an appropriate level of anaesthetic training should be attempting rapid-sequence induction and intubation.

Breathing Once the airway is opened and secure, an assessment of the casualty's breathing is made. If breathing is clearly adequate, oxygen is administered from a high flow, non-re-breathing reservoir mask. With a flow rate of 15 L/minute, approximately 85 per cent oxygen is delivered; there is no place for lower concentrations of oxygen in this situation. If there is any doubt that breathing is adequate, then ventilation must be supported with a bag–valve–mask (BVM) assembly. This should have a reservoir attached with oxygen flows of 15 L/minute. BVM ventilation is a difficult skill even in ideal situations, but chances of success can be improved with a two-person technique; one person holds the mask in place over the face with both hands and pulls the jaw up into the mask to open up the airway, whilst the second squeezes the bag.

Adequacy of oxygenation should be judged by clinical assessment of lip colour to detect cyanosis, or use of a pulse oximeter. Adequacy of ventilation can be judged by clinical assessment of chest expansion and breath sounds, or use of a chemical or electronic end-tidal carbon dioxide ($EtCO_2$) monitor, if a supraglottic airway device or tracheal tube is in place.

Absence of breath sounds indicates a pneumothorax or haemothorax, and when associated with deviation of the trachea and hyper-resonance, a tension pneumothorax. A *tension pneumothorax* is an immediately life-threatening injury, and is treated in the first instance by decompression with a large-bore (14-gauge) intravenous cannula through the second intercostal space in the mid-clavicular line. This converts the tension pneumothorax into a simple pneumothorax; definitive treatment of a simple pneumothorax in a spontaneously breathing casualty is to insert a wide-bore chest drain in the 5th intercostal space, anterior to the mid-axillary line, with the drain being connected to a Heimlich-type valve. However, if the casualty is breathing and stable with a simple pneumothorax, rapid transfer to hospital is preferable.

Open or sucking pneumothoraces should be covered with an occlusive dressing secured on three sides – the open fourth side prevents a tension pneumothorax developing.

Positive-pressure ventilation is likely to accelerate the conversion of a simple pneumothorax into a tension pneumothorax. If the casualty is intubated and ventilated, and a pneumothorax suspected, a simple thoracostomy is made in the 5th intercostal space, anterior to the mid-clavicular line. This allows a tension pneumothorax to decompress; however, the lung can still be inflated as the casualty is being ventilated. A thoracostomy is made by making a 3 cm horizontal incision immediately above the 6th rib, just anterior to the mid-axillary line, dissecting the subcutaneous tissues with large, straight Spencer Wells forceps until the chest cavity is entered. A finger is used to open up the thoracostomy and ensure no vital structures are felt.

Circulation External haemorrhage is controlled primarily by direct pressure with a dressing, and limb elevation if possible. Other methods used are wound packing, the windlass technique, indirect pressure and use of a tourniquet; haemostatic dressings can also be used at any stage (Lee et al., 2007).

The windlass technique involves the application of a dressing directly over the wound, which is then held in place with an appropriate bandage, knotted over the wound. A pen or similar object is placed under the knot, rotated to exert direct pressure over the site of the haemorrhage, and then secured.

Tourniquets have been discouraged in contemporary, civilian, pre-hospital care, due to the significant risk of serious complications. Inappropriately applied tourniquets can increase bleeding (from a venous tourniquet effect), result in distal limb ischaemia, and cause direct pressure damage to skin, muscle and nerves. However, with limb injuries resulting in catastrophic haemorrhage, judicious use of tourniquets can be life saving. Civilian indications include (Hodgetts et al., 2006):

- life-threatening limb haemorrhage due to shooting, stabbing and industrial or farming accidents;
- haemorrhagic, traumatic amputation;
- limb haemorrhage not controllable with direct pressure, or where direct pressure cannot be applied due to inaccessibility of wound from entrapment;
- multiple casualties with lack of manpower to apply direct pressure.

If possible, a wide-bore cannula should be sited in a large vein, or intraosseus access achieved with a placement device such as the EZ-IO®, FAST1™ or BIG Bone Injection Gun. Administration of intravenous fluids should be judicious in the pre-hospital environment; rapid infusion of large volumes of fluids can raise the blood pressure and bleeding can resume that has previously stopped due to low pressure. The blood pressure drops again, and more fluid administration causes increasing anaemia. Large volumes of intravenous fluid administered to casualties with haemorrhage have been shown to increase mortality, and current guidance in the UK (National Institute for Clinical Excellence, 2004) is to titrate fluids against the presence of a radial pulse in 250 mL boluses, with a crystalloid solution such as Ringer's lactate or Hartmann's compound sodium lactate being the preferred fluid (large, infused volumes of sodium chloride 0.9 per cent can be associated with the development of a hyperchloraemic acidosis and should be avoided).

Severe, unresponsive shock is likely to be the result of uncontrollable bleeding externally or into the chest, abdomen, pelvis and multiple long bones (embodied in the aperçu 'onto the floor and four more'). Loss of cardiac output can also be due to tension pneumothorax or cardiac tamponade. Cardiac tamponade is most commonly associated with penetrating trauma of the chest within the nipple lines anteriorly or scapulae posteriorly.

Severe shock leading to pulseless electrical activity (PEA) or asystolic cardiac arrest is an indication for bilateral thoracostomies and/or clam-shell opening of the chest and incision of the pericardium. These manoeuvres will treat the reversible causes of trauma cardiac arrest – hypoxia, hypovolaemia, tension pneumothorax and cardiac tamponade, and may precede intubation, ventilation and intravenous cannulation in this dire, pre-mortem situation.

Disability The casualty is quickly assessed for neurological disability using the Glasgow Coma Scale (GCS) and assessment for pupillary size and inequality.

Extrication and immobilization

More complex management is often impractical in an entrapped casualty, and so extrication becomes a priority. This should be done with regard to spinal protection, usually using spinal boards or other rigid immobilization devices. Fractured limbs should be splinted in an anatomical position to preserve neurovascular function. Analgesia may be necessary to extricate an injured casualty, and this can be achieved with inhalational or intravenous agents.

The initial manoeuvre in the extrication process is manual immobilization of the cervical spine. This can be done from behind the casualty (typically in seated casualties entrapped in vehicles with a rescuer in the rear of the vehicle), or from the front and side if access is limited. A stiff cervical collar is sized and fitted at the earliest opportunity, but manual immobilization is still mandatory until the casualty can be placed on a spinal board.

Further immobilization and extrication may be impossible until wreckage has been cleared enough to enable an extrication device to be positioned under the casualty. Managing wreckage is a specialist skill that is the province of the Fire and Rescue crews; however, the pre-hospital doctor should be familiar with the techniques used to advise how extrication can be managed without causing additional injury to the casualty. Common manoeuvres in road vehicle wreckage are removal of glass and doors, a dashboard roll to lift the dashboard off trapped limbs, and removal of the roof by cutting through the A, B and C pillars. The seat can then be carefully flattened, and a long spinal board slid under the casualty from the rear of the vehicle, minimizing movement of the spinal column. If a casualty is deteriorating fast, the rescue crews should be advised and a rapid extrication carried out.

Limb fractures and dislocations should be reduced and the limb returned, if possible, to its anatomical position with gentle traction and straightening. This may require analgesia. Note that some injuries such as posterior hip dislocations may prevent an anatomical alignment, and the limb must not be forced. The limb should then be splinted with traction, gutter or vacuum splints as appropriate. This reduces pain and haemorrhage, and minimizes neurovascular damage. Femoral traction splints such as the Thomas are effective for mid-shaft femur fractures, providing the pelvic ring is intact. The traction reduces the fracture, and the fusiform compression of the fracture haematoma reduces further bleeding. A unilateral, closed, femoral fracture can cause a 1.5 L blood loss – 30 per cent of the adult blood volume and enough to cause significant shock without other injury.

Open-book pelvic fractures cause uncontrollable retroperitoneal bleeding. Blood loss can be minimized by stabilizing and reducing the fracture using specialist, pelvic compression devices or a rolled sheet around the pelvis and twisted above.

Analgesia may be necessary to extricate an injured casualty. This can be administered by inhalation with Entonox, a 50:50 mixture of nitrous oxide and oxygen, delivered via a breath-actuated regulator valve and mask or mouthpiece. Parenteral analgesics should only be given intravenously, and titrated cautiously against effect. Other routes of administration are very unpredictable, especially in shocked casualties. Pure opioid agonists such as morphine, diamorphine and fentanyl are most effective, but it should be noted that there is a wide variation in response between individuals, and care should be taken not to cause respiratory depression by overdosage. Partial opioid agonists such as nalbuphine are used, but have a degree of narcotic antagonism that can make further administration of opioids unpredictable. Ketamine is a very useful drug that is a powerful analgesic in doses of 0.5 mg/kg intravenously, and a general anaesthetic in doses of 2–4 mg/kg. The advantage of ketamine is that it does not cause respiratory depression, and the casualty's airway is more predictably maintained. Doses and administration times of all drugs given should be noted.

Transfer to hospital

Delayed or prolonged transfer to hospital is associated with poor outcomes, and every effort should be made to minimize the on-scene times for injured casualties. There is a balance between 'scoop and run' and 'stay and play' management. The airway must be secured, and life-threatening chest injuries (e.g. tension pneumothorax) and catastrophic, external haemorrhage dealt with before transfer commences. Prolonged attempts at complex management on scene are disadvantageous, and should be limited to life-saving interventions where possible.

The appropriate method of transport should be chosen, with helicopters offering some advantage for long-distance transfers or rescue from remote and rough terrain. Police escorts can be used to aid ambulance progress, and a balance sought between speed of transfer and violent movement of the casualty and attendants.

The appropriate destination hospital should be chosen for the casualty's likely injuries, and this may mean bypassing a small unit that does not have the appropriate facilities. Wherever possible, the receiving medical team should be directly advised of the estimated time of arrival (ETA) and the identified injuries, enabling an appropriate trauma team to be standing by.

During the transfer, the casualty's vital signs should be monitored clinically and with available equipment. Conscious casualties should be constantly assessed by speaking to them, and a decrease in conscious level detected early. ECG and pulse should be continuously monitored, blood pressure measured with a non-invasive blood pressure (NIBP) monitor, and oxygen saturations measured if peripheral perfusion allows. $EtCO_2$ monitors are useful for gauging adequacy of ventilation in intubated and ventilated casualties.

The casualty's airway must be maintained at all times, and oxygenation and ventilation maintained. Oxygen saturations should be maintained above 95 per cent if possible, and ventilated casualties have their $EtCO_2$ maintained at a low normal level (4.0–4.5 kPa). Haemorrhage is controlled with direct pressure, and Hartmann's solution titrated intravenously to maintain a palpable radial pulse.

If the patient deteriorates *en route*, the medical attendant must decide whether to attempt resuscitation whilst on the move, stop and resuscitate or make a run for the nearest hospital. This decision will depend on the nature of the intervention required and the ETA at the hospital.

Contemporaneous records are almost impossible to maintain during a transfer, but electronic equipment can usually download a paper or electronic record. If not, notes should be made as soon as possible after arrival at the hospital. On arrival, the medical attendant should remain part of the resuscitation team until an effective handover can be made.

Helicopters and air ambulances

A helicopter emergency medical service (HEMS) is ideal, but is expensive to run. HEMS (London) data show that the primary life-saving benefit is the rapid delivery of advanced resuscitation skills to the scene. The most essential life-saving skill is advanced airway management, and this requires an anaesthetically trained doctor who can perform a rapid sequence anaesthetic induction and manage tracheal intubation in difficult circumstances. International data show that, as a result of these interventions, there is a reduction of 15 per cent in death from head injuries, and a reduction of between 5 and 7 days in intensive care stays.

However, the availability of appropriately trained doctors is variable; many HEMS are crewed by paramedics only, and this reduces the effectiveness of the service to less advanced life support and rapid delivery and evacuation of casualties to an appropriate facility. A common standard for response times in the UK and Europe is 12 minutes from call-out to arrival. This ability to transport casualties quickly over large distances also means that smaller, less well-equipped and well-staffed hospitals can be bypassed in favour of large, specialist centres.

A wide variety of helicopters are used internationally for HEMS work, ranging from large aircraft such as the Sikorsky S61-N to smaller craft like the Bolkow 105-DBS. A feature common to all HEMSs is that the helicopter is twin-engined for safety and flexibility of flight paths. As costs rise dramatically with increased size of the helicopter, HEMS aircraft are a compromise. With the exception of military and Coastguard craft, the size is usually restricted.

Cramped cabin space and poor patient access in these helicopters greatly restrict the patient interventions possible during flight. The aircraft are noisy and vibration considerable, so monitoring the patient's condition is difficult. These factors make it essential that the patient is stabilized and immobilized prior to transfer; the airway must be secured and protected, ventilation maintained, haemorrhage controlled and intravenous access for fluid administration preserved. Monitoring should be reliable, and the ECG, blood pressure, oxygen saturations and end-tidal carbon dioxide observed.

Safety is paramount for doctors working with helicopters, and all personnel should be trained and familiar with safety guidelines. The helicopter should not be exited until directed by the crew. If asked to disembark whilst the rotor blades are revolving, personnel must keep their heads down and be aware that the rotor disc droops as it slows and may come below head height, especially uphill if landing on an incline.

HOSPITAL MANAGEMENT

Upon reaching hospital, the following are important in hospital management:

1. Organization.
2. Trauma teams.
3. Assessment and management. The ATLS concept.
4. Initial management.
5. Systemic management.

Organization

The aim of any integrated EMS is to "get the right patient to the right hospital in the right amount of time" (Trunkey). Regional services were set up in the USA in 1973, with three levels of hospital designated as able to manage trauma to differing levels:

Level III centres: capable of treating most trauma victims, and stabilizing critically ill patients prior to transfer.

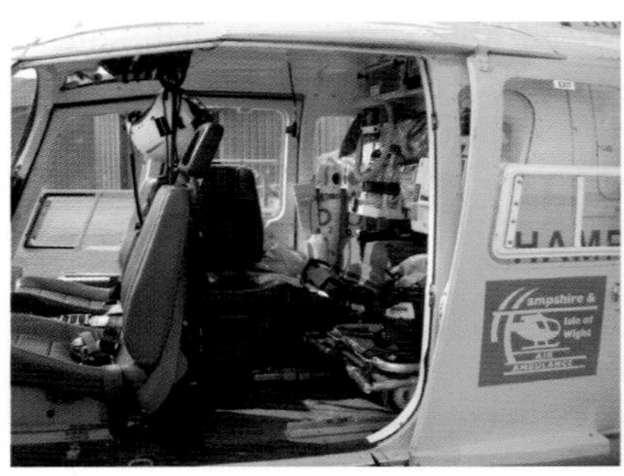

(a)

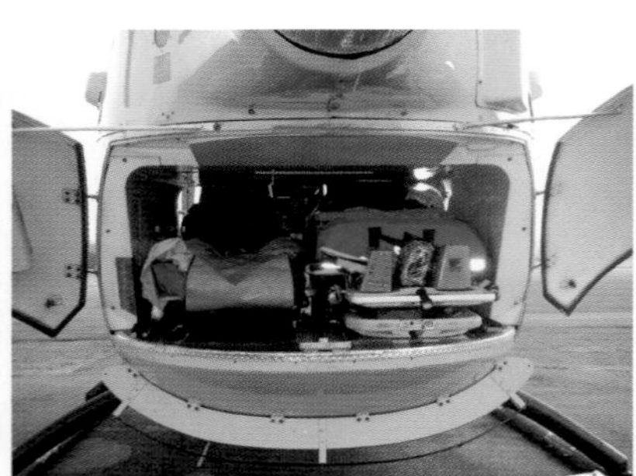

(b)

22.7 HEMS helicopter interior (a) Interior of Bolkow 105-DBS showing medical attendant seat (facing) and restricted patient access (stretcher on right). (b) Rear clam-shell doors for patient loading.

Level II centres: capable of managing almost all critically ill patients, but not offering all subspecialties.

Level I centres: able to manage all trauma patients with all specialist needs provided on site.

However, the development and integration of this system was patchy, and the expense of such a system prevents full development in many countries. There are also arguments as to whether such a system, which may be effective in a society with a high level of penetrating trauma, is appropriate for all environments.

In the UK, an experimental trauma centre and regional trauma system was set up in the Northwest Midlands in 1991–1992, and examined over the first 4 years. The assessment found little evidence of an integrated trauma system having developed, and there was no reliable evidence that survival rates from major trauma in the region had improved (Nicholl and Turner, 1997). However, after another 5 years, significant improvements in survival were noted (Oakley et al., 1998). This suggests that regional trauma systems take some time to develop to maximum effectiveness, but do demonstrate reductions in mortality. These findings are backed up by a meta-analysis of US and Canadian trauma centres.

Regionalized trauma systems are now operational in many countries, including the USA, Canada, Australia, and across Europe. In the UK, a nationally funded enquiry in 2007 advocated regionalization of trauma care and the establishment of Level 1 trauma centres (Findlay et al., 2007). However, in many or most health care economies, the majority of available hospitals will not have all the specialist staff and facilities to adequately manage major injuries. Each hospital must therefore have standard operating procedures (SOPs) for assessing, managing and if indicated, transferring trauma casualties, depending on the facilities available.

Trauma teams

Casualties who have survived their initial trauma and reached hospital alive need rapid assessment and appropriate resuscitation to avoid their dying during the 'golden hour'. Crucial to the effective management of seriously injured casualties is the immediate availability of appropriately trained and experienced doctors and healthcare professionals, and this need has led to the development of the trauma team concept.

The team is led by a senior doctor with advanced trauma skills, whose base specialty is less important than his or her training and experience. The trauma team is preferably activated by the pre-hospital practitioners according to a set of standard criteria, and should therefore be awaiting the casualty as they arrive at the hospital. Team members would normally include the following personnel:

- *First-tier response:*
  Emergency department physician
  Physician anaesthetist
  Emergency department nurses
  Radiographer
- *First- or second-tier response:*
  Surgeon from appropriate specialty
  Intensive care specialists
  Specific specialists, e.g. paediatric, obstetric, ear, nose and throat (ENT), maxillofacial etc.

The development of emergency medicine, and the increasing availability of experienced and senior emergency medicine doctors with sophisticated trauma imaging availability on a 'round the clock' basis, has enabled a two-tier call-out for trauma teams. Initial assessment and resuscitation rarely requires immediate specialist surgical skills; once the initial assessment and imaging has been completed, the appropriate specialist surgeon can be called in or stood by in the operating theatre for definitive surgical management of specific injuries.

Trauma teams should function in an appropriate environment, and most hospitals will have a resuscitation room with all required equipment immediately available. Personal protective equipment to include gowns, gloves and eye protection must be available. A sophisticated resuscitation room will have anaesthetic delivery systems, equipment and drugs for airway management, intravenous fluid and rapid administration systems for shock management, and a variety of surgical packs for specific interventions such as chest drain insertion etc. Patient trolleys should be compatible with the taking of x-rays, and the x-ray equipment can be built onto an overhead gantry. Ultrasound imaging equipment should be available for central venous cannulation and Focussed Assessment Sonography in Trauma (FAST). Both the environment and intravenous fluids should be warmed to minimize hypothermia.

The ATLS concept

Major musculoskeletal injuries can be dramatic and distracting, but it is rare for them to be immediately life-threatening in the absence of catastrophic haemorrhage. The classic mistake when treating trauma is to focus on the attention-grabbing compound fracture, and miss the obstructing airway, which is far more likely to cause a 'golden hour' death. Hence the most immediately life-threatening injuries should always be treated first. However, although this principle has been known for generations, in the stress of the moment a logical sequence may not be followed unless the treating doctor is trained and practised. To meet this need, a number of training systems have been developed over the years, of which the best known is the Advanced Trauma Life Support Program for Doctors (ATLS®) (American College of Surgeons Committee on Trauma, 2005), developed by the American College of Surgeons Committee on Trauma. The 2004 7th edition has been revised with updates from international ATLS subcommittees to reflect trauma developments across the world (Kortbeek et al., 2008).

ATLS originates from 1976, when James Styner, an orthopaedic surgeon, crashed his light aircraft in rural Nebraska with his wife and four children on board. His wife was killed instantly and three of his four children sustained critical injuries. Having arrived at the nearest hospital, Styner found that the care delivered to his family was inadequate and inappropriate, and this stimulated him to initiate a trauma care training programme that became ATLS. The course has since become an internationally recognized standard and is currently taught in over 40 countries worldwide.

The ATLS course is based on validated teaching techniques, and uses a system of core content lectures and practical skill stations to develop skills that are practised and finally tested in simulated trauma scenarios. The system taught is based on a three-stage approach:

1. *Primary survey and simultaneous resuscitation* – a rapid assessment and treatment of life-threatening injuries.
2. *Secondary survey* – a detailed, head-to-toe evaluation to identify all other injuries.
3. *Definitive care* – specialist treatment of identified injuries.

The primary and secondary surveys constitute the initial assessment and management, which leads to the definitive care of the casualty following transfer if required.

The intention of ATLS is to train doctors who do not manage major trauma on a regular basis, but it is applicable to any trauma situation as an underlying system on which to base management of an injured casualty. The sequence is taught assuming one non-specialist doctor supported by one nurse, working on a single casualty, but the various components can be performed simultaneously if a team is available. The training is didactic, but the use of specialist skills (e.g. anaesthetic) should not be excluded. Although the course is updated on a 4-yearly basis, there is an inevitable time lag, and fast-developing areas such as imaging may introduce changes to local trauma management not found in current ATLS courses. There are also national and local variations in practice that need to be taken into account, and these are discussed later in this chapter; however ATLS has stood the test of time and remains the most widely recognized basis for trauma management internationally.

Initial assessment and management

The initial assessment and management is part of a sequence leading to the transfer and definitive care of a casualty. During the primary and secondary surveys, a number of monitoring and investigative adjuncts are used alongside clinical examination as given in Figure 22.8 and the accompanying Box.

THE ABCs

The underlying principle of ATLS is to identify the most immediately life-threatening injuries first and start resuscitation. As a general rule, airway obstruction kills in a matter of minutes, followed by respiratory failure, circulatory failure and expanding intracranial mass lesions. This likely sequence of deterioration has led to the development of the trauma 'ABCs', a planned sequence of management predicated on treating the most lethal injuries first. Throughout this sequence, the assumption is made (until proved otherwise) that there may be an unrecognized and unstable cervical spine injury. Hence, the sequence is:

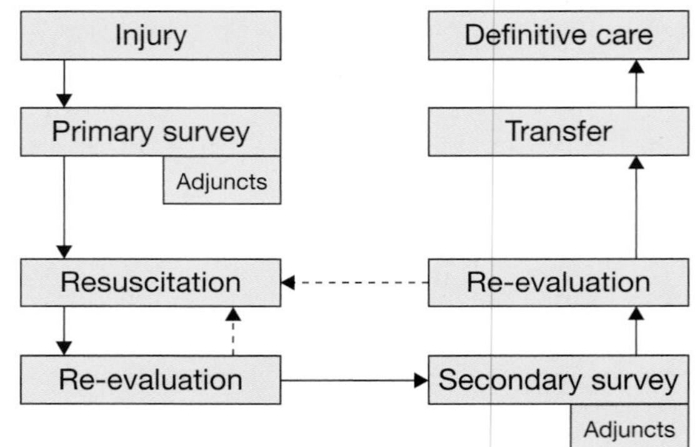

22.8 Algorithm of ATLS initial assessment and management

ADJUNCTS TO PRIMARY SURVEY
Vital signs
ECG
Pulse oximetry
End-tidal carbon dioxide
Arterial blood gases
Urinary output
Urethral catheter (unless contra-indicated)
Naso-gastric tube (unless contra-indicated)
Chest x-ray
Pelvic x-ray

A **A**irway with cervical spine protection.
B **B**reathing.
C **C**irculation with haemorrhage control.
D **D**isability or neurological status.
E **E**xposure and **E**nvironment – remove clothing, keep warm.

As previously described, catastrophic haemorrhage may be controlled before the airway, designated by the ABC sequence; however, death is ultimately caused by cerebral anoxia, regardless of whether the anoxia is a result of airway obstruction, respiratory failure, shock or old age. Hence, the goal of resuscitation is to preserve the perfusion of the brain with oxygenated blood.

TRIAGE

Triage, as described in the pre-hospital section of this chapter, is medical sorting to prioritize multiple casualties for resuscitation, and is used when the number of casualties outstrips the available resources. The initial two phases of triage, usually pre-hospital, are the *sieve* and the *sort*, to group casualties into the four priority groups of immediate, urgent, delayed or dead. Within the ATLS® system, multiple casualties are triaged by rapidly assessing each patient's **ABC**s. Those with the most immediately life-threatening injuries are treated first; these are injuries of the:

Airway:	Actual or impending obstruction	Priority 1
Breathing:	Hypoxia or ventilatory failure	Priority 2
Circulation:	External haemorrhage or shock	Priority 3

PRIMARY SURVEY AND RESUSCITATION

During the primary survey, life-threatening conditions are identified and resuscitation started simultaneously, again following the ABCDE sequence.

The Awareness Recognition Management system enables the treating doctor to focus rapidly on the likely problems; for example:

Awareness – a head injury is the most likely cause of unconsciousness and obstructed airway in trauma casualties.
Recognition – an obstructed airway is recognized by *looking, listening* and *feeling* for the diagnostic signs.
Management – the airway is established with simple 'bare hands' manoeuvres, airway adjuncts, advanced airway interventions or surgical airway techniques.

As each stage in the ABCs is completed, the casualty is re-evaluated for deterioration or improvement; on completion of the breathing assessment, the airway is re-examined and the airway and breathing reassessed before moving onto the circulation etc.

A – Airway and cervical spine control The cervical spine is stabilized immediately on the basis that an unstable injury cannot initially be ruled out. There are two techniques for this:

- manual, in-line immobilization
- cervical collar, head supports and strapping.

Simultaneously, the airway is examined for obstruction by *looking, listening* and *feeling* for signs such as respiratory distress, use of auxiliary muscles of respiration, decreased conscious level and lack of detectable breath on hand or cheek. The airway is supported initially by lifting the chin or thrusting the jaw forward from under the angles of the mandible. Secretions and blood are carefully suctioned, and oropharyngeal or NP airways used to hold the tongue forward. If these simple manoeuvres are unsuccessful, the options are supraglottic airway devices (e.g. the laryngeal mask airway), tracheal intubation or surgical airway. All these techniques can be performed without extending the neck.

B – Breathing A clear airway does not mean the casualty is breathing adequately enough to enable peripheral tissue oxygenation. As soon as the airway is

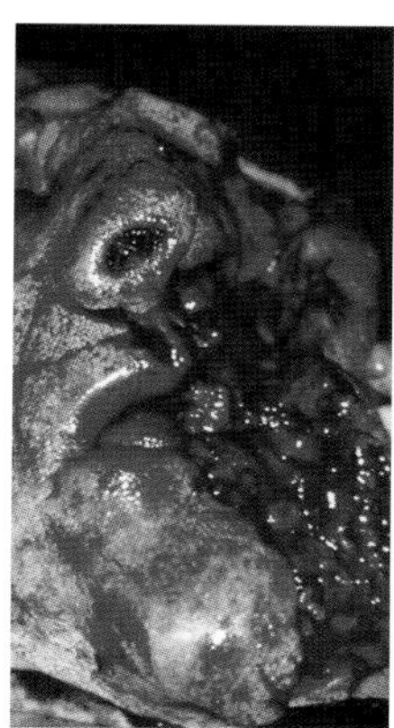
(a)

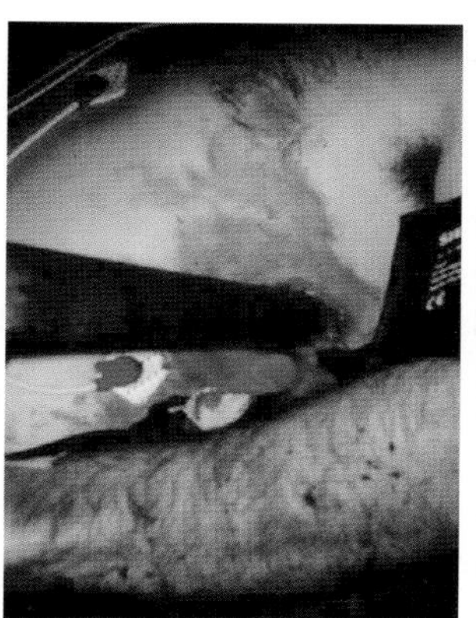
(b)

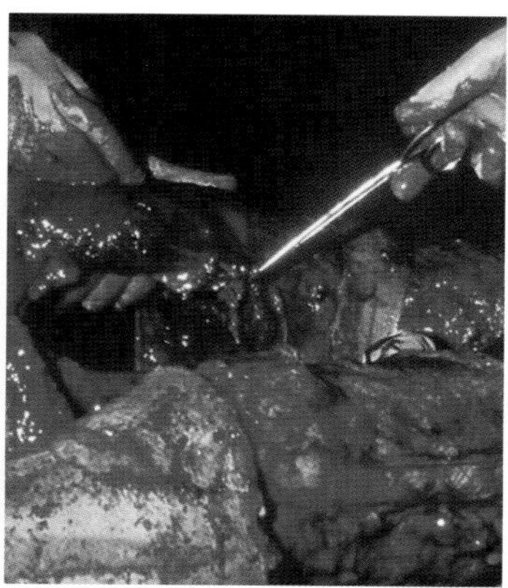
(c)

22.9 Triage priorities
(a) Priority 1 – Airway: severe face and neck wounds. (b) Priority 2 – Breathing: severe chest wounds; (c) Priority 3 – Circulation: severe bleeding and shock.

secured, the chest must be exposed and examined by *looking*, *listening* and *feeling*. Adequate and symmetrical excursion, bruising, open wounds and tachypnoea are looked for, and the chest is auscultated for abnormal or absent breath sounds, which indicate a pneumothorax or haemothorax. The trachea is palpated in the supra-sternal notch to detect the deviation caused by a tension pneumothorax, and the chest is percussed for the hyper-resonance of a tension pneumothorax or dullness of a haemothorax.

A tension pneumothorax must be treated immediately if the diagnostic signs of *absent breath sounds*, *hyper-resonance* and *deviated trachea* are found. Initial management is decompression with a 14-gauge cannula placed in the second intercostal space in the mid-clavicular line, followed by chest drain placement. If there is any doubt as to the adequacy of the casualty's breathing and oxygenation, ventilation should be started with a reservoir BVM assembly using high-flow oxygen. Any trauma casualty who has required intubation must be ventilated.

C – Circulation with haemorrhage control The circulation is assessed by looking for external bleeding and the visible signs of shock such as pallor, prolonged capillary refill and decreased conscious level. The heart is auscultated to detect the muffled sounds of cardiac tamponade, and poor perfusion assessed by feeling for clammy and cool skin. The peripheral and central pulses are palpated to detect tachycardia and diminished or absent pulse pressure.

External bleeding is controlled by pressure, and two 14-gauge cannulae sited for administration of in fluids and blood. Blood samples can be drawn from the cannulae for baseline diagnostic tests and transfusion cross-matching. As blood is available quickly in a hospital setting, warmed, crystalloid intravenous fluids can be given in an initial volume of 2 L to maintain cardiac output.

D – Disability The key element of assessing a patient's neurological status is the Glasgow Coma Score (GCS) (Table 22.1). This score records eye opening, the best motor response and the verbal response, giving a score of between 15 for normal responses, and 3 for no responses. Repeat GCS scoring can track deterioration in the conscious level, and indicate the need for elective intubation and ventilation. It is much more precise than the AVPU score (*A*ware, *V*erbally responsive, *P*ain responsive and *U*nresponsive). The classic pitfall of intoxication should be considered, but a lowered GCS is assumed to be secondary to a cerebral injury until proved otherwise.

The pupils are examined for any difference in size indicating raised intra-cerebral pressure, and unresponsive pupils, fixed at mid-point, which can indicate serious brain damage.

Table 22.1 Glasgow Coma Score

Response	Score
Eye opening:	
Spontaneous	4
On command	3
On pain	2
Nil	1
Best motor response:	
Obeys	6
Localizes pain	5
Normal flexor	4
Abnormal flexor	3
Extensor	2
Nil	1
Verbal response:	
Orientated	5
Confused	4
Words	3
Sounds	2
Nil	1

E – Exposure and environment The patient should have all clothing removed to enable a full examination of the entire body surface area to take place. This will require log rolling to examine the posterior aspects, and allow removal of any glass or debris. The casualty should be kept warm to maintain body temperature as close to 37°C as possible, and all fluids and ventilated gases warmed. Although patient cooling is used in some specialist situations, this is not indicated in the initial resuscitation. A hypothermic patient becomes peripherally shut down and acidotic, and if shivering, has greatly increased oxygen demands.

ADJUNCTS TO PRIMARY SURVEY

A number of monitoring and diagnostic adjuncts are used to supplement the primary survey and resuscitation, in addition to vital signs monitoring and haematological assays:

- *Electrocardiographic (ECG) monitoring* – used to monitor heart rate and detect arrhythmias and ischaemic changes.
- *Pulse oximetry* – measures arterial oxygen saturations (SaO_2) and monitors peripheral tissue perfusion (this is unreliable in low-output states, hypothermia and with motion artefact).
- *End-tidal carbon dioxide monitoring ($EtCO_2$)* – gives an estimation of arterial carbon dioxide partial pressure in intubated and ventilated patients, allowing optimization of lung ventilation. It also confirms tracheal intubation and alerts the practitioner to a drop in cardiac output.
- *Arterial blood gases (ABGs)* – allows quantification of arterial oxygen and carbon dioxide partial pressures with acid–base balance. This will also give the haemoglobin, sodium and potassium levels.

- *Urethral catheter* – allows measurement of hourly urine output (unless contraindicated, e.g. in the case of a ruptured urethra).
- *Nasogastric tube* – decompresses the stomach and helps prevent aspiration (unless contraindicated, e.g. because of a basal skull fracture).
- *Chest x-ray* – for diagnosis of life-threatening chest injuries such as pneumothorax, which will require early treatment.
- *Pelvic x-rays* – enable a fractured pelvis to be diagnosed, which will alert to the likelihood of retroperitoneal bleeding.

(**NOTE:** lateral cervical spine x-rays do not exclude fractures or unstable necks and so do not alter management; although important, they can be left until the secondary survey.)

SECONDARY SURVEY

The secondary survey is a detailed, head-to-toe evaluation to identify all injuries not recognized in the primary survey. It takes place after the primary survey has been completed, if the patient is stable enough and not in immediate need of definitive care; it may, in fact, take place after surgery, or on the intensive care unit (ICU). The importance of the secondary survey is that relatively minor injuries can be missed during the primary survey and resuscitation, but cause long-term morbidity if overlooked, for example small joint dislocations.

The components of the secondary survey are:

- history
- physical examination
- 'tubes and fingers in every orifice'
- neurological examination
- further diagnostic tests
- re-evaluation.

The history The patient's ongoing experience of his or her injuries, as well as details of events immediately before, during and after the injury should be recorded. Particularly important is to establish whether the trauma was subsequent to a medical collapse: did the patient suffer a myocardial infarct causing a car crash, or was the infarct a result of hypovolaemia? With the increasing proportion of the elderly in developed societies, more patients are receiving chronic treatment for hypertension etc., which can have a profound effect on their response to hypovolaemia. An example of this is a combination of beta-blockers and angiotensin-converting enzyme (ACE) inhibitors, which cause a profound drop in blood pressure if the patient's cardiac output is minimally compromised. A useful mnemonic is AMPLE: allergies; medications; past illnesses; last meal; events and environment.

Examination Examination follows a logical sequence from the head down to the extremities, including a log-roll to ensure that all the body surfaces are examined. The guiding injunctions are *look, listen* and *feel.*

The head is examined for contusions, lacerations and clinically detectable fractures. The eyes and ears are examined for local damage, and examined internally with an ophthalmoscope/otoscope for signs of bleeding etc. Bleeding from the ears can indicate a basal skull fracture. The GCS should be repeated.

The face is examined for signs of fractures with a consequent risk of airway obstruction – contusion, laceration, deformity, malocclusion of teeth and crepitus. Cerebrospinal fluid issuing from the nose (rhinorrhoea) is indicative of a basal skull fracture.

All aspects of the neck are examined for contusions, lacerations, swelling, tenderness, and a step in the cervical spine indicative of fracture/dislocation. Minor-looking contusions over the anterior neck can be indicative of underlying damage to the laryngeal and tracheal structures, which are associated with airway obstruction. A lateral cervical spine x-ray is taken at this stage.

The chest is inspected for deformity, contusions such as the classic 'seat belt' sign and open, possibly penetrating, wounds. A stethoscope is used to auscultate the lungs, comparing left and right apices and bases to identify the loss of breath sounds, indicating a pneumothorax. Feel for tenderness and crepitus due to fractured ribs and sternum, which may also be associated with underlying lung and heart contusions. Percussion can reveal the hyper-resonance of a tension pneumothorax, and the dullness of a haemothorax.

The abdomen is inspected for contusions and wounds, and auscultated for the absence of bowel sounds indicative of visceral damage. Palpation primarily detects rigidity and tenderness in the conscious patient, and percussion can identify gastric distension, but these are unreliable in many trauma casualties. The early use of specialist imaging such as ultrasound and computed tomography (CT) is indicated. Discrete areas such as the perineum, rectum and vagina should not be forgotten, and must be examined for bleeding, contusions, lacerations etc.

The key indicators for pelvic fracture are unequal leg length and pain or crepitus on palpation or gentle compression of the pelvis. If these signs are positive, a pelvic fracture is indicated, with the risk of profound haemorrhage. The examination should not be repeated.

All four limbs are examined for contusions, deformity and pallor. Pain and crepitus on palpation are indicative of underlying fracture or dislocation, and this examination should not be repeated if positive. Distal pallor and absence of pulses suggest a vascular injury, and sensory loss, neurological damage. X-rays that include the joint above and below the injury site are indicated.

Table 22.2 Palpable pulses at different blood pressures

Pulses palpable	Likely systolic blood pressure
Carotid, femoral, radial	> 80 mmHg
Carotid, femoral	> 70 mmHg
Carotid	> 60 mmHg
No pulse	< 60 mmHg

A rapid neurological assessment is carried out to detect lateralizing signs, loss of sensation and motor power, and abnormality of reflexes. Levels of sensory loss should be carefully documented to enable deterioration or improvement to be quantified. X-rays and CT may be indicated to detect spinal fractures.

Imaging Imaging techniques are developing rapidly, and changing practice. The use of *chest* and *pelvis x-rays* is still standard in the primary survey, but false-negative results with cervical spine radiographs limits their use. The incidence of spinal cord injury without radiographic abnormality (SCIWORA) is around 10 per cent of all spinal injuries, and is more common in children.

CT scans have in the past had the drawback that sending an unstable casualty for a lengthy procedure in a remote radiology department is too dangerous. However, modern spiral CT scanners are fast, and if located adjacent to the Emergency Department, a whole-body trauma CT can be completed in minutes. The risk of patient instability may therefore be outweighed by the benefit of a CT scan in enabling accurate diagnosis, and this technique is becoming a gold standard.

Magnetic resonance imaging (MRI) is not usually available as an emergency procedure, and is not safe with an unstable casualty. However, its ability to identify soft-tissue injuries is of use in diagnosing SCIWORA; removal of spinal precautions may not be safe until an MRI has excluded unstable spinal injuries.

Ultrasound scanning is often helpful, particularly for diagnosing intra-abdominal bleeding. In many departments *focussed assessment with sonography in trauma* (FAST) has largely supplanted diagnostic peritoneal lavage; however, its usefulness is limited to detecting fluid in the peritoneum, and it will not reliably enable diagnosis of specific visceral injuries. Though it remains a quick and useful Emergency Department adjunct, it does not provide the diagnostic information of CT.

PAIN MANAGEMENT

Pain management has in the past been underemphasized, due to concerns about masking surgical signs and the risks of sedation and respiratory depression. However, in expert hands, there are various techniques that can be used in the hospital setting.

Intravenous analgesia – This is the most commonly preferred technique, with morphine being the usual drug. Morphine is a pure agonist opioid and should be diluted and titrated against patient response as there is a wide variation in effect between individuals. It also provides a degree of mental detachment and euphoria useful in the trauma patient, but has the side effects associated with opioids of respiratory depression, sedation, hypotension, nausea and dysphoria. Being a pure agonist, its effects can be reversed with naloxone. Respiratory depression can be reversed whilst preserving analgesia with the respiratory stimulant doxapram. Partial agonists such as buprenorphine should be avoided as they are not fully reversed by naloxone. An anti-emetic such as cyclizine or ondansetron should be given with morphine to minimize nausea.

Inhalational analgesia – Nitrous oxide/oxygen 50:50 mix (Entonox) is useful for short-term analgesia when moving patients or aligning fractures. However, nitrous oxide diffuses into air-filled closed cavities such as a pneumothorax, and will expand the volume by a factor of four, potentially causing an undrained pneumothorax to tension.

Nerve blocks – Nerve blocks can be used with great effect in some limb injuries, but should only be administered after discussion with an orthopaedic surgeon due to the risk of masking a compartment syndrome. Femoral nerve blocks are technically straightforward and can be used for mid-shaft femur, anterior thigh and knee injuries.

INTRA-HOSPITAL AND INTER-HOSPITAL TRANSFER

Few hospitals enjoy the luxury of having the Emergency Department, radiology, operating theatres and ICUs all in the same location, and so transfer of seriously injured casualties is inevitable at some point. Transfer is indicated when the patient's needs exceed what can be delivered with the resources immediately available. The transfer may be between units within the same hospital, from a small hospital to a larger facility (e.g. a Level I trauma centre), or to a specialist unit (e.g. burns, neurosurgical or cardiothoracic). Even the shortest transfer within a hospital is fraught with hazard as monitoring and resuscitation are difficult on the move, and so must be carefully planned. A number of questions should be answered before the transfer is initiated: *When? Where? Who? What way? With?*

When to transfer is determined by the condition of the casualty and the urgency of definitive care. Patient outcome is directly related to time from injury to definitive care, so delays should be minimized. However, transferring partially assessed and unstable patients is dangerous, and so transfer is not usually contemplated until the primary survey and resuscitation have been completed. Ideally, the patient should be stable when transferred, but this may not be possible if bleeding is severe. Definitive care may be so urgent that intervention is required before the secondary survey is reached, e.g. for evacuation of an expanding intracerebral bleed. Transfer should not be delayed for investigations such as cervical spine x-ray, which will not change management. However, it is crucial that the ABCs are addressed; the airway should be secured and protected, the patient must be oxygenated and ventilated optimally, and shock should be addressed.

Where to transfer the casualty to is determined by the definitive care required and the best facility available that can offer that care. Multiply-injured patients may have injuries requiring input from differing surgical specialties such as neurosurgery and general surgery; in this situation, the definitive care surgeons must decide on the priorities, having assessed the patient. The back of the head should always be examined as injuries at the back of the head may sometimes be missed (Fig. 22.10). In life-threatening circumstances (e.g. with expanding intracerebral and intra-abdominal bleeds), the patient may require simultaneous management of both injuries.

Who conducts the transfer is determined by the staff available. The transferring physician should have an appropriate set of critical care competencies including advanced airway skills – this is not a job for the nearest junior doctor. Transfer should be authorized by the senior doctor with responsibility for the patient, and an appropriate team of nurses, technicians and paramedics should accompany the patient. The referring doctor should have direct communication with the receiving doctor, who should be briefed on the patient's condition, destination and ETA.

In which way the transfer is achieved depends on factors such as whether the transfer is between hospitals or within units of the same facility. The casualty must be secured and full spinal stabilization in place if spinal injury cannot be excluded. This may require immobilization on a spinal board with a cervical collar and head restraints; bear in mind that closely fitting cervical collars can raise intracerebral pressure, and prolonged restraint on a spinal board results in pressure injuries. The casualty should be transferred on an appropriate trolley, and a medical kit with equipment for ABC interventions must be carried. Full monitoring to include ECG, NIBP/intra-arterial BP, SaO_2 and $EtCO_2$ should be available. For transfers between hospitals, an appropriate form of transport must be available.

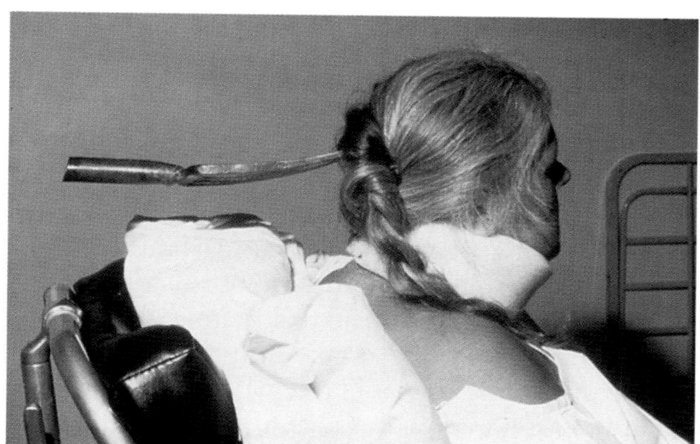

22.10 The head Failure to examine the back of the head may result in missed injuries!!

With the casualty should go a full set of paperwork to include patient identity and documentation of the full initial assessment; it is particularly important to note whether the secondary survey has been carried out, with any injuries duly noted. If the urgency of the transfer has taken precedence over the secondary survey, then this should be highlighted so the survey can be completed after the initial, life-saving, definitive care. Results of all blood tests and investigations such as x-rays must accompany the patient.

DEFINITIVE CARE

Definitive care describes the specialist care required to manage the injuries identified during the initial assessment and subsequent investigations. This may be specialist surgery to address a particular problem (e.g. neurosurgical evacuation of an intracerebral bleed), or critical care management on an ICU to provide systemic support (e.g. oxygenation and ventilation of patients with severe lung contusions).

SYSTEMIC MANAGEMENT

Accurate and effective management of a casualty with multiple injuries depends on a logical progression of examination, moving through the systems in a sequence most likely to identify the most immediately life-threatening injuries first. Using the ARM system described earlier helps structure the approach:

Awareness – use the history and accident mechanism to predict likely injuries and anticipate problems.
Recognition – examine the patient logically using the *look – listen – feel* sequence to identify the physical signs of injury.
Management – having identified injuries, implement the most effective and life-saving interventions first.

Systemic management may progress simultaneously in a hospital location with a trauma team; in the absence of a team, work through the systems following the ABCDE format. The exception to this would be control of catastrophic haemorrhage preceding airway management.

A – Airway and cervical spine

Management of the airway in all forms can be implemented whilst protecting the cervical spine. Until the airway is both secured and protected, this is best done by in-line immobilization, as use of a stiff cervical collar makes intubation difficult. Conventionally, in-line immobilization is performed with the practitioner standing at the head of the casualty, holding the head on both sides with the hands and maintaining it in a neutral position, in line with the neck and torso. This can make airway management difficult, with the in-line immobilizer squatting awkwardly to one side. An alternative and more effective stance is for the immobilizer to stand to one side of the casualty's shoulder and immobilize the head from below.

An additional technique is to stand at the casualty's head and support the head between the forearms whilst linking the hands behind the neck. This effectively immobilizes the cervical spine, but makes examination of the posterior neck difficult, and is uncomfortable for a tall practitioner.

Once the airway is secured and protected, the trinity of stiff collar, head blocks and tape should be implemented. Whatever techniques are used, the cervical spine should be immobilized at all times until an unstable injury is excluded – this may require CT or MRI scanning, and be after definitive care.

AIRWAY – AWARENESS

Head injury This is by far the most common cause of airway compromise in the trauma patient. As the level of consciousness decreases, so does muscle tone, and the pharynx collapses around the glottis, obstructing the airway. In the supine position, the tongue drops backwards, plugging the glottis anteriorly. Airway obstruction can be sudden or insidious, and partial or complete, but will result in damaging hypoxia and hypercarbia, which are particularly dangerous in a head-injured casualty.

Maxillofacial trauma Disruption of the facial bones allows the face to fall back, compressing and obstructing the pharynx. This is associated with soft tissue swelling and bleeding, which further obtund the airway. Typically, these patients need to sit up to allow the face to fall away from the pharynx and open up the airway.

Neck trauma Penetrating or blunt-force trauma results in haemorrhage and swelling, which compresses, distorts and obstructs the upper airway. This can progress rapidly and make tracheal intubation impossible and surgical airway difficult.

Laryngeal trauma Blunt force trauma from impact to the anterior neck (on a car steering wheel, for example) can disrupt the larynx and fracture the cartilaginous structures, leading to immediate or incipient airway obstruction. Signs can be subtle; contusion over the larynx with a hoarse voice, coughing of bright red blood and surgical emphysema should alert the practitioner to the likelihood of sudden airway obstruction.

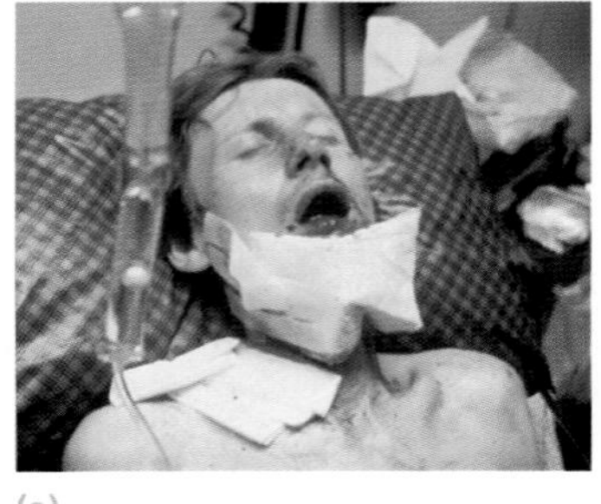

(a)

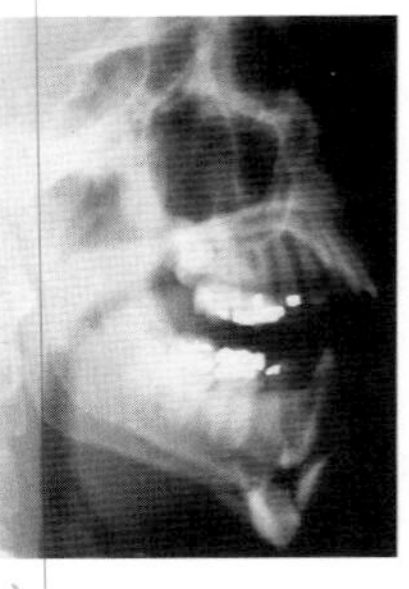

(b)

22.11 Mandibular fracture (a,b) Patient with a mandibular fracture showing the characteristic position to maintain the airway.

Inhalational burns Inhaling super-heated air burns the airway and can result in rapid development of swelling and airway obstruction. Signs such as facial burns, smoke staining and singed nasal hair suggest an inhalational burn, requiring early and expert intubation.

AIRWAY – RECOGNITION

Airway obstruction and respiratory failure may be obvious (to an experienced clinician), but early signs can sometimes be subtle and need systematic examination to detect:

Look

Agitation, aggression, anxiety – suggest hypoxia.
Obtunded conscious level – suggests hypercarbia.
Cyanosis – blue discoloration of nail beds and lips caused by hypoxaemia due to inadequate oxygenation.
Sweating – increased autonomic activity.
Use of accessory muscles of ventilation; casualty classically sitting forward splinting chest, and using neck and shoulder muscles to aid breathing. May also display flared nostrils.
Tracheal tug and intercostal retraction – caused by exaggerated intrathoracic pressure swings.

Listen

Noisy breathing – collapsing pharyngeal muscles obstruct airway leading to snoring sounds.
Stridor – air flow through an obstructing upper airway changes from laminar to turbulent, resulting in the typical hoarse wheeze of stridor – a sinister sign, as even minimal further reduction in the airway lumen can result in critical airway obstruction.

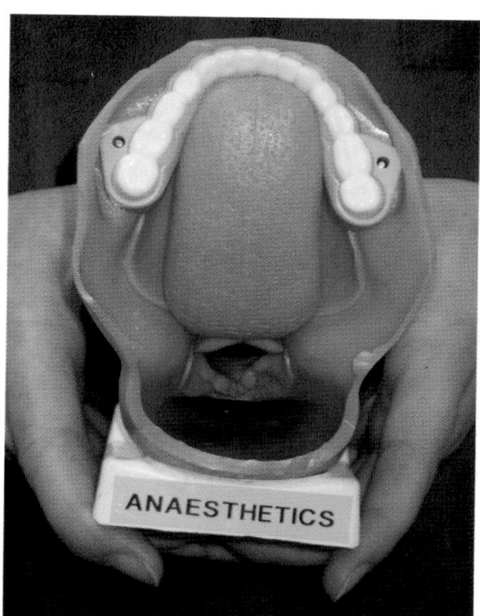

(a)

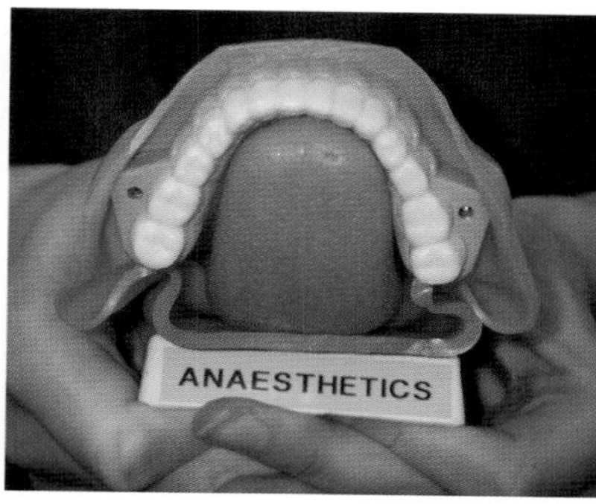

(b)

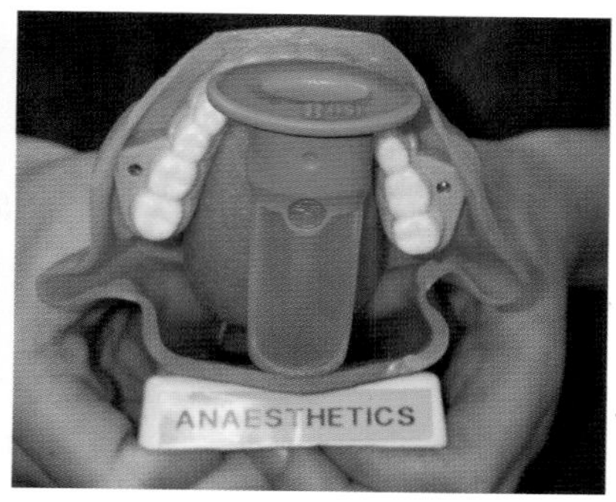

(c)

22.12 Pharyngeal airways preventing the tongue from falling back across the glottis (a) Open airway. (b) Obstructed airway. Collapse of pharynx and tongue across glottis. (c) Airway secured with oropharyngeal airway.

Hoarse voice (dysphonia) – functional damage to larynx.

Absence of noise – may indicate complete airway obstruction or apnoea.

Feel

Feel for passage of air through mouth and nose with palm of hand; very sensitive for detecting air flow.

Palpation of the trachea in supra-sternal notch will detect the deviation associated with a tension pneumothorax.

AIRWAY – MANAGEMENT

A range of manoeuvres is available to secure a patent airway, ranging from 'bare hands' techniques to a surgical airway. All these techniques can be performed without extending the head and compromising an unstable cervical spine. The anaesthetic 'sniffing the early morning air' position (head extended and neck flexed) should not be used in the trauma patient. Bare hands techniques and the use of pharyngeal airways are used together to pull the pharyngeal tissues and tongue off the posterior pharyngeal wall and away from the glottis, opening up the airway.

Supra-glottic airway devices (e.g. the laryngeal mask airway) provide more reliable airway maintenance, but only intubation and the surgical airway will provide a definitive airway that is both secured and protected.

All the non-surgical airway manoeuvres described are applicable to children, but require some modification in technique to accommodate their anatomical and physiological differences. Surgical cricothyroidotomy is not recommended in children under 12 years of age, as the cricoid cartilage can be damaged, leading to tracheal collapse.

Chin lift The chin is lifted forwards with the practitioner positioned at the casualty's head or side, using one hand. This pulls the jaw and pharyngeal structures forward off the posterior pharyngeal wall and glottis, and opens up the airway.

Jaw thrust This is a more assertive manoeuvre that is effective in patients with small jaws or thick necks, or who are edentulous. From the casualty's head, the thenar eminences are rested on the casualty's maxillae (assuming no obvious fracture), and the four fingers positioned under the angles of the mandible. Using the thenar eminences to provide a counterpoint on the maxillae, the mandible is lifted up and forwards to open up the airway as with chin lift. Considerable pressure can be exerted without displacing the head on the neck, and the manoeuvre can be combined with application of a BVM assembly for ventilation of the lungs.

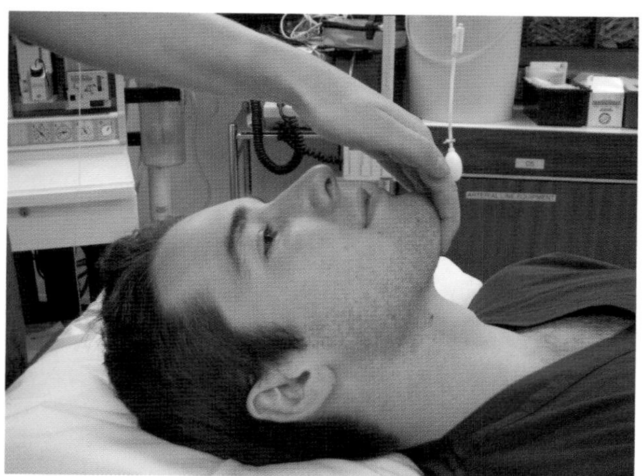

22.13 Chin lift

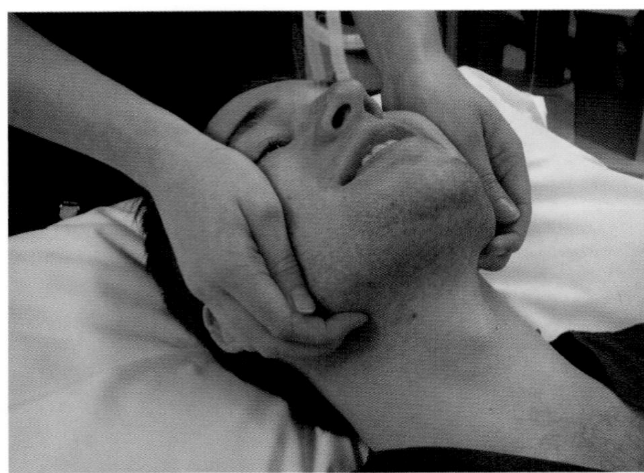

22.14 Jaw thrust

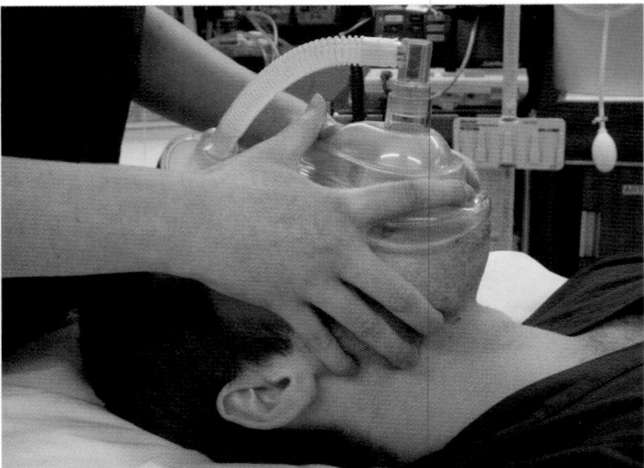

22.15 Jaw thrust with O_2 mask

Release of chin lift and jaw thrust almost inevitably results in loss of the airway, and progression to airway adjuncts will be required to free up the practitioner.

Oropharyngeal (OP) airway The oropharyngeal, or Guedel, airway is a curved and flattened, hard, plastic tube with a proximal flange, which is shaped and sized to hold the tongue and pharynx off the posterior pharyngeal wall. They are available in a range of sizes from neonate to large adult; selection of the correct size is important, as the pharyngeal tissues will collapse across the end of too small a device, whilst one too large will risk impinging on the glottis. The correct size is selected by lining up the OP airway alongside the patient's jaw; the flange to tip length of the OP airway should match the distance from the corner of the patient's mouth to the external auditory canal.

The OP airway is inserted above the tongue, initially with the concave aspect upwards. As the tip passes over the tongue, the OP airway is rotated so the concave aspect slides over the tongue, and slipped into the pharynx until the flange rests on the incisors. A correctly sized OP airway should neither project up beyond the teeth, nor disappear into the buccal cavity.

Use of the OP airway may need to be combined with chin lift or jaw thrust to maintain a patent airway, as they should only be used in obtunded patients with absent gag reflexes.

Nasopharyngeal (NP) airway The NP airway is a soft, plastic tube with a smooth, distal bevel and a proximal flange. Some makes have a safety pin to insert through the flange to prevent the NP airway disappearing into the nose. It is supplied in a number of internal diameter sizes, and should be selected according to the approximate size of the casualty's little finger. The NP airway is lubricated with aqueous jelly, and inserted along the floor of the nasal cavity into the nasopharynx. The NP airway should not be inserted up the nose as this risks haemorrhage from the mucosa and turbinates, further compromising the airway, and also introduces the possibility of entering the cranial cavity through a basal skull fracture.

NP airways are particularly useful as they can be tol-

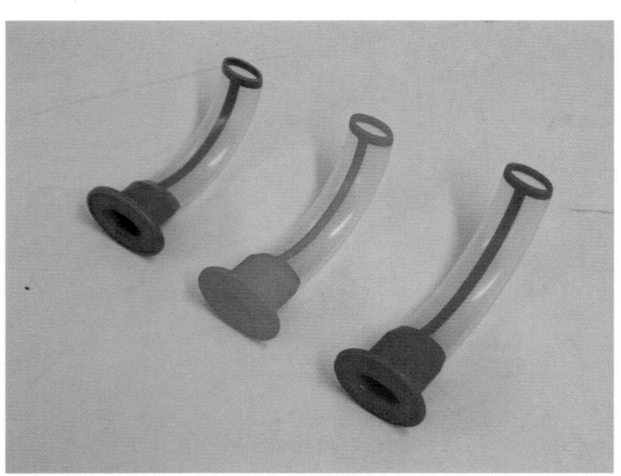

22.16 OP airway (Guedel)

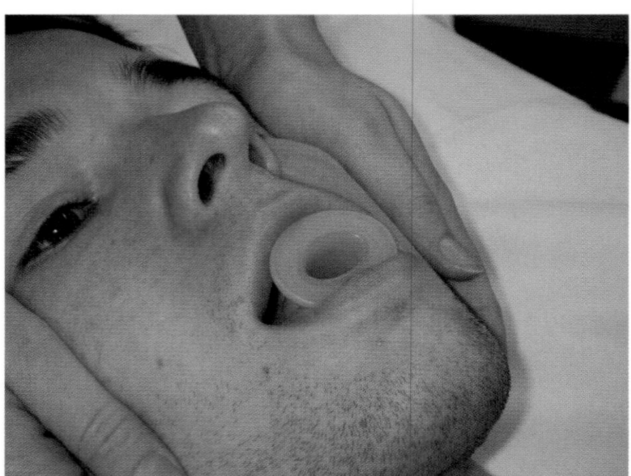

22.17 OP airway – correct position

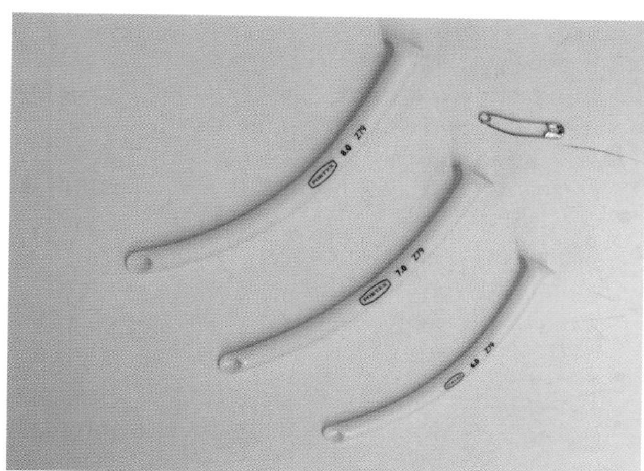

22.18 NP airway

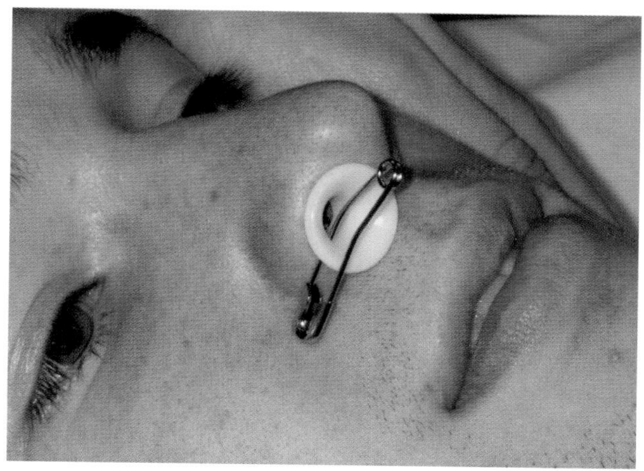

22.19 NP airway – correct position

erated by responsive casualties with obstructing airways. They also provide access to suction the nasopharynx with a soft suction catheter.

Oropharyngeal suction Secretions and blood should be cleared with a specialist pharyngeal sucker such as the Yankauer. Care should be taken not to damage the soft tissues, and as a general rule, the sucker should not be passed further than can be seen. Suction of the oro-nasopharynx with a Yankauer sucker, under direct vision using a laryngoscope, is effective in the obtunded patient.

Supra-glottic airway devices These are devices that function between an OP airway and a tracheal tube, and include multi-lumen oesophageal airway devices (e.g. Combitube), the laryngeal tube airway, and the laryngeal mask airway. The most commonly used device is the laryngeal mask airway (LMA). The LMA was developed by Dr Archie Brain and introduced initially in the UK for anaesthetic use in the late 1980s. Since then it has found an international role for resuscitation and trauma airway management, with the advantages that it is more effective than other airway devices, but does not require the skill and training required for successful tracheal intubation.

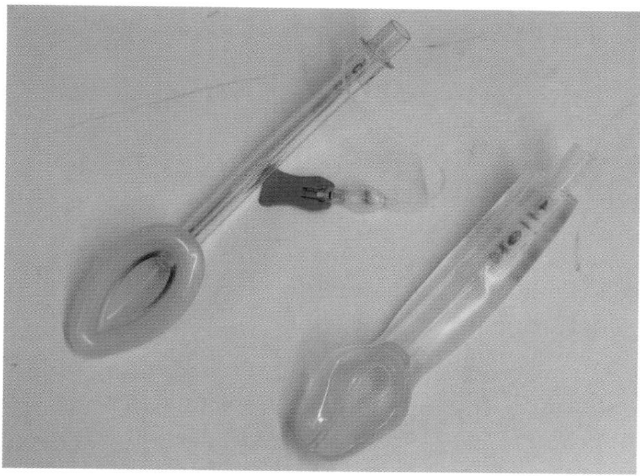

22.20 Supraglottic airways

Mounting international evidence suggests that intubation performed by practitioners without anaesthetic training can be detrimental to patient survival, and in the UK the ambulance service regulatory body (Joint Royal Colleges Ambulance Service Liaison Committee, 2008) has removed tracheal intubation as a core paramedic skill, and recommends the use of supra-glottic airway devices.

The LMA is available in a range of sizes from neonatal to large adult; for adult use, a size 3 will fit small women, size 4 larger women and smaller men, and size 5, larger men. The device consists of a cuffed distal portion shaped to fit into the oropharynx over the glottis. The cuff is inflated with air to fit snugly against the pharynx, but does not seal as does a tracheal tube cuff, and hence does not reliably protect the airway. The LMA is lubricated and inserted over the tongue with the open end of the cuffed distal portion positioned inferiorly. The device is slipped around the oropharynx until it is snugly positioned over the glottis, and the cuff inflated according to the size of the device (#3 20 mL, #4 30 mL, #5 40 mL).

As the laryngeal mask, in common with other supra-glottic airway devices, does not provide a definitive and protected airway, consideration should be given to its being replaced with a tracheal tube at the earliest opportunity.

Tracheal intubation Oro-tracheal intubation is the preferred method for securing and protecting the compromised airway in the trauma patient. However, it is a difficult procedure with minimal survival rates in un-anaesthetized, trauma casualties; un-anaesthetized casualties can normally only be intubated when protective reflexes are absent, allowing a view of the vocal cords on laryngoscopy. Lack of reflexes to this degree is associated with terminally deep levels of coma, when casualties are at the point of death. Casualties requiring a definitive airway should therefore be identified early, and expert assistance sought from an anaesthetist or critical care physician. The indications for oro-tracheal intubation are:

- apnoea
- inability to maintain airway by other means.
- need to protect airway from aspiration of blood and stomach contents
- impending airway obstruction, e.g. inhalational burn, expanding neck haematoma, facial fractures
- closed head injury with GCS below 8
- inability to maintain adequate oxygenation and ventilation with face mask or BVM assembly.

Nasotracheal intubation is indicated only in a spontaneously breathing patient, and has a poor success rate with a high incidence of complications such as nasal haemorrhage.

Trauma tracheal intubation should be performed with a rapid sequence induction (RSI) anaesthetic; after pre-oxygenation, anaesthesia is rapidly induced with an intravenous agent, cricoid pressure applied to hold the oesophagus closed and prevent passive reflux of stomach contents, the patient paralyzed with suxamethonium and a tracheal tube placed under direct vision with use of a laryngoscope. The tracheal tube cuff is inflated until no leak is detected, and the cricoid pressure not released until the anaesthetist confirms the tracheal tube is secure.

This procedure should not be performed by any practitioner without the necessary training and experience in anaesthetic techniques, as injudicious use of muscle relaxants can lead to immediate loss of the airway and a 'can't intubate, can't ventilate' scenario.

If a non-anaesthetically trained, trauma practitioner has to attempt intubation in extremis, the following sequence should be followed:

1. Select appropriately sized tracheal tube; size 8 (internal diameter) will be appropriate for most men and most women.
2. Leave tube uncut but ensure proximal connector is securely attached.
3. Have a smaller diameter tube available as back up.
4. Lubricate the cuff and test inflate, then deflate, to detect cuff leakage.
5. Have two functioning laryngoscopes available with bright lights.
6. Have intubating bougie or catheter available.
7. Maintain head and neck immobilized in neutral, in-line position.
8. Pre-oxygenate the patient, if possible, with a BVM assembly.
9. Use a laryngoscope in the left hand to visualize the vocal cords.
10. Insert, intubating the bougie through the cords and slide the tracheal tube over the bougie into the trachea, then remove the bougie.
11. Connect the self-inflating resuscitation bag to the tracheal tube directly or with a catheter mount, via a heat/moisture exchanger (HME) filter.
12. Inflate the cuff until no air leak is audible during ventilation.
13. Secure the tracheal tube with ties or tapes.
14. Confirm intubation with chest auscultation and $EtCO_2$ detection, and ventilate the patient with 100 per cent oxygen to normal $EtCO_2$ levels.

All intubated, trauma patients should be ventilated, as it is unlikely that they would be able to maintain adequate oxygenation and ventilation spontaneously.

Needle cricothyroidotomy Needle cricothyroidotomy is the insertion of a needle through the cricothyroid membrane into the trachea to allow jet insufflation of the lungs with oxygen. It is used in emergency 'can't intubate, can't ventilate' situations to buy time whilst expert assistance is sought, or a definitive surgical airway prepared. Oxygenation is achievable, but ventilation limited, so carbon dioxide accumulates and the $EtCO_2$ rises. Specialist equipment is available (e.g. ventilation with a Sanders injector driven from a high-pressure oxygen source, via a curved cricothyroid needle). However, a system can be rapidly assembled from routinely available components. The following sequence should be followed:

1. Prepare a 12- or 14-gauge, preferably unported, intravenous cannula, and attach it to a 10 mL syringe.
2. Prepare a length of oxygen tubing with a distal Y connector, three-way tap or cut side-hole, and attach it to a cylinder or wall oxygen source with a flow rate set at 15 L/minute.
3. Prepare skin with 2 per cent chlorhexidine in 70 per cent isopropyl alcohol, and insert the cannula through the patient's cricothyroid membrane in the midline, angled caudally at 45 degrees, aspirating air as the trachea is entered.
4. Slide the cannula fully into the trachea over the trochar and secure manually or with tape.
5. Attach the Y connector end of the oxygen tubing to the cannula.
6. Occlude the Y connector for 1 second to allow lung insufflation.
7. Allow a 4-second pause with the Y connector un-occluded to allow lung deflation.
8. Continue 1:4 cycles of insufflations until a definitive airway is secured.

Complications of needle cricothyroidotomy and jet insufflation are commonly misplacement, surgical emphysema and barotrauma. It should only be attempted if intubation and other airway maintenance techniques have failed.

Surgical cricothyroidotomy Surgical cricothyroidotomy is the insertion of a tracheal or tracheostomy tube through an incision in the cricothyroid membrane into the trachea. It is used in emergency situations when oro-tracheal intubation has been attempted, and failed, and will both secure and protect the airway. Adequate ventilation is just as achievable as with oro-tracheal intubation, and 100 per cent oxygen can be delivered. The following sequence should be followed:

1. Prepare skin over cricothyroid membrane with 2 per cent chlorhexidine in 70 per cent isopropyl alcohol, and infiltrate with local anaesthetic if the patient is aware.
2. Prepare an appropriate tracheal tube; a 6 mm internal diameter, reinforced/armoured tracheal tube is optimal, as this allows use of an intubating bougie and will not kink and obstruct. Alternatively, a tracheostomy tube with obturator can be used.
3. Prepare a scalpel, ideally with a curved No. 10 blade.
4. Prepare an intubating bougie or catheter, e.g. Cook Medical Frova intubation catheter.
5. Identify the cricothyroid membrane; place a finger on the thyroid cartilage prominence and roll it down onto a notch of cricothyroid membrane.
6. Tension skin over the cricothyroid membrane with the thumb and fore-finger on either side.
7. Make a single, 1–2 cm transverse incision through the skin and cricothyroid membrane into the trachea.
8. Without releasing skin tension, insert the intubation catheter through the incision and pass it inferiorly down the trachea.
9. Slide the tracheal tube over the intubation catheter into the trachea until the cuff is in the lumen of the trachea.
10. Inflate the cuff until the leak is sealed on ventilation.
11. Ventilate with a self-inflating bag and high-flow oxygen.
12. Secure the tracheal tube with ties or tape.
13. Confirm that both lungs are ventilated; if one-lung ventilation is detected (usually on the right), deflate the cuff, pull back the tracheal tube and re-inflate the cuff.

Surgical cricothyroidotomy can be a difficult procedure in casualties with challenging anatomy, and complications can be serious; this procedure should only be used if oro-tracheal intubation has been attempted and failed. Complications include haemorrhage, damage to laryngeal structures, false passage formation, misplacement of the tracheal tube, surgical emphysema and barotrauma.

Take-home message Whatever the means of airway management used, the goal is to secure and protect the airway. The focus should be on oxygenation and ventilation, not intubation. Casualties die from hypoxia and hypercarbia, not failure of intubation.

B – Breathing and chest injuries

Of severely injured patients admitted to hospital in the UK, 20 per cent have chest injuries (Joint Royal Colleges Ambulance Service Liaison Committee (JRCALC), 2008), and thoracic trauma is a significant cause of mortality (Findlay et al., 2007). However, the majority of chest injuries are not fatal and do not require specialist, surgical intervention.

BREATHING/CHEST INJURY – AWARENESS

The proportion of penetrating to blunt chest injuries varies between countries, and between rural and urban environments. Only 10 per cent of blunt chest injuries and 20 per cent of penetrating injuries require thoracotomy (Findlay et al., 2007; Joint Royal Colleges Ambulance Service Liaison Committee (JRCALC), 2008). Non-surgical management centres on supportive treatment of contused lungs and the insertion of chest drains. However with blunt trauma, the force of impact and energy transfer to the lung parenchyma should alert the clinician to the likelihood of severe intrathoracic damage and the potential for progressive cardiopulmonary problems.

Early recognition and management of immediately life-threatening injuries in the primary survey is imperative, with early imaging repeated as necessary. Potentially life-threatening injuries are sought during the secondary survey, and sophisticated imaging modalities such as CT and MRI may be indicated. Major chest injuries will require urgent referral to a specialist thoracic or cardiothoracic surgeon, and a surgeon capable of immediate thoracotomy must be available in hospitals designated as receiving major trauma cases.

BREATHING/CHEST INJURY – RECOGNITION

The patient's chest, neck and abdomen must be fully exposed to allow assessment of the chest. Examination should be systematic:

Look

- Respiratory rate – tachypnoea is indicative of hypoxia.
- Shallow, gasping or laboured breathing – suggests respiratory failure.
- Cyanosis – indicates hypoxia.
- Plethora and petechiae – suggest asphyxia and chest crushing.
- Paradoxical respiration; 'pendulum' breathing with asynchronization between chest and abdomen, resulting in a seesaw motion – indicates respiratory failure or structural damage.

- Unequal chest inflation – suggestive of pneumothorax or flail chest.
- Bruising and contusions – indicate significant energy transfer and consequent underlying lung contusion and potential hypoxia (e.g. 'seat belt' sign).
- Penetrating chest injuries – potential for pneumothorax and open, sucking pneumothorax.
- Distended neck veins – increased venous pressure secondary to a tension pneumothorax or cardiac tamponade.

Listen

- Absent breath sounds – indicate apnoea or tension pneumothorax.
- Noisy breathing/crepitations/stridor/wheeze – suggest a partially obstructed airway, blood and secretions in airways, tracheal or bronchial damage.
- Reduced air entry unilaterally – indicate a pneumothorax, haemothorax or haemo-pneumothorax, and flail chest.

Feel

- Tracheal deviation – indicative of tension pneumothorax, shifting the mediastinum (*Note*: the trachea is felt inferiorly in the suprasternal notch; do not confuse it with the larynx, which is extra-thoracic and hence does not shift.)
- Tenderness – suggests significant chest wall contusion and/or fractured ribs
- Crepitus/instability – underlying fractured ribs
- Surgical emphysema (classic 'bubble wrap' feel to subcutaneous tissues on palpation, due to presence of air forced into tissues under pressure) – tension pneumothorax, ruptured bronchi or trachea, and fractured larynx.

BREATHING/CHEST INJURY – MANAGEMENT

Immediate management is to stabilize the cervical spine, control catastrophic limb haemorrhage, secure the airway, administer oxygen at high flow and ventilate the lungs if breathing is absent or inadequate. It is vital to rapidly identify and manage immediately life-threatening chest injuries during the primary survey, as positive-pressure ventilation of the lungs can cause a rapid deterioration; a simple pneumothorax can be converted to a tension pneumothorax, and a tension pneumothorax will increase in pressure, leading to sudden collapse and cardiac arrest. Hence, if a patient is intubated and ventilated, signs of a pneumothorax must immediately be sought and, if present, decompressed and drained. Potentially life-threatening injuries can then be identified during the secondary survey.

IMMEDIATELY LIFE-THREATENING CHEST INJURIES (PRIMARY SURVEY)

1. Tension pneumothorax
2. Open pneumothorax (sucking chest wound)
3. Massive haemothorax
4. Cardiac tamponade
5. Flail chest
6. Disruption of tracheal–bronchial tree

TENSION PNEUMOTHORAX

A tension pneumothorax is the build-up of air under pressure in the pleural cavity, leading to compression and collapse of the underlying lung. The resultant ventilation–perfusion mismatch leads to hypoxia. However, the life-threatening, terminal event is a shift of the mediastinum away from the affected side, kinking the great vessels and obstructing venous return to the heart. This results in a deadly combination of hypoxia and loss of cardiac output, with a pulseless electrical activity (PEA) cardiac arrest.

Diagnosis should usually be clinical, not radiological, and the clinician should look specifically for the three cardinal signs:

- absent breath sounds – on the side of the pneumothorax
- deviated trachea – away from the side of the tension pneumothorax
- hyper-resonance – on the side of the pneumothorax.

The neck veins may be distended, as venous return is obstructed; however, this may not be readily visible, and is unreliable with concurrent hypovolaemia. There is an argument for radiological diagnosis if this is immediately available in the resuscitation room, and the patient is not exhibiting cardiovascular compromise; a tension pneumothorax can be mimicked by other conditions such as endo-bronchial intubation with distal lung collapse.

The immediate management is decompression (needle thoracocentesis) of the tensioning pneumothorax by insertion of a 14-gauge cannula into the pleural cavity through the second intercostal space, in the mid-clavicular line.

Diagnostically, a hiss is heard as air under pressure escapes. However, this is unreliable, and the relatively short 50 mm intravenous cannulae commonly used may not penetrate a thick chest wall in muscular or obese casualties. Presence of the cannula within the pleura is likely if air can be aspirated with a syringe, and use of the longer 140 mm cannulae will make correct placement more likely. Once sited, the cannula should be left open to reduce the risk of re-tensioning.

Needle decompression should not be performed if the only sign elicited is reduced or absent breath

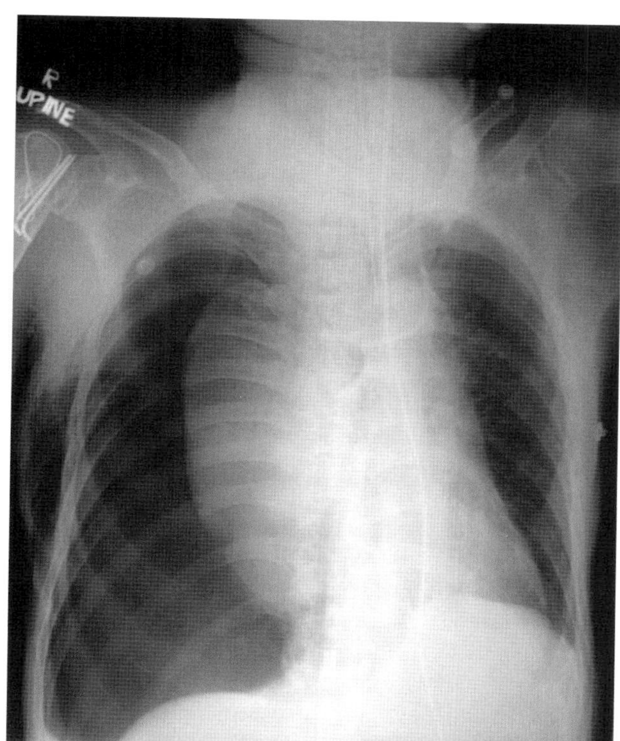

22.21 Left-sided tension pneumothorax

sounds, as there are associated complications such as misplacement and damage to the underlying lung. Insertion of a needle into the pleural cavity will convert a tension pneumothorax into a simple pneumothorax, which will in turn need draining. In an intubated and ventilated patient, immediate thoracostomies can be performed prior to formal chest drain insertion; the positive-pressure ventilation of the lungs will enable the lungs to be satisfactorily inflated. If immediately available, a controlled chest drain insertion is preferable to a blind needle decompression.

OPEN PNEUMOTHORAX (SUCKING CHEST WOUND)

An open wound in the chest wall will immediately result in a simple pneumothorax as intrathoracic pressure equilibrates with atmospheric pressure. If the defect is greater than some two-thirds of the diameter of the trachea (which has a lateral diameter of 20–25 mm), air is preferentially drawn into the pleural cavity rather than into the lungs via the trachea. This causes paradoxical respiration, where the lung deflates on inspiration, with resulting hypoventilation and hypoxia. If a flap valve effect occurs, the intra-pleural pressure will rise with each breath, leading to a tension pneumothorax.

Specific, immediate management is the application of an occlusive dressing, sealed on three sides, but leaving the third side open to allow any build up of positive intra-pleural pressure to vent. This can be ineffective in practice, and an occlusive dressing with immediate chest drain may be more reliable. The patient may need intubating and ventilating.

MASSIVE HAEMOTHORAX

The chest cavity presents an enormous potential space in which blood can accumulate following both blunt and penetrating chest injury (one of the four of 'bleeding onto the floor and four more'). 1500 mL or one-third of the patient's blood volume can rapidly accumulate, leading to a combination of hypoxia and shock. Smaller haemothoraces are usually due to lung parenchymal tears, fractured ribs and minor venous injuries and are self-limiting. Massive bleeds are usually due to arterial damage, which is more likely to require surgical repair and pulmonary lobectomy.

Diagnosis is based on the presence of hypoxia, reduced chest expansion, absent breath sounds and/or dullness to chest percussion, and hypovolaemic shock. Supine chest percussion may not demonstrate dullness, and supine x-rays may not reveal moderate haemothoraces. Specific management is by the insertion of a chest drain, correction of hypovolaemia and blood transfusion. If the total volume of blood initially drained is greater than 1500 mL, or the bleeding continues at 200 mL/hour, or the patient remains haemodynamically unstable, surgical referral and thoracotomy is indicated.

CARDIAC TAMPONADE

Cardiac tamponade is the accumulation of blood within the pericardium, restricting the ability of the heart to fill, and resulting in a progressive loss of cardiac output leading to PEA cardiac arrest. It is more commonly associated with penetrating rather than blunt trauma, especially stab wounds between the nipple lines or scapulae, and gunshot wounds.

Clinical diagnosis can be difficult, as the signs can be subtle and difficult to elicit in the trauma room. The three classic diagnostic criteria constitute Beck's Triad:

1. Distended neck veins due to elevated venous pressure.
2. Muffled heart sounds.
3. Fall in arterial blood pressure.

If an arterial line is present, a fall in systolic blood pressure may be seen on inspiration (pulsus paradoxus). If a central venous pressure (CVP) line is in situ, a rise in CVP may be seen on inspiration, in contrast to its normal fall on inspiration (Kussmaul's sign).

Reliable diagnosis may require sophisticated imaging. No change is seen on standard chest x-rays, but CT scanning, MRI scanning, FAST ultrasound and trans-oesophageal echo-cardiogram (TOE) can all be used to confirm the diagnosis.

Management has two components; relieving the pressure within the pericardium by draining the accumulated blood, and stopping the source of the bleeding to prevent re-accumulation. Since the bleeding is likely to come from the heart, immediate surgical repair to the myocardium may be required, and surgical assistance should be sought early.

Classically, aspiration of blood from the pericardium is achieved by needle peri-cardiocentesis, which should be viewed as a diagnostic procedure rather than curative. The ECG is monitored, and a long cannula (16–14 gauge, 14 cm as above) is attached to a syringe. The skin is prepared, pierced with the cannula to the left of the xiphisternum, and the cannula directed towards the pericardium in the direction of the left scapula tip. As the pericardium is entered, blood is aspirated. The needle can then be removed from the cannula, and a three-way tap attached to the cannula to allow further aspirations. Advancement too far will cause the tip of the cannula needle to enter the myocardium, which will be seen on the ECG as ventricular ectopics, widening QRS complexes or ST-T wave changes. Pericardiocentesis can be performed under ultrasound guidance.

Alternative and more definitive procedures are subxiphoid pericardial window, or emergency thoracotomy and pericardiotomy. These are optimally performed in the operating theatre if the patient's condition allows.

FLAIL CHEST

Massive impact to the chest wall can result in multiple rib fractures, and this is more common in older people who have less flexible rib cages. The multiple fractures, particularly if anterior and posterior, can result in a loss of the structural integrity of the chest wall, and a segment can 'float'; as the patient inspires, the flail segment is sucked in and the lung cannot inflate (paradoxical respiration). This results in hypoxia and ventilatory compromise. However, the force required to cause this injury inevitably causes a severe, underlying lung contusion, and this is the more significant cause of the hypoxia. The associated, severe pain further compromises the respiratory function, and respiratory failure can ensue.

Diagnosis is by clinical examination, chest x-rays to reveal the fractures and lung contusion, and arterial blood gases to quantify the hypoxia.

Management is initially supportive with administration of oxygen and analgesia. Advanced pain relieving methods such as epidurals may be required. Profound hypoxia may require that patients are intubated and ventilated until the contusion has adequately resolved, and pain can be controlled. Intravenous fluids may need to be restricted to avoid overload and worsening hypoxia. Very rarely, fractured ribs or costo-chondral disruption may require surgical stabilization.

DISRUPTION OF TRACHEOBRONCHIAL TREE

Major disruption of the tracheobronchial tree can result in a broncho-pleural fistula; the disrupted trachea or bronchus allows an air leak into the pleura which, if large enough, will not allow inflation of the lung, even with a large-bore chest drain in situ. Diagnosis is made by the presence of a persistent pneumothorax, pneumomediastinum, pneumopericardium or air below the deep fascia of the neck, often in patients who have suffered a deceleration injury.

Immediate management with tracheal intubation may not be successful, as the air leak may prevent inflation of either lung. In this situation, endobronchial intubation of the opposite lung or use of a bronchial blocker may be required before adequate lung ventilation can be achieved, and this may need the services of a thoracic anaesthetist.

SIMPLE PNEUMOTHORAX

A simple pneumothorax results from air entering the pleural cavity, causing collapse of the lung with a resulting ventilation–perfusion mismatch and hypoxia. As the air is at atmospheric pressure, and there is no one-way valve effect, no mediastinal shift develops, and cardiac output is maintained. The cause is usually a lung laceration, which can follow both blunt and penetrating chest trauma or thoracic spine fracture–dislocations.

The diagnosis is made during the primary or secondary survey, primarily by the absence or reduction of breath sounds. Hyper-resonance may not be obvious, and a chest x-ray may be required to confirm the pneumothorax. If the pneumothorax is stable, definitive treatment with a chest drain can be deferred to the secondary survey. However, a simple pneumothorax can develop into a tension pneumothorax at any time, and so a high index of suspicion should be maintained.

POTENTIALLY LIFE-THREATENING CHEST INJURIES (SECONDARY SURVEY)

1. Simple pneumothorax
2. Haemothorax
3. Pulmonary contusion
4. Tracheobronchial tree injury
5. Blunt cardiac injury
6. Traumatic aortic disruption
7. Traumatic diaphragmatic injury
8. Mediastinal traversing wounds
9. Simple pneumothorax

Intubation and ventilation in the presence of a pneumothorax predisposes to the development of a tension pneumothorax, and so chest drains should immediately be placed. Anaesthesia with a nitrous oxide-based anaesthetic will increase the air space by a factor of four, and can therefore cause rapid tensioning, as can air transport at altitude. In these situations, chest drains should be placed prophylactically, and it is good practice to insert chest drains in casualties prior to transfer in case a tension pneumothorax develops *en route*.

Chest drain insertion is a procedure with the potentially dangerous complication of visceral damage, and the classic chest drain technique using a pointed trochar should not be used. The appropriate technique is:

1. Confirm the correct side on the chest x-ray.
2. Identify the fifth intercostal space, just anterior to the mid-axillary line on the affected side.
3. Prepare the skin with 2 per cent chlorhexidine in 70 per cent isopropyl alcohol or alcoholic iodine.
4. Infiltrate the skin and subcutaneous tissues with lignocaine if the patient is aware.
5. Make a 2–3 cm, horizontal incision through the skin, just above the sixth rib (to avoid the intercostals vessels below the fifth rib).
6. Bluntly dissect through the subcutaneous tissues with a straight forceps, and puncture the parietal pleura with the tips.
7. Insert your gloved little finger through the incision into the chest cavity and sweep the finger around to ensure the cavity is empty and your incision is above the diaphragm (no viscus is felt).
8. Grasp the tip of an appropriately sized thoracostomy tube between the tips of the forceps and introduce through the incision into the chest cavity; unclamp the forceps and slide the tube posteriorly along the inside of the chest wall.
9. Attach the tube to an underwater drain or Heimlich valve and observe for tube fogging and underwater bubbling.
10. Suture the chest drain in place and apply a dressing.
11. Check lung reinflation with a chest x-ray.

The important steps are illustrated in Figure 22.22.

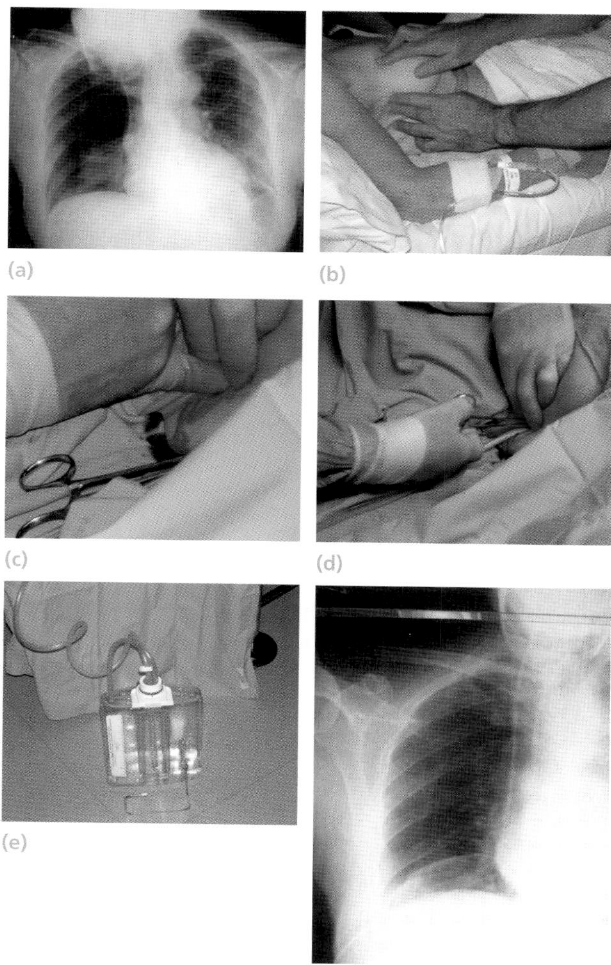

22.22 Chest drain insertion sequence (a) Chest x-ray to confirm correct side. (b) Identify the fifth intercostal space, just anterior to the mid-axillary line on affected side. (c) Insert gloved little finger through the incision into the chest cavity and finger sweep to ensure cavity is empty and the incision is above the diaphragm (no viscus is felt). (d) Grasp the tip of an appropriately sized thoracostomy tube between tips of forceps and introduce through incision into chest cavity. Unclamp forceps and slide tube posteriorly along inside of chest wall. (e) Attach tube to underwater drain or Heimlich valve and observe for tube fogging and underwater bubbling. (f) Check lung reinflation with chest x-ray.

Haemothorax Haemothoraces are primarily caused by lung lacerations or damage to intercostals and internal mammary vessels. Thoracic spine fracture dislocations can also result in haemothoraces. They are normally self-limiting, and rarely require operative intervention.

Diagnosis can be difficult in the supine patient as breath sounds will remain present. Dullness to percussion will be posterior and not reliable. Supine chest x-rays will not reveal moderate amounts of blood, although erect films are more sensitive; even with an erect film, 400–500 mL of blood are required to obliterate the costo-phrenic angle. The diagnosis may require the use of FAST or CT scanning.

An acute haemothorax visible on chest x-ray is treated with a large calibre chest drain, inserted using the technique described earlier. If more than 1500 mL are drained initially, or drainage continues at 200 mL/hour or faster, thoracotomy should be considered.

PULMONARY CONTUSION

Pulmonary contusion is the commonest potentially life-threatening chest injury, occurring in 20 per cent of casualties with an injury severity score (ISS) of > 15. Mortality ranges from 15–20 per cent and 40–60 per cent of patients will require ventilating. Blunt force trauma to the chest wall, or crushing injury, will contuse the underlying lung, which then becomes oedematous and haemorrhagic, with subsequent collapse and consolidation. This causes a ventilation–perfusion mismatch and hypoxia, dependant on the extent of the contusion and limitation of the patient's ventilation by pain. About half of these patients will develop bilateral acute respiratory distress syndrome (ARDS), a systemic inflammatory response to the injury.

Pulmonary contusion may not be associated with obvious rib fractures, particularly in children and teenagers with pliable rib cages. The initial chest x-ray may not reveal the extent of the contusion, which can develop over the following 48 hours. The diagnosis should be made taking into account the mechanism of injury and the degree of hypoxia revealed by oximeter saturation readings and arterial blood gas estimations.

Treatment is with supportive measures and oxygen administration. Patients with severe hypoxia despite inspired oxygen (e.g. $PaO_2 < 8.5$ kPa or $SaO_2 < 90$ per cent) should be considered for elective ventilation. Pre-existing pulmonary disease should be taken into account.

TRACHEOBRONCHIAL TREE INJURY

Tracheobronchial tree injuries are rare, but can easily be overlooked as signs can be subtle. Some 3 per cent of chest-crushing injuries are associated with upper airway injuries, but most trachea-bronchial tree injuries are within 1 inch of the carina. Patients frequently present with haemoptysis, surgical emphysema and a simple or tension pneumothorax. The pneumothorax may be resistant to re-inflation with a chest drain, and a post-drain and persistent air leak suggests the presence of a bronchopleural fistula. CT and MRI imaging may confirm the diagnosis, but bronchoscopy may be required.

Treatment is initially with one or more, large chest drains that may need a high-volume/low-pressure pump to allow lung re-inflation. Persistent bronchopleural fistulae may require operative intervention. Major tracheobronchial injuries are immediately life-threatening, and management is described earlier.

BLUNT CARDIAC INJURY

Blunt cardiac injury follows a direct blow to the anterior chest, and is associated with a fractured sternum. This can result in myocardial contusion, or more rarely, chamber rupture and valvular disruption. The myocardial damage can result in hypotension due to myocardial dysfunction, conduction abnormalities, and dysrhythmias. Sudden onset of dysrhythmias can result in death from ventricular fibrillation.

Management is supportive, and the patient should be monitored closely for a minimum of 24 hours, following which the risk of sudden dysrhythmias diminishes substantially.

TRAUMATIC AORTIC DISRUPTION

Blunt aortic injury is a deceleration injury commonly following high-speed road traffic crashes (RTCs) and falls from a height. Up to 15 per cent of deaths from road vehicle collisions are a result of damage to the thoracic aorta (Williams et al., 1994). Most injuries occur in the proximal thoracic aorta, where the relatively mobile aortic arch can move against the fixed descending aorta near the ligamentum arteriosum. Complete transection or rupture is immediately fatal, but the haematoma can be contained by the adventitial layer of the aortic wall, enabling the patient to survive to reach hospital.

Specific clinical signs and symptoms are often absent, and the mechanism of injury should provoke a high index of suspicion. Diagnosis is aided by chest x-ray findings, classically of a widened mediastinum (note that an anteroposterior (AP) film will magnify a normal width mediastinum), loss of the aortic knuckle

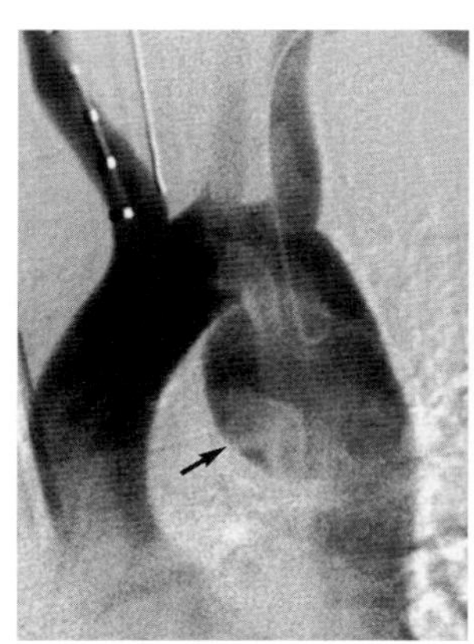

(a)

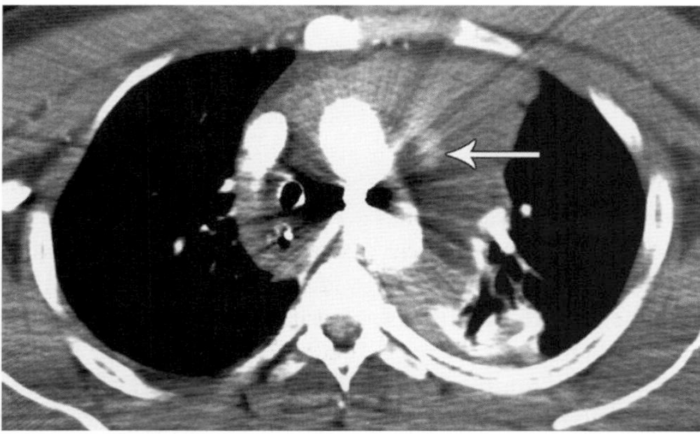

(b)

22.23 Ruptured aorta (a) Angiogram showing a rupture of the arch of the aorta. (b) CT scan showing the haematoma around the rupture.

and deviation of the trachea to the right. Whilst angiography has been the gold standard diagnostic tool, the advent of multidetector helical CT scanners has supplanted the more invasive technique. Modern CT scanning has an accuracy approaching 100 per cent, and is highly specific for detecting the injury.

Initial management is supportive, but a contained haematoma may rupture if the patient is hypertensive. Blood pressure should therefore be controlled in patients with suspected blunt aortic injury until CT scanning has excluded the injury. Once the injury is confirmed, the blood pressure must be controlled until the patient can be taken to the operating theatre for definitive cardiothoracic repair. Endovascular repair is possible for some blunt aortic injuries.

TRAUMATIC DIAPHRAGMATIC INJURY

Traumatic rupture of the diaphragm is associated with blunt and penetrating trauma to the abdomen. Blunt trauma is usually the result of a lateral or frontal vehicular collision, with distortion of the chest wall, shearing of the diaphragm and compressive rise in intra-abdominal pressure. Rupture is more common (in survivors) on the left side, probably because the severity of injury required to cause a right-sided rupture above the protective liver is more usually fatal. The injury is rarely found in isolation, and is associated with other chest, abdominal and pelvic injuries.

Diaphragmatic ruptures associated with penetrating trauma are usually due to gunshot and stab injuries, and result in a smaller tear with less visceral tissue protruding through the diaphragm.

Signs and symptoms can be subtle, and the injury missed, only becoming apparent years later as the herniation develops. The standard chest x-ray only may show an elevated but indistinct hemidiaphragm; however, the appearance of bowel gas or a nasogastric tube within the chest will help confirm the diagnosis. Contrast studies via a nasogastric tube, CT and MRI scanning are all useful adjuncts. Diaphragmatic rupture and visceral herniation may be mistaken for a haemothorax on the plain chest x-ray; however, the insertion of a finger into the chest during chest drain insertion may reveal the presence of stomach or bowel loops (hence the avoidance of sharp trochars to prevent visceral injury).

Initial management is supportive with careful assessment and management of the ABCs. Careful chest drain insertion is advisable prior to transfer or anaesthesia.

Definitive treatment is surgical – the diaphragmatic rupture can be repaired during a trauma laparotomy, but may require a thoracotomy or thoraco-abdominal approach.

MEDIASTINAL TRAVERSING WOUNDS

Penetrating objects that cross the mediastinum may cause damage to the lungs and to the major mediastinal structures (the heart, great vessels, tracheobronchial tree and oesophagus). The diagnosis is made by careful examination of the chest, backed up by chest x-ray and trauma CT imaging. The significant clinical finding is an entrance wound in one hemithorax and an exit wound or radiologically visible missile in the other. Bullets and shrapnel can tumble, so the trajectory is unpredictable. The presence of fragments adjacent to the mediastinum on x-ray should raise suspicion of a traversing injury.

Patients with symptomatic, haemodynamically unstable mediastinal traversing wounds should be assumed to have an ongoing haemothorax, tension pneumothorax or cardiac tamponade.

Initial management is ABC resuscitation with bilateral chest drains, prior to definitive surgical management. Stable patients should undergo extensive investigation with ultrasound, trauma CT, angiography, oesophagoscopy and bronchoscopy as indicated, and on early consultation with a cardiothoracic surgeon. Stable patients should be continually re-evaluated as they can suddenly deteriorate and require urgent surgical intervention; 50 per cent of patients with mediastinal traversing wounds are haemodynamically unstable on presentation, with a doubled mortality of 40 per cent over those who are stable (Findlay et al., 2007).

TAKE HOME MESSAGE

The primary goal in management of traumatic chest injuries is to rapidly identify and manage the six immediately life-threatening injuries within the primary survey. The eight potentially life-threatening injuries should be sought within the primary and secondary surveys, and may require sophisticated imaging to diagnose. Only 15 per cent of chest injuries require operative intervention.

C – Circulation and shock

For the healthcare professional 'shock' is not the commonly reported emotional condition in someone witnessing a disturbing incident. It can be broadly defined as circulatory failure, or inadequate perfusion of the tissues and organs with oxygenated blood.

Untreated, or inadequately treated, shock leads to organ damage and ultimately death from multi-organ failure. Recognition of shock, diagnosis of the cause and subsequent management are therefore important steps in the resuscitation and care of the seriously ill or traumatized patient. The C for circulation follows the A for airway and B for breathing, but in the presence of catastrophic, external bleeding from limb wounds, control of the bleeding takes precedence. This is the ABC sequence, and holds true in a hospital environment if the airway and catastrophic limb bleed cannot be managed simultaneously by the trauma team.

CIRCULATION AND SHOCK – AWARENESS

There are five main types of shock that can be grouped into two pathogenic groups:

1. *Vasoconstrictive:* hypovolaemic and cardiogenic shock.
2. *Vasodilative:* septic, neurogenic and anaphylactic shock.

The majority of patients presenting with shock following a major injury will be suffering from hypovolaemic shock; however, any patient can present with a combination of types of shock.

Hypovolaemic shock Hypovolaemic shock results from a loss of volume within the circulation; it may be due to whole blood loss from haemorrhage, or plasma and fluid loss from burns or severe medical conditions. As the circulating blood volume decreases, compensatory mechanisms are triggered to preserve blood pressure and vital organ perfusion. These mechanisms can maintain systolic blood pressure up to around 30 per cent blood loss in a fit patient. Above this, compensation increasingly fails until unconsciousness, followed by death at around 50 per cent blood loss.

Early compensatory mechanisms are tachycardia and peripheral vasoconstriction with a narrowed pulse pressure [vasoconstriction raises the diastolic blood pressure, bringing it closer to the systolic, e.g. 120/60 → 120/90]. Further compensations include tachypnoea, shift of fluid from tissues into circulation and reduced urine output.

Some injuries mimic hypovolaemic shock, classically tension pneumothorax and cardiac tamponade; the low-output state follows obstruction to the venous return and cardiac output, respectively. Peripheral vasoconstriction is not a feature of these conditions in the absence of hypovolaemia, unlike cardiogenic shock, and the veins remain full.

Cardiogenic shock Cardiogenic shock results from a decrease in myocardial contractility, and hence a reduction in stroke volume and cardiac output. This classically follows myocardial infarction or severe ischaemia, but can follow trauma damage to the myocardium from blunt or penetrating injury, e.g. fracture of the sternum. The disproportionate vasoconstriction is due not to hypovolaemia, but an outpouring of catecholamines and the profound autonomic stimulus, which can put further strain on the heart by causing vasoconstriction and increasing afterload. Trauma patients may present with cardiogenic shock if the cardiac event precedes, and indeed causes, the traumatic event.

Septic shock This results from the entry of toxins into the circulation, which poison the vasoconstrictive mechanisms within the blood vessels. These toxins usually come from infection, or are released from within the bowel secondary to bowel damage caused by ischaemia. The profound vasodilatation that results dramatically reduces afterload; even with a normal circulating blood volume and raised cardiac output, the patient's blood pressure falls and the pulse pressure widens, e.g. 110/70 → 90/30. Oxygen consumption increases, and despite the high cardiac output, tissue perfusion and oxygenation are reduced, and organ damage results. The toxins can also damage the myocardium and cause capillary leakage, complicating the presentation with elements of cardiogenic and hypovolaemic shock.

Neurogenic shock Neurogenic shock is produced by high spinal cord injury, which disrupts the sympathetic nerves controlling vasoconstriction. The peripheral vasculature relaxes and becomes profoundly dilated, reducing pre-load and afterload. Even with a raised cardiac output, the patient cannot maintain an adequate blood pressure, and shock ensues. Neurogenic shock is not caused by an isolated head injury, and is different from 'spinal shock', which is a temporary flaccidity following spinal damage. Since neurogenic shock is always related to traumatic spinal cord damage, it is likely to co-exist with a degree of hypovolaemia from associated trauma.

Anaphylactic shock This is a type of allergic reaction. Exposure to an antigen to which an individual has previously been sensitized triggers off a cascade reaction. The mast cells degranulate and release large quantities of histamine into the bloodstream. Other vasoactive substances are released, and profound vasodilatation is caused. Massive capillary leakage results in sudden oedema, which with loss of fluid into the bowel causes hypovolaemia [1 mm depth of oedema across the body surface equates to a 1.5 L fluid loss]. This picture is complicated by other effects such as bronchospasm.

Anaphylaxis can be triggered by many common antigens such as shellfish or peanuts. Of particular significance to the hospital practitioner are allergies to drugs and latex.

CIRCULATION AND SHOCK – RECOGNITION

Recognition of shock is relatively easy in the late stages when signs of underperfusion are obvious. Earlier stages of shock present with more subtle signs that require careful patient examination to elucidate; for example, the systolic blood pressure may not drop significantly until 30 per cent of the patient's blood volume has been lost. Hypovolaemic shock passes through a number of clinical stages as blood loss increases, and these have been grouped into four classes of shock, with increasingly apparent signs [adult blood volume is approximately 7 per cent of ideal body weight, or 5 L for a non-obese man weighing 70 kg]. It should be remembered, however, that the development and progression of shock is a continuum.

Blood loss of greater than 50 per cent (> 2500 mL) results in loss of consciousness, pulse and blood pressure, and finally respiration, causing a hypovolaemic PEA cardiac arrest.

The values shown in Table 22.1 relate to adults and children above the age of 12. Younger children compensate more effectively to a greater degree of blood loss, but they deteriorate very rapidly when they decompensate. The pulse rate is a good indicator of shock level, as is the respiratory rate; tables showing normal parameters for children at different ages are available.

A reasonable approximation of blood pressure can be gained from palpating pulses. However, practitioners tend to overestimate the blood pressure if pulses are palpable, although there is wide variation (Deakin and Low, 2000).

Recognition of shock therefore depends on a rapid clinical assessment of the patient, with measurement of the appropriate vital signs. The look, listen, feel sequence should be applied to identify the signs of *hypovolaemic* shock; blood pressure and pulse alone are not adequate.

CLASSES OF SHOCK

Class 1 – < 15 per cent loss blood volume (< 750 mL in a male weighing 70 kg)

(no change in BP, pulse pressure, respiratory rate or capillary refill)

- minimal tachycardia < 100 bpm
- skin pallor possible

Class 2 – 15–30 per cent loss blood volume (750–1500 mL)

(no change in systolic blood pressure)

- ↓ peripheral perfusion with cool, pale, clammy skin
- ↑ capillary refill > 2 seconds
- tachycardia > 100 bpm
- ↓ pulse pressure as diastolic BP rises
- increased respiratory rate (tachypnoea) of 20–30 bpm
- subtle mental status changes: anxiety, fear, aggression

Class 3 – 30–40 per cent loss blood volume (1500–2000 mL)

marked tachycardia > 120 bpm

- measurable fall in systolic blood pressure from patient's normal, e.g. < 100 mmHg
- thready peripheral pulses
- flat/empty veins
- marked tachypnoea > 30 bpm
- significant mental status changes: agitated ++
- dropping urine output

Class 4 – > 40 per cent loss blood volume (> 2000 mL)

- severe tachycardia > 140 bpm
- moribund, decreased conscious level
- significant drop in systolic blood pressure, e.g. < 70 mmHg
- impalpable peripheral pulses, weak central pulses
- respiratory distress
- central and peripheral cyanosis
- minimal urine output

Look and listen

- peripheral/central cyanosis and pallor
- sweating
- tachypnoea and respiratory distress
- change in mental status – anxiety, fear, aggression, agitation
- depressed level of consciousness or unconsciousness

Feel

- Peripheral perfusion poor – cool, clammy, shut down
- Capillary refill time > 2 seconds (this is unreliable in cold and frightened patients)
- Pulse rate and character – tachycardia and thready pulse
- Loss of pulses – radials, then femorals, then carotids as severity of shock increases
- Blood pressure – initially a raised diastolic with narrowed pulse pressure, then drop in systolic and diastolic, and finally an unrecordable blood pressure.

Observation of these factors will usually enable an assessment to be made of the presence and level of shock, and the likely degree of blood loss. This will act as a guide to whether volume replacement is indicated, and if so how much.

Hypovolaemic shock that remains unresponsive to treatment is likely to be due to bleeding into the body cavities or potential spaces, and evidence of this should be sought. Diagnosis may be helped by trauma imaging such as FAST or CT. A useful reminder of where to look is the catchy slogan: *bleeding onto the floor and four more* (i.e. external bleeding *and* chest, abdomen, pelvis/retroperitoneum, long bones). Bear in mind, though, that there are other forms of shock that need to be excluded.

Cardiogenic shock can mimic many of the signs of hypovolaemic shock. The history will give a good indication of the likely cause. The veins tend to be full in cardiogenic shock, and cyanosis more profound.

There may be other diagnostic signs present such as pulmonary oedema.

Septic, neurogenic and *anaphylactic shock* are characterized by vasodilatation as opposed to vasoconstriction. The veins tend to be full, and the peripheral pulses easily palpable and bounding. Peripheral perfusion may be good, with warm and flushed peripheries, but the skin may be mottled or cyanosed with sepsis.

CIRCULATION AND SHOCK – MANAGEMENT

Control of the airway (with cervical spine control), optimal oxygenation and ventilation are prerequisites to shock management. Immediate management of haemorrhagic shock depends on control of the bleeding and administration of intravenous fluids and blood to restore intravascular volume and haematocrit.

Control of haemorrhage This is achieved by direct pressure on the bleeding wounds with appropriate dressings, and elevation where practicable. Continuing developments from military experience have led to the introduction of additional measures to control external and limb bleeding. Wounds can be packed with a dressing, and a circumferential bandage applied around and over the packed wound. The bandage can then be twisted in a windlass technique to press the pack down into the wound. Specialist bandages have been designed for this purpose, such as the *Oales™ Modular Bandage*. This incorporates a gauze bandage for wound packing, with a plastic cup to compress into the packed wound beneath a circumferential, elastic bandage.

Tourniquets have been developed for controlling peripheral limb haemorrhage, with devices such as the *Combat Application Tourniquet (C-A-T™)*. The C-A-T™ is a single-handed device that uses a windlass system with a free moving internal band to provide circumferential pressure around the extremity. Once tightened and bleeding stopped, the windlass is locked in place. A Velcro® strap is then applied for further securing of the windlass during casualty evacuation.

Once in place and controlling the bleeding, the tourniquet should not be loosened or removed until a surgeon is available to definitively repair the injury.

Haemostatic dressings are useful for emergency control of arterial and venous haemorrhage from proximal sites where tourniquets cannot be applied (Mahoney et al., 2005). *Quikclot™* (granular zeolite, derived from volcanic rock) can effectively control devastating haemorrhage from large vessels, but generates tissue temperatures up to 570°C, potentially causing tissue necrosis. *HemCon™* (chitosan, derived from crushed shellfish) is an alternative, which has the advantage of not producing an exothermic reaction.

Clamping of bleeding points is difficult and can damage vessels; this should remain the province of the experienced surgeon.

Fracture of the pelvis can result in devastating retroperitoneal haemorrhage; this can be reduced by compressing the pelvis to approximate the bleeding fracture sites. Compression can be achieved manually, with a towel or blanket passed under the patient and tightened from both sides above the pelvis, or with specialized devices such as the *SAM Sling™*. This is a ratchet system compression belt for applying circumferential pressure around the pelvis. MAST trousers are impracticable and now rarely used.

Peripheral venous cannulation Intravenous access must be secured at the earliest opportunity; this can be very difficult in later stages of shock. The size of the cannula is important because of its effect on flow, which is directly proportional to the fourth power of the radius of the cannula (Poiseuille's Law). As an example, halving the radius of a cannula reduces the flow rate by a factor of 16. Flow is also reduced as the cannula lengthens.

Clearly it is difficult, if not impossible, to keep up with major haemorrhage without a minimum of two short, large-bore cannulae. Hence, the ATLS® guideline for in-hospital trauma cannulation is insertion of two cannulae, minimum size 16-gauge, but preferably 14-gauge, into large peripheral veins, typically in the antecubital fossae.

Central venous cannulation This is an option reserved for those with appropriate expertise; it can be very difficult and carries a significant risk of life-threatening complications (pneumothorax and arterial damage most commonly). In the UK, the use of two-

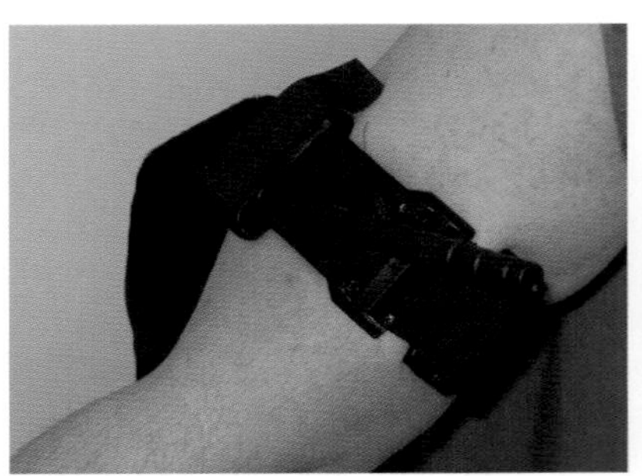

(a)

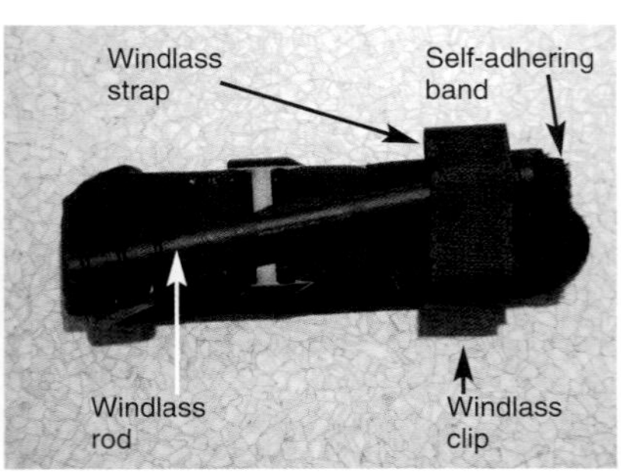

(b)

22.24 The C-A-T™ tourniquet (a) Tourniquet in use. (b) Tourniquet components.

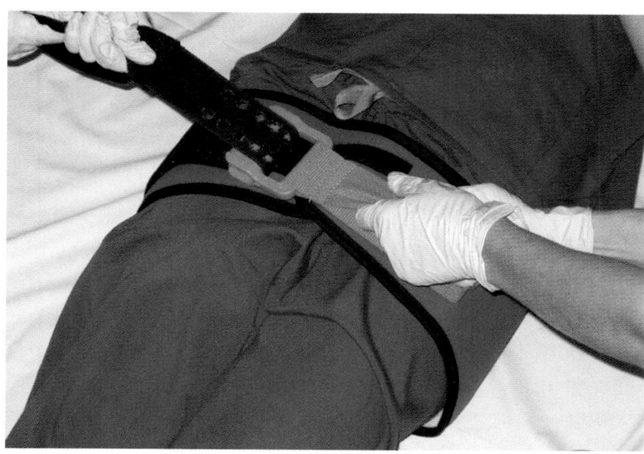

22.25 SAM Sling™ ratcheted compression belt in use

dimensional (2D) ultrasound imaging is strongly recommended in the routine siting of the CVP line. Access to the internal jugular can be difficult in a trauma patient, especially if he or she is immobilized with a stiff cervical collar and head blocks in place. The subclavian approach has the highest incidence of complications; femoral cannulation is a safer option than either central approach and a long cannula can often be sited in the femoral vein, medial to the femoral artery.

Intraosseus cannulation Intraosseous cannulation has previously been reserved for young children up to the age of about 5 years, where intravenous cannulation is not possible. The bone cortex is thin and relatively soft in children, and the marrow plentiful and vascular. A specialized 16-gauge intraosseus needle can be pushed or screwed into the bone of the tibia, below and medial to the knee joint. Response time to drug administration is close to IV administration, and entire resuscitations can be performed through intraosseus cannulae, including all anaesthetic drugs and fluids.

Intraosseus cannulation for adults has been validated, and specialist equipment is available for siting the cannulae through the thick and tough adult bone cortex. The Bone Injection Gun (BIG) is a spring-loaded device that fires a cannula through the cortex

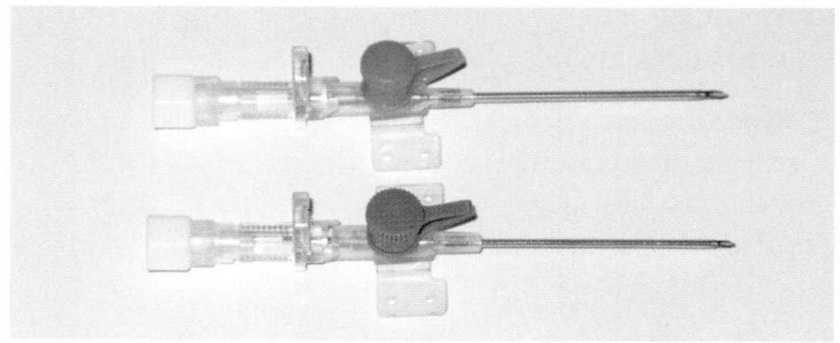

22.26 Cannulas A 16-gauge cannula (grey tap) has a 20 per cent smaller diameter but 40 per cent less flow than a 14-gauge cannula (orange tap).

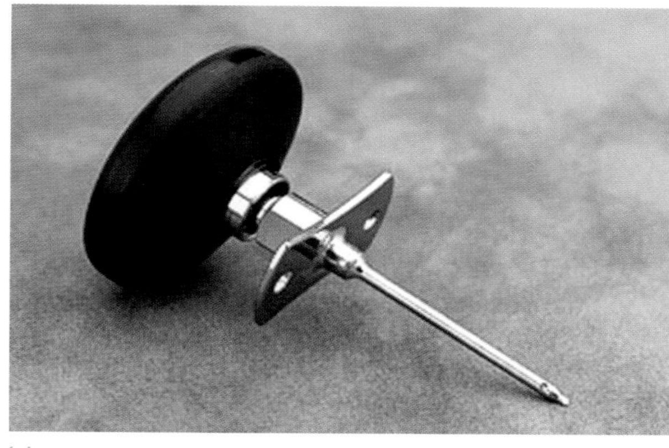

(a)

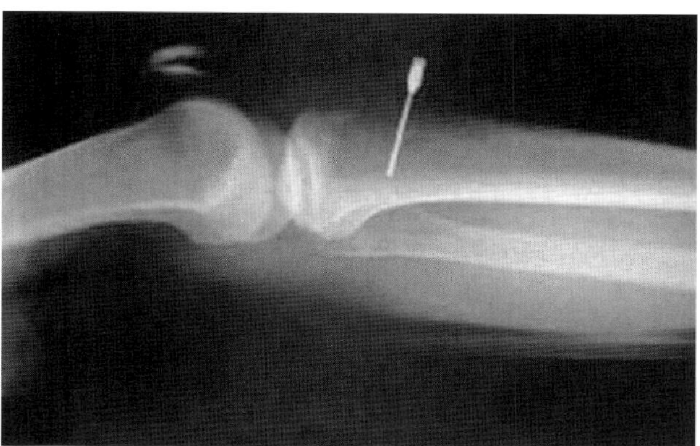

(b)

22.27 Intraosseous cannulation. (a) The Cook paediatric intraosseus needle. (b) Intraosseous needle in place in the medial proximal tibia.

of the tibia. The FAST1® is designed to manually push a cannula into the manubrium. The more recent EZ-IO® system consists of a hand-held electric drill to 'drill' a cannula through the cortex of the tibia or humeral head.

Fluid administration Fluid administration has for long been a controversial issue. The traditional ATLS approach for trauma circulation resuscitation, based on military experience, is to site two large-bore intravenous cannulae and administer an initial bolus of 2 L of warmed Ringer's lactate or Hartmann's solution. This is certainly successful in improving perfusion in bleeding patients, but is now not recommended for pre-hospital use where haemorrhage cannot be surgically controlled and blood is not available for transfusion. Casualties bleeding to a level 3 or 4 shock can reach a steady state as the blood pressure drops to a point where active bleeding may cease. Restoring vascular volume with crystalloids or colloids can restore the blood pressure to a point where bleeding resumes; further administration of clear fluids repeats the cycle until the haemoglobin level drops below a point where adequate oxygen can be carried.

Cardiac arrest and death then result from anaemic hypoxia.

In the UK, NICE guidance on Pre-hospital Initiation of Fluid Replacement Therapy in Trauma (National Institute for Clinical Excellence, 2004), relating to traumatized casualties with likely haemorrhage, is to titrate intravenous crystalloid fluids in 250 mL boluses against the radial pulse. If a radial pulse cannot be felt, the fluids are administered until the pulse returns, then withheld. NICE emphasizes the importance of not delaying transfer to hospital, and suggest fluids are administered if necessary *en route*. In penetrating chest wounds, fluids are titrated against a palpable central pulse. This strategy is known as *permissive hypotension*. Assuming O Rhesus-negative blood is immediately available in the Emergency Department, the blood pressure can be brought up with crystalloids pending rapid transfusion.

In UK practice, non-albumin colloid solutions are commonly used as plasma expanders (gelatine and starch formulations). These have a theoretical advantage in that they stay within an undamaged circulation for longer than crystalloids (saline and Hartmann's). However, there is little robust evidence that there is a practical advantage, particularly as any shocked patient will develop leaky capillaries and nullify the benefit of colloids. There is a risk of allergic reactions to these colloids, and NICE guidelines recommend the use of crystalloids only. Large volumes (> 2 L) of normal saline 0.9 per cent can cause a hyperchloraemic acidosis, and a lactated, balanced electrolyte solution such as Ringer's lactate or Hartmann's is preferable.

The dynamic response to a fluid challenge will give information as to whether bleeding is continuous or controlled. A 2 L volume of warmed Hartmann's is initially given (20 mL/kg in children), and the response in vital signs recorded:

Rapid responders – respond rapidly and remain haemodynamically normal, having lost < 20 per cent blood volume. No further fluid is required and surgical intervention may be required.

Transient responders – respond to the initial bolus, then deteriorate, having lost 20–40 per cent blood volume. These patients will need further fluid administration and blood transfusion, with probable surgical intervention.

Non-responders – show minimal or no response to the initial bolus. These patients are likely to require immediate transfusion and surgery to stop exsanguinating haemorrhage. There may be other causes such as tension pneumothorax, cardiac tamponade or non-haemorrhagic shock.

Fluids should be titrated against response, with optimum organ and peripheral tissue perfusion the goal. Blood pressure, pulse rate, peripheral perfusion and CVP are all used to assess response. Serial measurement of metabolic acidosis parameters such as bicarbonate, base deficit and lactate levels can be used to gauge adequate response to fluid therapy. More sophisticated methods such as oesophageal Doppler and arterial waveform analysis are also used in the critical care setting.

The use of *hypertonic saline* has been successfully demonstrated, and may have some benefits over the current use of isotonic fluids. Research with 7.5 per cent saline and dextran (as opposed to isotonic 0.9 per cent) suggests that mean arterial blood pressure and oxygen delivery are improved. Capillary damage is lessened, and organ perfusion improved, with a much larger increase in the intravascular volume. Short-term survival is improved, but the role of hypertonic solutions has yet to be determined.

The ultimate goal of synthetic, oxygen-carrying fluids has been researched for decades, but as yet nothing has effectively replaced the supremely efficient red blood cell. Blood transfusion should be given early if haemorrhagic shock is demonstrated, with O Rhesus-negative, type-specific or cross-matched blood. Transfusion should be titrated against the haematocrit, and blood products such as fresh-frozen plasma, platelet concentrates and clotting factors given during massive transfusions on the advice of the haematologists.

The information given earlier refers to resuscitation of hypovolaemic patients only. Most other forms of shock will respond initially to IV fluids pending accurate assessment and diagnosis. However, shock in elderly casualties without evidence of major trauma should raise a high index of suspicion for cardiogenic shock. Infusion of even small volumes of fluid can overload the circulation and cause collapse and cardiac arrest. Elderly patients may also be on medication for hypertension etc., which can severely limit their ability to maintain an adequate blood pressure and cardiac output. A drug history should be obtained as soon as possible; patients on vasodilator drugs such as ACE inhibitors and sartans may need inotropes to support the circulation, even if the patient is hypovolaemic.

Take home message In patients suffering from haemorrhagic, hypovolaemic shock the source of the bleeding must be identified and surgically or radiologically controlled. The priorities for restoring and maintaining adequate circulation are:

- control external bleeding
- restore intravascular volume
- transfuse blood
- turn off the tap – call a surgeon early.

D – Disability – head injury

The immediate management of the seriously head-injured patient is designed to prevent secondary injury and to provide the neurosurgeon with a live patient who has some hope of recovery. A significant number of fatalities from head injury are caused by the secondary and not the primary injury; prevention of this secondary brain injury is facilitated by following the ABC principles set out in ATLS®.

HEAD INJURIES – AWARENESS

In the UK, severe head injuries account for more than 50 per cent of trauma-related deaths, and these usually follow road traffic crashes, assaults and falls (Flannery and Buxton, 2001). Injury patterns differ between countries; in the UK patients experience predominantly closed injuries, with a peak incidence in males between the ages of 16 and 25 years. A second peak occurs in the elderly, with a high incidence of chronic subdural haematomas.

Only 10 per cent of head-injured patients presenting at Emergency Departments have a severe injury. The injuries can be classified into three groups based on the GCS (American College of Surgeons Committee on Trauma, 2004):

Mild (80 per cent)	GCS 13–15
Moderate (10 per cent)	GCS 9–12
Severe (10 per cent)	GCS 3–8

Investigation, management and outcomes depend on the severity of the injury; however, this is a continuum, and the classification given earlier is only a guideline. Even mild head injuries can be associated with prolonged morbidity in the form of headaches and memory problems; only 45 per cent are fully recovered 1 year later. With moderate head injuries, 63 per cent of patients remain disabled 1 year after the trauma, and this rises to 85 per cent with severe injuries (Royal College of Surgeons of England, 1999).

A knowledge of anatomy and pathophysiology is needed to understand and anticipate the development of a head injury.

The scalp comprises five layers of tissue, with the mnemonic SCALP: skin, connective tissue, aponeurosis, loose areolar tissue, and periosteum. It has a generous blood supply and serious scalp lacerations can result in major blood loss and shock if bleeding is not controlled.

The skull is composed of the cranial vault and the base. The vault has an inner and outer table of bone, and is particularly thin in the temporal regions, although protected by the temporalis muscle. The base of the skull is irregular, which may contribute to accelerative injuries. The floor of the cranial cavity has three distinct regions: the anterior, middle and posterior fossae:

The meninges cover the brain and consist of three layers:

1. *Dura mater* – a tough, fibrous layer, firmly adherent to the inner skull.
2. *Arachnoid mater* – a thin, transparent layer, not adherent to the overlying dura and so presenting a potential space. Cerebrospinal fluid (CSF) is contained and circulates within this space.
3. *Pia mater* – a thin, transparent layer, firmly adherent to the underlying surface of the brain.

The brain itself is divided into three main structures:

1. Cerebrum – composed of right and left hemispheres, divided into:
   - frontal lobes – emotions, motor function, speech
   - parietal lobes – sensory function, special orientation
   - temporal lobes – some memory and speech functions
   - occipital lobes – vision
2. Cerebellum – coordination and balance
3. Brainstem – composed of three main structures:
   - midbrain – reticular activating system (alertness)
   - pons – relays sensory information between cerebrum and cerebellum
   - medulla – vital cardiorespiratory centres.

The midbrain passes through a large opening in the tentorium, a fibrous membrane that divides the middle and posterior fossae. The third cranial nerve, which controls pupillary constriction, also runs through this opening, and is vulnerable to pressure damage if the cerebral hemispheres swell. This results in pupillary dilatation, an early sign of a significant rise in intracerebral pressure.

Pathophysiology The skull is in effect an enclosed, bony box containing the brain, blood vessels and the CSF. The intracerebral pressure (ICP) is normally maintained at approximately 10 mmHg, and is a balance of brain, intravascular and CSF volumes. Traumatic damage to the brain can cause swelling of the brain tissue itself, and bleeds from arteries and veins into the extradural space, subdural space or brain substance (intracerebral bleed) increase the intracerebral volume and raise the ICP. If the ICP is sustained at above 20 mmHg, permanent brain damage can result, with poor outcomes; this is the secondary brain injury. There is only limited, intracranial compensation for rising ICP, and this is largely achieved by a reduction in CSF volume (Monroe-Kelly doctrine). Once pressure compensation has reached its limits, the ICP rises rapidly in a breakaway exponential.

As the pressure rises, the conscious level decreases and the GCS falls. The medial part of the temporal lobe (the uncus) herniates through the tentorial

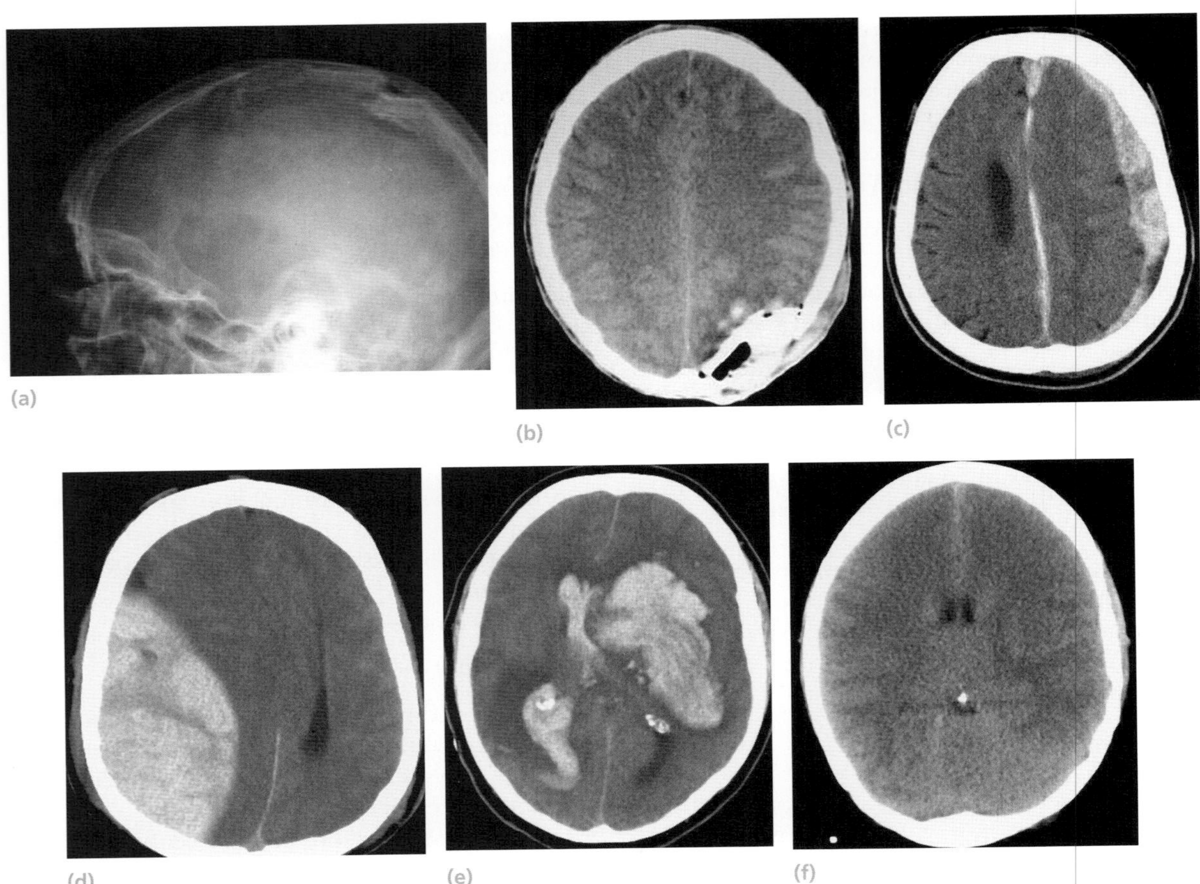

(a) (b) (c) (d) (e) (f)

22.28 Fractured skull – imaging (a) X-ray showing a depressed fracture of the skull. (b–f) CT scans showing various injuries: (b) a fracture; (c) an extradural haematoma; (d) a subdural haematoma and compression of the left ventricle; (e) an intracerebral haematoma; (f) diffuse brain injury with loss of both ventricles.

notch, compressing the third cranial nerve and the midbrain pyramidal tracts. This usually results in pupillary dilatation on the side of the injury, and hemiplegia on the opposite side. Pressure changes in the medulla cause a sympathetic discharge, with a rise in blood pressure and reflex bradycardia. With further pressure rise, cerebral blood flow is compromised, and ceases terminally when the ICP rises above the mean arterial pressure (MAP). Ultimately, the cerebellar tonsil is forced into the foramen magnum, resulting in a loss of vital cardiorespiratory function; this is known as brain stem or brain death, and is a terminal event.

Mechanism of brain injury Brain injury can be blunt or penetrating. The ***primary brain injury*** occurs at the time of the trauma, and results from sudden distortion and shearing of brain tissue within the rigid skull. The damage sustained may be focal, typically resulting from a localized blow or penetrating injury, or diffuse, typically resulting from a high-momentum impact. Sudden acceleration or deceleration can cause a contra-coup injury, as the brain impacts on the side of the skull away from the impact. High-velocity missile penetrating injuries will also cause a diffuse and severe brain injury as the resultant pressure wave moves across the brain. The ***secondary brain injury*** is pressure related, and is caused by swelling within the brain, causing a rise in ICP as described earlier. This is compounded by hypoxia, hypercarbia and hypotension.

Severity of brain injury The GCS is a well-tested and objective score for assessing the severity of brain injury: 13–15 is *mild;* 9–13 is *moderate*; 8 or less is *severe.*

Morphology of brain injury *Skull fractures* are seen in the cranial vault or skull base; they may be linear or stellate, and open or closed. The significance of a skull fracture is in the energy transfer to the brain tissue as a result of the considerable force required to fracture the bone. Open skull fractures may tear the underlying dura, resulting in a direct communication between the scalp laceration and the cerebral surface, which may be extruded as ICP rises.

Basal skull fractures are caused by a blow to the back of the head, or rapid deceleration of the torso with the head unrestrained, as in high-speed vehicular crashes. Fractures are rare, occurring in 4 per cent of severe head injuries, but can cause severe damage, and are a cause of death in front-end collisions and motor sport crashes. There are key physical signs pathognomic of basal skull fracture:

- peri-orbital ecchymosis (bruising – 'raccoon' or 'panda' eyes)
- retro-auricular ecchymosis (Battle sign – bruising behind ears)
- oto-rhinorrhea (CSF leakage from nose and ears)
- VIIth and VIIIth cranial nerve dysfunction (facial paralysis and hearing loss)

Basal skull fractures are not always visible on x-ray or CT, but blood in the sinus cavities and the clinical signs should suggest their presence.

Diffuse brain injury is due to axonal disruption of the neurones and varies from minor, resulting in mild concussion, to severe, resulting in an ultimately fatal hypoxic and ischaemic insult to the brain.

Extradural (epidural) haematomas are relatively uncommon, occurring in 0.5 per cent of all brain-injured patients, and 9 per cent of those who are comatose (Findlay et al., 2007). The haematoma is contained outside the dura but within the skull, and is typically biconvex or lenticular in shape. They are commonly located in the temporal or temporoparietal region, and usually result from a middle meningeal artery caused by a fracture.

Subdural haematomas are more common, and constitute 30 per cent of severe brain injuries (Findlay et al., 2007). They usually result from tearing of cortical surface vessels, and normally cover the entire surface of the hemisphere. Underlying brain damage is usually much more severe due to the greater energy transfer.

Contusions and *intracerebral haematomas* are fairly common (20–30 per cent of severe brain injuries). The majority occur in the frontal and temporal lobes. Inoperative contusions can evolve into haematomas requiring surgical evacuation over a period of hours or days, and repeat CT scanning within 24 hours may be indicated.

HEAD INJURIES – RECOGNITION

Initial recognition of a head injury takes place in the primary survey as part of the ABCDE sequence. The airway, cervical spine, breathing and circulation must all be assessed and resuscitation commenced before the brief neurological assessment takes place, as these measures will prevent the development of a secondary brain injury. The AVPU score is an instant and useful assessment but the level of consciousness should be assessed accurately at this point, using the GCS. The pupils are assessed for equality, diameter and response to light.

As there is a 5–10 per cent association of cervical spine fracture with head injury, the assumption is made that the neck is unstable until proved otherwise. As the cervical spine x-ray does not rule out a fracture, full immobilization should remain in place until the neck is cleared clinically or with further imaging such as CT.

A more thorough assessment of the neurological status takes place during the secondary survey. The GCS and pupils are re-evaluated, lateralizing signs are looked for, and the upper and lower limb motor and sensory function evaluated. If the patient is stable, further imaging may be indicated, and a number of guidelines exist to aid the decision.

CT scanning is the primary examination of choice for patients with a clinically important brain injury (National Institute for Health and Clinical Excellence, 2007). Modern, fast, spiral CT scanners are increasingly available adjacent to Emergency Departments, enabling rapid trauma CTs in the course of minutes. All patients suffering a severe head injury require an urgent CT scan. Specific indications for a head CT are (Royal College of Surgeons of England, 1999):

- GCS < 13 on first Emergency department assessment
- GCS < 15 2 hours after initial assessment
- suspected open or depressed skull fracture
- clinical basal skull fracture
- post-traumatic seizure
- focal neurological deficit
- > 1 episode of vomiting
- amnesia of events > 30 minutes before impact
- post-injury amnesia if:
  - age > 65 years
  - associated with coagulopathy
  - due to a dangerous mechanism of injury (pedestrian versus motor vehicle, ejection from motor vehicle, fall from height > 1 m).

HEAD INJURIES – MANAGEMENT

The management of head injuries depends on the severity, as assessed by the clinical examination, GCS and CT scan. Patients with a *mild head injury* should be admitted and monitored, with frequent neurological observations. Should there be any deterioration, CT scanning is indicated, and referral to the local neurosurgical unit is necessary. Discharge is when a complete neurological recovery has been made and provided the patient can be supervised at home by a responsible adult.

Patients sustaining moderate head injuries will need CT scanning and discussion with a neurosurgeon to decide on the need for transfer and definitive care. Other indications for neurosurgical referral, regardless of imaging findings, include:

- persistent coma after initial resuscitation (GCS < 8)
- unexplained confusion > 4 hours
- post-admission deterioration in GCS

- progressive, focal neurological signs
- seizure without full recovery
- definite or suspected penetrating injury
- CSF leak.

Patients with severe head injuries will require immediate resuscitation as described previously. The cervical spine must be immobilized whilst the airway is secured; this will require a competent, rapid sequence induction (RSI) of anaesthesia, and an anaesthetist must be involved early. Once the airway is secured and protected with a tracheal tube, the oxygenation and ventilation must be optimized. Hypoxia and hypercarbia must be avoided, but overventilation is equally damaging, as cerebral blood flow is compromised. Ventilation must be monitored with end-tidal carbon dioxide analysis, and the minute volume adjusted to maintain a low-normal $EtCO_2$ (4.5 kPa). Oxygen saturation levels should be maintained above 95 per cent, and sequential arterial blood gas estimations made to ensure the oxygen partial pressure is maintained in the normal range (> 13 kPa) as far as is possible.

The circulation should be monitored to maintain intravascular filling within an appropriate range. Overfilling will worsen cerebral oedema, but hypovolaemia will result in persistent shock. Central venous pressure should be monitored, and arterial pressures kept within a normal range for that patient, with reference to the ICP. This requires expert critical care skills, and patients with a severe brain injury must be managed in an appropriate critical care unit.

The rapid administration of intravenous mannitol at a dose of 0.5 mg/kg may be indicated to reduce ICP, and this should be given following discussion with the referral neurosurgeon. It can be a useful holding measure if signs of rising ICP (e.g. a dilated pupil) develop prior to or during transfer to a specialist centre.

Patients with significant head injuries in units without neurosurgical capability will require transfer, on discussion with the neurosurgeons. An expanding intracerebral haematoma will need to be evacuated within 4 hours of injury to prevent serious and permanent secondary brain injury.

TAKE HOME MESSAGE

Head-injured patients require early assessment and recognition of their brain injury. With severe head injuries, it should be remembered that:

1. A blow to the head causes a primary brain injury.
2. Hypoxia and hypercarbia cause cerebral swelling and a secondary brain injury.
3. Secondary brain injury should be minimized by optimal oxygenation, ventilation and blood pressure management.

E – Abdominal injuries

The abdomen is difficult to assess in the multiply injured trauma patient, especially when the patient is unconscious. The immediately life-threatening injury is bleeding into the abdominal cavity, and this is one of the 'onto the floor and four more' areas into which lethal volumes of blood may be sequestered. The abdomen is therefore examined in the primary survey as part of the circulation assessment.

ABDOMINAL INJURIES – AWARENESS

Abdominal injuries may be blunt or penetrating. Unrecognized abdominal injury is a cause of avoidable death after blunt trauma and may be difficult to detect. A direct blow from wreckage intrusion or crushing from restraints can compress and distort hollow viscera, causing rupture and bleeding. Deceleration causes differential movement of organs, and the spleen and liver are frequently lacerated at the site of supporting ligaments. In patients requiring laparotomy following blunt trauma, the organs most commonly injured are (Findlay et al., 2007):

- spleen (40–55 per cent)
- liver (35–45 per cent
- small bowel (5–10 per cent)
- retroperitoneum (15 per cent).

The mechanism of injury should lead to a high index of suspicion, e.g. flexion lap-belt injuries in car crashes can rupture the duodenum, with retroperitoneal leakage and subtle signs. Early imaging and exploratory laparotomy may be required.

Penetrating injuries between the nipples and the perineum may cause intra-abdominal injury, with unpredictable and widespread damage resulting from tumbling and fragmenting bullet fragments. High-velocity rounds transfer significant kinetic energy to the abdominal viscera, causing cavitation and tissue destruction. Gunshot wounds most commonly involve the:

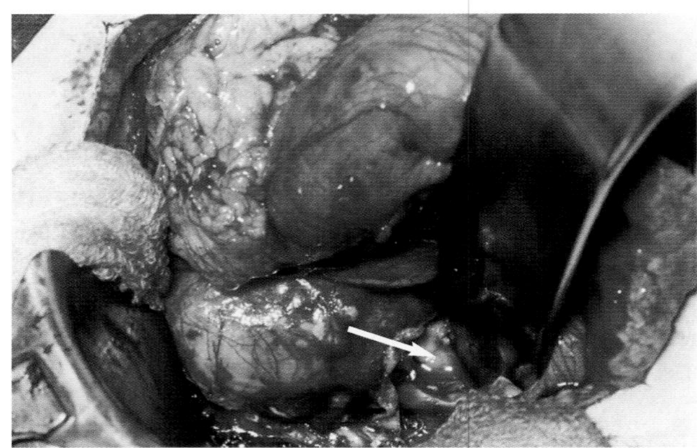

22.29 Abdominal injury Ruptured duodenum following flexion lap belt injury.

- small bowel (50 per cent)
- colon (40 per cent)
- liver (30 per cent)
- abdominal vasculature (25 per cent).

Stab wounds injure adjacent abdominal structures. Small wounds may result from thin-bladed knives that have penetrated deep and damaged several structures, with the most common injuries being:

- liver (40 per cent)
- small bowel (30 per cent)
- diaphragm (20 per cent)
- colon (15 per cent).

ABDOMINAL INJURIES – RECOGNITION

The abdomen is initially examined during the primary survey to determine if shock is due to an abdominal injury. A history from the patient, bystanders and paramedics is important, as the mechanism of injury can be identified and injuries predicted.

Examination of the abdomen follows the 'look, listen, feel' format. The patient must be fully exposed, and the anterior abdomen inspected for wounds, abrasions and contusions.

The flanks and posterior abdomen and back should be examined, and this may require log rolling to both sides. Auscultation is difficult in a noisy resuscitation room, but may reveal absence of bowel sounds caused by free intraperitoneal blood or gastrointestinal fluid. Percussion and palpitation may reveal tenderness or peritonism. The genitalia and perineum should be examined, and a rectal examination performed during the log roll.

Early imaging is indicated (a FAST examination will reveal the presence of intraperitoneal fluid) and can be performed in the resuscitation room; however, the technique has a high specificity but low sensitivity. Presence of fluid is an indication for laparotomy. CT scanning requires the patient to be stable, but is a much more effective diagnostic tool. Diagnostic peritoneal lavage is a technique largely supplanted by FAST and CT, but if these are unavailable it may still be used. It should be performed by the surgeon who would take the patient to the operating theatre.

ABDOMINAL INJURIES – MANAGEMENT

Initial management of an abdominal injury is to manage shock as described in circulation management. External bleeding is controlled with direct pressure, wound packing or haemostatic dressings. Intravenous access is established with two large-bore cannulae, and 2 L of warmed Hartmann's or Ringer's lactate infused at speed. If the shock remains unresponsive, further fluid is administered, and blood transfused. Confirmation of bleeding into the abdomen is an indication for immediate laparotomy, and imaging other than FAST may not be possible with an unstable patient. Other indications for laparotomy include:

- unexplained shock
- rigid silent abdomen
- evisceration
- radiological evidence of intraperitoneal gas
- radiological evidence of ruptured diaphragm
- gunshot wounds.

A naso- or oro-gastric tube should be passed in all multiple trauma patients; this should be passed orally in the presence of facial and basal skull fractures. A urinary catheter should be passed unless urethral bleeding or other signs of urethral injury such as genital bruising or a high-riding prostate are present.

Laparotomy is the definitive management and the province of the surgeon; general principles at initial operation are to:

- control haemorrhage with ligation of vessels and packing
- remove dead tissue
- control contamination with clamps, suturing and stapling devices
- lavage the abdominal cavity
- close the abdomen without tension.

Initial surgery may be for damage limitation rather than definitive treatment, and a second-look laparotomy at 24–48 hours may be indicated to allow:

- removal of packs
- removal of dead tissue
- definitive treatment of injuries
- restoration of intestinal continuity
- closure of musculofacial layers of the abdominal wall.

The patient will require supportive critical care, and may require ventilation on an ICU until after the second-look laparotomy.

TAKE HOME MESSAGE

Abdominal injuries are difficult to assess in the multiply injured patient. The immediate threat to life is bleeding into the peritoneal cavity, and early imaging with FAST and CT should be considered. Shock should be treated, and early consultation with a surgeon facilitated. Diagnostic or definitive treatment laparotomy may be required.

F – Musculoskeletal injuries

In the absence of catastrophic bleeding, musculoskeletal injuries are not immediately life-threatening. They are, however, limb threatening and potentially life-threatening. Definitive management is detailed elsewhere in this book, so this section will merely put these injuries into the context of the overall management of a severely injured casualty.

PELVIC FRACTURES

Awareness The pelvis and retroperitoneum constitute one of the 'onto the floor and four more' spaces into which blood can be sequestered to a level resulting in non-responsive shock. A haemorrhaging fracture of the pelvis therefore becomes a life-threatening emergency, and should be considered in every patient with a serious abdominal or lower limb injury. Potential causes are road accidents, falls from a height or crush injuries.

Recognition The pelvis is examined in the primary survey as part of the C – circulation assessment, once the airway and breathing have been assessed, and the cervical spine immobilized. Significant signs are swelling and bruising of the lower abdomen, thighs, perineum, scrotum or vulva, and blood at the urethral meatus. The pelvic ring should be gently palpated for tenderness side to side and front to back; however, if clinical suspicion is high, the pelvis should not be compressed for crepitus, as this can dislodge a clot from the fracture site and provoke further bleeding. If tenderness and crepitus are elicited, the examination should not be repeated.

An AP x-ray should be obtained during the primary survey, and in most cases will enable a preliminary diagnosis of pelvic fracture to be made. If the patient is stable, a trauma CT scan will give more detailed information, and also provide information on intra-abdominal and retroperitoneal bleeding.

Management The immediate management of a pelvic fracture resulting in shock is to control the bleeding and restore volume as described previously. There are a number of proprietary devices available to wrap around the pelvis and apply compression to approximate the bleeding fracture sites and allow clot formation. If these are not available, manual approximation can be used; this can be facilitated with a sheet wrapped around the pelvis and twisted anteriorly.

Once in place, the pelvic compression devices should not be removed until surgical interventions such as external fixation are available. Developments in interventional radiology and angiography have enabled embolization to be used to control haemorrhage from a fractured pelvis.

Take home message Pelvic fractures can result in life-threatening haemorrhage and should be recognized and managed as part of the circulation assessment during the primary survey. Pelvic compression devices should be used to minimize bleeding, and a rapid, surgical referral made for definitive management.

SPINAL INJURIES

Vertebral column injury, with or without neurological damage, must be considered in all patients with multiple injuries. A missed spinal injury can have devastating consequences. Immediate management therefore focuses on immobilization, recognition and referral for definitive care.

Awareness Spinal injuries can be stable or unstable, an unstable injury being one where there is a significant risk of fracture displacement and neurological sequelae. The mechanisms of injury are traction (avulsion), direct injury and indirect injury. Direct injuries are penetrating wounds usually associated with firearms and knives. Indirect injuries are the most common, and are typically the result of falls from a height or vehicular accidents where there is violent free movement of the neck or trunk. There is an association of cervical spinal damage with injuries above the clavicles, and some 5 per cent of head-injured patients have an associated spinal injury; 10 per cent of those with a cervical spine fracture have a second, non-contiguous spinal fracture. Regional occurrences of spinal injuries are approximately:

- cervical (55 per cent)
- thoracic (15 per cent)
- thoracolumbar junction (15 per cent)
- lumbosacral (15 per cent).

Spinal fractures with spinal cord transection also disrupt the sympathetic nerve supply and cause distal vasodilatation. A high spinal transection will therefore cause neurogenic shock – this is vasodilatory shock and is characterized by hypotension, a low diastolic blood pressure, widened pulse pressure, warm and well perfused peripheries and bradycardia. However, neurogenic shock can be complicated by hypovolaemic shock in multiply injured patients.

Recognition The spinal column and neurological function are examined in the secondary survey, with immobilization maintained throughout. Whilst the head is immobilized manually, and the patient log-rolled, the cervical spine and vertebral column from neck to sacrum are examined for:

- bruising, contusions and ecchymosis
- penetrating injury
- swelling or 'bogginess'
- tenderness on palpation
- step or misalignment between vertebrae.

A rectal examination is performed to assess anal tone. A neurological examination is carried out to identify loss of sensory and motor function.

If the casualty is conscious, has no neck pain, has no distracting painful injury, is not intoxicated and has not received any analgesia, the cervical spine can be examined and a fracture clinically excluded. Head blocks, cervical collar and tape are removed, and the patient taken through a full range of active movements (i.e. patient's voluntary movement). If there is neither pain nor neurological symptoms on movement, the cervical spine can be cleared.

X-rays are of limited use in the resuscitation phase as they do not reliably exclude unstable fracture-dislocations. Hence, they do not alter initial management. Plain x-rays of the spinal column are therefore taken during the secondary survey. Since cervical fractures cannot be radiologically excluded in patients who do not meet the criteria for clinical cervical spine clearance as above, CT or MRI may be required.

Management Initial management follows the ATLS® ABCDE sequence. The cervical spine must be immobilized at all times; deterioration of neurological function of even one myotome can cause a devastating loss of motor function, with absence of any useful function. However, only 5 per cent of multiply injured patients have cervical spine injuries, in contrast to the high percentage of patients with compromised airways; this is particularly significant with head injuries. In high spinal transections, the patient's respiratory function may be compromised, leading to ventilatory failure. The airway must be maintained without causing neck flexion or extension, and secured and protected with careful anaesthetic induction and intubation. This can be successfully done with specialist laryngoscopes such as the McCoy (lever activated, flexing tip to lift the epiglottis), in conjunction with an intubating catheter. The procedure should be carried out by an experienced anaesthetist.

Oxygenation and ventilation is optimized, monitoring SaO_2 and $EtCO_2$. The neurogenic shock will require judicious use of intravenous fluids, and may need circulatory support with vasoconstrictors and chronotropes.

The spinal fracture and neurological deficits are managed by immobilization and referral to a spinal surgeon.

Take home message Spinal injuries should be identified during the secondary survey and managed according to the ABCs. Immobilization is crucial throughout, and ventilatory and circulatory failure must be recognized and managed. Injuries should be excluded clinically, or with CT and MRI, as soon as possible.

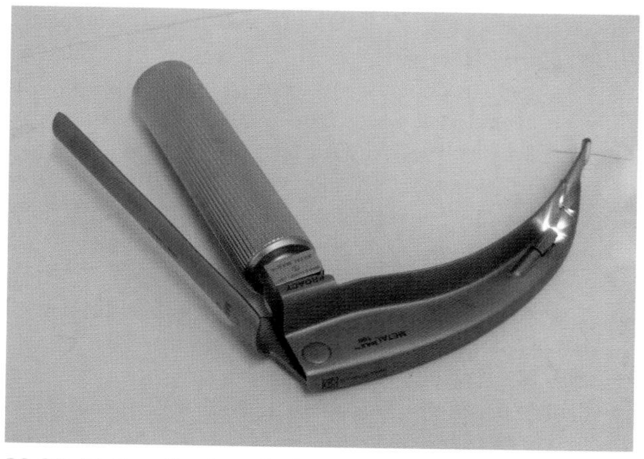

22.30 McCoy flexing tip laryngoscope

LONG-BONE INJURIES

Long bone injuries can be spectacular, but should not distract from the injuries compromising the airway, breathing or circulation. They are limb threatening, but not immediately life-threatening, and in the absence of catastrophic bleeding can be addressed in the secondary survey.

Awareness Musculoskeletal injuries occur in 85 per cent of patients sustaining blunt trauma (Findlay et al., 2007). Major injuries signify significant force applied to the body, and so are associated with an increased incidence of chest, abdomen and pelvis damage. Although not immediately-life threatening, they present a potential threat to life and prejudice the integrity and survival of the limb. Crush injuries can lead to compartment syndrome, and myoglobin release with the risk of renal failure. These injuries must therefore be addressed as soon as the resuscitation priorities have been addressed.

Recognition The casualty must be fully exposed, log-rolled and examined from head to toe in all planes. The limbs are examined visually for:

- colour and perfusion
- wounds
- deformity (angulation and shortening)
- swelling
- discoloration and bruising.

The extremities are then palpated to detect tenderness, swelling and deformity, indicating underlying fractures and dislocations. Crepitus may be felt, but should not be specifically elicited. Peripheral circulation is assessed with palpation of pulses and capillary refill. Doppler ultrasound examination may be needed to confirm the presence of pulses – however, the presence of a pulse does not exclude compartment syndrome. X-rays should be obtained as indicated as soon as the patient is stable.

Management The immediate management is to ensure the airway and ventilation are optimized, and then control limb haemorrhage with direct pressure, tourniquets, wound packing and haemostatic dressings as described previously. Large tissue deficits may need ongoing fluid and blood replacement as immediate haemorrhage control can be difficult.

Fractures and dislocations are splinted in the anatomical position where possible, to minimize neurovascular compromise, and significant analgesia may be required to facilitate this (e.g. Entonox, morphine or ketamine 0.5 mg/kg intravenously). The anatomical

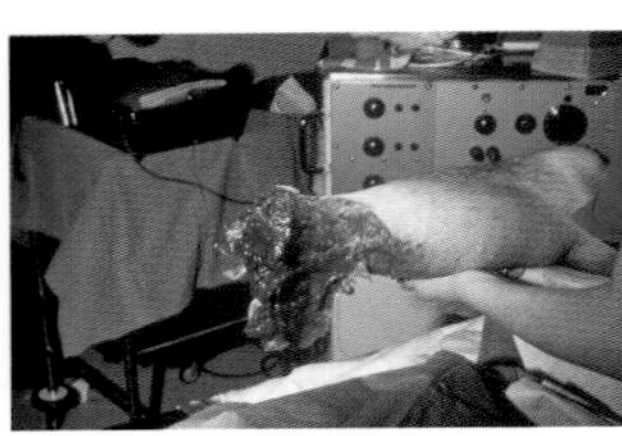

(a)

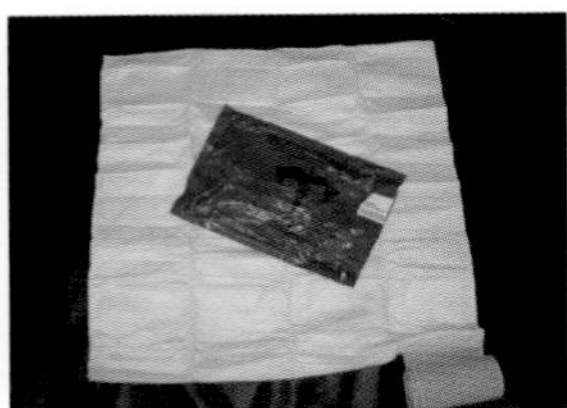

(b)

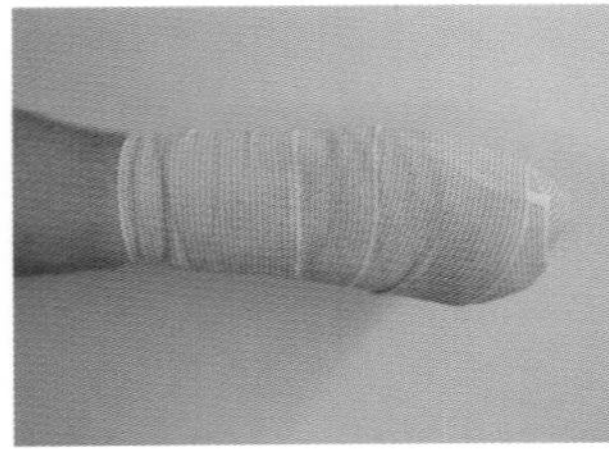

(c)

22.31 (a) Traumatic amputation, (b) blast dressing and (c) blast dressing in situ

position should not be forced if resistance is felt, e.g. posterior hip dislocation.

Tetanus toxoid should be given, and the patient referred urgently to an orthopaedic surgeon for definitive management. Significant fractures, compound fractures and dislocations may need operative intervention whilst life-saving abdominal or neurological surgery is taking place.

Take home message Limb injuries are not immediately life-threatening in the absence of catastrophic haemorrhage. They should be recognized and initially managed in the secondary survey. Splinting and immobilization are instituted before prompt surgical consultation.

Traumatic amputations, de-gloving injuries and blast injuries can be initially managed with specialist blast dressings.

G – Burns (thermal, chemical, electrical, cold injury)

A burn is a broad term that encompasses not only thermal injury to tissues from heat, but injury from electric shock, chemicals and cold. In the UK, some 250 000 burn victims attend hospital each year, of whom 16 000 are admitted; in the USA, about 1.25 million burns occur annually, with 51 000 patients hospitalized. The risk is highest in the 18–35 year age group, with a male to female ratio of 2:1 for both injury and death, and serious burns occur most frequently in children under 5 years of age. There are some 4500 burns deaths each year in the USA, and the death rate is much higher in those over the age of 65. The last two decades have seen much improvement in burns care, and the mortality rate is now 4 per cent in those treated in specialist burns centres (Schwartz and Balakrishnan, 2004).

THERMAL BURNS – AWARENESS

Major burns can present a threat to life through compromise of the airway, breathing and circulation. In addition, those burned may suffer other traumatic harm due to explosions etc. and can present with any of the systemic injuries described previously. Circumferential burns around the neck can cause tissue swelling and airway obstruction, and burns around the chest may cause restrictive respiratory failure. Large burns result in significant fluid shifts, and resultant shock. In combination with coma from toxin inhalation, burns present a potent mix of assaults on a casualty's life.

Cell damage occurs at a temperature greater than 45°C (113°F) owing to denaturation of cellular protein; a burn's size and depth are functions of the burning agent, its temperature and the duration of exposure. Thermal injury to the skin damages the skin's ability to function as a semi-permeable barrier to evaporative water loss, resulting in free water loss in moderate to large burns. Other functions such as protection from the environment, control of body temperature, sensation and excretion can also be harmed. Systemic effects include hormonal alterations, changes in tissue acid–base balance, haemodynamic changes and haematological derangement. Massive thermal injury results in an increase in haematocrit with increased blood viscosity during the early phase, followed by anaemia from erythrocyte extravasation and destruction. Vasoactive substances are released and a systemic inflammatory reaction can result.

Inhalational burns Inhalation of super-heated gases and inhalation of toxic smoke in entrapment result in inhalational burns and smoke inhalation. Inhalational injury is now the main cause of mortality in the burns patient, and half of all fire-related deaths are due to smoke inhalation. Direct thermal injury is usually limited to the upper airway above the vocal cords, and can result in rapid development of airway obstruction due to mucosal oedema. Smoke has two noxious components: particulate matter and toxic inhalants. The particles are due to incomplete combustion, are usually less than 0.5 μm in size and can reach the terminal bronchioles, where they initiate an inflammatory reaction, leading to bronchospasm, oedema and respiratory failure.

Toxic inhalants are divided into three main groups: (1) tissue asphyxiants; (2) pulmonary irritants; (3) systemic toxins. The two major tissue asphyxiants are carbon monoxide and hydrogen cyanide. Carbon monoxide poisoning is a well-known consequence of smoke inhalation injury. Severe carbon monoxide poisoning will produce brain hypoxia and coma, with loss of airway protective mechanisms, resulting in aspiration that exacerbates the pulmonary injury from smoke inhalation. The tight binding of the carbon monoxide to the haemoglobin, forming carboxy-haemoglobin, is resistant to displacement by oxygen, and so hypoxia is persistent. Hydrogen cyanide is formed when nitrogen-containing polymers such as wool, silk, polyurethane, or vinyl are burned. Cyanide binds to and disrupts mitochondrial oxidative phosphorylation, leading to profound tissue hypoxia.

Depth of burns The depth of a burn is classified according to the degree and extent of tissue damage:

First degree burns involve only the epidermis, and cause reddening and pain without blistering. They heal within 7 days and require only symptomatic treatment.

Second degree burns extend into the dermis, and can be subdivided into *superficial partial-thickness* and *deep partial-thickness burns.*

In *superficial partial-thickness burns*, the epidermis and the superficial dermis are injured. The deeper layers of the dermis, hair follicles, and sweat and sebaceous glands are spared. A common cause is hot water scalding. There is blistering of the skin and the exposed dermis is red and moist at the blister's base. These burns are very painful to touch. There is good perfusion of the dermis with intact capillary refill. Superficial partial-thickness burns heal in 14–21 days, scarring is usually minimal, and there is full return of function.

Deep partial-thickness burns extend into the deep dermis. There is damage to hair follicles as well as sweat and sebaceous glands, but their deeper portions usually survive. Hot liquids, steam, grease, or flame usually cause deep partial-thickness burns. The skin may be blistered and the exposed dermis is pale white to yellow. The burned area does not blanch, has no capillary refill and no pain sensation. Deep partial-thickness burns may be difficult to distinguish from full-thickness burns. Healing takes 3 weeks to 2 months. Scarring is common and is related to the depth of the injury. Surgical debridement and skin grafting may be necessary to obtain maximum function.

Third-degree or *full-thickness burns* involve the entire thickness of the skin, and all epidermal and dermal structures are destroyed. They are usually caused by flame, hot oil, steam, or contact with hot objects. The skin is charred, pale, painless, and leathery. These injuries will not heal spontaneously, as all dermal elements are destroyed. Surgical repair and skin grafting are necessary, and there will be significant scarring.

Fourth-degree burns are those that extend through the skin to the subcutaneous fat, muscle, and even bone. These are devastating, life-threatening injuries. Amputation or extensive reconstruction is sometimes required.

THERMAL BURNS – RECOGNITION

The initial assessment of burns takes place during the primary survey, and is designed to recognize immediately life-threatening injuries compromising the airway, breathing and circulation and conscious level. The likelihood of coincidental traumatic injuries should be remembered.

The patient is examined following the *look, listen, feel* format. Diagnosis of an inhalational burn is made from the history of a fire in an enclosed space and physical signs that include facial burns, singed nasal hair, soot in the mouth or nose, hoarseness, carbonaceous sputum, and expiratory wheezing. There is no single method capable of demonstrating the extent of inhalation injury. Stridor is a particularly sinister finding, as it indicates an imminent loss of the airway.

Carboxyhaemoglobin levels for carbon monoxide poisoning are useful to document prolonged exposure within an enclosed space with incomplete combustion, as the cherry red skin colour is rare.

Table 22.3 Diagnosis of carbon monoxide poisoning

Carbon monoxide level	Physical symptoms
< 20 per cent	No physical symptoms
20–30 per cent	Headache and nausea
30–40 per cent	Confusion
40–60 per cent	Coma
> 60 per cent	Death

The chest x-ray may be normal initially; bronchoscopy and radionuclide scanning are useful in determining the full extent of injury. Arterial blood gas analysis will track hypoxia, ventilatory failure and the development of metabolic acidosis. Signs of shock are looked for, as detailed previously, and the GCS and pupillary response assessed. The patient is fully exposed to allow evaluation of the whole-body surface area.

The burnt areas are assessed for depth of burn, as described earlier. This is a subjective clinical assessment. The extent of the burn is assessed and expressed as a percentage of body surface area (BSA). This can be done using the 'rule of nines', or with aids such as the Lund and Browder charts. The rule of nines is an approximate tool, and tends to overestimate the extent of a burn.

For irregular burns, the palmar surface of the patient's hand, including the fingers, represents approximately 1 per cent of the patient's body surface area.

Body surface areas are different in infants; they have a disproportionately larger head surface area and smaller lower limb surface area.

THERMAL BURNS – MANAGEMENT

The airway is secured as described previously. Inhalational burns can cause pharyngeal oedema and swelling, which can make tracheal intubation difficult if not impossible, leaving a surgical airway as the only

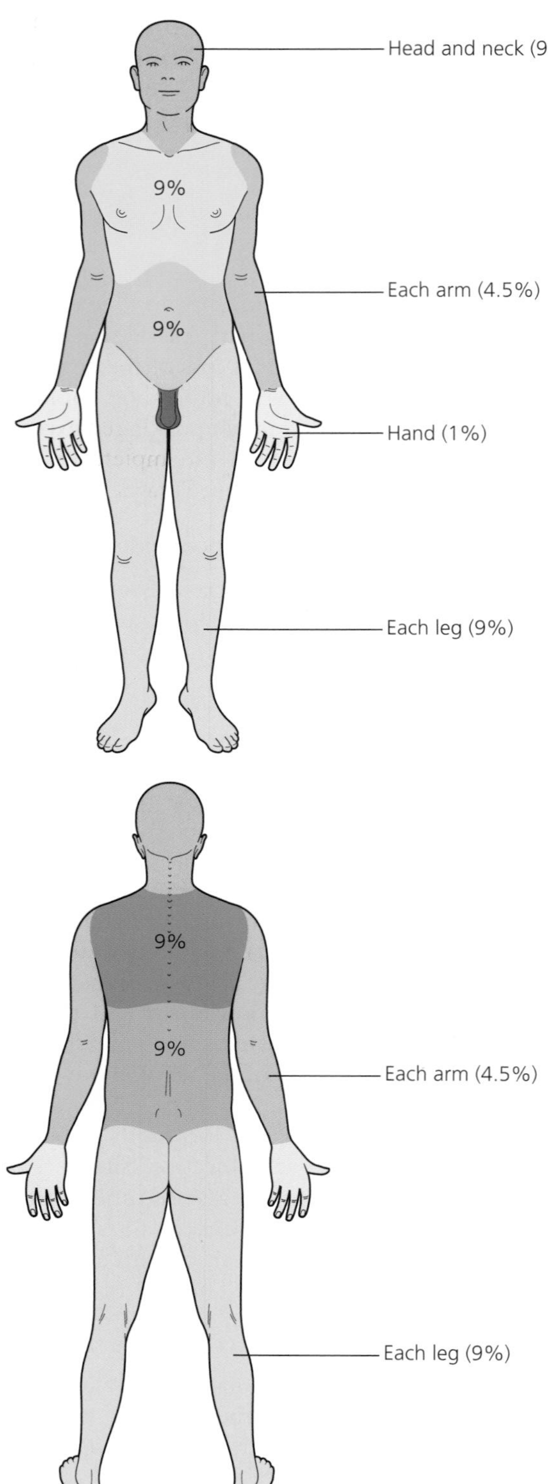

22.32 Burns. Rule of nines for assessment of extent of burns in adults.

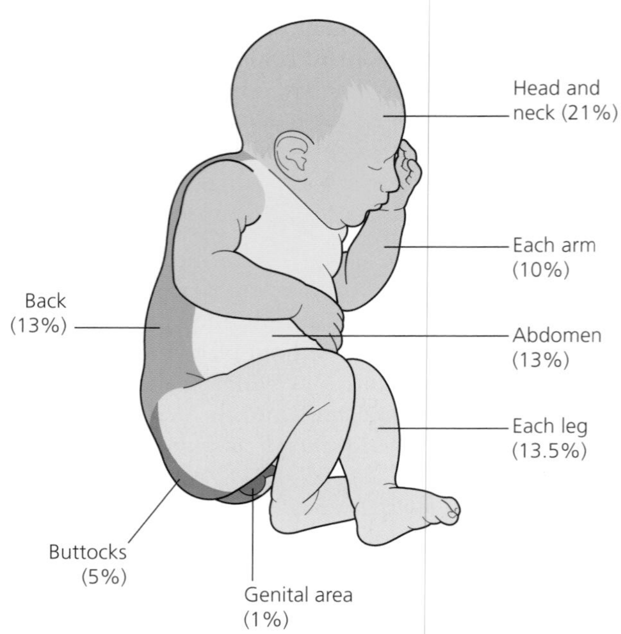

22.33 Burns in infants Surface areas differ markedly from those in adults.

recourse. The airway may need fibre-optic assessment, and warning signs such as stridor and respiratory distress indicate the need for early intubation. This should be performed under general anaesthesia by an experienced anaesthetist, with a range of difficult intubation equipment available. Needle cricothyroidotomy and surgical airway sets should be immediately accessible.

Breathing should be supported with high-flow oxygen administered via a non-rebreathing, reservoir mask that delivers 85 per cent at a flow rate of 15 L/min. The ventilation may need support using a BVM assembly with a reservoir and high-flow oxygen. Stridor can be eased, as a holding measure pending airway securement, by administering high-flow helium and oxygen, as this gas mixture has a low density that increases flow through the obstructing airway. However, heliox is only 21 per cent oxygen and will not address hypoxia and carbon monoxide poisoning. Once the airway has been secured by tracheal intubation, the inspired oxygen concentration and ventilation should be adjusted to give optimum SaO_2 levels (> 95 per cent) and low normal $EtCO_2$ (4.5 kPa).

The presence of an inhalational burn and pulmonary oedema may hinder oxygenation and ventilation, and a critical care physician should be involved early. Significant carbon monoxide levels may indicate the need for ventilation with 100 per cent oxygen and hyperbaric therapy, and an early referral should be made to a hyperbaric unit; these are often found located in diving and naval centres. Circumferential neck and chest burns may need to be incised to allow effective breathing and ventilation.

The circulation should be supported in any burn patient with signs of shock or a burn less than 20 per cent BSA. Two large-bore intravenous cannulae are sited, preferably, although not necessarily, through unburned skin. If intravenous cannulation or central venous cannulation are not possible, intraosseus or intravenous cut-down techniques should be used, as shock will develop rapidly in patients with large and deep burns.

Warmed Hartmann's or Ringer's lactate is the fluid of choice; large volumes of normal saline 0.9 per cent can cause a hyperchloraemic acidosis. Colloids and hypertonic saline have no proven beneficial role. If shock is present, 2 L should be administered as in the ATLS® guidelines for shock management. If haemorrhagic shock is excluded, the volume and rate of fluid administration is calculated according to the Parkland formula as given later. This regimen applies to partial- and full-thickness burns only; superficial burns do not require intravenous fluids. The administration time is calculated from the time of the burn, not from the time of admission or time of assessment. Deeper burns are likely to cause more tissue damage and consequent fluid shifts. The Parkland formula is a guide only, and fluid administration should be titrated against response. Blood pressure, central venous pressure, pulse, peripheral perfusion and urine outputs are used, but more sophisticated techniques such as oesophageal Doppler and arterial waveform analysis may aid optimization. Fluid overload should be avoided in patients with inhalational burns and systemic inflammatory reactions. Documented anaemia may indicate the need for blood transfusion.

Wound care starts in the pre-hospital environment with the removal of burnt clothing and the cooling and dressing of wounds. Rings, jewellery, watches and belts are removed as they retain heat and can cause compression as tissues swell. Wounds can initially be dressed with loose, clean, dry dressings. Alternatives are plastic sandwich wrap (known as cling film in the UK, plastic wrap in USA and cling wrap in Australia), specialized gel burns dressings or saline-moistened dressings. Cooling eases pain, but hypothermia should be avoided.

Patients with circumferential deep burns of the limbs may develop eschars (thick, black, dry and necrotic tissue that constricts) with compromise of the distal circulation. Distal pulses need to be monitored closely, with a Doppler probe if not easily palpable. If there is compromise to the circulation, surgical escharotomy will be needed. The eschar should be incised on the midlateral side of the limb, allowing the fat to bulge through. This may be extended to the hand and fingers. Escharotomy may cause substantial soft tissue bleeding.

Analgesia will be required for partial-thickness burns, which are most painful. Cooling and dressing will help, but opioids may be required. These should be administered intravenously, and can be given by infusion or patient-controlled analgesia (PCA) systems.

Consultation is important. A burns specialist should be involved from the outset for all patients with severe or unusual burns. Transfer will be required for these patients as outcomes are improved in specialist centres. Indications for transfer are:

- partial-thickness burns > 20 per cent BSA
- partial-thickness burns > 10 per cent BSA in ages 10–50 years
- full-thickness burns > 5 per cent any age
- partial- and full-thickness burns involving: face, eyes, ears, hands, feet, genitals, perineum, skin over major joints
- significant electrical burns (and lightning)
- significant chemical burns
- inhalational burns
- burns in patients with complicating illness, trauma, and long-term rehabilitation needs
- children.

CHEMICAL BURNS

Awareness Most chemical burns result from exposure of the skin to strong alkalis and acids, and phosphorus, phenol and petroleum products can also damage tissue. However, 25 000 products are capable of causing chemical burns, and they account for 5–10 per cent of US burns centre admissions. Full development of chemical burns is slower than thermal injury, so the true extent of the burn can be underestimated on initial evaluation. Alkali burns tend to be more serious and deeper, as the alkalis soften and penetrate tissue, whereas acids tend to form a protective eschar.

Recognition Definitive diagnosis depends on the history, and both the chemical involved and its

Table 22.4 Intravenous fluid requirements in partial- and full-thickness burn patients (Parkland formula)

Adults	Children
Hartmann's or Ringer's lactate:	Hartmann's or Ringer's lactate:
4 mL × weight (kg) × per cent BSA over initial 24 hours	3 mL × weight (kg) × per cent BSA over initial 24 hours plus maintenance
Half over first 8 hours from the time of burn (other half over subsequent 16 hours)	Half over first 8 hours from the time of burn (other half over subsequent 16 hours)

(Example: an adult weighing 70 kg with 40 per cent second- and third-degree burns would require 4 mL × 70 kg × 40 = 11 200 mL over 24 hours).

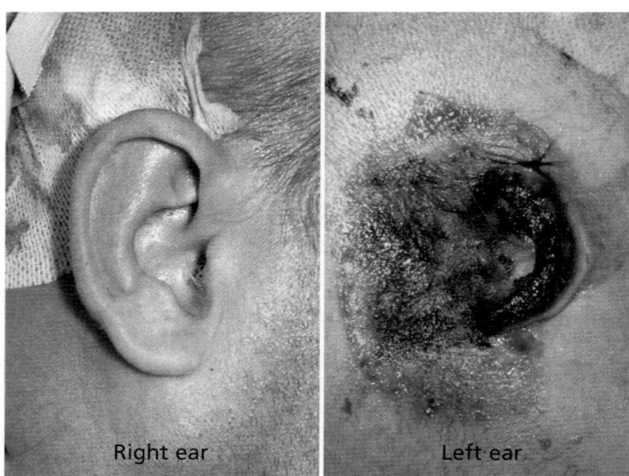

22.34 Chemical burns Sulphuric acid burn to left ear from car battery acid in roll-over traffic accident.

concentration should be determined if possible. Alkali burns are frequently full-thickness injuries, appear pale, and feel leathery and slippery. Acid burns are often partial-thickness injuries and are accompanied by erythema and erosion. Skin is stained black by hydrochloric acid, yellow by nitric acid, and brown by sulphuric acid.

Management The goal of treatment is to minimize any area of irreversible damage, and maximize salvage in the zone of reversible damage. If dry powder is present, it should be brushed off before irrigation with water, which is the mainstay of treatment. Irrigation should be commenced immediately when the injury is recognized, with copious amounts of tap water. Neutralizing agents (e.g. an acid to treat an alkali burn) should not be used, as there is a risk that heat generated by the neutralizing reaction will cause further thermal injury.

After copious water irrigation, some specific treatments are possible, e.g. calcium gluconate for hydrofluoric acid burns and polyethylene glycol for phenol. An urgent referral to a burns surgeon should be made; eschar formation may make irrigation ineffective and require emergency surgical excision.

ELECTRICAL BURNS

Awareness Electrical burns are caused when an individual makes contact between an electrical source and the earth, and severe, non-lethal electrical injuries constitute 3–5 per cent of admissions to US burns units. Current flows through the skin and variably through different tissues from the point of electrical contact to the ground contact, causing burns and necrosis. The physiological effects of an electric shock are related to the amount, duration, type (AC or DC), and path of current flow. Severe electrical skin burns are associated with high-voltage shocks, whereas most domestic, low-voltage shocks are not associated with skin burns even though they may cause death from ventricular fibrillation. Alternating current (AC) shocks produce tetanic muscle spasm, which can cause the victim's hand to clutch onto the electrical source, and the respiratory muscles can be paralyzed, resulting in respiratory arrest. Electrical muscle damage can result in rhabdomyolysis and renal failure.

Recognition The assessment of an electrical shock victim should follow the ABC principles of ATLS®. The airway may be obstructed if the victim is unconscious, and prolonged apnoea may follow paralysis of the respiratory muscles. The heart may be arrested in ventricular fibrillation or asystole depending on the nature of the shock. Of high voltage electrical shock victims, 50 per cent will have a neurological injury with coma, and spinal injuries can result from violent muscle spasms. The entry and exit points should be examined for burns that may be full thickness, and the true extent of underlying muscle damage may not be apparent. There may be musculoskeletal injuries from associated trauma or muscle spasm, and all long bones should be examined and x-rayed when indicated.

Management The immediate priority is to avoid personal injury if the casualty is in contact with or even adjacent to a high-voltage electrical source. Initial management is to secure the airway, protect the cervical spine and oxygenate and ventilate the casualty. Intravenous access is secured, and fluids administered if the casualty is shocked. If in cardiac arrest, advanced life support should be instituted, following the appropriate Advanced Life Support algorithms for VF/VT and non-shockable arrests as indicated.

The heart should be monitored for arrhythmias, which can occur in 30 per cent of high-voltage shock victims. Tissue damage may need surgical debridement, and compartment syndrome may develop, requiring fasciotomies. A urinary catheter is sited, and the urine observed for the brown discoloration indicative of development of myoglobinuria; this is treated by giving intravenous fluids to promote a diuresis, and administration of mannitol. Myoglobinuria should be considered present if a urine dipstick test registers positive for haemoglobin, but the freshly spun urine sediment shows no red blood cells.

As ongoing treatment will be complex in severe electrical injuries and burns, early consultation should be made with a burns surgeon and critical care specialist. Management on a critical care unit will be required.

COLD INJURY BURNS

Awareness Cold injury can be systemic, leading to hypothermia, or localized, leading to localized tissue damage to varying degrees dependent on the degree of freezing.

Hypothermia is defined as a core body temperature of below 35°C (95°F). The systemic effects depend on the severity of the drop in core temperature:

Mild hypothermia	35–32°C (95–89.6°F)
Moderate hypothermia	32–30°C (89.6–86°F)
Severe hypothermia	< 30°C (< 86°F)

As core temperature drops, the conscious level deteriorates, and the airway can obstruct as coma develops. Respiratory and cardiac functions deteriorate until respiratory and cardiac arrest result.

Localized cold injury is seen in three forms:

1. *Frostnip* – the mildest form, which is reversible on warming.
2. *Frostbite* – due to freezing of tissue and resultant damage from intracellular ice crystals and microvascular occlusion. There are four degrees of frostbite:
   - *First degree* – hyperaemia and oedema without skin necrosis.
   - *Second degree* – vesicle formation with partial-thickness skin necrosis.
   - *Third degree* – full-thickness and subcutaneous tissue necrosis, with haemorrhagic vesicle formation.
   - *Fourth degree* – full-thickness necrosis, including muscle and bone gangrene.
3. *Non-freezing injury* – trench foot or immersion foot, with microvascular endothelial damage, stasis and vascular occlusion.

Recognition Systemic cold injury is recognized in the primary survey as the airway, breathing and circulation and neurological function are assessed. The patient is cold to the touch, and looks gray and peripherally cyanosed. Strikingly, the expired breath can feel deathly cold on the hand. A low reading rectal or oesophageal temperature probe will be needed to accurately gauge the degree of hypothermia.

Local injuries are assessed during the secondary survey and the musculoskeletal survey. The affected part of the body initially appears hard, cold, white and anaesthetic, but the appearance changes frequently during treatment.

Management *Hypothermia* is treated by securing the airway, oxygenating and ventilating the patient to normal parameters, gaining intravenous access and treating shock with warmed intravenous fluids. In addition, the patient is re-warmed depending on the degree of hypothermia.

Mild and *moderate hypothermia* is treated by active external re-warming:

- heated blankets, warm baths, forced hot air. It is easier to monitor and perform diagnostic and therapeutic procedures using heated blankets
- warm bath re-warming is best done in a bath of 40–42°C moving water (re-warming rate: ~1–2°C/hour) The warming gradient should not be greater than this to avoid thermal injury. Re-warming should be slow to minimize peripheral dilation, which can cause hypovolaemic shock.

Severe hypothermia and *hypothermic cardiac arrest* require active internal (core) rewarming:

- extracorporeal blood rewarming (cardiopulmonary, venovenous, or arteriovenous femorofemoral bypass) is the treatment of choice, especially with cardiac arrest
- without equipment for extracorporeal re-warming, left-sided thoracotomy followed by pericardial cavity irrigation with warmed saline and cardiac massage is effective in systemic hypothermia < 28°C
- thoracic lavage or haemodialysis is also effective
- repeated peritoneal dialysis with 2 L of warm (43°C) potassium-free dialysate solution exchanged every 10–12 minutes until core temperature is raised to ~35°C
- parenteral fluids warmed to 43°C
- administer humidified air heated to 42°C through a face mask or tracheal tube
- (**NOTE:** warm colonic and gastrointestinal [GI] irrigations are of less value.)

Localized cold injury is initially managed in the field. The hypothermia and dehydration associated with frostbite should be addressed. Wet and constrictive clothing should be removed, the involved extremities should be elevated and wrapped carefully in dry sterile gauze, and affected fingers and toes separated. Further cold injury should be avoided. Rapid re-warming is the single most effective therapy for frostbite. As soon as possible, the injured extremity should be placed in gently circulating water at a temperature of 40–42°C (104–107.6°F) for approximately 10–30 minutes, until the distal extremity is pliable and erythematous. The current consensus is that clear blisters are aspirated or debrided and dressed. Early surgical intervention in the form of tissue debridement and amputation is not indicated; full demarcation of dead tissue can take 3–4 weeks to fully demarcate, and debridement at this point will avoid unnecessary tissue loss (Rabold, 2004).

Take home message *Thermal burns* are assessed by depth and extent, and managed by addressing the airway, breathing and circulation. Huge volumes of intravenous fluids may be required to maintain homeostasis. *Chemical burns* are treated primarily by copious irrigation with water. *Electrical burns* may be associated with severe tissue damage and systemic disturbance, and need treatment for the local burns and systemic cardiac, respiratory and renal complications. *Cold injury* can be systemic hypothermia, which is treated by active external and internal re-warming, depending on severity, or localized tissue damage. Localized tissue damage is treated by rapid re-warming and delayed surgical debridement.

INITIAL RESPONSE TO TRAUMA

The physiological effects of trauma are both widespread and predictable, invoking a range of hormonal and cellular mechanisms that have evolved to maximize the chances of survival following serious injury. These adaptations for survival can be considered as a whole body, fluid conservation and repair strategy.

Following injury the first survival offensive is a plan to prevent blood loss. Direct injury to blood vessels should induce an arterial vasospasm to reduce blood loss followed by the formation of a 'vascular patch' consisting of a fibrin-reinforced, aggregation of platelets.

If despite this strategy significant blood loss still occurs, some preservation of intravascular volume occurs by fluid redistribution between the vascular, cellular and interstitial fluid compartments. The resulting change in compartmental volumes will stimulate an endocrine response with the release of a number of renal, adrenal and pituitary hormones (renin, aldosterone, cortisol and antidiuretic hormone [ADH]). This hormonal response not only represents a secondary fluid conservation project but also heralds another survival strategy.

Serious injury, which in evolutionary terms would have limited the ability to hunt and feed, produces a metabolic re-conditioning. Under endocrine guidance, cellular metabolic priorities, and the type of substrate used, change with a falling basal metabolic rate. These marked changes in metabolism represent an approach to energy conservation, allowing a channelling of reserves to damage control and repair whilst still keeping the brain fuelled.

Ultimately a successful outcome following trauma (or major surgery) depends on the integration of these strategies *and* the maintenance of whole-body physiology. The integrity of the cardiorespiratory system is pivotal. Failure to maintain cellular (organ) perfusion, oxygenation and ATP regeneration will lead to cell apoptosis and death. Co-morbidities such as pre-existing lung disease or cardiac failure will increase complications and the chance of dying.

The normal physiological response to the increased metabolic demands of trauma, illness and surgery is to increase oxygen delivery in response to an increase in tissue oxygen consumption.

Failure to respond to this demand will generate an oxygen debt with metabolic consequences. This limitation of oxygen availability will favour anaerobic metabolism over aerobic, reducing metabolic efficiency

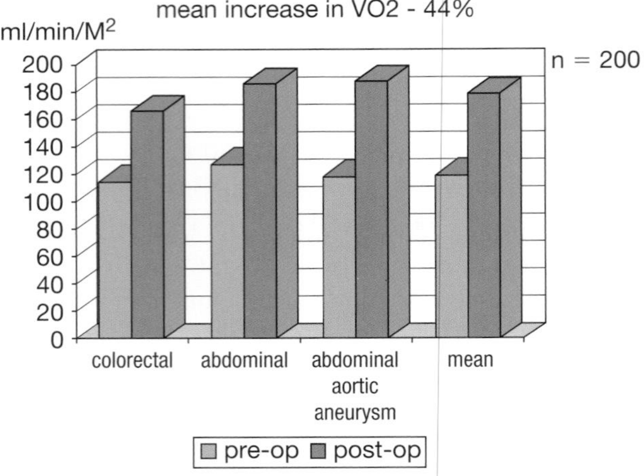

22.35 Oxygen consumption before and after surgery (Older and Smith, 1988).

and generating a lactic acidosis as a consequence. This is clearly unsustainable and clinical studies show that an inability to mount a sustained cardiovascular response is directly proportional to an increase in morbidity and mortality. Survival and outcome relies on the speed of repayment of this oxygen debt. The slower the payback, the greater the ensuing complications.

As a synopsis trauma and major surgery can be considered to be like running a marathon. To survive, cardiorespiratory function and cellular physiology have to remain intact. Systemic failure, for whatever reason, to maintain tissue perfusion leads to *shock*, which is one of the most frequently misused and misunderstood terms in medicine and the media. Correctly used it implies tissue hypoperfusion leading to cellular hypoxia and describes a medical emergency with a high mortality rate from multiple organ failure.

From an intensive care perspective, the recognition and appreciation of the type of shock is essential as other reasons for hypoperfusion may coexist.

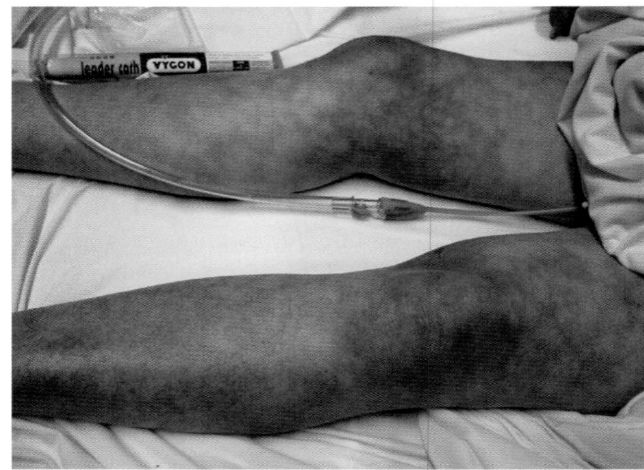

22.36 Hypoperfusion This 70-year-old man with severe sepsis developed hypoperfusion of the lower limbs. Note the typical marbling of the skin.

SHOCK

In health, cardiac output and the delivery of oxygen (global arterial blood flow multiplied by the blood oxygen content) and local tissue perfusion are closely matched to metabolic requirements. Shock follows a mismatch of metabolic demand to oxygen delivery at tissue level, leading to cellular hypoxia and (if uncorrected) to tissue and organ failure. The causes of circulatory shock can be classified as abnormalities of cardiac output, of systemic vascular resistance, or a combination of both.

Reduced cardiac output

Impaired performance *Cardiogenic shock* is an intrinsic failure of cardiac function despite adequate circulating volume and venous return, most commonly as a result of acute myocardial infarction. Cardiogenic shock may occur following an apparently minor insult to a heart with any pre-existing functional impairment.

Impaired venous return *Hypovolaemic shock* exists when a fall in circulating volume of sufficient magnitude occurs such that compensatory physiological mechanisms are unable to maintain adequate tissue flow, leading to critical hypoperfusion.

Obstructive shock *'Obstruction'* arises when venous return is compromised by raised intrathoracic or pericardial pressure (pneumothorax and cardiac tamponade), or if right ventricular ejection is blocked by a massive pulmonary embolus, resulting in right ventricular overload and impaired left heart filling. Plain x-rays may not show changes and CT angiography is the initial investigation of choice.

AETIOLOGY OF CIRCULATORY SHOCK

1. **Reduction in cardiac output**
   a. HYPOVOLAEMIC SHOCK:
      Reduced circulating volume causing a reduction in venous return and cardiac output (e.g. haemorrhage)
   b. OBSTRUCTIVE SHOCK:
      Mechanical obstruction to normal venous return or cardiac output, e.g. tension pneumothorax, cardiac tamponade or massive pulmonary embolism
   c. CARDIOGENIC SHOCK:
      Failure of cardiac pump to maintain cardiac output, e.g. post myocardial infarction.
2. **Reduction in peripheral resistance**
   a. DISTRIBUTIVE SHOCK:
      A drop in peripheral resistance due to vasodilatation, which is often associated with an increase in cardiac output but not sufficient to maintain blood pressure, e.g. anaphylaxis, neurogenic shock, SIRS, septic shock
   b. ENDOCRINE SHOCK:
      In the intensive care setting hypothyroidism, hyperthyroidism and adrenal insufficiency can all lead to reduced tissue perfusion.

Reduced systemic vascular resistance

Neurogenic shock This occurs when spinal cord injury – usually at a cervical or high thoracic level – leads to loss of sympathetic tone and hence peripheral vasodilatation, venous pooling and reduced venous return. This is aggravated by the absence of direct sympathetic nervous system connection into the heart, and hence impaired compensatory responses.

Anaphylactic shock A drug or parenteral fluid may be the trigger that provokes an immunological response with histamine release, resulting in cardiovascular instability and (potentially) respiratory distress.

Septic shock This condition is defined as severe sepsis with associated hypotension, evidence of tissue hypoperfusion that is unresponsive to fluid resuscitation. Various mechanisms are responsible for the vasodilatatory response and catecholamine resistance, which are characteristic of septic shock. It is becoming clearer that this host response does not appear to be determined by the infecting organism and there is a suggestion of genetic susceptibility being a contributory factor in dictating the severity of subsequent illness.

Diagnosis of shock

Early recognition, immediate resuscitation and treatment of the underlying cause are the cornerstones of successful therapy.

There may be an easily identifiable cause of shock, but often the aetiology is difficult to establish. Following massive trauma, shock may be hypovolaemic (blood loss), obstructive (tamponade or tension pneumothorax), cardiogenic (cardiac contusion), neurogenic (spinal cord injury) or anaphylactic (drug reaction).

Careful examination should clarify the aetiology in most cases, and will aid in determining severity by identifying end-organ effects. Examination should be thorough and structured to avoid missing useful signs.

Tests should include a full blood count and estimation of electrolytes as well as assessment of renal function, liver function, clotting and blood group/ cross-match, serum glucose, blood cultures and inflammatory markers (e.g. C-reactive protein, procal-

> **CLINICAL EXAMINATION IN SHOCK**
>
> **Cardiovascular system**
> - Pulse (rate/rhythm), blood pressure, JVP (or CVP if central line in situ), heart sounds (muffling/murmurs), peripheral perfusion (capillary refill time/skin colour)
>
> **Respiratory system**
> - Respiratory rate, work of breathing, tracheal deviation, air entry, added sounds, oxygen saturations (relative to inspired oxygen)
>
> **Abdomen**
> - Pain, distension, peritonitis, localizing signs, urine output
>
> **Central nervous system**
> - Level of consciousness, peripheral neurological signs (e.g. power, reflexes)
>
> **Other systems**
> - Temperature, skin signs (e.g. rashes), limbs (bony integrity/perfusion)

citonin). Arterial blood gas analysis provides rapid results, and the newer analyzers often measure a serum lactate level. This is a non-specific marker, but may indicate hypoperfusion if elevated.

X-ray examination, ultrasound scanning (e.g. a FAST scan) or CT may identify sources of blood loss and identify likely foci in the case of severe sepsis. An ECG and urgent echocardiography are obligatory if a cardiogenic cause of shock is suspected.

Careful and regularly repeated recording of vital signs (heart rate, respiratory rate, blood pressure, oxygen saturation) and indicators of end-organ perfusion (consciousness level, urine output) are crucial. The initial severity of illness at assessment, and subsequent response to initial resuscitative and treatment measures will dictate the need for more advanced and invasive monitoring tools. Continuous invasive blood pressure and central venous pressure monitoring are generally required, and are essential if vasoactive drugs are required, both to enable safe drug delivery and to allow titration of dosing.

Advanced monitoring systems

Invasive techniques that allow an estimation of cardiac output – and thereby tissue oxygen delivery – are used in the sickest patients, both as an aid to diagnosis and a guide to therapy.

PULMONARY ARTERY FLOTATION CATHETERIZATION

In pulmonary artery flotation catheterization (PAFC), a catheter is passed via a central vein through the right heart to rest within a branch of the pulmonary artery. Inflation of the distal balloon permits measurement of the pulmonary artery occlusion pressure (PAOP), which allows an estimate of left atrial pressure and hence (it is assumed) left ventricular preload. Many errors may, however, confound this measurement. The PAFC also allows measurement of cardiac output by way of thermodilution (either by cold injectate or by proximal heating coil, allowing semi-continuous data to be recorded). This is calculated from the area under a curve of distal temperature (recorded by a thermistor at the catheter tip) plotted against time. Cardiac output is inversely proportional to this area. PAFC use has declined in popularity recently due to concern regarding the complications of what is a highly invasive modality, failure to show outcome benefit in studies of patients monitored by PAFC, and the increasing availability of alternative, less invasive monitors that generate similar data.

CARDIAC OUTPUT FROM ANALYSIS OF ARTERIAL WAVEFORM

Pulse contour analysis The PiCCO® cardiac output monitor employs a mathematical analysis of the shape of the arterial waveform using a dedicated femoral arterial cannula to derive cardiac output data. It is calibrated by a transpulmonary thermodilution technique, following injection of cold saline into a central line.

Pulse power analysis The Lithium Dilution Cardiac Output (LiDCO®) monitor also employs the arterial

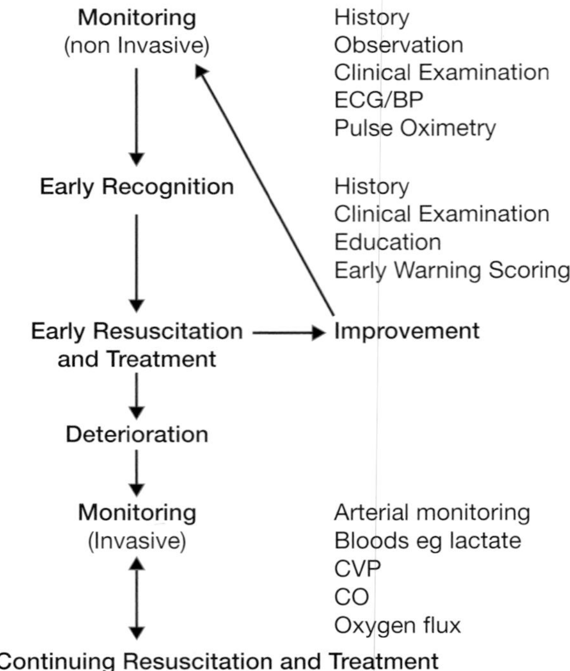

22.37 Investigation and monitoring shock

waveform to derive haemodynamic data but using a power algorithm that can be used in any artery, and thus does not require insertion of a proprietary arterial line. The monitor is calibrated using either the lithium dilution technique (LiDCO plus) or using a nomogram of patient demographics with the LiDCO Rapid monitor. As with pulse contour analysis, peripheral resistance and data indicating likely fluid responsiveness are calculated beat-to-beat. It does also have, unlike many other devices, positive outcome data in high-risk patients.

Management of shock

Initial approach Initially attention should be focussed on rapid assessment, with airway, breathing and circulation (ABC) addressed in the first instance. High-flow oxygen (F_IO_2 0.6 or greater) should be administered via a patent airway, and intravenous access obtained. *Definitive treatment of the underlying cause of shock should be commenced alongside resuscitative measures.* The aim should be to support the circulation to allow adequate tissue oxygen delivery, whilst mitigating or reversing the effects of the initial insult. This may be rapidly successful, for example in decompression of a tension pneumothorax; in other cases it may prove impossible to correct the underlying pathology (e.g. cardiogenic shock due to extensive myocardial infarction).

Fluid therapy Often large volumes are needed, guided by clinical response and monitored indicators of filling (e.g. central venous pressure). The response of these variables to a fluid challenge, and trends, are considerably more useful than 'snapshot' values. Indeed targeting a particular value of CVP or MAP is physiologically unsound and may be to the patient's detriment. It is always preferable to use fluid boluses or 'challenge techniques' to interpret volaemic status.

In ventilated patients, changes in intrathoracic pressure generate cyclical changes in systolic pressure and using the LiDCO or PiCCO monitors generates a stroke volume variation that is related to volaemic status under certain conditions. These variations in stroke volume may be more useful indicators of likely fluid responsiveness than other methods.

The choice of fluid is dictated by the underlying cause of the shock and local policies. There is an optimum amount of fluid to target resuscitation and it should be recognized that overenthusiastic transfusion, as with fluid restriction, is also associated with increased complications.

Inotropes/vasopressors This treatment should be instituted if the patient remains hypotensive despite adequate fluid resuscitation. Again, choice is determined by aetiology: vasopressor (e.g. norepinephrine) for distributive shock and inotrope (e.g. dobutamine) for cardiogenic shock. Combinations may be required, guided by haemodynamic data from monitoring equipment and clinical response. Significant doses of either inotropes or vasopressors should be mandatory. Cardiac output monitoring is much better than making decisions based on the arterial blood pressure.

TREATMENT OF UNDERLYING CAUSE OF SHOCK

Hypovolaemic

- Control of haemorrhage (may require surgery)
- Restoration of circulating volume (fluid and blood products)

Obstructive

- Needle decompression of tension pneumothorax
- Pericardiocentesis (tamponade)
- Thrombolysis or surgical removal of pulmonary embolus

Cardiogenic

- Inotropes
- Anti-arrhythmics
- Revascularization
- Aortic balloon counterpulsation
- Surgical repair of valve lesions

Distributive

- Early treatment of infection (source control, e.g. drainage, early antibiotic administration)

Endocrine support There is recent evidence that treatment with 'physiological' doses of corticosteroid in cases where adrenal response is inadequate may not improve outcomes as had previously been hoped. There is considered to be some benefit from the use of steroids with septic shock with an improvement in haemodynamic response but this is still the subject of considerable debate and there is a lack of cogent outcome data. The use of vasopressin has traditionally been reserved for patients with catecholamine-resistant septic shock but new evidence suggests that there may be some benefit for those requiring lower doses of noradrenaline.

Tight control of blood glucose levels has also been shown to lead to improved outcomes in the sickest patients in intensive care.

Systemic support Shock leads to multiple organ impairment or failure. Support of other organ systems may well be required during treatment.

Outcome Mortality is determined both by aetiology of circulatory shock and the response to treatment. Early recognition and prompt therapy are the most important factors.

MULTIPLE ORGAN FAILURE

Multiple organ failure or dysfunction syndrome (MODS) is the clinical appearance of a seemingly poorly controlled severe systemic inflammatory reaction, following a triggering event such as infection, inflammation or trauma. It represents the net result of altered host defence and deregulation of the inflammatory response and the immune system. The condition has emerged with medical advances as a result of increasing availability of intensive care facilities. Recognized as a syndrome in the early 1970s, progress in the management of critically ill patients has unmasked this frequently lethal cocktail of sequential pulmonary, hepatic and renal failure.

This pattern of progressive organ impairment and failure complicates illnesses with diverse aetiologies and, despite progress in understanding the underlying mechanisms involved, it carries a mortality rate that remains depressingly high. MODS has now become the commonest cause of stays in surgical ITUs of more than 5 days and (among these patients) the most frequent cause of death.

It is essential to differentiate MODS from postoperative or traumatic, isolated organ dysfunction, which has a different pathogenesis and markedly different survival outcomes.

Epidemiology

Definitions of organ failure use two types of criteria based on either measures of physiological derangement (e.g. hypotension, acidosis, serum creatinine concentration) or on the treatment methods (e.g. dialysis, ventilation, etc.).

The degrees of organ dysfunction, from covert physiological impairment to overt failure, coupled with the difficulties of monitoring the function of all the organs involved has led to controversies about the definition of organ failure and the clinical entities involved. This has hampered epidemiological surveys and the assessment of treatment outcomes. Confusion over the exact incidence of MODS stems from an absence of universal diagnostic criteria; many of the published studies have used differing clinical and temporal definitions of organ failure.

Review of the published studies suggests that MODS develops in 5–15 per cent of patients requiring ICU admission, depending on the diagnostic criteria used and the case-mix of the population of ICU patients studied. The outcome data is remarkably consistent between the studies, with mortality linked to the number of organs failed.

The appearance of MODS broadly follows two clinical courses, differing in onset relative to the initial event, time course and sequence of organ failure. The first pattern usually follows a direct pulmonary insult, such as trauma or aspiration. In this form the overall course of the disease may be relatively short and MODS occurs as a pre-terminal event, becoming evident just prior to death. The second type is the more classical form, as found in severe sepsis, with pulmonary manifestations of acute respiratory distress syndrome (ARDS). MODS is present early in the course of the illness but does not become progressive until after a 7–10-day delay, with manifestations of hepatic and subsequently renal failure becoming apparent.

The initiating events for MODS are many and diverse but by far the most common association is with severe sepsis and ARDS. The likelihood of occurrence and the progression of disease is related not only to the severity of the initiating event but also to the premorbid physiological reserve of the patient, i.e. old age and pre-existing disease such as cardiac failure, cirrhosis, drug abuse etc.

INITIATING EVENTS FOR MODS

Severe sepsis
- Peritonitis

Surgery
- Vascular
- Abdominal

Trauma
- Chest injury
- Burns

Medical
- Pancreatitis
- Aspiration

Shock
- Cardiogenic
- Haemorrhagic

Other
- Massive transfusion

Pathogenesis

MODS is now recognized as a systemic disorder resulting in widespread microvascular injury. Most of the initiating events can be characterized as infective, traumatic or ischaemic and mechanistically it is unravelling as a disorder of the host defence system, with an unregulated and exaggerated immune response, resulting in an excessive release of inflammatory mediators. It is these mediators that produce the widespread microvascular damage leading to organ failure.

As a syndrome, the classical form of MODS appears to progress through four clinical phases:

1. Shock (hypoperfusion).
2. Period of active resuscitation.
3. Stable hypermetabolism (systemic inflammatory response).
4. Organ failure.

Shock Common to all the initiating events associated with MODS are periods of relative or total ischaemia relating to regional or global perfusion deficits, which may go clinically unrecognized, i.e. cellular hypoperfusion as discussed earlier. The severity of these deficits, the passage of time to adequate resuscitation and the reserve functional capacity of the organs concerned, appear to provide the key to the path of organ dysfunction and eventual failure.

Active resuscitation If resuscitation is rapid and effective the sequence of events precipitating MODS may be aborted. However, in many cases, despite apparently adequate management the syndrome progresses, suggesting a genetic component.

Systemic inflammatory response If resuscitation fails to prevent further progression of the disease, the presence of widespread cellular damage manifests after several days with a picture of panendothelial dysfunction. This endothelial damage is manifest by increased microvascular permeability with the formation of protein-rich oedema fluid. This period of hypermetabolism has characteristic features that are a consequence of the host response. This has been referred to as the systemic inflammatory response (SIRS) in the absence of proven sepsis and the sepsis syndrome when associated with an identifiable invading pathogen. Once this phase is entered the mortality rises to the 25–40 per cent range.

Organ failure Failure adequately to control the inciting event and the inexorable progression of the disease is marked in this final stage by increasing organ dysfunction, failure and death. The appearance of clinically overt organ failure is a significant prognostic event signalling another leap in the mortality rate from the 25–40 per cent range to 40–60 per cent in the early stages and 90–100 per cent as the disease progresses with increasing hepatic and renal dysfunction.

CLINICAL FEATURES OF SIR
Fever
Tachycardia
Hyperdynamic circulation
Tachypnoea
Oliguria

MEDIATORS OF THE SIRS\SEPSIS RESPONSE AND MODS

The metabolic and physiological alterations found in the hyperdynamic\hypermetabolic phase and the subsequent cellular damage are caused by complex interactions of endogenous and exogenous mediators. These substances are mainly released from the host endothelial and reticulo-endothelial cells, principally macrophages, in response to provocation by a variety of stimuli including ischaemia, sepsis and cytokines. Experimental administration of endogenously produced mediators such as tumour necrosis factor (TNF), interleukins IL1, IL2 and IL6 and platelet-activating factor and exogenously produced mediators such as bacterial endotoxin produce not only similar physiological effects to those found in the SIRS\sepsis syndrome, but also organ dysfunction similar to that found in patients with MODS.

The wide variety of substances with vastly differing molecular structures implicated in the pathogenesis of the SIRS\sepsis syndrome, all producing the same characteristic physiological response, suggests a 'preprogrammed' or stereotyped host reaction. The effector systems involved in the translation of triggering injury to pathogenesis of MODS are additive and synergistic, and involve not only the endocrine and central nervous systems, but also the cellular and humoral components of the inflammatory responses. Following injury a local inflammatory response occurs resulting from the products of the damaged endothelium and platelets. Leucocytes and macrophages are presumably attracted to the area as a result of these products and secondary activation of complement, coagulation and other components of the inflammatory system occurs. If the injury is severe or persistent enough, this localized reaction may spill over into the systemic circulation, producing the systemic inflammatory response, or if identified with infection the sepsis syndrome. MODS may subsequently develop.

In health, cytokine production is strongly repressed since they are produced by immune cells following activation by foreign particles, e.g. bacteria. Cytokine induction and production is then closely regulated so as to benefit the host by localizing and destroying the foreign organisms. However in certain situations, this control system appears inadequate and cytokine production becomes both inappropriate and excessive, leading to destruction of normal cells with a generalized inflammatory response.

A decade of studies has underlined the importance of the immune system and these mediators in the sequence of events ultimately producing MODS. Interleukin-1 is the most extensively investigated cytokine; produced by macrophages, this polypeptide (as well as interleukin-6) can induce fever, hypermetabolism, muscle breakdown and hepatic acute phase protein synthesis. The interleukins, however, appear relatively late in the sequence of events as compared to TNF.

TNF appears early in the systemic circulation during critical infective illness, mediating directly or indirectly many of the major features of sepsis. It is probably one of the pivotal mediators with multiple effects, producing endothelial membrane permeability changes and cell death. Many of these effects appear to be secondarily mediated by prostaglandins and TNF-induced release of other cytokines; the full extent of its actions are poorly understood.

SPECIFIC ORGAN INVOLVEMENT IN MODS

Respiratory system

In the majority of critically ill patients who develop MODS the lungs are the first organ to fail, the other organs following in a sequential fashion. The lung appears to be a pivotal organ in the development of MODS, appearing either to generate inflammatory mediators that aggravate peripheral endothelial dysfunction or allow the persistence of mediators in the circulation following its decreased capacity to clear and metabolize inflammatory substances.

As with other organs, a spectrum of dysfunction exists ranging from minor demonstrable pathology, designated *acute lung injury* (ALI), to massive alterations in pulmonary pathophysiology – the so-called *adult respiratory distress syndrome* (ARDS).

ARDS has been defined as a condition characterized by severe hypoxia despite high concentrations of supplemental oxygen, with a radiographic appearance demonstrating diffuse infiltrates in the absence of infection or any other explanation for the respiratory distress. Included in this definition are clinical values reflecting the derangement of respiratory function.

FEATURES DEFINING ARDS
Hypoxia ($PaO_2/FiO_2 < 300$ mmHg)
Bilateral infiltrates on chest x-ray
Pulmonary capillary wedge pressure < 18 mmHg or no clinical evidence of increased left atrial pressure

ARDS is considered to be a more severe form of ALI, in which the same criteria apply except that the hypoxia is more severe [$PaO_2/FiO_2 < 200$ mmHg regardless of positive end-expiratory pressure (PEEP)]. The pathogenesis of this lung injury has in part been suggested to be endothelial damage initiated by complement activation with subsequent leucocyte aggregation and oxygen free radical formation. Platelet clumping and intravascular coagulation have also been implicated. Pathologically in ARDS pulmonary capillary endothelial damage causes fluid leakage and surfactant abnormalities resulting in alveolar and interstitial oedema and fibrosis. This damage to pulmonary architecture causes a reduction in functional residual capacity, increased ventilation\perfusion mismatching and a predilection for secondary infection. The net result is failure of gaseous exchange with hypoxia, hypercarbia and therefore an aggravation of the peripheral tissue hypoxia.

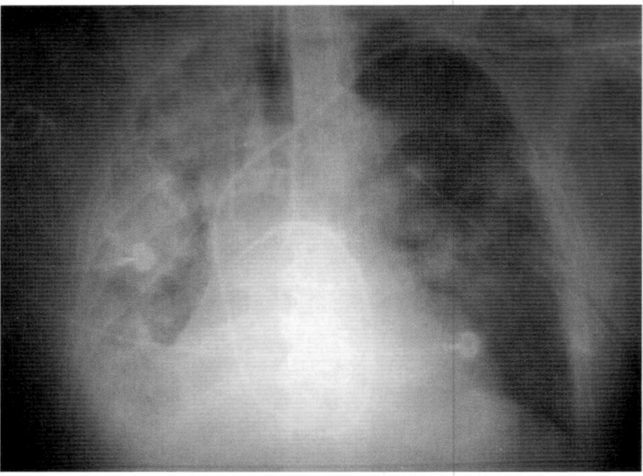

22.38 ARDS – x-ray Chest radiograph of a patient with ARDS following pulmonary contusion. Infiltrates and patchy consolidation are typical features. Note the pulmonary artery catheter in situ.

Cardiovascular system

Under normal physiological conditions, tissue oxygen utilization is closely matched by its delivery to the tissues. Oxygen uptake by cells is normally dictated by need. Cardiac output, minute ventilation and regional blood flow in the microcirculation are regulated to prevent cellular ischaemia. If stressed in this situation, cells cope with increasing metabolic demands by increasing oxygen extraction. However, under the pathological conditions found in patients with SIRS who are developing MODS, the tissues appear unable to extract oxygen efficiently from the blood, thus resulting in cellular oxygenation having to rely on increased oxygen delivery rather than extraction – the so-called pathological oxygen, supply or flow, dependency.

There may be a number of reasons for this. Microvascular inflammatory injury with endothelial and interstitial oedema hinders the diffusion of oxygen, and furthermore altered membrane characteristics of the erythrocytes render them less deformable and therefore less accessible to transit within the microcirculation.

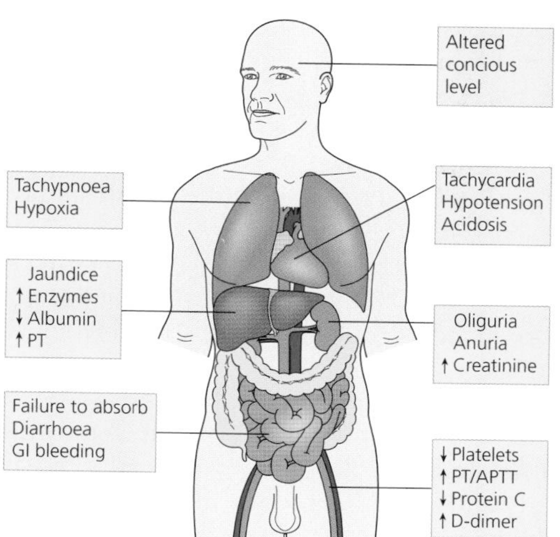

22.39 Physiological effects of MODS

In the hypermetabolic SIRS phase, the response to increased metabolic demands coupled with less effective utilization of oxygen must be met by an increased cardiac output. This increase, in conjunction with mediator-induced systemic vasodilation, gives rise to the hyperdynamic state characteristic of the SIRS–sepsis syndrome. Failure to meet this increased oxygen demand heralds a diminished likelihood of survival.

Poor cardiac performance may also contribute to the oxygen supply–utilization disequilibrium. It is well documented in sepsis that certain circulating factors adversely affect ventricular compliance and contractility. Furthermore, if pre-existing coronary artery disease co-exists with this hyperdynamic state, myocardial ischaemia and failure may progressively ensue. The effects of this may not only cause a decrease in organ perfusion but may also aggravate existing pulmonary dysfunction with raised left atrial pressures and the generation of pulmonary oedema, further aggravating oxygen delivery.

Gastrointestinal tract

The gastrointestinal tract is particularly vulnerable to the processes occurring in MODS. There is a growing body of evidence to suggest that the persistence of the SIRS–sepsis syndrome may be driven by abnormal colonization of the normally sterile upper gastrointestinal tract with pathogenic enteric bacteria. Some investigators believe that the development of MODS in the absence of a recognized focus of infection is caused by gut failure with translocation of bacteria and toxins from the gut eventually into the systemic circulation. This abnormal colonization of the gut, coupled with potentially toxic gut luminal contents, forms a deadly reservoir of pathogenic substances.

The body relies on the epithelial integrity of the gut wall to prevent seepage of these contents into the circulation. This epithelial barrier is, however, also involved in the systemic disease process, especially as preferential redistribution of the blood from the splanchnic circulation to muscle predisposes the gut mucosa to ischaemia and membrane reperfusion injury. The epithelial barrier is then likely to fail, allowing translocation of pathogenic bacteria, or endotoxins into the portal circulation. Under normal circumstances overspill of gut luminal toxic products into the portal circulation would be cleared by hepatic reticulo-endothelial system. In the presence of MODS the hepatic clearance of these substances is greatly reduced and spillage of toxins will be washed into the pulmonary microcapillary network. The appearance of endotoxin and bacteria in the lung will activate pulmonary alveolar macrophages with local damage occurring from macrophage-derived mediator release, adding to the destruction of pulmonary architecture already occurring in ARDS.

Kidney

The involvement of renal dysfunction and failure as part of classical MODS heralds a large increase in mortality. The explanation for this excess mortality is unknown; perhaps the failing kidneys act as a further source of inflammatory mediators 'fuelling' the systemic disease process further. The loss of intravascular volume control may exacerbate ARDS and heart failure with the potential for volume overload. In addition, institution of methods of renal support will have the potential for further activation of the reticulo-endothelial cells caused by bio-incompatibility problems of the extracorporeal circuit and haemofilter/dialyzer.

Haematological system

Coagulopathy is common after major trauma. Initially this may just reflect massive fluid replacement and transfusion. Massive transfusion, the replacement of greater than one circulating blood volume (approximately 10 u of blood) in less than 24 hours, may result in diffuse microvascular bleeding from surgical wounds, intravenous catheter sites and areas of minor trauma. The source of the coagulopathy, ignoring the presumed continuing consumption, is the dilution of coagulation factors through the infusion of products deficient in these factors (e.g. packed red blood cells, crystalloids and colloids). Laboratory tests demonstrate thrombocytopaenia, hypofibrinogenemia and prolongation of the prothrobin times.

An insidious complication of severe injury and blood loss is a widespread disorder of coagulation and haemostasis. This is due, at least in part, to the release of tissue thromboplastins into the circulation, endothelial damage and platelet activation. The result is a complex mixture of intravascular coagulation, depletion of clotting factors, fibrinolysis and thrombocytopaenia. Microvascular occlusion causes haemorrhagic infarctions and tissue necrosis, while deficient haemostasis leads to abnormal bleeding. This resulting coagulopathy is termed disseminated intravascular coagulation (DIC). The pathophysiology results from the generation of excessive amounts of thrombin. Thrombin generation in florid DIC is sufficiently intense that anticoagulant mechanisms such as antithrombin and activated protein C systems become ineffective. Fibrin deposition in the microvasculature undergoes fibrinolysis and promotes the consumption of clotting factors (especially fibrinogen, platelet factors V and VIII). This in turn leads to a consumptive coagulopathy characterized by thrombocytopaenia, hypofibrinogenaemia and ongoing thrombolysis.

The consequences of DIC are variable but include excessive bleeding due to consumption of haemostatic factors and secondary fibrinolysis, organ dysfunction, skin infarction, haemolysis, and disseminated thrombosis. The clinical features are those of diffuse microvascular thrombosis: restlessness, confusion, neurological dysfunction, skin infarcts, oliguria and renal failure. Abnormal haemostasis causes excessive bleeding at operation, oozing drip sites and wounds, spontaneous bruising, gastrointestinal bleeding and haematuria. The diagnosis is confirmed by finding a low haemoglobin concentration, prolonged prothrombin and thrombin times, thrombocytopaenia, hypofibrinogenaemia and raised levels of fibrinogen degradation products.

Management of MODS

Once the clinical syndrome of MODS is established, despite major advances in ITU technology and management strategies, the chances of survival dwindle. The best treatment for MODS remains prevention. This entails early aggressive resuscitation following insult, avoidance of hypotensive episodes and removal of risk factors, e.g. by early excision of necrotic tissue, early fracture stabilization and ambulation, and appropriate antibiotic usage following drainage of sources of sepsis.

Early circulatory resuscitation is of paramount importance and this should be guided by invasive monitoring. Oxygen delivery should be maximized to a point where oxygen consumption no longer rises or to the level where markers of anaerobic metabolism such as serum lactate fall. It appears that the use of less invasive clinical markers for the adequacy of the circulation, such as mean arterial pressure, temperature gradients and urine output, may not entirely reflect the success of microcirculatory resuscitation. Once the sequence of MODS is established, early appropriate institution of organ support, (e.g. endotracheal intubation and ventilation) is essential.

The treatment of ALI/ARDS remains mainly supportive and includes the management of precipitating causes. A large prospective study, supported by the National Heart Lung and Blood Institute in the USA has shown that the use of low tidal volume ventilatory strategies (6 mL/kg) and limited plateau pressure (< 30 cm H_2O) was effective in reducing the mortality rate from 40 per cent to 31 per cent. Other measures to improve oxygenation – e.g. prone positioning, high-frequency ventilation, nitrous oxide inhalation and extracorporeal life support – have limited success in improving overall outcome.

Renal and haematological management strategies are also largely supportive with renal replacement therapy and blood products frequently requiring expert involvement.

Malnutrition is a common and major contributing factor to MODS. Nutritional starvation combined with hypermetabolism leads to structural catabolism. Unlike starvation the substrates metabolized are mixed, with a significant increase in amino-acid oxidation. With the temporal progression of MODS, direct amino-acid oxidation increasingly becomes prevalent with rapid dissolution of skeletal muscle. Metabolic support in terms of providing adequate calories and maintaining nitrogen balance is essential if lean body mass is to be preserved and 'autocannabilism' slowed. This has led to recommendations for early parenteral feeding (this is still controversial). Providing a calorie source for these patients requires care and a balance of substrates has to be given to prevent adding iatrogenic problems to the metabolic mayhem already occurring. Whilst it is known that glucose has a protein-sparing effect, excessive amounts confers no additive advantages and may cause complications such as fatty liver, hyperosmolarity, hyperglycaemia, and increased CO_2 production, increasing the excretory load of the lungs and further exacerbating respiratory failure. The glucose load should not therefore exceed 4–5 mg/kg/minute, with a non-protein calorific load of 25–30 kcal/kg/day and 0.5–1.0 g/kg/day of lipids. Protein requirements run at 1–2 g/kg/day with modified amino acid preparations as these appear to be the most efficient protein source, producing less urea and better nitrogen retention.

Rigorous attention to these details has brought improvements in prevention and outcome in MODS. Other newer treatment strategies are still largely unproven in terms of outcome. Selective decontamination of the digestive tract (SDD) by administration of non-absorbable antimicrobial agents may reduce the incidence of nosocomial pneumonia by re-sterilizing the upper gastrointestinal tract. Trials of SDD have shown some benefit but large-scale effects on antibiotic resistance from widespread use of antiobiotics are awaited. The use of aggressive early enteral feeding in patients without an ileus may not only reduce the effects of catabolism but also prevent upper gut colonization by bacteria and hence nosocomial pneumonia by stimulation of bactericidal gastric acid secretion. Recent studies appear to suggest that this may have a positive effect on outcome.

Probably the most recent advances in treatment of MODS have been in relation to modulation of the hypermetabolic inflammatory response by use of specific agents. These include monoclonal antibodies against endotoxin and TNF inhibitors of nitric oxide synthase and receptor antagonists for interleukin-1. Unfortunately interim reports of the therapeutic effectiveness are conflicting and it would appear as yet that the 'magic bullet' remains elusive.

Again it must be emphasized that prevention is better than attempting cure for MODS, the major killer of critically ill patients in intensive care.

TETANUS

The tetanus organism *Clostridium tetani* flourishes only in dead tissue. The exotoxin released passes to the central nervous system via the blood and the perineural lymphatics from the infected region. The toxin is fixed in the anterior horn cells and therefore cannot be neutralized by antitoxin.

Established tetanus is characterized by tonic, and later clonic, contractions, especially of the muscles of the jaw and face (trismus, risus sardonicus), those near the wound itself, and later of the neck and trunk. Ultimately, the diaphragm and intercostal muscles may be 'locked' by spasm resulting in asphyxia.

TREATMENT

With established tetanus, intravenous antitoxin (human for choice) is advisable. Heavy sedation and muscle relaxant drugs may help; tracheal intubation and ventilation are the only options to treat respiratory muscle involvement.

Prophylaxis against tetanus by active immunization with tetanus toxoid vaccine is a valuable goal. If the patient has been immunized, booster doses of toxoid are given after all but trivial skin wounds. In the non-immunized patient prompt and thorough wound toilet together with antibiotics may be adequate, but if the wound is contaminated, and particularly with a delay before operation, antitoxin is advisable.

FAT EMBOLISM SYNDROME

Fat embolism is a common phenomenon following limb fractures. Circulating fat globules larger than 10 μm in diameter occur in most adults after closed fractures of long bones and histological traces of fat can be found in the lungs and other internal organs. A small percentage of these patients develop clinical features similar to those of ARDS; this was recognized as the *fat embolism syndrome* long before ARDS entered the medical literature. Whether the fat embolism syndrome is an expression of the same condition or whether it is an entirely separate entity is still uncertain.

The source of the fat emboli is probably the bone marrow, and the condition is more common in patients with multiple fractures.

Clinical features

Early warning signs of fat embolism (usually within 72 hours of injury) are a slight rise of temperature and pulse rate. In more pronounced cases there is breathlessness and mild mental confusion or restlessness. Pathognomonic signs are petechiae on the trunk, axillae and in the conjunctival folds and retinae. In more severe cases there may be respiratory distress and coma, due both to brain emboli and hypoxia from involvement of the lungs. The features at this stage are essentially those of ARDS.

There is no infallible test for fat embolism; however, urinalysis may show fat globules in the urine and the blood PO_2 should always be monitored; values below 8 kPa (60 mmHg or less) within the first 72 hours of any major injury must be regarded as suspicious. A chest x-ray may show classical changes in the lungs.

Management

Management of severe fat embolism is supportive. Symptoms of the syndrome can be reduced with the use of supplemental high inspired oxygen concentrations immediately after injury and the incidence appears to be reduced by the prompt stabilization of long-bone fractures. Intramedullary nailing is not thought to increase the risk of developing the syndrome. Fixation of fractures also allows the patient to be nursed in the sitting position, which optimizes the ventilation–perfusion match in the lungs.

CRUSH SYNDROME

This is seen when a limb is compressed for extended periods, e.g. following entrapment in a vehicle or rubble, but also after prolonged use of a pneumatic anti-shock garment.

The crushed limb is underperfused and myonecrosis follows, leading to the release of toxic metabolites when the limb is freed and so generating a *reperfusion injury*. Reactive oxygen metabolites create further tissue injury. Membrane damage and capillary fluid reabsorption failure result in swelling that may lead to a compartment syndrome, thus creating more tissue damage from escalating ischaemia. Tissue necrosis also causes systemic problems such as renal failure from free myoglobin, which is precipitated in the renal glomeruli. Myonecrosis may cause a metabolic acidosis with hyperkalaemia and hypocalcaemia.

Clinical features and treatment

The compromised limb is pulseless and becomes red, swollen and blistered; sensation and muscle power may be lost. The most important measure is prevention. From an intensive care perspective a high urine flow is encouraged with alkalization of the urine with sodium bicarbonate, which prevents myoglobin precipitating in the renal tubules. If oliguria or renal failure occurs then renal haemofiltration will be needed.

If a compartment syndrome develops, and is confirmed by pressure measurements, then a fasciotomy is indicated. Excision of dead muscle must be radical to avoid sepsis. Similarly, if there is an open wound then this should be managed aggressively. If there is no open wound and the compartment pressures are not high, then the risk of infection is probably lower if early surgery is avoided.

INTENSIVE CARE UNIT SCORING SYSTEMS

The role of scoring systems in medicine has expanded since the 1950s. There are now many scoring systems catering for most organ dysfunction, disease states, trauma and critical illness. New scoring systems are regularly being developed and older systems refined. This widespread use relates to their role in communication, audit and research as well as the clinical management of patients.

Scoring systems can theoretically be created from many types of variables. However, to be clinically useful, scoring systems must have predictive properties, and the information has to be unambiguous, reliable and easy to determine and collect. Ideally the variables should be frequently recorded or measured. Variables can be selected using clinical judgement and recognized physiological associations, or by using computerized searching of data collected from patient databases and relating it to outcome. The variables are then assigned a weighting in relation to their importance to the predictive power of the scoring system, again either by clinical relevance or from computerized databases.

Logical regression analysis, a multivariate statistical procedure, is used to convert a score to a predicted probability of the outcome measured, usually morbidity or mortality, using a large patient database suitable to the scoring system being developed. Finally the scoring system has to be validated on a population of patients independent from those used to develop the scoring system.

Patients form a heterogeneous population and differ in many respects including age, previous health status, reason for admission and severity of illness. When comparing patients on intensive care for the purpose of research or audit, it is often difficult to standardize for all physiological variables due to the diversity of patients and their conditions. Scoring systems are therefore used to standardize for the physiological variables, age and reason for admission, allowing comparisons to be made between patients with different severity of illness.

In the majority of scoring systems a high score reflects a patient who is more sick than one with a lower score (with the notable exception of the Glasgow Coma Score), but the score does not always follow a linear scale. Therefore a patient with a score of 20 is neither necessarily twice as sick nor has double the chance of dying than a patient with a score of 10. However, using logical regression it is possible to derive from the score a probability of morbidity, or mortality in hospital.

Audit

The most common use for scoring systems is for audit. This allows ICUs to assess their performance in comparison to other units and also their own performance from year to year. If an ICU admitted patients who were not very sick, then their actual mortality on that unit would be lower than on a unit that admitted extremely sick patients and therefore it would be difficult to compare the performance between those units. This has led to the comparisons of actual mortality to a predicted mortality. The ratio of the actual to predicted mortality gives a figure for the standardized mortality ratio (SMR). Therefore an ICU with an SMR of less than 1 is theoretically performing better than expected and a unit with an SMR of more than 1 is performing worse than expected. The SMR can then be used to compare performance between units. Also if the severity of illness of patients varies, or if different types of patients are admitted from year to year, the SMR can be used to assess the performance of a unit over time. Statistical significance of different SMRs can be evaluated using confidence intervals.

Research

The diversity of patients and different pathologies on the ICU makes comparisons between treatments or procedures difficult. Scoring systems can be used to adjust for the differences in case-mix in patients recruited for trials, so if an intervention is used on all patients, the scoring systems can standardize for any heterogenicity between the groups prior to the intervention being initiated. Stratification of the risk of death can also be inferred from the scoring systems, allowing for investigation in different subgroups of patients in the ITU, and allowing researchers to assess response to interventions in patients at different risk of mortality.

Clinical management

As well as quantifying the degree of physiological derangement or clinical intervention, and promoting better communication between clinicians, scoring systems can also be used to guide patient management. Some scoring systems lend themselves to sequential reassessment and thus can be used to monitor a patient's progress over time. Also, as most research conducted in ICUs use scoring systems, the recommendations from research can sometimes be applied to subsets of patients with a severity of illness score within a certain range. This allows therapies to be directed sensibly at patients with an appropriate severity of illness. As most ITU scoring systems are an assessment of risk of mortality they have also been used to trigger admission to high-dependency or intensive care.

Scoring systems on the ICU

Scoring systems are often classified into three subsets: (1) anatomical (e.g. the injury severity score); (2) physiological (e.g. the GCS) and therapeutic (e.g. therapeutic intervention scoring systems). Most intensive care scoring systems are based on physiological variables; however other data are also included in the score, making simple classification very difficult.

An ideal scoring system would be simple to use and be applicable to all intensive care patients irrespective of age, diagnosis and urgency of admission. It should also not be dependent upon treatment given prior to and on admission to ICU. The outcome prediction modelling should have a high sensitivity and specificity. The intensive care scoring systems are developed from large databases incorporating data from many ICUs. The data include physiological variables, co-morbidities, age, diagnoses, urgency of admission, and outcome at discharge from hospital.

Acute physiology and chronic health evaluation

Knaus et al (1981) introduced the first the Acute Physiology and Chronic Health Evaluation (APACHE) model in 1981 and revised it to APACHE II in 1985. APACHE III was presented in 1991 but as the regression analysis modelling is not in the public domain its uptake has been slow.

APACHE II is made up of four basic components: (1) acute physiology score; (2) chronic health evaluation; (3) age; (4) urgency of admission to critical care. The acute physiology score is composed of 12 variables, with the most deranged measurement during the first 24 hours of admission to critical care being used to calculate the score. The original data collection for APACHE II occurred between 1979 and 1982 from ICUs in North America, and the population studied included relatively few surgical and trauma patients. Also, there have been many advances in patient care since the1980s, which have made APACHE II dated, despite its continued popularity.

Simplified acute physiology score

The Simplified Acute Physiology Score (SAPS) initially used 14 variables, and did not provide any probability of survival. In 1993 it was revised to SAPS II with the data originating from European and North American ICUs. The score includes 12 physiological variables (the worst value within the first 24 hours), age, type of admission and three underlying disease variables (acquired immune deficiency syndrome (AIDS), metastatic cancer, and haematological malignancy). Using logistic regression, SAPS II can also be used to estimate the probability of survival. It is a simpler scoring system than APACHE and is also in the public domain, resulting in its widespread use, particularly in Europe. It suffers similar disadvantages to APACHE with regards to the timing of data collection, but is based on more recent and international data.

Mortality prediction model

The original mortality prediction model (MPM) was derived in the late 1980s with data from a single hospital, and differed from many of the scoring systems by not depending on physiological data but on the presence or absence of pathology. Therefore there was less of an impact by treatment on the physiology prior to and on admission to intensive care. In 1993 the MPM was revised to MPM II based on the same data set as SAPS II but with the inclusion of six extra ICUs. Initially the model was constructed of two time points: within 1 hour (MPM II_0) and the first 24 hours (MPM II_{24}) of admission. Now it can be used for 48- and 72-hour points as well, giving a prediction of mortality at those time points. Its variables include physiological parameters, age, acute diagnoses, chronic diseases, type of admission, as well as others. The MPM II_0 is useful as it is minimally affected by the treatment given in an ICU.

Therapeutic intervention scoring system

The original therapeutic intervention scoring system (TISS) was devised in 1976, consisting of 76 therapeutic activities and was used initially to stratify the severity of illness. Its use for this purpose has largely been superseded by the newer scoring systems, but it is still commonly used to assess nursing workload and in resource management, for which it was not designed. A simplified TISS was developed in 1996, which included only 28 therapeutic activities.

Limitations

Overall there is very little to choose between the third-generation scoring systems (APACHE III, SAPS II, MPM II) in terms of their predictive power. Despite this, APACHE II continues to dominate the literature and continues to be the most widely used score to date.

The APACHE II/III and SAPS I/II scoring systems measure physiological variables during the first 24 hours of ITU admission and there has been concern that this can lead to bias. If a patient is treated prior to admission to ITU, their physiological variables will have been improved and the patients will have lower scores. Similarly if a patient is admitted to the ITU and receives inappropriate treatment over the first 24 hours, their scores will suggest that the ITU is dealing with sicker patients. Lastly, if a patient dies within 24 hours their scores before death will be very high, and therefore skew the SMR of a unit to suggest that it is admitting very sick patients. MPM II measures variables during the first hour and within the first 24 hours, thereby reducing the bias that may occur in the score when measured over 24 hours.

Limitations and errors associated with the use of the scoring systems include missing data, observer error and interobserver variability. Even the method of data collection (manual data entry versus data collected automatically from monitoring systems) leads to wide variations in scores. Although the above scoring systems are useful to assess and compare outcomes in patient populations, such scores may not be appropriate to provide individual risk assessment in critically ill patients.

REFERENCES

American College of Surgeons Committee on Trauma. Advanced Trauma Life Support® Program for Doctors. (8th edition) American College of Surgeons, Chicago, 2008.

Calland V. *Safety at Scene. A Manual for Paramedics and Immediate Care Doctors.* Mosby, Edinburgh, 2000.

Clasper J, Rew D. Trauma life support in conflict. *Br Med J* 2003; **327:** 1178–9.

Commission on the Provision of Surgical Services. *The Management of Patients with Major Injuries.* The Royal College of Surgeons of England, 1988.

Deakin CD, Low JL. Do Advanced Trauma Life Support guidelines accurately predict systolic blood pressure by palpation of carotid, femoral and radial pulses? An observational study. *Br Med J* 2000; **321:** 674–5.

Earlam R. *Trauma Care.* Helicopter Emergency Medical Service (HEMS), London, 1997.

Findlay G *et al. Compilers. Trauma: Who cares?* A report of the National Confidential Enquiry into Patient Outcome and Death (2007). NCEPOD 2007.

Flannery T, Buxton N. Modern management of head injuries. *J R Coll Surg Edinb* 2001; **46:** 150–3.

Frankema SP, Ringburg AN, Steyerberg EW *et al.* Beneficial effect of helicopter emergency medical services on survival of severely injured patients. *Br J Surg* 2004; **91:** 1520–6.

Hodgetts T, Mahoney P, Russell M, Byers M. ABC to ABC: redefining the military trauma paradigm. *Emergency Med J* 2006; **23:** 745–6.

Hodgetts T, Porter C. *Major Incident Management System.* BMJ Books, London, 2002.

Joint Royal Colleges Ambulance Service Liaison Committee (JRCALC) 2008. A Joint Report from the Royal College of Surgeons of England and the British Orthopaedic Association. *Better Care for the Severely Injured.* The Royal College of Surgeons of England. London, 2000.

Knaus WA, Zimmerman JE, Wagner DP. APACHE: Acute Physiology and Chronic Health Evaluation, a physiologically based classification system. *Crit Care Med* 1981; **16:** 470–8.

Kortbeek JB, Al Turki SA, Ali J *et al. Advanced Trauma Life Support* (8th edition) The Evidence for Change. *J Trauma* 2008; **64:** 1638–50.

Lee C, Porter K, Hodgetts T. Tourniquet use in the civilian prehospital setting. *Emergency Med J* 2007; **24:** 584–7.

Mock C, Lormand JD, Goosen J, Joshipura M, Peden M. *Guidelines for Essential Trauma Care.* World Health Organization, Geneva, 2004.

Mahoney PF, Russell RJ, Russell MQ, Hodgetts TJ. Novel haemostatic techniques in military medicine. *J R Army Med Corps* 2005; **151:** 139–41.

National Institute for Clinical Excellence. *Pre-hospital initiation of fluid replacement therapy in trauma.* Technology Appraisal 74, January 2004.

National Institute for Health and Clinical Excellence. *Head injury. Triage, assessment, investigation and early management of head injury in infants, children and adults.* NICE clinical guideline 56, London, September 2007.

Nicholl J, Turner J. Effectiveness of a regional trauma system in reducing mortality from major trauma: before and after study. *Br Med J* 1997; **315:** 1349–54.

Oakley P, Kirby R, Redmond A, Templeton J. Effectiveness of regional trauma systems. Improvements have occurred since study. *Br Med J* 1998; **316:** 1383.

Peden M, Scurfield R, Sleet D *et al*. *The World Report on Road Traffic Injury Prevention*. World Health Organization, Geneva, 2004.

Rabold MB. Frostbite and other localized cold-related injuries In: Tintinalli JE, Kelen GD, Stapczynski JS, Ma OJ, Cline DM. *Tintinalli's Emergency Medicine: A Comprehensive Study Guide* (6th Edition) The American College of Emergency Physicians, Dallas, Texas, 2004.

Royal College of Surgeons of England. *Report of the Working Party on the Management of Patients with Head Injuries*. Royal College of Surgeons of England, London, 1999.

Schwartz LR, Balakrishnan C. Thermal burns. In: Tintinalli JE, Kelen GD, Stapczynski JS, Ma OJ, Cline DM: *Tintinalli's Emergency Medicine: A Comprehensive Study Guide* (6th Edition) The American College of Emergency Physicians, Dallas, Texas, 2004.

Williams JS, Graff JA, Uku JM, Steinig JP. Aortic injury in vehicular trauma. *Ann Thorac Surg* 1994; **57:** 726–30.

Principles of fractures 23

Selvadurai Nayagam

INTRODUCTION

A fracture is a break in the structural continuity of bone. It may be no more than a crack, a crumpling or a splintering of the cortex; more often the break is complete and the bone fragments are displaced. If the overlying skin remains intact it is a *closed* (or *simple) fracture;* if the skin or one of the body cavities is breached it is an *open* (or *compound*) *fracture*, liable to contamination and infection.

HOW FRACTURES HAPPEN

Bone is relatively brittle, yet it has sufficient strength and resilience to withstand considerable stress. Fractures result from: (1) injury; (2) repetitive stress; or (3) abnormal weakening of the bone (a 'patholog-ical' fracture).

FRACTURES DUE TO INJURY

Most fractures are caused by sudden and excessive force, which may be direct or indirect.

With a *direct force* the bone breaks at the point of impact; the soft tissues also are damaged. A direct blow usually splits the bone transversely or may bend it over a fulcrum so as to create a break with a 'butterfly' fragment. Damage to the overlying skin is common; if crushing occurs, the fracture pattern will be comminuted with extensive soft-tissue damage.

With an indirect force the bone breaks at a distance from where the force is applied; soft-tissue damage at

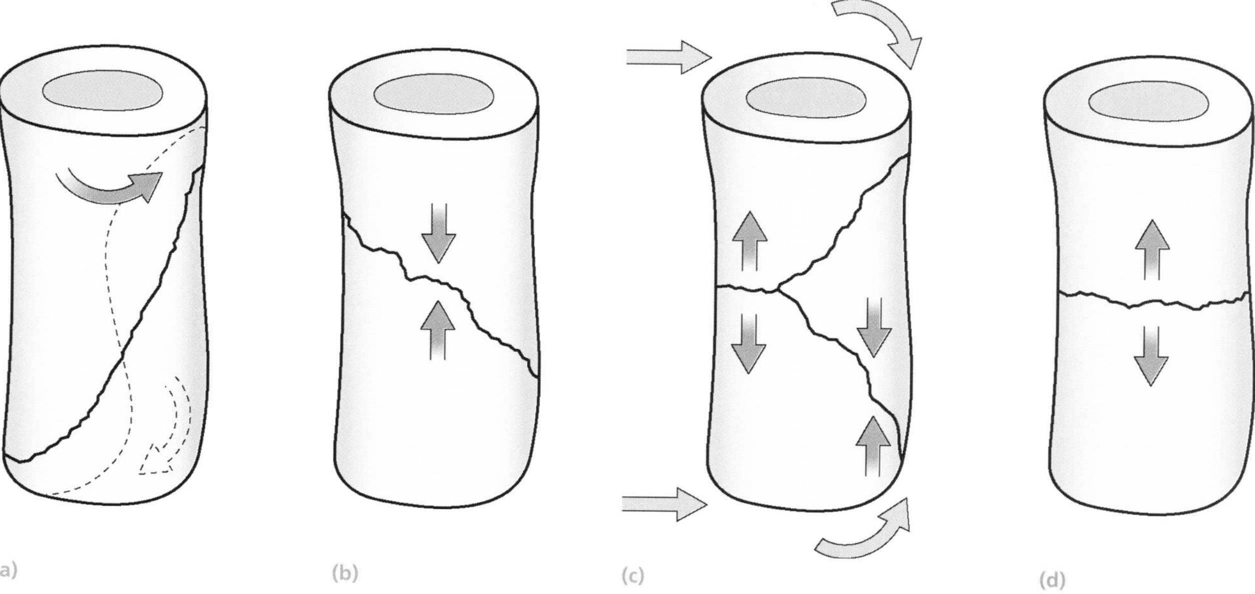

23.1 Mechanism of injury Some fracture patterns suggest the causal mechanism: (a) spiral pattern (twisting); (b) short oblique pattern (compression); (c) triangular 'butterfly' fragment (bending) and (d) transverse pattern (tension). Spiral and some (long) oblique patterns are usually due to low-energy indirect injuries; bending and transverse patterns are caused by high-energy direct trauma.

the fracture site is not inevitable. Although most fractures are due to a combination of forces (twisting, bending, compressing or tension), the x-ray pattern reveals the dominant mechanism:

- Twisting causes a spiral fracture;
- Compression causes a short oblique fracture.
- Bending results in fracture with a triangular 'butterfly' fragment;
- Tension tends to break the bone transversely; in some situations it may simply avulse a small fragment of bone at the points of ligament or tendon insertion.

NOTE: The above description applies mainly to the long bones. A cancellous bone, such as a vertebra or the calcaneum, when subjected to sufficient force, will split or be crushed into an abnormal shape.

Fatigue or stress fractures

These fractures occur in normal bone which is subject to repeated heavy loading, typically in athletes, dancers or military personnel who have gruelling exercise programmes. These high loads create minute deformations that initiate the normal process of remodelling – a combination of bone resorption and new bone formation in accordance with Wolff's law. When exposure to stress and deformation is repeated and prolonged, resorption occurs faster than replacement and leaves the area liable to fracture. A similar problem occurs in individuals who are on medication that alters the normal balance of bone resorption and replacement; stress fractures are increasingly seen in patients with chronic inflammatory diseases who are on treatment with steroids or methotrexate.

Pathological fractures

Fractures may occur even with normal stresses if the bone has been weakened by a change in its structure (e.g. in osteoporosis, osteogenesis imperfecta or Paget's disease) or through a lytic lesion (e.g. a bone cyst or a metastasis).

TYPES OF FRACTURE

Fractures are variable in appearance but for practical reasons they are divided into a few well-defined groups.

Complete fractures

The bone is split into two or more fragments. The fracture pattern on x-ray can help predict behaviour after reduction: in a *transverse fracture* the fragments usually remain in place after reduction; if it is *oblique* or *spiral,* they tend to shorten and re-displace even if the bone is splinted. In an *impacted fracture* the fragments are jammed tightly together and the fracture line is indistinct. A *comminuted fracture* is one in which there are more than two fragments; because there is poor interlocking of the fracture surfaces, these are often unstable.

Incomplete fractures

Here the bone is incompletely divided and the periosteum remains in continuity. In a *greenstick fracture* the bone is buckled or bent (like snapping a green

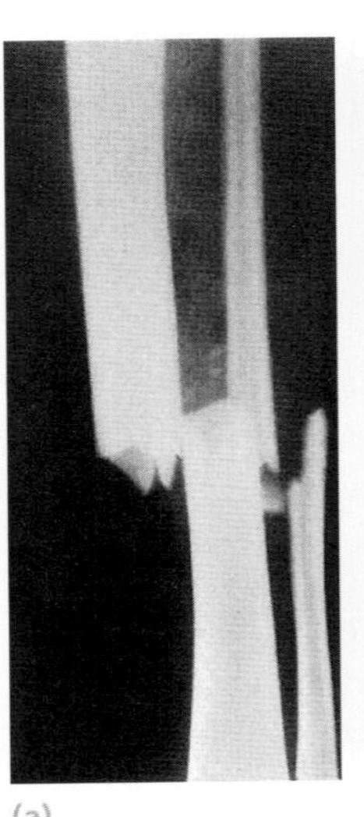
(a)

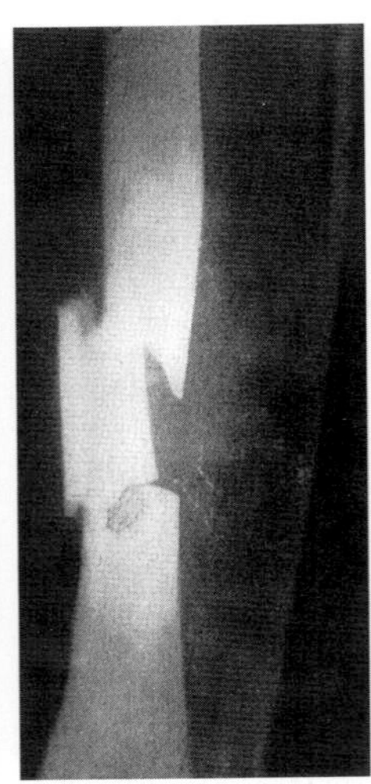
(b)

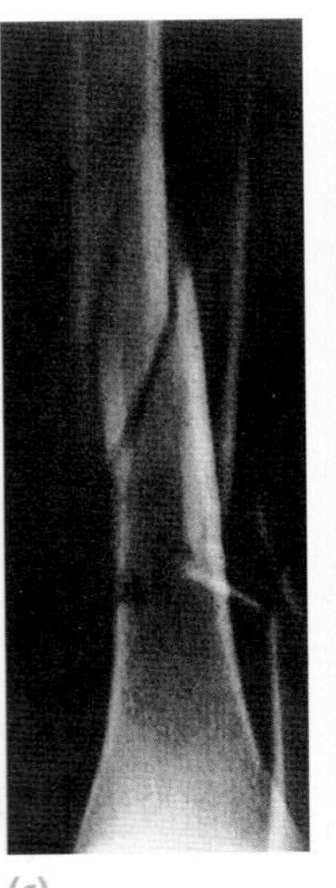
(c)

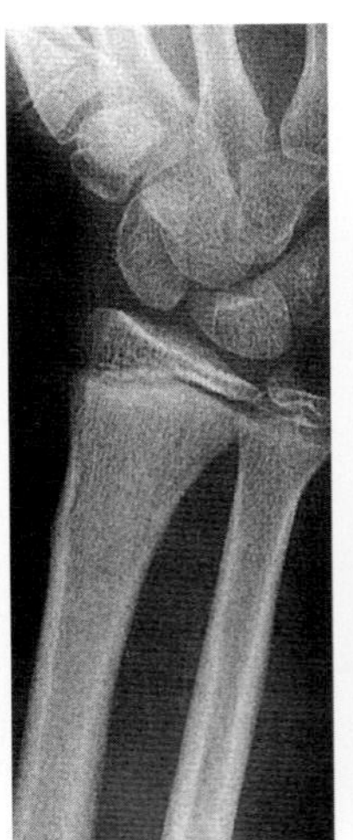
(d)

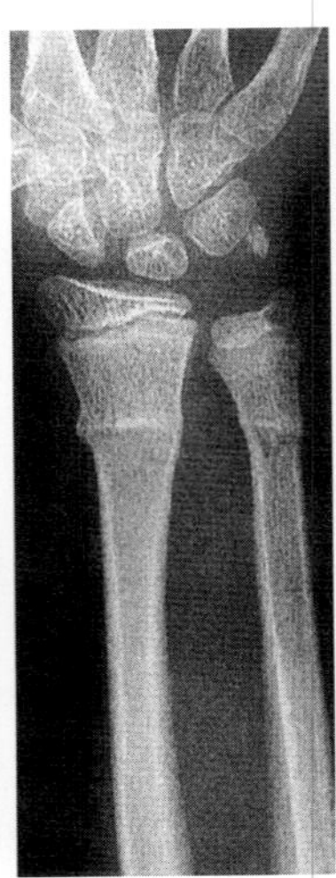
(e)

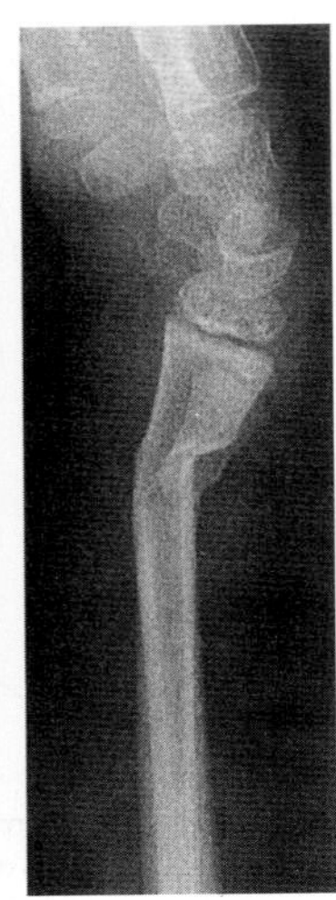
(f)

23.2 Varieties of fracture Complete fractures: (a) transverse; (b) segmental and (c) spiral. Incomplete fractures: (d) buckle or torus and (e,f) greenstick.

twig); this is seen in children, whose bones are more springy than those of adults. Children can also sustain injuries where the bone is plastically deformed (misshapen) without there being any crack visible on the x-ray. In contrast, *compression fractures* occur when cancellous bone is crumpled. This happens in adults and typically where this type of bone structure is present, e.g. in the vertebral bodies, calcaneum and tibial plateau.

CLASSIFICATION OF FRACTURES

Sorting fractures into those with similar features brings advantages: it allows any information about a fracture to be applied to others in the group (whether this concerns treatment or prognosis) and it facilitates a common dialogue between surgeons and others involved in the care of such injuries.

Traditional classifications, which often bear the originator's name, are hampered by being applicable to that type of injury only; even then the term is often inaccurately applied, famously in the case of Pott's fracture, which is often applied to any fracture around the ankle though that is not what Sir Percival Pott implied when he described the injury in 1765.

A universal, anatomically based system facilitates communication and the sharing of data from a variety of countries and populations, thus contributing to advances in research and treatment. An alphanumeric classification developed by Müller and colleagues has now been adapted and revised (Muller et al., 1990; Marsh et al., 2007; Slongo and Audige 2007). Whilst it has yet to be fully validated for reliability and reproducibility, it fulfils the objective of being comprehensive. In this system, the first digit specifies the bone (1 = humerus, 2 = radius/ulna, 3 = femur, 4 = tibia/fibula) and the second the segment (1 = proximal, 2 = diaphyseal, 3 = distal, 4 = malleolar). A letter specifies the fracture pattern (for the diaphysis: A = simple, B = wedge, C = complex; for the metaphysis: A = extra-articular, B = partial articular, C = complete articular). Two further numbers specify the detailed morphology of the fracture (Fig. 23.3).

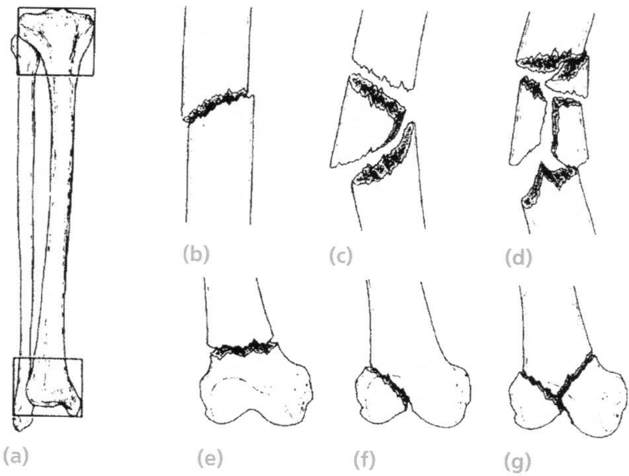

23.3 Müller's classification (a) Each long bone has three segments – proximal, diaphyseal and distal; the proximal and distal segments are each defined by a square based on the widest part of the bone. (b,c,d) Diaphyseal fractures may be simple, wedge or complex.
(e,f,g) Proximal and distal fractures may be extra-articular, partial articular of complete articular.

HOW FRACTURES ARE DISPLACED

After a complete fracture the fragments usually become displaced, partly by the force of the injury, partly by gravity and partly by the pull of muscles attached to them. Displacement is usually described in terms of translation, alignment, rotation and altered length:

- *Translation (shift)* – The fragments may be shifted sideways, backward or forward in relation to each other, such that the fracture surfaces lose contact. The fracture will usually unite as long as sufficient contact between surfaces is achieved; this may occur even if reduction is imperfect, or indeed even if the fracture ends are off-ended but the bone segments come to lie side by side.
- *Angulation (tilt)* – The fragments may be tilted or angulated in relation to each other. Malalignment, if uncorrected, may lead to deformity of the limb.
- *Rotation (twist)* – One of the fragments may be twisted on its longitudinal axis; the bone looks straight but the limb ends up with a rotational deformity.
- *Length* – The fragments may be distracted and separated, or they may overlap, due to muscle spasm, causing shortening of the bone.

HOW FRACTURES HEAL

It is commonly supposed that, in order to unite, a fracture must be immobilized. This cannot be so since, with few exceptions, fractures unite whether they are splinted or not; indeed, without a built-in mechanism for bone union, land animals could scarcely have evolved. It is, however, naive to suppose that union would occur if a fracture were kept moving indefinitely; the bone ends must, at some stage, be brought to rest relative to one another. But it is not mandatory for the surgeon to impose this immobility artificially – nature can do it with callus, and callus forms in response to movement, not to splintage.

Most fractures are splinted, not to ensure union but to: (1) alleviate pain; (2) ensure that union takes place in good position and (3) permit early movement of the limb and a return of function.

The process of fracture repair varies according to the type of bone involved and the amount of movement at the fracture site.

Healing by callus

This is the 'natural' form of healing in tubular bones; in the absence of rigid fixation, it proceeds in five stages:

1. *Tissue destruction and haematoma formation* – Vessels are torn and a haematoma forms around and within the fracture. Bone at the fracture surfaces, deprived of a blood supply, dies back for a millimetre or two.
2. *Inflammation and cellular proliferation* – Within 8 hours of the fracture there is an acute inflammatory reaction with migration of inflammatory cells and the initiation of proliferation and differentiation of mesenchymal stem cells from the periosteum, the breached medullary canal and the surrounding muscle. The fragment ends are surrounded by cellular tissue, which creates a scaffold across the fracture site. A vast array of inflammatory mediators (cytokines and various growth factors) is involved. The clotted haematoma is slowly absorbed and fine new capillaries grow into the area.
3. *Callus formation* – The differentiating stem cells provide chrondrogenic and osteogenic cell populations; given the right conditions – and this is usually the local biological and biomechanical environment – they will start forming bone and, in some cases, also cartilage. The cell population now also includes osteoclasts (probably derived from the new blood vessels), which begin to mop up dead bone. The thick cellular mass, with its islands of immature bone and cartilage, forms the callus or splint on the periosteal and endosteal surfaces. As the immature fibre bone (or 'woven' bone) becomes more densely mineralized, movement at the fracture site decreases progressively and at about 4 weeks after injury the fracture 'unites'.
4. *Consolidation* – With continuing osteoclastic and osteoblastic activity the woven bone is transformed into lamellar bone. The system is now rigid enough to allow osteoclasts to burrow through the debris at the fracture line, and close behind them. Osteoblasts fill in the remaining gaps between the fragments with new bone. This is a slow process and it may be several months before the bone is strong enough to carry normal loads.
5. *Remodelling* – The fracture has been bridged by a cuff of solid bone. Over a period of months, or even years, this crude 'weld' is reshaped by a continuous process of alternating bone resorption and formation. Thicker lamellae are laid down where the stresses are high, unwanted buttresses are carved away and the medullary cavity is reformed. Eventually, and especially in children, the bone reassumes something like its normal shape.

Healing by direct union

Clinical and experimental studies have shown that callus is the response to movement at the fracture site (McKibbin, 1978). It serves to stabilize the fragments as rapidly as possible – a necessary precondition for bridging by bone. If the fracture site is absolutely immobile – for example, an impacted fracture in cancellous bone, or a fracture rigidly immobilized by a metal plate – there is no stimulus for callus (Sarmiento et al., 1980). Instead, osteoblastic new bone formation occurs directly between the fragments. Gaps between the fracture surfaces are invaded by new capillaries and osteoprogenitor cells growing in from the edges, and new bone is laid down on the exposed surface (*gap healing*). Where the crevices are very narrow (less than 200 μm), osteogenesis produces lamellar bone; wider gaps are filled first by woven bone, which is then remodelled to lamellar bone. By 3–4 weeks the fracture is solid enough to allow penetration and bridging of the area by bone remodelling units, i.e. osteoclastic 'cutting cones' followed by osteoblasts. Where the exposed fracture surfaces are in intimate contact and held rigidly from the outset, internal bridging may occasionally occur without any intermediate stages (*contact healing*).

Healing by callus, though less direct (the term 'indirect' could be used) has distinct advantages: it ensures mechanical strength while the bone ends heal, and with increasing stress the callus grows stronger and stronger (an example of Wolff's law). With rigid metal fixation, on the other hand, the absence of callus means that there is a long period during which the bone depends entirely upon the metal implant for its integrity. Moreover, the implant diverts stress away from the bone, which may become osteoporotic and not recover fully until the metal is removed.

Union, consolidation and non-union

Repair of a fracture is a continuous process: any stages into which it is divided are necessarily arbitrary. In this book the terms 'union' and 'consolidation' are used, and they are defined as follows:

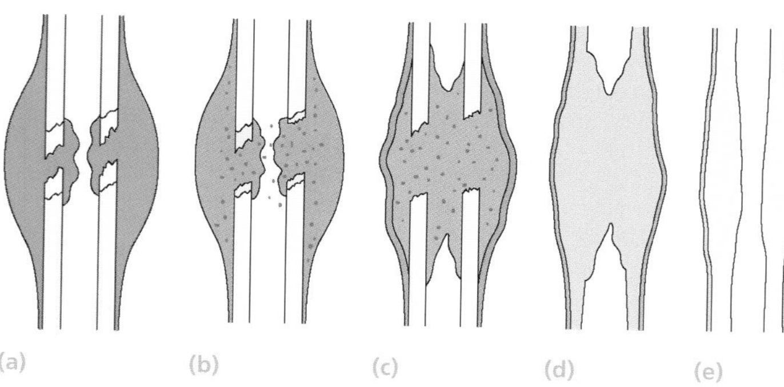

(a) (b) (c) (d) (e)

23.4 Fracture healing Five stages of healing: (a) Haematoma: there is tissue damage and bleeding at the fracture site; the bone ends die back for a few millimetres. (b) Inflammation: inflammatory cells appear in the haematoma. (c) Callus: the cell population changes to osteoblasts and osteoclasts; dead bone is mopped up and woven bone appears in the fracture callus. (d) Consolidation: woven bone is replaced by lamellar bone and the fracture is solidly united. (e) Remodelling: the newly formed bone is remodelled to resemble the normal structure.

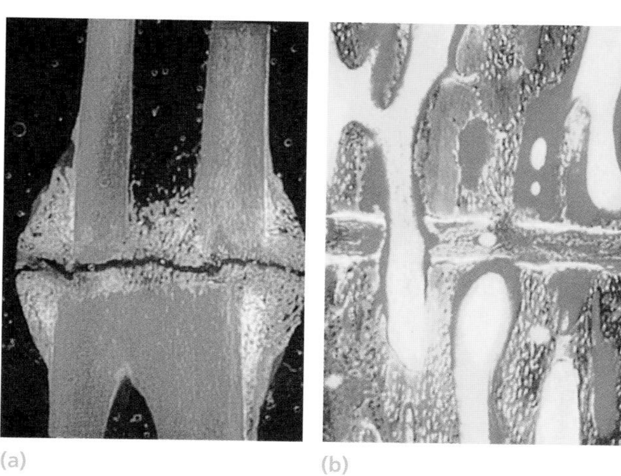

(a) (b)

23.5 Fracture healing – histology Experimental fracture healing: (a) by bridging callus and (b) by direct penetration of the fracture gap by a cutting cone.

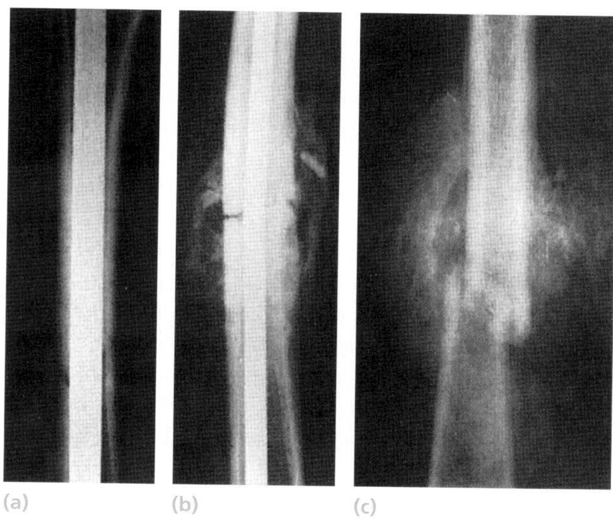

(a) (b) (c)

23.6 Callus and movement Three patients with femoral shaft fractures. (a) and (b) are both 6 weeks after fixation: in (a) the Kuntscher nail fitted tightly, preventing movement, and there is no callus; in (b) the nail fitted loosely, permitting some movement, so there is callus. (c) This patient had cerebral irritation and thrashed around wildly; at 3 weeks callus is excessive.

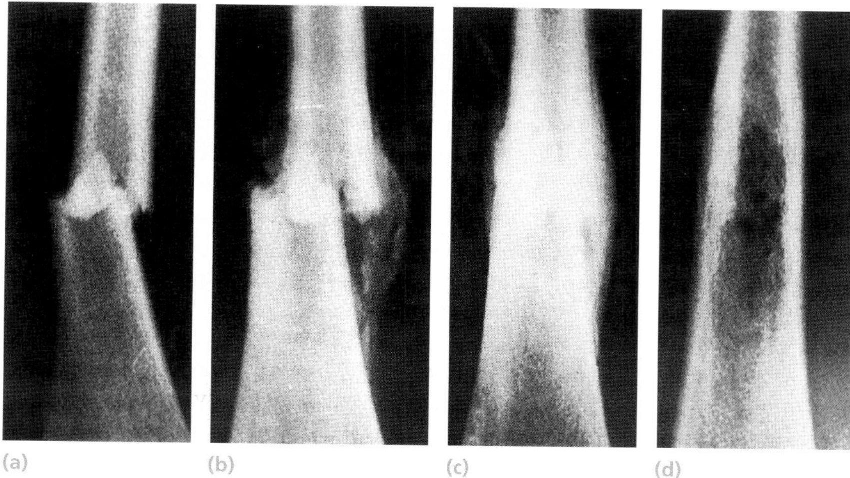

(a) (b) (c) (d)

23.7 Fracture repair (a) Fracture; (b) union; (c) consolidation; (d) bone remodelling. The fracture must be protected until consolidated.

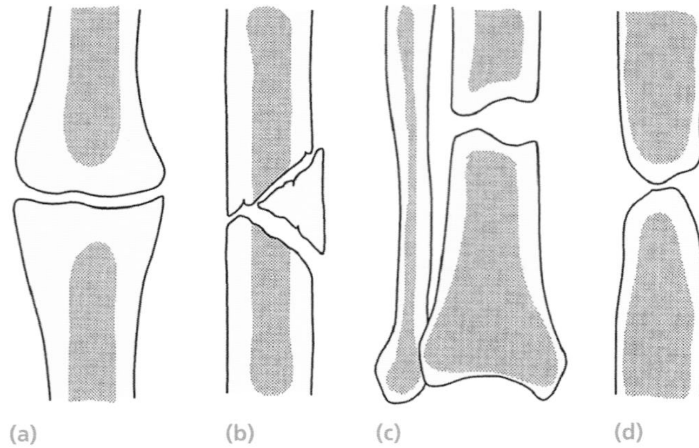

23.8 Non-unions Aseptic non-unions are generally divided into hypertrophic and atrophic types. Hypertrophic non-unions often have florid streams of callus around the fracture gap – the result of insufficient stability. They are sometimes given colourful names, such as: (a) elephant's foot. In contrast, atrophic non-unions usually arise from an impaired repair process; they are classified according to the x-ray appearance as (b) necrotic, (c) gap and (d) atrophic.

- *Union* – Union is incomplete repair; the ensheathing callus is calcified. Clinically the fracture site is still a little tender and, though the bone moves in one piece (and in that sense is united), attempted angulation is painful. X-Rays show the fracture line still clearly visible, with fluffy callus around it. Repair is incomplete and it is not safe to subject the unprotected bone to stress.
- *Consolidation* – Consolidation is complete repair; the calcified callus is ossified. Clinically the fracture site is not tender, no movement can be obtained and attempted angulation is painless. X-rays show the fracture line to be almost obliterated and crossed by bone trabeculae, with well-defined callus around it. Repair is complete and further protection is unnecessary.
- *Timetable* – How long does a fracture take to unite and to consolidate? No precise answer is possible because age, constitution, blood supply, type of fracture and other factors all influence the time taken.

  Approximate prediction is possible and Perkins' timetable is delightfully simple. A spiral fracture in the upper limb unites in 3 weeks; for consolidation multiply by 2; for the lower limb multiply by 2 again; for transverse fractures multiply again by 2. A more sophisticated formula is as follows. A spiral fracture in the upper limb takes 6–8 weeks to consolidate; the lower limb needs twice as long. Add 25% if the fracture is not spiral or if it involves the femur. Children's fractures, of course, join more quickly. These figures are only a rough guide; there must be clinical and radiological evidence of consolidation before full stress is permitted without splintage.
- *Non-union* – Sometimes the normal process of fracture repair is thwarted and the bone fails to unite. Causes of non-union are: (1) distraction and separation of the fragments, sometimes the result of interposition of soft tissues between the fragments; (2) excessive movement at the fracture line; (3) a severe injury that renders the local tissues nonviable or nearly so; (4) a poor local blood supply and (5) infection. Of course surgical intervention, if ill-judged, is another cause!

Non-unions are septic or aseptic. In the latter group, they can be either stiff or mobile as judged by clinical examination. The mobile ones can be as free and painless as to give the impression of a false joint (*pseudoarthrosis*). On x-ray, non-unions are typified by a lucent line still present between the bone fragments; sometimes there is exuberant callus trying – but failing – to bridge the gap (*hypertrophic non-union*) or at times none at all (*atrophic non-union*) with a sorry, withered appearance to the fracture ends.

CLINICAL FEATURES

HISTORY

There is usually a history of injury, followed by inability to use the injured limb – but beware! The fracture is not always at the site of the injury: a blow to the knee may fracture the patella, femoral condyles, shaft of the femur or even acetabulum. The patient's age and mechanism of injury are important. If a fracture occurs with trivial trauma, suspect a pathological lesion. Pain, bruising and swelling are common symptoms but they do not distinguish a fracture from a soft-tissue injury. *Deformity* is much more suggestive.

Always enquire about symptoms of associated injuries: pain and swelling elsewhere (it is a common mistake to get distracted by the main injury, particularly if it is severe), numbness or loss of movement, skin pallor or cyanosis, blood in the urine, abdominal pain, difficulty with breathing or transient loss of consciousness.

Once the acute emergency has been dealt with, ask about previous injuries, or any other musculoskeletal abnormality that might cause confusion when the x-ray is seen. Finally, a general medical history is important, in preparation for anaesthesia or operation.

General signs

Unless it is obvious from the history that the patient has sustained a localized and fairly modest injury, priority must be given to dealing with the general effects of trauma (see Chapter 22). Follow the ABCs: look for, and if necessary attend to, **A**irway obstruction, **B**reathing problems, **C**irculatory problems and **C**ervical spine injury. During the secondary survey it will also be necessary to exclude other previously unsuspected injuries and to be alert to any possible predisposing cause (such as Paget's disease or a metastasis).

Local signs

Injured tissues must be handled gently. To elicit crepitus or abnormal movement is unnecessarily painful; x-ray diagnosis is more reliable. Nevertheless the familiar headings of clinical examination should always be considered, or damage to arteries, nerves and ligaments may be overlooked. A systematic approach is always helpful:

- Examine the most obviously injured part.
- Test for artery and nerve damage.
- Look for associated injuries in the region.
- Look for associated injuries in distant parts.

Look

Swelling, bruising and deformity may be obvious, but the important point is whether the skin is intact; if the skin is broken and the wound communicates with the fracture, the injury is 'open' ('compound'). Note also the posture of the distal extremity and the colour of the skin (for tell-tale signs of nerve or vessel damage).

Feel

The injured part is gently palpated for localized tenderness. Some fractures would be missed if not specifically looked for, e.g. the classical sign (indeed the only clinical sign!) of a fractured scaphoid is tenderness on pressure precisely in the anatomical snuff-box. The common and characteristic associated injuries should also be felt for, even if the patient does not complain of them. For example, an isolated fracture of the proximal fibula should always alert to the likelihood of an associated fracture or ligament injury of the ankle, and in high-energy injuries always examine the spine and pelvis. Vascular and peripheral nerve abnormalities should be tested for both before and after treatment.

Move

Crepitus and abnormal movement may be present, but why inflict pain when x-rays are available? It is more important to ask if the patient can move the joints distal to the injury.

X-ray

X-ray examination is mandatory. Remember the *rule of twos*:

- *Two views* – A fracture or a dislocation may not be seen on a single x-ray film, and at least two views (anteroposterior and lateral) must be taken.
- *Two joints* – In the forearm or leg, one bone may be fractured and angulated. Angulation, however, is impossible unless the other bone is also broken, or a joint dislocated. The joints above and below the fracture must both be included on the x-ray films.
- *Two limbs* – In children, the appearance of immature epiphyses may confuse the diagnosis of a fracture; x-rays of the uninjured limb are needed for comparison.
- *Two injuries* – Severe force often causes injuries at more than one level. Thus, with fractures of the calcaneum or femur it is important to also x-ray the pelvis and spine.
- *Two occasions* – Some fractures are notoriously difficult to detect soon after injury, but another x-ray examination a week or two later may show the lesion. Common examples are undisplaced fractures of the distal end of the clavicle, scaphoid, femoral neck and lateral malleolus, and also stress fractures and physeal injuries wherever they occur.

Special imaging

Sometimes the fracture – or the full extent of the fracture – is not apparent on the plain x-ray. Computed tomography may be helpful in lesions of the spine or for complex joint fractures; indeed, these cross-sectional images are essential for accurate visualization of fractures in 'difficult' sites such as the calcaneum or acetabulum. Magnetic resonance imaging may be the only way of showing whether a fractured vertebra is threatening to compress the spinal cord. Radioisotope scanning is helpful in diagnosing a suspected stress fracture or other undisplaced fractures.

Description

Diagnosing a fracture is not enough; the surgeon should picture it (and describe it) with its properties: (1) Is it open or closed? (2) Which bone is broken, and where? (3) Has it involved a joint surface? (4) What is the shape of the break? (5) Is it stable or unstable? (6) Is it a high-energy or a low-energy

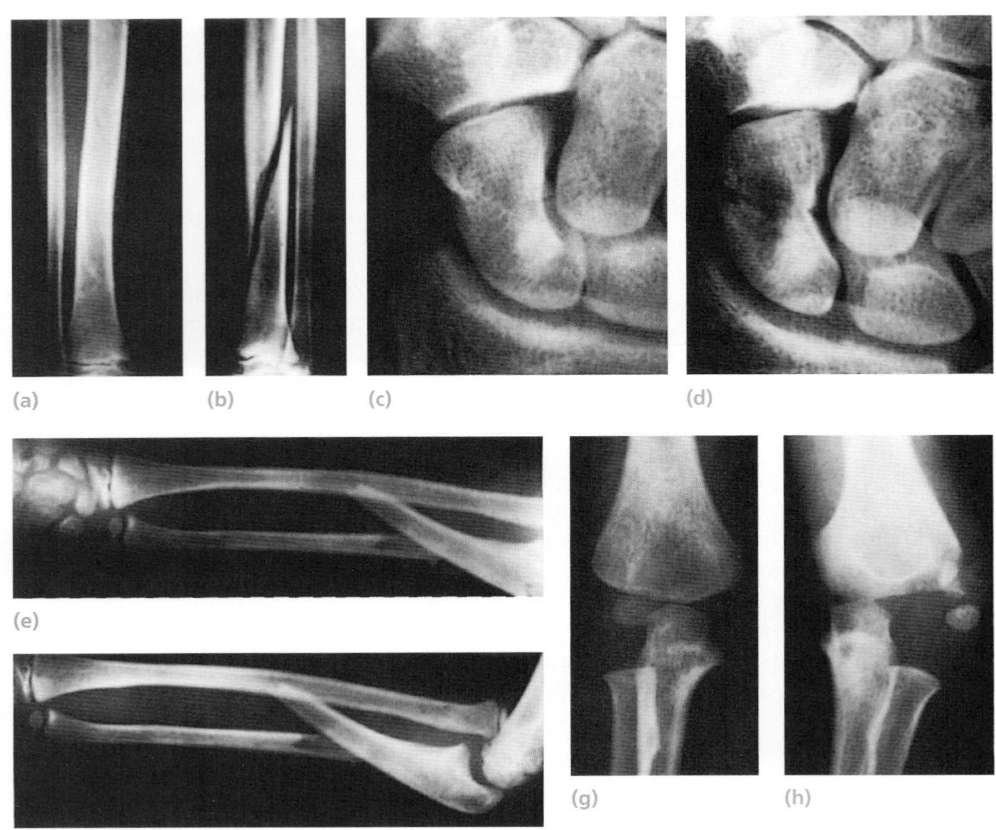

23.9 X-ray examination must be 'adequate' (a,b) Two films of the same tibia: the fracture may be 'invisible' in one view and perfectly plain in a view at right angles to that. (c,d) More than one occasion: A fractured scaphoid may not be obvious on the day of injury, but clearly seen 2 weeks later. (e,f) Two joints: The first x-ray (e) did not include the elbow. This was, in fact, a Monteggia fracture – the head of the radius is dislocated; (f) shows the dislocated radiohumeral joint. (g,h) Two limbs: Sometimes the abnormality can be appreciated only by comparision with the normal side; in this case there is a fracture of the lateral condyle on the left side (h).

injury? And last but not least (7) who is the person with the injury? In short, the examiner must learn to recognize what has been aptly described as the 'personality' of the fracture.

Shape of the fracture

A *transverse fracture* is slow to join because the area of contact is small; if the broken surfaces are accurately apposed, however, the fracture is stable on compression. A *spiral fracture* joins more rapidly (because the contact area is large) but is not stable on compression. *Comminuted fractures* are often slow to join because: (1) they are associated with more severe soft-tissue damage and (2) they are likely to be unstable.

Displacement

For every fracture, three components must be assessed:

1. *Shift or translation* – backwards, forwards, sideways, or longitudinally with impaction or overlap.
2. *Tilt or angulation* – sideways, backwards or forwards.
3. *Twist or rotation* – in any direction.

A problem often arises in the description of angulation. 'Anterior angulation' could mean that the apex of the angle points anteriorly or that the distal fragment is tilted anteriorly: in this text it is always the latter meaning that is intended ('anterior tilt of the distal fragment' is probably clearer).

SECONDARY INJURIES

Certain fractures are apt to cause secondary injuries and these should always be assumed to have occurred until proved otherwise:

- *Thoracic injuries* – Fractured ribs or sternum may be associated with injury to the lungs or heart. It is essential to check cardiorespiratory function.
- *Spinal cord injury* – With any fracture of the spine, neurological examination is essential to: (1) establish whether the spinal cord or nerve roots have been damaged and (2) obtain a baseline for later comparison if neurological signs should change.
- *Pelvic and abdominal injuries* – Fractures of the pelvis may be associated with visceral injury. It is especially important to enquire about urinary function; if a urethral or bladder injury is suspected, diagnostic urethrograms or cystograms may be necessary.
- *Pectoral girdle injuries* – Fractures and dislocations around the pectoral girdle may damage the brachial plexus or the large vessels at the base of the neck. Neurological and vascular examination is essential.

TREATMENT OF CLOSED FRACTURES

General treatment is the first consideration: *treat the patient, not only the fracture.* The principles are discussed in Chapter 22.

Treatment of the fracture consists of *manipulation* to improve the position of the fragments, followed by *splintage* to hold them together until they unite; meanwhile joint *movement* and function must be preserved. Fracture healing is promoted by physiological loading of the bone, so muscle activity and early *weightbearing* are encouraged. These objectives are covered by three simple injunctions:

- Reduce.
- Hold.
- Exercise.

Two existential problems have to be overcome. The first is how to hold a fracture adequately and yet permit the patient to use the limb sufficiently; this is a conflict (*Hold* versus *Move*) that the surgeon seeks to resolve as rapidly as possible (e.g. by internal fixation). However the surgeon also wants to avoid unnecessary risks – here is a second conflict (*Speed* versus *Safety*). This dual conflict epitomizes the four factors that dominate fracture management (the term 'fracture quartet' seems appropriate).

The fact that the fracture is closed (and not open) is no cause for complacency. The most important factor in determining the natural tendency to heal is the state of the surrounding soft tissues and the local blood supply. Low-energy (or low-velocity) fractures cause only moderate soft-tissue damage; high-energy (velocity) fractures cause severe soft-tissue damage, no matter whether the fracture is open or closed.

Tscherne (Oestern and Tscherne, 1984) has devised a helpful classification of closed injuries:

- *Grade 0* – a simple fracture with little or no soft-tissue injury.
- *Grade 1* – a fracture with superficial abrasion or bruising of the skin and subcutaneous tissue.
- *Grade 2* – a more severe fracture with deep soft-tissue contusion and swelling.
- *Grade 3* – a severe injury with marked soft-tissue damage and a threatened compartment syndrome.

The more severe grades of injury are more likely to require some form of mechanical fixation; good skeletal stability aids soft-tissue recovery.

REDUCTION

Although general treatment and resuscitation must always take precedence, there should not be undue delay in attending to the fracture; swelling of the soft parts during the first 12 hours makes reduction increasingly difficult. However, there are some situations in which reduction is unnecessary: (1) when there is little or no displacement; (2) when displacement does not matter initially (e.g. in fractures of the clavicle) and (3) when reduction is unlikely to succeed (e.g. with compression fractures of the vertebrae).

Reduction should aim for *adequate apposition* and *normal alignment* of the bone fragments. The greater the contact surface area between fragments the more likely healing is to occur. A gap between the fragment ends is a common cause of delayed union or non-union. On the other hand, so long as there is contact and the fragments are properly aligned, some overlap at the fracture surfaces is permissible. The exception is a fracture involving an articular surface; this should be reduced as near to perfection as possible because any irregularity will cause abnormal load distribution between the surfaces and predispose to degenerative changes in the articular cartilage.

There are two methods of reduction: closed and open.

Closed reduction

Under appropriate anaesthesia and muscle relaxation, the fracture is reduced by a three-fold manoeuvre: (1) the distal part of the limb is pulled in the line of the bone; (2) as the fragments disengage, they are repositioned (by reversing the original direction of force if this can be deduced) and (3) alignment is adjusted in each plane. This is most effective when the periosteum and muscles on one side of the fracture remain intact; the soft-tissue strap prevents over-reduction

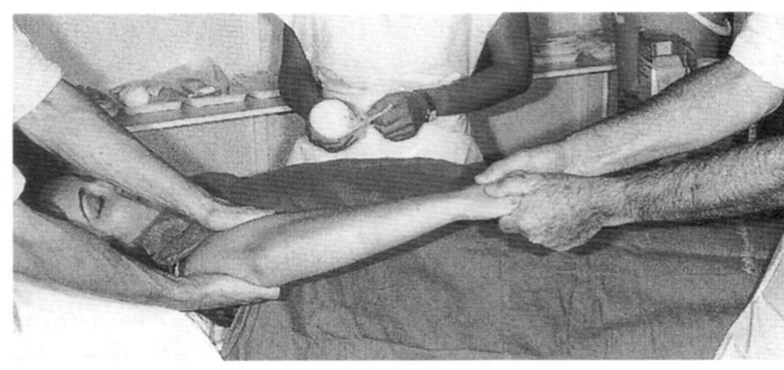
(a)

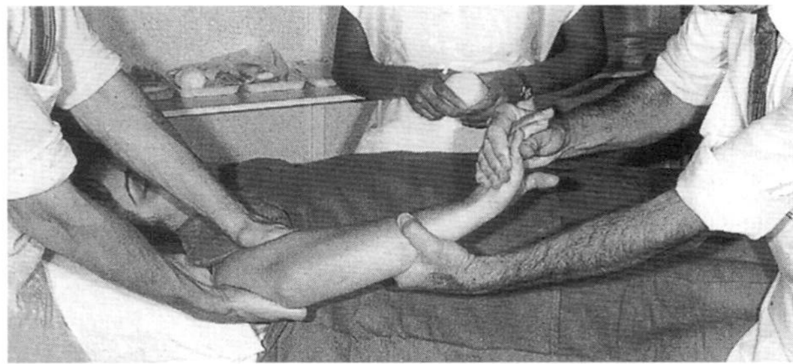
(b)

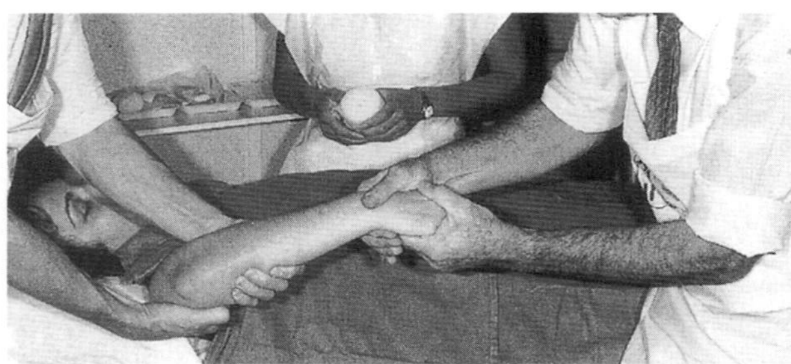
(c)

23.10 Closed reduction (a) Traction in the line of the bone. (b) Disimpaction. (c) Pressing fragment into reduced position.

and stabilizes the fracture after it has been reduced (Charnley 1961).

Some fractures are difficult to reduce by manipulation because of powerful muscle pull and may need prolonged traction. Skeletal or skin traction for several days allows for soft-tissue tension to decrease and a better alignment to be obtained; this practice is helpful for femoral and tibial shaft fractures and even supracondylar humeral fractures in children.

In general, closed reduction is used for all minimally displaced fractures, for most fractures in children and for fractures that are not unstable after reduction and can be held in some form of splint or cast. Unstable fractures can also be reduced using closed methods prior to stabilization with internal or external fixation. This avoids direct manipulation of the fracture site by open reduction, which damages the local blood supply and may lead to slower healing times; increasingly, surgeons resort to reduction manoeuvres that avoid fracture-site exposure, even when the aim is some form of internal or external fixation. Traction, which reduces fracture fragments through *ligamentotaxis* (ligament pull), can usually be applied by using a fracture table or bone distractor.

OPEN REDUCTION

Operative reduction of the fracture under direct vision is indicated: (1) when closed reduction fails, either because of difficulty in controlling the fragments or because soft tissues are interposed between them; (2) when there is a large articular fragment that needs accurate positioning or (3) for traction (avulsion) fractures in which the fragments are held apart. As a rule, however, open reduction is merely the first step to internal fixation.

HOLD REDUCTION

The word 'immobilization' has been deliberately avoided because the objective is seldom complete immobility; usually it is the prevention of displacement. Nevertheless, some restriction of movement is needed to promote soft-tissue healing and to allow free movement of the unaffected parts.

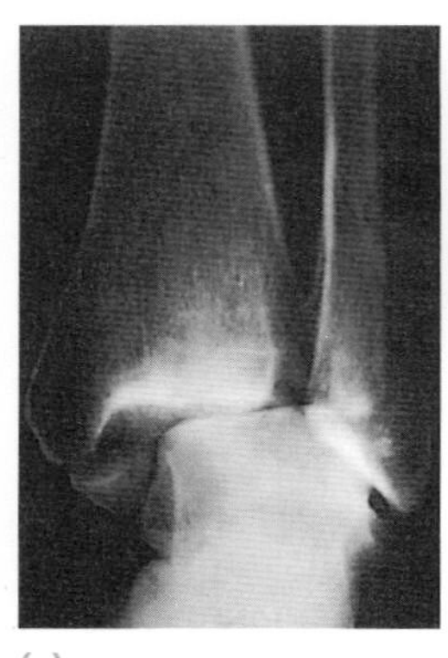
(a)

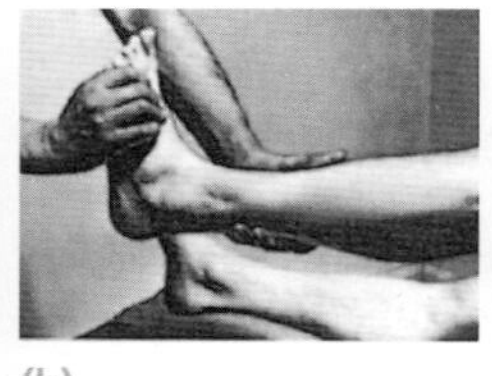
(b)

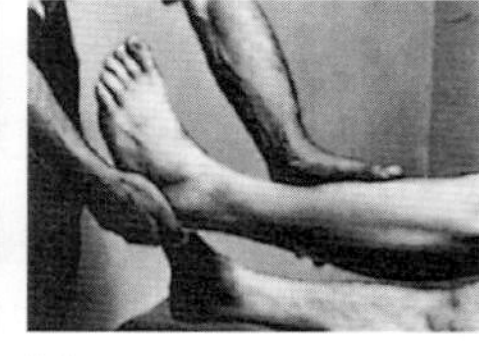
(c)

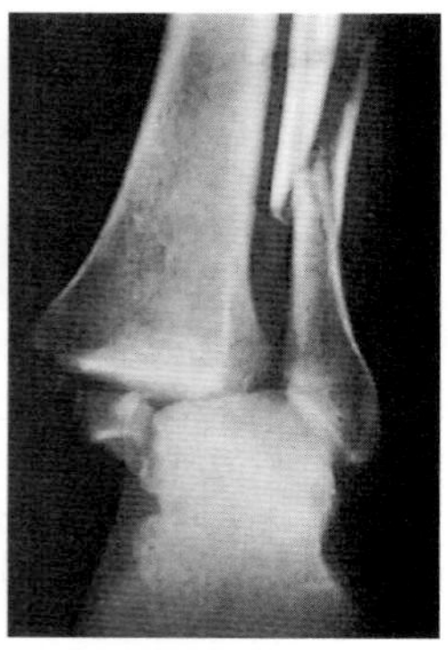
(d)

23.11 Closed reduction These two ankle fractures look somewhat similar but are caused by different forces. The causal force must be reversed to achieve reduction: (a) requires internal rotation (b); an adduction force (c) is needed for (d).

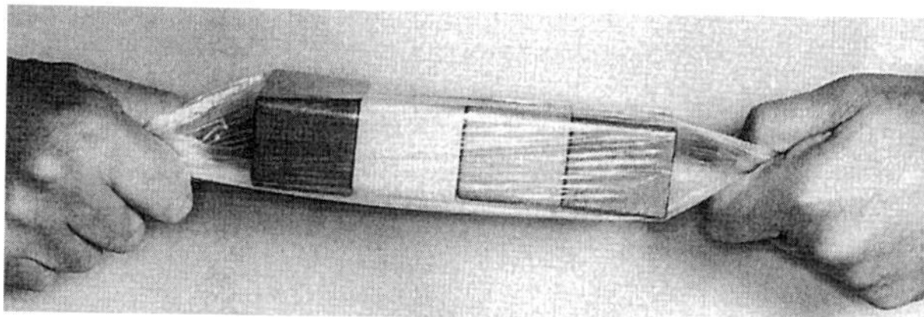

23.12 **Hold reduction** Showing how, if the soft tissues around a fracture are intact, traction will align the bony fragments.

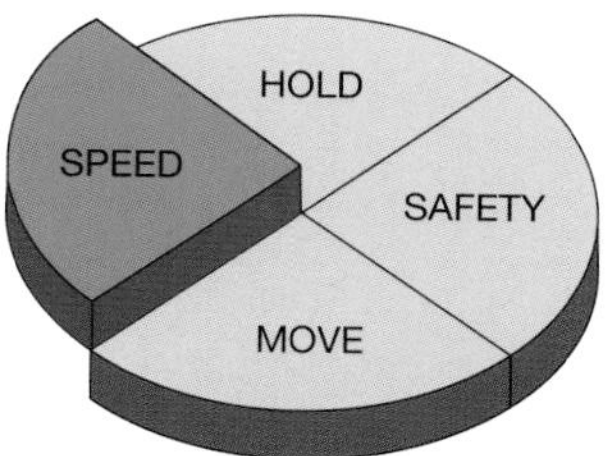

23.13 **Continuous traction** 'Speed' is the weak member of the quartet.

The available methods of holding reduction are:

- Continuous traction.
- Cast splintage.
- Functional bracing.
- Internal fixation.
- External fixation.

In the modern technological age, 'closed' methods are often scorned – an attitude arising from ignorance rather than experience. The muscles surrounding a fracture, if they are intact, act as a fluid compartment; traction or compression creates a hydraulic effect that is capable of splinting the fracture. Therefore closed methods are most suitable for fractures with intact soft tissues, and are liable to fail if they are used as the primary method of treatment for fractures with severe soft-tissue damage. Other contraindications to non-operative methods are inherently unstable fractures, multiple fractures and fractures in confused or uncooperative patients. If these constraints are borne in mind, closed reduction can be sensibly considered in choosing the most suitable method of fracture splintage. Remember, too, that the objective is to splint the fracture, not the entire limb!

CONTINUOUS TRACTION

Traction is applied to the limb distal to the fracture, so as to exert a continuous pull in the long axis of the bone, with a counterforce in the opposite direction (to prevent the patient being merely dragged along the bed). This is particularly useful for shaft fractures that are oblique or spiral and easily displaced by muscle contraction.

Traction cannot *hold* a fracture still; it can pull a long bone straight and hold it out to length but to maintain accurate reduction is sometimes difficult. Meanwhile the patient can *move* the joints and exercise the muscles.

Traction is safe enough, provided it is not excessive and care is taken when inserting the traction pin. The problem is *speed*: not because the fracture unites slowly (it does not) but because lower limb traction keeps the patient in hospital. Consequently, as soon as the fracture is 'sticky' (deformable but not displaceable), traction should be replaced by bracing, if this method is feasible. Traction includes:

- *Traction by gravity* – This applies only to upper limb injuries. Thus, with a wrist sling the weight of the arm provides continuous traction to the humerus. For comfort and stability, especially with a transverse fracture, a U-slab of plaster may be bandaged on or, better, a removable plastic sleeve from the axilla to just above the elbow is held on with Velcro.
- *Skin traction* – Skin traction will sustain a pull of no more than 4 or 5 kg. Holland strapping or one-way-stretch Elastoplast is stuck to the shaved skin and held on with a bandage. The malleoli are protected by Gamgee tissue, and cords or tapes are used for traction.
- *Skeletal traction* – A stiff wire or pin is inserted – usually behind the tibial tubercle for hip, thigh and knee injuries, or through the calcaneum for tibial fractures – and cords tied to them for applying traction. Whether by skin or skeletal traction, the fracture is reduced and held in one of three ways: fixed traction, balanced traction or a combination of the two.

Fixed traction

The pull is exerted against a fixed point. The usual method is to tie the traction cords to the distal end of a Thomas' splint and pull the leg down until the proximal, padded ring of the splint abuts firmly against the pelvis.

Balanced traction

Here the traction cords are guided over pulleys at the foot of the bed and loaded with weights; counter-traction is provided by the weight of the body when the foot of the bed is raised.

Combined traction

If a Thomas' splint is used, the tapes are tied to the end of the splint and the entire splint is then suspended, as in balanced traction.

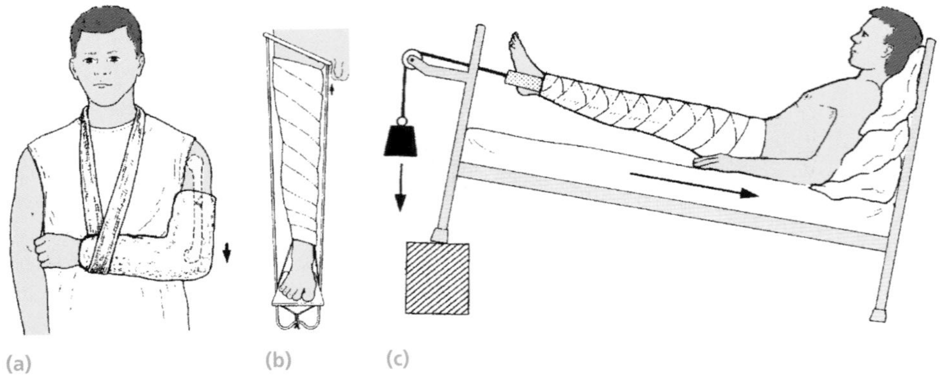

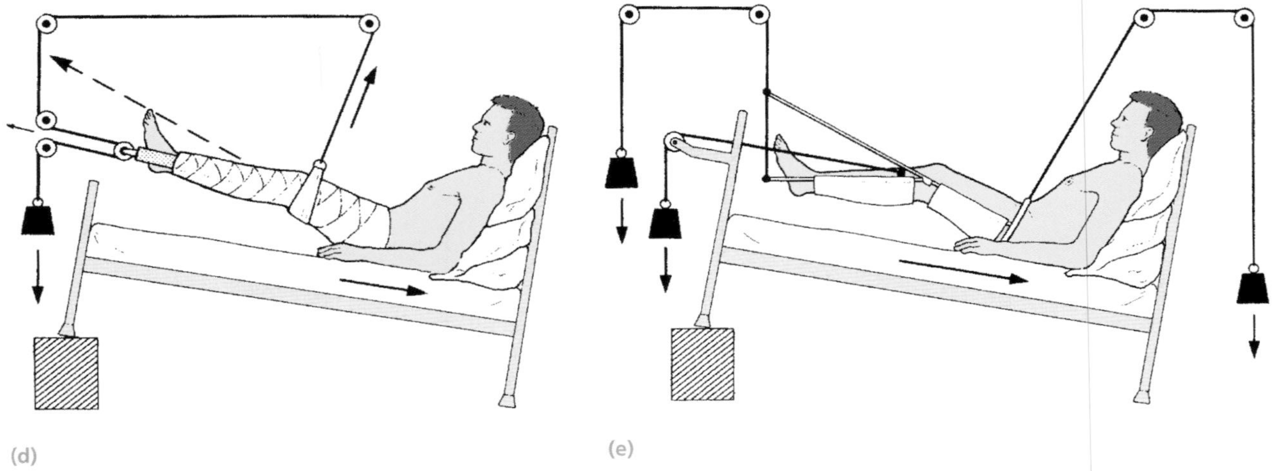

23.14 Methods of traction (a) Traction by gravity. (b,c,d) Skin traction: (b) fixed; (c) balanced; (d) Russell. (e) Skeletal traction with a splint and a knee-flexion piece.

Complications of traction

Circulatory embarrassment In children especially, traction tapes and circular bandages may constrict the circulation; for this reason 'gallows traction', in which the baby's legs are suspended from an overhead beam, should never be used for children over 12 kg in weight.

Nerve injury In older people, leg traction may predispose to peroneal nerve injury and cause a drop-foot; the limb should be checked repeatedly to see that it does not roll into external rotation during traction.

Pin site infection Pin sites must be kept clean and should be checked daily.

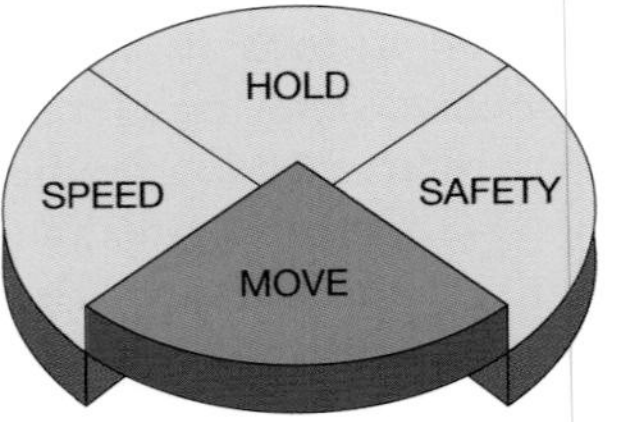

23.15 Casts 'Move' is the weakest member of the quartet.

Cast splintage

Plaster of Paris is still widely used as a splint, especially for distal limb fractures and for most children's fractures. It is safe enough, so long as the practitioner is alert to the danger of a tight cast and provided pressure sores are prevented. The speed of union is neither greater nor less than with traction, but the patient can go home sooner. Holding reduction is usually no problem and patients with tibial fractures can bear weight on the cast. However, joints encased in plaster cannot move and are liable to stiffen; stiffness, which has earned the sobriquet 'fracture disease', is the problem with conventional casts. While the swelling and haematoma resolve, adhesions may form that bind muscle fibres to each other and to the bone; with articular fractures, plaster perpetuates surface irregularities (closed reduction is seldom perfect) and lack of movement inhibits the healing of cartilage defects. Newer substitutes have some advantages over plaster (they are impervious to water, and also lighter) but as long as they are used as full casts the basic drawback is the same.

Stiffness can be minimized by: (1) delayed splintage – that is, by using traction until movement has been regained, and only then applying plaster; or (2)

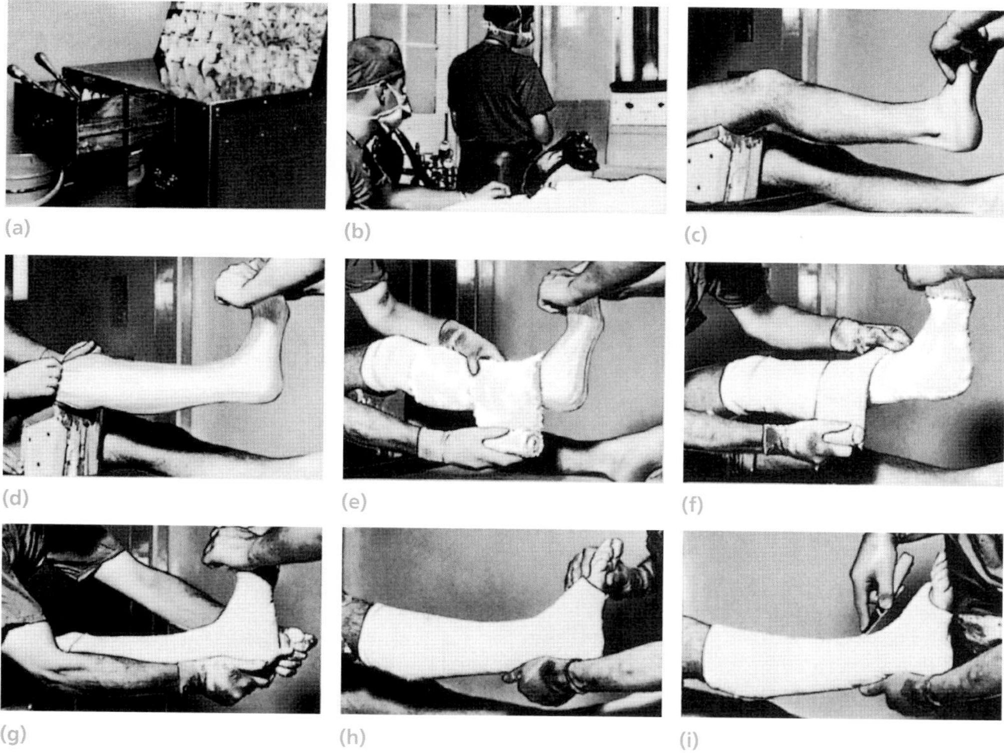

23.16 Plaster technique Applying a well-fitting and effective plaster needs experience and attention to detail. (a) A well-equipped plaster trolley is invaluable. (b) Adequate anaesthesia and careful study of the x-ray films are both indispensable. (c) For a below-knee plaster the thigh is best supported on a padded block. (d) Stockinette is threaded smoothly onto the leg. (e) For a padded plaster the wool is rolled on and it must be even. (f) Plaster is next applied smoothly, taking a tuck with each turn, and (g) smoothing each layer firmly onto the one beneath. (h) While still wet the cast is moulded away from the point points. (i) With a recent injury the plaster is then split.

starting with a conventional cast but, after a few weeks, when the limb can be handled without too much discomfort, replacing the cast by a functional brace which permits joint movement.

Technique

After the fracture has been reduced, stockinette is threaded over the limb and the bony points are protected with wool. Plaster is then applied. While it is setting the surgeon moulds it away from bony prominences; with shaft fractures three-point pressure can be applied to keep the intact periosteal hinge under tension and thereby maintain reduction.

If the fracture is recent, further swelling is likely; the plaster and stockinette are therefore split from top to bottom, exposing the skin. Check x-rays are essential and the plaster can be wedged if further correction of angulation is necessary.

With fractures of the shafts of long bones, rotation is controlled only if the plaster includes the joints above and below the fracture. In the lower limb, the knee is usually held slightly flexed, the ankle at a right angle and the tarsus and forefoot neutral (this 'plantigrade' position is essential for normal walking). In the upper limb the position of the splinted joints varies with the fracture. Splintage must not be discontinued (though a functional brace may be substituted) until the fracture is consolidated; if plaster changes are needed, check x-rays are essential.

Complications

Plaster immobilization is safe, but only if care is taken to prevent certain complications. These are tight cast, pressure sores and abrasion or laceration of the skin.

Tight cast The cast may be put on too tightly, or it may become tight if the limb swells. The patient complains of diffuse pain; only later – sometimes much later – do the signs of vascular compression appear. The limb should be elevated, but if the pain persists, the only safe course is to split the cast and ease it open: (1) throughout its length and (2) through all the padding down to skin. Whenever swelling is anticipated the cast should be applied over thick padding and the plaster

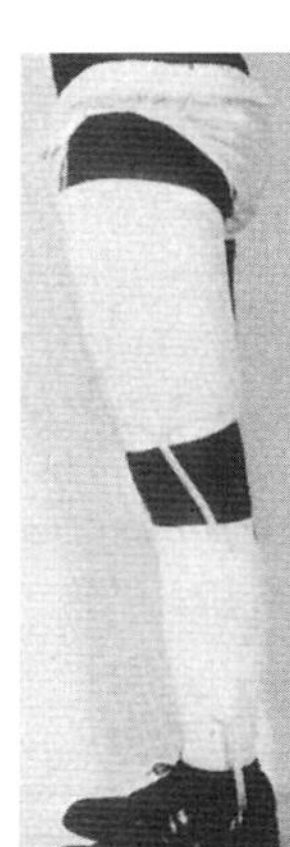
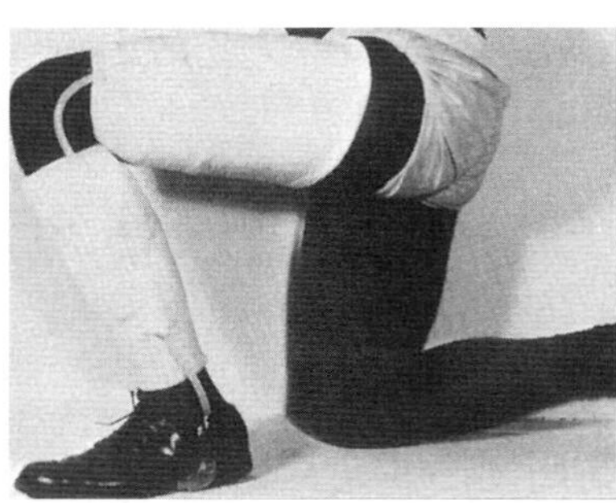
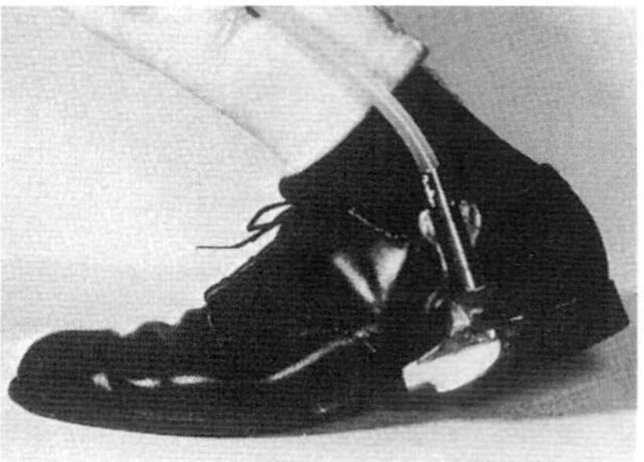

23.17 Functional bracing (cast bracing) Despite plaster the patient has excellent joint movement. (Courtesy of Dr John A Feagin).

should be split before it sets, so as to provide a firm but not absolutely rigid splint.

Pressure sores Even a well-fitting cast may press upon the skin over a bony prominence (the patella, heel, elbow or head of the ulna). The patient complains of localized pain precisely over the pressure spot. Such localized pain demands immediate inspection through a window in the cast.

Skin abrasion or laceration This is really a complication of removing plasters, especially if an electric saw is used. Complaints of nipping or pinching during plaster removal should never be ignored; a ripped forearm is a good reason for litigation.

Loose cast Once the swelling has subsided, the cast may no longer hold the fracture securely. If it is loose, the cast should be replaced.

FUNCTIONAL BRACING

Functional bracing, using either plaster of Paris or one of the lighter thermoplastic materials, is one way of preventing joint stiffness while still permitting fracture splintage and loading. Segments of a cast are applied only over the shafts of the bones, leaving the joints free; the cast segments are connected by metal or plastic hinges that allow movement in one plane. The splints are 'functional' in that joint movements are much less restricted than with conventional casts.

Functional bracing is used most widely for fractures of the femur or tibia, but since the brace is not very rigid, it is usually applied only when the fracture is beginning to unite, i.e. after 3–6 weeks of traction or conventional plaster. Used in this way, it comes out well on all four of the basic requirements: the fracture can be *held* reasonably well; the joints can be *moved*; the fracture joins at normal *speed* (or perhaps slightly quicker) without keeping the patient in hospital and the method is *safe*.

Technique

Considerable skill is needed to apply an effective brace. First the fracture is 'stabilized': by a few days on traction or in a conventional plaster for tibial fractures; and by a few weeks on traction for femoral fractures (until the fracture is sticky, i.e. deformable but not displaceable). Then a hinged cast or splint is applied, which holds the fracture snugly but permits joint movement; functional activity, including weight-bearing, is encouraged. Unlike internal fixation, functional bracing holds the fracture through compression of the soft tissues; the small amount of movement that occurs at the fracture site through using the limb encourages vascular proliferation and callus formation. Details of the rationale, technique and applications are given by Sarmiento and Latta (Sarmiento and Latta 1999, 2006).

INTERNAL FIXATION

Bone fragments may be fixed with screws, a metal plate held by screws, a long intramedullary rod or nail (with or without locking screws), circumferential bands or a combination of these methods.

Properly applied, internal fixation holds a fracture securely so that movement can begin at once; with early movement the 'fracture disease' (stiffness and

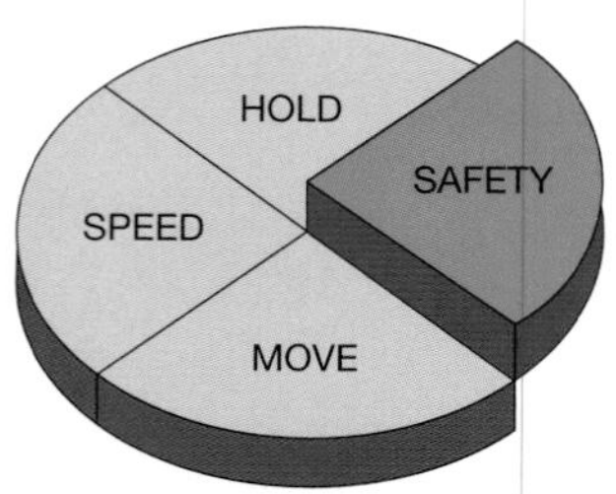

23.18 Internal fixation 'Safety' is the weak member of the quartet.

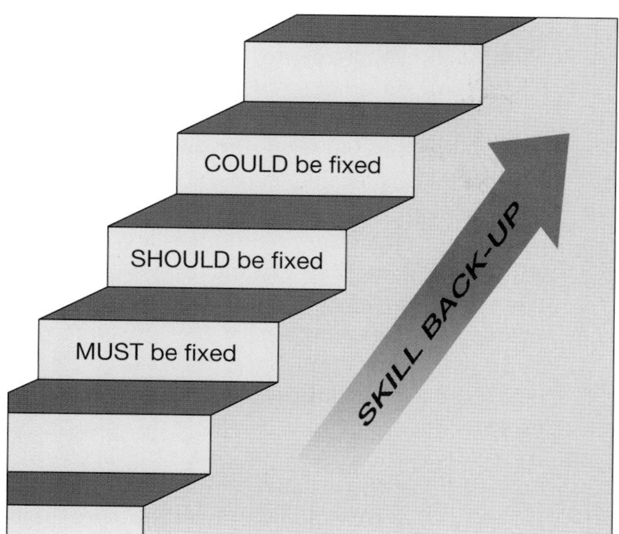

23.19 Indications staircase The indications for fixation are not immutable; thus, if the surgical skill or back-up facilities (staff, sterility and equipment) are of a low order, internal fixation is indicated only when the alternative is unacceptable (e.g. with femoral neck fractures). With average skill and facilities, fixation is indicated when alternative methods are possible but very difficult or unwise (e.g. multiple injuries). With the highest levels of skill and facilities, fixation is reasonable if it saves time, money or beds.

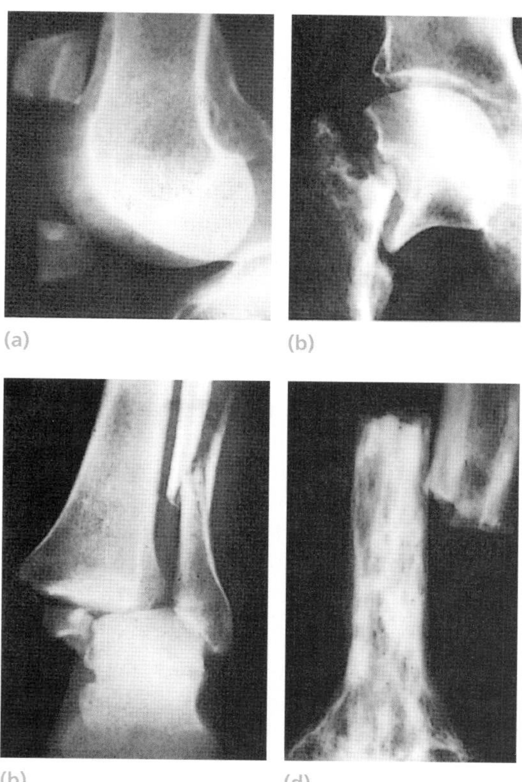

23.20 Indications for internal fixation (a) This patella has been pulled apart and can be held together only be internal fixation. (b) Fracture dislocation of the ankle is often unstable after reduction and usually requires fixation. (c) This patient was considered to be too ill for operation; her femoral neck fracture has failed to unite without rigid fixation. (d) Pathological fracture in Paget bone; without fixation, union may not occur.

oedema) is abolished. As far as speed is concerned, the patient can leave hospital as soon as the wound is healed, but he must remember that, even though the bone moves in one piece, the fracture is not united – it is merely held by a metal bridge and unprotected weightbearing is, for some time, unsafe.

The greatest danger, however, is sepsis; if infection supervenes, all the manifest advantages of internal fixation (precise reduction, immediate stability and early movement) may be lost. The risk of infection depends upon: (1) the patient – devitalized tissues, a dirty wound and an unfit patient are all dangerous; (2) the surgeon – thorough training, a high degree of surgical dexterity and adequate assistance are all essential and (3) the facilities – a guaranteed aseptic routine, a full range of implants and staff familiar with their use are all indispensable.

Indications

Internal fixation is often the most desirable form of treatment. The chief indications are:

1. Fractures that cannot be reduced except by operation.
2. Fractures that are inherently unstable and prone to re-displace after reduction (e.g. mid-shaft fractures of the forearm and some displaced ankle fractures). Also included are those fractures liable to be pulled apart by muscle action (e.g. transverse fracture of the patella or olecranon).
3. Fractures that unite poorly and slowly, principally fractures of the femoral neck.
4. Pathological fractures in which bone disease may prevent healing.
5. Multiple fractures where early fixation (by either internal or external fixation) reduces the risk of general complications and late multisystem organ failure (Pape et al., 2005; Roberts et al., 2005).
6. Fractures in patients who present nursing difficulties (paraplegics, those with multiple injuries and the very elderly).

Types of internal fixation

Interfragmentary screws Screws that are only partially threaded (a similar effect is achieved by overdrilling the 'near' cortex of bone) exert a compression or 'lag' effect when inserted across two fragments. The technique is useful for reducing single fragments onto the main shaft of a tubular bone or fitting together fragments of a metaphyseal fracture.

Wires (transfixing, cerclage and tension-band) Transfixing wires, often passed percutaneously, can hold major fracture fragments together. They are used in situations where fracture healing is predictably quick (e.g. in children or for distal radius fractures), and some form of external splintage (usually a cast) is applied as supplementary support.

Cerclage and tension-band wires are essentially loops of wire passed around two bone fragments and then tightened to compress the fragments together. When using cerclage wires, make sure that the wires hug the bone and do not embrace any of the close-lying nerves or vessels.

Both techniques are used for patellar fractures: the tension-band wire is placed such that the maximum compressive force is over the tensile surface, which is usually the convex side of the bone.

Plates and screws This form of fixation is useful for treating metaphyseal fractures of long bones and diaphyseal fractures of the radius and ulna. Plates have five different functions:

1. *Neutralization* – when used to bridge a fracture and supplement the effect of interfragmentary lag screws; the plate is to resist torque and shortening.
2. *Compression* – often used in metaphyseal fractures where healing across the cancellous fracture gap may occur directly, without periosteal callus. This technique is less appropriate for diaphyseal fractures and there has been a move towards the use of long plates that span the fracture, thus achieving some stability without totally sacrificing the biological (and callus producing) effect of movement.
3. *Buttressing* – here the plate props up the 'overhang' of the expanded metaphyses of long bones (e.g. in treating fractures of the proximal tibial plateau).
4. *Tension-band* – using a plate in this manner, again on the tensile surface of the bone, allows compression to be applied to the biomechanically more advantageous side of the fracture.
5. *Anti-glide* – by fixing a plate over the tip of a spiral or oblique fracture line and then using the plate as a reduction aid, the anatomy is

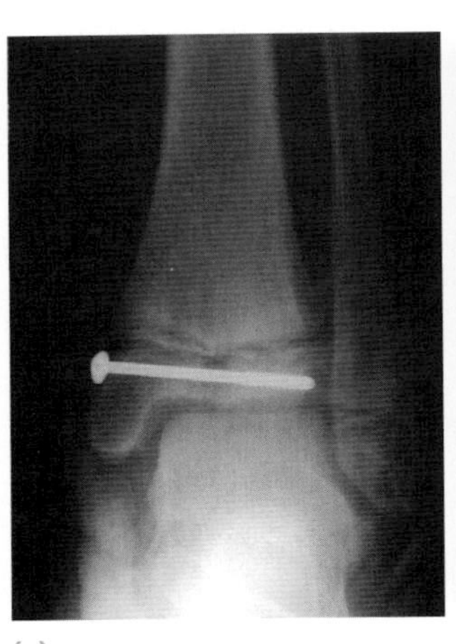

(a)

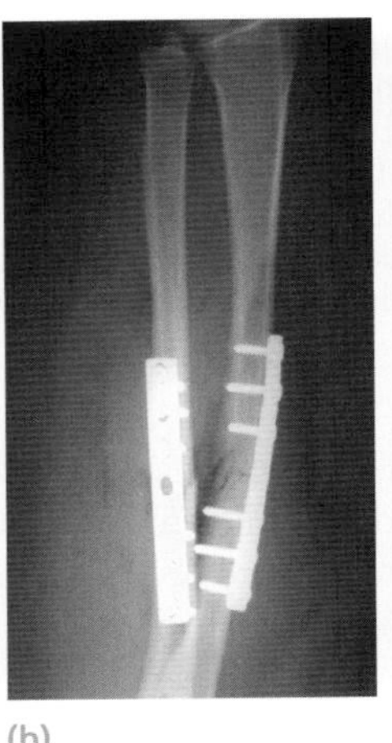

(b)

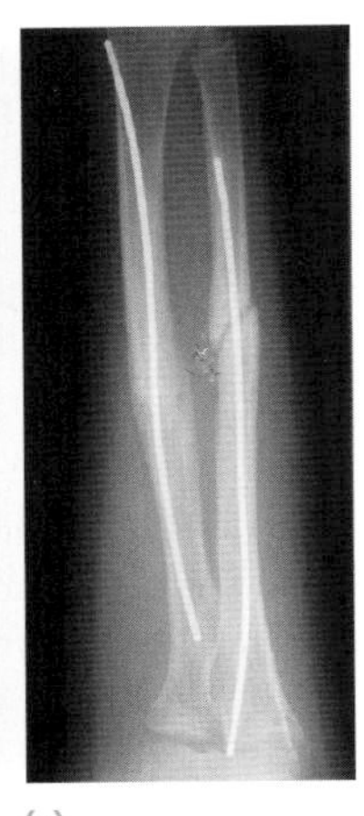

(c)

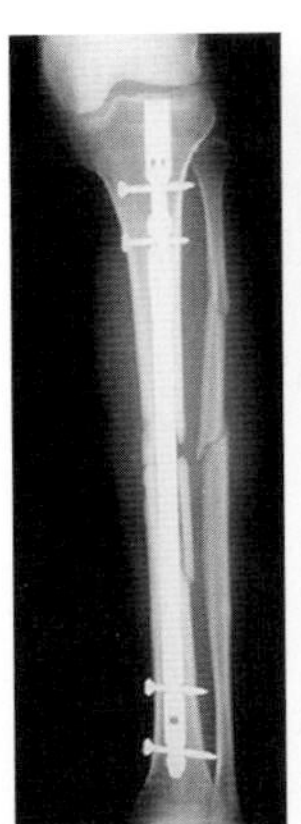

(d)

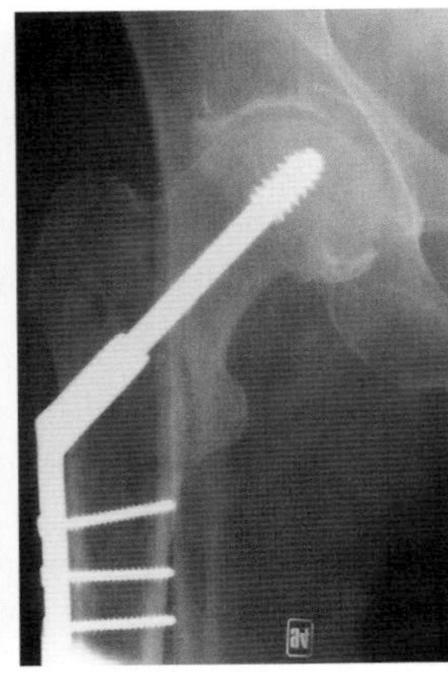

(e)

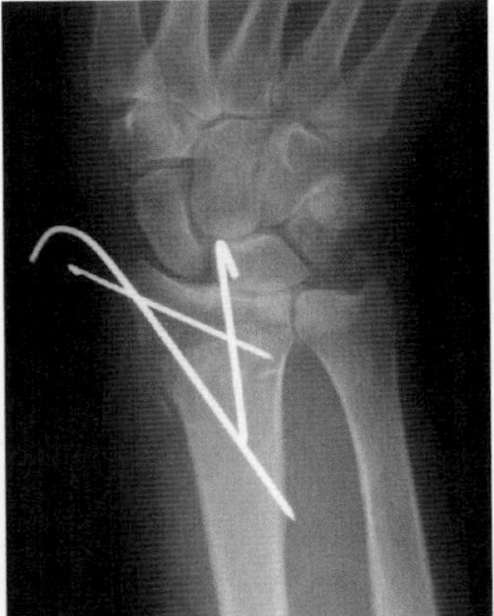

(f)

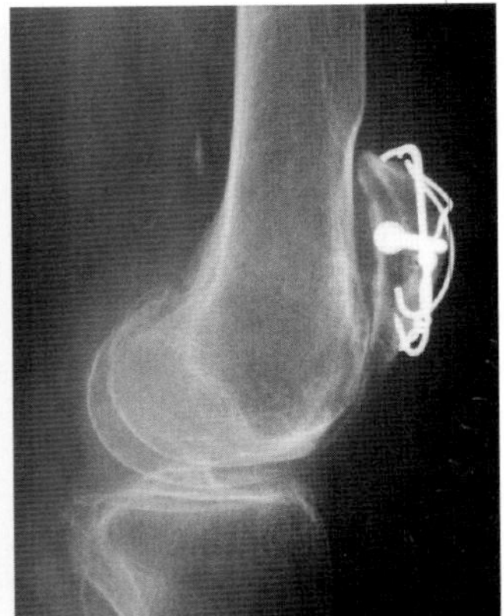

(g)

23.21 Internal fixation The method used must be appropriate to the situation: (a) screws – interfragmentary compression; (b) plate and screws – most suitable in the forearm or around the metaphysis; (c) flexible intramedullary nails – for long bones in children, particularly forearm bones and the femur; (d) interlocking nail and screws – ideal for the femur and tibia; (e) dynamic compression screw and plate – ideal for the proximal and distal ends of the femur; (f) simple K-wires – for fractures around the elbow and wrist and (g) tension-band wiring – for olecranon or fractures of the patella.

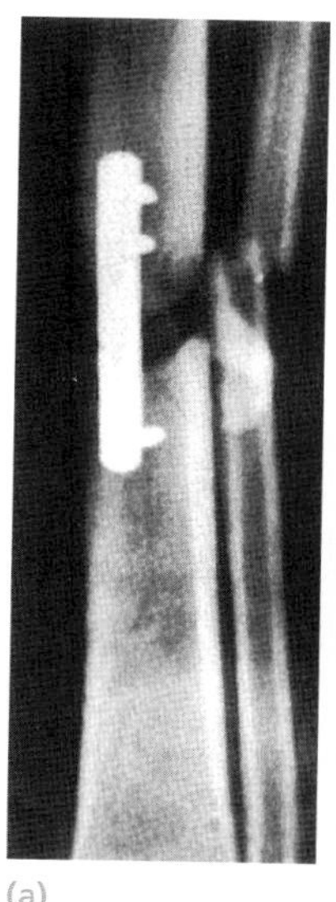
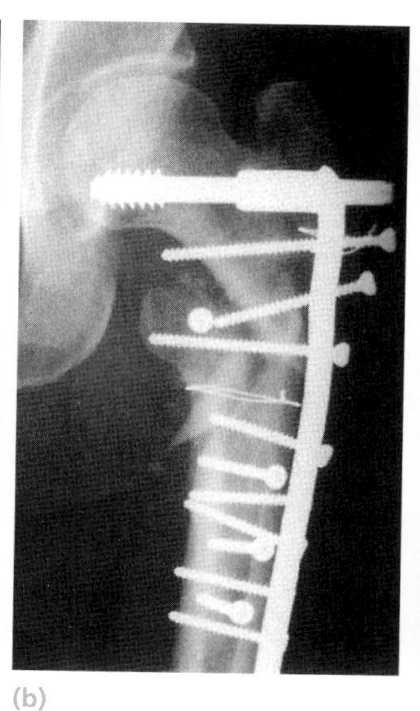
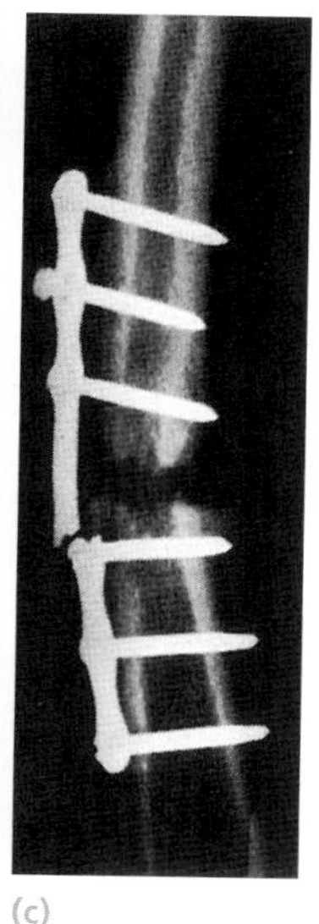
(a) (b) (c)

23.22 Bad fixation (how not to do it) (a) Too little. (b) Too much. (c) Too weak.

restored with minimal stripping of soft tissues. The position of the plate acts to prevent shortening and recurrent displacement of the fragments.

Intramedullary nails These are suitable for long bones. A nail (or long rod) is inserted into the medullary canal to splint the fracture; rotational forces are resisted by introducing transverse *interlocking screws* that transfix the bone cortices and the nail proximal and distal to the fracture. Nails are used with or without prior reaming of the medullary canal; reamed nails achieve an interference fit in addition to the added stability from interlocking screws, but at the expense of temporary loss of the intramedullary blood supply.

Complications of internal fixation

Most of the complications of internal fixation are due to poor technique, poor equipment or poor operating conditions:

Infection Iatrogenic infection is now the most common cause of chronic osteomyelitis; the metal does not predispose to infection but the operation and quality of the patient's tissues do.

Non-union If the bones have been fixed rigidly with a gap between the ends, the fracture may fail to unite. This is more likely in the leg or the forearm if one bone is fractured and the other remains intact. Other causes of non-union are stripping of the soft tissues and damage to the blood supply in the course of operative fixation.

Implant failure Metal is subject to fatigue and can fail unless some union of the fracture has occurred. Stress must therefore be avoided and a patient with a broken tibia internally fixed should walk with crutches and stay away from partial weightbearing for 6 weeks or longer, until callus or other radiological sign of fracture healing is seen on x-ray. Pain at the fracture site is a danger signal and must be investigated.

Refracture It is important not to remove metal implants too soon, or the bone may refracture. A year is the minimum and 18 or 24 months safer; for several weeks after removal the bone is weak, and care or protection is needed.

External fixation

A fracture may be held by transfixing screws or tensioned wires that pass through the bone above and below the fracture and are attached to an external frame. This is especially applicable to the tibia and pelvis, but the method is also used for fractures of the femur, humerus, lower radius and even bones of the hand.

Indications

External fixation is particularly useful for:

1. Fractures associated with severe soft-tissue damage (including open fractures) or those that are contaminated, where internal fixation is risky and repeated access is needed for wound inspection, dressing or plastic surgery.
2. Fractures around joints that are potentially suitable for internal fixation but the soft tissues are too swollen to allow safe surgery; here, a spanning external fixator provides stability until soft-tissue conditions improve.
3. Patients with severe multiple injuries, especially if there are bilateral femoral fractures, pelvic fractures with severe bleeding, and those with limb and associated chest or head injuries.

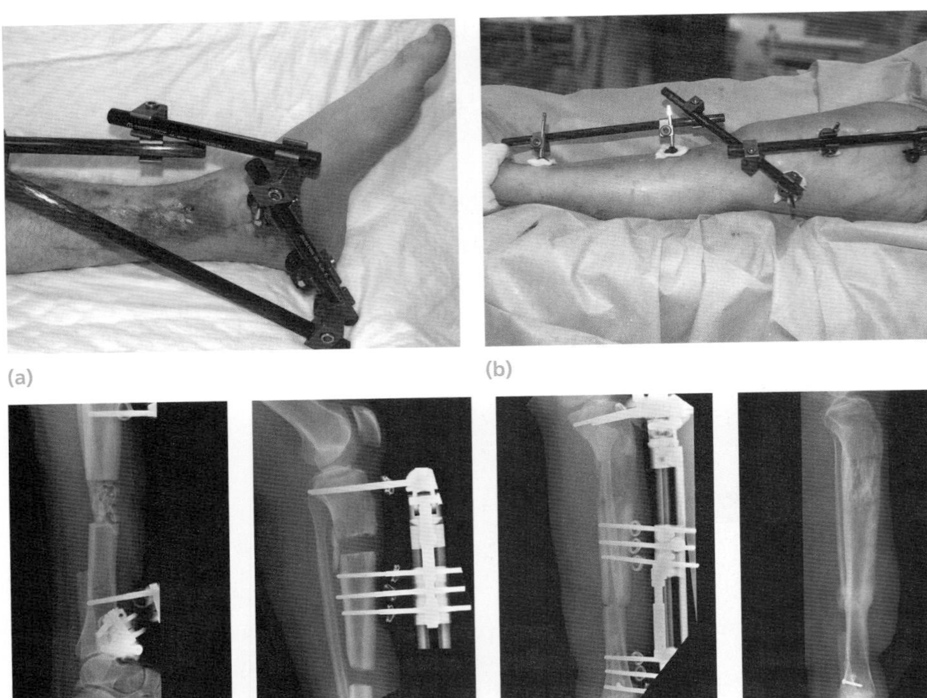

23.23 External fixation of fractures External fixation is widely used for 'damage control' **(a,b)** temporary stabilization of fractures in order to allow the patient's general condition or the state of soft tissues to improve prior to definitive surgery or **(c–f)** reconstruction of limbs using distraction osteogenesis. **(c)** A bone defect after surgical resection with gentamicin beads used to fill the space temporarily. **(d)** Bone transport from a more proximal osteotomy. **(e)** 'Docking' of the transported segment and **(f)** final union and restoration of structural integrity.

4. Ununited fractures, which can be excised and compressed; sometimes this is combined with bone lengthening to replace the excised segment.
5. Infected fractures, for which internal fixation might not be suitable.

Technique

The principle of external fixation is simple: the bone is transfixed above and below the fracture with screws or tensioned wires and these are then connected to each other by rigid bars. There are numerous types of external fixation devices; they vary in the technique of application and each type can be constructed to provide varying degrees of rigidity and stability. Most of them permit adjustment of length and alignment after application on the limb.

The fractured bone can be thought of as broken into segments – a simple fracture has two segments whereas a two-level (segmental) fracture has three and so on. Each segment should be held securely, ideally with the half-pins or tensioned wires straddling the length of that segment.

The wires and half-pins must be inserted with care. Knowledge of 'safe corridors' is essential so as to avoid injuring nerves or vessels; in addition, the entry sites should be irrigated to prevent burning of the bone (a temperature of only 50°C can cause bone death).

The fracture is then reduced by connecting the various groups of pins and wires by rods.

Depending on the stability of fixation and the underlying fracture pattern, weightbearing is started as early as possible to 'stimulate' fracture healing. Some fixators incorporate a telescopic unit that allows 'dynamization'; this will convert the forces of weightbearing into axial micromovement at the fracture site, thus promoting callus formation and accelerating bone union (Kenwright et al., 1991).

Complications

Damage to soft-tissue structures Transfixing pins or wires may injure nerves or vessels, or may tether ligaments and inhibit joint movement. The surgeon must be thoroughly familiar with the cross-sectional anatomy before operating.

Overdistraction If there is no contact between the fragments, union is unlikely.

Pin-track infection This is less likely with good operative technique. Nevertheless, meticulous pin-site care is essential, and antibiotics should be administered immediately if infection occurs.

EXERCISE

More correctly, restore function – not only to the injured parts but also to the patient as a whole. The objectives are to reduce oedema, preserve joint movement, restore muscle power and guide the patient back to normal activity:

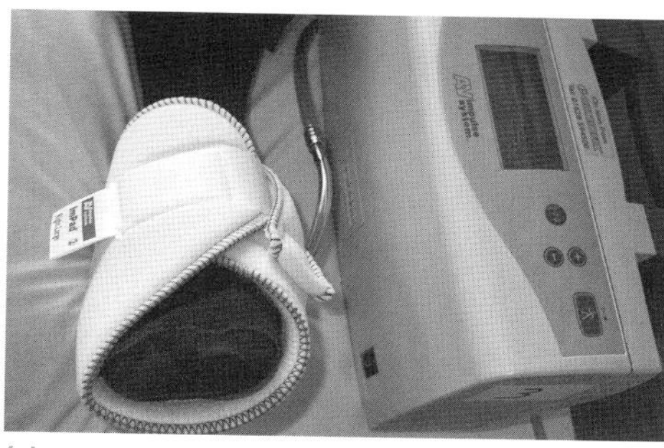

(a)

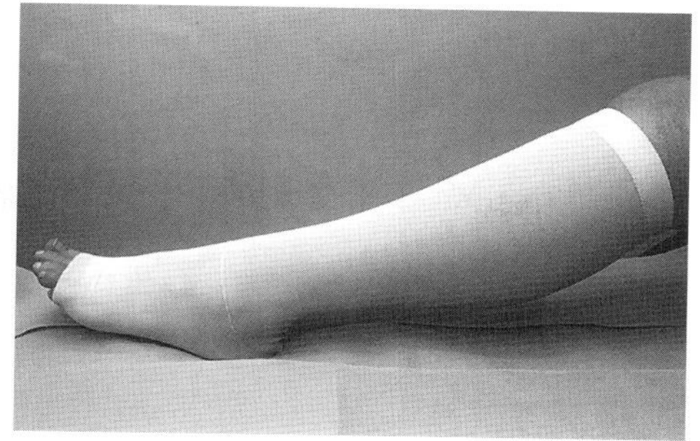

(b)

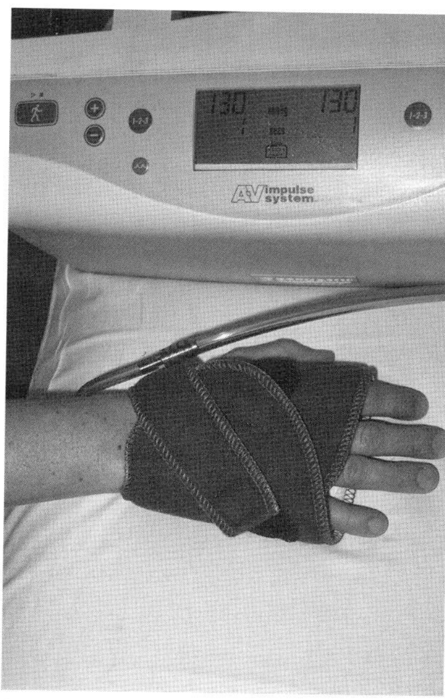

(c)

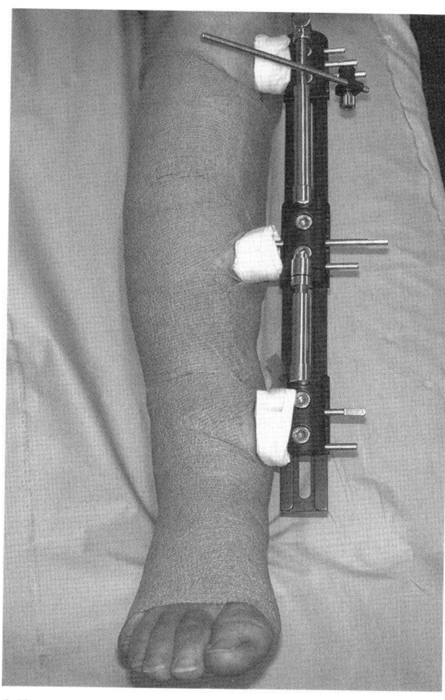

(d)

23.24 Some aspects of soft tissue treatment Swelling is minimized by improving venous drainage. This can be accomplished by: (1) elevation and (2) firm support. Stiffness is minimized by exercise. **(a,c)** Intermittent venous plexus pumps for use on the foot or palm to help reduce swelling. **(b)** A made-to-measure pressure garment that helps reduce swelling and scarring after treatment. **(d)** Coban wrap around a limb to control swelling during treatment.

Prevention of oedema Swelling is almost inevitable after a fracture and may cause skin stretching and blisters. Persistent oedema is an important cause of joint stiffness, especially in the hand; it should be prevented if possible, and treated energetically if it is already present, by a combination of elevation and exercise. Not every patient needs admission to hospital, and less severe injuries of the upper limb are successfully managed by placing the arm in a sling; but it is then essential to insist on active use, with movement of all the joints that are free. As with most closed fractures, in all open fractures and all fractures treated by internal fixation it must be assumed that swelling will occur; the limb should be elevated and active exercise begun as soon as the patient will tolerate this. The essence of soft-tissue care may be summed up thus: elevate and exercise; never dangle, never force.

Elevation An injured limb usually needs to be elevated; after reduction of a leg fracture the foot of the bed is raised and exercises are begun. If the leg is in plaster the limb must, at first, be dependent for only short periods; between these periods, the leg is elevated on a chair. The patient is allowed, and encouraged, to exercise the limb actively, but not to let it dangle. When the plaster is finally removed, a similar routine of activity punctuated by elevation is practised until circulatory control is fully restored.

Injuries of the upper limb also need elevation. A sling must not be a permanent passive arm-holder; the limb must be elevated intermittently or, if need be, continuously.

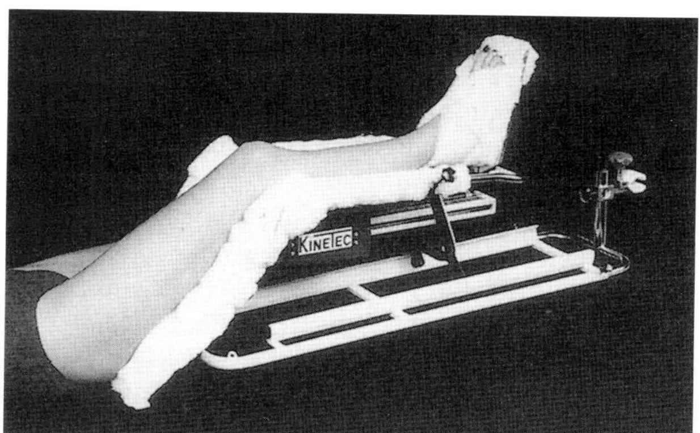

23.25 Continuous passive motion The motorized frame provides continuous flexion and extension to pre-set limits.

Active exercise Active movement helps to pump away oedema fluid, stimulates the circulation, prevents soft-tissue adhesion and promotes fracture healing. A limb encased in plaster is still capable of static muscle contraction and the patient should be taught how to do this. When splintage is removed the joints are mobilized and muscle-building exercises are steadily increased. Remember that the unaffected joints need exercising too; it is all too easy to neglect a stiffening shoulder while caring for an injured wrist or hand.

Assisted movement It has long been taught that passive movement can be deleterious, especially with injuries around the elbow, where there is a high risk of developing myositis ossificans. Certainly forced movements should never be permitted, but gentle assistance during active exercises may help to retain function or regain movement after fractures involving the articular surfaces. Nowadays this is done with machines that can be set to provide a specified range and rate of movement ('continuous passive motion').

Functional activity As the patient's mobility improves, an increasing amount of directed activity is included in the programme. He may need to be taught again how to perform everyday tasks such as walking, getting in and out of bed, bathing, dressing or handling eating utensils. Experience is the best teacher and the patient is encouraged to use the injured limb as much as possible. Those with very severe or extensive injuries may benefit from spending time in a special rehabilitation unit, but the best incentive to full recovery is the promise of re-entry into family life, recreational pursuits and meaningful work.

TREATMENT OF OPEN FRACTURES

INITIAL MANAGEMENT

Patients with open fractures may have multiple injuries; a rapid general assessment is the first step and any life-threatening conditions are addressed (see Chapter 22).

The open fracture may draw attention away from other more important conditions and it is essential that the step-by-step approach in advanced trauma life support not be forgotten.

When the fracture is ready to be dealt with, the wound is first carefully inspected; any gross contamination is removed, the wound is photographed with a Polaroid or digital camera to record the injury and the area then covered with a saline-soaked dressing under an impervious seal to prevent desiccation. This is left undisturbed until the patient is in the operating theatre. The patient is given antibiotics, usually co-amoxiclav or cefuroxime, but clindamycin if the patient is allergic to penicillin. Tetanus prophylaxis is administered: toxoid for those previously immunized, human antiserum if not. The limb is then splinted until surgery is undertaken.

The limb circulation and distal neurological status will need checking repeatedly, particularly after any fracture reduction manoeuvres. Compartment syndrome is not prevented by there being an open fracture; vigilance for this complication is wise.

CLASSIFYING THE INJURY

Treatment is determined by the type of fracture, the nature of the soft-tissue injury (including the wound size) and the degree of contamination. Gustilo's classification of open fractures is widely used (Gustilo et al., 1984):

Type I – The wound is usually a small, clean puncture through which a bone spike has protruded. There is little soft-tissue damage with no crushing and the fracture is not comminuted (i.e. a low-energy fracture).
Type II – The wound is more than 1 cm long, but there is no skin flap. There is not much soft-tissue damage and no more than moderate crushing or comminution of the fracture (also a low- to moderate-energy fracture).
Type III – There is a large laceration, extensive damage to skin and underlying soft tissue and, in the most severe examples, vascular compromise. The injury is caused by high-energy transfer to the bone and soft tissues. Contamination can be significant.

There are three grades of severity. In *type III A* the fractured bone can be adequately covered by soft tissue despite the laceration. In *type III B* there is extensive periosteal stripping and fracture cover is not possible without use of local or distant flaps. The fracture is classified as *type III C* if there is an arterial injury that needs to be repaired, regardless of the amount of other soft-tissue damage.

The incidence of wound infection correlates directly with the extent of soft-tissue damage, rising from less than 2 per cent in type I to more than 10 per cent in type III fractures.

PRINCIPLES OF TREATMENT

All open fractures, no matter how trivial they may seem, must be assumed to be contaminated; it is important to try to prevent them from becoming infected. The four essentials are:

- Antibiotic prophylaxis.
- Urgent wound and fracture debridement.
- Stabilization of the fracture.
- Early definitive wound cover.

Sterility and antibiotic cover

The wound should be kept covered until the patient reaches the operating theatre. In most cases co-amoxiclav or cefuroxime (or clindamycin if penicillin allergy is an issue) is given as soon as possible, often in the Accident and Emergency department. At the time of debridement, gentamicin is added to a second dose of the first antibiotic. Both antibiotics provide prophylaxis against the majority of Gram-positive and Gram-negative bacteria that may have entered the wound at the time of injury. Only co-amoxiclav or cefuroxime (or clindamycin) is continued thereafter; as wounds of Gustilo grade I fractures can be closed at the time of debridement, antibiotic prophylaxis need not be for more than 24 hours. With Gustilo grade II and IIIA fractures, some surgeons prefer to delay closure after a 'second look' procedure. Delayed cover is also usually practised in most cases of Grade IIIB and IIIC injuries. As the wounds have now been present in a hospital environment for some time, and there are data to indicate infections after such open fractures are caused mostly by hospital-acquired bacteria and not seeded at the time of injury, gentamicin and vancomycin (or teicoplanin) are given at the time of definitive wound cover. These antibiotics are effective against methicillin-resistant Staphylococcus aureus and Pseudomonas, both of which are near the top of the league table of responsible bacteria. The total period of antibiotic use for these fractures should not be greater than 72 hours (Table 23.1).

Debridement

The operation aims to render the wound free of foreign material and of dead tissue, leaving a clean surgical field and tissues with a good blood supply throughout. Under general anaesthesia the patient's clothing is removed, while an assistant maintains traction on the injured limb and holds it still. The dressing previously applied to the wound is replaced by a sterile pad and the surrounding skin is cleaned. The pad is then taken off and the wound is irrigated thoroughly with copious amounts of physiological saline. The wound is covered again and the patient's limb then prepped and draped for surgery.

Many surgeons prefer to use a tourniquet as this provides a bloodless field. However this induces ischaemia in an already badly injured leg and can make it difficult to recognize which structures are devitalized. A compromise is to apply the tourniquet but not to inflate it during the debridement unless absolutely necessary.

Because open fractures are often high-energy injuries with severe tissue damage, the operation should be performed by someone skilled in dealing with both skeletal and soft tissues; ideally this will be a joint effort by orthopaedic and plastic surgeons. The following principles must be observed:

Table 23.1 Antibiotics for open fractures[1]

	Grade I	Grade II	Grade IIIA	Grade IIIB/IIIC
As soon as possible (within 3 hours of injury)	Co-amoxiclav[2]	Co-amoxiclav[2]	Co-amoxiclav[2]	Co-amoxiclav[2]
At debridement	Co-amoxiclav[2] and gentamicin	Co-amoxiclav[2] and gentamicin	Co-amoxiclav[2] and gentamicin	Co-amoxiclav[2] and gentamicin
At definitive fracture cover	Wound cover is usually possible at debridement; delayed closure unnecessary	Wound cover is usually possible at debridement. If delayed, gentamicin and vancomycin (or teicoplanin) at the time of cover	Wound cover is usually possible at debridement. If delayed, gentamicin and vancomycin (or teicoplanin) at the time of cover	Gentamicin and vancomycin (or teicoplanin)
Continued prophylaxis	Only co-amoxiclav[2]* continued after surgery	Only co-amoxiclav[2] continued between procedures and after final surgery	Only co-amoxiclav[2] continued between procedures and after final surgery	Only co-amoxiclav[2] continued between procedures and after final surgery
Maximum period	24 hours	72 hours	72 hours	72 hours

[1]Based on the Standards for the Management of Open Fractures of the Lower Limb, British Orthopaedic Association and British Association of Plastic, Reconstructive and Aesthetic Surgeons, 2009
[2]Or cefuroxime (clindamycin for those with penicillin allergy).

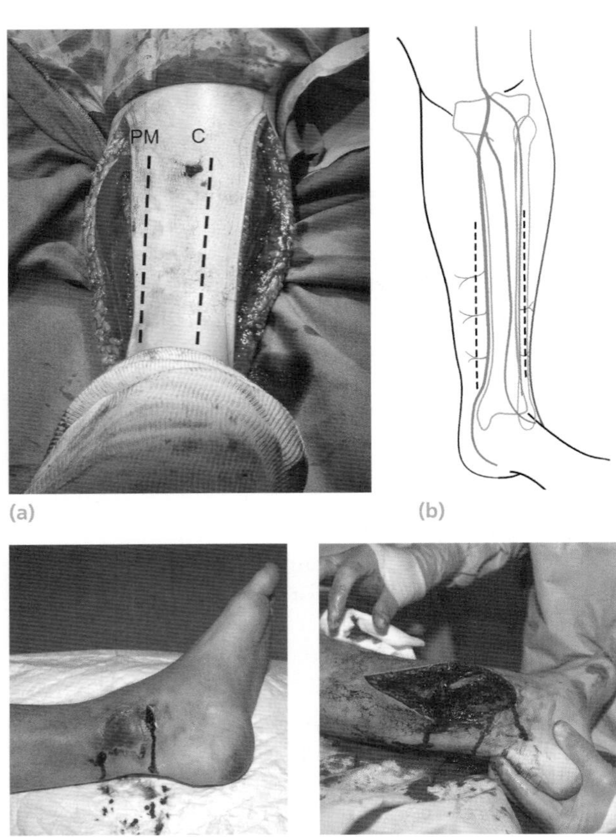

23.26 Wound extensions for access in open fractures of the tibia Wound incisions (extensions) for adequate access to an open tibial fracture are made along standard fasciotomy incisions: 1 cm behind the posteromedial border of the tibia and 2–3 cm lateral to the crest of the tibia as shown in this example of a two-incision fasciotomy. The dotted lines mark out the crest (C) and posteromedial corner (PM) of the tibia (a). These incisions avoid injury to the perforating branches that supply areas of skin that can be used as flaps to cover the exposed fracture (b). This clinical example shows how local skin necrosis around an open fracture is excised and the wound extended proximally along a fasciotomy incision (c,d).

Wound excision The wound margins are excised, but only enough to leave healthy skin edges.

Wound extension Thorough cleansing necessitates adequate exposure; poking around in a small wound to remove debris can be dangerous. If extensions are needed they should not jeopardize the creation of skin flaps for wound cover if this should be needed. The safest extensions are to follow the line of fasciotomy incisions; these avoid damaging important perforator vessels that can be used to raise skin flaps for eventual fracture cover.

Delivery of the fracture Examination of the fracture surfaces cannot be adequately performed without extracting the bone from within the wound. The simplest (and gentlest) method is to bend the limb in the manner in which it was forced at the moment of injury; the fracture surfaces will be exposed through the wound without any additional damage to the soft tissues. Large bone levers and retractors should not be used.

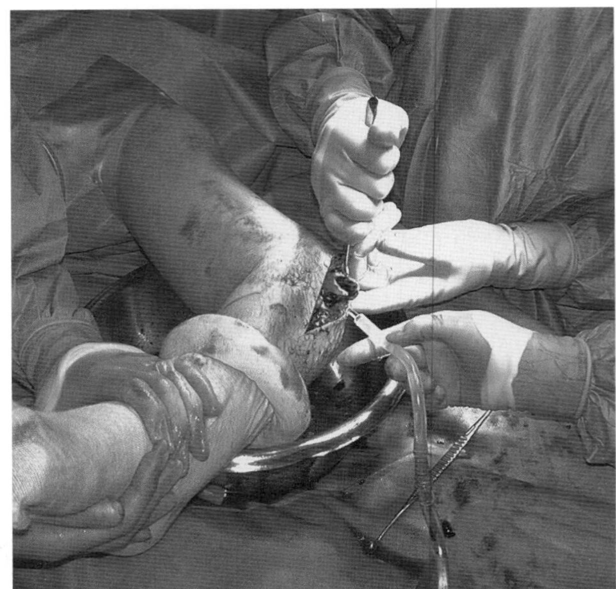

23.27 Delivering the fracture Debridement is only possible if the fracture is adequately seen; for this, the fracture ends have to be delivered from within.

Removal of devitalized tissue Devitalized tissue provides a nutrient medium for bacteria. Dead muscle can be recognized by its purplish colour, its mushy consistency, its failure to contract when stimulated and its failure to bleed when cut. All doubtfully viable tissue, whether soft or bony, should be removed. The fracture ends can be nibbled away until seen to bleed.

Wound cleansing All foreign material and tissue debris is removed by excision or through a wash with copious quantities of saline. A common mistake is to inject syringefuls of fluid through a small aperture – this only serves to push contaminants further in; 6–12 L of saline may be needed to irrigate and clean an open fracture of a long bone. Adding antibiotics or antiseptics to the solution has no added benefit.

Nerves and tendons As a general rule it is best to leave cut nerves and tendons alone, though if the wound is absolutely clean and no dissection is required – and provided the necessary expertise is available – they can be sutured.

Wound closure

A small, uncontaminated wound in a Grade I or II fracture may (after debridement) be sutured, provided this can be done without tension. In the more severe grades of injury, immediate fracture stabilization and wound cover using split-skin grafts, local or distant

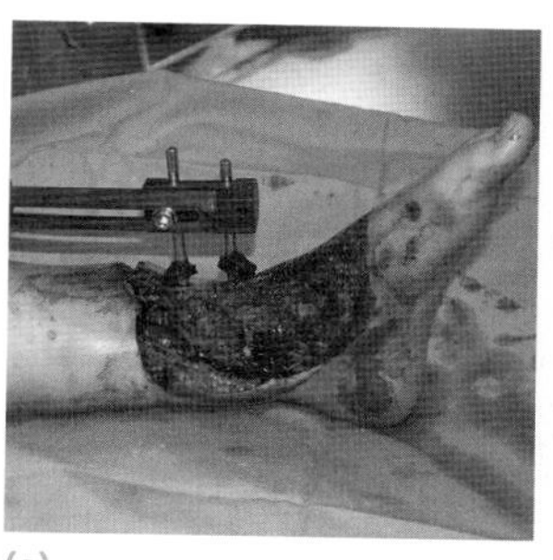
(a)

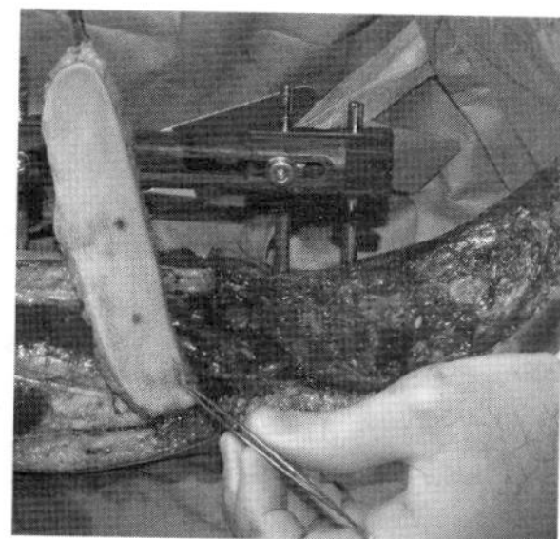
(b)

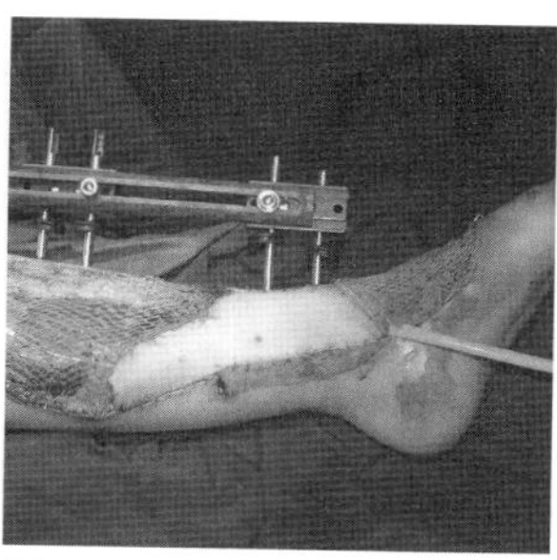
(c)

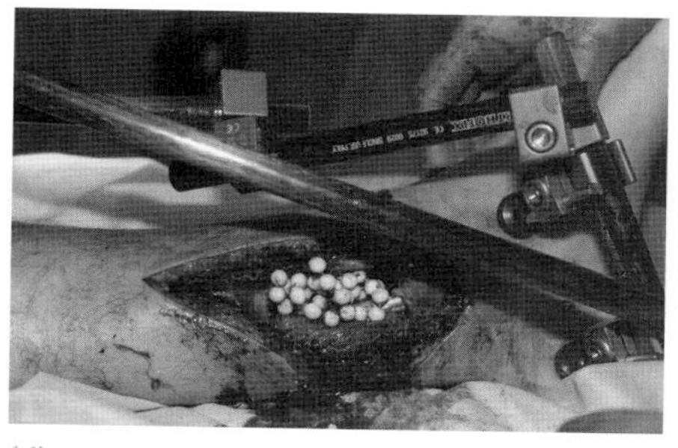
(d)

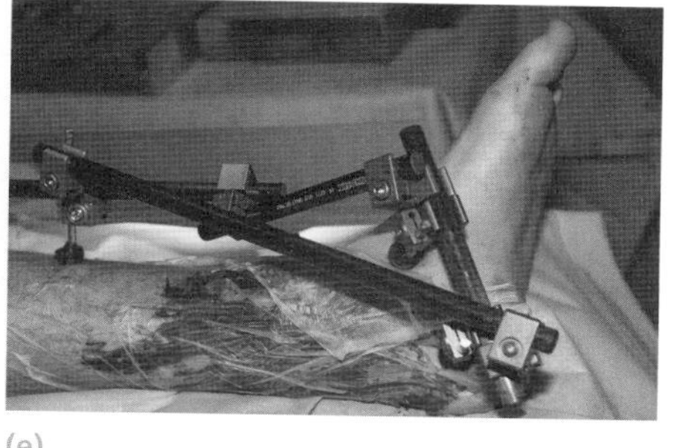
(e)

23.28 Covering the fracture The best fracture cover is skin or muscle – with the help of a plastic surgeon (a–c). If none is available, gentamicin beads can be inserted and sealed with an impervious dressing until the second operation, where a further debridement and, ideally, definitive fracture cover is obtained (d,e).

flaps is ideal, provided both orthopaedic and plastic surgeons are satisfied that a clean, viable wound has been achieved after debridement. In the absence of this combined approach at the time of debridement, the fracture is stabilized and the wound left open and dressed with an impervious dressing. Adding gentamicin beads under the dressing has been shown to help, as has the use of vacuum dressings. Return to surgery for a 'second look' should have definitive fracture cover as an objective. It should be done by 48–72 hours, and not later than 5 days. Open fractures do not fare well if left exposed for long and multiple debridement can be self-defeating.

Stabilizing the fracture

Stabilizing the fracture is important in reducing the likelihood of infection and assisting recovery of the soft tissues. The method of fixation depends on the degree of contamination, length of time from injury to operation and amount of soft-tissue damage. If there is no obvious contamination and definitive wound cover can be achieved at the time of debridement, open fractures of all grades can be treated as for a closed injury; internal or external fixation may be appropriate depending on the individual characteristics of the fracture and wound. This ideal scenario of judicious soft-tissue and bone debridement, wound cleansing, immediate stabilization and cover is only possible if orthopaedic and plastic surgeons are present at the time of initial surgery.

If wound cover is delayed, then external fixation is safer; however, the surgeon must take care to insert the fixator pins away from potential flaps needed by the plastic surgeon!

The external fixator may be exchanged for internal

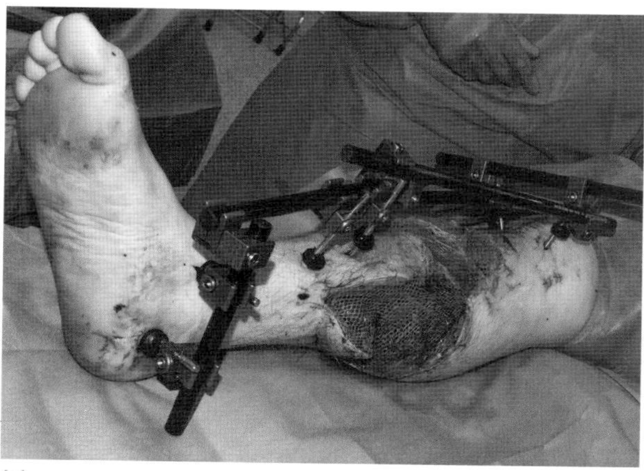
(a)

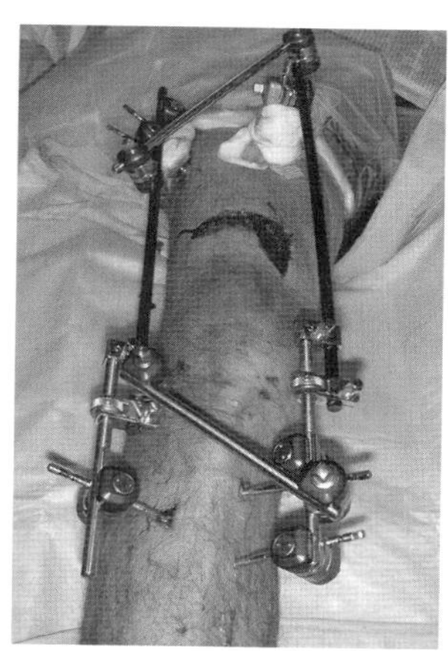
(b)

23.29 Stabilizing the limb in open fractures Spanning external fixation is a useful method of holding the fracture in the first instance (a,b). When definitive fracture cover is carried out, this can be substituted with internal fixation, provided the wound is clean and the interval between the two procedures is less than 7 days.

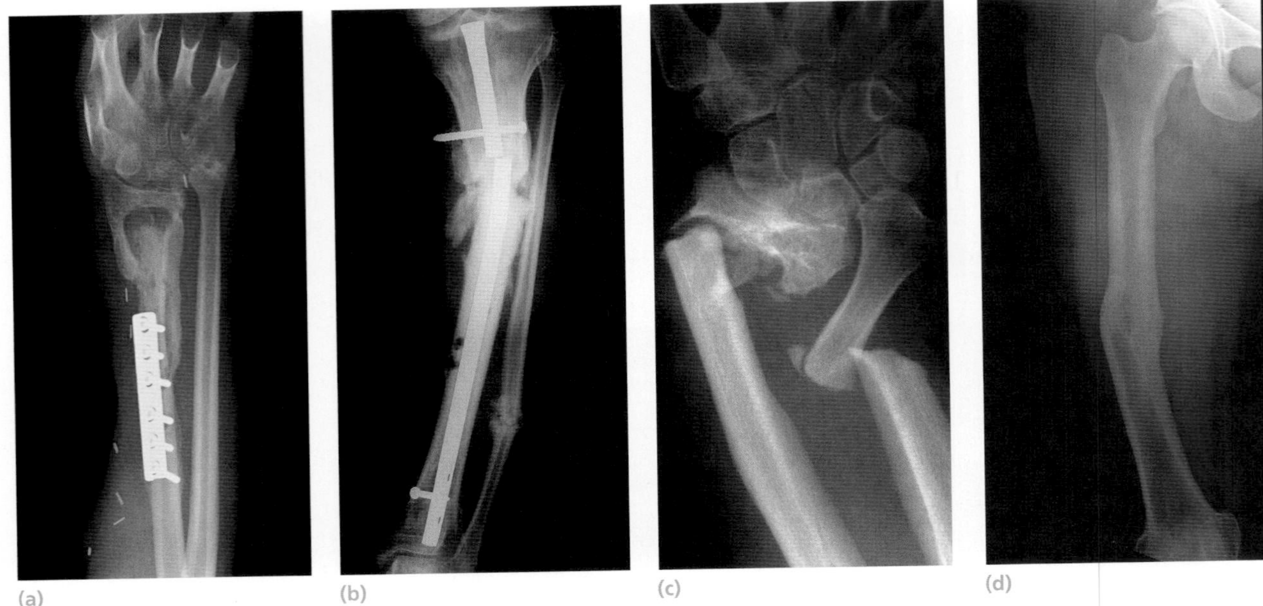

(a) (b) (c) (d)

23.30 Complications of fractures Fractures can become infected (a,b), fail to unite (c) or (d) unite in poor alignment.

fixation at the time of definitive wound cover as long as (1) the delay to wound cover is less than 7 days; (2) wound contamination is not visible and (3) internal fixation can control the fracture as well as the external fixator. This approach is less risky than introducing internal fixation at the time of initial surgery and leaving both metalwork and bone exposed until definitive cover several days later.

Aftercare

In the ward, the limb is elevated and its circulation carefully watched. Antibiotic cover is continued but only for a maximum of 72 hours in the more severe grades of injury. Wound cultures are seldom helpful as osteomyelitis, if it were to ensue, is often caused by hospital-derived organisms; this emphasizes the need for good debridement and early fracture cover.

SEQUELS TO OPEN FRACTURES

Skin

If split-thickness skin grafts are used inappropriately, particularly where flap cover is more suited, there can be areas of contracture or friable skin that breaks down intermittently. Reparative or reconstructive surgery by a plastic surgeon is desirable.

Bone

Infection involves the bone and any implants that may have been used. Early infection may present as wound inflammation without discharge. Identifying the causal organism without tissue samples is difficult but, at best guess, it is likely to be *S. aureus* (including methicillin-resistant varieties) or *Pseudomonas*. Suppression by appropriate antibiotics, as long as the fixation remains stable, may allow the fracture to proceed to union, but further surgery is likely later, when the antibiotics are stopped.

Late presentation may be with a sinus and x-ray evidence of sequestra. The implants and all avascular pieces of bone should be removed; robust soft tissue cover (ideally a flap) is needed. An external fixator can be used to bridge the fracture. If the resulting defect is too large for bone grafting at a later stage, the patient should be referred to a centre with the necessary experience and facilities for limb reconstruction.

Joints

When an infected fracture communicates with a joint, the principles of treatment are the same as with bone infection, namely debridement and drainage, drugs and splintage. On resolution of the infection, attention can be given to stabilizing the fracture so that joint movement can recommence. Permanent stiffness is a real threat; where fracture stabilization cannot be achieved to allow movement, the joint should be splinted in the optimum position for ankylosis, lest this should occur.

GUNSHOT INJURIES

Missile wounds are looked upon as a special type of open injury. Tissue damage is produced by: (1) direct injury in the immediate path of the missile; (2) contusion of muscles around the missile track and (3) bruising and congestion of soft tissues at a greater distance from the primary track. The exit wound (if any) is usually larger than the entry wound.

With high-velocity missiles (bullets, usually from rifles, travelling at speeds above 600 m/s) there is marked cavitation and tissue destruction over a wide area. The splintering of bone resulting from the transfer of large quantities of energy creates secondary missiles, causing greater damage. With low-velocity missiles (bullets from civilian hand-guns travelling at speeds of 300–600 m/s) cavitation is much less, and with smaller weapons tissue damage may be virtually confined to the bullet track. However, with all gunshot injuries debris is sucked into the wound, which is therefore contaminated from the outset.

Emergency treatment

As always, the arrest of bleeding and general resuscitation take priority. The wounds should each be covered with a sterile dressing and the area examined for artery or nerve damage. Antibiotics should be given immediately, following the recommendations for open fractures (see Table 23.1).

Definitive treatment

Traditionally, all missile injuries were treated as severe open injuries, by exploration of the missile track and formal debridement. However, it has been shown that low-velocity wounds with relatively clean entry and exit wounds can be treated as Gustilo type I injuries, by superficial debridement, splintage of the limb and antibiotic cover; the fracture is then treated as for similar open fractures. If the injury is to soft tissues only with minimal bone splinters, the wound may be safely treated without surgery but with local wound care and antibiotics.

High-velocity injuries demand thorough cleansing of the wound and debridement, with excision of deep damaged tissues and, if necessary, splitting of fascial compartments to prevent ischaemia; the fracture is stabilized and the wound is treated as for a Gustilo type III fracture. If there are comminuted fractures, these are best managed by external fixation. The method of wound closure will depend on the state of tissues after several days; in some cases delayed primary suture is possible but, as with other open injuries, close collaboration between plastic and orthopaedic surgeons is needed (Dicpinigaitis et al., 2006).

Close-range shotgun injuries, although the missiles may be technically low velocity, are treated as high-velocity wounds because the mass of shot transfers large quantities of energy to the tissues.

COMPLICATIONS OF FRACTURES

The general complications of fractures (blood loss, shock, fat embolism, cardiorespiratory failure etc.) are dealt with in Chapter 22.

Local complications can be divided into *early* (those that arise during the first few weeks following injury) and *late*.

EARLY COMPLICATIONS

Early complications may present as part of the primary injury or may appear only after a few days or weeks.

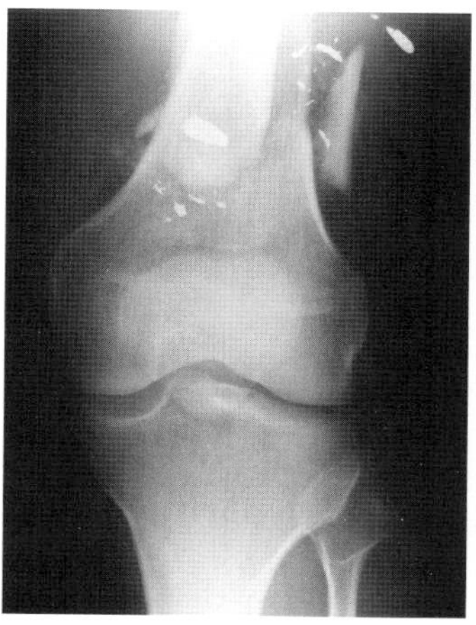
(a)

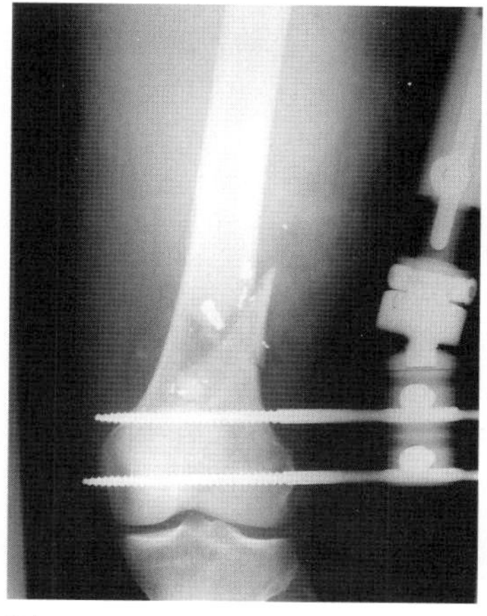
(b)

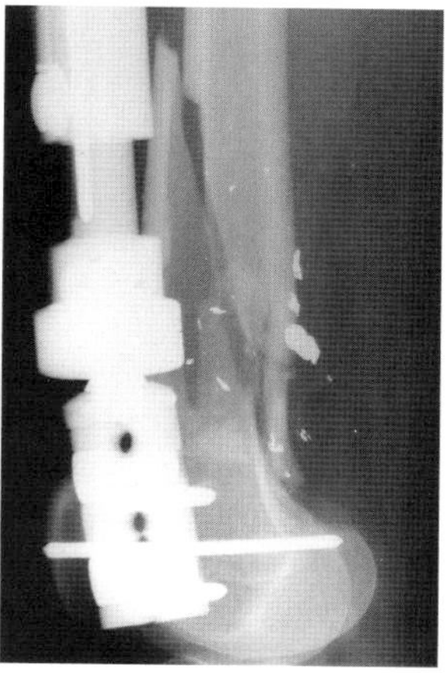
(c)

23.31 Gunshot injuries (a) Close-range shotgun blasts, although technically low velocity, transfer large quantities of destructive force to the tissues due to the mass of shot. They should be treated like high-energy open fractures (b,c).

Table 23.2 Local complications of fractures

Urgent	Less urgent	Late
Local visceral injury	Fracture blisters	Delayed union
Vascular injury	Plaster sores	Malunion
Nerve injury	Pressure sores	Non-union
Compartment syndrome	Nerve entrapment	Avascular necrosis
Haemarthrosis	Myositis ossificans	Muscle contracture
Infection	Ligament injury	Joint instability
Gas gangrene	Tendon lesions	Osteoarthritis
	Joint stiffness	
	Algodystrophy	

Visceral injury

Fractures around the trunk are often complicated by injuries to underlying viscera, the most important being penetration of the lung with life-threatening pneumothorax following rib fractures and rupture of the bladder or urethra in pelvic fractures. These injuries require emergency treatment.

Table 23.3 Common vascular injuries

Injury	Vessel
First rib fracture	Subclavian
Shoulder dislocation	Axillary
Humeral supracondylar fracture	Brachial
Elbow dislocation	Brachial
Pelvic fracture	Presacral and internal iliac
Femoral supracondylar fracture	Femoral
Knee dislocation	Popliteal
Proximal tibial	Popliteal or its branches

Vascular injury

The fractures most often associated with damage to a major artery are those around the knee and elbow, and those of the humeral and femoral shafts. The artery may be cut, torn, compressed or contused, either by the initial injury or subsequently by jagged bone fragments. Even if its outward appearance is normal, the intima may be detached and the vessel blocked by thrombus, or a segment of artery may be in spasm. The effects vary from transient diminution of blood flow to profound ischaemia, tissue death and peripheral gangrene.

Clinical features

The patient may complain of paraesthesia or numbness in the toes or the fingers. The injured limb is cold and pale, or slightly cyanosed, and the pulse is weak or absent. X-rays will probably show one of the 'high-risk' fractures listed above. If a vascular injury is suspected an angiogram should be performed immediately; if it is positive, emergency treatment must be started without further delay.

Treatment

All bandages and splints should be removed. The fracture is re-x-rayed and, if the position of the bones suggests that the artery is being compressed or kinked, prompt reduction is necessary. The circulation is then reassessed repeatedly over the next half hour. If there is no improvement, the vessels must be explored by operation – preferably with the benefit of preoperative or peroperative angiography. A cut vessel can be sutured, or a segment may be replaced by a vein graft; if it is thrombosed, endarterectomy may restore the blood flow. If vessel repair is undertaken, stable fixation is a must and where it is practicable, the fracture should be fixed internally.

Nerve injury

Nerve injury is particularly common with fractures of the humerus or injuries around the elbow or the knee

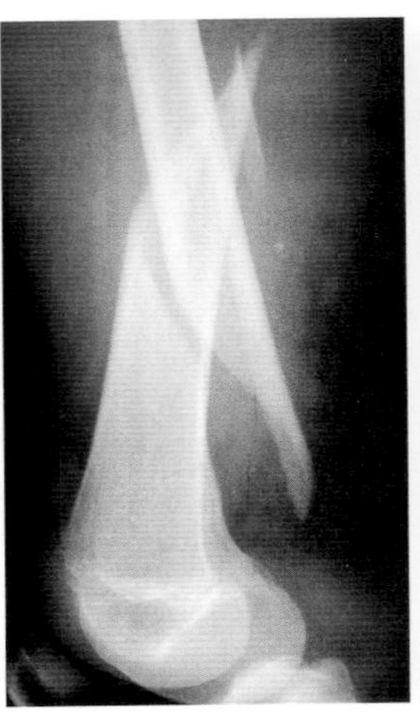
(a)

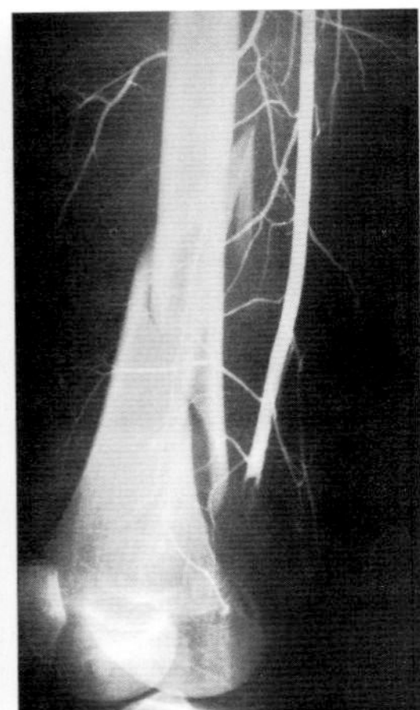
(b)

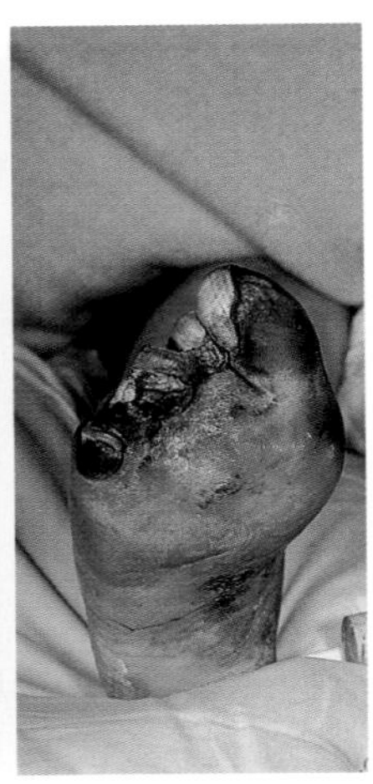
(c)

23.32 Vascular injury This patient was brought into hospital with a fractured femur and early signs of vascular insufficiency. The plain x-ray (a) looked as if the proximal bone fragment might have speared the popliteal artery. The angiogram (b) confirmed these fears. Despite vein grafting the patient developed peripheral gangrene (c).

Table 23.4 Common nerve injuries

Injury	Nerve
Shoulder dislocation	Axillary
Humeral shaft fracture	Radial
Humeral supracondylar fracture	Radial or median
Elbow medial condyle	Ulnar
Monteggia fracture–dislocation	Posterior-interosseous
Hip dislocation	Sciatic
Knee dislocation	Peroneal

(see also Chapter 11). The telltale signs should be looked for (*and documented*) during the initial examination and again after reduction of the fracture.

Closed nerve injuries

In closed injuries the nerve is seldom severed, and spontaneous recovery should be awaited – it occurs in 90 per cent within 4 months. If recovery has not occurred by the expected time, and if nerve conduction studies and EMG fail to show evidence of recovery, the nerve should be explored.

Open nerve injuries

With open fractures the nerve injury is more likely to be complete. In these cases the nerve should be explored at the time of debridement and repaired at the time or at wound closure.

Acute nerve compression

Nerve compression, as distinct from a direct injury, sometimes occurs with fractures or dislocations around the wrist. Complaints of numbness or paraesthesia in the distribution of the median or ulnar nerves should be taken seriously and the patient monitored closely; if there is no improvement within 48 hours of fracture reduction or splitting of bandages around the splint, the nerve should be explored and decompressed.

INDICATIONS FOR EARLY EXPLORATION

- Nerve injury associated with open fracture
- Nerve injury with fractures that need internal fixation
- Presence of a concomitant vascular injury
- Nerve damage diagnosed after manipulation of the fracture

COMPARTMENT SYNDROME

Fractures of the arm or leg can give rise to severe ischaemia, even if there is no damage to a major vessel. Bleeding, oedema or inflammation (infection) may increase the pressure within one of the osseofascial compartments; there is reduced capillary flow, which results in muscle ischaemia, further oedema, still greater pressure and yet more profound ischaemia – a vicious circle that ends, after 12 hours or less, in necrosis of nerve and muscle within the compartment. Nerve is capable of regeneration but muscle, once infarcted, can never recover and is replaced by inelastic fibrous tissue (*Volkmann's ischaemic contracture*). A similar cascade of events may be caused by swelling of a limb inside a tight plaster cast.

Clinical features

High-risk injuries are fractures of the elbow, forearm bones, proximal third of the tibia, and also multiple

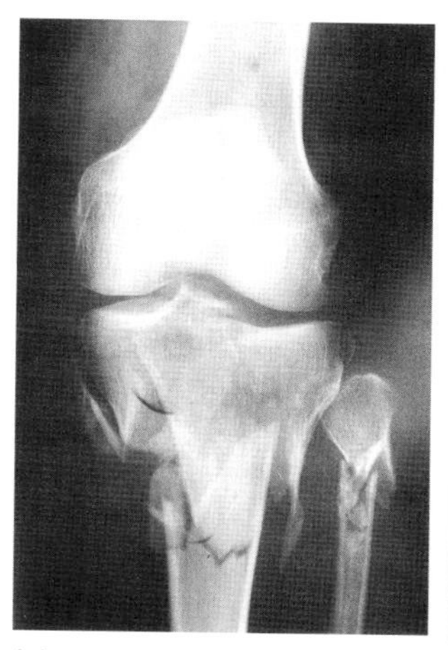

(a)

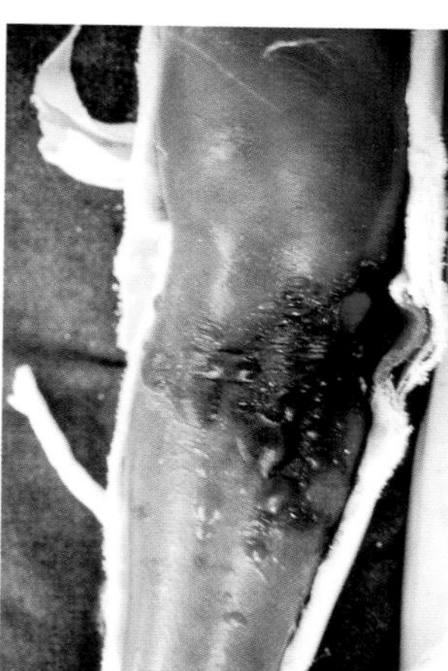

(b)

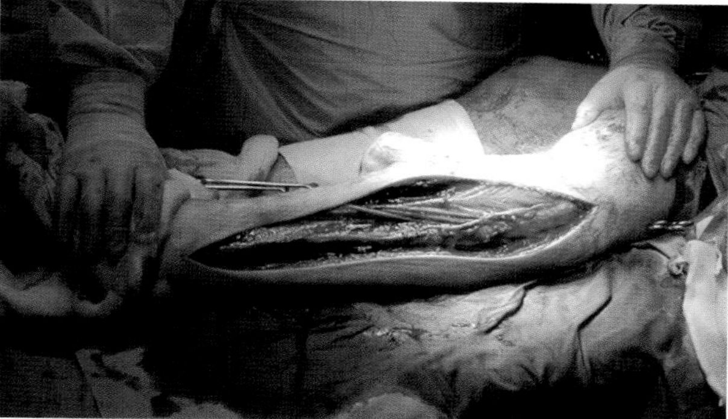

(c)

23.33 Compartment syndrome (a) A fracture at this level is always dangerous. This man was treated in plaster. Pain became intense and when the plaster was split (which should have been done immediately after its application), the leg was swollen and blistered (b). Tibial compartment decompression (c) requires fasciotomies of *all* the compartments in the leg.

fractures of the hand or foot, crush injuries and circumferential burns. Other precipitating factors are operation (usually for internal fixation) or infection.

The classic features of ischaemia are the five Ps:

- Pain
- Paraesthesia
- Pallor
- Paralysis
- Pulselessness.

However in compartment syndrome the ischaemia occurs at the capillary level, so pulses may still be felt and the skin may not be pale! The earliest of the 'classic' features are pain (or a 'bursting' sensation), altered sensibility and paresis (or, more usually, weakness in active muscle contraction). Skin sensation should be carefully and repeatedly checked.

Ischaemic muscle is highly sensitive to stretch. If the limb is unduly painful, swollen or tense, the muscles (which may be tender) should be tested by stretching them. When the toes or fingers are passively hyperextended, there is increased pain in the calf or forearm.

Confirmation of the diagnosis can be made by measuring the intracompartmental pressures. So important is the need for early diagnosis that some surgeons advocate the use of continuous compartment pressure monitoring for high-risk injuries (e.g. fractures of the tibia and fibula) and especially for forearm or leg fractures in patients who are unconscious. A split catheter is introduced into the compartment and the pressure is measured close to the level of the fracture. A differential pressure (ΔP) – the difference between diastolic pressure and compartment pressure – of less than 30 mmHg (4.00 kilopascals) is an indication for immediate compartment decompression.

Treatment

The threatened compartment (or compartments) must be promptly decompressed. Casts, bandages and dressings must be completely removed – merely splitting the plaster is utterly useless – and the limb should be nursed flat (elevating the limb causes a further decrease in end capillary pressure and aggravates the muscle ischaemia). The ΔP should be carefully monitored; if it falls below 30 mmHg, immediate open fasciotomy is performed. In the case of the leg, 'fasciotomy' means opening all four compartments through medial and lateral incisions. The wounds should be left open and inspected 2 days later: if there is muscle necrosis, debridement can be carried out; if the tissues are healthy, the wounds can be sutured (without tension) or skin-grafted.

NOTE: If facilities for measuring compartmental pressures are not available, the decision to operate will have to be made on clinical grounds. If three or more signs are present, the diagnosis is almost certain (Ulmer, 2002). If the clinical signs are 'soft', the limb should be examined at 30-minute intervals and if there is no improvement within 2 hours of splitting the dressings, fasciotomy should be performed. Muscle will be dead after 4–6 hours of total ischaemia – there is no time to lose!

Haemarthrosis

Fractures involving a joint may cause acute haemarthrosis. The joint is swollen and tense and the patient resists any attempt at moving it. The blood should be aspirated before dealing with the fracture.

Infection

Open fractures may become infected; closed fractures hardly ever do unless they are opened by operation. Post-traumatic wound infection is now the most common cause of chronic osteitis. The management of early and late infection is summarized under the section *Sequels to open fractures* *(page 710)*.

Gas gangrene

This terrifying condition is produced by clostridial infection (especially *Clostridium welchii*). These are anaerobic organisms that can survive and multiply only in tissues with low oxygen tension; the prime site for infection, therefore, is a dirty wound with dead muscle that has been closed without adequate debridement. Toxins produced by the organisms destroy the cell wall and rapidly lead to tissue necrosis, thus promoting the spread of the disease.

Clinical features appear within 24 hours of the injury: the patient complains of intense pain and swelling around the wound and a brownish discharge may be seen; gas formation is usually not very marked. There is little or no pyrexia but the pulse rate is increased and a characteristic smell becomes evident (once experienced this is never forgotten). Rapidly the patient becomes toxaemic and may lapse into coma and death.

It is essential to distinguish gas gangrene, which is characterized by myonecrosis, from anaerobic cellulitis, in which superficial gas formation is abundant but toxaemia usually slight. Failure to recognize the difference may lead to unnecessary amputation for the non-lethal cellulitis.

Prevention

Deep, penetrating wounds in muscular tissue are dangerous; they should be explored, all dead tissue

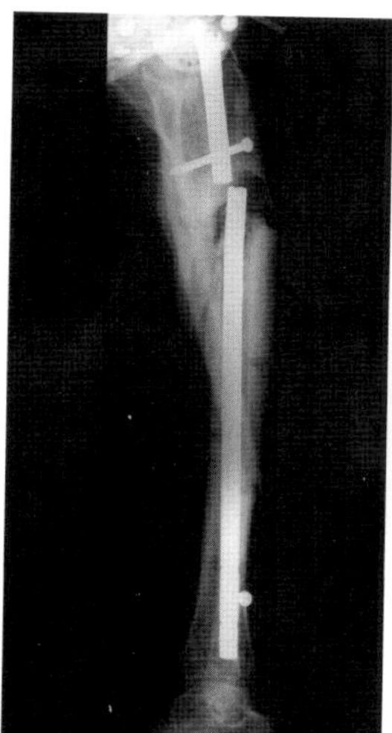

(a)

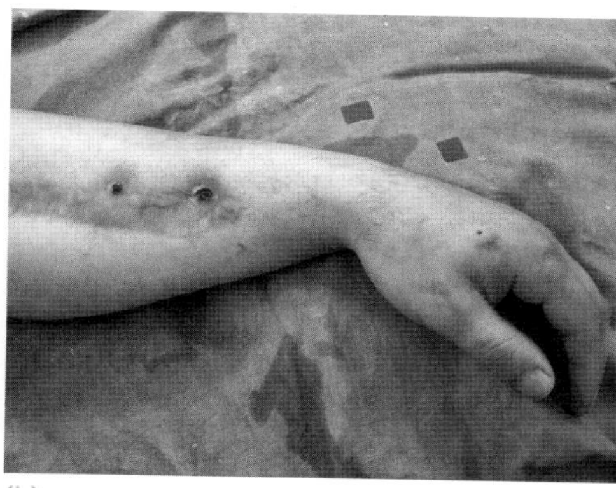

(b)

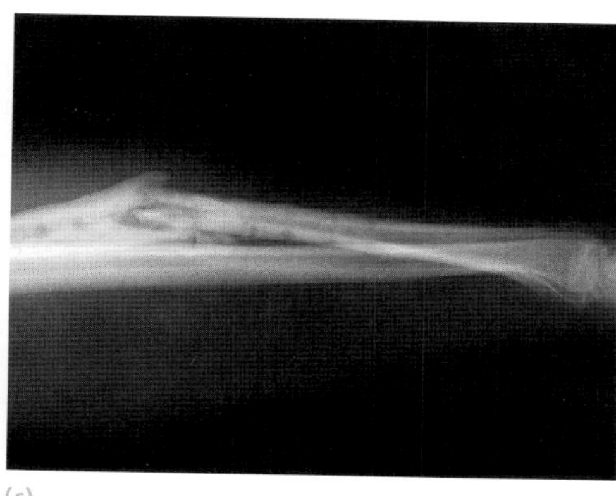

(c)

23.34 Infection after fracture treatment Operative fixation is one of the commonest causes of infection in closed fractures. Fatigue failure of implants is inevitable if infection hinders union (a). Deep infection can lead to development of discharging sinuses (b,c).

should be completely excised and, if there is the slightest doubt about tissue viability, the wound should be left open. Unhappily there is no effective antitoxin against *C. welchii*.

Treatment

The key to life-saving treatment is early diagnosis. General measures, such as fluid replacement and intravenous antibiotics, are started immediately. Hyperbaric oxygen has been used as a means of limiting the spread of gangrene. However, the mainstay of treatment is prompt decompression of the wound and removal of all dead tissue. In advanced cases, amputation may be essential.

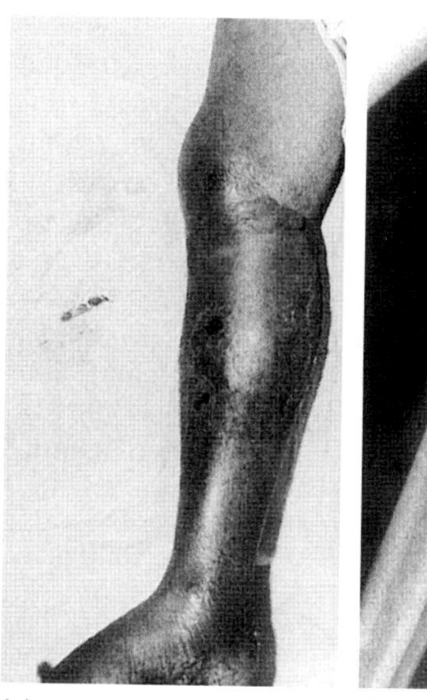

(a)

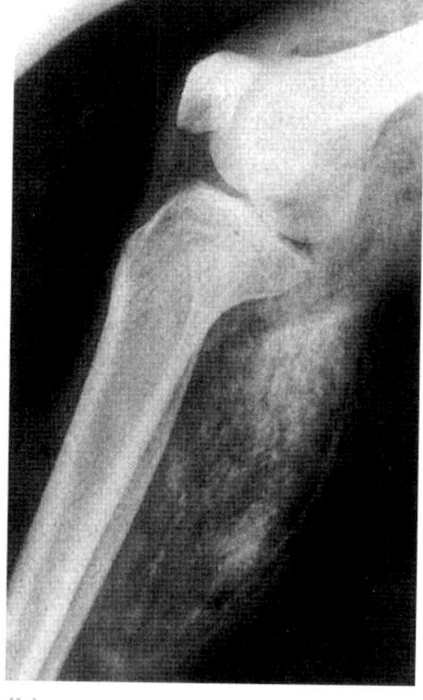

(b)

23.35 Gas gangrene (a) Clinical picture of gas gangrene. (b) X-rays show diffuse gas in the muscles of the calf.

Fracture blisters

Two distinct blister types are sometimes seen after fractures: clear fluid-filled vesicles and blood-stained ones. Both occur during limb swelling and are due to elevation of the epidermal layer of skin from the dermis (Giordano et al., 1994). There is no advantage to puncturing the blisters (it may even lead to increased local infection) and surgical incisions through blisters, whilst generally safe, should be undertaken only when limb swelling has decreased.

Plaster and pressure sores

Plaster sores occur where skin presses directly onto bone. They should be prevented by padding the bony points and by moulding the wet plaster so that pressure is distributed to the soft tissues around the bony points. While a plaster sore is developing the patient feels localized burning pain. A window must

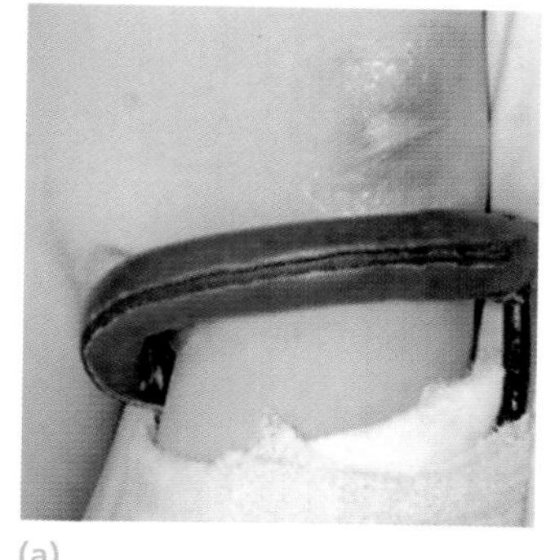

(a)

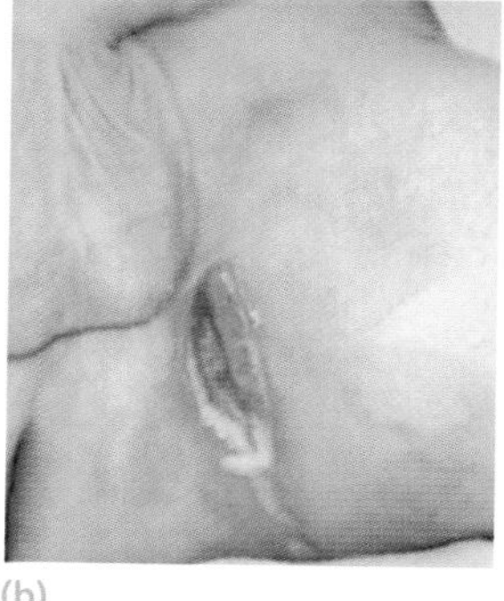

(b)

23.36 Pressure sores Pressure sores are a sign of carelessness. (a,b) Sores from poorly supervised treatment in a Thomas splint.

immediately be cut in the plaster, or warning pain quickly abates and skin necrosis proceeds unnoticed.

Even traction on a Thomas splint requires skill in nursing care; careless selection of ring size, excessive fixed (as opposed to balanced) traction, and neglect can lead to pressure sores around the groin and iliac crest.

LATE COMPLICATIONS

DELAYED UNION

The timetable on page 692 is no more than a rough guide to the period in which a fracture may be expected to unite and consolidate. It must never be relied upon in deciding when treatment may be discontinued. If the time is unduly prolonged, the term 'delayed union' is used.

Causes

Factors causing delayed union can be summarized as: *biological, biomechanical or patient-related*.

BIOLOGICAL

Inadequate blood supply A badly displaced fracture of a long bone will cause tearing of both the periosteum and interruption of the intramedullary blood supply. The fracture edges will become necrotic and dependent on the formation of an ensheathing callus mass to bridge the break. If the zone of necrosis is extensive, as might occur in highly comminuted fractures, union may be hampered.

Severe soft tissue damage Severe damage to the soft tissues affects fracture healing by: (1) reducing the effectiveness of muscle splintage; (2) damaging the local blood supply and (3) diminishing or eliminating the osteogenic input from mesenchymal stem cells within muscle.

Periosteal stripping Over-enthusiastic stripping of periosteum during internal fixation is an avoidable cause of delayed union.

BIOMECHANICAL

Imperfect splintage Excessive traction (creating a fracture gap) or excessive movement at the fracture site will delay ossification in the callus. In the forearm and leg a single-bone fracture may be held apart by an intact fellow bone.

Over-rigid fixation Contrary to popular belief, rigid fixation delays rather than promotes fracture union. It is only because the fixation device holds the fragments so securely that the fracture seems to be 'uniting'. Union by primary bone healing is slow, but provided stability is maintained throughout, it does eventually occur.

Infection Both biology and stability are hampered by active infection: not only is there bone lysis, necrosis and pus formation, but implants which are used to hold the fracture tend to loosen.

PATIENT RELATED

In a less than ideal world, there are patients who are:

- Immense
- Immoderate
- Immovable
- Impossible.

These factors must be accommodated in an appropriate fashion.

Clinical features

Fracture tenderness persists and, if the bone is subjected to stress, pain may be acute.

On x-ray, the fracture line remains visible and there is very little or incomplete callus formation or periosteal reaction. However, the bone ends are not sclerosed or atrophic. The appearances suggest that, although the fracture has not united, it eventually will.

Treatment

CONSERVATIVE

The two important principles are: (1) to eliminate any possible cause of delayed union and (2) to promote healing by providing the most appropriate environment. Immobilization (whether by cast or by internal fixation) should be sufficient to prevent shear at the fracture site, but fracture loading is an important stimulus to union and can be enhanced by: (1) encouraging muscular exercise and (2) by weightbearing in the cast or brace. The watchword is patience; however, there comes a point with every fracture where the ill-effects of prolonged immobilization outweigh the advantages of non-operative treatment, or where the risk of implant breakage begins to loom.

OPERATIVE

Each case should be treated on its merits; however, if union is delayed for more than 6 months and there is no sign of callus formation, internal fixation and bone grafting are indicated. The operation should be planned in such a way as to cause the least possible damage to the soft tissues.

NON-UNION

In a minority of cases delayed union gradually turns into non-union – that is it becomes apparent that the fracture will never unite without intervention. Movement can be elicited at the fracture site and pain

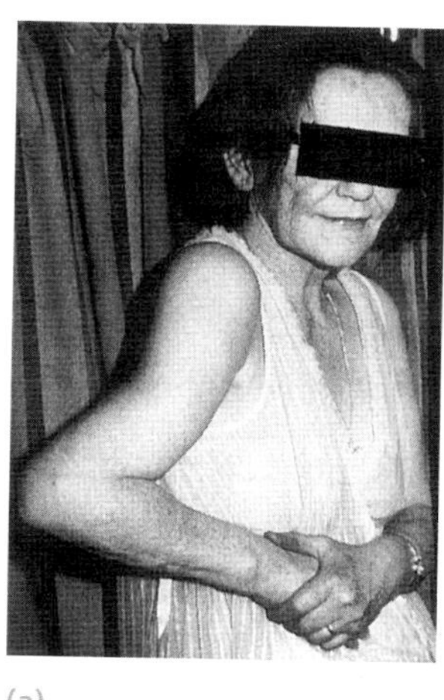
(a)

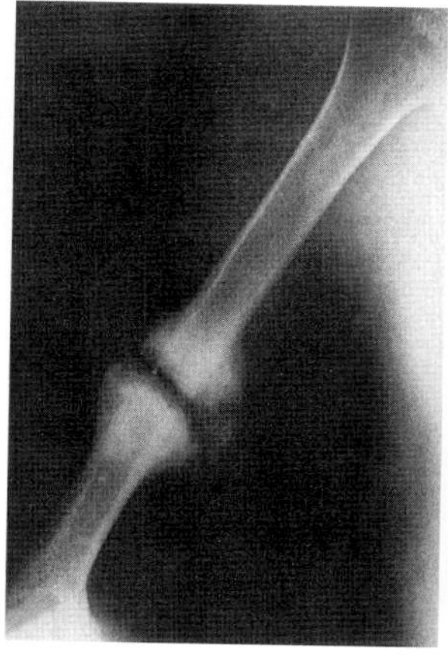
(b)

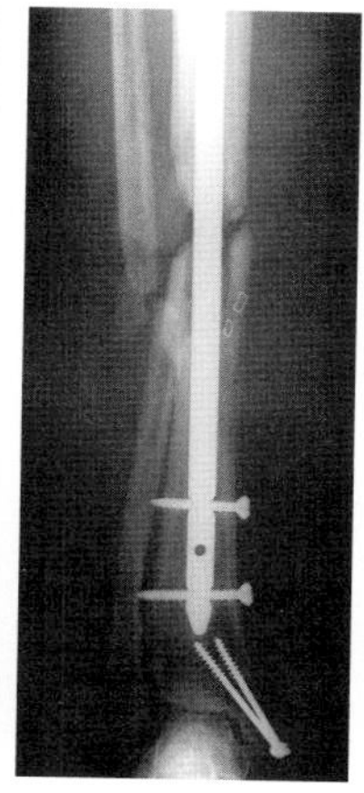
(c)

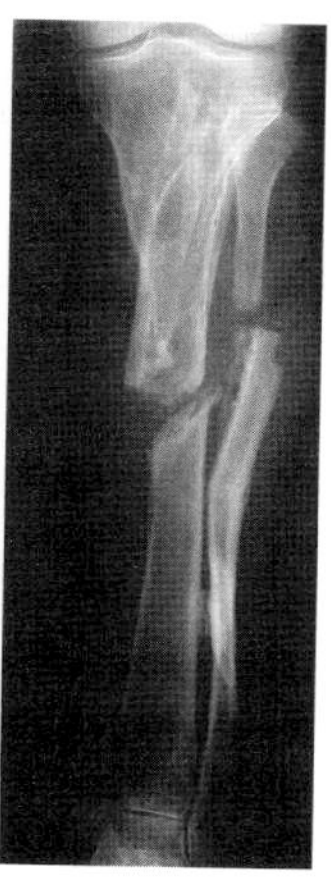
(d)

23.37 Non-union (a) This patient has an obvious pseudarthrosis of the humerus. The x-ray (b) shows a typical hypertrophic non-union. (c,d) Examples of atrophic non-union.

diminishes; the fracture gap becomes a type of pseudoarthrosis.

X-ray The fracture is clearly visible but the bone on either side of it may show either exuberant callus or atrophy. This contrasting appearance has led to non-union being divided into hypertrophic and atrophic types. *In hypertrophic non-union* the bone ends are enlarged, suggesting that osteogenesis is still active but not quite capable of bridging the gap. In *atrophic non-union*, osteogenesis seems to have ceased. The bone ends are tapered or rounded with no suggestion of new bone formation.

Causes

When dealing with the problem of non-union, four questions must be addressed. They have given rise to the acronym *CASS*:

1. *Contact* – Was there sufficient contact between the fragments?
2. *Alignment* – Was the fracture adequately aligned, to reduce shear?
3. *Stability* – Was the fracture held with sufficient stability?
4. *Stimulation* – Was the fracture sufficiently 'stimulated'? (e.g. by encouraging weightbearing).

There are, of course, also biological and patient-related reasons that may lead to non-union: (1) poor soft tissues (from either the injury or surgery); (2) local infection; (3) associated drug abuse, anti-inflammatory or cytotoxic immunosuppressant medication and (4) non-compliance on the part of the patient.

Treatment

CONSERVATIVE

Non-union is occasionally symptomless, needing no treatment or, at most, a removable splint. Even if symptoms are present, operation is not the only

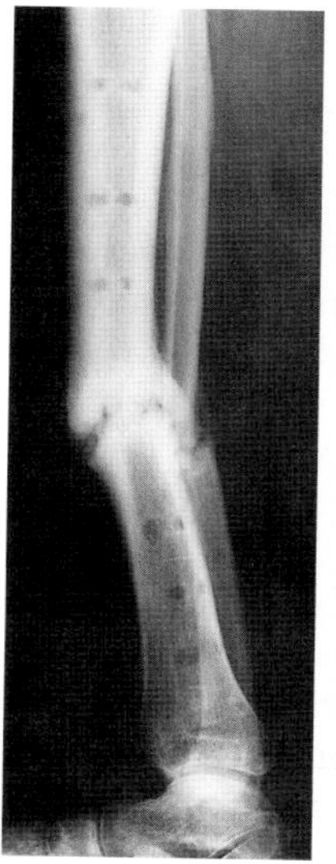
(a)

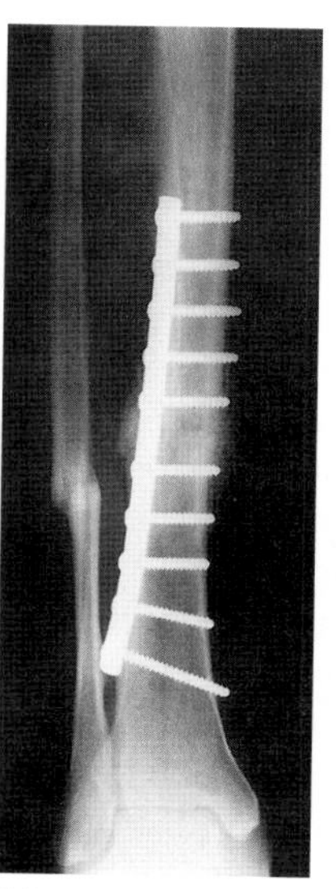
(b)

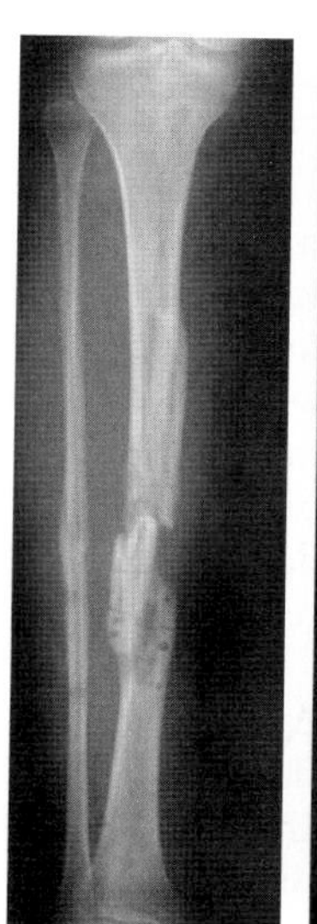
(c)

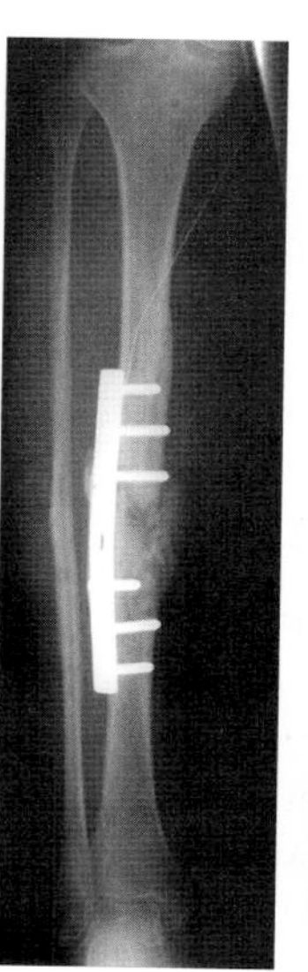
(d)

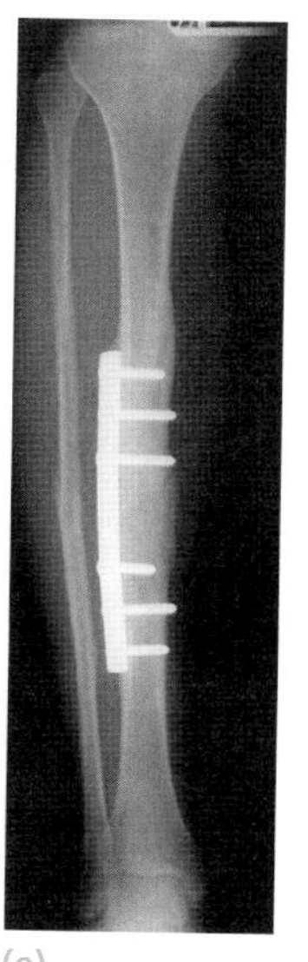
(e)

23.38 Non-union – treatment (a) This patient with fractures of the tibia and fibula was initially treated by internal fixation with a plate and screws. The fracture failed to heal, and developed the typical features of hypertrophic non-union. (b) After a further operation, using more rigid fixation (and no bone grafts), the fractures healed solidly. (c,d) This patient with atrophic non-union needed both internal fixation and bone grafts to stimulate bone formation and union (e).

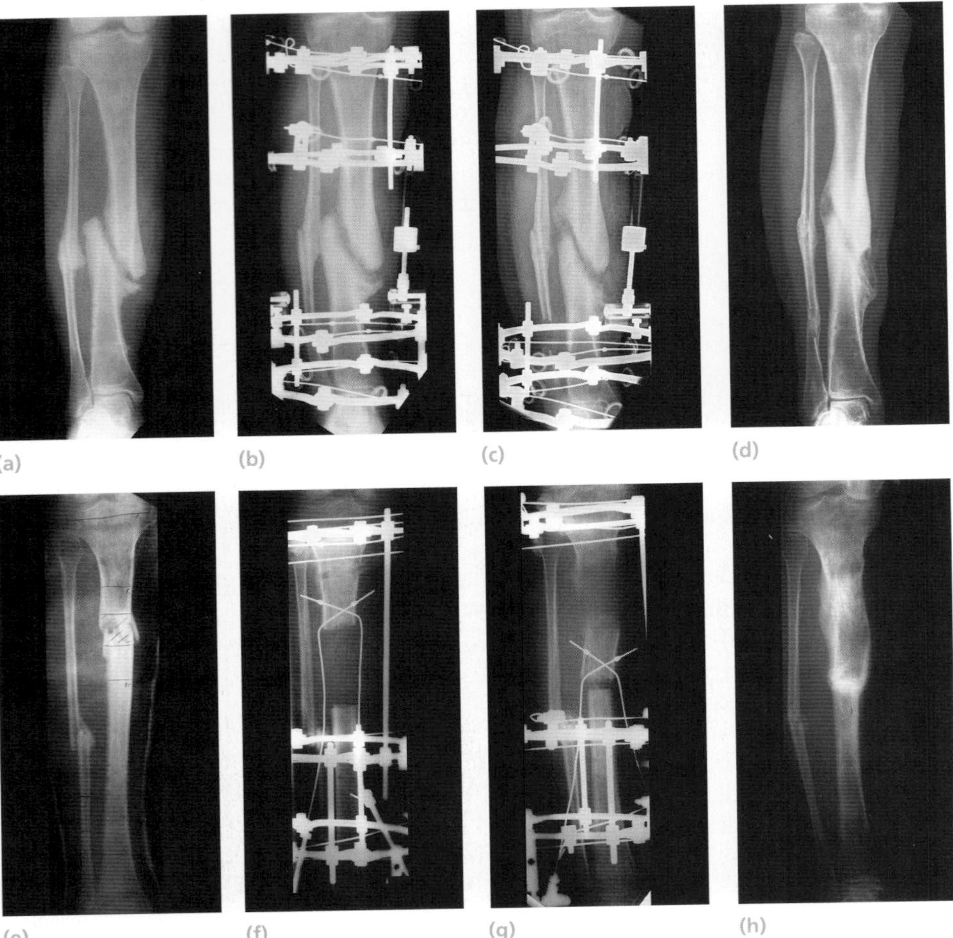

(a) (b) (c) (d) (e) (f) (g) (h)

23.39 Non-union – treatment by the Ilizarov technique Hypertrophic non-unions can be treated by gradual distraction and realignment in an external fixator (a–d). Atrophic non-unions will need more surgery; the poor tissue is excised (e,f) and replaced through bone transport (g,h).

answer; with hypertrophic non-union, functional bracing may be sufficient to induce union, but splintage often needs to be prolonged. Pulsed electromagnetic fields and low-frequency, pulsed ultrasound can also be used to stimulate union.

OPERATIVE

With hypertrophic non-union and in the absence of deformity, very rigid fixation alone (internal or external) may lead to union. With atrophic non-union, fixation alone is not enough. Fibrous tissue in the fracture gap, as well as the hard, sclerotic bone ends is excised and bone grafts are packed around the fracture. If there is significant 'die-back', this will require more extensive excision and the gap is then dealt with by bone advancement using the Ilizarov technique.

MALUNION

When the fragments join in an unsatisfactory position (unacceptable angulation, rotation or shortening) the fracture is said to be malunited. Causes are failure to reduce a fracture adequately, failure to hold reduction while healing proceeds, or gradual collapse of comminuted or osteoporotic bone.

Clinical features

The deformity is usually obvious, but sometimes the true extent of malunion is apparent only on x-ray. Rotational deformity of the femur, tibia, humerus or forearm may be missed unless the limb is compared with its opposite fellow. Rotational deformity of a metacarpal fracture is detected by asking the patient to flatten the fingers onto the palm and seeing whether the normal regular fan-shaped appearance is reproduced (Chapter 26).

X-rays are essential to check the position of the fracture while it is uniting. This is particularly important during the first 3 weeks, when the situation may change without warning. At this stage it is sometimes difficult to decide what constitutes 'malunion'; acceptable norms differ from one site to another and these are discussed under the individual fractures.

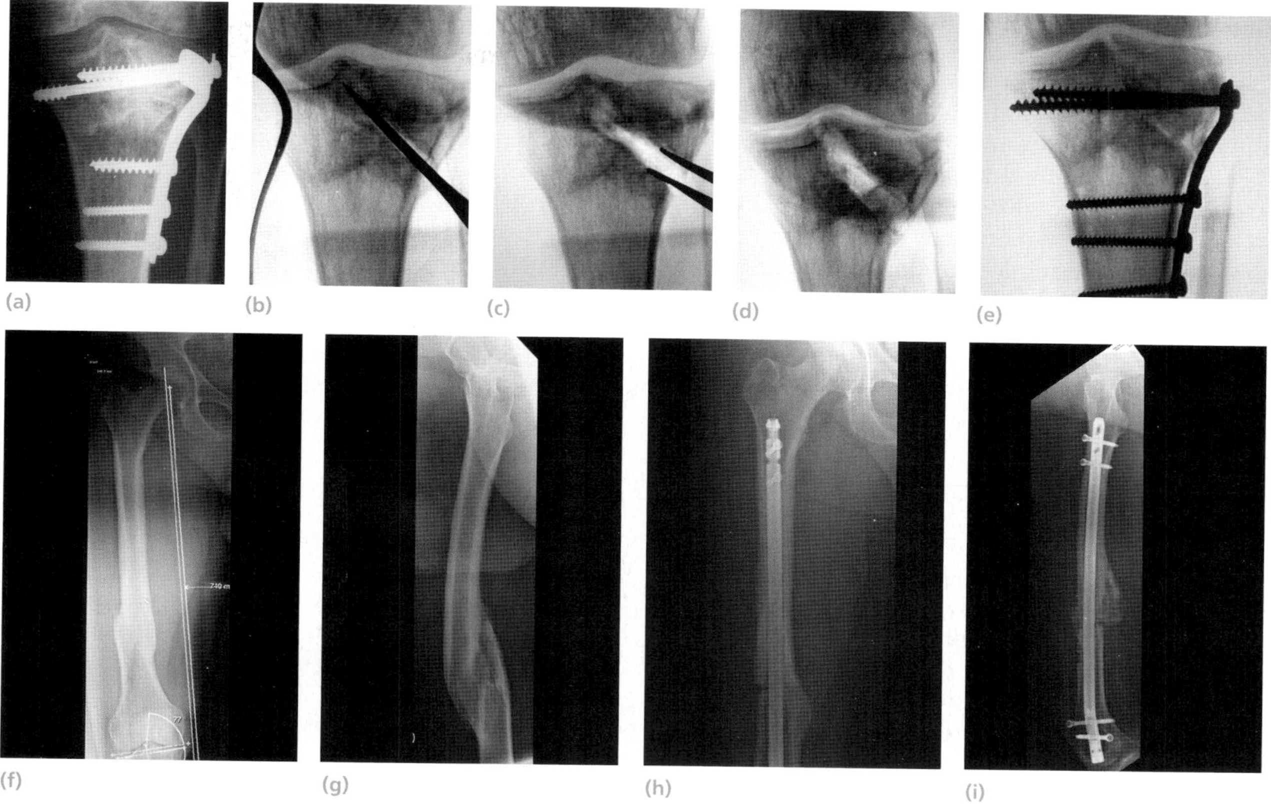

(a) (b) (c) (d) (e)

(f) (g) (h) (i)

23.40 Malunion – treatment by internal fixation An osteotomy, correction of deformity and internal fixation can be used to treat both intra-articular deformities (a–e) and those in the shaft of a long bone (f–i).

Treatment

Incipient malunion may call for treatment even before the fracture has fully united; the decision on the need for re-manipulation or correction may be extremely difficult. A few guidelines are offered:

1. In adults, fractures should be reduced as near to the anatomical position as possible. Angulation of more than 10–15 degrees in a long bone or a noticeable rotational deformity may need correction by re-manipulation, or by osteotomy and fixation.
2. In children, angular deformities near the bone ends (and especially if the deformity is in the same plane as that of movement of the nearby joint) will usually remodel with time; rotational deformities will not.
3. In the lower limb, shortening of more than 2.0 cm is seldom acceptable to the patient and a limb length equalizing procedure may be indicated.
4. The patient's expectations (often prompted by cosmesis) may be quite different from the surgeon's; they are not to be ignored.

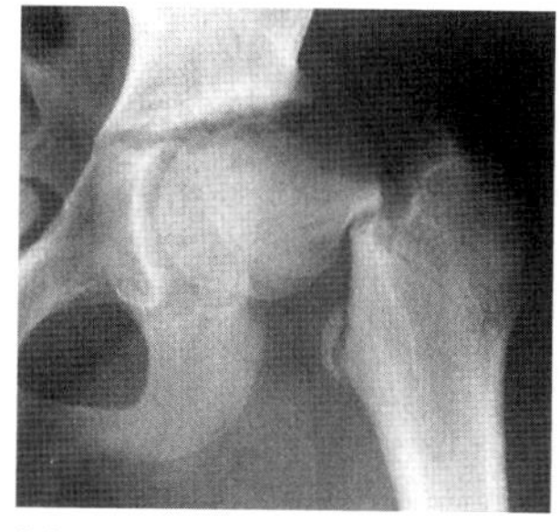

(a)

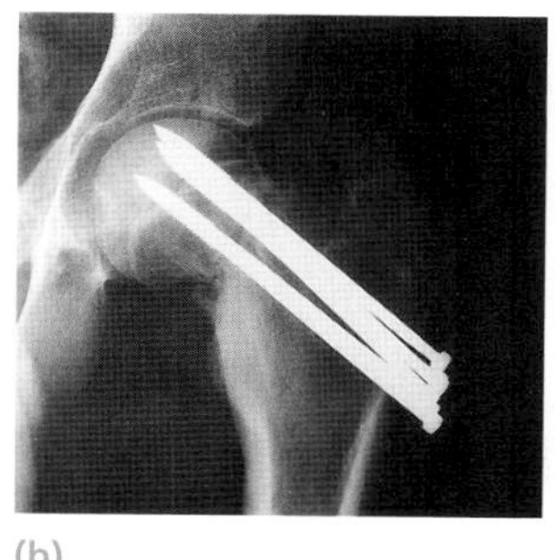

(b)

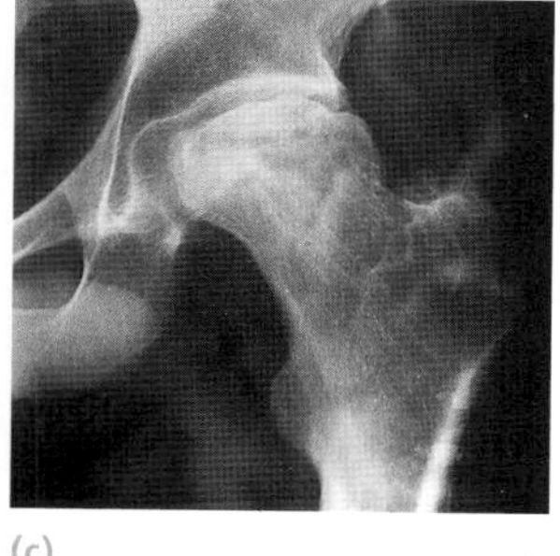

(c)

23.41 Avascular necrosis (a) Displaced fractures of the femoral neck are at considerable risk of developing avascular necrosis. Despite internal fixation within a few hours of the injury (b), the head-fragment developed avascular necrosis. (c) X-ray after removal of the fixation screws.

5. Early discussion with the patient, and a guided view of the x-rays, will help in deciding the need for treatment and may prevent later misunderstanding.
6. Very little is known of the long-term effects of small angular deformities on joint function. However, it seems likely that malalignment of more than 15 degrees in any plane may cause asymmetrical loading of the joint above or below and the late development of secondary osteoarthritis; this applies particularly to the large weightbearing joints.

Avascular necrosis

Certain regions are notorious for their propensity to develop ischaemia and bone necrosis after injury (see also Chapter 6). They are: (1) the head of the femur (after fracture of the femoral neck or dislocation of the hip); (2) the proximal part of the scaphoid (after fracture through its waist); (3) the lunate (following dislocation) and (4) the body of the talus (after fracture of its neck).

Accurately speaking, this is an early complication of bone injury, because ischaemia occurs during the first few hours following fracture or dislocation. However, the clinical and radiological effects are not seen until weeks or even months later.

Clinical features

There are no symptoms associated with avascular necrosis, but if the fracture fails to unite or if the bone collapses the patient may complain of pain. X-ray shows the characteristic increase in x-ray density, which occurs as a consequence of two factors: disuse osteoporosis in the surrounding parts gives the impression of 'increased density' in the necrotic segment, and collapse of trabeculae compacts the bone and increases its density. Where normal bone meets the necrotic segment a zone of increased radiographic density may be produced by new bone formation.

Treatment

Treatment usually becomes necessary when joint function is threatened. In old people with necrosis of the femoral head an arthroplasty is the obvious choice; in younger people, realignment osteotomy (or, in some cases, arthrodesis) may be wiser. Avascular necrosis in the scaphoid or talus may need no more than symptomatic treatment, but arthrodesis of the wrist or ankle is sometimes needed.

Growth disturbance

In children, damage to the physis may lead to abnormal or arrested growth. A transverse fracture through the growth plate is not always disastrous; the fracture runs through the hypertrophic and calcified layers and not through the germinal zone, so provided it is accurately reduced, there may not be any disturbance of growth. However fractures that split the epiphysis inevitably traverse the growing portion of the physis, and so further growth may be asymmetrical and the bone end characteristically angulated; if the entire physis is damaged, there may be slowing or complete cessation of growth. The subject is dealt with in more detail on page 727.

Bed sores

Bed sores occur in elderly or paralysed patients. The skin over the sacrum and heels is especially vulnerable. Careful nursing and early activity can usually prevent bed sores; once they have developed, treatment is difficult – it may be necessary to excise the necrotic tissue and apply skin grafts. In recent years vacuum-assisted closure (a form of negative pressure dressing) has been used for sacral bed sores.

Myositis ossificans

Heterotopic ossification in the muscles sometimes occurs after an injury, particularly dislocation of the elbow or a blow to the brachialis, deltoid or quadriceps. It is thought to be due to muscle damage, but it also occurs without a local injury in unconscious or paraplegic patients.

Clinical features

Soon after the injury, the patient (usually a fit young man) complains of pain; there is local swelling and

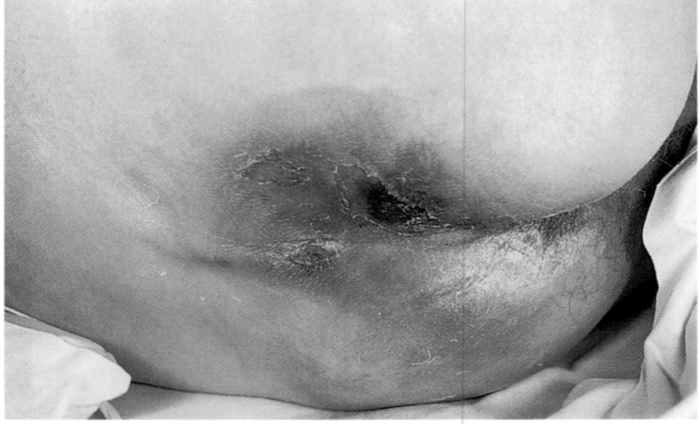

23.42 Bed sores Bed sores in an elderly patient, which kept her in hospital for months.

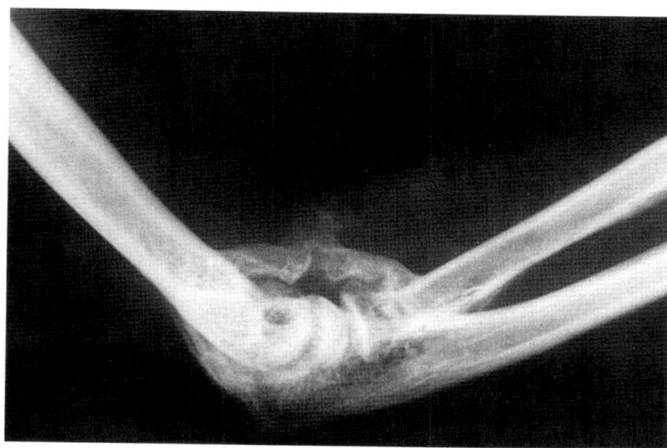

23.43 Myositis ossificans This followed a fractured head of the radius.

soft-tissue tenderness. X-ray is normal but a bone scan may show increased activity. Over the next 2–3 weeks the pain gradually subsides, but joint movement is limited; x-ray may show fluffy calcification in the soft tissues. By 8 weeks the bony mass is easily palpable and is clearly defined in the x-ray.

Treatment

The worst treatment is to attack an injured and slightly stiff elbow with vigorous muscle-stretching exercises; this is liable to precipitate or aggravate the condition. The joint should be rested in the position of function until pain subsides; gentle active movements are then begun.

Months later, when the condition has stabilized, it may be helpful to excise the bony mass. Indomethacin or radiotherapy should be given to help prevent a recurrence.

Tendon lesions

Tendinitis may affect the tibialis posterior tendon following medial malleolar fractures. It should be prevented by accurate reduction, if necessary at surgery. Rupture of the extensor pollicis longus tendon may occur 6–12 weeks after a fracture of the lower radius. Direct suture is seldom possible and the resulting disability is treated by transferring the extensor indicis proprius tendon to the distal stump of the ruptured thumb tendon. Late rupture of the long head of biceps after a fractured neck of humerus usually requires no treatment.

Nerve compression

Nerve compression may damage the lateral popliteal nerve if an elderly or emaciated patient lies with the leg in full external rotation. Radial palsy may follow the faulty use of crutches. Both conditions are due to lack of supervision.

Bone or joint deformity may result in local nerve entrapment with typical features such as numbness or paraesthesia, loss of power and muscle wasting in the distribution of the affected nerve. Common sites are: (1) the ulnar nerve, due to a valgus elbow following a malunited lateral condyle or supracondylar fracture; (2) the median nerve, following injuries around the wrist and (3) the posterior tibial nerve, following fractures around the ankle. Treatment is by early decompression of the nerve; in the case of the ulnar nerve this may require anterior transposition.

Muscle contracture

Following arterial injury or compartment syndrome, the patient may develop ischaemic contractures of the affected muscles (*Volkmann's ischaemic contracture*). Nerves injured by ischaemia sometimes recover, at least partially; thus the patient presents with deformity and stiffness, but numbness is inconstant. The sites most commonly affected are the forearm and hand, leg and foot.

In a severe case affecting the forearm, there will be wasting of the forearm and hand, and clawing of the fingers. If the wrist is passively flexed, the patient can extend the fingers, showing that the deformity is largely due to contracture of the forearm muscles. Detachment of the flexors at their origin and along the interosseous membrane in the forearm may improve the deformity, but function is no better if sensation and active movement are not restored. A pedicle nerve graft, using the proximal segments of the median and ulnar nerves may restore protective sensation in the hand, and tendon transfers (wrist extensors to finger and thumb flexors) will allow active grasp. In less severe cases, median nerve sensibility may be quite good and, with appropriate tendon releases and transfers, the patient regains a considerable degree of function.

Ischaemia of the hand may follow forearm injuries, or swelling of the fingers associated with a tight forearm bandage or plaster. The intrinsic hand muscles fibrose and shorten, pulling the fingers into flexion at the metacarpophalangeal joints, but the interphalangeal joints remain straight. The thumb is adducted across the palm (Bunnell's 'intrinsic-plus' position).

Ischaemia of the calf muscles may follow injuries or operations involving the popliteal artery or its divisions. This is more common than is usually supposed. The symptoms, signs and subsequent contracture are similar to those following ischaemia of the forearm. One of the causes of late claw-toe deformity is an undiagnosed compartment syndrome.

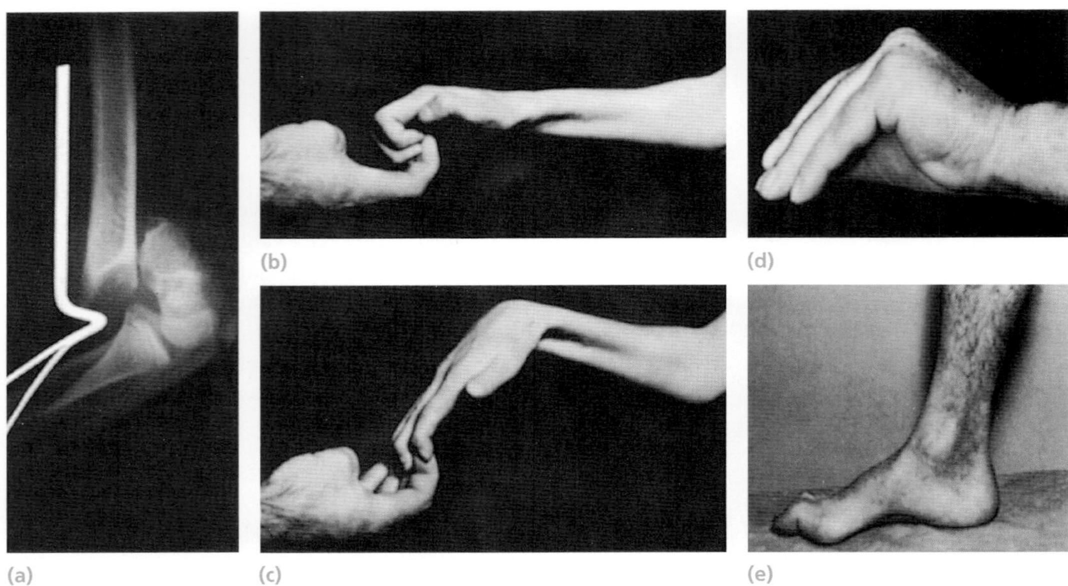

(a) (b) (c) (d) (e)

23.44 Volkmann's ischaemia (a) Kinking of the main artery is an important cause, but intimal tears may also lead to blockage from thrombosis. A delayed diagnosis of compartment syndrome carries the same sorry fate. (b,c) Volkmann's contracture of the forearm. The fingers can be straightened only when the wrist is flexed (the constant length phenomenon). (d) Ischaemic contracture of the small muscles of the hand. (e) Ischaemic contracture of the calf muscles with clawing of the toes.

JOINT INSTABILITY

Following injury a joint may give way. Causes include the following:

- *Ligamentous laxity* – especially at the knee, ankle and metacarpophalangeal joint of the thumb.
- *Muscle weakness* – especially if splintage has been excessive or prolonged, and exercises have been inadequate (again the knee and ankle are most often affected).
- *Bone loss* – especially after a gunshot fracture or severe compound injury, or from crushing of metaphyseal bone in joint depression fractures.

Injury may also lead to *recurrent dislocation*. The commonest sites are: (1) the shoulder – if the glenoid labrum has been detached (a Bankart lesion) and (2) the patella – if, after traumatic dislocation, the restraining patellofemoral ligament heals poorly.

A more subtle form of instability is seen after fractures around the wrist. Patients complaining of persistent discomfort or weakness after wrist injury should be fully investigated for *chronic carpal instability* (see Chapters 15 and 25).

JOINT STIFFNESS

Joint stiffness after a fracture commonly occurs in the knee, elbow, shoulder and (worst of all) small joints of the hand. Sometimes the joint itself has been injured; a haemarthrosis forms and leads to synovial adhesions. More often the stiffness is due to oedema and fibrosis of the capsule, ligaments and muscles around the joint, or adhesions of the soft tissues to each other or to the underlying bone. All these conditions are made worse by prolonged immobilization; moreover, if the joint has been held in a position where the ligaments are at their shortest, no amount of exercise will afterwards succeed in stretching these tissues and restoring the lost movement completely.

In a small percentage of patients with fractures of the forearm or leg, early post-traumatic swelling is accompanied by tenderness and progressive stiffness of the distal joints. These patients are at great risk of developing a *complex regional pain syndrome*; whether this is an entirely separate entity or merely an extension of the 'normal' post-traumatic soft-tissue reaction is uncertain. What is important is to recognize this type of 'stiffness' when it occurs and to insist on skilled physiotherapy until normal function is restored.

Treatment

The best treatment is prevention – by exercises that keep the joints mobile from the outset. If a joint has to be splinted, make sure that it is held in the 'position of safety' (page 431).

Joints that are already stiff take time to mobilize, but prolonged and patient physiotherapy can work wonders. If the situation is due to intra-articular adhesions, arthroscopic-guided releases may free the joint sufficiently to permit a more pliant response to further exercise. Occasionally, adherent or contracted tissues need to be released by operation (e.g. when knee flexion is prevented by adhesions in and around the quadriceps).

Complex regional pain syndrome (algodystrophy)

Sudeck, in 1900, described a condition characterized by painful osteoporosis of the hand. The same condition sometimes occurs after fractures of the extremities and for many years it was called *Sudeck's atrophy*. It is now recognized that this advanced atrophic disorder is the late stage of a post-traumatic *reflex sympathetic dystrophy* (also known as *algodystrophy*), which is much more common than originally believed (Atkins, 2003) and that it may follow relatively trivial injury. Because of continuing uncertainty about its nature, the term *complex regional pain syndrome* (CRPS) has been introduced (see page 261).

Two types of CRPS are recognized:

- Type 1 –a reflex sympathetic dystrophy that develops after an injurious or noxious event.
- Type 2 – causalgia that develops after a nerve injury.

The patient complains of continuous pain, often described as 'burning' in character. At first there is local swelling, redness and warmth, as well as tenderness and moderate stiffness of the nearby joints. As the weeks go by the skin becomes pale and atrophic, movements are increasingly restricted and the patient may develop fixed deformities. X-rays characteristically show patchy rarefaction of the bone.

The earlier the condition is recognized and treatment begun, the better the prognosis. Elevation and active exercises are important after all injuries, but in CRPS they are essential. In the early stage of the condition anti-inflammatory drugs and adequate analgesia are helpful. Involvement of a pain specialist who has familiarity with desensitization methods, regional anaesthesia, and use of drugs like amitriptyline, carbamazepine and gabapentin may help; this, combined with prolonged and dedicated physiotherapy, is the mainstay of treatment.

Osteoarthritis

A fracture involving a joint may severely damage the articular cartilage and give rise to post-traumatic osteoarthritis within a period of months. Even if the cartilage heals, irregularity of the joint surface may

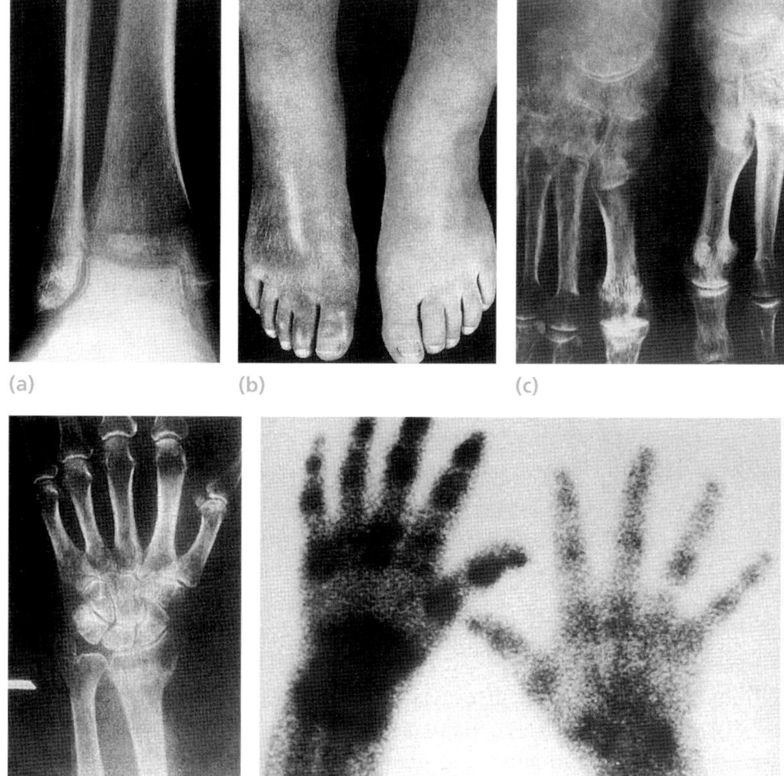

23.45 Complex regional pain syndrome (a) Regional osteoporosis is common after fractures of the extremities. The radiolucent bands seen here are typical. (b) In algodystrophy the picture is exaggerated and the soft tissues are also involved: here the right foot is somewhat swollen and the skin has become dusky, smooth and shiny. (c) In the full-blown case, x-rays show a typical patchy osteoporosis. (d) Similar changes may occur in the wrist and hand; they are always accompanied by (e) increased activity in the radionuclide scan.

cause localized stress and so predispose to secondary osteoarthritis years later. If the step-off in the articular surface involves a large fragment in a joint that is readily accessible to surgery, intra-articular osteotomies and re-positioning of the fragment may help. Often though the problem arises from areas that were previously comminuted and depressed – little can be done once the fracture has united.

Malunion of a metaphyseal fracture may radically alter the mechanics of a nearby joint and this, too, can give rise to secondary osteoarthritis. It is often asserted that malunion in the shaft of a long bone (e.g. the tibia) may act in a similar manner; however, there is little evidence to show that residual angulation of less than 15 degrees can cause proximal or distal osteoarthritis.

STRESS FRACTURES

A stress or fatigue fracture is one occurring in the normal bone of a healthy patient, due not to any specific traumatic incident but to small repetitive stresses of two main types: bending and compression.

Bending stress causes deformation and bone responds by changing the pattern of remodelling. With repeated stress, osteoclastic resorption exceeds osteoblastic formation and a zone of relative weakness develops – ultimately leading to a breach in the cortex. This process affects young adults undertaking strenuous physical routines and is probably due to muscular forces acting on bone. Athletes in training, dancers and military recruits build up muscle power quickly but bone strength only slowly; this accounts for the high incidence of stress fractures in these groups.

Compressive stresses act on soft cancellous bone; with frequent repetition an impacted fracture may result.

A combination of compression and shearing stresses may account for the osteochondral fracures that characterize some of the so-called osteochondritides.

'Spontaneous fractures' occur with even greater ease in people with osteoporosis or osteomalacia and in patients treated with drugs that affect bone remodelling in a similar way (e.g. corticosteroids and methotrexate). These are often referred to as *insufficiency fractures*.

Sites affected

Least rare are the following: shaft of humerus (adolescent cricketers); pars interarticularis of fifth lumbar vertebra (causing spondylolysis); pubic rami (inferior in children, both rami in adults); femoral neck (at any age); femoral shaft (chiefly lower third); patella (children and young adults); tibial shaft (proximal third in children, middle third in athletes and trainee paratroopers, distal third in the elderly); distal shaft of the fibula (the 'runner's fracture'); calcaneum (adults); navicular (athletes) and metatarsals (especially the second).

Clinical features

There may be a history of unaccustomed and repetitive activity or one of a strenuous physical exercise programme. A common sequence of events is: *pain after exercise – pain during exercise – pain without exercise*. Occasionally the patient presents only after the fracture has healed and may then complain of a lump (the callus).

The patient is usually healthy. The affected site may be swollen or red. It is sometimes warm and usually tender; the callus may be palpable. 'Springing' the bone (attempting to bend it) is often painful.

Imaging

X-RAY

Early on, the fracture is difficult to detect, but radioscintigraphy will show increased activity at the painful spot. Plain x-rays taken a few weeks later may show a small transverse defect in the cortex and/or localized periosteal new-bone formation. These appearances have, at times, been mistaken for those of an osteosarcoma, a horrifying trap for the unwary. Compression stress fractures (especially of the femoral neck and upper tibia) may show as a hazy transverse band of sclerosis with (in the tibia) peripheral callus.

Another typical picture is that of a small osteoarticular fracture – most commonly of the dome of the medial femoral condyle at the knee or the upper surface of the talus at the ankle. Later, ischaemic necrosis of the detached fragment may render the lesion even more obvious.

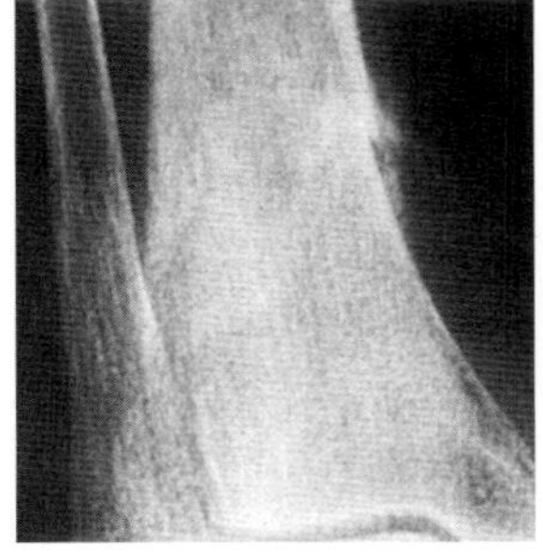

(a)

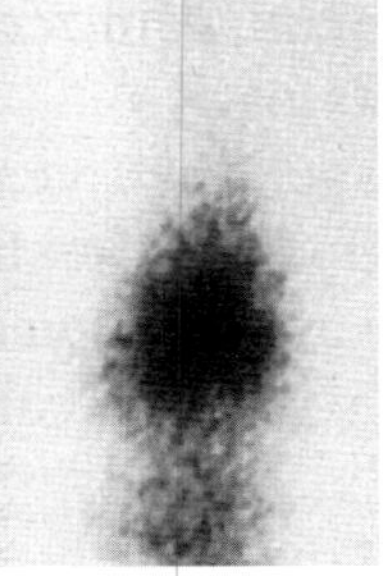

(b)

23.46 Stress fracture (a) The stress fracture in this tibia is only just visible on x-ray, but it had already been suspected 2 weeks earlier when the patient first complained of pain and a radioisotope scan revealed a 'hot' area just above the ankle **(b)**.

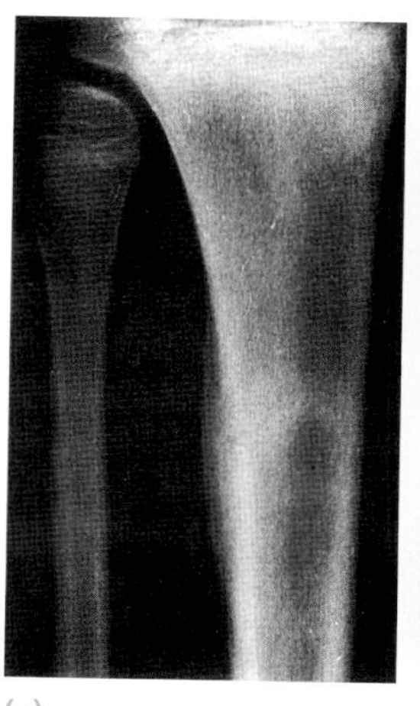

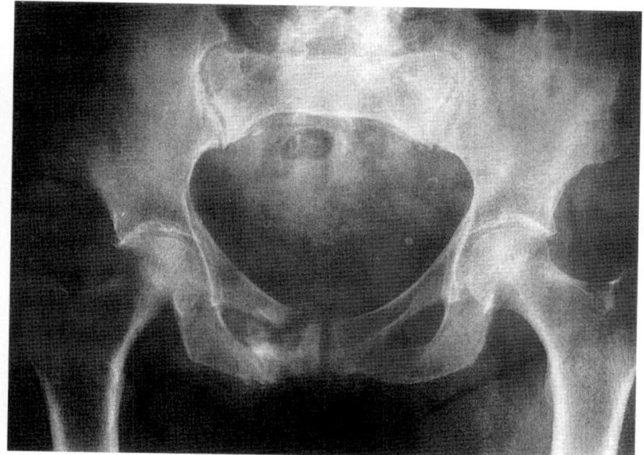

(a) (b)

23.47 Stress fractures Stress fractures are often missed or wrongly diagnosed. (a) This tibial fracture was at first thought to be an osteosarcoma. (b) Stress fractures of the pubic rami in elderly women can be mistaken for metastases.

MRI

The earliest changes, particularly in 'spontaneous' undisplaced osteoarticular fractures, are revealed by MRI. This investigation should be requested in older patients (possibly with osteoporosis) complaining of sudden onset of pain over the anteromedial part of the knee.

Diagnosis

Many disorders, including osteomyelitis, scurvy and battered baby syndrome, may be confused with stress fractures. The great danger, however, is a mistaken diagnosis of osteosarcoma; scanning shows increased uptake in both conditions and even biopsy may be misleading.

Treatment

Most stress fractures need no treatment other than an elastic bandage and avoidance of the painful activity until the lesion heals; surprisingly, this can take many months and the forced inactivity is not easily accepted by the hard-driving athlete or dancer.

An important exception is stress fracture of the femoral neck. This should be suspected in all elderly people who complain of pain in the hip for which no obvious cause can be found. If the diagnosis is confirmed by bone scan, the femoral neck should be internally fixed with screws as a prophylactic measure.

PATHOLOGICAL FRACTURES

When abnormal bone gives way this is referred to as a pathological fracture. The causes are numerous and varied; often the diagnosis is not made until a biopsy is examined (Table 23.5).

Table 23.5 Causes of pathological fracture

Generalized bone disease	Primary malignant tumours
1. Osteogenesis imperfecta 2. Postmenopausal osteoporosis 3. Metabolic bone disease 4. Myelomatosis 5. Polyostotic fibrous dysplasia 6. Paget's disease	1. Chondrosarcoma 2. Osteosarcoma 3. Ewing's tumour
Local benign conditions	**Metastatic tumours**
1. Chronic infection 2. Solitary bone cyst 3. Fibrous cortical defect 4. Chondromyxoid fibroma 5. Aneurysmal bone cyst 6. Chondroma 7. Monostotic fibrous dysplasia	Carcinoma in breast, lung, kidney, thyroid, colon and prostate

History

Bone that fractures spontaneously, or after trivial injury, must be regarded as abnormal until proved otherwise. Older patients should always be asked about previous illnesses or operations. A malignant tumour, no matter how long ago it occurred, may be the source of a late metastatic lesion; a history of gastrectomy, intestinal malabsorption, chronic alcoholism or prolonged drug therapy should suggest a metabolic bone disorder.

Symptoms such as loss of weight, pain, a lump, cough or haematuria suggest that the fracture may be through a secondary deposit.

In younger patients, a history of several previous fractures may suggest a diagnosis of osteogenesis imperfecta, even if the patient does not show the classic features of the disorder.

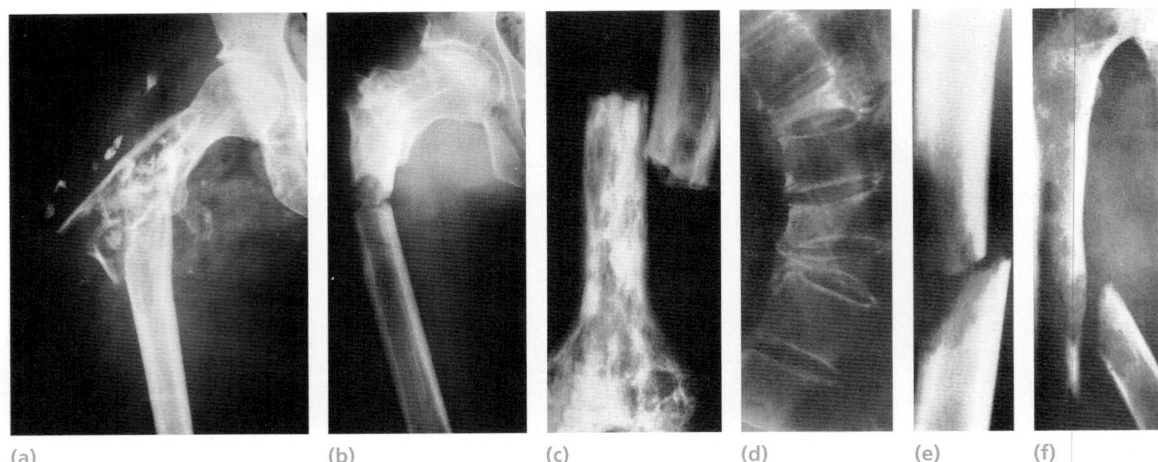

(a) (b) (c) (d) (e) (f)

23.48 Pathological fractures Six examples of pathological fractures, due to: (a) primary chondrosarcoma; (b) postoperative bone infection at a screw-hole following plating of an intertrochanteric fracture; (c) Paget's disease; (d) vertebral metastases; (e) metastasis from carcinoma of the breast and (f) myelomatosis.

Examination

Local signs of bone disease (an infected sinus, an old scar, swelling or deformity) should not be missed. The site of the fracture may suggest the diagnosis: patients with involutional osteoporosis develop fractures of the vertebral bodies and corticocancellous junctions of long bones; a fracture through the shaft of the bone in an elderly patient, especially in the subtrochanteric region, should be regarded as a pathological fracture until proved otherwise.

General examination may be informative. Congenital dysplasias, fibrous dysplasia, Cushing' syndrome and Paget' disease all produce characteristic appearances. The patient may be wasted (possibly due to malignant disease). The lymph nodes or liver may be enlarged. It should be noted whether there is a mass in the abdomen or pelvis. Old scars should not be overlooked and rectal and vaginal examinations are mandatory.

Under the age of 20 the common causes of pathological fracture are benign bone tumours and cysts. Over the age of 40 the common causes are multiple myeloma, secondary carcinoma and Paget's disease.

X-ray

Understandably, the fracture itself attracts most attention but the surrounding bone must also be examined, and features such as cyst formation, cortical erosion, abnormal trabeculation and periosteal thickening should be sought. The type of fracture, too, is important: vertebral compression fractures may be due to severe osteoporosis or osteomalacia, but they can also be caused by skeletal metastases or myeloma. Middle-aged men, unlike women, do not normally become osteoporotic: x-ray signs of bone loss and vertebral compression in a male younger than 75 years should be regarded as 'pathological' until proven otherwise.

Additional investigations

Local radionuclide imaging may help elucidate the diagnosis, and whole-body scanning is important in revealing or excluding other deposits.

X-ray of other bones, the lungs and the urogenital tract may be necessary to exclude malignant disease.

Investigations should always include a full blood count, ESR, protein electrophoresis, and tests for syphilis and metabolic bone disorders.

Urine examination may reveal blood from a tumour, or Bence–Jones protein in myelomatosis.

Biopsy

Some lesions are so typical that a biopsy is unnecessary (solitary cyst, fibrous cortical defect, Paget's disease). Others are more obscure and a biopsy is essential for diagnosis. If open reduction of the fracture is indicated, the biopsy can be carried out at the same time; otherwise a definitive procedure should be arranged.

Treatment

The principles of fracture treatment remain the same: *reduce, hold, exercise*. However the choice of method is influenced by the condition of the bone; and the underlying pathological disorder may need treatment in its own right (see Chapter 9).

Generalized bone disease In most of these conditions (including Paget's disease) the bones fracture more easily, but they heal quite well provided the fracture is

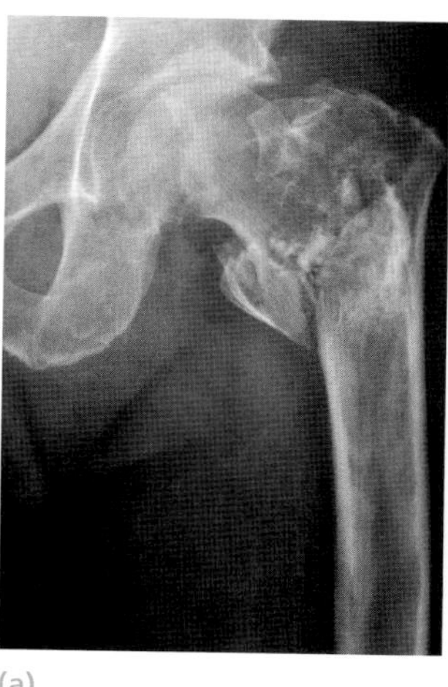
(a)

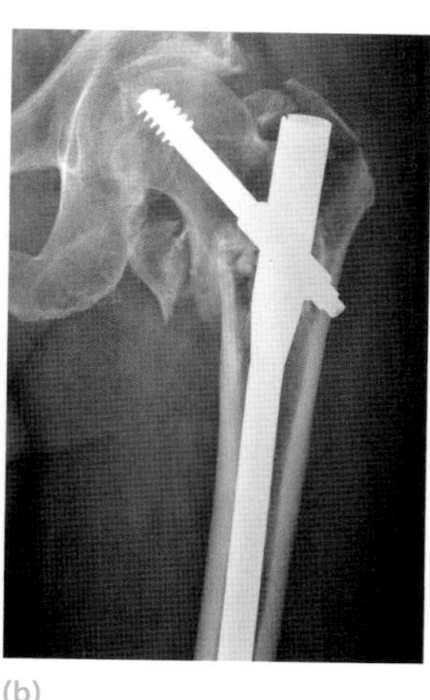
(b)

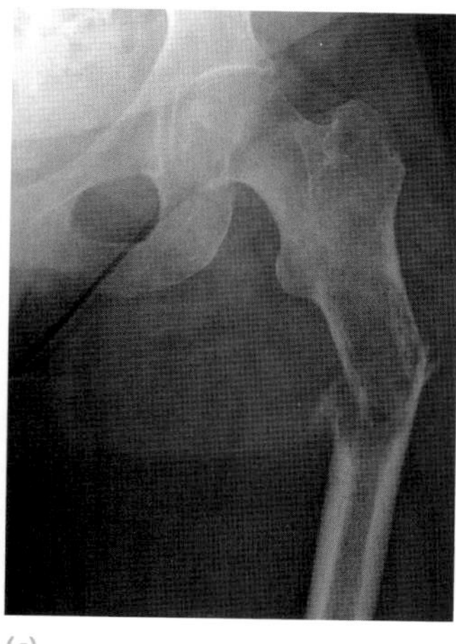
(c)

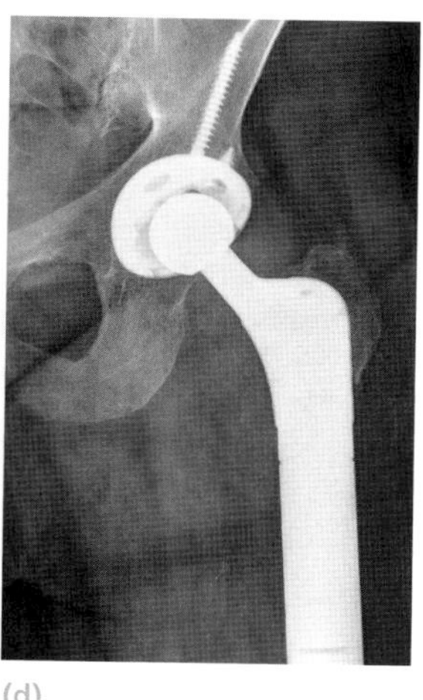
(d)

23.49 Pathological fractures – treatment (a,b) Paget's disease of the femur increases the brittleness of bone, making it more likely to fracture. Intramedullary fixation allows the entire femur to be supported. (c,d) A fracture through a solitary metastasis from a previously excised renal cell carcinoma can be resected in order to achieve cure. In this case replacement of the proximal femur with an endoprosthesis is needed.

properly immobilized. Internal fixation is therefore advisable (and for Paget's disease almost essential). Patients with osteomalacia, hyperparathyroidism, renal osteodystrophy and Paget's disease will need systemic treatment as well.

Local benign conditions Fractures through benign cyst-like lesions usually heal quite well and they should be allowed to do so before tackling the local lesion. Treatment is therefore the same as for simple fractures in the same area, although in some cases it will be necessary to take a biopsy before immobilizing the fracture. When the bone has healed, the tumour can be dealt with by curettage or local excision.

Primary malignant tumour The fracture may need splinting but this is merely a prelude to definitive treatment of the tumour, which by now will have spread to the surrounding soft tissues. The prognosis is almost always very poor.

Metastatic tumours Metastasis is a frequent cause of pathological fracture in older people. Breast cancer is the commonest source and the femur the commonest site. Nowadays cancer patients (even those with metastases) often live for several years and effective treatment of the fracture will vastly improve their quality of life.

Fracture of a long-bone shaft should be treated by internal fixation; if necessary the site is also packed with acrylic cement. Bear in mind that the implant will function as a load-*bearing* and not a load-*sharing* device; intramedullary nails are more suitable than plates and screws.

Fracture near a bone end can often be treated by excision and prosthetic replacement; this is especially true of femoral neck fractures.

Preoperatively, imaging studies should be performed to detect other bone lesions; these may be amenable to prophylactic fixation. Once the wound has healed, local irradiation should be applied to reduce the risk of progressive osteolysis.

Pathological compression fractures of the spine cause severe pain. This is due largely to spinal instability and treatment should include operative stabilization. If there are either clinical or imaging features of actual or threatened spinal cord or cauda equina compression, the segment should also be decompressed. Postoperative irradiation is given as usual.

With all types of metastatic lesion, the primary tumour should be investigated and treated as well.

INJURIES OF THE PHYSIS

In children over 10 per cent of fractures involve injury to the growth plate (or physis). Because the physis is a relatively weak part of the bone, joint strains that might cause ligament injuries in adults are liable to result in separation of the physis in children. The fracture usually runs transversely through the hypertrophic or the calcified layer of the growth plate, often veering off into the metaphysis at one of the edges to include a triangular lip of bone. This has little effect on longitudinal growth, which takes place in the germinal and proliferating layers of the physis. However, if the fracture traverses the cellular 'reproductive' layers of the physis, it may result in premature ossification of the injured part and serious disturbances of bone growth.

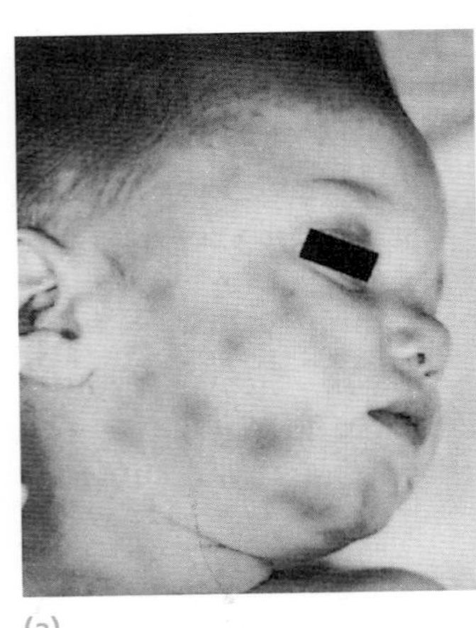

(a)

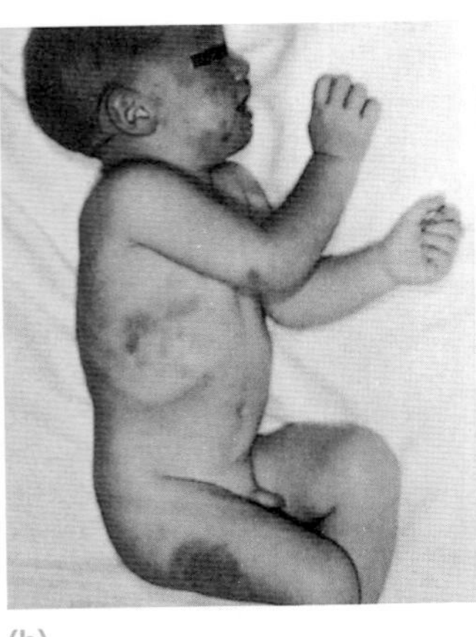

(b)

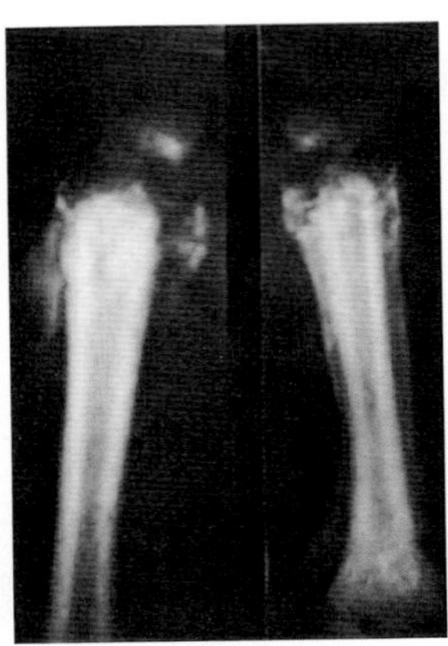

(c)

23.50 Battered baby syndrome (a–c) The fractures are not pathological but the family is. The metaphyseal lesions in each humerus are characteristic.

Classification

The most widely used classification of physeal injuries is that of Salter and Harris (Salter and Harris, 1963), which distinguishes five basic types of injury:

- *Type 1* – A transverse fracture through the hypertrophic or calcified zone of the plate. Even if the fracture is quite alarmingly displaced, the growing zone of the physis is usually not injured and growth disturbance is uncommon.
- *Type 2* – This is essentially similar to type 1, but towards the edge the fracture deviates away from the physis and splits off a triangular metaphyseal fragment of bone (sometimes referred to as the *Thurston– Holland* fragment).
- *Type 3* – A fracture that splits the epiphysis and then veers off transversely to one or the other side, through the hypertrophic layer of the physis. Inevitably it damages the 'reproductive' layers of the physis (as these layers are closer to the epiphysis than the metaphysis) and may result in growth disturbance.
- *Type 4* – As with type 3, the fracture splits the epiphysis, but it extends into the metaphysis. These fractures are liable to displacement and a consequent misfit between the separated parts of the physis, resulting in asymmetrical growth.
- *Type 5* – A longitudinal compression injury of the physis. There is no visible fracture but the growth plate is crushed and this may result in growth arrest.

Rang (Rang, 1969) has added a *Type 6,* an injury to the perichondrial ring (the peripheral zone of Ranvier), which carries a significant risk of growth disturbance. The diagnosis is made usually in retrospect after development of deformity.

Mechanism of injury

Physeal fractures usually result from falls or traction injuries. They occur mostly in road accidents and during sporting activities or playground tumbles.

Clinical features

These fractures are more common in boys than in girls and are usually seen either in infancy or between the ages of 10 and 12. Deformity is usually minimal,

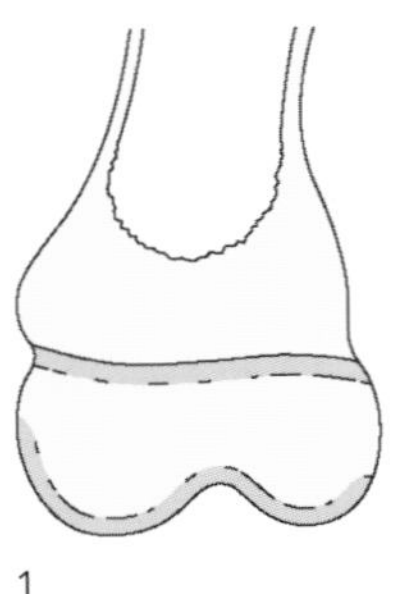

1

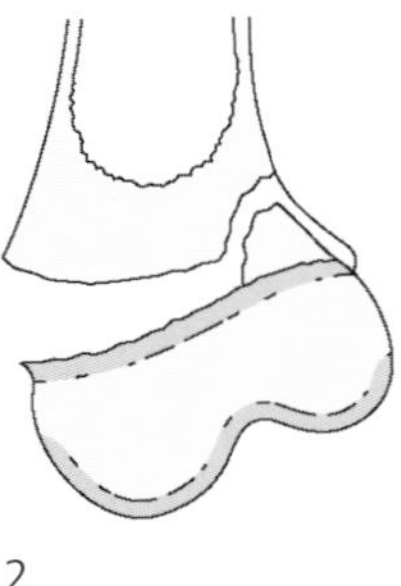

2

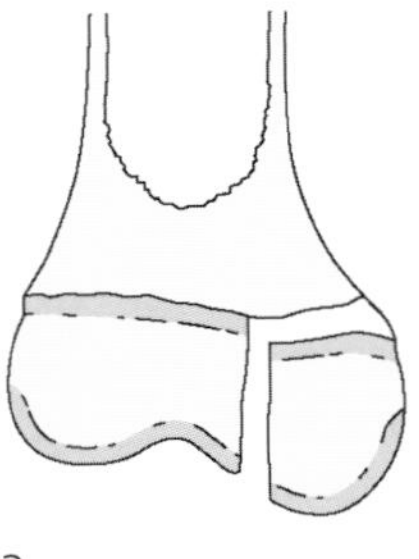

3

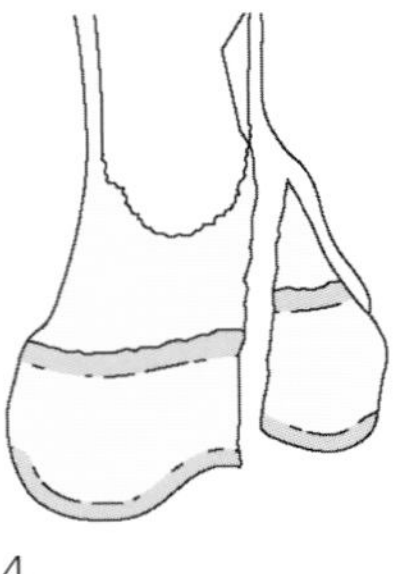

4

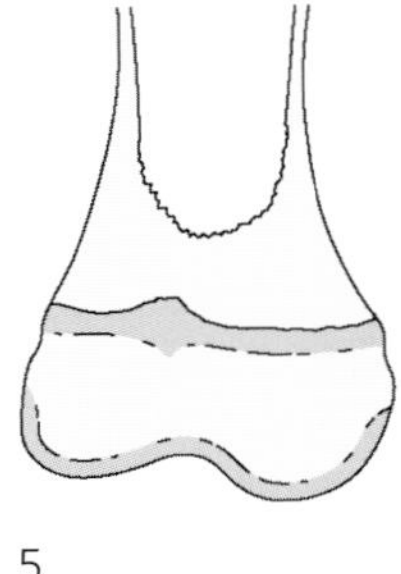

5

23.51 Physeal injuries Type 1 – separation of the epiphysis – which usually occurs in infants but is also seen at puberty as a slipped femoral epiphysis. Type 2 – fracture through the physis and metaphysis – is the commonest; it occurs in older children and seldom results in abnormal growth. Type 3 – an intra-articular fracture of the epiphysis – needs accurate reduction to restore the joint surface. Type 4 – splitting of the physis and epiphysis – damages the articular surface and may also cause abnormal growth; if it is displaced it needs open reduction. Type 5 – crushing of the physis – may look benign but ends in arrested growth.

but any injury in a child followed by pain and tenderness near the joint should arouse suspicion, and x-ray examination is essential.

X-rays

The physis itself is radiolucent and the epiphysis may be incompletely ossified; this makes it hard to tell whether the bone end is damaged or deformed. The younger the child, the smaller the 'visible' part of the epiphysis and thus the more difficult it is to make the diagnosis; comparison with the normal side is a great help. Telltale features are widening of the physeal 'gap', incongruity of the joint or tilting of the epiphyseal axis. If there is marked displacement the diagnosis is obvious, but even a type 4 fracture may at first be so little displaced that the fracture line is hard to see; if there is the faintest suspicion of a physeal fracture, a repeat x-ray after 4 or 5 days is essential. Types 5 and 6 injuries are usually diagnosed only in retrospect.

Treatment

Undisplaced fractures may be treated by splinting the part in a cast or a close-fitting plaster slab for 2–4 weeks (depending on the site of injury and the age of the child). However, with undisplaced types 3 and 4 fractures, a check x-ray after 4 days and again at about 10 days is mandatory in order not to miss late displacement.

Displaced fractures should be reduced as soon as possible. With types 1 and 2 this can usually be done closed; the part is then splinted securely for 3–6 weeks. Types 3 and 4 fractures demand perfect anatomical reduction. An attempt can be made to achieve this by gentle manipulation under general anaesthesia; if this is successful, the limb is held in a cast for 4–8 weeks (the longer periods for type 4 injuries). If a type 3 or 4 fracture cannot be reduced accurately by closed manipulation, immediate open reduction and internal fixation with smooth K-wires is essential. The limb is then splinted for 4–6 weeks, but it takes that long again before the child is ready to resume unrestricted activities.

Complications

Types 1 and 2 injuries, if properly reduced, have an excellent prognosis and bone growth is not adversely affected. Exceptions to this rule are injuries around the knee involving the distal femoral or proximal tibial physis; both growth plates are undulating in shape, so a transverse fracture plane may actually pass through more than just the hypertrophic zone but also damage the proliferative zone. Complications such as malunion or non-union may also occur if the diagnosis is missed and the fracture remains unreduced (e.g. fracture separation of the medial humeral epicondyle).

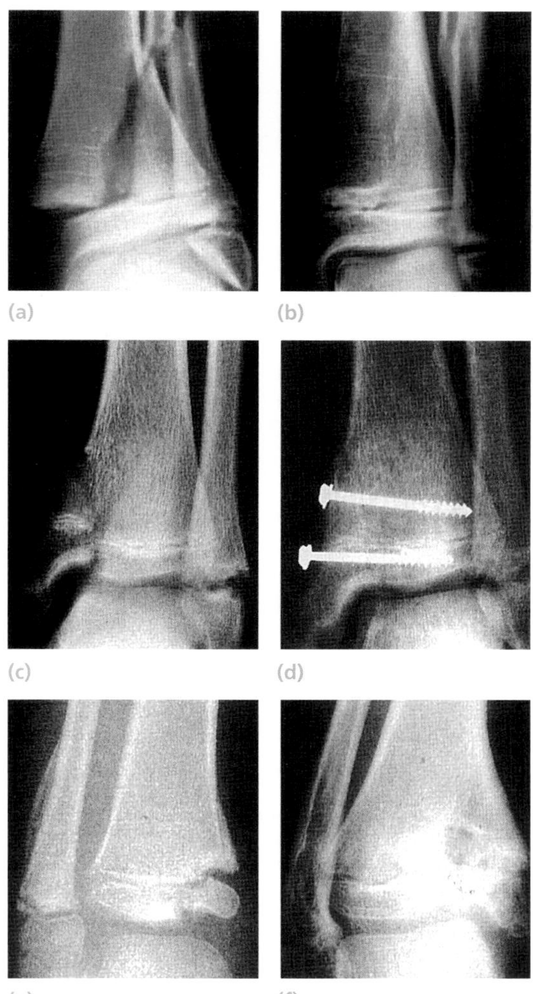

23.52 Physeal injuries (a) Type 2 injury. The fracture does not traverse the width of the physis; after reduction (b) bone growth is not distorted. (c,d) This type 4 fracture of the tibial physis was treated immediately by open reduction and internal fixation and a good result was obtained. (e,f) In this case accurate reduction was not achieved and the physeal fragment remained displaced; the end result was partial fusion of the physis and severe deformity of the ankle.

Types 3 and 4 injuries may result in premature fusion of part of the growth plate or asymmetrical growth of the bone end. Types 5 and 6 fractures cause premature fusion and retardation of growth. The size and position of the bony bridge across the physis can be assessed by tomography or magnetic resonance imaging (MRI). If the bridge is relatively small (less than one-third the width of the physis) it can be excised and replaced by a fat graft, with some prospect of preventing or diminishing the growth disturbance (Langenskiold, 1975; 1981). However, if the bone

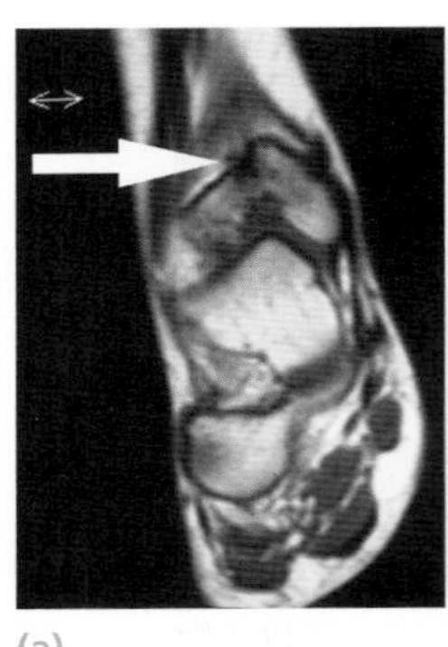

(a)

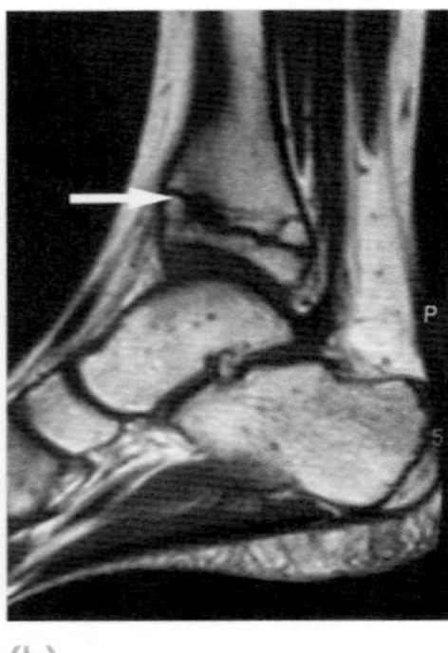

(b)

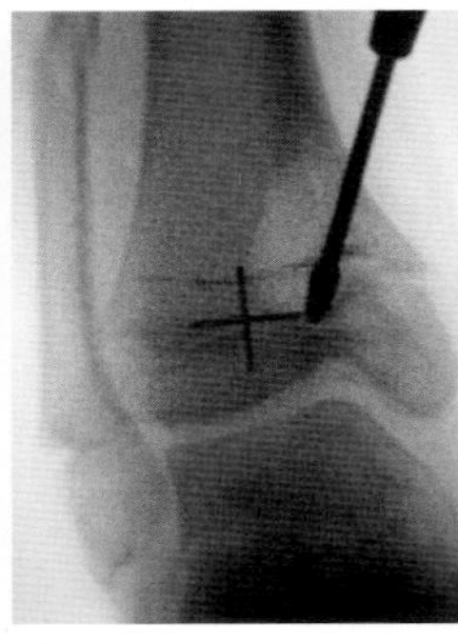

(c)

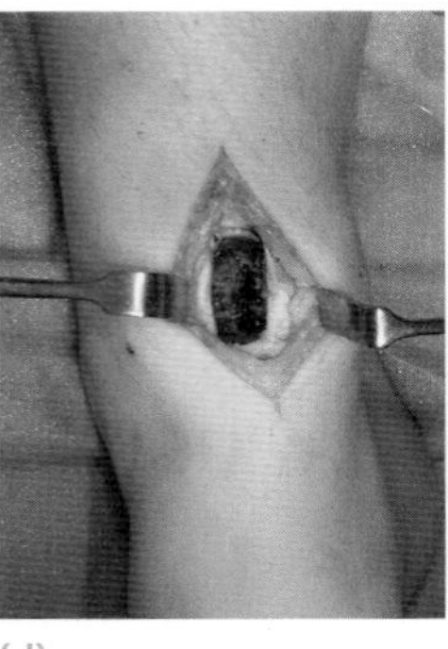

(d)

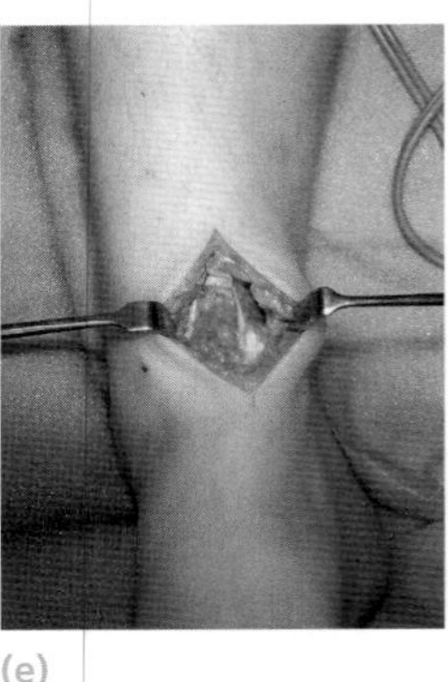

(e)

23.53 Langenskiold procedure for physeal arrest Small tethers across the physis can be mapped out by MRI (a,b), then surgically removed by drilling out and curettage (c) and filling the defect with fat graft (d,e).

bridge is more extensive the operation is contraindicated as it can end up doing more harm than good.

Established deformity, whether from asymmetrical growth or from malunion of a displaced fracture (e.g. a valgus elbow due to proximal displacement of a lateral humeral condylar fracture) should be treated by corrective osteotomy. If further growth is abnormal, the osteotomy may have to be repeated.

INJURIES TO JOINTS

Joints are usually injured by twisting or tilting forces that stretch the ligaments and capsule. If the force is great enough the ligaments may tear, or the bone to which they are attached may be pulled apart. The articular cartilage, too, may be damaged if the joint surfaces are compressed or if there is a fracture into the joint.

As a general principle, forceful angulation will tear the ligaments rather than crush the bone, but in older people with porotic bone the ligaments may hold and the bone on the opposite side of the joint is crushed instead, while in children there may be a fracture-separation of the physis.

Sprains, strains and ruptures

There is much confusion about the use of the terms 'sprain', 'strain' and 'rupture'. Strictly speaking, a *sprain* is any painful wrenching (twisting or pulling) movement of a joint, but the term is generally reserved for joint injuries less severe than actual tearing of the capsule or ligaments. *Strain* is a physical effect of stress, in this case tensile stress associated with some stretching of the ligaments; in colloquial usage, 'strained ligament' is often meant to denote an injury somewhat more severe than a 'sprain', which possibly involves tearing of some fibres. If the stretching or twisting force is severe enough, the ligament may be strained to the point of complete *rupture*.

STRAINED LIGAMENT

Only some of the fibres in the ligament are torn and the joint remains stable. The injury is one in which the joint is momentarily twisted or bent into an abnormal position. The joint is painful and swollen and the tissues may be bruised. Tenderness is localized to the injured ligament and tensing the tissues on that side causes a sharp increase in pain.

Treatment

The joint should be firmly strapped and rested until the acute pain subsides. Thereafter, active movements are encouraged, and exercises practised to strengthen the muscles.

RUPTURED LIGAMENT

The ligament is completely torn and the joint is unstable. Sometimes the ligament holds and the bone to which it is attached is avulsed; this is effectively the same lesion but easier to deal with because the bone fragment can be securely reattached.

As with a strain, the joint is suddenly forced into an abnormal position; sometimes the patient actually hears a snap. The joints most likely to be affected are the ones that are insecure by virtue of their shape or least well protected by surrounding muscles: the knee, ankle and finger joints.

Pain is severe and there may be considerable bleeding under the skin; if the joint is swollen, this is probably due to a haemarthrosis. The patient is unlikely to permit a searching examination, but under general anaesthesia the instability can be demonstrated; it is this that distinguishes the lesion from a strain. X-ray

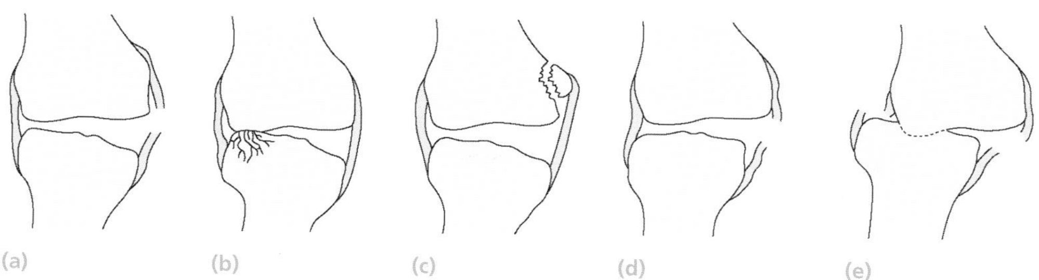

23.54 Joint injuries Severe stress may cause various types of injury. (a) A ligament may rupture, leaving the bone intact. If the soft tissues hold, the bone on the opposite side may be crushed (b), or a fragment may be pulled off by the taut ligament (c). Subluxation (d) means the articular surfaces are partially displaced; dislocation (e) refers to complete displacement of the joint.

may show a detached flake of bone where the ligament is inserted.

Treatment

Torn ligaments heal by fibrous scarring. Previously this was thought inevitable and the surgeon's task was to ensure that the torn ends were securely sutured so as to restore the ligament to its normal length. In some injuries, e.g. rupture of the ulnar collateral ligament of the metacarpophalangeal joint of the thumb, this approach is still valid. In others, however, it has changed; thus, solitary medial collateral ligament ruptures of the knee, even complete ruptures, are often treated non-operatively in the first instance. The joint is splinted and local measures are taken to reduce swelling. After 1–2 weeks, the splint is exchanged for a functional brace that allows joint movement but at the same time prevents repeat injury to the ligament, especially if some instability is also present. Physiotherapy is applied to maintain muscle strength and later proprioceptive exercises are added. This non-operative approach has shown better results not only in the strength of the healed ligament but also in the nature of healing – there is less fibrosis (Woo et al., 2000). An exception to this non-operative approach is when the ligament is avulsed with an attached fragment of bone; reattachment of the fragment is indicated if the piece is large enough. Occasionally non-operative treatment may result in some residual instability that is clinically detectable; often this is not symptomatic, but if it is then surgical reconstruction should be considered.

DISLOCATION AND SUBLUXATION

'Dislocation' means that the joint surfaces are completely displaced and are no longer in contact; 'subluxation' implies a lesser degree of displacement, such that the articular surfaces are still partly apposed.

Clinical features

Following an injury the joint is painful and the patient tries at all costs to avoid moving it. The shape of the joint is abnormal and the bony landmarks may be displaced. The limb is often held in a characteristic position; movement is painful and restricted. X-rays will usually clinch the diagnosis; they will also show whether there is an associated bony injury affecting joint stability – i.e. a fracture-dislocation.

Apprehension test If the dislocation is reduced by the time the patient is seen, the joint can be tested by stressing it as if almost to reproduce the suspected dislocation: the patient develops a sense of impending disaster and violently resists further manipulation.

Recurrent dislocation If the ligaments and joint margins are damaged, repeated dislocation may occur. This is seen especially in the shoulder and patellofemoral joint.

Habitual (voluntary) dislocation Some patients acquire the knack of dislocating (or subluxating) the joint by voluntary muscle contraction. Ligamentous laxity may make this easier, but the habit often betrays a manipulative and neurotic personality. It is important to recognize this because such patients are seldom helped by operation.

Treatment

The dislocation must be reduced as soon as possible; usually a general anaesthetic is required, and sometimes a muscle relaxant as well. The joint is then rested or immobilized until soft-tissue swelling reduces – usually after 2 weeks. Controlled movements then begin in a functional brace; progress with physiotherapy is monitored. Occasionally surgical reconstruction for residual instability is called for.

Complications

Many of the complications of fractures are seen also after dislocations: vascular injury, nerve injury, avascular necrosis of bone, heterotopic ossification, joint stiffness and secondary osteoarthritis. The principles of diagnosis and management of these conditions have been discussed earlier.

REFERENCES AND FURTHER READING

Atkins RM. Complex regional pain syndrome. *J Bone Joint Surg* 2003; **85B:** 1100–6.

Charnley J. *The Closed Treatment of Common Fractures.* Churchill Livingstone, Edinburgh, 1961.

Dicpinigaitis PA, Koval KJ, Tejwani NC, Egol KA. Gunshot wounds to the extremities. *Bull NYU Hosp Jt Dis* 2006; **64:** 139–55.

Giordano CP, Koval KJ, Zuckerman JD, Desai P. Fracture blisters. *Clin Orthop* 1994; **307:** 214–21.

Gustilo RB, Mendoza RM, Williams DN. Problems in the management of type III (severe) open fractures: a new classification of type III open fractures. *J Trauma* 1984; **24:** 742–6.

Kenwright J, Richardson JB, Cunningham JL *et al.* Axial movement and tibial fractures. A controlled randomised trial of treatment. *J Bone Joint Surg* 1991; **73B:** 654–9.

Langenskiold A. An operation for partial closure of an epiphysial plate in children, and its experimental basis. *J Bone Joint Surg* 1975; **57B:** 325–30.

Langenskiold A. Surgical treatment of partial closure of the growth plate. *J Pediatr Orthop* 1981; **1:** 3–11.

Marsh JL, Slongo TF, Agel J *et al.* Fracture and dislocation classification compendium – 2007: Orthopaedic Trauma Association classification, database and outcomes committee. *J Orthop Trauma* 2007; **21(Suppl):** S1–133.

McKibbin B. The biology of fracture healing in long bone. *J Bone Joint Surg* 1978; **60B:** 150–62.

Müller M., Nazarian S, Koch P, Schatzker J. *The Comprehensive Classification of Fractures of Long Bones.* Springer Verlag, Berlin, Heidelberg, New York, 1990.

Oestern H, Tscherne H. Pathophysiology and classification of soft tissue injuries associated with fractures. In: H. Tscherne and L. Gotzen (eds) *Fractures with Soft Tissue Injuries.* Springer Verlag, Berlin, 1984.

Pape HC, Giannoudis PV, Kretteck C, Trentz O. Timing of fixation of major fractures in blunt polytrauma: role of conventional indicators in clinical decision making. *J Orthop Trauma* 2005; **19:** 551–62.

Rang M. *The growth plate and its disorders.* Churchill Livingstone, Edinburgh, 1969.

Roberts CS, Pape HC, Jones AL *et al.* Damage control orthopaedics. Evolving concepts in the treatment of patients who have sustained orthopaedic trauma. *J Bone Joint Surg* 2005; **87A:** 434–49.

Salter RB, Harris WR. Injuries involving the epiphyseal plate. *J Bone Joint Surg* 1963; **45A:** 587–622.

Sarmiento A, Latta L. Functional fracture bracing. *J Am Acad Orthop Surg* 1999; **7:** 66–75.

Sarmiento A, Latta L. The evolution of functional bracing of fractures. *J Bone Joint Surg* 2006; **88B:** 141–8.

Sarmiento A, Mullis DL, Latta L *et al.* A quantitative comparative analysis of fracture healing under the influence of compression plating vs. closed weight-bearing treatment. *Clin Orthop* 1980; **149:** 232–9.

Slongo TF, Audige L. Fracture and dislocation classification compendium for children: the AO pediatric comprehensive classification of long bone fractures (PCCF). *J Orthop Trauma* 2007; **21(Suppl):** S135–60.

Ulmer T. The clinical diagnosis of compartment syndrome of the lower leg: Are clinical findings predictive of the disorder? *J Orthop Trauma* 2002; **16:** 572–577.

Woo SL, Vogrin TM, Abramowitch SD. Healing and repair of ligament injuries in the knee. *J Am Acad Orthop Surg* 2000; **8:** 364–72.

Injuries of the shoulder, upper arm and elbow

24

Andrew Cole, Paul Pavlou, David Warwick

The great bugbear of upper limb injuries is stiffness – particularly of the shoulder but sometimes of the elbow and hand as well. Two points should be constantly borne in mind:

- Whatever the injury, and however it is treated, all the joints that are not actually immobilized – and especially the finger joints – should be exercised from the start.
- In elderly patients it is sometimes best to disregard the fracture and concentrate on regaining movement.

FRACTURES OF THE CLAVICLE

In children the clavicle fractures easily, but it almost invariably unites rapidly and without complications. In adults this can be a much more troublesome injury.

In adults clavicle fractures are common, accounting for 2.6–4 per cent of fractures and approximately 35 per cent of all shoulder girdle injuries. Fractures of the mid-shaft account for 69–82 per cent, lateral fractures for 21–28 per cent and medial fractures for 2–3 per cent.

Mechanism of injury

A fall on the shoulder or the outstretched hand may break the clavicle. In the common mid-shaft fracture, the outer fragment is pulled down by the weight of the arm and the inner half is held up by the sternomastoid muscle. In fractures of the outer end, if the ligaments are intact there is little displacement; but if the coracoclavicular ligaments are torn, or if the fracture is just medial to these ligaments, displacement may be severe and closed reduction impossible.

Clinical features

The arm is clasped to the chest to prevent movement. A subcutaneous lump may be obvious and occasionally a sharp fragment threatens the skin. Though vascular complications are rare, it is prudent to feel the pulse and gently to palpate the root of the neck. Outer third fractures are easily missed or mistaken for acromioclavicular joint injuries.

Imaging

Radiographic analysis requires at least an anteroposterior view and another taken with a 30 degree cephalic tilt. The fracture is usually in the middle third of the bone, and the outer fragment usually lies below the inner. Fractures of the outer third may be missed, or the degree of displacement underestimated, unless additional views of the shoulder are obtained. With medial third fractures it is also wise to obtain x-rays of the sterno-clavicular joint. In assessing clinical progress, remember that 'clinical' union usually precedes 'radiological' union by several weeks.

CT scanning with three-dimensional reconstructions may be needed to determine accurately the degree of shortening or for diagnosing a sterno-clavicular fracture-dislocation, and also to establish whether a fracture has united.

Classification

Clavicle fractures are usually classified on the basis of their location: Group I (middle third fractures), Group II (lateral third fractures) and Group III (medial third fractures). Lateral third fractures can be further sub-classified into (a) those with the coraco-clavicular ligaments intact, (b) those where the coracoclavicular ligaments are torn or detached from the medial segment but the trapezoid ligament remains intact to the distal segment, and (c) factures which are intra-articular. An even more detailed classification proposed by Robinson (1998) is useful for managing data and comparing clinical outcomes.

Treatment

MIDDLE THIRD FRACTURES

There is general agreement that undisplaced fractures should be treated non- operatively. Most will go on to

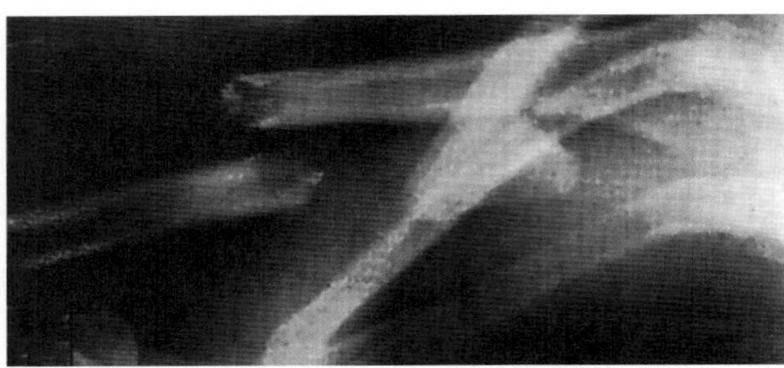

(a)

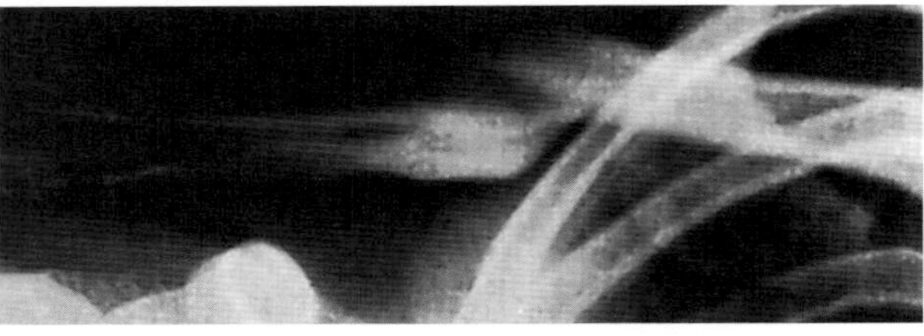

(b)

24.1 Fracture of the clavicle (a) Displaced fracture of the middle third of the clavicle – the most common injury. (b) The fracture usually unites in this position, leaving a barely noticable 'bump'.

unite uneventfully with a non-union rate below 5 per cent and a return to normal function.

Non-operative management consists of applying a simple sling for comfort. It is discarded once the pain subsides (between 1–3 weeks) and the patient is then encouraged to mobilize the limb as pain allows. There is no evidence that the traditional figure-of-eight bandage confers any advantage and it carries the risk of increasing the incidence of pressures sores over the fracture site and causing harm to neurological structures; it may even increase the risk of non-union.

There is less agreement about the management of displaced middle third fractures. Treating those with shortening of more than 2 cm by simple splintage is now believed to incur a considerable risk of symptomatic mal-union – mainly pain and lack of power during shoulder movements (McKee et al., 2006) – and an increased incidence of non-union. There is, therefore, a growing trend towards internal fixation of acute clavicular fractures associated with severe displacement. Methods include plating (specifically contoured locking plates are available) and intramedullary fixation.

LATERAL THIRD FRACTURES

Most lateral clavicle fractures are minimally displaced and extra-articular. The fact that the coracoclavicular ligaments are intact prevents further displacement and non-operative management is usually appropriate. Treatment consists of a sling for 2–3 weeks until the pain subsides, followed by mobilization within the limits of pain.

Displaced lateral third fractures are associated with disruption of the coracoclavicular ligaments and are therefore unstable injuries. A number of studies have shown that these particular fractures have a higher than usual rate of non-union if treated non-operatively. Surgery to stabilize the fracture is often recom-

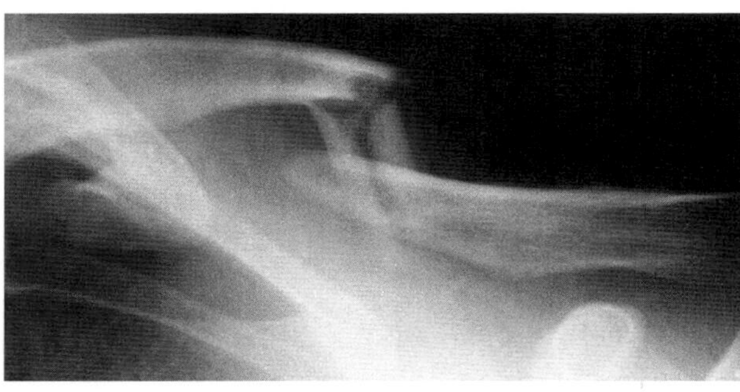

(a)

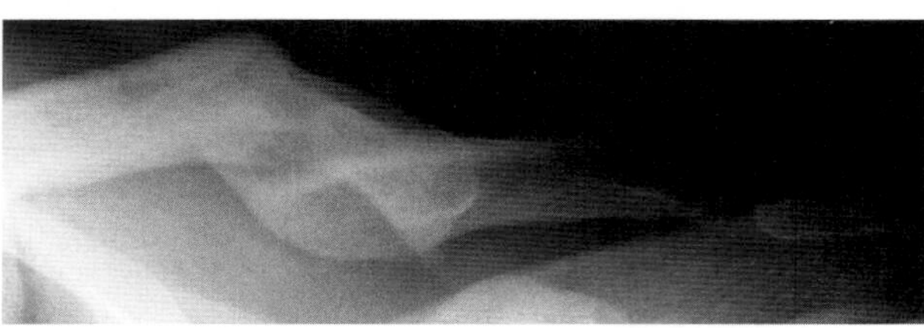

(b)

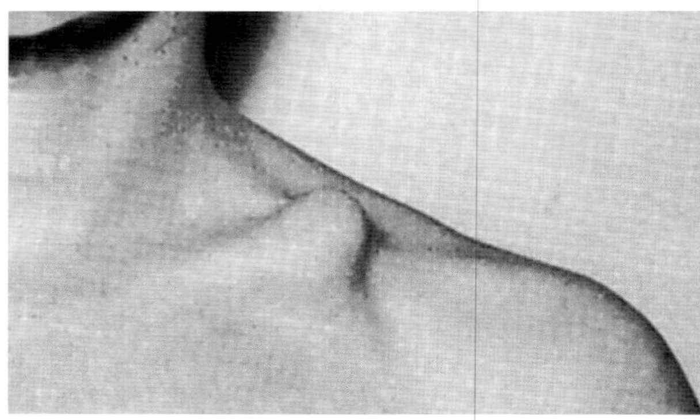

(c)

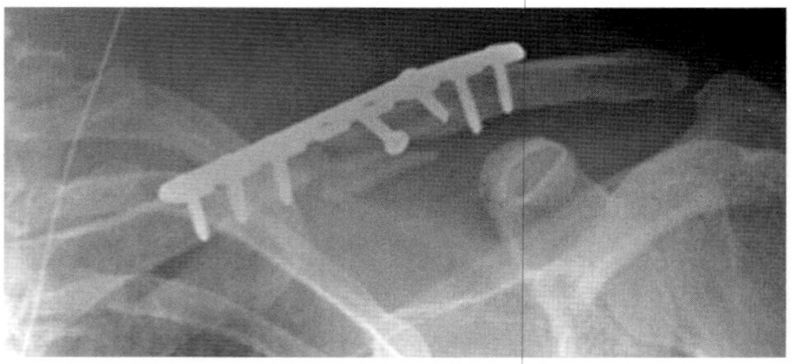

(d)

24.2 Severely displaced fracture (a) A comminuted fracture which united in this position (b) leaving an unsightly deformity (c). This fracture would have been better managed by (d) open reduction and internal fixation.

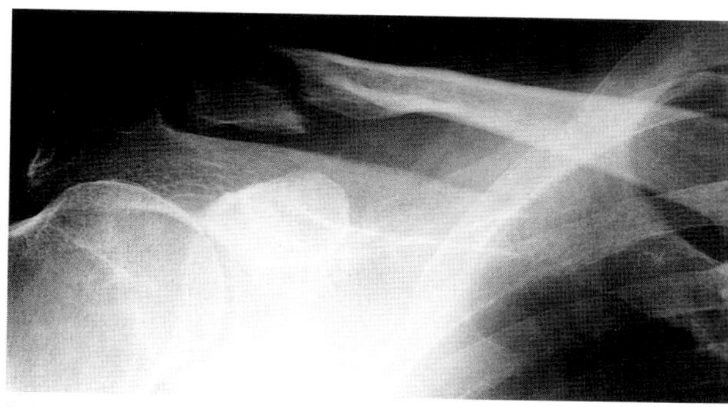

(a)

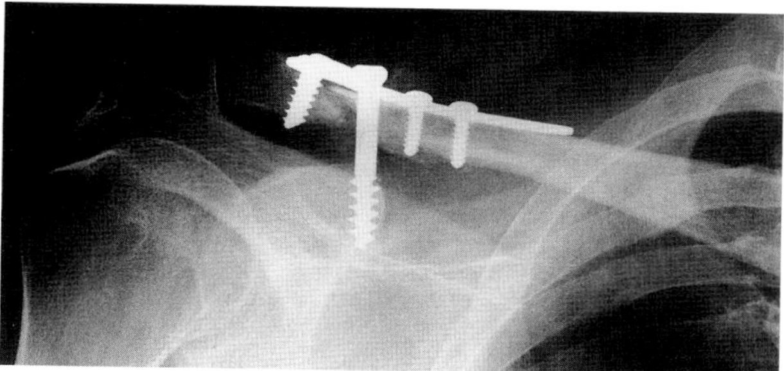

(b)

24.3 Fracture of the outer (lateral) third (a) The shaft of the clavicle is elevated, suggesting that the medial part of the coracoclavicular ligament is ruptured. (b) This was treated by open reduction and internal fixation, using a long screw to fix the clavicle to the coracoid process temporarily while the soft tissues healed.

mended. However the converse argument is that many of the fractures that develop non-union do not cause any symptoms and surgery can therefore be reserved for patients with symptomatic non-union. Operations for these fractures have a high complication rate and no single procedure has been shown to be better than the others. Techniques include the use of a coracoclavicular screw, plate and hook plate fixation and suture and sling techniques with Dacron graft ligaments.

MEDIAL THIRD FRACTURES

Most of these rare fractures are extra-articular. They are mainly managed non-operatively unless the fracture displacement threatens the mediastinal structures. Initial fixation is associated with significant complications, including migration of the implants into the mediastinum, particularly when K-wires are used. Other methods of stabilization include suture and graft techniques and the newer locking plates.

Complications

EARLY

Despite the close proximity of the clavicle to vital structures, a pneumothorax, damage to the subclavian vessels and brachial plexus injuries are all very rare.

LATE

Non-union In displaced fractures of the shaft non-union occurs in 1–15 per cent. Risk factors include increasing age, displacement, comminution and female sex. However accurate prediction of those fractures most likely to go on to non-union remains difficult.

Symptomatic non-unions are generally treated with plate fixation and bone grafting if necessary. This procedure usually produces a high rate of union and satisfaction.

Lateral clavicle fractures have a higher rate of non-union (11.5–40 per cent). Treatment options for symptomatic non-unions are excision of the lateral part of the clavicle (if the fragment is small and the coracoclavicular ligaments are intact) or open reduction, internal fixation and bone grafting if the fragment is large. Locking plates and hooked plates are used.

Malunion All displaced fractures heal in a non-anatomical position with some shortening and angulation, however most do not produce symptoms. Some may go on to develop periscapular pain and this is more likely with shortening of more than 1.5cm. In these circumstances the difficult operation of corrective osteotomy and plating can be considered.

Stiffness of the shoulder This is common but temporary; it results from fear of moving the fracture. Unless the fingers are exercised, they also may become stiff and take months to regain movement.

FRACTURES OF THE SCAPULA

Mechanisms of injury

The body of the scapula is fractured by a crushing force, which usually also fractures ribs and may dislocate the sternoclavicular joint. The neck of the scapula may be fractured by a blow or by a fall on the shoulder; the attached long head of triceps may drag the glenoid downwards and laterally. The coracoid process may fracture across its base or be avulsed at the tip. Fracture of the acromion is due to direct force. Fracture of the glenoid fossa usually suggests a medially directed force (impaction of the joint) but may occur with dislocation of the shoulder.

Clinical features

The arm is held immobile and there may be severe bruising over the scapula or the chest wall. Because of the energy required to damage the scapula, fractures of the body of the scapula are often associated with severe injuries to the chest, brachial plexus, spine, abdomen and head. Careful neurological and vascular examinations are essential.

X-Ray

Scapular fractures can be difficult to define on plain x-rays because of the surrounding soft tissues. The films may reveal a comminuted fracture of the body of the scapula, or a fractured scapular neck with the outer fragment pulled downwards by the weight of the arm. Occasionally a crack is seen in the acromion or the coracoid process. CT is useful for demonstrating glenoid fractures or body fractures.

Classification

Fractures of the scapula are divided anatomically into scapular body, glenoid neck, glenoid fossa, acromion and coracoid processes. Scapular neck fractures are the most common. Further subdivisions are shown in Table 24.1.

Table 24.1

Fractures of the scapular body
Fractures of the glenoid neck
Intra-articular glenoid fossa fractures (Ideberg modified by Goss)
Type I Fractures of the glenoid rim
Type II Fractures through the glenoid fossa, inferior fragment displaced with subluxed humeral head
Type III Oblique fracture through glenoid exiting superiorly (may be associated with acromioclavicular dislocation or fracture)
Type IV Horizontal fracture exiting through the medial border of the scapula
Type V Combination of Type IV and a fracture separating the inferior half of the glenoid
Type VI Severe comminution of the glenoid surface
Fractures of acromion process
Type I Minimally displaced
Type II Displaced but not reducing subacromial space
Type III Inferior displacement and reduced subacromial space
Fractures of coracoid process
Type I Proximal to attachment of the coracoclavicular ligaments and usually associated with acromioclavicular separation
Type II Distal to the coraco-acromial ligaments

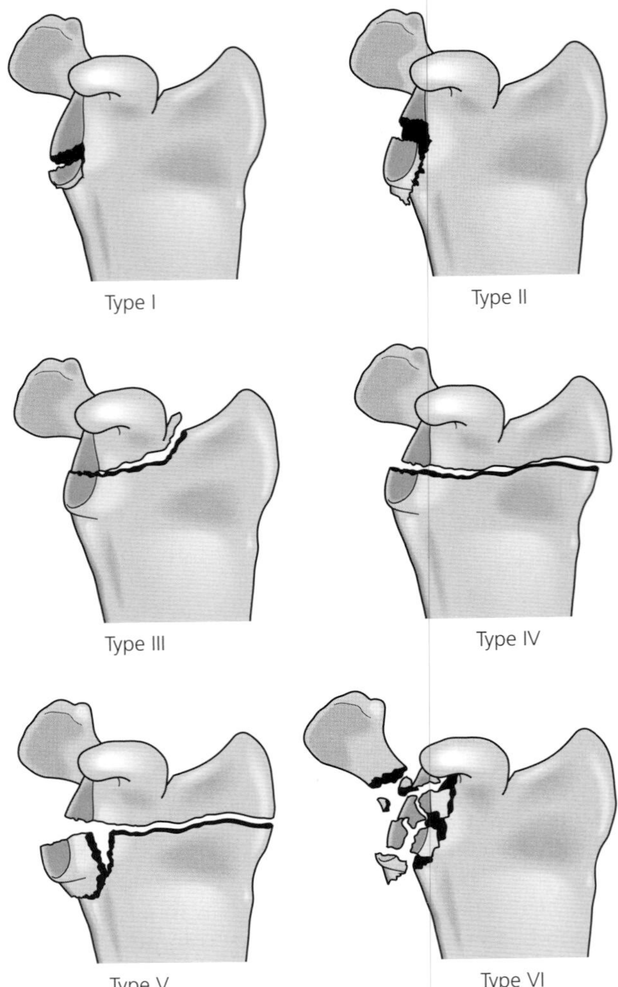

24.4 Fractures of the glenoid – classification Diagrams showing the main types of glenoid fracture.

Treatment

Body fractures Surgery is not necessary. The patient wears a sling for comfort, and from the start practises active exercises to the shoulder, elbow and fingers.

Isolated glenoid neck fractures The fracture is usually impacted and the glenoid surface is intact. A sling is worn for comfort and early exercises are begun.

Intra-articular fractures Type I glenoid fractures, if displaced, may result in instability of the shoulder. If the fragment involves more than a third of the glenoid surface and is displaced by more than 5 mm surgical fixation should be considered. Anterior rim fractures are approached through a delto-pectoral incision and posterior rim fractures through the posterior approach. Type II fractures are associated with inferior subluxation of the head of the humerus and require open reduction and internal fixation. Types III, IV, V and VI fractures have poorly defined indications for surgery. Generally speaking, if the head is centred on the major portion of the glenoid and the shoulder is stable a non-operative approach is adopted. Comminuted fractures of the glenoid fossa are likely to lead to osteoarthritis in the longer term.

Fractures of the acromion Undisplaced fractures are treated non-operatively. Only Type III acromial fractures, in which the subacromial space is reduced, require operative intervention to restore the anatomy.

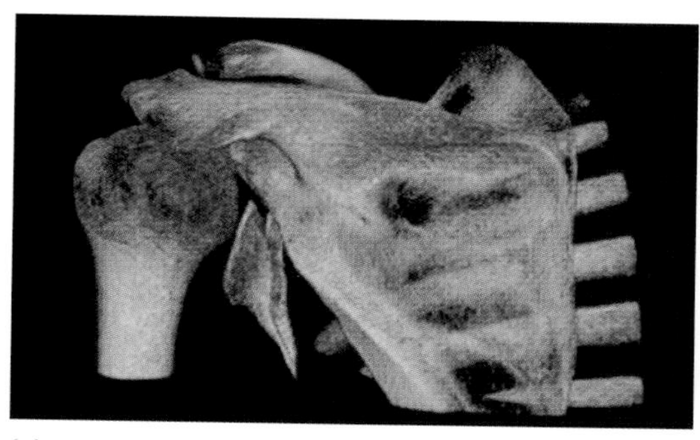
(a)

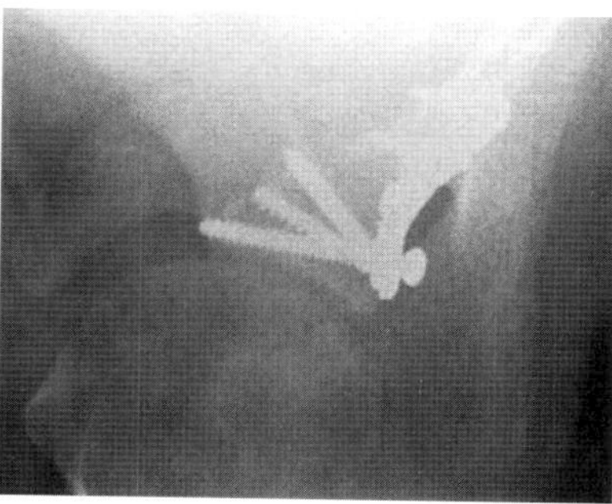
(b)

24.5 Glenoid fracture – imaging (a) Three-dimentional CT of a Type II glenoid fracture. (b) X-ray after open reduction and internal fixation.

Fractures of the coracoid process Fractures distal to the coracoacromial ligaments do not result in serious anatomical displacement; those proximal to the ligaments are usually associated with acromioclavicular separations and may need operative treatment.

Combined fractures Whereas an isolated fracture of the glenoid neck is stable, if there is an associated fracture of the clavicle or disruption of the acromioclavicular ligament the glenoid mass may become markedly displaced giving rise to a 'floating shoulder' (Williams et al, 2001). Diagnosis can be difficult and may require advanced imaging and three-dimensional reconstructions. At least one of the injuries (and sometimes both) will need operative fixation before the fragments are stabilized.

SCAPULOTHORACIC DISSOCIATION

This is a high energy injury. The scapula and arm are wrenched away from the chest, rupturing the subclavian vessels and brachial plexus. Many patients die.

Clinical features

The limb is flail and ischaemic. The diagnosis is usually made on the chest x-ray. There is swelling above the clavicle from an expanding haematoma. A distraction of more than 1 cm of a fractured clavicle should give rise to suspicion of this injury.

Treatment

The patient is resuscitated. The outcome for the upper limb is very poor. Neither vascular reconstruction nor brachial plexus exploration and repair are likely to give a functional limb.

ACROMIOCLAVICULAR JOINT INJURIES

Acute injury of the acromioclavicular joint is common and usually follows direct trauma. Chronic sprains, often associated with degenerative changes, are seen in people engaged in athletic activities like weightlifting or occupations such as working with jack-hammers and other heavy vibrating tools.

Mechanism of injury

A fall on the shoulder with the arm adducted may strain or tear the acromioclavicular ligaments and upward subluxation of the clavicle may occur; if the force is severe enough, the coracoclavicular ligaments will also be torn, resulting in complete dislocation of the joint.

Pathological anatomy and classification

The injury is graded according to the type of ligament injury and the amount of displacement of the joint.

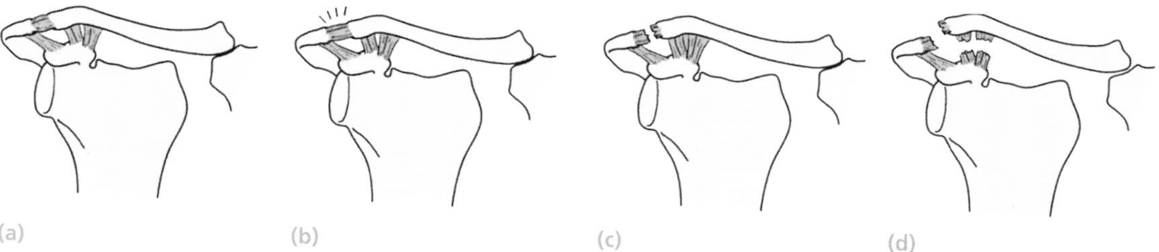

24.6 Acromioclavicular joint injuries (a) Normal joint. (b) Sprained acromioclavicular joint; no displacement. (c) Torn capsule and subluxation but coracoclavicular ligaments intact. (d) Dislocation with torn coracoclavicular ligaments.

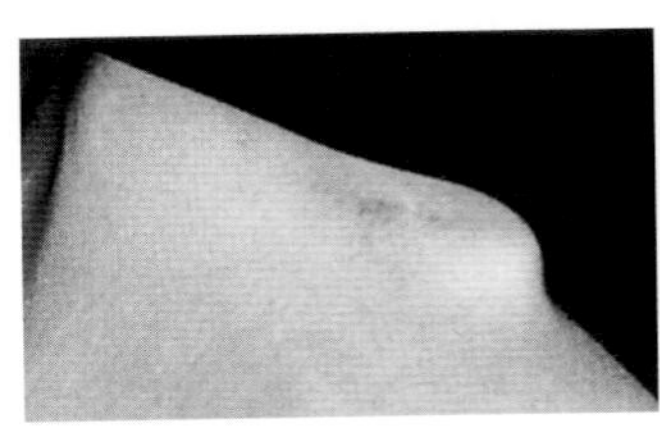
(a)

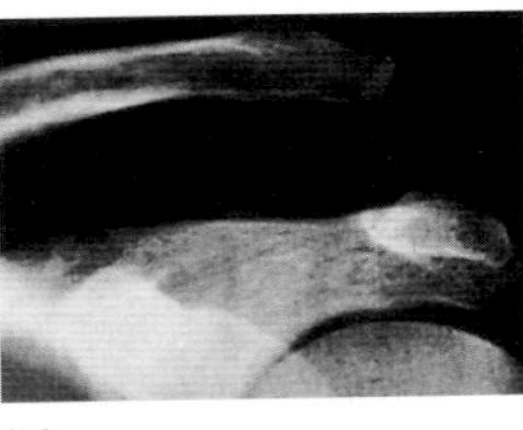
(b)

24.7 Acromioclavicular dislocation (a) Clinically one sees a definite 'step' in the contour at the lateral end of the clavicle. (b) The x-ray shows complete separation of the acromioclavicular joint.

Type I is an acute sprain of the acromioclavicular ligaments; the joint is undisplaced. In Type II the acromioclavicular ligaments are torn and the joint is subluxated with slight elevation of the clavicle. In Type III the acromioclavicular and coracoclavicular ligaments are torn and the joint is dislocated; the clavicle is elevated (or the acromion depressed) creating a visible and palpable 'step'. Other types of displacement are less common, but occasionally the clavicle is displaced posteriorly (Type IV), very markedly upwards (Type V) or inferiorly beneath the coracoid process (Type VI).

Clinical features

The patient can usually point to the site of injury and the area may be bruised. If there is tenderness but no deformity, the injury is probably a sprain or a subluxation. With dislocation the patient is in severe pain and a prominent 'step' can be seen and felt. Shoulder movements are limited.

X-ray

The acromioclavicular joint is not always easily visualized; anteroposterior, cephalic tilt and axillary views are advisable. In addition, a stress view is sometimes helpful in distinguishing between a Type II and Type III injury: this is an anteroposterior x-ray including both shoulders with the patient standing upright, arms by the side and holding a 5 kg weight in each hand. The distance between the coracoid process and the inferior border of the clavicle is measured on each side; a difference of more than 50 per cent is diagnostic of acromioclavicular dislocation.

Treatment

Sprains and subluxations do not affect function and do not require any special treatment; the arm is rested in a sling until pain subsides (usually no more than a week) and shoulder exercises are then begun.

Dislocations are poorly controlled by padding and bandaging, yet the role of surgery is controversial. The large number of operations suggests that none is ideal. There is no convincing evidence that surgery provides a better functional result than conservative treatment for a straightforward Type III injury. Operative repair should be considered only for patients with extreme prominence of the clavicle, those with posterior or inferior dislocation of the clavicle and those who aim to resume strenuous overarm or overhead activities.

Whilst there is no consensus regarding the best surgical solution, there are a number of underlying principles to consider if surgery is contemplated. Accurate reduction should be the goal. The ligamentous stability can be recreated either by transferring existing ligaments (the coracoacromial or conjoined tendons), or by using a free graft (e.g., autogenous semitendinosis or a synthetic ligament). This reconstruction must have sufficient stability to prevent re-dislocation during recovery. Any rigid implants which cross the joint will need to be removed at a later date to prevent loosening or fracture.

In the modified Weaver–Dunn procedure the lateral end of the clavicle is excised and the coracoacromial ligament is transferred to the outer end of the clavicle and attached by trans-osseous sutures. Tension on the repair can be reduced either by anchoring the clavicle to the coracoid with a Bosworth coracoclavicular screw (which has to be removed after 8 weeks) or by employing a Dacron sling – looped round the coracoid and the clavicle – for the same purpose. Great care is needed to avoid entrapment or damage to a nerve or vessel. Elbow and forearm exercises are begun on the day after operation and active-assisted shoulder movements 2 weeks later, increasing gradually to active movements at 4–6 weeks. Strenuous lifting movements are avoided for 4–6 months.

Recent advances in instrumentation have made it

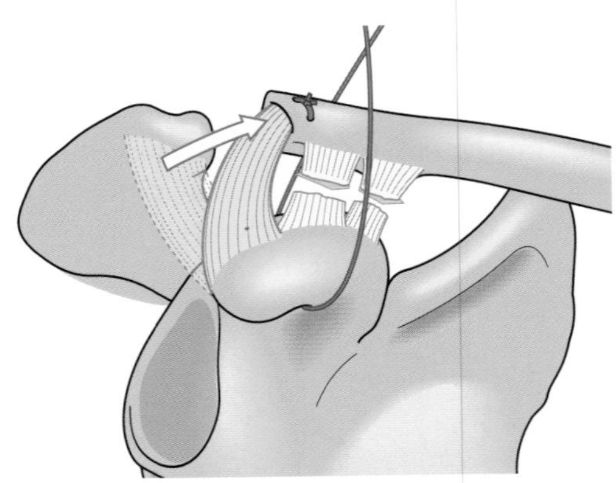

24.8 Modified Weaver Dunn operation The lateral end of the clavicle is excised; the acromial end of the coracoacromial ligament is detached and fastened to the lateral end of the clavicle. Tension on the ligament is lessened by placing a 'sling' around the clavicle and the coracoid process. (Dotted lines show former position of coracoacromial ligament).

feasible to perform this type of reconstructive surgery arthroscopically (Snow and Funk, 2006).

Complications

Rotator cuff syndrome An acute strain of the acromioclavicular joint is sometimes followed by supraspinatus tendinitis. Whether this is directly due to the primary injury or whether it results from post-traumatic oedema or inflammation of the overlying acromioclavicular joint is unclear. Treatment with anti-inflammatory preparations may help.

Unreduced dislocation An unreduced dislocation is ugly and sometimes affects function. Simple excision of the distal clavicle will only make matters worse. An attempt should be made to reconstruct the coracoclavicular ligament. The Weaver–Dunn procedure may be suitable (See Figure 24.8).

Ossification of the ligaments The more severe injuries are quite often followed by ossification of the coracoclavicular ligaments. Bony spurs may predispose to later rotator cuff dysfunction, which may require operative treatment.

Secondary osteoarthritis A late complication of Type I and II injuries is osteoarthritis of the acromioclavicular joint. This can usually be managed conservatively, but if pain is marked the outer 2 cm of the clavicle can be excised. The patient will be aware of some weakness during strenuous over-arm activities and pain is often not completely abolished.

STERNOCLAVICULAR DISLOCATIONS

Mechanism of injury

This uncommon injury is usually caused by lateral compression of the shoulders; for example, when someone is pinned to the ground following a road accident or an underground rock-fall. Rarely, it follows a direct blow to the front of the joint. Anterior dislocation is much more common than posterior. The joint can be sprained, subluxed or dislocated.

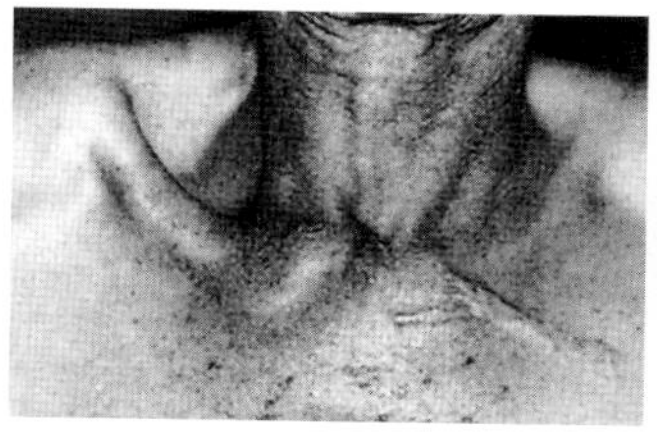
(a)

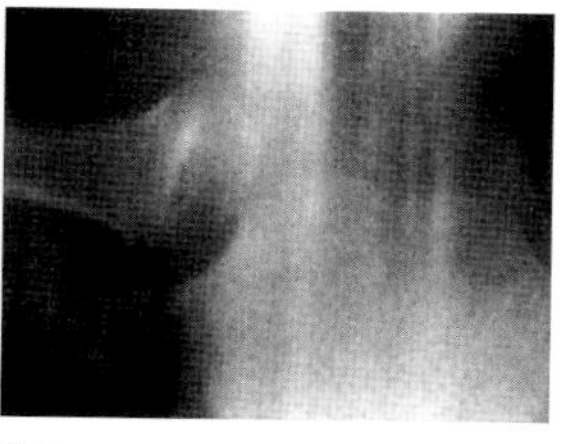
(b)

24.9 Sternoclavicular dislocation (a) The bump over the sternoclavicular joint may be obvious, though this is difficult to demonstrate on plain x-ray. (b) Tomography (or, better still, CT) will show the lesion.

Clinical features

Anterior dislocation is easily diagnosed; the dislocated medial end of the clavicle forms a prominent bump over the sternoclavicular joint. The condition is painful but there are usually no cardiothoracic complications.

Posterior dislocation, though rare, is much more serious. Discomfort is marked; there may be pressure on the trachea or large vessels, causing venous congestion of the neck and arm and circulation to the arm may be decreased.

X-Ray

Because of overlapping shadows, plain x-rays are difficult to interpret. Special oblique views are helpful and CT is the ideal method.

Treatment

Sprains and subluxations do not require specific treatment.

Anterior dislocation can usually be reduced by exerting pressure over the clavicle and pulling on the arm with the shoulder abducted. However, the joint usually redislocates. Not that this matters much; full function will be regained, though this may take several months.

Internal fixation is unnecessary and very dangerous (because of the large vessels behind the sternum).

Posterior dislocation should be reduced as soon as possible. This can usually be done closed (if necessary under general anaesthesia) by lying the patient supine with a sandbag between the scapulae and then pulling on the arm with the shoulder abducted and extended. The joint reduces with a snap and stays reduced. If this manoeuvre fails, the medial end of the clavicle is grasped with bone forceps and pulled forwards. If this too, fails (a very rare occurrence) open reduction is justified, but great care must be taken not to damage the mediastinal structures. After reduction, the shoulders are braced back with a figure-of-eight bandage, which is worn for 3 weeks.

DISLOCATION OF THE SHOULDER

Of the large joints, the shoulder is the one that most commonly dislocates. This is due to a number of factors: the shallowness of the glenoid socket; the extraordinary range of movement; underlying conditions such as ligamentous laxity or glenoid dysplasia; and the sheer vulnerability of the joint during stressful activities of the upper limb.

In this chapter, acute anterior and posterior dislocations are described. Chronic instability is described in Chapter 13.

ANTERIOR DISLOCATION

Mechanism of injury

Dislocation is usually caused by a fall on the hand. The head of the humerus is driven forward, tearing the capsule and producing avulsion of the glenoid labrum (the Bankart lesion). Occasionally the posterolateral part of the head is crushed. Rarely, the acromion process levers the head downwards and the joint dislocates with the arm pointing upwards (*luxatio erecta*); nearly always the arm then drops, bringing the head to its subcoracoid position.

Clinical features

Pain is severe. The patient supports the arm with the opposite hand and is loathe to permit any kind of examination. The lateral outline of the shoulder may be flattened and, if the patient is not too muscular, a bulge may be felt just below the clavicle. The arm must always be examined for nerve and vessel injury before reduction is attempted.

X-Ray

The anteroposterior x-ray will show the overlapping shadows of the humeral head and glenoid fossa, with the head usually lying below and medial to the socket. A lateral view aimed along the blade of the scapula will show the humeral head out of line with the socket.

If the joint has dislocated before, special views may show flattening or an excavation of the posterolateral contour of the humeral head, where it has been indented by the anterior edge of the glenoid socket, the Hill–Sachs lesion.

Treatment

Various methods of reduction have been described, some of them now of no more than historical interest. In a patient who has had previous dislocations, simple traction on the arm may be successful. Usually, sedation and occasionally general anaesthesia is required.

With Stimson's technique, the patient is left prone with the arm hanging over the side of the bed. After 15 or 20 minutes the shoulder may reduce.

In the Hippocratic method, gently increasing traction is applied to the arm with the shoulder in slight abduction, while an assistant applies firm countertraction to the body (a towel slung around the patient's chest, under the axilla, is helpful).

With Kocher's method, the elbow is bent to 90° and held close to the body; no traction should be applied. The arm is slowly rotated 75 degrees laterally, then the point of the elbow is lifted forwards, and finally the arm is rotated medially. This technique carries the risk of nerve, vessel and bone injury and is not recommended.

Another technique has the patient sitting on a reduction chair and with gentle traction of the arm over the back of the padded chair the dislocation is reduced.

An x-ray is taken to confirm reduction and exclude

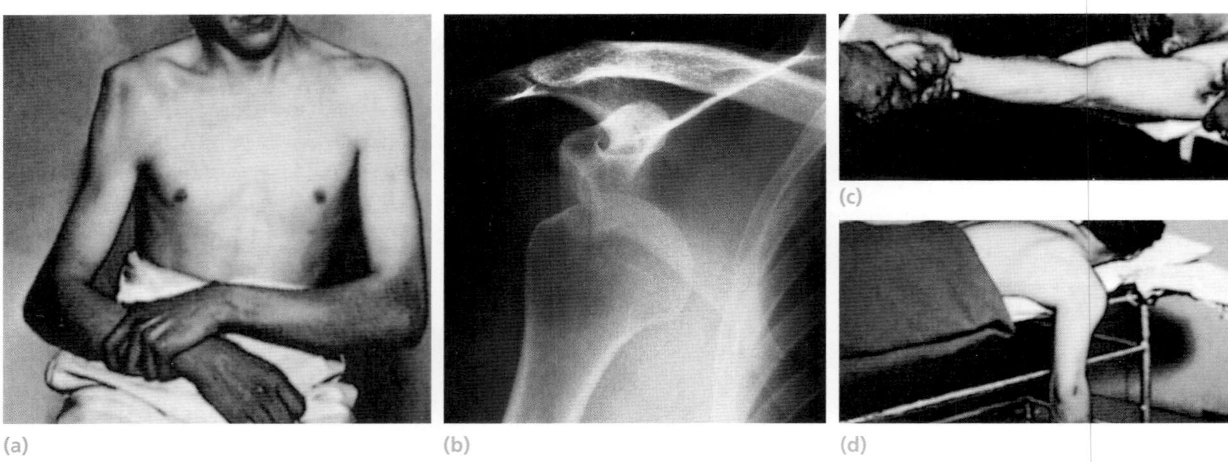

(a) (b) (c) (d)

24.10 Anterior dislocation of the shoulder (a) The prominent acromion process and flattening of the contour over the deltoid are typical signs. (b) X-ray confirms the diagnosis of anterior dislocation. (c,d) Two methods of reduction.

a fracture. When the patient is fully awake, active abduction is gently tested to exclude an axillary nerve injury and rotator cuff tear. The median, radial, ulnar and musculocutaneous nerves are also tested and the pulse is felt.

The arm is rested in a sling for about three weeks in those under 30 years of age (who are most prone to recurrence) and for only a week in those over 30 (who are most prone to stiffness). Then movements are begun, but combined abduction and lateral rotation must be avoided for at least 3 weeks. Throughout this period, elbow and finger movements are practised every day.

There has been some interest in the use of external rotation splints, based on the theory that this would reduce the Bankart lesion into a better position for healing. However a recent Cochrane review has concluded that there is insufficient evidence to inform on the choices for conservative treatment and that further trials are needed to compare different types and duration of immobilization.

Young athletes who dislocate their shoulder traumatically and who continue to pursue their sports (particularly contact sports) are at a much higher risk of re-dislocation in the future. With increasing advances and techniques of arthroscopy and arthroscopic anterior stabilization surgery, some are now advocating early surgery in this group of patients to repair the Bankart lesion of the anterior labrum. However a consensus on early surgery has still not been reached.

Complications

EARLY

Rotator cuff tear This commonly accompanies anterior dislocation, particularly in older people. The patient may have difficulty abducting the arm after reduction; palpable contraction of the deltoid muscle excludes an axillary nerve palsy. Most do not require surgical attention, but young active individuals with large tears will benefit from early repair.

Nerve injury The axillary nerve is most commonly injured; the patient is unable to contract the deltoid muscle and there may be a small patch of anaesthesia over the muscle. The inability to abduct must be distinguished from a rotator cuff tear. The nerve lesion is usually a neuropraxia which recovers spontaneously after a few weeks; if it does not, then surgery should be considered as the results of repair are less satisfactory if the delay is more than a few months.

Occasionally the radial nerve, musculocutaneous nerve, median nerve or ulnar nerve can be injured. Rarely there is a complete infra-clavicular brachial plexus palsy. This is somewhat alarming, but fortunately it usually recovers with time.

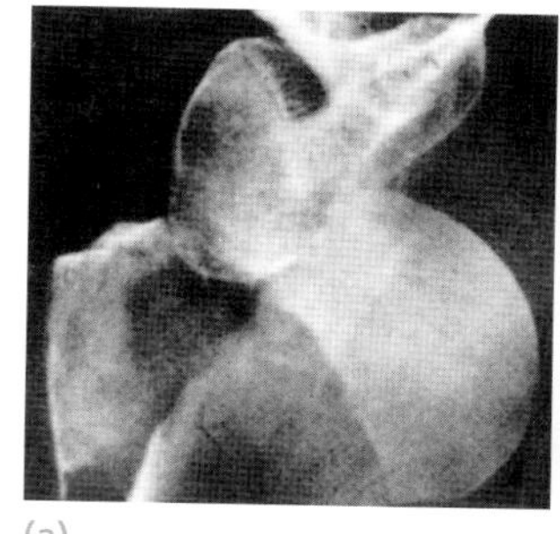
(a)

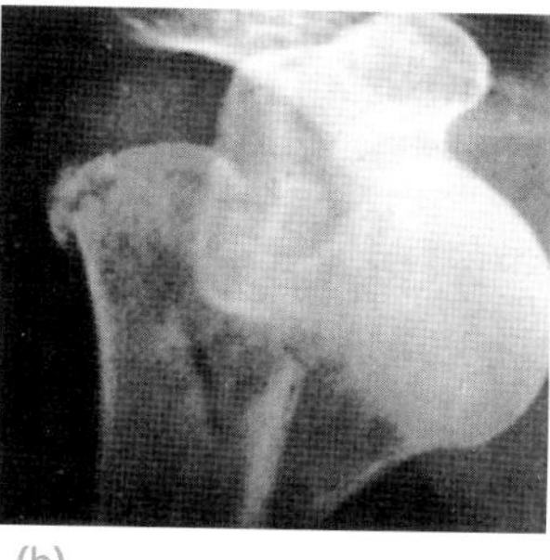
(b)

24.11 Anterior fracture-discloation Anterior dislocation of the shoulder may be complicated by fracture of (a) the greater tuberosity or (b) the neck of the humerus – this often needs open reduction and internal fixation.

Vascular injury The axillary artery may be damaged, particularly in old patients with fragile vessels. This can occur either at the time of injury or during overzealous reduction. The limb should always be examined for signs of ischaemia both before and after reduction.

Fracture-dislocation If there is an associated fracture of the proximal humerus, open reduction and internal fixation may be necessary. The greater tuberosity may be sheared off during dislocation. It usually falls into place during reduction, and no special treatment is then required. If it remains displaced, surgical reattachment is recommended to avoid later subacromial impingement.

LATE

Shoulder stiffness Prolonged immobilization may lead to stiffness of the shoulder, especially in patients over the age of 40. There is loss of lateral rotation, which automatically limits abduction. Active exercises will usually loosen the joint. They are practised vigorously, bearing in mind that full abduction is not possible until lateral rotation has been regained. Manipulation under anaesthesia or arthroscopic capsular release is advised only if progress has halted and at least 6 months have elapsed since injury.

Unreduced dislocation Surprisingly, a dislocation of the shoulder sometimes remains undiagnosed. This is more likely if the patient is either unconscious or very old. Closed reduction is worth attempting up to 6 weeks after injury; manipulation later may fracture the bone or tear vessels or nerves. Operative reduction is indicated after 6 weeks only in the young, because it is difficult, dangerous and followed by prolonged stiffness. An anterior approach is used, and the vessels and nerves are carefully identified before the dislocation is reduced. 'Active neglect' summarizes the treatment of unreduced dislocation in the elderly. The dislocation is disregarded and gentle active movements are encouraged. Moderately good function is often regained.

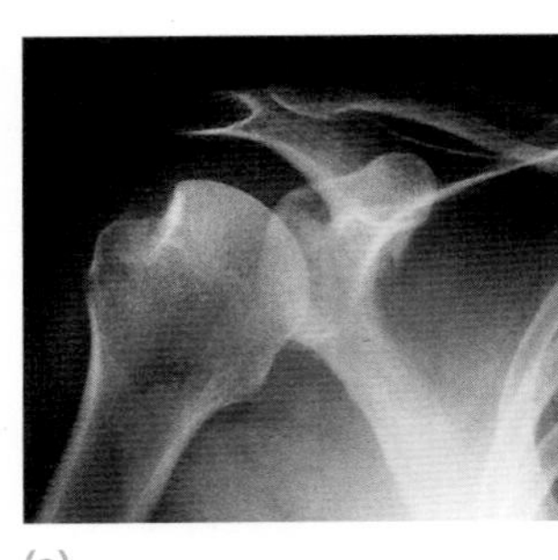

(a)

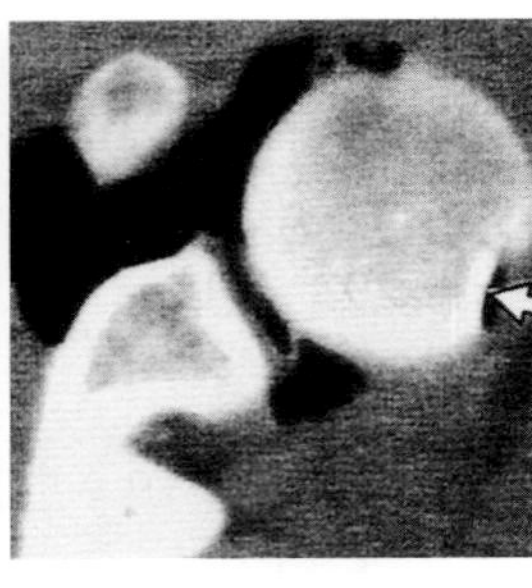

(b)

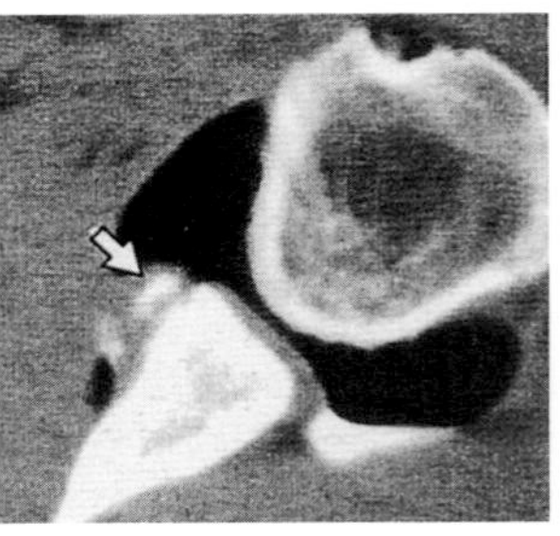

(c)

24.12 Recurrent dislocation of the shoulder (a) The classic x-ray sign is a depression in the posterosuperior part of the humeral head (the Hill-Sachs lesion). (b,c) MRI scans showing both the Hill–Sachs lesion and a Bankart lesion of the glenoid rim (arrows).

Recurrent dislocation If an anterior dislocation tears the shoulder capsule, repair occurs spontaneously following reduction and the dislocation may not recur; but if the glenoid labrum is detached, or the capsule is stripped off the front of the neck of the glenoid, repair is less likely and recurrence is more common. Detachment of the labrum occurs particularly in young patients, and, if at injury a bony defect has been gouged out of the posterolateral aspect of the humeral head, recurrence is even more likely. In older patients, especially if there is a rotator cuff tear or greater tuberosity fracture, recurrent dislocation is unlikely. The period of post-operative immobilization makes no difference.

The history is diagnostic. The patient complains that the shoulder dislocates with relatively trivial everyday actions. Often he can reduce the dislocation himself. Any doubt as to diagnosis is quickly resolved by the apprehension test: if the patient's arm is passively placed behind the coronal plane in a position of abduction and lateral rotation, his immediate resistance and apprehension are pathognomonic. An anteroposterior x-ray with the shoulder medially rotated may show an indentation in the back of the humeral head (the Hill–Sachs lesion).

Even more common, but less readily diagnosed, is recurrent subluxation. The management of both types of instability is dealt with in Chapter 13.

POSTERIOR DISLOCATION OF THE SHOULDER

Posterior dislocation is rare, accounting for less than 2 per cent of all dislocations around the shoulder.

Mechanism of injury

Indirect force producing marked internal rotation and adduction needs be very severe to cause a dislocation. This happens most commonly during a fit or convulsion, or with an electric shock. Posterior dislocation can also follow a fall on to the flexed, adducted arm, a direct blow to the front of the shoulder or a fall on the outstretched hand.

Clinical features

The diagnosis is frequently missed – partly because reliance is placed on a single anteroposterior x-ray (which may look almost normal) and partly because those attending to the patient fail to think of it. There are, in fact, several well-marked clinical features. The arm is held in internal rotation and is locked in that position. The front of the shoulder looks flat with a prominent coracoid, but swelling may obscure this deformity; seen from above, however, the posterior displacement is usually apparent.

X-Ray

In the anteroposterior film the humeral head, because it is medially rotated, looks abnormal in shape (like an

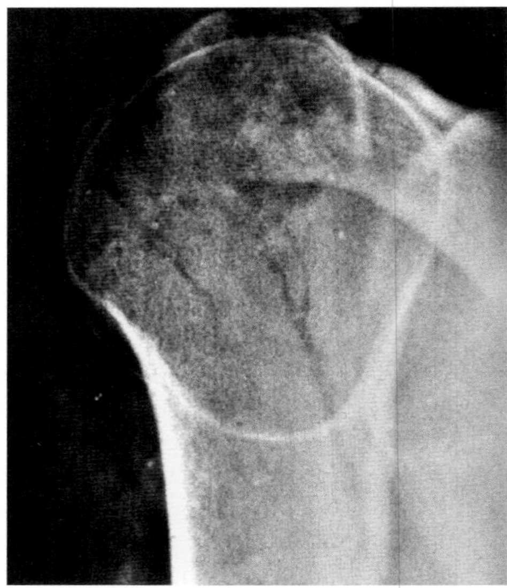

24.13 Posterior dislocation of the shoulder The characteristic x-ray image. Because the head of the humerus is internally rotated, the anteroposterior x-ray shows a head-on projection giving the classic 'electric light-bulb' appearance.

electric light bulb) and it stands away somewhat from the glenoid fossa (the 'empty glenoid' sign). A lateral film and axillary view is essential; it shows posterior subluxation or dislocation and sometimes a deep indentation on the anterior aspect of the humeral head. Posterior dislocation is sometimes complicated by fractures of the humeral neck, posterior glenoid rim or lesser tuberosity. Sometimes the patient is too uncomfortable to permit adequate imaging and in these difficult cases CT is essential to rule out posterior dislocation of the shoulder.

Treatment

The acute dislocation is reduced (usually under general anaesthesia) by pulling on the arm with the shoulder in adduction; a few minutes are allowed for the head of the humerus to disengage and the arm is then gently rotated laterally while the humeral head is pushed forwards. If reduction feels stable the arm is immobilized in a sling; otherwise the shoulder is held widely abducted and laterally rotated in an airplane type splint for 3–6 weeks to allow the posterior capsule to heal in the shortest position. Shoulder movement is regained by active exercises.

Complications

Unreduced dislocation At least half the patients with posterior dislocation have 'unreduced' lesions when first seen. Sometimes weeks or months elapse before the diagnosis is made and up to two thirds of posterior dislocations are not recognised initially. Typically the patient holds the arm internally rotated; he cannot abduct the arm more than 70–80 degrees, and if he lifts the extended arm forwards he cannot then turn the palm upwards. If the patient is young, or is uncomfortable and the dislocation fairly recent, open reduction is indicated. This is a difficult procedure. It is generally done through a delto-pectoral approach; the shoulder is reduced and the defect in the humeral head can then be treated by transferring the subscapularis tendon into the defect (McLaughlin procedure). Alternatively, the defect on the humeral head can be bone grafted. A useful technique for treating a defect smaller than 40 per cent of the humeral head is to transfer of the lesser tuberosity together with the subscapularis into the defect. For defects larger than this a hemiarthroplasty may be considered.

Late dislocations, especially in the elderly, are best left, but movement is encouraged.

Recurrent dislocation or subluxation Chronic posterior instability of the shoulder is discussed in Chapter 13.

INFERIOR DISLOCATION OF THE SHOULDER (*LUXATIO ERECTA*)

Inferior dislocation is rare but it demands early recognition because the consequences are potentially very serious. Dislocation occurs with the arm in nearly full abduction/elevation. The humeral head is levered out of its socket and pokes into the axilla; the arm remains fixed in abduction.

Mechanism of injury and pathology

The injury is caused by a severe hyper-abduction force. With the humerus as the lever and the acromion as the fulcrum, the humeral head is lifted across the inferior rim of the glenoid socket; it remains in the subglenoid position, with the humeral shaft pointing upwards. Soft-tissue injury may be severe and includes avulsion of the capsule and surrounding tendons, rupture of muscles, fractures of the glenoid or proximal humerus and damage to the brachial plexus and axillary artery.

Clinical features

The startling picture of a patient with his arm locked in almost full abduction should make diagnosis quite easy. The head of the humerus may be felt in or below the axilla. Always examine for neurovascular damage.

X-ray

The humeral shaft is shown in the abducted position with the head sitting below the glenoid. It is important to search for associated fractures of the glenoid or proximal humerus.

NOTE: True inferior dislocation must not be confused with postural downward displacement of the humerus, which results quite commonly from weakness and laxity of the muscles around the shoulder, especially after trauma and shoulder splintage; here

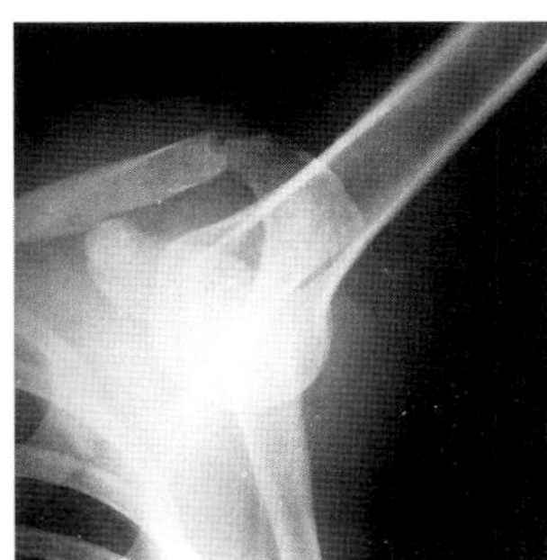

24.14 Inferior dislocation of the shoulder You can see why the condition is called *luxatio erecta*. The shaft of the humerus points upwards and the humeral head is displaced downwards.

the shaft of the humerus lies in the normal anatomical position at the side of the chest. The condition is harmless and resolves as muscle tone is regained.

Treatment

Inferior dislocation can usually be reduced by pulling upwards in the line of the abducted arm, with counter-traction downwards over the top of the shoulder. If the humeral head is stuck in the soft tissues, open reduction is needed. It is important to examine again, after reduction, for evidence of neurovascular injury.

The arm is rested in a sling until pain subsides and movement is then allowed, but avoiding abduction for 3 weeks to allow the soft tissues to heal.

SHOULDER DISLOCATIONS IN CHILDREN

Traumatic dislocation of the shoulder is exceedingly rare in children. Children who give a history of the shoulder 'slipping out' almost invariably have either voluntary or involuntary (atraumatic) dislocation or subluxation. With voluntary dislocation, the child can demonstrate the instability at will. With involuntary dislocation, the shoulder slips out unexpectedly during everyday activities. Most of these children have generalized joint laxity and some have glenoid dysplasia or muscle patterning disorders (Chapter 13). Examination may show that the shoulder subluxates in almost any direction; x-rays may confirm the diagnosis.

Treatment

Atraumatic dislocation should be viewed with great caution. Some of these children have behavioural or muscle patterning problems and this is where treatment should be directed. A prolonged exercise programme may also help. Only if the child is genuinely distressed by the disorder, and provided psychological factors have been excluded, should one consider reconstructive surgery.

FRACTURES OF THE PROXIMAL HUMERUS

Fractures of the proximal humerus usually occur after middle age and most of the patients are osteoporotic, postmenopausal women. Fracture displacement is usually not marked and treatment presents few problems. However, in about 20 per cent of cases there is considerable displacement of one or more fragments and a significant risk of complications due to bone fragility, damage to the rotator cuff and the prevailing co-morbidities. Deciding between operative and non-operative treatment can be very difficult.

Mechanism of injury

Fracture usually follows a fall on the out-stretched arm – the type of injury which, in younger people, might cause dislocation of the shoulder. Sometimes, indeed, there is both a fracture and a dislocation.

Classification and pathological anatomy

The most widely accepted classification is that of Neer (1970) who drew attention to the four major segments involved in these injuries: the head of the humerus, the lesser tuberosity, the greater tuberosity and the shaft. Neer's classification distinguishes between the number of displaced fragments, with displacement defined as greater than 45 degrees of angulation or 1 cm of separation. Thus, however many fracture lines there are, if the fragments are undisplaced it is regarded as a one-part fracture; if one segment is sep-

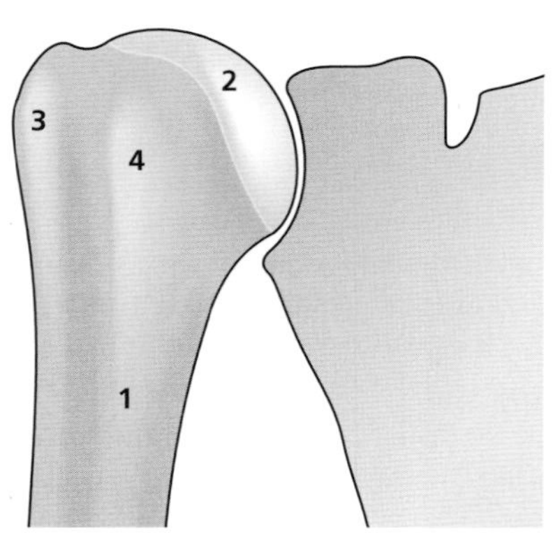

(a)

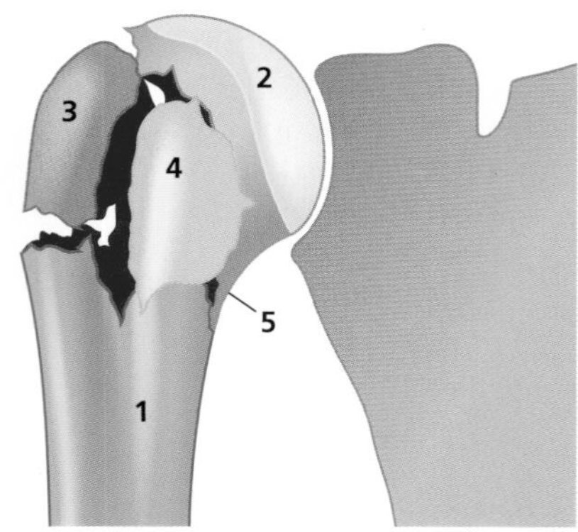

(b)

24.15 Fractures of the proximal humerus Diagram of (a) the normal and (b) a fractured proximal humerus, showing the four main fragments, two or more of which are seen in almost all proximal humeral fractures. 1=shaft of humerus; 2=head of humerus; 3=greater tuberosity; 4=lesser tuberosity. In this figure there is a sizeable medial calcar spike; 5=suggesting a low risk of avascular necrosis.

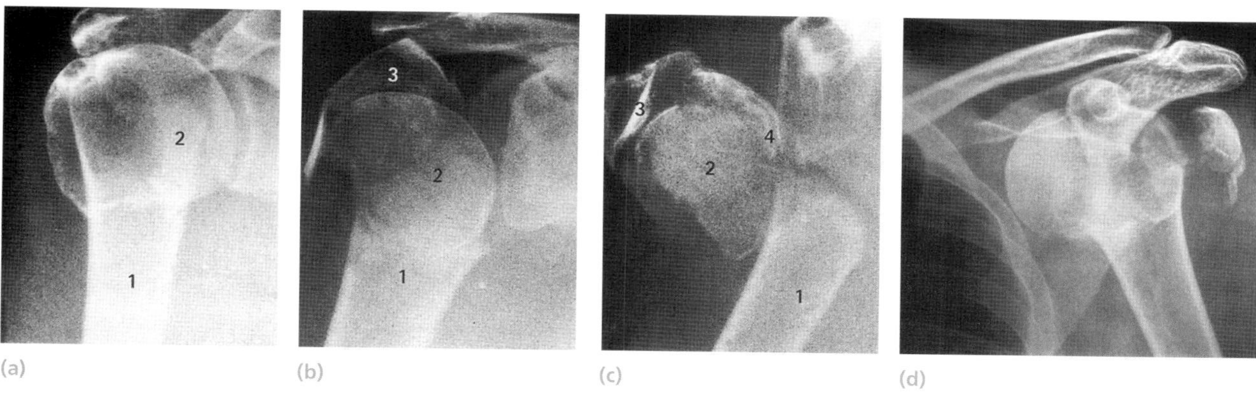

24.16 X-rays of proximal humeral fractures Classification is all very well, but x-rays are more difficult to interpret than line drawings. (a) Two-part fracture. (b) Three-part fracture involving the neck and the greater tuberosity. (c) Four-part fracture. (1=shaft of humerus; 2=head of humerus; 3=greater tuberosity; 4=lesser tuberosity). (d) X-ray showing fracture-dislocation of the shoulder.

arated from the others, it is a two-part fracture; if two fragments are displaced, that is a three-part fracture; if all the major parts are displaced, it is a four-part fracture. Furthermore, a fracture-dislocation exists when the head is dislocated and there are two, three or four parts. This grading is based on x-ray appearances, although observers do not always agree with each other on which class a particular fracture falls into.

Clinical features

Because the fracture is often firmly impacted, pain may not be severe. However, the appearance of a large bruise on the upper part of the arm is suspicious. Signs of axillary nerve or brachial plexus injury should be sought.

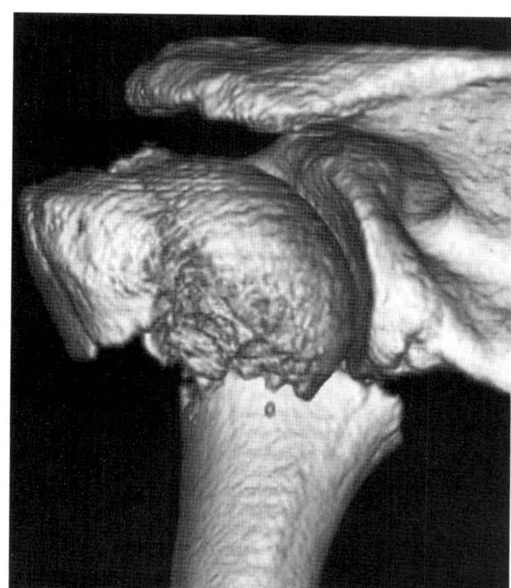

24.17 CT with three-dimensional reconstruction Advanced imaging provides a much clearer picture of the injury, allowing better pre-operative planning.

X-ray

In elderly patients there often appears to be a single, impacted fracture extending across the surgical neck. However, with good x-rays, several undisplaced fragments may be seen. In younger patients, the fragments are usually more clearly separated. Axillary and scapular-lateral views should always be obtained, to exclude dislocation of the shoulder.

It has always been difficult to apply Neer's classification when based on plain x-rays and not surprisingly there is a relatively high level of both inter- and intra-observer disagreement. Neer himself later noted that when this classification was developed the criteria for displacement (distance >1 cm, angulation >45 degrees) were set arbitrarily. The classification was not intended to dictate treatment, but simply to help clarify the pathoanatomy of the different fracture patterns.

The advent of three-dimensional CT reconstruction has helped to reduce the degree of inter- and intra-observer error, enabling better planning of treatment than in the past.

As the fracture heals, the humeral head is sometimes seen to be subluxated downwards (inferiorly); this is due to muscle atony and it usually recovers once exercises are begun.

Treatment

MINIMALLY DISPLACED FRACTURES

These comprise the vast majority. They need no treatment apart from a week or two period of rest with the arm in a sling until the pain subsides, and then gentle passive movements of the shoulder. Once the fracture has united (usually after 6 weeks), active exercises are encouraged; the hand is, of course, actively exercised from the start.

TWO-PART FRACTURES

Surgical neck fractures The fragments are gently manipulated into alignment and the arm is immobilized in a sling for about four weeks or until the fracture feels stable and the x-ray shows some signs of healing. Elbow and hand exercises are encouraged throughout this period; shoulder exercises are commenced at about four weeks. The results of conservative treatment are generally satisfactory, considering that most of these patients are over 65 and do not demand perfect function. However, if the fracture cannot be reduced closed or if the fracture is very unstable after closed reduction, then fixation is required. Options include percutaneous pins, bone sutures, intramedullary pins with tension band wiring or a locked intramedullary nail. Plate fixation requires a wider exposure and the newer locking plates offer a stable fixation without the need for extensive periosteal stripping.

Greater tuberosity fractures Fracture of the greater tuberosity is often associated with anterior dislocation and it reduces to a good position when the shoulder is relocated. If it does not reduce, the fragment can be re-attached through a small incision with interosseous sutures or, in young hard bone, cancellous screws.

Anatomical neck fractures These are very rare. In young patients the fracture should be fixed with a screw. In older patients prosthetic replacement (hemiarthroplasty) is preferable because of the high risk of avascular necrosis of the humeral head.

THREE-PART FRACTURES

These usually involve displacement of the surgical neck and the greater tuberosity; they are extremely difficult to reduce closed. In active individuals this injury is best managed by open reduction and internal fixation. There is little evidence that one technique is better than another although the newer implants with locked plating and nailing are biomechanically superior in osteoporotic bone.

FOUR-PART FRACTURES

The surgical neck and both tuberosities are displaced. These are severe injuries with a high risk of complications such as vascular injury, brachial plexus damage, injuries of the chest wall and (later) avascular necrosis of the humeral head. The x-ray diagnosis is difficult (how many fragments are there, and are they displaced?). Often the most one can say is that there are 'multiple displaced fragments', sometimes together with glenohumeral dislocation. In young patients an attempt should be made at reconstruction. In older patients, closed treatment and attempts at open reduction and fixation can result in continuing pain and stiffness and additional surgical treatment can compromise the blood supply still further. If the fracture pattern is such that the blood-supply is likely to be compromised, or that reconstruction and internal fixation will be extremely difficult, then the treatment of choice is prosthetic replacement of the proximal humerus.

The results of hemiarthroplasty are somewhat unpredictable. Anatomical reduction, fixation and healing of the tuberosities are prerequisites for a satisfactory outcome; even then, secondary displacement of the tuberosities may result in a poor functional outcome. In addition the prosthetic implant should be perfectly positioned. Be warned – these are operations for the expert; the subject is well covered by Boileau et al. (2006).

FRACTURE-DISLOCATION

Two-part fracture-dislocations (greater tuberosity with anterior dislocation and lesser tuberosity with posterior) can usually be reduced by closed means.

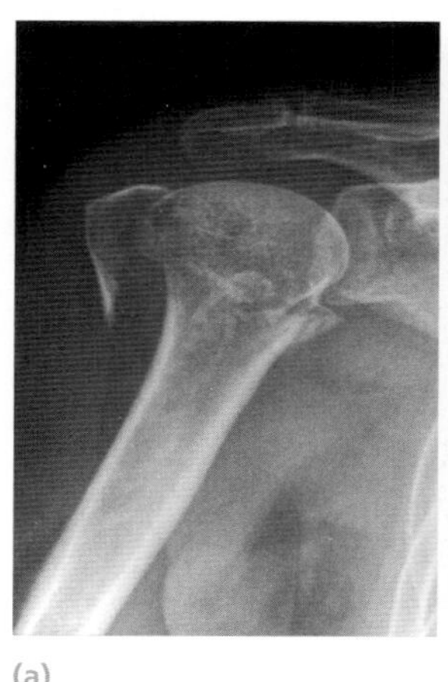
(a)

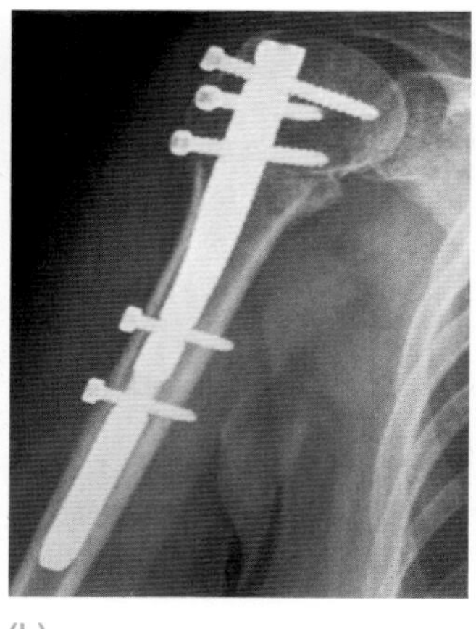
(b)

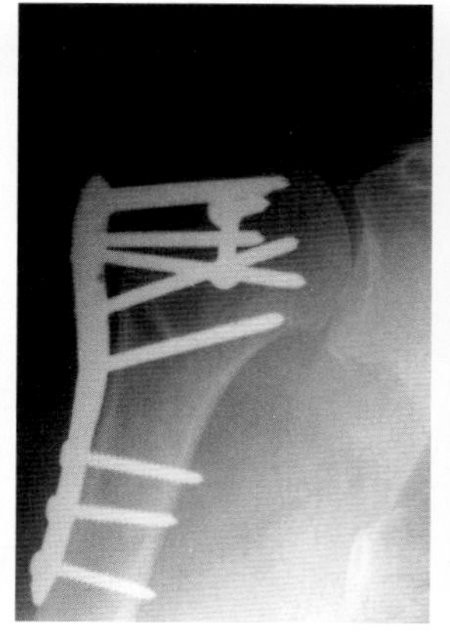
(c)

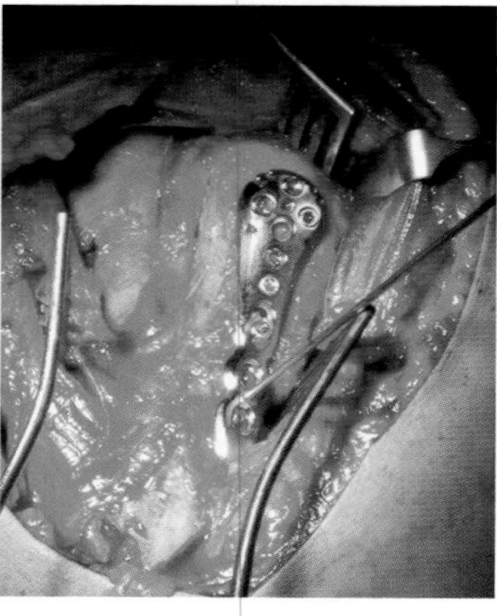
(d)

24.18 Proximal humerus fractures – treatment (a) Three-part fracture, treated by (b) locked nail fixation. (c) Four-part fracture fixed with a locked plate; the intra-operative picture (d) shows how the plate was positioned.

Three-part fracture-dislocations, when the surgical neck is also broken, usually require open reduction and fixation; the brachial plexus is at particular risk during this operation.

Four-part fracture-dislocations have a poor prognosis; prosthetic replacement is recommended in all but young and very active patients.

Complications

Vascular injuries and nerve injuries The patient should always be carefully assessed for signs of vascular and nerve injuries, both at the initial examination and again after any operation. The axillary nerve is at particular risk, both from the injury and from surgery.

Avascular necrosis The reported incidence of avascular necrosis (AVN) of the humeral head ranges from 10–30 per cent in three-part fractures and 10 to over 50 per cent in four-part fractures. The ability to predict the likelihood of this outcome is important in making the choice between internal fixation and hemiarthroplasty for complex fractures.

The blood-supply of the humeral head is provided mainly by the anterior circumflex artery and its ascending branch (the arcuate artery) which penetrates into the humeral head and arches across subchondrally. Additional blood-supply is provided by vessels entering the posteromedial aspect of the proximal humerus, metaphyseal vessels and vessels of the greater and lesser tuberosities that anastomose with the intraosseous arcuate artery. Thus, in three- and four-part fractures with the only supply coming from the posteromedial vessels, there may still be sufficient perfusion of the humeral head if the head fragment includes a sizeable part of the calcar on the medial side of the anatomical neck. Hertel et al. (2004) have made the point that fractures at the anatomical neck with a medial metaphyseal (calcar) spike shorter than 8 mm carry a high risk of developing humeral head avascular necrosis (see Fig. 24.15). Disruption of the medial periosteal hinge is another predictor of avascular necrosis and the presence of these two factors combined has a positive predictive value of 98 per cent for avascular necrosis of the humeral head. Contrariwise, fractures with an intact medial hinge and/or a large posteromedial metaphyseal spike carry a much better prognosis. The mere number of fracture parts, their degree of displacement and split-head fractures are rated as poor predictors of avascular necrosis, as is the presence of dislocation.

Stiffness of the shoulder This is a common complication, particularly in elderly patients. Unlike a frozen shoulder, the stiffness is maximal at the outset. It can be prevented, or at least minimized, by starting exercises early.

Malunion Malunion usually causes little disability, but loss of rotation may make it difficult for the patient to reach behind the neck or up the back.

FRACTURES OF THE PROXIMAL HUMERUS IN CHILDREN

At birth, the shoulder is sometimes dislocated or the proximal humerus fractured. Diagnosis is difficult and a clavicular fracture or brachial plexus injury should also be considered.

In infancy, the physis can separate (Salter–Harris I); reduction does not have to be perfect and a good outcome is usual.

In older children, metaphyseal fractures or Type II physeal fractures occur. Considerable displacement and angulation can be accepted; because of the marked growth and remodelling potential of the proximal humerus, malunion is readily compensated for during the remaining growth period.

Pathological fractures are not unusual, as the proximal humerus is a common site of bone cysts and tumours in children. Fracture through a simple cyst usually unites and the cyst often heals spontaneously; all that is needed is to rest the arm in a sling for 4–6 weeks. Other lesions require treatment in their own right (See Chapter 9).

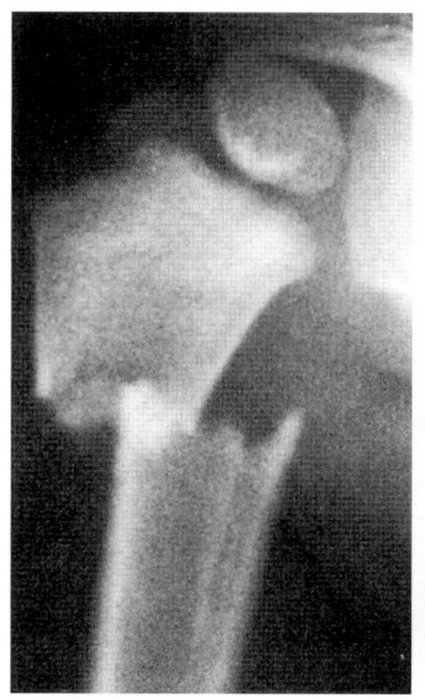
(a)

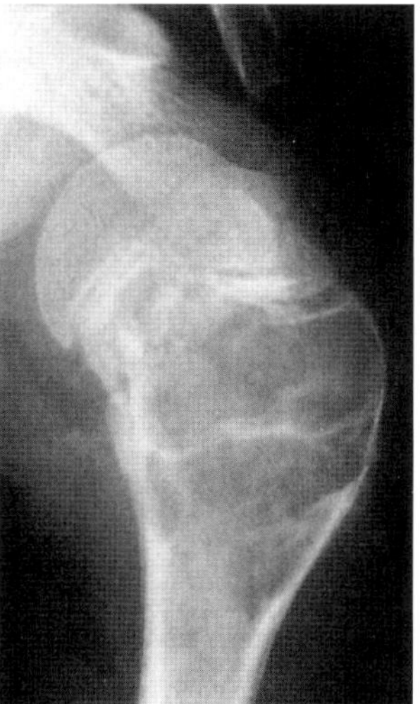
(b)

24.19 Fractures of the proximal humerus in children (a) The typical metaphyseal fracture. Reduction need not be perfect as remodelling will compensate for malunion. (b) Fracture through a benign cyst.

FRACTURED SHAFT OF HUMERUS

Mechanism of injury

A fall on the hand may twist the humerus, causing a spiral fracture. A fall on the elbow with the arm abducted exerts a bending force, resulting in an oblique or transverse fracture. A direct blow to the arm causes a fracture which is either transverse or comminuted. Fracture of the shaft in an elderly patient may be due to a metastasis.

Pathological anatomy

With fractures above the deltoid insertion, the proximal fragment is adducted by pectoralis major. With fractures lower down, the proximal fragment is abducted by the deltoid. Injury to the radial nerve is common, though fortunately recovery is usual.

Clinical features

The arm is painful, bruised and swollen. It is important to test for radial nerve function before and after treatment. This is best done by assessing active extension of the metacarpophalangeal joints; active extension of the wrist can be misleading because extensor carpi radialis longus is sometimes supplied by a branch arising proximal to the injury.

X-ray

The site of the fracture, its line (transverse, spiral or comminuted) and any displacement are readily seen. The possibility that the fracture may be pathological should be remembered.

Treatment

Fractures of the humerus heal readily. They require neither perfect reduction nor immobilization; the weight of the arm with an external cast is usually enough to pull the fragments into alignment. A 'hanging cast' is applied from shoulder to wrist with the elbow flexed 90 degrees, and the forearm section is suspended by a sling around the patient's neck. This cast may be replaced after 2–3 weeks by a short (shoulder to elbow) cast or a functional polypropylene brace which is worn for a further 6 weeks.

The wrist and fingers are exercised from the start. Pendulum exercises of the shoulder are begun within a week, but active abduction is postponed until the fracture has united (about 6 weeks for spiral fractures but often twice as long for other types); once united, only a sling is needed until the fracture is consolidated.

OPERATIVE TREATMENT

Patients often find the hanging cast uncomfortable, tedious and frustrating; they can feel the fragments moving and that is sometimes quite distressing. The temptation is to 'do something', and the 'something' usually means an operation. It is well to remember (a) that the complication rate after internal fixation of the humerus is high and (b) that the great majority of humeral fractures unite with non-operative treatment. (c) There is no good evidence that the union rate is higher with fixation (and the rate may be lower if there is distraction with nailing or periosteal stripping with plating). There are, nevertheless, some well defined indications for surgery:

- severe multiple injuries
- an open fracture

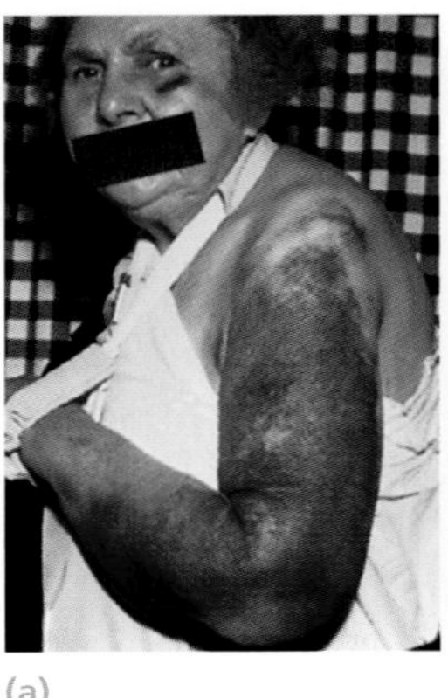
(a)

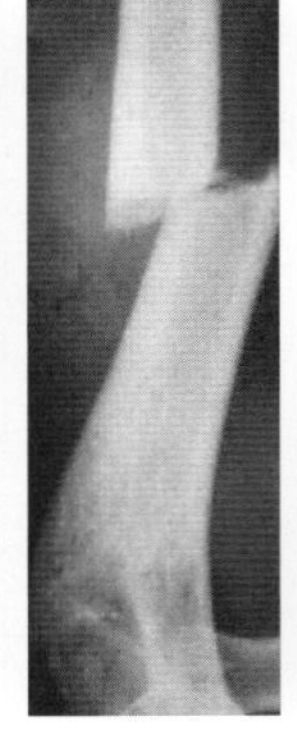
(b)

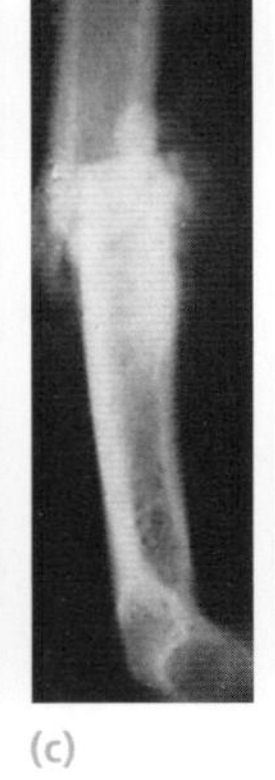
(c)

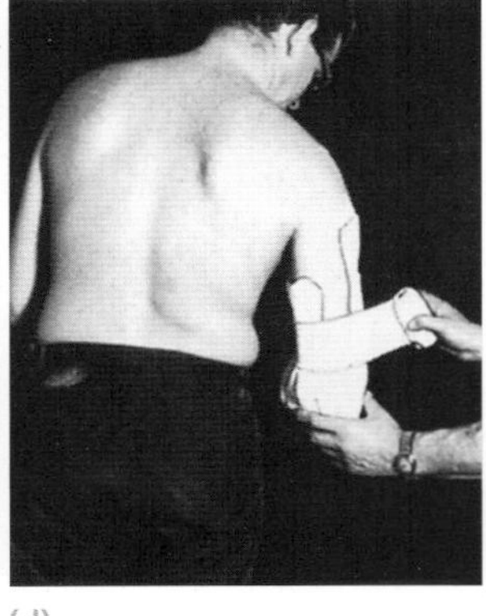
(d)

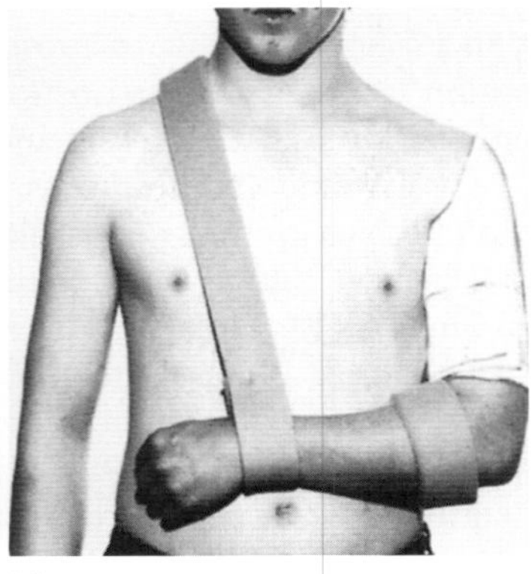
(e)

24.20 Fractured shaft of humerus (a) Bruising is always extensive. (b,c) Closed transverse fracture with moderate displacement. (d) Applying a U-slab of plaster (after a few days in a shoulder-to-wrist hanging cast) is usually adequate. (e) Ready-made braces are simpler and more comfortable, though not suitable for all cases. These conservative methods demand careful supervision if excessive angulation and malunion are to be prevented.

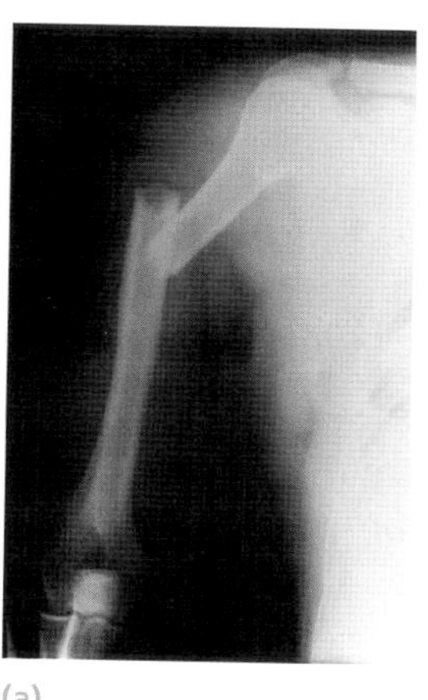
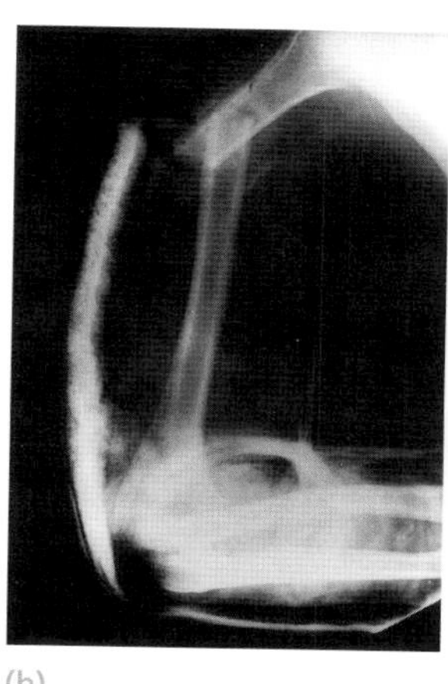
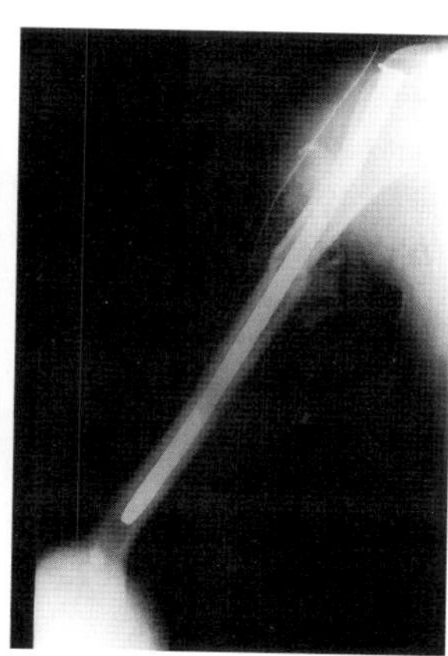

(a) (b) (c)

24.21 Fractured shaft of humerus – treatment (a,b) Most shaft fractures can be treated in a hanging cast or functional brace, but beware the upper third fracture which tends to angulate at the proximal border of a short cast. This fracture would have been better managed by (c) intramedullary nailing (and better still with a locking nail).

- segmental fractures
- displaced intra-articular extension of the fracture
- a pathological fracture
- a 'floating elbow' (simultaneous unstable humeral and forearm fractures)
- radial nerve palsy after manipulation
- non-union
- problems with nursing care in a dependent person.

Fixation can be achieved with either (1) a compression plate and screws, (2) an interlocking intramedullary nail or semi-flexible pins, or (3) an external fixator.

Plating permits excellent reduction and fixation, and has the added advantage that it does not interfere with shoulder or elbow function. However, it requires wide dissection and the radial nerve must be protected. Too much periosteal stripping or inadequate fixation will probably increase the risk of non-union.

Antegrade nailing is performed with a rigid interlocking nail inserted through the rotator cuff under fluoroscopic control. It requires minimal dissection but has the disadvantage that it causes rotator cuff problems in a significant proportion of cases (the reported incidence ranges from 5–40 per cent). The nail can also distract the fracture which will inhibit union; if this happens, exchange nailing and bone grafting of the fracture may be needed.

Retrograde nailing with multiple flexible rods is not entirely stable. Retrograde nailing with an interlocking nail is suitable for some fractures of the middle third.

External fixation may be the best option for high-energy segmental fractures and open fractures. However, great care must be taken in placing the pins as the radial nerve is vulnerable.

Complications

EARLY

Vascular injury If there are signs of vascular insufficiency in the limb, brachial artery damage must be excluded. Angiography will show the level of the injury. This is an emergency, requiring exploration and either direct repair or grafting of the vessel. In these circumstances, internal fixation is advisable.

Nerve injury Radial nerve palsy (wrist drop and paralysis of the metacarpophalangeal extensors) may occur with shaft fractures, particularly oblique fractures

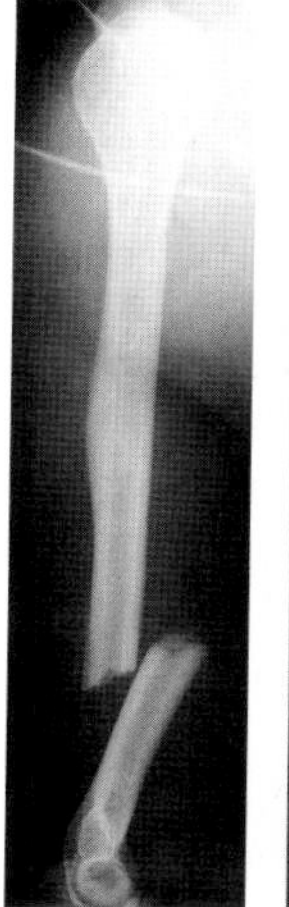
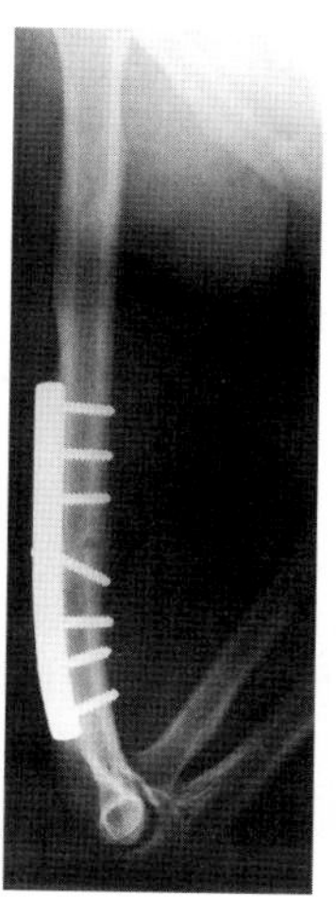
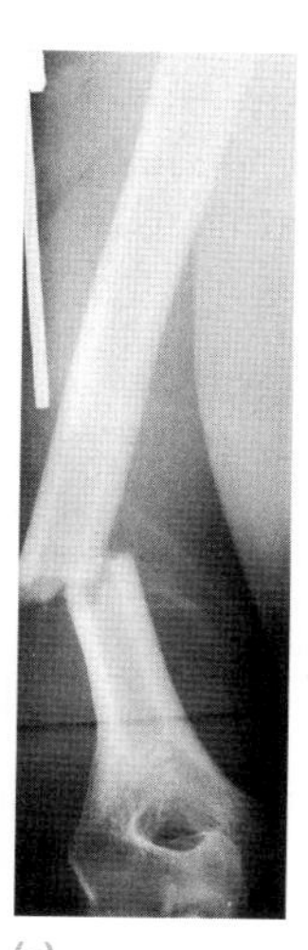
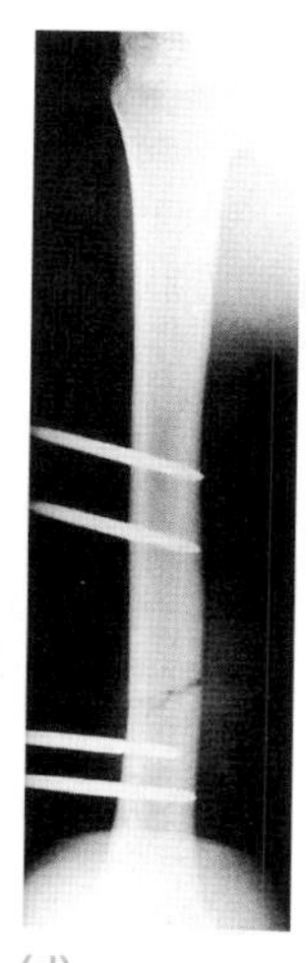
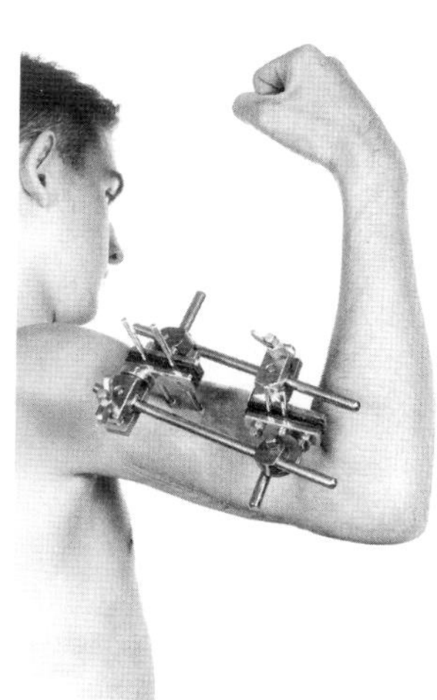

(a) (b) (c) (d) (e)

24.22 Fractured humerus – other methods of fixation (a,b) Compression plating, and (c,d,e) external fixation.

at the junction of the middle and distal thirds of the bone (Holstein–Lewis fracture). If nerve function was intact before manipulation but is defective afterwards, it must be assumed that the nerve has been snagged and surgical exploration is necessary. Otherwise, in closed injuries the nerve is very seldom divided, so there is no hurry to operate as it will usually recover. The wrist and hand must be regularly moved through a full passive range of movement to preserve joint motion until the nerve recovers. If there is no sign of recovery by 12 weeks, the nerve should be explored. It may just need a neurolysis, but if there is loss of continuity of normal-looking nerve then a graft is needed. The results are often satisfactory but, if necessary, function can be largely restored by tendon transfers (see Chapter 11).

LATE

Delayed union and non-union Transverse fractures sometimes take months to unite, especially if excessive traction has been used (a hanging cast must not be too heavy). Simple adjustments in technique may solve the problem; as long as there are signs of callus formation it is worth persevering with non-operative treatment, but remember to keep the shoulder moving. The rate of non-union in conservatively treated low-energy fractures is less than 3 per cent. Segmental high energy fractures and open fractures are more prone to both delayed union and non-union.

Intramedullary nailing may contribute to delayed union, but if rigid fixation can be maintained (if necessary by exchange nailing) the rate of non-union can probably be kept below 10 per cent.

A particularly vicious combination is incomplete union and a stiff joint. If elbow or shoulder movements are forced before consolidation of the fracture, or if an intramedullary nail is removed too soon (e.g., because of shoulder problems), the humerus may re-fracture and non-union is then more likely.

The treatment of established non-union is operative. The bone ends are freshened, cancellous bone graft is packed around them and the reduction is held with an intramedullary nail or a compression plate.

Joint stiffness Joint stiffness is common. It can be minimized by early activity, but transverse fractures (in which shoulder abduction is ill-advised) may limit shoulder movement for several weeks.

SPECIAL FEATURES IN CHILDREN

Fractures of the humerus are uncommon; in children under 3 years of age the possibility of child abuse should be considered and tactful examination for other injuries performed.

Taking advantage of the robust periosteum and the power of rapid healing in children, the humeral fracture can usually be treated by applying a collar and cuff bandage for 3 or 4 weeks. If there is gross shortening, manipulation may be needed. Older children may require a short plaster splint.

FRACTURES OF THE DISTAL HUMERUS IN ADULTS

Fractures around the elbow in adults – especially those of the distal humerus – are often high-energy injuries which are associated with vascular and nerve damage. Some can be reduced and stabilized only by complex surgical techniques; and the tendency to stiffness of the elbow means that with all severe injuries the striving for anatomical perfection has to be weighed up against the realities of imperfect post-operative function.

The AO-ASIF Group have defined three types of distal humeral fracture:

Type A – an extra-articular supracondylar fracture;
Type B – an intra-articular unicondylar fracture (one condyle sheared off);
Type C – bicondylar fractures with varying degrees of comminution.

TYPE A – SUPRACONDYLAR FRACTURES

These extra-articular fractures are rare in adults. When they do occur, they are usually displaced and unstable – probably because there is no tough periosteum to tether the fragments. In high-energy injuries there may be comminution of the distal humerus.

Treatment

Closed reduction is unlikely to be stable and K-wire fixation is not strong enough to permit early mobilization. Open reduction and internal fixation is therefore the treatment of choice. The distal humerus is approached through a posterior exposure. It is sometimes possible to fix the fracture without recourse to an olecranon osteotomy or triceps reflection. A simple transverse or oblique fracture can usually be reduced and fixed with a pair of contoured plates and screws.

TYPES B AND C – INTRA-ARTICULAR FRACTURES

Except in osteoporotic individuals, intra-articular condylar fractures should be regarded as high-energy injuries with soft-tissue damage. A severe blow on the point of the elbow drives the olecranon process upwards, splitting the condyles apart. Swelling is considerable, but if the bony landmarks can be felt the elbow is found to be distorted. The patient should be carefully examined for evidence of vascular or nerve injury; if there are signs of vascular insufficiency, this must be addressed as a matter of urgency.

X-Ray

The fracture extends from the lower humerus into the elbow joint; it may be difficult to tell whether one or both condyles are involved, especially with an undisplaced condylar fracture. There is often also comminution of the bone between the condyles, the extent of which is usually underestimated. Sometimes the fracture extends into the metaphysis as a T- or Y-shaped break, or else there may be multiple fragments (comminution). The lesson is: 'Prepare for the worst before operating'. CT scans can be helpful in planning the surgical approach.

Treatment

These are severe injuries associated with joint damage; prolonged immobilization will certainly result in a stiff elbow. Early movement is therefore a prime objective.

Undisplaced fractures These can be treated by applying a posterior slab with the elbow flexed almost 90 degrees; movements are commenced after 2 weeks. However, great care should be taken to avoid the dual pitfalls of underdiagnosis (displacement and comminution are not always obvious on the initial x-ray) and late displacement (always obtain check x-rays a week after injury).

Displaced Type B and C fractures If the appropriate expertise and facilities are available, open reduction and internal fixation is the treatment of choice for displaced fractures (some would say for all Type B and C fractures – minor displacement is easily overlooked in the early post-injury x-rays). The danger with conservative treatment is the strong tendency to stiffening of the elbow and persistent pain.

Good exposure of the joint is needed, if necessary by performing an intra-articular olecranon osteotomy. The ulnar nerve should be identified and protected throughout. The fragments are reduced and held temporarily with K-wires. A unicondylar fracture without comminution can then be fixed with screws; if the fragment is large, a contoured plate is added to prevent re-displacement. First the articular block is reconstructed with a transverse screw; bone graft is sometimes needed. The distal block is then fixed to the humeral shaft with medial and lateral plates. Pre-contoured plates with locking screws are now available. These hold the distal fragments more effectively.

Postoperatively the elbow is held at 90 degrees with the arm supported in a sling. Movement is encouraged but should never be forced. Fracture healing usually occurs by 12 weeks. Despite the best efforts, the patient often does not regain full extension and in the most severe cases movement may be severely restricted.

A description of this sort fails to convey the real difficulty of these operations. Unless the surgeon is more than usually skilful, the elbow may end up stiffer than if treated by activity (see below).

ALTERNATIVE METHODS OF TREATMENT

If it is anticipated that the outcome of operative treatment will be poor (either because of the degree of comminution and soft-tissue damage or because of lack of expertise and facilities) other options can be considered.

Elbow replacement The elderly patient with a comminuted fracture, a low transverse fracture or osteopaenic bone, may be best served by replacement of the elbow.

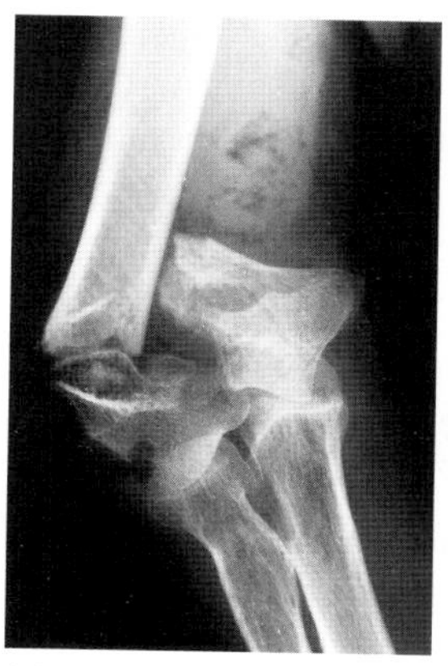
(a)

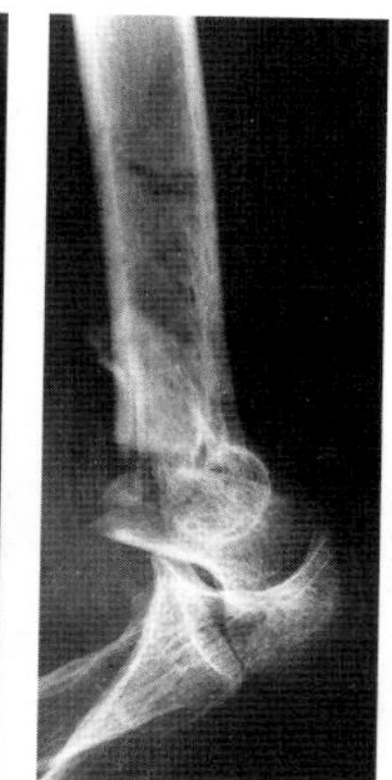
(b)

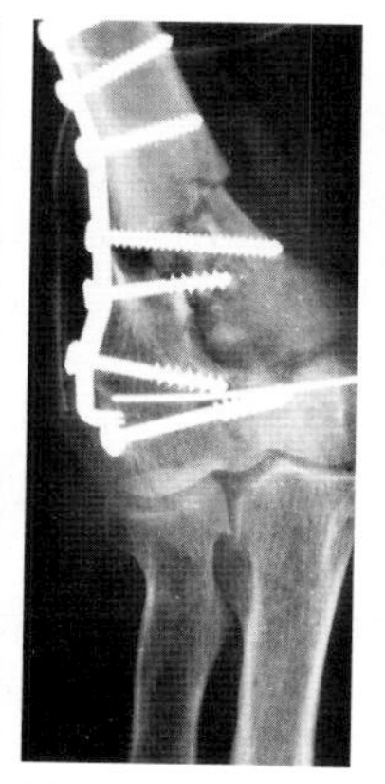
(c)

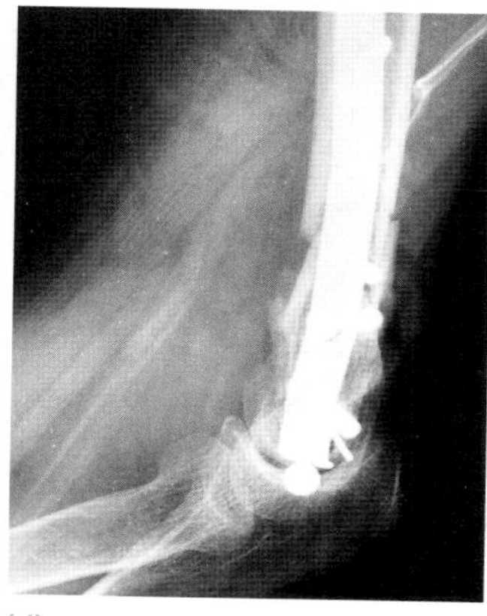
(d)

24.23 Bicondylar fractures X-rays taken (a,b) before and (c,d) after open reduction and internal fixation. An excellent reduction was obtained in this case; however, the elbow sometimes ends up with considerable loss of movement even though the general anatomy has been restored.

The 'bag of bones' technique The arm is held in a collar and cuff or, better, a hinged brace, with the elbow flexed above a right angle; active movements are encouraged as soon as the patient is willing. The fracture usually unites within 6–8 weeks, but exercises are continued far longer. A useful range of movement (45–90 degrees) is often obtained.

Skeletal traction An alternative method of treating either moderately displaced or severely comminuted fractures is by skeletal traction through the olecranon (beware the ulnar nerve!); the patient remains in bed with the humerus held vertical, and elbow movements are encouraged. Again, meticulous internal fixation or elbow replacement are usually preferable.

Complications

EARLY

Vascular injury Always check the circulation (repeatedly!). Vigilance is required to make the diagnosis and institute treatment as early as possible.

Nerve injury There may be damage to either the median or the ulnar nerve. It is important to examine the hand and record the findings before treatment is commenced. The ulnar nerve is particularly vulnerable during surgery.

LATE

Stiffness Comminuted fractures of the elbow always result in some degree of stiffness. However, the disability may be reduced by encouraging an energetic exercise programme. Late operations to improve elbow movement are difficult but can be rewarding.

Heterotopic ossification Severe soft-tissue damage may lead to heterotopic ossification. Forced movement should be avoided.

FRACTURED CAPITULUM

This is a rare articular fracture which occurs only in adults. The patient falls on the hand, usually with the elbow straight. The anterior part of the capitulum is sheared off and displaced proximally.

Clinical features

Fullness in front of the elbow is the most notable feature. The lateral side of the elbow is tender and flexion is grossly restricted.

X-Ray

In the lateral view the capitulum (or part of it) is seen in front of the lower humerus, and the radial head no longer points directly towards it. Bryan and Morrey classify these as:

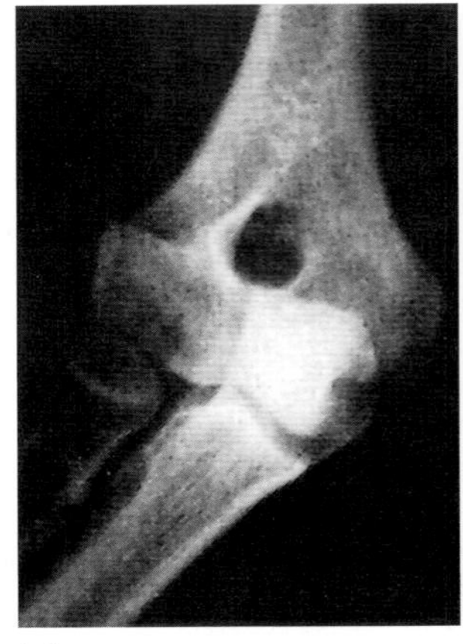
(a)

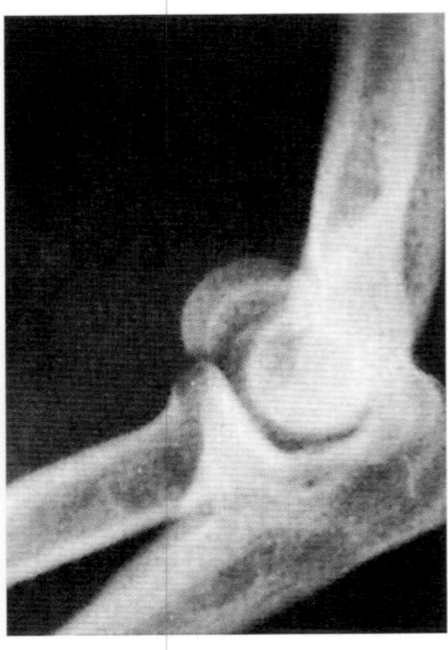
(b)

24.24 Fractured capitulum Anteroposterior and lateral x-rays showing proximal displacement and tilting of the capitular fragment.

Type I	Complete fracture
Type II	Cartilaginous shell
Type III	Comminuted fracture.

CT scans can be helpful in clarifying the diagnosis.

Treatment

Undisplaced fractures can be treated by simple splintage for 2 weeks.

Displaced fractures should be reduced and held. Closed reduction is feasible, but prolonged immobilization may result in a stiff elbow. Operative treatment is therefore preferred. The fragment is always larger than expected. If it can be securely replaced, it is fixed in position with a small screw. Headless bone screws are ideally passed from front to back; alternatively, if the fragment is large enough, lag screws can be passed from back to front. If this proves too difficult, the fragment is best excised. Movements are commenced as soon as discomfort permits. The longer term outcome is not always good because of stiffness and sometimes instability.

FRACTURED HEAD OF RADIUS

Radial head fractures are common in adults but are hardly ever seen in children (probably because the proximal radius is mainly cartilaginous) whereas radial neck fractures occur in children more frequently.

Mechanism of injury

A fall on the outstretched hand with the elbow extended and the forearm pronated causes impaction of the radial head against the capitulum. The radial head may be split or broken. In addition, the articular cartilage of the capitulum may be bruised or chipped; this cannot be seen on x-ray but is an important complication. The radial head is also sometimes fractured during elbow dislocation.

Clinical features

This fracture is sometimes missed, but tenderness on pressure over the radial head and pain on pronation and supination should suggest the diagnosis.

X-ray

Three types of fracture are identified and classified by Mason as:

Type I	An undisplaced vertical split in the radial head
Type II	A displaced single fragment of the head
Type III	The head broken into several fragments (comminuted).

An additional Type IV has been proposed, for those fractures with an associated elbow dislocation.

Special radial head views, rather than simple PA and lateral views are needed to fully assess the fracture. The wrist also should be x-rayed to exclude a concomitant injury of the distal radioulnar joint, which would signify damage to the interosseous membrane (acute longitudinal radioulnar dissociation).

Treatment

An undisplaced split (Type I) Worthwhile pain relief can be achieved by aspirating the haematoma and injecting local anaesthetic. The arm is held in a collar and cuff for 3 weeks; active flexion, extension and rotation are encouraged. The prognosis for this injury is very good, although there is often some loss of elbow extension.

A single large fragment (Type II) If the fragment is displaced, it should be reduced and held with one or two small headless screws.

A comminuted fracture (Type III) This is a challenging injury. Always assess for an associated soft tissue injury:

Rupture of the medial collateral ligament;
Rupture of the interosseous membrane (Essex Lopresti lesion);
Combined fractures of the radial head and coronoid process plus dislocation of the elbow – the 'terrible triad'.

If any of these is present, excision of the radial head is contra-indicated; this may lead to intractible instability of the elbow or forearm. The head must be meticulously reconstructed with small headless screws or replaced with a metal spacer. A medial collateral rupture, if unstable after replacing or fixing the radial head, should be repaired.

Radial head excision usually gives a good long-term result if there are no contra-indications; however, wrist pain from ulnar head impaction, valgus instability of the elbow and trochleo-olecranon arthritis can develop.

Complications

Joint stiffness is common and may involve both the elbow and the radioulnar joints. Even with minimally displaced fractures the elbow can take several months to recover, and stiffness may occur whether the radial head has been excised or not.

Myositis ossificans is an occasional complication.

Recurrent instability of the elbow can occur if the medial collateral ligament was also injured and the radial head excised.

FRACTURE OF THE RADIAL NECK

In adults, a displaced fracture of the radial neck may need open reduction; if so, a mini-plate can be

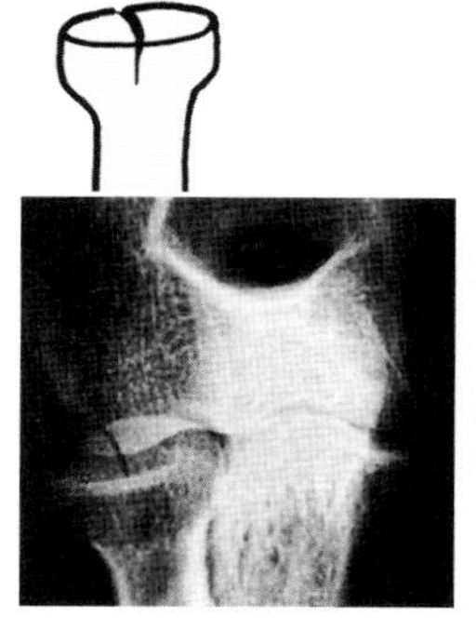
(a)

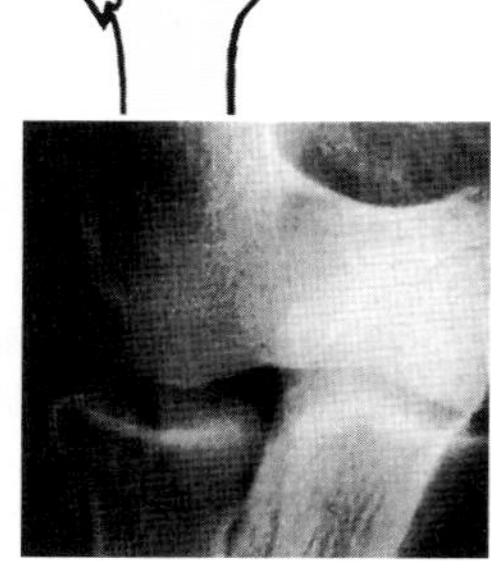
(b)

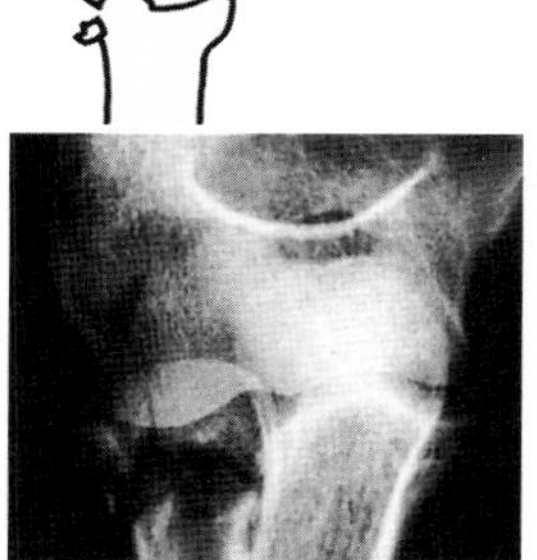
(c)

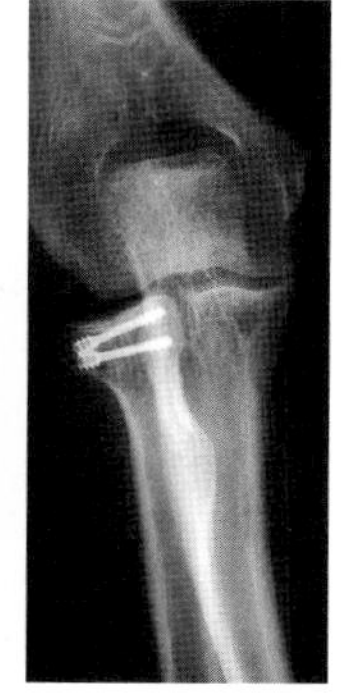
(d)

24.25 Fractured head of radius There are three main types of adult radial head fracture: (a) a chisel-like split of head, (b) a marginal fracture or (c) a comminuted fracture. Displaced marginal fractures can often be treated by (d) internal fixation.

applied, making sure not to damage the articular surface. An alternative is to use oblique headless screws.

FRACTURES OF THE OLECRANON

Two broad types of injury are seen: (1) a comminuted fracture which is due to a direct blow or a fall on the elbow; and (2) a transverse break, due to traction when the patient falls onto the hand while the triceps muscle is contracted. These two types can be further sub-classified into (a) displaced and (b) undisplaced fractures. More severe injuries may be associated also with subluxation or dislocation of the ulno-humeral joint.

The fracture always enters the elbow joint and therefore damages the articular cartilage. With transverse fractures, the triceps aponeurosis sometimes remains intact, in which case the fracture fragments stay together.

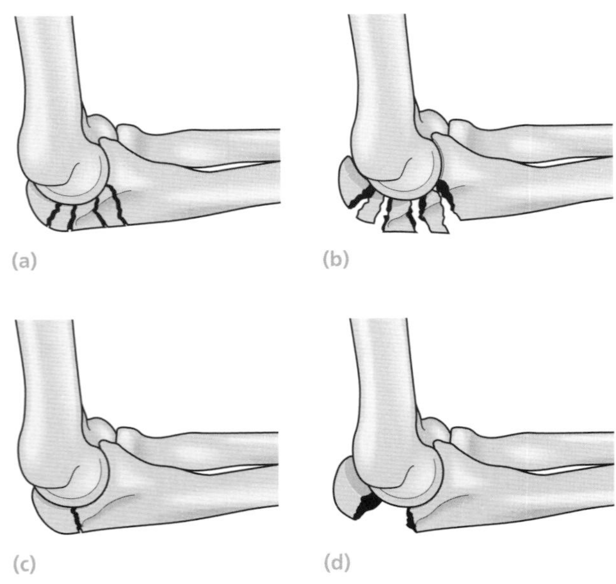

24.26 Fractured olecranon **(a,b)** Comminuted fractures, undisplaced and displaced. **(c,d)** Transverse fractures, undisplaced and displaced.

Clinical features

A graze or bruise over the elbow suggests a comminuted fracture; the triceps is intact and the elbow can be extended against gravity. With a transverse fracture there may be a palpable gap and the patient is unable to extend the elbow against resistance.

X-ray

A properly orientated lateral view is essential to show details of the fracture, as well as the associated joint damage. Always check the position of the radial head – it may be dislocated.

Treatment

A comminuted fracture with the triceps intact should be treated as a severe 'bruise'. Many of these patients are old and osteoporotic, and immobilizing the elbow will lead to stiffness. The arm is rested in a sling for a week; a further x-ray is obtained to ensure that there is no displacement and the patient is then encouraged to start active movements.

An undisplaced transverse fracture that does not separate when the elbow is x-rayed in flexion can be treated closed. The elbow is immobilized by a cast in about 60 degrees of flexion for 2–3 weeks and then exercises are begun. Repeat x-rays are needed to exclude displacement.

Displaced transverse fractures can be held only by splinting the arm absolutely straight – but stiffness in that position would be disastrous. Operative treatment is therefore strongly recommended. The fracture is reduced and held by tension band wiring. Oblique fractures may need a lag screw, neutralised by a tension band system or plate.

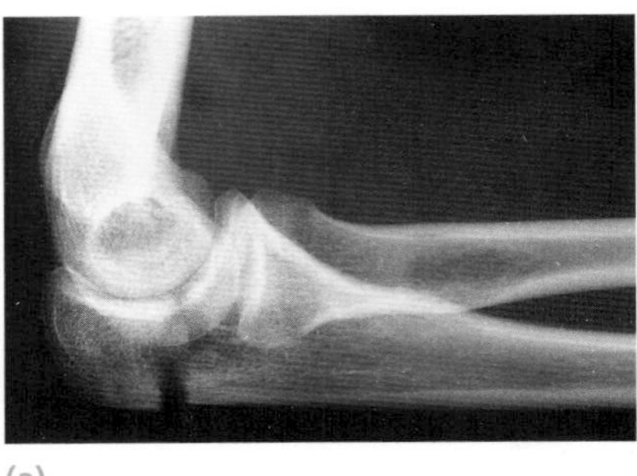
(a)

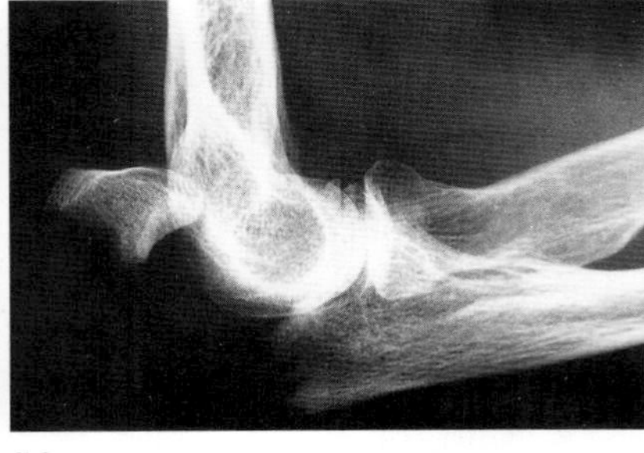
(b)

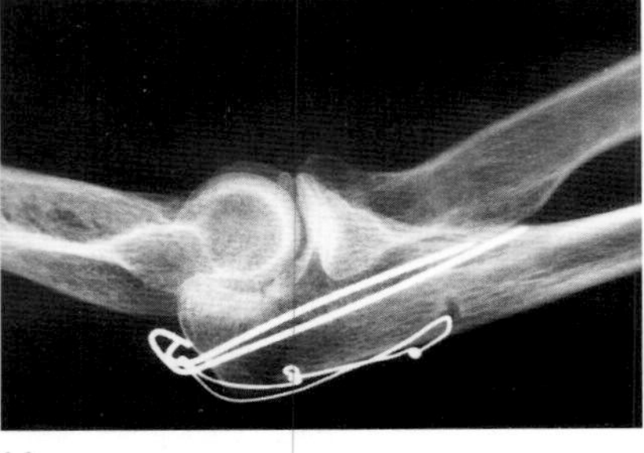
(c)

24.27 Fractured olecranon **(a)** Slightly displaced transverse fracture. **(b)** Markedly displaced transverse fracture – the extensor mechanism is no longer intact. Treatment in this case was by open reduction and tension-band wiring **(c)**.

Displaced comminuted fractures need a plate and often bone graft. In the osteoporotic bone of low-demand elderly patients, good results can be achieved with excision of fragments and re-attachment of triceps to the ulna. If the coronoid portion of the joint is intact it will reduce the risk of instability. Following operation, early mobilization should be encouraged.

Complications

Stiffness used to be common, but with secure internal fixation and early mobilization the residual loss of movement should be minimal.

Non-union sometimes occurs after inadequate reduction and fixation. If elbow function is good, it can be ignored; if not, rigid internal fixation and bone grafting will be needed.

Ulnar nerve symptoms can develop. These usually settle spontaneously.

Osteoarthritis is a late complication, especially if reduction is less than perfect. This can usually be treated symptomatically.

DISLOCATION OF THE ELBOW

Dislocation of the ulno-humeral joint is fairly common – more so in adults than in children. Injuries are usually classified according to the direction of displacement. However, in 90% of cases the radioulnar complex is displaced posteriorly or posterolaterally, often together with fractures of the restraining bony processes.

Mechanism of injury and pathology

The cause of posterior dislocation is usually a fall on the outstretched hand with the elbow in extension. Disruption of the capsule and ligaments structures alone can result in posterior or posterolateral dislocation. However, provided there is no associated fracture, reduction will usually be stable and recurrent dislocation unlikely. The combination of ligamentous disruption and fracture of the radial head, coronoid process or olecranon process (or, worse still, several fractures) will render the joint more unstable and, unless the fractures are reduced and fixed, liable to re-dislocation.

Once posterior dislocation has taken place, lateral shift may also occur. Soft tissue disruption is often considerable and surrounding nerves and vessels may be damaged. Although certain common patterns of fracture-dislocation are recognized (based on the particular combination of structures involved), high-energy injuries do not necessarily follow any rules. A classic example is the so-called side-swipe injury which occurs, typically, when a car-driver's elbow, protruding through the window, is struck by another vehicle. The result is forward dislocation with fractures of any or all of the bones around the elbow; soft-tissue damage (including neurovascular injury) is usually severe.

Clinical features

The patient supports his forearm with the elbow in slight flexion. Unless swelling is severe, the deformity is obvious. The bony landmarks (olecranon and epicondyles) may be palpable and abnormally placed.

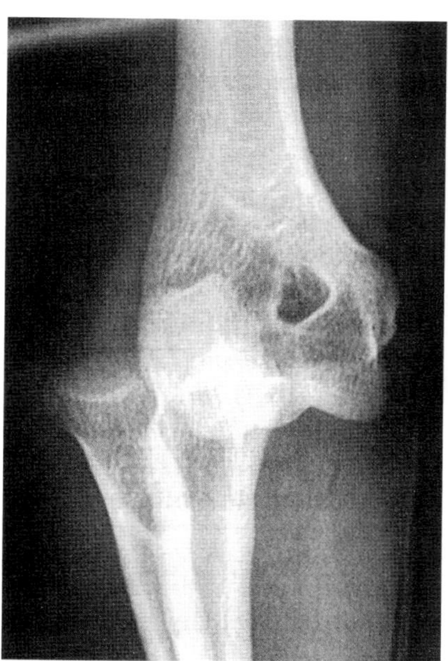

(a)

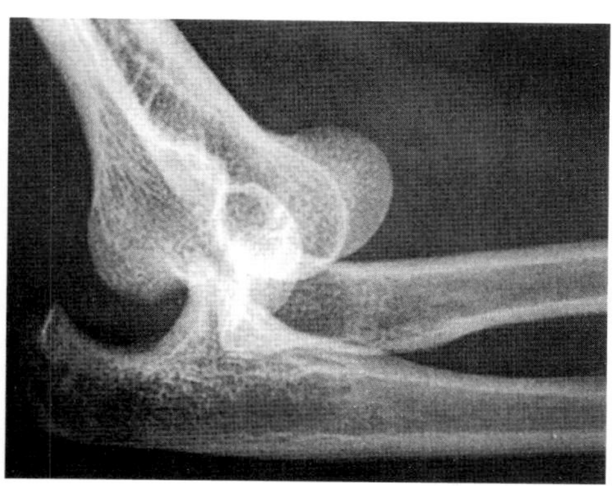

(b)

24.28 Dislocation of the elbow X-rays showing (a) lateral and (b) posterior displacement.

However, in severe injuries pain and swelling are so marked that examination of the elbow is impossible. Nevertheless, the hand should be examined for signs of vascular or nerve damage.

X-ray

X-ray examination is essential (a) to confirm the presence of a dislocation and (b) to identify any associated fractures. It is often only when the elbow is screened at the time of surgery that the full extent of the injury can be established.

Treatment

UNCOMPLICATED DISLOCATION

The patient should be fully relaxed under anaesthesia. The surgeon pulls on the forearm while the elbow is slightly flexed. With one hand, sideways displacement is corrected, then the elbow is further flexed while the olecranon process is pushed forward with the thumbs. Unless almost full flexion can be obtained, the olecranon is not in the trochlear groove.

After reduction, the elbow should be put through a full range of movement to see whether it is stable. The distal nerves and circulation are checked again. In addition, an x-ray is obtained to confirm that the joint is reduced and to disclose any associated fractures.

The arm is held in a collar and cuff with the elbow flexed above 90 degrees. After 1 week the patient gently exercises his elbow; at 3 weeks the collar and cuff is discarded. Elbow movements are allowed to return spontaneously and are never forced. The long-term results are usually good.

DISLOCATION WITH ASSOCIATED FRACTURES

Coronoid process Coronoid fractures have been classified by Regan and Morrey as:

Type I	Avulsion of the tip. A benign enough injury, but it can represent a substantial soft-tissue injury of the elbow
Type II	A single or comminuted fracture of the coronoid with 50 per cent or less involved. This is usually not repaired surgically, as the elbow remains stable
Type III	A single or comminuted fracture involving more than 50 per cent. If the elbow is unstable after reduction, then fixation is usually needed.

Medial epicondyle An avulsed medial epicondyle is, for practical purposes, a medial ligament disruption. If the epicondylar fragment is displaced, it must be reduced and fixed back in position. The arm and wrist are splinted with the elbow at 90 degrees; after 3 weeks movements are begun under supervision.

Head of radius The combination of ligament disruption and a type II or III radial head fracture is an unstable injury; stability is restored only by healing or repair of the ligaments and restoration of the radial pillar – either by fracture fixation or (in the case of a comminuted fracture) by prosthetic replacement of the radial head. The medial collateral ligament may also be repaired to protect the radial head fixation or implant from undue valgus stress.

Olecranon process In the rare forward dislocation of the elbow, the olecranon process may fracture; a large piece of the olecranon is left behind as a separate fragment. Open reduction with internal fixation is the best treatment.

Side-swipe injuries These severe fracture-dislocations are often associated with damage to the large vessels of the arm. The priorities are repair of any vascular injury, skeletal stabilization and soft tissue coverage. This is demanding surgery, necessitating a high level of expertise, and is best undertaken in a unit specialising in upper limb injuries.

Persistent instability In cases where the elbow remains unstable after the bone and joint anatomy has been restored, a hinged external fixator can be applied in order to maintain mobility while the tissues heal.

Complications

Complications are common; some are potentially so serious that the patient with a dislocation or a fracture-dislocation of the elbow must be observed with the closest attention.

EARLY

Vascular injury The brachial artery may be damaged. Absence of the radial pulse is a warning. If there are other signs of ischaemia, this should be treated as an emergency. Splints must be removed and the elbow should be straightened somewhat. If there is no improvement, an arteriogram is performed; the brachial artery may have to be explored.

Nerve injury The median or ulnar nerve is sometimes injured. Spontaneous recovery usually occurs after 6–8 weeks.

LATE

Stiffness Loss of 20 to 30 degrees of extension is not uncommon after elbow dislocation; fortunately this is usually of little functional significance. The most common cause of undue stiffness is prolonged immobilization. In the management of all elbow injuries the joint should be moved as soon as possible, with due consideration to stability of the fractures and soft tissues and without undue passive stretching of the soft tissues. For injuries requiring prolonged splintage, a hinged elbow brace, or on some occasions a hinged external fixator, can allow some movement in the flexion-extension plane whilst protecting against collateral stress.

Persistent stiffness of severe degree can often be improved by anterior capsular release. However, operative treatment should not be rushed; remember that sometimes the stiffness is due to myositis ossificans, which is usually undetectable on plain x-ray examination until a month or more after injury.

Heterotopic ossification (myositis ossificans) Heterotopic bone formation may occur in the damaged soft tissues in front of the joint. It is due to muscle bruising or haematoma formation; however the precise pathogenesis is not known. In former years 'myositis ossificans' was a fairly common complication of elbow injury, usually associated with forceful reduction and overenthusiastic passive movement of the elbow. Nowadays it is rarely seen, but it is as well to be alert for signs such as slight swelling, excessive pain and tenderness around the front of the elbow, along with tardy recovery of active movements.

X-ray examination is initially unhelpful; soft-tissue ossification is usually not visible until 4–6 weeks after injury. If the condition is suspected, exercises are stopped and the elbow is splinted in comfortable flexion until pain subsides; gentle active movements and continuous passive motion are then resumed. Anti-inflammatory drugs may help to reduce stiffness; they are also used prophylactically to reduce the risk of heterotopic bone formation.

A bone mass which markedly restricts movement and elbow function can be excised, though not before the bone is fully 'mature', i.e. has well-defined cortical margins and trabeculae (as seen on x-ray).

Unreduced dislocation A dislocation may not have been diagnosed; or only the backward displacement corrected, leaving the olecranon process still displaced sideways. Up to 3 weeks from injury, manipulative reduction is worth attempting but care is needed to avoid fracturing one of the bones. Other than this, there is no satisfactory treatment. Open reduction can be considered, but a wide soft tissue release is required, which predisposes to yet further stiffness. Alternatively, the condition can be left, in the hope that the elbow will regain a useful range of movement. If pain is a problem, the patient can be offered an arthrodesis or an arthroplasty.

Recurrent dislocation This is rare unless there is a large coronoid fracture or radial head fracture. If recurrent elbow instability occurs, the lateral ligament and capsule can be repaired or re-attached to the lateral condyle. A cast with the elbow at 90 degrees is worn for 4 weeks.

Osteoarthritis Secondary osteoarthritis is quite common after severe fracture-dislocations. In older patients, total elbow replacement can be considered.

ISOLATED DISLOCATION OF THE RADIAL HEAD

A true isolated dislocation of the radial head is very rare; if it is seen, search carefully for an associated fracture of the ulna (the Monteggia injury). In a child, the ulnar fracture may be difficult to detect if it is incomplete, either green-stick or plastic deformation of the shaft; it is very important to identify these incomplete fractures because even a minor deformity, if it is allowed to persist, may prevent full reduction of the radial head dislocation.

FRACTURES AROUND THE ELBOW IN CHILDREN

The elbow is second only to the distal forearm for frequency of fractures in children. Most of these injuries are supracondylar fractures, the remainder being divided between condylar, epicondylar and proximal radial and ulnar fractures. Boys are injured more often than girls and more than half the patients are under 10 years old.

The usual accident is a fall directly on the point of the elbow or – more often – onto the outstretched hand with the elbow forced into valgus or varus. Pain and swelling are often marked and examination is difficult. X-ray interpretation also has its problems: The bone ends are largely cartilaginous and therefore radiographically incompletely visualized. A good knowledge of the normal anatomy is essential if fracture displacements are to be recognized.

Points of anatomy

The elbow is a complex hinge, providing sufficient mobility to permit the upper limb to reach through wide ranges of flexion, extension and rotation, yet also enough stability to support the necessary gripping, pushing, pulling and carrying activities of daily life. Its stability is due largely to the shape and fit of the bones that make up the joint – especially the humero-ulnar component – and this is liable to be compromised by any break in the articulating structures. The surrounding soft-tissue structures also are important, especially the capsular and collateral ligaments and, to a lesser extent, the muscles. Ligament disruption is also, therefore, a destabilizing factor.

The forearm is normally in slight valgus in relation to the upper arm, the average carrying angle in children being about 15 degrees. (Published measurements range from 5 to 25 degrees). When the elbow is flexed, the forearm comes to lie directly upon the upper arm. Doubts about the normality of these features can usually be resolved by comparing the injured with the normal arm.

With the elbow flexed, the tips of the medial and lateral epicondyles and the olecranon prominence form an isosceles triangle; with the elbow extended, they lie transversely in line with each other.

Though all the epiphyses are in some part cartilaginous, the secondary ossific centres can be seen on x-ray; they should not be mistaken for fracture fragments! The average ages at which the ossific centres appear are easily remembered by the mnemonic CRITOE: Capitulum – 2 years. Radial head – 4 years. Internal (medial) epicondyle – 6 years. Trochlea – 8 years. Olecranon – 10 years. External (lateral) epicondyle – 12 years. Obviously epiphyseal displacements will not be detectable on x-ray before these ages. Fracture displacement and accuracy of reduction can be inferred from radiographic indices such as Baumann's angle (see Fig. 24.30).

SUPRACONDYLAR FRACTURES

These are among the commonest fractures in children. The distal fragment may be displaced either posteriorly or anteriorly.

Mechanism of injury

Posterior angulation or displacement (95 per cent of all cases) suggests a hyperextension injury, usually due to a fall on the outstretched hand. The humerus breaks just above the condyles. The distal fragment is pushed backwards and (because the forearm is usually in pronation) twisted inwards. The jagged end of the proximal fragment pokes into the soft tissues anteriorly, sometimes injuring the brachial artery or median nerve.

Anterior displacement is rare; it is thought to be due to direct violence (e.g. a fall on the point of the elbow) with the joint in flexion.

Classification

Type I is an undisplaced fracture.
Type II is an angulated fracture with the posterior cortex still in continuity.
- IIA – a less severe injury with the distal fragment merely angulated.
- IIB – a severe injury; the fragment is both angulated and malrotated.

Type III is a completely displaced fracture (although the posterior periosteum is usually still preserved, which will assist surgical reduction).

Clinical features

Following a fall, the child is in pain and the elbow is swollen; with a posteriorly displaced fracture the S-deformity of the elbow is usually obvious and the bony landmarks are abnormal. It is essential to feel the pulse and check the capillary return; passive extension of the flexor muscles should be pain-free. The wrist and the hand should be examined for evidence of nerve injury.

X-ray

The fracture is seen most clearly in the lateral view. In an undisplaced fracture the 'fat pad sign' should raise suspicions: there is a triangular lucency in front of the distal humerus, due to the fat pad being pushed forwards by a haematoma.

In the common posteriorly displaced fracture the fracture line runs obliquely downwards and forwards and the distal fragment is tilted backwards and/or shifted backwards. In the anteriorly displaced fracture the crack runs downwards and backwards and the

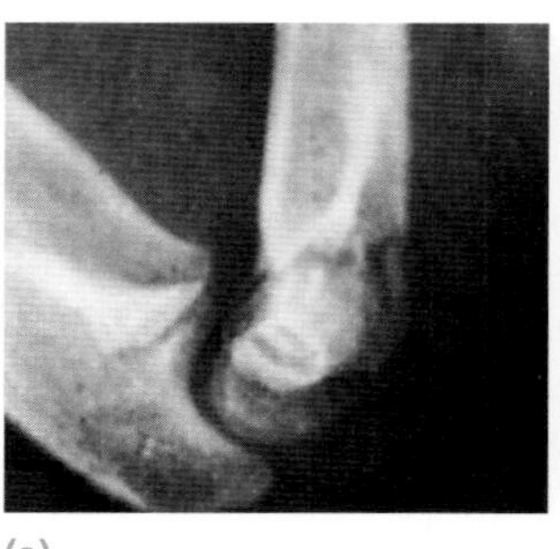
(a)

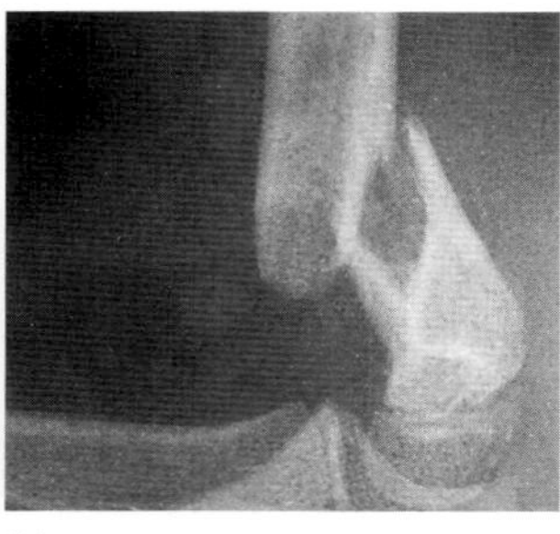
(b)

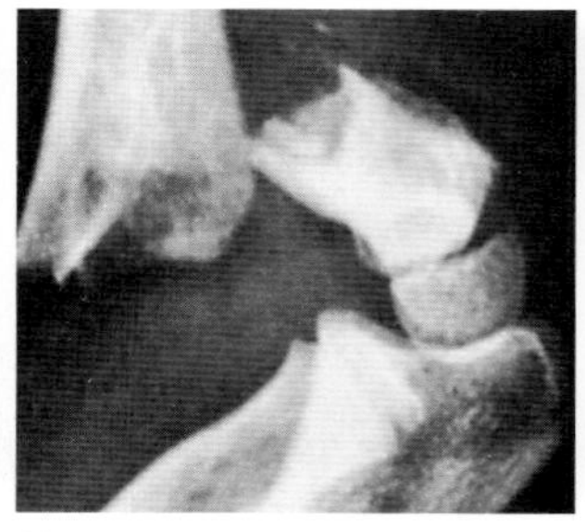
(c)

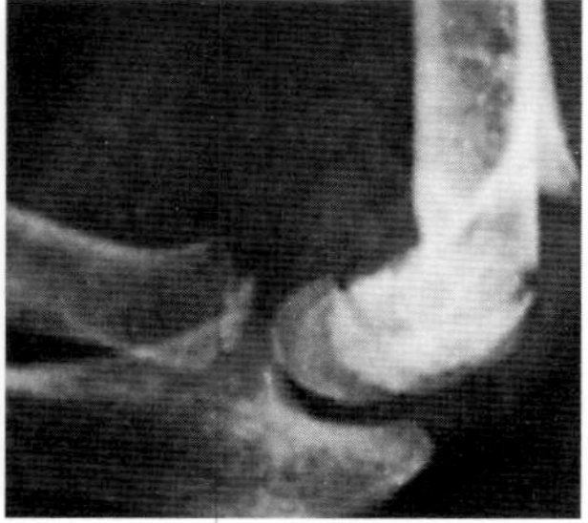
(d)

24.29 Supracondylar fractures X-rays showing supracondylar fractures of increasing severity. (a) Undisplaced. (b) Distal fragment posteriorly angulated but in contact. (c) Distal fragment completely separated and displaced posteriorly. (d) A rarer variety with anterior angulation.

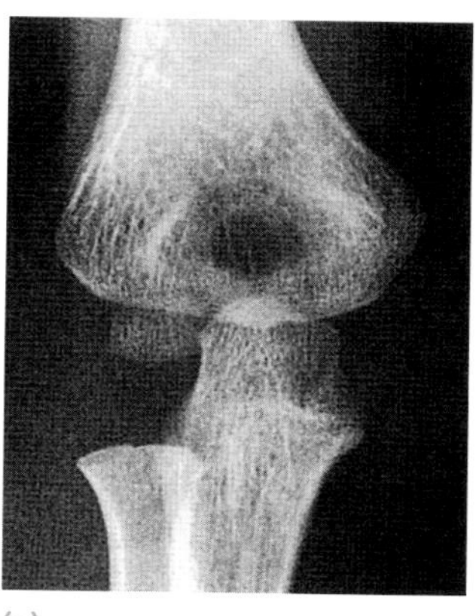

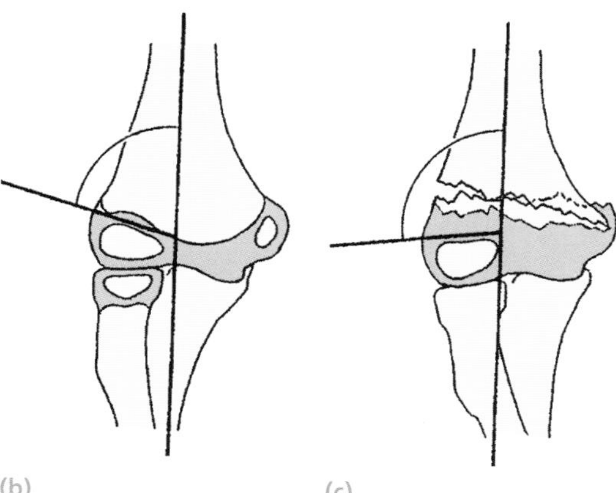

(a) (b) (c)

24.30 Baumann's angle Anteroposterior x-rays are sometimes difficult to make out, especially if the elbow is held flexed after reduction of the supracondylar fracture. Measurement of Baumann's angle is helpful. This is the angle subtended by the longitudinal axis of the humeral shaft and a line through the coronal axis of the capitellar physis, as shown in (a) the x-ray of a normal elbow and the accompanying diagram (b). Normally this angle is less than 80 degrees. If the distal fragment is tilted in varus, the increased angle is readily detected (c).

distal fragment is tilted forwards. On a normal lateral x-ray, a line drawn along the anterior cortex of the humerus should cross the middle of the capitulum. If the line is anterior to the capitulum then a Type II fracture is suspected.

An anteroposterior view is often difficult to obtain without causing pain and may need to be postponed until the child has been anaesthetized. It may show that the distal fragment is shifted or tilted sideways, and rotated (usually medially). Measurement of Baumann's angle is useful in assessing the degree of medial angulation before and after reduction (Fig. 24.30).

Treatment

If there is even a suspicion of a fracture, the elbow is gently splinted in 30 degrees of flexion to prevent movement and possible neurovascular injury during the x-ray examination.

TYPE I: UNDISPLACED FRACTURE

The elbow is immobilized at 90 degrees and neutral rotation in a light-weight splint or cast and the arm is supported by a sling. It is essential to obtain an x-ray 5–7 days later to check that there has been no displacement. The splint is retained for 3 weeks and supervised movement is then allowed.

The capitulum normally angles forward about 30 degrees; if the capitulum is in a straight line with the humerus on the lateral x-ray, it will still remodel.

Even with Type I fractures, care must be taken to recognise any medial tilt of the distal fragment on the anteroposterior x-ray, otherwise cubitus varus can result. Measure Baumann's angle.

TYPE II A: POSTERIORLY ANGULATED FRACTURE – MILD

In these cases swelling is usually not severe and the risk of vascular injury is low. If the posterior cortices are in continuity, the fracture can be reduced under general anaesthesia by the following step-wise manoeuvre: (1) traction for 2–3 minutes in the length of the arm with counter-traction above the elbow; (2) correction of any sideways tilt or shift and rotation (in comparison with the other arm); (3) gradual flexion of the elbow to 120 degrees, and pronation of the forearm, while maintaining traction and exerting finger pressure behind the distal fragment to correct posterior tilt. Then feel the pulse and check the capillary return – if the distal circulation is suspect, immediately relax the amount of elbow flexion until it improves. X-rays are taken to confirm reduction, checking carefully to see that there is no varus or valgus angulation and no rotational deformity. The anteroposterior view is confusing and unreliable with the elbow flexed, but the important features can be inferred by noting Baumann's angle. *Again, subtle medial tilt and rotation of the distal fragment must be recognised.* If the acutely flexed position cannot be maintained without disturbing the circulation, or if the reduction is unstable, (and most of these fractures are unstable!) the fracture should be fixed with percutaneous crossed K-wires (take care not to skewer the ulnar nerve!).

Following reduction, the arm is held in a collar and cuff; the circulation should be checked repeatedly during the first 24 hours. An x-ray is obtained after 3–5 days to confirm that the fracture has not slipped. The splint is retained for 3 weeks, after which movements are begun.

TYPES II B AND III: ANGULATED AND MALROTATED OR POSTERIORLY DISPLACED

These are usually associated with severe swelling, are difficult to reduce and are often unstable; moreover, there is a considerable risk of neurovascular injury or circulatory compromise due to swelling. The fracture should be reduced under general anaesthesia as soon as possible, by the method described above, and then held with percutaneous crossed K-wires; this obviates the necessity to hold the elbow acutely flexed.

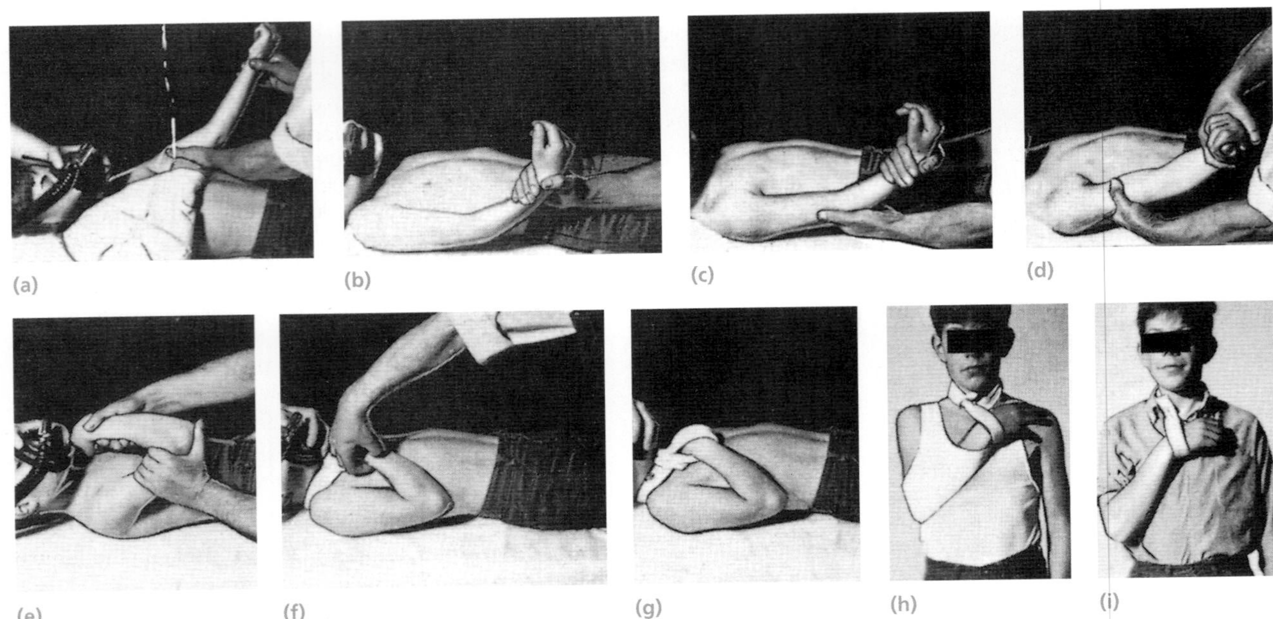

24.31 Supracondylar fractures – treatment (a) The uninjured arm is examined first; (b) traction of the fractured arm; (c) correcting lateral shift and tilt; (d) correcting rotation; (e) correcting backwards shift and tilt; (f) feeling the pulse; the elbow is kept well flexed while x-ray films are taken. (h) For the first 3 weeks the arm is kept under the clothes; after this (i) it is outside the clothes.

Smooth wires should be used (this lessens the risk of physeal injury) and great care should be taken not to injure the ulnar, radial and median nerves. Postoperative management is the same as for Type II A.

OPEN REDUCTION
This is sometimes necessary for (1) a fracture which simply cannot be reduced closed; (2) an open fracture; or (3) a fracture associated with vascular damage. The fracture is exposed (preferably through two incisions, one on each side of the elbow), the haematoma is evacuated and the fracture is reduced and held by two crossed K-wires.

CONTINUOUS TRACTION
Traction through a screw in the olecranon, with the arm held overhead, can be used (1) if the fracture is severely displaced and cannot be reduced by manipulation; (2) if, with the elbow flexed 100 degrees, the pulse is obliterated and image intensification is not available to allow pinning and then straightening of the elbow; or (3) for severe open injuries or multiple injuries of the limb. Once the swelling subsides, a further attempt can be made at closed reduction.

TREATMENT OF ANTERIORLY DISPLACED FRACTURES
This is a rare injury (less than 5 per cent of supracondylar fractures). However, 'posterior' fractures are sometimes inadvertently converted to 'anterior' ones by excessive traction and manipulation.

The fracture is reduced by pulling on the forearm with the elbow semi-flexed, applying thumb pressure over the front of the distal fragment and then extending the elbow fully. Crossed percutaneous pins are used if unstable. A posterior slab is bandaged on and retained for 3 weeks. Thereafter, the child is allowed to regain flexion gradually.

Complications

EARLY

Vascular injury The great danger of supracondylar fracture is injury to the brachial artery, which, before the introduction of percutaneous pinning, was reported as occurring in over 5 per cent of cases. Nowadays the incidence is probably less than 1 per cent. Peripheral ischaemia may be immediate and severe, or the pulse may fail to return after reduction. More commonly the injury is complicated by forearm oedema and a mounting compartment syndrome which leads to necrosis of the muscle and nerves without causing peripheral gangrene. Undue pain plus one positive sign (pain on passive extension of the fingers, a tense and tender forearm, an absent pulse, blunted sensation or reduced capillary return on pressing the finger pulp) demands urgent action. The flexed elbow must be extended and all dressings removed. If the circulation does not promptly improve, then angiography (on the operating table if it saves time) is carried out, the vessel repaired or grafted and a forearm fasciotomy performed. If angiography is not available, or would cause much delay, then Doppler imaging should be used. In extreme cases, operative exploration would be justified on clinical criteria alone.

Nerve injury The radial nerve, median nerve (particularly the anterior interosseous branch) or the ulnar nerve may be injured. Tests for nerve function are described in Chapter 11. Fortunately loss of function is usually temporary and recovery can be expected in 3 to 4 months. If there is no recovery the nerve should be explored. However, if a nerve, documented as intact prior to manipulation, is then found to have failed after manipulation, then entrapment in the fracture is suspected and immediate exploration should be arranged.

The ulnar nerve may be damaged by careless pinning. If the injury is recognized, and the pin removed, recovery will usually follow.

LATE

Malunion Malunion is common. However, backward or sideways shifts are gradually smoothed out by modelling during growth and they seldom give rise to visible deformity of the elbow. Forward or backward tilt may limit flexion or extension, but consequent disability is slight.

Uncorrected sideways tilt (angulation) and rotation are much more important and may lead to varus (or rarely valgus) deformity of the elbow; this is permanent and will not improve with growth (Fig. 24.32). The fracture is extra-physeal and so physeal damage should not be blamed for the deformity; usually it is faulty reduction which is responsible. Cubitus varus is disfiguring and cubitus valgus may cause late ulnar palsy. If deformity is marked, it will need correction by supracondylar osteotomy usually once the child approaches skeletal maturity.

Elbow stiffness and myositis ossifficans Stiffness is an ever-present risk with elbow injuries. Extension in particular may take months to return. It must not be hurried. Passive movement (which includes carrying weights) or forced movement is prohibited – this will only make matters worse and may contribute to the development of myositis ossificans. As it is, myositis ossificans is extremely rare, and should remain so if rehabilitation is properly supervised.

Fractures of the lateral condyle

The lateral condylar (or capitellar) epiphysis begins to ossify during the first year of life and fuses with the shaft at 12–16 years. Between these ages it may be sheared off or avulsed by forceful traction.

Mechanism of injury and pathology

The child falls on the hand with the elbow extended and forced into varus. A large fragment, which includes the lateral condyle, breaks off and is pulled upon by the attached wrist extensors. Sometimes there is a compression, rather than avulsion, mechanism of injury. The fracture line usually runs along the physis and into the trochlea; less often it continues through the medial epiphysis and exits through the capitulatrochlear groove. It crosses the growth plate and so is a Salter Harris Type IV injury. In severe injuries the elbow may dislocate posterolaterally; the condyle is 'capsized' by muscle pull and remains capsized while the elbow reduces spontaneously.

The extent of this injury is often not appreciated. Because the condylar epiphysis is largely cartilaginous, the bone fragment may look deceptively small on

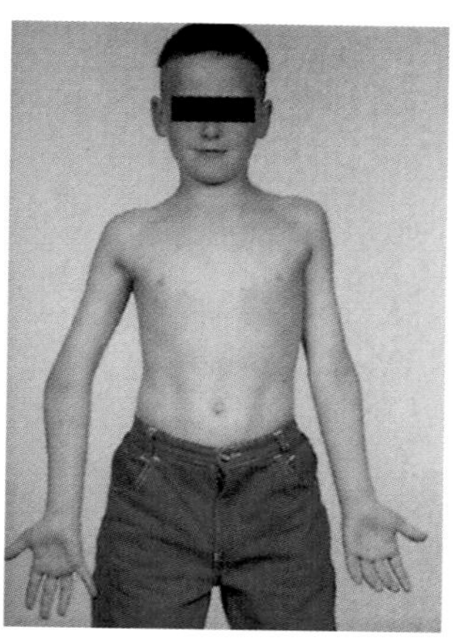
(a)

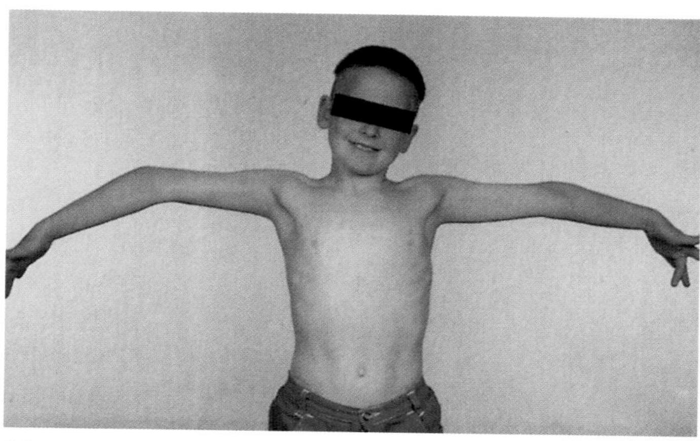
(b)

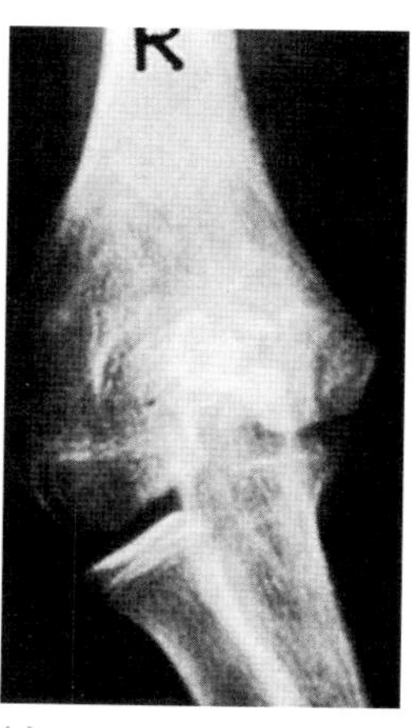

(c)

24.32 Supracondylar fracture – malunion (a) Varus deformity of the right elbow, due to incomplete correction of the varus and rotational displacements in a supracondylar fracture. (b) It is most obvious when the boy raises his arms, displaying the typical 'gunstock deformity'. (c) X-ray showing the characteristic malunion.

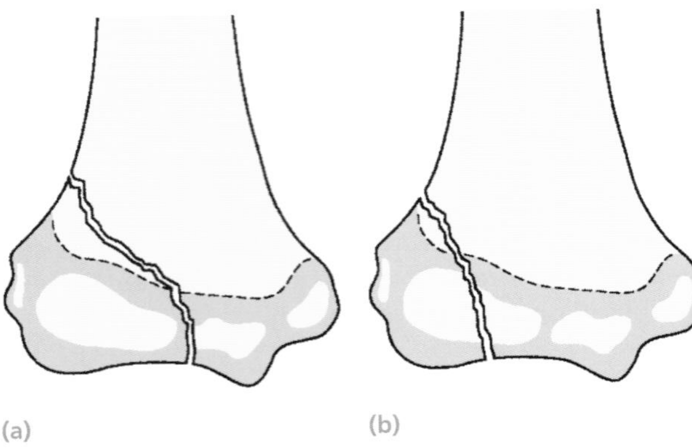

24.33 Physeal fractures of the lateral condoyle (a) The commonest is a fracture starting in the metaphysi and running along the physis of the lateral condyle into the trochlea (Salter–Harris Type II injury). (b) Less common is a fracture running right through the lateral condyle to reach the articular surface in the capitulotrochlear groove (Salter–Harris Type IV): though uncommon, this latter injury is important because of its potential for causing growth defects.

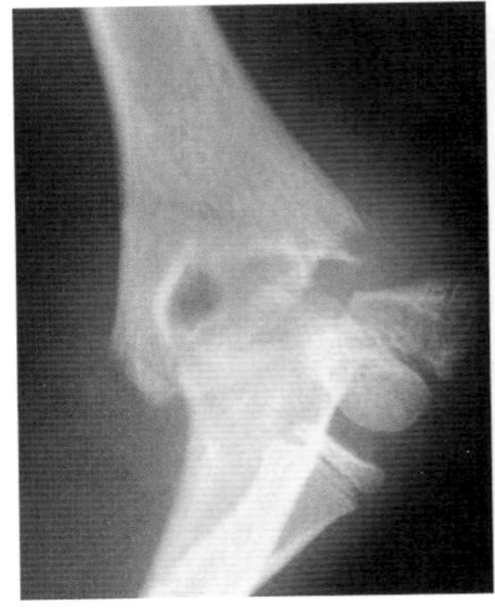

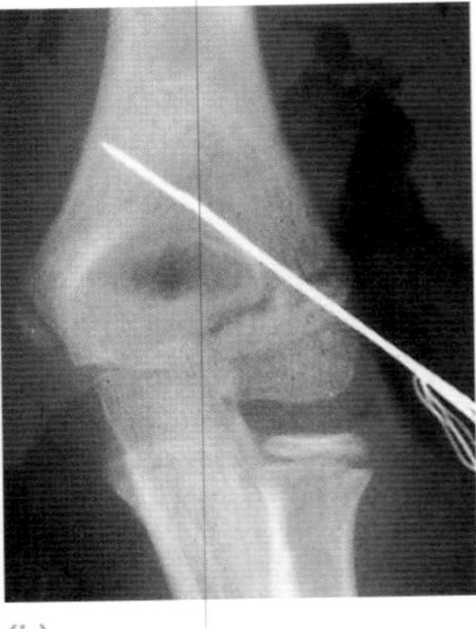

24.34 Fractured lateral condyle If displacement is more than 2 mm, open reduction and internal fixation is the treatment of choice.

x-ray. Displacement can be quite marked due to muscle pull. The fracture is important for two reasons: (a) it may damage the growth plate and (b) it always involves the joint. Early recognition and accurate reduction are therefore essential if a poor outcome is to be avoided.

Clinical features

The elbow is swollen and deformed. There is tenderness over the lateral condyle. Passive flexion of the wrist (pulling on the extensors) may be painful.

X-ray

X-ray examination must include oblique views or else the full extent of the fracture may be missed. Two types of fracture are recognized and classified by Milch:

Type I: A fracture lateral to the trochlea: the elbow joint is not involved and is stable.

Type II: A fracture through the middle of the trochlea: this injury is more common; the elbow is unstable as the radius and ulna are carried along with the fragment.. The fragment is often grossly displaced and capsized, and it may carry with it a triangular piece of the metaphysis. Remember that the fragment (partly cartilaginous) is much larger than it seems on x-ray.

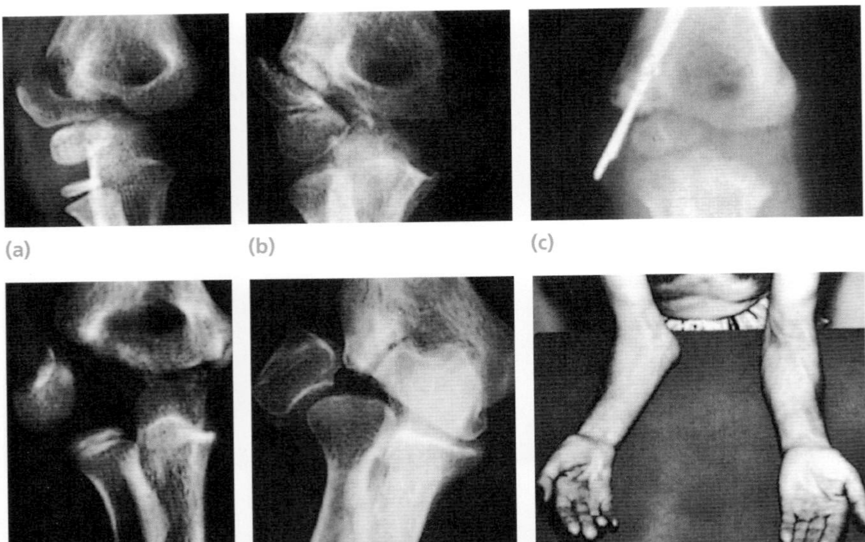

24.35 Fractured lateral condyle – complications (a,b) A large fragment of bone and cartilage is avulsed; even with reasonable reduction, union is not inevitable. (c) Open reduction with fixation is often wise. (d) Sometimes the condyle is capsized; if left unreduced non-union is inevitable (e) and a valgus elbow with delayed ulnar palsy (f) the likely sequel.

Treatment

If there is no displacement the arm can be splinted in a backslab with the elbow flexed 90 degrees, the forearm neutral and the wrist extended (this position relaxes the extensor mechanism which attaches to the fragment). However, it is essential to repeat the x-ray after 5 days to make sure that the fracture has not displaced. The splint is removed after 2 weeks and exercises are encouraged.

A displaced fracture requires accurate reduction and internal fixation. If the fragment is only moderately displaced (hinged), it may be possible to manipulate it into position by extending the elbow and pressing upon the condyle, and then fixing the fragment with percutaneous pins. If this fails, and for all separated fractures, open reduction and internal fixation with pins is required. The arm is immobilized in a cast; cast and pins are removed after 3 or 4 weeks.

Complications

Non-union and malunion If the condyle is left capsized, non-union is inevitable; with growth the elbow becomes increasingly valgus, and ulnar nerve palsy is then likely to develop. Stiffness and pain can result. Even minor displacements sometimes lead to non-union, and even slight malunion may lead to ulnar palsy in later life; it is for these reasons that open reduction (and internal fixation) is preferred for any displaced fracture. The fracture is a Salter Harris Type IV injury and so imperfect reduction can result in growth arrest. Even if a fracture presents late (e.g. up to 3 months) open reduction and fixation should be attempted.

Recurrent dislocation Occasionally condylar displacement results in posterolateral dislocation of the elbow. The only effective treatment is reconstruction of the bony and soft tissues on the lateral side.

Separation of the medial epicondyle

Mechanism of injury and pathology

The medial epicondyle begins to ossify at the age of about 5 years and fuses to the shaft at about 16; between these ages it may be avulsed by a severe muscle or ligament strain. The child falls on the outstretched hand with the wrist and elbow extended; the elbow is wrenched into valgus. The unfused epicondylar apophysis is avulsed by tension on either the wrist flexor muscles or the medial ligament of the elbow. If the elbow subluxates (even momentarily), the small apophyseal fragment may be dragged into the joint. With more severe injuries the joint dislocates laterally.

Clinical features

The diagnosis should be suspected if injury is followed by pain, swelling and bruising on the medial side of the elbow. If the joint is dislocated, deformity is of course obvious. Sensation and power in the fin-

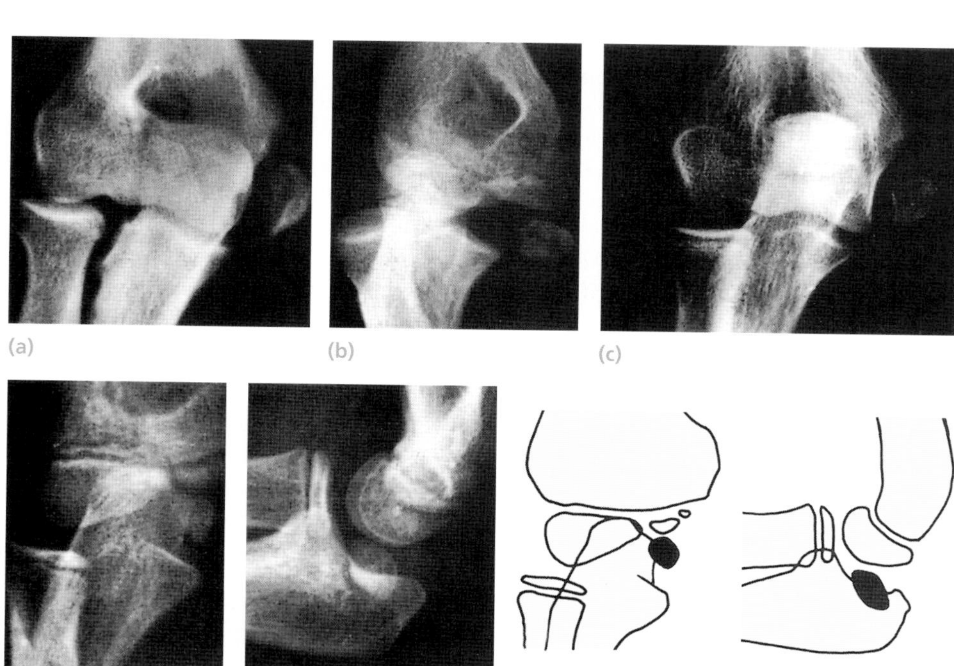

24.36 Fractured medial epicondyle (a) Avulsion of the medial epicondyle following valgus train. (b) Avulsion associated with dislocation of the elbow; (c) after reduction. Sometimes the epicondylar fragment is trapped in the joint (d,e); the serious nature is then liable to be missed unless the surgeon specifically looks for the trapped fragment, which is emphasized in the tracings (f,g).

gers should be tested to exclude concomitant ulnar nerve damage.

X-ray

In the anteroposterior view the medial epicondylar epiphysis may be tilted or shifted downwards; if the joint is dislocated the fragment lies distal to the lower humerus. A lateral view may show the epicondyle looking like a loose body in the joint. If in any doubt, the normal side should be x-rayed for comparison (see Fig. 24.36 d–g).

Treatment

Minor displacement may be disregarded. This is an extra-articular fracture, so the elbow can be mobilized as soon as the child wishes.

If the epicondyle is trapped in the joint it must be freed. Manipulation with the elbow in valgus and the wrist hyperextended (to pull on the flexor muscles) may be successful; if this fails, the joint must be opened (the ulnar nerve must be visualized and protected) and the fragment retrieved and fixed back in position.

Displaced fractures which are not trapped in the joint usually do not need to be operated upon: however, if there is valgus instability (because the medial collateral ligament complex is attached to the fragment) then reduction and pinning is recommended.

Complications

EARLY

Ulnar nerve damage is not uncommon. Mild symptoms recover spontaneously; even a complete palsy will usually recover but, if there is the possibility that the nerve is kinked in the joint, exploration should be considered.

LATE

Stiffness of the elbow is common and extension often limited for months; but, provided movement is not forced, it will eventually return.

Fractures of the medial condyle

This is much rarer than either a fracture of the lateral condyle or a separation of the medial epicondylar apophysis.

Mechanism of injury

The injury is usually caused by a fall from a height, involving either a direct blow to the point of the elbow or a landing on the outstretched hand with the elbow forced into valgus; in the latter case it would be an avulsion injury. The fracture line runs through the physis, exiting in the trochlear notch or even further laterally, and the medial fragment may be displaced by the pull of the flexor muscle group.

Clinical features and x-ray

This is an intra-articular fracture, resulting in considerable pain and swelling. In older children the metaphyseal component is usually easily visualized on x-ray. However, in young children much of the medial condylar epiphysis is cartilaginous and therefore not visible on x-ray, so the full extent of the fracture may not be recognized; seeing only the epicondylar ossific centre in a displaced position on the x-ray may mislead the surgeon into thinking that this is only an epicondylar fracture. In doubtful cases an arthrogram may be helpful.

Treatment

Undisplaced fractures are treated by splintage; x-rays are repeated until the fracture has healed, so as to ensure that it does not become displaced.

Displaced fractures are treated by either closed reduction (sometimes with percutaneous pinning) or by open reduction and fixation with pins.

Postoperative management is similar to that of lateral condyle fractures.

Complications

EARLY

Lateral dislocation of the elbow occasionally occurs with a severe valgus strain and avulsion of the medial condyle. Early reduction of both the dislocation and the fracture, if necessary by open operation and pinning, is important.

Ulnar nerve damage is not uncommon, but recovery is usual unless the nerve is left kinked in the joint.

LATE

Stiffness of the elbow is common and extension often limited for months; but, provided movement is not forced, it will eventually return.

FRACTURE-SEPARATION OF THE DISTAL HUMERAL PHYSIS

Up to the age of 7 years the distal humeral epiphysis is a solid cartilaginous segment with maturing centres of ossification. With severe injury it may separate *en bloc*. This is likely to occur with fairly severe violence; for example, in birth injuries or child abuse.

Clinical features

The child is in pain and the elbow is markedly swollen. The history may be deceptively uninformative.

X-ray

In a very young child, in whom the bony outlines are still unformed, the x-ray may look normal. All that can be seen of the epiphysis is the pea-like ossification centre of the capitulum; its position should be compared with that of the normal side. Medial displacement of either the capitellar ossification centre or the proximal radius and ulna is very suspicious. In the older child the deformity is usually obvious.

Treatment

If the diagnosis is uncertain, arthrography or ultrasound can help. If the fracture is undisplaced, the elbow is merely splinted for 3 weeks; if displaced then the fracture should be accurately reduced and held with smooth percutaneous wires (otherwise there is a high incidence of cubitus varus). The wires are removed at 3 weeks.

Fractured neck of radius

Mechanism of injury and pathology

A fall on the outstretched hand forces the elbow into valgus and pushes the radial head against the capitulum. In children the bone fractures through the neck of the radius; in adults the injury is more likely to fracture the radial head.

Clinical features

Following a fall, the child complains of pain in the elbow. There may be localized tenderness over the radial head and pain on rotating the forearm.

X-ray

The fracture line is transverse. It is either situated immediately distal to the physis or there is true separation of the epiphysis with a triangular fragment of shaft (a Salter-Harris II injury). The proximal fragment is tilted distally, forwards and outwards. Sometimes the upper end of the ulna is also fractured or there may be a posterior dislocation of the elbow.

Treatment

In children there is considerable potential for remodelling after these fractures. Up to 30 degrees of radial head tilt and up to 3 mm of transverse displacement are acceptable. The arm is rested in a collar and cuff, and exercises are commenced after a week.

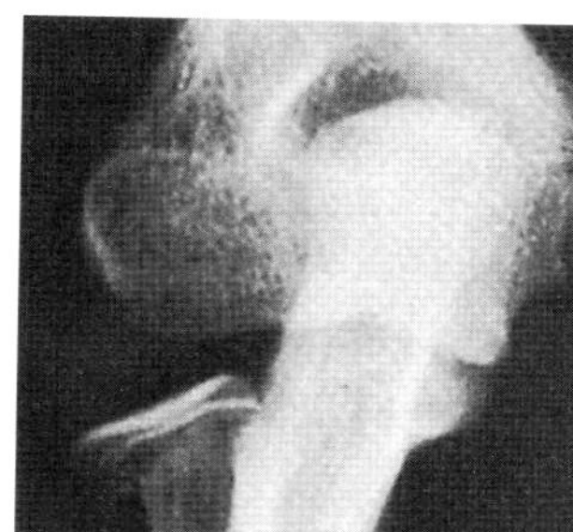

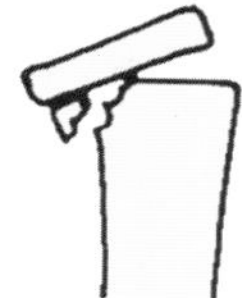

24.37 Fractured neck of radius in a child Up to 30° of tilt is acceptable. Greater degrees of angulation should be reduced; never excise the radial head in a child.

Displacement of more than 30 degrees requires reduction. With the patient's elbow extended, traction and varus force are applied; the surgeon then pushes the displaced radial fragment into position with his thumb. If this fails, a percutaneous implement can be used to push the fragment back into place. Open reduction is occasionally performed if significant displacement persists. The radial head tilt is corrected but internal fixation is unnecessarily meddlesome. The head of the radius must never be excised in children because this will interfere with the synchronous growth of radius and ulna.

Fractures that are seen a week or longer after injury should be left untreated (except for light splintage).

Following operation, the elbow is splinted in 90 degrees of flexion for a week or two and then movements are encouraged.

Subluxation of the radial head ('pulled elbow')

In young children the elbow may be injured by pulling on the arm, usually with the forearm pronated. It is sometimes called subluxation of the radial head; more accurately, it is a subluxation of the orbicular ligament which slips up over the head of the radius into the radiocapitellar joint.

A child aged 2 or 3 years is brought with a painful, dangling arm: there is usually a history of the child being jerked by the arm and crying out in pain. The forearm is held in pronation and extension, and any attempt to supinate it is resisted. There are no x-ray changes.

A dramatic cure is achieved by forcefully supinating and then flexing the elbow; the ligament slips back with a snap.

Fracture of the olecranon in children

This is rare. When it does occur it is usually due to a direct blow onto the tip of the flexed elbow or a fall onto the outstretched hand. Most are undisplaced and are treated in a splint for 3 or 4 weeks. If displaced, then they should be reduced and held with wires.

REFERENCES AND FURTHER READING

Boileau P, Sinnerton RJ, Chuinard C, Walch G. Arthroplasty of the shoulder. *J Bone Joint* Surg 2006; **88B:** 562–75.

Goss TP. Fractures of the glenoid cavity. *J Bone Joint Surg* 1992; **74A:** 299–305.

Hertel R, Hempfing A, Stiehler M, Leunig M. Predictors of humeral head ischemia after intracapsular fracture of the proximal humerus. *J Shoulder Elbow Surg*, 2004; **13:** 427–33.

Jupiter JB. Complex fractures of the distal part of the humerus *J Bone Joint Surg* 1994; **76A:** 1252–63.

McKee MD, Pedersen EM, Jones C. Deficits following nonoperative treatment of displaced midshaft clavicular fractures. *J Bone Joint Surg* 2006; **88A:** 35–40.

Modabber MR, Jupiter JB. Reconstruction for post-traumatic conditions of the elbow joint. *J Bone Joint Surg* 1995; **77A:** 1431–46.

Morrey BF. Current concepts in the treatment of fractures of the radial head, the olecranon and coronoid. *J Bone Joint Surg* 1995; **77A:** 316–27.

Neer CS II. Displaced proximal humeral fractures. Classification and evaluation. *J Bone Joint Surg* 1970; **52A:** 1077–89.

O'Hara LJ, Barlow JW, Clarke NMP. Displaced supracondylar fractures of the humerus in children. *J Bone Joint Surg* 2000; **82B:** 204–210.

Ring D, Jupiter JB. Fracture-dislocation of the elbow. *J Bone Joint Surg* 1998; **80A:** 566–80.

Robinson CM. Fractures of the clavicle in the adult. Epidemiology and classification. *J Bone Joint Surg* 1998; **80B:** 476–84.

Rockwood CA Jr, Green DP, Bucholz RW, Heckman JD (eds). Rockwood and Green's Fractures in Adults, 4th Edition. 1996 Lippincott-Raven, Philadelphia.

Snow M, Funk L. Technique of arthroscopic Weaver–Dunn in chronic acromioclavicular joint dislocation. *Techniques in Shoulder and Elbow Surgery* 2006; **7:** 155–9.

Williams GR, Naranja J, Klimkiewcz J *et al.* The floating shoulder: a biomechanical basis for classification and management. *J Bone Joint Surg* 2001; **83A:** 1182–7.

Injuries of the forearm and wrist 25

David Warwick

FRACTURES OF THE RADIUS AND ULNA

Mechanism of injury and pathology

Fractures of the shafts of both forearm bones occur quite commonly. A twisting force (usually a fall on the hand) produces a spiral fracture with the bones broken at different levels. An angulating force causes a transverse fracture of both bones at the same level. A direct blow causes a transverse fracture of just one bone, usually the ulna. Additional rotation deformity may be produced by the pull of muscles attached to the radius: they are the biceps and supinator muscles to the upper third, the pronator teres to the middle third, and the pronator quadratus to the lower third. Bleeding and swelling of the muscle compartments of the forearm may cause circulatory impairment.

Clinical features

The fracture is usually quite obvious, but the pulse must be felt and the hand examined for circulatory or neural deficit. Repeated examination is necessary in order to detect an impending compartment syndrome.

X-RAY

Both bones are broken, either transversely and at the same level or obliquely with the radial fracture usually at a higher level. In children, the fracture is often incomplete (greenstick) and only angulated. In adults, displacement may occur in any direction – shift, overlap, tilt or twist. In low-energy injuries, the fracture tends to be transverse or oblique; in high-energy injuries it is comminuted or segmental.

Treatment

CHILDREN

In children, closed treatment is usually successful because the tough periosteum tends to guide and then control the reduction. The fragments are held in a well-moulded full-length cast, from axilla to metacarpal shafts (to control rotation). The cast is applied with the elbow at 90 degrees. If the fracture is proximal to pronator teres, the forearm is supinated; if it is distal to pronator teres, then the forearm is held

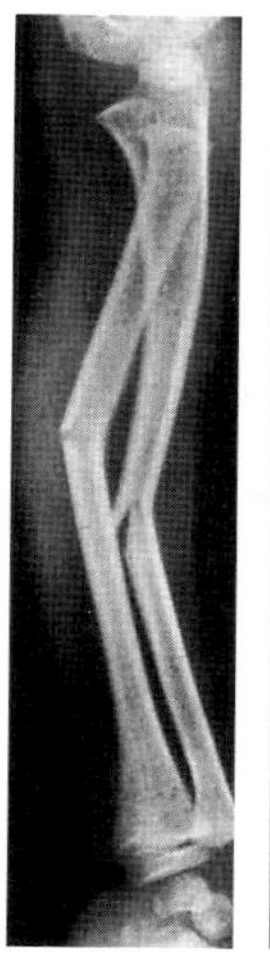
(a)

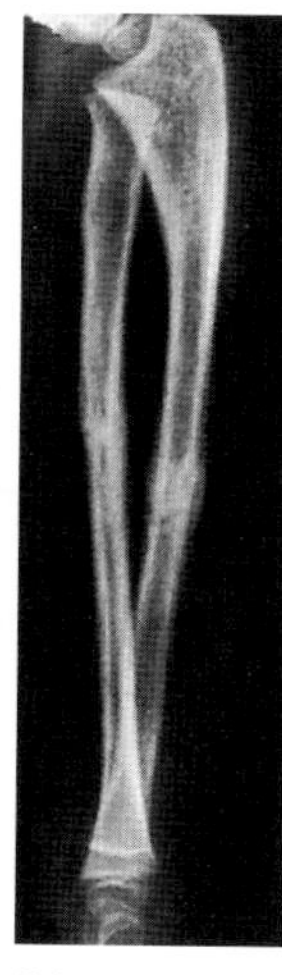
(b)

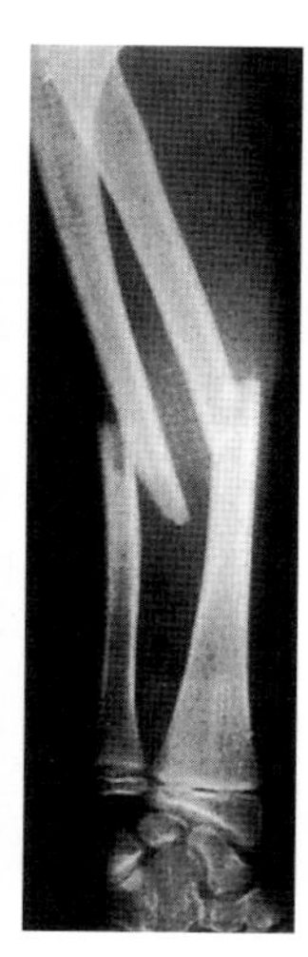
(c)

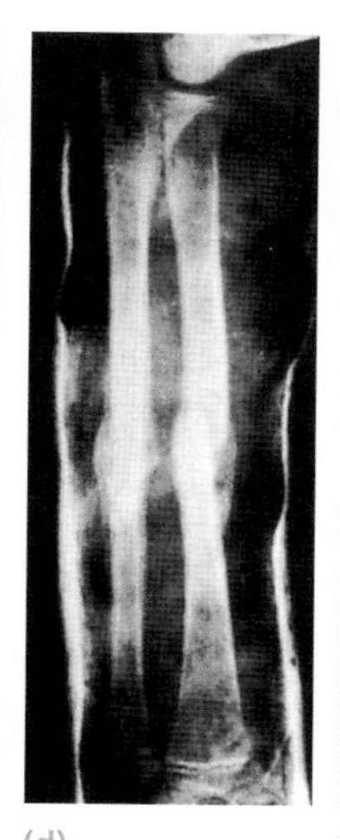
(d)

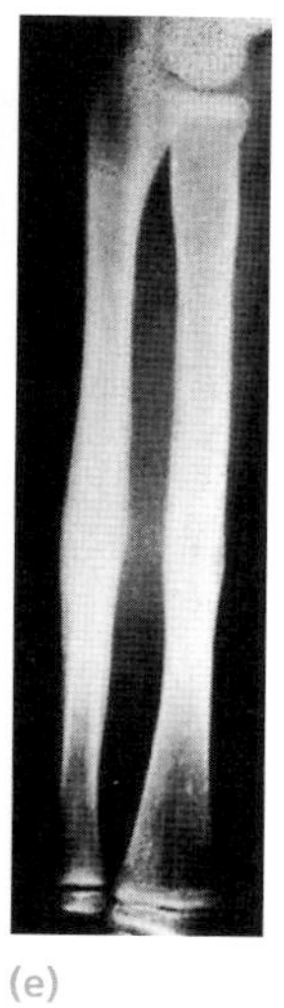
(e)

25.1 Fractured radius and ulna in children Greenstick fractures (a) need only correction of angulation (b), and plaster splintage. Complete fractures (c) are harder to reduce; but provided alignment is corrected and held in plaster (d), slight lateral shift remodels with growth (e).

in neutral. The position is checked by x-ray after a week and, if it is satisfactory, splintage is retained until both fractures are united (usually 6–8 weeks). Throughout this period hand and shoulder exercises are encouraged. The child should avoid contact sports for a few weeks to prevent re-fracture.

Occasionally an operation is required, either if the fracture cannot be reduced or if the fragments are unstable. Fixation with intramedullary rods is preferred, but they should be inserted with great care to avoid injury to the growth plates. Alternatively, a plate or K-wire fixation can be used.

Childhood fractures usually remodel well, but not if there is any rotational deformity or an angular deformity of more than 15 degrees in children under 6 years or 10 degrees in children between 6 and 12. In those over 12 years old even slight angular deformities are unlikely to remodel satisfactorily.

ADULTS

Unless the fragments are in close apposition, reduction is difficult and re-displacement in the cast almost invariable. So predictable is this outcome that most surgeons opt for open reduction and internal fixation from the outset. The fragments are held by interfragmentary compression with plates and screws. Bone grafting is advisable if there is comminution. The deep fascia is left open to prevent a build-up of pressure in the muscle compartments, and only the skin is sutured.

After the operation the arm is kept elevated until the swelling subsides, and during this period active exercises of the hand are encouraged. If the fracture is not comminuted and the patient is reliable, early range of movement exercises are commenced but lifting and sports are avoided. It takes 8–12 weeks for the bones to unite. With comminuted fractures or unreliable patients, immobilization in plaster is safer.

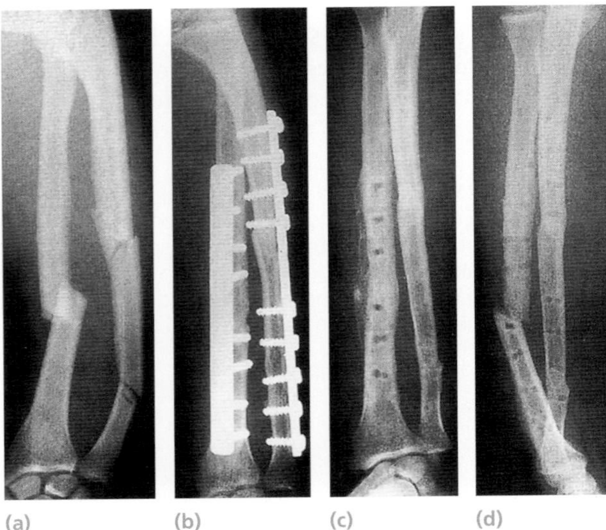

(a) (b) (c) (d)

25.2 Fractured radius and ulna in adults (a, b) These fractures are usually treated by internal fixation with sturdy plates and screws. However, removal of the implants is not without risk. **(c,d)** In this case, the radius fractured through one of the screw holes.

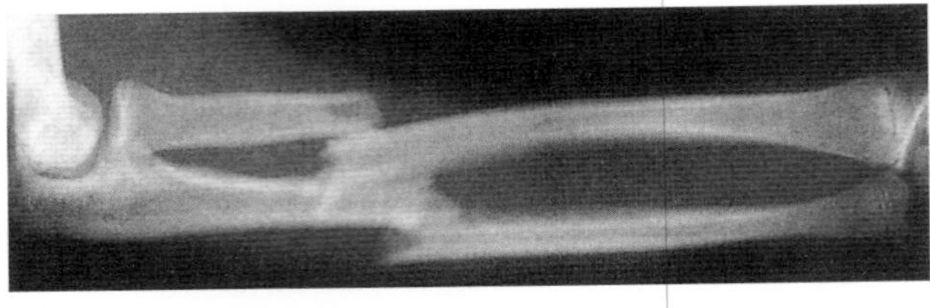

(a)

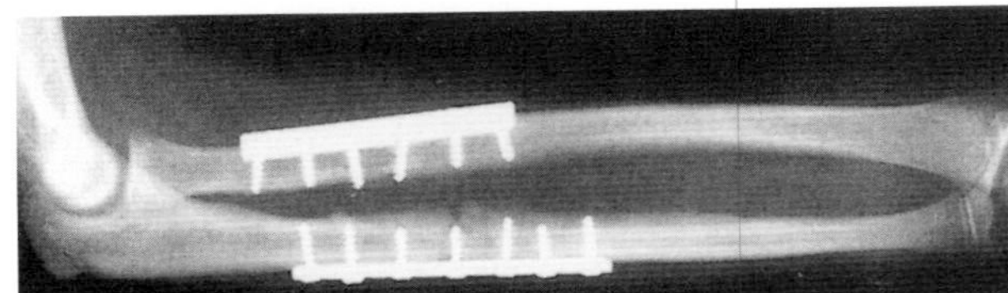

(b)

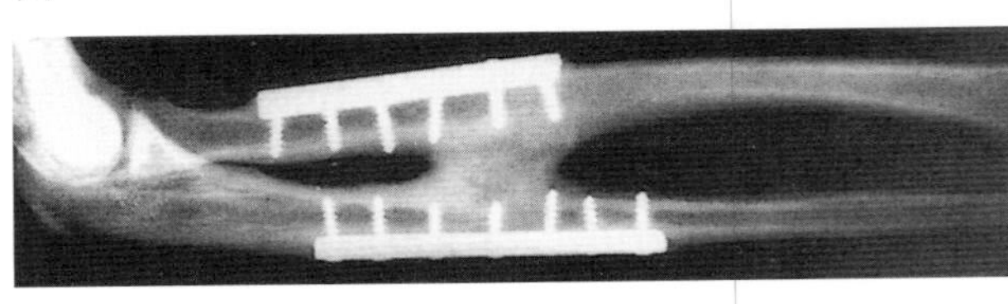

(c)

25.3 Fractured radius and ulna – cross-union If the interosseous membrane is severely damaged, even successful plating **(a,b)** cannot guarantee that cross-union will not occur **(c)**.

OPEN FRACTURES

Open fractures of the forearm must be managed meticulously. Antibiotics and tetanus prophylaxis are given as soon as possible; the wounds are copiously washed and nerve function and circulation are checked. At operation the wounds are excised and extended and the bone ends are exposed and thoroughly cleaned. The fractures are primarily fixed with compression screws and plates; if the wounds are absolutely clean, the soft tissues can be closed. If bone grafting is necessary, this is best deferred until the wounds are healed. If there is major soft-tissue loss, the bones are better stabilized by external fixation. The aim is to obtain skin cover as soon as possible; if plastic surgery services are available, these should be enlisted from the outset.

If there is any question of a compartment syndrome, the wounds should be left open and closed 24–48 hours later, with a skin graft if needed.

Complications

EARLY

Nerve injury Nerve injuries are rarely caused by the fracture, but they may be caused by the surgeon!

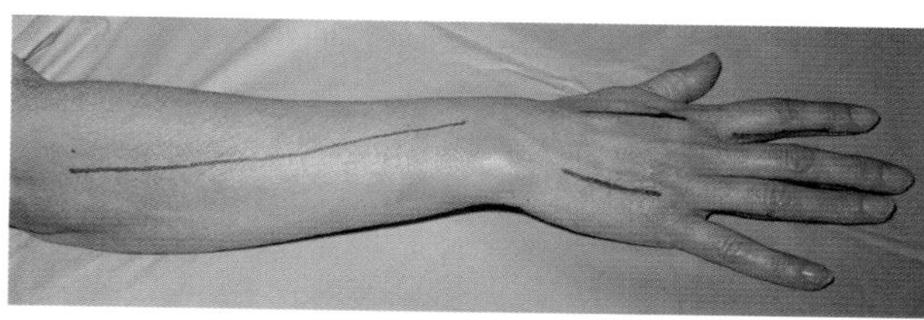

(a)

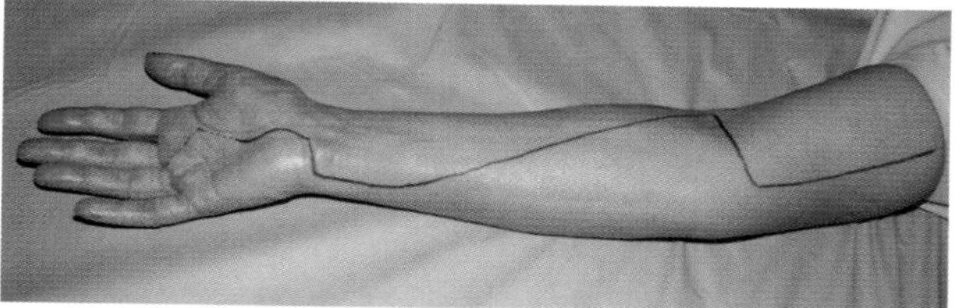

(b)

25.4 Compartment syndrome Incisions to relieve a compartment syndrome in the forearm.

Exposure of the radius in its proximal third risks damage to the posterior interosseous nerve where it is covered by the superficial part of the supinator muscle. The proximal fragment of radius may have rotated so the nerve may not be where it is expected. Surgical technique is particularly important here; the anterior Henry approach is safest.

Vascular injury Injury to the radial or ulnar artery seldom presents any problem, as the collateral circulation is excellent.

Compartment syndrome Fractures (and operations) of the forearm bones are always associated with swelling of the soft tissues, with the attendant risk of a compartment syndrome. The threat is even greater, and the diagnosis more difficult, if the forearm is wrapped up in plaster. A distal pulse does not exclude compartment syndrome! The byword is 'watchfulness'; if there are any signs of circulatory embarrassment, treatment must be prompt and uncompromising.

LATE

Delayed union and non-union Most fractures of the radius and ulna heal within 8–12 weeks; high energy fractures and open fractures are less likely to unite. Delayed union of one or other bone (usually the ulna) is not uncommon; immobilization may have to be continued beyond the usual time. Non-union will require bone grafting and internal fixation.

Malunion With closed reduction there is always a risk of malunion, resulting in angulation or rotational deformity of the forearm, cross-union of the fragments, or shortening of one of the bones and disruption of the distal radio-ulnar joint. If pronation or supination is severely restricted, and there is no cross-union, mobility may be improved by corrective osteotomy. However, it can be very difficult to calculate the deformity and subsequent correction.

Complications of plate removal Removal of plates and screws is often regarded as a fairly innocuous procedure. Beware! Complications are common and they include damage to vessels and nerves, infection and fracture through a screw-hole.

FRACTURE OF A SINGLE FOREARM BONE

Fracture of the radius alone is very rare and fracture of the ulna alone is uncommon. These injuries are usually caused by a direct blow – the 'nightstick fracture'. They are important for two reasons:

- An associated dislocation may be undiagnosed; if only one forearm bone is broken along its shaft and there is displacement, then either the proximal or the distal radio-ulnar joint must be dislocated. The entire forearm, elbow and wrist should always be x-rayed.
- Non-union is liable to occur unless it is realized that one bone takes just as long to consolidate as two.

Clinical features

Ulnar fractures are easily missed – even on x-ray. If there is local tenderness, a further x-ray a week or two later is wise.

X-ray The fracture may be anywhere in the radius or ulna. The fracture line is transverse and displacement is slight. In children, the intact bone sometimes bends without actually breaking ('plastic deformation').

Treatment

Isolated fracture of the ulna The fracture is rarely displaced; a forearm brace leaving the elbow free can be sufficient. However, it takes about 8 weeks before full activity can be resumed. Rigid internal fixation will allow earlier activity and avoids the risk of displacement or non-union.

Isolated fracture of the radius Radius fractures are prone to rotary displacement; to achieve reduction in children the forearm needs to be supinated for upper third fractures, neutral for middle third fractures and pronated for lower third fractures. The position is sometimes difficult to hold in children and just about impossible in adults; if so, then internal fixation with a compression plate and screws in adults, and preferably intramedullary rods in children, is better.

Middle/distal third fractures of the radius in children These are particularly unstable, being deformed by the pull of the thumb abductors and pronator quadratus. They

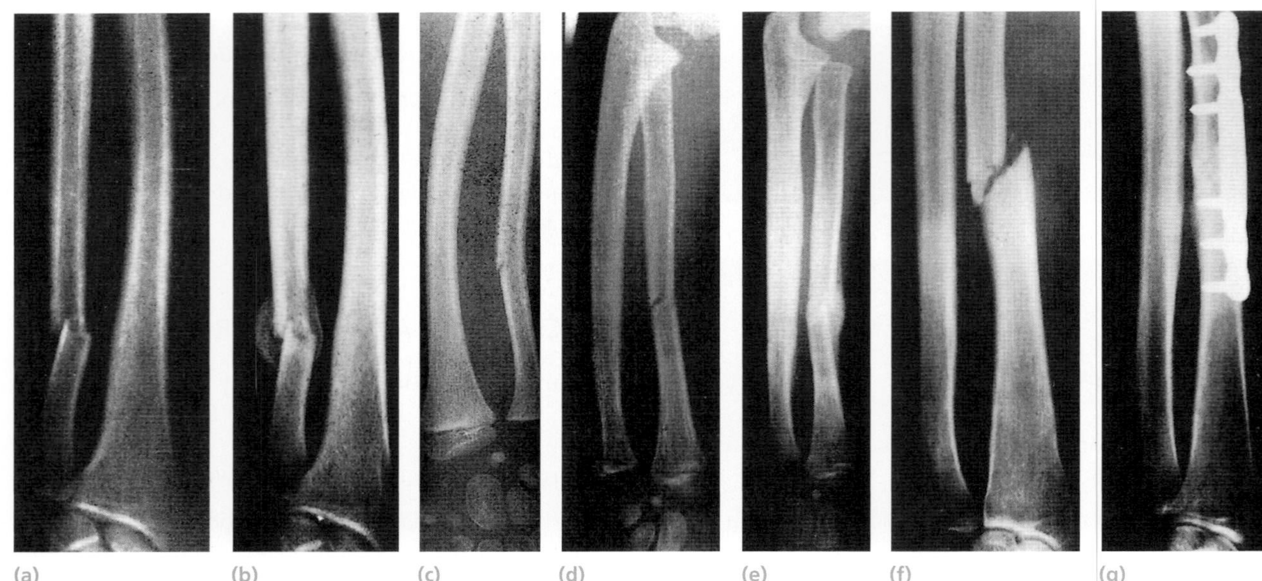

25.5 Fracture of one forearm bone *Fracture of the ulna*: A fracture of the ulna alone (a) usually joins satisfactorily (b); in children the intact radius may be bowed (c). *Fracture of the radius*: In a child, fracture of the radius alone (d) may join in plaster (e), but in adults a fractured radius (f) is better treated by plating (g).

can be treated with an above-elbow cast in supination but, failing that, fixation with an intramedullary rod, Kirschner (K-) wires or a plate is advisable.

MONTEGGIA FRACTURE-DISLOCATION OF THE ULNA

The injury described by Monteggia in the early nineteenthth century (without benefit of x-rays!) was a fracture of the shaft of the ulna associated with dislocation of the proximal radio-ulnar joint; the radio-capitellar joint is inevitably dislocated or subluxated as well. More recently the definition has been extended to embrace almost any fracture of the ulna associated with dislocation of the radio-capitellar joint, including trans-olecranon fractures in which the proximal radio-ulnar joint remains intact. If the ulnar shaft fracture is angulated with the apex anterior (the commonest type) then the radial head is displaced anteriorly; if the fracture apex is posterior, the radial dislocation is posterior; and if the fracture apex is lateral then the radial head will be laterally displaced. In children, the ulnar injury may be an incomplete fracture (greenstick or plastic deformation of the shaft).

Mechanism of injury

Usually the cause is a fall on the hand; if at the moment of impact the body is twisting, its momentum may forcibly pronate the forearm. The radial head usually dislocates forwards and the upper third of the ulna fractures and bows forwards. Sometimes the causal force is hyperextension.

Clinical features

The ulnar deformity is usually obvious but the dislocated head of radius is masked by swelling. A useful clue is pain and tenderness on the lateral side of the elbow. The wrist and hand should be examined for signs of injury to the radial nerve.

X-ray With isolated fractures of the ulna, it is essential to obtain a true anteroposterior and true lateral view of the elbow. In the usual case, the head of the radius (which normally points directly to the capitulum) is dislocated forwards, and there is a fracture of the upper third of the ulna with forward bowing. Backward or lateral bowing of the ulna (which is much less common) is likely to be associated with, respectively, posterior or lateral displacement of the radial head. Trans-olecranon fractures, also, are often associated with radial head dislocation.

Treatment

The key to successful treatment is to restore the length of the fractured ulna; only then can the dislocated joint be fully reduced and remain stable. In adults, this means an operation through a posterior approach. The ulnar fracture must be accurately reduced, with the bone restored to full length, and then fixed with a plate and screws; bone grafts may be added for safety.

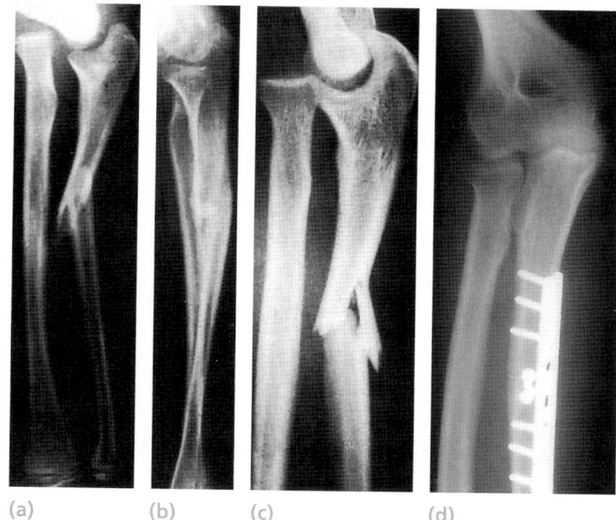

25.6 Monteggia fracture-dislocation (a) The ulna is fractured and the head of the radius no longer points to the capitulum. In a child, closed reduction and plaster (b) is usually satisfactory; in the adult (c) open reduction and plating (d) is preferred.

The radial head usually reduces once the ulna has been fixed. Stability must be tested through a full range of flexion and extension. If the radial head does not reduce, or is not stable, open reduction should be performed.

If the elbow is completely stable, then flexion–extension and rotation can be started after very soon after surgery. If there is doubt, then the arm should be immobilized in plaster with the elbow flexed for 6 weeks.

Complications

Nerve injury Nerve injuries can be caused by over-enthusiastic manipulation of the radial dislocation or during the surgical exposure. Always check for nerve function after treatment. The lesion is usually a neurapraxia, which will recover by itself.

Malunion Unless the ulna has been perfectly reduced, the radial head remains dislocated and limits elbow flexion. In children, no treatment is advised. In adults, osteotomy of the ulna or perhaps excision of the radial head may be needed.

Non-union Non-union of the ulna should be treated by plating and bone grafting.

Special features in children

The general features of Monteggia fracture-dislocations are similar to those in adults. However, it is important to remember that the ulnar fracture may be incomplete (greenstick or plastic deformation); if this is not detected, and corrected, the child may end up with chronic subluxation of the radial head. Because of incomplete ossification of the radial head and capitellar epiphysis in children, these landmarks may not be easily defined on x-ray and a proximal dislocation could be missed. The x-rays should be studied very carefully and if there is any doubt, x-rays should be taken of the other side for comparison.

Incomplete ulnar fractures can often be reduced closed, although considerable force is needed to straighten the ulna with plastic deformation. The position of the radial head is then checked; if it is not perfect, closed reduction can be completed by flexing and supinating the elbow and pressing on the radial head. The arm is then immobilized in a cast with the elbow in flexion and supination, for 3 weeks.

Complete fractures are best treated by open reduction and fixation using an intramedullary rod or a small plate.

GALEAZZI FRACTURE-DISLOCATION OF THE RADIUS

Mechanism of injury

This injury was first described in 1934 by Galeazzi. The usual cause is a fall on the hand; probably with a superimposed rotation force. The radius fractures in its lower third and the inferior radio-ulnar joint subluxates or dislocates.

Clinical features

The Galeazzi fracture is much more common than the Monteggia. Prominence or tenderness over the lower end of the ulna is the striking feature. It may be possible to demonstrate the instability of the radio-ulnar joint by 'ballotting' the distal end of the ulna (the 'piano-key sign') or by rotating the wrist. It is important also to test for an ulnar nerve lesion, which may occur.

X-ray A transverse or short oblique fracture is seen in the lower third of the radius, with angulation or overlap. The distal radio-ulnar joint is subluxated or dislocated.

Treatment

As with the Monteggia fracture, the important step is to restore the length of the fractured bone. In children, closed reduction is often successful; in adults, reduction is best achieved by open operation and compression plating of the radius. An x-ray is taken to ensure that the distal radio-ulnar joint is reduced. There are three possibilities:

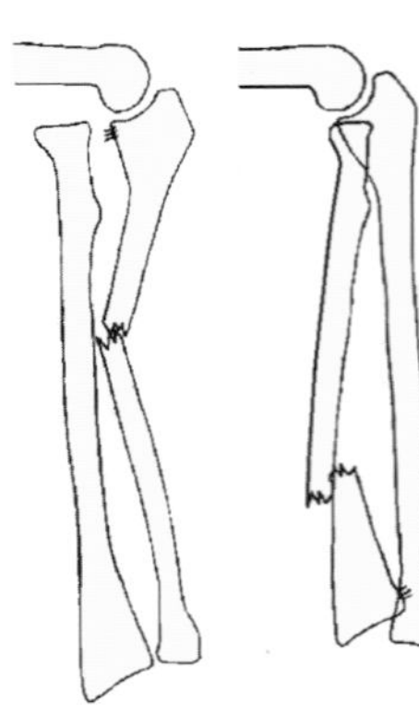

(a) (b)

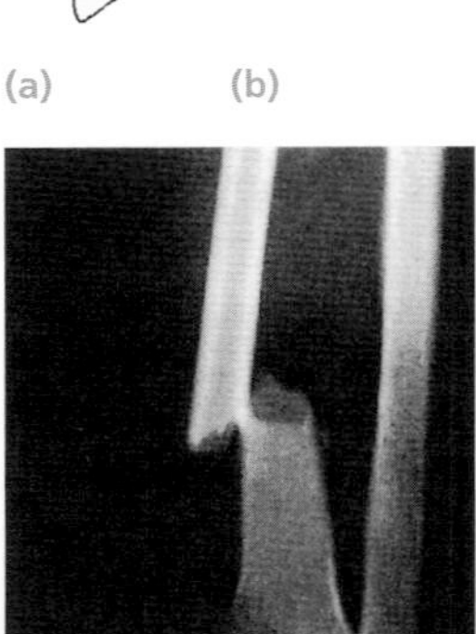

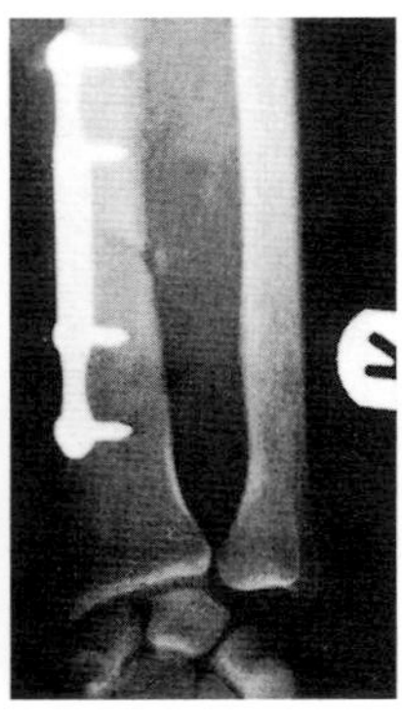

(c) (d)

25.7 Galeazzi fracture-dislocation The diagrams show the contrast between (a) Monteggia and (b) Galeazzi fracture-dislocations. (c,d) Galeazzi type before and after reduction and plating.

The distal radio-ulnar joint is reduced and stable No further action is needed. The arm is rested for a few days, then gentle active movements are encouraged. The radio-ulnar joint should be checked, both clinically and radiologically, during the next 6 weeks.

The distal radio-ulnar joint is reduced but unstable The forearm should be immobilized in the position of stability (usually supination), supplemented if required by a transverse K-wire. The forearm is splinted in an above-elbow cast for 6 weeks. If there is a large ulnar styloid fragment, it should be reduced and fixed.

The distal radio-ulnar joint is irreducible This is unusual. Open reduction is needed to remove the interposed soft tissues. The triangular fibrocartilage complex (TFCC) and dorsal capsule are then carefully repaired and the forearm immobilized in the position of stability (again, usually supination, supported by a wire if needed) for 6 weeks.

FRACTURES OF THE DISTAL RADIUS IN ADULTS

The distal end of the radius is subject to many different types of fracture, depending on factors such as age, transfer of energy, mechanism of injury and bone quality.

With any of these fractures, the wrist also can suffer substantial ligamentous injury causing instability to the carpus or distal radio-ulnar joint. These injuries are easily missed because the x-rays may look normal.

COLLES' FRACTURE

The injury that Abraham Colles described in 1814 is a transverse fracture of the radius just above the wrist, with dorsal displacement of the distal fragment. It is the most common of all fractures in older people, the high incidence being related to the onset of post-menopausal osteoporosis. Thus the patient is usually an older woman who gives a history of falling on her outstretched hand.

Mechanism of injury and pathological anatomy

Force is applied in the length of the forearm with the wrist in extension. The bone fractures at the cortico-cancellous junction and the distal fragment collapses into extension, dorsal displacement, radial tilt and shortening.

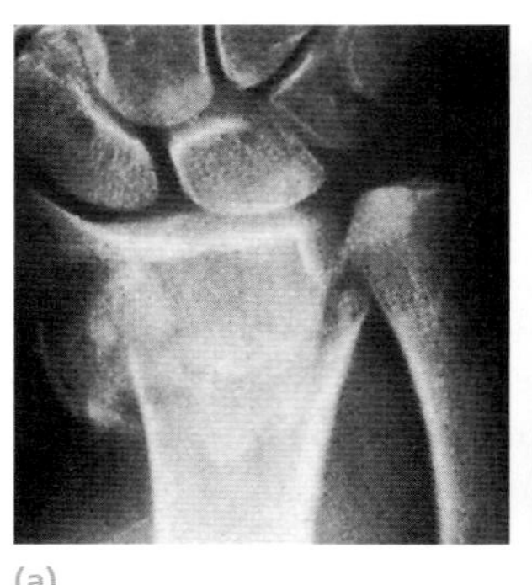

(a)

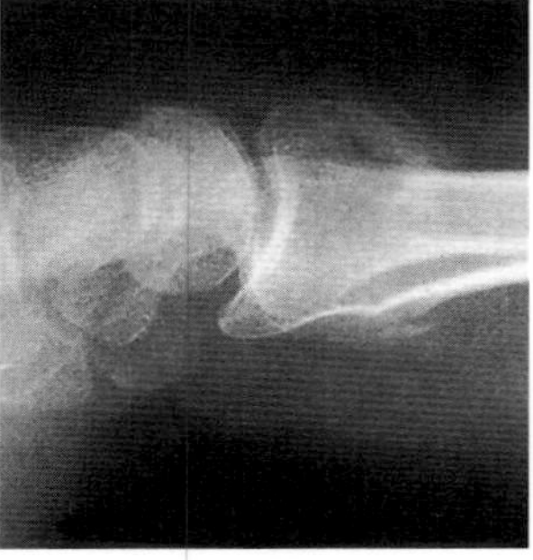

(b)

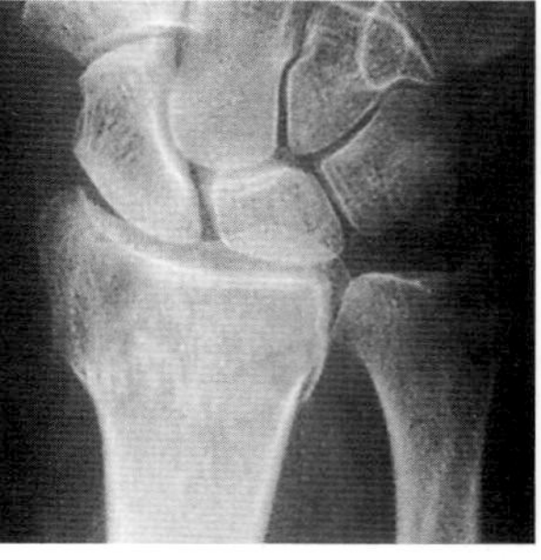

(c)

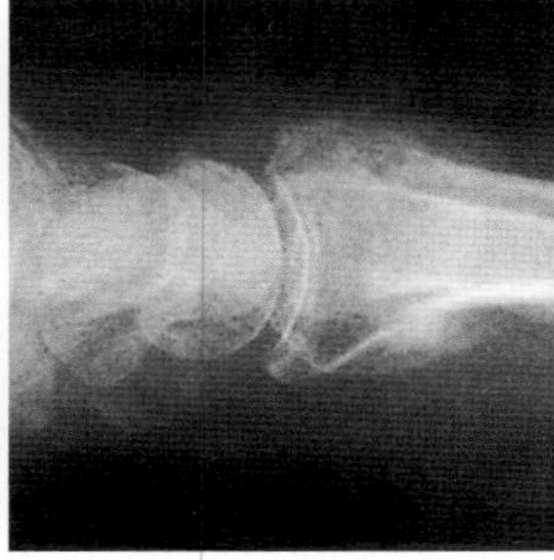

(d)

25.8 Colles' fracture (a,b) The typical Colles' fracture is both displaced and angulated towards the dorsum and towards the radial side of the wrist. (c,d) Note, how, after successful reduction, the radial articular surface faces correctly both distally and slightly volarwards.

Clinical features

We can recognize this fracture (as Colles did long before radiography was invented) by the 'dinner-fork' deformity, with prominence on the back of the wrist and a depression in front. In patients with less deformity there may only be local tenderness and pain on wrist movements.

X-ray There is a transverse fracture of the radius at the corticocancellous junction, and often the ulnar styloid process is broken off. The radial fragment is impacted into radial and backward tilt. Sometimes there is an intra-articular fracture; sometimes it is severely comminuted.

Treatment

UNDISPLACED FRACTURES

If the fracture is undisplaced (or only very slightly displaced), a dorsal splint is applied for a day or two until the swelling has resolved, then the cast is completed. An x-ray is taken at 10–14 days to ensure that the fracture has not slipped; if it has, surgery may be required; if not, the cast can usually be removed after four weeks to allow mobilization.

DISPLACED FRACTURES

Displaced fractures must be reduced under anaesthesia (haematoma block, Bier's block or axillary block). The hand is grasped and traction is applied in the length of the bone (sometimes with extension of the wrist to disimpact the fragments); the distal fragment is then pushed into place by pressing on the dorsum while manipulating the wrist into flexion, ulnar deviation and pronation. The position is then checked by x-ray. If it is satisfactory, a dorsal plaster slab is applied, extending from just below the elbow to the metacarpal necks and two-thirds of the way round the circumference of the wrist. It is held in position by a crepe bandage. *Extreme positions of flexion and ulnar deviation must be avoided*; 20 degrees in each direction is adequate.

The arm is kept elevated for the next day or two; shoulder and finger exercises are started as soon as possible. If the fingers become swollen, cyanosed or painful, there should be no hesitation in splitting the bandage.

At 7–10 days fresh x-rays are taken; re-displacement is not uncommon and should be treated, if the patient's functional demands are high, by re-manipulation and internal fixation. However, in some elderly patients with low functional demands, modest degrees of displacement should be accepted because (a) outcome in these patients is not so dependent upon anatomical perfection, and (b) fixation of the fragile bone can be very difficult.

The fracture unites in about 6 weeks and, even in the absence of radiological proof of union, the slab may safely be discarded and exercises begun.

IMPACTED OR COMMINUTED COLLES' FRACTURES

With substantial impaction or comminution in osteoporotic bone, manipulation and plaster immobilization alone may be insufficient. The fracture can sometimes be reduced and held with percutaneous wires, but if impaction is severe even this may not be enough to maintain length; in that case, an external fixator is used to neutralize the compressive force of the 25 tendons crossing the wrist, and bone graft or bone substitute is placed into the gap. The fixator is attached to the distal radius and the second metacarpal shaft. *It should be used only as a neutralizing device; too much distraction will lead to stiffness.* The fixation is removed after 5–6 weeks and exercises begun.

Plate fixation is increasingly being used for some Colles' fractures. The so-called 'volar locking plate' is

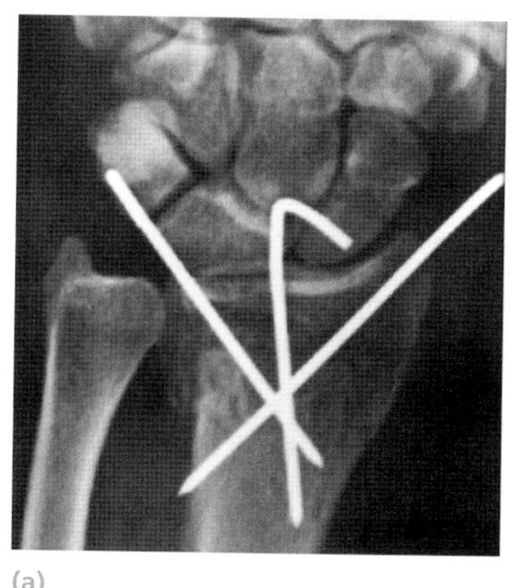

(a)

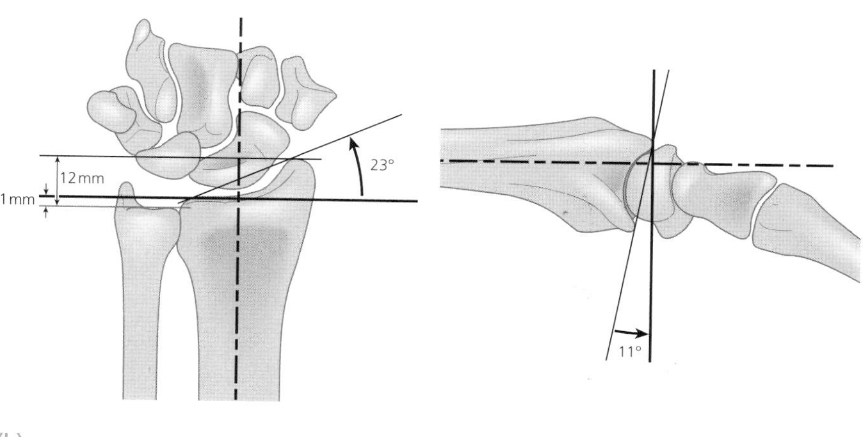

(b) (c)

25.9 Colles' fracture – operative fixation (a) Comminuted Colles' fracture reduced and held with percutaneous wires. Make sure that the articular surface angles are correctly restored (b,c).

applied to the front of the radius through the bed of flexor carpi radialis. The screws are fixed to the plate itself and are passed into the relatively stronger subchondral bone distally. These devices, which are flourishing in the orthopaedic marketplace, allow stable fixation and thus early mobilization of the forearm. Other devices, such as a locked intramedullary nail or crossed K-wires, are also suitable for the distal radius.

Outcome

As Colles himself recognized, the outcome of these fractures in an older age group with lower functional demands is usually good, regardless of the cosmetic or the radiographic appearance. Poor outcomes can often be improved by performing a corrective osteotomy. The amount of displacement that can be accepted depends on patient factors such as age, co-morbidity, functional demands, handedness, and quality of bone, and treatment factors such as surgical skill and implants available. As a rule, shortening of more than 2 mm at the distal radio-ulnar joint, dorsal tilt of more than 10 degrees and dorsal translation of more than 30 per cent are likely to lead to a poor outcome and early correction should be considered. This advice applies to older osteopaenic fractures; in younger patients the tolerances are far less!

Complications

EARLY

Circulatory problems The circulation in the fingers must be checked; the bandage holding the slab may need to be split or loosened.

Nerve injury Direct injury is rare, but compression of the median nerve in the carpal tunnel is fairly common. If it occurs soon after injury and the symptoms are mild, they may resolve with release of the dressings and elevation. If symptoms are severe or persistent, the transverse ligament should be divided.

Reflex sympathetic dystrophy This condition is probably quite common, but fortunately it seldom progresses to the full-blown picture of Sudeck's atrophy. There may be swelling and tenderness of the finger joints, a warning not to neglect the daily exercises. In about 5 per cent of cases, by the time the plaster is removed the hand is stiff and painful and there are signs of vasomotor instability. X-rays show osteoporosis and there is increased activity on the bone scan.

TFCC injury TFCC injury is more common than is generally appreciated. As the distal radius displaces dorsally, the TFCC is damaged; the ulnar styloid fracture which commonly accompanies a Colles' fracture illustrates the forces which are transmitted to the TFCC, which attaches in part to it.

LATE

Malunion Malunion is common, either because reduction was not complete or because displacement within the plaster was overlooked. The appearance is ugly, and weakness and loss of rotation may persist. In most cases treatment is not necessary. Where the disability is severe and the patient relatively young, the lower 1.5 cm of the ulna may be excised to restore rotation, and the radial deformity corrected by osteotomy.

Delayed union and non-union Non-union of the radius is rare, but the ulnar styloid process often joins by fibrous tissue only and remains painful and tender for several months.

Stiffness Stiffness of the shoulder, elbow and fingers from neglect is a common complication. Stiffness of the wrist may follow prolonged splintage.

Tendon rupture Rupture of extensor pollicis longus occasionally occurs a few weeks after an apparently trivial undisplaced fracture of the lower radius. The patient should be warned of the possibility and told that operative treatment is available.

SMITH'S FRACTURE

Smith (a Dubliner, like Colles) described a similar fracture about 20 years later. However, in this injury the distal fragment is displaced anteriorly (which is

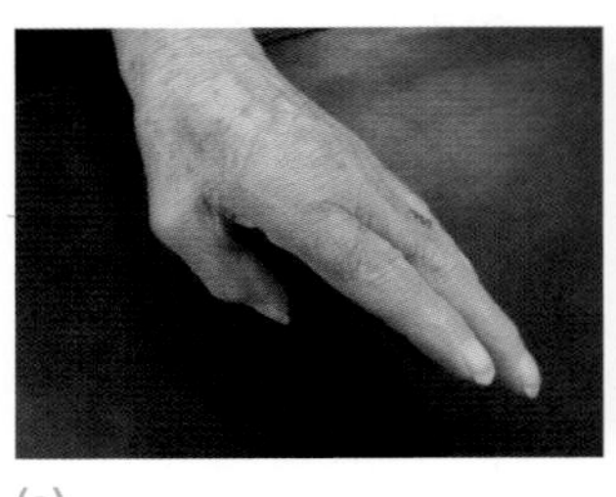

(a)

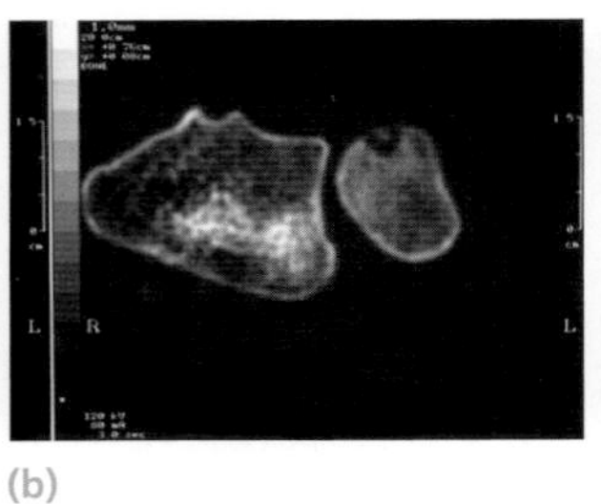

(b)

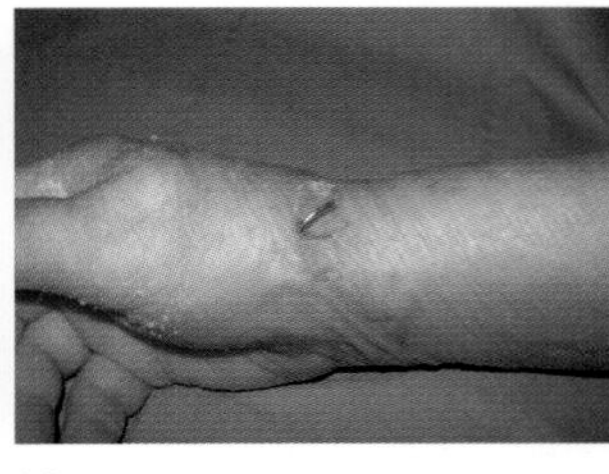

(c)

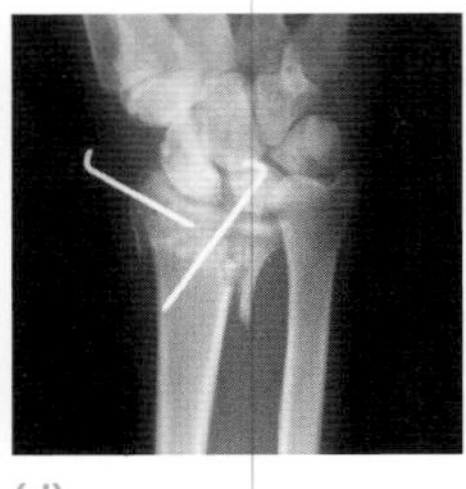

(d)

25.10 Colles' fracture-complications (a) Rupture of extensor pollicis longus; (b) malunion – CT scan showing incongruity of the distal radio-ulnar joint; (c) infected K-wire; (d) failed fixation as the wires have cut through the osteoporotic bone.

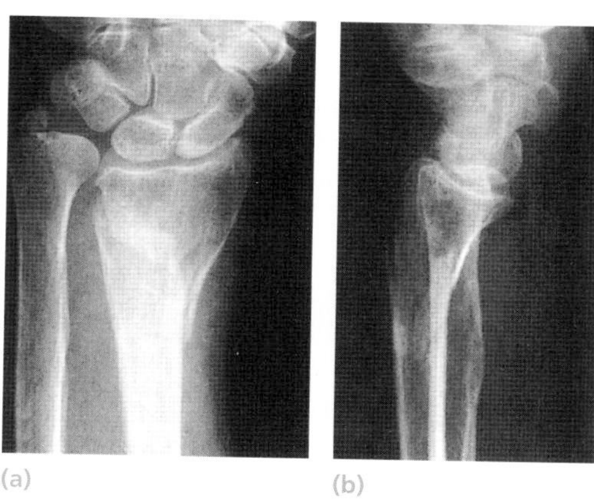

(a) (b)

25.11 Smith's fracture (a,b) Here, in contrast to Colles' fracture, the displacement of the lower radial fragment is forwards – not backwards.

why it is sometimes called a 'reversed Colles'). It is caused by a fall on the back of the hand.

Clinical features

The patient presents with a wrist injury, but there is no dinner-fork deformity. Instead, there is a 'garden spade' deformity.

X-ray There is a fracture through the distal radial metaphysis; a lateral view shows that the distal fragment is displaced and tilted anteriorly – the opposite of a Colles' fracture. The entire metaphysis can be fractured, or there can be an oblique fracture exiting at the dorsal or volar rim of the radius.

Treatment

The fracture is reduced by traction, supination and extension of the wrist, and the forearm is immobilized in a cast for 6 weeks. X-rays should be taken at 7–10 days to ensure the fracture has not slipped. Unstable fractures should be fixed with percutaneous wires or a plate.

DISTAL FOREARM FRACTURES IN CHILDREN

The distal radius and ulna are among the commonest sites of childhood fractures. The break may occur through the distal radial physis or in the metaphysis of one or both bones. Metaphyseal fractures are often incomplete or greenstick.

Mechanism of injury

The usual injury is a fall on the outstretched hand with the wrist in extension; the distal fragment is forced posteriorly (this is often called a 'juvenile Colles' fracture'). However, sometimes the wrist is in flexion and the fracture is angulated anteriorly. Lesser force may do no more than buckle the metaphyseal cortex (a type of compression fracture, or torus fracture).

Clinical features

There is usually a history of a fall, though this may be passed off as one of many childhood spills. The wrist is painful, and often quite swollen; sometimes there is an obvious 'dinner-fork' deformity.

X-ray The precise diagnosis is made on the x-ray appearances.

Physeal fractures are almost invariably Salter–Harris type I or II, with the epiphysis shifted and tilted backwards and radially. Type V injuries are unusual; sometimes they are diagnosed in retrospect when premature epiphyseal fusion occurs.

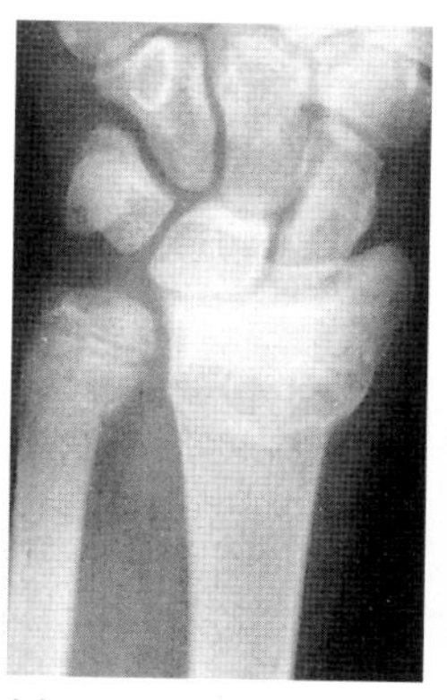

(a)

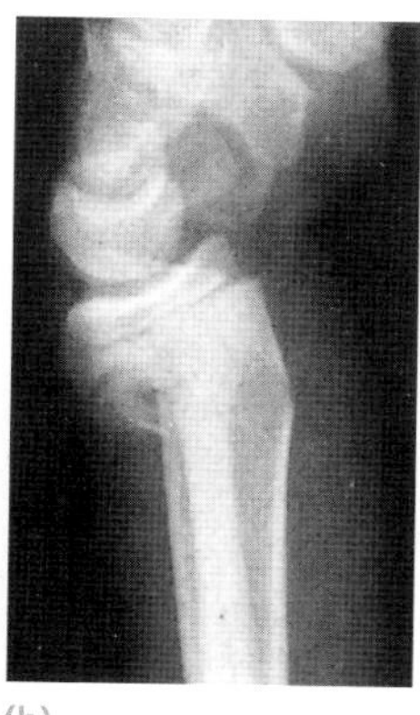

(b)

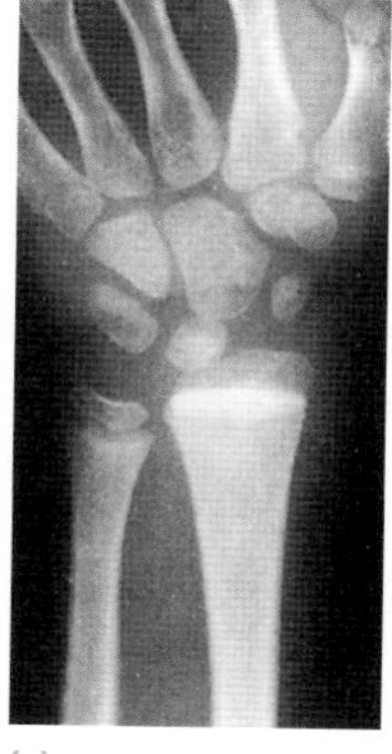

(c)

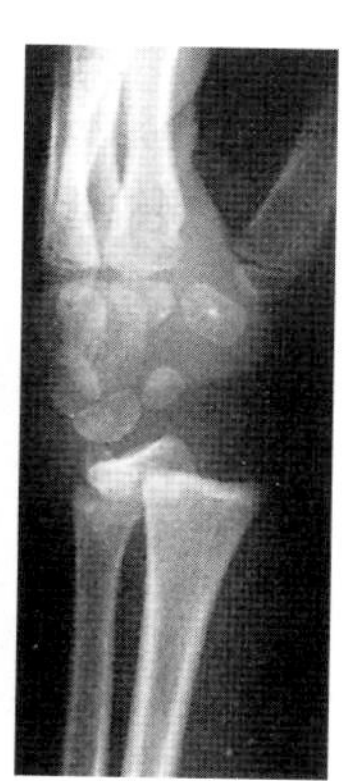

(d)

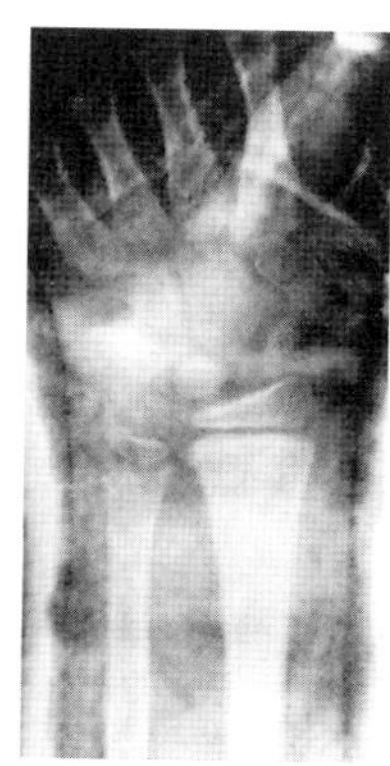

(e)

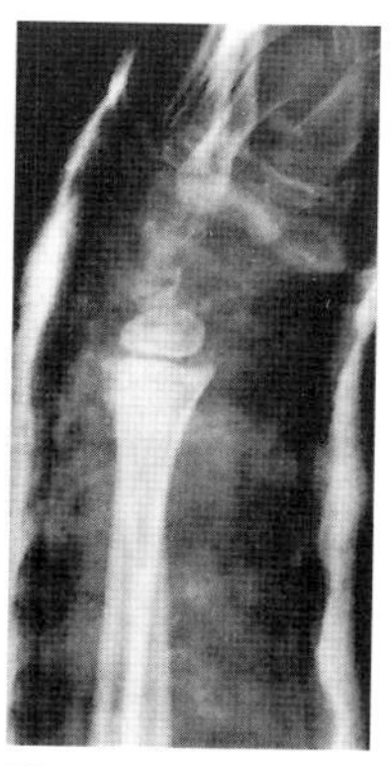

(f)

25.12 Distal forearm fractures in children (a,b) In older children the fracture is usually slightly more proximal than a true Colles', and often merely a greenstick or buckling injury. (c,d) In young children physeal fractures are usually Salter–Harris type I or II. In this case, accurate reduction has been achieved (e,f).

Metaphyseal injuries may appear as mere buckling of the cortex (easily missed unless appropriate views are obtained), as angulated greenstick fractures or as complete fractures with displacement and shortening. If only the radius is fractured, the ulna may be bent though not fractured.

Treatment

Physeal fractures are reduced, under anaesthesia, by pressure on the distal fragment. The arm is immobilized in a full-length cast with the wrist slightly flexed and ulnar deviated, and the elbow at 90 degrees. The cast is retained for 4 weeks. These fractures very rarely interfere with growth. Even if reduction is not absolutely perfect, further growth and modelling will obliterate any deformity. Patients seen more than 2 weeks after injury are best left untreated.

Buckle fractures require no more than 2 weeks in plaster, followed by another 2 weeks of restricted activity.

Greenstick fractures are usually easy to reduce – but apt to re-displace in the cast! Some degree of angulation can be accepted: in children under 10, up to 30 degrees and in children over 10, up 15 degrees. If the deformity is greater, the fracture is reduced by thumb pressure and the arm is immobilized with three-point fixation in a full-length cast with the wrist and forearm in neutral and the elbow flexed 90 degrees. The cast is changed and the fracture re-x-rayed at 2 weeks; if it has re-displaced a further manipulation can be carried out. The cast is finally discarded after 6 weeks.

Complete fractures can be embarrassingly difficult to reduce – especially if the ulna is intact. The fracture is manipulated in much the same way as a Colles' fracture; the reduction is checked by x-ray and a full-length cast is applied with the wrist neutral and the forearm supinated. After 2 weeks, a check x-ray is obtained; the cast is kept on for 6 weeks. If the fracture slips, especially if the ulna is intact, it should be stabilized with a percutaneous K-wire.

Complications

EARLY

Forearm swelling and threatened compartment syndrome This dire combination can be prevented by avoiding over-forceful or repeated manipulations, splitting the plaster, elevating the arm for the first 24–48 hours and encouraging exercises.

LATE

Malunion This late sequel is uncommon in children under 10 years of age. Deformity of as much as 30 degrees will straighten out with further growth and remodelling over the next 5 years. This should be carefully explained to the worried parents.

Radio-ulnar discrepancy Premature fusion of the radial epiphysis may result in bone length disparity and subluxation of the radio-ulnar joint. If this is troublesome, the radius can be lengthened and, if the child is near to skeletal maturity, the ulnar physis fused surgically.

RADIO-CARPAL FRACTURES

FRACTURED RADIAL STYLOID

This injury is caused by forced radial deviation of the wrist and may occur after a fall, or when a starting handle 'kicks back' – the so-called 'chauffeur's fracture'. The fracture line is transverse, extending laterally from the articular surface of the radius; the fragment, much more than the radial styloid, is often undisplaced. The radial styloid can also be fractured as part of the far more serious trans-scaphoid perilunate fracture dislocation.

Treatment

If there is displacement it is reduced, and the wrist is held in ulnar deviation by a plaster slab round the outer forearm extending from below the elbow to the metacarpal necks. Imperfect reduction may lead to osteoarthritis; therefore if closed reduction is imperfect the fragment should be screwed back, or held with K-wires.

FRACTURE-SUBLUXATION (BARTON'S FRACTURE)

VOLAR SUBLUXATION

The true Barton's injury is a volar fracture of the distal radius associated with volar subluxation of the carpus.

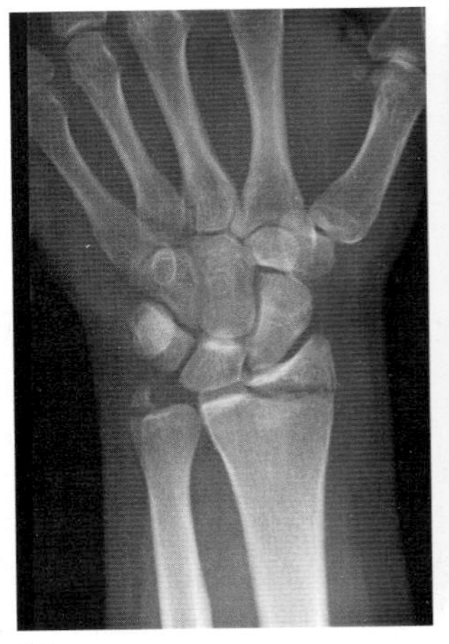

(a)

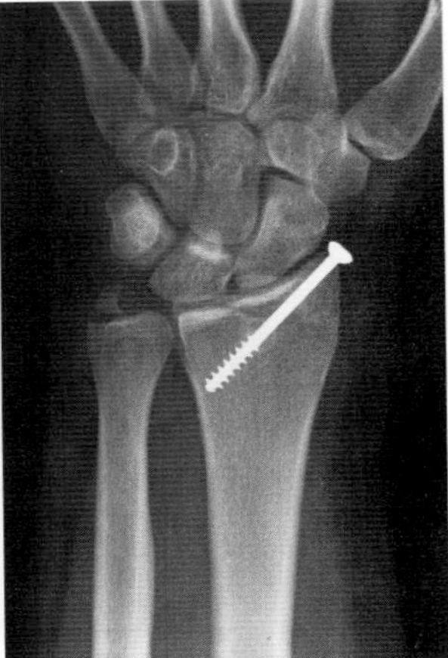

(b)

25.13 Fractured radial styloid (a) X-ray; (b) fixation with cannulated percutaneous screw.

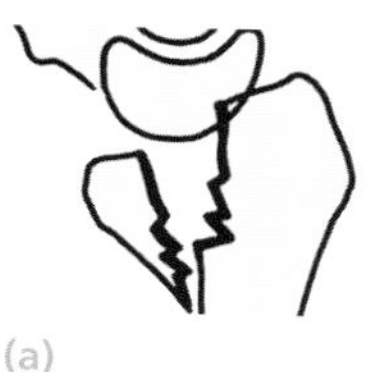

(a)

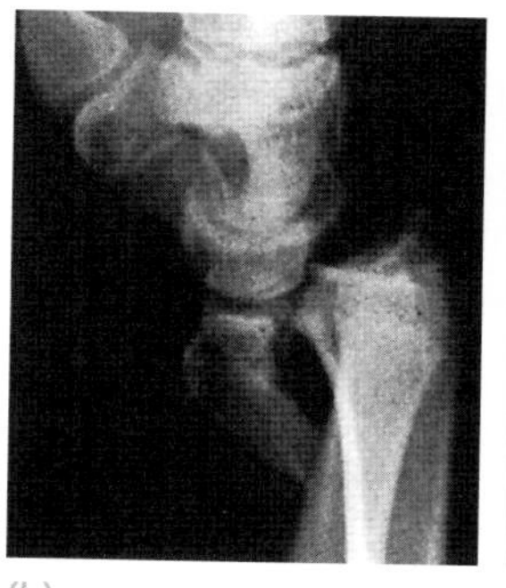

(b)

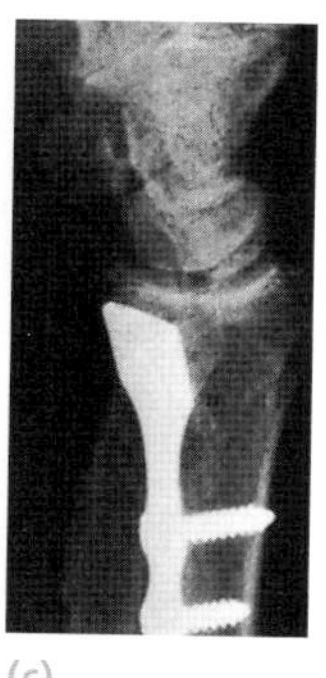

(c)

25.14 Fracture-subluxation (Barton's fracture) (a,b) The true Barton's fracture is a split of the volar edge of the distal radius with anterior (volar) subluxation of the wrist. This has been reduced and held (c) with a small anterior plate.

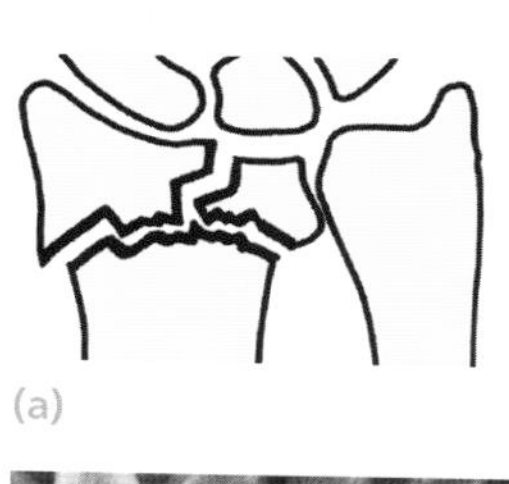

(a)

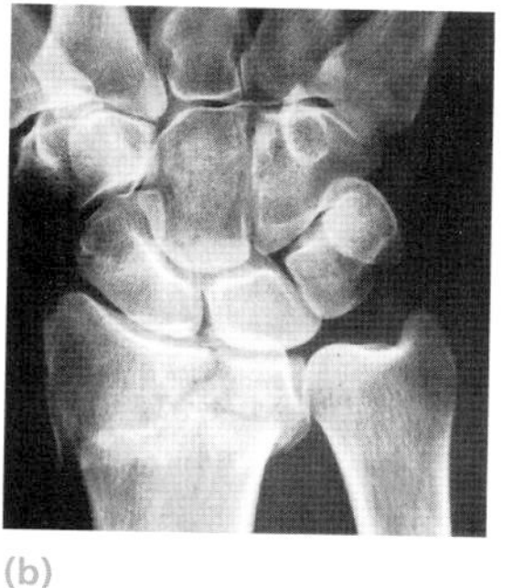

(b)

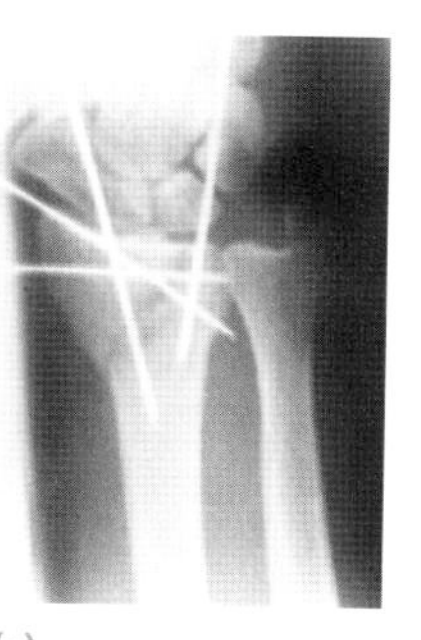

(c)

25.15 Comminuted fracture of the distal radius The 'die punch fragment' of the lunate fossa of the distal radius (a,b) must be perfectly reduced and fixed; here this has been achieved by closed reduction and percutaneous K-wire fixation (c). The wires can be used as 'joy sticks' to manipulate the fragment back before fixation.

It is sometimes mistaken for a Smith's fracture, but it differs from the latter in that the fracture line runs obliquely across the volar lip of the radius into the wrist joint; the distal fragment is displaced anteriorly, carrying the carpus with it. Because the fragment is small and unsupported, the fracture is inherently unstable.

Treatment The fracture can be easily reduced, but it is just as easily re-displaced. Internal fixation, using a small anterior buttress plate, is recommended.

DORSAL SUBLUXATION

This is sometimes called a 'dorsal Barton's fracture'. Here the line of fracture runs obliquely across the dorsal lip of the radius and the carpus is carried posteriorly.

Treatment The fracture is easier to control than the volar Barton's. It is reduced closed and the forearm is immobilized in a cast for 6 weeks. If it re-displaces, closed K-wiring or open reduction and plating is advisable.

COMMINUTED INTRA-ARTICULAR FRACTURES IN YOUNG ADULTS

In the young adult, a comminuted intra-articular fracture is a high energy injury. A poor outcome will result unless intra-articular congruity, fracture alignment and length are restored and movements started as soon as possible. For these patients a much higher standard must be set than would be accepted for the typical osteoporotic fracture. In addition to the usual posteroanterior and lateral x-rays, oblique views and often CT scans are useful to show the fragment alignment.

The simplest option is a manipulation and cast. If the anatomy is not restored, then an open reduction

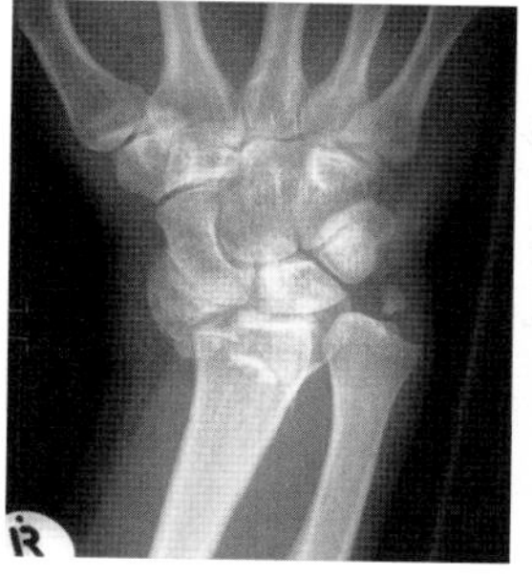

(a)

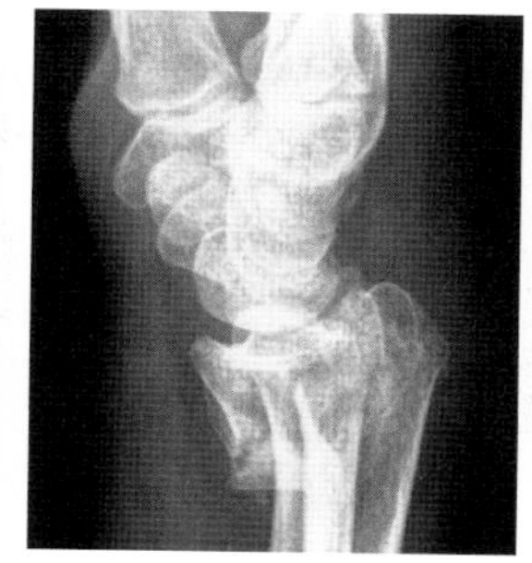

(b)

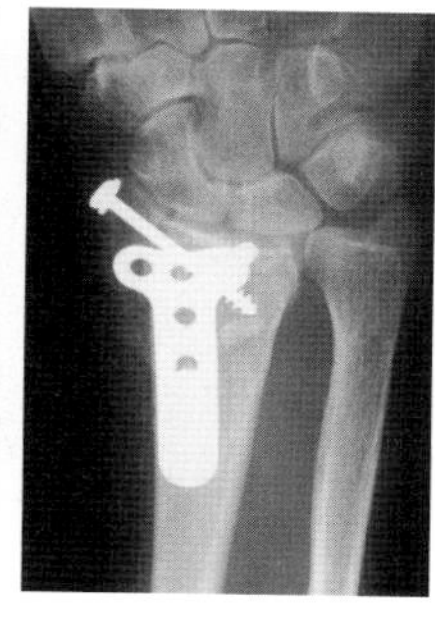

(c)

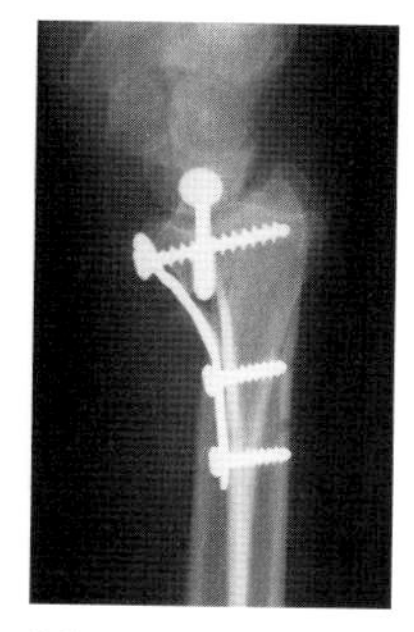

(d)

25.16 High energy injuries in younger patients Perfect reduction is required.

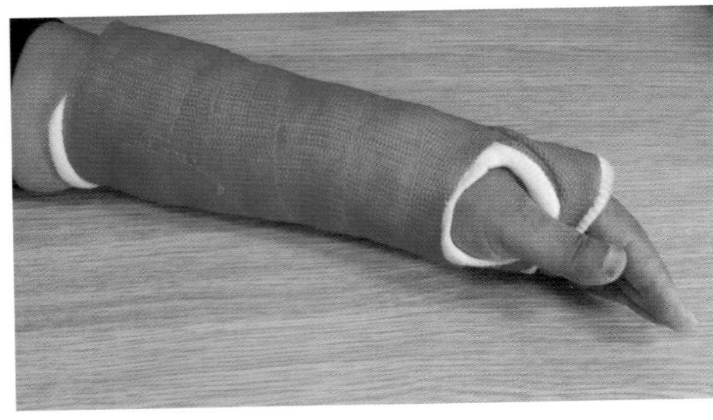

(a)

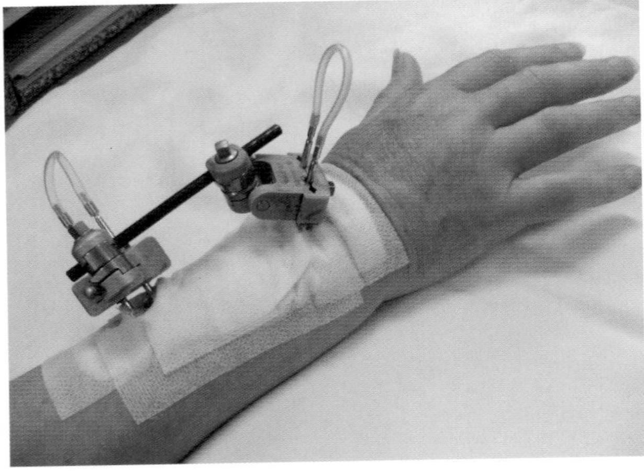

(b)

25.17 Distal radius fracture Options include simple plaster (a) or external fixation (b) depending on the amount of comminution, stability of the fracture and patient demands.

may be necessary. The medial complex must be anatomically reduced, which may require open reduction through dorsal and palmar approaches and a combination of wires, plates, screws and bone grafts.

Complications of radio-carpal fractures

Associated injuries of the carpus Injuries of the carpus are easily overlooked while attention is focussed on the radius. Carpal injuries must be excluded by careful clinical and x-ray examination, occasionally supplemented by MRI or arthroscopy.

Re-displacement There is a strong tendency for Barton's fracture to re-displace if it is held in a cast; hence our preference for internal fixation.

Carpal instability The patient may present years later with chronic carpal instability. The wrist injury may have been overlooked at the time.

Secondary osteoarthritis Fractures into the joint and carpal instability may eventually lead to secondary osteoarthritis. It is difficult to predict when (or even whether) this is likely to occur; symptoms develop slowly and disability is often not severe. Warning symptoms are restricted wrist movement and loss of grip strength. If pain and weakness interfere significantly with function, arthrodesis of the wrist may be need, especially if it is the dominant side which is affected.

CARPAL INJURIES

Fractures and dislocations of the carpal bones are common. They vary greatly in type and severity. *These should never be regarded as isolated injuries; the entire carpus suffers*, and sometimes, long after the fracture has healed, the patient still complains of pain and weakness in the wrist.

The commonest wrist injuries are: sprains of the capsule and ligaments; fracture of a carpal bone

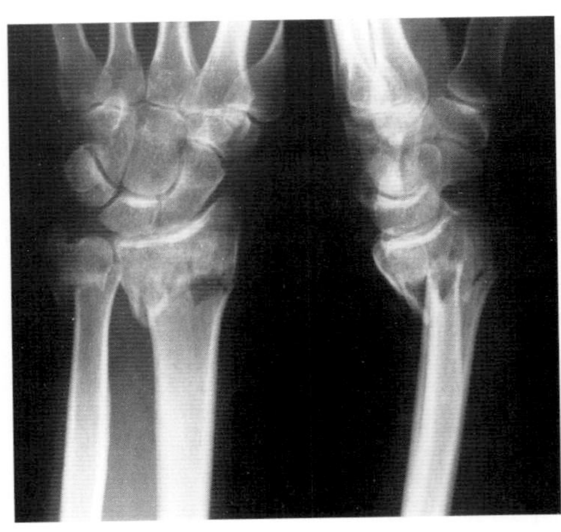

(a)

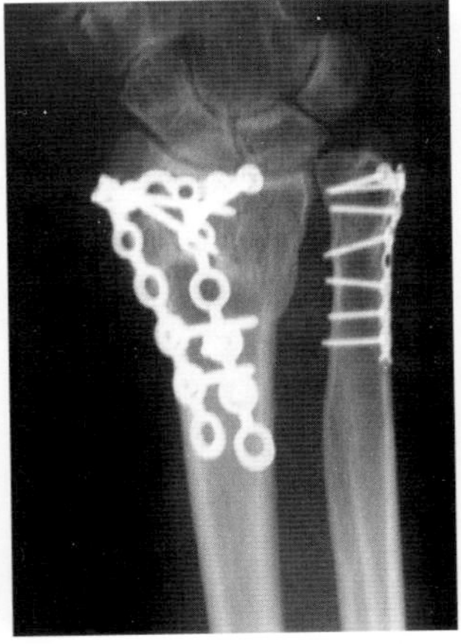

(b)

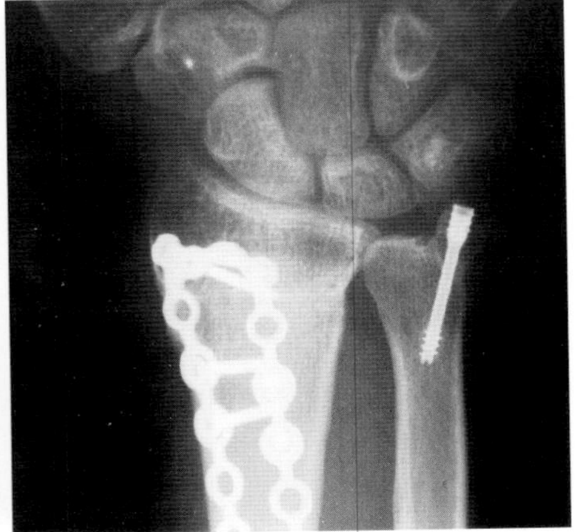

(c)

25.18 Don't forget the ulna (a) Fracture of radius and ulna, both unstable. (b) Both bones fixed. (c) Ulnar styloid fracture fixed to prevent instability of distal radio-ulnar joint.

(usually the scaphoid); injury of the triangular fibrocartilage complex (TFCC) and distal radio-ulnar joint; dislocations of the lunate or the bones around it; and subluxations and 'carpal collapse', which may be acute or chronic.

Clinical assessment

Following a fall, the patient complains of pain in the wrist. There may be swelling or well-marked deformity of the joint. Tenderness should be carefully localized; undirected prodding will confuse both the patient and the examiner. The blunt end of a pencil is helpful in testing for point tenderness. For scaphoid fractures, the 'jump spot' is in the anatomical snuffbox and scaphoid tubercle; for scapho-lunate injuries, just beyond Lister's tubercle; for lunate dislocation, in the middle of the wrist; for triquetral injuries, beyond the head of the ulna; for hamate fractures, at the base of the hypothenar eminence; for triangular fibrocartilage complex injuries, over the dorsum of the ulnocarpal joint. Movements are often limited (more by pain than by stiffness) and they may be accompanied by a palpable catch or an audible clunk.

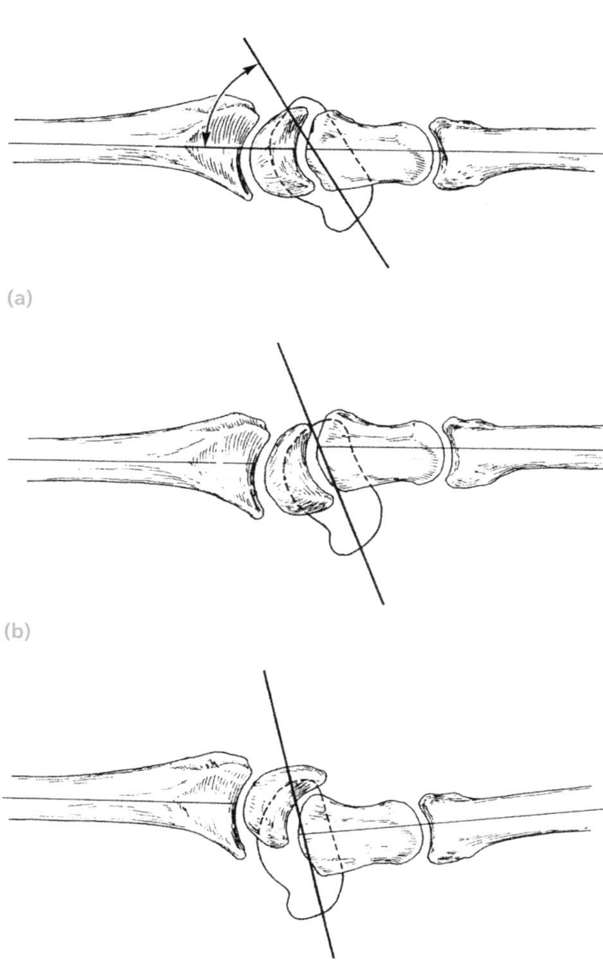

25.19 Carpal instability – x-ray patterns (a) Normal lateral view. The radius, capitate and middle metacarpal lie in a straight line and the scaphoid axis is angled at 45° to the line of the radius. (b) Dorsal intercalated segmental instability (DISI). The lunate is tilted dorsally and the scaphoid is tilted somewhat volarwards; the axes of the capitate and metacarpals now lie behind (dorsal to) that of the radius. (c) Volar intercalated segmental instability (VISI). The lunate and scaphoid are tilted somewhat volarwards and the capitate and metacarpals lie anterior (volar) to the radius.

Imaging

X-rays are the key to diagnosis. There are three golden rules:

- Accept only high-quality films
- If the initial x-rays are 'normal', treat the clinical diagnosis
- Repeat the x-ray examination 2 weeks later.

Initially three standard views are obtained: anteroposterior and lateral with the wrist neutral, and an oblique 'scaphoid' view. If these are normal and clinical features suggest a carpal injury, further views are obtained: anteroposterior x-rays with the wrist first in maximum ulnar and then in maximum radial deviation, and an anteroposterior view with the fist clenched.

The examiner should be familiar with the normal x-ray anatomy of the carpus in all the standard views, so that he or she can visualize a three-dimensional picture from the two-dimensional, overlapping images of the carpal bones.

In the anteroposterior x-rays note the shape of the carpus, whether the individual bones are clearly outlined and whether there are any abnormally large gaps suggesting disruption of the ligaments. The scaphoid may be fractured; or it may have lost its normal bean shape and look squat and foreshortened, sometimes with an inner circular density (the cortical ring sign) – features of an end-on view when the bone is hyperflexed because of damage to the restraining scapholunate ligament. The lunate is normally quadrilateral in shape, but if it is dislocated it looks triangular.

In the lateral x-ray the axes of the radius, lunate, capitate and third metacarpal are co-linear, and the scaphoid projects at an angle of about 45 degrees to this line. With traumatic instability the linked carpal segments collapse (like the buckled carriages of a derailed train). Two patterns are recognized: dorsal intercalated segment instability (DISI), in which the lunate is torn from the scaphoid and tilted backwards; and volar intercalated segment instability (VISI), in which the lunate is torn from the triquetrum and turns towards the palm; the capitate shows a complementary dorsal tilt. There may be a flake fracture off the back of a carpal bone (usually the triquetrum).

Special x-ray studies are sometimes helpful: a *carpal*

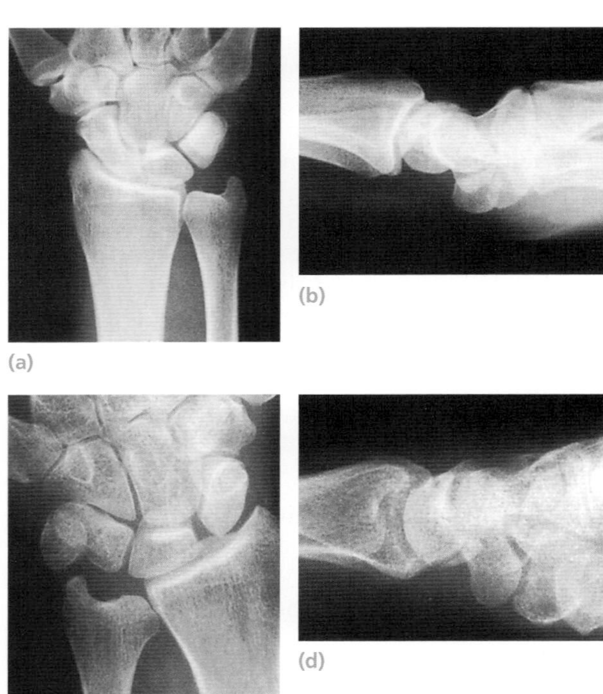

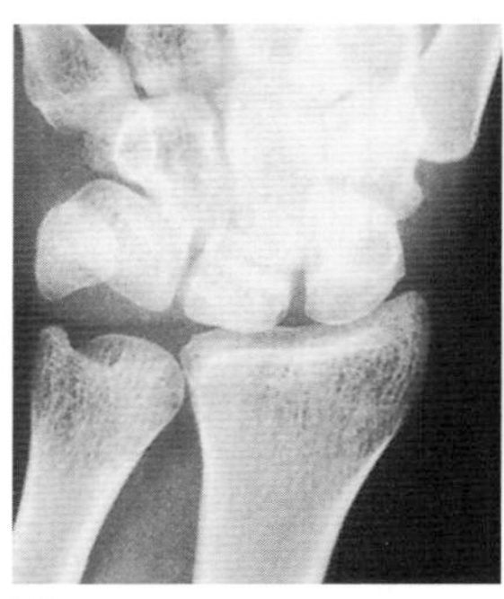

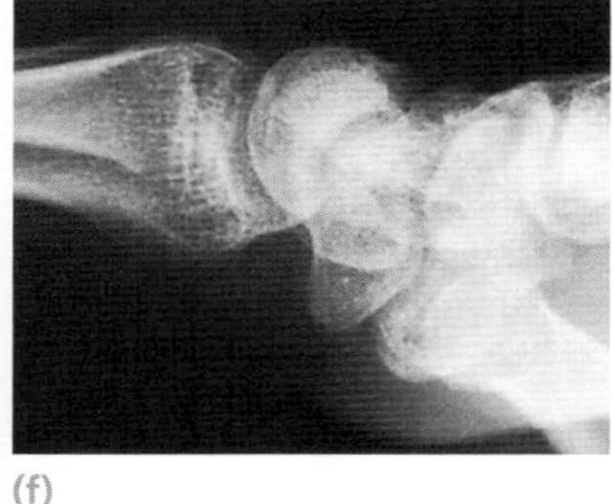

25.20 Carpal injuries **(a,b)** Normal appearances in antero-posterior and lateral x-rays. **(c,d)** Following a 'sprained wrist' this patient developed persistent pain and weakness. X-rays showed **(c)** scapho-lunate dissociation and **(d)** dorsal rotation of the lunate (the typical DISI pattern). **(e,f)** This patient, too, had a sprained wrist. The anteroposterior and lateral x-rays show foreshortening of the scaphoid and volar rotation of the lunate (VISI).

tunnel view may show a fractured hook of hamate, and *motion studies* in different positions may reveal a subluxation. A *radioisotope scan* will confirm a wrist injury although it may not precisely localize it.

MRI is sensitive and specific (especially for detecting undisclosed fractures or Kienböck's disease), but unless very fine cuts are taken it may miss TFCC and interosseous ligament tears.

Arthroscopy

Wrist arthroscopy is the best way of demonstrating TFCC or interosseous ligament tears.

Principles of management

'Wrist sprain' should not be diagnosed unless a more serious injury has been excluded with certainty. Even with apparently trivial injuries, ligaments are sometimes torn and the patient may later develop carpal instability.

If the x-rays are normal but the clinical signs strongly suggest a carpal injury, a splint or plaster should be applied for 2 weeks, after which time *the x-rays are repeated*. A fracture or dislocation may become more obvious after a few weeks, but a second negative x-ray still does not exclude a serious injury. A bone scan or MRI at this stage will confirm the diagnosis and avoid an unnecessary period of immobilization and time from work. If these tests are not readily available, then the patient should be re-examined repeatedly until the symptoms settle or a firm diagnosis is made.

The more common lesions are dealt with below.

Fractured scaphoid

Scaphoid fractures account for almost 75 per cent of all carpal fractures although they are rare in the elderly and in children. With unstable fractures there may also be disruption of the scapho-lunate ligaments and dorsal rotation of the lunate.

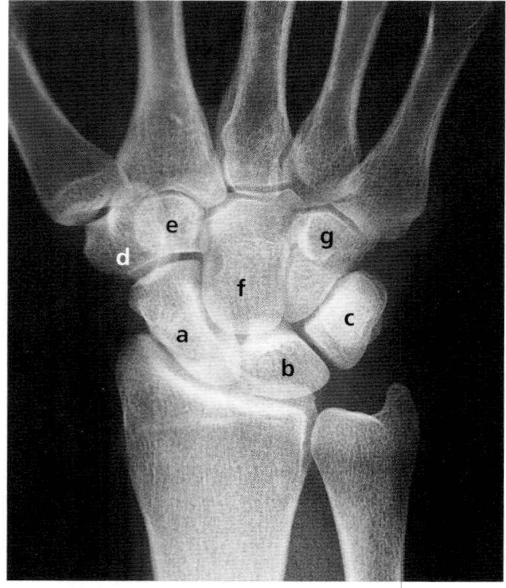

25.21 X-ray appearance of the normal carpus X-ray of a normal wrist showing the shape and disposition of the eight carpal bones: **(a)** scaphoid; **(b)** lunate; **(c)** triquetrum overlain by pisiform; **(d)** trapezium; **(e)** trapezoid; **(f)** capitate; and **(g)** hamate.

Mechanism of injury and pathological anatomy

The scaphoid lies obliquely across the two rows of carpal bones, and is also in the line of loading between the thumb and forearm. The combination of forced carpal movement and compression, as in a fall on the dorsiflexed hand, exerts severe stress on the bone and it is liable to fracture. Most scaphoid fractures are stable; with unstable fractures the fragments may become displaced. The distal fragment, unrestrained by the scapho-lunate ligament, flexes and the proximal fragment tilts dorsally with the lunate (a DISI deformity); the hump-backed deformity of the scaphoid is permanent.

The blood supply of the scaphoid diminishes proximally. This accounts for the fact that 1 per cent of distal third fractures, 20 per cent of middle third fractures and 40 per cent of proximal fractures result in non-union or avascular necrosis of the proximal fragment.

Clinical features

The appearance may be deceptively normal, but the astute observer can usually detect fullness in the anatomical snuffbox; precisely localized tenderness in the same place is an important diagnostic sign; the scaphoid can of course also be palpated from the front and back of the wrist and it may be tender there as well. Proximal pressure along the axis of the thumb may be painful.

X-ray

Anteroposterior, lateral and oblique views are all essential; often a recent fracture shows only in the oblique view. Usually the fracture line is transverse, and through the narrowest part of the bone (waist), but it may be more proximally situated (proximal pole fracture). Sometimes only the tubercle of the scaphoid is fractured.

It is very important to look for subtle signs of displacement or instability: e.g. obliquity of the fracture line, opening of the fracture line, angulation of the distal fragment and foreshortening of the scaphoid image.

A few weeks after the injury the fracture may be more obvious; if union is delayed, cavitation appears on either side of the break. Old, un-united fractures have 'hard' borders, making it seem as if there is an extra carpal bone. Relative sclerosis of the proximal fragment is pathognomonic of avascular necrosis.

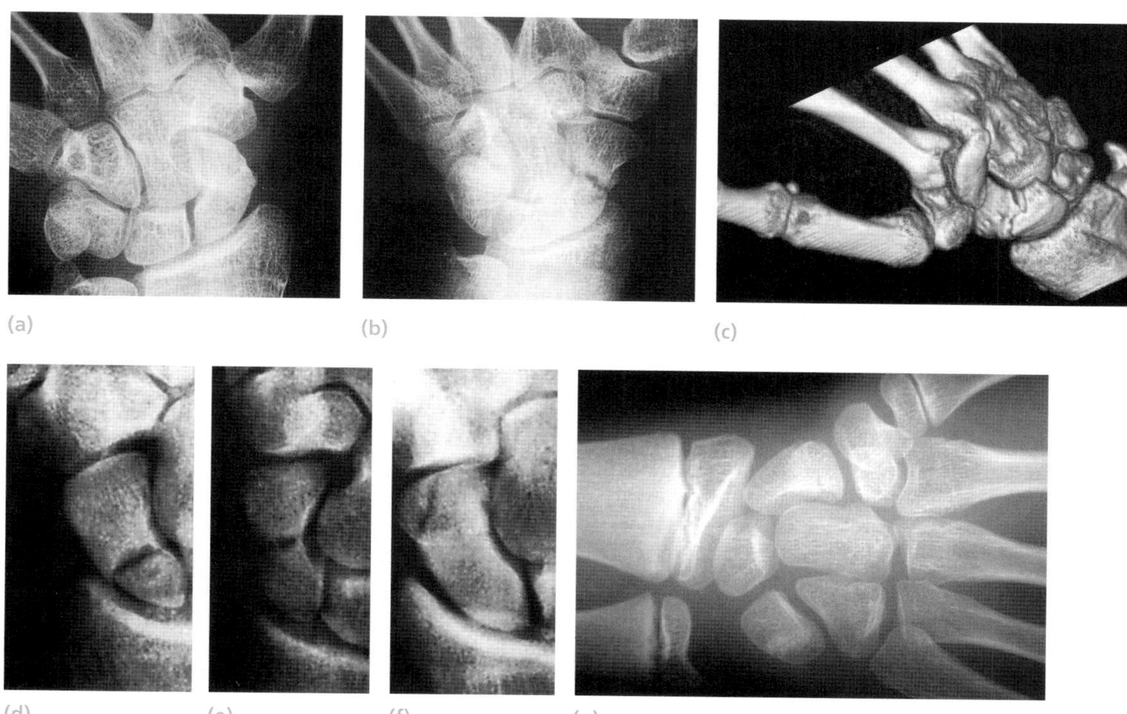

25.22 Fractures of the scaphoid – diagnosis (a) The initial anteroposterior view often fails to show the fracture; (b) always ask for a 'scaphoid series', including two oblique views. If the clinical features are suggestive of a fracture, then immobilize the wrist and repeat the x-ray 2 weeks later when the fracture is more likely to be apparent. (c) A CT scan is useful for showing the fracture configuration. The fracture may be (d) through the proximal pole, (e) the waist, or (f) the scaphoid tubercle. Occasionally these fractures are seen in children (g).

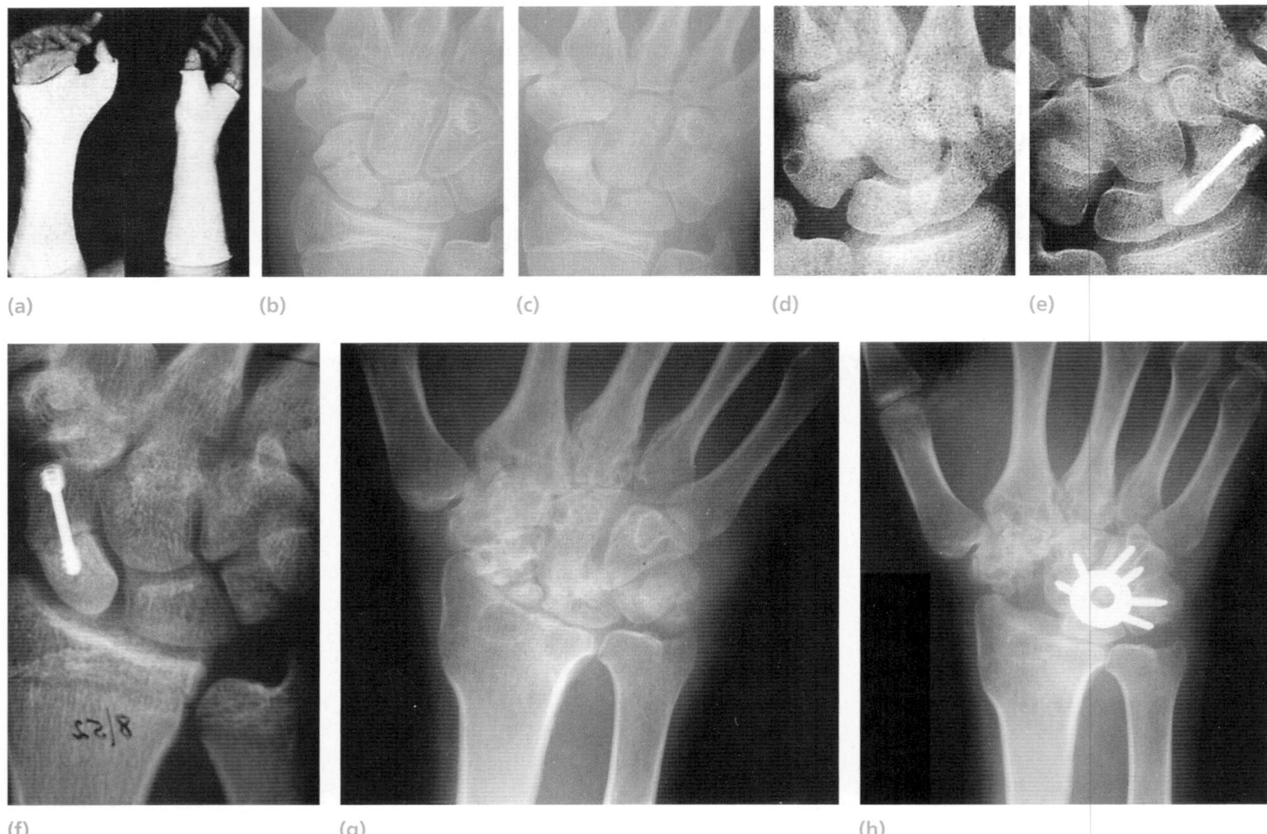

(a) (b) (c) (d) (e)

(f) (g) (h)

25.23 Fractures of the scaphoid –treatment (a) Scaphoid plaster – position and extent. (b,c) Before and after treatment: in this case radiological union was visible at 10 weeks. (d) Delayed union, treated successfully by (e) bone grafting and screw fixation. (f) Long-standing stable non-union. (g) Non-union with avascular necrosis and secondary osteoarthritis treated by (h) scaphoid excision and four-corner fusion.

Treatment

Fracture of the scaphoid tubercle needs no splintage and should be treated as a wrist sprain; a crepe bandage is applied and movement is encouraged. *Other scaphoid fractures* are treated as follows.

Undisplaced fractures need no reduction and are treated in plaster; 90 per cent of waist fractures should heal. The cast is applied from the upper forearm to just short of the metacarpo-phalangeal joints of the fingers, but incorporating the proximal phalanx of the thumb. The wrist is held dorsiflexed and the thumb forwards in the 'glass-holding' position. The plaster must be carefully moulded into the hollow of the hand, and is not split. It is retained (and if necessary repaired or renewed) for 8 weeks.

After 8 weeks the plaster is removed and the wrist examined clinically and radiologically. If there is no tenderness and the x-ray shows signs of healing, the wrist is left free; a CT scan is the most reliable means of confirming union if in doubt.

If the scaphoid is tender, or the fracture still visible on x-ray, the cast is reapplied for a further 4 weeks. At that stage, one of two pictures may emerge: (a) the wrist is painless and the fracture has healed – the cast can be discarded; (b)the x-ray shows signs of delayed healing (bone resorption and cavitation around the fracture) – union can be hastened by bone grafting and internal fixation.

Displaced fractures can also be treated in plaster, but the outcome is less predictable. It is better to reduce the fracture openly and to fix it with a compression screw. This should increase the likelihood of union and reduce the time of immobilization.

Some patients may not want to endure a prolonged period in plaster. Early percutaneous fixation with a compression screw, though technically demanding, can dramatically reduce the time away from work and the difficulties associated with personal care.

Complications

Avascular necrosis The proximal fragment may die, especially with proximal pole fractures, and then at 2–3 months it appears dense on x-ray. Although revascularization and union are theoretically possible, they take years and meanwhile the wrist collapses and arthritis develops. Bone grafting, as for delayed union, may be successful, in which case the bone, though abnormal, is structurally intact. If the wrist becomes painful, the dead fragment can be excised. However, the wrist tends to collapse after this procedure; a better option would be to remove the entire proximal row of carpal bones or else to remove the scaphoid and fuse the proximal to the distal row (four-corner fusion: capitate–hamate–triquetrum–lunate).

Non-union By 3 months it may be obvious that the fracture will not unite. Bone grafting should be attempted, especially in the younger, more vigorous type of patient, because this probably reduces the chance of later, symptomatic osteoarthritis. Two types of graft are used. If the scaphoid has folded into a flexed 'humpback' shape, then it is approached from the front and a wedge of cortico-cancellous iliac crest graft is inserted to restore the shape of the bone. The graft is fixed with a buried screw and/or K-wires. If the scaphoid has not collapsed, the graft is inserted into a trough carved into the front of the scaphoid and again stabilized with a screw or wires. If these techniques fail to achieve union then the options are a vascularized bone graft, scaphoidectomy with proximal-to-distal-row (four-corner) fusion, proximal row carpectomy or radio-carpal arthrodesis.

In older patients, and those who are completely asymptomatic, non-union may be left untreated. Sometimes a patient is seen for the first time with a 'sprain', but x-rays show an old, un-united fracture with sclerosed edges; 3–4 weeks in plaster may suffice to make him or her comfortable once again, and no further treatment is required.

Osteoarthritis Non-union or avascular necrosis may lead to secondary osteoarthritis of the wrist. If the arthritis is localized to the distal pole, excising the radial styloid may help. As the arthritis progresses, changes appear in the scapho-capitate joint then the capitate-lunate joint. The lunate-radius joint is never affected, thus allowing salvage procedures – either proximal row carpectomy or four-corner fusion.

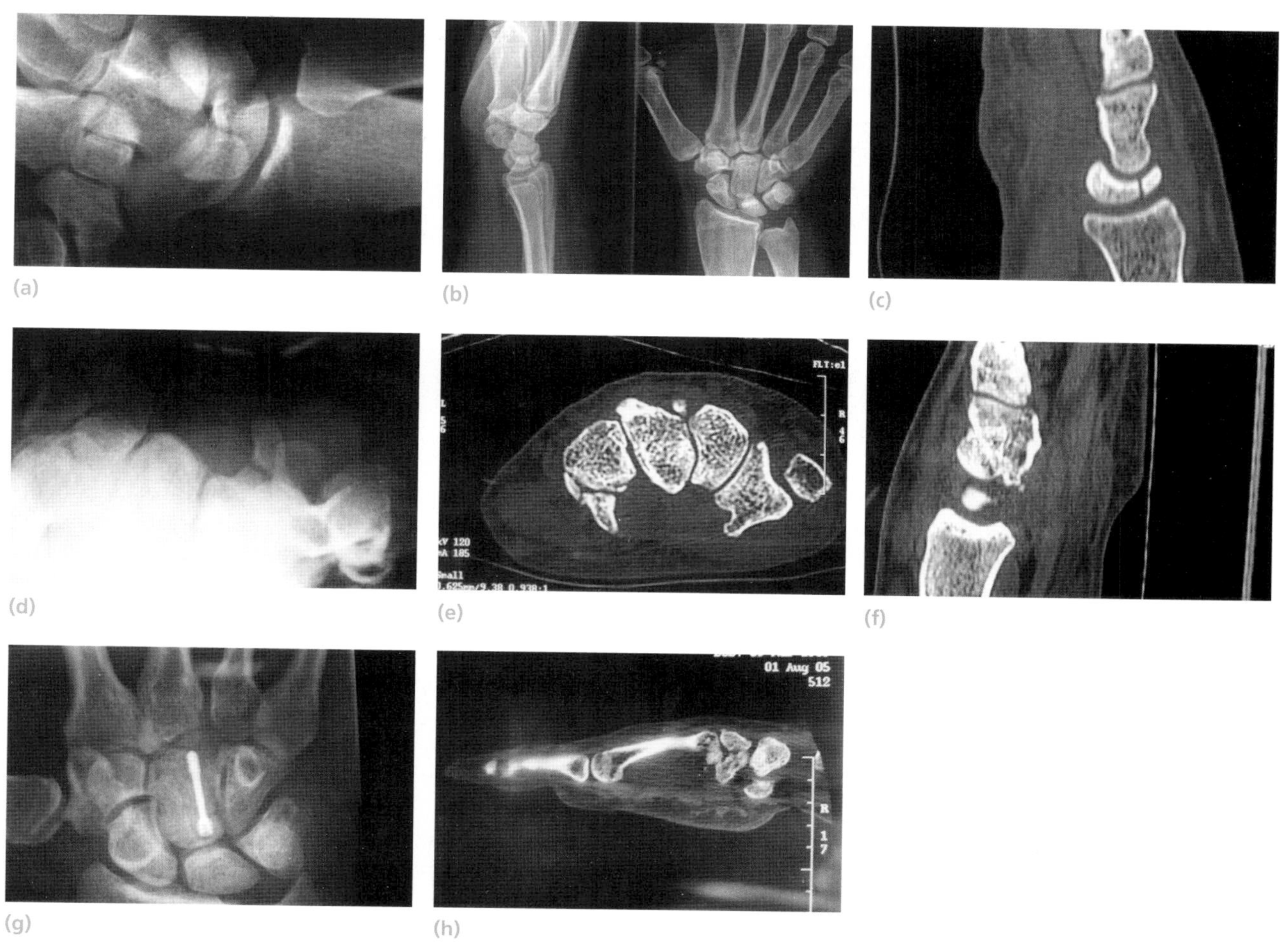

25.24 Fractures of other carpal bones (a) Fracture of body of trapezium; (b) lunate fracture; (c) lunate fracture; (d) hook of hamate; (e) hook of hamate CT; (f) capitate fracture fixed (g) with a screw; (h) fracture of body of hamate.

Fractures of other carpal bones

Triquetrum

Avulsion of the dorsal ligaments is not uncommon; analgesics and splintage for a few days are all that is required. Occasionally the body is fractured; it usually heals after 4–6 weeks in plaster.

Hamate

A fracture of the hook of hamate follows a direct blow to the palm of the hand. These fractures cannot be seen on routine x-rays; a carpal tunnel view, CT or MRI is needed. The fracture does not heal readily; if symptoms are prolonged then the fragment is excised, taking care not to damage the ulnar nerve. Fractures of the body are rare. They are also difficult to define on plain x-rays. If the CT scan shows a fracture, fixation may occasionally be needed.

Trapezium

The body of the trapezium can be fractured if the shaft of the first metacarpal impacts onto it; the ridge (to which the transverse carpal ligament attaches) can be fractured by a direct blow. The latter fracture can usually be seen on a carpal tunnel view rather than standard x-rays. The body fracture may need open reduction and internal fixation if displaced; the ridge fracture usually settles with splintage for a week or two.

Capitate

The capitate is relatively protected within the carpus. However, in severe trauma the wrist can be fractured; the distal fragment can rotate, in which case open reduction and internal fixation is required.

Lunate

Fractures of the lunate are rare and follow a hyperextension injury to the wrist. There is a real risk of non-union; undisplaced fractures should be immobilized in a cast for 6 weeks; displaced fractures should be reduced and fixed with a screw.

ULNAR-SIDE WRIST INJURIES

(see also Chapter 16)

The distal radio-ulnar joint is often injured with a radial fracture; it can also be damaged in isolation, particularly after hyperpronation. The triangular fibrocartilage complex (TFCC) can be torn, the ulnar styloid avulsed or the articular surfaces of the ulnocarpal joint or distal radio-ulnar joint damaged.

Clinical features

There is tenderness over the distal radio-ulnar joint and pain on rotation of the forearm. The distal ulna may be unstable; the *piano-key sign* is elicited by holding the patient's forearm pronated and pushing sharply forwards on the head of the ulna.

Imaging and arthroscopy

A lateral x-ray in pronation and supination shows incongruity of the distal radio-ulnar joint. The anteroposterior view may show an avulsed ulnar styloid. Arthrography, MRI and arthroscopy may be needed to confirm the diagnosis.

Treatment

Instability usually resolves if the arm is held in supination for 6 weeks; occasionally a K-wire is needed to maintain the reduction. If the dislocation is irreducible, this may be due to trapped soft tissue, which will have to be removed. Chronic instability may require reconstructive surgery.

A TFCC tear should be repaired and the ulnocarpal capsule reefed. A displaced fracture at the base of the ulnar styloid, if painful or associated with instability of the radio-ulnar joint, should be fixed with a small screw.

CARPAL DISLOCATIONS, SUBLUXATIONS AND INSTABILITY

The wrist functions as a system of intercalated segments or links, stabilized by the intercarpal ligaments and the scaphoid which acts as a bridge between the proximal and distal rows of the carpus. Fractures and dislocations of the carpal bones, or even simple ligament tears and sprains, may seriously disturb this system so that the links collapse into one of several well-recognized patterns (see Chapter 16).

Lunate and perilunate dislocations

A fall with the hand forced into dorsiflexion may tear the tough ligaments that normally bind the carpal bones. The lunate usually remains attached to the radius and the rest of the carpus is displaced backwards (*perilunate dislocation*). Usually the hand immediately snaps forwards again but, as it does so, the lunate may be levered out of position to be displaced anteriorly (*lunate dislocation*). Sometimes the scaphoid remains attached to the radius and the force of the perilunar dislocation causes it to fracture through the waist (*trans-scaphoid perilunate dislocation*).

Clinical features

The wrist is painful and swollen and is held immobile. If the carpal tunnel is compressed there may be paraesthesia or blunting of sensation in the territory of the median nerve, and weakness of palmar abduction of the thumb.

X-ray

Most dislocations are perilunate. In the antero-posterior view the carpus is diminished in height and the bone shadows overlap abnormally. One or more of the carpal bones may be fractured (usually the scaphoid and radial styloid). If the lunate is dislocated, it has a characteristic triangular shape instead of the normal quadrilateral appearance.

In the lateral view it is easy to distinguish a lunate from a perilunate dislocation. The *dislocated lunate* is tilted forwards and is displaced in front of the radius, while the capitate and metacarpal bones are in line with the radius. With a *perilunate dislocation* the lunate is tilted only slightly and is not displaced forwards, and the capitate and metacarpals lie behind the line of the radius (DISI pattern); if there is an associated *scaphoid fracture*, the distal fragment may be flexed.

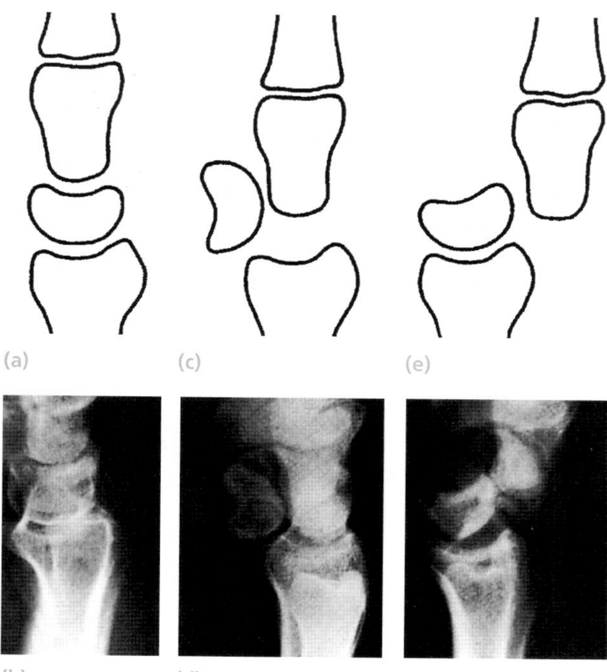

25.25 Lunate and perilunate dislocations.
(a,b) Lateral x-ray of normal wrist; (c,d) lunate dislocation; (e,f) perilunate dislocation.

Treatment

Closed reduction The surgeon pulls strongly on the dorsiflexed hand; then, while maintaining traction, he or she slowly palmarflexes the wrist, at the same time squeezing the lunate backwards with his or her other thumb. These manoeuvres usually effect reduction; they also prevent conversion of a perilunate to a lunate dislocation. A plaster slab is applied holding the wrist neutral. Percutaneous K-wires may be needed to hold the reduction.

Open reduction Reduction is imperative, and if closed reduction fails, or if a later x-ray shows that the wrist has collapsed into the familiar DISI pattern, open reduction is performed. The carpus is exposed by an anterior approach which has the advantage of decompressing the carpal tunnel. While an assistant pulls on the hand, the lunate is levered into place and kept there by a K-wire which is inserted through the lunate into the capitate. If the scaphoid is fractured, this too can be reduced and fixed with a Herbert screw or K-wires. Where possible, the torn soft tissues should be repaired through palmar and dorsal approaches. At the end of the procedure, the wrist is splinted in a plaster slab, which is retained for 3 weeks. Finger, elbow and shoulder exercises are practised throughout this period. The K-wires are removed at 6 weeks.

This injury is frequently accompanied by severe compression of the median nerve, which should be released.

SCAPHO-LUNATE DISSOCIATION

A wrist sprain may be followed by persistent pain and tenderness over the dorsum just distal to Lister's tubercle.

X-rays show an excessively large gap between the scaphoid and the lunate. The scaphoid may appear foreshortened, with a typical cortical ring sign. In the lateral view, the lunate is tilted dorsally and the scaphoid anteriorly (DISI pattern).

Treatment

Scapho-lunate instability causes weakness of the wrist and recurrent discomfort. If seen early (i.e. less than 4 weeks after injury) the scapho-lunate ligament should be repaired directly with interosseous sutures, protected by K-wires for 6 weeks and a cast for 8–12 weeks. If seen between 4 and 24 weeks, then the

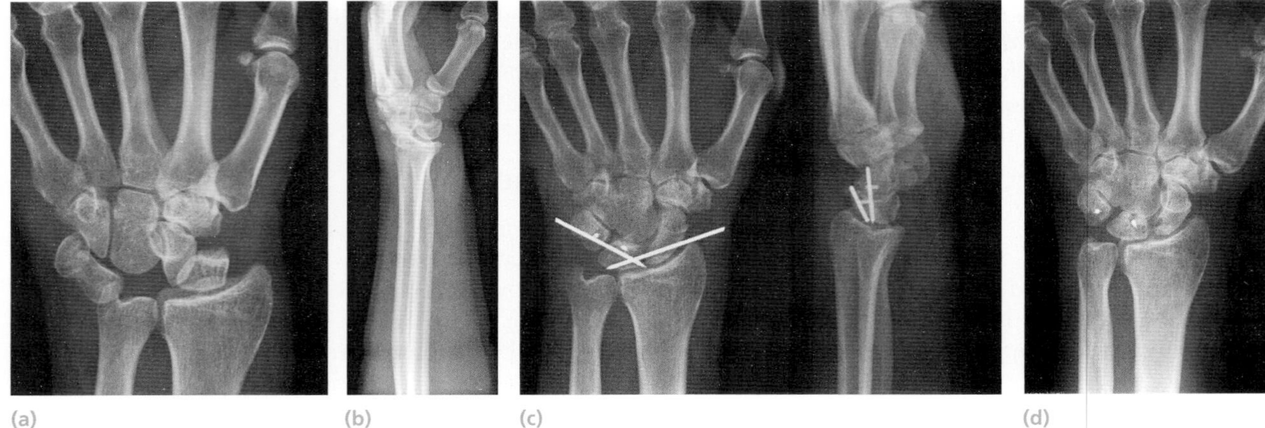

(a) (b) (c) (d)

25.26 Perilunate dislocation (a,b) Lunate still in its original position while the rest of the carpus is dislocated around it. (c) The dislocation has been reduced and held with K-wires. (d) The luno-triquetral ligament is re-attached with ligament anchors.

ligament is unlikely to heal. Blatt's capsulodesis is helpful: a proximally based flap of dorsal capsule is attached to the back of the scaphoid to haul it back from flexion into a normal position. In chronic lesions without secondary osteoarthritis, a capsulodesis or ligament reconstruction is attempted. If there is severe symptomatic osteoarthritis then a limited intercarpal arthrodesis or radio-carpal arthrodesis is performed.

Triquetro-lunate dissociation

A medial sprain followed by weakness of grip and tenderness distal to the head of the ulna should suggest disruption of the triquetro-lunate ligaments.

X-rays show a noticeable gap between the triquetrum and the lunate, with a VISI carpal collapse pattern in the lateral view.

Treatment

Acute tears should be repaired with interosseous sutures, supported by temporary K-wires for 6 weeks and a cast for 8–12 weeks. In chronic injuries, a ligament substitution (e.g. a slip of extensor carpi ulnaris) or a limited intercarpal fusion may be considered.

Radio-carpal dislocation

The most common injuries of this type involve a fracture of the anterior or posterior rim of the distal radius (Barton's fracture – see page 776). However, occasionally the ligaments which bind the carpus to the distal radius can rupture; the carpus tends to translate medially. Repair of the ligaments and temporary K-wire stabilization is needed.

Midcarpal dislocation

The extrinsic ligaments which bind the proximal to the distal row can rupture (there are, by definition, no intrinsic ligaments between these two rows). The diagnosis is difficult but is more readily suggested in those with generalized ligament laxity and a chronic wrist problem. The patient complains of a painful, recurrent snap in the wrist; the two rows can be passively 'clunked' apart when shifted backwards and forwards. If an acute ligament rupture is diagnosed, then repair and temporary K-wire stabilization should be carried out. In a chronic lesion, fusion of the proximal row to the distal row is the most effective treatment but this operation will restrict wrist movement and may predispose to later arthritis.

Hand injuries

26

David Warwick

Hand injuries – the commonest of all injuries – are important out of all proportion to their apparent severity, because of the need for perfect function. Nowhere else do painstaking evaluation, meticulous care and dedicated rehabilitation yield greater rewards. The outcome is often dependent upon the judgement of the doctor who first sees the patient.

If there is skin damage the patient should be examined in a clean environment with the hand displayed on sterile drapes.

A brief but searching history is obtained; often the mechanism of injury will suggest the type and severity of the trauma. The patient's age, occupation and 'handedness' should be recorded.

Superficial injuries and severe fractures are obvious, but deeper injuries are often poorly disclosed. It is important in the initial examination to assess the circulation, soft-tissue cover, bones, joints, nerves and tendons.

X-rays should include at least three views (postero-anterior, lateral and oblique), and with finger injuries the individual digit must be x-rayed.

GENERAL PRINCIPLES OF TREATMENT

Most hand injuries can be dealt with under local or regional anaesthesia; a general anaesthetic is only rarely required.

Circulation If the circulation is threatened, it must be promptly restored, if necessary by direct repair or vein grafting.

Swelling Swelling must be controlled by elevating the hand and by early and repeated active exercises.

Splintage Incorrect splintage is a potent cause of stiffness; it must be appropriate and it must be kept to a minimum length of time. If a finger has to be splinted, it may be possible simply to tape it to its neighbour so that both move as one; if greater security is needed, only the injured finger should be splinted. If the entire hand needs splinting, this must always be in the 'position of safety' – with the metacarpo-phalangeal joints flexed at least 70 degrees and the interphalangeal joints almost straight. Sometimes an external splint, to be effective, would need to immobilize undamaged fingers or would need to hold the joints of the injured finger in an unfavourable position (e.g. flexion of the interphalangeal joints). If so, internal fixation may be required (K-wires, screws or plates).

Skin cover Skin damage demands wound toilet followed by suture, skin grafting, local flaps, pedicled flaps or (occasionally) free flaps. Treatment of the skin takes precedence over treatment of the fracture.

Nerve and tendon injury Generally, the best results will follow primary repair of tendons and nerves. Occasionally grafts are required.

METACARPAL FRACTURES

The metacarpal bones are vulnerable to blows and falls upon the hand, or the longitudinal force of the boxer's punch. Injuries are common and the bones may fracture at their *base*, in the *shaft* or through the *neck*.

Angular deformity is usually not very marked, and even if it persists, it does not interfere much with

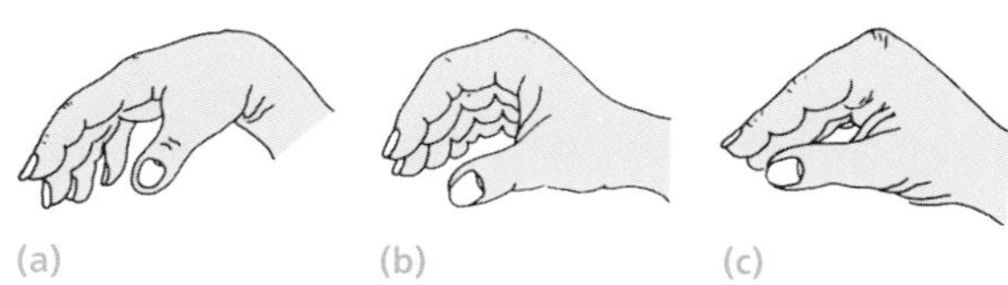

26.1 Splintage of the hand Three positions of the hand: (a) The position of relaxation, (b) the position of function (ready for action) and (c) the position of safe immobilization, with the ligaments taut.

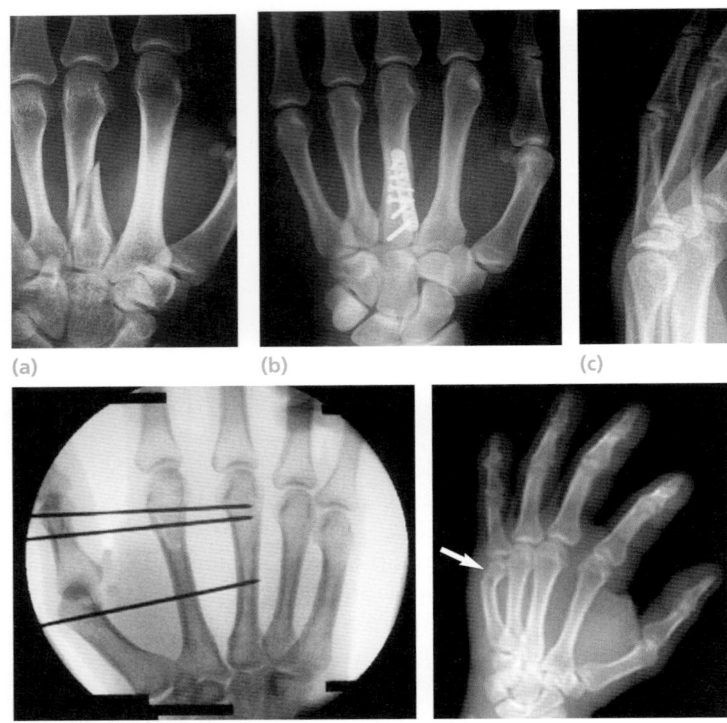

26.2 Metacarpal fractures (a) A spiral fracture (especially an 'inboard' one) can be adequately held by the surrounding muscles and ligaments but internal fixation (b) allows early mobilization. A displaced fracture (c), especially an 'outboard' one, can be held by a plate or transverse wires to allow early mobilization (d); multiple metacarpal fractures should be fixed with rigid plates for wires (e). A boxer's fracture (f) should be treated by early mobilization.

function. Rotational deformity, however, is serious. Close your hand with the distal phalanges extended, and look: the fingers converge across the palm to a point above the thenar eminence; malrotation of the metacarpal (or proximal phalanx) will cause that finger to diverge and overlap one of its neighbours. Thus, with a fractured metacarpal it is important to regain normal rotational alignment.

The fourth and fifth metacarpals are more mobile at their base than the second and third, and therefore are better able to compensate for residual angular deformity.

Fractures of the thumb metacarpal usually occur near the base and pose special problems. They are dealt with separately below.

Fractures of the metacarpal shaft

A direct blow may fracture one or several metacarpal shafts transversely, often with associated skin damage. A twisting or punching force may cause a spiral fracture of one or more shafts. There is local pain and swelling, and sometimes a dorsal 'hump'.

Treatment

Oblique or transverse fractures with slight displacement require no reduction. Splintage also is unnecessary, but a firm crepe bandage may be comforting; this should not be allowed to discourage the patient from active movements of the fingers, which should be practised assiduously. As the patient moves the fingers, the fracture may shorten until the intertacarpal ligaments between the metacarpal necks tighten, thus limiting further shortening and rotational deformity.

Transverse fractures with considerable displacement are reduced by traction and pressure. Reduction can sometimes be held by a plaster slab extending from the forearm over the fingers (only the damaged ones). The slab is maintained for 3 weeks and the undamaged fingers are exercised. However, these fractures are usually unstable and should be fixed surgically with compression plates or percutaneous K-wires placed either across the fracture or transversely through the neighbouring undamaged metacarpals.

Spiral fractures are liable to rotate; if so, they should be perfectly reduced and fixed with lag screws and a plate, or percutaneous wires.

Fractures of the metacarpal neck

A blow may fracture the metacarpal neck, usually of the fifth finger (the 'boxer's fracture') and occasionally one of the others. There may be local swelling, with flattening of the knuckle. X-rays show an impacted transverse fracture with volar angulation of the distal fragment.

Treatment

The main function of the *fifth and fourth fingers* is firm flexion ('power grip') and, as can be readily

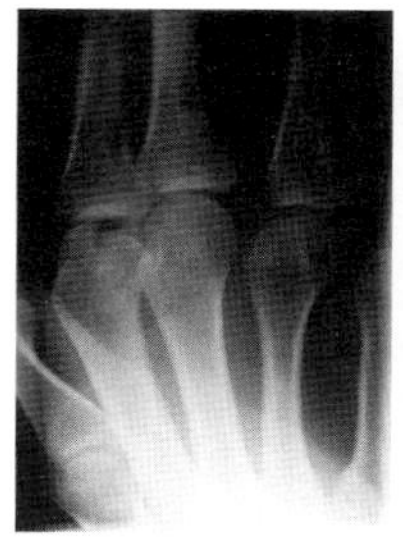

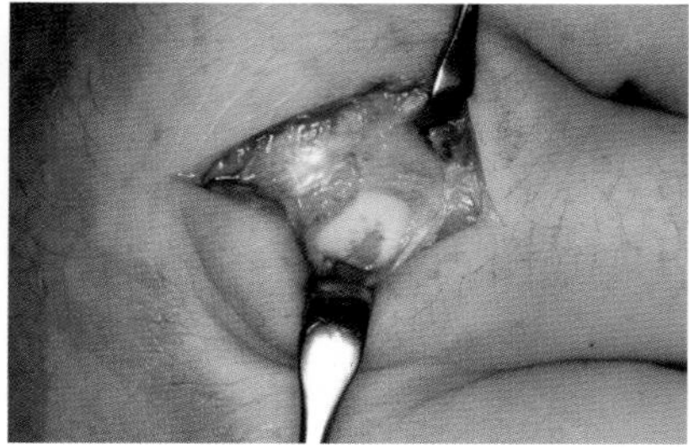

(a) (b)

26.3 Fracture of the metacarpal head (a) Depressed head fracture which was reduced and held with buried mini-screws. (b) A 'fight-bite', with metacarpal head damage from an opponent's tooth.

demonstrated on a normal hand, there is 'spare' extension available at the metacarpo-phalangeal (MCP) joint. Therefore in these digits, a flexion deformity of up to 40 degrees can be accepted; as long as there is no rotational deformity, a good outcome can be expected. The hand is immobilized in a gutter splint with the MCP joint flexed and the interphalangeal (IP) joints straight until discomfort settles – a week or two – and then the hand is mobilized. The patient is warned that the knuckle profile may be permanently lost. In the *index and middle fingers*, which function mainly in extension, no more than 20 degrees of flexion at the fracture is acceptable.

If the fracture needs reduction, this can be done under a local block. The reduced finger is held with a gutter splint moulded at three points to support the fracture; the MCP joints are flexed and the IP joints are straight. Unfortunately, these fractures are usually fairly unstable because of the tone of the flexor tendons and the palmar comminution of the fracture. If there is a tendency to redisplacement, fixation should be used. Plates are not really suitable because the fracture is so distal. A bouquet of two or three bent wires passed distally through a hole in the styloid process of the fifth metacarpal base is particularly effective.

Complications

Malunion, with volar angulation of the distal fragment, is poorly tolerated if this occurs in the second or third rays. The patient may be aware of a bump in the palm from the prominent metacarpal head and the digit may take on a 'Z' appearance as the knuckle joint hyperextends to compensate for the deformity.

FRACTURES OF THE METACARPAL HEAD

These fractures occur after a direct blow. They are often quite comminuted and sometimes 'open'. Operative reduction is usually required and fixation with small headless buried screws is ideal. Occasionally the joint is so badly damaged that primary replacement is considered (Silastic, pyrocarbon or polythene–metal).

FRACTURES OF THE METACARPAL BASE

Excepting fractures of the thumb metacarpal, these are usually stable injuries which can be treated by ensuring that rotation is correct and then splinting the digit in a volar slab extending from the forearm to the proximal finger joint. The splint is retained for 3 weeks and exercises are then encouraged.

Displaced intra-articular fractures of the base of the fourth or fifth metacarpal may cause marked incongruity of the joint. This is a mobile joint and it may, therefore, be painful. The fracture should be reduced by traction on the little finger and then held with a percutaneous K-wire or compression screw. In the long term, if painful arthritis supervenes, treatment would be with either arthrodesis or joint excision.

FRACTURE OF THE THUMB METACARPAL

Three types of fracture are encountered: impacted fracture of the metacarpal base; Bennett's fracture-dislocation of the carpo-metacarpal (CMC) joint; and Rolando's comminuted fracture of the base.

Impacted fracture

A boxer may, while punching, sustain a fracture of the base of the first metacarpal. Localized swelling and tenderness are found, and x-ray shows a transverse fracture about 6 mm distal to the CMC joint, with outward bowing and impaction.

Treatment If the angulation is less than 20–30 degrees and the fragments are impacted, the thumb is rested in a plaster of Paris cast extending from the forearm to just short of the interphalangeal thumb joint with the thumb fully abducted and extended. The cast is removed after 2–3 weeks and the thumb is mobilized.

If the angulation is greater than 30 degrees, then the reduced thumb web span will be noticeable and so the fracture should be reduced. The surgeon pulls on the abducted thumb and, by levering the metacarpal outwards against his own thumb, corrects the bowing. A plaster cast is applied. If the fracture is still unstable, then a percutaneous K-wire is inserted. An alternative would be a low profile plate.

Bennett's fracture-dislocation

This fracture, too, occurs at the base of the first metacarpal bone and is commonly due to punching; however the fracture is oblique, extends into the CMC joint and is unstable.

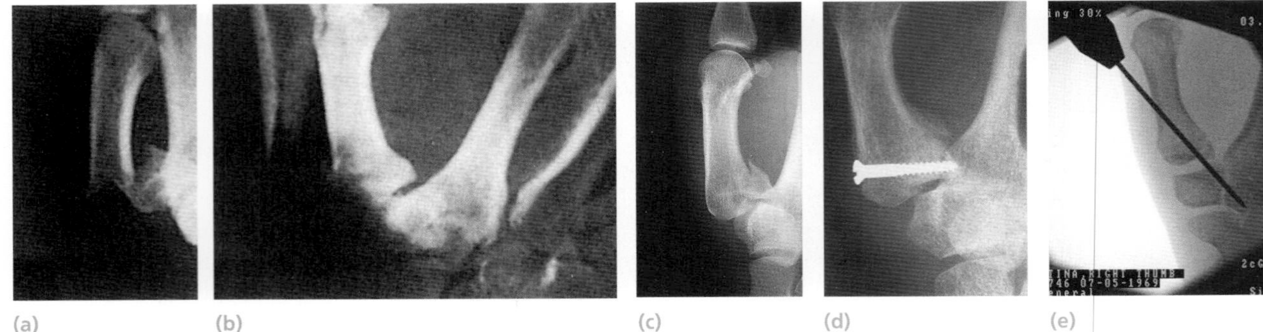

26.4 Fractures of the first metacarpal base A transverse fracture (a) can be reduced and held in plaster (b). Bennett's fracture-dislocation (c) is best held with a small screw (d) or a percutaneous K-wire (e).

The thumb looks short and the carpo-metacarpal region swollen. X-rays show that a small triangular fragment has remained in contact with the medial edge of the trapezium, while the remainder of the thumb has subluxated proximally, pulled upon by the abductor pollicis longus tendon.

Treatment It is widely supposed (with little evidence) that perfect reduction is essential. It should, however, be attempted and can usually be achieved by pulling on the thumb, abducting it and extending it. Reduction can then be held in one of two ways: plaster or internal fixation.

Plaster may be applied with a felt pad over the fracture, and the first metacarpal held abducted and extended (usually best achieved by *flexing* the MCP joint). However, plaster only works if it is applied with great skill, and the pressure required to maintain a reduction can cause skin damage; it has, therefore, generally been abandoned in favour of surgery.

Surgical fixation is achieved by passing a K-wire across the metacarpal base into the carpus. If the fragment is large and cannot be reduced and held with a wire, then open reduction and fixation with a lag screw is effective.

ROLANDO'S FRACTURE

This is an intra-articular comminuted fracture of the base of the first metacarpal with a T or Y configuration. Closed reduction and K-wiring or open reduction and plate fixation can be used. With more severe comminution, external fixation is needed.

METACARPAL FRACTURES IN CHILDREN

Metacarpal fractures are less common in children than in adults. In general they also present fewer problems: the vast majority can be treated by manipulation and plaster splintage; angular deformities will almost always be remodelled with further growth. However, rotational alignment is as important as it is in adults.

Bennett's fracture is rare; but when it does occur it usually requires open reduction. This is, by definition, a Salter-Harris type III fracture-separation of the physis; it must be accurately reduced and fixed with a K-wire.

FRACTURES OF THE PHALANGES

The fingers are usually injured by direct violence, and there may be considerable swelling or open wounds. Injudicious treatment may result in a stiff finger which, in some cases, can be worse than no finger.

FRACTURES OF THE PROXIMAL AND MIDDLE PHALANGEAL SHAFTS

The phalanx may fracture in various ways:

- *Transverse fracture of the shaft*, often with forward angulation.
- *Spiral fracture of the shaft*, from a twisting injury.
- *Comminuted fracture*, usually due to a crush injury and often associated with significant tendon damage and skin loss.
- *Avulsion* of a small fragment of bone.
- *Metaphyseal fracture* at the base of the proximal phalanx, commonly seen in osteopaenic bone. The shaft is pulled into extension and at the distal end the entire head may displace. This is most commonly seen in children.
- *Intra-articular fractures:* At the distal end of the phalanx, the entire head may rotate or, more commonly, one condyle rotates through a longitudinal midline fracture into the joint. At the proximal end, displacement tends to lead to an angular deformity.

Treatment

UNDISPLACED FRACTURES

These can be treated by 'functional splintage'. The finger is strapped to its neighbour ('buddy strapping')

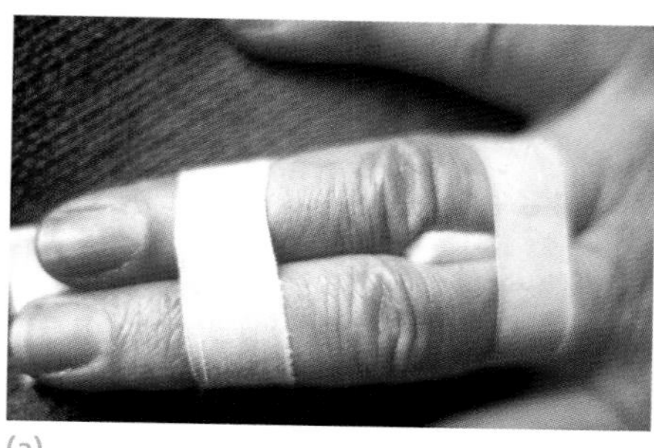
(a)

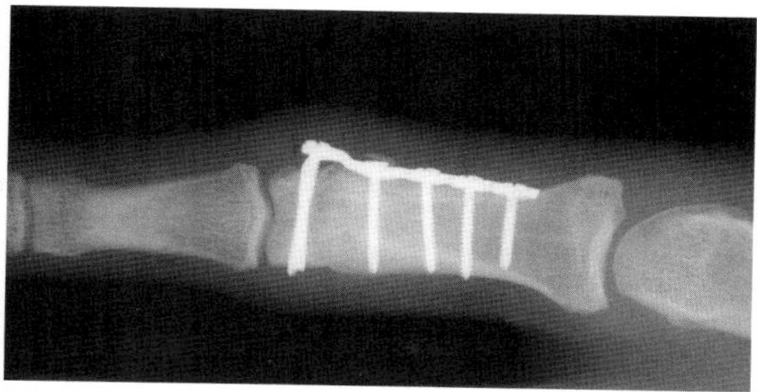
(b)

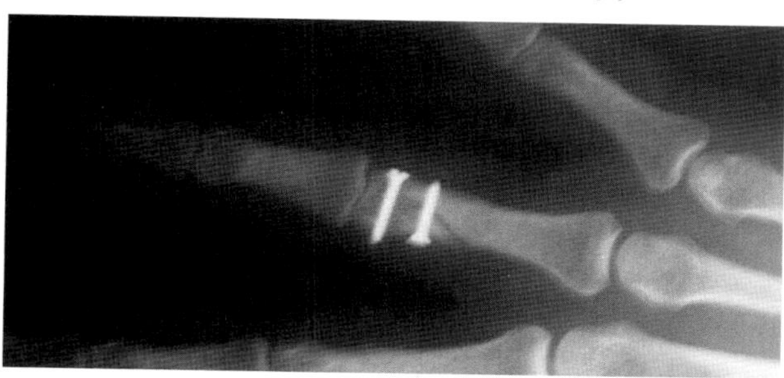
(c)

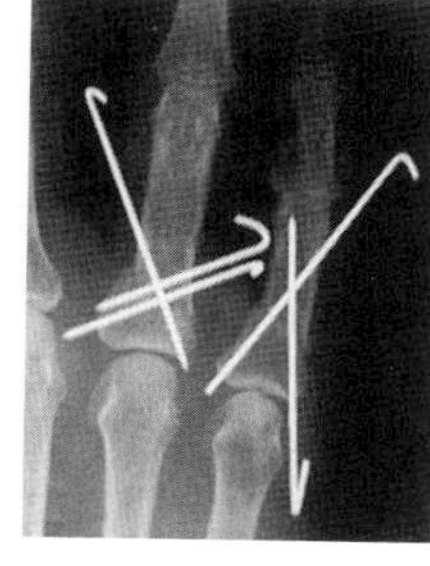
(d)

26.5 Phalangeal fractures These can be treated, depending on the 'personality' of the fracture, experience of the surgeon and equipment available, with neighbour strapping (a), plate fixation (b), percutaneous screw fixation (c) or percutaneous wires (d).

and movements are encouraged from the outset. Splintage is retained for 2–3 weeks, but during this time it is wise to check the position by x-ray in case displacement has occurred.

DISPLACED FRACTURES

Displaced fractures must be reduced and immobilized. *It is essential to check for rotational correction* by (1) noting the convergent position of the finger when the MCP joint is flexed, and (2) seeing that the fingernails are all in the same plane. The technique depends on the fracture pattern. Most need simple manipulation and can then be held in a splint. *Basal fractures* with extension are manipulated and held with a dorsal blocking splint with the MCP joint at 90 degrees. *Angulated basal fractures* are manipulated with a pencil between the digits as a lever and then held with neighbour strapping which pulls the injured finger to the next one. *Spiral fractures* are held with 'de-rotation taping' to the next digit, using tension in the tape to unwind the fracture. Transverse fractures may be held in a gutter splint or neighbour splint.

If a reduction cannot be achieved, or if it is unstable and the position slips, then surgery is needed. The technique depends upon the configuration of the fracture. *K-wires* are less invasive and are perfect for some fractures; other techniques include *percutaneous lag screw* fixation (for spiral fractures and distal condylar fractures) and *plate fixation* (which risks stiffness in the proximal phalanx due to the soft-tissue exposure and subsequent tendon adhesion). *External fixation* may be needed for comminuted fractures.

CHILDHOOD FRACTURES

In children the phalangeal neck can be broken, often after a crush injury. The distal fragment displaces dorsally and extends. These are serious injuries and should be reduced as soon as possible and then held with a percutaneous wire.

Fractures of the terminal phalanx

The terminal phalanx, small though it is, is subject to five different types of fracture.

Fracture of the tuft

The tip of the finger may be struck by a hammer or caught in a door, and the bone shattered. The fracture is disregarded and treatment is focused on controlling swelling and regaining movement. The painful haematoma beneath the finger nail should be drained by piercing the nail with a hot paper clip. If the nail bed is shattered and cosmesis is important, it should be meticulously repaired under magnification.

Mallet finger injury

After a sudden flexion injury (e.g. stubbing the tip of the finger) the terminal phalanx droops and cannot be straightened actively. Three types of injury are recognized: avulsion of the most distal part of the extensor tendon; avulsion of a small flake of bone from the base of the terminal phalanx; and avulsion of a large dorsal

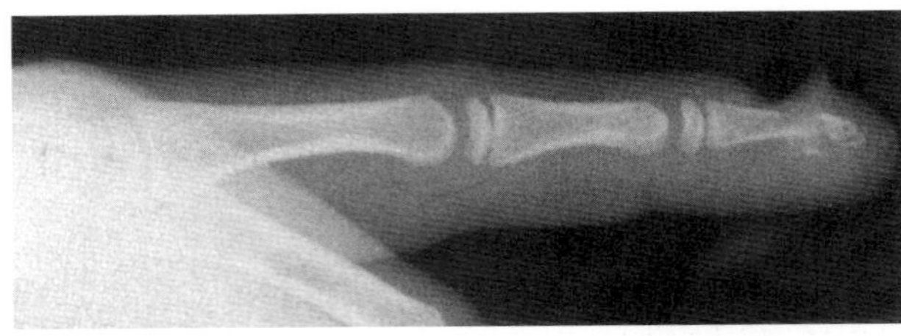

(a)

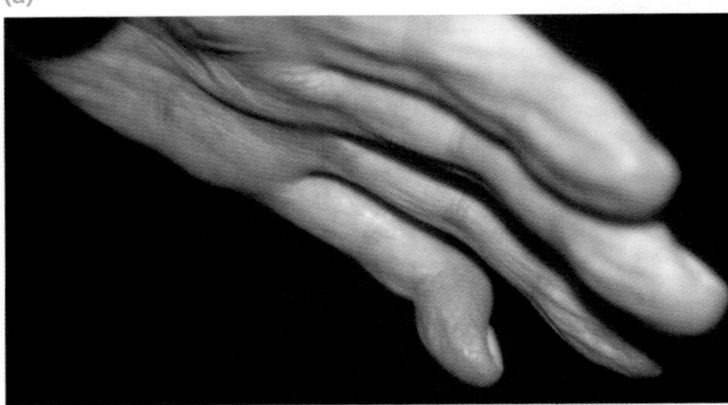

(c)

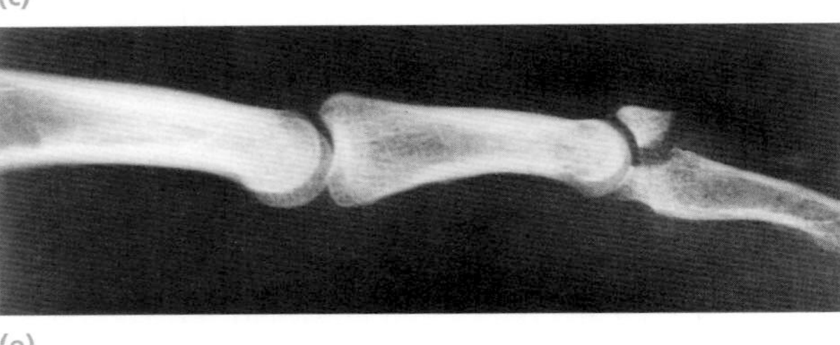

(e)

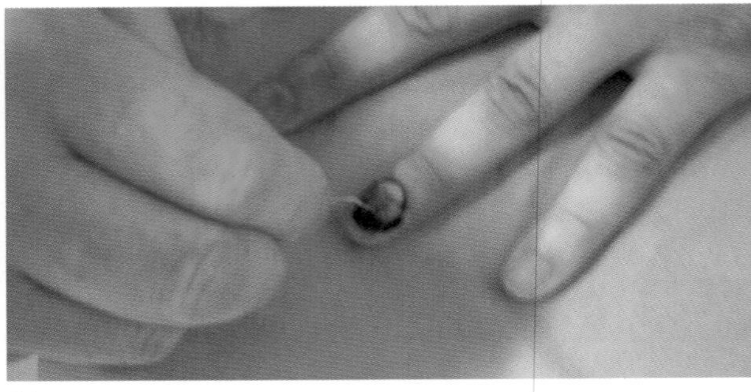

(b)

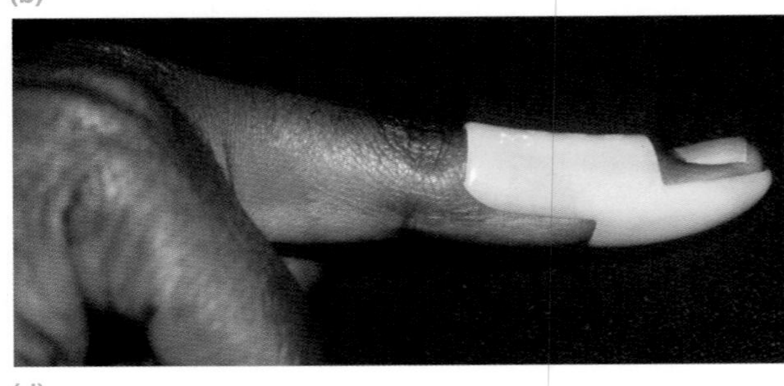

(d)

26.6 Distal phalangeal injury A fracture of the tuft (a), caused by a hammer blow, is treated by a protective dressing. The subungual haematoma should be evacuated using a red-hot paper clip tip (b) or a small drill. A mallet finger (c) is best treated with a splint for 6 weeks (d). Mallet fractures (e) are also better splinted – surgery can make the outcome worse.

bone fragment, sometimes with subluxation of the terminal interphalangeal (TIP) joint.

TREATMENT

The TIP joint should be immobilized in slight hyperextension, using a special mallet-finger splint which fixes the distal joint but leaves the proximal joints free.

For tendinous avulsions (which usually occur painlessly) the splint should be kept in place constantly for 8 weeks and then only at night for another 4 weeks. Even if there has been a delay of 3 or 4 weeks after injury, this prolonged splintage is usually successful.

Bone avulsions are also treated in a splint, but 6 weeks should suffice as bone heals quicker than tendon. Operative treatment is generally avoided, even for large bone fragments, unless there is subluxation. Surgery carries a high complication rate (wound failure, metalwork problems) without evidence that the outcome is improved. However, if there is subluxation then K-wires or small screws are used to fix the fragment in place.

COMPLICATIONS OF MALLET FINGER

Non-union This is usually painless and treatment is not needed.

Persistent droop About 85 per cent of mallet fingers recover full extension. If there is a persistent droop this can be treated by tendon repair supported by K-wire fixation of the joint, but the results are often disappointing. The alternative would be joint arthrodesis, best achieved with a buried intramedullary double-pitch screw.

Swan neck deformity Imbalance of the extensor mechanism can cause this in lax-jointed individuals. A central slip tenotomy is straightforward and can give a very good result.

Fracture of the terminal shaft

Undisplaced fractures of the shaft need no treatment apart from analgesia. If angulated, they should be reduced and held with a longitudinal K-wire through the pulp for 4 weeks. The nail is often dislocated from its fold; if so it must be carefully tucked back in and held with a suture in each corner.

Avulsion of the flexor tendon

This injury is caused by sudden hyperextension of the distal joint, typically when a game player catches his

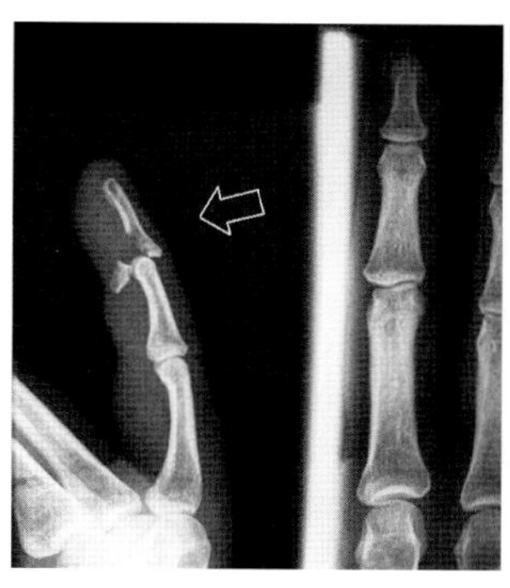

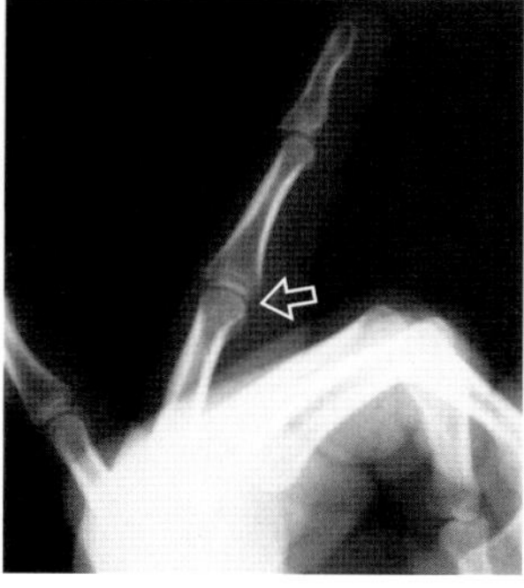

(a) (b)

26.7 Flexor tendon avulsion (a) Large fragment and (b) smaller fragment lodged in front of the PIP joint.

finger on an opponent's shirt. The ring finger is most commonly affected. The flexor digitorum profundus tendon is avulsed, either rupturing the tendon itself or taking a fragment of bone with it. If the bone fragment is small, or if only the tendon is ruptured, it can recoil into the palm. If the lesion is detected within a few days (and the diagnosis is easily missed if not thought about), then the tendon can be re-attached. If the diagnosis is much delayed, repair is likely to be unsuccessful. Two-stage tendon reconstruction is possible but difficult, and the finger may end up stiff. Thus, for late cases, tenodesis or fusion of the distal joint is usually preferable.

Physeal fracture

The basal physis can break, usually producing a Salter–Harris I fracture (Seymour fracture). The nail may be dislocated from its fold and the germinal matrix can be trapped in the fracture. The injury is easily overlooked if the finger is very swollen. The nail must be cleaned and carefully replaced into its bed.

JOINT INJURIES

Any finger joint may be injured by a direct blow (often the overlying skin is damaged), or by an angulation force, or by the straight finger being forcibly stubbed. The affected joint is swollen, tender and too painful to move. X-rays may show that a fragment of bone has been sheared off or avulsed.

Carpo-metacarpal dislocation

The thumb is most frequently affected and clinically the injury then resembles a Bennett's fracture-dislocation; however, x-rays reveal proximal subluxation or dislocation of the first metacarpal bone without a fracture. The displacement is easily reduced by traction and hyperpronation, but reduction is unstable and can be held only by a K-wire driven through the metacarpal into the carpus. The wire is removed after 5 weeks but a protective splint should be worn for 8 weeks because of the risk of instability.

Chronic instability can occur. This is treated prior to arthritis developing, by using part of the flexor carpi radialis tendon to reconstruct the ruptured and incompetent palmar ligament of the CMC joint.

The other carpo-metacarpal joints are also sometimes dislocated, typically when a motorcyclist, holding the handlebars, strikes an object and the hand is driven backwards. The hand swells up rapidly and the diagnosis is easily missed unless a true lateral x-ray is carefully examined. Closed manipulation is usually successful, although a K-wire is recommended to prevent the joint from dislocating again.

Late presentation Late presentation or secondary arthritis is treated by joint fusion. However, if just the fifth CMC joint is involved, a neat operation is to fuse the base of the fourth to the fifth metacarpal and then excise the articular surface of the fifth. This will maintain movement at the fourth CMC, so allowing the ulnar side of the hand to 'cup' around during grip.

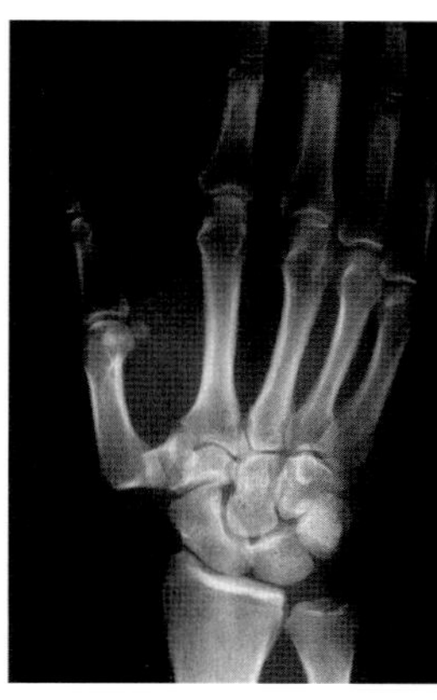

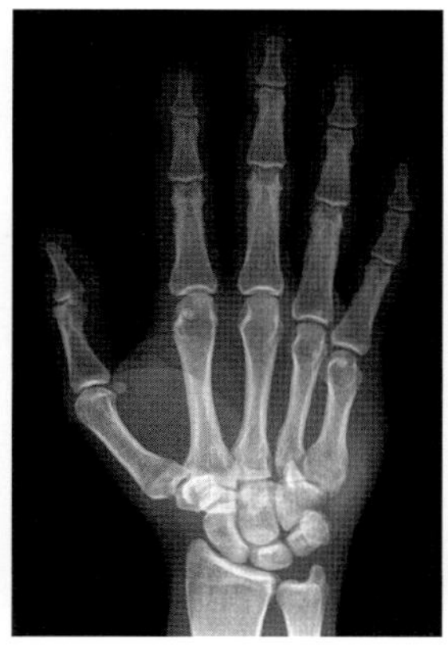

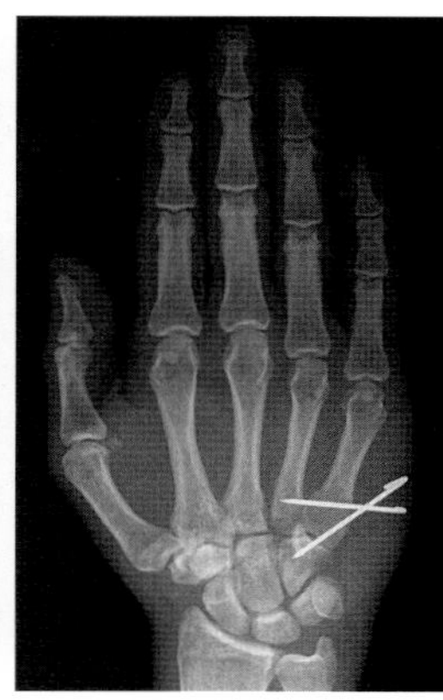

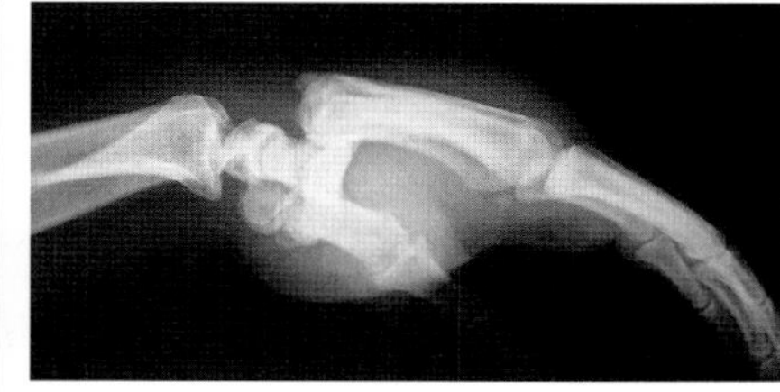

(a) (b) (c) (d)

26.8 Carpo-metacarpal dislocation (a) Thumb dislocation. (b) Dislocation of the fourth and fifth CMC joints treated by closed reduction and K-wires (c). Complete carpo-metacarpal dislocation (d).

METACARPO-PHALANGEAL DISLOCATION

Usually the thumb is affected, sometimes the fifth finger, and rarely the other fingers. The entire finger is suddenly forced into hyperextension and the capsule and muscle insertions in front of the joint may be torn. There are two types of dislocation:

Simple dislocation The finger is extended about 75 degrees. It is easily reduced by traction, firstly in hyperextension then pulling the finger around. The finger is strapped to its neighbour and early mobilization is encouraged.

Complex dislocation The avulsed palmar plate sits in the joint, blocking reduction. Furthermore, the metacarpal head can be clasped between the flexor tendon and lumbrical tendon. The finger is extended only about 30 degrees and there is usually a tell-tale dimple in the palm. Very occasionally the fracture can be reduced closed by hyperextending the MCP joint and flexing the IP joints to release the clasp. If this fails, open reduction is required. A dorsal approach is safest. After reduction the joint is stable and should be mobilized in a neighbour-splint.

Chronic instability in the thumb MCP joint This is treated by a sesamoid arthrodesis. The abductor sesamoid is fused to the underside of the metacarpal neck. This preserves some flexion yet prevents hyperextension. An alternative is formal arthrodesis. The use of a low-profile compression plate allows early mobilization. The functional result is usually very good.

INTERPHALANGEAL JOINT DISLOCATION

Distal joint dislocation is rare; proximal joint dislocation is more common. The dislocation is easily reduced by pulling. The joint is strapped to its neighbour for a few days and movements are begun immediately. The lateral x-ray may show a small flake of bone, representing a palmar plate avulsion; this should be ignored. The patient must be warned that it can take many months (and sometimes forever) for the spindle-like swelling of the joint to settle and for full extension to recover. If there is a large palmar fragment with displacement, then this should be reduced and fixed. If closed reduction is successful, then an extension splint or temporary transarticular wire is used. If it cannot be reduced or remains unstable then screw fixation or a small wire loop can be used. If there is marked comminution and instability, the joint is exposed from the palmar surface, the damaged fragments are excised and the palmar plate is reattached to the base of the proximal phalanx ('palmar-plate arthroplasty').

'PILON' FRACTURES OF THE MIDDLE PHALANX

These are quite common injuries and can be very troublesome. The head of the proximal phalanx impacts into the base of the middle phalanx, causing the latter to splay open in several pieces. These injuries are best treated with dynamic distraction using a spring-loaded external fixator which rotates around the head of the proximal phalanx and disimpacts the distal fragment. The results can be surprisingly good.

CONDYLAR FRACTURE

The basal joint surface or distal joint surface of the phalanges can be fractured, usually by an angulation force. If the fragment is not displaced, it is best to disregard the fracture, strap the finger to its neighbour and concentrate on regaining movement. An x-ray should be taken after a week to ensure there is no displacement.

If the fracture is displaced, there is a risk of permanent angular deformity and loss of movement at the joint. The fracture should be anatomically reduced, either closed or by open operation and fixed with small K-wires or mini-screws. The finger is splinted for a few days and then supervised movements are commenced.

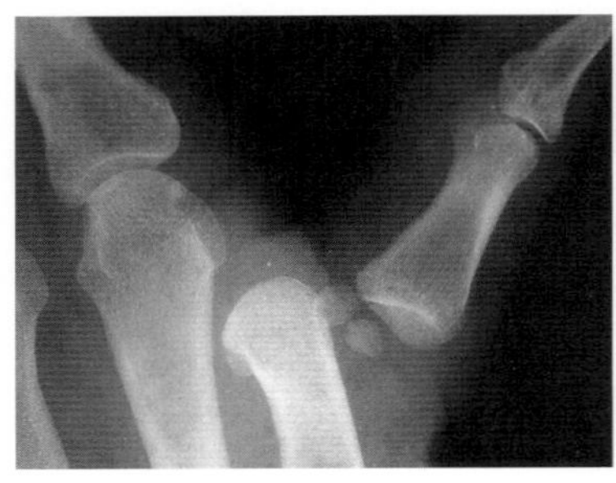
(a)

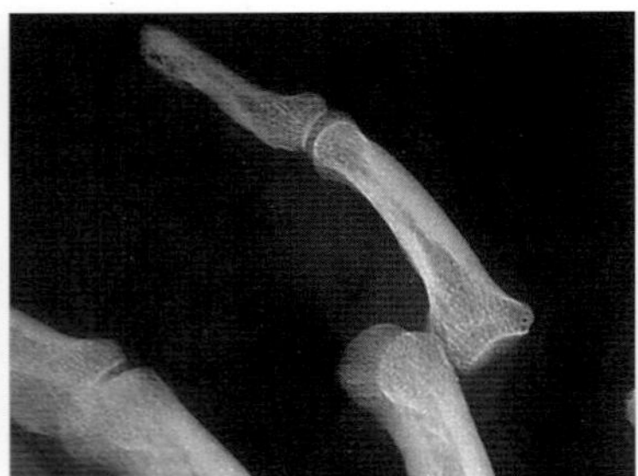
(b)

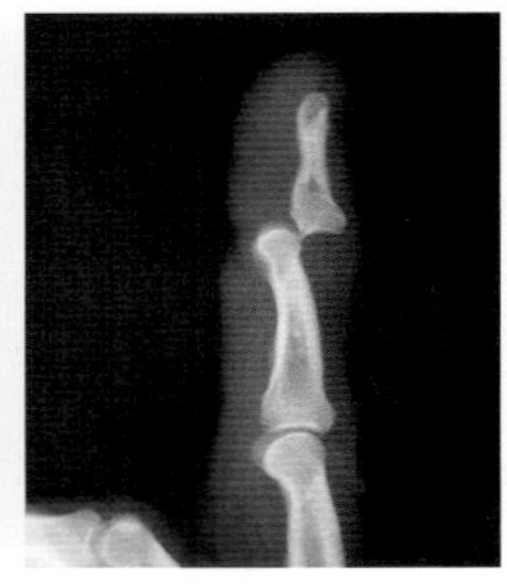
(c)

26.9 Finger dislocation **(a)** Metacarpo-phalangeal dislocation in the thumb occasionally buttonholes and needs open reduction; **(b,c)** interphalangeal dislocations are easily reduced (and easily missed if not x-rayed!).

Volar fracture-dislocations

When the proximal interphalangeal joint dislocates, a fragment of bone may be avulsed from the base of the middle phalanx. If this fragment is large, the joint can subluxate forwards. Surgical fixation is very difficult and can lead to permanent stiffness of the joint. The fracture can be reduced by flexing the joint to 40 degrees. The joint is then held in a splint which allows flexion but not extension. The amount of extension block is reduced over the next 4 weeks and the splint is then discarded. If the fragment is large enough, then miniscrew fixation may be attempted, but failure of fixation, tendon adhesion or joint stiffness are risks.

LIGAMENT INJURIES

Proximal interphalangeal ligaments

Partial or complete tears of the proximal interphalangeal ligaments are quite common, due to forced angulation of the joint. *Mild sprains* require no treatment but with more severe injuries the finger should be splinted in extension for 2 or 3 weeks, If the joint is frankly unstable, especially the index and middle which oppose load from the thumb, repair is considered.

Occasionally, the bone to which the ligament is attached is avulsed; if the fragment is markedly displaced (and large enough), it should be re-attached. The patient must be warned that the joint is likely to remain swollen and slightly painful for at least 6–12 months. If the instability persists – which is rare – it can be treated by using spare tendon (e.g. palmaris longus) for reconstruction.

Metacarpo-phalangeal joints

The radial collateral ligament of the index finger is most vulnerable, although with a suitable force any ligament can be injured. The tension of the ligament is tested with the MP joint flexed (if extended, even a normal ligament is very lax!).

In children, the injury may be accompanied by a Salter–Harris III fracture at the base of the proximal phalanx.

A large bone fragment, if displaced, can be re-attached from a palmar approach, using a tension band suture or small screw. Smaller fragments are treated by splintage with the MP joints flexed.

Ulnar collateral ligament of the thumb metacarpo-phalangeal joint ('gamekeeper's thumb'; 'skier's thumb')

In former years, gamekeepers who twisted the necks of little animals ran the risk of tearing the ulnar collateral ligament of the thumb metacarpo-phalangeal joint, either acutely or as a chronic injury. Nowadays this injury is seen in skiers who fall onto the extended thumb, forcing it into hyperabduction. A small flake of bone may be pulled off at the same time. The resulting loss of stability may interfere markedly with prehensile (pinching) activities.

The ulnar collateral ligament inserts partly into the palmar plate. In a *partial rupture*, only the ligament proper is torn and the thumb is unstable in flexion but still more or less stable in full extension because the palmar plate is intact. In a *complete rupture*, both the ligament proper and the palmar plate are torn and the thumb is unstable in all positions. If the ligament ruptures completely (usually at its distal attachment to the base of the proximal phalanx), it will not heal unless it is repaired; this is because the proximal end gets trapped in front of the adductor pollicis aponeurosis (the Stener lesion).

Clinical assessment

On examination there is tenderness and swelling precisely over the ulnar side of the thumb metacarpo-

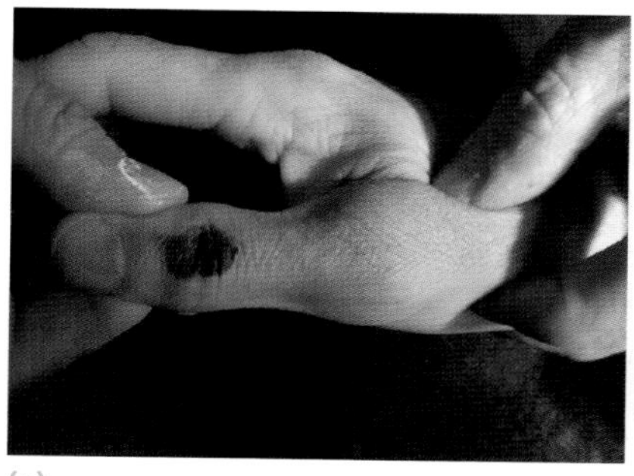
(a)

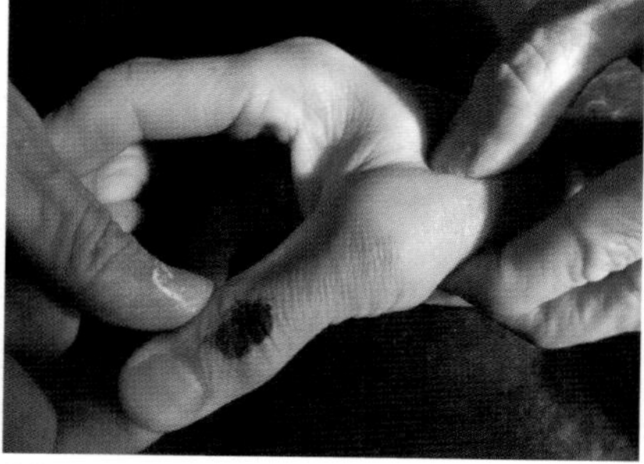
(b)

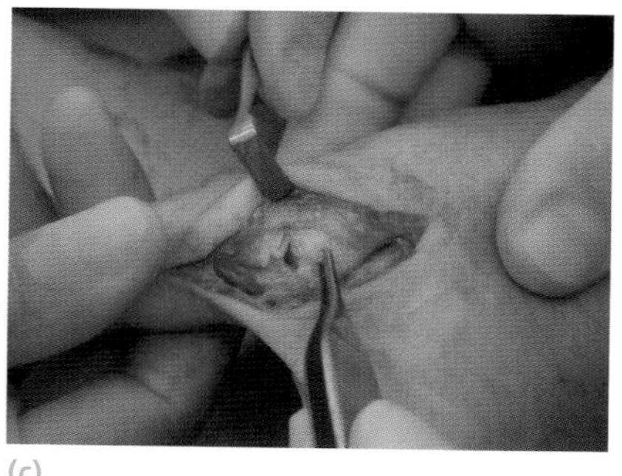
(c)

26.10 Skier's thumb (a,b) The ulnar collateral ligament has ruptured. Urgent repair is indicated (c).

phalangeal joint. *An x-ray is essential, to exclude a fracture before carrying out any stress tests.* Laxity is often obvious but if in doubt, then the joint can be examined under local anaesthetic. If there is no undue laxity (compare with the normal side) in both extension and 30 degrees flexion, then a serious injury can be excluded. If there is more than a few degrees of laxity there is probably a complete rupture which will require operative repair.

Treatment

Partial tears can be treated by a short period (2–4 weeks) of immobilization in a splint followed by increasing movement. Pinch should be avoided for 6–8 weeks.

Complete tears need operative repair. Care should be taken during the exposure not to injure the superficial radial nerve branches. The Stener lesion is found at the proximal edge of the adductor aponeurosis. The aponeurosis is incised and retracted to expose the ligaments and capsule and the torn structures are then carefully repaired. Postoperatively, the joint is immobilized in a thumb splint for 6 weeks, but can be moved early in the flexion–extension plane as the ligament is isometric (i.e. the same length in flexion and extension). The thumb interphalangeal joint should be left free from the outset to avoid the adductor aponeurosis becoming adherent (which would limit flexion). A neglected tear leads to weakness of pinch. In early cases without articular damage, stability may be restored by using a free tendon graft. If this fails, or if the joint is painful, MP joint arthrodesis is reliable and leaves minimal functional deficit.

In children, the injury may be accompanied by a Salter–Harris Type III fracture through the physis. This should be reduced and fixed with smooth K-wires which should not cross the growth plate.

OPEN INJURIES OF THE HAND

Over 75 per cent of work injuries affect the hands; inadequate treatment costs the patient (and society) dear in terms of functional disability.

Clinical assessment

Open injuries comprise tidy or 'clean' cuts, lacerations, crushing and injection injuries, burns and pulp defects.

The precise *mechanism of injury* must be understood. Was the instrument sharp or blunt? Clean or dirty? The position of the fingers (flexed or extended) at the time of injury will influence the relative damage to the deep and superficial flexor tendons. A history of high pressure injection predicts major soft-tissue damage, however innocuous the wound may seem. What are the patient's occupation, hobbies and aspirations? Is he or she right-handed or left-handed?

Examination should be gentle and painstaking. *Skin damage* is important, but it should be remembered that even a tiny, clean cut may conceal nerve or tendon damage.

The circulation to the hand and each digit must be assessed. The Allen test can be applied to the hand as a whole or to an individual finger. The radial and ulnar arteries at the wrist are simultaneously compressed by the examiner while the patient clenches his fist for several seconds before relaxing; the hand should now be pale. The radial artery is then released; if the hand flushes it means that the radial blood supply is intact. The test is repeated for the ulnar artery. An injured finger can be assessed in the same way. The digital arteries are occluded by pinching the base of the finger. When blood is squeezed out of the finger the pulp will become noticeably pale; one digital artery is then released and the pulp should pink up; the test is repeated for the other digital artery.

Sensation is tested in the territory of each nerve. *Two-point discrimination* may be reduced in partial injuries. In children, who are more difficult to examine, the *plastic pen* test is helpful: if a plastic pen is brushed along the skin it will tend to 'stick' due to the normal thin layer of sweat on the surface; absence of sweating (due to a nerve injury) is revealed by noting that the pen does not adhere as it should (compared to the normal side). Another observation is that the skin in the territory of a divided nerve will not *wrinkle* if immersed in water.

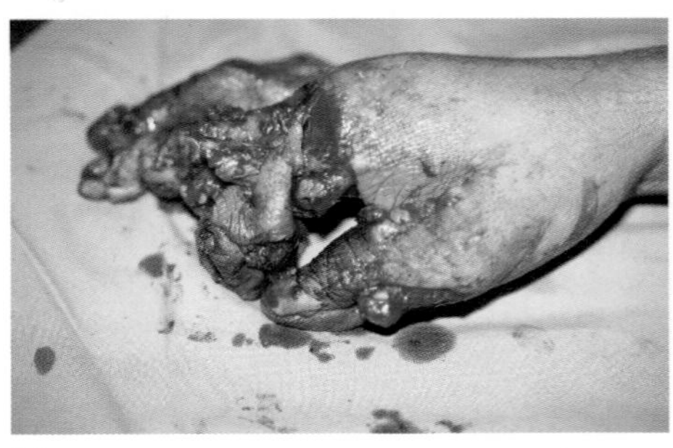

(a)

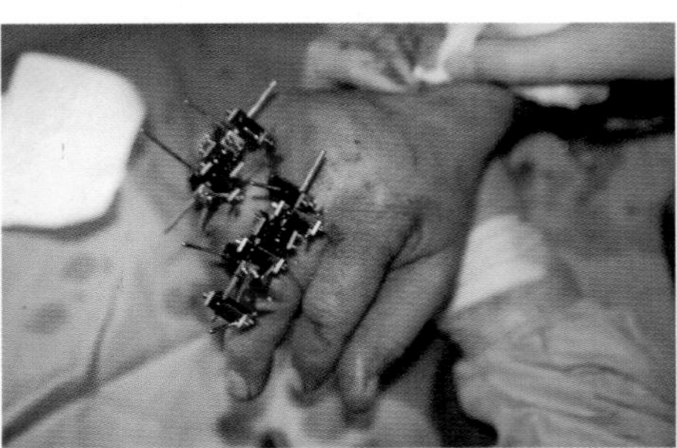

(b)

26.11 Open injuries (a) A mangled hand; **(b)** open finger fracture treated with external fixation.

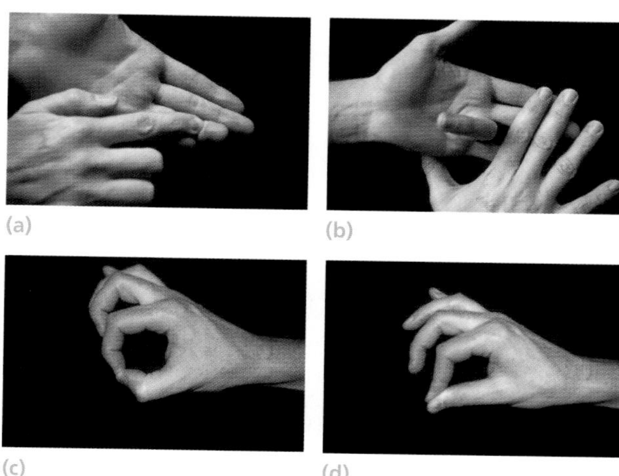

26.12 Testing the flexor tendons Testing for (a) flexor digitorum profundus (FDP) lesser fingers, (b) flexor digitorum superficialis (FDS) lesser fingers, (c) FDP index, (d) FDS index.

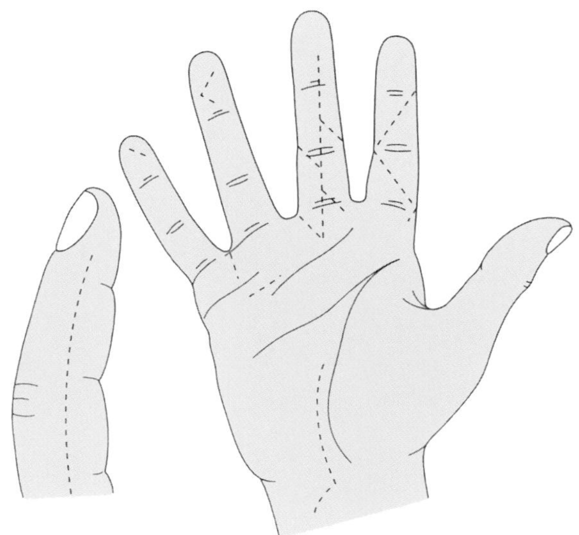

26.13 Hand incisions 'Permissable' incisions in hand surgery. Incisions must not cross a skin crease or an interdigital web or else scarring may cause contracture and deformity.

Tendons must be examined with similar care. Start by testing for 'passive tenodesis'. When the wrist is extended passively, the fingers automatically flex in a gentle and regular cascade; when the wrist is flexed, the fingers fall into extension. These actions rely upon the balanced tension of the opposing flexor and extensor tendons to the fingers; if a tendon is cut, the cascade will be disturbed.

Active movements are then tested for each individual tendon. Flexor digitorum profundus is tested by holding the proximal finger joint straight and instructing the patient to bend the distal joint. Flexor digitorum superficialis is tested by the examiner holding all the fingers together out straight, then releasing one and asking the patient to bend the proximal joint. Holding the fingers out straight 'immobilizes' all the deep flexors (including that of the finger being tested) which have a common muscle belly. However, in the index finger this test is not 100 per cent reliable because the deep flexor is sometimes separate. It is better to ask the patient to make a 'circle' between thumb and index (FDP intact) and a 'buttonhole' (FDS intact).

If a tendon is only partly divided, it will still work although it may be painful. In full thickness skin lacerations, if there is any doubt about the integrity of the tendons, the wound should be explored.

X-rays may show fractures, foreign bodies, air or paint.

Primary treatment

PREOPERATIVE CARE

The patient may need treatment for pain and shock. If the wound is contaminated, it should be rinsed with sterile crystalloid; antibiotics should be given as soon as possible. Prophylaxis against tetanus and gas gangrene may also be needed. The hand is lightly splinted and the wound is covered with an iodine-soaked dressing.

WOUND EXPLORATION

Under general or regional anaesthesia, the wound is cleaned and explored. A pneumatic tourniquet is essential unless there is a crush injury where muscle viability is in doubt. Skin is too precious to waste and only obviously dead skin should be excised. For adequate exposure the wound may need enlarging, but incisions must not cross a skin crease or an interdigital web. Through the enlarged wound, loose debris is picked out, dead muscle is excised and the tissues are thoroughly irrigated with isotonic crystalloid solution. A further assessment of the extent of the injury is then undertaken.

TISSUE REPAIR

Fractures are reduced and held appropriately (splintage, K-wires, external fixator or plate and screws) unless there is some specific contraindication.

Joint capsule and ligaments are repaired.

Artery and vein repair may be needed if the hand or finger is ischaemic. This done with the aid of an operating microscope. Any gap should be bridged with a vein graft.

Severed nerves are sutured under an operating microscope (or at least loupe magnification) with the finest, non-reactive material. If the repair cannot be achieved without tension then a nerve graft (e.g. from the posterior interosseous nerve at the wrist) should

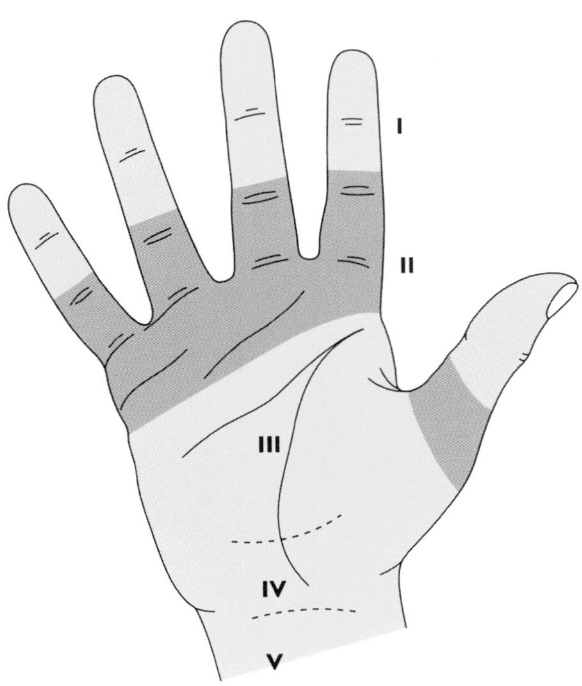

26.14 The zones of injury I – Distal to the insertion of flexor digitorum superficialis. II – Between the opening of the flexor sheath (the distal palmar crease) and the insertion of flexor superficialis. IIII – Between the end of the carpal tunnel and the beginning of the flexor sheath. IV – Within the carpal tunnel. V – Proximal to the carpal tunnel.

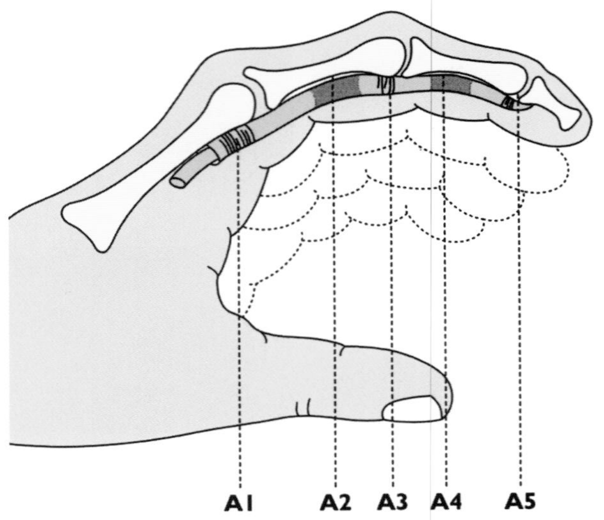

26.15 The flexor tendon sheath and pulleys Fibrous pulleys – designated A1 to A5 – hold the flexor tendons to the phalanges and prevent bowstringing during movement. A1, 3 and 5 are attached to the palmar plate near each joint; A2 and 4 have a crucial tethering effect and must always be preserved or reconstructed.

be performed. More recently, dissolvable nerve guides have been used to bridge the gap, allowing a biological regeneration across the gap).

Extensor tendon repair is not as easy and the results not as reliable as some have suggested. Repair and postoperative management should be meticulous.

Flexor tendon repair is even more challenging, particularly in the region between the distal palmar crease and the flexor crease of the proximal interphalangeal joint where both the superficial and deep tendons run together in a tight sheath (Zone II or, more dramatically, 'no man's land' because injuries in this zone are the most dangerous). Primary repair with fastidious postoperative supervision gives the best outcome but calls for a high level of expertise and specialized physiotherapy. If the necessary facilities are not available, then the wound should be washed out and loosely closed, and the patient transferred to a special centre. A delay of several days, with a clean wound, is unlikely to affect the outcome. The tendon repair must be strong and accurate enough to allow early mobilization (usually passive) so that the tendons can glide freely and independently from each other and the sheath. Four strands of locked core suture are placed

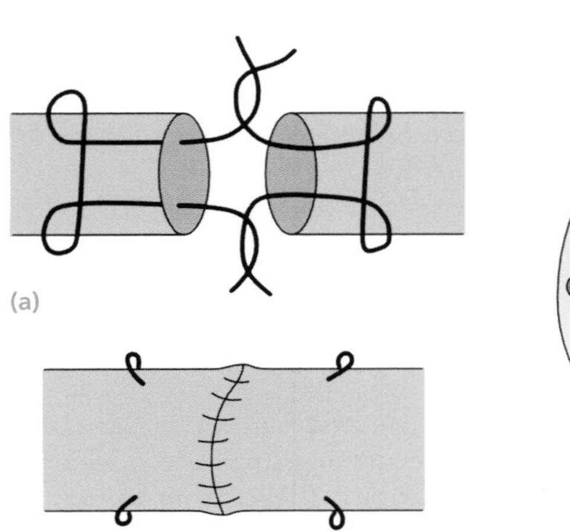

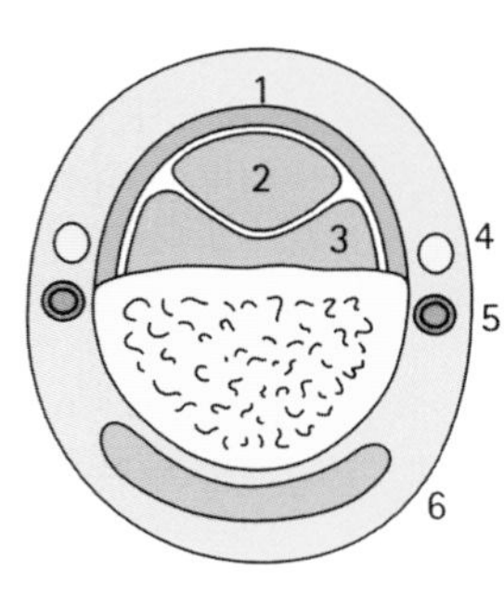

26.16 Flexor tendon repair A core suture (a) is supplemented by circumferential sutures (b). (c) The relationship of the important structures in 'no man's land': 1 – the tendon sheath; 2 – flexor digitorum profundus; 3 – flexor digitorum superficialis; 4 – digital nerve; 5 – artery; 6 – extensor tendon.

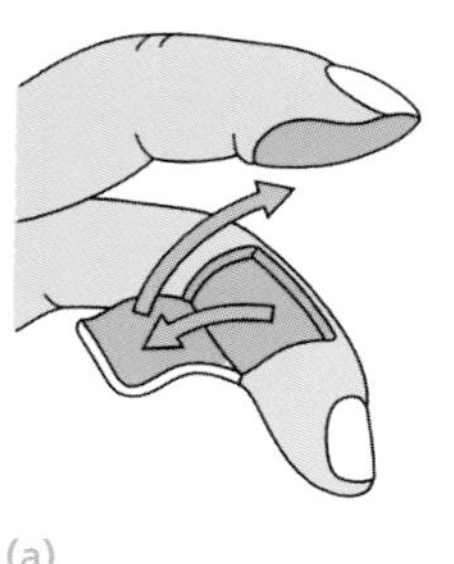

(a)

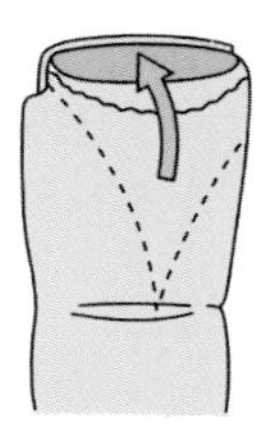

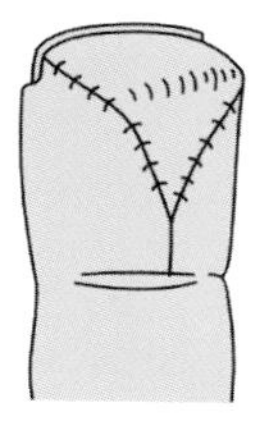

(b)

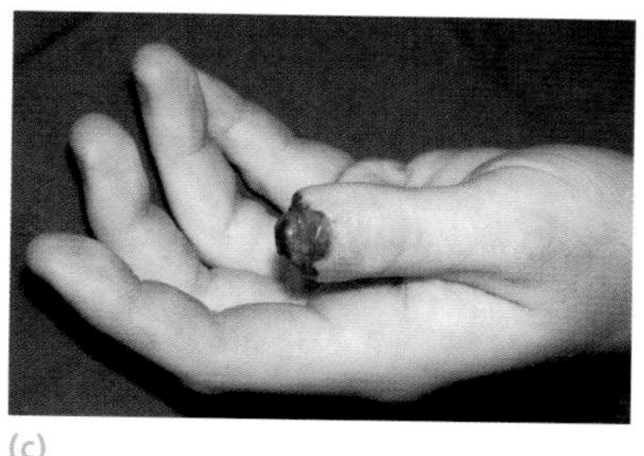

(c)

26.17 Pulp and finger-tip injuries (a) Cross-finger graft for a palmar oblique finger-tip injury with exposed bone. (b) V-to-Y advancement for a transverse finger-tip injury with exposed bone. Thumb tip loss (c) must always be reconstructed – never amputate.

without handling the tendon any more than is absolutely necessary; this is supplemented by a continuous circumferential suture which strengthens the repair and smoothes it, thus making the gliding action through the sheath easier. The A2 and A4 pulleys must be repaired or reconstructed, otherwise the tendons will bowstring. Cuts above the wrist (Zone V), in the palm (Zone III) or distal to the superficialis insertion (Zone I) generally have a better outcome than injuries in the carpal tunnel (Zone IV) or flexor sheath (Zone II). Division of the superficialis tendon noticeably weakens the hand and a swan neck deformity can develop in those with lax ligaments. At least one slip should therefore always be repaired.

Amputation of a finger as a primary procedure should be avoided unless the damage involves many tissues and is clearly irreparable. Even when a finger has been amputated by the injury, the possibility of reattachment should be considered (see below).

Ring avulsion is a special case. When a finger is caught by a ring, the soft tissues are sheared away from the underlying skeleton. Depending on the amount of damage, skin reattachment, microvascular reconstruction or even amputation may be required.

CLOSURE

The tourniquet is deflated and bipolar diathermy is used to stop bleeding. Haematoma formation leads to poor healing and tendon adhesions. Unless the wound is contaminated, the skin is closed – either by direct suture without tension or, if there is skin loss, by skin grafting. Skin grafts are conveniently taken from the inner aspect of the upper arm. If tendon or bare bone is exposed, this must be covered by a rotation or pedicled flap. Sometimes a severely mutilated finger is sacrificed and its skin used as a rotation flap to cover an adjacent area of loss.

Pulp and finger-tip injuries In full thickness wounds without bone exposure, the wound should be thoroughly cleaned and then covered with a non-adherent dressing. This is left well alone for 7 days; the accumulation of fluid beneath the dressing is not usually a sign of infection and antibiotics should be avoided. The wound is inspected only infrequently, then re-covered with the non-adherent dressing, until it heals.

If the open area is greater than 1 cm in diameter, healing will be quicker with a split-skin or full thickness graft but the residual pulp cover may not be as satisfactory as a wound that has been left to heal naturally by granulation and re-epithelialization.

If bone is exposed and length of the digit is important for the individual patient, then an advancement flap or neurovascular island flap should be considered. The precise type of flap depends on the orientation of the cut. Otherwise, primary cover can be achieved by shortening the bone and tailoring the skin flaps ('terminalization').

In young children, the finger-tips recover extraordinarily well from injury and they should be treated with dressings rather than grafts or terminalization. *Thumb length should never be sacrificed lightly* and every effort should be made to provide a long, sensate digit.

Nail bed injuries Nail bed injuries are often seen in association with fractures of the terminal phalanx. If appearance is important, meticulous repair of the nail bed under magnification, replacing any loss with a split thickness nail bed graft from one of the toes, will give the best cosmetic result. In children, these injuries are associated with a physeal fracture.

DRESSING AND SPLINTAGE

The wound is covered with a single layer of paraffin gauze and ample wool roll. A light plaster slab holds the wrist and hand in the *position of safety* (wrist extended, metacarpo-phalangeal joints flexed to 90 degrees, interphalangeal joints straight, thumb abducted). This is the position in which the metacarpo-phalangeal and interphalangeal ligaments are fully stretched and fibrosis therefore least likely to cause contractures. *Failure to appreciate this point is the commonest cause of irrecoverable stiffness after injury* (see Fig 16.26).

This position is modified in two circumstances. (1) After primary flexor tendon suture, the wrist is held with a dorsal splint in about 20 degrees of flexion to take tension off the repair (too much wrist flexion invites wrist stiffness and carpal tunnel symptoms) but the interphalangeal joints must remain straight. There should be minimal restriction at the front of the fingers, otherwise the resistance can precipitate rupture of the tendon. (2) After extensor tendon repair, the metacarpo-phalangeal joints are flexed to only about 30 degrees so that there is less tension on the repair; the wrist is extended to 30 degrees and the interphalangeal joints remain straight.

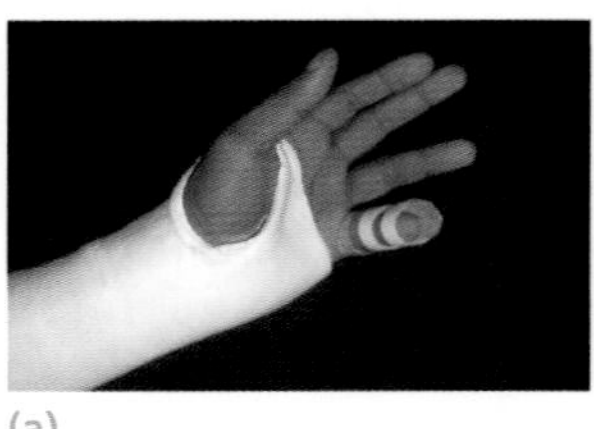
(a)

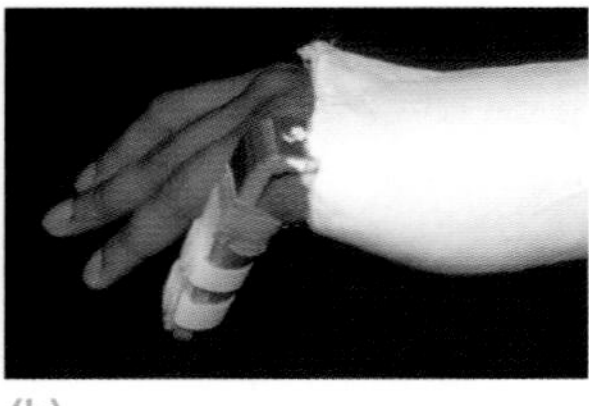
(b)

26.18 Splintage Always splint in the safe position (wrist slightly extended, MP joint flexed, PIP extended). Only immobilize the affected ray if there is a metacarpal or phalangeal injury.

Postoperative management

IMMEDIATE AFTERCARE

Following an operation, the hand is kept elevated in a roller towel or high sling. If the latter is used, the sling must be removed several times a day to exercise the elbow and shoulder. Too much elbow flexion can stop venous return and make swelling worse. Antibiotics are continued as necessary.

REHABILITATION

Movements of the hand must be commenced within a few days at most. Splintage should allow as many joints as possible to be exercised, consistent with protecting the repair. Most extensor tendon injuries are splinted for about 4 weeks. Dynamic splintage can be used, particularly for injuries at the level of the extensor retinaculum and the metacarpo-phalangeal joint. Various protocols are followed for flexor tendon injuries, including passive, active or elastic-band assisted flexion. Early movement promotes tendon healing and excursion. In all cases the risk of rupture is balanced against the need for early mobilization. Close supervision and attention to detail are essential.

Once the tissues have healed, the hand is increasingly used for more and more arduous and complex tasks, especially those that resemble the patient's normal job, until he or she is fit to start work; if necessary, his or her work is modified temporarily. If secondary surgery is required, tendon or nerve repair is postponed until the skin is healthy, there is no oedema and the joints have regained a normal range of passive movement.

Replantation

With modern microsurgical techniques and appropriate skill, amputated digits or hands can be replanted. An amputated part should be wrapped in sterile saline gauze and placed in a plastic bag, which is itself placed in watery ice. The 'cold ischaemic time' for a *finger*, which contains so little muscle, is about 30 hours, but the 'warm time' less than six. For a *hand or forearm*, the cold ischaemic time is only about 12 hours and the warm time much less. After resuscitation and attention to other potentially life-threatening injuries, the patient and the amputated part should be transferred to a centre where the appropriate surgical skills and facilities are available.

INDICATIONS

The decision to replant depends on the patient's age, his or her social and professional requirements, the condition of the part (whether clean-cut, mangled, crushed or avulsed), and the warm and cold ischaemic time. Furthermore, and perhaps most importantly, it depends on whether the replanted part is likely to give better function than an amputation.

The *thumb* should be replanted whenever possible. Even if it functions only as a perfused 'post' with protective sensation, it will give useful service. *Multiple dig-*

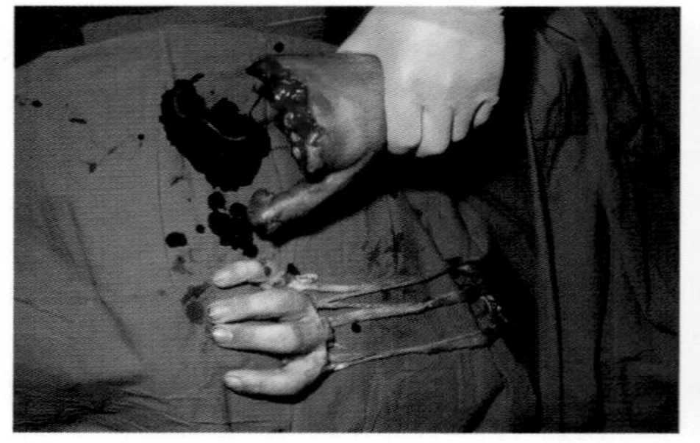
(a)

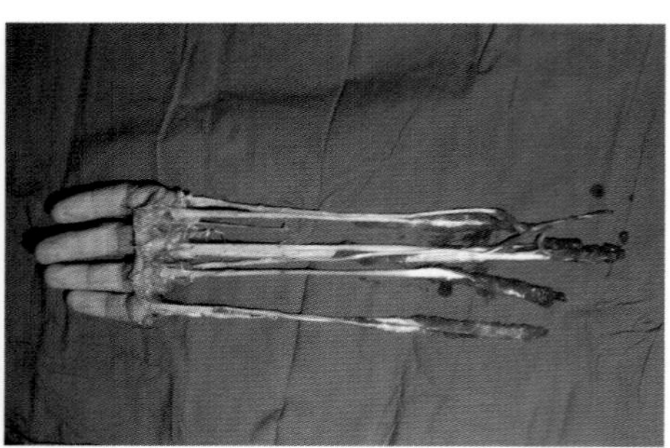
(b)

26.19 Avulsion This is not replantable.

its also should be replanted, and in a child even a single digit. *Proximal amputations* (through the palm, wrist or forearm) likewise merit an attempt at replantation.

RELATIVE CONTRAINDICATIONS

Single digits do badly if replanted. There is a high complication rate, including stiffness, non-union, poor sensation, and cold intolerance; a replanted single finger is likely to be excluded from use. The exception is an amputation beyond the insertion of flexor digitorum superficialis, when a cosmetic, functioning finger-tip can be retrieved. Severely *crushed, mangled or avulsed* parts may not be replantable; and parts with a *long ischaemic time* may not survive. *General medical disorders* or *other injuries* may engender unacceptable risks from the prolonged anaesthesia needed for replantation.

MANAGEMENT OF BURNS

Generally, hand burns should be dealt with in a specialized unit. *Superficial burns* are covered with moist non-adherent dressings; the hand is elevated and finger movements are encouraged. *Partial thickness burns* can usually be allowed to heal spontaneously; the hand is dressed with an antimicrobial cream and splinted in the position of safety.

Full thickness burns will not heal. Devitalized tissue should be excised; the wound is cleaned and dressed and 2–5 days later skin-grafted. Full thickness circumferential burns may need early escharotomy to preserve the distal circulation. Skin flaps are sometimes needed in sites such as the thumb web which are prone to contracture. The hand should be splinted in the position of safety; K-wires may be needed to maintain this position.

Electric burns may cause extensive damage and thrombosis which become apparent only after several days. The patient may of course need resuscitation (treating cardiac anomalies and myoglobinuria). The arm needs to be monitored and fasciotomy with debridement of dead tissue is often needed.

Chemical burns should be irrigated copiously for 20 or 30 minutes, usually with water or saline but sometimes with a specific reagent (calcium gluconate for hydrogen fluoride burns, soda lime or magnesium solution for hydrochloric acid, mineral oil for sodium).

MANAGEMENT OF INJECTION INJURIES

Oil, grease, solvents, hydraulic fluid or paint injected under pressure are damaging because of tension, toxicity or both. The thumb or index finger is usually involved. Substances can gain entry even through intact skin. Air or lead paint may show on x-ray.

Immediate decompression and removal of the foreign substance offers the best hope. This means an extensive dissection. The outcome is often poor, with amputation sometimes being necessary.

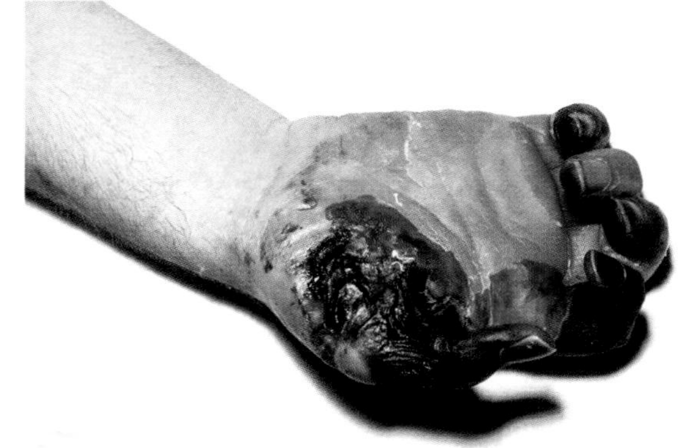

26.20 Frostbite

FROSTBITE

Frostbite requires special treatment. The limb is rewarmed in a water bath at 40–42 degrees for 30 minutes. Oedema is minimized by elevation, and blisters are drained. Digits sometimes need amputation.

SECONDARY OPERATIONS

The primary treatment of hand injuries should always be carried out with an eye to any future reconstructive procedures that might be necessary. These are of three kinds:

- secondary repair or replacement of damaged structures
- amputation of fingers
- reconstruction of a mutilated hand.

Delayed repair

SKIN

If the skin cover is unsuitable for primary closure or has broken down it is replaced by a graft or flap. As always, the skin creases must be respected. Contractures are dealt with by Z-plasty, skin grafting, or local flaps, regional flaps or free flaps. When important volar surfaces such as the thumb or index tip are insensate, a flap of skin complete with its neurovascular supply may be transposed.

Split thickness skin contracts and so full thickness grafts are preferred. The upper inner arm can provide a fair amount of skin leaving a reasonable cosmetic defect. Larger amounts of skin can be harvested from the groin or abdomen. Bear in mind that grafts will not adhere to raw tendon or bone.

TENDONS

Primary suture may have been contraindicated by wound contamination, undue delay between injury and repair, massive skin loss or inadequate operating facilities. In these circumstances secondary repair or tendon grafting may be necessary.

In a late-presenting *injury of the profundus tendon with an intact superficialis*, advancement of a retracted tendon can cause a flexion deformity of the entire finger. Tendon grafting also is risky: the finger could end up even stiffer. Unless the patient's work or hobby demands flexion of the distal joint and maximum power in the finger, fusion or tenodesis of the distal interphalangeal joint is a more reliable option.

If *both the superficialis and profundus tendons* have been divided and have retracted, a tendon graft is needed. Full passive joint movement is a prerequisite.

If the pulley system is in good condition and there are no adhesions, the tendons are excised from the flexor sheath and replaced with a tendon graft (palmaris longus, plantaris or a toe extensor). Rehabilitation is the same as for a primary repair.

If the pulleys are damaged, the skin cover poor, the passive range of movement limited or the sheath scarred, a two-stage procedure is preferred. The tendons are excised and the pulleys reconstructed with extensor retinaculum or excised tendon. A Silastic rod is sutured to the distal stump of the profundus tendon and left free proximally either in the palm or distal forearm. Rehabilitation is planned to maintain a good passive range of movement. A smooth gliding surface forms around the rod. At least 3 months later, the rod is removed through two smaller incisions and a tendon graft (palmaris longus, plantaris or a lesser toe extensor) is sutured to the proximal and distal stumps of flexor digitorum profundus. Rehabilitation is the same as that for a primary repair.

Tenolysis is sometimes indicated. After flexor tendon repair in Zone II, a poor excursion is not infrequent because of adhesions between the tendons and the sheath. There is some active movement – indicating that the tendon is intact – but not enough for good function. The passive range of movement should be good if the tenolysis is to succeed. The tendons are painstakingly freed through small windows in the flexor sheath. Postoperatively an intensive programme of movement is essential, otherwise there will be even more scar tissue than before and the tenolysis will have made matters worse.

NERVES

Late-presenting nerve injuries must be carefully assessed. The results of repair deteriorate with time, particularly for motor nerves where the end plate begins to fail and the muscle begins to fibrose. If several months have passed, tendon transfer may be a more reliable alternative. If nerve repair is attempted, the scar is excised and the stumps pared back until healthy nerve is found proximally and distally; a nerve graft or tubular nerve guide is usually needed to avoid tension at the suture line.

JOINTS

The proximal interphalangeal joint is most prone to a flexion contracture. Active and passive exercises can be supplemented by serial static splints or dynamic splints. Surgery (capsulotomy, palmar plate and collateral ligament release) may be required but these operations themselves can invite further stiffness. Unstable or painful joints are best fused.

BONES

Malunion, especially if rotational, may require treatment. Non-union is very uncommon, but if present grafting may be required. Extensor tendons may stick to bone, most commonly after plate fixation of the proximal phalanx.

Plate removal and tenolysis is followed by aggressive active and passive movements: a fair result is usually achieved.

AMPUTATION

Indications A finger is amputated only if it remains painful or unhealed, or if it is a nuisance (i.e. the patient cannot bend it, straighten it or feel with it), and then only if repair is impossible or uneconomic.

Technique In the finger-tip, the aim is a mobile digit covered by healthy skin with normal sensation. This can be achieved by local advancement flaps or neurovascular island flaps, or by bone shortening ('terminalization'). A cross-finger flap is fairly straightforward and provides good skin cover, but sensation is limited and a flexion contracture can develop in the donor finger. The final choice depends on the patient's requirements and the surgeon's skill.

In the thumb every millimetre is worth preserving; even a stiff or deformed thumb is worth keeping.

The middle and ring fingers should not be amputated through the knuckle joint because cosmetically this is unsatisfactory and small objects will fall through the gap ('incontinence of grip'). If the proximal phalanx can be left, the appearance is still abnormal but function is better. The extensor tendon must never be sutured to the flexor tendon; this will act as a tether on the common belly of flexor digitorum profundus and prevent the other digits from flexing fully (the 'Quadriga effect'). If the middle phalanx is amputated distal to the flexor digitorum superficialis insertion, the profundus tendon continues to pull, but now through the lumbrical, making the proximal interphalangeal joint paradoxically extend rather than flex. This irritating anomaly is avoided by suturing the superficialis stump to the flexor sheath or by dividing the lumbrical.

For more proximal injuries, the entire finger with most of its metacarpal may be amputated; the hand is weakened but the appearance is usually satisfactory. If the middle ray is amputated through the metacarpal, the index finger may 'scissor' across it in flexion; this can be overcome by dividing the adjacent index metacarpal and transposing it to the stump of the middle metacarpal.

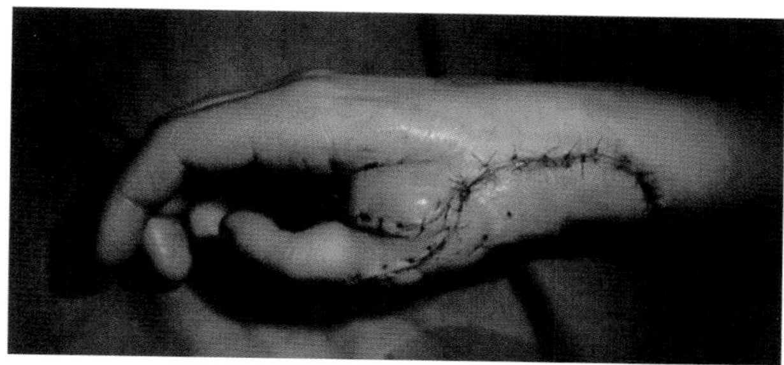

26.21 Late reconstruction The second toe has been transferred to replace the thumb, which was severed in an accident.

LATE RECONSTRUCTION

A severely mutilated hand should be dealt with by a hand expert. Certain options may be considered in exceptional cases. If all the fingers have been lost but the thumb is present, a new finger can sometimes be constructed with cortical bone, covered by a tubular flap of skin; an alternative is a neurovascular microsurgical transfer from the second toe. If the thumb has been lost, the options include pollicization (rotating a finger to oppose the other fingers), second toe transfer and osteoplastic reconstruction (a cortical bone graft surrounded by a skin flap).

Injuries of the spine 27

Stephen Eisenstein, Wagih El Masry

PATHOPHYSIOLOGY OF SPINE INJURIES

Stable and unstable injuries

Spinal injuries carry a double threat: damage to the vertebral column and damage to the neural tissues. While the full extent of the damage may be apparent from the moment of injury, there is always the fear that movement may cause or aggravate the neural lesion; hence the importance of establishing whether the injury is stable or unstable and treating it as unstable until proven otherwise.

A stable injury is one in which the vertebral components will not be displaced by normal movements; in a stable injury, if the neural elements are undamaged there is little risk of them becoming damaged.

An unstable injury is one in which there is a significant risk of displacement and consequent damage – or further damage – to the neural tissues.

In assessing spinal stability, three structural elements must be considered: the *posterior osseoligamentous complex (or posterior column)* consisting of the pedicles, facet joints, posterior bony arch, interspinous and supraspinous ligaments; the *middle column* comprising the posterior half of the vertebral body, the posterior part of the intervertebral disc and the posterior longitudinal ligament; and the *anterior column* composed of the anterior half of the vertebral body, the anterior part of the intervertebral disc and the anterior longitudinal ligament (Denis, 1983). All fractures involving the middle column and at least one other column should be regarded as unstable. Fortunately, only 10 per cent of spinal fractures are unstable and less than 5 per cent are associated with cord damage.

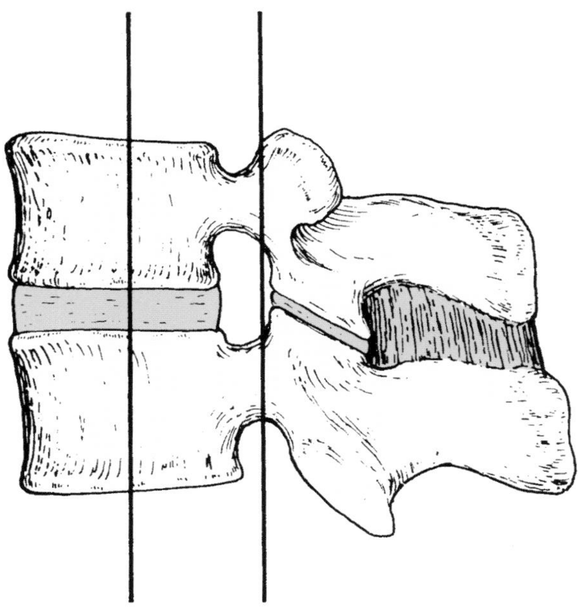

27.1 Structural elements of the spine The vertical lines show Denis' classification of the structural elements of the spine. The three elements are: the posterior complex, the middle component and the anterior column. This concept is particularly useful in assessing the stability of lumbar injuries.

Pathophysiology

Primary changes Physical injury may be limited to the *vertebral column*, including its soft-tissue components, and varies from ligamentous strains to vertebral fractures and fracture-dislocations. The *spinal cord and/or nerve roots* may be injured, either by the initial trauma or by ongoing structural instability of a vertebral segment, causing direct compression, severe energy transfer, physical disruption or damage to its blood supply.

Secondary changes During the hours and days following a spinal injury biochemical changes may lead to more gradual cellular disruption and extension of the initial neurological damage.

Mechanism of injury

There are three basic mechanisms of injury: traction (avulsion), direct injury and indirect injury.

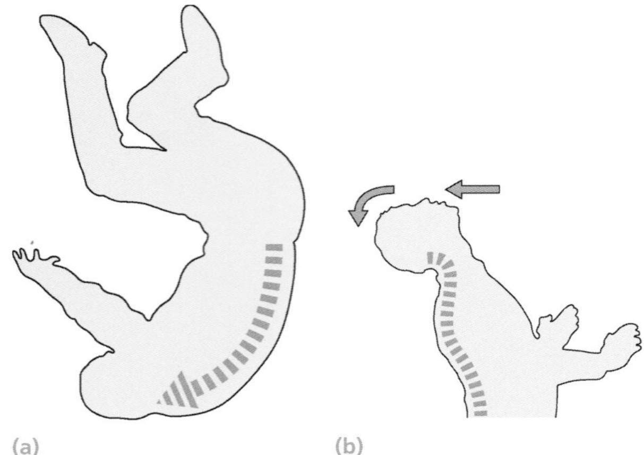

27.2 Mechanism of injury The spine is usually injured in one of two ways: (a) a fall onto the head or the back of the neck; and (b) a blow on the forehead, which forces the neck into hyperextension.

Traction injury In the lumbar spine resisted muscle effort may avulse transverse processes; in the cervical spine the seventh spinous process can be avulsed ('clay-shoveller's fracture').

Direct injury Penetrating injuries to the spine, particularly from firearms and knives, are becoming increasingly common.

Indirect injury This is the most common cause of significant spinal damage; it occurs most typically in a fall from a height when the spinal column collapses in its vertical axis, or else during violent free movements of the neck or trunk. A variety of forces may be applied to the spine (often simultaneously): axial compression, flexion, lateral compression, flexion-rotation, shear, flexion-distraction and extension.

NOTE: *Insufficiency fractures* may occur with minimal force in bone which is weakened by osteoporosis or a pathological lesion.

Healing

Spinal injuries may damage both bone and soft tissue (ligaments, facet joint capsule and intervertebral disc). Non-union of fractures is very rare while malunion is common. The bone injury will usually heal; however, if the bone structures heal in an abnormal position the healed soft tissues may not always protect against progressive deformity. This may occur with flexion injuries in which there is anterior wedging of the vertebral body of more than 40 per cent. An increasing flexion-deformity (kyphosis) may occur. Injuries with a predominant soft-tissue element – for example flexion-distraction with bilateral facet dislocation and disruption of the posterior ligaments and disc – heal with fibrous tissue and can become completely stable; sometimes, however, they do not regain stability.

PRINCIPLES OF DIAGNOSIS AND INITIAL MANAGEMENT

Diagnosis and management go hand in hand; inappropriate movement and examination can irretrievably change the outcome for the worse.

Early management

The adherence to the resuscitation protocol (airway with cervical spine control, breathing, circulation and haemorrhage control) supersedes the assessment of the spinal injury. Adequate oxygenation, ventilation and circulation will minimize secondary spinal cord injury. The essential principle is that if there is the slightest possibility of a spinal injury in a trauma patient, the spine must be immobilized until the patient has been resuscitated and other life-threatening injuries have been identified and treated. Immobilization is abandoned only when spinal injury has been excluded by clinical and radiological assessment.

Methods of temporary immobilization

CERVICAL SPINE

In-line immobilization The head and neck are supported in the neutral position.

QUADRUPLE IMMOBILIZATION

A backboard, sandbags, a forehead tape and a semirigid collar are applied. Because children have a relatively prominent occiput, care must be taken to ensure that the neck is not flexed: padding may be required behind the shoulders.

Thoracolumbar spine The patient should be moved without flexion or rotation of the thoracolumbar spine. A scoop stretcher and spinal board are very useful; however in the paralysed patient, there is a high risk of pressure sores – adequate padding is essential and transfer to a special bed must be undertaken as soon as possible.

If the back is to be examined, or if the patient is to be placed onto a scoop stretcher or spinal board, the *logrolling technique* should be used.

DIAGNOSIS

History

A high index of suspicion is essential; symptoms and signs may be minimal; the history is crucial. Every patient with a blunt injury above the clavicle, a head injury or loss of consciousness should be considered to have a cervical spine injury until proven otherwise. Every patient who is involved in a fall from a height or a high-speed deceleration accident should similarly be considered to have a thoracolumbar injury. The safe approach is to consider the presence of a vertebral column injury in all patients with multiple injuries. Lesser injuries also should arouse suspicion if they are followed by pain in the neck or back or neurological symptoms in the limbs.

Examination

NECK

The patient may be supporting his or her head with their hands – a warning to the examiner to be equally careful! The head and face are thoroughly inspected for bruises or grazes which could indicate indirect trauma to the cervical spine. The neck is inspected for deformity, bruising or penetrating injury. The bones and soft tissues of the neck are gently palpated for tenderness and areas of 'bogginess', or increased space between the spinous processes, suggesting instability due to posterior column failure. The back of the neck must also be examined but throughout the entire examination *the cervical spine must not be moved* because of the risk of injuring the cord in an unstable injury (see below).

BACK

The patient is 'log-rolled' (i.e. turned over 'in one piece') to avoid movement of the vertebral column. The back is inspected for deformity, penetrating injury, haematoma or bruising. The bone and soft-tissue structures are palpated, again with particular reference to the interspinous spaces. A haematoma, a gap or a step are signs of instability.

GENERAL EXAMINATION – 'SHOCK'

Early examination of the severely injured patent is considered in Chapter 22. The ABC sequence of advanced trauma life support (ATLS) always takes precedence.

Three types of shock may be encountered in patients with spinal injury:

Hypovolaemic shock is suggested by tachycardia, peripheral shutdown and, in later stages, hypotension.

Neurogenic shock reflects loss of the sympathetic pathways in the spinal cord; the peripheral vessels dilate causing hypotension but the heart, deprived of its sympathetic innervation, does not respond by increasing its rate. The combination of paralysis, warm and well-perfused peripheral areas, bradycardia and hypotension with a low diastolic blood pressure suggests neurogenic shock. Over-enthusiastic use of fluids can cause pulmonary oedema; atropine and vasopressors may be required.

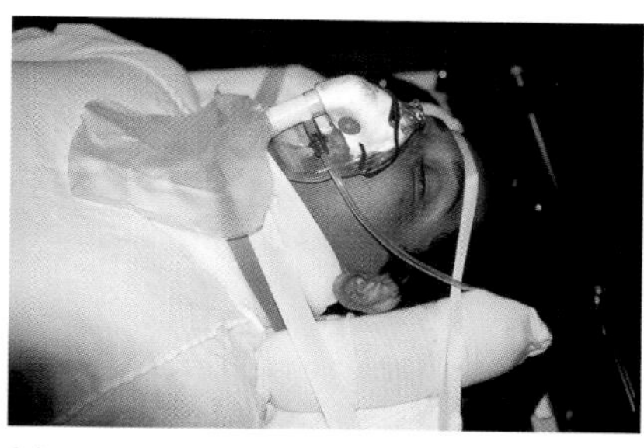
(a)

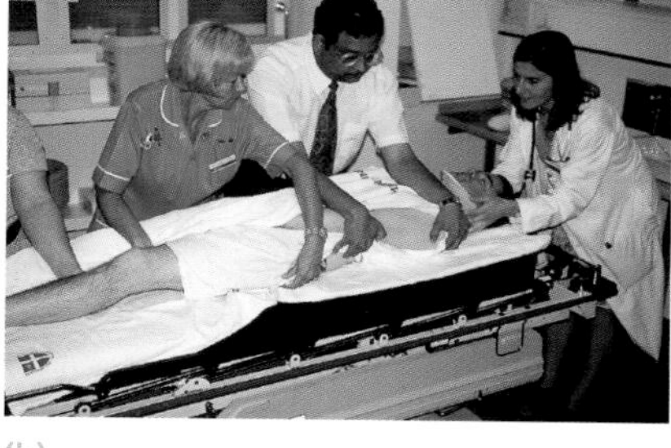
(b)

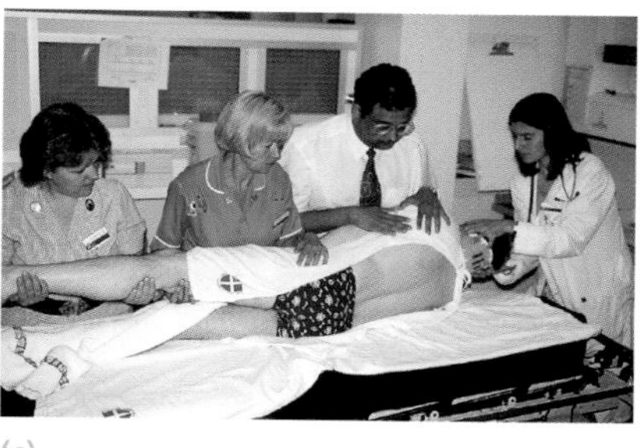
(c)

27.3 Spinal injuries – early management (a) Quadruple immobilization: the patient is on a backboard, the head is supported by sandbags and held with tape across the forehead, and a semi-rigid collar has been applied. (b,c) The log-rolling technique for exposure and examination of the back.

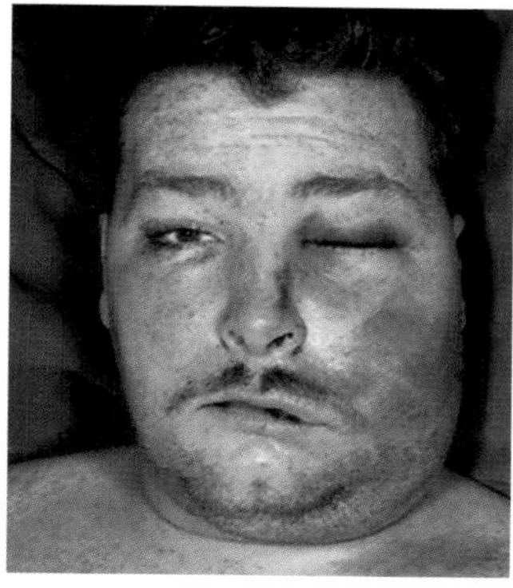
(a)

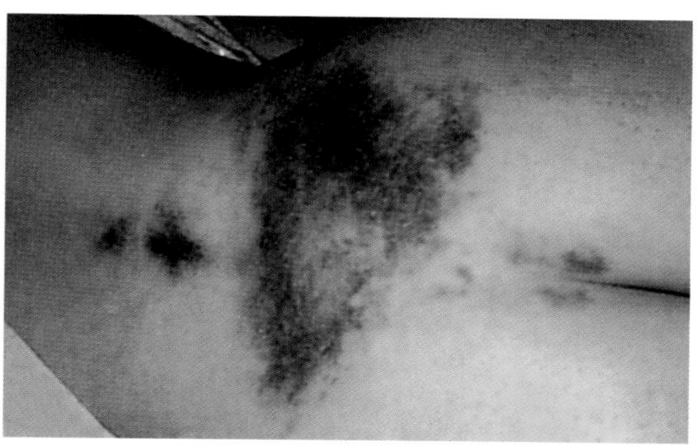
(b)

27.4 Spinal injuries – suspicious signs First appearances do matter. (a) With severe facial bruising always suspect a hyperextension injury of the neck. (b) Bruising over the lower back should raise the suspicion of a lumbar vertebral fracture.

'Spinal shock' occurs when the spinal cord fails temporarily following injury. Even parts of the cord without structural damage may not function. Below the level of the injury, the muscles are flaccid, the reflexes absent and sensation is lost. This rarely lasts for more than 48 hours and during this period it is difficult to tell whether the neurological lesion is complete or incomplete. If the primitive reflexes (anal 'wink' and the bulbocavernosus reflex) are absent, their return usually does not mark the end of 'spinal shock'; some neurological improvement can occur as time passes.

NEUROLOGICAL EXAMINATION

A full neurological examination is carried out in every case; this may have to be repeated several times during the first few days. Each dermatome, myotome and reflex is tested.

Cord longitudinal column functions are assessed: corticospinal tract (posterolateral cord, ipsilateral motor power), spinothalamic tract (anterolateral cord, contralateral pain and temperature) and posterior columns (ipsilateral proprioception).

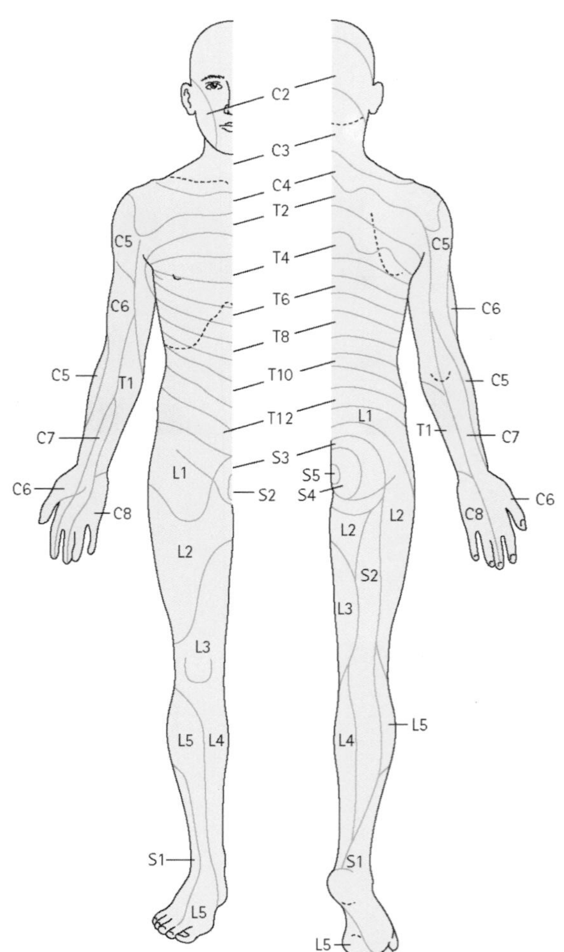

27.5 Spine injuries – neurological examination Dermatomes supplied by the spinal nerve roots.

Sacral sparing should be tested for. Preservation of active great toe flexion, active anal squeeze (on digital examination) and intact peri-anal sensation suggest a partial rather than complete lesion. Further recovery may occur.

The unconscious patient is difficult to examine; a spinal injury must be assumed until proven otherwise. Clues to the existence of a spinal cord lesion are a history of a fall or rapid deceleration, a head injury, diaphragmatic breathing, a flaccid anal sphincter, hypotension with bradycardia and a pain response above, but not below, the clavicle.

IMAGING

- X-ray examination of the spine is mandatory for all accident victims complaining of pain or stiffness in the neck or back or peripheral paraesthesiae, all patients with head injuries or severe facial injuries (cervical spine), patients with rib fractures or severe seat-belt bruising (thoracic spine), and those with severe pelvic or abdominal injuries (thoracolumbar spine). This is performed during the secondary survey.
- Accident victims who are unconscious should have spine x-rays as part of the routine work-up.
- Elderly people and patients with known vertebral pathology (e.g. ankylosing spondylitis) may suffer fractures after comparatively minor back injury. The spine should be x-rayed even if pain is not marked.

Table 27.1 Tests for nerve root motor function

Nerve root	Test
C5	Elbow flexion
C6	Wrist extension
C7	Wrist flexion, finger extension
C8	Finger flexion
T1	Finger abduction
L1,2	Hip abduction
L3,4	Knee extension
L5,S1	Knee flexion
L5	Great toe extension
S1	Great toe flexion

Table 27.2 Root values for tendon reflexes

Root value	Tendon reflex
C5	Biceps
C6	Brachioradialis
C7	Triceps
L3,4	Quadriceps
L5,S1	Achilles tendon

- Pain is often poorly localized; views should include several segments above and below the painful area.
- X-ray examination should be carried out with a minimum of movement and manipulation. No attempt should be made to obtain 'flexion-and-extension' views during the initial work-up.
- 'Difficult' areas, such as the upper cervical spine, the cervico-thoracic junction and the upper thoracic segments which are often obscured by shoulder and rib images, may require plain film tomography, CT or MRI. Odontoid fractures also are sometimes better shown on axial tomograms than on routine CT.
- In addition to anteroposterior and lateral views, open-mouth views are needed for the upper two cervical vertebrae and oblique views may be needed for the cervical as well as the thoracolumbar region.
- CT is ideal for showing structural damage to individual vertebrae and displacement of bone fragments into the vertebral canal. In fact, screening CT is employed routinely in many centres; the drawback is its high level of radiation exposure.
- MRI is the method of choice for displaying the intervertebral discs, ligamentum flavum and neural structures, and is indicated for all patients with neurological signs and those who are considered for surgery.
- CT myelography, with the intrathecal introduction of contrast agent, provides information on the dimensions of the spinal canal, impingement by fracture fragments or intervertebral disc, and root avulsion. This investigation has been largely replaced by MRI.
- Three-dimensional reconstruction of CT images defines certain complex fracture patterns. Spiral CT allows high resolution sagittal reconstruction and, when available, is useful for displaying fractures of the odontoid process.
- Remember that the spine may be damaged in more than one place.
- Do not accept poor quality images.
- Consult with the radiologist.

PRINCIPLES OF DEFINITIVE TREATMENT

The objectives of treatment are:

- to preserve neurological function;
- to minimize a perceived threat of neurological compression;
- to stabilize the spine;
- to rehabilitate the patient.

The *indications for urgent surgical stabilization* are: (a) an unstable fracture with progressive neurological deficit and MRI signs of likely further neurological deterioration; and (b) controversially an unstable fracture in a patient with multiple injuries.

Patients with no neurological injury

Stable injuries If the spinal injury is stable, the patient is treated by supporting the spine in a position that will cause no further strain; a firm collar or lumbar brace will usually suffice, but the patient may need to rest in bed until pain and muscle spasm subside. The exception is a burst fracture of the vertebral body: a CT should be arranged which may show displaced fragments within the spinal canal; however, even if a retropulsed fragment is identified, operative treatment is not imperative, though rehabilitation may be easier if surgery is performed. Furthermore, these patients are potentially 'neurologically unstable'. A progressive neurological deficit may occasionally develop, which could be an indication for decompression and fusion.

The correction of *deformity* by surgery is also controversial. It is not clear that symptoms are related to minor deformity, although a kyphosis of greater than 30 degrees may on occasions be associated with back pain in the long term. The patient should be given the choice between surgery for early mobilization and discharge, and conservative management which is likely to take longer.

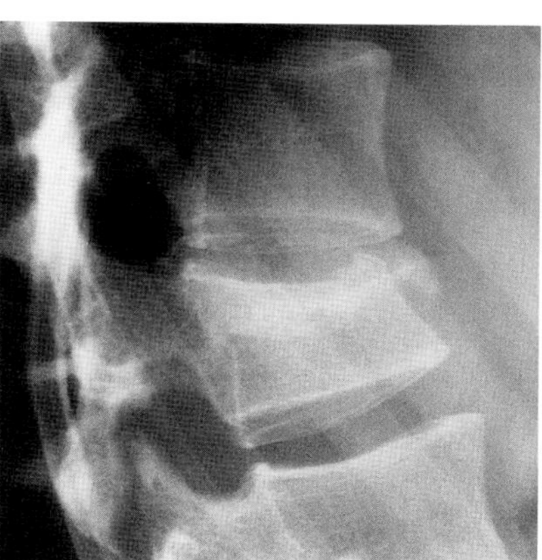

(a)

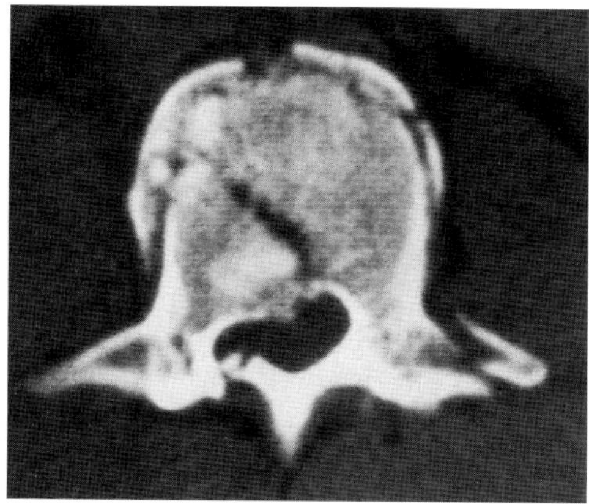

(b)

27.6 X-ray diagnosis Plain x-ray alone may be insufficient to show the true state of affairs. (a) This x-ray showed the fracture, but it needed a CT scan (b) to reveal the large fragment encroaching on the spinal canal.

Unstable injuries If the spinal injury is unstable it should be held secure until the tissues heal and the spine becomes stable. In the cervical spine this should be done as soon as possible by traction, using tongs or a halo device attached to the skull. If the halo is attached to a body cast the combination can be used as an external fixator for prolonged immobilization (see below). Alternatively (particularly in the thoracolumbar spine) internal fixation can be carried out. Attempts to reduce dislocations and subluxations should be made whether by adjusting the posture, by traction or by open operation if the patient so chooses.

Patients with a neurological injury

Once spinal shock has recovered, the full extent of the neurological injury is assessed. Caring for patients with neurological injury requires the infrastructure of an experienced multidisciplinary team that can optimally manage their multisystem physiological impairment and malfunction, including the spinal injury. Whenever feasible, they should be transferred to a Spinal Injury Centre as soon as possible after injury.

If the spinal injury is stable (which is rare), the patient can be treated conservatively and rehabilitated as soon as possible.

With the usual unstable injury, conservative treatment can be still be used; this is highly demanding and is best carried out in a special unit equipped for round-the-clock nursing, 2-hourly turning routines, skin toilet, bladder care and specialized physiotherapy and occupational therapy. After a few weeks the injury stabilizes spontaneously and the patient can be got out of bed for intensive rehabilitation. This approach is applicable to almost all injuries. Early operative stabilization is preferred by many; it facilitates nursing by inexperienced carers and reduces the risk of spinal deformity.

The benefit of surgery on ease and speed of rehabilitation, total period of hospitalization and neurological recovery is uncertain. A positive indication for early operative reduction or decompression and stabilization is *progressive neurological deterioration with evidence (or a serious risk) of further neural compression on MRI.*

Patients with incomplete lesions are also sometimes considered for operation, but there is little enthusiasm for this approach in specialized centres. Significant neurological recovery occurs without surgery in the majority of those who present with sensory and/or motor sparing in the first 48–72 hours. Furthermore, such recovery can theoretically be endangered by operative manoeuvres, arterial injury, hypoxia, hypotension, hypothermia, further damage to the blood–brain barrier or sepsis associated with spinal surgery.

'Medical treatment' to counteract the secondary pathophysiological changes associated with cord injury has been (and still is being) pursued. Of the various methods the one that gained most attention was the use of corticosteroids. However, after several trials in the USA and elsewhere, the use of intravenous methylprednisolone is considered to be of dubious benefit and is currently viewed as an 'option' for patients seen within the first few hours of injury, rather than a 'recommendation' (Short et al., 2000; Molano et al., 2002; Hugenholtz et al., 2002).

TREATMENT METHODS

Cervical spine

Collars *Soft collars* offer very little biomechanical support to the cervical spine and their use is restricted to minor sprains for the first few days after injury. *Semi-rigid collars* limit motion quite effectively and are widely used in the acute setting. They are not adequate for very unstable injury patterns. *Four-poster braces* are more stable, applying pressure to the mandible, occiput, sternum and upper thoracic spine. They can be uncomfortable.

Tongs A pin is inserted into the outer table on each side of the skull; these are mounted on a pair of tongs and traction is applied to reduce the fracture or dislocation and to maintain the reduced position.

Halo ring At least four pins are inserted into the outer table of the skull and a ring is applied. The use of titanium pins and graphite ring allows an MRI scan to be performed. The halo ring can be used for initial traction and reduction of the fracture or dislocation, and then can be attached to a plaster vest. Proper positioning and torque-pressure of the pins is essential. Bear in mind that the use of a halo-vest carries a significant risk of complications such as pin loosening, pin-site infection and (in elderly patients) respiratory distress.

Fixation Various operative procedures are available, depending on the level and pattern of injury. *Odontoid fractures* can be fixed with lag screws, *burst fractures* can be decompressed through an anterior approach, and *facet dislocations* can be reduced through a posterior approach. The spine can be stabilized anteriorly with plates between the vertebral bodies or posteriorly with wires between the spinous processes, or with small plates between the lateral masses.

Thoracolumbar spine

Beds Special beds are used in the management of spinal injuries. They are designed to avoid pressure

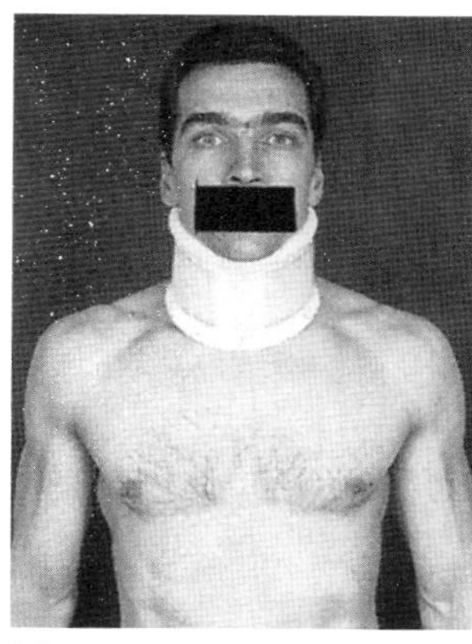
(a)

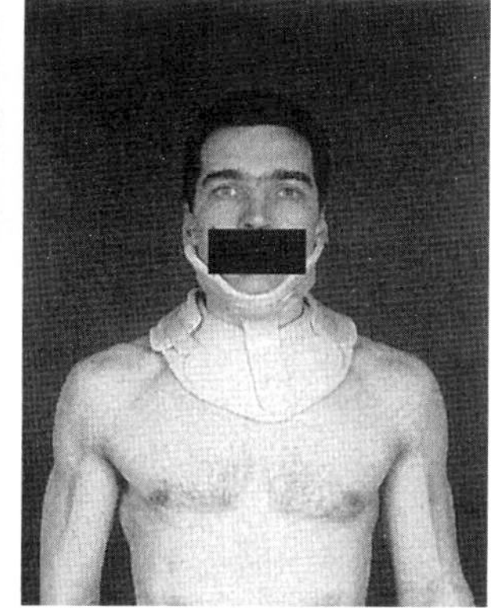
(b)

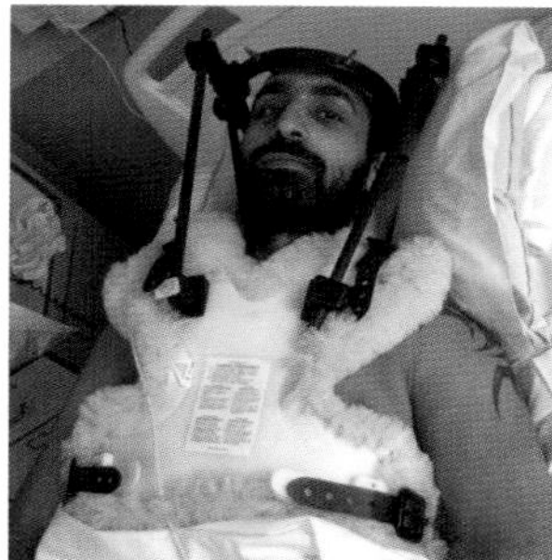
(c)

27.7 Spine injuries – treatment (a) Standard cervical collar. (b) More rigid variety. (c) Halo-body cast.

sores (with special mattresses or the facility to turn the patient frequently). Some beds allow postural reduction of fractures.

Brace A thoracolumbar brace avoids flexion by three-point fixation. It is suitable for some burst fractures, seat-belt injuries and compression fractures.

Decompression and stabilization The aim of surgery is to reduce the fracture, hold the reduction and decompress the neural elements. The surgical approach can be either anterior or posterior.

The anterior approach is suitable for burst fractures with significant canal impingement or as a supplement to posterior fixation in those compression fractures with considerable loss of anterior bone stock. With an anterior approach, the spine is exposed through a transthoracic, transdiaphragmatic or transperitoneal approach depending on the level of the fracture. The vertebral body is removed so that the spinal canal is decompressed; a bone graft (rib, fibula or iliac crest) is then inserted and special plates are applied between the intact vertebral bodies above and below the injured level.

The posterior approach is more suitable for flexion-compression injuries, seat-belt injuries and fracture-dislocations. Some burst fractures can also be reduced indirectly from a posterior approach using implants that apply distraction to the fracture. Hook and rod systems provide fixation between intact vertebrae several segments above and below the injury. The advent of *segmental spinal instrumentation*, with the fixation device attached to the spinal column through pedicle screws, allows secure fixation of a much shorter implant, reaching only one or two segments away from the injury. These devices also allow correction of the deformity by distraction and extension. Bone graft is required so that a biological fusion can supplement the implants.

CERVICAL SPINE INJURIES

The patient will usually give a history of a fall from a height, a diving accident or a vehicle accident in which the neck is forcibly moved. In a patient unconscious from a head injury, a fractured cervical spine should be assumed (and acted upon) until proved otherwise.

An abnormal position of the neck is suggestive, and careful palpation may elicit tenderness. Movement is best postponed until the neck has been x-rayed. Pain or paraesthesia in the limbs is significant, and the patient should be examined for evidence of spinal cord or nerve root damage.

Imaging

Plain x-rays must be of high quality and should be inspected methodically.

- In the anteroposterior view the lateral outlines should be intact, and the spinous processes and tracheal shadow in the midline. An open-mouth view is necessary to show C1 and C2 (for odontoid and lateral mass fractures).

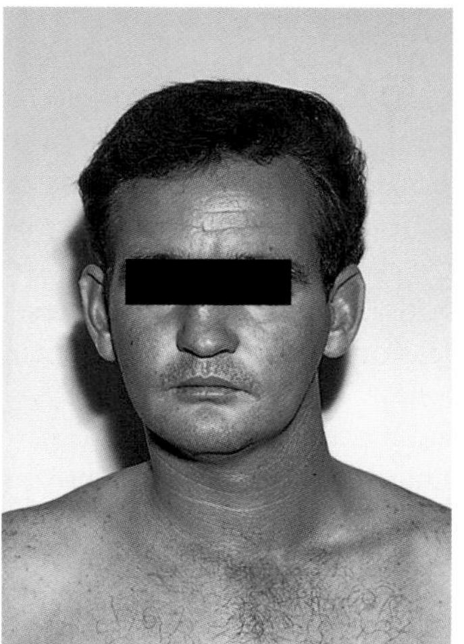

27.8 Cervical spine injury Look at the position of this patient's neck. He complained of pain and stiffness after a fall. It could have been no more than a soft-tissue strain, but x-ray examination revealed an odontoid fracture.

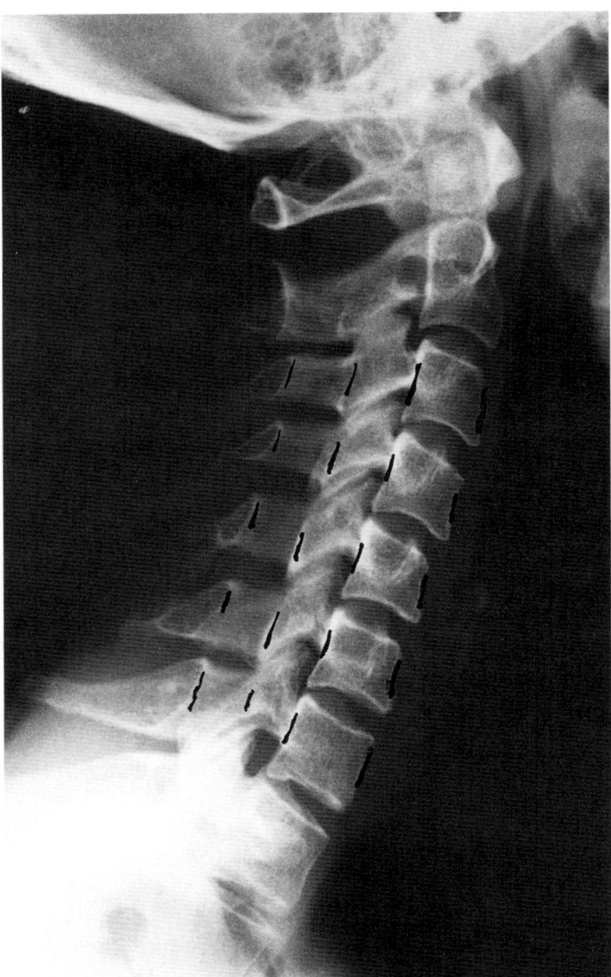

27.9 Cervical spine – normal x-ray In the lateral projection, four parallel lines can be traced unbroken from C1 to C7. They are formed by: (1) the anterior surfaces of the vertebral bodies; (2) the posterior surfaces of the bodies; (3) the posterior borders of the lateral masses; and (4) the bases of the spinous processes.

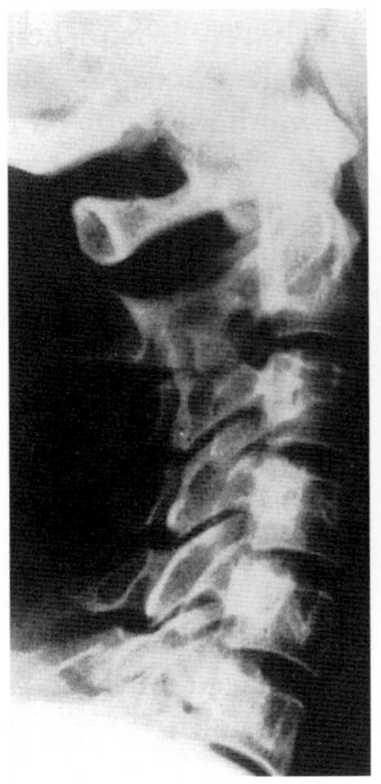

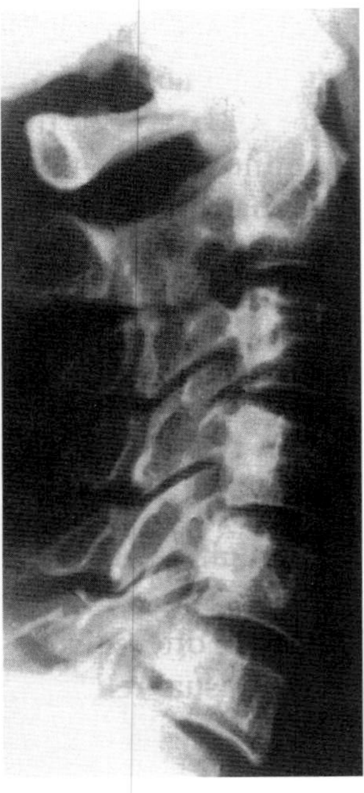

(a) (b)

27.10 Cervical spine injuries – x-ray diagnosis (a) Following a traffic accident this patient had a painful neck and consulted her doctor three times; on each occasion she was told 'the x-rays are normal'. But count the vertebrae! There are only six in this film. (b) When a shoulder 'pull-down view' was obtained to show the entire cervical spine, a dislocation of C6 on C7 could be seen at the very bottom of the film.

- In the lateral view the smooth lordotic curve should be followed, tracing four parallel lines formed by the front of the vertebral bodies, the back of the bodies, the posterior borders of the lateral masses and the bases of the spinous processes; any irregularity suggests a fracture or displacement. Forward shift of the vertebral body by 25 per cent suggests a unilateral facet dislocation and by 50 per cent a bilateral facet dislocation.
- The lateral view must include all seven cervical vertebrae and the upper half of T1, otherwise a serious injury at the cervico-thoracic junction will be missed. If the cervico-thoracic junction cannot be seen, then the lateral view should be repeated while the patient's shoulders are pulled down. If this fails, then a 'swimmer's view' is obtained. If this, too, fails, then tomography or a CT scan is required.
- The distance between the odontoid peg and the back of the anterior arch of the atlas should be no more than 3 mm in adults and 4.5 mm in children.
- Compare the shape of each vertebral body with that of the others; note particularly any loss of height, fragmentation or backward displacement of the posterior border of the vertebral body.
- Examine the soft-tissue shadows. The retropharyngeal space may contain a haematoma; the prevertebral soft-tissue shadow should be less than 5 mm in thickness above the level of the trachea and less than one vertebral body's width in thickness below. The interspinous space may be widened after ligament rupture.

Diagnostic pitfalls in children

Children are often distressed and difficult to examine; more than usual reliance may be placed on the x-rays. It is well to recall some common pitfalls.

An increased atlanto-dental interval (up to 4.5mm)

may be quite normal; this is because the skeleton is incompletely ossified and the ligaments relatively lax during childhood. There may also be apparent subluxation of C2 on C3 (*pseudosubluxation*).

An increased retropharyngeal space can be brought about by forced expiration during crying.

Growth plates and synchondroses can be mistaken for *fractures*. The normal synchondrosis at the base of the dens has usually fused by the age of 6 years, but it can be mistaken for an undisplaced fracture; the spinous process growth plates also resemble fractures; and the growth plate at the tip of the odontoid can be taken for a fracture in older children.

SCIWORA is an acronym for spinal cord injury without obvious radiographic abnormality. Normal radiographs in children do not exclude the possibility of spinal cord injury.

Upper cervical spine

Occipital condyle fracture

This is usually a high-energy fracture and associated skull or cervical spine injuries must be sought. The diagnosis is likely to be missed on plain x-ray examination and CT is essential.

Impacted and undisplaced fractures can be treated by brace immobilization for 8–12 weeks. Displaced fractures are best managed by using a halo-vest or by operative fixation.

Occipito-cervical dislocation

This high-energy injury is almost always associated with other serious bone and/or soft-tissue injuries, including arterial and pharyngeal disruption, and the outcome is often fatal. Patients are best dealt with by a multidisciplinary team of surgeons and physicians.

The diagnosis can sometimes be made on the lateral cervical radiograph: the tip of the odontoid should be no more than 5mm in vertical alignment and 1mm in horizontal alignment from the basion (anterior rim of the foramen magnum). Greater distances are allowable in children. CT scans are more reliable.

The injury is likely to be unstable and requires immediate reduction (without traction!) and stabilization with a halo-vest, pending surgical treatment. After appropriate attention to the more serious soft-tissue injuries and general resuscitation, the dislocation should be internally fixed; specially designed occipito-cervical plates and screws are available for the purpose. In severely unstable injuries, halo-vest stabilization should be retained for another 6–8 weeks.

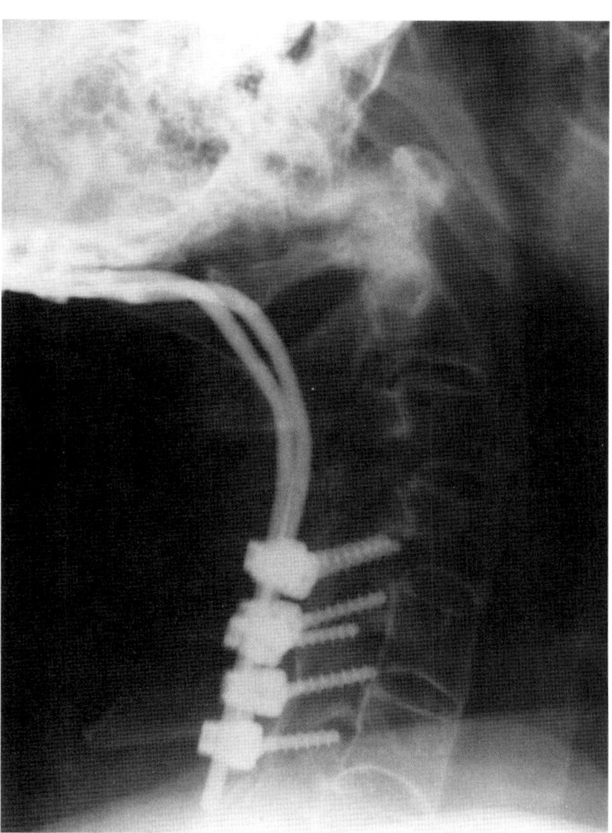

27.11 Occipito–cervical fusion X-ray showing one of the devices used for internal fixation in occipito-cervical fusion operations.

C1 ring fracture

Sudden severe load on the top of the head may cause a 'bursting' force which fractures the ring of the atlas (Jefferson's fracture). There is no encroachment on the neural canal and, usually, no neurological damage. The fracture is seen on the open-mouth view (if the lateral masses are spread away from the odontoid peg) and the lateral view. A CT scan is particularly helpful in defining the fracture. If it is undisplaced, the injury

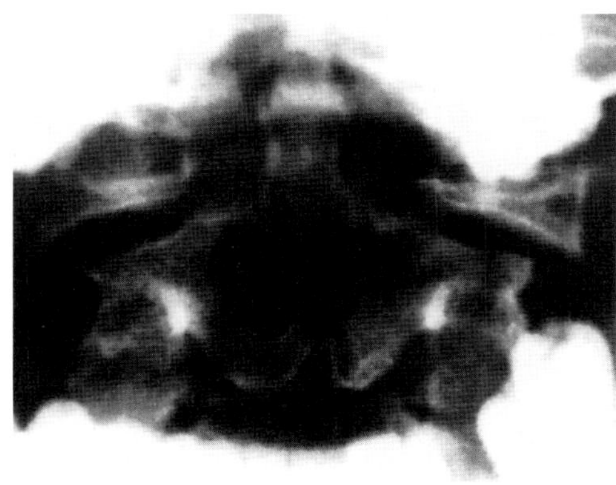

27.12 Fracture of C1 ring Jefferson's fracture – bursting apart of the lateral masses of C1.

is stable and the patient wears a semi-rigid collar or halo-vest until the fracture unites. If there is sideways spreading of the lateral masses (more than 7 mm on the open-mouth view), the transverse ligament has ruptured; this injury is unstable and should be treated by a halo-vest for several weeks. If there is persisting instability on x-ray, a posterior C1/2 fixation and fusion is needed.

A hyperextension injury can fracture either the anterior or posterior arch of the atlas. These injuries are usually relatively stable and are managed with a halo-vest or semi-rigid collar until union occurs.

Fractures of the atlas are associated with injury elsewhere in the cervical spine in up to 50 per cent of cases.

C2 pars interarticularis fractures

In the true judicial 'hangman's fracture' there are bilateral fractures of the pars interarticularis of C2 and the C2/3 disc is torn; the mechanism is extension with distraction. In civilian injuries, the mechanism is more complex, with varying degrees of extension, compression and flexion. This is one cause of death in motor vehicle accidents when the forehead strikes the dashboard. Neurological damage, however, is unusual because the fracture of the posterior arch tends to decompress the spinal cord. Nevertheless the fracture is potentially unstable.

Undisplaced fractures which are shown to be stable on supervised flexion–extension views (less than 3mm of C2/3 subluxation) can be treated in a semi-rigid orthosis until united (usually 6–12 weeks).

Fractures with more than 3mm displacement but no kyphotic angulation may need reduction; *however, because the mechanism of injury usually involves distraction, traction must be avoided*. After reduction, the neck is held in a halo-vest until union occurs. C2/3 fusion is sometimes required for persistent pain and instability ('traumatic spondylolisthesis').

Occasionally, the 'hangman's fracture' is associated with a C2/3 facet dislocation. This is a severely unstable injury; open reduction and stabilization is required.

C2 Odontoid process fracture

Odontoid fractures are uncommon. They usually occur as flexion injuries in young adults after high-velocity accidents or severe falls. However, they also occur in elderly, osteoporotic people as a result of low-energy trauma in which the neck is forced into hyperextension, e.g. a fall onto the face or forehead.

27.13 Fracture of C2 'Hangman's fracture' – fracture of the pars interarticularis of C2.

A displaced fracture is really a fracture-dislocation of the atlanto-axial joint in which the atlas is shifted forwards or backwards, taking the odontoid process with it. At this level about a third of the internal diameter of the atlas is free space, a third filled with the odontoid and a third with the cord; thus there is room for displacement without neurological injury. However, cord damage is not uncommon and in old people there is a considerable mortality rate.

Classification

Odontoid fractures have been classified by Anderson and D'Alonzo (1974) as follows:

- *Type I* – An avulsion fracture of the tip of the odontoid process due to traction by the alar ligaments. The fracture is stable (above the transverse ligament) and unites without difficulty.
- *Type II* – A fracture at the junction of the odontoid process and the body of the axis. This is the most common (and potentially the most dangerous) type. The fracture is unstable and prone to non-union.
- *Type III* – A fracture through the body of the axis. The fracture is stable and almost always unites with immobilization.

Clinical features

The history is usually that of a severe neck strain followed by pain and stiffness due to muscle spasm. The diagnosis is confirmed by high quality x-ray examination; it is important to rule out an associated

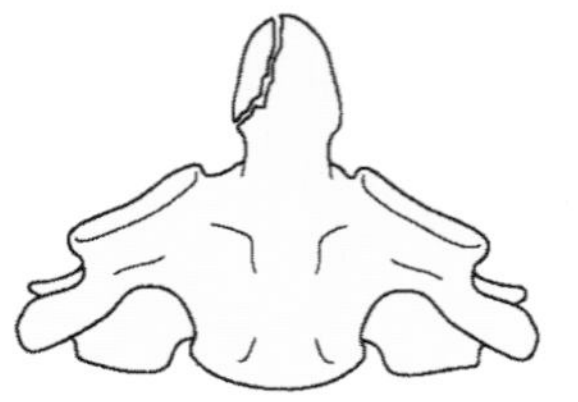
(a)

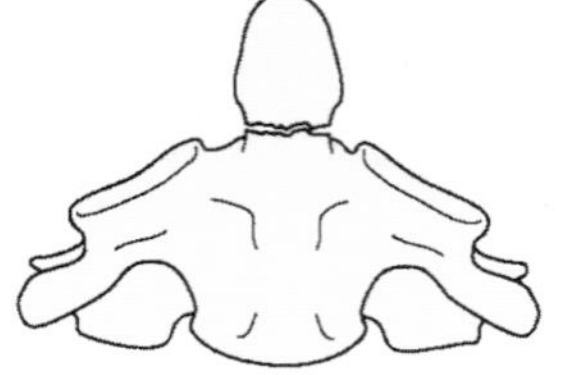
(b)

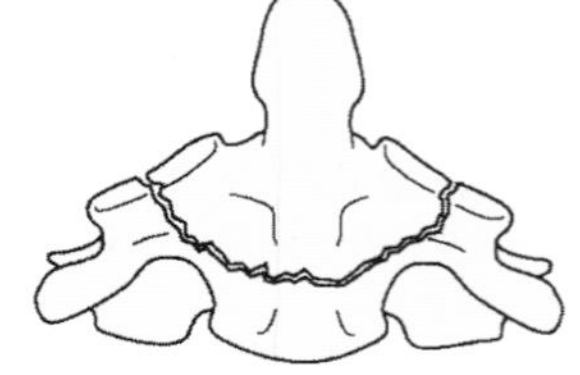
(c)

27.14 Odontoid fractures – classification (a) Type I – fracture through the tip of the odontoid process. (b) Type II – fracture at the junction of the odontoid process and the body. (c) Type III – fracture through the body of the axis. (Anderson and D'Alonzo, 1974.)

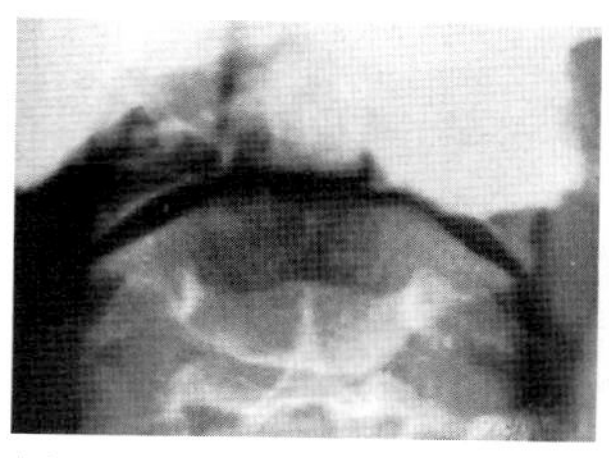
(a)

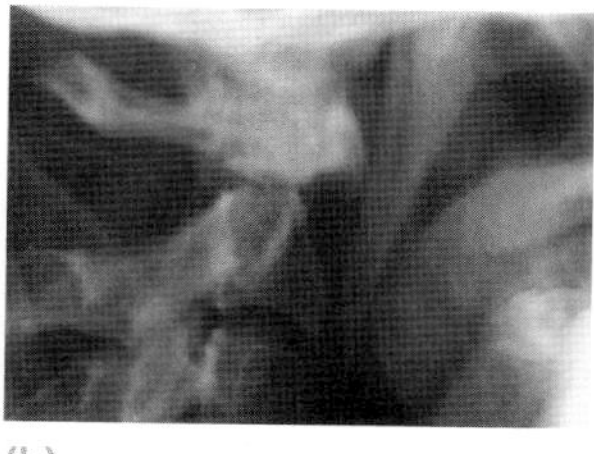
(b)

27.15 Fractured odontoid process (a) Anteroposterior 'open-mouth' x-ray showing a Type II odontoid fracture. (b) Lateral x-ray of the same patient.

occipito-cervical injury which commands immediate attention. In some cases the clinical features are mild and continue to be overlooked for weeks on end. Neurological symptoms occur in a significant number of cases.

Imaging

Plain x-rays usually show the fracture, although the extent of the injury is not always obvious – e.g. there may be an associated fracture of the atlas or displacement at the occipito-atlanto level. Tomography is helpful but MRI has the advantage that it may reveal rupture of the transverse ligament; this can cause instability in the absence of a fracture.

Treatment

Type I fractures Isolated fractures of the odontoid tip are uncommon. They need no more than immobilization in a rigid collar until discomfort subsides.

Type II fractures These are often unstable and prone to non-union, especially if displaced more than 5 mm. *Undisplaced fractures* can be held by fitting a halo-vest or – in elderly patients – a rigid collar. *Displaced fractures* should be reduced by traction and can then be held by operative posterior C1/2 fusion; a drawback is that neck rotation will be restricted. Anterior screw fixation is suitable for Type II fractures that run from anterior-superior to posterior-inferior, provided the fracture is not comminuted, that the transverse ligament is not ruptured, that the fracture is fully reduced and the bone solid enough to hold a screw; in that case neck rotation is retained. If full operative facilities are not available, immobilization can be applied by using a halo-vest with repeated x-ray monitoring to check for stability.

Type III fractures If undisplaced, these are treated in a halo-vest for 8–12 weeks. If displaced, attempts should be made at reducing the fracture by halo traction, which will allow positioning in either flexion or extension, depending on whether the displacement is forward or backward; the neck is then immobilized in a halo-vest for 8–12 weeks. For elderly patients with poor bone a collar may suffice, though this carries a higher risk of non-union.

LOWER CERVICAL SPINE

Fractures of the cervical spine from C3 to C7 tend to produce characteristic fracture patterns, depending on the mechanism of injury: flexion, axial compression, flexion–rotation or hyperextension.

Posterior ligament injury

Sudden flexion of the mid-cervical spine can result in damage to the posterior ligament complex (the interspinous ligament, facet capsule and supraspinous ligament). The upper vertebra tilts forward on the one below, opening up the interspinous space posteriorly.

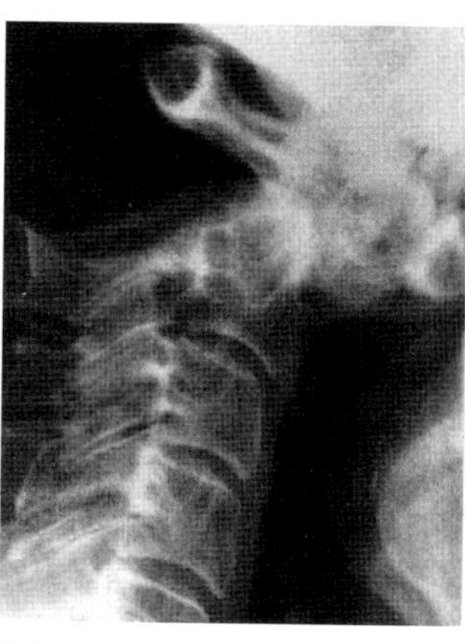
(a)

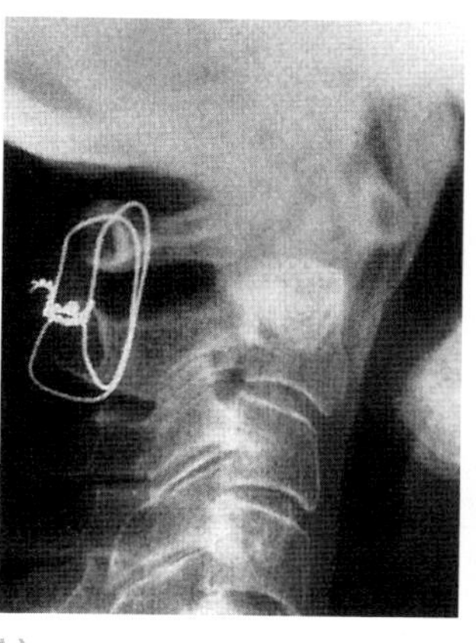
(b)

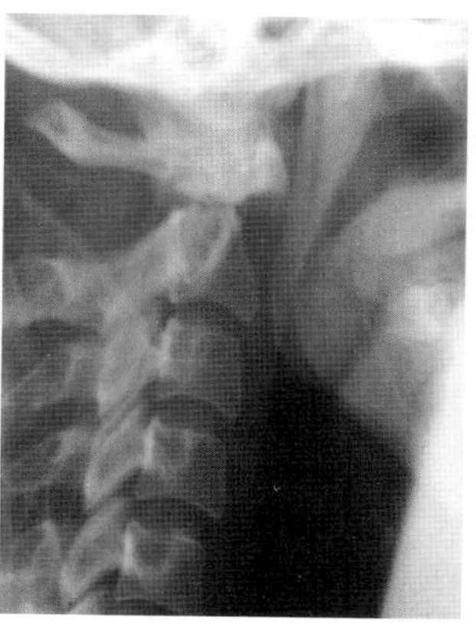
(c)

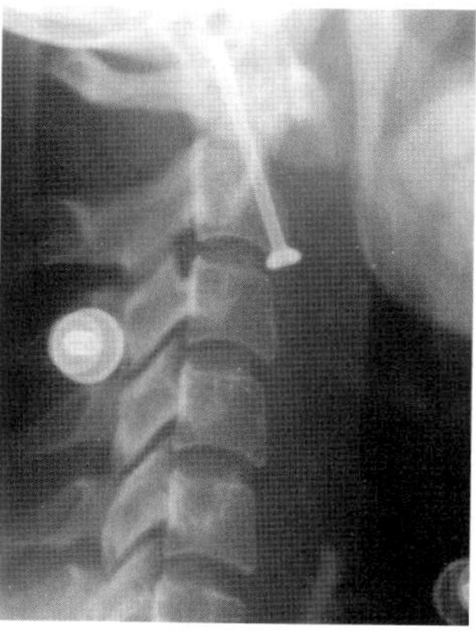
(d)

27.16 Fractured odontoid – treatment (a) A severely displaced Type II odontoid fracture. (b) The fracture was reduced by skull traction and held by fixing the spinous process of C1 to that of C2 with wires. (c) An undisplaced Type II fracture, which was suitable for (d) anterior screw fixation.

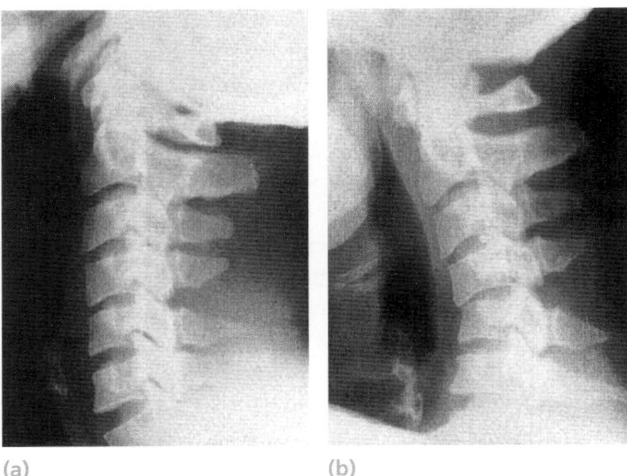

(a) (b)

27.17 Cervical spine – posterior ligament injury (a) The film taken in extension shows no displacement of the vertebral bodies, but there is an unduly large gap between the spinous processes of C4 and 5. (b) With the neck slightly flexed the subluxation is obvious. *NB: flexion–extension views are potentially dangerous and should be used only in specific situations under direct supervision of an experienced surgeon.*

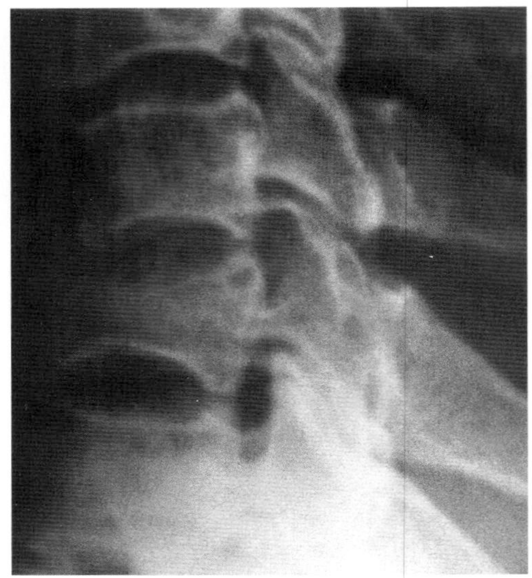

27.18 Cervical compression fracture A wedge compression fracture of a single cervical vertebral body. This is a stable injury because the middle and posterior elements are intact. Compare and contrast with Figure 27.19.

The patient complains of pain and there may be localized tenderness posteriorly. *X-ray* may reveal a slightly increased gap between the adjacent spines; however, if the neck is held in extension this sign can be missed, so it is always advisable to obtain a lateral view with the neck in the neutral position. A flexion view would, of course, show the widened interspinous space more clearly, *but flexion should not be permitted in the early post-injury period*. This is why the diagnosis is often made only some weeks after the injury, when the patient goes on complaining of pain.

The assessment of stability is essential in these cases. If the angulation of the vertebral body with its neighbour exceeds 11 degrees, if there is anterior translation of one vertebral body upon the other of more than 3.5 mm or if the facets are fractured or displaced, then the injury is unstable and it should be treated as a subluxation or dislocation. If it is certain that the injury is stable, a semi-rigid collar for 6 weeks is adequate; if the injury is unstable then posterior fixation and fusion is advisable.

Wedge compression fracture

A pure flexion injury results in a wedge compression fracture of the vertebral body (Fig. 27.18). The middle and posterior elements remain intact and the injury is stable. All that is needed is a comfortable collar for 6–12 weeks.

A note of warning: The x-ray should be carefully examined to exclude damage to the middle column and posterior displacement of the vertebral body fragment, i.e. features of a burst fracture (see below) which is potentially dangerous. If there is the least doubt, an axial CT or MRI should be obtained.

Burst and compression-flexion ('tear-drop') fractures

These severe injuries are due to axial compression of the cervical spine, usually in diving or athletic accidents (Fig. 27.19). If the vertebral body is crushed in neutral position of the neck the result is a '**burst fracture**'. With combined axial compression and flexion, an antero-inferior fragment of the vertebral body is sheared off, producing the eponymous '**tear-drop**' on the lateral x-ray. *In both types of fracture there is a risk of posterior displacement of the vertebral body fragment and spinal cord injury.*

Plain x-rays show either a crushed vertebral body (burst fracture) or a flexion deformity with a triangular fragment separated from the antero-inferior edge of the fractured vertebra (the innocent-looking 'tear-drop'). The x-ray images should be carefully examined for evidence of middle column damage and posterior displacement (even very slight displacement) of the main body fragment. Traction must be applied immediately and *CT* or *MRI* should be performed to look for retropulsion of bone fragments into the spinal canal.

TREATMENT

If there is no neurological deficit, the patient can be treated surgically or by confinement to bed and traction for 2–4 weeks, followed by a further period of

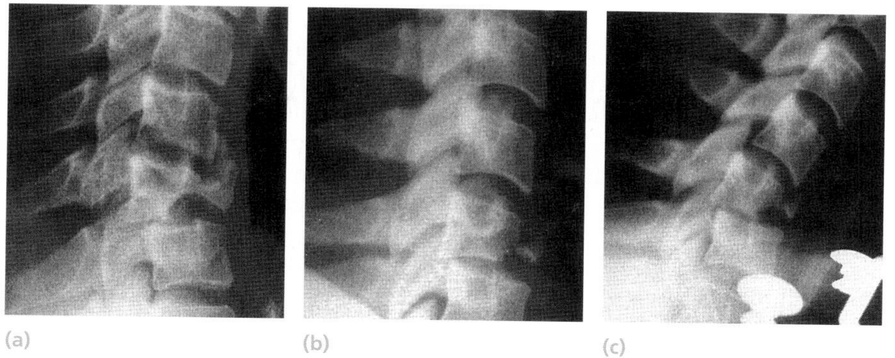

27.19 Tear-drop fracture (a) This comminuted vertebral body fracture has produced a large anterior fragment and obvious posterior displacement of the posterior fragment. (b) In this case the anterior 'tear-drop' was noted but the severity of the injury was underestimated; careful examination shows that the main body fragment is displaced slightly posteriorly. The patient was treated in a collar; 3 weeks later (c) the fracture had collapsed and the large body fragment was now very obviously tilted and displaced posteriorly. By then he was complaining of tingling and weakness in his right arm. Beware the innocent tear-drop!

immobilization in a halo-vest for 6–8 weeks. (The halo-vest is unsuitable for initial treatment because it does not provide axial traction).

If there is any deterioration of neurological status while the fracture is believed to be unstable, and the MRI shows that there is a threat of cord compression, then urgent anterior decompression is considered – anterior corpectomy, bone grafting and plate fixation, and sometimes also posterior stabilization.

Fracture-dislocations

Bilateral facet joint dislocations are caused by severe flexion or flexion–rotation injuries. The inferior articular facets of one vertebra ride forward over the superior facets of the vertebra below. One or both of the articular masses may be fractured or there may be a pure dislocation – 'jumped facets'. The posterior ligaments are ruptured and the spine is unstable; often there is cord damage.

The lateral x-ray shows forward displacement of a vertebra on the one below of greater than half the vertebra's antero-posterior width.

The displacement must be reduced as a matter of urgency. Skull traction is used, starting with 5 kg and increasing it step-wise by similar amounts up to about 30kg; intravenous muscle relaxants and a bolster beneath the shoulders may help. The entire procedure should be done without anaesthesia (or under mild sedation only) and neurological examination should be repeated after each incremental step. If neurological symptoms or signs develop, or increase, further attempts at closed reduction should be stopped.

When x-rays show that the dislocation has been reduced, traction is diminished to about 5 kg and then maintained for 6 weeks. During this time MRI can be performed to rule out the presence of an associated disc disruption. At the end of that period the patient should still wear a collar for another 6 weeks;

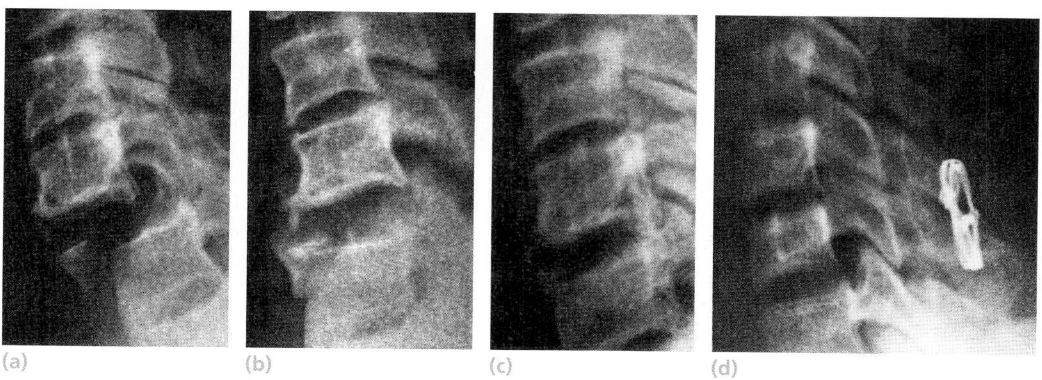

27.20 Cervical fracture-dislocation (a) Fracture-dislocation in the lower cervical spine. (b,c) Stages in the reduction of this fracture-dislocation by skull traction; (d) subsequent posterior wiring to ensure stability.

however, it may be more convenient to immobilize the neck in a halo-vest for 12 weeks.

Another alternative is to carry out a posterior fusion as soon as reduction has been achieved; the patient is then allowed up in a cervical brace which is worn for 6–8 weeks. Posterior open reduction and fusion is also indicated if closed reduction fails.

The need for pre-reduction MRI is controversial. In its favour is the ability to diagnose an extruded disc fragment which may further compromise any neurological lesion but can be dealt with by anterior decompression. This is particularly applicable to elderly patients in whom immediate closed reduction may be hazardous and long periods on their backs can lead to pressure sores. An argument against pre-reduction MRI is that there is insufficient correlation between various degrees of disc extrusion and neurological deterioration to justify another surgical assault on the traumatized patient.

Unilateral facet dislocation This is a flexion–rotation injury in which only one apophyseal joint is dislocated. There may be an associated fracture of the facet. On the lateral x-ray the vertebral body appears to be partially displaced (less than one-half of its width); on the anteroposterior x-ray the alignment of the spinous processes is distorted. Cord damage is unusual and the injury is stable.

Management is the same as for bilateral dislocation. Sometimes complete reduction is prevented by the upper facet becoming perched upon the lower. When no further progress occurs, it is tempting to assist in the final reduction by gently manipulating the patient's head in extension and rotation; this should be attempted only by an experienced operator. As a general rule, if closed reduction fails, open reduction and posterior fixation are advisable.

After reduction, if the patient is neurologically intact the neck is immobilized in a halo-vest for 6–8 weeks. However, in about 50 per cent of the patients surgery may still have to be considered at the end of this period. If there is an associated facet fracture or recurrent dislocation in the external fixator, then posterior fusion again becomes necessary. Patients left with an unreduced unilateral facet dislocation may develop neck pain and nerve root symptoms long-term if poorly managed.

Remember that halo vests can cause pressure sores over the scapula in sensory impaired patients.

Hyperextension injury

Hyperextension strains of soft-tissue structures are common and may be caused by comparatively mild acceleration forces. Bone and joint disruptions, however, are rare.

The more severe injuries are suggested by the history and the presence of facial bruising or lacerations. The posterior bone elements are compressed and may fracture; the anterior structures fail in tension, with tearing of the anterior longitudinal ligament or an avulsion fracture of the anterosuperior or anteroinferior edge of the vertebral body, opening up of the anterior part of the disc space, fracture of the back of the vertebral body and/or damage to the intervertebral disc. In patients with pre-existing cervical spondylosis, the cord can be pinched between the bony spurs or disc and the posterior ligamentum flavum; oedema and haematomyelia may cause an acute central cord syndrome (quadriplegia, sacral sparing and more upper limb than lower limb deficit, a flaccid upper limb paralysis and spastic lower limb paralysis).

These injuries are stable in the neutral position, in which they should be held by a collar for 6–8 weeks. Healing may lead to spontaneous fusion between adjacent vertebral bodies.

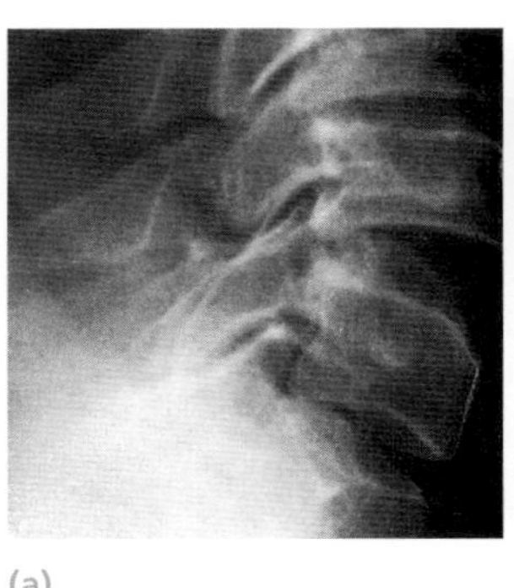
(a)

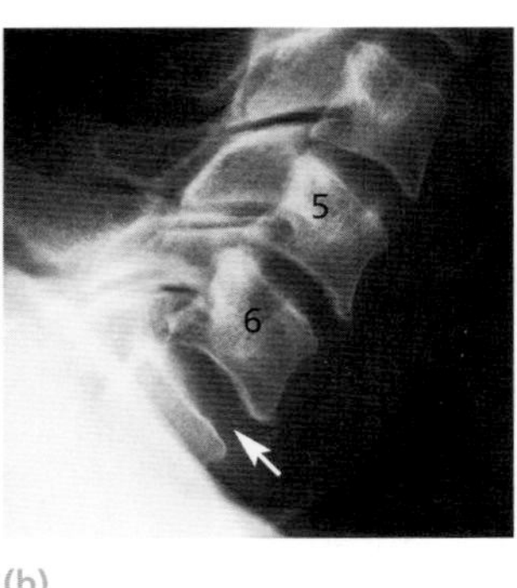

(b)

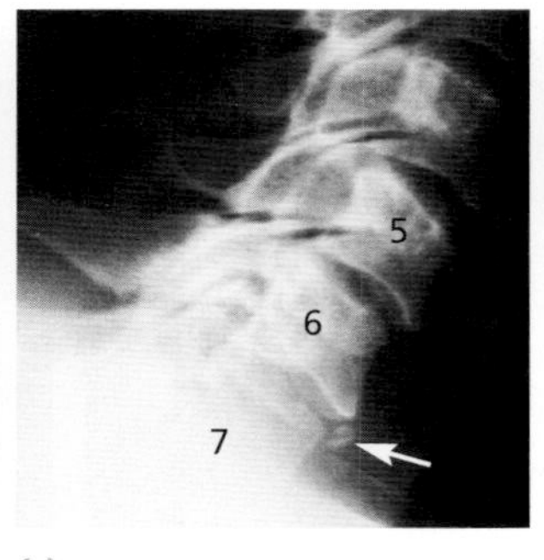

(c)

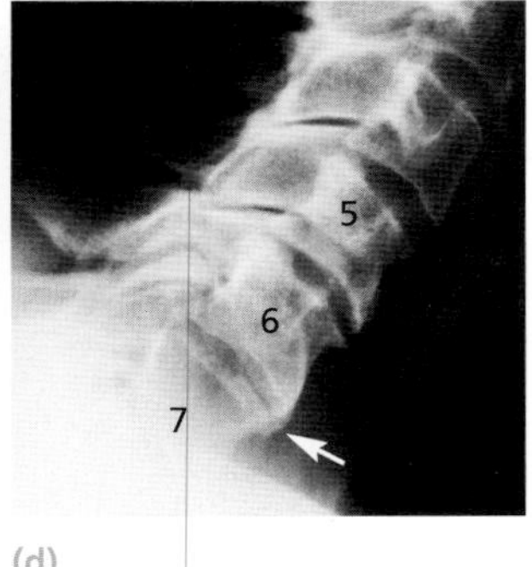

(d)

27.21 Hyperextension injuries (a) The anterior longitudinal ligament has been torn; in the neutral position the gap will close and reduction will be stable, but a collar or brace will be needed until the soft tissues are healed. (b) X-ray in this case showed a barely visible flake of bone anteriorly at the C6/7 disc space. (c) 1 month later the traction fracture at C6/7 was more obvious, as was the disc lesion at C5/6. (d) A year later C6/7 has fused anteriorly; the patient still has neck pain due to the C5/6 disc degeneration.

Double injuries

With high-energy trauma the cervical spine may be injured at more than one level. Discovery of the most obvious lesion is no reason to drop one's guard. Two salutary examples are shown in Figures 27.22 and 27.23.

Avulsion injury of the spinous process

Fracture of the C7 spinous process may occur with severe voluntary contraction of the muscles at the back of the neck; it is known as the *clay-shoveller's fracture*. The injury is painful but harmless. No treatment is required; as soon as symptoms permit, neck exercises are encouraged.

Cervical disc herniation

Acute post-traumatic disc herniation may cause severe pain radiating to one or both upper limbs, and neurological symptoms and signs ranging from mild paraesthesia to weakness, loss of a reflex and blunted sensation. Rarely a patient presents with full-blown paresis. The diagnosis is confirmed by MRI or CT-myelography.

Sudden paresis will need immediate surgical decompression. With lesser symptoms and signs, one can afford to wait a few days for improvement; if this does not occur, then anterior discectomy and interbody fusion will be needed.

Neurapraxia of the cervical cord

Accidents causing sudden, severe axial loading with the neck in hyperflexion or hyperextension are occasionally followed by transient pain, paraesthesia and weakness in the arms or legs, all in the absence of any x-ray or MRI abnormality. Symptoms may last for as little as a few minutes or as long as two or three days. The condition has been called neurapraxia of the cervical cord and is ascribed to pinching of the cord by the bony edges of the mobile spinal canal and/or local compression by infolding of the posterior longitudinal ligament or the ligamentum flavum (Thomas et al., 1999). Congenital narrowing of the spinal canal may be a predisposing factor.

Treatment consists of reassurance (after full neurological investigation) and graded exercises to improve strength in the neck muscles.

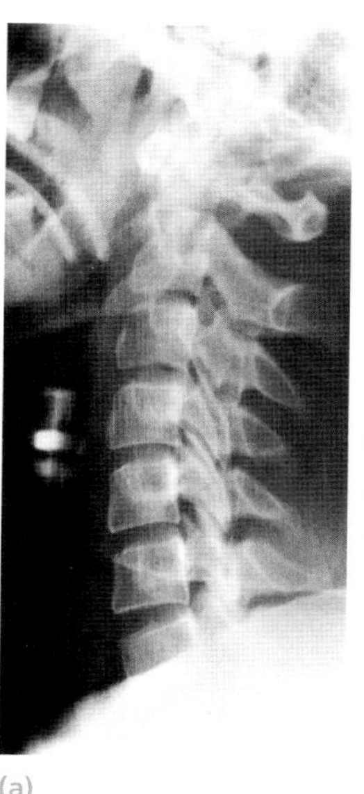
(a)

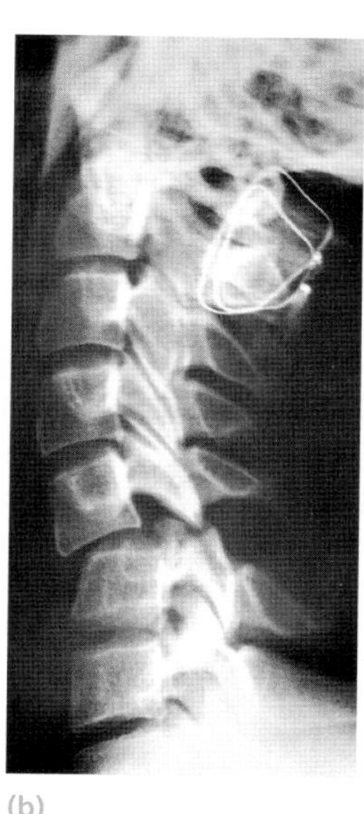
(b)

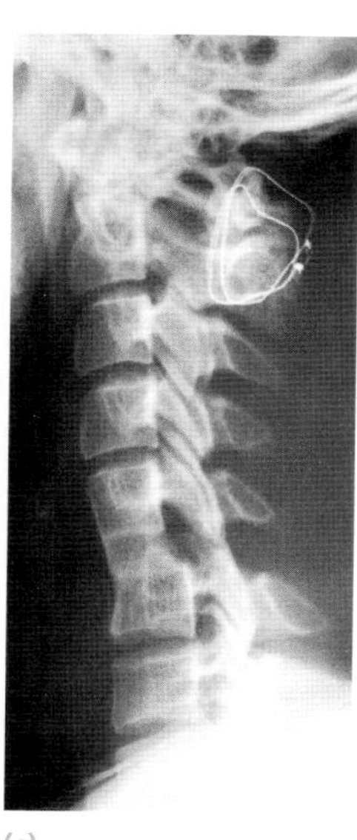
(c)

27.22 Double cervical injuries (a) This patient with a neck injury was suspected of having an odontoid fracture. This was confirmed and a posterior stabilization was performed. Only when the brace was removed and he started flexing his neck did the x-ray show an obvious subluxation lower down (b). This was treated by anterior fusion (c).

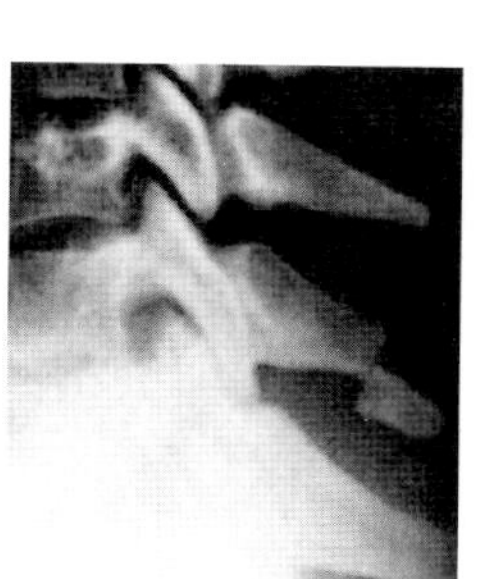
(a)

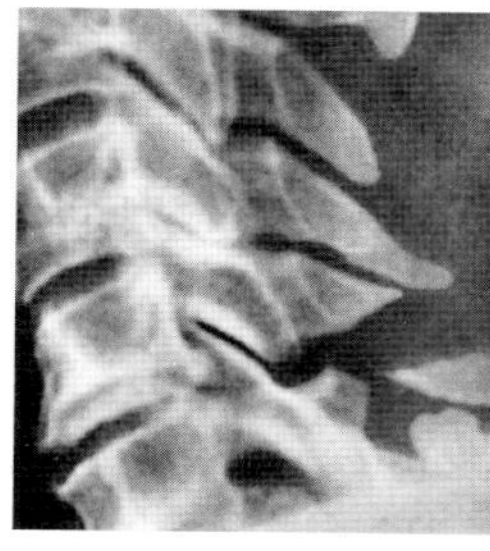
(b)

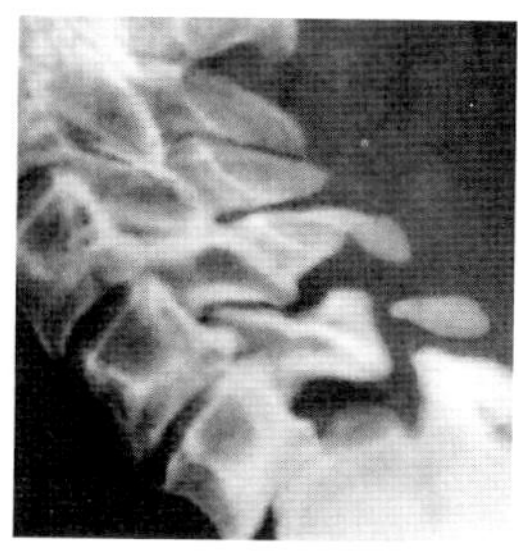
(c)

27.23 Avulsions (a) The clay-shoveller's fracture. Jerking the neck backwards has resulted in avulsion of one of the spinous processes – a benign injury. (b) This patient might be thought to have a similar fracture, but a subsequent flexion film (c) shows the serious nature of the injury – a severe fracture-dislocation.

SPRAINED NECK (WHIPLASH INJURY)

Soft-tissue sprains of the neck are so common after motor vehicle accidents that they now constitute a veritable epidemic. There is usually a history of a low-velocity rear-end collision in which the occupant's body is forced against the car seat while his or her head flips backwards and then recoils in flexion. This mechanism has generated the imaginative term whiplash injury, which has served effectively to enhance public apprehension at its occurrence. However, similar symptoms are often reported with flexion and rotation injuries. Women are affected more often than men, perhaps because their neck muscles are more gracile. There is disagreement about the exact pathology but it has been suggested that the anterior longitudinal ligament of the spine and the capsular fibres of the facet joints are strained and in some cases the intervertebral discs may be damaged in some unspecified manner. There is no correlation between the amount of damage to the vehicle and the severity of complaints.

Clinical features

Often the victim is unaware of any abnormality immediately after the collision. Pain and stiffness of the neck usually appear within the next 12–48 hours, or occasionally only several days later. Pain sometimes radiates to the shoulders or interscapular area and may be accompanied by other, more ill-defined, symptoms such as headache, dizziness, blurring of vision, paraesthesia in the arms, temporomandibular discomfort and tinnitus. Neck muscles are tender and movements often restricted; the occasional patient may present with a 'skew neck'. Other physical signs – including neurological defects – are uncommon.

X-ray examination may show straightening out of the normal cervical lordosis, a sign of muscle spasm; in other respects the appearances are usually normal. In some cases, however, there are features of long-standing intervertebral disc degeneration or degenerative changes in the uncovertebral joints; it may be that these patients suffer more, and for longer spells, than others.

Table 27.3 Proposed grading of whiplash-associated injuries

Grade	Clinical pattern
0	No neck symptoms or signs
1	Neck pain, stiffness and tenderness No physical signs
2	Neck symptoms and musculoskeletal signs
3	Neck symptoms and neurological signs
4	Neck symptoms and fracture or dislocation

MRI may show early degenerative changes, but no more commonly than in the age-matched population at large; the examination is not indicated except in patients with convincing neurological signs.

For purposes of comparison, the severity grading system proposed by the Quebec Task Force on Whiplash-Associated Disorders is useful.

Differential diagnosis

The diagnosis of sprained neck is reached largely by a process of exclusion, i.e. the inability to demonstrate any other credible explanation for the patient's symptoms. X-rays should be carefully scrutinized to avoid missing a vertebral fracture or a mid-cervical subluxation. The presence of neurological signs such as muscle weakness and wasting, a depressed reflex or definite loss of sensibility should suggest an acute disc lesion and is an indication for MRI.

Seat-belt injuries often accompany neck sprains. They do not always cause bruising of the chest, but they can produce pressure or traction injuries of the suprascapular nerve or the brachial plexus, either of which may cause symptoms resembling those of a whiplash injury. The examining doctor should be familiar with the clinical features of these conditions.

Treatment

Collars are more likely to hinder than help recovery. Simple pain-relieving measures, including analgesic medication, may be needed during the first few weeks. However, the emphasis should be on graded exercises, beginning with isometric muscle contractions and postural adjustments, then going on gradually to active movements and lastly movements against resistance. The range of movement in each direction is slowly increased without subjecting the patient to unnecessary pain. Many patients find osteopathy and chiropractic treatment to be helpful.

Progress and outcome

The natural history of whiplash injury is reflected in the statistics appearing in the medical literature on this subject. Details and references are presented in a recent review by Bannister et al. (2009).

Many people who are involved in road collisions do not seek medical attention at all; this is particularly the case in countries where medical and legal costs are not compensated. Some patients start improving within a few weeks and reports in the medical literature suggest that 50–60 per cent eventually make a full recovery; in most cases symptoms diminish after about 3 months and go on improving over the next year or two; however, 2–5 per cent continue to complain of symptoms and loss of functional capacity more or less indefinitely (Bannister et al., 2009). Negative prognostic indicators are increasing age, severity of symptoms at the outset, prolonged duration of symptoms and the presence of pre-existing intervertebral disc degeneration. Other factors that presage a poor outcome are a history of pre-accident psychological dysfunction, unduly frequent attendance with unrelated physical complaints, a record of unemployment and a general tendency to underachievement.

It should be borne in mind that outcome studies are almost invariably based on a selected group of patients, namely those who attend for medical treatment after the accident, and little is known of the natural progress in the thousands of people who experience similar injuries and either do not develop symptoms or do not report them.

Chronic whiplash-associated disorder

Those patients who, in the absence of any objective clinical or imaging signs, continue almost indefinitely to complain of pain, restriction of movement, loss of function, depression and inability to work constitute a sizeable problem in terms of medical resources, compensation claims, legal costs and – not least – personal suffering. As yet, no convincing evidence of a new pathological lesion has been adduced to account for this long-lasting disorder and it cannot be said with certainty how much of it is due to a physical abnormality and how much is an expression of a behavioural disorder. The subject is well reviewed in the Current Concepts monograph edited by Gunzburg and Szpalski (1997).

THORACOLUMBAR INJURIES

Most injuries of the thoracolumbar spine occur in the transitional area – T11 to L2 – between the somewhat rigid upper and middle thoracic column and the flexible lumbar spine. The upper three-quarters of the thoracic segments are also protected to some extent by the rib-cage and fractures in this region tend to be mechanically stable. However, the spinal canal in that area is relatively narrow so cord damage is not uncommon and when it does occur it is usually complete (Bohlman, 1985). The spinal cord actually ends at L1 and below that level it is the lower nerve roots that are at risk.

Pathogenesis

Pathogenetic mechanisms fall into three main groups: *low-energy insufficiency fractures* arising from comparatively mild compressive stress in osteoporotic bone; *minor fractures of the vertebral processes* due to compressive, tensile or tortional strains; and *high-energy fractures or fracture-dislocations* due to major injuries sustained in motor vehicle collisions, falls or diving from heights, sporting events, horse-riding and collapsed buildings. It is mainly in the third group that one encounters neurological complications, but lesser fractures also sometimes cause nerve damage. The common mechanisms of injury are:

- *Flexion–compression* – failure of the anterior column and wedge-compression of the vertebral body. Usually stable, but greater than 50 per cent loss of anterior height suggests some disruption of the posterior ligamentous structures.
- *Lateral compression* – lateral wedging of the vertebral body resulting in a localized 'scoliotic' deformity.
- *Axial compression* – failure of anterior and middle columns causing a 'burst' fracture and the danger of retropulsion of a posterior fragment into the spinal canal. Often unstable.
- *Flexion–rotation* – failure of all three columns and a risk of displacement or dislocation. Usually unstable.
- *Flexion–distraction* – the so-called 'jack-knife' injury causing failure of the posterior and middle columns and sometimes also anterior compression.
- *Extension* – tensile failure of the anterior column and compression failure of the posterior column. Unstable.

Examination

Patients complaining of back pain following an injury or showing signs of bruising and tenderness over the spine, as well as those suffering head or neck injuries, chest injuries, pelvic fractures or multiple injuries elsewhere, should undergo a careful examination of the spine and a full neurological examination, including rectal examination to assess sphincter tone.

Imaging

X-rays The *anteroposterior x-ray* may show loss of height or splaying of the vertebral body with a crush fracture. Widening of the distance between the pedicles at one level, or an increased distance between two adjacent spinous processes, is associated with posterior column damage. The *lateral view* is examined for alignment, bone outline, structural integrity, disc space defects and soft-tissue shadow abnormalities. Always look carefully for evidence of fragment retropulsion towards the spinal canal. Plain x-rays, while showing the lower thoracic and lumbar spine quite clearly, are less revealing of the upper thoracic vertebrae because the scapulae and shoulders get in the way

CT and MRI *Rapid screening CT* scans are now routine in many accident units. Not only are they more reliable than x-rays in showing bone injuries throughout the spine, and indispensable if axial views are necessary, but they also eliminate the delay, discomfort and anxiety so often associated with multiple attempts at 'getting the right views' with plain x-rays. In some cases *MRI* also may be needed to evaluate neurological or other soft-tissue injuries.

Treatment

Treatment depends on: (a) the type of anatomical disruption; (b) whether the injury is stable or unstable; (c) whether there is neurological involvement or not; and (d) the presence or absence of concomitant injuries. Details are discussed under each fracture type.

Minor injuries

Fractures of the transverse processes

The transverse processes can be avulsed with sudden muscular activity. Isolated injuries need no more than symptomatic treatment. More ominous than usual is a fracture of the transverse process of L5; this should alert one to the possibility of a vertical shear injury of the pelvis.

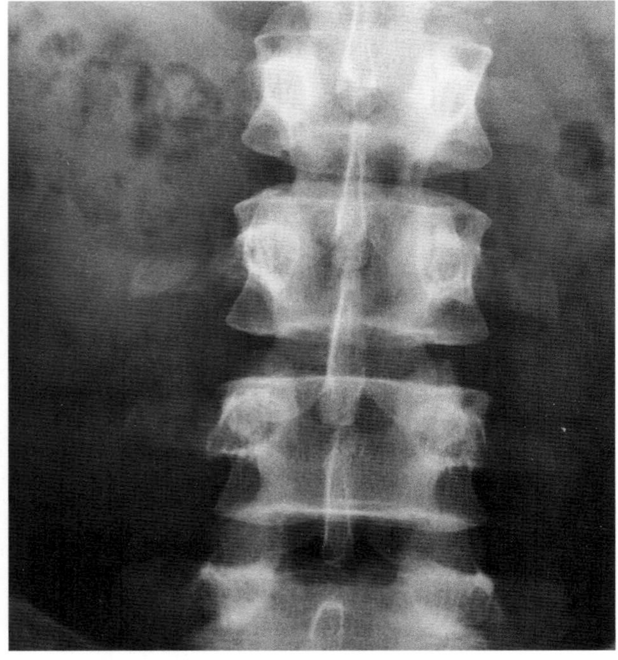

27.24 Thoracolumbar injuries – minor fractures Fracture of the transverse processes on the right at L3 and L4.

Fracture of the pars interarticularis

A stress fracture of the pars interarticularis should be suspected if a gymnast or athlete or weight-lifter complains of the sudden onset of back pain during the course of strenuous activity. The injury is often ascribed to a disc prolapse, whereas in fact it may be a stress fracture of the pars interarticularis (*traumatic spondylolysis*). This is best seen in the oblique x-rays, but a thin fracture line is easily missed; a week or two later, an isotope bone scan may show a 'hot' spot. Bilateral fractures occasionally lead to spondylolisthesis. The fracture usually heals spontaneously, provided the patient is prepared to forego his (more often her) athletic passion for several months.

Major injuries

Flexion–compression injury

This is by far the most common vertebral fracture and is due to severe spinal flexion, though in osteoporotic individuals fracture may occur with minimal trauma. The posterior ligaments usually remain intact, although if anterior collapse is marked they may be damaged by distraction. CT shows that the posterior part of the vertebral body (middle column) is unbroken. Pain may be quite severe but the fracture is usually stable. Neurological injury is extremely rare.

Patients with minimal wedging and a stable fracture pattern are kept in bed for a week or two until pain subsides and are then mobilized; no support is needed.

Those with moderate wedging (loss of 20–40 per cent of anterior vertebral height) and a stable injury can be allowed up after a week, wearing a thoracolumbar brace or a body cast applied with the back in extension. At 3 months, flexion–extension x-rays are obtained with the patient out of the orthosis; if there is no instability, the brace is gradually discarded. If the deformity increases and neurological signs appear, or if the patient cannot tolerate the orthosis, surgical stabilization is indicated.

If loss of anterior vertebral height is greater than 40 per cent, it is likely that the posterior ligaments have been damaged by distraction and will be unable to resist further collapse and deformity. If the patient is neurologically intact, surgical correction and internal fixation is the preferred treatment, though if necessary even these patients can be treated conservatively with vigilant monitoring of their neurological status.

In the rare cases of patients with a wedge compression fracture and neurological impairment treatment will depend on the degree of dysfunction and the risk of progression. If nerve loss is incomplete there is the potential for further recovery; any increase in kyphotic deformity or MRI signs of impending cord

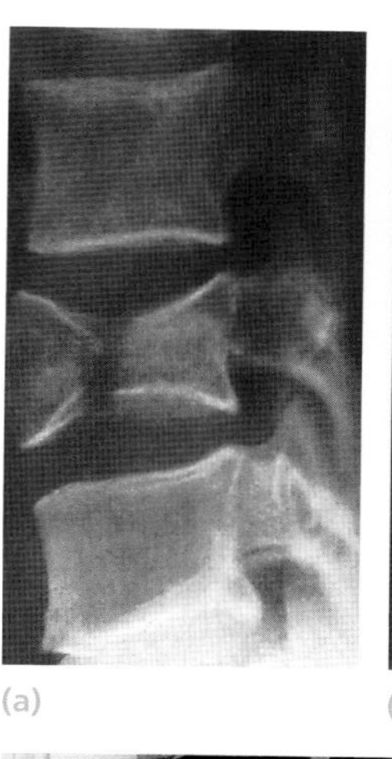
(a)

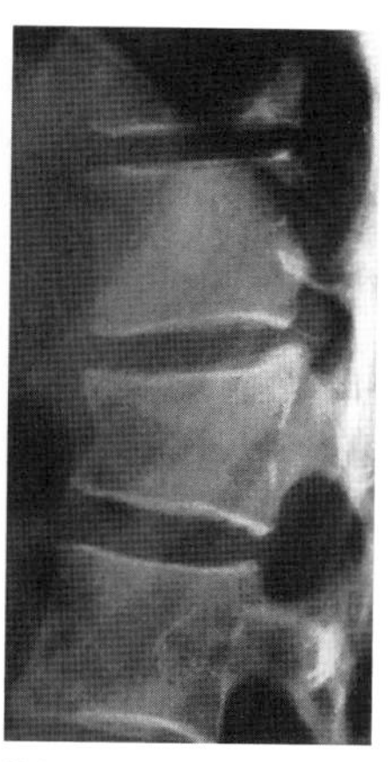
(b)

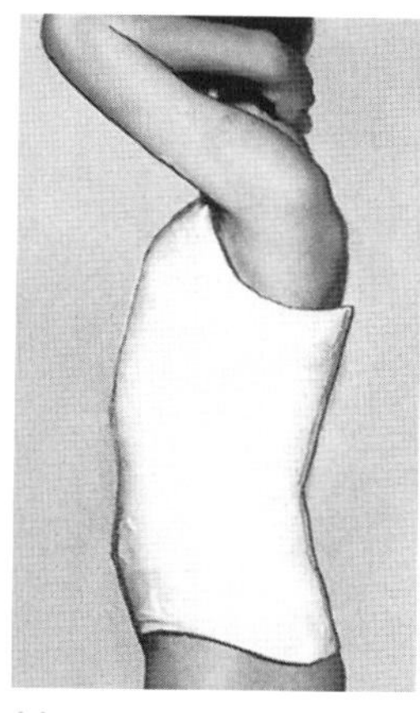
(c)

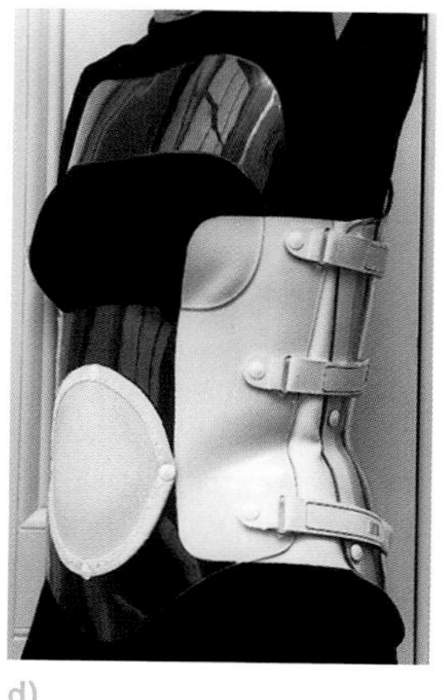
d)

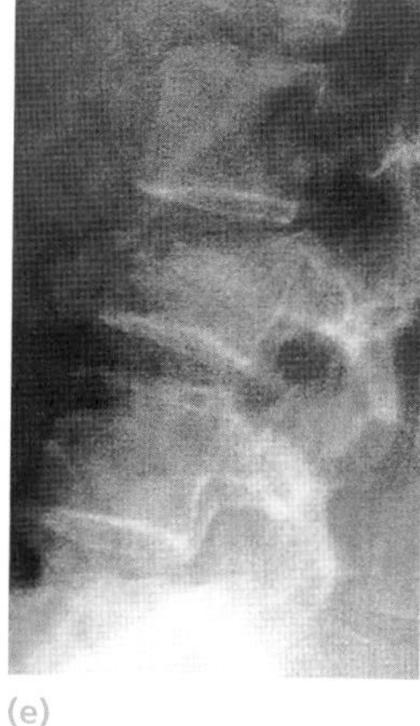
(e)

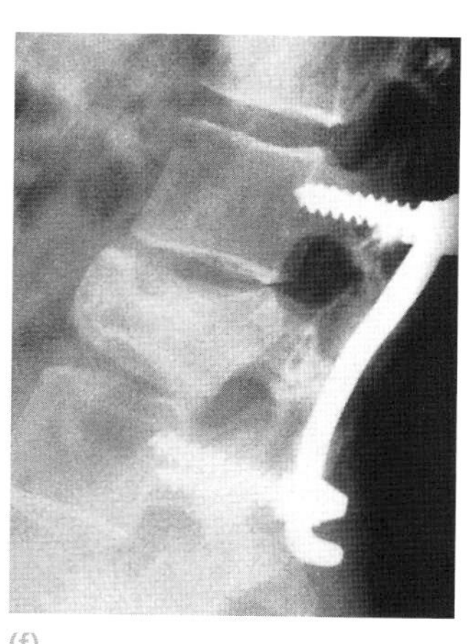
(f)

27.25 Wedge-compression fractures (a) Central compression fracture of the vertebral body and (b) anterior wedge-compression fracture with less than 20 per cent loss of vertebral body height. In both cases the middle and posterior columns are intact; further collapse can be prevented by immobilization for 8–12 weeks in (c) a plaster 'jacket' or (d) a lightweight removable orthosis. (e,f) More severe and potentially unstable compression fractures may need posterior internal fixation.

neurological compression would be an indication for operative decompression and stabilization through a trans-thoracic approach.

If there is complete paraplegia with no improvement after 48 hours, conservative management is adequate; the patient can be rested in bed for 5–6 weeks, then gradually mobilized in a brace. With severe bony injury, however, increasing kyphosis may occur and internal fixation should be considered.

Axial compression or burst injury

Severe axial compression may 'explode' the vertebral body, causing failure of both the anterior and the middle columns. The posterior column is usually, but not always, undamaged. The posterior part of the vertebral body is shattered and fragments of bone and disc may be displaced into the spinal canal. The injury is usually unstable.

Anteroposterior x-rays may show spreading of the vertebral body with an increase of the interpedicular distance. Posterior displacement of bone into the spinal canal (retropulsion) is difficult to see on the plain lateral radiograph; a CT is essential.

If there is minimal anterior wedging and the fracture is stable with no neurological damage, the patient is kept in bed until the acute symptoms settle (usually under a week) and is then mobilized in a thoracolumbar brace or body cast which is worn for about 12 weeks. Wood et al. (2003) carried out a prospective randomized trial comparing operative and non-operative treatment of stable thoracolumbar burst fractures with no neurological impairment; they found no difference in the long-term results in the two groups, but complications were more frequent in the surgical group.

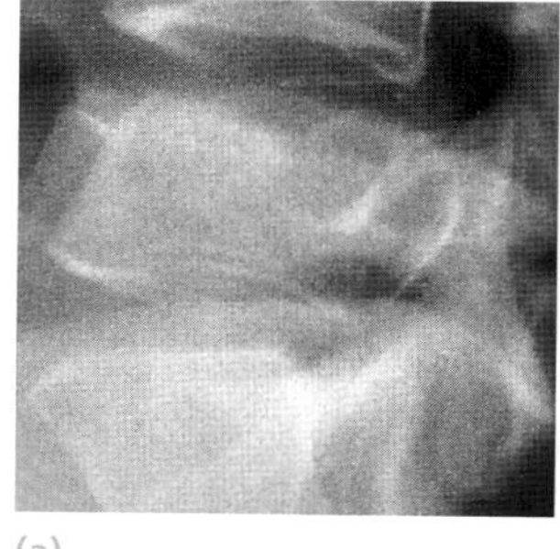
(a)

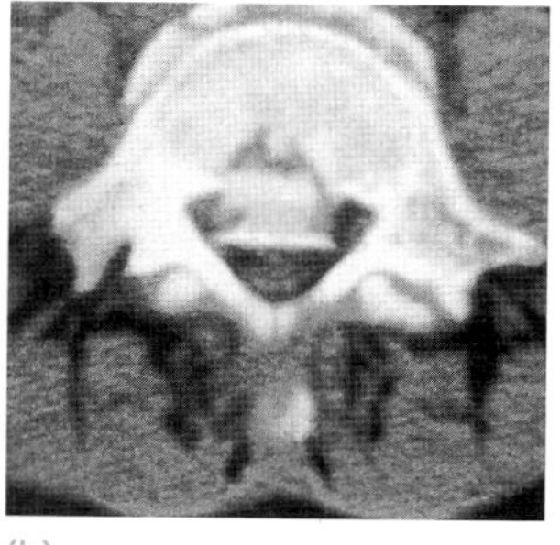
(b)

27.26 Lumbar burst fracture Severe compression may shatter the middle column and cause retropulsion of the vertebral body (a). The extent of spinal canal encroachment is best shown by CT (b).

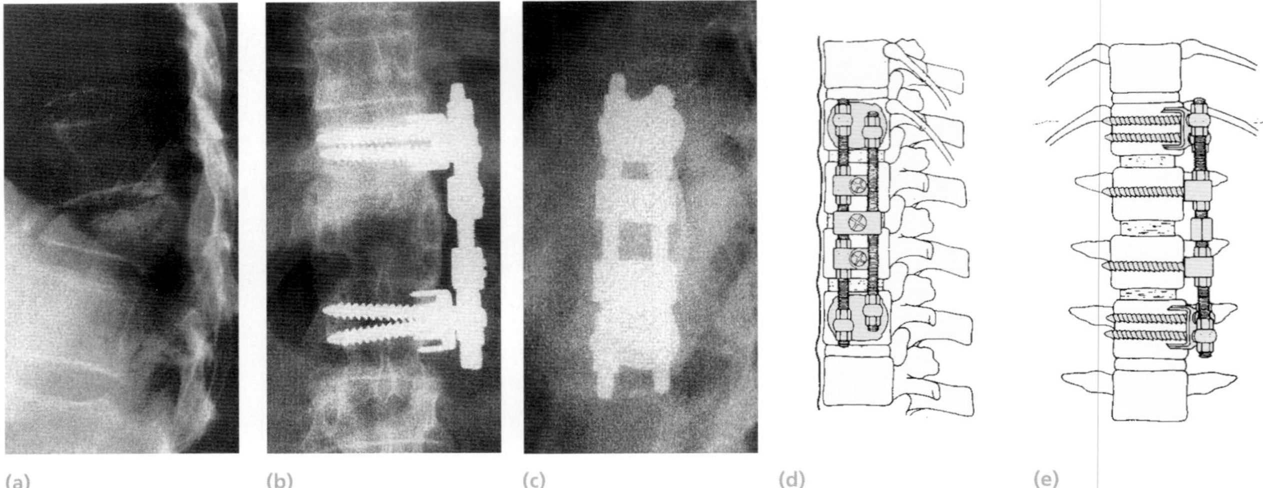

(a) (b) (c) (d) (e)

27.27 Burst fracture – treatment (a) Burst fracture in a 44-year-old man who fell from his horse; 3 months later he developed paraesthesia in both legs. (b–e) Internal fixation and grafting through a transthoracic transdiaphragmatic approach provided total stability (the Kaneda method).

Even if CT shows that there is considerable compromise of the spinal canal, provided there are no neurological symptoms or signs non-operative treatment is still appropriate; the fragments usually remodel. However, any new symptoms such as tingling, weakness or alteration of bladder or bowel function must be reported immediately and should call for further imaging by MRI; anterior decompression and stabilization may then be needed if there are signs of present or impending neurological compromise.

Jack-knife injury

Combined flexion and posterior distraction may cause the mid-lumbar spine to jack-knife around an axis that is placed anterior to the vertebral column. This is seen most typically in *lap seat-belt injuries*, where the body is thrown forward against the restraining strap. There is little or no crushing of the vertebral body, but the posterior and middle columns fail in distraction; thus these fractures are unstable in flexion.

The tear passes transversely through the bones or the ligament structures, or both. The most perfect example of tensile failure is the injury described by Chance in 1948, in which the split runs through the spinous process, the transverse processes, pedicles and the vertebral body. Neurological damage is uncommon, though the injury is (by definition) unstable. X-rays may show horizontal fractures in the pedicles or transverse processes, and in the anteroposterior view the apparent height of the vertebral body may be increased. In the lateral view there may be opening up of the disc space posteriorly.

The Chance fracture (being an 'all bone' injury) heals rapidly and requires 3 months in a body cast or well-fitting brace. Flexion–extension lateral views should then be taken to ensure that there is no unstable deformity.

Severe ligamentous injuries are less predictable and posterior spinal fusion is advisable.

Fracture-dislocation

Segmental displacement may occur with various combinations of flexion, compression, rotation and shear. All three columns are disrupted and the spine is

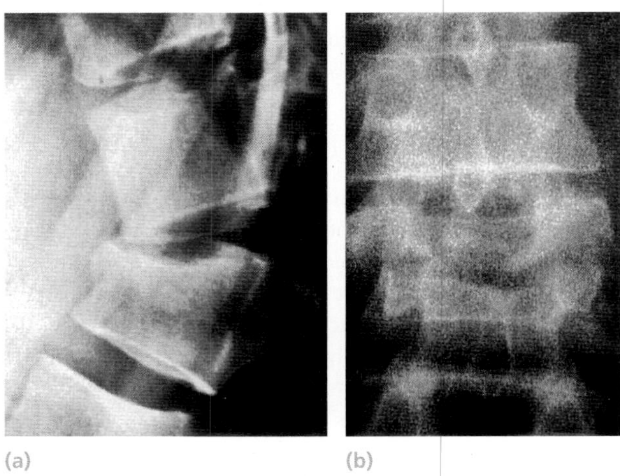

(a) (b)

27.28 Jack-knife injuries (a) Whereas flexion usually crushes the vertebral body and leaves the posterior ligaments intact, the jack-knife injury disrupts the posterior ligaments causing only slight anterior compression. (b) The rare Chance fracture.

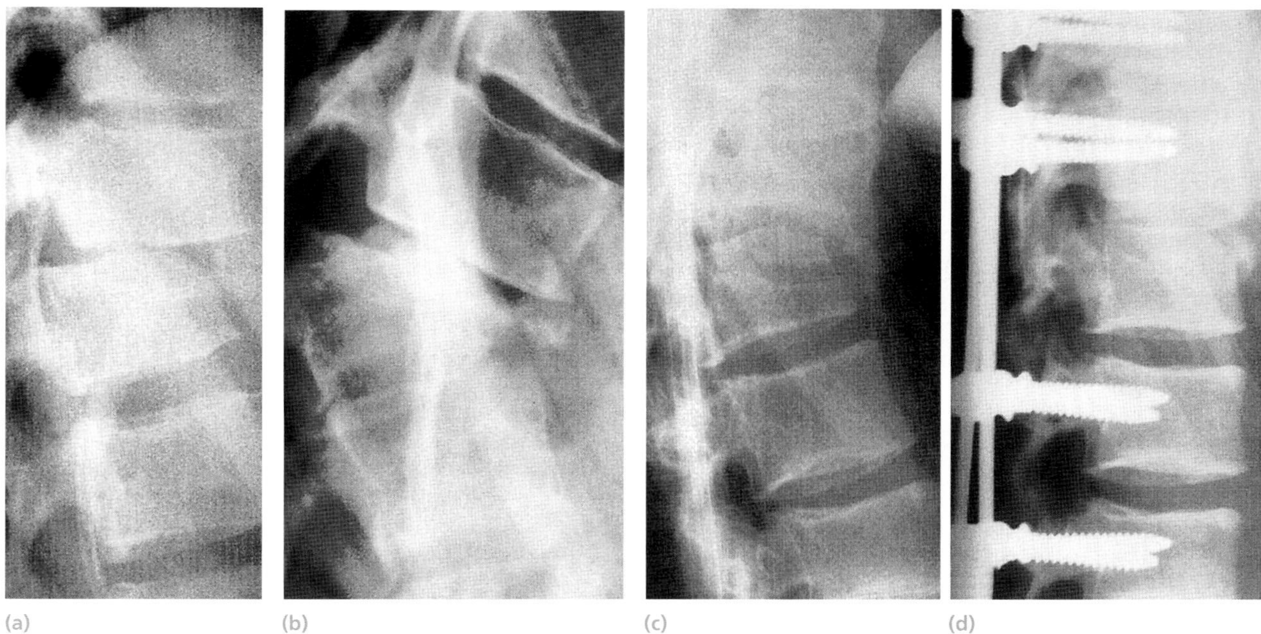

27.29 Thoracolumbar fracture-dislocation (a) Fracture-dislocation at T11/12 in a 32-year-old woman who was a passenger in a truck that overturned. She was completely paraplegic and operation was not thought worthwhile. (b) Four weeks later the deformity has increased, leaving her with a marked gibbus. (c,d) A similar injury in a 17-year-old man, treated by open reduction and internal fixation.

grossly unstable. These are the most dangerous injuries and are often associated with neurological damage to the lowermost part of the cord or the cauda equina.

The injury most commonly occurs at the thoracolumbar junction. X-rays may show fractures through the vertebral body, pedicles, articular processes and laminae; there may be varying degrees of subluxation or even bilateral facet dislocation. Often there are associated fractures of transverse processes or ribs. CT is helpful in demonstrating the degree of spinal canal occlusion.

In neurologically intact patients, most fracture-dislocations will benefit from early surgery.

In *fracture-dislocation with paraplegia*, there is no convincing evidence that surgery will facilitate nursing, shorten the hospital stay, help the patient's rehabilitation or reduce the chance of painful deformity. In *fracture-dislocation with a partial neurological deficit*, there is also no evidence that surgical stabilization and decompression provides a better neurological outcome than conservative treatment. If surgical decompression and stabilization are performed, this may require a combined posterior and anterior approach.

In *fracture-dislocation without neurological deficit*, surgical stabilization will prevent future neurological complications and allow earlier rehabilitation.

When specialized surgery cannot be performed, these injuries can be managed non-operatively with postural reduction, bed rest and bracing. For patients with neurological impairment who have the benefit of being treated in a specialized spinal injuries unit, a strong case can be made for managing them also by non-operative methods.

NEURAL INJURIES

In spinal injuries the displaced structures may damage the cord or the nerve roots, or both; cervical lesions may cause quadriplegia, thoracolumbar lesions paraplegia. The damage may be partial or complete. Three varieties of lesion occur: neurapraxia, cord transection and root transection.

Neurapraxia

Motor paralysis (flaccid), burning paraesthesia, sensory loss and visceral paralysis below the level of the cord lesion may be complete, but within minutes or a few hours recovery begins and soon becomes full. The condition is most likely to occur in patients who, for some reason other than injury, have a small-diameter anteroposterior canal; there is, however, no radiological evidence of recent bony damage.

Cord transection

Motor paralysis, sensory loss and visceral paralysis occur below the level of the cord lesion; as with cord concussion, the motor paralysis is at first flaccid. This is a temporary condition known as cord shock, but the injury is anatomical and irreparable.

After a time the cord below the level of transection recovers from the shock and acts as an independent structure; that is, it manifests reflex activity. Within 48 hours the primitive anal wink and bulbocavernosus reflexes return. Within 4 weeks of injury tendon reflexes return and the flaccid paralysis becomes spastic, with increased tone, increased tendon reflexes and clonus; flexor spasms and contractures may develop with inadequate management.

Root transection

Motor paralysis, sensory loss and visceral paralysis occur in the distribution of the damaged roots. Root transection, however, differs from cord transection in two ways: recovery may occur and residual motor paralysis remains permanently flaccid.

ANATOMICAL LEVELS

Cervical spine With cervical spine injuries the segmental level of cord transection nearly corresponds to the level of bony damage. Not more than one or two additional roots are likely to be transected. High cervical cord transection is fatal because all the respiratory muscles are paralysed. At the level of the C5 vertebra, cord transection isolates the lower cervical cord (with paralysis of the upper limbs), the thoracic cord (with paralysis of the trunk) and the lumbar and sacral cord (with paralysis of the lower limbs and viscera). With injury below the C5 vertebra, the upper limbs are partially spared and characteristic deformities result.

Between T1 and T10 vertebrae The first lumbar cord segment in the adult is at the level of the T10 vertebra. Consequently, cord transection at that level spares the thoracic cord but isolates the entire lumbar and sacral cord, with paralysis of the lower limbs and viscera. The lower thoracic roots may also be transected but are of relatively little importance.

Below T10 vertebra The cord forms a slight bulge (the conus medullaris) between the T10 and L1 vertebrae, and tapers to an end at the interspace between the L1 and L2 vertebrae. The L2 to S4 nerve roots arise from the conus medullaris and stream downwards in a bunch (the cauda equina) to emerge at successive levels of the lumbosacral spine. Therefore, spinal injuries above the T10 vertebra cause cord transection, those between the T10 and L1 vertebrae cause cord and nerve root lesions, and those below the L1 vertebra only root lesions.

The *sacral roots* innervate:

- sensation in the 'saddle' area (S3, S4), a strip down the back of the thigh and leg (S2) and the outer two-thirds of the sole (S1);
- motor power to the muscles controlling the ankle and foot;
- the anal and penile reflexes, plantar responses and ankle jerks;
- bladder and bowel continence.

The *lumbar roots* innervate:

- sensation to the groins and entire lower limb other than that portion supplied by the sacral segment;
- motor power to the muscles controlling the hip and knee;
- the cremasteric reflexes and knee jerks.

It is essential, when the bony injury is at the thoracolumbar junction, to distinguish between cord transection with root escape and cord transection with root transection. A patient with root escape is much better off than one with cord and root transection.

DIAGNOSIS

Clinical examination of the back nearly always shows the signs of an unstable fracture; however, a 'burst' fracture with paraplegia is stable as long as the patient is in recumbency or very well braced until the fracture heals. The nature and level of the bone lesion are demonstrated by x-ray, and that of the neural lesion by CT or MRI.

Neurological examination should be painstaking. Without detailed information, accurate diagnosis and prognosis are impossible; rectal examination is mandatory.

Complete cord lesions Complete paralysis and anaesthesia below the level of injury suggest cord transection. During the stage of spinal shock when the anal reflex is absent (seldom longer than the first 24 hours) the diagnosis cannot be absolutely certain; if the anal reflex returns and the neural deficit (sensory and motor) persists, the cord lesion is complete. Complete lesions lasting more than 72 hours have only a small chance of neurological recovery.

Incomplete cord lesions Persistence of any sensation distal to the injury (peri-anal pinprick is most important) suggests an incomplete lesion.

The commonest is the *central cord syndrome* where the initial flaccid weakness is followed by lower motor neuron paralysis of the upper limbs with upper motor neuron (spastic) paralysis of the lower limbs, and intact peri-anal sensation (sacral sparing). Bladder control may or may not be preserved from an early stage.

With the less common *anterior cord syndrome* there is complete paralysis and anaesthesia but deep pressure and position sense are retained in the lower limbs (dorsal column sparing).

The *posterior cord syndrome* is rare; only deep pressure and proprioception are lost.

The *Brown-Séquard syndrome* (due to cord hemisection) is usually associated with penetrating thoracic injuries. There is loss of motor power on the side of the injury and loss of pain and temperature sensation on the opposite side. Most of these patients improve and regain bowel and bladder function and some walking ability.

High root lesions sometimes cause confusion. Below the T10 vertebra, discrepancies between neurological and skeletal levels are due to transection of roots descending from cord segments higher than the vertebral lesion.

FRANKEL GRADING

A well-established method of recording the functional deficit after an incomplete spinal cord injury was that described by Frankel:

Grade A = Absent motor and sensory function.
Grade B = Sensation present, motor power absent.
Grade C = Sensation present, motor power present but not useful.
Grade D = Sensation present, motor power present and useful (grade 4 or 5).
Grade E =Normal motor and sensory function.

Frankel observed that 60 per cent of patients with partial cord lesions (Grades B, C or D) improved (spontaneously) by one grade regardless of the treatment type and a significant number are able to walk again. Although many of the patients who present in Frankel Grade A improve to B or C, only 5 per cent of these patients improve to Frankel D or E.

MANAGEMENT OF TRAUMATIC PARAPLEGIA AND QUADRIPLEGIA

With *both* complete and *incomplete paralysis* it is the overall management of the patient that is most important – from the early stages onwards.

The patient must be transported with great care to prevent further damage, and preferably taken to a spinal centre. The strategy is outlined below.

Skin Within a few hours anaesthetic skin may develop large pressure sores; this can be prevented by meticulous nursing. Creases in the sheets and crumbs in bed are not permitted. Every 2 hours the patient is gently rolled onto his or her side and the back is carefully washed (without rubbing), dried and powdered. After a few weeks the skin becomes a little more tolerant and the patient can turn him- or herself. Later he or she should be taught how to relieve skin pressure intermittently during periods of sitting. If sores have been allowed to develop, they may never heal without surgical closure.

Bladder and bowel For the first 24 hours the bladder distends only slowly, but, if the distension is allowed to progress, overflow incontinence occurs and infection is probable. In special centres it is usual to manage the patient from the outset by intermittent catheterization under sterile conditions. If early transfer to a paraplegia centre is not possible, continuous drainage through a fine Silastic catheter is advised. The catheter drains in a closed manner into a disposable bag, and is changed twice weekly to prevent urethral and bladder complications, catheter blockage and infection. When infection supervenes, antibiotics are given.

Bladder training is begun as early as possible. Although retention is complete to begin with, partial recovery may lead to either an automatic bladder which works reflexly or an expressible bladder which is emptied by manual suprapubic pressure.

A few patients are left with a high residual urine after emptying the bladder. They need special investigations, including cystography and cystometry; transurethral resection of the bladder neck or sphincterotomy may be indicated but should not be performed until at least 3 months of bladder training have been completed.

The bowel is more easily trained, with the help of enemas, aperients and abdominal exercises.

Muscles and joints The paralysed muscles, if not treated, may develop severe flexion contractures. These are usually preventable by moving the joints passively through their full range twice daily. Later, splints may be necessary.

With lesions below the cervical cord, the patient should be up within 6 weeks; standing and walking are valuable in preventing contractures.

Callipers are usually necessary to keep the knees straight and the feet plantigrade. The callipers are removed at intervals during the day while the patient lies prone, and while he or she is having physiotherapy. The upper limbs must be trained until they develop sufficient power to enable the patient to use crutches and a wheelchair.

If flexion contractures have been allowed to develop, tenotomies may be necessary. Painful flexor spasms are rare unless skin or bladder infection occurs. They can sometimes be relieved by tenotomies, neurectomies, rhizotomies or the intrathecal injection of alcohol.

Heterotopic ossification is a common and disturbing complication. It is more likely to occur with high lesions and complete lesions. It may restrict or abolish movement, especially at the hip. Once the new bone is mature it should be considered for excision if it interferes with function.

Tendon transfers Some function can be regained in the upper limb by the use of tendon transfers. The aim with patients who have a low cervical cord injury is to use the limited number of functioning muscles in the arm to provide a primitive pinch mechanism (normally powered by C8 or T1 which, being below the level of injury, are lost). One must establish which muscles are working, which are not and which are available for transfer.

- *If only deltoid and biceps are working (C5, C6)* then a posterior-deltoid to triceps transfer using interposition tendon grafts will replace the lost C7 function of elbow extension; this will enable the patient to orient his or her hand in space.
- *If brachioradialis (C6) is working,* this can be transferred to become a wrist extensor (since its prime function as an elbow flexor is duplicated by biceps). A primitive thumb pinch can be achieved by the Moberg procedure in which the thumb interphalangeal joint is fused and the basal joint of the thumb is tenodesed with a loop of the redundant flexor pollicis longus. On active extension of the wrist, the basal joint of the thumb is passively flexed.
- *If extensor carpi radialis longus and brevis (C7) are both available,* one of them can be transferred into the flexor pollicis longus to provide active thumb flexion (normally supplied by C8).

Morale The morale of a paraplegic patient is liable to reach a low ebb, and the restoration of his or her self-confidence is an important part of treatment. Constant enthusiasm and encouragement by doctors, physiotherapists and nurses is essential. Their scrupulous attention to the patient's comfort and toilet are of primary importance; the unpleasant smells of bowel accidents, or those associated with skin or urinary infection must be prevented. The patient should find a hobby or be trained for a new job as quickly as possible.

REFERENCES AND FURTHER READING

Advanced Trauma Life Support. American College of Surgeons 1997.

Anderson LD, D'Alonzo RT. Fractures of the odontoid process of the axis. *J Bone Joint Surg* 1974; **56A:** 1663–74.

Bannister G, Amirfeyz R, Kelley S, Gargan M. Whiplash injury. *J Bone Joint Injury* 2009; **91B:** 845–50.

Bohlman HH. Treatment of fractures and dislocations of the thoracic and lumbar spine – current concepts review. *J Bone Joint Surg* 1985; **67A:** 165–9.

Chance CQ. Note on a type of flexion fracture of the spine. *Br J Radiol* 1948; **21:** 452–3.

Denis F. The three column spine and its significance in the classification of acute thoracolumbar spinal injuries. *Spine* 1983; **8:** 817–31.

El Masry WS. Management of Traumatic Spinal Cord Injuries: current standard of care revisited. *Ad Clin Neuroscience Rehab.* 2010; **10:** 37–40.

El Masry WS. Traumatic spinal cord injury: the relationship between pathology and clinical implications. *Trauma* 2006; **8:** 29–46.

El Masri WS. Physiological instability of the spinal cord following injury. *Paraplegia* 1993; **31:** 273–5.

Gunzburg R, Szpalski M. Whiplash injuries. Current concepts in prevention, diagnosis and treatment of the cervical whiplash syndrome. Philadelphia, Lippincott-Raven, 1997.

Hugenholtz H, Cass DE, Dvorak MF. High-dose methylprednisolone for acute closed spinal cord injury: Only a treatment option. *Can J Neurol Sci* 2002; **29:** 227–35.

Katoh S, El Masry WS, Jaffray D *et al*. The neurologic outcome in conservatively treated patients with incomplete closed traumatic cervical spinal cord injuries. *Spine*; **21:** 2345–2351.

Molano M, Broton JG, Bean JA *et al*. Complications associated with prophylactic use of methylprednisolone during surgical stabilization after spinal cord injury. *J Neurosurg* 2002; **96:** 267–72.

Short DJ, El Masry WS, Jones PW. High dose methylprednisolone in the management of acute spinal cord injury: A systematic review from a clinical perspective. *Spinal Cord* 2000; **38:** 273–86.

Slucky AV, Eismont FJ. Treatment of acute injury of the cervical spine. *J Bone Joint Surg* 1994; **76A:** 1882–95.

Solomon L, Pearse MF. Osteonecrosis following low-dose short-course corticosteroids. *J Orthop Rheumatol* 1994; **7:** 203–5.

Spitzer WO, Skovron ML, Salmi LR *et al*. Scientific monograph of the Quebec Task Force on whiplash-associated disorders: redefining whiplash and its management. *Spine* 1995; **20(8):** 1S–73S.

Thomas BE, McCullen GM, Yuan HA. Cervical spine injuries in football players. J *Am Acad Orthop Surg* 1999; **7:** 338–47.

Wood K, Butterman G, Mehbod A *et al*. Operative compared with non-operative treatment of a thoracolumbar burst fracture without neurological deficit. *J Bone Joint Surg* 2003; **85A:** 773–81.

Injuries of the pelvis

28

Louis Solomon

Fractures of the pelvis account for less than 5 per cent of all skeletal injuries, but they are particularly important because of the high incidence of associated soft-tissue injuries and the risks of severe blood loss, shock, sepsis and adult respiratory distress syndrome (ARDS). Like other serious injuries, they demand a combined approach by experts in various fields.

About two-thirds of all pelvic fractures occur in road accidents involving pedestrians; over 10 per cent of these patients will have associated visceral injuries, and in this group the mortality rate is probably in excess of 10 per cent.

Surgical anatomy

The pelvic ring is made up of the two innominate bones and the sacrum, articulating in front at the symphysis pubis (the anterior or pubic bridge) and posteriorly at the sacroiliac joints (the posterior or sacroiliac bridge). This basin-like structure transmits weight from the trunk to the lower limbs and provides protection for the pelvic viscera, vessels and nerves.

The stability of the pelvic ring depends upon the rigidity of the bony parts and the integrity of the strong ligaments that bind the three segments together across the symphysis pubis and the sacroiliac joints. The strongest and most important of the tethering ligaments are the sacroiliac and iliolumbar ligaments; these are supplemented by the sacrotuberous and sacrospinous ligaments and the ligaments of the symphysis pubis. As long as the bony ring and the ligaments are intact, load-bearing is unimpaired.

The major branches of the common iliac arteries arise within the pelvis between the level of the sacroiliac joint and the greater sciatic notch. With their accompanying veins they are particularly vulnerable in fractures through the posterior part of the pelvic ring. The nerves of the lumbar and sacral plexuses, likewise, are at risk with posterior pelvic injuries.

The bladder lies behind the symphysis pubis. The trigone is held in position by the lateral ligaments of the bladder and, in the male, by the prostate. The prostate lies between the bladder and the pelvic floor. It is held laterally by the medial fibres of the levator ani, whilst anteriorly it is firmly attached to the pubic bones by the puboprostatic ligament. In the female the trigone is attached also to the cervix and the anterior vaginal fornix. The urethra is held by both the pelvic floor muscles and the pubourethral ligament. Consequently in females the urethra is much more mobile and less prone to injury.

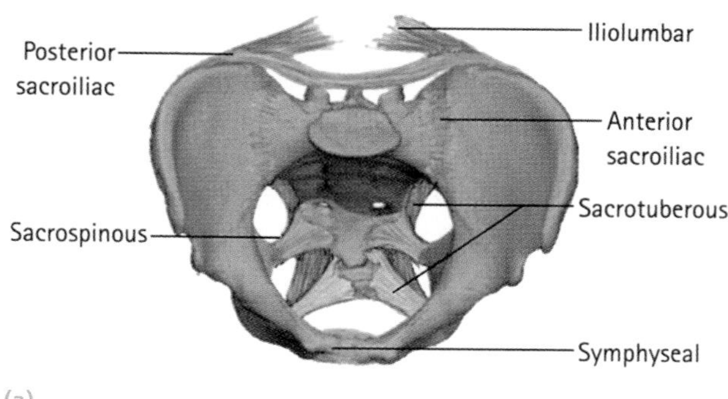

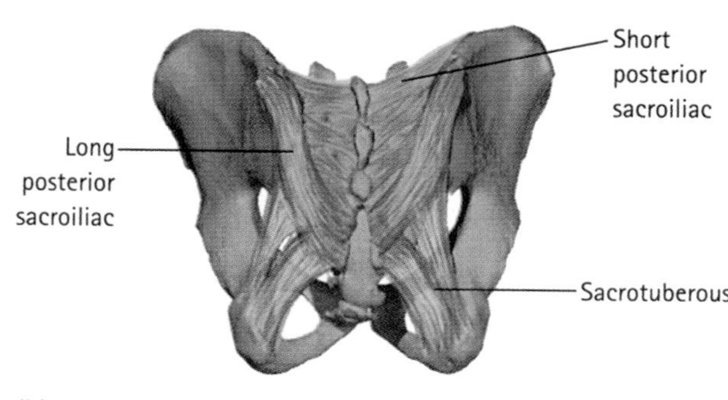

28.1 Ligaments supporting the pelvis (a) Anterior view. (b) Posterior view. Some ligaments run transversely and will resist rotational forces which separate the two halves (the posterior sacroiliac and iliolumbar ligaments can be thought of as a posterior band), whilst those that are oriented longitudinally tend to resist vertical shear.

In severe pelvic injuries the membranous urethra is damaged when the prostate is forced backwards whilst the urethra remains static. When the puboprostatic ligament is torn, the prostate and base of the bladder can become grossly dislocated from the membranous urethra.

The pelvic colon, with its mesentery, is a mobile structure and therefore not readily injured. However, the rectum and anal canal are more firmly tethered to the urogenital structures and the muscular floor of the pelvis and are therefore vulnerable in pelvic fractures.

Pelvic instability

If the pelvis can withstand weightbearing loads without displacement, it is stable; this situation exists only if the bony and key ligamentous structures are intact.

An anterior force applied to both halves of the pelvis forces apart the symphysis pubis. If a diastasis occurs because of capsular rupture, the extent of separation is checked by the anterior sacroiliac and sacrospinous ligaments. Should these restraints fail through the application of a still greater force, the pelvis opens like a book until the posterior iliac spines abut; because the more vertically oriented long posterior sacroiliac and sacrotuberous ligaments remain intact, the pelvis will still resist vertical shear but it is rotationally unstable. If, however, the posterior sacroiliac and sacrotuberous ligaments are damaged, then the pelvis is not only rotationally and vertically unstable, but there will also be posterior translation of the injured half of the pelvis. Vertical instability is therefore ominous as it suggests complete loss of the major ligamentous support posteriorly.

It should be remembered that some fracture patterns can cause instability which mimics that of ligamentous disruption; e.g. fractures of both pubic rami may behave like symphyseal disruptions, and fractures of the iliac wing combined with ipsilateral pubic rami fractures are unstable to vertical shear.

Clinical assessment

Fracture of the pelvis should be suspected in every patient with serious abdominal or lower limb injuries. There may be a history of a road accident or a fall from a height or crush injury. Often the patient complains of severe pain and feels as if he has fallen apart, and there may be swelling or bruising of the lower abdomen, the thighs, the perineum, the scrotum or the vulva. All these areas should be rapidly inspected, looking for evidence of extravasation of urine. *However, the first priority, always, is to assess the patient's general condition and look for signs of blood loss. It may be necessary to start resuscitation before the examination is completed.*

The abdomen should be carefully palpated. Signs of irritation suggest the possibility of intraperitoneal bleeding. The pelvic ring can be gently compressed from side to side and back to front. Tenderness over the sacroiliac region is particularly important and may signify disruption of the posterior bridge.

A rectal examination is then carried out in every case. The coccyx and sacrum can be felt and tested for tenderness. If the prostate can be felt, which is often difficult due to pain and swelling, its position should be gauged; an abnormally high prostate suggests a urethral injury.

Enquire when the patient passed urine last and look for bleeding at the external meatus. An inability to void and blood at the external meatus are the classic features of a ruptured urethra. However, the absence of blood at the meatus does not exclude a urethral injury, because the external sphincter may be in spasm, halting the passage of blood from the site of injury. Thus every patient who has a pelvic fracture must be considered to be at risk.

The patient can be encouraged to void; if he is able to do so, either the urethra is intact or there is only minimal damage which will not be made worse by the passage of urine. *No attempt should be made to pass a catheter, as this could convert a partial to a complete tear of the urethra.* If the urethral injury is suspected, this can be diagnosed more accurately and more safely by retrograde urethrography.

A ruptured bladder should be suspected in patients who do not void or in whom a bladder is not palpable after adequate fluid replacement. This palpation is often difficult because of abdominal wall haematoma. The physical findings initially can be minimal, with normal bowel sounds, as extravasation of sterile urine produces little peritoneal irritation. Only a very small

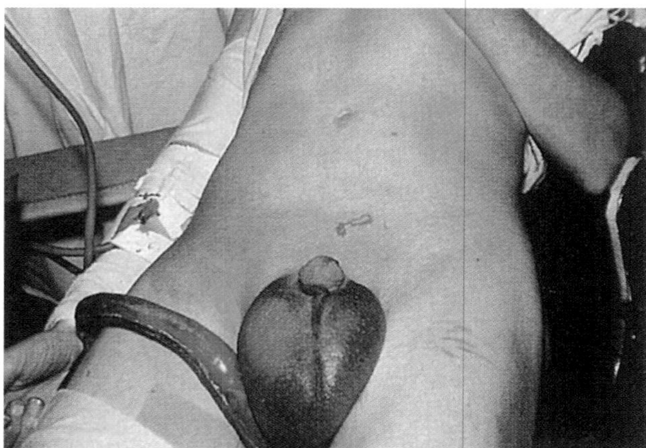

28.2 Fractures of the pelvis This young man crashed on his motorcycle and was brought into the Accident and Emergency Department with a fractured femur. His perineum and scrotum were swollen and bruised, he was unable to pass urine and a streak of blood appeared at the external meatus. X-rays confirmed that he had a fractured pelvis.

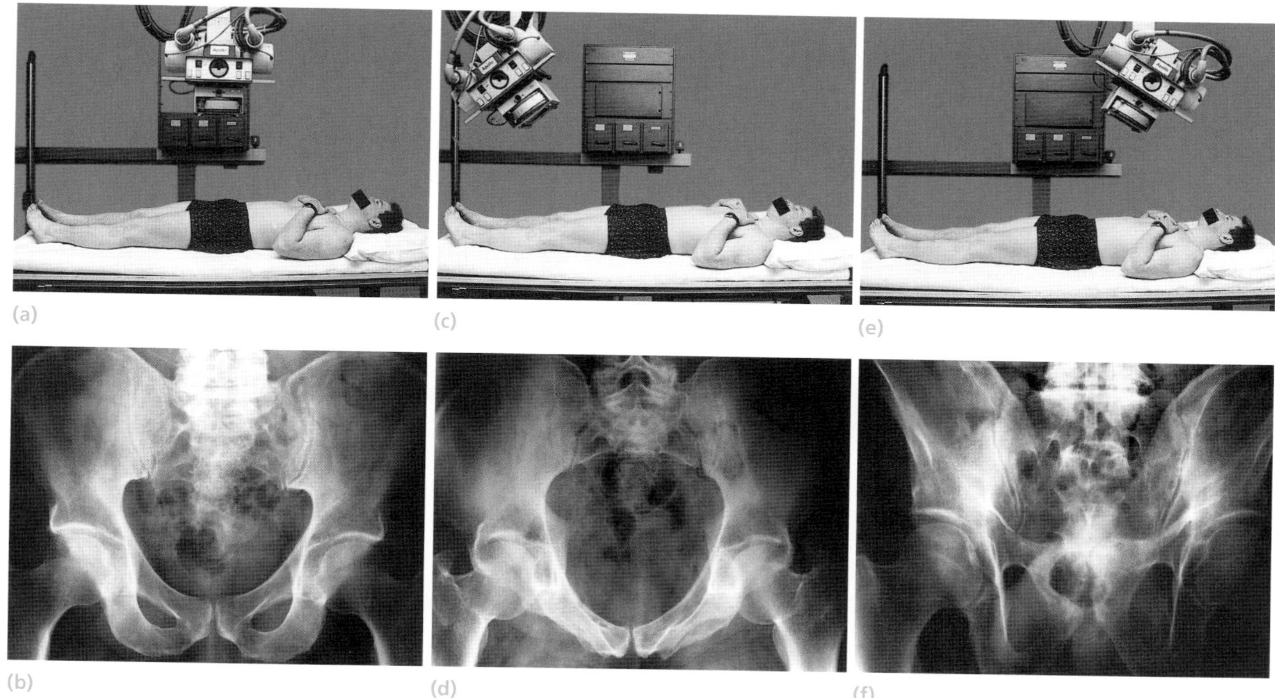

28.3 Pelvic fractures – x-ray diagnosis (1) (a,b) The anteroposterior view is usually taken during the initial assessment of the multiply-injured patient as part of a 'trauma series'. It is useful in quickly diagnosing gross disruptions or fractures. The x-ray should be read systematically: Is the picture well centred? Look for asymmetry in the pubic symphysis, the pubic rami, the iliac blades, the sacroiliac joints and the sacral foramina. If the patient's condition permits, at least two additional views should be obtained: (c,d) an *inlet* view with the tube titled 30° downwards and (e,f) an *outlet* view with the tube titled 40° upwards.

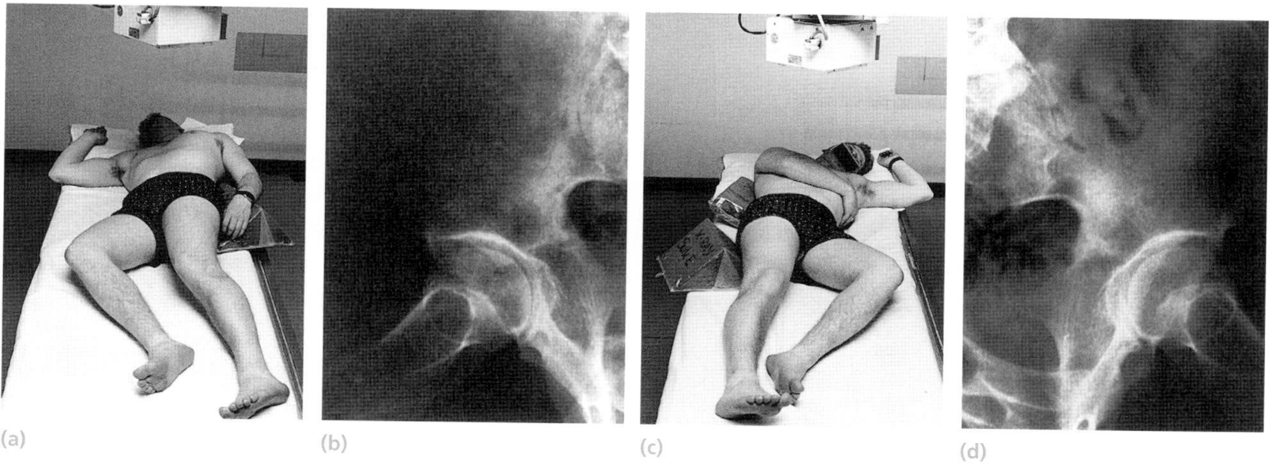

28.4 Pelvic fractures – x-ray diagnosis (2) Oblique views are helpful for defining the ilium and acetabulum on each side. (a,b) the *right oblique* view; and (c,d) the *left oblique* view. These can be omitted if facilities for CT are available.

proportion of patients with a ruptured bladder are hypotensive, so if a patient is hypotensive another cause must be sought.

Neurological examination is important; there may be damage to the lumbar or sacral plexus.

If the patient is unconscious, the same routine is followed. However, early x-ray examination is essential in these cases.

Imaging of the pelvis

During the initial survey of every severely injured patient, a plain anteroposterior x-ray of the pelvis should be obtained at the same time as the chest x-ray. In most cases this film will give sufficient information to make a preliminary diagnosis of pelvic fracture. The exact nature of the injury can be clarified by more

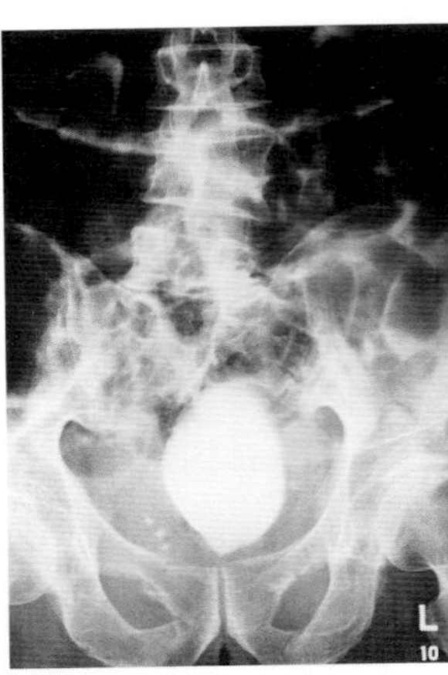

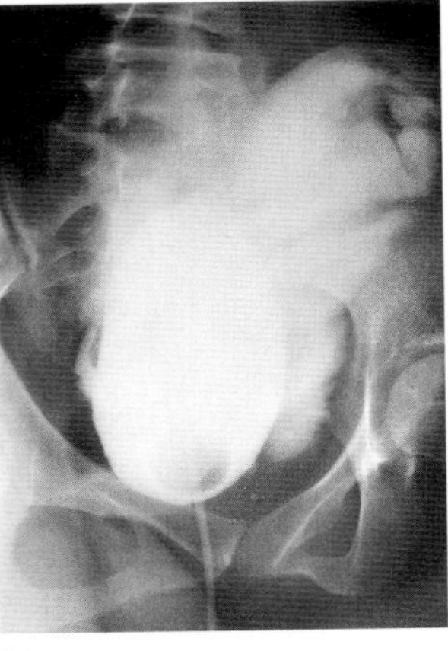

(a) (b)

28.5 Pelvic fractures and bladder injury
(a) Intravenous urogram outlining the bladder and showing the typical globular appearance due to compression by blood and extravasated urine. There is also marked gastric dilation suggesting retroperitoneal bleeding. (b) Cystogram showing extravasation of radio-opaque material. This patient had a ruptured bladder.

detailed radiography once it is certain that the patient can tolerate an extended period of positioning and repositioning on the x-ray table. Five views are necessary: anteroposterior, an inlet view (tube cephalad to the pelvis and tilted 30° downwards), an outlet view (tube caudad to the pelvis and tilted 40° upwards), and right and left oblique views.

If any serious injury is suspected, a CT scan at the appropriate level is extremely helpful (some would say essential). This is particularly true for posterior pelvic ring disruptions and for complex acetabular fractures, which cannot be properly evaluated on plain x-rays.

Three-dimensional CT re-formation of the pelvic image gives the most accurate picture of the injury; however, with practice almost as much information can be gleaned from a good set of plain radiographs and standard CT images.

Imaging of the urinary tract

If there is evidence of upper abdominal injury, and the patient has haematuria, an intravenous urogram is performed to exclude renal injury. This will also show whether there is any ureteric or major bladder damage. In a case of urethral rupture, the base of the bladder may be riding high (dislocated prostate) or there may be a teardrop deformity of the bladder owing to compression by blood and extravasated urine (prostate-in-situ).

When a urethral injury is considered likely, an urethrogram should be undertaken using 25–30ml of water-soluble contrast agent with suitable aseptic technique. A film must be taken during injection of the contrast agent to ensure that the urethra is fully distended. This technique will confirm a urethral tear and will show whether it is complete or incomplete.

In a patient with possible rupture of the bladder (so long as there is no evidence of a urethral injury) a cystogram should be performed.

Types of injury

Injuries of the pelvis fall into four groups: (1) isolated fractures with an intact pelvic ring; (2) fractures with a broken ring – these may be stable or unstable; (3) fractures of the acetabulum – although these are ring fractures, involvement of the joint raises special problems and therefore they are considered separately; and (4) sacrococcygeal fractures.

ISOLATED FRACTURES

Avulsion fractures

A piece of bone is pulled off by violent muscle contraction; this is usually seen in sportsmen and athletes. The sartorius may pull off the anterior superior iliac spine, the rectus femoris the anterior inferior iliac spine, the adductor longus a piece of the pubis, and the hamstrings part of the ischium. All are essentially muscle injuries, needing only rest for a few days and reassurance.

Pain may take months to disappear and, because there is often no history of impact injury, biopsy of the callus may lead to an erroneous diagnosis of a tumour. Rarely, avulsion of the ischial apophysis by the hamstrings may lead to persistent symptoms, in which case open reduction and internal fixation is indicated (Wootton, Cross and Holt, 1990).

Direct fractures

A direct blow to the pelvis, usually after a fall from a height, may fracture the ischium or the iliac blade. Bed rest until pain subsides is usually all that is needed.

Stress fractures

Fractures of the pubic rami are fairly common (and often quite painless) in severely osteoporotic or osteomalacic patients. More difficult to diagnose are stress fractures around the sacroiliac joints; this is an uncommon cause of 'sacroiliac' pain in elderly osteoporotic individuals and long distance runners. Obscure stress fractures are best demonstrated by radioisotope scans.

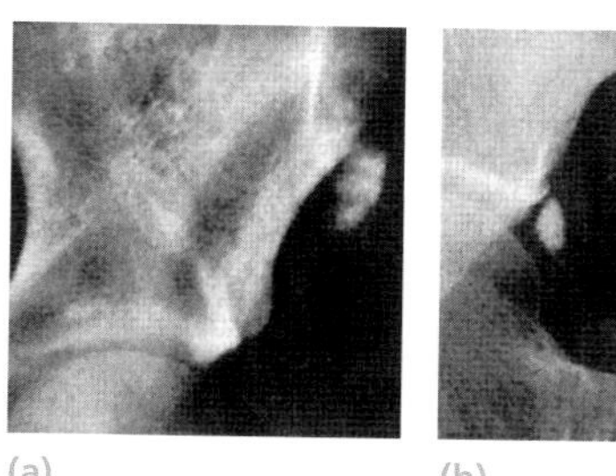

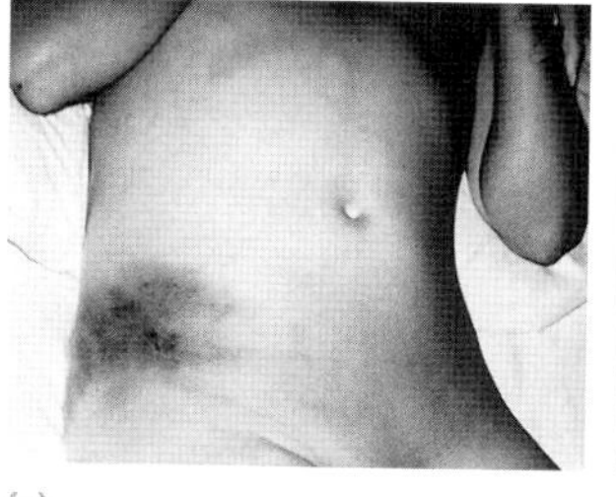

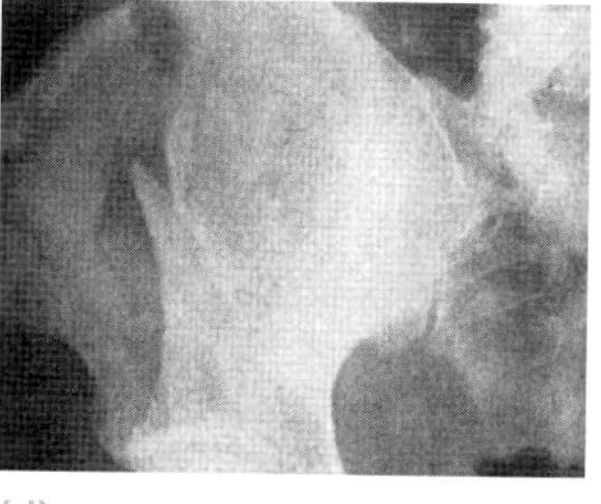

28.6 Isolated injuries (a,b) Avulsion fractures. Unusually powerful muscle contraction may tear off a piece of bone at its attachment. Two examples are shown here: (a) avulsion of sartorius attachment; (b) avulsion of rectus femoris origin. (c,d) Fractured iliac blade. The bruise suggests the site of the injury. The fracture looks alarming and is certainly painful but, if the remainder of the bony pelvis is intact, it poses no threat to the patient.

FRACTURES OF THE PELVIC RING

It has been cogently argued that, because of the rigidity of the pelvis, a break at one point in the ring must be accompanied by disruption at a second point; exceptions are fractures due to direct blows (including fractures of the acetabular floor), or ring fractures in children, whose symphysis and sacroiliac joints are springy. Often, however, the second break is not visible – either because it reduces immediately or because the sacroiliac joints are only partially disrupted.

Mechanisms of injury

The basic mechanisms of pelvic ring injury are anteroposterior compression, lateral compression, vertical shear and combinations of these.

Anteroposterior compression This injury is usually caused by a frontal collision between a pedestrian and a car. The pubic rami are fractured or the innominate bones are sprung apart and externally rotated, with disruption of the symphysis – the so-called 'open book' injury. The anterior sacroiliac ligaments are strained and may be torn, or there may be a fracture of the posterior part of the ilium.

Lateral compression Side-to-side compression of the pelvis causes the ring to buckle and break. This is usually due to a side-on impact in a road accident or a fall from a height. Anteriorly the pubic rami on one or both sides are fractured, and posteriorly there is a severe sacroiliac strain or a fracture of the sacrum or ilium, either on the same side as the fractured pubic rami or on the opposite side of the pelvis. If the sacroiliac injury is much displaced, the pelvis is unstable.

Vertical shear The innominate bone on one side is displaced vertically, fracturing the pubic rami and disrupting the sacroiliac region on the same side. This occurs typically when someone falls from a height onto one leg. These are usually severe, unstable injuries with gross tearing of the soft tissues and retroperitoneal haemorrhage.

Combination injuries In severe pelvic injuries there may be a combination of the above.

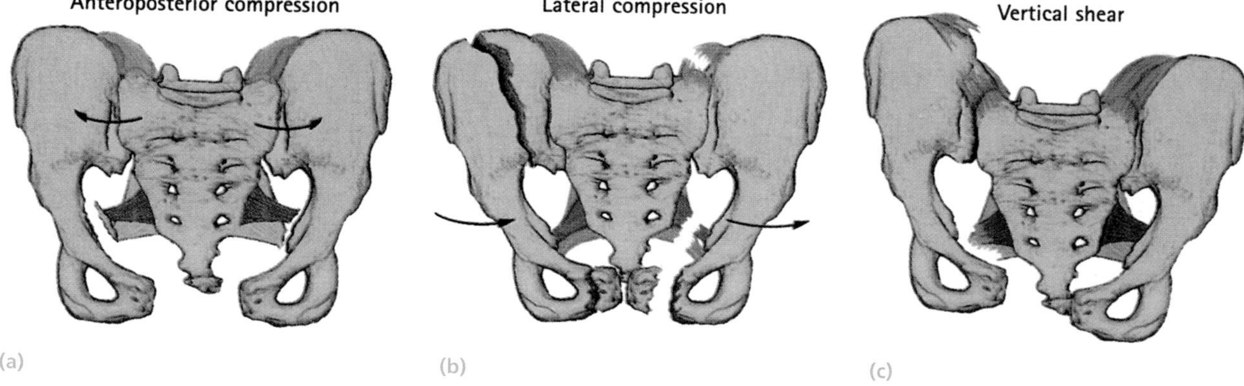

28.7 Types of pelvic ring fracture The three important types of injury are shown. (a) Anteroposterior compression with lateral rotation may cause the 'open book' injury, the hallmark of which is diastasis of the pubic symphysis. Widening of the anterior portion of the sacroiliac joint is best seen on an inlet view. (b) Lateral compression causing the ring to buckle and break; the pubic rami are fractured, sometimes on both sides. Posteriorly the iliac blade may break or the sacrum is crushed. (c) Vertical shear, with disruption of both the sacroiliac and symphyseal regions on one side.

Stable and unstable fractures

A stable pelvic ring injury is usually defined as one that will (theoretically) allow full weightbearing without the risk of pelvic deformity. Of course one cannot actually perform the test in an acutely injured patient. However, because the mechanisms which cause these injuries are fairly consistent, typical patterns and displacements are defined which make it possible to deduce the mechanism of injury, the type of ligament damage and the degree of pelvic instability. Occasionally the decision on stability cannot be made until the patient is examined under anaesthesia.

Several classifications are in use. The one presented here is based on that of Young and Burgess (1986; 1987).

ANTEROPOSTERIOR COMPRESSION (APC) INJURIES

The 'open book' pattern appears as either diastasis of the pubic symphysis or fracture(s) of the pubic rami; as the pelvis is sprung open, the posterior (sacroiliac) elements also are strained. This general pattern is subclassified according to the severity of the injury:

In *APC-I injuries* there may be only slight (less than 2 cm) diastasis of the symphysis; however, although invisible on x-ray, there will almost certainly be some strain of the anterior sacroiliac ligaments. The pelvic ring is stable.

In *APC-II injuries* diastasis is more marked and the anterior sacroiliac ligaments (often also the sacrotuberous and sacrospinous ligaments) are torn. CT may show slight separation of the sacroiliac joint on one side. Nevertheless, the pelvic ring is still stable.

In *APC-III injuries* the anterior and posterior sacroiliac ligaments are torn. CT shows a shift or separation of the sacroiliac joint; the one hemi-pelvis is effectively disconnected from the other anteriorly and from the sacrum posteriorly. The ring is unstable.

LATERAL COMPRESSION (LC) INJURIES

The hallmark of this injury is a transverse fracture of the pubic ramus (or rami), often best seen on an inlet view x-ray. There may also be a compression fracture of the sacrum. In its simplest form this would be classified as a *LC-I injury*. The ring is stable.

The *LC-II injury* is more severe; in addition to the anterior fracture, there may be a fracture of the iliac wing on the side of impact. However, the ring remains stable.

The *LC-III injury* is worse still. As the victim is run over, the lateral compression force on one iliac wing results in an opening anteroposterior force on the opposite ilium, causing injury patterns typical for that mechanism.

VERTICAL SHEAR (VS) INJURIES

The hemi-pelvis is displaced in a cranial direction, and often posteriorly as well, producing a typically asymmetrical appearance of the pelvis. As with APC-III injuries, the hemi-pelvis is totally disconnected and the pelvic ring is unstable.

COMBINATION INJURIES

Combination patterns do occur but, in the main, the above classification defines the most common types of injury. The LC-II pattern is linked to abdominal, head and chest injuries; all the unstable patterns carry a high risk of severe haemorrhage and are life-threatening (Dalal *et al.*, 1989).

Clinical features

Stable ring injuries The patient is not severely shocked but has pain on attempting to walk. There is localized tenderness but seldom any damage to pelvic viscera. Plain x-rays reveal the fractures.

Unstable ring injuries The patient is severely shocked, in great pain and unable to stand. He or she may also be unable to pass urine and there may be blood at the external meatus. Tenderness is widespread, and attempting to move one or both blades of the ilium is very painful. Clinical assessment for stability is difficult; few patients will allow pulling or pushing to reveal abnormal vertical movement (Olson and Pollack, 1996). One leg may be partly anaesthetic because of sciatic nerve injury.

Haemodynamic instability High-energy fractures of the pelvis are extremely serious injuries, carrying a great risk of associated visceral damage, intra-abdominal and retroperitoneal haemorrhage, shock, sepsis and ARDS; the mortality rate is considerable. The patient should be repeatedly assessed and re-assessed for signs of blood loss and hypovolaemia. Bear in mind that, although the pelvis may be the main focus of attention, haemorrhage may occur also in areas outside the pelvis.

Imaging

This may show fractures of the pubic rami, ipsilateral or contralateral fractures of the posterior elements, separation of the symphysis, disruption of the sacroiliac joint or combinations of these injuries. The films are often difficult to interpret and CT scans are much the best way of visualizing the nature of the injury.

Management

EARLY MANAGEMENT

Treatment should not await full and detailed diagnosis. It is vital to keep a sense of priorities and to act on any information that is already available while moving along to the next diagnostic hurdle. 'Management' in this context is a combination of assessment and treatment, following the ATLS protocols.

Six questions must be asked and the answers acted upon as they emerge:

- Is there a clear airway?
- Are the lungs adequately ventilated?
- Is the patient losing blood?
- Is there an intra-abdominal injury?
- Is there a bladder or urethral injury?
- Is the pelvic fracture stable or unstable?

With any severely injured patient, the first step is to make sure that the airway is clear and ventilation is unimpaired. Resuscitation must be started immediately and active bleeding controlled. The patient is rapidly examined for multiple injuries and, if necessary, painful fractures are splinted. A single anteroposterior x-ray of the pelvis is obtained.

A more careful examination is then carried out, paying attention to the pelvis, the abdomen, the perineum and the rectum. The urethral meatus is inspected for signs of bleeding. The lower limbs are examined for signs of nerve injury.

If the patient's general condition is stable, further x-rays can then be obtained. If a urethral tear is suspected, an urethrogram is gently performed. The findings up to that stage may dictate the need for an intravenous urogram.

By now the examining doctor will have a good idea of the patient's general condition, the extent of the pelvic injury, the presence or absence of visceral injury and the likelihood of continued intra-abdominal or retroperitoneal bleeding. Ideally, a team of experts will be on hand to deal with the individual problems or undertake further investigations.

MANAGEMENT OF SEVERE BLEEDING

Severe bleeding is the main cause of death following high-energy pelvic fractures. The general treatment of shock is described in Chapter 22. If there is an unstable fracture of the pelvis, haemorrhage will be reduced by rapidly applying an external fixator.

If either the expertise or the necessary equipment is lacking, unstable APC injuries can initially be managed by applying a pelvic binder to achieve side-to-side compression; the rationale is to try and close the 'open book' and reduce the internal pelvic volume.

The diagnosis of persistent bleeding is often difficult, and even when it seems clear that continuing shock is due to haemorrhage, it is not easy to determine the source of the bleeding. Patients with suspicious abdominal signs should be further investigated by peritoneal aspiration or lavage. If there is a positive diagnostic tap, the abdomen should be explored in an attempt to find and deal with the source of bleeding. However, if there is a large retroperitoneal haematoma, it should not be evacuated as this may release the tamponade effect and lead to uncontrollable haemorrhage.

If there is no evidence of intra-abdominal bleeding and laparotomy is not contemplated, but the patient shows signs of continuing blood loss, then angiography should be performed with a view to carrying out embolization. If blood loss continues after embolization, angiography can again be performed to seek other sites of bleeding. However, angiography will not reveal any source of *venous* bleeding and repeated procedures are time-wasting.

An alternative approach is the application of pelvic packing to provide a tamponade effect (Ertel et al., 2001).

The management of severe haemorrhage in pelvic injuries is well-described in a recent review paper by Hak et al. (2009).

MANAGEMENT OF THE URETHRA AND BLADDER

Urological injury occurs in about 10 per cent of patients with pelvic ring fractures. As these patients are often seriously ill from other injuries, a urinary catheter may be required to monitor urinary output, and therefore the urologist is placed under pressure to make a rapid diagnosis of urethral damage.

There is no place for passing a diagnostic catheter as this will most probably convert any partial tear to a complete tear. For an incomplete tear, the insertion of a suprapubic catheter as a formal procedure is all that is required. Around half of all incomplete tears will heal and require little long-term management.

The treatment of a complete urethral tear is controversial. Primary realignment of the urethra may be achieved by performing suprapubic cystostomy, evacuating the pelvic haematoma and then threading a catheter across the injury to drain the bladder. If the bladder is floating high it is repositioned and held down by a sling suture passed through the lower anterior part of the prostatic capsule, through the perineum on either side of the bulbar urethra and anchored to the thighs by elastic bands. An alternative – and much simpler – approach is to perform the cystostomy as soon as possible, making no attempt to drain the pelvis or dissect the urethra, and to deal with the resulting stricture 4–6 months later. The latter method is contraindicated if there is severe prostatic dislocation or severe tears of the rectum or bladder neck. With both methods there is a significant incidence of late stricture formation, incontinence and impotence.

TREATMENT OF THE FRACTURE

For patients with very severe injuries, early external fixation is one of the most effective ways of reducing haemorrhage and counteracting shock (Poka and Libby, 1996; Hak et al., 2009). If there are no life-threatening complications, definitive treatment is as follows.

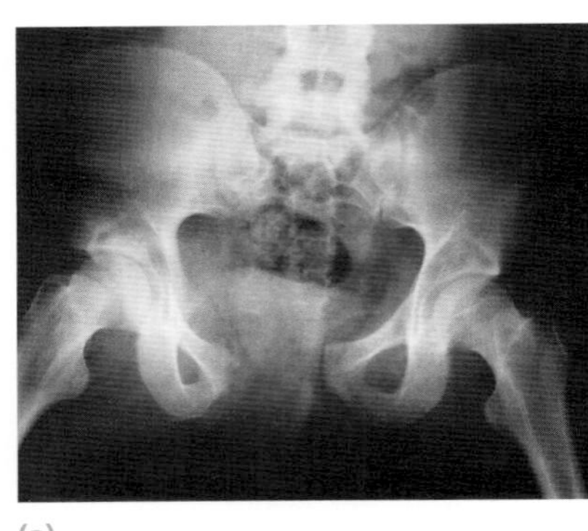
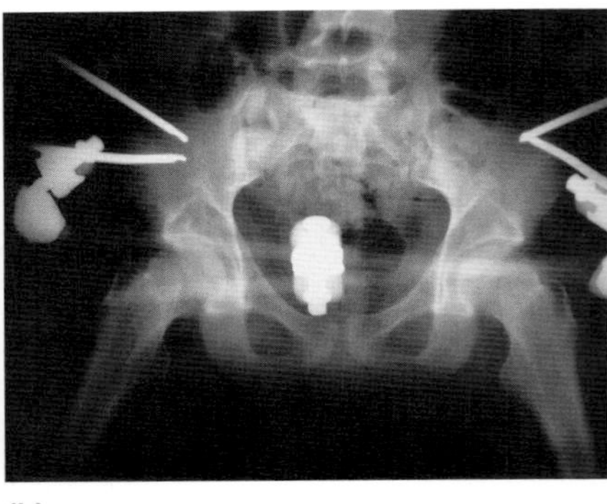
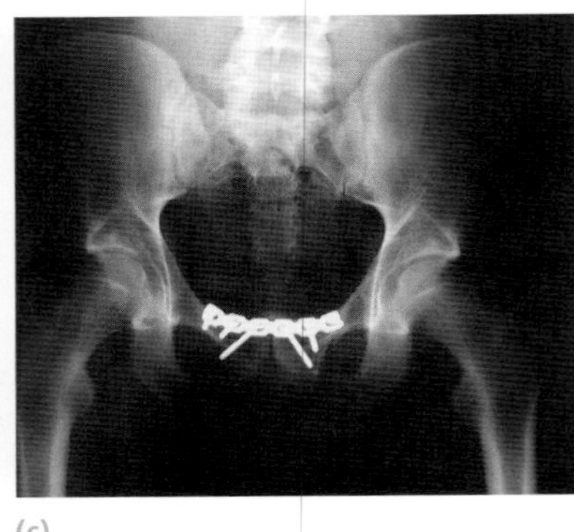

(a) (b) (c)

28.8 Internal fixation (a) Severe open-book injury with complete disruption of the symphysis pubis. (b) Reduction and stabilization by external fixator. (c) The symphysis was then firmly held by internal fixation with a plate and screws.

Isolated fractures and minimally displaced fractures These injuries need only bed rest, possibly combined with lower limb traction. Within 4–6 weeks the patient is usually comfortable and may then be allowed up using crutches.

Open-book injuries Provided the anterior gap is less than 2 cm and it is certain that there are no displaced posterior disruptions, these injuries can usually be treated satisfactorily by bed rest; a posterior sling or a pelvic binder helps to 'close the book'.

The most efficient way of maintaining reduction is by external fixation with pins in both iliac blades connected by an anterior bar; 'closing the book' may also reduce the amount of bleeding. Placing the pins is made easier if two temporary pins are first inserted hugging the medial and lateral surfaces of each iliac blade and then directing the fixing pins between them. Internal fixation by attaching a plate across the symphysis should be performed: (1) during the first few days after injury only if the patient needs a laparotomy; and (2) later on if the gap cannot be closed by less radical methods.

Fractures of the iliac blade can often be treated with bed rest. However, if displacement is marked, or if there is an associated anterior ring fracture or symphysis separation, then open reduction and internal fixation with plates and screws will need to be considered (e.g. in displaced LC-II injuries causing a leg length discrepancy greater than 1.5 cm). It is also possible to reduce and hold some of these fractures by external fixation.

APC-III and VS injuries These are the most dangerous injuries and the most difficult to treat. It may be possible to reduce some or all of the vertical displacement by skeletal traction combined with an external fixator; even so, the patient needs to remain in bed for at least 10 weeks. This prolonged recumbency is not without risk. As these injuries represent loss of both anterior and posterior support, both areas will need to be stabilized. Two techniques are used: (a) anterior external fixation and posterior stabilization using screws across the sacroiliac joint, or (b) plating anteriorly and iliosacral screw fixation posteriorly. Posterior operations are hazardous (the dangers include massive haemorrhage, neurological damage and infection)

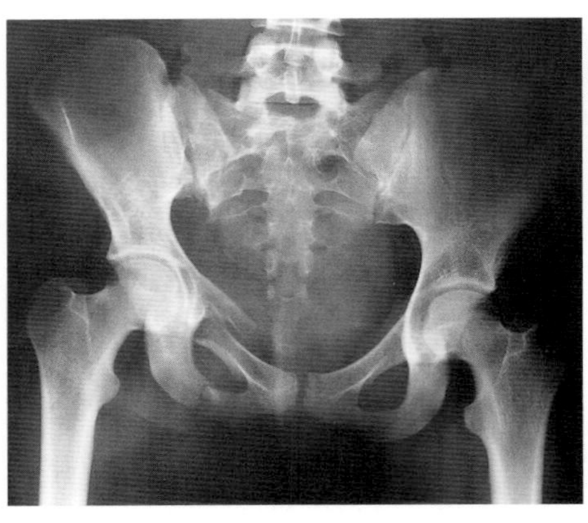
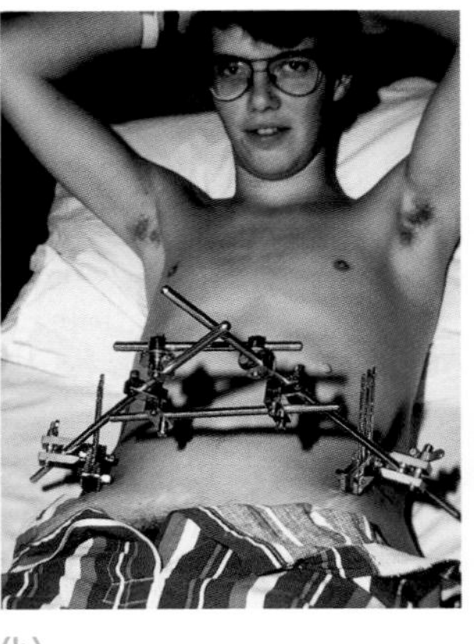
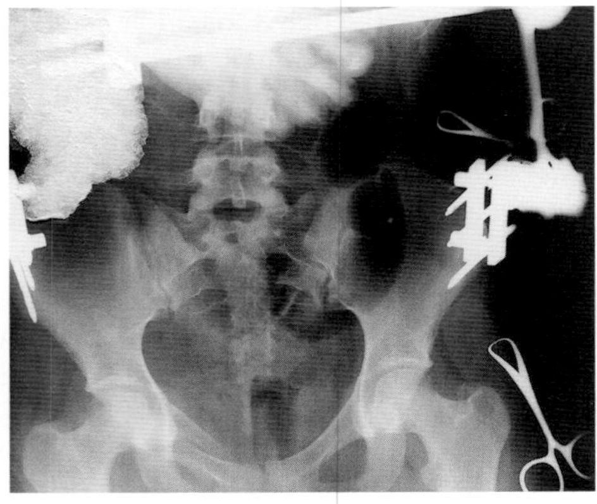

(a) (b) (c)

28.9 Treatment of vertical sheer fracture (a) X-ray showing a fractured superior pubic ramus and disruption of the right sacroiliac joint. (b) This was initially treated by traction and external fixation. (c) X-ray showing the pelvic ring restored. Thereafter, the sacroiliac joint was stabilized with plates and screws.

and should be attempted only by surgeons with considerable experience in this field.

Persisting with skeletal traction and external fixation is probably safer, though the malposition is likely to leave a legacy of posterior pain. It should be emphasized that more than 60 per cent of pelvic fractures need no fixation.

Open pelvic fractures *Open fractures* are best managed by external fixation. A diversion colostomy may be necessary.

Complications

Thromboembolism A careful watch should be kept for signs of deep vein thrombosis or pulmonary embolism (Montgomery *et al.*, 1996). Prophylactic anticoagulants are advocated in some hospitals.

Sciatic nerve injury It is essential to test for sciatic nerve function both before and after treating the pelvic fracture. If the nerve is injured it is usually a neuropraxia and one can afford to wait several weeks for signs of recovery. Occasionally, though, nerve exploration is necessary.

Urogenital problems Urethral injuries sometimes result in *stricture, incontinence* or *impotence* and may require further treatment.

Persistent sacroiliac pain Unstable pelvic fractures are often associated with partial or complete sacroiliac joint disruption, and this can lead to persistent pain at the back of the pelvis. Occasionally arthrodesis of the sacroiliac joint is needed.

FRACTURES OF THE ACETABULUM

Fractures of the acetabulum occur when the head of the femur is driven into the pelvis. This is caused either by a blow on the side (as in a fall from a height) or by a blow on the front of the knee, usually in a dashboard injury when the femur also may be fractured.

Acetabular fractures combine the complexities of pelvic fractures (notably the frequency of associated soft-tissue injury) with those of joint disruption (namely, articular cartilage damage, noncongruent loading and secondary osteoarthritis).

Patterns of fracture

Several classifications of acetabular fractures are currently popular (Letournel, 1981; Müller *et al.*, 1991; Tile, 1995). All use similar anatomical descriptions, but Tile's universal classification has much to commend it for simplicity.

The fractures are divided into four major types; though they are distinguished on anatomical grounds, it is important to recognize that they also differ in their ease of reduction, their stability after reduction and their long-term prognosis.

Acetabular wall fractures Fractures of the anterior or posterior part of the acetabular rim affect the depth of the socket and may lead to hip instability unless they are properly reduced and fixed.

COLUMN FRACTURES

The *anterior column* extends from the pubic symphysis, along the superior pubic ramus, across the acetabulum to the anterior part of the ilium. On the x-ray it is shown in profile by the iliopectineal line in the oblique view. Anterior column fractures are uncommon, do not involve the weightbearing area and have a good prognosis.

The *posterior column* extends from the ischium, across the posterior aspect of the acetabular socket to the sciatic notch and the posterior part of the innominate bone. In an iliac oblique x-ray it is seen in

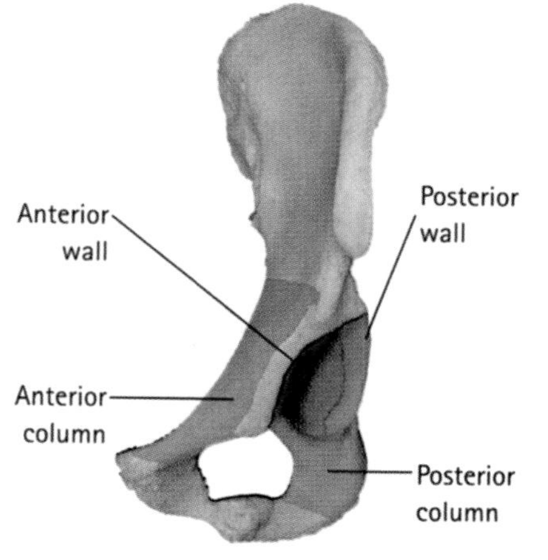

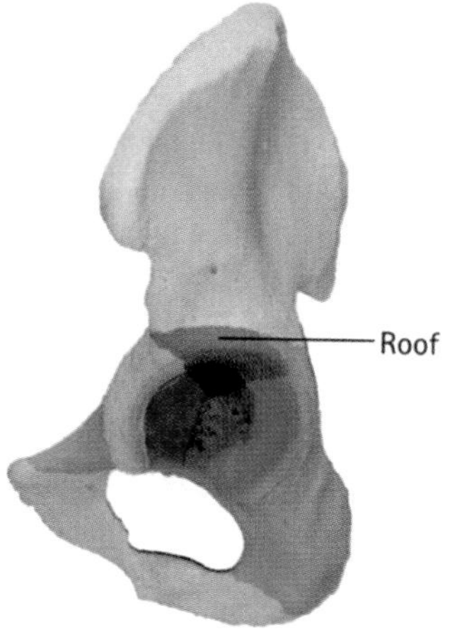

28.10 Acetabular fractures (a) Fractures occur through the wall (rim) or supporting columns. (b) Of particular importance is the roof (superior dome – which carries a high proportion of the load in walking).

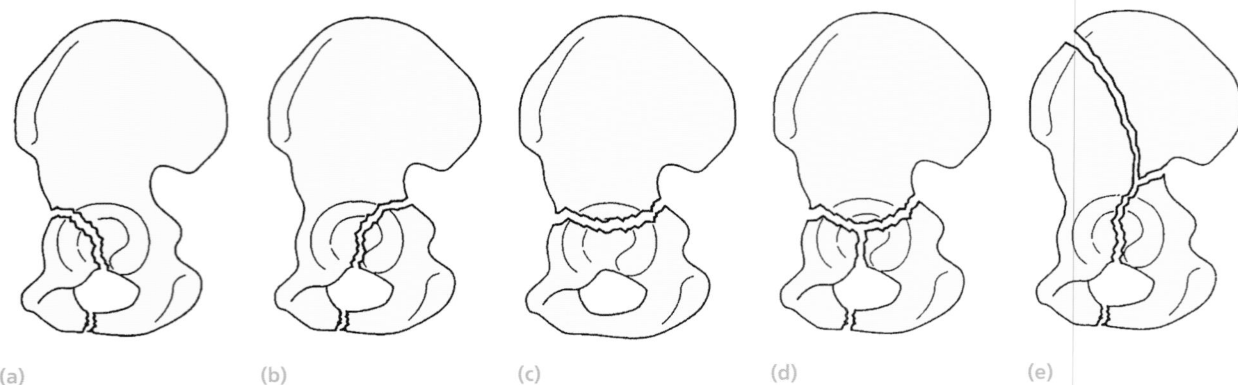

28.11 The classification of acetabular fractures There are four types of injury: (a,b) a simple fracture involving either the anterior or the posterior wall or column; (c) a transverse or (d) a T-type fracture involving two columns; (e) the both-column fracture, resulting in a 'floating' acetabulum with no part of the socket attached to the ilium (compare this with the transverse or T-type fractures).

profile as the ilioischial line. A posterior column fracture usually runs upwards from the obturator foramen into the sciatic notch, separating the posterior ischiopubic column of bone and breaking the weightbearing part of the acetabulum. It is usually associated with a posterior dislocation of the hip and may injure the sciatic nerve. Treatment is more urgent and usually involves internal fixation to obtain a stable joint.

TRANSVERSE FRACTURE

This fracture runs transversely through the acetabulum, involving both the anterior and posterior columns, and separating the iliac portion above from the pubic and ischial portions below. A vertical split into the obturator foramen may coexist, resulting in a T-fracture. Note that in both transverse and T-type fractures, a portion of the acetabulum remains attached to the ilium. These fractures are usually difficult to reduce and to hold reduced.

COMPLEX FRACTURES

Many acetabular fractures are complex injuries which damage either the anterior or the posterior columns (or both) as well as the roof or the walls of the acetabulum. Of particular note, and sometimes a cause of confusion, is the '*both-column fracture*' – this is really a variant of the T-fracture in that the two columns are involved but the transverse part of the 'T' lies just *above* the acetabulum; effectively, no portion of the acetabulum remains connected to the rest of the pelvis. Understandably, the confusion arises when the term 'both-column' is used to refer to a transverse

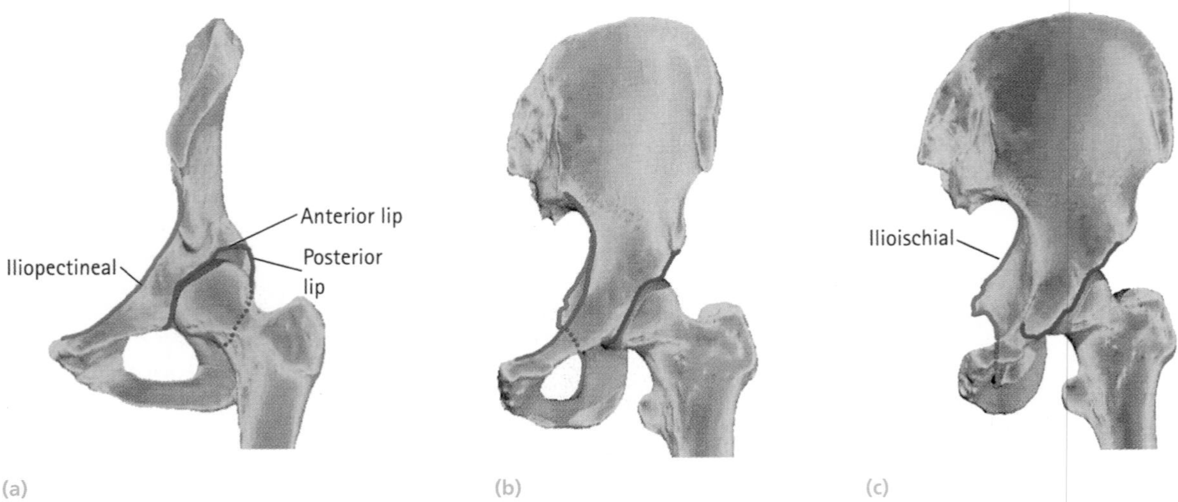

28.12 Imaging the pelvis for acetabular fractures Although CT scans have become the standard in assessing acetabular fractures, plain x-rays have much to offer. The obturator oblique (a), standard anteroposterior (b) and iliac oblique (c) views will allow the trained eye to picture the structures involved in the injury. The iliopectineal line represents a profile of the anterior column whereas the ilioischial line defines the posterior column. The margins of the anterior and posterior walls are usually seen in all three views.

fracture – perhaps the term 'high T' would have been better!

Complex fracture patterns share the following features: (1) the injury is severe; (2) the joint surface is disrupted; (3) they usually need operative reduction and internal fixation; and (4) the end result is likely to be less than perfect, unless surgical restoration has been exact.

Clinical features

There has usually been a severe injury; either a traffic accident or a fall from a height. Associated fractures are not uncommon and, because they may be more obvious, are liable to divert attention from the more urgent pelvic injuries. Whenever a fractured femur, a severe knee injury or a fractured calcaneum is diagnosed, the hips also should be x-rayed.

The patient may be severely shocked, and the complications associated with all pelvic fractures should be excluded. Rectal examination is essential. There may be bruising around the hip and the limb may lie in internal rotation (if the hip is dislocated). No attempt should be made to move the hip.

Careful neurological examination is important, testing the function of the sciatic, femoral, obturator and pudendal nerves.

Imaging

At least four *x-ray views* should be obtained in every case: a standard anteroposterior view, the pelvic inlet view and two 45 degrees oblique views. Each view shows a different profile of the acetabulum; with practice the various landmarks (iliopectineal line, ilioischial line and the boundaries of the anterior and posterior walls) can be identified, thus providing a fairly good mental picture of the fracture type, the degree of comminution and the amount of displacement. *CT scans* and *three-dimensional re-formations* are added refinements, and are particularly helpful if surgical reconstruction is planned.

Treatment

EMERGENCY TREATMENT

The first priority is to counteract shock and reduce a dislocation. Skeletal traction is then applied to the distal femur (10 kg will suffice) and during the next 3–4 days the patient's general condition is brought under control. Occasionally, additional lateral traction through the greater trochanter is needed for central hip dislocations. Definitive treatment of the fracture is delayed until the patient is fit and operation facilities are optimal.

NON-OPERATIVE TREATMENT

In recent years opinion has moved in favour of operative treatment for displaced acetabular fractures. However, conservative treatment is still preferable in certain well-defined situations: (1) acetabular fractures with minimal displacement (in the weightbearing zone, less than 3 mm); (2) displaced fractures that do not involve the superomedial weightbearing segment (roof) of the acetabulum – usually distal anterior column and distal transverse fractures; (3) a both-column fracture that retains the ball and socket congruence of the hip by virtue of the fracture line lying in the coronal plane and displacement being limited by an intact labrum; (4) fractures in elderly patients, where closed reduction seems feasible; (5) patients with 'medical' contraindications to operative treatment (including local sepsis). Comminution in itself is not a contraindication to operative treatment, provided adequate facilities and expertise are available.

Matta and Merritt (1988) have listed certain criteria which should be met if conservative treatment is expected to succeed: (1) when traction is released, the

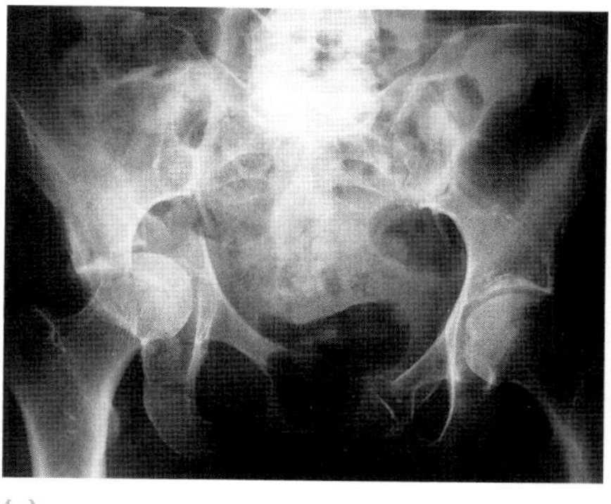
(a)

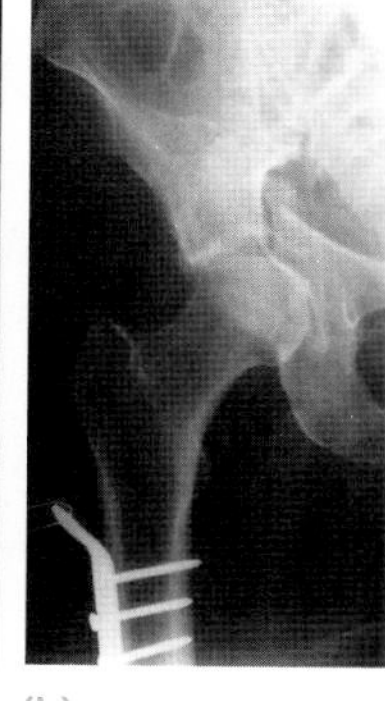
(b)

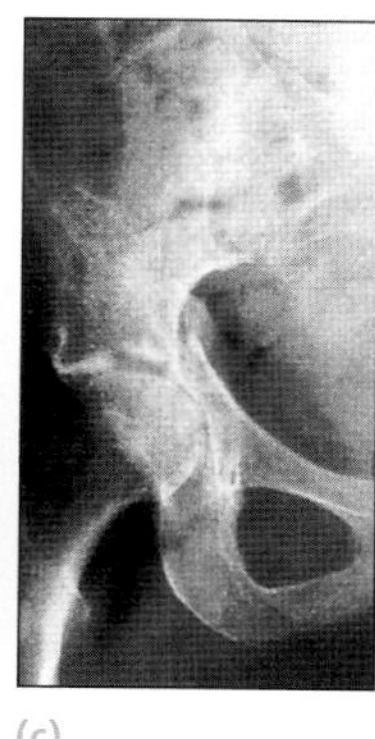
(c)

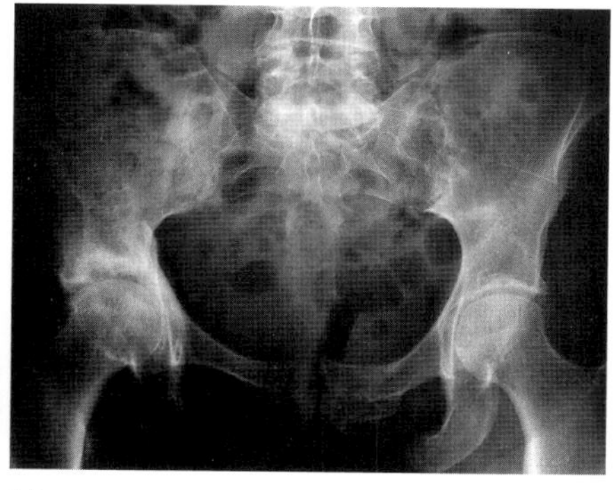
(d)

28.13 Fractured acetabulum – conservative treatment This severely displaced acetabular fracture (a) was almost completely reduced by (b) longitudinal and lateral traction. (c) The fracture healed and the patient regained a congruent joint with a fairly good range of movement. (d) X-ray two years later.

hip should remain congruent; (2) the weightbearing portion of the acetabular roof should be intact; and (3) associated fractures of the posterior wall should be excluded by CT. Non-operative treatment is more suitable for patients aged over 50 years than for adolescents and young adults.

If there are medical contraindications to operative treatment, closed reduction under general anaesthesia is attempted. In all patients treated conservatively, longitudinal traction, if necessary supplemented by lateral traction, is maintained for 6–8 weeks; this will unload the articular cartilage and will help to prevent further displacement of the fracture. During this period, hip movement and exercises are encouraged. The patient is then allowed up, using crutches with minimal weightbearing for a further 6 weeks.

OPERATIVE TREATMENT

Operative treatment is indicated for all unstable hips and fractures resulting in significant distortion of the ball and socket congruence. The hip may be dislocated centrally, anteriorly or posteriorly. Patients with isolated posterior wall fractures and dislocation may require immediate open reduction and stabilization. In other cases operation is usually deferred for 4 or 5 days.

Matta and Merritt (1988) have made the important point that open reduction is an operation on the pelvis and not merely the acetabular socket. Adequate exposure is essential, if possible through a single approach which is selected according to the type of fracture. The posterior Kocher–Langenbach exposure allows good access to the posterior wall and column but may have to be combined with a trochanteric osteotomy to gain adequate sight in transverse fractures. The anterior ilioinguinal approach is suited for anterior wall and column fractures. Both exposures are usually needed in T-type and both-column fractures – this is a considerable undertaking, encouraging some surgeons to adopt the singular triradiate or extended iliofemoral approaches instead. The fracture (or fractures) is fixed with lag screws or special buttressing plates which can be shaped in the operating theatre. It is useful to monitor somatosensory evoked potentials during the operation, in order to avoid damaging the sciatic nerve (separate electrodes are required for medial and lateral popliteal branches).

Prophylactic antibiotics are used, and postoperatively hip movements are started as soon as possible. Some prophylaxis against heterotopic ossification is often used, usually indomethacin. The patient is allowed up, partial weightbearing with crutches, after 7 days. Exercises are continued for 3–6 months; it may take a year or longer for full function to return.

Complications

Operative treatment should aim for a perfect anatomical reduction and is best undertaken in centres that specialize in this form of treatment.

Iliofemoral venous thrombosis This is potentially serious and in some clinics prophylactic anticoagulation is used.

Sciatic nerve injury Nerve injury may occur either at the time of fracture or during the subsequent operation. Unless the nerve is seen to be unharmed during the operation, there can be no certainty about the prognosis. Intra-operative somatosensory monitoring is advocated as a means of preventing serious nerve damage. For an established lesion, it is worth waiting for 6 weeks to see if there is any sign of recovery. If there is none, the nerve should be explored in order to establish the diagnosis and ensure that the nerve is not being compressed.

Hereterotopic bone formation Periarticular ossification is common after severe soft-tissue injury and extended surgical dissections. In cases where this is anticipated, prophylactic indomethacin is useful.

Avascular necrosis Osteonecrosis of the femoral head may occur even if the hip is not fully dislocated. The condition is probably overdiagnosed because of erroneous interpretation of the x-ray appearances following impacted marginal fractures of the acetabulum (Gruen, Mears and Tauxe, 1988).

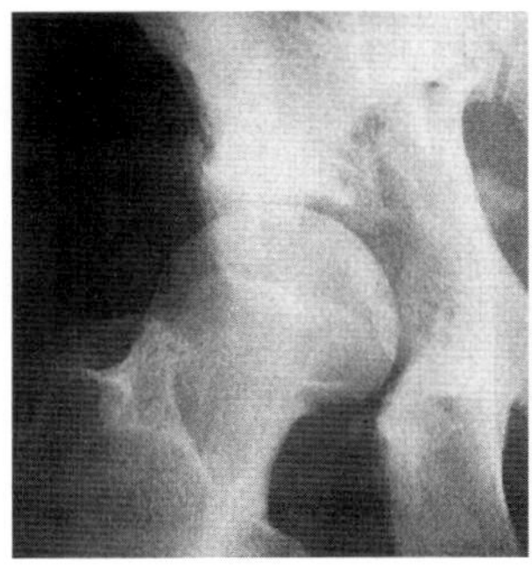
(a)

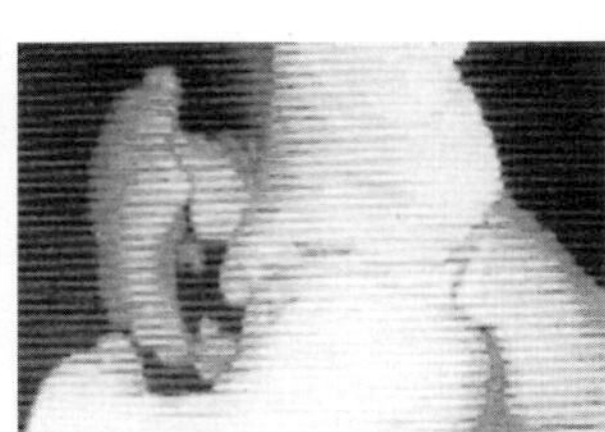
(b)

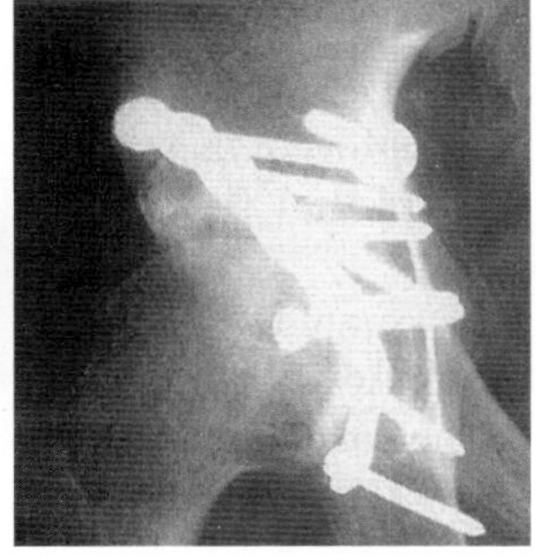
(c)

28.14 Fractured acetabulum – internal fixation **(a)** X-ray and **(b)** three-dimensional CT before reduction, showing a large posterior fragment which needed accurate repositioning and internal fixation **(c)**. (Courtsey of Mr RN Brueton and Dr RL Guy).

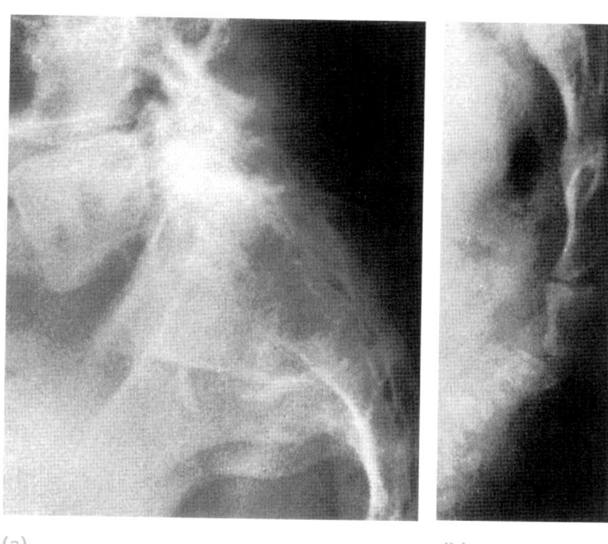

(a) (b)

28.15 Sacrococcygeal fractures (a) Fractured sacrum; (b) fractured coccyx.

Loss of joint movement and secondary osteoarthritis Displaced fractures involving the weightbearing portion of the joint may result in loss of movement and early onset osteoarthritis. If a joint replacement operation is contemplated it should be deferred until the fractures have consolidated; the acetabular implant is bound to work loose if there is any movement of the innominate segments.

INJURIES TO THE SACRUM AND COCCYX

A blow from behind, or a fall onto the 'tail' may fracture the sacrum or coccyx, or sprain the joint between them. Women seem to be affected more commonly than men.

Bruising is considerable and tenderness is elicited when the sacrum or coccyx is palpated from behind or per rectum. Sensation may be lost over the distribution of sacral nerves.

X-rays may show: (1) a transverse fracture of the sacrum, in rare cases with the lower fragment pushed forwards; (2) a fractured coccyx, sometimes with the lower fragment angulated forwards; or (3) a normal appearance if the injury was merely a sprained sacrococcygeal joint.

Treatment If the fracture is displaced, reduction is worth attempting. The lower fragment may be pushed backwards by a finger in the rectum. The reduction is stable, which is fortunate. The patient is allowed to resume normal activity, but is advised to use a rubber ring cushion when sitting. Occasionally, sacral fractures are associated with urinary problems, necessitating sacral laminectomy.

Persistent pain, especially on sitting, is common after coccygeal injuries. If the pain is not relieved by the use of a cushion or by the injection of local anaesthetic into the tender area, excision of the coccyx may be considered.

REFERENCES AND FURTHER READING

Dalal SA, Burgess AR, Siegel JH, *et al.* Pelvic fracture in multiple trauma. *J Trauma* 1989; **29:** 981–1000.

Ertel W, Keel M, Eid K, *et al.* Control of severe haemorrhage using C-clamp and pelvic packing in multiply injured patients with pelvic ring disruption. *J Orthop Trauma* 2001; **15:** 468–74.

Gruen GS, Mears DC, Tauxe WN. Distinguishing avascular necrosis from segmental impaction of the femoral head following an acetabular fracture. *J Orthop Trauma* 1988; **2:** 5–9.

Hak DJ, Smith WR, Suzuki T. Management of haemorrhage in life-threatening pelvic fracture. *J Am Acad Orthop Surg* 2009; **17:** 447–57.

Letournel E. Fractures of the Acetabulum 1981. Springer, Berlin, 1981.

Matta JM, Merritt PO. Displaced acetabular fractures. *Clin Orthop Relat Res* 1988; **230:** 83–97.

Montgomery KD, Geerts WH, Potter HG, Helfet DL. Thromboembolic complications in patients with pelvic trauma. *Clin Orthop Relat Res* 1996; **329:** 68–87.

Müller ME, Allgower M, Schneider R, Willeneger H. *Manual of Internal Fixation*, 3rd edition. Springer Verlag. Berlin, Heidelberg, New York, 1991.

Olson SA, Pollak AN. Assessment of pelvic ring stability after injury. Indications for surgical stabilisation. *Clin Orthop Relat Res* 1996; **329:** 15–27.

Poka A, Libby EP. Indications and techniques for external fixation of the pelvis. *Clin Orthop Relat Res* 1996; **329:** 54–9.

Tile M. Fractures of the pelvis and acetabulum. 2nd edition. Williams and Wilkins, Baltimore, 1995.

Wootton JR, Cross MJ, Holt KWG. Avulsion of the ischial apophysis. *J Bone Joint Surg* 1990; **72B:** 625–7.

Young JWR, Burgess AR, Brumback RJ, Poka A. Lateral compression fractures of the pelvis: the importance of plain radiographs in the diagnosis and surgical management. *Skeletal Radiol* 1986; **15:** 103–9.

Young JWR, Burgess AR. Radiologic management of pelvic ring fractures: Systematic radiographic diagnosis. Urban and Schwarzenberg. Baltimore, 1987.

Injuries of the hip and femur

29

Selvadurai Nayagam

DISLOCATION OF THE HIP

The magnitude of force needed to dislocate the hip, a joint particularly well-contained by virtue of its bony and soft-tissue anatomy, is so great that the dislocation is often associated with fractures – either around the joint or elsewhere in the same limb. Small fragments of bone are often chipped off, usually from the femoral head or from the wall of the acetabulum. If there is a major fragment, the injury is regarded as a fracture-dislocation.

Hip dislocations are classified according to the direction of the femoral head displacement: *posterior* (by far the commonest variety), *anterior* and *central* (a comminuted or displaced fracture of the acetabulum).

POSTERIOR DISLOCATION

Mechanism of injury

This is a posterior dislocation, usually occurring in a road accident when someone seated in a truck or car is thrown forward, striking the knee against the dashboard. The femur is thrust upwards and the femoral head is forced out of its socket; often a piece of bone at the back of the acetabulum (usually the posterior wall) is sheared off, making it a fracture-dislocation. Seat-belt restraints can reduce the number of posterior hip dislocations.

Clinical features

In a straightforward case the diagnosis is easy; the leg is short and lies adducted, internally rotated and slightly flexed. However, if one of the long bones is fractured – usually the femur – the injury can easily be missed as the limb can adopt almost any position. The golden rule is to x-ray the pelvis in every case of severe injury and, with femoral fractures, to insist on an x-ray that includes both the hip and knee. The lower limb should be examined for signs of sciatic nerve injury (Figure 29.1).

X-ray

In the anteroposterior film the femoral head is seen out of its socket and above the acetabulum. A

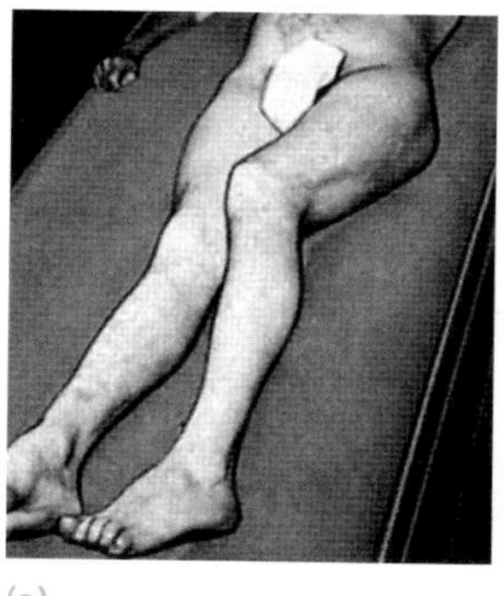
(a)

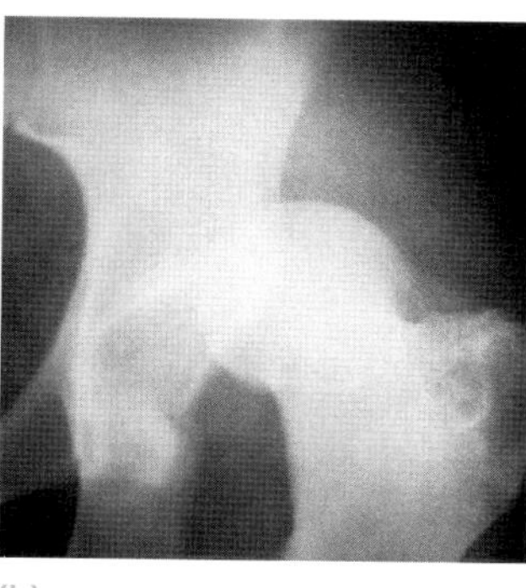
(b)

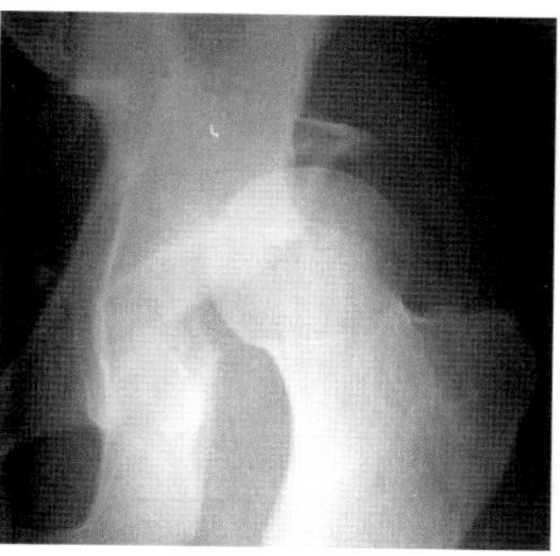
(c)

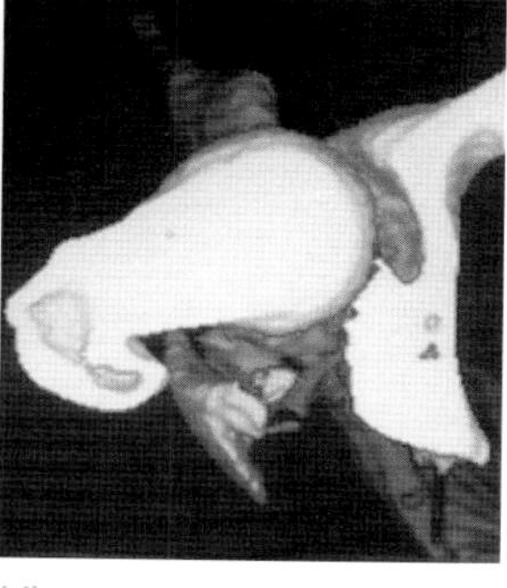
(d)

29.1 Posterior dislocation of the hip (a) This is the typical posture in a patient with posterior dislocation: the left hip is slightly flexed and internally rotated. (b) The x-ray in this case showed a simple dislocation, with the femoral head lying above and behind the acetabulum. (c) Another patient with dislocation and an associated acetabular rim fracture. However, in some cases it may need a CT scan and three-dimensional image reconstruction to appreciate the full extent of the associated acetabular injury (d).

Table 29.1 Classification of hip dislocation (Thompson and Epstein).

Types	Thompson and Epstein classification of hip dislocations
I	Dislocation with no more than minor chip fractures
II	Dislocation with single large fragment of posterior acetabular wall
III	Dislocation with comminuted fragments of posterior acetabular wall
IV	Dislocation with fracture through acetabular floor
V	Dislocation with fracture through acetabular floor and femoral head

segment of acetabular rim or femoral head may have been broken off and displaced; oblique films are useful in demonstrating the size of the fragment. If any fracture is seen, other bony fragments (which may need removal) must be suspected. A CT scan is the best way of demonstrating an acetabular fracture (or any bony fragment) but detailed imaging at this stage should be undertaken only if it does not delay reduction of the dislocation unduly.

Thompson and Epstein (1951) suggested a classification which is helpful in planning treatment. Types I and II are relatively simple dislocations; these are associated with either minor chip fractures (small fragments of the acetabular wall or fovea centralis) or a single large fragment from the posterior acetabular wall. In Type III the posterior wall is comminuted. type IV has an associated fracture of the acetabular floor, and Type V an associated fracture of the femoral head, which can be further subdivided according to Pipkin's (1957) classification. (Figure 29.2)

Treatment

The dislocation must be reduced as soon as possible under general anaesthesia. In the vast majority of cases this is performed closed, but if this is not achieved after two or three attempts an open reduction is required. An assistant steadies the pelvis; the surgeon starts by applying traction in the line of the femur as it lies (usually in adduction and internal rotation), and then gradually flexes the patient's hip and knee to 90 degrees, maintaining traction throughout. At 90 degrees of hip flexion, traction is steadily increased and sometimes a little rotation (either internal or external) is required to accomplish reduction. Another assistant can help by applying direct medial and anterior pressure to the femoral head through the buttock. A satisfying 'clunk' terminates the manoeuvre. An important test follows, to assess the stability of the reduced hip. By flexing the hip to 90 degrees and applying a longitudinal and posteriorly-directed force, the hip is screened on an image-intensifier looking for signs of subluxation. Evidence of this should prompt a repair to the posterior wall of the acetabulum.

Reduction is usually stable in type I injuries, but the hip has been severely injured and needs to be rested. The simplest way is to apply traction and maintain it for a few days. Movement and exercises are begun as soon as pain allows; continuous passive movement machines are helpful. The terminal ranges of hip movements are avoided to allow healing of the capsule and ligaments. As soon as active limb control is achieved, and this may take about 2 weeks, the patient is allowed to walk with crutches but without taking weight on the affected side. The rationale for not bearing weight is to prevent collapse of femoral head due to an unsuspected avascular change.

The period of hip 'protection' varies according to

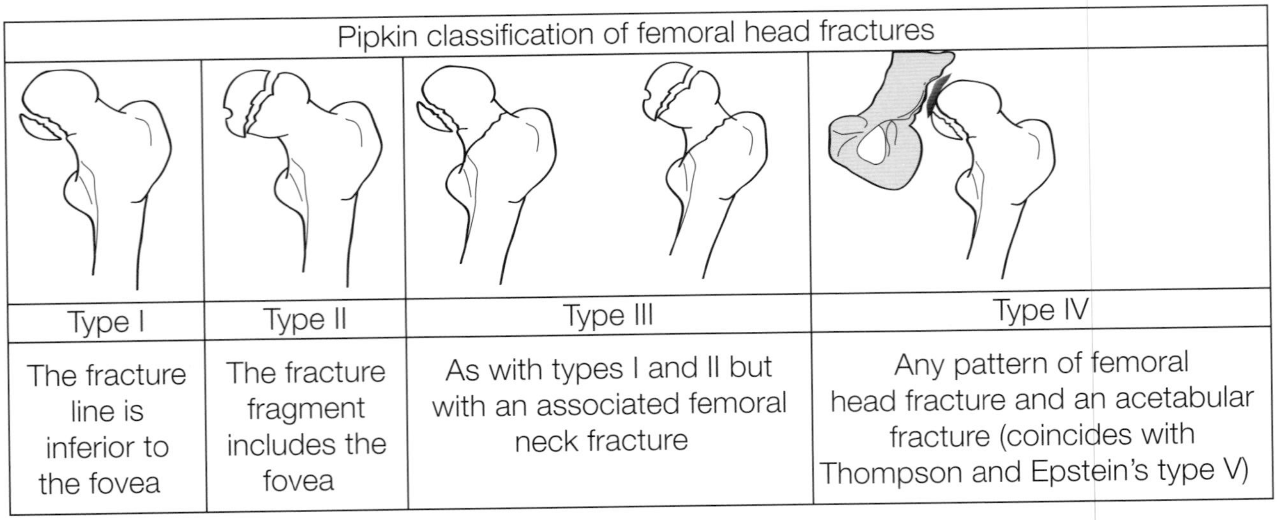

Pipkin classification of femoral head fractures			
Type I	Type II	Type III	Type IV
The fracture line is inferior to the fovea	The fracture fragment includes the fovea	As with types I and II but with an associated femoral neck fracture	Any pattern of femoral head fracture and an acetabular fracture (coincides with Thompson and Epstein's type V)

29.2 Pipkin classification of femoral head fractures

the risk of avascular necrosis: if the reduction was performed promptly (within 6 hours), then no more than 6 weeks should suffice, but if there was a longer delay then an extended period of 12 weeks may be wiser. Progression of weightbearing should be graduated and the hip joint monitored by x-ray (Tornetta and Mostafavi 1997).

If the post-reduction x-rays or CT scans show the presence of intra-articular bone fragments or larger femoral head pieces that are incompletely reduced, an open procedure should be planned. The approach is dictated by the location of the fragment on CT scan; however, the operation is not an emergency and can be done once the patient's condition has stabilized. The joint needs to be thoroughly washed out at the conclusion of the procedure to remove bone 'grit'.

Type II fracture-dislocations are often treated by immediate open reduction and anatomical fixation of the detached fragment, the rationale being that many large posterior wall fragments either do not reduce well or remain as a cause of instability even after reduction. However, if the patient's general condition is suspect, or the necessary surgical skills are not available, the hip is reduced closed, as described above. Traction can be applied until conditions are appropriate for surgery – open reduction and internal fixation will remedy the source of instability, return congruity to the joint and remove any trapped bone fragments.

Type III injuries are treated closed, but there may be retained fragments and these should be removed by open operation. Fixation of a comminuted posterior wall is sometimes impossible – if persistent instability is present, referral to a specialist centre, where reconstruction using a segment of iliac crest could be undertaken, is advisable.

Types IV and V are treated initially by closed reduction. The indications for surgery follow the principles already outlined: instability, retained fragments or joint incongruity. In type V injuries, a femoral head fragment may automatically fall into place, and this can be confirmed by post-reduction CT. If the fragment remains unreduced, operative treatment is indicated: a small fragment can simply be removed, but a large fragment should be replaced; the joint is opened, the femoral head dislocated and the fragment fixed in position with a countersunk screw. Postoperatively, traction is maintained for 2–4 weeks and full weightbearing is deferred for 12 weeks.

Complications

EARLY

Sciatic nerve injury The sciatic nerve is damaged in 10–20 per cent of cases but it usually recovers. *Nerve function must be tested and documented before reduction is attempted.* If, after reducing the dislocation, a sciatic nerve lesion is diagnosed, the nerve should be explored to ensure it is not trapped by the reduction manoeuvre. Recovery often takes months and in the meantime the limb must be protected from injury and the ankle splinted to overcome the foot drop.

Vascular injury Occasionally the superior gluteal artery is torn and bleeding may be profuse. If this is suspected, an arteriogram should be performed. The torn vessel may need to be ligated.

Associated fractured femoral shaft When this occurs at the same time as the hip dislocation, the dislocation is often missed. *It should be a rule that with every femoral shaft fracture, the buttock and trochanter are palpated, and the hip clearly seen on x-ray.* Even if this precaution has been omitted, a dislocation should be suspected if the proximal fragment of a transverse shaft fracture is seen to be adducted. Closed reduction of the dislocation will be much more difficult. A prompt open reduction of the hip followed by internal fixation of the shaft fracture should be undertaken.

LATE

Avascular necrosis Avascular necrosis of the femoral head has been reported in about 10 per cent of traumatic hip dislocations; if reduction is delayed by more than 12 hours, the figure rises to over 40 per cent. Changes are seen first on MRI or isotope bone scans. X-ray features such as increased density of the femoral head may not be seen for at least 6 weeks, and sometimes very much later (up to 2 years), depending on the rate of bone repair.

Ischaemia is due to interruption of femoral head blood supply when the hip is dislocated. There is evidence to suggest that this results from compression, traction and arterial spasm rather than actual disruption of blood vessels (Shim 1979), which means that the consequences of ischaemia are proportional to the delay in starting treatment; blood flow is restored on reduction of the hip, especially if this is performed early – which highlights the need for emergency treatment with a target of less than 12 hours (preferably less than 6) from the time of injury.

If the femoral head develops signs of fragmentation, an operation may be needed. If the necrotic segment is small, realignment osteotomy is the method of choice; for extensive femoral head collapse, usually with accompanying degenerative arthritis, the choice is between joint replacement and hip arthrodesis (never an easy procedure).

Myositis ossificans This is an uncommon complication, probably related to the severity of the injury. During recovery, movements should never be forced and in severe injuries the period of rest and non-weightbearing may need to be prolonged. Small areas of ossification seen on x-ray usually bear no clinical significance.

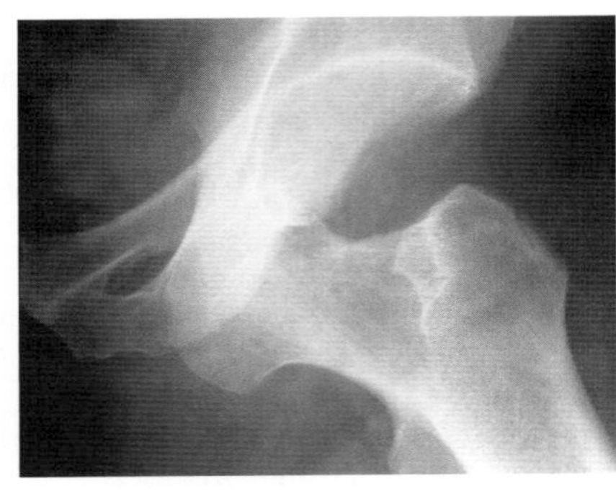

(a)

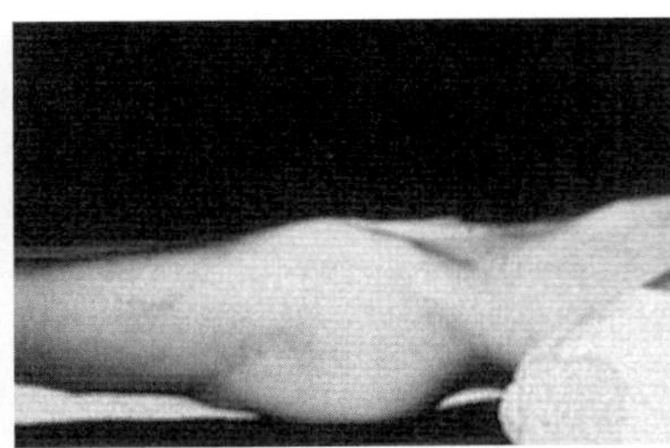

(b)

29.3 Anterior hip dislocation (a,b) The usual appearance of an anterior dislocation: the hip is only slightly abducted and the head shows clinically as a prominent lump.

Unreduced dislocation After a few weeks an untreated dislocation can seldom be reduced by closed manipulation and open reduction is needed. The incidence of stiffness or avascular necrosis is considerably increased and the patient may later need reconstructive surgery.

Osteoarthritis Secondary osteoarthritis is not uncommon and is due to (1) cartilage damage at the time of the dislocation, (2) the presence of retained fragments in the joint or (3) ischaemic necrosis of the femoral head. In young patients treatment presents a difficult problem.

ANTERIOR DISLOCATION

Anterior dislocation is rare compared with posterior. Dislocation of one or even both hips may occur when a weight falls onto the back of a miner or building labourer who is working with his legs wide apart, knees straight and back bent forwards. However, nowadays the usual cause is a road accident or air crash – even a posteriorly directed force on an abducted and externally rotated hip may cause the neck to impinge on the acetabular rim and lever the femoral head out in front of its socket. The femoral head will then lie superiorly (type I - *pubic*) or inferiorly (type II - *obturator*).

Clinical features

The leg lies externally rotated, abducted and slightly flexed. It is not short, because the attachment of rectus femoris prevents the head from displacing upwards. Occasionally the leg is abducted almost to a right angle. Seen from the side, the anterior bulge of the dislocated head is unmistakable, especially when the head has moved anteriorly and superiorly. The prominent head is easy to feel, either anteriorly (superior type) or in the groin (inferior type). Hip movements are impossible (Figure 29.3).

X-ray

In the anteroposterior view the dislocation is usually obvious, but occasionally the head is almost directly in front of its normal position; any doubt is resolved by a lateral film.

Treatment and complications

The manoeuvres employed are similar to those used to reduce a posterior dislocation, except that while the flexed knee is being pulled and the hip gently flexed upwards, it should be kept adducted; an assistant then helps by applying lateral pressure to the inside of the thigh. The point of reduction is usually heard and felt. The subsequent treatment is similar to that employed for posterior dislocation.

Avascular necrosis occurs in less than 10 per cent of cases.

CENTRAL DISLOCATION

A fall on the side, or a blow over the greater trochanter, may force the femoral head medially

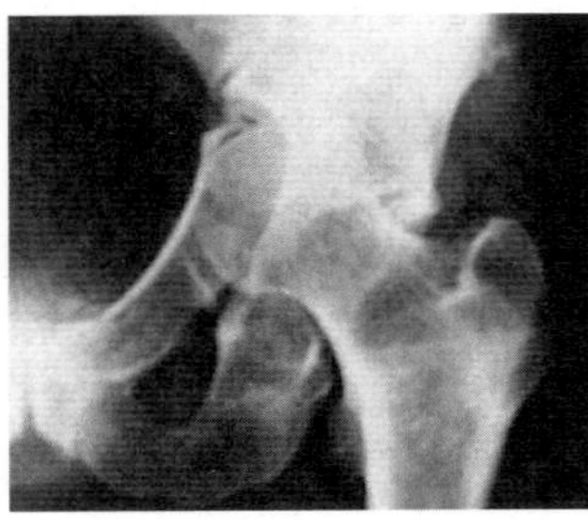

(a)

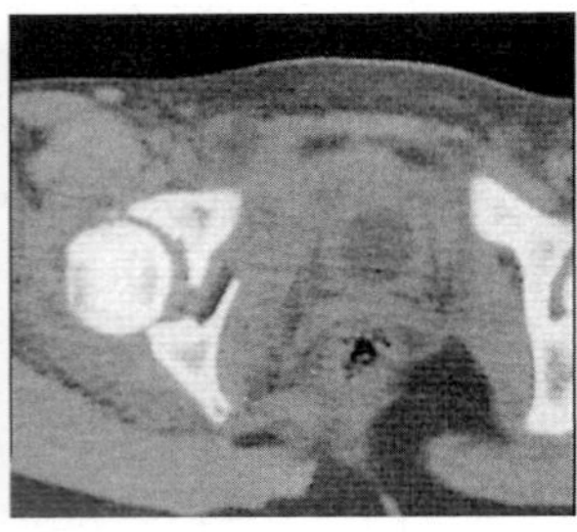

(b)

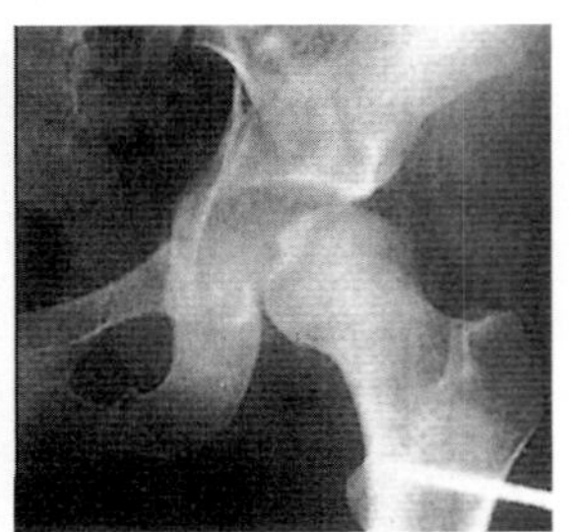

(c)

29.4 Central dislocation (a) The plain x-ray gives a good picture of the displacement, but (b) a CT scan shows the pelvic injury more clearly. (c) Skeletal traction, which often needs both longitudinal and lateral vectors, is an effective method of reduction.

through the floor of the acetabulum. Although this is called 'central dislocation', it is really a fracture of the acetabulum (Figure 29.4). The condition is dealt with in the chapter on *'Injuries of the pelvis'*.

FRACTURES OF THE FEMORAL NECK

The femoral neck is the commonest site of fractures in the elderly. The vast majority of patients are Caucasian women in the seventh and eighth decades, and the association with osteoporosis is so manifest that the incidence of femoral neck fractures has been used as a measure of age-related osteoporosis in population studies. Other risk factors include bone-losing or bone-weakening disorders such as osteomalacia, diabetes, stroke (disuse), alcoholism and chronic debilitating disease. In addition, old people often have weak muscles and poor balance resulting in an increased tendency to fall.

The association of femoral neck fracture with postmenopausal bone loss has stimulated renewed interest in screening for osteoporosis and prophylactic measures in the 'at risk' population (see Chapter 7). By contrast, this injury is much less common among people whose bone mass is above that of the population average, e.g. those with osteoarthritis of the hip.

Femoral neck fractures are also much less common in black (Negroid) peoples than in whites and Asians. The reasons for this phenomenon are poorly understood. Slightly higher bone mass and a slower rate of bone loss after the menopause may be significant, but a *qualitative* difference in bone structure has also been suggested: even among people with the *same* bone mass, those with greater loss of trabecular interconnectivity (typical in elderly whites) will suffer fractures more easily than those with firmer structure.

The incidence of femoral neck fractures is set to double over the next 30 years; this is a reflection of a higher number of individuals living beyond 65 years and a parallel rise in those affected with osteoporosis. The economic impact of treating, rehabilitating and caring for this group of patients is increasingly being recognized, with many governments and healthcare administration bodies focusing on preventive strategies.

Mechanism of injury

The fracture usually results from a simple fall; however, in very osteoporotic people, less force is required — perhaps no more than catching a toe in the carpet and twisting the hip into external rotation. Some patients may have experienced minor symptoms of a preceding stress fracture of the femoral neck.

In younger individuals, the usual cause is a fall from a height or a blow sustained in a road accident. These patients often have multiple injuries and in 20 per cent there is an associated fracture of the femoral shaft. Occasionally, stress fractures of the femoral neck occur in runners or military personnel.

Pathological anatomy and classification

The most useful classification is that of Garden, which is based on the amount of displacement apparent in the pre-reduction x-rays (Garden 1961). Once fractured, the head and neck become displaced in progressively severe stages. *Stage I* is an incomplete impacted fracture, including the so-called abduction fracture in which the femoral head is tilted into valgus in relation to the neck. *Stage II* is a complete but undisplaced fracture. *Stage III* is a complete fracture with moderate displacement. And *Stage IV* is a severely displaced fracture. This is essentially a radiographic classification; the distinctive x-ray features are described below.

Garden I and II fractures, which are only slightly displaced, have a much better prognosis for union and for viability of the femoral head than the more severely displaced Garden III and IV fractures (Barnes, Brown et al. 1976). This has an important influence on the choice of treatment for the various stages. However, there is little room for complacency with any of these fractures; left untreated, a comparatively benign-looking Stage I fracture may rapidly disintegrate to Stage IV.

Healing of femoral neck fractures is bedevilled by two problems: the threat of bone ischaemia and tardy union. The femoral head gets its blood supply from three sources: (1) intramedullary vessels in the femoral neck; (2) ascending cervical branches of the medial and lateral circumflex anastomoses, which run within the capsular retinaculum before entering the bone at the articular margin of the femoral head; and (3) the vessels of the ligamentum teres. The intramedullary supply is always interrupted by the fracture; the retinacular vessels, also, may be kinked or torn if the fracture is displaced. In elderly people, the remaining supply in the ligamentum teres is at best fairly meagre and, in 20 per cent of cases, nonexistent. Hence the high incidence of avascular necrosis in displaced femoral neck fractures.

Transcervical fractures are, by definition, intracapsular. They have a poor capacity for healing because: (1) by tearing the retinacular vessels the injury deprives the head of its main blood supply; (2) intra-articular bone has only a flimsy periosteum and no contact with soft tissues which could promote callus formation; and (3) synovial fluid prevents clotting of the fracture haematoma. Accurate apposition and impaction of bone fragments are therefore of more importance than usual. There is evidence that aspirating a haemarthrosis increases the blood flow in the femoral head by relieving tension in the capsule, and the practice is encouraged at the time of surgery (Harper, Barnes et al. 1991; Bonnaire and Weber 2002).

Clinical features

There is usually a history of a fall, followed by pain in the hip. If the fracture is displaced, the patient lies with the limb in lateral rotation and the leg looks short.

Beware, not all hip fractures are so obvious. With an impacted fracture the patient may still be able to walk, and debilitated or mentally handicapped patients may not complain at all – even with bilateral fractures.

In contrast, femoral neck fractures in young adults result from road traffic accidents or falls from heights and are often associated with multiple injuries. A good rule is that young adults with severe injuries – whether they complain of hip pain or not – should always be examined for an associated femoral neck fracture.

X-ray

Two questions must be answered: is there a fracture, and is it displaced? Usually the break is obvious, but an impacted fracture can be missed by the unwary. Displacement is judged by the abnormal shape of the bone outlines and the degree of mismatch of the trabecular lines in the femoral head and neck and the supra-acetabular (innominate) part of the pelvis (Figure 29.5). This assessment is important because impacted or undisplaced fractures do well after internal fixation, whereas displaced fractures have a high rate of non-union and avascular necrosis.

In *Garden I fractures* the femoral head is in its normal position or tilted into valgus and impacted on the femoral neck stump. The medial cortex may be intact. The femoral head stress trabeculae are normally aligned with the innominate trabeculae.

In *Garden II fractures* the femoral head is normally placed and the fracture line may be difficult to discern.

In *Garden III fractures* the anteroposterior x-ray shows that the femoral head is tilted out of position and the trabecular markings are not in line with those of the innominate bone; this is because the proximal fragment retains some contact with the neck stump and is pushed out of alignment.

In *Garden IV fractures* the femoral head trabeculae are normally aligned with those of the innominate bone; the reason is that the proximal fragment has lost contact with the femoral neck and lies in its normal position in the acetabular socket.

Diagnosis

There are four situations in which a femoral neck fracture may be missed, sometimes with dire consequences.

- *Stress fractures* The elderly patient with unexplained pain in the hip should be considered to have a stress fracture until proved otherwise. A similar cautionary note is raised for young athletes who do regular impact-loading sports and military personnel on marching routines. The x-ray is usually normal but a bone scan, or better still an MRI, will show the lesion (Figure 29.6).

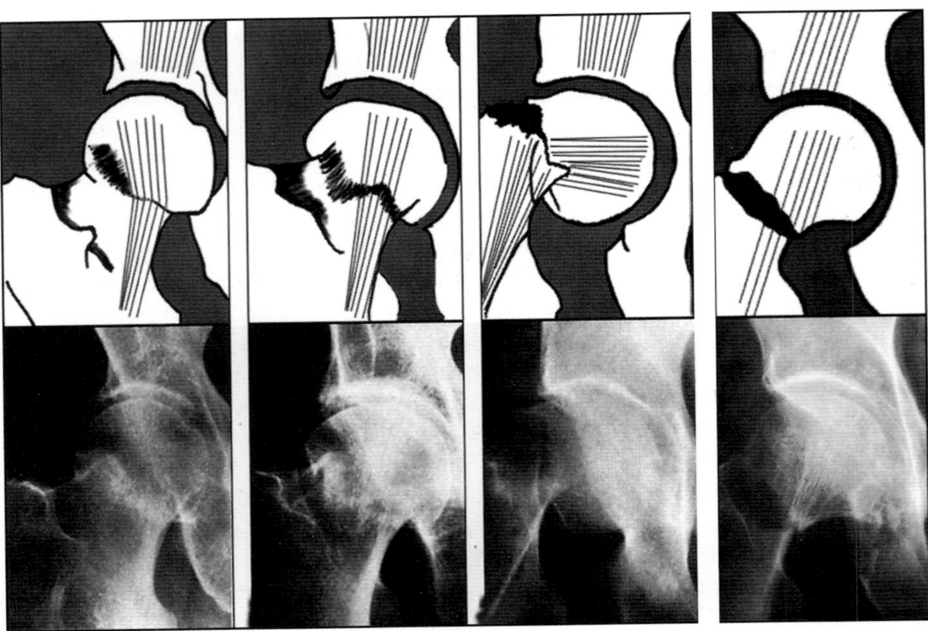

29.5 Garden's classification of femoral neck fractures (a) *Stage I*: incomplete (so-called abducted or impacted) – the femoral head in this case is in slight valgus. (b) *Stage II:* complete without displacement. (c) *Stage III:* complete with partial displacement – the fragments are still connected by the posterior retinacular attachment; the femoral head trabeculae are no longer in line with those of the innominate bone. (d) *Stage IV*: complete with full displacement – the proximal fragment is free and lies correctly in the acetabulum so that the trabeculae appear normally aligned with those of the innominate.

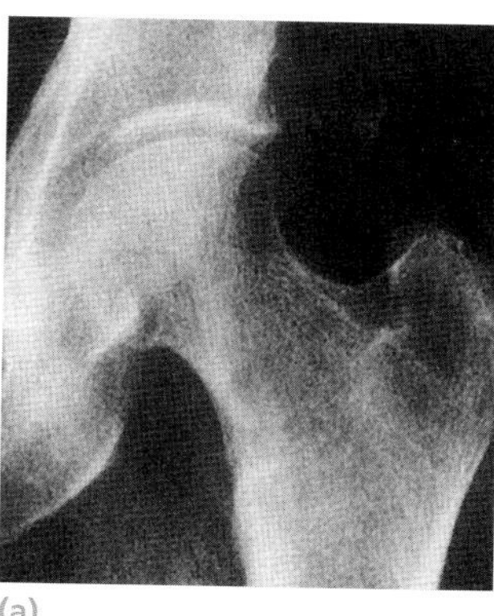

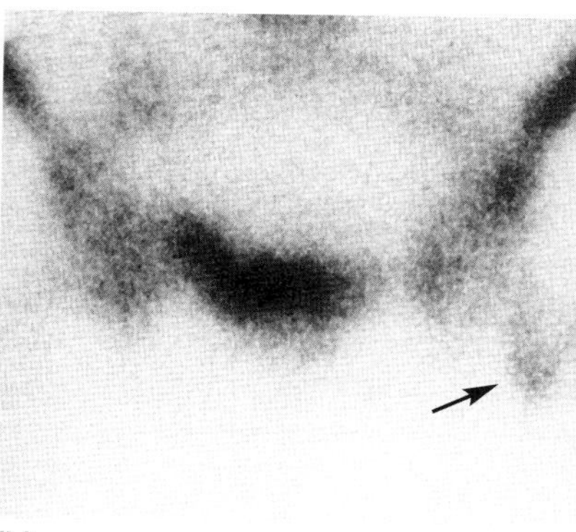

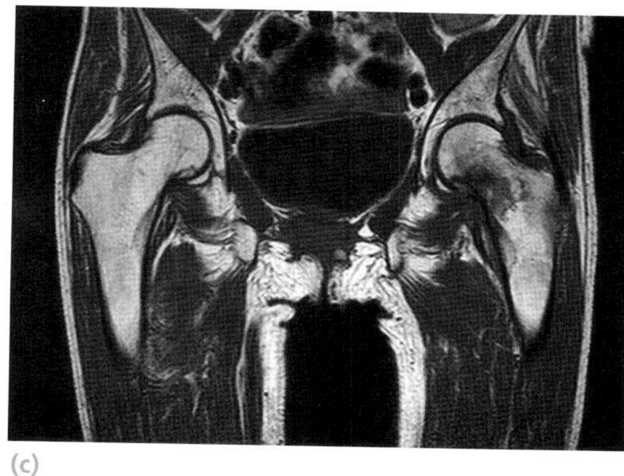

(a) (b) (c)

29.6 Fractures of the femoral neck – diagnosis (a) An elderly woman tripped on the pavement and complained of pain in the left hip. The plain x-ray showed no abnormality. Two weeks later she was still in pain; (b) a bone scan showed a 'hot' area medially at the base of the femoral neck. MRI, if available, is an alternative investigation to confirm suspicions of a femoral neck fracture (c).

- *Undisplaced fractures* Impacted fractures may be extremely difficult to discern on plain x-ray. If there is a fracture it will show up on MRI or a bone scan after a few days.
- *Painless fractures* A bed-ridden patient may develop a 'silent' fracture. Even a fit patient occasionally walks about without pain if the fracture is impacted. If the context suggests an injury, investigate – whether the patient complains or not.
- *Multiple fractures* The patient with a femoral shaft fracture may also have a hip fracture, which is easily missed unless the pelvis is x-rayed.

Treatment

Initial treatment consists of pain-relieving measures and simple splintage of the limb. If operation is delayed, a femoral nerve block may be helpful.

A case for non-operative treatment of undisplaced (Garden Stages I and II) fractures can be made in treating patients with advanced dementia and little discomfort. For all others, operative treatment is almost mandatory. Displaced fractures will not unite without internal fixation, and in any case elderly people should be got up and kept active without delay if pulmonary complications and bed sores are to be prevented. Impacted fractures can be left to unite, but there is always a risk that they may become displaced, even while lying in bed, so fixation is safer.

Another indication for non-operative management is an impacted Garden I fracture that is an 'old' injury, where the diagnosis is made only after the patient has been walking about for several weeks without deleterious effect on the fracture position.

When should the operation be performed? In young patients operation is urgent; interruption of the blood supply will produce irreversible cellular changes after 12 hours and, to prevent this, an accurate reduction and stable internal fixation is needed as soon as possible. In older patients, also, the longer the delay, the greater is the likelihood of complications. However, here speed is tempered by the need for adequate preparation, especially in the very elderly, who are often ill and debilitated.

What if operation is considered too dangerous? Lying in bed on traction may be even more dangerous, and leaving the fracture untreated too painful; the patient least fit for operation may need it most.

Internal fixation Notwithstanding the advances in joint replacement, for most patients the principles of treatment are as of old: accurate reduction, secure internal fixation and early activity. Displaced fractures must first be reduced: with the patient under anaesthesia, the fracture is disimpacted by applying traction with the hip held in 45 degrees of flexion and slight abduction; the limb is then slowly brought into extension and finally internally rotated; as traction is released, the fracture re-impacts in the reduced position.

The reduction is assessed by x-ray. The femoral head should be positioned correctly with the stress trabeculae in the femoral head and those in the femoral neck aligned close to their normal position in both anteroposterior and lateral views, as shown in Figure 29.7. In the AP x-ray the trabeculae in the femoral head and a line along the medial border of the femoral shaft should subtend an angle of 155–180 degrees.

To fix an imperfectly reduced fracture is to risk failure. If a stage III or IV fracture cannot be reduced closed, and the patient is under 60 years of age, open reduction through an anterolateral approach is advisable. However, in older patients (and certainly in those over 70) this may not be justified; if two careful attempts at closed reduction fail, prosthetic

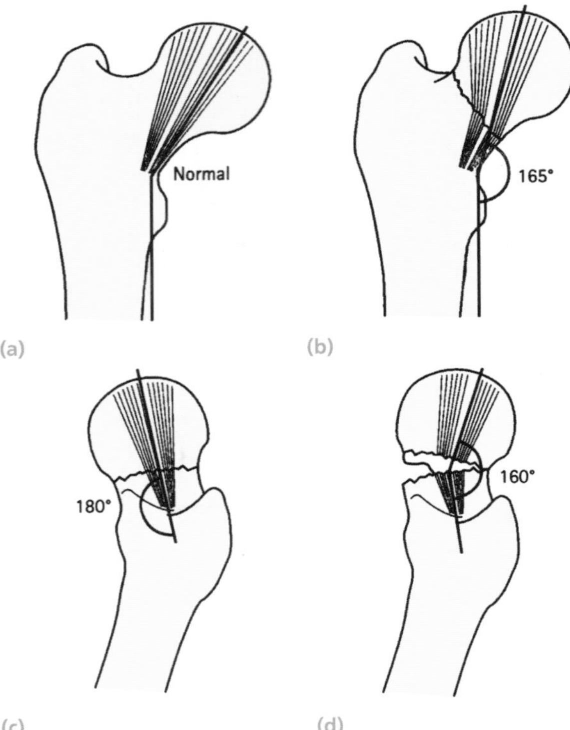

29.7 Garden's index for assessing reduction in subcapital fractures On the anteroposterior x-ray (a,b), the medial femoral shaft and the axis of trabecular markings over the medial aspect of the femoral neck lie at an angle of 160°; an acceptable reduction is deemed to lie between 155° and 180°. On the lateral view (c,d), the trabecular markings would be in line (i.e. 180°) if the fracture was perfectly reduced; an acceptable reduction is within 20° of this ideal. Garden (1974) noted that there was a higher association with complications such as avascular necrosis, non-union and osteoarthritis if the quality of reduction was outside these acceptable limits.

replacement is preferable. Some may even argue that prosthetic replacement is always a preferable option for this older group as it carries a much lower risk of needing revision surgery.

Once the fracture is reduced, it is held with cannulated screws or a sliding screw and side-plate which attaches to the femoral shaft. A lateral incision is used to expose the upper femur. When using cannulated screws, guide wires — inserted under fluoroscopic control – are used to ensure correct placement of the fixing device. Usually three cannulated screws will suffice; they should lie parallel and extend to within 5 mm of the subchondral bone plate. It is usual to start with an inferior screw that skirts the inferior cortex of the neck but remains centred in the lateral x-ray view. This screw should be inserted through the lateral cortex of the femur at a level proximal to the lesser trochanter lest a stress riser is created and produces a subtrochanteric fracture. Two further screws are inserted more proximally, this time centred in the femoral neck on the anteroposterior x-ray but straddling the anterior and posterior margins of the femoral neck on the lateral x-ray (Figure 29.8). If a sliding screw is used, the femoral neck will first have to be reamed; a temporary guidewire should always be introduced before reaming so as to prevent the femoral head from rotating with the reamer and tearing the remaining soft-tissue attachments. Once the sliding screw is fixed, the guidewire is replaced by a single screw to reduce the risk of femoral head rotation during fracture healing – this screw must be parallel to the sliding screw or else impaction of the fracture will not occur!

From the first day patients should sit up in bed or in a chair. They are taught breathing exercises, and

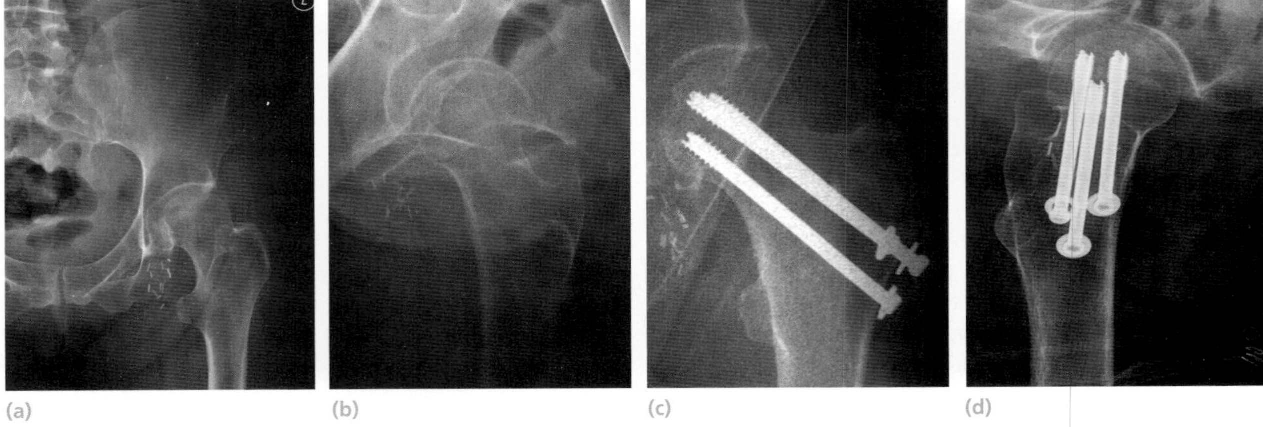

29.8 Femoral neck injuries – treatment (a,b) This Garden stage II fracture has been stabilized with 3 cannulated screws. (c,d) An optimum position for the screws is: one to support the inferior portion of the neck (centrally); and another two, central in level, skirting the anterior and posterior cortices of the femoral neck on the lateral x-ray. It is important the most inferior screw enters the lateral cortex of the femur proximal to the level of the inferior margin of the lesser trochanter.

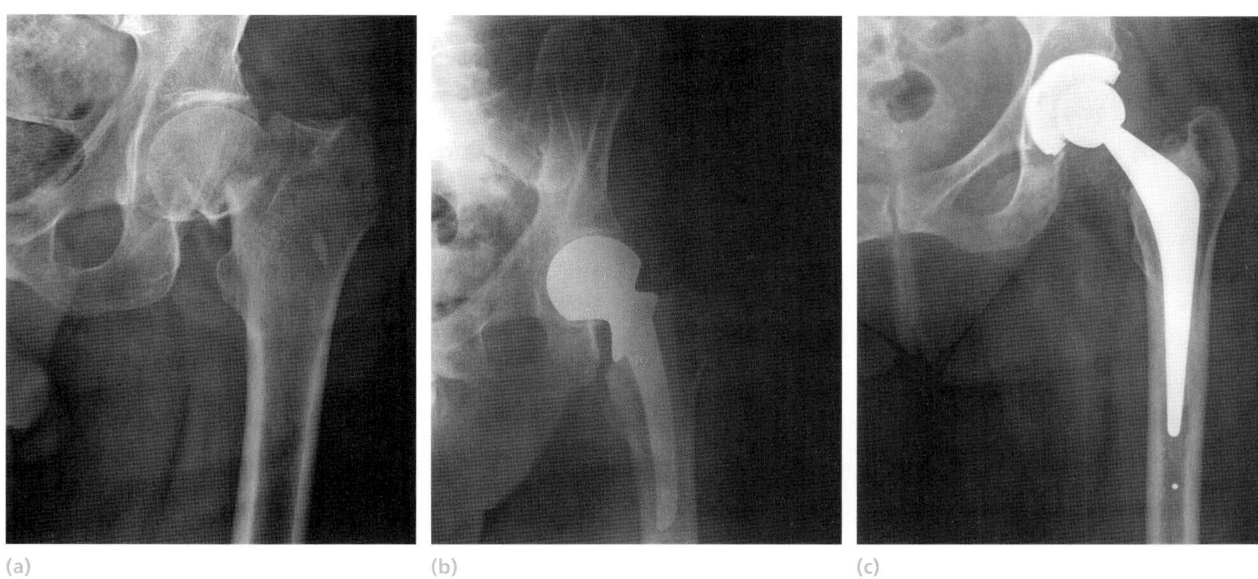

29.9 Fracture of the femoral neck – treatment (a) A fracture as severely displaced as this (Stage IV), if treated by reduction and internal fixation, will probably end up needing revision surgery; instead it could be treated by performing a hemiarthroplasty using a cemented femoral prostheses (b). A total hip replacement (c) provides a better outcome for younger patients (50–60 year olds) with this type of fracture.

encouraged to help themselves and to begin walking (with crutches or a walker) as soon as possible. To delay weightbearing may be theoretically appropriate but is rarely practicable.

Prosthetic replacement This procedure carries a longer operating time, greater blood loss and a higher infection rate than internal fixation. However, in its favour is a much lower need for revision surgery (nearly four times less) when compared to internal fixation for stage III and IV fractures. The mortality rates are equivalent for the two groups but there is insufficient data to be certain there is a difference in morbidity (Masson, Parker et al. 2003). Some argue that prosthetic replacement is always preferable for stage III and IV fractures so that patients, particularly the elderly, are subject to one single surgical intervention (Figure 29.9). This is also true for patients with pathological fractures and those in whom closed reduction cannot be achieved.

Hip prostheses used for femoral neck fractures are usually of the femoral part only (hemiarthroplasty) and may be inserted with or without cement. Cemented prostheses have better mobility and less thigh pain; uncemented prostheses should be reserved for the very frail where the pre-injury status suggests that mobility is unlikely to be attained after operation and those who will benefit significantly from the reduced operating time. There is little evidence to support use of bipolar prostheses over unipolar types for the elderly group; the mortality, morbidity and functional recovery following use of either are similar. However, some studies suggest a longer survivorship of bipolar implants and an argument can be made for their use in younger patients.

Total hip replacement for femoral neck fractures may be indicated: (1) if treatment has been delayed for some weeks and acetabular damage is suspected, or (2) in patients with metastatic disease or Paget's disease. Hip function and quality of life are reported to be better with total hip replacement, even when compared with hemiarthroplasty, and there is some justification for using this as a preferred option in the healthy, active person who needs treatment for a stage III or IV fracture (Keating, Grant et al. 2006).

Postoperatively, breathing exercises and early mobilization are important. Speed of recovery depends largely on how active the patient was before the fracture; after 2–4 months, further improvement is unlikely.

Complications

General complications These patients, most of whom are elderly, are prone to general complications such as deep vein thrombosis, pulmonary embolism, pneumonia and bed sores; not to mention disorders that might have been present before the fracture and which lead to death in a substantial proportion of cases. Notwithstanding the advances in perioperative care, the mortality rate in elderly patients may be as high as 20 per cent at 4 months after injury. Among the survivors over 80 years, about half fail to resume independent walking.

Avascular necrosis Ischaemic necrosis of the femoral head occurs in about 30 per cent of patients with displaced fractures and 10 per cent of those with undisplaced fractures. There is no way of diagnosing this at the time of fracture. A few weeks later, an isotope bone scan may show diminished vascularity. X-ray changes may not become apparent for months or even years. Whether the fracture unites or not, collapse of the femoral head will cause pain and progressive loss of function (Figure 29.10). In patients over 45 years, treatment is by total joint replacement.

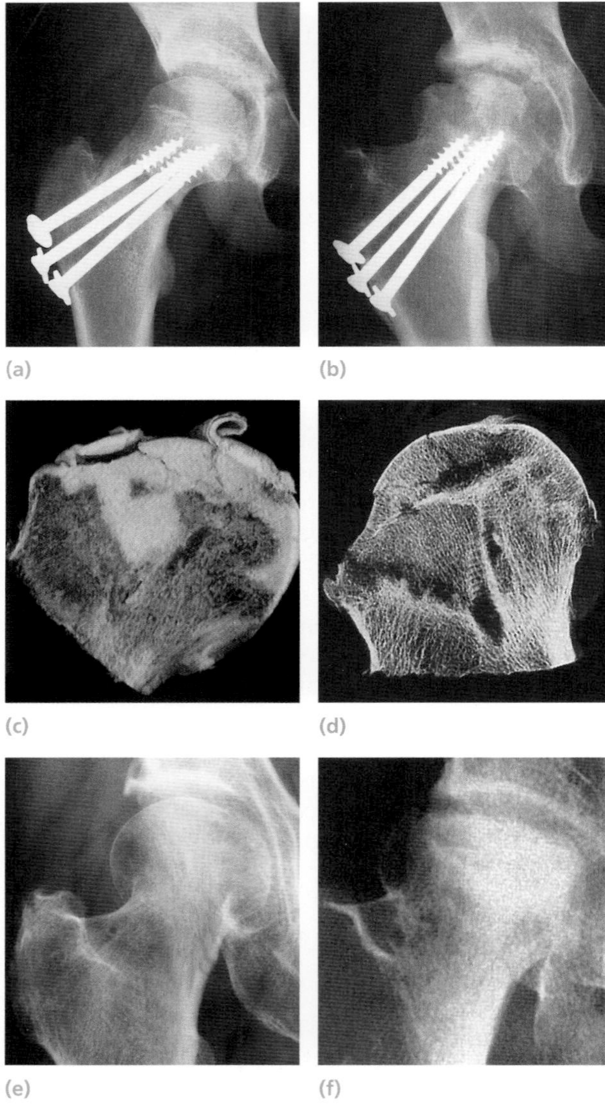

29.10 Fracture of the femoral neck – avascular necrosis (a) The post-reduction x-ray may look splendid but the blood supply is compromised and 6 months later (b) there is obvious necrosis of the femoral head. (c) Section across the excised femoral head, showing the large necrotic segment and splitting of the articular cartilage. (d) Fine detail x-ray of the same. (e,f) Even an impacted fracture, if it is displaced in valgus, can lead to avascular necrosis.

In younger patients, the choice of treatment is controversial. Core decompression has no place in the management of traumatic osteonecrosis. Realignment or rotational osteotomy is suitable for those with a relatively small necrotic segment. Arthrodesis is often mentioned in armchair discussions, but in practice it is seldom carried out. Provided the risks are carefully explained, including the likelihood of at least one revision procedure, joint replacement may be justifiable even in this group.

Non-union More than 30 per cent of all femoral neck fractures fail to unite, and the risk is particularly high in those that are severely displaced. There are many causes: poor blood supply, imperfect reduction, inadequate fixation, and the tardy healing that is characteristic of intra-articular fractures. The bone at the fracture site is ground away, the fragments fall apart and the screw cuts out of the bone or is extruded laterally. The patient complains of pain, shortening of the limb and difficulty with walking. The x-ray shows the sorry outcome.

The method of treatment depends on the cause of the non-union and the age of the patient. In the relatively young, three procedures are available: (1) if the fracture is nearly vertical but the head is alive, subtrochanteric osteotomy with internal fixation changes the fracture line to a more horizontal angle; (2) if the reduction or fixation was faulty and there are no signs of necrosis, it is reasonable to remove the screws, reduce the fracture, insert fresh screws correctly and also to apply a bone graft across the fracture, either a segment of fibula or a muscle pedicle graft; and (3), if the head is avascular but the joint unaffected, prosthetic replacement may be suitable; if the joint is damaged or arthritic, total replacement is indicated.

In elderly patients, only two procedures should be considered: (1) if pain is considerable then the femoral head, no matter whether it is avascular or not, is best removed and (provided the patient is reasonably fit) total joint replacement is performed; (2) if the patient is old and infirm and pain not unbearable, a raised heel and a stout stick or elbow crutch are often sufficient.

Osteoarthritis Avascular necrosis or femoral head collapse may lead, after several years, to secondary osteoarthritis of the hip. If there is marked loss of joint movement and widespread damage to the articular surface, total joint replacement will be needed.

Combined fractures of the neck and shaft

Young patients with high-energy fractures of both the femoral neck and the ipsilateral femoral shaft present a special problem. Both fractures must be fixed, and there are several ways of doing this. The femoral neck fracture takes priority as complications following this fracture are generally more difficult to address than those of the shaft fracture. Anatomic reduction and stable fixation of the femoral neck fracture must not be compromised in order to accommodate fixation of the shaft fracture. The femoral neck fracture is reduced using closed or, if necessary, open methods. The fracture is fixed using multiple screws. The femoral shaft fracture can then be managed with a retrograde locked intramedullary nail (inserted through the knee) or by a lateral plate inserted in a submuscular fashion.

INTERTROCHANTERIC FRACTURES

Intertrochanteric fractures are, by definition, extracapsular. As with femoral neck fractures, they are common in elderly, osteoporotic people; most of the patients are women in the 8th decade. However, in contrast to intracapsular fractures, extracapsular trochanteric fractures unite quite easily and seldom cause avascular necrosis.

Mechanism of injury

The fracture is caused either by a fall directly onto the greater trochanter or by an indirect twisting injury. The crack runs up between the lesser and greater trochanter and the proximal fragment tends to displace in varus.

Pathological anatomy

Intertrochanteric fractures are divided into stable and unstable varieties. In essence, unstable fractures are those where:

1. there is poor contact between the fracture fragments, as in four-part intertrochanteric types (greater and lesser trochanter, proximal and distal femoral fragments), or if the posteromedial cortex is comminuted.
2. the fracture pattern is such that forces of weightbearing continually displace the fragments further, as in those with a reverse oblique pattern or with a subtrochanteric extension.
3. osteoporosis leading to poor quality grip by the fixation implants.

The importance of fracture pattern is detailed in the classification by Kyle (1994) which distinguishes four basic patterns that reflect increasing instability and increasing difficulty at reduction and fixation (Figure 29.11).

Clinical features

The patient is usually old and is unable to stand. The leg is shorter and more externally rotated than with a transcervical fracture (because the fracture is extracapsular) and the patient cannot lift his or her leg.

X-ray

Undisplaced, stable fractures may show no more than a thin crack along the intertrochanteric line; indeed, there is often doubt as to whether the bone is fractured and the diagnosis may have to be confirmed by scintigraphy or MRI.

More often the fracture is displaced and there may be considerable comminution. The lesser and greater trochanters may be identifiable as separate fragments and this calls for caution; surgery is technically more difficult and, even with modern implants, stable fixation may be hindered because of poor bone quality.

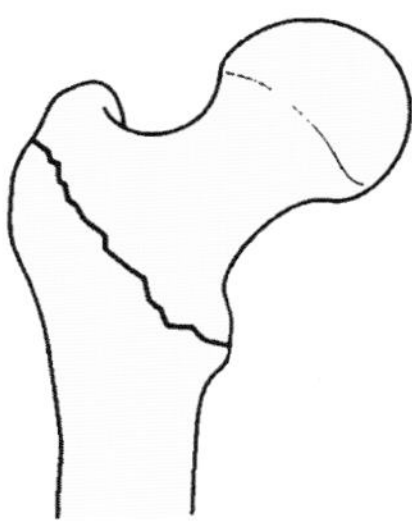

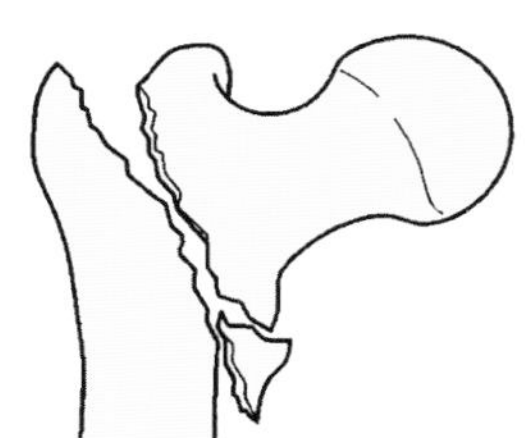

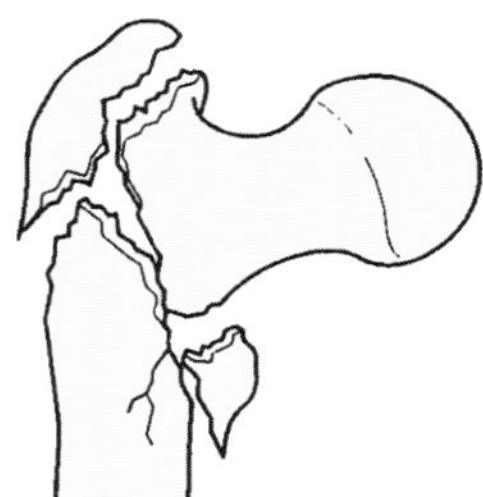

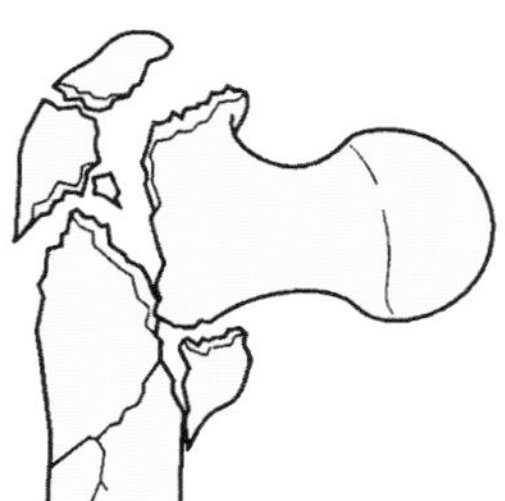

29.11 Intertrochanteric fractures – classification Types 1 to 4 are arranged in increasing degrees of instability and complexity. Types 1 and 2 account for the majority (nearly 60 per cent). The reverse oblique type of intertrochanteric fracture represents a subgroup of Type 4; it causes similar difficulties with fixation.

Treatment

Intertrochanteric fractures are almost always treated by early internal fixation – not because they fail to unite with conservative treatment (they unite quite readily), but (a) to obtain the best possible position and (b) to get the patient up and walking as soon as possible and thereby reduce the complications associated with prolonged recumbency. Non-operative treatment may be appropriate for a small group who are too ill to undergo anaesthesia; traction in bed until there is sufficient reduction of pain to allow mobilization can yield reasonable results but much depends on the quality of nursing care and physical therapy (Kaplan, Miyamoto et al. 2008).

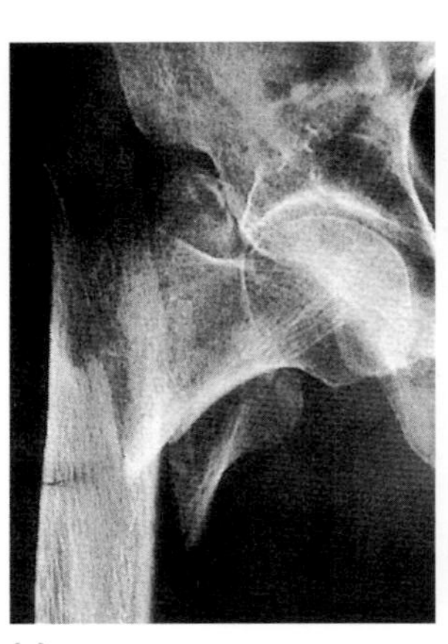

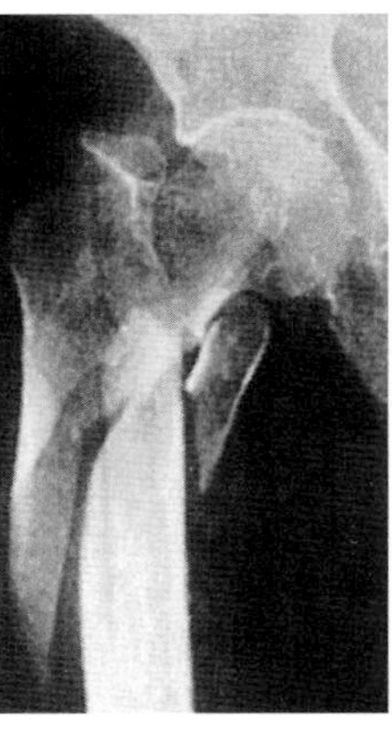

(a) (b)

29.12 Intertrochanteric features Two contrasting types of intertrochanteric fracture. (a) Type 2 fracture: the fracture runs obliquely downwards from the lateral to medial cortex, in this case associated with a lesser trochanter fracture and resulting in a typical varus deformity. This is an unstable fracture. (b) Type 4 'reverse oblique' fracture: here the fracture line runs downwards from medial to lateral cortex, to give an even more unstable geometry.

Fracture reduction at surgery is performed on a fracture table that provides slight traction and internal rotation; the position is checked by x-ray and the fracture is fixed with an angled device – preferably a sliding screw in conjunction with a plate or intramedullary nail. Positioning the screw is important if it is to be prevented from cutting out of the osteoporotic bone. It should pass up the femoral neck to end within the centre of the femoral head, with the tip resting about 5 mm from the subchondral bone plate. A 'tip-apex' distance is described to identify a 'sweet-spot' for positioning this sliding screw: if within 25 mm, there is a lower risk of the screw cutting out of the femoral head (Figure 29.13). The side plate should be long enough to accommodate at least 4 screws below the fracture line. A small lesser trochanteric fragment may be 'caught' with additional screws.

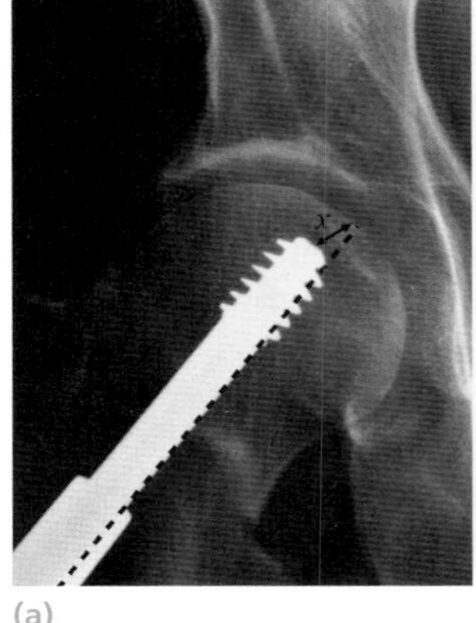

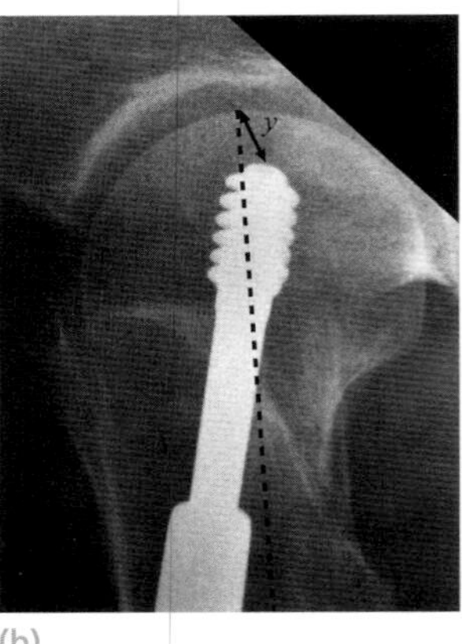

(a) (b)

29.13 Risk of screw cut-out The tip-apex distance is a measure that estimates the risk of screw cut-out from the femoral head. (a,b) It is the sum of the measured distances (after adjustment for magnification on the x-ray) from the tip of the screw to the apex of the femoral head – on both the AP (x) and lateral views (y). The risk of cut-out is low if the sum is less than 25 mm.

With the less common 'reversed oblique' fracture (where the fracture line runs downwards obliquely from medial to lateral cortex) there is a tendency for the distal fragment to shift medially under the proximal fragment as the hip screw slides in the barrel; often the screws from the slide plate lose their purchase from the femoral shaft. In these cases a 95 degree screw-plate device or an intramedullary device with a hip screw gives more stable fixation.

If closed reduction fails to achieve a satisfactory position, open reduction and manipulation of the fragments will be necessary. A large posteromedial fragment (often including the lesser trochanter) may need additional fixation. The addition of bone grafts may hasten union of the medial cortex. On the occasion that anatomical reduction proves impossible, a valgus osteotomy may be needed to allow the proximal fragment to abut securely against the femoral shaft (Dimon and Hughston 1967) (Figure 29.14 c,d).

Postoperatively, exercises are started on the day after operation and the patient allowed up and partial weightbearing as soon as possible.

Complications

EARLY

Early complications are the same as with femoral neck fractures, reflecting the fact that most of these patients are in poor health.

LATE

Failed fixation Screws may cut out of the osteoporotic bone if reduction is poor or if the fixation device is incorrectly positioned. If union is delayed, the implant

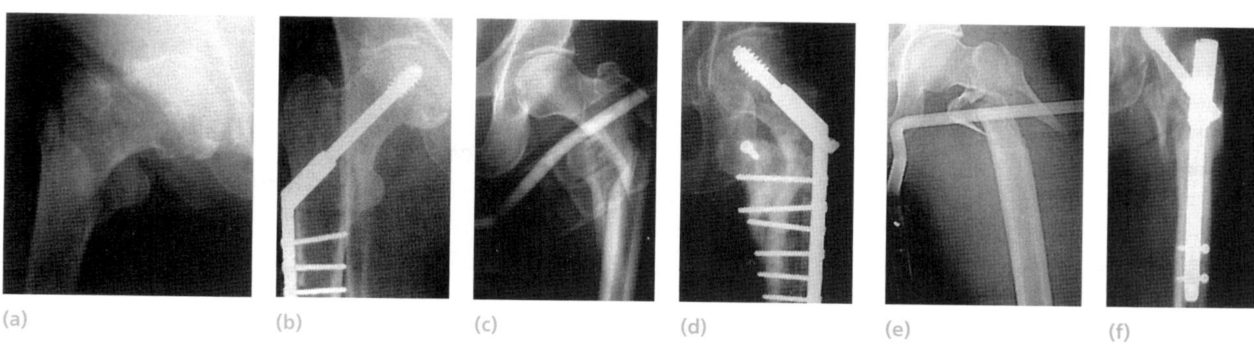

(a) (b) (c) (d) (e) (f)

29.14 Intertrochanteric fractures – treatment Anatomic reduction is the ideal; but stable fixation is equally important. Types 1 and 2 fractures (a,b) can usually be held in good position with a compression screw and plate. If this is not possible, an osteotomy of the lateral cortex (c,d) will allow a screw to be inserted up to the femoral neck and into the head of the femur; this can be used as a lever to reduce the fracture so that the medial spike of the proximal fragment engages securely into the femoral canal; fixation is completed with a side plate. Reverse oblique fractures (e,f) are inherently unstable even after perfect reduction; here one can use an intramedullary device with an oblique screw that engages the femoral head. (Courtesy of Mr M Manning and Mr JS Albert).

itself may break. In either event, reduction and fixation may have to be re-done.

Malunion Varus and external rotation deformities are common. Fortunately they are seldom severe and rarely interfere with function.

Non-union Intertrochanteric fractures seldom fail to unite. If healing is delayed (say beyond 6 months) the fracture probably will not join and further operation is advisable; the fragments are repositioned as anatomically as is feasible, the fixation device is applied more securely and bone grafts are packed around the fracture (Figure 29.15).

Pathological fractures

Intertrochanteric fractures may be due to metastatic disease or myeloma. Unless patients are terminally ill, fracture fixation is essential in order to ensure an acceptable quality of life for their remaining years. In addition to internal fixation, methylmethacrylate cement may be packed in the defect to improve stability.

If there is involvement of the femoral neck, replacement with a cemented prosthesis may be preferable.

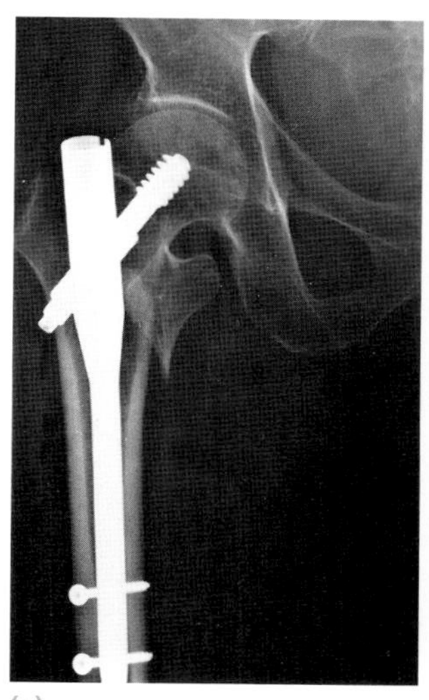

(a)

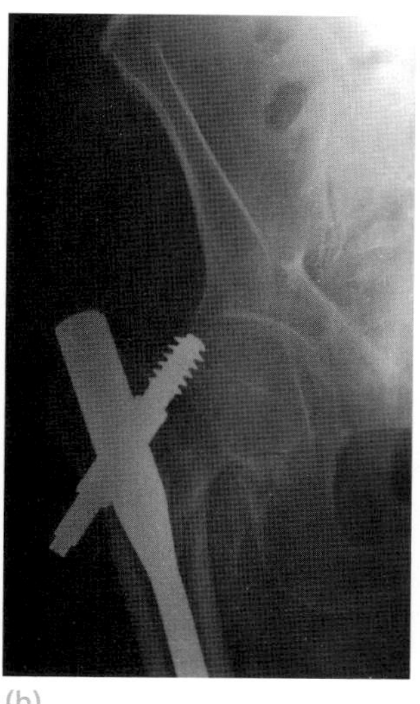

(b)

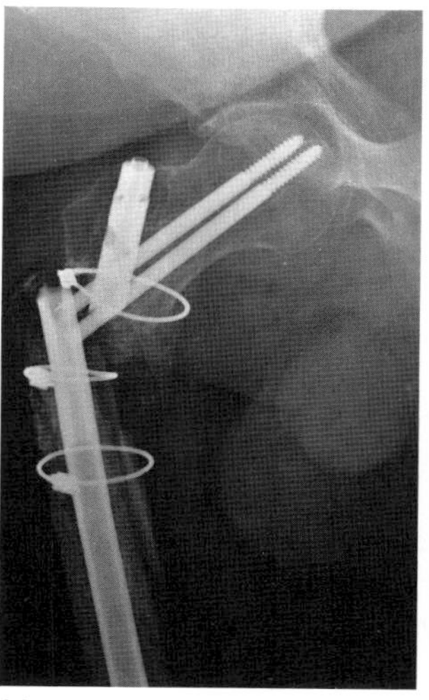

(c)

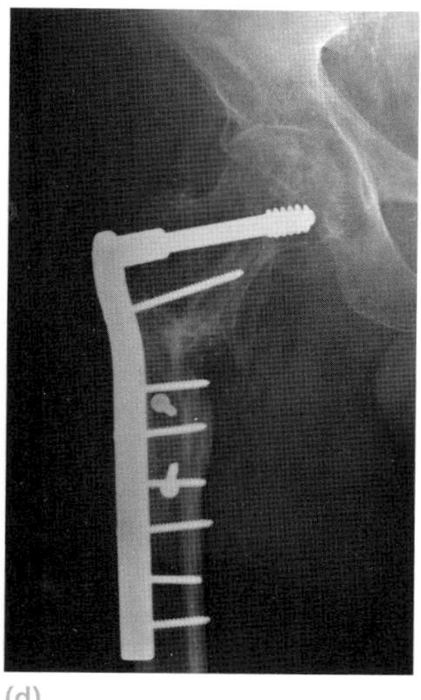

(d)

29.15 Complications of treatment of intertrochanteric fractures (a,b) Failure to maintain reduction, which can be early – usually in osteoporotic bone or from poor implant seating (c,d). The implant may fracture if union is not timely. Revision surgery is complex and may involve bone grafts and a new implant.

PROXIMAL FEMORAL FRACTURES IN CHILDREN

Hip fractures rarely occur in children but when they do they are potentially very serious.

The fracture is usually due to high velocity trauma; for example, falling from a height or a car accident. Pathological fractures sometimes occur through a bone cyst or benign tumour. In children under two years, the possibility of child abuse should be considered.

There is a high risk of complications, such as avascular necrosis, premature physeal closure and coxa vara.

At birth the proximal end of the femur is entirely cartilaginous and for several years, as ossification proceeds, the area between the capital epiphysis and greater trochanter is unusually vulnerable to trauma. Moreover, between the ages of 4 and 8 the ligamentum teres contributes very little to the blood supply of the epiphysis; hence its susceptibility to post-traumatic ischaemia.

Classification

The most useful classification is that of Delbet, which is based on the level of the fracture (Hughes and Beaty 1994). *Type I* is a fracture-separation of the epiphysis; sometimes the epiphyseal fragment is dislocated from the acetabulum. *Type II* is a transcervical fracture of the femoral neck; this is the commonest variety, accounting for almost half of the injuries. *Type III* is a basal (cervico-trochanteric) fracture, the second most common injury. *Type IV* is an intertrochanteric fracture (Figure 29.16).

Clinical features

Diagnosis can be difficult, especially in infants where the epiphysis is not easily defined on x-ray. Type I fractures are easily mistaken for hip dislocation. Ultrasonography, MRI and arthrography may help. In older children the diagnosis is usually obvious on plain x-ray examination.

It is important to establish whether the fracture is displaced or undisplaced; the former carries a much higher risk of complications. Type IV fractures are the least likely to give rise to complications.

Treatment

These fractures should be treated as a matter of urgency, and certainly within 24 hours of injury. Initially the hip is supported or splinted while investigations are carried out. Early aspiration of the intracapsular haematoma is advocated by some authors as a means of reducing the risk of epiphyseal ischaemia; however, the benefits are uncertain and the matter is controversial.

Undisplaced fractures may be treated by immobilization in a plaster spica for 6–8 weeks. However, fracture position is not always maintained and there is a considerable risk of late displacement and malunion or non-union.

Displaced type IV fractures also can be treated non-operatively: closed reduction, traction and spica immobilization. Careful follow-up is essential; if position is lost, operative fixation will be needed.

Type I, II and III fractures are treated by closed reduction and then internal fixation with smooth pins or cannulated screws. 'Closed reduction' means one gentle manipulation; if this fails, open reduction is performed. In small children, operative fixation is supplemented by a spica cast for 6–12 weeks.

Complications

Avascular necrosis of the femoral head This is the most common (and most feared) complication; it occurs in

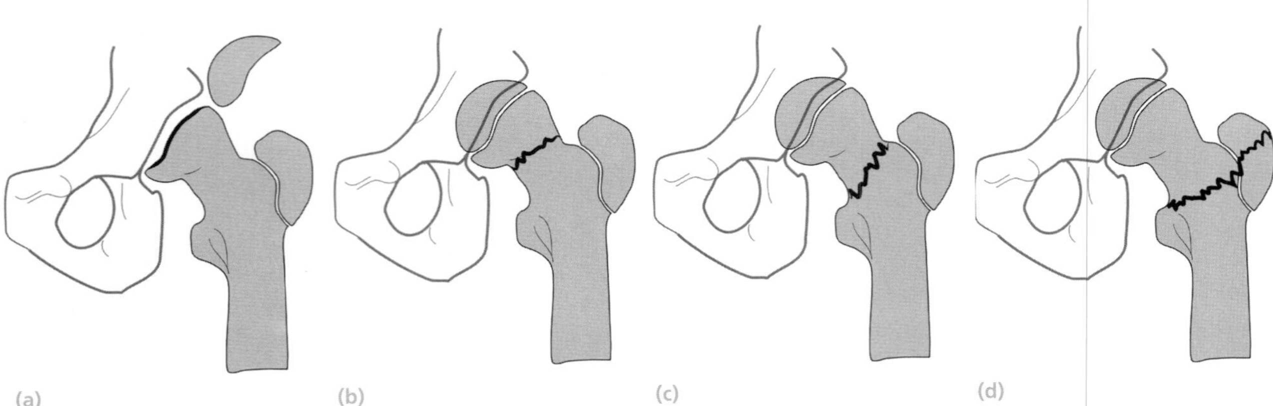

29.16 Proximal femoral fractures in children These are the result of strong forces or weak bone, e.g. through cysts. There are 4 types (the Delbet classification), depending on the level of the fracture: (a) Type 1 at the physeal level; (b) Type 2 through the middle of the neck; (c) Type 3 at the base of the neck and (d) Type 4 at the intertrochanteric level.

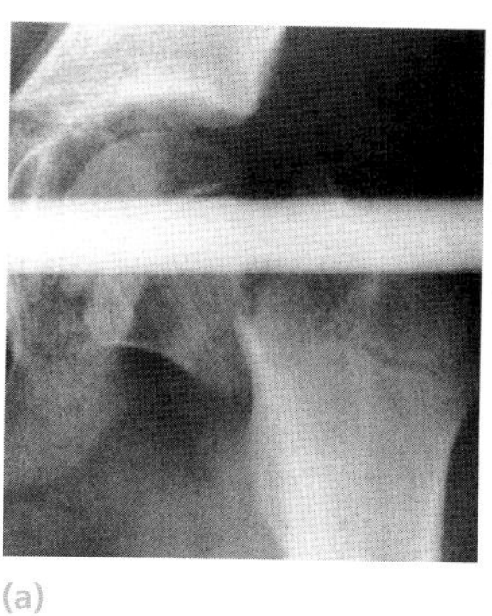
(a)

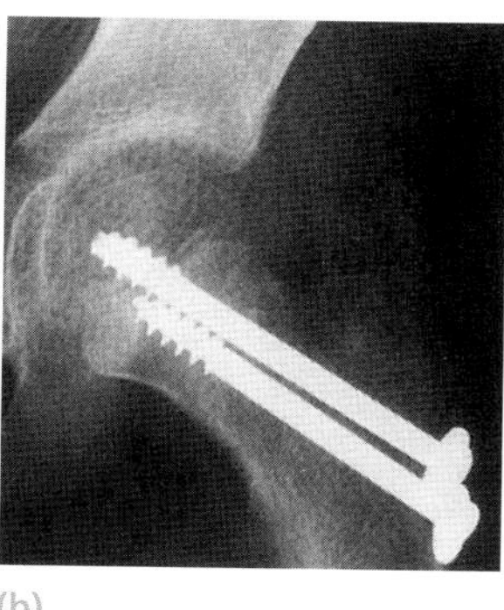
(b)

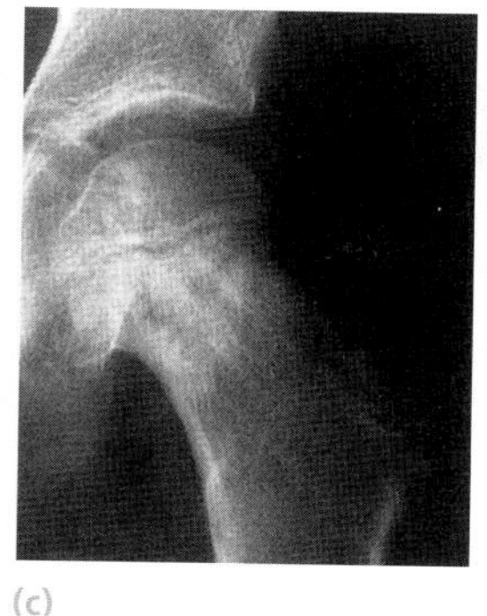
(c)

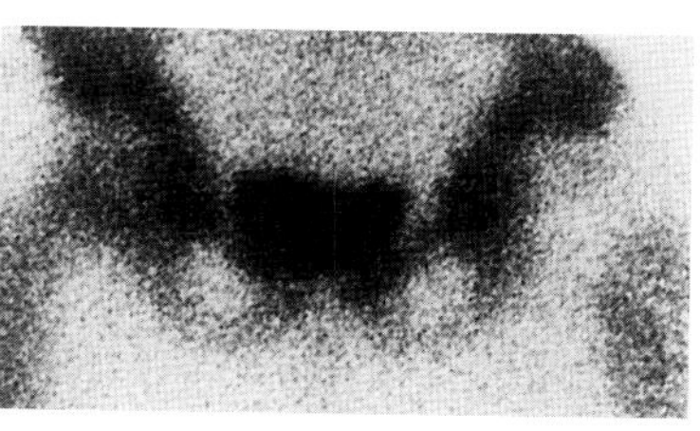
(d)

29.17 Femoral neck fractures in children: (a) Fracture of the femoral neck in a child is particularly worrying because, even with perfect fixation (b), there is often ischaemia of the femoral head. This fracture united and the screws were removed (c), but the radioisotope scan shows no activity in the left femoral head (d) i.e. ischaemic necrosis.

about 30 per cent of all cases. Important risk factors are (1) an age of more than 10; (2) a high velocity injury; (3) a type I or II fracture; and (4) displacement. The child complains of pain and loss of movement; x-ray changes usually appear within 3 months of injury. Treatment is problematic. Non-weightbearing, or 'containment splintage' in abduction and internal rotation, is sometimes advocated but there is little evidence that this makes any difference. The outcome depends largely on the size of the necrotic area; unfortunately most end up with intrusive pain and marked restriction of movement. Arthrodesis may be advisable, as a late salvage procedure.

Coxa vara Femoral neck deformity may result from malunion, avascular necrosis or premature physeal closure. If the deformity is mild, remodelling may take care of it. If the neck-shaft angle is less than 110 degrees, subtrochanteric valgus osteotomy will probably be needed.

Diminished growth Physeal damage may result in retarded femoral growth. Limb length equalization may be needed.

ISOLATED FRACTURES OF THE TROCHANTERS

In adolescents, the *lesser trochanter* apophysis may be avulsed by the pull of the psoas muscle; the injury nearly always occurs during hurdling. Treatment is rest, followed by return to activity when comfortable. In the elderly, separation of the lesser trochanter should arouse suspicions of metastatic malignant disease.

In the elderly, part of the *greater trochanter* can be fractured by a direct blow after a fall. The x-ray should be scrutinised for a subtle associated intertrochanteric fracture. In the event this is absent, treatment is non-operative and functional recovery is usually good. Occasionally, the greater trochanter is fractured and the fragment widely separated in a young individual. It can be fixed back in position with cancellous screws or tension band wiring. Full weightbearing is prohibited for 6–8 weeks.

SUBTROCHANTERIC FRACTURES

The part of the femoral shaft around the lesser trochanter is substantially strengthened by a widening cortex and that stout pillar of bone posteromedially, the calcar femorale. Therefore, large forces are needed to cause fractures in this area – and that is usually the case when this injury is diagnosed in young adults. By contrast, in the elderly, who are the second group who sustain this fracture quite frequently, the injury is relatively trivial; here the reason is a weakening of bone in this area by osteoporosis, osteomalacia, Paget's disease or a secondary deposit.

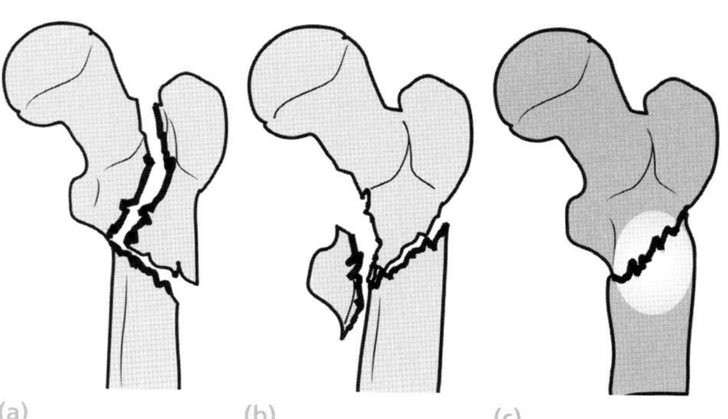

29.18 Subtrochanteric fractures of the femur – warning signs on the x-ray X-ray findings that should caution the surgeon: (a) comminution, with extension into the piriform fossa; (b) displacement of a medial fragment including the lesser trochanter and, (c) lytic lesions in the femur.

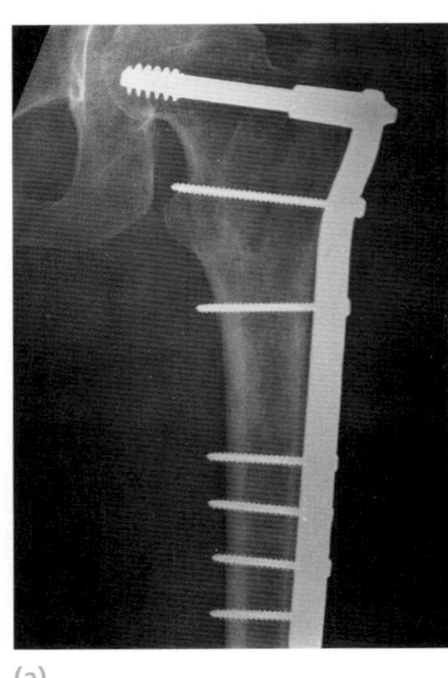

(a)

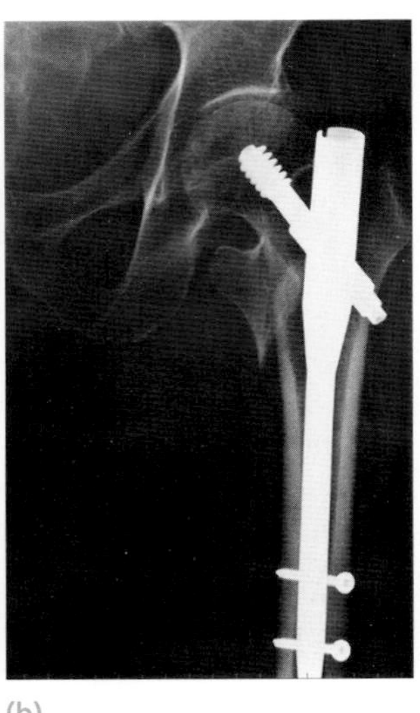

(b)

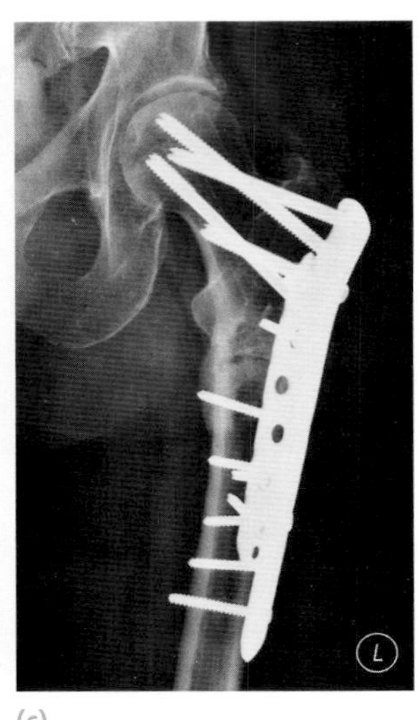

(c)

29.19 Subtrochanteric fractures – internal fixation Several methods of fixation are in use: (a) a 95° screw and plate device; (b) an intramedullary nail with proximal interlocking screw into the femoral head; and (c) a proximal femoral plate with locking screws.

Subtrochanteric fractures have several features which make them interesting (and challenging to treat):

1. Blood loss is greater than with femoral neck or trochanteric fractures – the region is covered with anastomosing branches of the medial and lateral circumflex femoral arteries which come off the profunda femoris trunk.
2. There may be subtle extensions of the fracture into the intertrochanteric region, which may influence the manner in which internal fixation can be performed.
3. The proximal part is abducted and externally rotated by the gluteal muscles, and flexed by the psoas. The shaft of the femur has to be brought into a position to match the proximal part or else a malunion is created by internal fixation.

Clinical features

The leg lies in neutral or external rotation and looks short; the thigh is markedly swollen. Movement is excruciatingly painful.

X-ray

The fracture is through or below the lesser trochanter. It may be transverse, oblique or spiral, and is frequently comminuted. The upper fragment is flexed and appears deceptively short; the shaft is adducted and is displaced proximally.

Three important features should be looked for, as the presence of any one will influence treatment: (1) an unusually long fracture line extending proximally towards the greater trochanter and piriform fossa; (2) a large, displaced fragment which includes the lesser trochanter; and (3) lytic lesions in the femur.

Treatment

Traction may help to reduce blood loss and pain. It is an interim measure until the patient, especially if elderly and with multiple medical problems, is stabilized and prepared for surgery.

Open reduction and internal fixation is the treatment of choice. Two main types of implant are used for fracture fixation: (a) an intramedullary nail with a proximal interlocking screw that can be directed into the femoral head or placed in the standard manner, and (b) a 95 degree hip screw-and-plate device. Both implants are suitable but there are circumstances where one may be preferable:

1. Intramedullary nails are generally stronger and can tolerate stresses for longer if healing is slow; this may be the case if the fracture is very comminuted or unstable, or if one suspects that operative dissection may have compromised bone viability.
2. An intramedullary nail is also preferable for a pathological fracture; a full-length nail should be used as there may be tumour deposits in the distal part of the femur.

Key points to bear in mind when operating on these fractures are: (a) an anatomic reduction will provide the greatest surface area of contact between the fragments and reduce stresses on the implant; with intramedullary nails this has to be achieved *before* reaming is commenced; (b) as little soft-tissue dissection as possible to accomplish reduction should be performed; and (c) it is important that the integrity of the medial cortex (around the lesser trochanter) be established, particularly if a hip screw-and-plate device is used.

Proximal interlocking screws with intramedullary nails should be directed into the femoral head if the fracture pattern extends above the lesser trochanter. If the fracture enters the piriformis fossa, then an intramedullary nail designed to be inserted at the tip of the greater trochanter is better; alternatively a 95 degree hip screw-and-plate device can be used.

Postoperatively the patient is allowed partial weightbearing (with crutches) until union is secure. It is rarely feasible to impose significant weightbearing restrictions on the elderly and it would be better to choose a stronger implant (and ensure a near-anatomic reduction of the fracture) so that early loading can be tolerated.

Complications

Malunion Varus and rotational malunions are fairly common. This can be prevented by careful attention to accurate reduction before internal fixation is applied. If the degree of malunion produces symptoms, it may need operative correction.

Non-union This occurs in about 5 per cent of cases; it will require operative correction of any deformity, renewed fixation and bone grafting.

FEMORAL SHAFT FRACTURES

The femoral shaft is circumferentially padded with large muscles. This provides advantages and disadvantages: reduction can be difficult as muscle contraction displaces the fracture; however, healing potential is improved by having this well-vascularized sleeve containing a source of mesenchymal stem cells, and open fractures often need no more than split thickness skin grafts to obtain satisfactory cover.

Mechanism of injury

This is usually a fracture of young adults and results from a high energy injury. Diaphyseal fractures in elderly patients should be considered 'pathological' until proved otherwise. In children under 4 years the possibility of physical abuse must be kept in mind.

Fracture patterns are clues to the type of force that produced the break. A *spiral fracture* is usually caused by a fall in which the foot is anchored while a twisting force is transmitted to the femur. *Transverse* and *oblique fractures* are more often due to angulation or direct violence and are therefore particularly common in road accidents. With severe violence (often a combination of direct and indirect forces) the fracture may be *comminuted*, or the bone may be broken in more than one place (*a segmental fracture*).

Pathological anatomy

Most fractures of the femoral shaft have some degree of comminution, although it is not always apparent on x-ray. Small bone fragments, or a single large 'butterfly' fragment, may separate at the fracture line but usually remain attached to the adjacent soft tissue and retain their blood supply. With more extensive comminution there is no point of firm contact between proximal and distal fragments and the fracture is completely unstable (Figure 29.20). This is the basis of a helpful classification (Winquist, Hansen et al. 1984).

Fracture displacement often follows a predictable pattern dictated by the pull of muscles attached to each fragment.

- In *proximal shaft fractures* the proximal fragment is flexed, abducted and externally rotated because of gluteus medius and iliopsoas pull; the distal fragment is frequently adducted.
- In *mid-shaft fractures* the proximal fragment is again flexed and externally rotated but abduction is less marked.
- In *lower third fractures* the proximal fragment is adducted and the distal fragment is tilted by gastrocnemius pull.

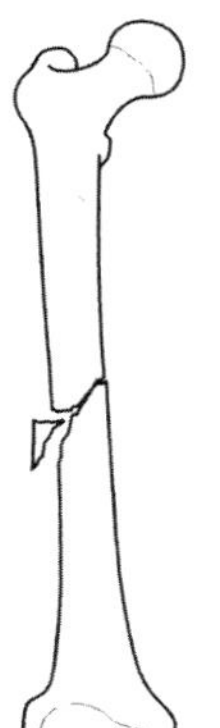
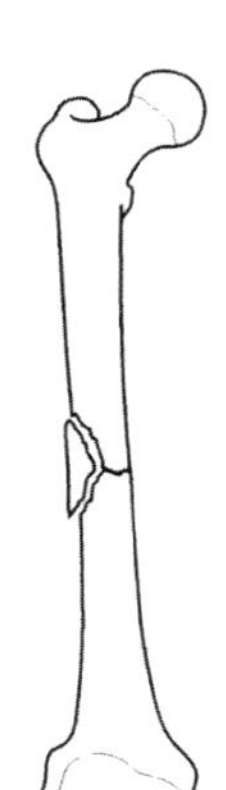
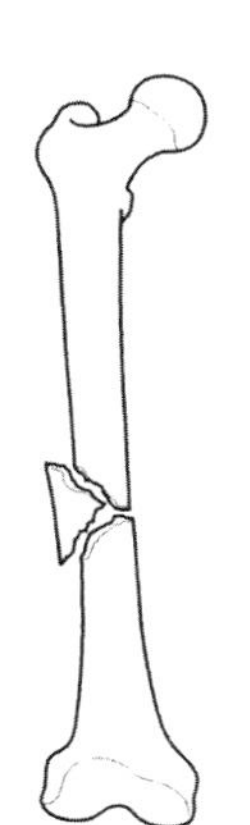
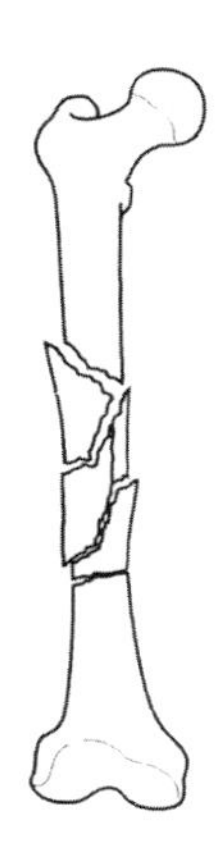

29.20 Femoral shaft fractures – classification Winquist's classification reflects the observation that the degrees of soft-tissue damage and fracture instability increase with increasing grades of comminution. In *Type 1* there is only a tiny cortical fragment. In *Type 2* the 'butterfly fragment' is larger but there is still at least 50 per cent cortical contact between the main fragments. In *Type 3* the butterfly fragment involves more than 50 per cent of the bone width. *Type 4* is essentially a segmental fracture.

The soft tissues are always injured and bleeding from the perforators of the profunda femoris may be severe. Over one litre may be lost into the tissues and, in the case of bilateral femoral shaft fractures, the patient can become hypotensive quickly if not adequately resuscitated. Beware of the fracture at the junction of the middle and distal thirds of the femoral shaft – it can be responsible for damaging the femoral artery in the adductor canal.

Clinical features

There is swelling and deformity of the limb, and any attempt to move the limb is painful. With the exception of a fracture through pathological bone, the large forces needed to break the femur usually produce accompanying injuries nearby and sometimes further afield. Careful clinical scrutiny is necessary to exclude neurovascular problems and other lower limb or pelvic fractures. An ipsilateral femoral neck fracture occurs in about 10 per cent of cases and, if present, there is a one in three chance of a significant knee injury as well. The combination of femoral shaft and tibial shaft fractures on the same side, producing a 'floating knee', signals a high risk of multi-system injury in the patient. The effects of blood loss and other injuries, some of which can be life-threatening, may dominate the clinical picture.

X-ray

It may be difficult to obtain adequate views in the Accident and Emergency Room setting, especially views that provide reliable information on proximal or distal fracture extensions or joint involvement; these can be postponed until better facilities and easier patient positioning are possible. *But never forget to x-ray the hip and knee as well* (Figure 29.21). A baseline chest x-ray is useful as there is a risk of adult respiratory distress syndrome (ARDS) in those with multiple injuries.

The fracture pattern should be noted; it will form a guide to treatment.

Emergency treatment

Traction with a splint is first aid for a patient with a femoral shaft fracture. It is applied at the site of the accident, and before the patient is moved. A Thomas' splint, or one of the modern derivations of this practical device, is ideal: the leg is pulled straight and threaded through the ring of the splint; the shod foot is tied to the cross-piece so as to maintain traction and the limb and splint are firmly bandaged together. This temporary stabilization helps to control pain, reduces bleeding and makes transfer easier. Shock should be treated; blood volume is restored and maintained, and

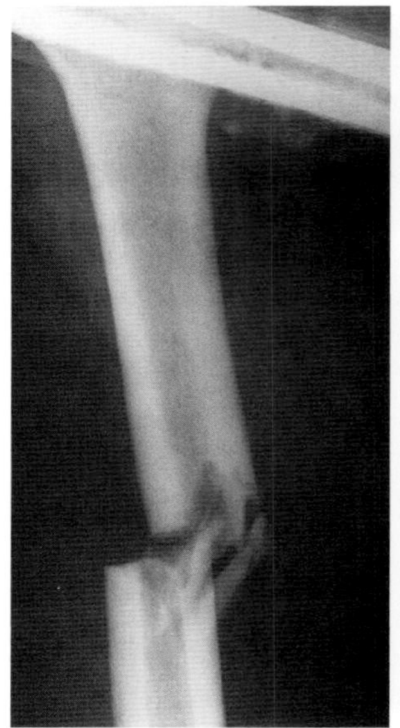

(a)

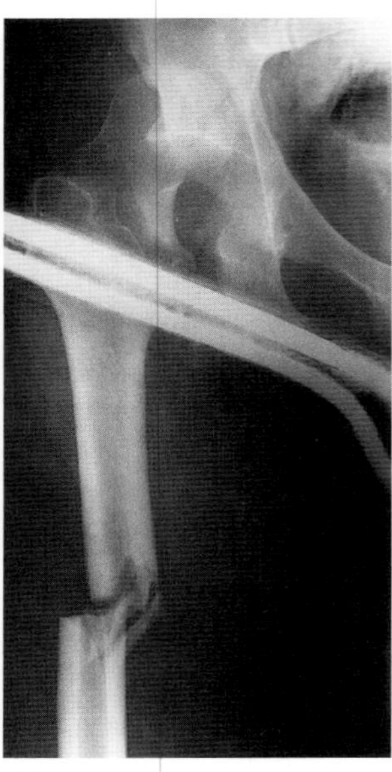

(b)

29.21 Femoral shaft fractures – diagnosis (a) The upper fragment of this femur is adducted, which should alert the surgeon to the possibility of (b) an associated hip dislocation. With this combination of injuries the dislocation is frequently missed; the safest plan is to *x-ray the pelvis with every fracture of the femoral shaft.*

a definitive plan of action instituted as soon as the patient's condition has been fully assessed.

Definitive treatment

The patient with multiple injuries The association of femoral shaft fractures with other injuries, including head, chest, abdominal and pelvic trauma, increases the potential for developing fat embolism, ARDS and multi-organ failure. The risk of systemic complications can be significantly reduced by early stabilization of the fracture, usually by a locked intramedullary nail. However, surgery to introduce a reamed intramedullary nail may produce untoward effects in those with severe chest injuries, especially when carried out within 24 hours of the fracture. It is thought the trauma of surgery and blood loss induces inflammatory changes that may increase both morbidity and mortality – this phenomenon is called *'the second hit'*, referring to a second episode of trauma, albeit surgical, on the patient. Consequently, in the multiply-injured patient, particularly one with severe chest trauma, prompt stabilization with an external fixator may be wise; the fixator can be exchanged for an intramedullary nail when the patient's condition stabilizes. The timing of this second procedure is problematic. Some guidance can be sought from measurement of circulating levels of interleukin-6, a pro-inflammatory cytokine (Pape, van Griensven et al.

2001); when the levels start to decrease, it should be safe to perform 'second hit' interventions. Clinically this occurs around 5–7 days after admission, but this window is by no means applicable to all patients nor is it conclusive at this time.

Performing the exchange to an intramedullary nail also carries the risk of transferring contaminants from pin sites to the intramedullary nail; the earlier the operation is performed, the lower the risk. In the patient who spends a protracted period in the intensive care unit, it may be safer to use external fixation as definitive treatment, perhaps with a return to theatre later to allow insertion of new pins to increase the stability of the construct.

THE ISOLATED FEMORAL SHAFT FRACTURE

Traction, bracing and spica casts Traction can reduce and hold most fractures in reasonable alignment, except those in the upper third of the femur. Joint mobility can be ensured by active exercises. The chief drawback is the length of time spent in bed (10–14 weeks for adults) with the attendant problems of keeping the femur aligned until sufficient callus has formed plus reducing patient morbidity and frustration. Some of these difficulties are overcome by changing to a plaster spica or – in the case of lower third fractures – functional bracing when the fracture is 'sticky', usually around 6–8 weeks.

The main indications for traction are (1) fractures in children; (2) contraindications to anaesthesia; and (3) lack of suitable skill or facilities for internal fixation. It is a poor choice for elderly patients, for pathological fractures and for those with multiple injuries.

The various methods of traction are described in Chapter 23. For young children, *skin traction* without a splint is usually all that is needed. Infants less than 12 kg in weight are most easily managed by suspending the lower limbs from overhead pulleys (*'gallows traction'*), but no more than 2 kg weight should be used and the feet must be checked frequently for circulatory problems. Older children are better suited to *Russell's traction* (Chapter 23) or use of a *Thomas' splint*. Fracture union will have progressed sufficiently by 2–4 weeks (depending on the age of the child) to permit a *hip spica* to be applied and the child is then allowed up. Consolidation is usually complete by 6–12 weeks.

Adults (and older adolescents) require *skeletal traction* through a pin or a tightly strung Kirschner wire behind the tibial tubercle. Traction (8–10 kg for an adult) is applied over pulleys at the foot of the bed. The limb is usually supported on a *Thomas' splint* and a flexion piece allows movement at the knee (Figure 29.22). However, a splint is not essential; indeed, *skeletal traction without a splint* (Perkins' traction) has the advantages of producing less distortion of the fracture and allowing freer movement in bed (Figure 29.23). Exercises are begun as soon as possible.

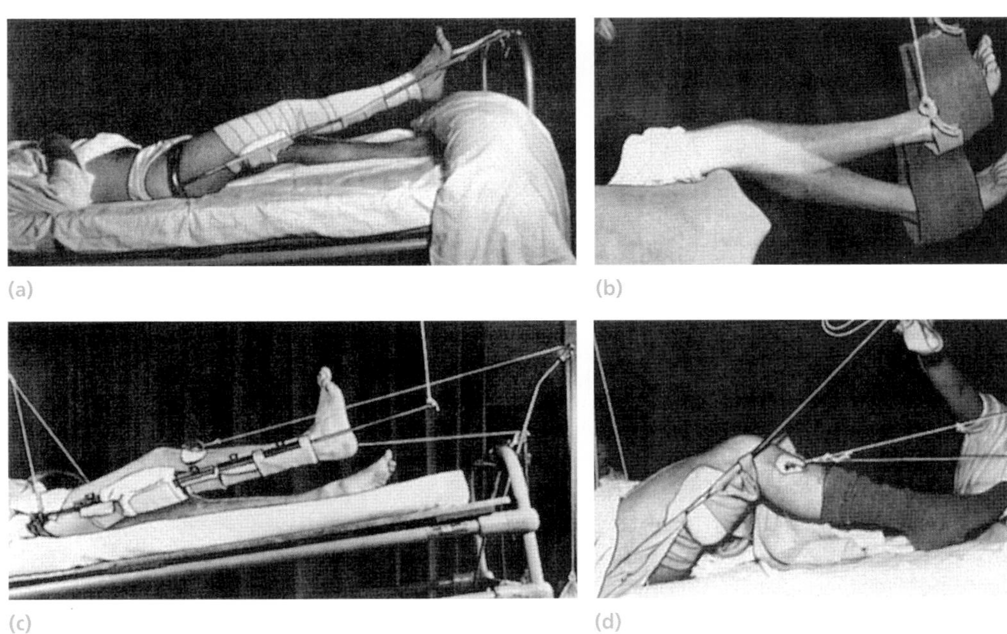

29.22 Femoral fractures – treatment by traction (a) *Fixed traction on a Thomas' splint:* the splint is tied to the foot of the bed which is elevated. This method should be used only rarely because the knee may stiffen; (b) this was the range in such a case when the fracture had united. (c,d) *Balanced traction:* one way to minimize stiffness is to use skeletal balanced traction; the lower slings can be removed to permit knee flexion while traction is still maintained.

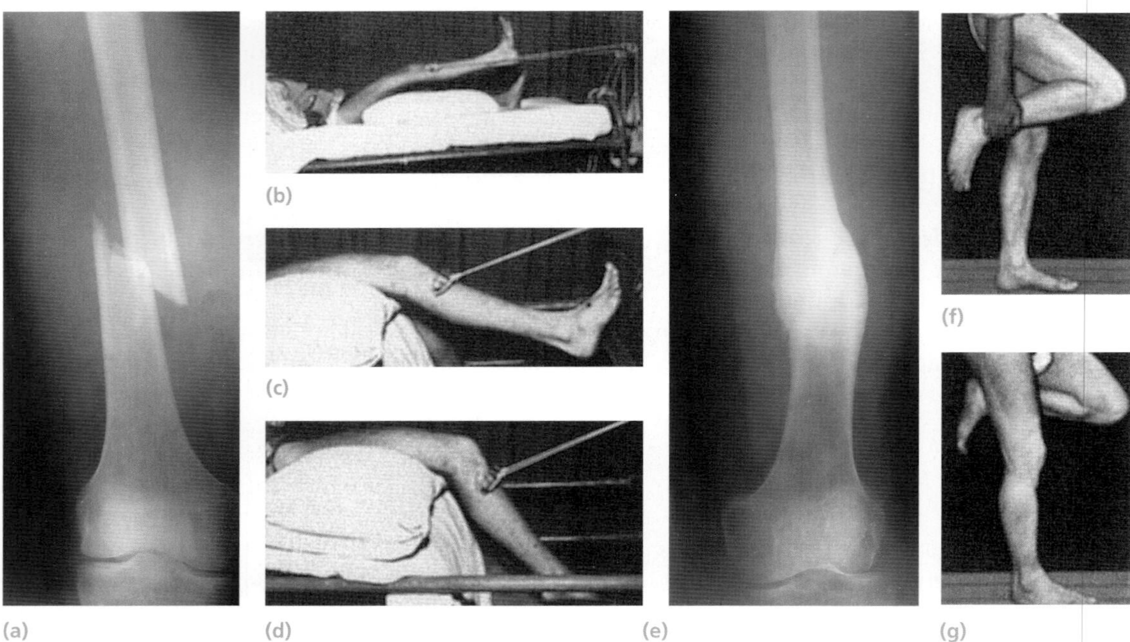

(a) (b) (c) (d) (e) (f) (g)

29.23 Femoral fractures – treatment by traction Even in the adult, traction without a splint can be satisfactory, but skeletal traction is essential. The patient with this rather unstable fracture (a) can lift his leg and exercise his knee (b,c,d). At no time was the leg splinted, but clearly the fracture has consolidated (e), and the knee range (f) is only slightly less than that of the uninjured left leg (g).

Once the fracture is sticky (at about 8 weeks in adults) traction can be discontinued and the patient allowed up and partial weightbearing in a *cast or brace*. For fractures in the upper half of the femur, a *plaster spica* is the safest but it will almost certainly prolong the period of knee stiffness. For fractures in the lower half of the femur, *cast-bracing* is suitable. This type of protection is needed until the fracture has consolidated (16–24 weeks).

Plate and screw fixation Plating is a comparatively easy way of obtaining accurate reduction and firm fixation. The method was popular at one time but went out of favour because of a high complication rate. This occurred when plates were applied through a wide open exposure of the fracture site and perfect anatomical reduction of all bone pieces. Such extensive surgery damaged the healing potential and led to tardy union and implant failure. However, plates have encountered resurgence: today, they are inserted through short incisions and placed in a submuscular plane, rather than deep to periosteum; an indirect (closed) reduction of the fracture is done; fewer screws are used, and usually placed at the ends of the plate, leading to a less rigid hold on the fracture. This technique of *minimally invasive plate osteosynthesis (MIPO)* has led to better union rates. However, postoperative weightbearing will need to be modified as the implant is not as strong as an intramedullary nail. The main indications for plates are (1) fractures at either end of the femoral shaft, especially those with extensions into the supracondylar or pertrochanteric areas, (2) a shaft fracture in a growing child, and (3) a fracture with a vascular injury which requires repair (Figure 29.24).

Intramedullary nailing Intramedullary nailing is the method of choice for most femoral shaft fractures. However, it should not be attempted unless the appropriate facilities and expertise are available. The basic implant system consists of an intramedullary nail (in a range of sizes) which is perforated near each end so that locking screws can be inserted transversely at the proximal and distal ends; this controls rotation and length, and ensures stability even for subtrochanteric and distal third fractures (Figure 29.25).

These important details should be remembered when using locked intramedullary nails:

1. Reamed nails have a lower need for revision surgery when compared to unreamed nails.
2. Select a nail that is approximately the size of the medullary isthmus so that it fills the canal reasonably well (after reaming) and adds to stability – small diameter nails are quicker to insert but more frequently lead to the need for revision surgery.
3. Consider alternative means of fracture fixation if the isthmus is so narrow that a large amount of canal reaming will have to be done in order to fit the smallest diameter nail available.

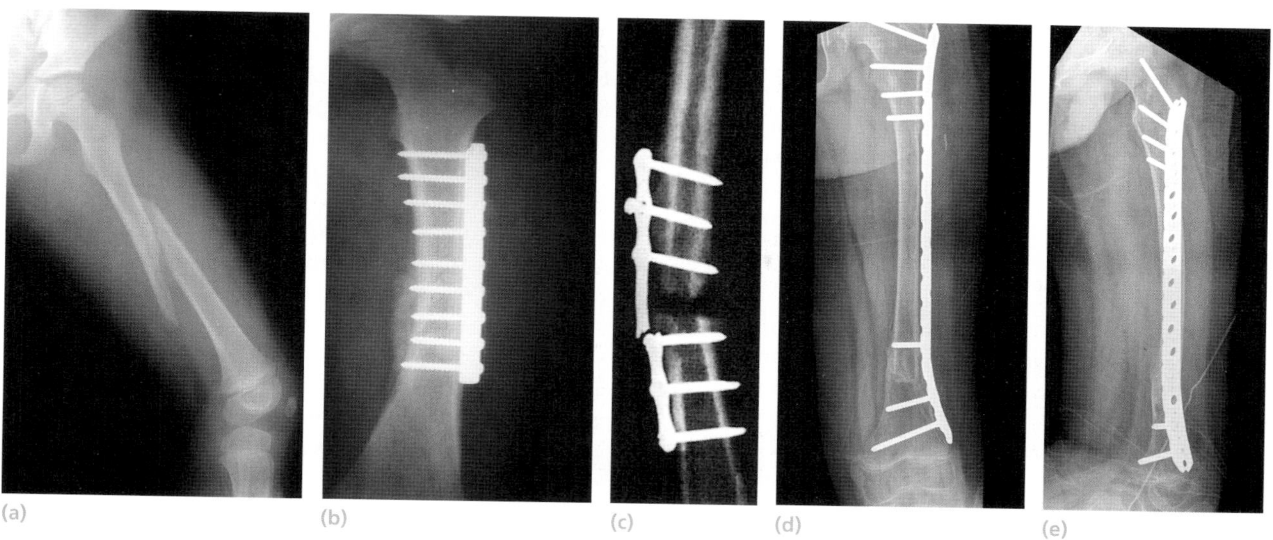

(a) (b) (c) (d) (e)

29.24 Plate fixation – past and present (a,b) Plate fixation was popular in the past, but it fell out of favour because of the high complication rate (c). Modern techniques of minimally invasive plate osteosynthesis (d,e) have shown that it still has place in the treatment of certain types of femoral shaft fracture.

4. Use a nail of sufficient length to fully span the canal.
5. Antegrade insertion (through either the piriformis fossa or the tip of the greater trochanter, depending on the design of nail) or retrograde insertion (through the intercondylar notch distally) are equally suitable techniques to use; there is a small incidence of hip and thigh pain with antegrade nails, whereas there is a small problem with knee pain with retrograde nails. Retrograde insertion of intramedullary nails is particularly useful for: obese patients; when there are bilateral femoral shaft fractures (as the procedure can be performed without the need for a fracture table and the added time for setting up for each side); when there is a tibial shaft fracture on the same side; and if there is a femoral neck fracture more proximally, as screws can be inserted to hold this fracture without being impeded by the nail.

Stability is improved by using interlocking screws; all locking holes in the nail should be used. Often there is enough shared stability between the nail and fracture ends to allow some weightbearing early on. The fracture usually heals within 20 weeks and the complication rate is low; sometimes malunion (more likely malrotation) or delayed union (from leaving the fracture site over-distracted) occurs.

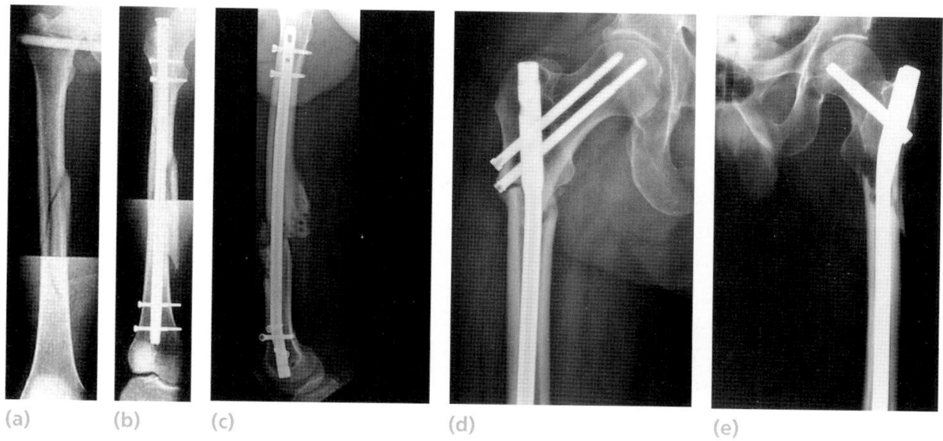

(a) (b) (c) (d) (e)

29.25 Intramedullary nailing Nowadays this is the commonest way of treating femoral shaft fractures. Ideally a range of designs to suit different types of fracture should be available. (a,b) Antegrade nailing with insertion of the nail through the pyriform fossa and transverse locking screws proximally and distally. (c) Retrograde nailing with insertion of the nail through the intercondylar notch at the knee – useful for obese patients and those with bilateral femoral fractures. (d,e) Proximal locking can be achieved in other ways e.g. by using parallel screws or a sliding hip screw.

Open medullary nailing is a feasible alternative where facilities for closed nailing are lacking. A limited lateral exposure of the femur is made; the fracture is reduced and a guidewire is passed between the main proximal and distal fragments. A small exposure to achieve reduction does not significantly affect the risk of complications or fracture healing as compared to 'closed' nailing.

External fixation The main indications for external fixation are (1) treatment of severe open injuries; (2) management of patients with multiple injuries where there is a need to reduce operating time and prevent the 'second hit'; and (3) the need to deal with severe bone loss by the technique of bone transport. External fixation is also useful for (4) treating femoral fractures in adolescents (Figure 29.26).

Like closed intramedullary nailing, it has the advantage of not exposing the fracture site and small amounts of axial movement can be applied to the bone by allowing a telescoping action in the fixator body (with some designs of external fixator). As the callus increases in volume and quality, the fixator can be adjusted to increase stress transfer to the fracture site, thus promoting quicker consolidation. However, there are still problems with pin-site infection, pin loosening and (if the half-pins are applied close to joints) limitation of movement due to interference with sliding structures.

The patient is allowed up as soon as he or she is comfortable and knee movement exercises are encouraged to prevent tethering by the half pins. Partial weightbearing is usually possible immediately but this will depend on the x-ray appearance of callus – this may take some time (more than 6 weeks) if the fixator is a rigid device. Most femoral shaft fractures will unite in under 5 months but some take longer if the fracture is badly comminuted or contact between fracture ends is poor.

Treatment of open fractures

Open femoral fractures should be carefully assessed for (1) skin loss; (2) wound contamination; (3) muscle ischaemia; and (4) injury to vessels and nerves.

The immediate treatment is similar to that of closed fractures; in addition, the patient is started on intravenous antibiotics. The wound will need cleansing: it should be extended to give unhindered access, contaminated areas and dead tissue must be excised and the entire area should be washed thoroughly.

Stabilization of open femoral shaft fractures is best achieved with locked intramedullary nails unless there is heavy contamination or bone loss – in which case external fixation (if necessary with the capacity to deal with bone loss through distraction osteogenesis) is preferable.

Complex injuries

FRACTURES ASSOCIATED WITH VASCULAR INJURY

Warning signs of an associated vascular injury are (1) excessive bleeding or haematoma formation; and (2) paraesthesia, pallor or pulselessness in the leg and foot. *Do not accept 'arterial spasm' as a cause of absent pulses; the fracture level on x-ray will indicate the region of arterial damage and arteriography may only delay surgery to re-establish perfusion.* Most femoral fractures with vascular injuries will have had warm ischaemia times greater than 2–3 hours by the time the patient arrives in the operating theatre; when this exceeds 4–6 hours, salvage may not be possible and the risk of amputation rises. This means that diagnosis must be prompt and re-establishing perfusion a priority; fracture stabilization is secondary.

A recommended sequence for treatment, particularly if the warm ischaemia time is approaching the salvage threshold, is (a) *to create a shunt* from the femoral vessels in the groin to beyond the point of

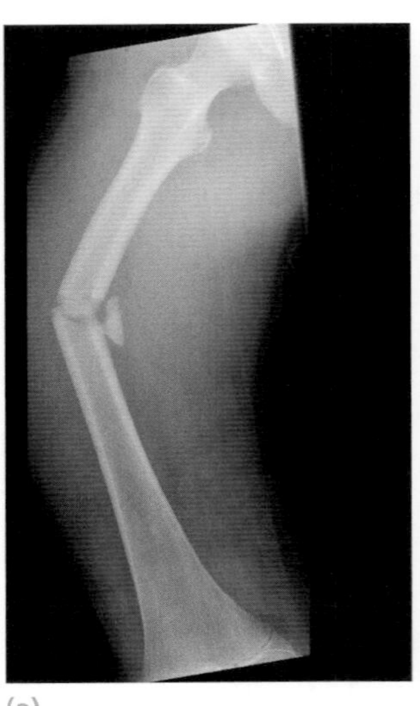
(a)

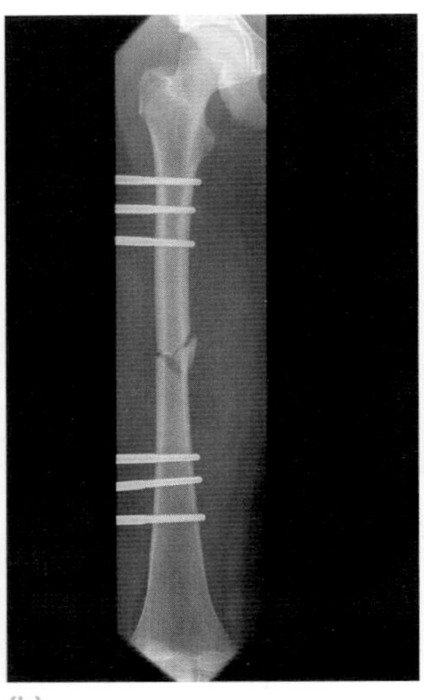
(b)

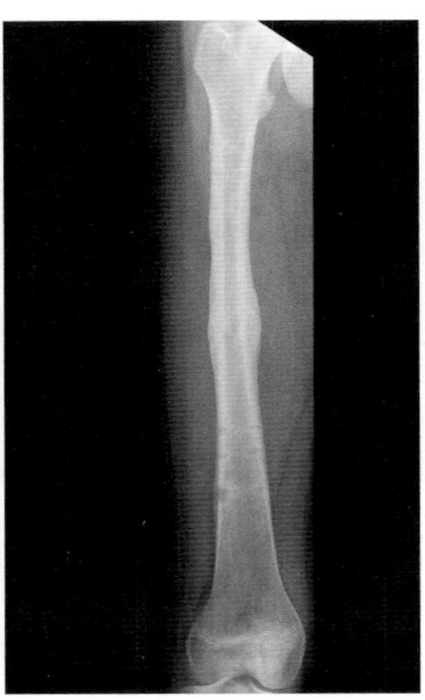
(c)

29.26 External fixation for femoral shaft fractures in older children (a–c) External fixation is an option for treating femoral shaft fractures in adolescents. Elastic stable intramedullary nails shown in Fig 29.31 may not be strong enough for this heavier group of teenagers.

injury using plastic catheters; (b) *to stabilize the fracture* (usually by plating or external fixation) and then (c) *to carry out definitive vascular repair*. This sequence establishes blood flow quickly and permits fracture fixation and vascular repair to be carried out without pressure of time.

FRACTURE ASSOCIATED WITH KNEE INJURY

Femoral fractures are frequently accompanied by injury to the ligaments of the knee. Direct blows to the knee from the dashboard of a car in an accident will damage knee ligaments as well as break the femoral shaft and femoral neck – this triad of problems should be recognized. With attention focused on the femur, the knee injury is easily overlooked, only to re-emerge as a persistent complaint weeks or months later. As soon as the fracture has been stabilized, the knee should be carefully examined and any associated abnormality treated.

'FLOATING KNEE'

Ipsilateral fractures of the femur and tibia may leave the knee joint 'floating'. This is a very serious situation, and other injuries are often present. Both fractures will need immediate stabilization – an anterior approach to the knee joint will allow both fractures to be stabilized by intramedullary nails – retrograde for the femur and antegrade for the tibia. It is usual to fix the femur first.

COMBINED NECK AND SHAFT FRACTURES

This is dealt with on page 850. The most important thing is diagnosis: always examine the hip and obtain an x-ray of the pelvis. Both sites must be stabilized, first the femoral neck and then the femur. Parallel screw fixation of the femoral neck followed by retrograde femoral nailing is a useful way to treat this problem.

PATHOLOGICAL FRACTURES

Fractures through metastatic lesions should be fixed by intramedullary nailing. Provided the patient is fit enough to tolerate the operation, a short life expectancy is not a contraindication. 'Prophylactic fixation' is also indicated if a lytic lesion is (a) greater than half the diameter of the bone; (b) longer than 3 cm on any view, or (c) painful, irrespective of its size.

Paget's disease, fibrous dysplasia or rickets may present a problem. The femur is likely to be bowed and, in the case of Paget's disease, abnormally hard. An osteotomy to straighten the femur may be necessary to allow a nail to be inserted fully (Figure 29.27).

PERIPROSTHETIC FRACTURES

Femoral shaft fractures around a hip implant are uncommon; they may happen during primary hip surgery when reaming or preparing the medullary canal, or when forcing in an over-sized uncemented prosthesis, or during revision surgery while extracting cement or attempting to dislocate the hip if the soft tissue release has been insufficient. Sometimes the fracture occurs much later, and there are usually x-ray signs of osteolysis or implant loosening suggesting a reason for bone weakness.

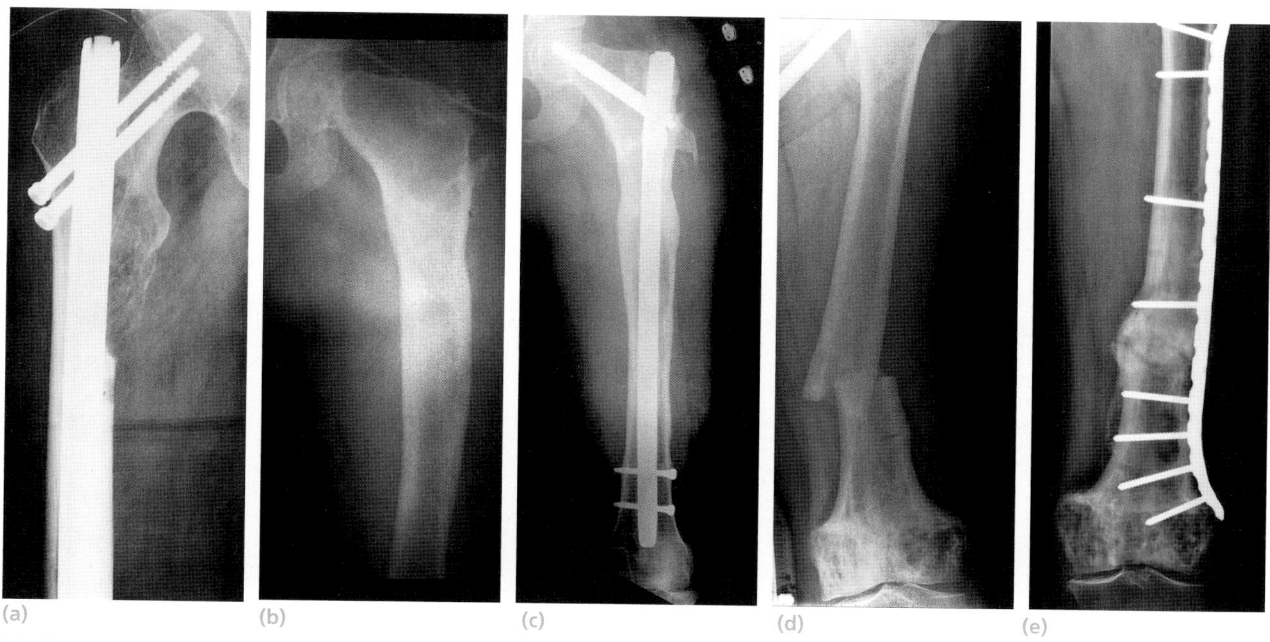

(a) (b) (c) (d) (e)

29.27 Pathological fractures – internal fixation (a) Metastatic tumour, nailed before it actually causes a fracture. (b) Fibrous dysplasia with a stress fracture; (c) nailing provided the opportunity to correct the deformity. (d,e) Paget's disease, with a fracture; in this case (because of its site) treated by fixation with a plate and screws.

If the prosthesis is worn or loose, it should be removed and replaced by one with a long stem, thereby treating both problems. If the primary implant is neither loose nor worn it can be left in place and the fracture treated by plate fixation with structural allografts bridging the fracture (Figure 29.28).

Complications of femoral shaft fractures

All the complications described in Chapter 23, with the exception of visceral injury and avascular necrosis, are encountered in femoral shaft fractures. The more common ones are as follows.

EARLY

Shock One or two litres of blood can be lost even with a closed fracture, and if the injury is bilateral shock may be severe. Prevention is better than cure; most patients will require a transfusion.

Fat embolism and ARDS Fracture through a large marrow-filled cavity almost inevitably results in small showers of fat emboli being swept to the lungs. This can usually be accommodated without serious consequences, but in some cases (and especially in those with multiple injuries and severe shock, or in patients with associated chest injuries) it results in progressive respiratory distress and multi-organ failure (adult respiratory distress syndrome). Blood gases should be measured if this is suspected and signs such as shortness of breath, restlessness or a rise in temperature or pulse rate should prompt a search for petechial haemorrhages over the upper body, axillae and conjunctivae. Treatment is supportive, with the emphasis on preventing hypoxia and maintaining blood volume.

Thromboembolism Prolonged traction in bed predisposes to thrombosis. Movement and exercise are important in preventing this, but high-risk patients should be given prophylactic anticoagulants as well. Vigilance is needed and full anticoagulant treatment is started immediately if thigh or pelvic vein thrombosis is diagnosed.

Infection In open injuries, and following internal fixation, there is always a risk of infection. Prophylactic antibiotics and careful attention to the principles of fracture surgery should keep the incidence below 2 per cent. If the bone does become infected, the patient should be treated as for an acute osteomyelitis. Antibiotic treatment may suppress the infection until the fracture unites, at which time the femoral nail can be removed and the canal reamed and washed out. However, if there is pus or a sequestrum, a more radical approach is called for: the wound is explored, all dead and infected tissue is removed and the nail as well; the

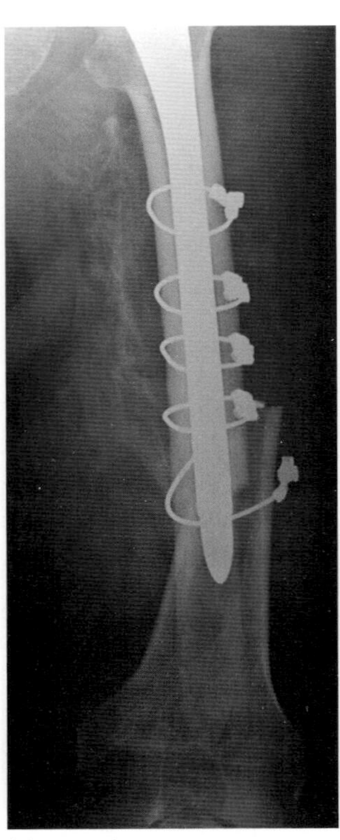
(a)

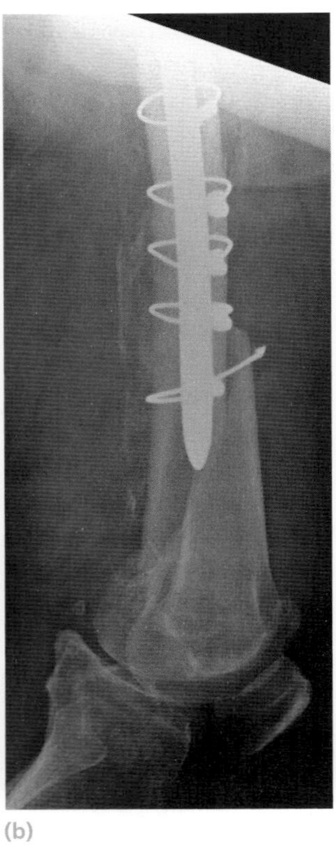
(b)

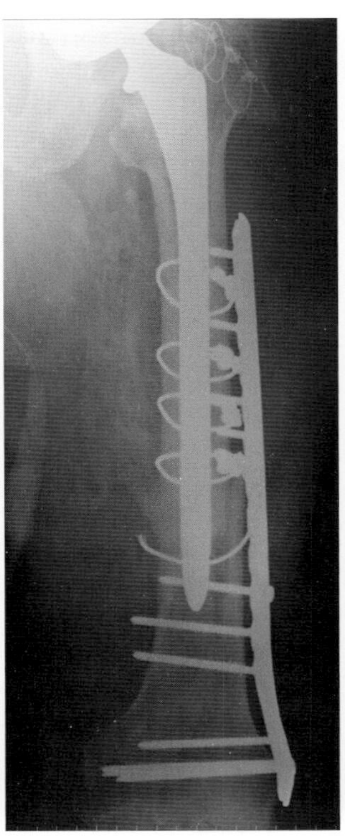
(c)

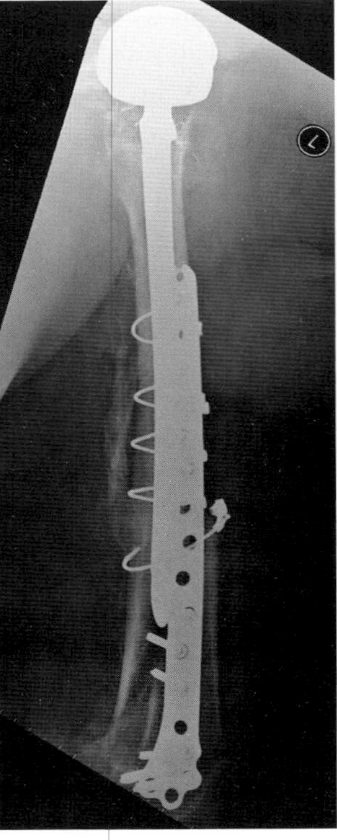
(d)

29.28 Periprosthetic fracture This patient had two successive fractures around his hip prosthesis. The first was held with cerclage wires **(a,b)**. As the prosthesis was secure in the femur the second fracture was fixed with a plate and screws **(c,d)**.

canal is reamed and washed out and the fracture is then stabilized by an external fixator. Replacement of the external fixator by another intramedullary nail can be risky, and much depends of the nature of the infecting organism (its sensitivity or resistance to antibiotics), the length of time during which the infection has been present and the quality of the surgical debridement.

The long-term management of chronic osteomyelitis is discussed in Chapter 2.

LATE

Delayed union and non-union The time-scale for declaring a delayed or non-union can vary with the type of injury and the method of treatment. If there is failure to progress by 6 months, as judged by serial x-rays, then intervention may be needed. A common practice is to remove locking screws from the intramedullary nail to enable the fracture to 'collapse' (*'dynamise'* in modern orthopaedic parlance). This can be successful in a small proportion of cases; more often it fails and results in pain as rotational control of the fracture is lost (the femur is often subject to torsional forces in walking). A better course is to remove the nail, ream the medullary canal and introduce a larger diameter nail – *exchange nailing*. Bone grafts should be added to the fracture site if there are gaps not closed at the revision procedure.

Malunion Fractures treated by traction and bracing often develop some deformity; no more than 15 degrees of angulation should be accepted (Figure 29.29). Even if the initial reduction was satisfactory, until the x-ray shows solid union the fracture is too insecure to permit weightbearing; the bone will bend and what previously seemed a satisfactory reduction may end up with lateral or anterior bowing.

Malunion is much less likely in those treated with static interlocked nails; yet it does still occur – especially malrotation – and this can be prevented only by meticulous intra-operative and post-operative assessment followed, where necessary, by immediate correction. Shortening is seldom a major problem unless there was bone loss; if it does occur, treatment will depend on the amount and its clinical impact – sometimes all that is needed is a built-up shoe.

Joint stiffness The knee is often affected after a femoral shaft fracture. The joint may be injured at the same time, or it stiffens due to soft-tissue adhesions during treatment; hence the importance of repeated evaluation and early physiotherapy.

Refracture and implant failure Fractures which heal with abundant callus are unlikely to recur. By contrast, in those treated by internal fixation, callus formation is often slow and meagre. With delayed union or non-

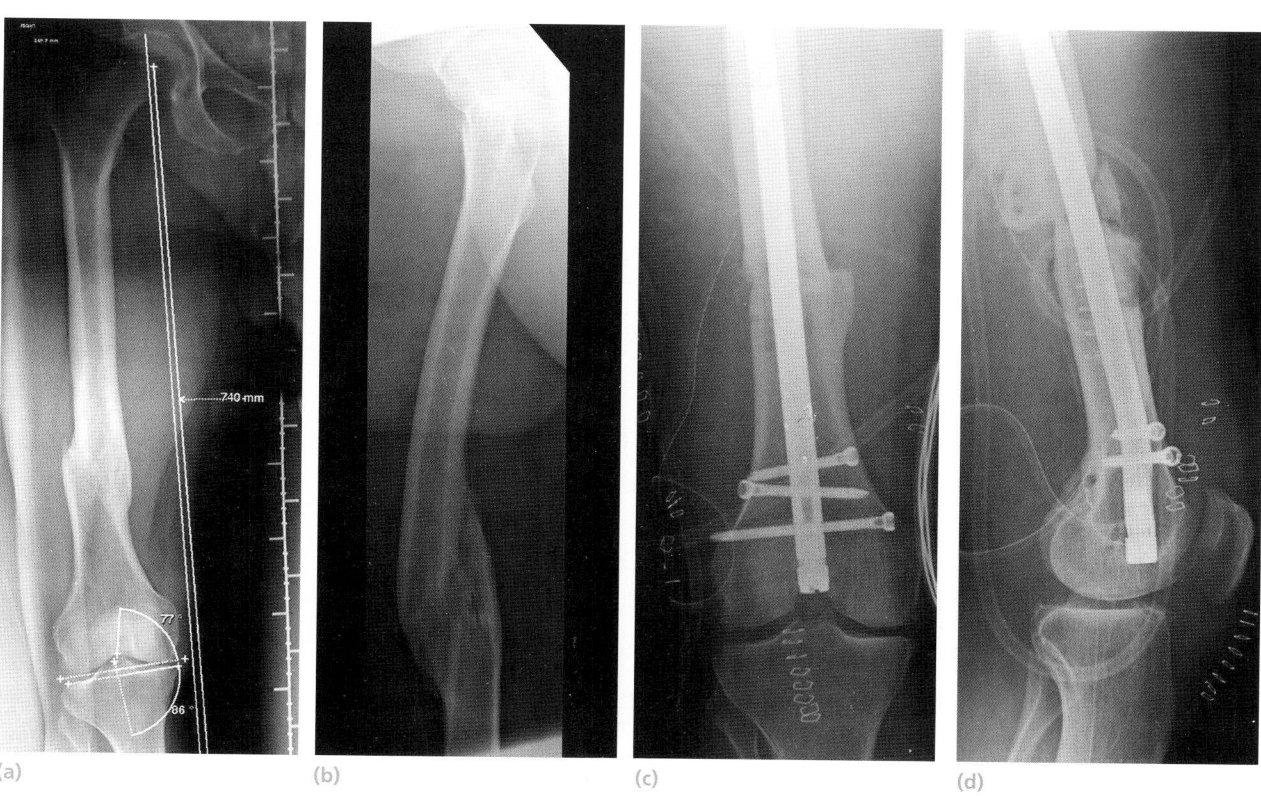

(a) (b) (c) (d)

29.29 Malalignment after treatment Treatment of femoral shaft fractures by traction can produce good results but, in some, a malunion can lead to symptoms. In this patient (a,b) the varus deformity produced knee symptoms from overloading of the medial compartment; this was relieved by corrective osteotomy and intramedullary nailing (c,d).

union, the integrity of the femur may be almost wholly dependent on the implant and sooner or later it will fail. If a comminuted fracture is plated, bone grafts should be added and weightbearing delayed so as to protect the plate from reaching its fatigue limit too soon. Intramedullary nails are less prone to break. However, sometimes they do, especially with a slow-healing fracture of the lower third and a static locked nail; the break usually occurs through the screw-hole closest to the fracture. Treatment consists of replacing the nail and adding bone grafts. In resistant cases, the fracture site may need excising (as viability of the bone ends is poor) followed by distraction osteogenesis which simultaneously stabilizes the limb and deals with the length discrepancy (Figure 29.30).

FEMORAL SHAFT FRACTURES IN CHILDREN

Mechanism

Fractures of the femur are quite common in older children and are usually due to *direct violence* (e.g. a road accident) or a *fall* from a height. However, in children under 2 years of age the commonest cause is child abuse; if there are several fractures in different stages of healing, this is very suspicious.

Pathological fractures are common in generalized disorders such as spina bifida and osteogenesis imperfecta, and with local bone lesions (e.g. a benign cyst or tumour).

Treatment

The principles of treatment in children are the same as in adults but it should be emphasized that in young children open treatment is rarely necessary. The choice of closed method depends largely on the age and weight of the child. As children get older (and larger), fractures take longer to heal and conservative treatment is more likely to result in problems associated with long hospitalization and a greater risk of malunion (Poolman, Kocher et al. 2006). Coupled to this is the cost of protracted bed occupancy. Consequently there has been a trend towards treating femoral shaft fractures in older children by operation, but the argument is flawed if this is based on cost alone – many of these children will have to return for implant removal. Perhaps it is the risk of malunion, particularly in unstable fracture patterns, that renders

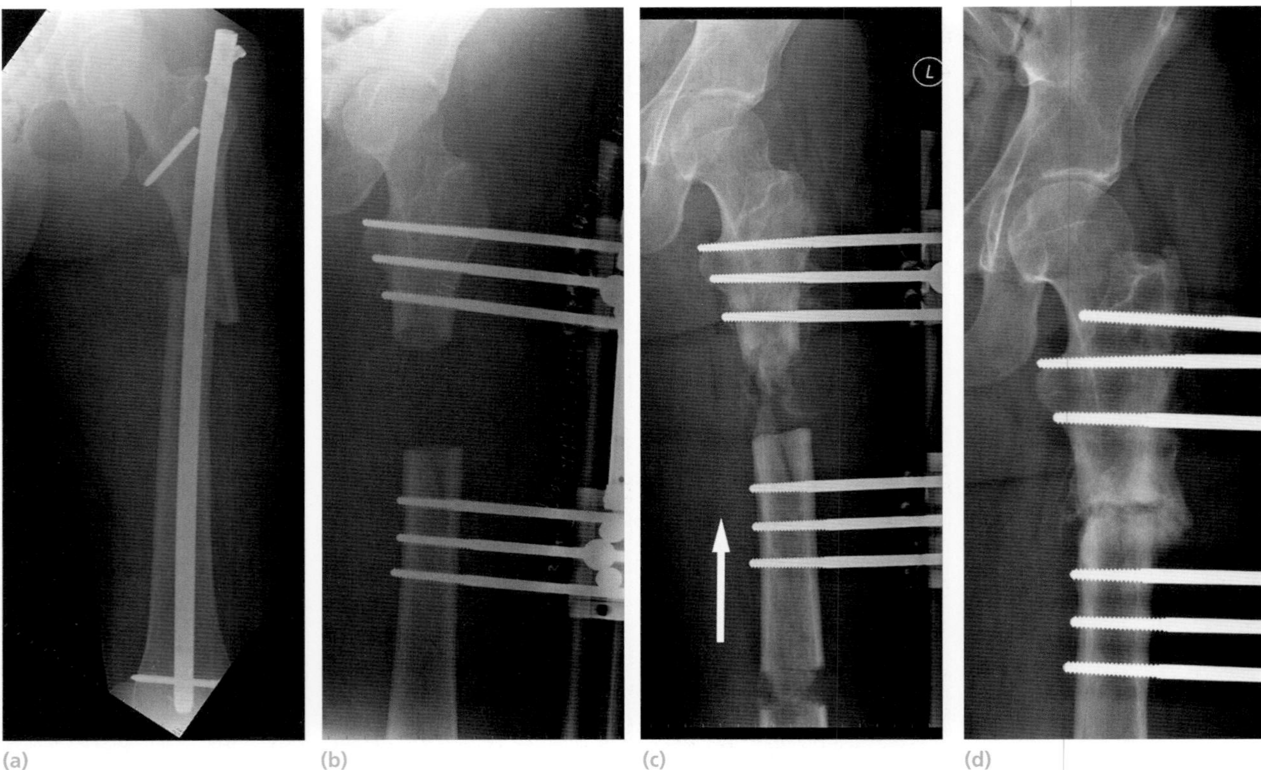

29.30 Implant failure and non-union (a) This was an open injury with poor vascularity of the fracture ends. It was fixed with an intramedullary nail in the hope that it might unite. It didn't, and one of the proximal screws broke. The fracture ends were excised; an external fixator was applied (b); and an osteotomy was performed lower down (c); then the fracture ends were brought together with distraction osteogenesis at the osteotomy site. The fracture united (d).

surgery a better option for older children and adolescents.

Traction and casts *Infants* need no more than a few days in balanced traction, followed by a spica cast for another 3–4 weeks. Angulation of up to 30 degrees can be accepted, as the bone remodels quite remarkably with growth. Immediate spica casting has also found favour and this approach does not appear to increase the risk of complications.

Children between 2 and 10 years of age can be treated either with balanced traction for 2–3 weeks followed by a spica cast for another 4 weeks, or by early reduction and a spica cast from the outset. Shortening of 1–2 cm and angulation of up to 20 degrees are acceptable.

Teenagers require somewhat longer (4–6 weeks) in balanced traction, and those aged over 15 (or even younger adolescents if they are large and muscular) may need skeletal traction. Once the fracture feels firm, traction is exchanged for either a spica cast (in the case of upper third and mid-shaft fractures) or a cast-brace (for lower third fractures), which is retained for a further 6 weeks. The position should be checked every few weeks; the limit of acceptable angulation in this age group is 15 degrees in the anteroposterior x-ray and 25 degrees in the lateral.

If a satisfactory reduction cannot be achieved by traction, internal (plates or flexible intramedullary nails) or external fixation is justified. This applies to older children and those with multiple injuries.

Operative treatment This is growing in popularity as there is: (1) a shorter in-patient stay (and for the child, a quick return home); (2) a lower incidence of malunion. Against this is the added risk of surgery, taking into account that many such fractures have good results when treated non-operatively. The tendency to adopt this approach in older children and adolescents may be justified. Surgical options include fixation with flexible intramedullary nails or trochanteric entry-point rigid nails with interlocking screws (neither of which damages the physes), plates inserted by the *MIPO* technique and external fixation (Figure 29.31).

Complications

Shortening Overlapping and comminution of the bone fragments may shorten the femur. However, anything up to 2 cm is quite acceptable in young children; indeed, some surgeons regard this as an advantage because there is a tendency for the fractured bone to grow faster for up to 2 years after the injury. This may be related to stimulation of the physes

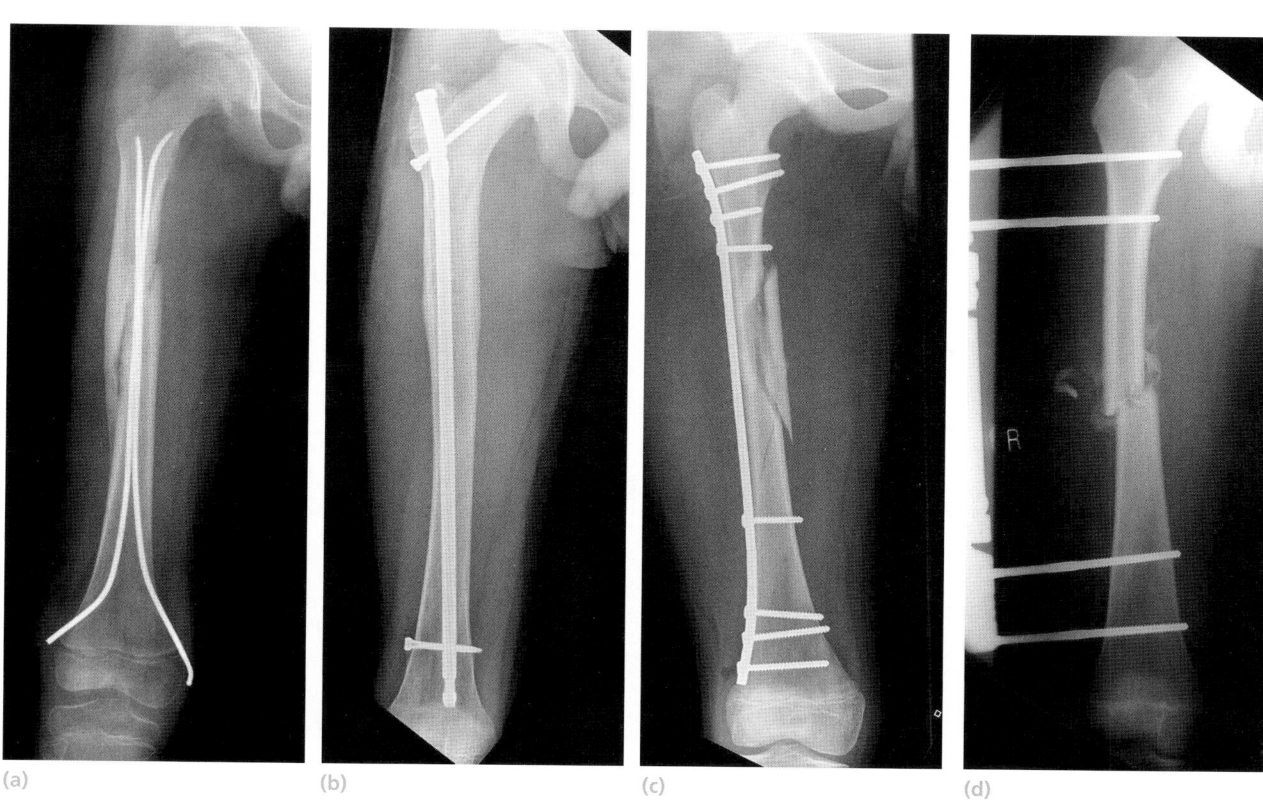

(a) (b) (c) (d)

29.31 Fixation techniques for femoral shaft fractures in children Non-operative treatment is safest for children. If surgery is indicated, options include: (a) flexible nailing; (b) trochanteric entry-point rigid nails; (c) plates and screws inserted by the minimally invasive percutaneous osteosynthesis (MIPO) technique and, (d) external fixation.

derived from the increased blood flow that accompanies fracture healing. Unfortunately, the effect on growth is unpredictable.

Malunion Angulation can usually be tolerated within the limits mentioned above. However, the fact that bone modelling is excellent in children is no excuse for casual management; bone may be forgiving but parents are not! Certainly rotational malunion is not corrected by growth or remodelling. It is probably wise to observe a malunited fracture for 2 years before offering corrective osteotomy.

SUPRACONDYLAR FRACTURES OF THE FEMUR

Supracondylar fractures of the femur are encountered (a) in young adults, usually as a result of high energy trauma, and (b) in elderly, osteoporotic individuals.

Mechanism and pathological anatomy

Direct violence is the usual cause. The fracture line is just above the condyles, but may extend between them. In the worst cases the fracture is severely comminuted. A useful classification is from the AO group: *type A fractures* have no articular splits and are truly 'supracondylar'; *type B fractures* are simply shear fractures of one of the condyles; and *type C fractures* have supracondylar and intercondylar fissures (Figure 29.32). Gastrocnemius, arising from the posterior surface of the distal femur, will tend to pull the distal segment into extension, thus risking injury to the popliteal artery.

Clinical features

The knee is swollen because of a haemarthrosis – this can be severe enough to cause blistering later. Movement is too painful to be attempted. The tibial pulses should always be checked to ensure the popliteal artery was not injured in the fracture.

X-RAY The entire femur should be x-rayed so as not to miss a proximal fracture or dislocated hip. The supracondylar fracture pattern will vary. Of importance are: (a) whether there is a fracture into the joint and if it is comminuted; (b) the size of the distal segment; and (c) whether the bone is osteoporotic. These factors influence the type of internal fixation required, if that is the chosen mode of treatment.

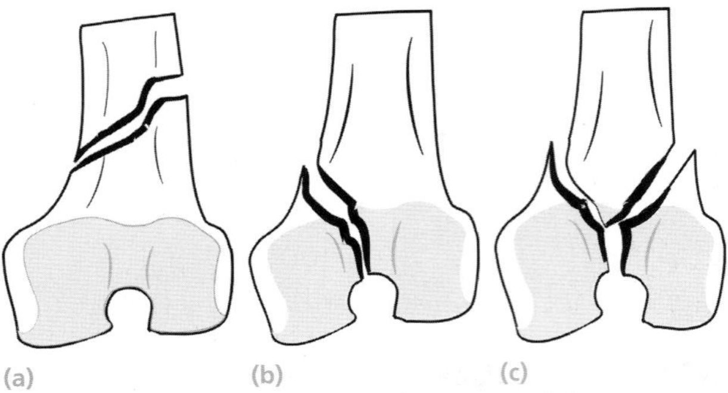

(a) (b) (c)

29.32 The AO classification of supracondylar fractures (a) Type A fractures do not involve the joint surface; (b) type B fractures involve the joint surface (one condyle) but leave the supracondylar region intact; (c) type C fractures have supracondylar and condylar components.

Treatment

Non-operative If the fracture is only slightly displaced and extra-articular, or if it reduces easily with the knee in flexion, it can be treated quite satisfactorily by traction through the proximal tibia; the limb is cradled on a Thomas' splint with a knee flexion piece and movements are encouraged. If the distal fragment is displaced by gastrocnemius pull, a second pin above the knee, and vertical traction, will correct this. At 4–6 weeks, when the fracture is beginning to unite, traction can be replaced by a cast-brace and the patient allowed up and partially weightbearing with crutches. Non-operative treatment should be considered as an option if the patient is young or the facilities and skill to treat by internal fixation are absent. Elderly patients tend not do as well with the 6 weeks of enforced recumbency.

Surgery Operative treatment with internal fixation can enable accurate fracture reduction, especially of the joint surface, and early movement. If the necessary facilities and skill are available, this is the treatment of choice. For the elderly, early mobilization is so important that internal fixation is almost obligatory. Sometimes the hold on osteoporotic bone is poor (despite modern implant designs) or the patient may be old and frail, making early mobilization difficult or risky, but nursing in bed is made easier and knee movements can be started sooner.

Several different devices are available:

1. *Locked intramedullary nails* which are introduced retrograde through the intercondylar notch – these are suitable for the type A and simpler type C fractures
2. *Plates that are applied to the lateral surface of the femur*: traditional angled blade-plates or 95 degree condylar screw-plates. They are suitable for type A and the simpler type C fractures. For severely comminuted type C fractures, the newer plate designs with locking screws appear to offer an advantage over other implants; they provide adequate stability, even in the presence of osteoporotic bone, but (as with compression plates) unprotected weightbearing is best avoided until union is assured.

3. *Simple lag screws* – these suffice for type B fractures and are inserted in parallel, with the screw heads buried within the articular cartilage to avoid abrading the opposing joint surface. They are also used to hold the femoral condyles together in type C fractures before intramedullary nails or lateral plates are used to hold the main supracondylar break (Figure 29.33).

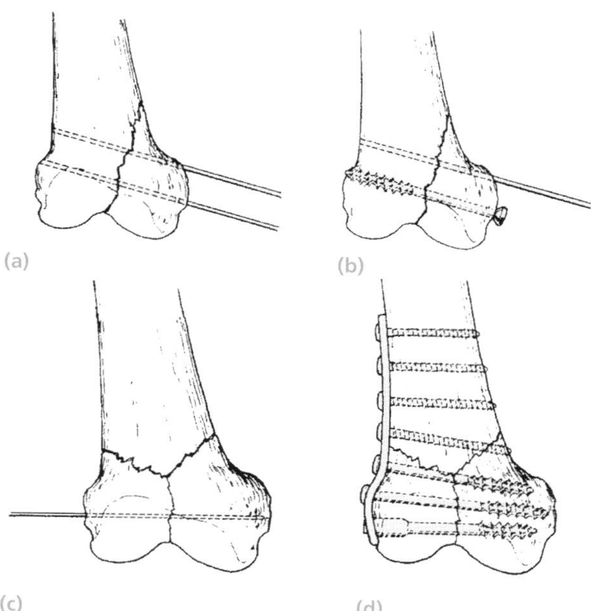

29.33 Femoral condyle fractures – treatment (a) A single condylar fracture can be reduced open and held with Kirschner wires preparatory to (b) inserting compression screws. (c) T- or Y-shaped fractures are best fixed with a dynamic condylar screw and plate (d).

Knee movements are started soon after operation, if wound healing allows. This limits adhesions forming within the knee joint.

Complications

EARLY

Arterial damage There is a small but definite risk of arterial damage and distal ischaemia. Careful assessment of the leg and peripheral pulses is essential, even if the x-ray shows only minimal displacement.

LATE

Joint stiffness Knee stiffness – probably due to scarring from the injury and the operation – is almost inevitable. A long period of exercise is needed in all cases, and even then full movement is rarely regained. For marked stiffness, arthroscopic division of adhesions in the joint or even a quadricepsplasty may be needed.

Malunion Internal fixation of these fractures is difficult and malunion – usually varus and recurvatum – is not uncommon. Corrective osteotomy may be needed for patients who are still physically active.

Non-union Modern surgical techniques of internal fixation recognize the importance of minimizing damage to the soft tissues around the fracture; where possible, only those parts that are essential for fracture reduction are exposed. The knee joint may need to be opened for reduction of articular fragments but the metaphyseal area is left untouched in order to preserve its vitality. If these precautions are taken, non-union is unlikely. If non-union does occur, autogenous bone grafts and a revision of internal fix-

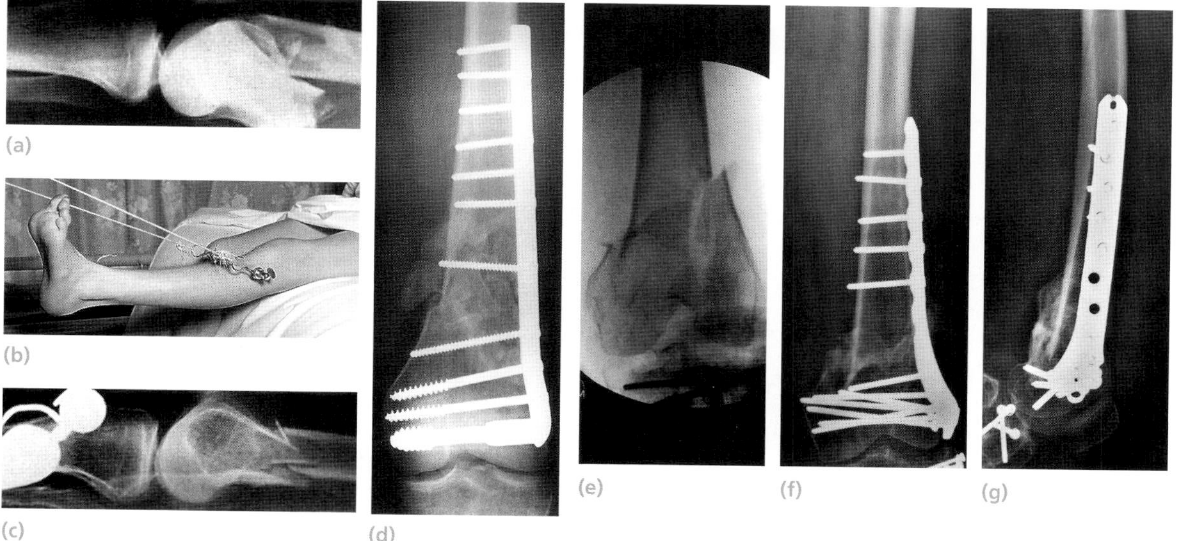

29.34 Supracondylar fractures (a–c) These fractures can sometimes be treated successfully by traction through the upper tibia. (d–g) If the bone is not too osteoporotic, internal fixation is often preferable and the patient can get out of bed sooner: a dynamic condylar screw and plate for a Type A fracture (d) and a combination of lag screws and a lateral side plate for more complex fracture patterns (e,f,g).

ation will be needed – particularly if there are signs that the fixation is working loose or has failed.

Knee stiffness is another threat. Unless great care is exercised during mobilization, the ultimate range of movement at the knee may be less than that at the fracture!

FRACTURE-SEPARATION OF DISTAL FEMORAL EPIPHYSIS

In the childhood or adolescent equivalent of a supracondylar fracture, the lower femoral epiphysis may be displaced – either to one side (usually laterally) by forced angulation of the straight knee or forwards by a hyperextension injury. Although not nearly as common as physeal fractures at the elbow or ankle, this injury is important because of its potential for causing abnormal growth and deformity of the knee.

The fracture is usually a Salter–Harris type 2 lesion – i.e. physeal separation with a large triangular metaphyseal bone fragment (Figure 29.35). Although this type of fracture usually has a good prognosis, asymmetrical growth arrest is not uncommon and the child may end up with a valgus or varus deformity. All grades of injury, but especially Salter–Harris types 3 and 4, may result in femoral shortening. Nearly 70 per cent of the femur's length is derived from the distal physis, so an early arrest can present a major problem.

Clinical features

The knee is swollen and perhaps deformed. The pulses in the foot should be palpated because, with forward displacement of the epiphysis, the popliteal artery may be obstructed by the lower femur.

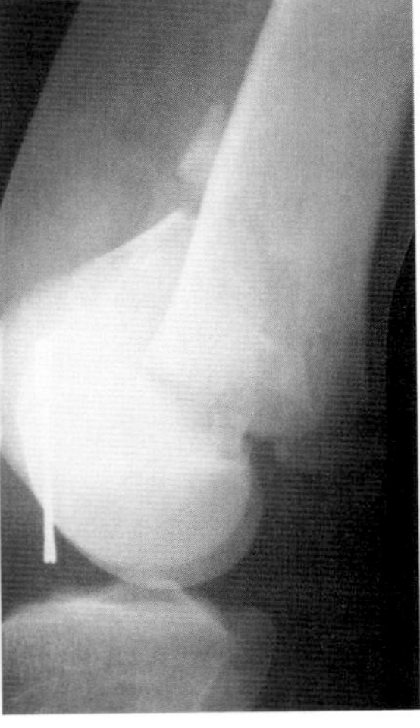

(a) (b)

29.35 Fracture-separation of the epiphysis These fractures are not difficult to reduce and can usually be held adequately in plaster, but they must be watched carefully for several weeks.

Treatment

The fracture can usually be perfectly reduced manually, but further x-ray checks will be needed over the next few weeks to ensure that reduction is maintained. Occasionally open reduction is needed; a flap of periosteum may be trapped in the fracture line. Salter–Harris types 3 and 4 should be accurately reduced and fixed. If there is a tendency to redisplacement, the fragments may be stabilized with percutaneous Kirschner wires or lag screws driven across the metaphyseal spike. The limb is immobilized in plaster and the patient is allowed partial weightbearing on crutches. The cast can be removed after 6–8 weeks and physiotherapy started.

Complications

EARLY

Vascular injury There is danger of gangrene unless the hyperextension injury is reduced without delay.

LATE

Physeal arrest Damage to the physis is not uncommon and residual deformity may require corrective osteotomy at the end of the growth period. Small areas of tethering across the growth plate can sometimes be successfully removed and normal growth restored. Shortening, if it is marked, can be treated by femoral lengthening.

REFERENCES AND FURTHER READING

Barnes R, Brown JT, Garden RS, *et al.* Subcapital fractures of the femur. A prospective review. *J Bone Joint Surg* 1976; **58B:** 2–24.

Bonnaire FA, Weber AT. The influence of haemarthrosis on the development of femoral head necrosis following intracapsular femoral neck fractures. *Injury* 2002; **33 Suppl 3:** C33–40.

Dimon JH III, Hughston JC. Unstable Intertrochanteric Fractures of the Hip. *J Bone Joint Surg* 1967; **49A:** 440–50.

Garden RS. Low angle fixation in fractures of the femoral neck. *J Bone Joint Surg* 1961; **43B:** 647–63.

Harper WM, Barnes MR, Gregg PJ. Femoral head blood flow in femoral neck fractures. An analysis using intraosseous pressure measurement. *J Bone Joint Surg* 1991; **73B:** 73–5.

Hughes LO, Beaty JH. Fractures of the head and neck of the femur in children. *J Bone Joint Surg* 1994; **76A:** 283–92.

Kaplan K, Miyamoto R, Levine BR, *et al*. Surgical Management of Hip Fractures: An Evidence-based Review of the Literature. II: Intertrochanteric Fractures. *J Am Acad Orthop Surg* 2008; **16(11):** 665–73.

Keating JF, Grant A, Masson M, *et al*. Randomized comparison of reduction and fixation, bipolar hemiarthroplasty, and total hip arthroplasty. Treatment of displaced intracapsular hip fractures in healthy older patients. *J Bone Joint Surg* 2006; **88A:** 249–60.

Kyle RF. Fractures of the Proximal Part of the Femur. *J Bone Joint Surg* 1994; **76A:** 924–50.

Masson M, Parker MJ, Fleischer S. Internal fixation versus arthroplasty for intracapsular proximal femoral fractures in adults. *Cochrane Database of Systematic Reviews* 2003; **(2):** CD001708.

Pape HC, van Griensven M, Rice J, *et al*. Major secondary surgery in blunt trauma patients and perioperative cytokine liberation: determination of the clinical relevance of biochemical markers. *J Trauma* 2001; **50(6):** 989–1000.

Pipkin G. Treatment of grade IV fracture dislocation of the hip. *J Bone Joint Surg* 1957; **39:** 1027–42.

Poolman RW, Kocher MS, Bhandari M. Pediatric femoral fractures: a systematic review of 2422 cases. *J Orthop Trauma* 2006; **20(9):** 648–54.

Shim SS. Circulatory and vascular changes in the hip following traumatic hip dislocation. *Clin Orthop Relat Res* 1979; **140:** 255–61.

Thompson VP, Epstein VP. Traumatic dislocation of the hip. *J Bone Joint Surg* 1951; **33A:** 746–78.

Tornetta P III, Mostafavi HR. Hip Dislocation: Current Treatment Regimens. *J Am Acad Orthop Surg* 1997; **5(1):** 27–36.

Winquist RA, Hansen ST Jnr, Clawson DK. Closed intramedullary nailing of femoral fractures. A report of five hundred and twenty cases. *J Bone Joint Surg* 1984; **66A:** 529–39.

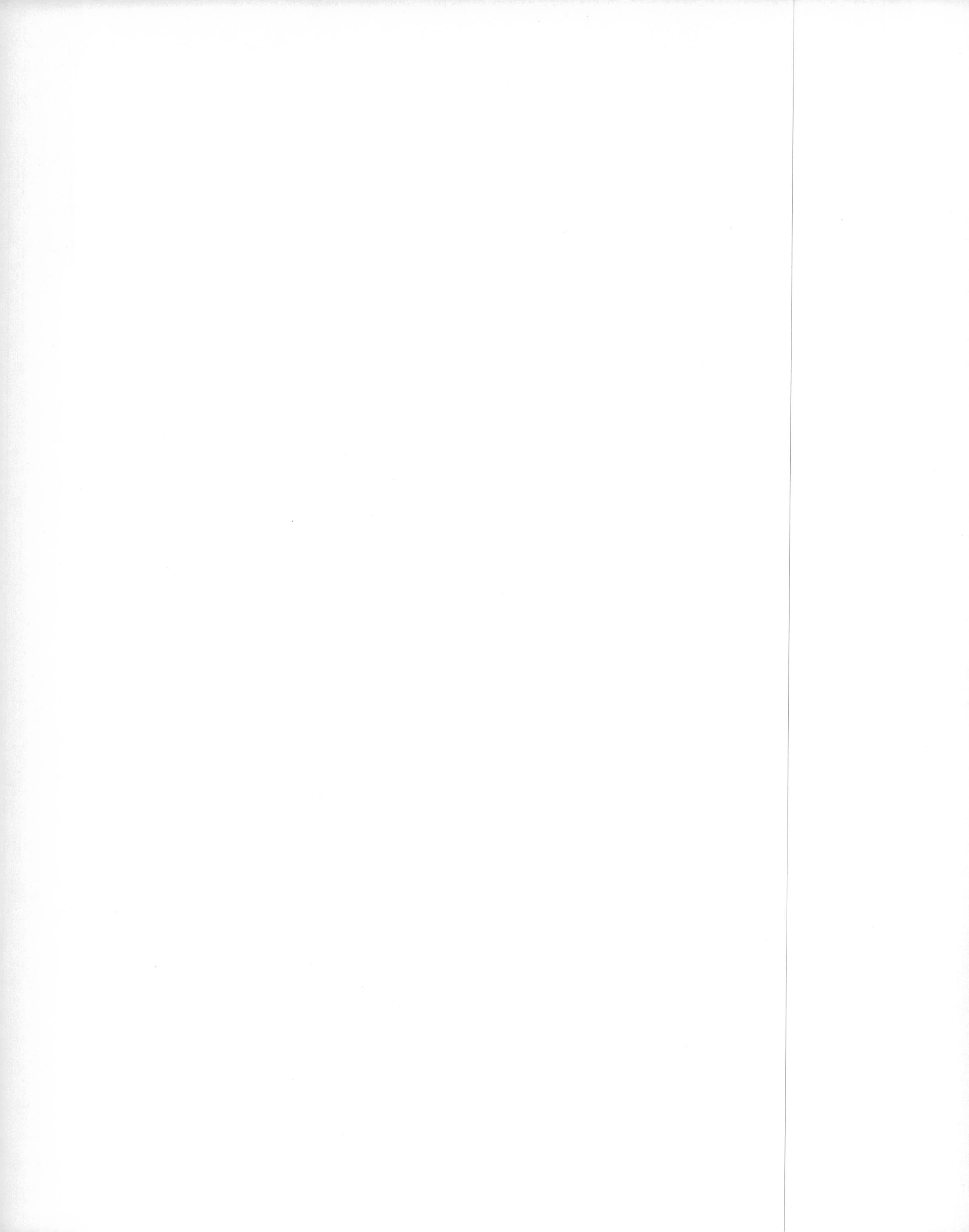

Injuries of the knee and leg 30

Selvadurai Nayagam

ACUTE KNEE LIGAMENT INJURIES

The bony structure of the knee joint is inherently unstable; were it not for the strong capsule, intra- and extra-articular ligaments and controlling muscles, the knee would not be able to function effectively as a mechanism for support, balance and thrust.

Valgus stresses are resisted by the superficial and deep layers of the medial collateral ligament (MCL), semimembranosus tendon and its expansions, the tough posteromedial part of the capsule (referred to as the posterior oblique ligament) as well as the cruciate ligaments (Fig. 30.1a).

Depending on the position of the knee, some will act as primary and others as secondary stabilizers. At 30 degrees of flexion, the MCL is the primary stabilizer.

The main checks to varus angulation are the iliotibial tract and the lateral collateral ligament (LCL). Structures forming the posterolateral corner of the knee also make an important contribution to stability; they comprise the popliteus tendon, the capsule and the arcuate ligament – a condensation of fibres lying posterior to the LCL and running from the fibula over popliteus tendon to the posterior capsule (Fig. 30.1b). The iliotibial band and LCL are the primary stabilizers to a varus stress between full extension and 30 degrees of flexion; however, as flexion increases, the LCL relaxes and the posterolateral structures come into play to provide additional stability.

The cruciate ligaments provide both anteroposterior and rotary stability; they also help to resist excessive valgus and varus angulation. Both cruciate ligaments have a double bundle structure and some fibres of each bundle are taut in all positions of the knee (Petersen and Zantop, 2007). The anterior cruciate has anteromedial and posterolateral bundles, whereas the posterior cruciate has anterolateral and posteromedial bundles. Anterior displacement of the tibia (as in the anterior drawer test) is resisted by the anteromedial bundle of the anterior cruciate ligament

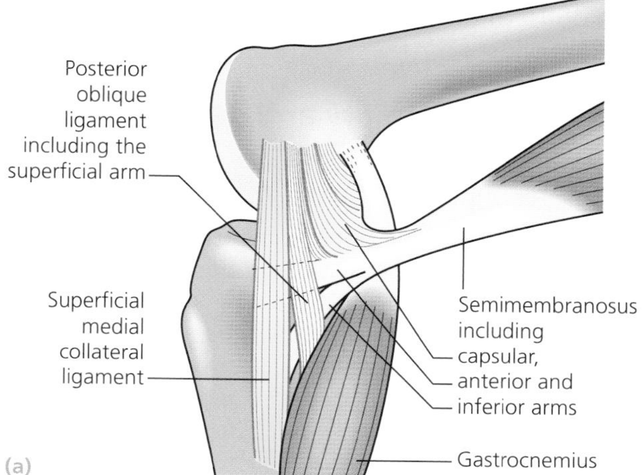

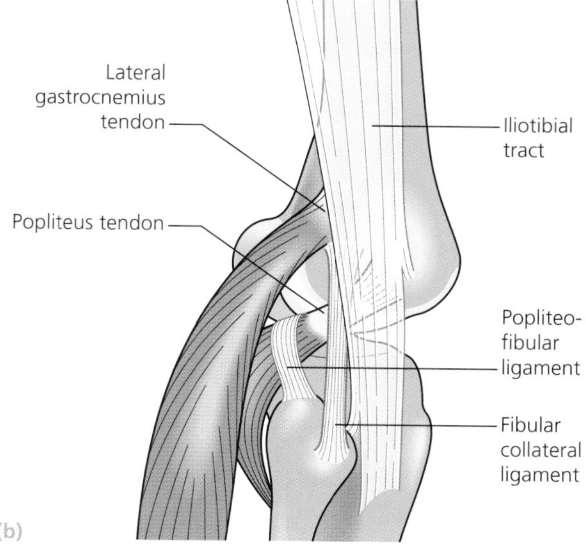

30.1 Extracapsular restraints to valgus and varus stresses on the knee (a) Restraints on valgus stresses: the deep and superficial parts of the medial collateral ligament, semimembranosus and the posterior oblique ligament. (b) Extracapsular restraints on varus stresses: lateral collateral ligament, popliteus tendon, popliteofibular ligament and the capsule.

(ACL) whilst the posterolateral part tightens as the knee extends. Posterior displacement is prevented by the posterior cruciate ligament (PCL), specifically by the anterolateral bundle when the knee is in near 90 degree flexion and by the posteromedial bundle when the knee is straight (Fig. 30.2).

Injuries of the knee ligaments are common, particularly in sporting pursuits but also in road accidents, where they may be associated with fractures or dislocations. They vary in severity from a simple sprain to complete rupture. It is important to recognize that these injuries are seldom 'unidirectional'; they often involve more than one structure and it is therefore useful to refer to them in functional terms (e.g. 'anteromedial instability') as well as anatomical terms (e.g. 'torn MCL and ACL').

Mechanism of injury and pathological anatomy

Most ligament injuries occur while the knee is bent, i.e. when the capsule and ligaments are relaxed and the femur is allowed to rotate on the tibia. The damaging force may be a straight thrust (e.g. a dashboard injury forcing the tibia backwards) or, more commonly, a combined rotation and thrust as in a football tackle. The medial structures are most often affected but if the injury involves a twist in addition to a valgus force, the ACL also may be damaged. This twisting force in a weightbearing knee often tears the medial meniscus, causing the well-recognized triad of MCL, ACL and medial meniscal injury described by O'Donoghue. A solitary MCL injury, if sufficiently severe, can be shown to cause the knee joint to 'open' on the medial side when the joint is flexed to 30 degrees a valgus stress is applied, but if this is still detectable when the knee is extended, then it is likely the expansions of the semimembranosus tendon, capsule and ACL are also damaged.

Forces that push the tibia into varus will damage the lateral structures, but these forces are relatively uncommon; as with medial injuries, the cruciate ligaments are at risk if there is a twisting component, and a clinically detectable opening on varus stressing in an extended knee suggests that there is, in addition to a rupture of the LCL, capsular and cruciate damage.

Cruciate ligament injuries occur in isolation or in combination with damage to other structures. The ACL is the more commonly affected. Solitary cruciate ligament injuries result in instability in the sagittal plane, i.e. the tibia can be pushed backwards or pulled forwards in relation to the femoral condyles. If there is accompanying damage to a collateral ligament or the capsule, then the direction of instability is often oblique and there may be a problem in controlling rotation. These oblique plane and rotatory instabilities are complex; in essence, one of the cruciate ligaments is ruptured and there is also laxity in one part of the capsule – this causes movement of the tibia on the femur, usually around an axis of the remaining intact capsule or other supporting ligament. Thus, in the more common anterolateral instability, where the ACL, lateral capsule and LCL are injured, the lateral plateau of the tibia can be made to sublux anteriorly when the tibia is rotated internally. If this is done with the knee fully extended whilst maintaining a valgus force, and the knee is then gradually flexed, a palpable reduction of this subluxation is felt at 20–30 degrees. This is the basis of the *pivot shift test*; it is thought the tibia rotates around the axis of an intact MCL.

The common rotational instability patterns are summarized in Table 30.1, showing the likely ligaments involved and the clinical tests for assessment.

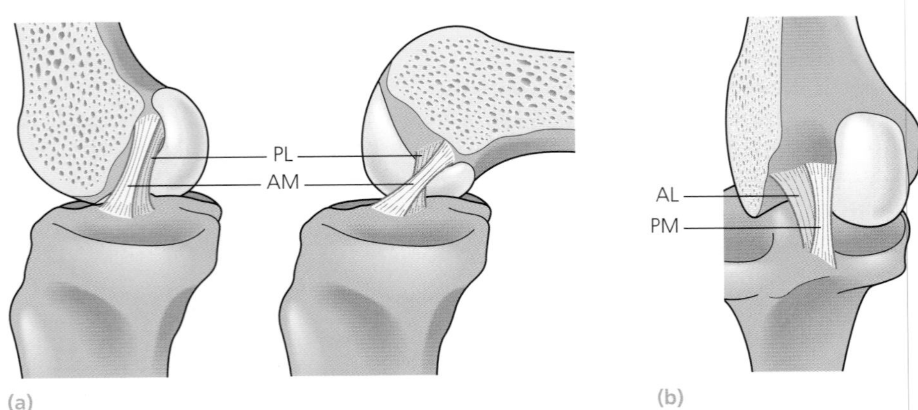

30.2 Dual-bundle structure of the anterior and posterior cruciate ligaments (a) The anteromedial (AM) bundle of an anterior cruciate ligament is taut in 90° of knee flexion whereas the posterolateral (PL) bundle tightens in extension. (b) In contrast, it is the anterolateral (AL) bundle of the posterior cruciate ligament that is tight in 90° flexion and the posteromedial (PM) bundle tightens in extension (and therefore resists hyperextension).

Table 30.1 Rotational instabilities of the knee

Type of instability	Test	Positive result	Probable structures damaged
Anterolateral rotatory instability	Perform an anterior drawer test but with the foot internally rotated 30 degrees	The tibia subluxes forward to an equal or greater extent as when the foot is in a neutral position	ACL LCL Lateral aspect of knee capsule
	Perform the pivot shift manoeuvre	The tibia is subluxed when the knee is extended and felt to reduce as it is gradually flexed	
Anteromedial rotatory instability	Perform an anterior drawer test but with the foot externally rotated 15 degrees	The tibia subluxes forward	ACL MCL Posteromedial aspect of knee capsule (including the posterior oblique ligament and expansions of semimembranosus
Posterolateral rotatory instability	Perform a reverse (external rotation) pivot shift manoeuvre	The tibia subluxes posteriorly in the extended knee but is felt to reduce as flexion is gradually increased	PCL Popliteus tendon Arcuate ligament
	Pick up the foot by grasping the medial forefoot	The knee hyperextends and tibia externally rotates. The tibia appears to be in varus	

ACL, anterior cruciate ligament; LCL, lateral collateral ligament, MCL, medial collateral ligament; PCL, posterior cruciate ligament.

Clinical features

The patient gives a history of a twisting or wrenching injury and may even claim to have heard a 'pop' as the tissues snapped. The knee is painful and (usually) swollen – and, in contrast to meniscal injury, the swelling appears almost immediately. Tenderness is most acute over the torn ligament, and stressing one or other side of the joint may produce excruciating pain. The knee may be too painful to permit deep palpation or much movement.

For all the apparent consistency, the findings can be somewhat perverse: thus, with a complete tear the patient may have little or no pain, whereas with a partial tear the knee is painful. Swelling also is worse with partial tears, because haemorrhage remains confined within the joint; with complete tears the ruptured capsule permits leakage and diffusion. With a partial tear attempted movement is always painful; the abnormal movement of a complete tear is often painless or prevented by spasm.

Abrasions suggest the site of impact, but bruising is more important and indicates the site of damage. The doughy feel of a haemarthrosis distinguishes ligament injuries from the fluctuant feel of the synovial effusion of a meniscus injury. Tenderness localizes the lesion, but the sharply defined tender spot of a partial tear (usually medial and 2.5 cm above the joint line) contrasts with the diffuse tenderness of a complete one. The entire limb should be examined for other injuries and for vascular or nerve damage.

The most important aspect of the examination is to test for joint stability. Partial tears permit no abnormal movement, but the attempt causes pain. Complete tears permit abnormal movement, which sometimes is almost painless. To distinguish between the two is critical because their treatment is different; *if there is doubt, examination under anaesthesia is mandatory.*

Sideways tilting (varus/valgus) is examined, first with the knee at 30 degree of flexion and then with the knee straight. Movement is compared with the normal side. If the knee angulates only in slight flexion, there is probably an isolated tear of the collateral ligaments; if it angulates in full extension, there is almost certainly rupture of the capsule and cruciate ligaments as well.

Anteroposterior stability is assessed first by placing the knees at 90 degrees with the feet resting on the couch and looking from the side for posterior sag of the proximal tibia; when present, this is a reliable sign of posterior cruciate damage. Next, the drawer test is carried out in the usual way; a positive drawer sign is diagnostic of a tear, but a negative test does not exclude one. The Lachman test is more reliable; anteroposterior glide is tested with the knee flexed 15–20 degrees. Rotational stability arising from acute injuries can usually be tested only under anaesthesia.

Imaging

Plain x-rays may show that the ligament has avulsed a small piece of bone:

- from the medial edge of the femur by the medial ligament
- from the fibula by the lateral ligament
- from the *tip* of the fibula, probably by a postero-lateral corner injury
- from the tibial spine by the anterior cruciate ligament
- from the back of the upper tibia by the posterior cruciate
- from the near edge of the lateral tibial condyle by the iliotibial tract or capsule (a *Segond fracture,* which is often associated with anterior cruciate ligament and meniscal injuries).

Stress films (if necessary under anaesthesia) show whether the joint hinges open on one side (Fig. 30.3).

Magnetic resonance imaging (*MRI*) is helpful in distinguishing partial from complete ligament tears. This may also reveal 'bone bruising', a hitherto poorly recognized source of pain.

Arthroscopy

With severe tears of the collateral ligaments and capsule, arthroscopy should not be attempted; fluid extravasation will hamper diagnosis and may complicate further procedures. The main indication for arthroscopy, which is usually conducted after capsular healing has occurred and knee motion recovered, is for reconstruction of cruciate ligament tears in those individuals who would benefit, and to deal with other internal injuries such as meniscal tears.

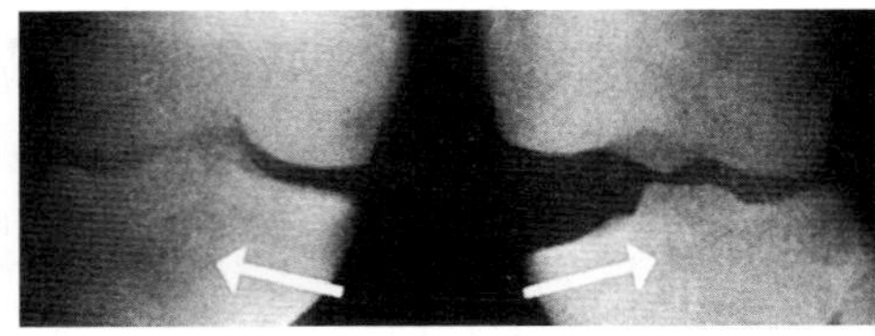

(a)

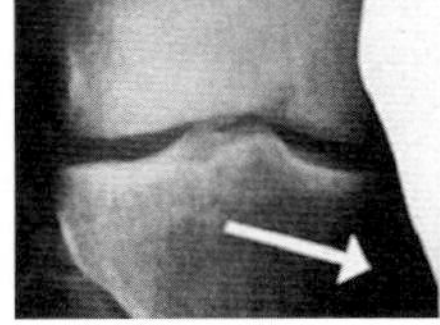
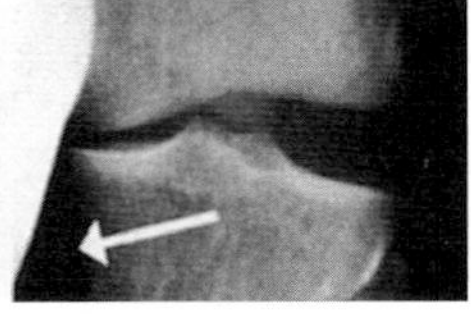

(b)

30.3 Stress x-rays Stress films show: **(a)** complete tear of medial ligament, left knee; **(b)** complete tear of lateral ligament. In both, the anterior cruciate also was torn.

Treatment

SPRAINS AND PARTIAL TEARS

The intact fibres splint the torn ones and spontaneous healing will occur. The hazard is adhesions, so active exercise is prescribed from the start, facilitated by aspirating a tense effusion, applying ice-packs to the knee and, sometimes, by injecting local anaesthetic into the tender area. Weightbearing is permitted but the knee is protected from rotational or angulatory strain by a heavily padded bandage or a functional brace. A complete plaster cast is unnecessary and disadvantageous; it inhibits movement and prevents weekly reassessment – an important precaution if the occasional error is to be avoided. With a dedicated exercise programme, the patient can usually return to sports training by 6–8 weeks.

COMPLETE TEARS

Isolated tears of the MCL, i.e. where the knee is stable in full extension, usually heal well enough to permit near-normal function. Operative repair is unnecessary. A long cast-brace is worn for 6 weeks and thereafter graded exercises are encouraged.

Isolated tears of the LCL are rare. If the diagnosis is certain, these can be treated conservatively as for MCL tears. If the fibular styloid is avulsed, the injury is probably more severe and involves part of the posterolateral capsule and arcuate complex. Examination for posterolateral instability should be done and, if confirmed, these injuries may benefit from repair. In contrast, a fibular head fracture indicates an avulsion of the LCL as a solitary injury.

Isolated tears of the ACL should, in theory, be treated by early operative reconstruction. Indeed, such are the pressures on professional sportspersons that this is often demanded. Operation may also be indicated for non-professionals if the tibial spine is avulsed; the bone fragment, with the attached ACL, is replaced and fixed under arthroscopic control and the knee is braced for 6 weeks. In all other cases it is more prudent to follow the conservative regime described earlier; the cast-brace is worn only until symptoms subside and thereafter movement and muscle-strengthening exercises are encouraged. About half of these patients regain sufficiently good function not to need further treatment. The remainder complain of varying degrees of instability; late assessment will identify those who are likely to benefit from ligament reconstruction.

Isolated tears of the PCL are treated conservatively. Most patients end up with little or no loss of function.

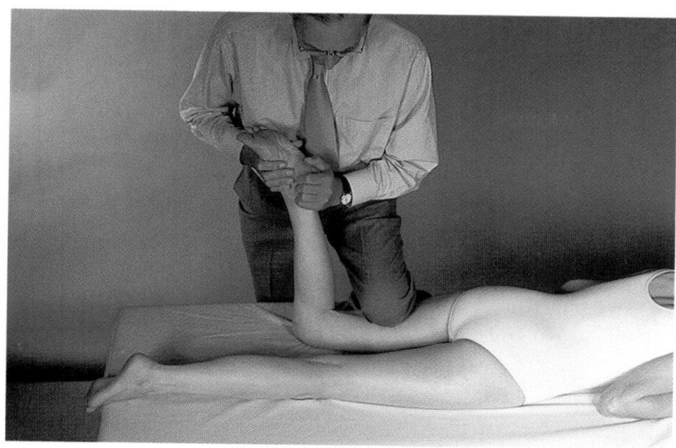

30.4 Apley's test The knee is flexed to 90° and rotated while applying first a compression force and then a distraction force. Pain and/or clicking on compression is suggestive of a meniscal lesion.

However, some experience instability whilst walking up stairs and are sufficiently disabled to warrant late reconstruction.

Combined injuries may result in significant loss of function. With concurrent ACL and collateral ligament injury, reconstruction of the ACL often obviates the need for collateral ligament treatment; however, early operation carries the risk of postoperative joint fibrosis, so it is wiser to start treatment with joint support and physiotherapy in order to restore a good range of movement before following on with ACL reconstruction. A similar approach is adopted for combined injuries involving the PCL, but here all damaged structures will need to be repaired.

Complications

Adhesions If the knee with a partial ligament tear is not actively exercised, torn fibres stick to intact fibres and to bone. The knee 'gives way' with catches of pain; localized tenderness is present and there is pain on medial or lateral rotation. The obvious confusion with a torn meniscus can be resolved by the grinding test (Fig. 30.4) or, better still, by MRI. Physiotherapy will resolve the problem caused by adhesions and rarely is manipulation under anaesthesia needed.

Ossification in the ligament (Pellegrini–Stieda's disease) Occasionally, an abduction injury is followed by ossification near the upper attachment of the medial ligament. This is usually discovered as a chance finding in x-rays of the knee and carries no prognostic significance.

Instability The knee may continue to give way. The instability tends to get worse and the repeated injury predisposes to osteoarthritis. This important subject is discussed under a separate heading later.

CHRONIC LIGAMENTOUS INSTABILITY

Instability ('giving way') of the knee may be obvious soon after the acute injury has healed, or it may only become apparent much later. It is usually progressive (a partial meniscectomy for a meniscal tear is likely to make it worse and create new tears) but, except in people engaged in strenuous sport, dancing or certain work activities, the disability is often tolerated without complaint. In more severe and longstanding cases, osteoarthritis may eventually supervene.

Functional pathology

Unstable tibiofemoral relationships may result in abnormal sideways tilt (varus or valgus), excessive glide (forwards, backwards or even in an oblique direction), unnatural rotation (internal or external), or combinations of these.

Seldom is only one ligament at fault. As described at the beginning of this chapter, stability is normally maintained by both primary and secondary stabilizers (not to mention the dynamic forces of surrounding muscles). In different positions, different structures come into play as primary stabilizers. *Therefore, when testing for medial and lateral stability, valgus and varus stresses should be applied with the knee first in 30 degrees of flexion and then in full extension.*

Abnormal translation or rotation of the tibia on the femur is even more complex. A positive anterior drawer sign is the result of a torn ACL, but a *solitary* cruciate injury is unusual. More commonly there is *anterolateral rotatory instability* where, in addition to a torn ACL, the lateral capsule and LCL are torn or 'stretched'. In this instance, not only will the anterior drawer test be positive, but the lateral tibial condyle can be made to sublux forwards as the tibia rotates abnormally around an axis through the medial condyles; this is the basis of the *pivot shift phenomenon* (Galway and MacIntosh, 1980).

A positive posterior tibial sag and drawer sign means that the posterior cruciate ligament is torn (Fig. 30.5).

Soon after injury, however, this sign is difficult to elicit unless the ligaments of the arcuate complex and popliteus also are torn. Chronic deficiency of the arcuate ligament complex causes a type of *posterolateral rotatory instability* that is a counterpart of the pivot shift phenomenon (Bahk and Cosgarea, 2006; Ranawat et al., 2008). Complete tears of all the posterior structures also allow the knee to hyperextend.

Clinical features

The patient complains of a feeling of insecurity and of giving way. With collateral ligament instability the

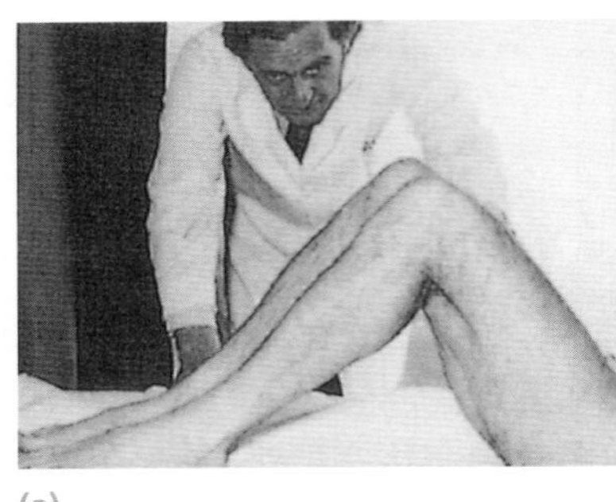

(a)

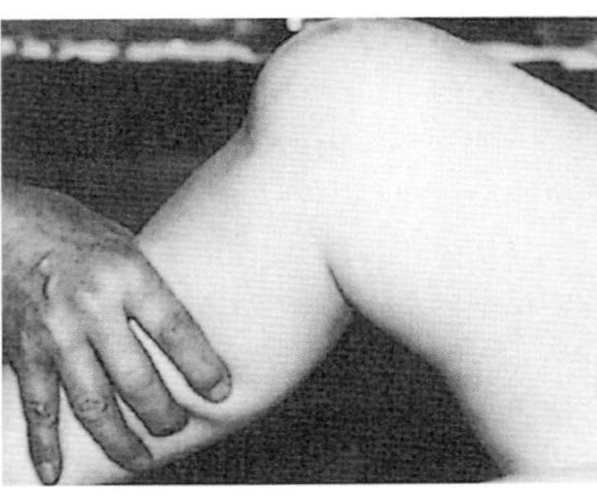

(b)

30.5 Cruciate ligaments (a) Viewed from the side, any backwards displacement of the upper tibia is plainly visible and can be confirmed by (b) pushing the tibia backwards.

cause is obvious even to the patient, but with anterolateral rotatory instability the symptoms are more subtle – the knee suddenly gives way as the patient pivots on the affected side (effectively causing a pivot shift to occur). Some patients describe this jerking sensation by grinding the knuckles of clenched fists upon each other. The explanation is that, with the knee just short of full extension, the lateral tibial condyle slips forward (subluxes); then, as the knee is flexed, the iliotibial band pulls the condyle back into the reduced position with a 'clunk'. For a sportsman, 'cutting' is particularly troublesome. Locking is not a feature of instability and always suggests an associated meniscal tear.

In the less common posterior cruciate insufficiency, symptoms are mild unless the arcuate ligament complex also is torn or stretched; instability is sometimes felt only on climbing stairs.

The joint looks normal apart from slight wasting; there is rarely tenderness but excessive movement in one or more directions can usually be demonstrated. Comparison with the normal knee is essential. A useful routine is to observe gait and knee posture in standing, then to examine for hyperextension, then for increased tilting into varus or valgus (at 0 and 30 degrees knee flexion), followed by the drawer tests and the more specific Lachman test (see later), and finally to perform special tests for rotational instability.

Start by watching the patient walk and noting knee posture and movement in the stance phase. Then ask the patient to stand on one leg – those with severe instabilities may not be able to achieve this task, whereas others who do may demonstrate the problem.

Hyperextension is tested with the patient supine and the knee straight; with the patient relaxed, lift each heel in turn. Repeat the test, but this time grasp the medial forefoot – if the tibia sags posteriorly and externally rotates, this suggests that both posterior cruciate and posterolateral capsule are torn (*posterolateral rotatory instability*).

To test stability in the coronal plane, the patient's ankle is tucked under the examiner's armpit whilst both hands support the knee by straddling it on either side (Fig. 30.6a).

The examiner is then able to control both knee flexion and the amount of varus or valgus thrust applied;

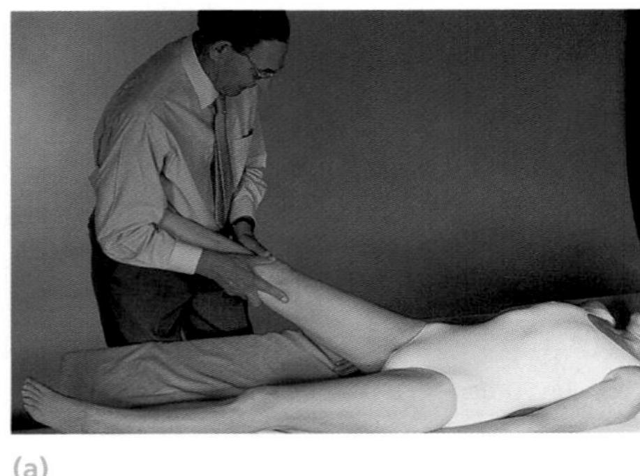

(a)

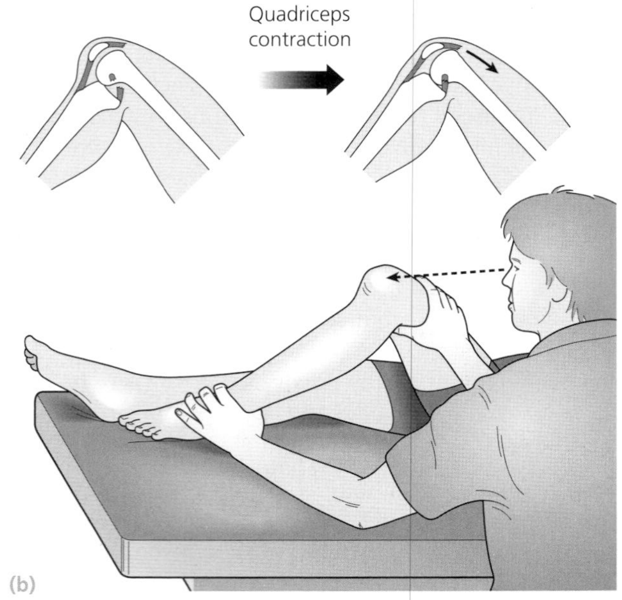

(b)

30.6 Testing collateral ligaments (a) Side-to-side stability of the knee can be checked by holding the foot between the upper arm and body and moving the joint between supporting hands. This method is useful if the leg is large. (b) The quadriceps active test. Note the position of the examiner's hands in supporting the thigh and resisting knee extension by the ankle. At 90° of knee flexion, a posterior sag caused by a damaged posterior cruciate ligament is corrected when the quadriceps contracts.

perform the test first with the knee straight and then flexed at 30 degrees. This manner of performing varus and valgus stressing enables even large limbs to be held and examined.

Next, place the knees at 90 degrees with the soles of the feet flat on the couch and the heels lined up; the quadriceps should be relaxed. Looking from the side, note if there is any posterior sag of the upper tibia by checking the levels of the tibial tuberosities on each leg – a posterior sag is a sure sign of posterior cruciate laxity. Then support the patient's thigh in this position to ensure the hamstring muscles are relaxed, and use the other hand to grasp the patient's ankle (Fig. 30.6b). Ask the patient to slide the foot slowly down the couch while resisting this movement by holding on to the ankle as the quadriceps contracts, the posterior sag is pulled up and the proximal tibia shifts forward. This is the *quadriceps active test* (Daniel et al., 1988).

Again with the knees flexed at 90 degrees and both feet resting on the couch (it is useful to sit across the couch to prevent the feet sliding forward), grasp the upper tibia with both hands, and making sure the hamstrings are relaxed, test for anterior and posterior laxity (*the drawer sign*). A more reliable test for anterior cruciate laxity is to examine for anterior–posterior displacement with the knee flexed to 20 degrees (*the Lachman test*). Hold the calf with one hand and the thigh with the other, and try to displace the joint backwards and forwards.

Rotational stability can be tested in several ways:

Modified drawer test The anterior drawer test is performed with the tibia in 30 degrees of internal rotation; if positive, it suggests anterolateral rotatory instability. Likewise, a positive drawer sign with the knee in external rotation (about 15 degrees) suggests anteromedial rotatory instability (Slocum and Larson, 1968).

Dial test The leg is dangled over the edge of the couch. The examiner steadies the distal femur with one hand and holds the heel firmly in the other. The knee is flexed at 30 degrees. External rotation is applied through the heel and the position of the tibial tuberosity is noted. If external rotation is greater by 15 degrees as compared to the other side, a posterolateral corner injury is suspected. If the test is repeated with the knee flexed further to 90 degrees and the external rotation is noted to increase, a posterior cruciate injury is likely too (LaPrade and Wentorf, 2002).

Pivot shift test The examiner supports the knee in extension with the tibia internally rotated (the subluxed position – the lateral tibial condyle is drawn in front of the femoral condyle); the knee is then gradually flexed while a valgus stress is applied. In a positive test, as the knee reaches 20 or 30 degrees, there is a sudden jerk as the tibial condyle slips backwards and reduces. The valgus stress compresses the lateral femoral condyle against the tibia and, through a jamming effect, amplifies the sudden 'jerk' when the condyle drops back. Another way to show this is MacIntosh's test (Fig. 30.8). A positive pivot shift test indicates *anterolateral rotatory instability*. A modification of this test can be used to diagnose *posterolateral rotatory instability*; the tibia is held in external rotation while the knee is extended and, similarly, a valgus stress is applied as the knee is gradually flexed – a characteristic 'clunk' signals the change from a subluxed to a reduced position (*the reverse pivot shift*).

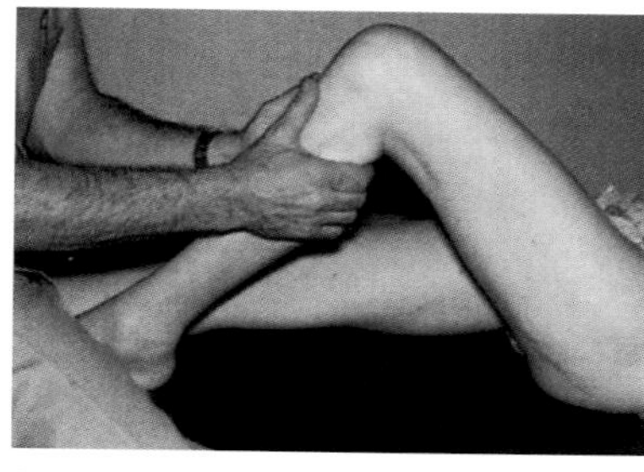

(a)

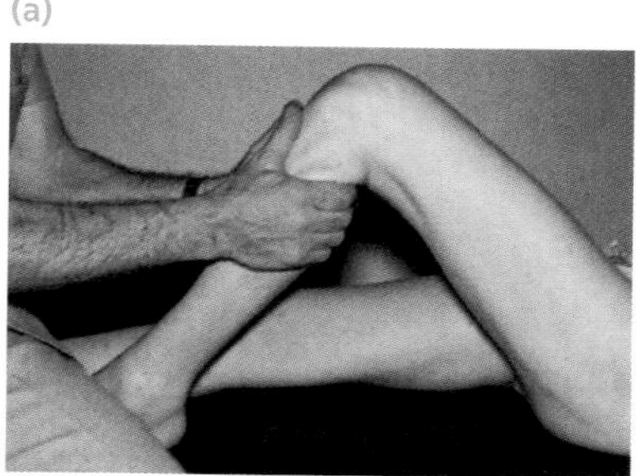

(b)

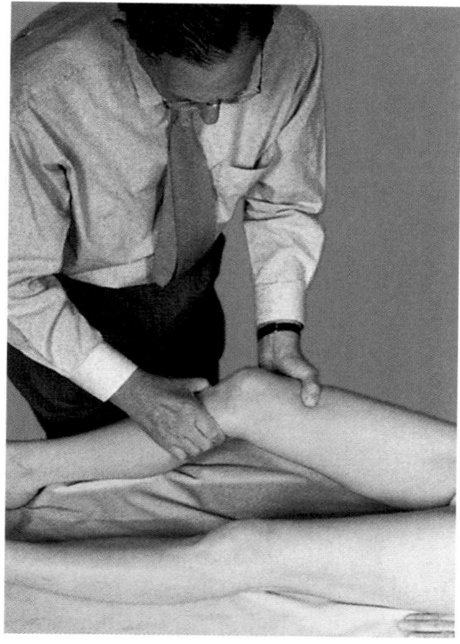

(c)

30.7 Tests for cruciate ligament instability (a) *Drawer test*: Wth the knee at 90° and the hamstrings relaxed, grasp the top of the patients leg and try to shift it forwards and backwards. (b) Note that there is some anterior shift when the tibia is pulled forwards (slight anterior cruciate laxity. (c) *Lachman test*: This is more sensitive than the drawer test. Note the position of the knee and the examiner's hands.

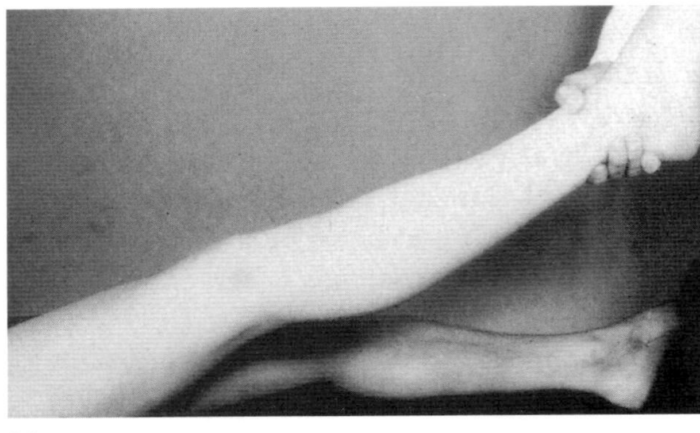

(a)

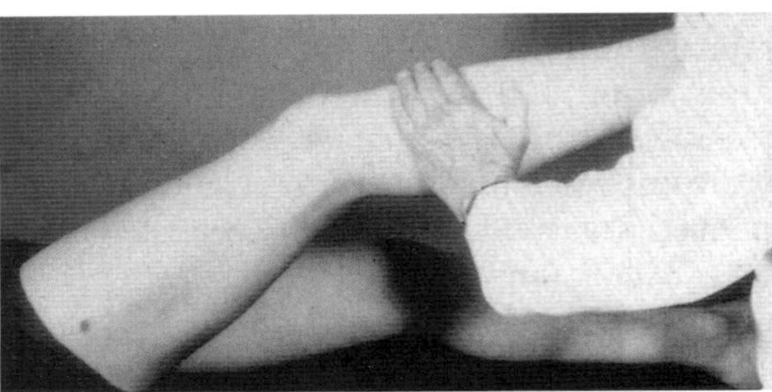

(b)

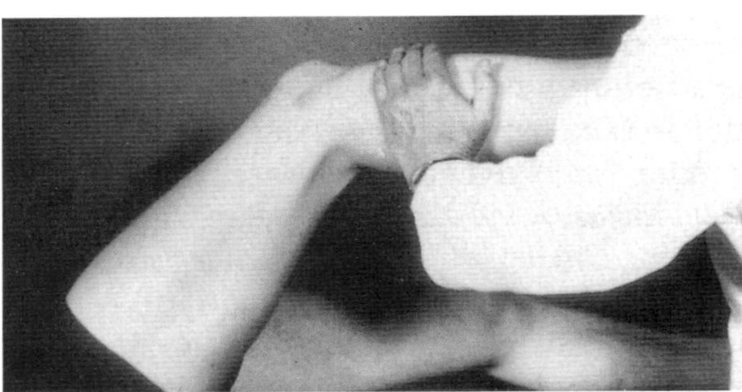

(c)

30.8 Cruciate ligament tears – MacIntosh's test (a) The leg is lifted with the knee straight. (b) The fibula is pushed forwards – if the anterior cruciate is torn the lateral tibial condyle is now subluxed forwards. (c) It is held forwards while the knee is flexed; at 30–40° the condyle reduces with a jerk. This may be painful and an alternative method is to lift the straight leg by holding it with both hands just above the ankle, rotating the leg inwards, then flexing the knee. The jerk is often visible and usually painless.

Imaging

MRI is a reliable method of diagnosing cruciate ligament and meniscal injuries, providing almost 100 per cent sensitivity and over 90 per cent accuracy (Fig. 30.9).

Arthroscopy

Arthroscopy is indicated if: (1) the diagnosis, or the extent of the ligament injury, remains in doubt; (2)

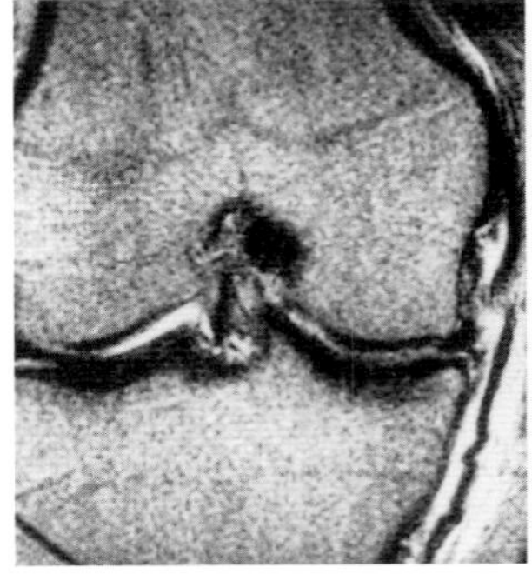

(a)

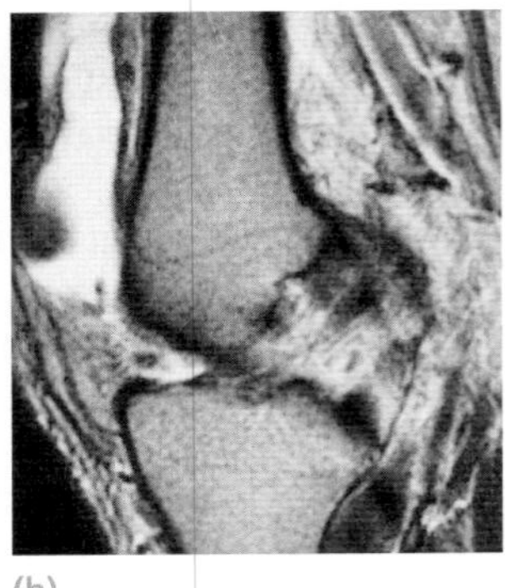

(b)

30.9 Torn knee ligaments – MRI (a) Coronal T2-weighted image showing a medial collateral ligament tear with surrounding oedema and joint effusion. (b) Sagittal T2-weighted image showing an intrasubstance tear of the anterior cruciate ligament with a large joint effusion.

other lesions, such as meniscal tears or cartilage damage, are suspected; (3) surgical treatment is anticipated. Partial meniscectomy and removal of loose cartilage tags can be performed at the same time.

Treatment

Most patients with chronic instability have reasonably good function and will not require an operation. The first approach should always be a supervised, disciplined and progressively vigorous exercise programme to strengthen the quadriceps and the hamstrings. At the end of 6 months the patient should be re-examined.

The indications for operation are:

1. Recurrent locking, with MRI or arthroscopic confirmation of a meniscal tear (arthroscopic meniscectomy alone may alleviate the patient's symptoms, though this may later lead to increased instability);
2. intolerable symptoms of giving way;
3. suboptimal function in a sportsperson or others with similarly demanding occupations (even in this group, some patients will accept the use of a knee brace for specific activities that are known to cause trouble);
4. ligament injuries in adolescents (the long-term effects of chronic instability in this group are more marked).

Partial tears of the anterior cruciate ligament are more problematic and there is still much controversy about the need for surgery in these cases. The decision should be based on an assessment of the patient's symptoms and functional capacity rather than the appearance of the ligament. Young adults with chronic anterior cruciate insufficiency and proven partial tears show diminished activity and run the risk of developing secondary problems such as meniscal lesions, cartilage damage, increasing instability and (eventually) secondary osteoarthritis. With careful follow-up and reassessment, those most at risk can usually be identified and advised to undergo reconstructive surgery.

Operative treatment

Medial collateral ligament insufficiency seldom causes much disability unless there is an associated anterior cruciate tear. However, if valgus instability is marked, and particularly if it is progressive, ligament reconstruction, by advancing the proximal or distal end of the ligament, restoring the tension of the posteromedial capsule and reinforcing the medial structures with the semimembranosus tendon, is justified.

Isolated lateral instability is uncommon and symptoms are rarely troublesome enough to warrant surgery. If operative reconstruction is attempted, it should follow the lines described earlier.

Isolated PCL insufficiency rarely causes loss of function. Conservative treatment (mainly quadriceps strengthening exercises) will usually suffice.

Isolated ACL insufficiency is uncommon and can usually be managed by physiotherapy. Splints or braces may be used to speed the return to weightbearing. Patients seeking to resume competitive sport may need something more; reconstructive surgery involves replacing the torn ACL with an autologous graft, usually a strip of patellar tendon with bone attachments at either end or with hamstring tendons.

Combined injuries such as anterolateral or anteromedial rotatory instability are the commonest reasons for reconstructive surgery. When the ACL is damaged together with either the medial or lateral collateral ligament, reconstruction of the ACL alone often suffices. The torn ACL is replaced by an autograft (usually from the patellar tendon or from hamstring tendons) or by an allograft. Some surgeons advocate replicating the dual bundle arrangement of the original ligament. The ideal synthetic graft has yet to be developed. Postoperative care will depend on the fixation of the new ligament; in many cases a short period of splintage can be followed by regular physiotherapy to avoid joint stiffness and improve muscle control. Many patients return to sports within 6 months.

The treatment of combined injuries in which the PCL is involved is changing; until recently, it was thought that most of these patients had good function and therefore did not need reconstructive surgery. Newer studies have shown that there is an increased risk of osteoarthritis (especially of the medial compartment) and this is seen as an indication for PCL reconstruction in patients who have more than 10–15 mm of posterior tibial translation in the drawer test. Unlike injuries involving the ACL, combination injuries involving the PCL require all damaged structures to be repaired.

FRACTURED TIBIAL SPINE

Severe valgus or varus stress, or twisting injuries, may damage the knee ligaments and fracture the tibial spine. This is, in fact, a type of traction injury – the adolescent variant of a cruciate ligament tear.

Pathological anatomy

The detached bone fragment may remain almost undisplaced, held in position by the soft tissues; it may be partially displaced, the anterior end lifted away on

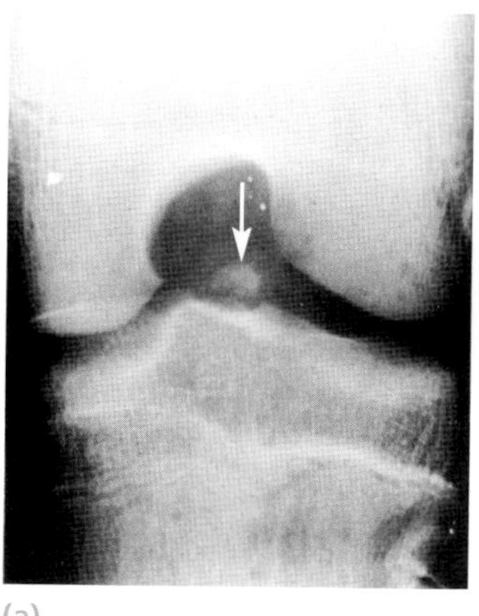
(a)
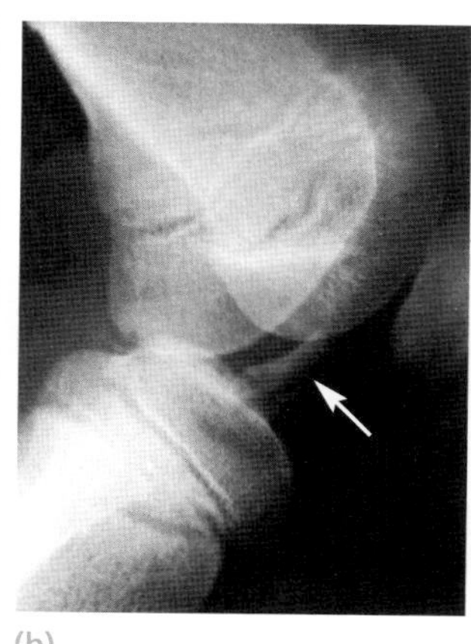
(b)
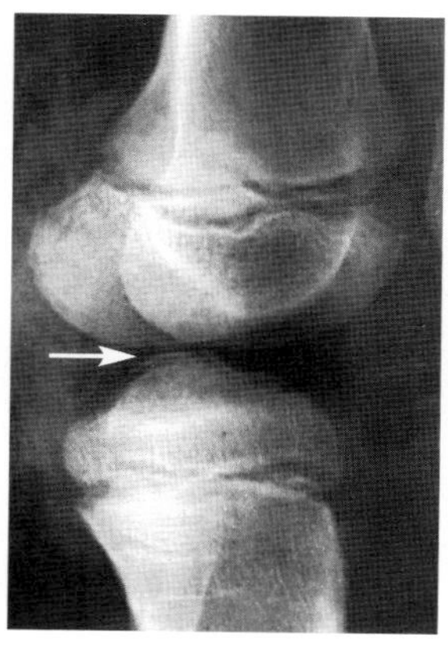
(c)
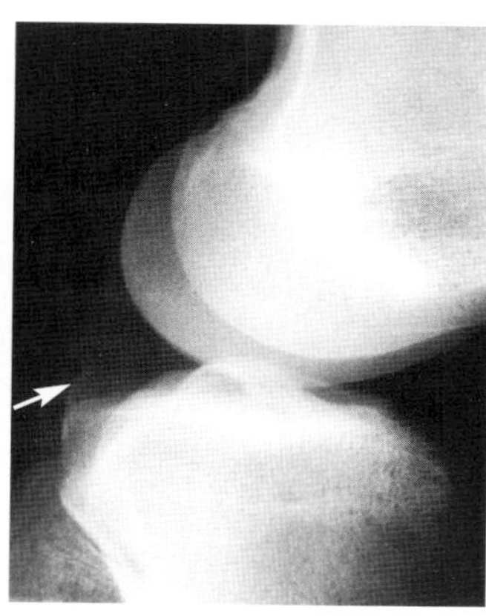
(d)

30.10 Tibial spine fracture (a,b) This young man injured his knee while playing football; x-rays showed a large, displaced avulsion fracture of the tibial spine. (c) An undisplaced tibial spine fracture. (d) Posterior fractures, with avulsion of the posterior cruciate ligament, are often missed.

a posterior hinge, or it may be completely detached and displaced. Because its articular surface is covered with cartilage – invisible on x-ray – the image seen on x-ray is smaller than the actual fragment.

Clinical features

The patient – usually an older child or adolescent – presents with a swollen, immobile knee. The joint feels tense, tender and 'doughy' and aspiration will reveal a haemarthrosis. Examination under anaesthesia may show that extension is blocked. There may also be associated ligament injuries; always test for varus and valgus stability and cruciate laxity.

X-ray The fracture is not always obvious and a small posterior fracture may be missed unless the x-rays are carefully examined. The fragment – often including part of the intercondylar eminence – may be undisplaced, tilted upwards or completely detached (Fig. 30.10).

Treatment

Under anaesthesia the joint is aspirated and gently manipulated into full extension. Often the fragment falls back into position and the x-ray shows that the fracture is reduced. As long as the knee extends fully, small amounts of fragment elevation can be accepted. If there is a block to full extension or if the bone fragment remains displaced, operative reduction is essential. The fragment – often larger than suspected – is restored to its bed and anchored by small screws, taking care to avoid the physis.

After either closed or open reduction, a long plaster cylinder is applied with the knee almost straight; it is worn for 6 weeks and then movements are encouraged.

The outcome is usually good and full movement regained; there may be some residual laxity on examination, but this rarely causes symptoms.

DISLOCATION OF KNEE

The knee can be dislocated only by considerable violence, as in a road accident. The cruciate ligaments and one or both lateral ligaments are torn.

Clinical features

Rupture of the joint capsule produces a leak of the haemarthrosis, leading to severe bruising and swelling. This may be the only clue on inspection, especially if the dislocated joint has reduced spontaneously. Otherwise, the diagnosis is straightforward as there is gross deformity (Fig. 30.11). The circulation in the foot must be examined because the popliteal artery may be torn or obstructed. Repeated examination is necessary as compartment syndrome is also a risk. Common peroneal nerve injury occurs in nearly 20 per cent of cases; distal sensation and movement should be tested.

X-ray In addition to the dislocation, the films occasionally reveal a fracture of the tibial spine or posterior part of the plateau (cruciate ligament avulsion), avulsion of the fibular styloid or avulsion of a fragment from the near the edge of the lateral tibial condyle (the *Segond fracture*).

Arteriograpy is not essential if the clinical assessment of the circulation is normal. The ankle/brachial arterial pressure index (ratio of systolic pressure at the ankle relative to systolic pressure at the elbow) is a useful measure and should not be less than 0.9, but if there is any doubt an arteriogram should be obtained (Robertson et al., 2006).

Treatment

Reduction under anaesthesia is urgent; this is usually achieved by pulling directly in the line of the leg, but hyperextension must be avoided because of the danger to the popliteal vessels. If reduction is achieved,

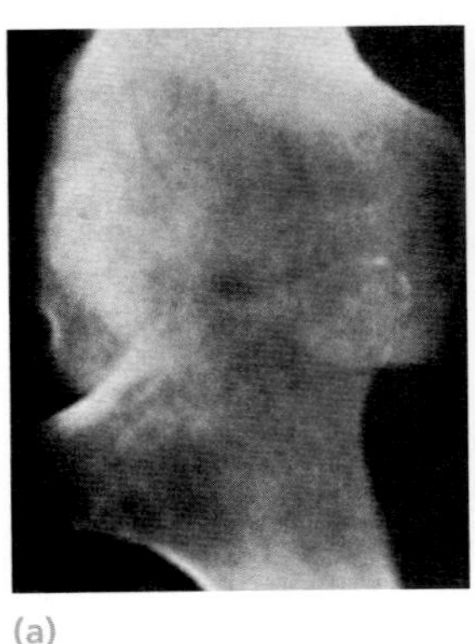
(a)

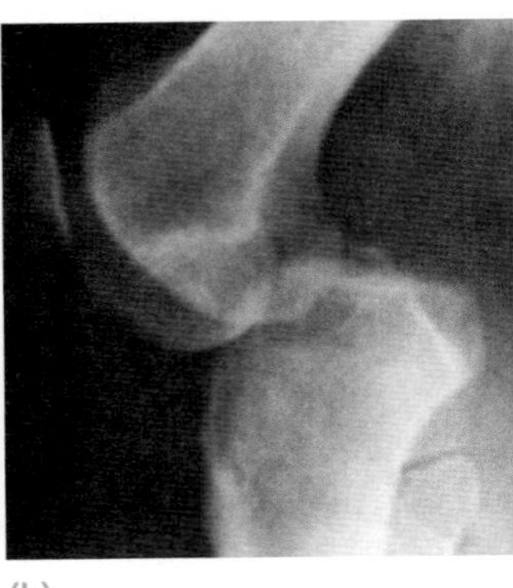
(b)

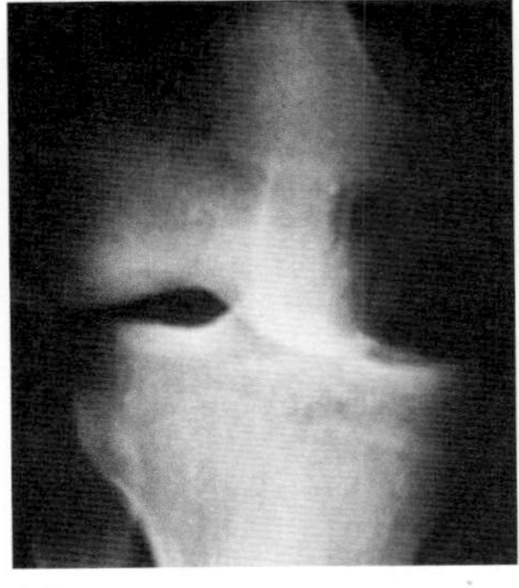
(c)

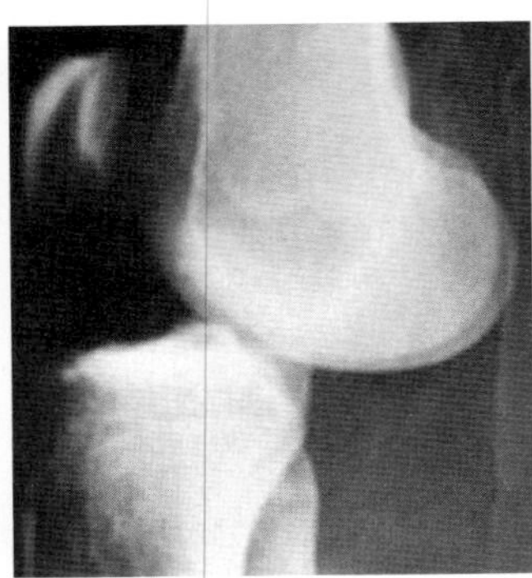
(d)

30.11 Dislocations of the knee (a,b) Posterolateral dislocation; (c,d) anteromedial dislocation.

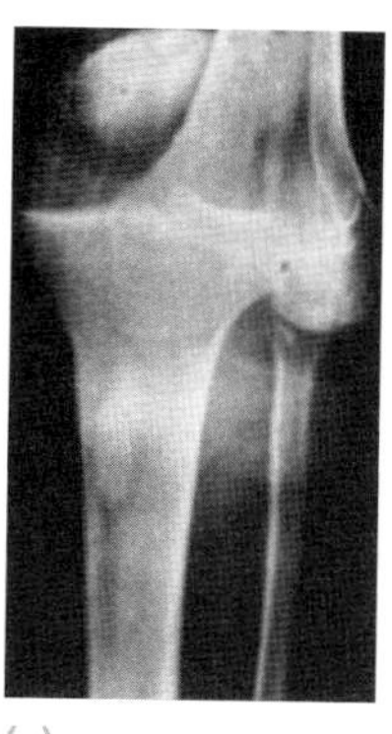
(a)
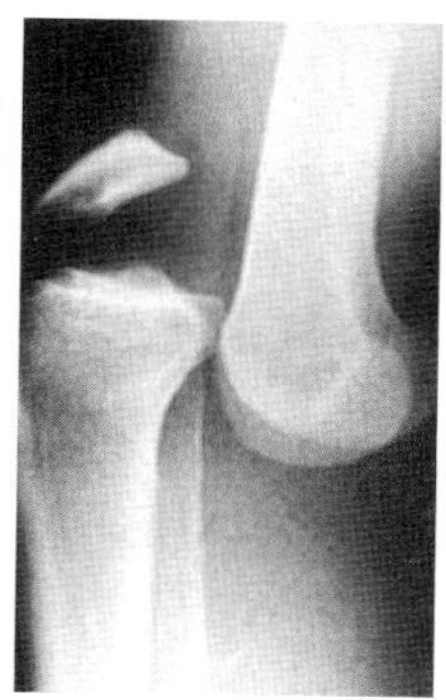
(b)
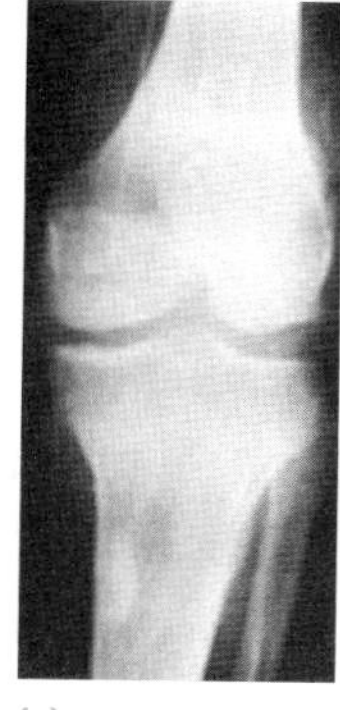
(c)
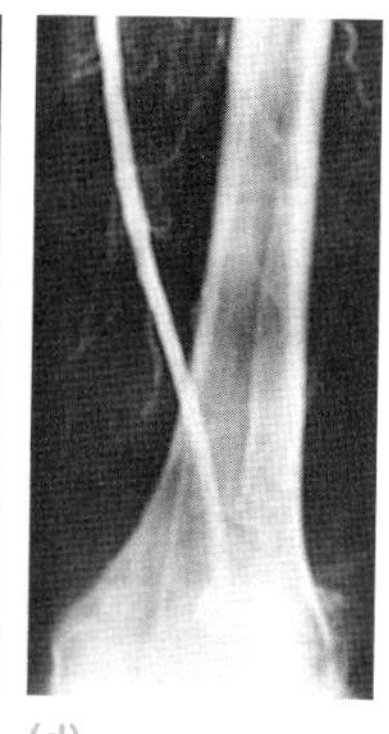
(d)

30.12 Knee dislocation and vascular trauma (a,b) This patient was admitted with a dislocated knee. After reduction (c) the x-ray looked satisfactory, but the circulation did not. (d) An arteriogram showed vascular cut-off just above the knee; had this not been recognized and treated, amputation might have been necessary.

the limb is rested on a back-splint and the circulation is checked repeatedly during the 48 hours. Because of swelling, a plaster cylinder is dangerous.

A vascular injury will need immediate repair and the limb is then more conveniently splinted with an anterior external fixator (Fig. 30.12). If possible, repair or reconstruction of the capsule and collateral ligaments should be undertaken at the same time – this may involve simple suture or reattachment of the avulsed portions to bone – in order to enable early movement of the knee with the support of a hinged knee brace. If the direct repair is tenuous, augmentation using tendon grafts may be needed.

In general, early reconstruction of the torn ligaments followed by protected movement of the joint reduces the severity of joint stiffness. The cruciate ligaments can be reconstructed after knee movement has recovered, usually some 6–12 months later. Prolonged cast immobilization (usually 12 weeks) is no longer recommended as it has been shown to be less good at preserving knee function.

Complications

EARLY

Arterial damage Popliteal artery damage occurs in nearly 20 per cent of patients and needs immediate repair. Delay and an extended warm ischaemic period can result in amputation.

Nerve injury The lateral popliteal nerve may be injured. Spontaneous recovery is possible if the nerve is not completely disrupted – about 20 per cent of patients can be expected to improve. If nerve conduction studies or clinical examination shows no sign of recovery, a transfer of tibialis posterior tendon through the interosseous membrane to the lateral cuneiform may help restore ankle dorsiflexion.

LATE

Joint instability Anteroposterior glide or a lateral wobble often remains but, provided the quadriceps muscle is sufficiently powerful, the disability is not severe.

Stiffness Loss of movement, due to prolonged immobilization, is a common problem and may be even more troublesome than instability. Even with early surgical reconstruction, normal knee function is elusive.

ACUTE INJURIES OF EXTENSOR APPARATUS

Disruption of the extensor apparatus may occur: in the quadriceps tendon, at the attachment of the quadriceps tendon to the proximal surface of the patella, through the patella and retinacular expansions, at the junction of the patella and the patellar ligament, in the patellar ligament or at the insertion of the patellar ligament to the tibial tubercle. (*Note*: The patellar ligament is often called the patellar tendon).

In all but direct fractures of the patella, the mechanism of injury is the same: sudden resisted extension of the knee or (essentially the same thing) sudden passive flexion of the knee while the quadriceps is contracting. The patient gives a history of stumbling on a stair, catching the foot while running, or kicking hard at a muddy football.

The lesion tends to occur at progressively higher levels with increasing age: adolescents suffer avulsion fractures of the tibial tubercle; young adult sportspeople tear the patellar ligament, middle-aged adults fracture their patellae; and older people (as well as those whose tissues are weakened by chronic illness or steroid medication) suffer acute tears of the quadriceps tendon.

RUPTURE OF QUADRICEPS TENDON

The patient is usually elderly, may have a history of diabetes or rheumatoid disease, or may have been treated with corticosteroids. Occasionally acute rupture is seen in a young athlete. The typical injury is followed by tearing pain and giving way of the knee.

There is bruising and local tenderness; sometimes a gap can be felt proximal to the patella. Active knee extension is either impossible (suggesting a complete rupture) or weak (partial rupture). The diagnosis can be confirmed by MRI.

Treatment

Partial tears Non-operative treatment will suffice: a plaster cylinder is applied for 6 weeks, followed by physiotherapy that concentrates on restoring knee flexion and quadriceps strength.

Complete tears Early operation is needed, or else the ruptured fibres will retract and repair will be more difficult. End-to-end suturing can be reinforced by turning down a partial-thickness triangular flap of quadriceps tendon proximal to the repair (Scuderi). If the tendon has been avulsed from the proximal pole of the patella, it should be re-attached to a trough created at that site using pull-through sutures. Postoperatively the knee is held in extension in hinged brace. Early supervised movement through the brace is important to prevent adhesions; limits to the amount of flexion can be controlled through the brace and increased as the repair heals over the next 12 weeks (Fig. 30.13).

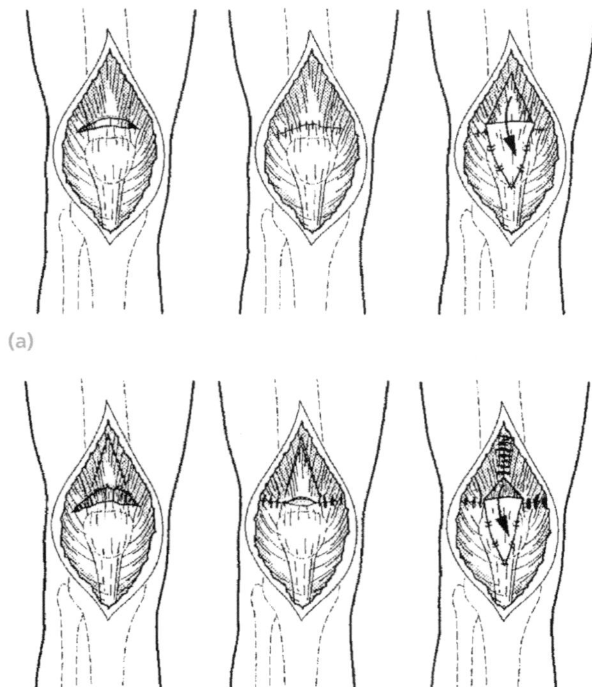

30.13 Repairing ruptures of the quadriceps tendon (a) Acute ruptures can usually be sutured and reinforced with a partial-thickness flap of the quadriceps tendon (Scuderi). When the patient presents late (b), the retracted ends may have to be bridged by a full-thickness V-shaped flap (Codivilla).

'Chronic' ruptures (usually the result of delayed presentations or missed diagnoses) are difficult to repair because the ends have retracted. The gap can often be made smaller by closing the medial and lateral ends, and the remaining central gap is then covered by a full-thickness V-flap turned down from the proximal quadriceps tendon (Codivilla). A pull-out or cerclage wire protects the repair.

The results of acute repairs are good, with most patients regaining full power, a good range of movement and little or no extensor lag. Late repairs are less predictable.

Rupture of patellar ligament

This is an uncommon injury; it is usually seen in young athletes and the tear is almost always at the proximal or distal attachment of the ligament. There may be a previous history of 'tendinitis' and local injection of corticosteroid.

The patient gives a history of sudden pain on forced extension of the knee, followed by bruising, swelling and tenderness at the lower edge of the patella or more distally.

X-rays may show a high-riding patella and a tell-tale flake of bone torn from the proximal or distal attachment of the ligament.

MRI will help to distinguish a partial from a complete tear.

Treatment

ACUTE TEARS

Partial tears can be treated by applying a plaster cylinder. *Complete tears* need operative repair or re-attachment to bone. Tension on the suture line can be lessened by inserting a temporary pull-out wire to keep the distance between the inferior pole and attachment to the tibial tuberosity constant. Immobilization in full extension may precipitate stiffness – it is, after all, a joint injury – and it may be better to support the knee in a hinged brace with limits to the amount of flexion permitted. This range can be gradually increased after 6 weeks.

Early repair of acute ruptures gives excellent results. Late repairs are less successful and the patient may be left with a permanent extension lag.

LATE CASES

Late cases are difficult to manage because of proximal retraction of the patella. A two-stage operation may be needed: first to release the contracted tissues and apply traction directly to the patella, then at a later stage to repair the patellar ligament and reinforce it with grafts of tendon from gracilis or semitendinosus. Here, again, a tension-relieving pull-out wire is helpful. Postoperatively a hinged brace is used to hold the knee in extension with supervised knee movement and limits to the amount of flexion until the repair is healed, usually at 12 weeks.

FRACTURES OF TIBIAL TUBERCLE

Fracture or avulsion of the tibial tubercle usually occurs as a sports injury in young people. If the knee is suddenly forced into flexion while the quadriceps is contracting, a fragment of the tubercle – or sometimes the entire apophysis – may be wrenched from the bone. The diagnosis is suggested by the history. The area over the tubercle is swollen and tender; active extension causes pain.

The lateral x-ray shows the fracture. Sometimes the patella is abnormally high, having lost part of its distal attachment.

An incomplete fracture can be treated by applying a long-leg cast with the knee in extension for 6 weeks. Complete separation requires open reduction and fixation with lag screws; a cast or hinged brace is applied for 6 weeks.

Osgood–Schlatter disease Repetitive strain on the patellar ligament may give rise to a painful, tender swelling over the tibial tubercle. The condition is fairly common in adolescents who are keen on sport. Treatment consists of restricting sports activities until the symptoms subside (see page 576).

FRACTURED PATELLA

The patella is a sesamoid bone in continuity with the quadriceps tendon and the patellar ligament (also called the patellar tendon). There are additional insertions from the vastus medialis and lateralis into the medial and lateral edges of the patella. The extensor 'strap' is completed by the medial and lateral extensor retinacula (or quadriceps expansions), which bypass the patella and insert into the proximal tibia.

The mechanical function of the patella is to hold the entire extensor 'strap' away from the centre of rotation of the knee, thereby lengthening the anterior lever arm and increasing the efficiency of the quadriceps.

The key to the management of patellar fractures is the state of the entire extensor mechanism. If the extensor retinacula are intact, active knee extension is still possible, even if the patella itself is fractured.

Mechanism of injury and pathological anatomy

The patella may be fractured, either by a direct force that cracks the bone like a tile under the blow of a hammer or by an indirect traction force that pulls the bone apart (and often tears the extensor expansions as well).

Direct injury – usually a fall onto the knee or a blow against the dashboard of a car – causes either an undisplaced crack or else a comminuted ('stellate') fracture without severe damage to the extensor expansions.

Indirect injury occurs, typically, when someone catches the foot against a solid obstacle and, to avoid falling, contracts the quadriceps muscle forcefully. This is a transverse fracture with a gap between the fragments.

Clinical features

Following one of the typical injuries, the knee becomes swollen and painful. There may be an abrasion or bruising over the front of the joint. The patella is tender and sometimes a gap can be felt.

Active knee extension should be tested. If the patient can lift the straight leg, the quadriceps mechanism is still intact. If this manoeuvre is too painful, active extension can be tested with the patient lying on his side.

If there is an effusion, aspiration may reveal the presence of blood and fat droplets.

X-ray The x-ray may show one or more fine fracture lines without displacement, multiple fracture lines with irregular displacement or a transverse fracture with a gap between the fragments (Fig. 30.14). Comparative x-rays of the opposite knee may help to distinguish normal from abnormal appearances in undisplaced fractures.

Patellar fractures are classified as transverse, longitudinal, polar or comminuted (stellate). Any of these may be either undisplaced or displaced. Separation of the fragments is significant if it is sufficient to create a step on the articular surface of the patella or, in the case of a transverse fracture, if the gap is more than 3 mm wide.

A fracture line running obliquely across the superolateral corner of the patella should not be confused with the smooth, regular line of a (normal) bipartite patella. Check the opposite knee; bipartite patella is often bilateral.

Treatment

Undisplaced or minimally displaced fractures If there is a haemarthrosis it should be aspirated. The extensor mechanism is intact and treatment is mainly protective. A plaster cylinder holding the knee straight should be worn for 3–4 weeks, and during this time quadriceps exercises are to be practised every day.

Comminuted (stellate) fracture The extensor expansions are intact and the patient may be able to lift the leg.

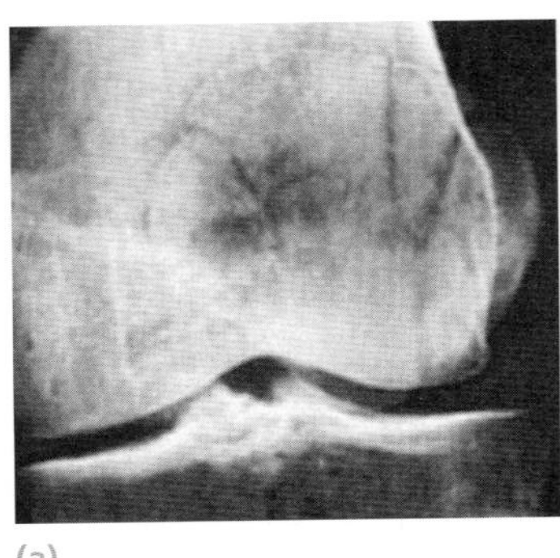
(a)

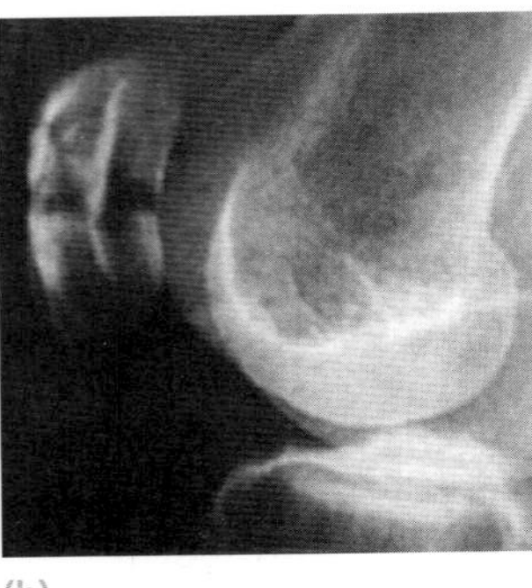
(b)

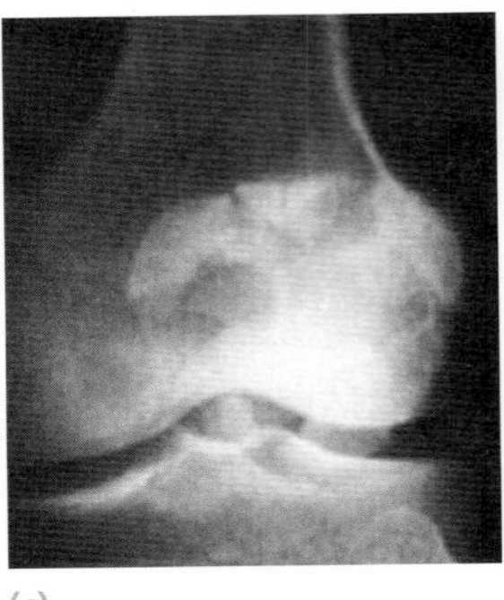
(c)

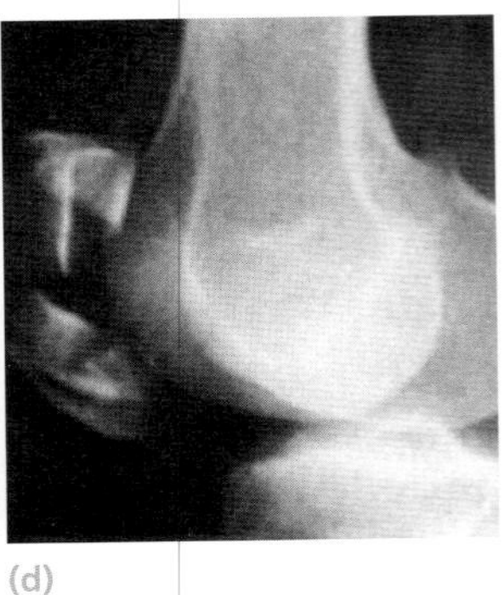
(d)

30.14 Fractured patella – stellate (a,b) A fracture with little or no displacement can be treated conservatively by a posterior slab of plaster that is removed several times a day for gentle active exercises. (c,d) With severe comminutions, patellectomy is arguably the best treatment, although some surgeons would consider preserving as many useful fragments as possible.

However, the undersurface of the patella is irregular and there is a serious risk of damage to the patellofemoral joint. For this reason some people advocate patellectomy, whatever the degree of displacement. To others it seems reasonable to preserve the patella if the fragments are not severely displaced (or to remove only those fragments that obviously distort the articular surface); a hinged brace is used in extension but unlocked several times daily for exercises to mould the fragments into position and to maintain mobility.

Displaced transverse fracture The lateral expansions are torn and the entire extensor mechanism is disrupted. Operation is essential.

Through a longitudinal incision the fracture is exposed and the patella repaired by the tension-band principle. The fragments are reduced and transfixed with two stiff K-wires; flexible wire is then looped tightly around the protruding K-wires and over the front of the patella (Fig. 30.15). The tears in the extensor expansions are then repaired. A plaster backslab or hinged brace is worn until active extension of the knee is regained; either may be removed every day to permit active knee-flexion exercises.

(a) (b)

30.15 Fractured patella – transverse The separated fragments (a) are transfixed by K-wires; (b) malleable wire is then looped around the protruding ends of the K-wires and tightened over the front of the patella.

Outcome

Patients usually regain good function but, depending on the severity of the injury, there is a significant incidence of late patellofemoral osteoarthritis.

DISLOCATION OF PATELLA

Because the knee is normally angled in slight valgus, there is a natural tendency for the patella to pull towards the lateral side when the quadriceps muscle contracts. Lateral deviation of the patella during knee extension is prevented by a number of factors: the patella is seated in the intercondylar groove, which has a high lateral 'embankment'; the force of extensor muscle contraction pulls it firmly into the groove; and the extensor retinacula and patellofemoral ligaments guide it centrally as it tracks along the intercondylar runway. The most important static check-rein on the medial side is the medial patellofemoral ligament, a more or less distinct structure extending from the superomedial border of the patella towards the medial femoral condyle deep to vastus medialis (Conlan et al., 1993). Additional restraint is provided by the medial patellomeniscal and patellotibial ligaments and the associated medial retinacular fibres. In the normal knee, considerable force is required to wrench the patella out of its track. However, if the intercondylar groove is unusually shallow, or the patella seated higher than usual, or the ligaments are abnormally lax, dislocation is not that difficult.

Mechanism of injury

While the knee is flexed and the quadriceps muscle relaxed, the patella may be forced laterally by direct violence; this is rare. More often traumatic dislocation is due to indirect force: sudden, severe contraction of the quadriceps muscle while the knee is stretched in valgus and external rotation. Typically this occurs in field sports when a runner dodges to one side. The patella dislocates laterally and the medial patellofemoral ligament and retinacular fibres may be torn. Predisposing factors are anatomical variations such as genu valgum, tibial torsion, high-riding patella (patella alta) and a shallow intercondylar groove, as well as patellar hypermobility due to generalized ligamentous laxity or localized muscle weakness.

Clinical features

In a 'first-time' dislocation the patient may experience a tearing sensation and a feeling that the knee has gone 'out of joint'; when running, he or she may collapse and fall to the ground. Often the patella springs back into position spontaneously; however, if it remains unreduced there is an obvious (if somewhat misleading) deformity: the displaced patella, seated on the lateral side of the knee, is not easily noticed but the uncovered medial femoral condyle is unduly prominent and may be mistaken for the patella. Neither active nor passive movement is possible (Fig. 30.16). In the rare intra-articular (downward) dislocation the patella is stuck between the condyles and there is a marked prominence on the front of the knee.

If the dislocation has reduced spontaneously, the knee may be swollen and there may be bruising and tenderness on the medial side. If there is fluid in the joint, aspiration may show that it is bloodstained; the presence of fat droplets suggests a concurrent osteochondral fracture.

With recurrent dislocation the symptoms and signs are much less marked, though still unpleasant. After spontaneous reduction the knee looks normal, but the apprehension test is positive.

Imaging

Anteroposterior, lateral and tangential ('skyline') *x-ray views* are needed. In an unreduced dislocation, the patella is seen to be laterally displaced and tilted or rotated. In 5 per cent of cases there is an associated osteochondral fracture.

MRI may reveal a soft-tissue lesion (e.g. disruption of the medial patellofemoral ligament) as well as articular cartilage and/or bone damage.

Treatment

In most cases the patella can be pushed back into place without much difficulty and anaesthesia is not always necessary; the exception is an intra-articular (intercondylar) dislocation, which may need open reduction.

If there are no signs of soft tissue rupture – i.e. there is minimal swelling, no bruising and little tenderness – cast splintage alone will usually suffice. The knee is aspirated and then immobilized in almost full extension; a small pad along the lateral edge of the patella may help to keep the medial soft tissues relaxed. The cast is retained for 2 or 3 weeks and the patient then undergoes a long period (2–3 months) of quadriceps strengthening exercises.

The same approach has been advocated for more severe forms of dislocation. However, if there is much bruising, swelling and tenderness medially, the patellofemoral ligaments and retinacular tissues are probably torn and immediate operative repair will reduce the likelihood of later recurrent dislocation.

OPERATIVE TREATMENT

The area is approached through a medial incision. If the patellofemoral ligament is avulsed from the femur, it is reattached with suitable anchors. Mid-substance tears of the ligaments are sutured directly. At the same time, if the lateral retinaculum is tight it is released. Osteochondral fragments are removed – unless they are single, large and amenable to reattachment. Postoperatively a padded cylinder cast is applied with the knee in extension; this can be renewed when the swelling has subsided. A hinged brace is substituted, which provides control for weightbearing and allows knee movement. Quadriceps exercises are encouraged.

Complications

Recurrent dislocation Patients treated non-operatively for a first-time dislocation have a 15–20 per cent chance of suffering further dislocations. This depends

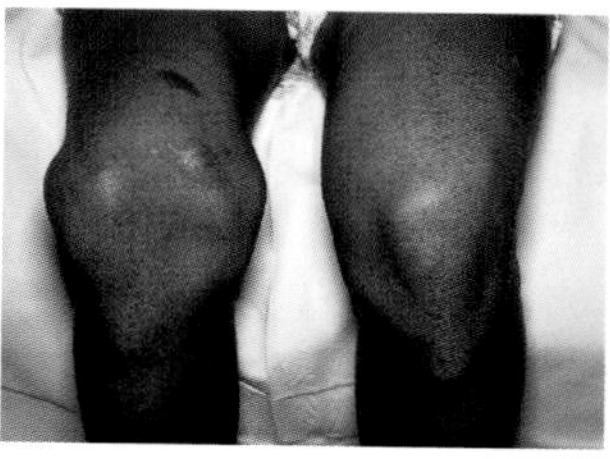
(a)

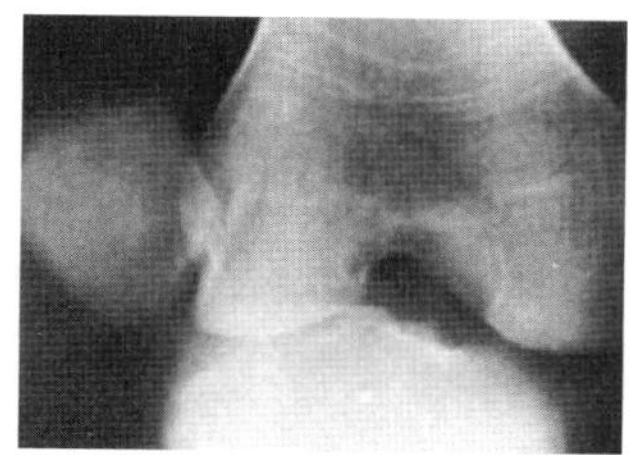
(b)

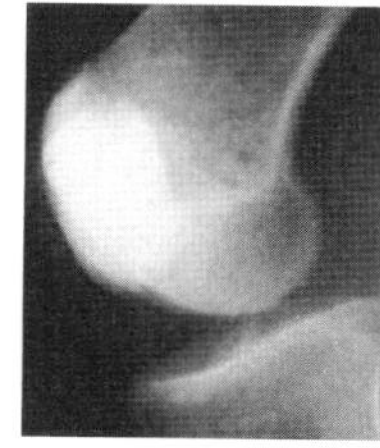
(c)

30.16 Dislocation of the patella (a) The right patella has dislocated laterally; the flattened appearance is typical. **(b,c)** Anteroposterior and lateral films of traumatic dislocation of the patella.

also on whether there are other predisposing abnormalities, and prevention consists of dealing with all these conditions (the subjects of recurrent dislocation, subluxation, chronic patellar instability and patellar mal-tracking are dealt with in Chapter 20).

OSTEOCHONDRAL INJURIES

Osteochondral fractures and osteochondritis dissecans are similar injuries of the articular cartilage and subchondral bone. The knee joint is a common site for both conditions. The lesion is usually located on one of the femoral condyles, the intercondylar groove or the medial facet of the patella, and is thought to be due to the patella striking the opposed articular surface.

OSTEOCHONDRAL FRACTURES

The patient gives a history of patellar dislocation or a blow to the front of the knee. The joint is swollen and aspiration yields blood-stained fluid mixed with fat globules.

Standard anteroposterior and lateral x-rays seldom show the abnormality; if the diagnosis is suspected, tunnel and patellar skyline views are needed, and even then the fracture may be hard to see because the damaged area consists largely of articular cartilage. MRI or arthroscopy will be more helpful.

Treatment

Small fragments should be removed as they may cause symptoms. Larger fragments, and especially those from loadbearing areas, can be reattached with screws (counter-sunk or 'headless' small fragment screws). Postoperatively a long-leg cast is applied for 2 weeks before movement is allowed.

Sometimes a large area of cartilage damage, or even a crater, is discovered on the anterior intercondylar surface. In the past this was treated by trimming any ragged parts and drilling through the crater to stimulate an inflammatory response ('micro-fracturing'). More recently, cartilage transplantation into these defects has shown promising results.

OSTEOCHONDRITIS DISSECANS

Teenagers and young adults who complain of intermittent pain in the knee are sometimes found to have developed a small segment of osteochondral necrosis, usually on the lateral aspect of the medial femoral condyle. This is probably a traumatic lesion, caused by repetitive contact with the overlying patella or an adjacent ridge on the tibial plateau. The condition is described in Chapter 6.

TIBIAL PLATEAU FRACTURES

Mechanism of injury

Fractures of the tibial plateau are caused by a varus or valgus force combined with axial loading (a pure valgus force is more likely to rupture the ligaments). This is sometimes the result of a car striking a pedestrian (hence the term 'bumper fracture'); more often it is due to a fall from a height in which the knee is forced into valgus or varus. The tibial condyle is crushed or split by the opposing femoral condyle, which remains intact.

Pathological anatomy

The fracture pattern and degree of displacement depend on the type and direction of force as well as the quality of the bone at the upper end of the tibia. A useful classification is that of Schatzker (Fig. 30.17):

Type 1 – a vertical split of the lateral condyle This is a fracture through dense bone, usually in younger people. It may be virtually undisplaced, or the condylar fragment may be pushed inferiorly and tilted; the damaged lateral meniscus may be trapped in the crevice.

Type 2 – a vertical split of the lateral condyle combined with depression of an adjacent loadbearing part of the condyle The wedge fragment, which varies in size from a portion of the rim to a sizeable part of the lateral condyle, is displaced laterally; the joint is widened and, if the fracture is not reduced, may later develop a valgus deformity.

Type 3 – depression of the articular surface with an intact condylar rim Unlike type 2, the split to the edge of the plateau is absent. The depressed fragments may be wedged firmly into the subchondral bone. The joint is usually stable and may tolerate early movement.

Type 4 – fracture of the medial tibial condyle Two types of fracture are seen: (1) a depressed, crush fracture of osteoporotic bone in an elderly person (a low-energy lesion), and (2) a high-energy fracture resulting in a condylar split that runs obliquely from the intercondylar eminence to the medial cortex. The momentary varus angulation may be severe enough to cause a rupture of the lateral collateral ligament and a traction injury of the peroneal nerve. The severity of these injuries should not be underestimated.

Type 5 – fracture of both condyles Both condyles are split but there is a column of the metaphysis wedged in between that remains in continuity with the tibial shaft.

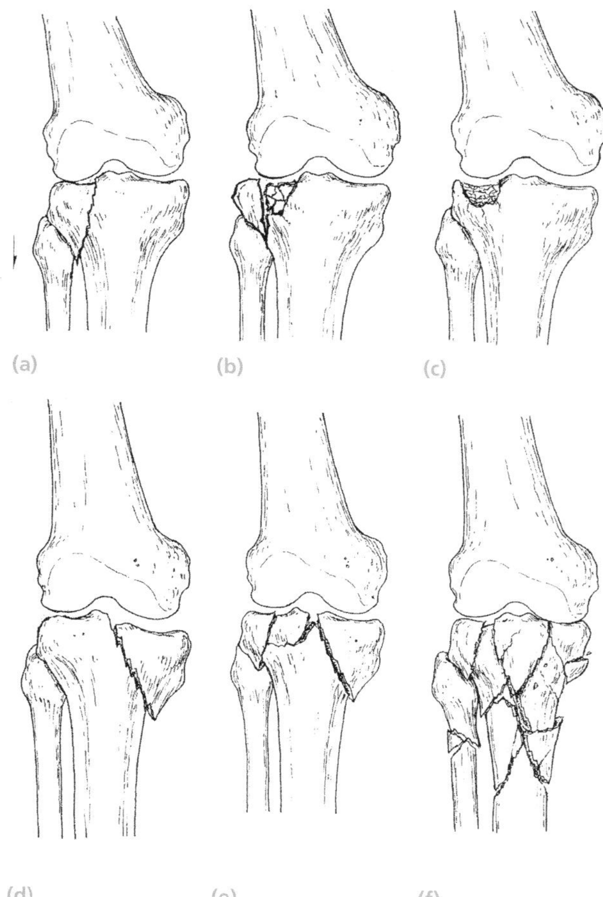

30.17 Tibial plateau fractures (a) Type 1 – simple split of the lateral condyle. (b) Type 2 – a split of the lateral condyle with a more central area of depression. (c) Type 3 – depression of the lateral condyle with an intact rim. (d) Type 4 – a fracture of the medial condyle. (e) Type 5 – fractures of both condyles, but with the central portion of the metaphysis still connected to the tibial shaft. (f) Type 6 – combined condylar and subcondylar fractures; effectively a disconnection of the shaft from the metaphysis.

Type 6 – combined condylar and subcondylar fractures This is a high-energy injury that may result in severe comminution. Unlike type 5 fractures, the tibial shaft is effectively disconnected from the tibial condyles.

Clinical features

The knee is swollen and may be deformed. Bruising is usually extensive and the tissues feel 'doughy' because of haemarthrosis. Examining the knee may suggest medial or lateral instability but this is usually painful and adds little to the x-ray diagnosis. More importantly, the leg and foot should be carefully examined for signs of vascular or neurological injury. Traction injury of the peroneal or tibial nerves is not uncommon and it is important to establish whether this is present at the time of admission and before operation.

Imaging

Anteroposterior, lateral and oblique x-rays will usually show the fracture, but the amount of comminution or plateau depression may not be appreciated without computer tomography (CT). This provides information on the location of the main fracture lines, the site and size of the portion of condyle that is depressed and the position of major parts of articular surface that have been displaced. Software-generated re-assembly of the axial images can provide sagittal and coronal views that aid in surgical planning (Fig. 30.18). It is important not to miss a posterior condylar component in high-energy fractures because this may require a separate posteromedial or posterolateral exposure for internal fixation. With a crushed lateral condyle the medial ligament is often intact, but with a crushed medial condyle the lateral ligament is often torn.

Treatment

Treatment by traction is simple and often produces a well-functioning knee, but residual angulation is not

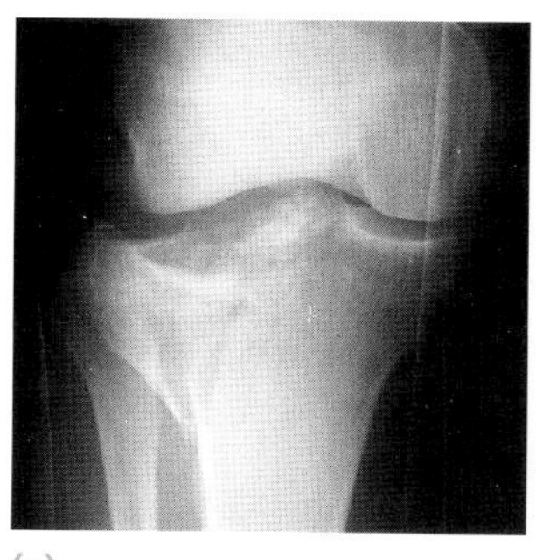
(a)

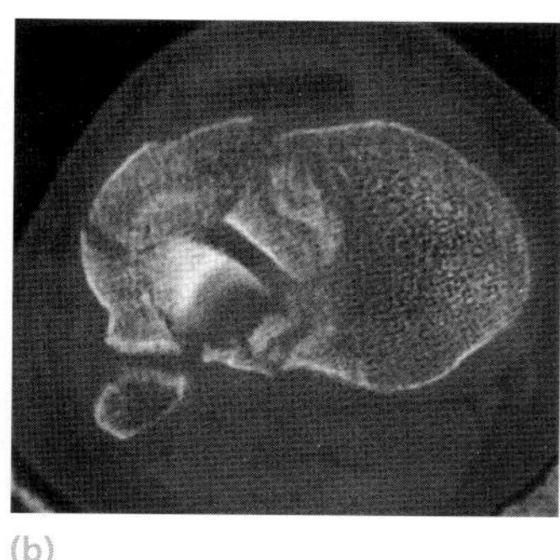
(b)

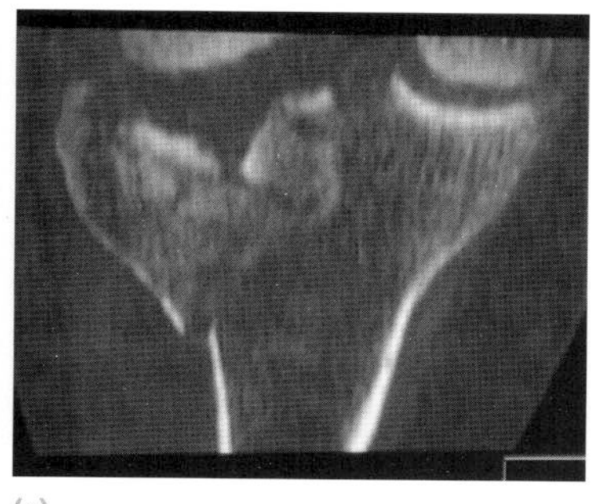
(c)

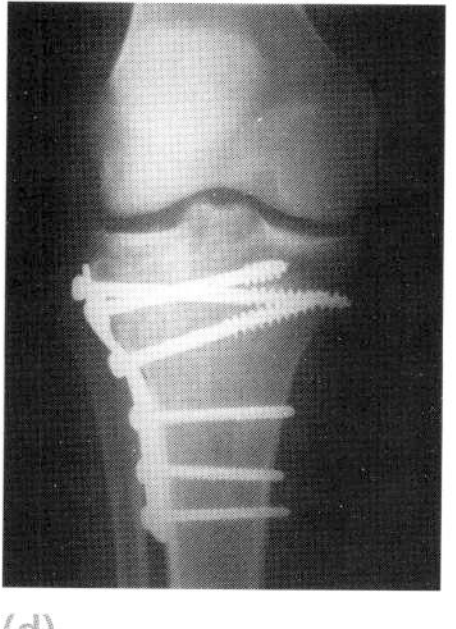
(d)

30.18 Tibial plateau fractures – imaging (a) X-rays provide information about the position of the main fracture lines and areas of articular surface depression. (b,c) CT reconstructions reveal the extent and direction of displacements, vital information for planning the operation. (d) The postoperative x-ray shows that perfect reduction has been achieved.

uncommon (Apley, 1979). On the other hand, obsessional surgery to restore the shattered surface may produce a good x-ray appearance – and a stiff knee, especially if the operation is followed by prolonged immobilization (Fig. 30.19).

Type 1 fractures Undisplaced type 1 fractures can be treated conservatively. The haemarthrosis is aspirated and a compression bandage is applied. The limb is rested on a continuous passive motion (CPM) machine and knee movements are begun. As soon as the acute pain and swelling have subsided (usually within 1 week), a hinged cast-brace is fitted and the patient is allowed up; however, weightbearing is not allowed for another 3 weeks. Thereafter, partial weightbearing is permitted but full weightbearing is delayed until the fracture has healed (usually around 8 weeks).

Displaced fractures should be treated by open reduction and internal fixation.

The condylar surface is examined and trapped fragments are released or removed. The aim is for an accurate reduction; two lag screws or a buttress plate are usually sufficient for fixation.

Type 2 fractures If depression is slight (less than 5 mm) and the knee is not unstable, or if the patient is old and frail or osteoporotic, the fracture is treated closed with the aim of regaining mobility and function rather than anatomical restitution. After aspiration and compression bandaging, skeletal traction is applied via a threaded pin passed through the tibia 7 cm below the fracture. An attempt is made to squeeze the condyle into shape; the knee is then flexed and extended several times to 'mould' the upper tibia on the opposing femoral condyle. The leg is cradled on pillows and, with 5 kg traction in place, active exercises are carried out every day. As soon as the fracture is 'sticky' (usually at 3–4 weeks), the traction pin is removed, a hinged cast-brace is applied and the patient is allowed up on crutches. Full weightbearing is deferred for another 6 weeks.

In younger patients, and more so in those with a central depression of more than 5 mm, open reduction with elevation of the plateau and internal fixation is often preferred. A midline incision offers good exposure – together with a limited transverse arthrotomy beneath the lateral meniscus; the joint is seen to allow a check on the quality of reduction. Bone graft or a similar substitute is needed to support the elevated fragments. Small 3.5 mm screws placed in parallel just beneath the subchondral bone hold up the elevated fragments well (these are sometimes referred to as 'raft' screws, describing the arrangement of parallel screws, Fig. 30.20).

Alternatively cannulated screws can be used. The wedge of lateral condyle is then fixed with a buttress plate – newer designs of contoured and angle-stable plates (using screws that lock into the plate) are available but are not always necessary – and early knee movement is encouraged after surgery (Fig. 30.21). A CPM machine can help with the regime of passive exercise to complement the active work; at 2 weeks the patient is allowed up in a cast-brace, which is retained until the fracture has united.

Type 3 fractures The principles of treatment are similar to those applying to type 2 fractures. However, the fact that the lateral rim of the condyle is intact means that the knee is usually stable and a satisfactory outcome is more predictable. The depressed fragments may need to be elevated through a window in the metaphysis; reduction should be checked by x-ray or arthroscopy. The elevated fragments are supported with bone grafts and the whole segment is fixed in position with 'raft' screws. Postoperatively, exercises are begun as soon as possible and the patient is allowed up in a cast-brace, which is retained until the fracture has united.

Type 4 fracture of the medial condyle Osteoporotic *crush fractures* of the medial plateau are difficult to reduce; in the long term the patient is likely to be left with some degree of varus deformity. The principles of treatment are the same as for type 2 fractures of the lateral plateau.

Medial condylar *split fractures* usually occur in younger people and are caused by high-energy trauma. The fracture itself is often more complex than is appreciated at first sight; there may be a second, posterior split in the coronal plane that cannot be fixed through the standard anterior approach. Good lateral x-rays or CT are needed to define the fracture pattern. There is often an underlying ligament injury on the lateral side. Stable fixation of the medial side, along the lines described for the type 2 fracture will

(a)

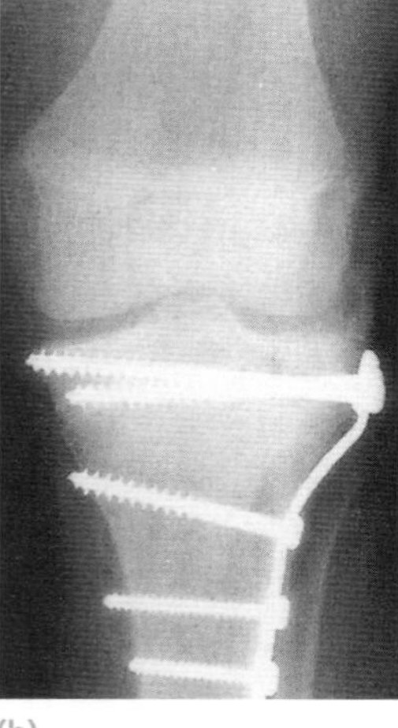

(b)

3.19 Tibial plateau fractures – fixation **(a)** Tomography showed significant depression and some lateral displacement of the lateral condyle. **(b)** Open reduction and internal fixation with a buttress plate.

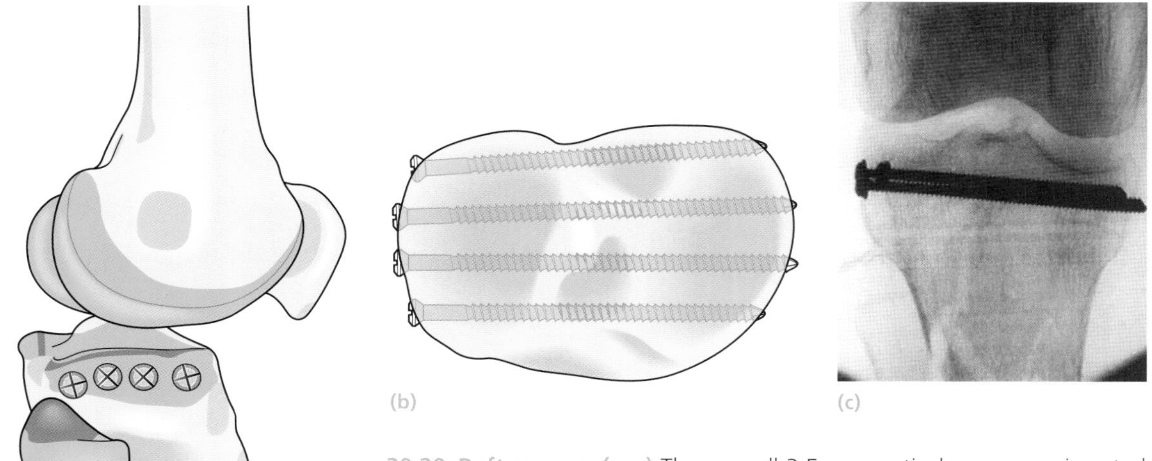

30.20 Raft screws (a–c) These small 3.5 mm cortical screws are inserted just beneath the subchondral surface and form a 'raft' above which the elevated fragments of the plateau are supported. In types 2, 5 or 6 injuries, they need to be supplemented by a buttress plate.

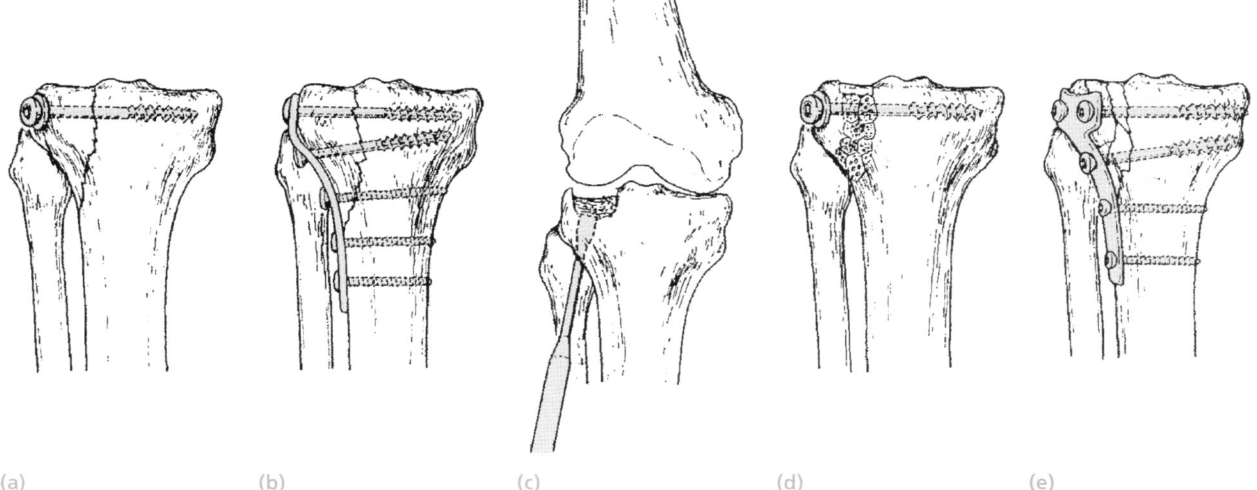

30.21 Tibial plateau fractures – fixation (a) Two or three lag screws may be sufficient for simple split fractures (type 1), though (b) a buttress plate and screws may be more secure. (c) Depression of more than 5 mm in a type 3 fracture can be treated by elevation from below and (d) supported by bone grafts and fixation. (e) Type 2 fractures require a combination of both techniques – direct reduction, elevation of depressed areas, bone grafting and buttress plate fixation.

then allow an assessment of the ligament injury. If the joint is unstable after fracture fixation, the torn structures on the lateral side may need repair.

Types 5 and 6 fractures These are severe injuries that carry the added risk of a compartment syndrome. A simple bicondylar fracture, in an elderly patient, can often be reduced by traction and the patient then treated as for a type 2 injury – some residual angulation may follow (Fig. 30.22). However, it is more usual to consider stable internal fixation and early joint movement for these injuries, but surgery is not without significant risk. The danger is that the wide exposure necessary to gain access to both condyles may strip the supporting soft tissues, thus increasing the risk of wound breakdown and delayed union or non-union.

New strategies involve spanning the knee joint with an external fixator, thereby providing provisional stability, and waiting for the soft-tissue conditions to improve – sometimes as long as 2–3 weeks. Then a double incision approach (anterior and posteromedial usually) is made, which provides access to the main fracture fragments and limits the amount of subperiosteal elevation carried out if both condyles are approached through a single anterior incision only. Buttress plates placed in a submuscular fashion are used (Fig. 30.23). An alternative method is to perform the articular reduction through a limited surgi-

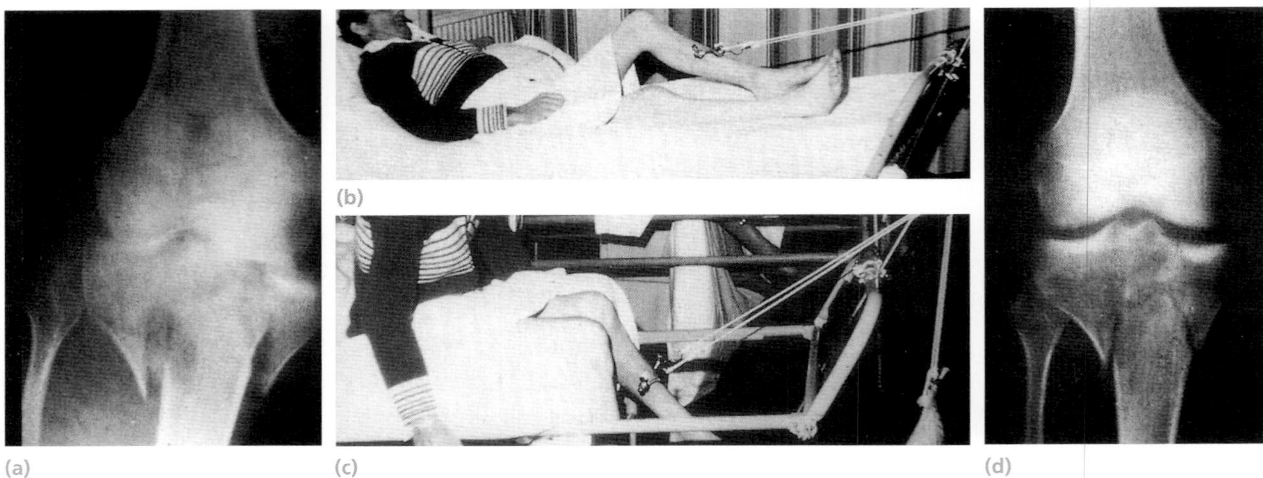

30.22 Complex plateau fractures – non-operative treatment (a) Even in this complex bicondylar fracture, non-operative treatment (b,c) with a low-traction pin makes early movement possible. (d) 10 days later the x-ray shows reasonably good reduction and the functional result was excellent.

cal exposure (this can often be done percutaneously) and to stabilize the metaphysis to the diaphysis using a circular external fixator (Fig. 30.24). This approach is less risky and can produce better results (Canadian Orthopaedic Trauma Society, 2006).

Principles in reduction and fixation Traction is used to achieve reduction; many of the fragments that have soft-tissue attachments will reduce spontaneously (*ligamentotaxis*). This is done by applying bone distractors across the knee joint or by traction on a traction table.

If open reduction is needed or intended, the operation should be carefully planned. High-quality imaging is needed to define the fracture pattern accurately. The difficulty of fixing plateau fractures should not be underestimated; operative treatment should be undertaken only if the full range of implants and the necessary expertise are available.

The standard approach to the lateral part of the joint is through a longitudinal parapatellar incision. The aim is to preserve the meniscus while fully exposing the fractured plateau; this is best done by entering the joint through a transverse capsular incision beneath the meniscus. If exposure of the medial compartment is needed, a separate posteromedial incision and approach is made. Dividing the patellar ligament in a Z-fashion – whilst giving good access across the entire joint – limits the extent of knee flexion exercises after surgery, even if the ligament is repaired.

A single large fragment may be re-positioned and held with lag screws and washers; a buttress plate is

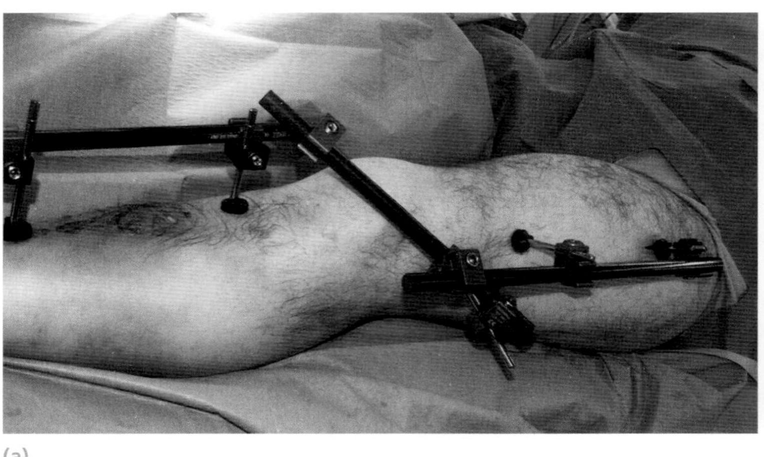

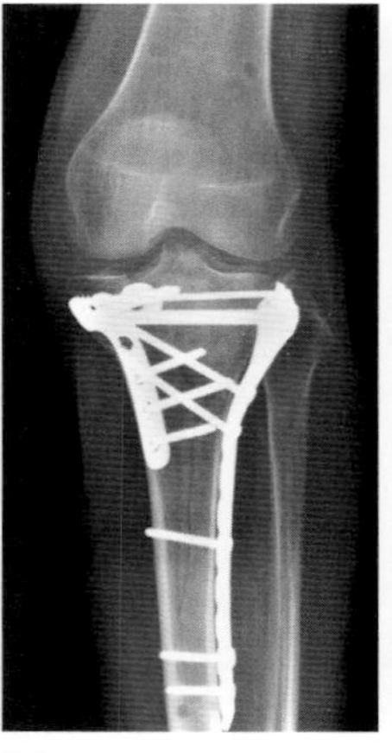

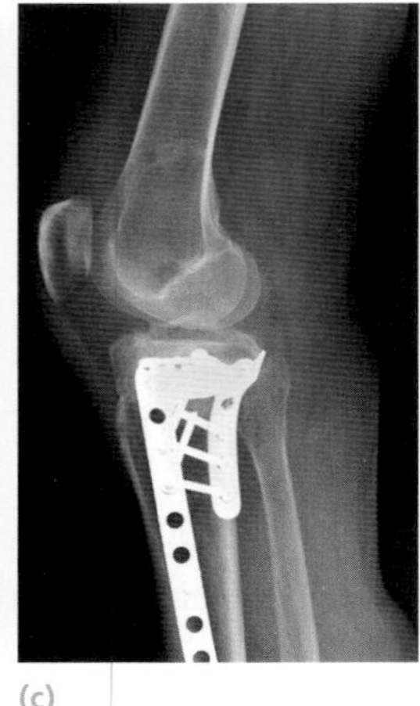

(a) (b) (c)

30.23 Complex tibial plateau fractures – internal fixation Soft tissue trauma in high-energy complex fractures of the tibial plateau usually makes it unsafe to undertake extensive open surgery early on. Provisional stabilization by a spanning external fixator allows the swelling to reduce and the patient to rest comfortably (a). When conditions improve, and this may take as long as 2 weeks, open surgery can be undertaken. In this example two buttress plates were used to shore up the lateral and posteromedial aspects of the tibial plateau (b,c).

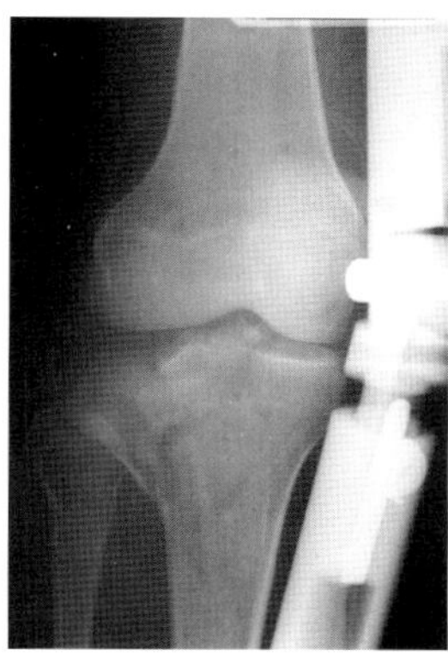
(a)

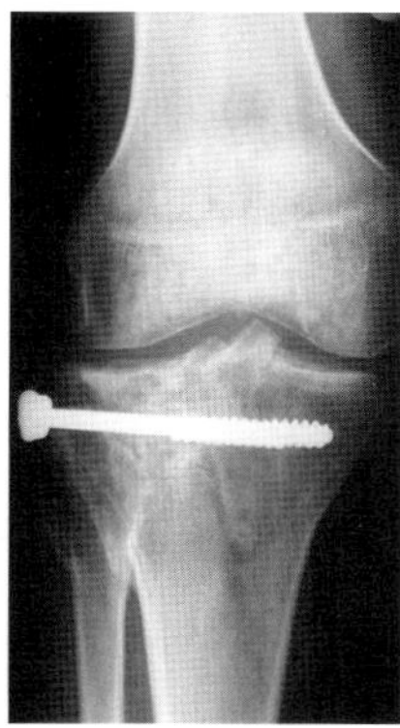
(b)

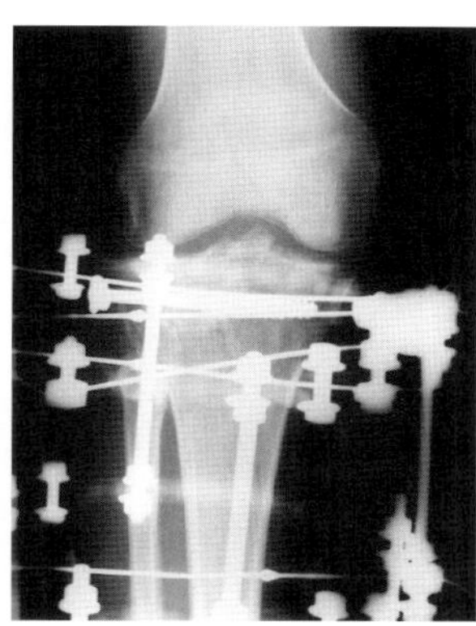
(c)

30.24 Complex tibial plateau fractures – external fixation Rather than expose the joint formally in order to reduce the fracture, this can be done percutaneously, albeit with x-ray control, and the articular fragments held with multiple screws (a,b). The tibial metaphysis is then held to the shaft using a circular external fixator (c).

added for security. Comminuted, depressed fractures must be elevated by pushing the fragmented mass upwards from below; the osteoarticular surface is then supported by packing the subchondral area with cortico-cancellous grafts (obtained from the iliac crest) and held in place by inserting 'raft' screws and a suitably contoured buttress plate. Unless it is torn, the meniscus should be preserved and sutured back in place when the capsule is repaired.

Displaced fractures with splits in both the sagittal and the coronal plane may be impossible to reduce and fix through the anterior approach; a second, posteromedial or posterolateral approach is the answer.

Extensive exposure and manipulation of highly comminuted fractures can sometimes be self-defeating. These injuries may be better treated by percutaneous manipulation of the fragments (under traction) and circular-frame external fixation.

Stability is all-important; no matter which method is used, fixation must be secure enough to permit early joint movement. There is little point in ending up with a pleasing x-ray and a stiff knee.

Postoperatively the limb is elevated and splinted until swelling subsides; movements are begun as soon as possible and active exercises are encouraged. The patient is allowed up as swelling subsides, and at the end of 6 weeks the patient can partial weightbear with crutches; full weightbearing is resumed when healing is complete, usually after 12–16 weeks.

Complications

EARLY

Compartment syndrome – With closed types 4 and 5 fractures there is considerable bleeding and swelling of the leg – and a risk of developing a compartment syndrome. The leg and foot should be examined repeatedly for signs.

LATE

Joint stiffness With severely comminuted fractures, and after complex operations, there is a considerable risk of developing a stiff knee. This is prevented by avoiding prolonged immobilization and encouraging movement as early as possible.

Deformity Some residual valgus or varus deformity is quite common – either because the fracture was incompletely reduced or because, although adequately reduced, the fracture became re-displaced during treatment. Fortunately, moderate deformity is compatible with good function, although constant overloading of one compartment may predispose to osteoarthritis in later life.

Osteoarthritis If, at the end of treatment, there is marked depression of the plateau, or deformity of the knee or ligamentous instability, secondary osteoarthritis is likely to develop after 5 or 10 years. This may eventually require reconstructive surgery.

FRACTURE-SEPARATION OF PROXIMAL TIBIAL EPIPHYSIS

This uncommon injury is usually caused by a severe hyperextension and valgus strain. The epiphysis displaces forwards and laterally, often taking a small fragment of the metaphysis with it (a Salter–Harris type 2 injury). There is a risk of popliteal artery damage where the vessel is stretched across the step at the back of the tibia.

Clinical features

The knee is tensely swollen and extremely tender. If the epiphysis is displaced, there may be a valgus or hyperextension deformity. All movements are resisted. The swelling may extend into the calf and a careful watch for compartment syndrome, particularly if the fracture was caused by hyperextension, is important.

X-ray Salter–Harris type 1 and 2 injuries may be undisplaced and difficult to define on x-ray; a few small bone fragments near the epiphysis may be the only clue. In the more serious injuries the entire upper tibial epiphysis may be tilted forwards or sideways. The fracture is categorized by the direction of displacement, so there are hyperextension, flexion, varus or valgus types.

Treatment

Under anaesthesia, closed manipulative reduction can usually be achieved. The direction of tilt may suggest the mechanism of injury; the fragment can be reduced by gentle traction and manipulation in a direction opposite to that of the fracturing force. Fixation using smooth K-wires or screws may be needed if the fracture is unstable. Occasionally, when the entire tibial epiphysis cannot be accurately reduced by closed manipulation, it is repositioned at operation and held by a screw (Figure 30.25). The rare Salter–Harris type 3 or 4 fractures also may need open reduction and fixation.

Following reduction, whether closed or open, a long-leg cast is applied. For the usual hyperextension injury the knee is held flexed at 30 degrees; for the less common flexion and varus injuries the knee is kept straight. The cast is worn for 6–8 weeks, with partial weightbearing from the outset. Knee movement quickly returns when the cast is removed.

Complications

Epiphyseal fractures in young children sometimes result in angular *deformity* of the proximal tibia. This may later require operative correction.

With the higher grades of injury there is a risk of complete *growth arrest* at the proximal tibia. If the predicted leg length discrepancy is greater than 2.5 cm, tibial lengthening (or epiphyseodesis of the opposite limb) may be needed.

FRACTURE OF PROXIMAL END OF FIBULA

Fracture of the proximal end of the fibula may be caused by either direct injury or an indirect twisting injury of the lower limb. *Beware:* an isolated fracture of the proximal fibula is rare; it may be merely the most visible part of a more extensive rotational injury of the leg involving a serious fracture or ligament injury of the ankle (the Maisonneuve fracture) or a major disruption of the posterolateral corner of the knee. *Always x-ray the ankle and check for knee stability!*

The fracture itself is of little consequence and it requires no treatment. However, associated injuries are frequent and they may result in prolonged disability.

Complications

Associated injuries Associated lesions, which should be looked for in every case, are: (1) the ankle injury mentioned earlier; (2) peroneal nerve injury; (3) lateral collateral ligament injury – more usually a disruption of this ligament and the posterolateral corner – especially if the fibula styloid is avulsed; (4) peroneal nerve entrapment – an occasional late complication. Each of these conditions requires specific treatment.

DISLOCATION OF PROXIMAL TIBIO-FIBULAR JOINT

A blow or twisting injury may cause subluxation or dislocation of the proximal tibio-fibular joint. Isolated injuries are rare; they usually occur in parachuting or

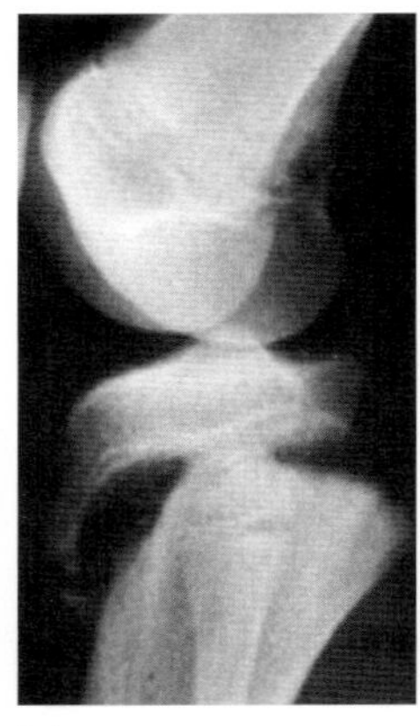
(a)

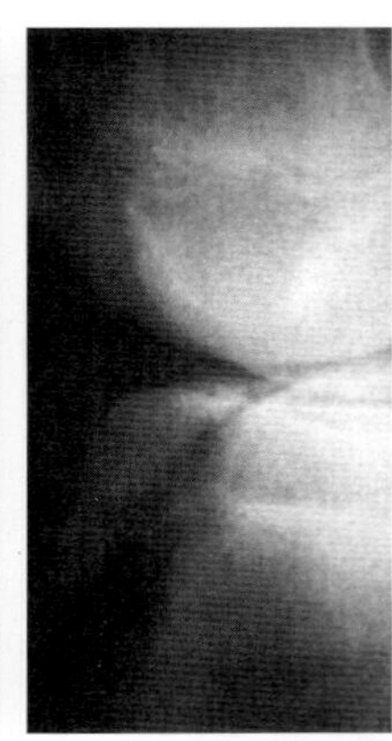
(b)

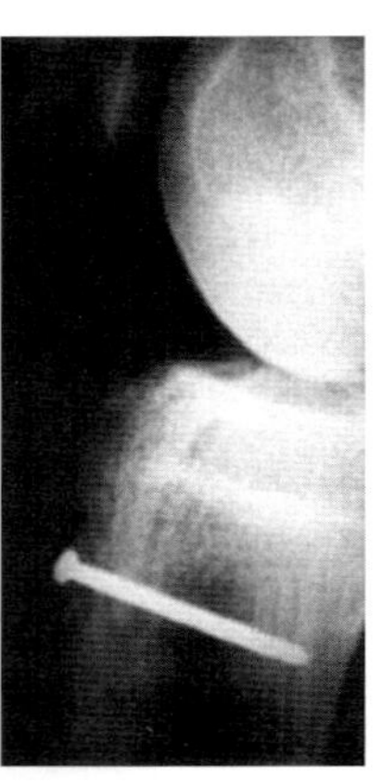
(c)

30.25 Fracture-separation of proximal tibial epiphysis (a) This hyperextension type of fracture needs urgent reduction because the popliteal vessels are endangered. (b) A flexion type of fracture-separation, but essentially a Salter–Harris type 4 pattern; in this case reduction was held with internal fixation (c).

similar activities. Occasionally the condition is habitual and associated with generalized ligamentous laxity.

The fibular head displaces upwards, and either anterolaterally or posteromedially. There is usually pain and local tenderness; the abnormal contour over the lateral aspect of the knee is best seen when the two knees are flexed to 90 degrees on the examination couch. Always check for peroneal nerve injury.

X-ray In the normal anteroposterior x-ray of the knee the fibular head overlaps the lateral tibial condyle; in a dislocation the fibular head stands clear of the tibia, and in the lateral view the fibular head is displaced either forwards or backwards.

Manual reduction is carried out by flexing the knee to 90 degrees (to relax the lateral collateral ligament) and pressing upon the fibular head; reductions are usually stable and a plaster cylinder is applied for 4 weeks. Recurrent subluxation may call for excision of the fibular head.

FRACTURES OF TIBIA AND FIBULA

Because of its subcutaneous position, the tibia is more commonly fractured, and more often sustains an open fracture, than any other long bone.

Mechanism of injury

A twisting force causes a spiral fracture of both leg bones at different levels; an angulatory force produces transverse or short oblique fractures, usually at the same level.

Indirect injury is usually low energy; with a spiral or long oblique fracture one of the bone fragments may pierce the skin from within.

Direct injury crushes or splits the skin over the fracture; this is usually a high-energy injury and the most common cause is a motorcycle accident.

Pathological anatomy

The behaviour of these injuries – and therefore the choice of treatment – depends on the following factors:

1. *The state of the soft tissues* – The risk of complications and the progress to fracture healing are directly related to the amount and type of soft-tissue damage. Closed fractures are best described using Tscherne's (Oestern and Tscherne, 1984) method; for open injuries, Gustilo's grading (Table 30.2) is more useful (Gustilo et al., 1984). The incidence of tissue breakdown and/or infection ranges from 1 per cent for Gustilo type I to 30 per cent for type IIIC.
2. *The severity of the bone injury* – High-energy fractures are more damaging and take longer to heal than low-energy fractures; this is regardless of whether the fracture is open or closed. Low-energy breaks are typically closed or Gustilo I or II, and spiral. High-energy fractures are usually caused by direct trauma and tend to be open (Gustilo III A–C), transverse or comminuted.
3. *Stability of the fracture* – Consider whether it will displace if weightbearing is allowed. Long oblique fractures tend to shorten; those with a butterfly fragment tend to angulate towards the butterfly. Severely comminuted fractures are the least stable of all, and the most likely to need mechanical fixation.
4. *Degree of contamination* – In open fractures this is an important additional variable.

TSCHERNE'S CLASSIFICATION OF SKIN LESIONS IN CLOSED FRACTURES

IC1	No skin lesion
IC2	No skin laceration but contusion
IC3	Circumscribed degloving
IC4	Extensive, closed degloving
IC5	Necrosis from contusion

Clinical features

The limb should be carefully examined for signs of soft-tissue damage: bruising, severe swelling, crushing or tenting of the skin, an open wound, circulatory

Table 30.2 Gustilo's classification of open fractures

Grade	Wound	Soft-tissue injury	Bone injury
I	<1 cm long	Minimal	Simple low-energy fractures
II	>1 cm long	Moderate, some muscle damage	Moderate comminution
IIIA	Usually >1 cm long	Severe deep contusion; + compartment syndrome	High-energy fracture patterns; comminuted but soft-tissue cover possible
IIIB	Usually >10 cm long	Severe loss of soft-tissue cover	Requires soft-tissue reconstruction for cover
IIIC	Usually >10 cm long	As IIIB, with need for vascular repair	Requires soft-tissue reconstruction for cover

changes, weak or absent pulses, diminution or loss of sensation and inability to move the toes. Any deformity should be noted before splinting the limb. *Always be on the alert for signs of an impending compartment syndrome.*

X-ray The entire length of the tibia and fibula, as well as the knee and ankle joints, must be seen. The type of fracture, its level and the degree of angulation and displacement are recorded. Rotational deformity can be gauged by comparing the width of the tibio-fibular interspace above and below the fracture.

Spiral fractures without comminution are low-energy injuries. Transverse, short oblique and comminuted fractures, especially if displaced or associated with a fibular fracture at a similar level, are high-energy injuries.

Management

The main objectives are: (1) to limit soft-tissue damage and preserve (or restore, in the case of open fractures) skin cover; (2) to prevent – or at least recognize – a compartment syndrome; (3) to obtain and hold fracture alignment; (4) to start early weightbearing (loading promotes healing); (5) to start joint movements as soon as possible.

The first step is to gain a clear idea of the character of the injury – what some have called the 'fracture personality' – which is a combination of the soft tissue condition and fracture pattern. Uncomminuted, spiral fractures with minimal soft-tissue damage (including open injuries like Gustilo I) are likely to heal with a minimum of trouble; they can be treated conservatively unless there is a definite indication for surgery (see later). Fractures associated with severe soft-tissue damage (whether open or closed) and unstable fracture patterns need much more careful attention if complications are to be avoided.

LOW-ENERGY FRACTURES

Most low-energy fractures, including Gustilo I injuries after attention to the wounds, can be treated by non-operative methods.

If the fracture is *undisplaced or minimally displaced*, a full-length cast from upper thigh to metatarsal necks is applied with the knee slightly flexed and the ankle at a right angle (Fig. 30.26). Displacement of the fibular fracture, unless it involves the ankle joint, is unimportant and can be ignored.

If the fracture is *displaced*, it is reduced under general anaesthesia with x-ray control. Apposition need not be complete but alignment must be near-perfect (no more than 7 degrees of angulation) and rotation absolutely perfect. A full-length cast is applied as for undisplaced fractures (note, however, that if placing the ankle at 0 degrees causes the fracture to displace, a few degrees of equinus are acceptable). The position is checked by x-ray; minor degrees of angulation can still be corrected by making a transverse cut in the plaster and wedging it into a better position.

The limb is elevated and the patient is kept under

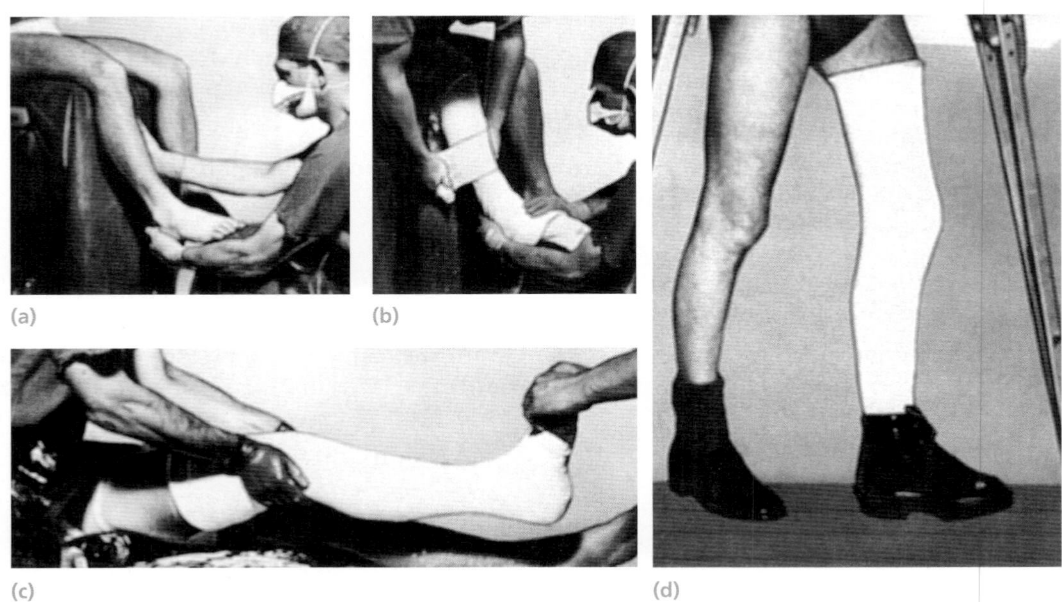

30.26 Fractured tibia and fibula – closed treatment (1) Reduction is facilitated by bending the knee over the end of the table, with the normal leg alongside for comparison (a). The surgeon holds the position while an assistant applies plaster from the knee downwards (b). When the plaster has set, the leg is lifted and the above-knee plaster completed (c); note that the foot is plantigrade, the knee slightly bent, and the plaster moulded round the patella. A rockered boot is fitted for walking (d).

observation for 48–72 hours. If there is excessive swelling, the cast is split. Patients are usually allowed up (and home) on the second or third day, bearing minimal weight with the aid of crutches. The immediate application of plaster may be unwise if skin viability is doubtful, in which case a few days on skeletal traction is useful as a preliminary measure (Fig. 30.27).

After 2 weeks the position is checked by x-ray. A change from an above- to a below-the-knee cast is possible around 4–6 weeks, when the fracture becomes 'sticky'. The cast is retained (or renewed if it becomes loose) until the fracture unites, which is around 8 weeks in children but seldom under 12 weeks in adults.

Exercise From the start, the patient is taught to exercise the muscles of the foot, ankle and knee. When he gets up, an overboot with a rocker sole is fitted and he is taught to walk correctly. When the plaster is removed, a crepe bandage or elasticated support is applied and the patient is told that he may either elevate and exercise the limb or walk correctly on it, but he must not let it dangle idly.

Functional bracing With stable fractures the full-length cast may be changed after 4–6 weeks to a functional below-knee brace that is carefully moulded to bear upon the upper tibia and patellar tendon. This liberates the knee and allows full weightbearing (Sarmiento and Latta, 2006). A snug fit is important and the fastening straps will need to be tightened as the swelling subsides.

Indications for skeletal fixation If follow-up x-rays show unsatisfactory fracture alignment, and wedging fails to correct this, the plaster is abandoned and the fracture is reduced and fixed at surgery. Indeed, many surgeons would hold that unstable fractures are better treated by skeletal fixation from the outset.

Closed intramedullary nailing This is the method of choice for internal fixation. The fracture is reduced under x-ray control and image intensification. The proximal end of the tibia is exposed; a guide-wire is passed down the medullary canal and the canal is reamed. A nail of appropriate size and shape is then introduced from the proximal end across the fracture site. Transverse locking screws are inserted at the proximal and distal ends (Fig. 30.28). Postoperatively, partial weightbearing is started as soon as possible, progressing to full weightbearing when this is comfortable.

For diaphyseal fractures, union can be expected in over 95 per cent of cases. However, the method is less suitable for fractures near the bone ends.

Plate fixation Plating is best for metaphyseal fractures that are unsuitable for nailing. It is also sometimes used for unstable tibial shaft fractures in children. Previously, the disadvantages of plate fixation included the need to expose the fracture site and, in so doing, stripping the soft tissues around the fracture. This may increase the risk of introducing infection and delaying union. Newer techniques of plating overcome these disadvantages. The plate is slid across the fracture through proximal and distal 'access incisions' on the anterolateral aspect of the tibia and then fixed to the bone *only at these levels*. This method of 'submuscular' plating preserves the soft tissues around the fracture site better than conventional open plating, and provides a relative stability that appears to hasten

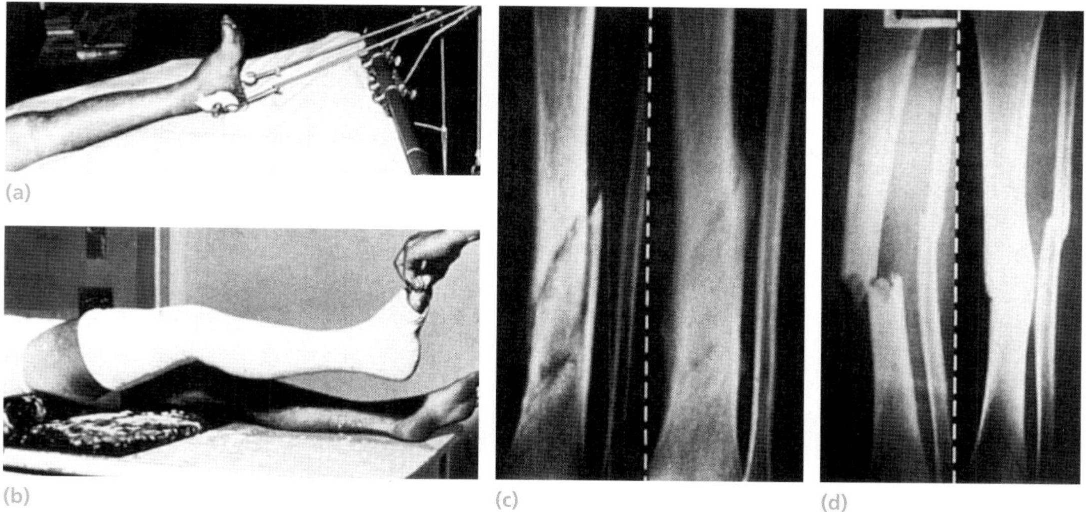

30.27 Fractured tibia and fibula – closed treatment (2) (a) Skeletal traction is used to reduce overlap, and also as provisional treatment when skin viability is doubtful. Plaster is applied 10–14 days later (b), using the technique shown in Figure 30.26, except that the skeletal pin is retained until the plaster has set. Examples of spiral and transverse fractures treated in this way are shown in (c) and (d).

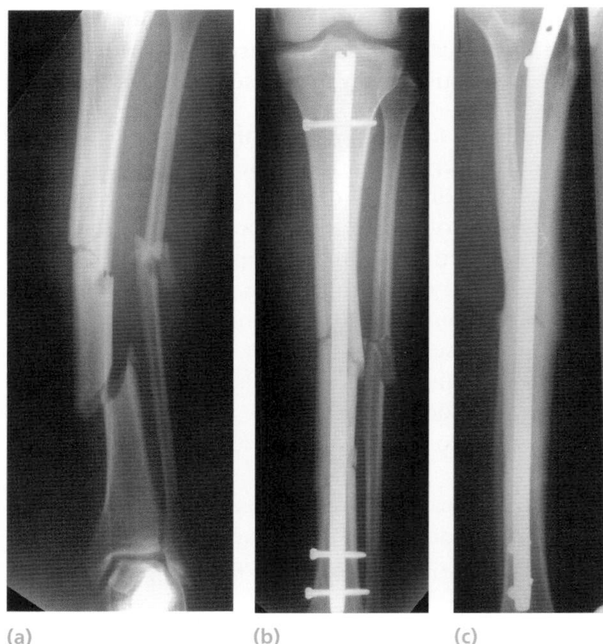

(a) (b) (c)

30.28 Fractured tibia and fibula – intramedullary nailing Closed intramedullary nailing is now the preferred treatment for unstable tibial fractures. This series of x-rays shows the fracture before (a) and after (b,c) nailing. Active movements and partial weightbearing were started soon after operation.

union. Even so, full weightbearing will need to be deferred until some callus formation is evident on x-ray, usually at 6–8 weeks.

External fixation This is an alternative to closed nailing; it avoids exposure of the fracture site and allows further adjustments to be made if this should be needed. Partial weightbearing is permitted from the start and the external fixator can be replaced by a functional brace once there are signs of union (although, with modern fixators, this is usually unnecessary because fracture loading can be controlled and adjusted in the fixator).

HIGH-ENERGY FRACTURES

Initially, the most important consideration is the viability of the damaged soft tissues and underlying bone. Tissues around the fracture should be disturbed as little as possible and open operations should be avoided unless there is already an open wound.

Transverse fractures are usually stable after reduction; they can be treated 'closed', provided a careful watch is kept for symptoms and signs of complications (excessive pain, swelling, tightness or sensory change).

Comminuted and segmental fractures, those associated with bone loss, and indeed any high-energy fracture that is inherently unstable, require early surgical stabilization. For closed fractures, external fixation and closed nailing are equally suitable; in both cases the tissues around the fracture are left undisturbed (Fig. 30.29). For open fractures, the use of internal fixation has to be accompanied by judicious and expert debridement and prompt cover of the exposed bone and implant; alternatively, external fixation can be safer if these pre-requisites cannot be met.

In cases of bone loss, small defects can be treated by delayed bone grafting; larger defects will need either bone transport or compression-distraction (acute shortening to close the defect, with subsequent lengthening at a different level) with an external fixator (Chapter 12).

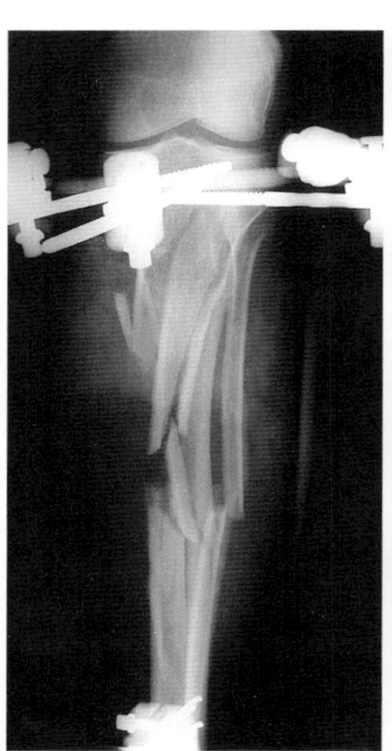

(a)

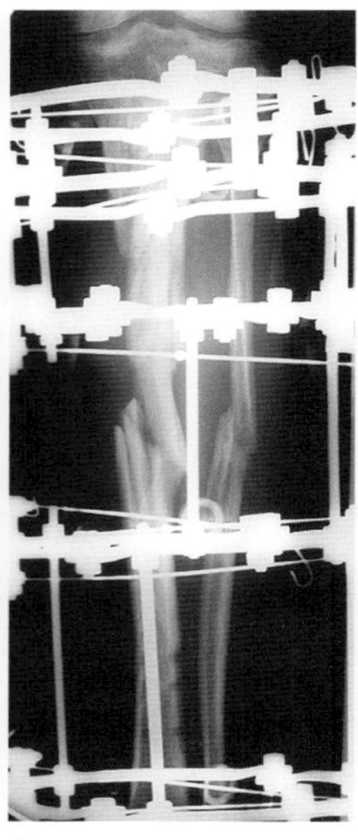

(b)

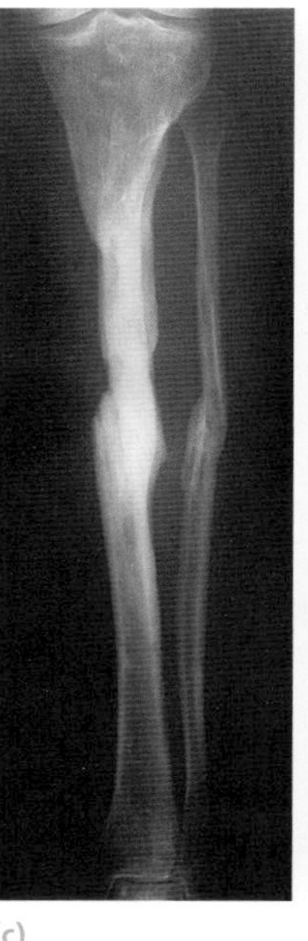

(c)

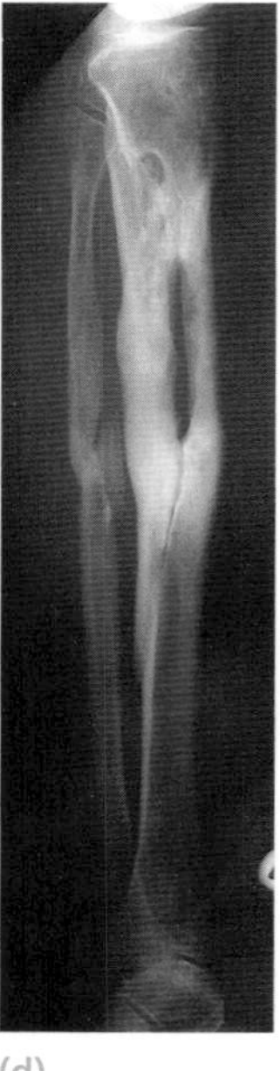

(d)

30.29 Fixation (a–d) This method of fixation offers the benefit of multilevel stability and can be carried out with little additional damage to the soft tissues around the injury.

OPEN FRACTURES

A suitable mantra for the treatment of open tibial fractures is:

- antibiotics
- debridement
- stabilization
- prompt soft-tissue cover
- rehabilitation.

Antibiotics are started immediately. A first- or second-generation cephalosporin is suitable for Gustilo grades I–IIIA wounds but more severe grades may benefit from Gram-negative cover as well (an aminoglycoside such as gentamicin is often used). With an adequate debridement, the antibiotics are continued for 24 hours in a grade 1 fracture and 72 hours in more severe grades. However, the evidence for prolonged antibiotic use is lacking and, not surprisingly, most infections from delayed closure of open tibial wounds tend to be by nosocomial hospital-acquired bacteria. These can be multiresistant organisms that are not covered by standard antibiotics, thus good debridement of the fracture and prompt cover remain the strongest defence against infection.

The wound should be photographed on first inspection in the emergency department using a Polaroid or digital camera, and then covered with a sterile dressing. The photograph can then be printed for inclusion in the patient's case notes to serve as a record and prevent further disturbance to the wound.

Adequate debridement is possible only if the original wound is extended. However, excise as little skin as possible and discuss wound extensions with a plastic surgeon, especially if there appears to be a need for local or free skin or muscle flaps. Ideally the debridement should be performed jointly with the plastic surgeon. All dead and foreign material is removed; this includes bone without significant soft-tissue attachments. Tissue of doubtful viability may be left for a second look in 48 hours. The wound and fracture site are then washed out with large quantities of normal saline.

Gustilo grade I injuries can be closed primarily – being a low-energy injury with a small wound, closure should be possible without skin tension – and the fracture then treated as for closed injuries. More severe wounds should, ideally, be closed at primary surgery as long as the debridement has been thorough and the skills of a plastic surgeon are at hand. If there is tissue of doubtful viability that requires another look, or a local flap cover deemed to be inappropriate, a second planned operation is needed. This allows further debridement and, hopefully, sufficient time to plan cover by free tissue transfer. Temporary cover of the exposed bone by using antibiotic beads sealed with an impervious plastic film can help reduce bacterial colonization. In general the aim should be to close the wound in the first 3–5 days.

It is important to stabilize the fracture. For Gustilo I, II and IIIA injuries, locked intramedullary nailing is permissible as definitive wound cover is usually possible at the time of debridement. For more severe grades of open tibial fracture, internal fixation should be performed only at the time of definitive soft tissue cover. If this is not feasible at the time of primary debridement, the fracture should be stabilized temporarily with a spanning external fixator. Exchange of the fixator for an intramedullary nail can be done at the point when definitive soft tissue cover is carried out – ideally within 5 days of the injury. Alternatively, definitive fracture management can be carried out using external fixation.

Severe grades of open fractures should, whenever possible, be managed from the outset under the combined care of an orthopaedic surgeon and a plastic surgeon.

Postoperative management

Swelling is common after tibial fractures; even after skeletal fixation the soft tissues continue to swell for several days. The limb should be elevated and frequent checks made for signs of compartment syndrome (see later).

After intramedullary nailing of a transverse or short oblique fracture, weightbearing can be started within a few days and increased to full weight when this is comfortable. If the fracture is comminuted or segmental, meaning that almost the entire load will be taken by the nail initially, only partial weightbearing is permitted until some callus is seen on x-ray.

With plate fixation, additional support with a cast may be needed if partial weightbearing is to start soon after surgery; otherwise weightbearing is delayed for 6 weeks. Unlike fractures treated with intramedullary nails, callus formation is not seen as rapidly and this may give a poor signal for increasing the amount of weightbearing.

Patients with fractures stabilized with external fixators can usually weightbear early unless there is major bone loss. Weightbearing through the fractured tibia is increased when callus is visible on x-ray; the fixator is later 'dynamized' to allow greater load transfer through the bone and help the callus bridge to mature. This does away with the need for exchanging the external fixator for a functional brace. However, if the pin sites are in poor condition or there is loosening of the hold on the tibia, a change to functional bracing is helpful.

Early complications

VASCULAR INJURY

Fractures of the proximal half of the tibia may damage the popliteal artery. This is an emergency of the first order, requiring exploration and repair. Damage to one of the two major tibial vessels may also occur and go unnoticed if there is no critical ischaemia.

COMPARTMENT SYNDROME

Tibial fractures – both open and closed – are among the commonest causes of compartment syndrome in the leg. The combination of tissue oedema and bleeding (oozing) causes swelling in the muscle compartments and this may precipitate ischaemia. Additional risk factors are proximal tibial fractures, severe crush injury, a long ischaemic period before revascularization (in type IIIC open fractures), a long delay to treatment, haemorrhagic shock, difficult and prolonged operation and a fracture fixed in distraction.

The diagnosis is usually suspected on clinical grounds. Warning symptoms are increasing pain, a feeling of tightness or 'bursting' in the leg and numbness in the leg or foot. These complaints should always be taken seriously and followed by careful and repeated examination for pain provoked by muscle stretching and loss of sensibility and/or muscle strength.

Heightened awareness is all! The diagnosis can be confirmed by measuring the compartment pressures in the leg. Indeed, so important is the need for early diagnosis that some surgeons advocate the use of continuous compartment pressure monitoring for *all* tibial fractures (McQueen et al., 1996). This deals admirably with patients who are unconscious or uncooperative, and those with multiple injuries. It also serves as an 'early warning system' in less problematic cases. A split-tip 20-gauge catheter is introduced into the anterior compartment of the leg and the pressure is measured close to the level of the fracture (Heckman et al., 1994). A differential pressure (ΔP) – the difference between diastolic pressure and compartment pressure – of less than 30 mmHg (4.00 kPA) is regarded as critical and an indication for compartment decompression. Ideally the pressure should be measured in all four compartments but this is often impractical; however, if the clinical features suggest a compartment syndrome and the anterior compartment pressure is normal or borderline, pressures should be measured in the other compartments.

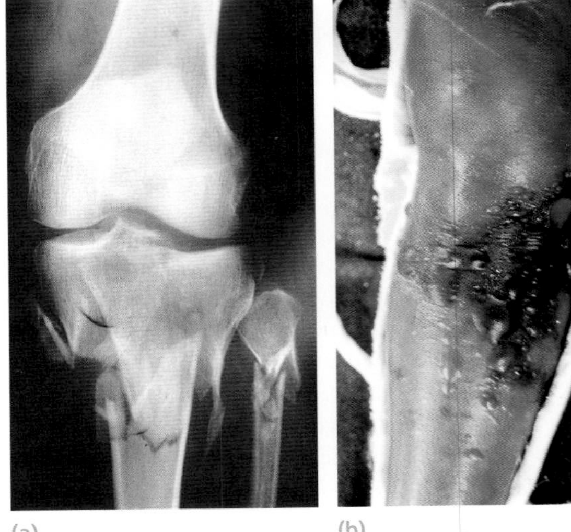

(a) (b)

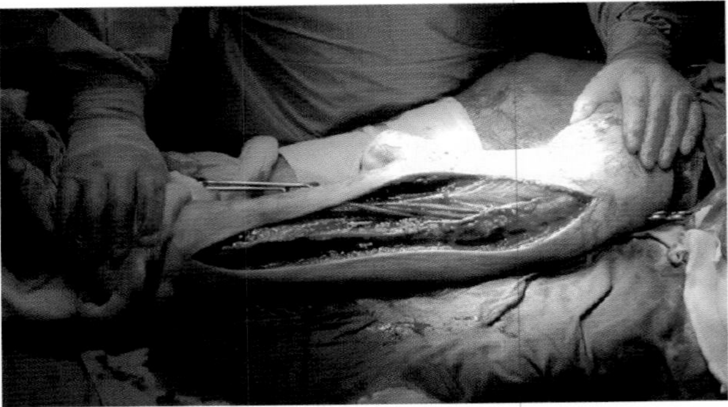

(c)

30.30 Compartment syndrome (a) With a fracture at this level the surgeon should be constantly on the alert for symptoms and signs of a compartment syndrome. This patient was treated in plaster. Pain became intense and when the plaster was split (which should have been done immediately after its application), the leg was swollen and blistered (b). Tibial compartment decompression (c) requires fasciotomies of all the compartments in the leg.

Fasciotomy and decompression Once the diagnosis is made, decompression should be carried out with the minimum delay – *and that means decompression of all four compartments at the first operation.* This is best and most safely accomplished through two incisions, one anterolateral and one posteromedial. The anterolateral incision is made about 2–3 cm lateral to the crest of the tibia and extends from the level of the tibial tuberosity to just above the ankle (Fig. 30.30). The fascia is split along the length of the anterior and lateral compartments taking care not to damage the superficial peroneal nerve. A second, similar incision is made just posterior to the posteromedial border of the tibia; the fascial covering of the superficial posterior compartment is split. The deep posterior compartment is identified just above the ankle (where its fascial covering is absent) and traced proximally; the muscle bulk of the superficial compartment needs to be retracted posteriorly, exposing the fascial envelope of the deep posterior compartment, which is likewise split down its entire length. Segmental arteries that perforate the fascia from the posterior tibial artery should be preserved for possible use in local skin flaps (Fig. 30.31). The incisions are left open, a well-padded dressing is applied and the leg is splinted with the ankle in the neutral position. The fracture is treated as a grade III open injury requiring a spanning external fixator and prompt return for wound closure or skin grafting.

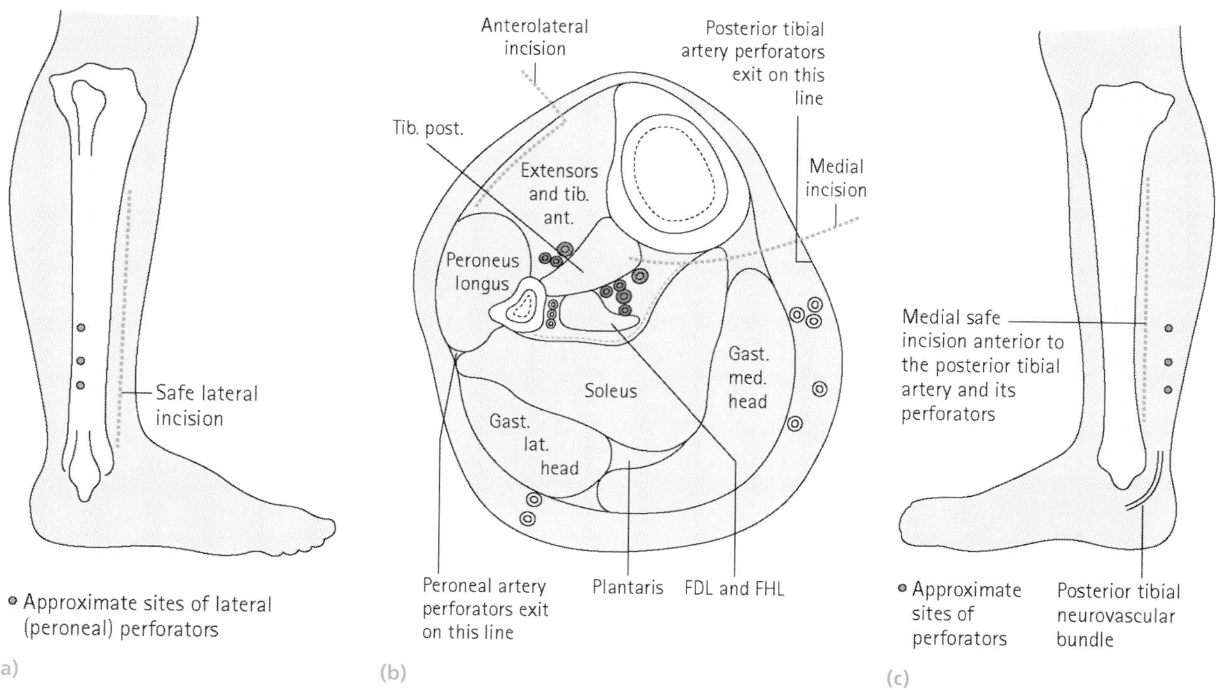

30.31 Fasciotomies for compartment decompression (a) The first incision is usually anterolateral, giving access to the anterior and lateral compartments. *But this is not enough.* The superficial and deep posterior compartments also must be opened; their position is shown in (b), a cross-section of the leg. This requires a second incision (b,c), which is made a finger's breadth behind the posteromedial border of the tibia; care must be taken not to damage the deep perforators of the posterior tibial artery. Note that the two incisions should be placed at least 7 cm apart so as to ensure a sufficient skin bridge without risk of sloughing.

Outcome Compartment decompression within 6 hours of the onset of symptoms (or critical pressure measurement) should result in full recovery. Delayed decompression carries the risk of permanent dysfunction, the extent of which varies from mild sensory and motor loss to severe muscle and nerve damage, joint contractures and trophic changes in the foot.

INFECTION

Open fractures are always at risk; even a small perforation should be treated with respect and debridement carried out before the wound is closed.

If the diagnosis is suspected, wound swabs and blood samples should be taken and antibiotic treatment started forthwith, using a 'best guess' intravenous preparation; once the laboratory results are obtained, a more suitable antibiotic may be substituted.

With established infection, skeletal fixation should not be abandoned if the system is stable; infection control and fracture union are more likely if fixation is secure. However, if there is a loose implant it should be removed and replaced by external fixation.

Late complications

Malunion Slight shortening (up to 1.5 cm) is usually of little consequence, but rotation and angulation deformity, apart from being unsightly, can be disabling because the knee and ankle no longer move in the same plane.

Angulation should be prevented at all stages; anything more than 7 degrees in either plane is unacceptable. Angulation in the sagittal plane, especially if accompanied by a stiff equinus ankle, produces a marked increase in sheer forces at the fracture site during walking; this may result in either refracture or non-union.

Varus or valgus angulation will alter the axis of loading through the knee or ankle, causing increased stress in some part of the joint. This is often cited as a cause of secondary osteoarthritis; however while this may be true for angular deformities close to the joint, long-term studies have failed to show that it applies to moderate deformities in the middle third of the bone.

Rotational alignment should be near-perfect (as compared with the opposite leg). This may be difficult to achieve with closed methods, but it should be possible with locked intramedullary nailing.

Late deformity, if marked, should be corrected by tibial osteotomy.

Delayed union High-energy fractures are slow to unite and liable to non-union or fatigue failure if a nail has been used. If there is insufficient contact at the fracture site, either through bone loss or comminution, 'prophylactic' bone grafting as soon as the soft tissues have healed is recommended (Watson, 1994). If there is a failure of union to progress on x-ray by 6 months, secondary intervention should be considered. The first nail is removed, the canal reamed and a larger nail re-inserted. If the fibula has united before the tibia, it should be osteotomized so as to allow better apposition and compression of the tibial fragments.

Non-union This may follow bone loss or deep infection, but a common cause is faulty treatment. Either the risks and consequences of delayed union have not been recognized, or splintage has been discontinued too soon, or the patient with a recently united fracture has walked with a stiff equinus ankle.

Hypertrophic non-union can be treated by intramedullary nailing (or exchange nailing) or compression plating. Atrophic non-union needs bone grafting in addition. If the fibula has united, a small segment should be excised so as to permit compression of the tibial fragments. Intractable cases will respond to nothing except radical Ilizarov techniques (Fig. 30.32).

Joint stiffness Prolonged cast immobilization is liable to cause stiffness of the ankle and foot, which may persist for 12 months or longer in spite of active exercises. This can be avoided by changing to a functional brace as soon as it is safe to do so, usually by 4–6 weeks.

Osteoporosis Osteoporosis of the distal fragment is so common with all forms of treatment as to be regarded as a 'normal' consequence of tibial fractures. Axial loading of the tibia is important and weightbearing should be re-established as soon as possible. After prolonged external fixation, special care should be taken to prevent a distal stress fracture.

Regional complex pain syndrome With distal third fractures, this is not uncommon. Exercises should be encouraged throughout the period of treatment. The management of the established condition is discussed in Chapter 10.

FRACTURE OF TIBIA ALONE

A direct injury, such as a kick or blow with a club, may cause a transverse or slightly oblique fracture of the tibia alone at the site of impact. In children, the fracture is usually caused by an indirect injury; the fibula is intact or may show plastic deformation.

Local bruising and swelling are usually evident, but knee and ankle movements are possible. Transverse or slightly oblique fractures are easy to spot on x-ray even if displacement is slight. The child with a spiral fracture may be able to stand on the leg, and as the fracture may be almost invisible in an anteroposterior film, the injury can be missed unless two views are obtained; a few days later an angry mother brings the child back with a lump that proves to be callus!

Treatment

If the fracture is displaced, reduction should be attempted. An above-knee plaster is applied as with a fracture of both bones; first a split plaster and then, when swelling has subsided, a complete one. A fracture of the tibia alone takes just as long to unite as if both bones were broken, so at least 12 weeks is needed for consolidation and sometimes much longer. The child with a spiral fracture, however, can be safely released after 6 weeks; and with a mid-shaft transverse fracture the surgeon may (if he or she is a skilled plasterer and reduction is perfect) replace the above-knee plaster by a short plaster gaiter.

Complications

Delayed union Isolated tibial fractures, especially in the lower third, may be slow to join and the temptation is to discard splintage too soon. Even slight displacement and loss of contact at the fracture level may delay union, so internal fixation is often preferred as primary treatment. This fracture also has a tendency to drift

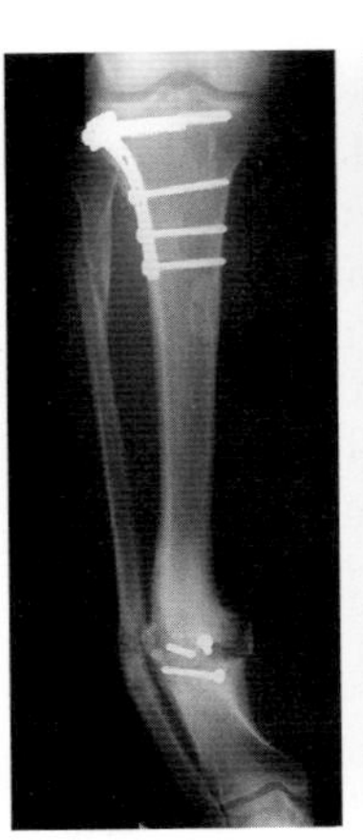

(a)

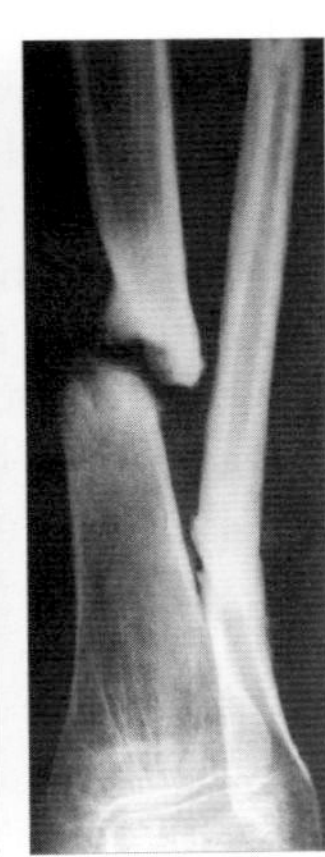

(b)

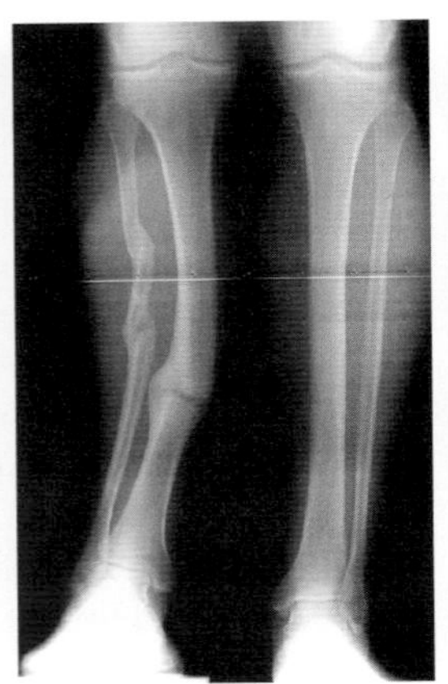

(c)

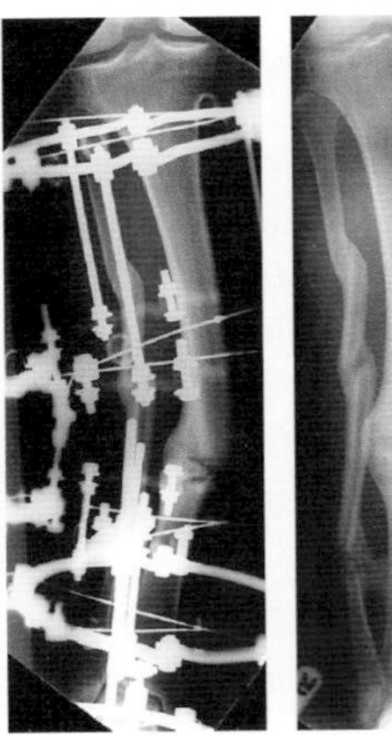

(d)

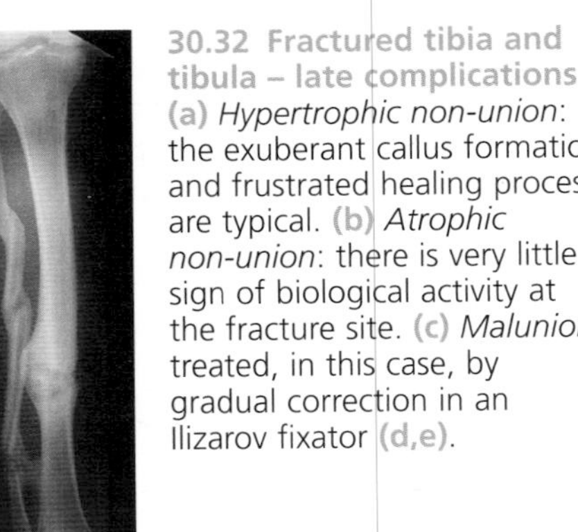

(e)

30.32 Fractured tibia and tibula – late complications (a) *Hypertrophic non-union*: the exuberant callus formation and frustrated healing process are typical. (b) *Atrophic non-union*: there is very little sign of biological activity at the fracture site. (c) *Malunion*: treated, in this case, by gradual correction in an Ilizarov fixator (d,e).

into varus in the later stages of healing; sometimes a fibular osteotomy is needed to allow correction of the deformity at surgery.

FRACTURE OF FIBULA ALONE

Isolated spiral fractures should be regarded with suspicion: they are often associated with other injuries and it is wise to obtain x-rays of the ankle and knee.

A transverse or short oblique fracture may be due to a direct blow. There is local tenderness, but the patient is able to stand and to move the knee and ankle. Pain can usually be controlled by analgesic medication and the patient will need no more than an elastic bandage, from knee to toes, for 2 or 3 weeks. In the occasional case where pain is more severe, a below-knee walking cast may be necessary.

Pathological fractures sometimes occur in patients with osteomyelitis or bone tumours. Treatment is that of the underlying condition.

FATIGUE FRACTURES

Repetitive stress may cause a fatigue fracture of the tibia (usually in the upper half of the bone) or the fibula (most often in the lower third). This injury is seen in army recruits, mountaineers, runners and ballet dancers, who complain of pain in the leg. There is local tenderness and slight swelling. The condition may be mistaken for a chronic compartment syndrome.

X-ray For the first 4 weeks there may be nothing abnormal about the x-ray, but a bone scan shows increased activity. After some weeks periosteal new bone may be seen, with a small transverse defect in the cortex.

There is a danger that these appearances may be mistaken for those of an osteosarcoma, with tragic consequences. If the diagnosis of stress fracture is kept in mind, such mistakes are unlikely.

Treatment

The patient is told to avoid the stressful activity. Usually after 8–10 weeks the symptoms settle down. A short leg gaiter can be applied for comfort during weightbearing.

REFERENCES AND FURTHER READING

Apley AG. Fractures of the tibial plateau. *Orthop Clin North Am* 1979; **10:** 61–74.

Bahk MS, Cosgarea AJ. Physical examination and imaging of the lateral collateral ligament and posterolateral corner of the knee. *Sports Med Arthrosc* 2006; **14:** 12–19.

Canadian Orthopaedic Trauma Society. Open reduction and internal fixation compared with circular fixator application for bicondylar tibial plateau fractures. Results of a multicenter, prospective, randomized clinical trial. *J Bone Joint Surg* 2006; **88A:** 2613–23.

Conlan T, Garth WP, Lemons JE. Evaluation of the medial soft-tissue restraints of the extensor mechanism of the knee. *J Bone Joint Surg* 1993; **75A:** 682–93.

Daniel DM, Stone ML, Barnett P, Sachs R. Use of the quadriceps active test to diagnose posterior cruciate-ligament disruption and measure posterior laxity of the knee. *J Bone Joint Surg* 1988; **70A:** 386–91.

Galway HR, MacIntosh DL. The lateral pivot shift: a symptom and sign of anterior cruciate ligament insufficiency. *Clin Orthop Relat Res* 1980; **147:** 45–50.

Gustilo RB, Mendoza RM, Williams DN. Problems in the management of type III (severe) open fractures: a new classification of type III open fractures. *J Trauma* 1984; **24:** 742–6.

Heckman MM, Whitesides TE Jr, Grewe SR, Rooks MD. Compartment pressure in association with closed tibial fractures. The relationship between tissue pressure, compartment, and the distance from the site of the fracture. *J Bone Joint Surg* 1994; **76A:** 1285–92.

LaPrade RF, Wentorf F. Diagnosis and treatment of posterolateral knee injuries. *Clin Orthop Relat Res* 2002; **402:** 110–21.

McQueen MM, Christie J, Court-Brown CM. Acute compartment syndrome in tibial diaphyseal fractures. *J Bone Joint Surg* 1996; **78B:** 95–8.

O'Donoghue D. Surgical treatment of fresh injuries to the major ligaments of the knee. *J Bone Joint Surg* 1950; **32A:** 721–38.

Oestern H, Tscherne H. *Pathophysiology and classification of soft tissue injuries associated with fractures.* In: Tscherne H, Gotzen L (Eds) Fractures with Soft Tissue Injuries. Springer Verlag, Berlin, 1984.

Petersen WMD, Zantop TMD. Anatomy of the anterior cruciate ligament with regard to its two bundles. *Clin Orthop Relat Res* 2007; **454:** 35–47.

Ranawat A, Baker CL 3rd, Henry S, Harner CD. Posterolateral corner injury of the knee: evaluation and management. *J Am Acad Orthop Surg* 2008; **16:** 506–18.

Robertson A, Nutton RW, Keating JF. Dislocation of the knee. *J Bone Joint Surg* 2006; **88B:** 706–11.

Sarmiento A, Latta L. The evolution of functional bracing of fractures. *J Bone Joint Surg* 2006; **88B:** 141–8.

Slocum DB, Larson RL. Rotatory instability of the knee: Its pathogenesis and a clinical test to demonstrate its presence. *J Bone Joint Surg* 1968; **50A:** 211–25.

Watson JT. Treatment of unstable fractures of the shaft of the tibia. *J Bone Joint Surg* 1994; **76A:** 1575–84.

Injuries of the ankle and foot

31

Gavin Bowyer

INTRODUCTION

The foot and ankle act to both support and propel the body and are well adapted for these roles. During running and jumping, loads well in excess of 10 times body weight are transmitted through the ankle and foot. If this loading is excessive, or excessively repeated, it can lead to foot and ankle injuries.

The ankle is a close-fitting hinge-like joint of which the two parts interlock like a mortise (the box formed by the distal ends of the tibia and fibula) and tenon (the upward projecting talus). The mortise bones are held together as a syndesmosis by the distal (inferior) tibiofibular and interosseous ligaments, and the talus is prevented from slipping out of the mortise by the medial and lateral collateral ligaments and joint capsule. The peroneal tendons provide additional stability.

The ankle moves only in one plane (flexion/extension), but with a complex axis of rotation, actually rolling forward as the talus goes into plantar flexion; sideways movement is prevented by the malleolar buttresses and the collateral ligaments, but the bony constraint lessens as the ankle flexes. If the talus is forced to tilt or rotate, something must give: the ligaments, the malleoli or both. Movements of the talus into internal or external rotation come about from a rotatory force upon the foot, or more commonly inversion/supination of the foot, which, through the orientation of the subtalar joint, causes external rotation of the talus. Whenever a fracture of the malleolus is seen, it is important to ask about the associated ligament injury.

ANKLE LIGAMENT INJURIES

Ankle sprains are the most common of all sports-related injuries, accounting for over 25 per cent of cases. They are probably even more common in pedestrians and country walkers who stumble on stairways, pavements and potholes.

In more than 75 per cent of cases it is the lateral ligament complex that is injured, in particular the anterior talofibular and calcaneofibular ligaments. Medial ligament injuries are usually associated with a fracture or joint injury.

A sudden twist of the ankle momentarily tenses the structures around the joint. This may amount to no more than a painful wrenching of the soft tissues – what is commonly called a *sprained ankle*. If more severe force is applied, the ligaments may be strained to the point of rupture. With a *partial tear*, most of the ligament remains intact and, once it has healed, it is able to support the weight of the body. With a *complete tear*, the ligament may still heal but it never regains its original form and the joint will probably be unstable.

Functional anatomy

The *lateral collateral ligaments* consist of the anterior talofibular, the posterior talofibular and (between them) the calcaneofibular ligaments. The anterior talofibular ligament (ATFL) runs almost horizontally from the anterior edge of the lateral malleolus to the neck of the talus; it is relaxed in dorsiflexion and tense in plantarflexion. In plantarflexion the ligament essentially changes its orientation from horizontal with respect to the floor, to almost vertical. Thus the ligament at greatest stretch, and most vulnerable, with the foot plantar-flexed is the ATFL – hence the propensity for ATFL injury with the plantar-flexed, inverting, foot (down a pot-hole, off a kerb, etc). The calcaneofibular ligament stretches from the tip of the lateral malleolus to the posterolateral part of the calcaneum, thus it helps also to stabilize the subtalar joint. Maximum tension is produced by inversion and dorsiflexion of the ankle. The posterior talofibular ligament runs from the posterior border of the lateral malleolus to the posterior part of the talus.

The *medial collateral (deltoid) ligament* consists of superficial and deep portions. The superficial fibres spread like a fan from the medial malleolus as far

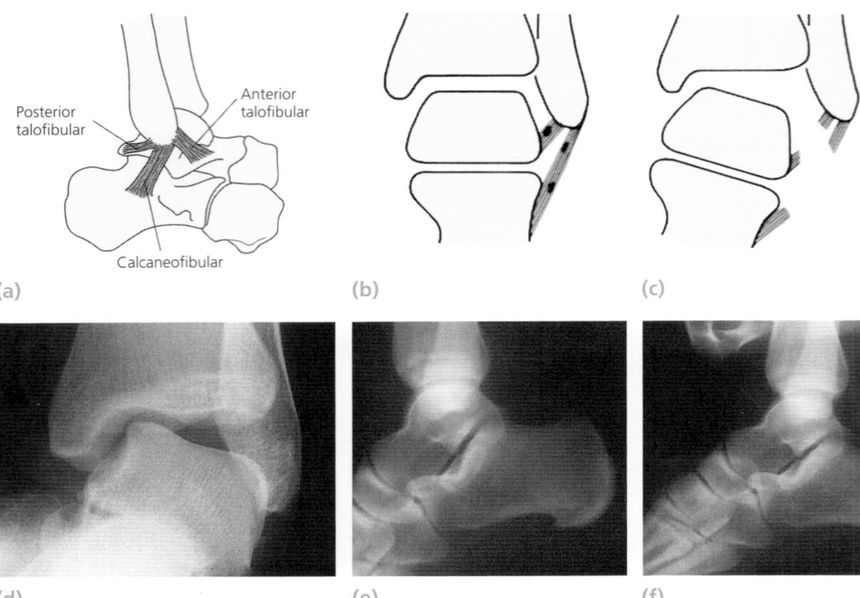

31.1 Ankle ligament injuries (a) Schematic diagram showing the mortise-and-tenon articulation and main ligaments of the ankle. (b) The three components of the lateral collateral ligament. (c) The commonest injury is a partial tear of one or other component of the lateral ligament. Following a complete tear, the talus may be displaced in the ankle mortise; the tibiofibular ligament may have ruptured as well, shown here in somewhat exaggerated form. (d) Stress x-ray showing talar tilt. (e,f) X-rays demonstrating anteroposterior instability. Pulling the foot forward under the tibia causes the talus to shift appreciably at the ankle joint; this is usually seen after recurrent sprains.

anteriorly as the navicular and inferiorly to the calcaneum and talus. Its chief function is to resist eversion of the hindfoot. The deep portion is intra-articular, running directly from the medial malleolus to the medial surface of the talus. Its principal effect is to prevent external rotation of the talus. The combined action of restraining eversion and external rotation makes the deltoid ligament the major stabilizer of the ankle.

The *distal tibiofibular joint* is held by four ligaments: anterior, posterior, inferior transverse and the interosseous 'ligament', which is really a thickened part of the interosseous membrane. This strong ligament complex still permits some movement at the tibiofibular joint during flexion and extension of the ankle.

Pathology

The common 'twisted ankle' is due to unbalanced loading with the ankle inverted and plantarflexed. First the anterior talofibular and then the calcaneofibular ligament is strained; sometimes the talocalcaneal ligaments also are injured. If fibres are torn there is bleeding into the soft tissues. The tip of the malleolus may be avulsed and in some cases the peroneal tendons are injured. There may be a small fracture of an adjacent tarsal bone or (on the lateral side) the base of the fifth metatarsal.

Acute injury of lateral ligaments

Clinical features

A history of a twisting injury followed by pain and swelling could suggest anything from a minor sprain to a fracture. If the patient is able to walk, and bruising is only faint and slow to appear, it is probably a sprain; if bruising is marked and the patient unable to put any weight on the foot, this suggests a more severe injury. Tenderness is maximal just distal and slightly anterior to the lateral malleolus. The slightest attempt at passive inversion of the ankle is extremely painful. It is impossible to test for abnormal mobility without using local or general anaesthesia.

With all ankle injuries it is essential to examine the entire leg and foot; undisplaced fractures of the fibula or the tarsal bones, or even the fifth metatarsal bone are easily missed and injuries of the distal tibiofibular joint and the peroneal tendon sheath cause features that mimic those of a lateral ligament strain.

Imaging

About 15 per cent of ankle sprains reaching the Emergency Department are associated with an ankle fracture. This complication can be excluded by obtaining an x-ray, but there are doubts as to whether all patients with ankle injuries should be subjected to x-ray examination. Almost 2 decades ago The Ottawa Ankle Rules were developed to assist in making this decision. X-ray examination is called for if there is: (1) pain around the malleolus; (2) inability to take weight on the ankle immediately after the injury; (3) inability to take four steps in the Emergency Department; (4) bone tenderness at the posterior edge or tip of the medial or lateral malleolus or the base of the fifth metatarsal bone.

If x-ray examination is considered necessary, anteroposterior, lateral and 'mortise' (30-degree oblique) views of the ankle should be obtained. Localized soft tissue swelling and, in some cases, a small avulsion fracture of the tip of the lateral malleolus or the anterolateral surface of the talus may be the only corroborative signs of a lateral ligament injury. However, it is important to exclude other injuries, such as an undisplaced fibular fracture or diastasis of the tibiofibular syndesmosis. If tenderness extends onto the foot, or if swelling is so severe that the area cannot be properly examined, additional x-rays of the foot are essential.

Persistent inability to weightbear over 1 week or longer should call for re-examination and review of all the initial 'negative' x-rays. For patients who have had persistent pain, swelling, instability and impaired function over 6 weeks or longer, despite appropriate early treatment, magnetic resonance imaging (MRI) or computed tomography (CT) will be required to assess the extent of soft tissue injury or subtle bony changes.

Treatment

Initial treatment consists of **r**est, **i**ce, **c**ompression and **e**levation (RICE), which is continued for 1–3 weeks depending on the severity of the injury and the response to treatment. Cold compresses should be applied for about 20 minutes every 2 hours, and after any activity that exacerbates the symptoms.

More recently the acronym has been extended to 'PRICE' by adding **p**rotection (crutches, splint or brace) and still further to 'PRICER', adding **r**ehabilitation (supported return to function). The principles remain the same – a phased approach, to support the injured part during the first few weeks and then allow early mobilization and a supported return to function. An advice leaflet for patients is probably helpful.

The use of non-steroidal anti-inflammatory drugs (NSAIDs) in the acute phase can be helpful, with the usual contraindications and caveats. There is evidence that in acute injuries topical non-steroidal anti-inflammatory (NSAI) gels or creams might be as beneficial as oral preparations, probably with a better risk profile.

Functional treatment, i.e. 'protected mobilization', leads to earlier recovery of all grades of injury – without jeopardizing stability – than either rigid immobilization or early operative treatment.

OPERATIVE TREATMENT

If the ankle does not start to settle within 1 or 2 weeks of starting RICE, further review and investigation are called for. Persistent problems at 12 weeks after injury, despite physiotherapy, may signal the need for operative treatment. Residual complaints of ankle pain and stiffness, a sensation of instability or giving way and intermittent swelling are suggestive of cartilage damage or impinging scar tissue within the ankle. Arthroscopic repair or ligament substitution is now effective in many cases, allowing a return to full function and sports.

RECURRENT LATERAL INSTABILITY

Recurrent sprains are potentially associated with added cartilage damage, and warrant careful investigation by MRI, arthroscopy and examination under anaesthesia.

Clinical features

The patient gives a history of a 'sprained ankle' that never quite seems to recover and is followed by recurrent 'giving way' or a feeling of instability when walking on uneven surfaces. This is said to occur in about 20 per cent of cases after acute lateral collateral ligament tears (Colville, 1994).

The ankle looks normal and passive movements are full, however stress tests for abnormal lateral ligament laxity may show either excessive talar tilting in the sagittal plane or anterior displacement (an anterior drawer sign) in the coronal plane. In the chronic phase these tests are painless and can be performed either manually or with the use of special mechanical stress devices. Both ankles are tested, so as to allow comparison of the abnormal with the normal side.

Talar tilt test With the ankle held in the neutral position, the examiner stabilizes the tibia by grasping the leg with one hand above the ankle; the other hand is then used to force the heel into maximum inversion. The range of movement can be estimated clinically and compared with that of the normal ankle. The exact degree of talar tilt can also be measured by x-rays, which should be taken with the ankles in 30 degrees of internal rotation (mortise views); 15 degrees of talar tilt (or 5 degrees more than in the normal ankle) is regarded as abnormal. Inversion laxity suggests injury to both the calcaneofibular and anterior talofibular ligaments.

Anterior drawer test The patient should be sitting with the knee flexed to 90 degrees and the ankle in 10 degrees of plantarflexion. The lower leg is stabilized with one hand while the other hand forces the patient's heel forward under the tibia. In a positive test the talus can be felt sliding forwards and backwards. The position of the talus is verified by lateral x-rays; anterior displacement of 10 mm (or 5 mm more than on the normal side) indicates abnormal laxity of the anterior talofibular ligament. With an isolated tear of the anterior talofibular ligament, the anterior drawer test may be positive in the absence of abnormal talar tilt. (*Note*: A positive anterior drawer test can sometimes be obtained in normal, asymptomatic individuals; the finding should always be considered in conjunction with other symptoms and signs).

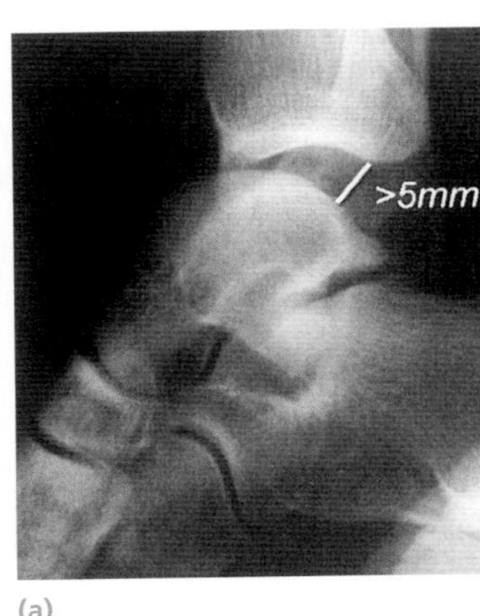

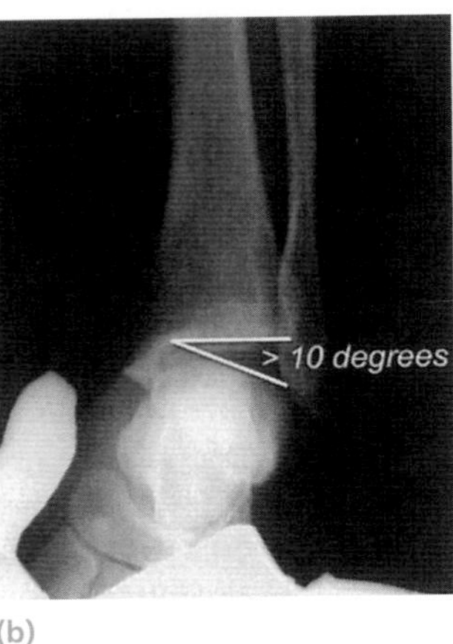

(a) (b)

31.2 Recurrent lateral instability – special tests (a) *Anterior drawer test*: When the heel is drawn forwards under the tibia, the abnormally lax ligaments allow the talus to displace anteriorly. (b) *Talar tilt test*: Forcibly inverting the ankle causes the talus to tilt abnormally in the mortise. For both tests comparison with the normal side is important.

Treatment

Recurrent 'giving way' can sometimes be prevented by modifying shoe-wear, raising the outer side of the heel and extending it laterally. More effectively, the secondary dynamic ankle stabilizers, the peronei, can be strengthened and brought into play by specific physiotherapy regimes. Ankle exercises to strengthen the peroneal muscles are helpful, and a light brace can be worn during stressful activities.

If, in spite of these measures, the patient continues to experience mechanical instability (true giving way) during everyday activities, reconstruction of the lateral ligament should be considered. More commonly the persisting problem will be functional instability, in which the patient does not trust the ankle, and there are recurrent episodes in which the patient has rapidly or suddenly to unload the ankle, probably because of inhibitory feedback from the injured ankle.

Most patients with functional instability can be improved and returned to sport by arthroscopic debridement of the impinging tissue within the ankle joint, followed by physiotherapy.

Various operations for mechanical stabilization are described; they fall mainly into two groups: (1) those that aim to repair or tighten the ligaments, (2) those that are designed to construct a 'check-rein' against the unstable movement. The *Broström–Karlsson* or *Gould operation* is an example of the first type: the anterior talofibular and calcaneofibular ligaments are exposed and repaired, usually by an overlapping – or 'double-breasting' – technique (Karlsson et al., 1988). In the second type of operation a substitute ligament is constructed by using peroneus brevis to act as a tenodesis and prevent sudden movements into varus (Chrisman and Snook, 1969). The disadvantages of the non-anatomic reconstructions are that they sacrifice or partially sacrifice the secondary stabilizers, the peroneal tendons.

Postoperatively the ankle is immobilized in eversion for 2 weeks; a below-knee cast is then applied for another 4 weeks, during which time the patient can

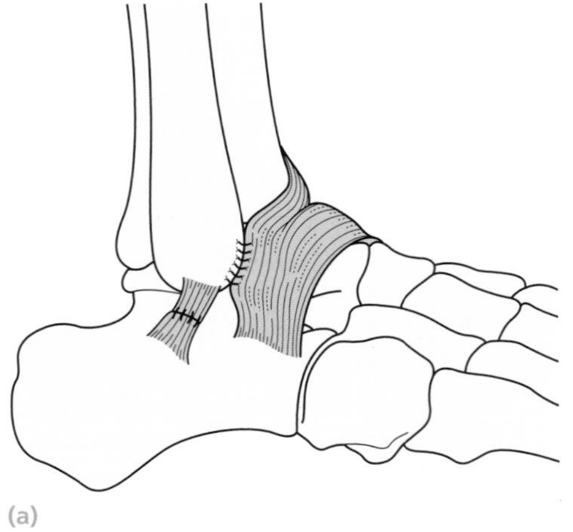

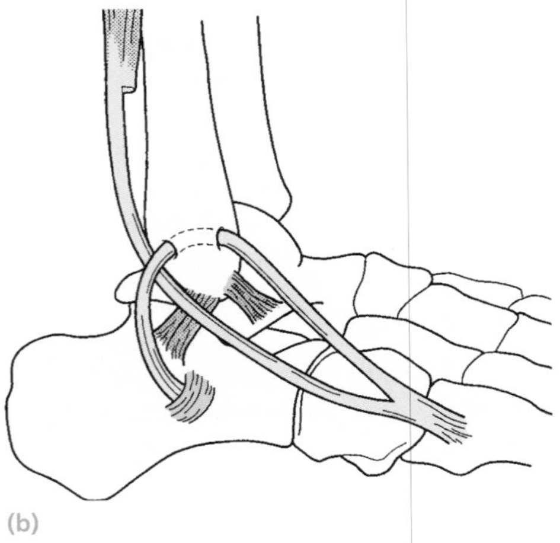

(a) (b)

31.3 Recurrent lateral instability – operative treatment (a) The lax anterior talofibular and calcaneofibular ligaments can be reinforced by a double-breasting technique (the Broström–Karlsson operation). (b) Another way of augmenting the lateral ligament is to re-route part of the peroneus brevis tendon so that is acts as a check-rein (tenodesis) (The Chrisman operation).

bear weight. Thereafter, a removable brace is worn and exercises are encouraged. The brace can usually be discarded after 3 months but it may need to be used from time to time for sports activities.

Deltoid ligament tears

Rupture of the deltoid ligament is usually associated with either a fracture of the distal end of the fibula or tearing of the distal tibiofibular ligaments (or both). The effect is to destabilize the talus and allow it to move into eversion and external rotation. The diagnosis is made by x-ray: there is widening of the medial joint space in the mortise view; sometimes the talus is tilted, and diastasis of the tibiofibular joint may be obvious.

When there is a deltoid ligament or medial malleolar injury but no apparent lateral disruption at the ankle, it is important to look for a fracture or dislocation of the proximal fibula – the highly unstable *Maissoneuve injury.*

Treatment

Provided the medial joint space is completely reduced, the ligament will heal. The fibular fracture or diastasis must be accurately reduced, if necessary by open operation and internal fixation. Occasionally the medial joint space cannot be reduced; it should then be explored in order to free any soft tissue trapped in the joint. A below-knee cast is applied with the foot plantigrade and is retained for 8 weeks.

Dislocation of peroneal tendons

Acute dislocation of the peroneal tendons may accompany – or may be mistaken for – a lateral ligament strain. Tell-tale signs on x-ray are an oblique fracture of the lateral malleolus (the so-called 'rim fracture') or a small flake of bone lying lateral to the lateral malleolus (avulsion of the retinaculum). Treatment in a below-knee cast for 6 weeks will help in a proportion of cases; the remainder will complain of residual symptoms.

Recurrent subluxation or *dislocation* is unmistakable; the patient can demonstrate that the peroneal tendons dislocate forwards over the fibula during dorsiflexion and eversion. Treatment is operative and is based on the observation that the attachment of the retinaculum to the periosteum on the front of the fibula has come adrift, creating a pouch into which the tendons displace. Using non-absorbable sutures through drill holes in the bone, the normal anatomy is recreated (Das De and Balasubramaniam, 1985). An alternative approach is to modify the morphology of the distal fibula, posteriorly translating a shelf of bone to constrain the tendons mechanically in a deepened posterior channel. Whichever method of stabilization is used, it is important to also assess the state of the tendons themselves, as an associated longitudinal split tear is commonly found, and this will lead to continuing pain and dysfunction around the lateral border of the ankle if it is not repaired.

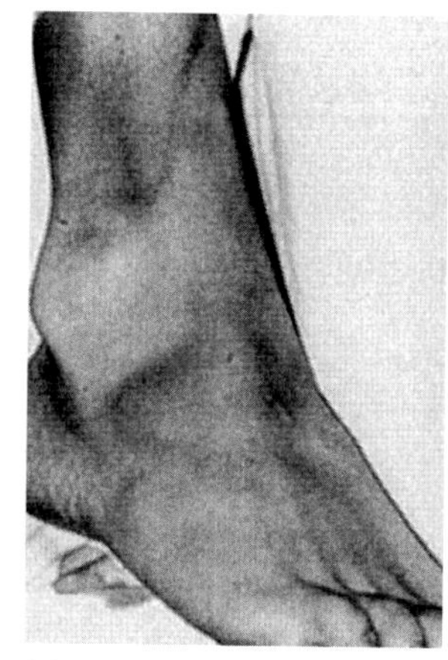

(a)

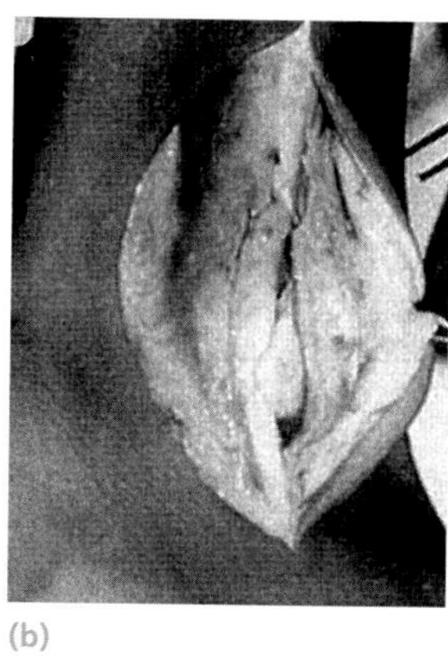

(b)

31.4 Dislocation of peroneal tendons (a) On movement of the ankle, the peroneal tendons slip forwards over the lateral malleolus. (b) The anterior part of the retinaculum is being reconstructed.

Tears of inferior tibiofibular ligaments

The inferior tibiofibular ligaments may be torn, allowing partial or complete separation of the tibiofibular joint (diastasis). *Complete diastasis,* with tearing of both the anterior and posterior fibres, follows a severe abduction strain. *Partial diastasis,* with tearing of only the anterior fibres, is due to an external rotation force. These injuries may occur in isolation, but they are usually associated with fractures of the malleoli or rupture of the collateral ligaments.

Clinical features

Following a twisting injury, the patient complains of pain in the front of the ankle. There is swelling and marked tenderness directly over the inferior tibiofibular joint. A 'squeeze test' has been described by Hopkinson et al. (1990); when the leg is firmly compressed some way above the ankle, the patient experiences pain over the syndesmosis. Be sure, though, to exclude a fracture before carrying out the test.

X-ray

With a partial tear the fibula usually lies in its normal position and the x-ray looks normal. With a complete tear the tibiofibular joint is separated and the ankle mortise is widened; sometimes this becomes apparent only when the ankle is stressed in abduction. There may be associated fractures of the distal tibia or fibula, or an isolated fracture more proximally in the fibula.

Treatment

Partial tears can be treated by strapping the ankle firmly for 2–3 weeks. Thereafter exercises are encouraged.

Complete tears are best managed by internal fixation with a transverse screw just above the joint. This must be done as soon as possible so that the tibiofibular space does not become clogged with organizing haematoma and fibrous tissue. If the patient is seen late and the ankle is painful and unstable, open clearance of the syndesmosis and transverse screw fixation may be warranted. The ankle is immobilized in plaster for 8 weeks, after which the screw is removed. However, some degree of instability usually persists.

MALLEOLAR FRACTURES OF THE ANKLE

Fractures and fracture dislocations of the ankle are common. Most are low-energy fractures of one or both malleoli, usually caused by a twisting mechanism. Less common are the more severe fractures involving the tibial plafond, the pilon fractures, which are high-energy injuries often caused by a fall from a height.

The patient usually presents with a history of a twisting injury, usually with the ankle going into inversion, followed by immediate pain, swelling and difficulty weightbearing. Bruising often comes out soon after injury.

One such injury was described by Percival Pott in 1768, and the group as a whole was for a long time referred to as Pott's fracture – although as with many eponyms, he was not the first to notice or describe it, and what became known by this eponym was not what he described anyway!

The most obvious injury is a fracture of one or both malleoli; often, though, the 'invisible' part of the injury – rupture of one or more ligaments – is just as serious.

Mechanism of injury

The patient stumbles and falls. Usually the foot is anchored to the ground while the body lunges forward. The ankle is twisted and the talus tilts and/or rotates forcibly in the mortise, causing a low-energy fracture of one or both malleoli, with or without associated injuries of the ligaments. If a malleolus is pushed off, it usually fractures obliquely; if it is pulled off, it fractures transversely. The precise fracture pattern is determined by: (1) the position of the foot; (2) the direction of force at the moment of injury. The foot may be either pronated or supinated and the force upon the talus is towards adduction, abduction or external rotation, or a combination of these.

Pathological anatomy

There is no completely satisfactory classification of ankle fractures. Lauge-Hansen (1950) grouped these injuries according to the likely position of the foot and the direction of force at the moment of fracture. This is useful as a guide to the method of reduction (reverse the pathological force); it also gives a pointer to the associated ligament injuries. However, some people find this classification overly complicated. For a detailed description the reader is referred to the original paper by Lauge-Hansen (1950).

A simpler (perhaps too simple) classification is that of *Danis* and *Weber* (Müller et al., 1991), which focuses on the fibular fracture. Type A is a transverse fracture of the fibula below the tibiofibular syndesmosis, perhaps associated with an oblique or vertical fracture of the medial malleolus; this is almost certainly an adduction (or adduction and internal rotation) injury. Type B is an oblique fracture of the fibula in the sagittal plane (and therefore better seen in the lateral x-ray) at the level of the syndesmosis; often there is also an avulsion injury on the medial side (a torn deltoid ligament or fracture of the medial malleolus). This is probably an external rotation injury and it may be associated with a tear of the anterior tibiofibular ligament. Type C is a more severe injury, above the level of the syndesmosis, which means that the tibiofibular ligament and part of the interosseous membrane must have been torn. This is due to severe abduction or a combination of abduction and external rotation. Associated injuries are an avulsion fracture of the medial malleolus (or rupture of the medial collateral ligament), a posterior malleolar fracture and diastasis of the tibiofibular joint.

Clinical features

Ankle fractures are seen in skiers, footballers and climbers; an older group includes women with postmenopausal osteoporosis.

A history of a severe twisting injury, followed by intense pain and inability to stand on the leg suggests something more serious than a simple sprain. The ankle is swollen and deformity may be obvious. The site of tenderness is important; if both the medial and lateral sides are tender, a double injury (bony or ligamentous) must be suspected.

X-ray

At least three views are needed: anteroposterior, lateral and a 30-degree oblique 'mortise' view. The level of the fibular fracture is often best seen in the lateral view; diastasis may not be appreciated without the mortise view. Further x-rays may be needed to exclude a proximal fibular fracture.

From a careful study of the x-rays it should be possible to reconstruct the mechanism of injury. The four most common patterns are shown in Figure 31.5.

Treatment

Swelling is usually rapid and severe, particularly in the higher energy injuries. If the injury is not dealt with within a few hours, definitive treatment may have to be deferred for several days while the leg is elevated so that the swelling can subside; this can be hastened by using a foot pump (which also reduces the risk of deep-vein thrombosis).

Fractures are visible on x-ray; ligaments are not. Always look for clues to the invisible ligament injury – widening of the tibiofibular space, asymmetry of the talotibial space, widening of the medial joint space, or tilting of the talus – before deciding on a course of action.

Like other intra-articular injuries, ankle fractures must be accurately reduced and held if later mechanical dysfunction is to be prevented. Persistent displacement of the talus, or a step in the articular surface, leads to increased stress and predisposes to secondary osteoarthritis.

In assessing the accuracy of reduction, four objectives must be met: (1) the fibula must be restored to its full length; (2) the talus must sit squarely in the mortise, with the talar and tibial articular surfaces parallel; (3) the medial joint space must be restored to its normal width, i.e. the same width as the tibio-talar space (about 4 mm); (4) oblique x-rays must show that there is no tibiofibular diastasis.

Ankle fractures are often unstable. Whatever the method of reduction and fixation, the position must be checked by x-ray during the period of healing.

UNDISPLACED FRACTURES

The first step is to decide whether the injury is stable or unstable. An isolated, *undisplaced Danis–Weber*

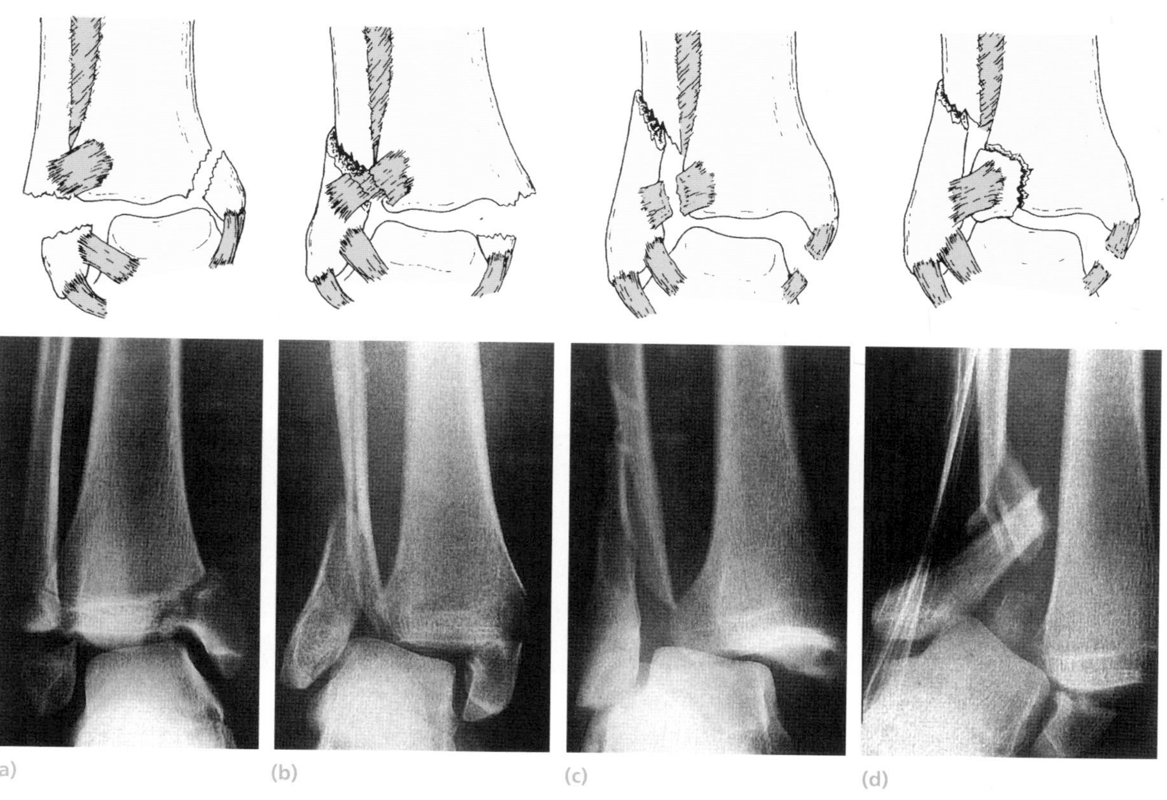

31.5 Ankle fractures – classification The Danis–Weber classification is based on the level of the fibular fracture. (a) Type A – a fibular fracture below the syndesmosis and an oblique fracture of the medial malleolus (caused by forced supination and adduction of the foot). (b) Type B – fracture at the syndesmosis, often associated with disruption of the anterior fibres of the tibiofibular ligament and fracture of the posterior and/or medial malleolus, or disruption of the medial ligament (caused by forced supination and external rotation). (c) Type C – a fibular fracture above the syndesmosis; the tibiofibular ligament must be torn, or else (d) the ligament avulses a small piece of the tibia. Here, again, there must also be disruption on the medial side of the joint – either a medial malleolar fracture or rupture of the deltoid ligament.

type A fracture is stable and will need minimal splintage: a firm bandage or stirrup brace is applied mainly for comfort until the fracture heals.

Undisplaced type B fractures are potentially unstable only if the tibiofibular ligament is torn or avulsed, or if there is a significant medial-sided injury. X-rays will show if the syndesmosis or mortise is intact; if it is, a below-knee cast is applied with the ankle in the neutral (anatomical) position. The plaster may need to be split and, if so, it must be completed or replaced when swelling has subsided. A check x-ray is taken at 2 weeks to confirm that the fracture remains undisplaced. An overboot is fitted and the patient is taught to walk correctly as soon as possible. The cast can usually be discarded after 6–8 weeks. Ankle and foot movements are regained by active exercises when the plaster is removed. As with any lower limb fracture, the leg must not be allowed to dangle idly – it must be exercised and elevated.

Undisplaced type C fractures are deceivingly innocent-looking but are often accompanied by disruption of the medial joint structures as well as the tibiofibular syndesmosis and interosseous membrane. These defects may become apparent only when the fracture displaces in a cast; arguably, therefore, type C fractures are better fixed from the outset.

DISPLACED FRACTURES

Reduction of these joint disruptions is a prerequisite to all further treatment; knowledge of the causal mechanism (and this is where the Lauge-Hansen classification is useful) helps to guide the method of closed reduction. Although internal fixation is usually performed to stabilize the reduction, not all such fractures require surgery.

Displaced Weber type A fractures The medial malleolar fracture is nearly vertical and after closed reduction it often remains unstable; internal fixation of the malleolar fragment with one or two screws directed almost parallel to the ankle joint is advisable. A perfect reduction should be aimed for, with accurate restoration of the tibial articular surface. Loose bone fragments are removed. The lateral malleolar fracture, unless it is already perfectly reduced and stable, should be fixed with a plate and screws or tension-band wiring. Postoperatively a 'walking cast' or removable splintage boot is applied for 6 weeks; the advantage of removable splintage is that early physiotherapy can be commenced.

Displaced Weber type B fractures The most common fracture pattern is a spiral fracture of the fibula and an oblique fracture of the medial malleolus. The causal mechanism is external rotation of the ankle when the foot is caught in a supinated position. Closed reduction therefore needs traction (to disimpact the fracture) and then internal rotation of the foot. If closed reduction succeeds, a cast is applied, following the same routine as for undisplaced fractures. Failure of closed reduction (sometimes a torn medial ligament is caught in between the talus and medial malleolus) or late redisplacement calls for operative treatment.

Type B fractures may also be caused by abduction; often the lateral aspect of the fibula is comminuted and the fracture line more horizontal. Despite accurate reduction (the ankle is adducted and the foot supinated), these injuries are unstable and often poorly controlled in a cast; internal fixation is therefore preferred.

Displaced Weber type C fractures The fibular fracture is well above the syndesmosis and frequently there are

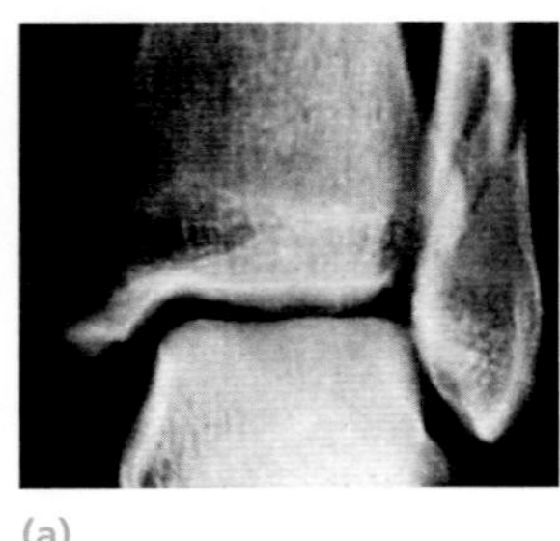

(a)

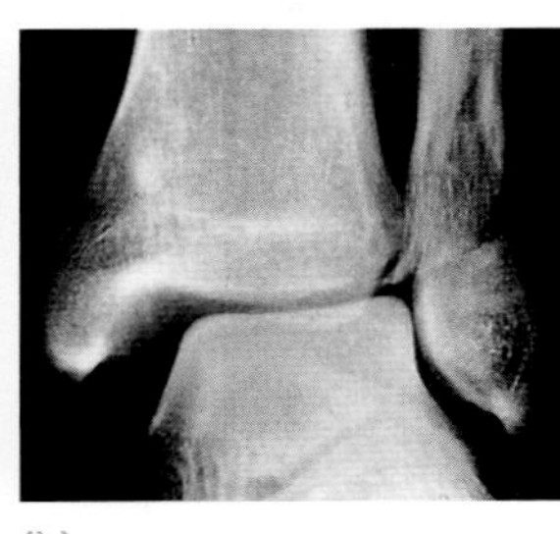

(b)

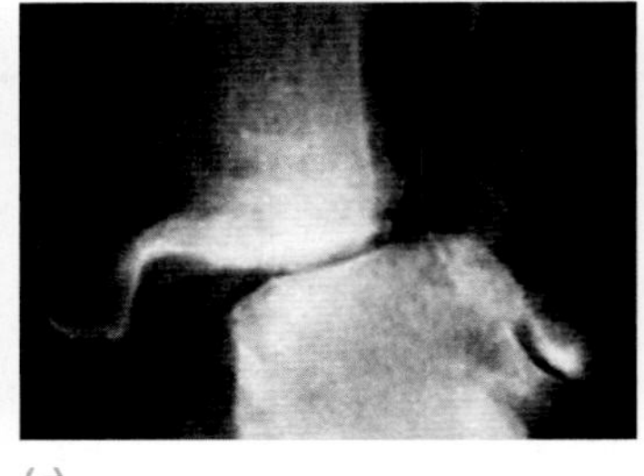

(c)

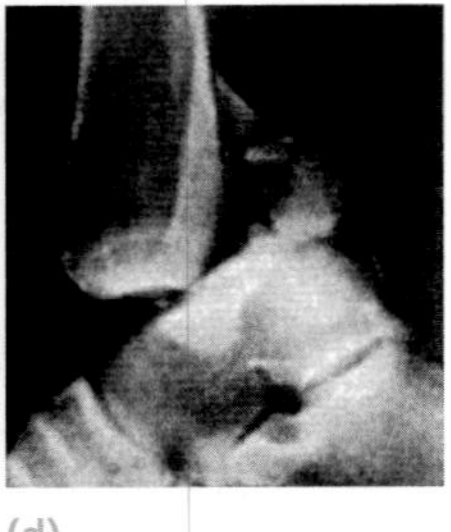

(d)

31.6 Ankle fractures – stable or unstable? (a) Stable fracture: in this Danis–Weber type B fracture the tibiofibular syndesmosis has held; the surfaces of the tibia and talus are precisely parallel and the width of the joint space is regular both superiorly and medially. (b) *Slight subluxation*: the syndesmosis is intact but the talus has moved laterally with the distal fibular fragment; the medial joint space is too wide, signifying a deltoid ligament rupture. It is vital, after reduction of the fibular fracture, to check that the medial joint space is normal; if it is not, the ligament has probably been trapped in the joint and it must be freed so as to allow perfect re-positioning of the talus. (c) *Fracture–dislocation*: in this high fibular fracture the syndesmosis has given way, the medial collatoral ligament has been torn and the talus is displaced and tilted. The fibula must be fixed to full length and the tibiofibular joint secured before the ankle can be stabilized. (d) *Posterior fracture–dislocation*: if the posterior margin of the tibia is fractured, the talus may be displaced upwards. The fragment must be replaced and fixed securely.

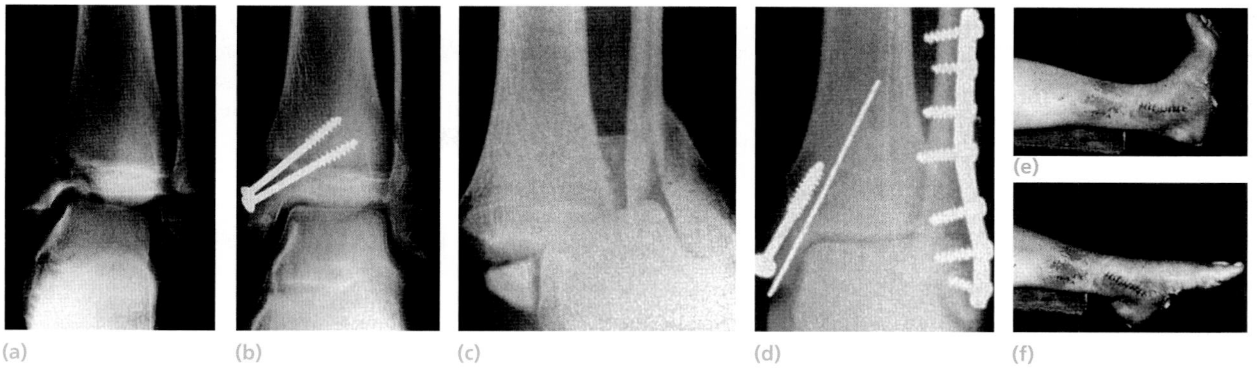

31.7 Ankle fractures – open treatment (1) (a,b) Danis–Weber type A fractures can often be treated conservatively, but if the medial malleolar fragment involves a large segment of the articular surface, it is best treated by accurate open reduction and internal fixation with one or two screws. (c,d) An unstable fracture–dislocation such as this almost always needs open reduction and internal fixation. The fibula should be restored to full length and fixed securely; in this case the medial malleolus also needed internal fixation; (e) and (f) show the range of ankle movement a few days after operation and before a 'walking plaster' was applied.

associated medial and posterior malleolar fragments. An isolated type C fibular fracture should raise strong suspicions of major ligament damage to the syndesmosis and medial side of the joint. Almost all type C fractures are unstable and will need open reduction and internal fixation. The first step is to reduce the fibula, restoring its length and alignment; the fracture is then stabilized using a plate and screws. If there is a medial fracture, this also is fixed. The syndesmosis is then checked, using a hook to pull the fibula laterally. If the joint opens out, it means that the ligaments are torn; the syndesmosis is stabilized by inserting a transverse screw across from the fibula into the tibia (the ankle should be held in 10 degrees of dorsiflexion when the screw is inserted).

Fracture subluxations more than 1 or 2 weeks old may prove difficult to reduce because of clot organization in the syndesmosis. Granulation tissue should be removed from the syndesmosis and transverse tibiofibular fixation secured.

Postoperative management After open reduction and fixation of ankle fractures, movements should be regained before applying a below-knee plaster cast, or removable support boot. The patient is then allowed partial weightbearing with crutches; the support is retained until the fractures have consolidated (anything from 6–12 weeks).

Management of the syndesmosis- or diastasis-screw remains controversial. Some advocate removal of the screw when the syndesmosis has healed, and before weightbearing has commenced (6 weeks is too early, 10 weeks is probably more appropriate). Others are happy to allow early weightbearing with the screw still

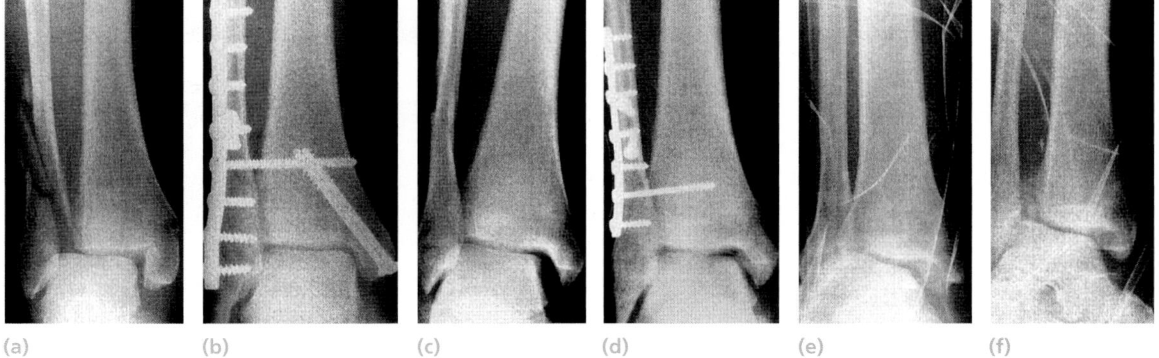

31.8 Ankle fractures with diastasis – open treatment (2) (a) In this type B fracture there is partial disruption of the distal tibiofibular syndesmosis. Treatment (b) required medial and lateral fixation as well a tibiofibular screw. (c) A type C fracture must, inevitably, disrupt the tibiofibular ligament; in this case the medial malleolus was intact but the deltoid ligament was torn (look at the wider than normal medial joint space). (d) By fixing the fibular fracture and using a tibiofibular screw, the ankle was completely reduced and it was therefore unnecessary to explore the deltoid ligament. (e) This patient presented 5 days after his injury; he, too, had a diastasis with disruption of the deltoid ligament (f). In this case the tibiofibular joint as well as the deltoid ligament had to be explored before the ankle could be reduced.

in place, accepting that the screw may break (especially if four cortices are engaged).

OPEN FRACTURES

Open fractures of the ankle pose special problems. If the fracture is not reduced and stabilized at an early stage, it may prove impossible to restore the anatomy. For this reason unstable injuries should be treated by internal fixation even in the presence of an open wound, provided the soft tissues are not too severely damaged and the wound is not contaminated. If internal fixation seems too risky, an external fixator can be used, often as a temporary spanning option. Treatment in other respects follows the principles outlined in chapter 23.

Complications

EARLY

Vascular injury With a severe fracture-subluxation the pulses may be obliterated. The ankle should be immediately reduced and held in a splint until definitive treatment has been initiated.

Wound breakdown and infection Diabetic patients are at greater than usual risk of developing wound-edge necrosis and deep infection. In dealing with displaced fractures, these risks should be carefully weighed against the disadvantages of conservative treatment; casts may also cause skin problems if not well padded and are less effective in preventing malunion.

LATE

Incomplete reduction Incomplete reduction is common and, unless the talus fits the mortise accurately, degenerative changes may occur. This can sometimes be prevented by a corrective osteotomy.

Non-union The medial malleolus occasionally fails to unite because a flap of periosteum is interposed between it and the tibia. It should be prevented by operative reduction and screw fixation.

Joint stiffness Swelling and stiffness of the ankle are usually the result of neglect in treatment of the soft tissues. The patient must walk correctly in plaster and, when the plaster is removed, he or she must, until circulatory control is regained, wear a crepe bandage and elevate the leg whenever it is not being used actively. Physiotherapy is always helpful.

Algodystrophy This often follows fractures of the ankle. The patient complains of pain in the foot; there may be swelling and diffuse tenderness, with gradual development of trophic changes and severe osteoporosis. Management is discussed in Chapter 10.

Osteoarthritis Malunion and/or incomplete reduction may lead to secondary osteoarthritis of the ankle in later years. Unless the ankle is unstable, symptoms can often be managed by judicious analgesic treatment and the use of firm, comfortable footwear. However, in the longer term if symptoms become severe arthrodesis may be necessary.

PILON FRACTURES

Unlike the twisting injuries that cause the common ankle fractures, this injury to the ankle joint occurs when a large force drives the talus upwards against the tibial plafond, like a pestle (pilon) being struck into a mortar. There is considerable damage to the articular cartilage and the subchondral bone may be broken into several pieces; in severe cases, the comminution extends some way up the shaft of the tibia.

Clinical features

There may be little swelling initially but this rapidly changes and fracture blisters are common. The ankle may be deformed or even dislocated; prompt approximate reduction is mandatory.

X-rays

This is a comminuted fracture of the distal end of the tibia, extending into the ankle joint. The fracture may

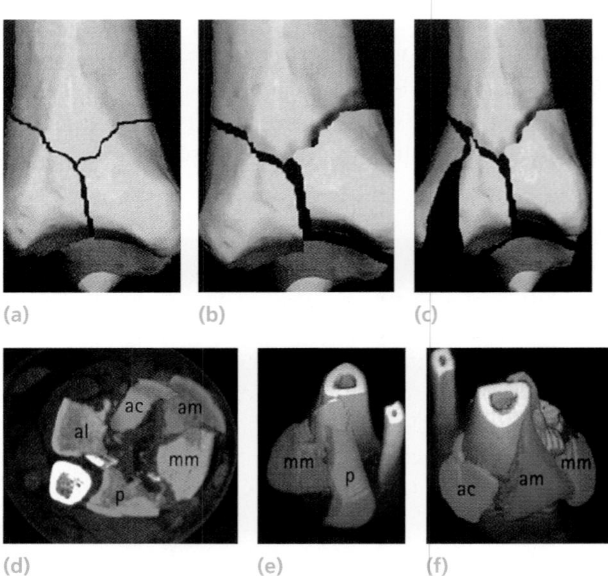

31.9 Pilon fractures – imaging These are either (a) undisplaced (type 1), (b) minimally displaced (type 2); (c) markedly displaced (type 3). CT (d) shows that there are usually five major tibial fragments: anterolateral (al), anterocentral (ac), anteromedial (am), the medial malleolus (mm) and the posterior fragment (p). These elements are better defined by three-dimensional CT reconstruction (e,f).

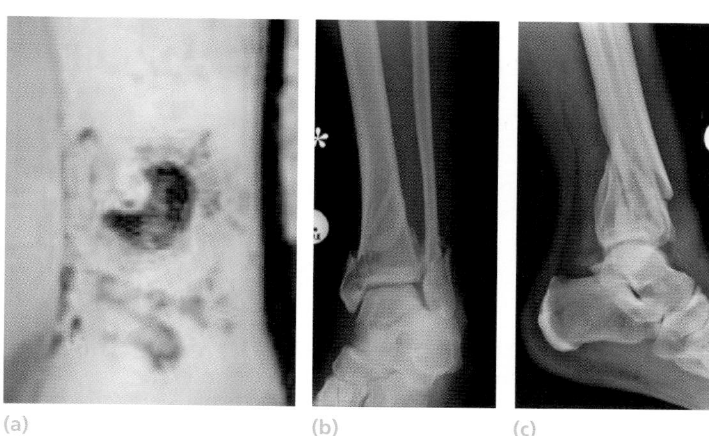

(a) (b) (c)

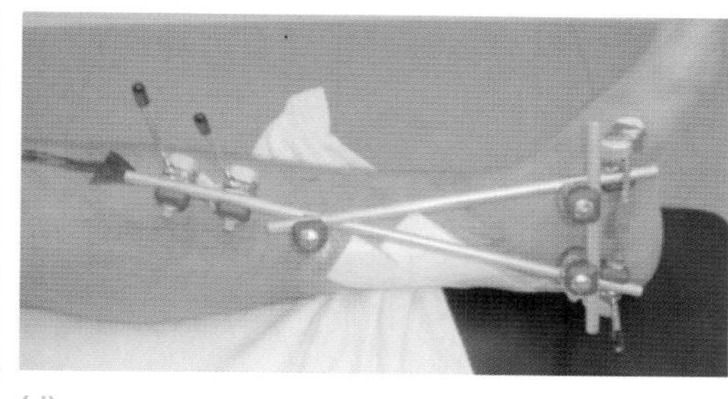

(d)

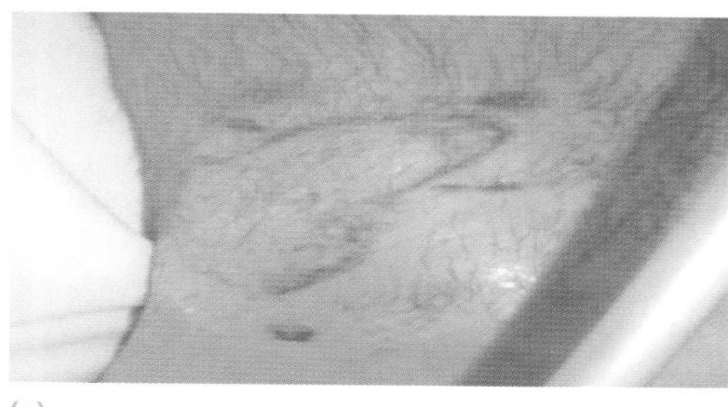

(e)

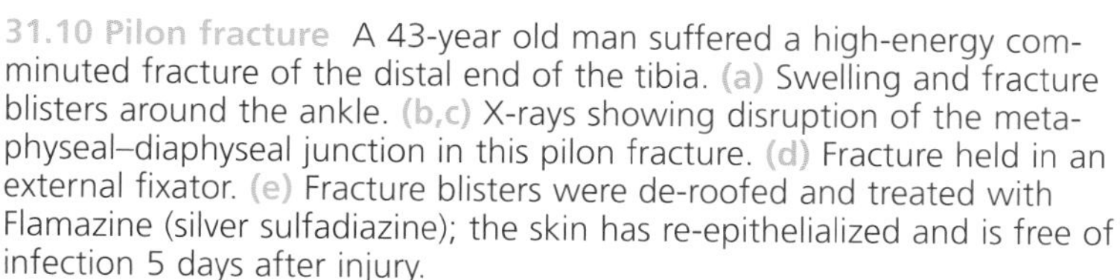

31.10 Pilon fracture A 43-year old man suffered a high-energy comminuted fracture of the distal end of the tibia. (a) Swelling and fracture blisters around the ankle. (b,c) X-rays showing disruption of the metaphyseal–diaphyseal junction in this pilon fracture. (d) Fracture held in an external fixator. (e) Fracture blisters were de-roofed and treated with Flamazine (silver sulfadiazine); the skin has re-epithelialized and is free of infection 5 days after injury.

be classified according to the amount of displacement and comminution (Rüedi and Allgöwer, 1979), though this will usually require accurate definition by CT. Rüedi *type 1* is an intra-articular fracture with little or no displacement of the fragments; in *type 2* there is more severe disruption of the articular surface but without very marked comminution. *Type 3* is a severely comminuted fracture with displacement of the fragments and gross articular irregularity.

In all cases, assessment is far better with CT scanning (preferably including three-dimensional reconstruction) than with plain x-ray examination.

Treatment

The three points of early management of these injuries are: *span*, *scan*, *plan*. Staged treatment has reduced the complication rate in these injuries.

Control of soft tissue swelling is a priority; this is best achieved either by elevation and applying an external fixator across the ankle joint (the spanning external fixator, or travelling traction). It may take 2–3 weeks before the soft tissues improve, and fracture blisters can be actively managed rather than hidden under plaster. Surgery can be planned, based on the CT scan.

Once the skin has recovered, an open reduction and fixation with plates and screws (usually with bone grafting) may be possible. However, the more severe injuries (types 2 and 3) do not readily tolerate large surgical exposures for plating and significant wound breakdown and infection rates have been reported. Better results have followed wider use of indirect reduction techniques (e.g. applying a bone distractor or utilizing the spanning fixator across the joint to obtain as much reduction as possible through ligamentotaxis) and plating through limited exposures. Recently, these injuries have been successfully treated by using a combination of indirect reduction methods and small screws to hold the articular fragments, coupled with axially stable locking plates. Circular frame fixation has also been successful.

The soft-tissue swelling following these injuries is substantial. After fixation, elevation and early movement help to reduce the oedema; arterio-venous impulse devices applied to the sole of the foot are also helpful.

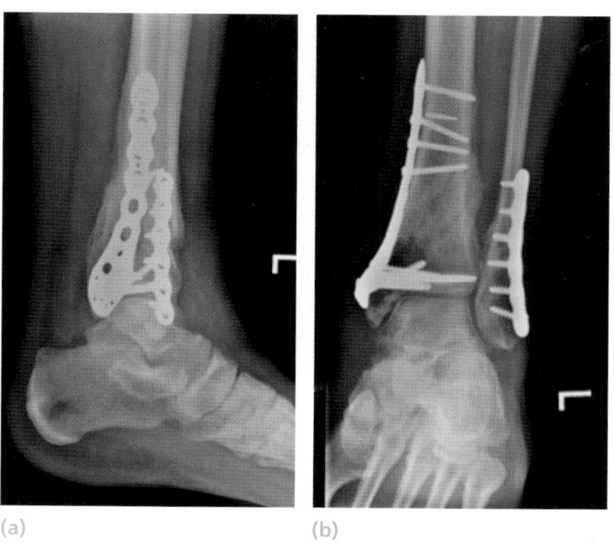

(a) (b)

31.11 Same case as 31.10 – Outcome At 3 months after minimal approach reduction and fixation with distal locking plates the fractures have healed and the joint is congruent and normally aligned.

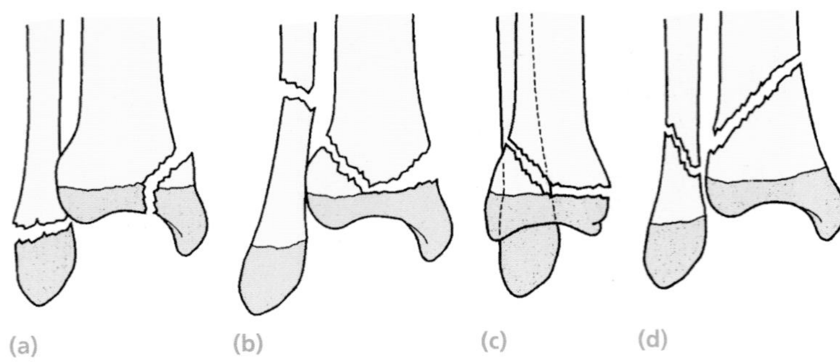

31.12 Physeal injuries of the distal tibia The classification suggested by Dias and Tachdjian (1978) has the merit of pointing to the required reduction manoeuvre – the reverse of the causal mechanism. (a) *Supination–inversion*: the fibular fracture is usually an avulsion (Salter–Harris type 1) whereas the medial malleolar fracture can be variable. (b) *Pronation–eversion–external rotation*: the fibular fracture is often high and transverse. (c) *Supination–plantarflexion*: a fracture of the distal tibia only (Salter–Harris type 1 or 2) with posterior displacement. (d) *Supination–external rotation*: an oblique fibular fracture coupled with a fracture of the distal tibia.

Outcome

Pilon fractures usually take several months to heal. Postoperatively, physiotherapy is focused on joint movement and reduction of swelling. There remains, however, a challenging problem with poor functional results in these complex fractures, which represent a significant soft tissue injury as well as bony jigsaw. Although bony union may be achieved, the fate of the joint is decided by the degree of cartilage injury – the 'invisible' factor on x-rays. Secondary osteoarthritis, stiffness and pain are still frequent late complications.

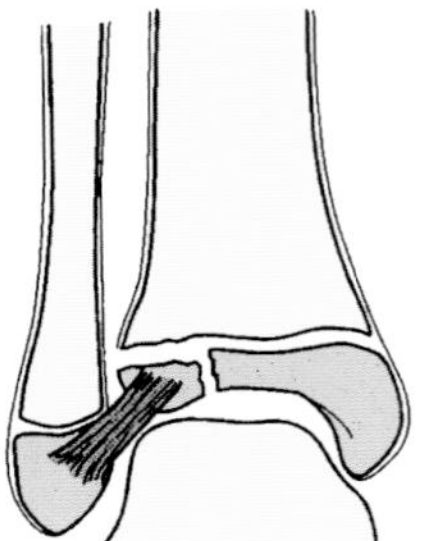

31.13 Tillaux fracture Diagram illustrating the elements of this unusual injury.

ANKLE FRACTURES IN CHILDREN

Physeal injuries are quite common in children and almost a third of these occur around the ankle.

Mechanism of injury

The foot is fixed to the ground or trapped in a crevice and the leg twists to one or the other side. The tibial (or fibular) physis is wrenched apart, usually resulting in a *Salter–Harris type 1 or 2 fracture*. With severe external rotation or abduction the fibula may also fracture more proximally. The tibial metaphyseal spike may come off posteriorly, laterally or posteromedially; its position is determined by the mechanism of injury and suggests the method of reduction. With adduction injuries the tip of the fibula may be avulsed.

Type 3 and 4 fractures are uncommon. They are due to a supination–adduction force. The epiphysis is split vertically and one piece of the epiphysis (usually the medial part) may be displaced.

Two unusual injuries of the growing ankle are the *Tillaux fracture* and the notorious *triplane fracture*. The Tillaux fracture is an avulsion of a fragment of tibia by the anterior tibiofibular ligament; in the child or adolescent this fragment is the lateral part of the epiphysis and the injury is therefore a Salter–Harris type 3 fracture.

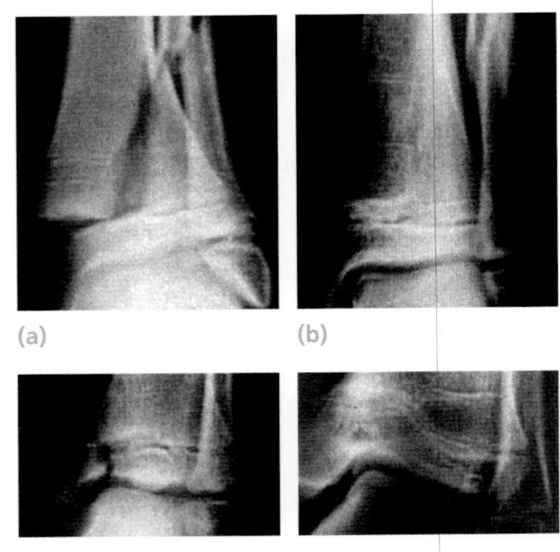

31.14 Ankle fractures in children (a) Salter–Harris type 2 injury; after reduction (b) growth has proceeded normally. (c) Salter–Harris type 3 injury; (d) the medial side of the physis has fused prematurely, resulting in distorted growth.

The *triplane fracture* occurs on the medial side of the tibia and is a combination of Salter–Harris types 2

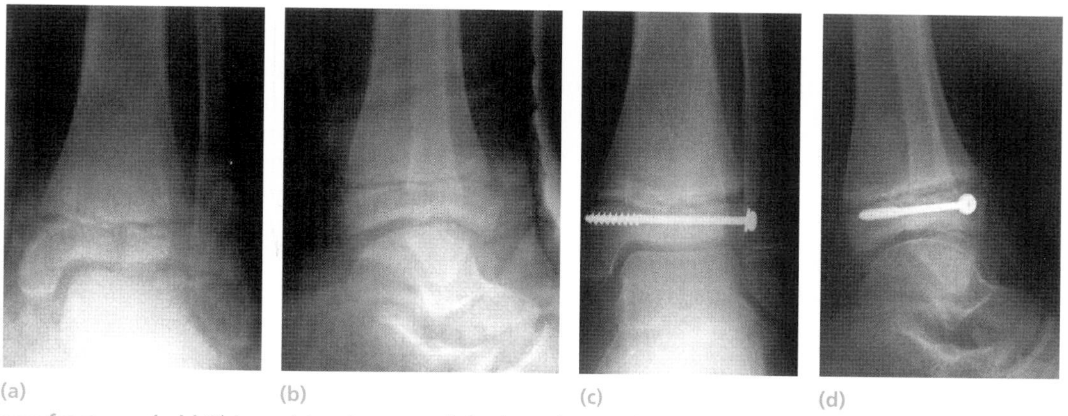

31.15 Tillaux fracture (a,b) This avulsion fracture of the lateral part of the physis was reduced and fixed percutaneously (c,d).

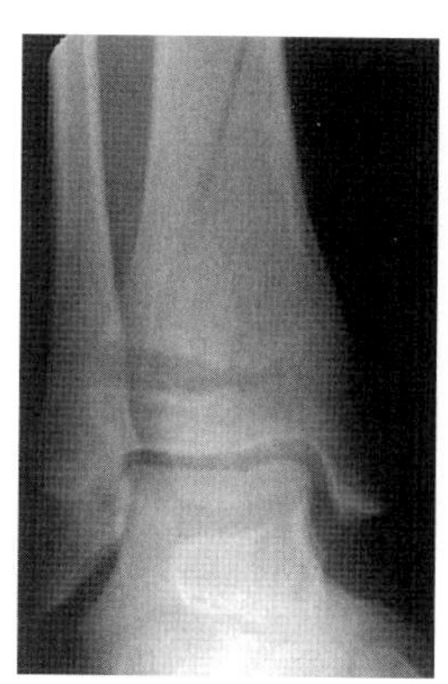

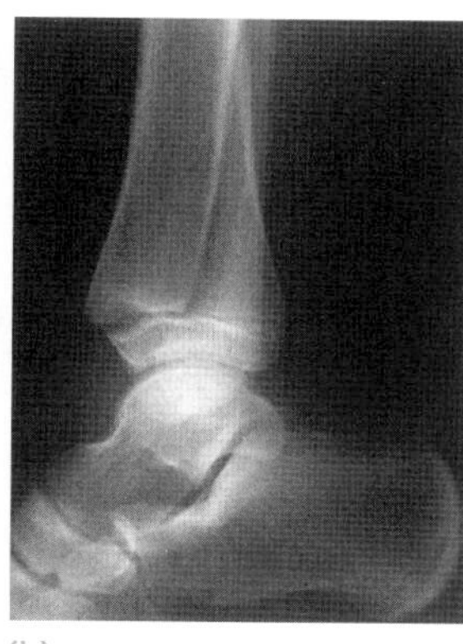

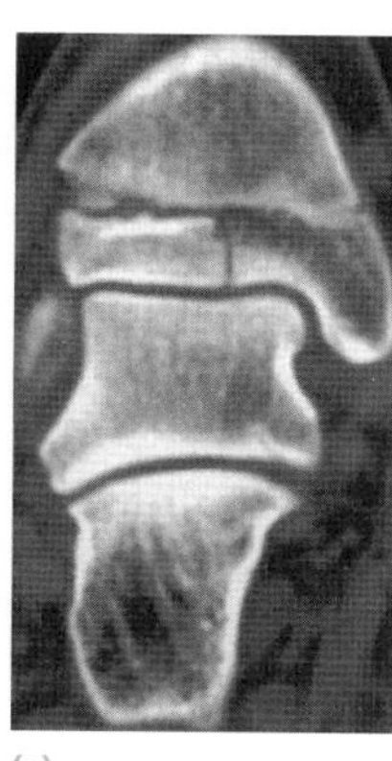

31.16 Triplane fracture The three fracture planes may not be seen in a single x-ray, but can be visualized from a combination of images. In this case the epiphyseal fracture is clearly seen only in the coronal plane CT scan (c).

and 3 injuries. Fracture lines appear in the coronal, sagittal and transverse planes. Injury to the physis may result in either asymmetrical growth or arrested growth.

Clinical features

Following a sprain the ankle is painful, swollen, bruised and acutely tender. There may be an obvious deformity, but sometimes the injury looks deceptively mild.

Imaging

Undisplaced physeal fractures – especially those in the distal fibula – are easily missed. Even a hint of physeal widening should be regarded with great suspicion and the child x-rayed again after 1 week. In an infant the state of the physis can sometimes only be guessed at, but a few weeks after injury there may be extensive periosteal new bone formation.

In triplane fractures the tibial epiphysis may be split in one plane and the metaphysis in another, thus making it difficult to see both fractures in the same x-ray. CT scans are particularly helpful in these and other type 3 injuries.

Treatment

Salter–Harris types 1 and 2 injuries are treated closed. If it is displaced, the fracture is gently reduced under general anaesthesia; the limb is immobilized in a full-length cast for 3 weeks and then in a below-knee walking cast for a further 3 weeks. Occasionally, surgery is needed to extract a periosteal flap, which prevents an adequate reduction.

Type 3 or 4 fractures, if undisplaced, can be treated in the same manner, but *the ankle must be re-x-rayed after 5 days to ensure that the fragments have not slipped*. Displaced fractures can sometimes be reduced closed by reversing the forces that produced the injury. However, unless reduction is near-perfect, the fracture should be reduced open and fixed with interfragmentary screws, which are inserted parallel to the physis. Postoperatively the leg is immobilized in a below-knee cast for 6 weeks.

Tillaux fractures are treated in the same way as type 3 fractures. Triplane fractures, if undisplaced, can be managed closed but require vigilant monitoring for late displacement. Displaced fractures must be reduced and fixed.

Complications

Malunion Imperfect reduction may result in angular deformity of the ankle – usually valgus. In children under 10 years old, mild deformities may be accommodated by further growth and modelling. In older children the deformity should be corrected by a supramalleolar closing-wedge osteotomy.

Asymmetrical growth Fractures through the epiphysis (Salter–Harris type 3 or 4) may result in localized fusion of the physis. The bony bridge is usually in the medial half of the growth plate; the lateral half goes on growing and the distal tibia gradually veers into varus. MRI and CT are helpful in showing precisely where physeal arrest has occurred. If the bony bridge is small (less than 30 per cent of the physeal width) it can be excised and replaced by a pad of fat in the hope that physeal growth may be restored. If more than half of the physis is involved, or the child is near the end of the growth period, a supramalleolar closing-wedge osteotomy is indicated.

Shortening Early physeal closure occurs in about 2 per cent of children with distal tibial injuries. Fortunately the resulting limb length discrepancy is usually mild. If it promises to be more than 2 cm and the child is young enough, proximal tibial epiphysiodesis in the opposite limb may restore equality. If the discrepancy is marked, or the child near the end of the growth period, leg lengthening is indicated.

PRINCIPLES IN MANAGING INJURIES OF THE FOOT

Injuries of the foot are apt to be followed by residual symptoms and loss of function, which seem out of proportion to the initial trauma. Severe injuries affect the foot as a whole, whatever the particular bone that might be fractured. A global approach is therefore essential in dealing with these injuries, the objective being a return to full weightbearing without pain, with an appropriate propulsive gait.

Identification of these injuries is particularly challenging in the patient with multiple trauma, where the more subtle foot injuries might be missed as the life-threatening truncal injuries and limb-threatening long bone injuries distract attention from the more subtle injuries to the foot, which may nonetheless impair eventual function.

Clinical assessment

The entire foot should be examined systematically, no matter that the injury may appear to be localized to one spot. Multiple fractures, or combinations of fractures and dislocations, are easily missed. The circulation and nerve supply must be carefully assessed; a well-reduced fracture is a useless achievement if the foot becomes ischaemic or insensitive. Similarly, attention must be paid to the soft tissues and functional movement of the foot; the stiff, painful foot is impaired for propulsion, and maybe even for stance.

Fractures and dislocations may cause tenting of the skin; this is always a bad sign because there is a risk of skin necrosis if reduction is delayed.

Imaging

Imaging routinely begins with anteroposterior, lateral and oblique x-rays of the foot. If a fracture of the talus or calcaneum, or fracture–dislocation of the midtarsal joints is suspected then special views may be helpful, but a more rewarding approach is to carry out a CT scan of the foot.

CT is especially useful for evaluating fractures of the calcaneum, and MRI is helpful in diagnosing osteochondral fractures of the talus. *Familiarity with the talocalcaneal anatomy is essential if fractures of the hindfoot are to be diagnosed properly.*

Treatment

Swelling is always a problem. Not only does it make clinical examination difficult, but more importantly it may lead to definitive treatment being delayed; fractures and dislocations are more difficult to reduce in a swollen foot. The principles are:

- realign and splint the foot, keep it elevated and apply Cryo-Cuff or ice-packs and intermittent pneumatic compression foot pumps;

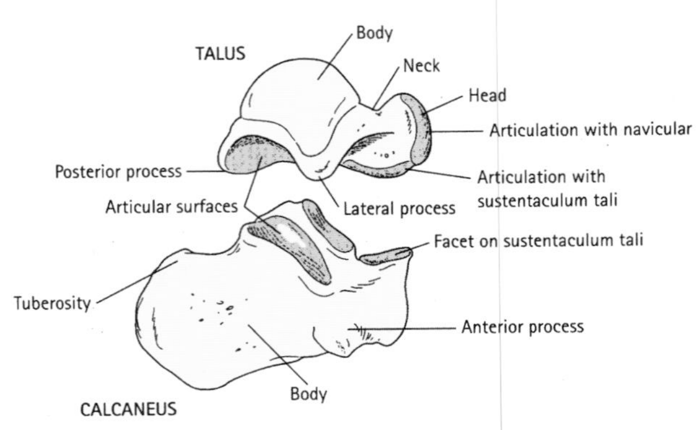

31.17 Talus and calcaneum The main features of these two bones, and their relationship to each other, are shown here.

- make the diagnosis, defining the extent of injury;
- start definitive treatment as soon as the fracture pattern is properly defined and swelling permits.

In the rehabilitation phase, if the foot has to be immobilized, exercise those joints that can be left free. Start weightbearing as soon as the patient will tolerate it, provided this will not jeopardize the reduction. If a removable splint will fit the purpose, use it so that non-weightbearing exercises can be started as soon as possible. Prolonged immobilization predisposes to stiffness, impaired function, localized osteoporosis and complex regional pain syndrome.

INJURIES OF THE TALUS

Talar fractures and dislocations are relatively uncommon. They usually involve considerable violence – car accidents in which the occupants are thrown against the resistant frame of the vehicle, falls from a height, or severe wrenching of the ankle. The injuries include fractures of the neck, body, head or bony processes of the talus, dislocations of the talus or the joints around the talus, osteochondral fractures of the superior articular surface, and a variety of chip or avulsion fractures.

The significance of the more serious injuries is enhanced by two important facts: (1) the talus is a major weightbearing structure (the superior articular surface carries a greater load per unit area than any other bone in the body); (2) it has a vulnerable blood supply and is a relatively common site for post-traumatic ischaemic necrosis.

Blood vessels enter the bone from the anterior tibial, posterior tibial and peroneal arteries, as well as anastomotic vessels from the surrounding capsule and ligaments. The head of the talus is richly supplied by intraosseous vessels. However, the body of the talus is supplied mainly by vessels that enter the talar neck from the tarsal canal and then run retrograde from distal to proximal. In fractures of the talar neck these vessels are divided; if the fracture is displaced, the extraosseous plexus too may be damaged and the body of the talus is at risk of ischaemia.

Mechanism of injury

Fracture of the talar neck is produced by violent hyperextension of the ankle. The neck of the talus is forced against the anterior edge of the tibia, which acts like a cleaver. If the force continues, the fracture is displaced and the surrounding joints may sublux or dislocate.

Fracture of the body is usually a compression injury due to a fall from a height, or an everting force across the body, fracturing the lateral process (the snowboarders' fracture). Avulsion fractures are associated with ligament strains around the ankle and hindfoot.

Clinical features

The patient has most commonly been involved in a motor vehicle accident or has fallen from a height. The foot and ankle are painful and swollen; if the fracture is displaced, there may be an obvious deformity, or the skin may be tented or split. Tenting is a dangerous sign; if the fracture or dislocation is not promptly reduced, the skin may slough and become

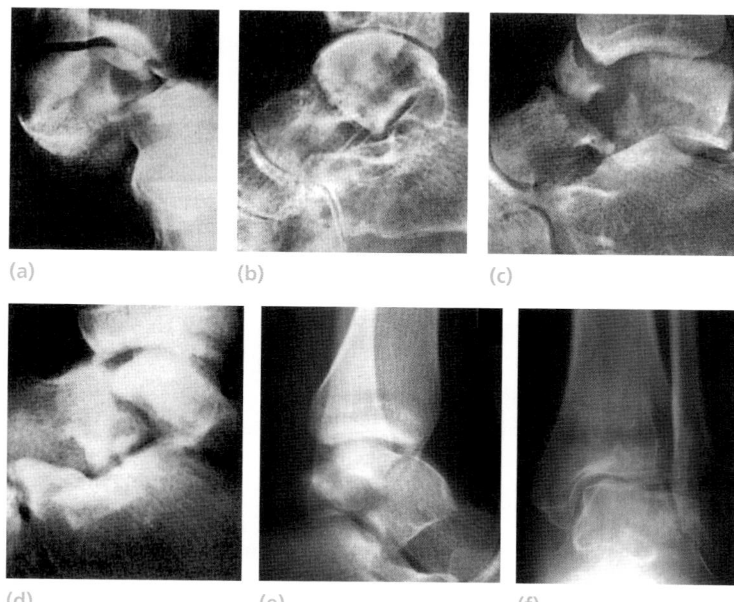

31.18 Injuries of the talus–x-rays (a) Talocalcaneal fracture–dislocation. (b) Undisplaced fracture of the talar neck. (c) Type III fracture of the neck. (d) Displaced fracture of the body of the talus. (e) This fracture of the body was thought to be well reduced; however, in the AP view (f) it is possible to see two overlapping outlines, indicating that the fragments are malrotated.

infected. The pulses should be checked and compared with those in the opposite foot.

X-ray

Anteroposterior, lateral and oblique views are essential; CT scanning helps to identify associated injuries of the ankle and foot. Both malleoli, the ankle mortise, the talus and all the adjacent tarsal bones should be carefully assessed. Undisplaced fractures are not always easy to see, and sometimes even severely displaced fractures are missed in the initial assessment because of unfamiliarity with the normal appearance – sad but true.

Classification

Fractures of the neck of the talus These fractures are classified according to the system devised by Hawkins (1970) and modified by Canale (1978):

- Group I – undisplaced
- Group II – displaced (however little) and associated with subluxation or dislocation of the subtalar joint
- Group III – displaced, with dislocation of the body of the talus from the ankle joint
- Type IV – displaced vertical talar neck fracture with associated talonavicular joint disruption.

Fractures of the head of the talus This is a rare injury; the fracture usually involves the talonavicular joint.

Fractures of the body of the talus These are also uncommon. The fracture is often displaced and may cause distortion of the talocalcaneal joint. Rotational malalignment of the fragments is difficult to diagnose on plain x-ray examination; the deformity is best visualized by three-dimensional CT reconstruction.

Fractures of the lateral and posterior processes These are usually associated with ankle ligament strains. It is sometimes difficult to distinguish between a fracture of the posterior process and a normal os trigonum. A simple rule is 'if it's not causing symptoms it doesn't really matter'.

Osteochondral fractures Osteochondral fractures following acute trauma usually occur on the lateral part of the dome of the talus. The diagnosis is often missed when the patient is first seen and may come to light only after CT or MRI scan.

Treatment

The general principles set out on page 920 should be observed.

UNDISPLACED FRACTURES

A split below-knee plaster is applied and, when the swelling has subsided, is replaced by a complete cast with the foot plantarflexed. Weightbearing is not permitted for the first 4 weeks; thereafter, the plaster is removed, the fracture position is checked by x-ray, a new cast is applied and weightbearing is gradually introduced. Further plaster changes or use of an adjustable splintage boot will allow the foot to be brought up, slowly, to plantigrade; physiotherapy is commenced. At 8–12 weeks the splintage is discarded and function is regained by normal use.

DISPLACED FRACTURES OF THE NECK

Even the slightest displacement makes it a type II fracture, which needs to be reduced. If the skin is tight, reduction becomes urgent because of the risk of skin necrosis. Reduction must be *perfect*: (1) in order to ensure that the subtalar joint is mechanically sound; (2) to lessen the chance – or at any rate lessen the effects – of avascular necrosis.

With *type II fractures*, closed manipulation under general anaesthesia can be tried first. Traction is applied with the ankle in plantarflexion; the foot is then steered into inversion or eversion to correct the displacement shown on the x-ray. The reduction is checked by x-ray; nothing short of 'anatomic' is acceptable. A below-knee cast is applied (with the foot still in equinus) and this is retained, non-weightbearing, for 4 weeks. Cast changes after that will allow the foot to be gradually brought up to plantigrade; however, weightbearing is not permitted until there is evidence of union (8–12 weeks).

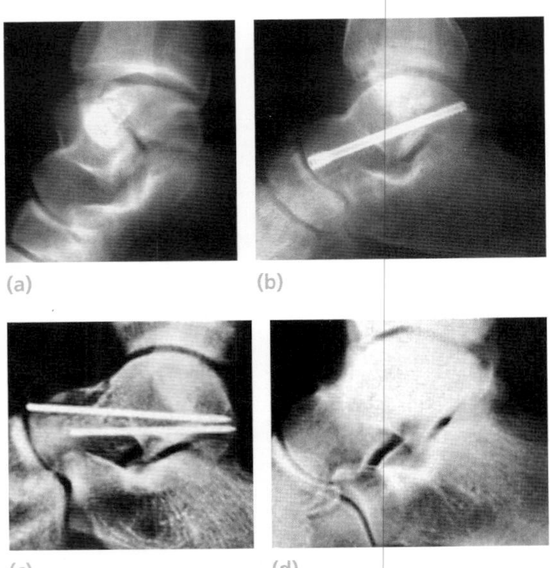

31.19 Fractures of the talus – treatment (a) This displaced fracture of the body was reduced and fixed with a countersunk screw (b), giving a perfect result. Fractures of the neck, even if well reduced (c) are still at risk of developing ischaemic necrosis (d).

If closed reduction fails (which it often does), open reduction is essential; indeed, some would say that *all* type II fractures should be managed by open reduction and internal fixation without attempting closed treatment. Through an anteromedial incision the fracture is exposed and manipulated into position. Wider access can be obtained by pre-drilling and then osteotomizing the medial malleolus; after the talar fracture has been reduced, the malleolar fragment is fixed back in position with a screw. The position is checked by x-ray and the fracture is then fixed with two K-wires or a lag screw. Postoperatively a below-knee cast is applied; weightbearing is not permitted until there are signs of union (8–12 weeks).

Type III fracture–dislocations need urgent open reduction and internal fixation. The approach will depend on the fracture pattern and position of displaced fragments. Osteotomy of the medial malleolus might help; the malleolus is pre-drilled for screw fixation and osteotomized and retracted distally without injuring the deltoid ligament. This wide exposure is essential to permit removal of small fragments from the ankle joint and perfect reduction of the displaced talar body under direct vision; even then, it is difficult! The position is checked by x-ray and the fracture is then fixed securely with screws. If there is the slightest doubt about the condition of the skin, the wound is left open and delayed primary closure carried out 5 days later. Postoperatively the foot is splinted and elevated until the swelling subsides; a below-knee cast or splintage boot is then applied, following the same routine as for type II injuries.

DISPLACED FRACTURES OF THE BODY

Fractures through the body of the talus are usually displaced or comminuted and involve the ankle and/or the talocalcaneal joint; occasionally the fragments are completely dislocated.

Minimal displacement can be accepted; a below-knee non-weightbearing cast is applied for 6–8 weeks; this is then replaced by a weightbearing cast for another 4 weeks.

Horizontal fractures that do not involve the ankle or subtalar joint are treated by closed reduction and cast immobilization (as earlier).

Displaced fractures with dislocation of the adjacent joints should be accurately reduced. In almost all cases open reduction and internal fixation will be needed. An osteotomy of the medial malleolus is useful for adequate exposure of the talus; the malleolus is predrilled before the osteotomy and fixed back into position after the talar fracture has been dealt with. The prognosis for these fractures is poor: there is a considerable incidence of malunion, joint incongruity, avascular necrosis and secondary osteoarthritis of the ankle or talocalcaneal joint.

DISPLACED FRACTURES OF THE HEAD

The main problem is injury to the talonavicular joint. If the fragments are large enough, open reduction and internal fixation with screws is the recommended treatment. If there is much comminution, it may be better simply to excise the smaller fragments. Postoperative immobilization is the same as for other talar fractures.

FRACTURES OF THE TALAR PROCESSES

If the fragment is large enough, open reduction and fixation with K-wires or small screws is advisable. Tiny fragments are left but can be removed later if they become symptomatic.

OSTEOCHONDRAL FRACTURES

These small surface fractures of the dome of the talus usually occur with severe ankle sprains or subtalar dislocations. Most acute lesions can be treated by cast immobilization for 4–6 weeks. Occasionally a displaced fragment is large enough to warrant operative replacement and internal fixation – easier said than done! More often it is separated from its bed and is excised: the exposed bone is then drilled to encourage repair by fibrocartilage.

OPEN FRACTURES

Fractures of the talus are often associated with burst skin wounds. In some cases the fracture becomes 'open' when stretched or tented skin starts sloughing. There is a high risk of infection in these wounds and prophylactic antibiotics are advisable.

The injury is treated as an emergency. Under general anaesthesia, the wound is cleaned and debrided and all necrotic tissue is removed. The fracture is then dealt with as for closed injuries, except that the wound is left open and closed by delayed primary suture or skin grafting 5–7 days later, when swelling has subsided and it is certain that there is no infection.

Sometimes, in open injuries, the talus is completely detached and lying in the wound. After adequate debridement and cleansing, the talus should be replaced in the mortise and stabilized, if necessary with crossed K-wires. Later definitive fixation is then performed.

Complications

Malunion The importance of accurate reduction has been stressed. Malunion may lead to distortion of the joint surface, limitation of movement and pain on weightbearing. If early follow-up x-rays show redisplacement of the fragments, a further attempt at reduction is justified. Persistent malunion predisposes to osteoarthritis.

Avascular necrosis Avascular necrosis of the body of the talus occurs in displaced fractures of the talar neck. The incidence varies with the severity of displacement: in type 1 fractures it is less than 10 per cent; in type 2 about 30–40 per cent; and in type 3 more than 90 per cent. The earliest x-ray sign (often present by the sixth week) is apparent increased density of the avascular segment; in reality it is the rest of the tarsus that has become slightly porotic with disuse, but the avascular portion remains unaffected and therefore looks more 'dense'. The opposite is also true: if the dome of the talus becomes osteoporotic, this means that it has a blood supply and it will not develop osteonecrosis. This is the basis of Hawkins' sign, which should be looked for 6–8 weeks after injury.

If osteonecrosis does occur, the body of the talus will eventually appear on x-ray to be more dense than the surrounding bones. Despite necrosis, the fracture may heal, so treatment should not be interrupted by this event; if anything, weightbearing should be delayed in the hope that the bone is not unduly flattened. Function may yet be reasonable. However, if the talus becomes flattened or fragmented, or pain and disability are marked, the ankle may need to be arthrodesed.

Secondary osteoarthritis Osteoarthritis of the ankle and/or subtalar joints occurs some years after injury in over 50 per cent of patients with talar neck fractures. There are a number of causes: (1) articular damage due to the initial trauma; (2) malunion and distortion of the articular surface; (3) avascular necrosis of the talus. Pain and stiffness may be managed by judicious analgesic medication and orthotic adjustments, but in some cases the painful hindfoot will simply not allow a return to function; arthrodesis of the affected joints can help to relieve symptoms. Operative fusion of one joint may predispose to overload of the associated foot joints, and hence to later arthritis, but this should be accepted.

FRACTURES OF THE CALCANEUM

The calcaneum is the most commonly fractured tarsal bone, and in 5–10 per cent of cases both heels are injured simultaneously. Crush injuries, although they always heal in the biological sense, are likely to be followed by long-term disability. The general attitude to these injuries at the beginning of the twentieth century (at least from an industrial point of view) was that "the man who breaks his heel-bone is finished". This was followed by attempts, throughout the latter part of that century, to modify the outcome through open reduction and internal fixation of these fractures.

Mechanism of injury

In most cases the patient falls from a height, often from a ladder, onto one or both heels. The calcaneum is driven up against the talus and is split or crushed. Over 20 per cent of these patients suffer associated injuries of the spine, pelvis or hip.

Avulsion fractures sometimes follow traction injuries of the tendo Achillis or the ankle ligaments. Occasionally the bone is shattered by a direct blow.

Pathological anatomy

Based largely on the work of Palmer (1948) and Essex-Lopresti (1952), it has been customary to divide calcaneal fractures into *extra-articular fractures* (those involving the various calcaneal processes or the body posterior to the talocalcaneal joint) and *intra-articular fractures* (those that split the talocalcaneal articular facet).

EXTRA-ARTICULAR FRACTURES

These account for 25 per cent of calcaneal injuries. They usually follow fairly simple patterns, with shearing or avulsion of the anterior process, the sustentaculum tali, the tuberosity or the inferomedial process. Fractures of the posterior (extra-articular) part of the body are caused by compression. Extra-articular fractures are usually easy to manage and have a good prognosis.

INTRA-ARTICULAR FRACTURES

These injuries are much more complex and unpredictable in their outcome. They are best understood by imagining the impact of the talus cleaving the bone from above to produce a *primary fracture line* that runs obliquely across the posterior articular facet and the body from posteromedial to anterolateral. Where it splits, the posterior articular facet depends upon the position of the foot at impact: if the heel is in valgus (abducted), the fracture is in the lateral part of the facet; if the heel is in varus (adducted), the fracture is more medial.

The upward displacement of the body of the calca-

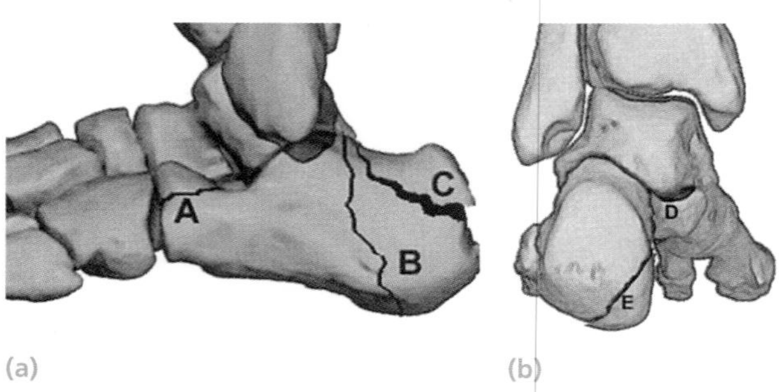

31.20 Extra-articular fractures of the calcaneum Fractures may occur through (**A**) the anterior process, (**B**) the body, (**C**) the tuberosity, (**D**) the sustentaculum tali or (**E**) the medial tubercle. Treatment is closed unless the fragment is large and badly displaced, in which case it will need to be fixed back in position.

neum produces one of the classic x-ray signs of a 'depressed' fracture: flattening of the angle subtended by the posterior articular surface and the upper surface of the body posterior to the joint (Böhler's angle).

The advent of CT, and the trend towards operative reduction and fixation of displaced calcaneal fractures, have sharpened our understanding of these complex injuries. There are two important ways of assessing or classifying these injuries that are of relevance to the treating surgeon (and the patient). The work of Sanders and Gregory (1995) has helped to define the intra-articular fracture pattern and the associated outcome and prognosis. Knowledge of the variations in fracture pattern, particularly in relation to the lateral wall of the calcaneum (Eastwood et al., 1993) has improved our understanding of the anatomy that is likely to be encountered at operation, approaching from an extended L-shaped incision; the lateral joint fragment may sometimes be trapped within the body of the calcaneum and can only be reduced if the lateral wall of the body is osteotomized so as to gain access to it (Eastwood et al., 1993).

Clinical features

There is usually a history of a fall from a height, or a road traffic accident; in elderly osteoporotic people even a comparatively minor injury may fracture the calcaneum.

The foot is painful and swollen and a large bruise appears on the lateral aspect of the heel. The heel may look broad and squat. The surrounding tissues are thick and tender, and the normal concavity below the lateral malleolus is lacking. The subtalar joint cannot be moved but ankle movement is possible.

Always check for signs of a compartment syndrome of the foot (intense pain, very extensive bruising and diminished sensation, with pain on passive toe movement).

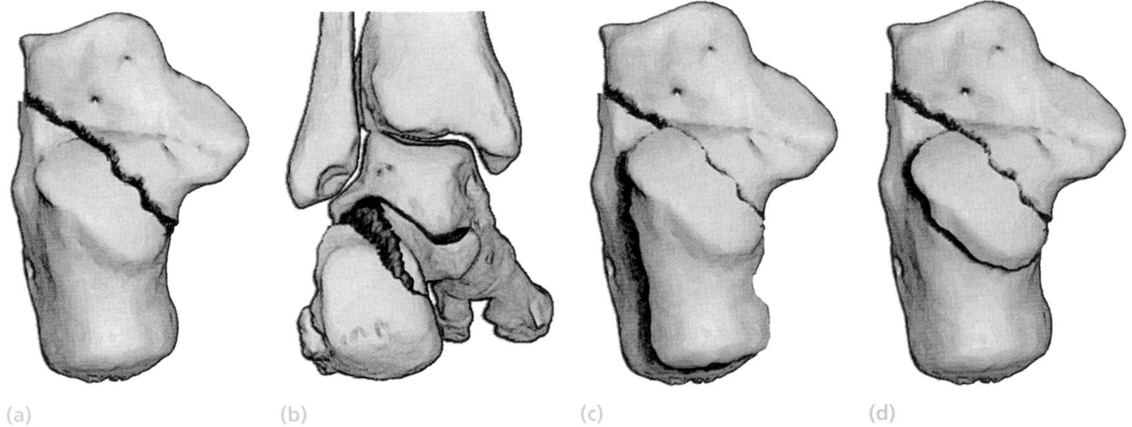

(a) (b) (c) (d)

31.21 Intra-articular fractures of the calcaneum The primary fracture line (a,b) is created by the impact of the talus on the calcaneum – it runs from posteromedial to anterolateral. Secondary fracture lines may create 'tongue' (c) or 'joint depression' (d) variants to the fracture pattern.

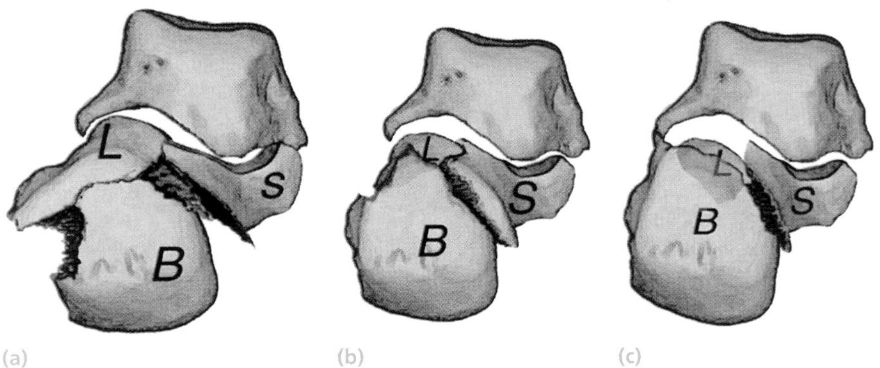

(a) (b) (c)

31.22 Intra-articular fractures of the calcaneum CT scans have allowed a better understanding of the fracture anatomy. A coronal CT scan enables the identification of three major fragments in most intra-articular fractures: the lateral joint fragment (L), the sustentaculum tali (S) and the body fragment (B). In type 1 fractures (a) the lateral joint fragment is in valgus whereas the body is in varus. In type 2 fractures (b), the sustentaculum tali is in varus and the lateral joint is elevated in relation to it. In type 3 fractures (c) the lateral joint fragment is impacted and buried within the body fragment (Eastwood et al., 1993).

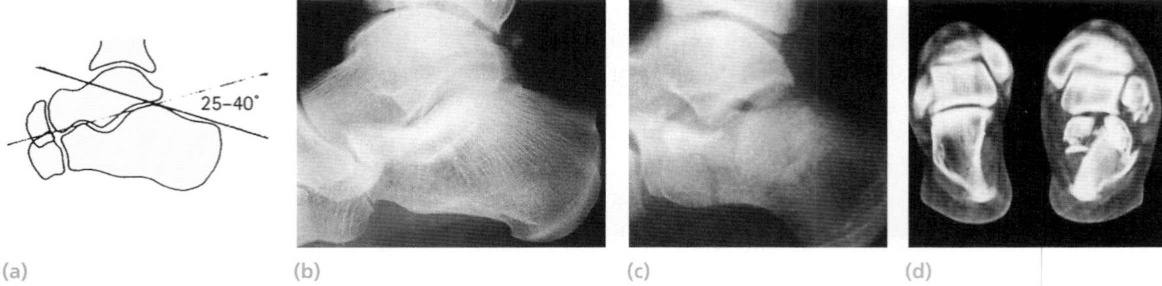

31.23 Fracture of the calcaneum – imaging (a,b) Measurement of Böhler's angle and the x-ray appearance in a normal foot. (c) Flattening of Böhler's angle in a fractured calcaneum. (d) The CT scan in this case shows how the articular fragments have been split apart.

X-ray

Plain x-rays should include lateral, oblique and axial views. Extra-articular fractures are usually fairly obvious. Intra-articular fractures, also, can often be identified in the plain films and if there is displacement of the fragments the lateral view may show flattening of the tuber-joint angle (Böhler's angle).

For accurate definition of intra-articular fractures, CT is essential and three-dimensional reconstruction views even better. Coronal sections will show the fracture 'geometry' clearly enough to permit accurate diagnosis of most intra-articular fractures (Lowrie et al., 1988).

With severe injuries – and especially with bilateral fractures or in the unconscious patient – *it is essential to assess the knees, spine and pelvis as well.*

Treatment

For all except the most minor injuries, the patient is admitted to hospital so that the leg and foot can be elevated and treated with cold (ice or Cryo-Cuff) and compression until swelling subsides. This also gives time to obtain the necessary CT scans.

EXTRA-ARTICULAR FRACTURES

The byword for the management of extra-articular fractures is 'mobility and function are more important than anatomical repositioning'. The vast majority are treated closed: (1) compression bandaging, ice packs and elevation until the swelling subsides; (2) exercises as soon as pain permits; (3) no weightbearing for 4 weeks and partial weightbearing for another 4 weeks. Variations from this routine relate to specific injuries.

Fractures of the anterior process Most of these are avulsion fractures and many are mistaken for an ankle sprain. Oblique x-rays will show the fracture, which almost always involves the calcaneocuboid joint. If there is a large displaced fragment, internal fixation may be needed; this is followed by the usual 'closed' routine.

Fractures of the tuberosity These are usually due to avulsion by the tendo Achillis; clinical signs are similar to those of a torn Achilles tendon. If the fragment is displaced, it should be reduced and fixed with cancellous screws; the foot is then immobilized in slight equinus to relieve tension on the tendo Achillis. Weightbearing can be permitted after 4 weeks.

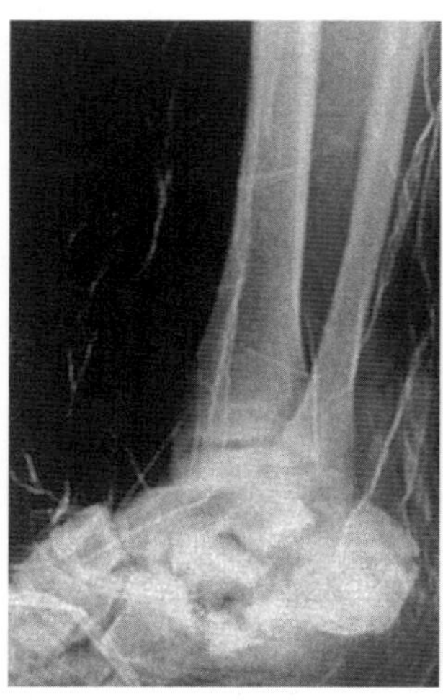
(a)

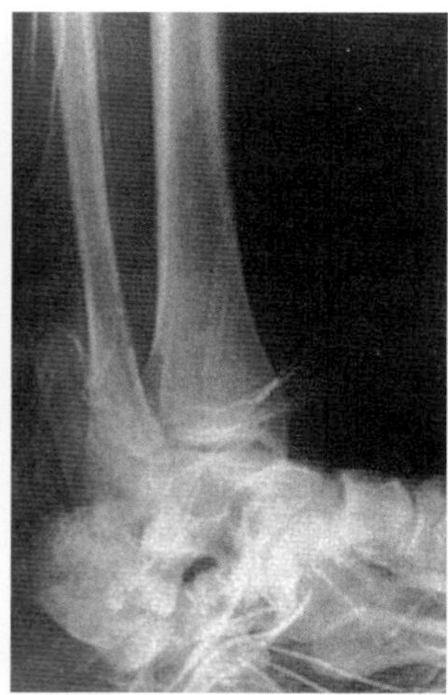
(b)

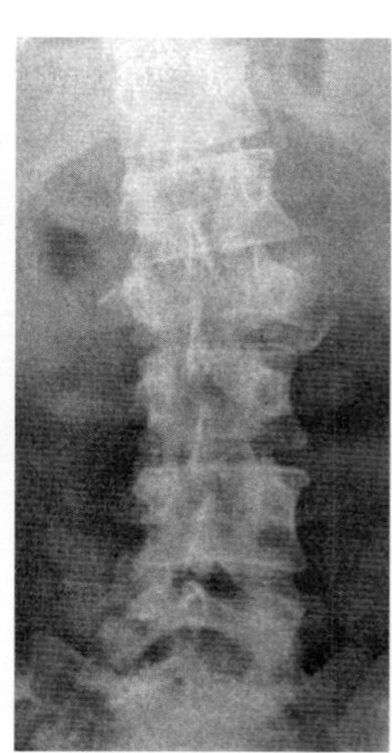
(c)

31.24 Calcaneal fractures – imaging Bilateral calcaneal fractures (a,b) are caused by a fall on the heels from a height or by an explosion from below. In either case the spine also may be fractured, as it was in this patient (c). With bilateral heel fractures, always x-ray the spine.

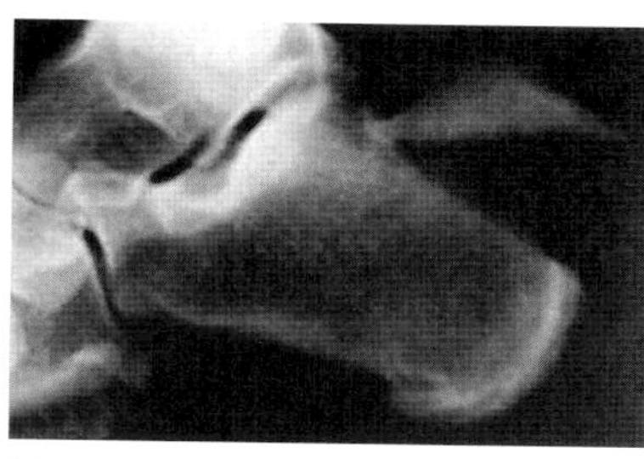

(a)

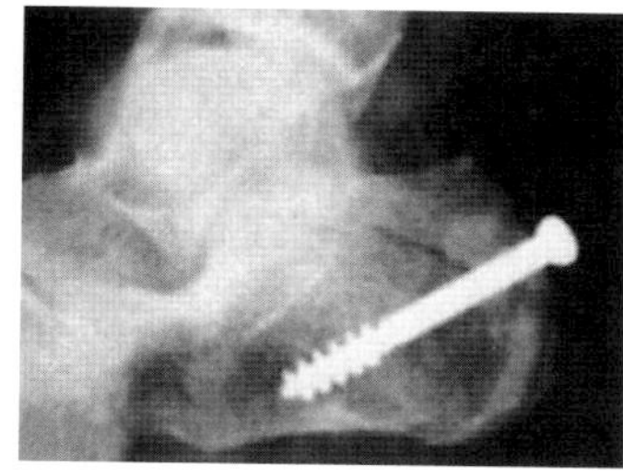

(b)

31.25 Extra-articular calcaneal fractures – treatment (a) Avulsion fracture of posterosuperior corner (b) fixed by a screw.

Fractures of the body If it is certain that the subtalar joint is not involved, the prognosis is good and the fracture can be treated by the usual 'closed' routine. However, if there is much sideways displacement and widening of the heel, closed reduction by manual compression should be attempted. Weightbearing is avoided for 6–8 weeks; however, cast immobilization is unnecessary except if both heels are fractured or if the patient simply cannot manage a one-legged gait with crutches (e.g. those who are elderly or frail).

INTRA-ARTICULAR FRACTURES

Undisplaced fractures are treated in much the same way as extra-articular fractures: compression bandaging, ice-packs and elevation followed by exercises and non-weightbearing for 6–8 weeks. As long as vertical stress is avoided, the fracture will not become displaced; cast immobilization is therefore unnecessary and it may even be harmful in that it increases the risk of stiffness and algodystrophy. Good or excellent results can be expected in most patients with undisplaced intra-articular fractures.

Displaced intra-articular fractures are best treated by open reduction and internal fixation as soon as the swelling subsides. CT has greatly facilitated this approach; the medial and lateral fragments can be clearly defined and, with suitable drawings or models, the surgical procedure can be carefully planned and rehearsed.

The operation is usually performed through a single, wide lateral approach; access to the posterior facet and medial fragment is achieved by taking down the lateral aspect of the calcaneum, performing the reduction, and then rebuilding this wall. The various fragments are held with interfragmentary screws – bone grafts are sometimes added to fill in defects. The anterior part of the calcaneum and the calcaneocuboid joint also need attention; the fragments are similarly reduced and fixed. Finally a contoured plate is placed on the lateral aspect of the calcaneum to buttress the entire assembly. The wound is then closed and drained.

Postoperatively the foot is lightly splinted and elevated. Exercises are begun as soon as pain subsides and after about 2 weeks the patient can be allowed up non-weightbearing on crutches. Partial weightbearing is permitted only when the fracture has healed (seldom before 8 weeks) and full weightbearing about 4 weeks after that. Restoration of function may take 6–12 months.

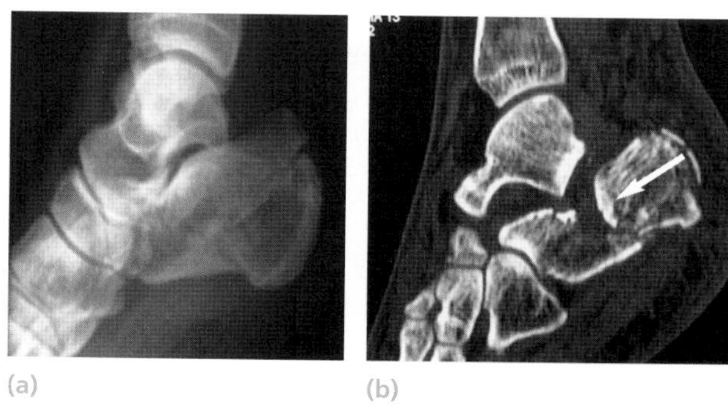

(a) (b)

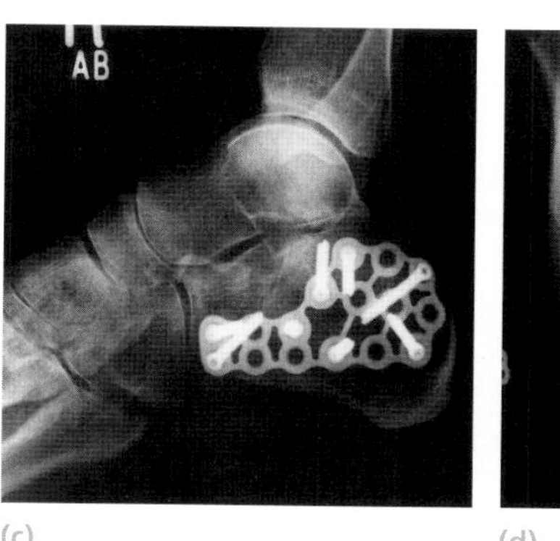

(c)

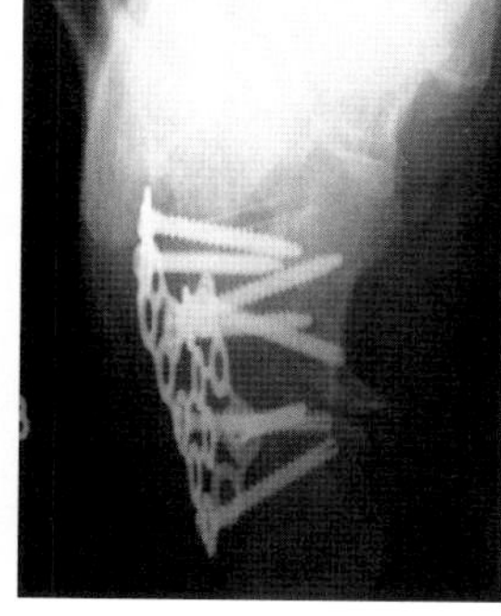

(d)

31.26 Intra-articular calcaneal fracture – treatment (a) X-ray gives limited information, but the CT (b) shows the severe depression of the posterior calcaneal facet. This was treated operatively with a calcaneal locking plate, to reconstitute the posterior facet (arrow) and restore the height of the calcaneum (c,d).

Outcome

Extra-articular fractures and *undisplaced intra-articular fractures*, if properly treated, usually have a good result. However, the patient should be warned that it may take 6–12 months before full function is regained, and in about 10 per cent of cases there will be residual symptoms that might preclude a return to their previous job if this involved walking on uneven surfaces or balancing on ladders.

The outcome for *displaced intra-articular fractures* is much less predictable. The results of operative treatment are heavily dependent on the severity of the fracture and the experience of the surgeon (Buckley et al., 1992; Sanders et al., 1995). The Canadian multicentre study showed a shorter time off work and lower requirement for subtalar arthrodesis in those managed operatively. Results were particularly favourable with internal fixation in younger men and those not working with heavy loads or receiving workmen's compensation. In experienced hands, for selected fractures, this is a rational treatment. However, it is not an enterprise for the tyro and unless the appropriate skills and facilities are available the patient should be referred to a specializing centre.

Closed treatment, though it may be the only alternative, has a bad reputation. Crosby and Fitzgibbons (1990), in a follow up of 30 patients who had undergone closed treatment, found that 50 per cent of those with uncomplicated displaced intra-articular fractures were contemplating having an arthrodesis within 4 years of injury; only two out of 10 patients had a 'good' result. Those with comminuted fractures fared even worse: all of them were assessed as having a poor result.

The fact remains that the heel fracture is a serious and disabling injury in many patients with heavy or physically demanding jobs; mechanical reconstruction of the bony anatomy does not necessarily improve the functional outcome.

Complications

EARLY

Swelling and blistering Intense swelling and blistering may jeopardize operative treatment. The limb should be elevated with the minimum of delay.

Compartment syndrome About 10 per cent of patients develop intense pressure symptoms. The risk of a full-blown compartment syndrome can be minimized by starting treatment early. If operative decompression is carried out, this will delay any definitive procedure for the fracture.

LATE

Malunion Closed treatment of displaced fractures, or injudicious weightbearing after open reduction, may result in malunion. *The heel is broad and squat*, and the patient has a problem fitting shoes. Usually the foot is in valgus and walking may be impaired.

Peroneal tendon impingement Lateral displacement of the body of the calcaneum may cause painful compression of the peroneal tendons against the lateral malleolus. Treatment consists of operative paring down of protuberant bone on the lateral wall of the calcaneum.

Insufficiency of the tendo Achillis The loss of heel height may result in diminished tendo Achillis action. If this interferes markedly with walking, subtalar arthrodesis with insertion of a bone block may alleviate the problem.

Talocalcaneal stiffness and osteoarthritis Displaced intra-articular fractures may lead to joint stiffness and, eventually, osteoarthritis. This can usually be managed conservatively but persistent or severe pain may necessitate subtalar arthrodesis. If the calcaneocuboid joint is also involved, a triple arthrodesis is better.

MIDTARSAL INJURIES

Injuries in this area vary from minor sprains, often incorrectly labelled as 'ankle' sprains, to severe fracture–dislocations that can threaten the survival of the foot. The mechanism differs accordingly, from benign twisting injuries to crushing forces that produce severe soft tissue damage; bleeding into the fascial compartments of the foot may cause a typical compartment syndrome.

Isolated injuries of the navicular, cuneiform or cuboid bones are rare. Fractures in this region should be assumed to be 'combination' fractures or fracture–subluxations, until proved otherwise.

Remember that small flakes of bone on x-ray often have large ligaments attached to them, and that 'mid-foot sprain' (like 'partial Achilles tendon rupture') is a dangerous diagnosis to make.

Pathological anatomy

The most useful classification is that of Main and Jowett (1975), which is based on the mechanism of injury.

Medial stress injuries are caused by violent inversion of the foot and vary in severity from sprains of the midtarsal joint to subluxation or fracture–subluxation of the talonavicular or midtarsal joints.

Longitudinal stress injuries are the most common. They are caused by a severe longitudinal force with the foot in plantarflexion. The navicular is compressed between the cuneiforms and the talus, resulting in fracture of the navicular and subluxation of the midtarsal joint.

Lateral stress injuries are usually due to falls in which the foot is forced into valgus. Injuries include fractures and fracture–subluxations of the cuboid and the anterior end of the calcaneum as well as avulsion injuries on the medial side of the foot.

Plantar stress injuries result from falls in which the foot is twisted and trapped under the body; they usually present as dorsal avulsion injuries or fracture–subluxation of the calcaneocuboid joint.

Crush injuries usually cause open comminuted fractures of the midtarsal region.

Clinical features

The foot is bruised and swollen. Tenderness is usually diffuse across the midfoot. A medial midtarsal dislocation looks like an 'acute club-foot' and a lateral dislocation produces a valgus deformity; with longitudinal stress injuries there is often no obvious deformity. Any attempt at movement is painful. It is important to exclude distal ischaemia or a compartment syndrome.

X-ray

Multiple views are necessary to determine the extent of the injury; be sure that *all* the tarsal bones are clearly shown. Tarso-metatarsal dislocation may be missed if the forefoot falls back into place; fractures of the tarsal bones or bases of the metatarsals should alert the surgeon to this possibility. Abnormality of alignment, or fracture, on any view should lead to CT scanning to better assess the extent of injury.

Treatment

Ligamentous strains The foot may be bandaged until acute pain subsides. Thereafter, movement is encouraged. Be prepared to re-examine and re-x-ray the foot that does not settle within a few weeks.

Undisplaced fractures The foot is elevated to counteract swelling. After 3 or 4 days a below-knee cast or removeable splintage boot is applied and the patient is allowed up on crutches with limited weightbearing. The plaster is retained for 4–6 weeks.

Displaced fractures An isolated navicular or cuboid fracture is sometimes displaced and, if so, may need open reduction and screw fixation.

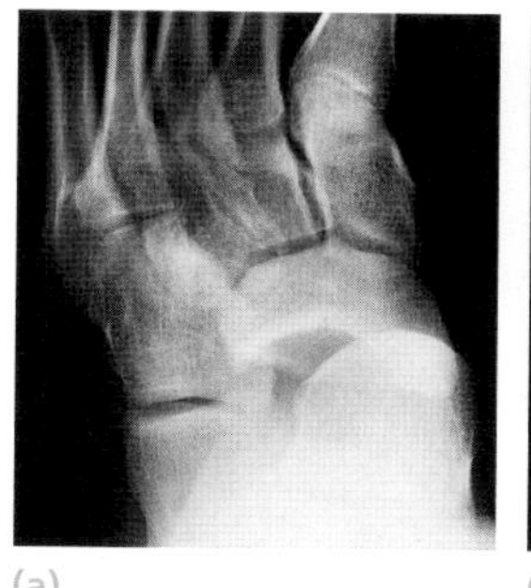

(a)

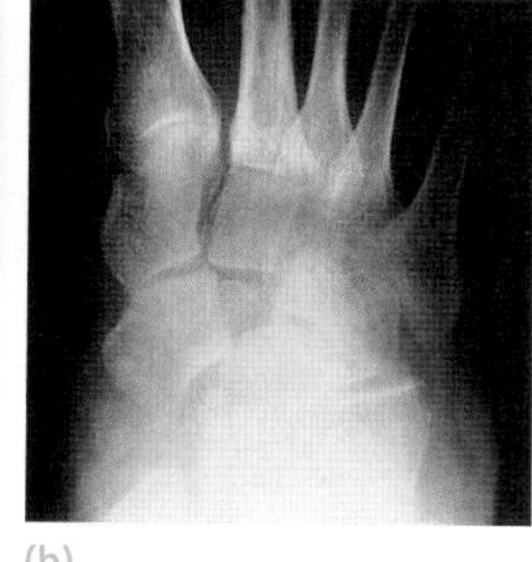

(b)

31.27 Midtarsal injuries (a) X-ray showing dislocation of the talonaviclar joint. (b) X-ray on another patient showing longitudinal compression fracture of the navicular bone and subluxation of the head of the talus. This injury is often difficult to demonstrate accurately on plain x-ray.

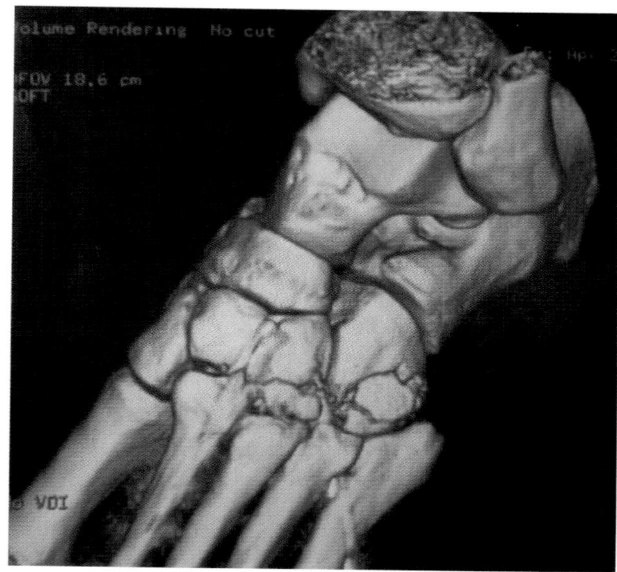

31.28 Midtarsal injuries Reconstructed CT after reduction of a severe tarso-metatarsal injury reveals associated injuries of the cuboid and the lateral cuneiform.

Fracture–dislocation These are severe injuries. Under general anaesthesia, the dislocation can usually be reduced by closed manipulation but holding it is a problem. If there is the least tendency to redisplacement, percutaneous K-wires are run across the joints to fix them in position.

The foot is immobilized in a below-knee cast for 6–8 weeks. Exercises are then begun and should be practised assiduously; it may be 6–8 months before function is regained.

If accurate reduction cannot be achieved by closed manipulation, then open reduction and screw fixation is necessary; the importance of anatomical reduction cannot be overemphasized. However, missed fractures are a lost cause and open reduction will seldom improve the situation in those who present late (more than 3 weeks after injury).

Comminuted fractures Severely comminuted fractures defy accurate reduction. Attention should be paid to the soft tissues; there is a risk of ischaemia. The foot is splinted in the best possible position and elevated until swelling subsides. Early arthrodesis, with restoration of the longitudinal arch, is advisable, with stable fixation and interpositional bone graft block.

OUTCOME

A major problem with midtarsal injuries is the frequency with which fractures and dislocations are missed at the first examination, resulting in undertreatment and a poor outcome. Even with accurate reduction of midtarsal fracture–dislocations, post-traumatic osteoarthritis may develop and about 50 per cent of patients fail to regain normal function. If symptoms are persistent and intrusive, arthrodesis may be indicated.

TARSO-METATARSAL INJURIES

The five tarso-metatarsal (TMT) joints form a structural complex that is held intact partly by the interdigitating joints and partly by the strong ligaments that bind the metatarsal bones to each other and to the tarsal bones of the midfoot.

An appreciation of the anatomy across the TMT joints is important in understanding these injuries. The second metatarsal base is set into a recess formed by the medial, intermediate and lateral cuneiforms. There is no ligament between the first and second metatarsal bases, but the plantar ligament between second metatarsal base and medial cuneiform is short and thick. In the coronal plane, the second metatarsal base forms the apex or keystone in the arch.

Dislocation is rare, but important not to miss; twisting and crushing injuries are the usual causes, with the foot buckling or twisting at the midfoot–forefoot junction. The term *Lisfranc injury* is often used for the disruptions that occur at the midfoot–forefoot junction. Classifying these by direction of forefoot dislocation is, however, pointless – it is neither a guide to treatment nor an indication of outcome. These are often high-energy injuries with extensive damage to the whole region of the foot, and simply to assess the direction of metatarsal displacement is to miss the complexity of the injury pattern.

Clinical features

TMT dislocation or fracture–dislocation should always be suspected in patients with pain and swelling of the foot after high-velocity car accidents and falls. Unfortunately about 20–30 per cent of these injuries are initially missed. Only with severe injury is there an obvious deformity.

X-rays may be difficult to interpret; something looks wrong but it is often difficult to tell what. A systematic method for examining the foot x-rays can help to improve the pick-up rate for these injuries. Concentrate on the second and fourth metatarsals in the oblique views: the medial edge of the second should be in line with the medial edge of the second cuneiform, and the medial edge of the fourth should line up with the medial side of the cuboid. A true lateral may show the dorsal displacement of the second metatarsal base. If a fracture–dislocation is suspected (the displacement may reduce spontaneously and not be immediately detectable), stress views may reveal the abnormality, but a CT scan is a more efficient way of showing the extent of injury.

Treatment

The method of treatment depends on the severity of the injury. Undisplaced sprains require cast immobilization for 4–6 weeks. Subluxation or dislocation calls for accurate reduction. This can often be achieved by traction and manipulation under anaesthesia; the position is then held with percutaneous K-wires or screws and cast immobilization. The cast is changed after a few days when swelling has subsided; the new cast is retained, non-weightbearing, for 6–8 weeks. The K-wires are then removed and rehabilitation exercises begun.

If closed reduction fails, open reduction is essential. The key to success is the second TMT joint. Through a longitudinal incision, the base of the second metatarsal is exposed and the joint manipulated into position. Reduction of the remaining parts of the tarso-metatarsal articulation will not be too difficult. The bones are fixed with percutaneous K-wires or screws and the foot is immobilized as described earlier.

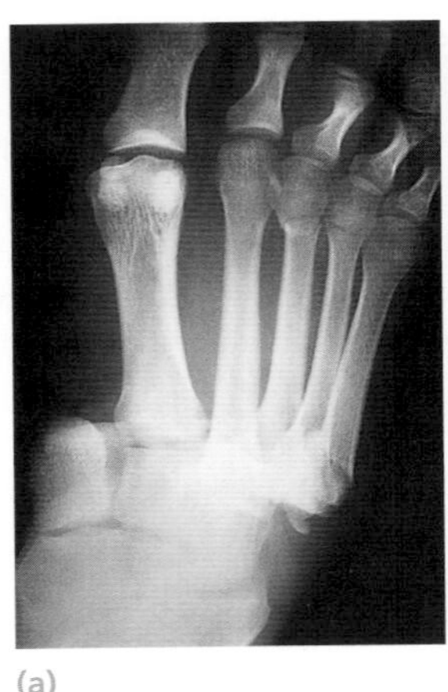
(a)

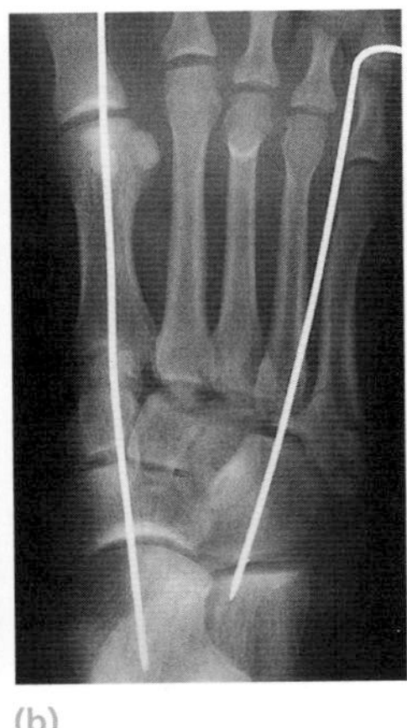
(b)

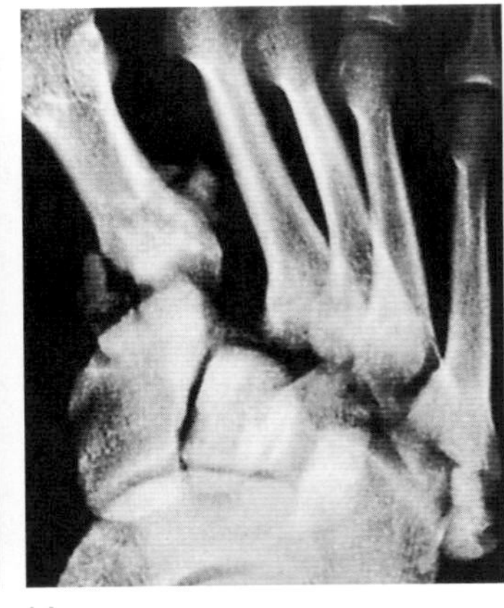
(c)

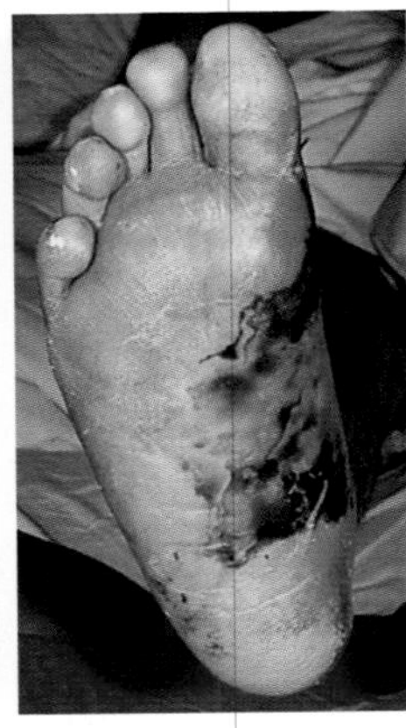
(d)

31.29 TMT injuries (a) Dislocation of the TMT joints. (b) X-ray after reduction and stabilization with K-wires. (c) X-ray showing a high-energy fracture–dislocation involving the TMT joints. These are serious injuries that may be complicated by (d) compartment syndrome of the foot.

Complications

Compartment syndrome A tensely swollen foot may hide a serious compartment syndrome that could result in ischaemic contractures. If this is suspected, intracompartmental pressures should be measured (see Chapter 23). Treatment should be prompt and effective: through a medial longitudinal incision, or two well-spaced dorsal incisions, all the compartments can be decompressed; the wound is left open until swelling subsides and the skin can be closed without tension.

INJURIES OF METATARSAL BONES

Metatarsal fractures are relatively common and are of four types: (1) crush fractures due to a direct blow; (2) a spiral fracture of the shaft due to a twisting injury; (3) avulsion fractures due to ligament strains; (4) insufficiency fractures due to repetitive stress.

Clinical features

In acute injuries pain, swelling and bruising of the foot are usually quite marked; with stress fractures, the symptoms and signs are more insidious.

X-rays should include routine anteroposterior, lateral and oblique views of the entire foot; multiple injuries are not uncommon. Undisplaced fractures may be difficult to detect and stress fractures usually show nothing at all until several weeks later.

Treatment

Treatment will depend on the type of fracture, the site of injury and the degree of displacement.

UNDISPLACED AND MINIMALLY DISPLACED FRACTURES

These can be treated by support in a below-knee cast or removable boot splint; the foot is elevated and active movements are started immediately, partial weightbearing for about 4–6 weeks. At the end of that period, exercise is very important and the patient is encouraged to resume normal activity. Slight malunion rarely results in disability once mobility has been regained.

DISPLACED FRACTURES

Displaced fractures can usually be treated closed. The foot is elevated until swelling subsides. The fracture may be reduced by traction under anaesthesia and the leg immobilized in a cast – non-weightbearing – for 4 weeks. Alternatively the fracture position might be accepted, depending on the degree of displacement. For the second to fifth metatarsals, displacement in the coronal plane can be accepted and closed treatment, as above, is satisfactory. However, for the first metatarsal and for all fractures with significant displacement in the sagittal plane (i.e. depression or elevation of the displaced fragment) open reduction and internal fixation with K-wires, or better with stable fixation using a plate and small screws, is advisable. A below-knee cast is applied and weightbearing is avoided for 3 weeks; this is then replaced by a weightbearing cast for another 4 weeks.

Fractures of the metatarsal neck have a tendency to displace, or re-displace, with closed immobilization. It is therefore important to check the position repeatedly if closed treatment is used. If the fracture is unstable, it may be possible to maintain the position by percutaneous K-wire or screw fixation. The wire is removed after 4 weeks; cast immobilization is retained for 4–6 weeks.

FRACTURES OF THE FIFTH METATARSAL BASE

Forced inversion of the foot (the 'pot-hole injury') may cause avulsion of the base of the fifth metatarsal, with pull-off by the peroneus brevis tendon or the

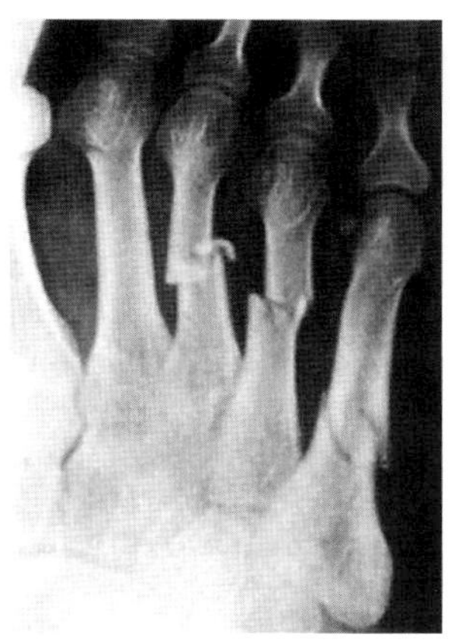
(a)

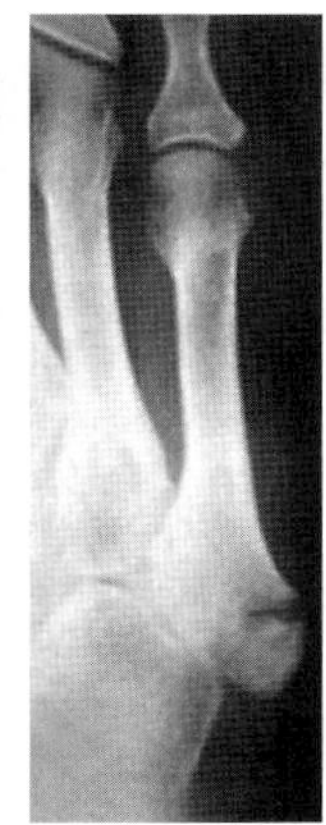
(b)

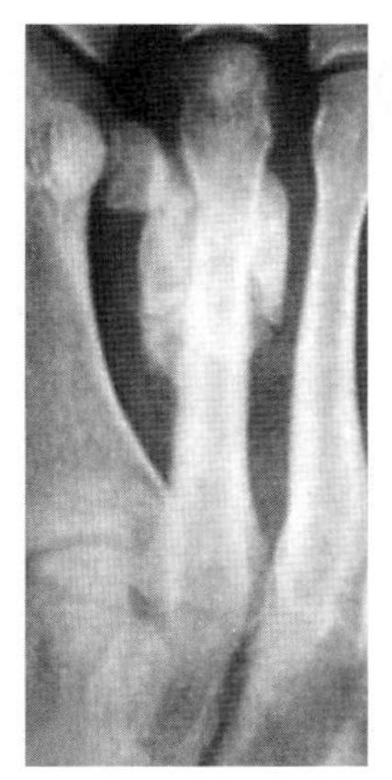
(c)

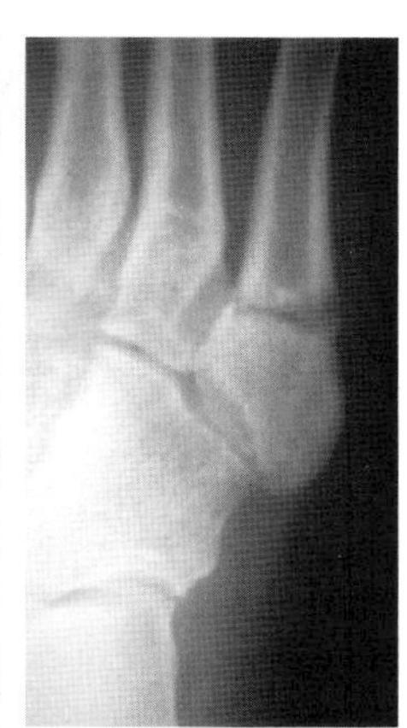
(d)

31.30 Metatarsal injuries (a) Transverse fractures of three metatarsal shafts. (b) Avulsion fracture of the base of the fifth metatarsal – the pot-hole injury, or Robert Jones fracture. (c) Florid callus in a stress fracture of the second metatarsal. (d) Jones' fracture of the fifth metatarsal.

lateral band of the plantar fascia. Pain due to a sprained ankle may overshadow pain in the foot. Examination will disclose a point of tenderness directly over the prominence at the base of the fifth metatarsal bone.

A careful assessment of the fracture pattern will provide a guide to prognosis and treatment. Again, an appreciation of the patho-anatomy explains these factors.

The fifth metatarsal base extends much more proximal into the midfoot region, compared to the other metatarsal bases. It articulates with the cuboid and with the fourth metatarsal. The peroneus brevis tendon and lateral band of the plantar fascia insert onto the base of the fifth metatarsal. There is a relative watershed in the blood supply to the fifth metatarsal at the junction between the diaphysis and metaphysis.

Robert Jones, a founding father and doyen of orthopaedics, described his own fracture (sustained whilst dancing), as a fracture of the fifth metatarsal about three-fourths of an inch from its base. Unfortunately, as observed above with Pott's fractures, what has passed into history as this eponymous fracture is often not what was actually described, and the term 'Jones fracture' is now sometimes used for any fracture of the proximal fifth metatarsal. A more useful classification system takes account of the fracture line, and whether it is proximal, affecting the tuberosity, in the region of articulation with the fourth metatarsal, or at the metaphyseal/diaphyseal junction – the latter has a higher rate of non-union, probably as a consequence of the relatively poor blood supply in that region.

Occasionally a normal peroneal ossicle in this area may be mistaken for a fracture; there is also an apophyseal ossification centre in the tuberosity.

Treatment

The proximal avulsion fractures can usually be treated symptomatically, with initial rest and support, but with early mobilization and return to function.

The intra-articular injuries and those at the metaphyseal–diaphyseal junction may also be treated non-operatively, but there is a greater risk of non-union and slower return to function. The role of fixation with an interfragmentary screw or screws and plate is therefore an issue for discussion between the surgeon and the patient, depending to a large extent on the patient's functional demands and expectations with respect to sport, activity, and time away from these.

Stress injury (March fracture)

In a young adult (often a military recruit or a nurse) the foot may become painful and slightly swollen after overuse. A tender lump is palpable just distal to the midshaft of a metatarsal bone. Usually the second metatarsal is affected, especially if it is much longer than an 'atavistic' first metatarsal. The x-ray appearance may at first be normal but a radioisotope scan will show an area of intense activity in the bone. Later a hairline crack may be visible and later still (4–6 weeks) a mass of callus is seen.

Unaccountable pain in elderly osteoporotic people may be due to the same lesion; x-ray diagnosis is more difficult because callus is minimal and there may be no more than a fine linear periosteal reaction along the metatarsal. If osteoporosis has not already been diagnosed, then this should be considered and assessed with bone densitometry.

Metatarsal pain after forefoot surgery may also be due to stress fractures of the adjacent metatarsals, a consequence of redistributed stresses in the foot.

No displacement occurs and neither reduction nor splintage is necessary. The forefoot may be supported with an elastic bandage and normal walking is encouraged.

INJURIES OF METATARSOPHALANGEAL JOINTS

Sprains and dislocations of the metatarsophalangeal (MTP) joints are common in dancers and athletes. A simple sprain requires no more than light splinting; strapping a lesser toe (second to fifth) to its neighbour for a week or two is the easiest way. If the toe is dislocated, it should be reduced by traction and manipulation; the foot is then protected in a short walking cast for a few weeks.

FRACTURED TOES

A heavy object falling on the toes may fracture phalanges. If the skin is broken it must be covered with a sterile dressing, and antibiotics are given; a contaminated wound will require formal surgical washout and exploration. The fracture is disregarded and the patient encouraged to walk in a supportive boot or shoe. If pain is marked, the toe may be splinted by strapping it to its neighbour for 2–3 weeks.

FRACTURED SESAMOIDS

One of the sesamoids (usually the medial) may fracture from either a direct injury (landing from a height on the ball of the foot) or sudden traction; chronic, repetitive stress is more often seen in dancers and runners.

The patient complains of pain directly over the sesamoid. There is a tender spot in the same area and sometimes pain can be exacerbated by passively hyperextending the big toe. X-rays will usually show the fracture (which must be distinguished from a smooth-edged bipartite sesamoid).

Treatment is often unnecessary, though a local injection of lignocaine helps for pain. If discomfort is marked, the foot can be supported in a removable boot/splint for 2–3 weeks. An insole with differential padding or cut-out under the sesamoid might also speed a return to sporting activities. Occasionally, intractable symptoms call for excision of the offending ossicle; care should be taken not to disrupt the flexor attachment to the proximal phalanx as this may result in great toe deformity.

REFERENCES AND FURTHER READING

Ajis A, Younger AS, Maffulli N. Anatomic repair for chronic lateral ankle instability. *Foot Ankle Clin* 2006; **11:** 539–45.

Bajammal S, Tornetta P 3rd, Sanders D, Bhandari M. Displaced intra-articular calcaneal fractures. *J Orthop Trauma* 2005; **19:** 360–4.

Blauth M, Bastian L, Krettek C, Knop C, Evans S. Surgical options for the treatment of severe tibial pilon fractures: a study of three techniques. *J Orthop Trauma* 2001; **15:** 153–60.

Bosse MJ, McCarthy ML, Jones AL *et al.* Lower Extremity Assessment Project (LEAP) Study Group. The insensate foot following severe lower extremity trauma: an indication for amputation? *J Bone Joint Surg* 2005; **87A:** 2601–8.

Broström L. Sprained ankles. Surgical treatment of 'chronic' ligament ruptures. *Acta Chir Scand* 1966; **132:** 551–65.

Buckley R, Tough S, McCormack R *et al.* Operative compared with nonoperative treatment of displaced intra-articular calcaneal fractures: a prospective, randomized, controlled multicenter trial. *J Bone Joint Surg* 2002; **84A:** 1733–44.

Canale ST, Kelly FB Jr. Fractures of the neck of the talus. Long-term evaluation of seventy-one cases. *J Bone Joint Surg* 1978; **60A:** 143–56.

Chrisman OD, Snook GA. Reconstruction of lateral ligament tears of the ankle: an experimental study and clinical evaluation of seven patients treated by a new modification of the Elmslie procedure. *J Bone Joint Surg* 1969; **51A:** 904–12.

Clare MP, Sanders RW. Preoperative considerations in ankle replacement surgery. *Foot Ankle Clin* 2002; **7:** 709–20.

Coetzee JC, Ly TV. Treatment of primarily ligamentous Lisfranc joint injuries: primary arthrodesis compared with open reduction and internal fixation. Surgical technique. *J Bone Joint Surg* 2007; **89A(Suppl 2 Pt 1):** 122–7.

Coetzee JC. Making sense of Lisfranc injuries. *Foot Ankle Clin* 2008; **13:** 695–704.

Colville MR. Reconstruction of the lateral ankle ligaments. *J Bone Joint Surg* 1994; **76A:** 1092–102.

Crosby LA, Fitzgibbons T. Intra-articular calcaneal fractures: Results of closed treatment. *Clin Orthop* 1993; **290:** 46–54.

Das De S, Balasubramaniam P. A repair operation for recurrent dislocation of the peroneal tendons. *J Bone Joint Surg* 1985; **67B:** 585–7.

Dattani R, Patnaik S, Kantak A, Srikanth B, Selvan TP. Injuries to the tibiofibular syndesmosis. *J Bone Joint Surg* 2008; **90B:** 405–10.

Dias LS, Tachdjian MO. Physeal injuries of the ankle in children. *Clinical Orthopaedics and Related Research* 1978; **136:** 230.

Eastwood DM, Gregg PJ, Atkins RM. Intra-articular fractures of the calcaneum. Part 1: Pathological anatomy and classification. *J Bone Joint Surg* 1993; **75B:** 183–8.

Eastwood DM, Langkamer VG, Atkins RM. Intra-articular fractures of the calcaneum. Part 2: Open reduction and internal fixation by the extended lateral transcalcaneal approach. *J Bone Joint Surg* 1993; **75B:** 189–95.

Egol KA, Wolinsky P, Koval KJ. Open reduction and internal fixation of tibial pilon fractures. *Foot Ankle Clin* 2000; **5:** 873–85.

Eiff M, Smith A, Smith G. Early mobilization versus immobilization in the treatment of lateral ankle sprains. *Am J Sports Med* 1994; **22:** 83–8.

Espinosa N, Smerek JP, Myerson MS. Acute and chronic syndesmosis injuries: pathomechanisms, diagnosis and management. *Foot Ankle Clin* 2006; **11:** 639–57.

Essex-Lopresti P. The mechanism, reduction technique and results in fractures of the os calcis. *Br J Surg* 1952; **39:** 395–419.

Goel DP, Buckley R, deVries G, Abelseth G, Ni A, Gray R. Prophylaxis of deep-vein thrombosis in fractures below the knee: a prospective randomised controlled trial. *J Bone Joint Surg* 2009; **91B:** 388–94.

Harris AM, Patterson BM, Sontich JK, Vallier HA. Results and outcomes after operative treatment of high-energy tibial plafond fractures. *Foot Ankle Int* 2006; **27:** 256–65.

Hawkins LG. Fractures of the neck of the talus. *J Bone Joint Surg* 1970; **52A:** 991–1002.

Helfet DL, Koval K, Pappas J, Sanders RW, DiPasquale T. Intraarticular 'pilon' fracture of the tibia. *Clin Orthop Relat Res* 1994; **298:** 221–8.

Hopkinson WJ, St Pierre P, Ryan JB *et al.* Syndesmosis sprains of the ankle. *Foot Ankle* 1990; **10:** 325.

Karlsson J, Bergsten T, Lansinger O, Peterson L. Reconstruction of the lateral ligaments of the ankle for chronic-lateral instability. *J Bone Joint Surg* 1988; **70A:** 581–588.

Konradsen L, Homer P, Sondergaard L. Early mobilization treatment for grade III ankle ligament injuries. *Foot Ankle* 1992; **12:** 69–73.

Kuo RS, Tejwani NC, Digiovanni CW *et al*. Outcome after open reduction and internal fixation of Lisfranc joint injuries. *J Bone Joint Surg Am* 2000; **82A:** 1609–18.

Langdon IJ, Kerr PS, Atkins RM. Fractures of the calcaneum: the anterolateral fragment. *J Bone Joint Surg* 1994; **76B:** 303–5.

Lauge-Hansen N. Fractures of the ankle. II. Combined experimental-surgical and experimental-roentgenologic investigations. *Arch Surg* 1950; **60:** 957–85.

Li X, Killie H, Guerrero P, Busconi BD. Anatomical reconstruction for chronic lateral ankle instability in the high-demand athlete: functional outcomes after the modified Broström repair using suture anchors. *Am J Sports Med* 2009; **37:** 488–94.

Lowrie IG, Finlay DB, Brenkel IJ, Gregg PJ. Computerised tomographic assessment of the subtalar joint in calcaneal fractures. *J Bone Joint Surg Am* 1988; **70B:** 247–50.

Main BJ, Jowett RL. Injuries of the midtarsal joint. *J Bone Joint Surg* 1975; **57B:** 89–97.

Michelson JD. Ankle fractures resulting from rotational injuries. *J Am Acad Orthop Surg* 2003; **11:** 403–12.

Muller ME, Allgöwer M, Schneider R, Willeneger H. *Manual of Internal Fixation*. (3rd edition) Springer, Berlin, 1991, pp 598–600.

Nunn T, Baird C, Robertson D, Gray I, Gregori A. Fitness to drive in a below knee plaster? An evidence based response. *Injury* 2007; **38:** 1305–07.

Palmer I. The mechanism and treatment of fractures of the calcaneus. *J Bone Joint Surg* 1948; **30A:** 2–8.

Papadokostakis G, Kontakis G, Giannoudis P, Hadjipavlou A. External fixation devices in the treatment of fractures of the tibial plafond: a systematic review of the literature. *J Bone Joint Surg Br* 2008; **90:** 1–6.

Pearse EO, Klass B, Bendall SP. The 'ABC' of examining foot radiographs. *Ann R Coll Surg Engl* 2005; **87:** 449–51.

Philbin T, Rosenberg G, Sferra JJ. Complications of missed or untreated Lisfranc injuries. *Foot Ankle Clin* 2003; **8:** 61–71.

Porter DA. Evaluation and treatment of ankle syndesmosis injuries. *Instr Course Lect* 2009; **58:** 575–81.

Quill GE Jr. Fractures of the proximal fifth metatarsal. *Orthop Clin North Am* 1995; **26:** 353–61.

Rammelt S, Heineck J, Zwipp H. Metatarsal fractures. *Injury* 2004; **35(Suppl 2):** SB77–86.

Ruedi TP, Allgöwer M. The operative treatment of intra-articular fractures of the lower end of the tibia. *Clin Orthop* 1979; **138:** 105–10.

Sanders R, Gregory P. Operative treatment of intra-articular fractures of the calcaneus. *Orthop Clin N Am* 1995; **26:** 203–14.

Schnetzler KA, Hoernschemeyer D. The pediatric triplane ankle fracture. *J Am Acad Orthop Surg* 2007; **15:** 738–47.

Sirkin M, Sanders R, DiPasquale T, Herscovici D Jr. A staged protocol for soft tissue management in the treatment of complex pilon fractures. *J Orthop Trauma* 1999; **13:** 78–84.

Sirkin MS. Plating of tibial pilon fractures. *Am J Orthop* 2007; **36(Suppl 2):** 13–17.

SooHoo NF, Krenek L, Eagan MJ, Gurbani B, Ko CY, Zingmond DS. Complication rates following open reduction and internal fixation of ankle fractures. *J Bone Joint Surg* 2009; **91A:** 1042–9.

Tarkin IS, Clare MP, Marcantonio A, Pape HC. An update on the management of high-energy pilon fractures. *Injury* 2008; **39:** 142–54.

Teeny SM, Wiss DA. Open reduction and internal fixation of tibial plafond fractures. *Clin Orthop* 1993; **292:** 108–17.

Tezval M, Dumont C, Stürmer KM. Prognostic reliability of the Hawkins sign in fractures of the talus. *J Orthop Trauma* 2007; **21:** 538–43.

Thordarson DB. Complications after treatment of tibial pilon fractures: prevention and management strategies. *J Am Acad Orthop Surg* 2000; **8:** 253–65.

Vallier HA, Nork SE, Barei DP, Benirschke SK, Sangeorzan BJ. Talar neck fractures: results and outcomes. *J Bone Joint Surg* 2004; **86A:** 1616–24.

Vander Griend R, Michelson JD, Bone LB. Fractures of the ankle and distal part of the tibia. *J Bone Joint Surg* 1996; **78A:** 1772–83.

Weinfeld SB, Haddad SL, Myerson MS. Metatarsal stress fractures. *Clin Sports Med* 1997; **16:** 319–38.

Epilogue – Global Orthopaedics

Christopher Lavy, Felicity Briggs

Textbooks tend to project an idealised version of the medical world: they assume, for a start, that there is a doctor, or at least a qualified medical attendant, and a hospital or clinic where patients can be examined and treated as prescribed on the printed page; that basic equipment such as x-ray machines and CT scanners are accessible; that there are facilities for essential laboratory investigations; that the recommended drugs and surgical implants are available; that the environment is clean if not actually sterile; that a variety of operations can be performed and that an appropriate level of postoperative care will be applied.

It is right that a book such as this should teach what is considered to be 'best practice' at the time of writing. However, we should also recognise that for the majority of people in the world these high standards are out of reach and compromises have to be made at every level of healthcare provision.

It is beyond the scope of this book to discuss ways of improving conditions in disadvantaged countries. Here we simply offer a brief reminder of what exists in the wider world.

GLOBAL DISTRIBUTION OF RESOURCES

Modern orthopaedic surgery is expensive by virtue of the equipment and hospital facilities required and the training of surgeons and allied medical staff. Table 1 shows the disparities among a number of representative countries in terms of per capita expenditure on health per year, the number of doctors per hundred thousand population and Gross Domestic Product (GDP). The situation in poorer countries threatens to be made even worse by the migration of doctors to relatively richer countries that offer better working facilities, economic benefits and living conditions.

GENERAL EFFECTS OF POVERTY AND MALNUTRITION

Poverty is linked to malnutrition, which contributes to reduced immune function and increased susceptibility to infection – including osteomyelitis, septic arthritis and tuberculosis of bones and joints. The strain on resources is considerable and the incidence of chronic infection requiring long-term care is high.

Table 1 Variation in health expenditure and number of doctors compared to GDP

	GDP per capita in US$	Per capita total expenditure on health in US$	Doctors/ 1000 population
Malawi	600	58	0.02
Egypt	4,200	258	0.54
China	7,800	277	1.06
Thailand	9,200	293	0.37
Mexico	10,700	655	1.98
Mauritius	13,700	516	1.06
Latvia	16,000	852	3.01
Kuwait	23,100	538	1.53
New Zealand	26,200	2,081	2.37
UK	31,800	2,560	2.30
USA	43,800	6,096	2.56

Cases such as the one shown in Figure 1 are rarely seen in affluent countries.

Specific nutritional deficiencies also take their toll and conditions such as calcium deficiency rickets and scurvy, seldom seen in affluent countries, are not uncommon in Africa.

EFFECTS OF THE HIV PANDEMIC

HIV infection rates are unusually high in some parts of the world, particularly in Africa. The virus causes a de-

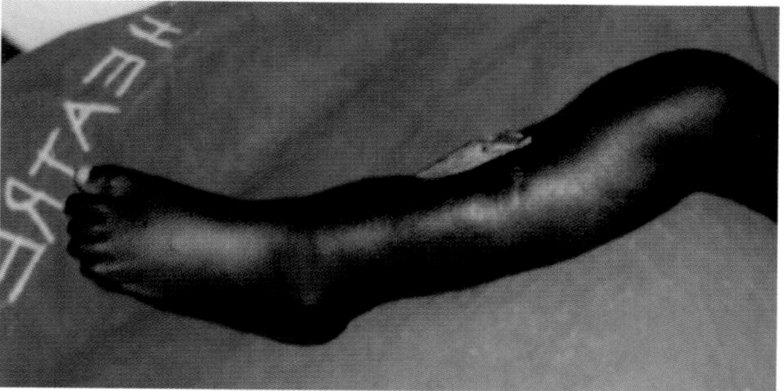

1 Chronic osteomyelitis with massive sequestrum

crease in helper CD4 cells, thus predisposing the patient to opportunistic local and systemic infections. On a global level one of the most important outcomes is the rise in the number of patients with tuberculosis. Though the skeleton is involved in only 1 per cent of cases, treatment (especially for spinal tuberculosis) is demanding, prolonged and expensive. If paraplegia develops, the outlook – more often than not – is hopeless.

EFFECTS OF WAR INJURIES

Conventional warfare is usually attended by more or less skilled medical services, advanced surgical facilities and efficient transfer of the wounded to hospitals. Small-scale conflicts that flare up in under-resourced civilian populations may cause fewer casualties but lack of experienced personnel and field services results in a proportionately greater number of serious complications and poor outcomes among the wounded. Were it not for voluntary medical organizations the death toll would be much greater than it is. Even after these conflicts have ended, people continue to suffer injuries inflicted by abandoned anti-personnel weapons, and health services in poor countries continue to be substandard. In Cambodia and Angola, for example, the presence of unexploded mines in populated areas has resulted in a high percentage of amputees among civilians. Facilities for treating these patients are poor and provision of prostheses inadequate. Knock-on effects can also be serious. In Northern Uganda, where there has been low-level conflict for many years, polio vaccination services have broken down, resulting in an increased number of children with poliomyelitis and the resulting deformities.

FRACTURE MANAGEMENT

For a given fracture there is no universal 'best practice' method of management as so much depends on facilities, resources and personnel. A closed mid-shaft femoral fracture in a rich country where there is an available clean operating theatre, a full set of intramedullary nail sizes, an image intensifier and a fully trained operating theatre staff, may be appropriately treated by internal fixation. The patient has a low risk of complications and will return to full mobility in a short time. In a poor country with no dedicated orthopaedic theatre or team, a small number of implants and limited imaging facilities, it might be wiser to treat the same fracture conservatively because the risk of complications associated with surgery is unacceptably high. Moreover, treating a femoral fracture by traction for many weeks might well be cheaper than internal fixation, because of the lower cost of running a hospital and the lower daily cost of occupying a hospital bed.

ELECTIVE ORTHOPAEDICS

Elective orthopaedic treatment is also affected. In rich countries joint replacement for osteoarthritis is taken for granted. In poor countries conservative treatment and operations that do not involve the use of expensive implants and instrumentation are all that can be afforded. Similarly, the unavailability of arthroscopic equipment forces surgeons to set a higher threshold for operating on knees and shoulders. Surgical treatment of bone tumours is particularly problematic. Ideal investigative procedures are often unavailable for lack of imaging equipment and experienced pathology services. Limb salvage procedures by endoprosthetic replacement are usually out of the question because of the need for high quality prostheses, a tissue bank and specialized postoperative care. In these circumstances malignant tumours are more often treated by amputation.

In organizing elective orthopaedic treatment knock-on effects must also be considered. A good example is in the management of a common condition such as congenital club-foot. In countries with well-supported child health services treatment is started soon after birth and usually follows Ponseti's method of repeated manipulation and splintage, perhaps followed by limited surgery. This requires a level of parental participation and medical supervision that is simply not available in resource poor countries where treatment is usually started much later, return visits are sporadic and many do not get treated at all. The outcome is often severe deformity which requires prolonged and highly skilled surgical management (Fig. 2).

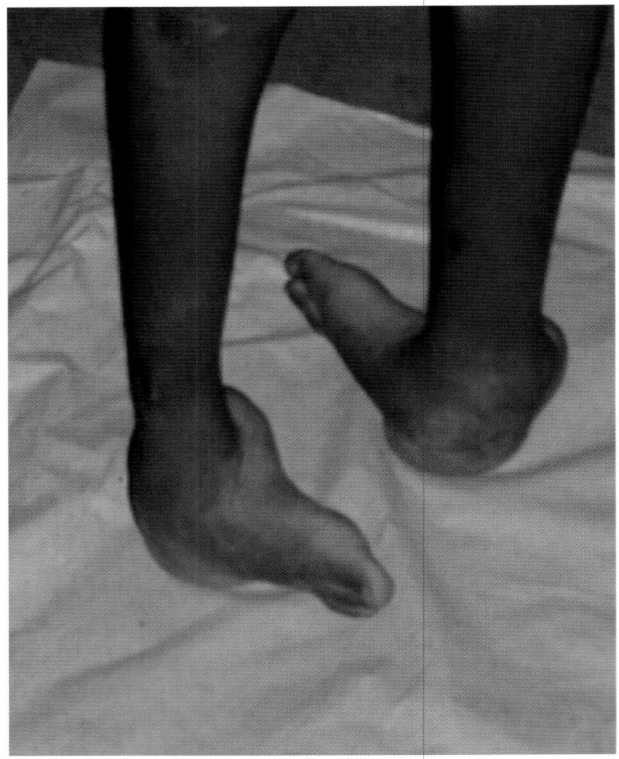

2 Untreated club-foot

PERSONNEL ISSUES

Surgeons working in countries with a high workload are often required to treat a much wider spectrum of pathology than those operating in more specialised hospitals. Indeed, in many cases a single surgeon covers the entire range of surgical specialties. This obviously reduces the level of expertise that he or she can develop in a particular field. In many countries throughout the developing world non-medically qualified assistants ('clinical officers') are being trained to deal with common simple conditions such as closed fractures. On the one hand this practice carries an increased risk of late complications but on the other hand the regular management of these conditions can lead to a higher degree of skill in methods of manual fracture reduction than that possessed by the qualified surgeon who does not have time to master everything!

Training is a crucial part of surgery and it is important that surgeons are taught to deal with the pathology that they are eventually going to encounter, using the methods that will be available where they work. The scenario of a poor country sending its surgical trainees to better resourced centres where they learn only high cost methods of treatment is common. It often results in a trainee who returns to his or her own country with a certificate of completion of training, but no knowledge or experience of how to function in a resource limited environment. This is a problem that deserves the attention of both those who send aspiring surgeons to other countries for training, and those in recipient countries organizing training for them.

ETHICAL AND LEGAL ISSUES

The practice of orthopaedic surgery is expensive, and in Western countries continues to get more expensive as better and more complex treatments and implants are devised. Poorer countries do not have the economic capability to afford such treatments and are forced into a dilemma over treatment rationing that has both moral and legal implications. If a limited number of modern products, for example hip replacements, are available, then the decision as to which of many clinically deserving patients receives them is difficult. There is no correct solution to this problem, but often the decision is made on economic grounds: the patient who can pay has first call on the resources. This is clearly wrong, but one must also beware of having the decision taken out of the hands of the clinician and made by politicians.

A related legal and ethical issue arises when less than best but cheaper than best treatment options are on offer. For example a country may not be able to afford fracture implants made of the highest quality titanium, but may have low quality fracture plates available. The decision about whether to use equipment that is not perfect is a hard one; similarly the decision about whether to use donated or previously used, but still effective, implants, or implants, sutures and sterile supplies that are past their 'use by' dates. It is easy to take the moral high ground and decry such practices, but where the options are limited the practical choice – and the choice of many surgeons in the world – is between second best or nothing.

CONSENT TO TREATMENT

It is always essential that the patient receives an easily understandable description of any operative procedure you have advised, as well as an honest opinion about the likely outcome and the foreseeable complications that might arise from the operation. When working in a disadvantaged community, where the patient may be poorly educated, it is much more difficult than usual to convey this information, and be sure that it has been understood, when seeking consent. The difficulty is increased if the surgeon and patient do not speak the same language and information is conveyed via an interpreter. The solution is to ask the patient to repeat the message to you in small portions, and to ensure that it is still intelligible.

THE FUTURE

It is not possible in a chapter to cover all the differences between orthopaedic practice in different parts of the world. What is clear is that although there are some real differences in pathology in the different geographical regions, the key differences are those of economic inequality. They are differences that have always existed, and differences that are not likely to disappear in the near future. Indeed they might well grow as international donor funds tend to be spent on public health and infectious diseases rather than on orthopaedics and fractures. The World Health Organization estimates that by 2020 road trauma will be the third biggest global cause of morbidity for males. It may be that this will cause an improvement in global funding of orthopaedic care. Whether or not this occurs it is important for those who practise orthopaedics in all countries to maintain and increase their understanding of the global issues, for training programme organizers to keep their eyes on a horizon that is not limited to their own part of the world, and for those responsible for planning and funding research to be aware of the world's real orthopaedic problems. Best of all is for aspiring orthopaedic surgeons to spend some time working in one of the poor countries of the world.

Index

Note 'vs' indicates the differential diagnosis of two conditions.

INDEX